Principles and Practice of Neuro-Oncology

Principles and Practice of Neuro-Oncology

A Multidisciplinary Approach

EDITOR-IN-CHIEF

Minesh P. Mehta, MD, FASTRO
Professor
Department of Human Oncology
University of Wisconsin
Madison, Wisconsin

EDITORS

Susan M. Chang, MD
Professor
Vice Chair, Neurological Surgery
Director, Division of Neuro-Oncology
University of California, San Francisco
San Francisco, California

Abhijit Guha, MSc, MD, FRCSC, FACS
Professor of Surgery (Neurosurgery)
Toronto Western Hospital
Senior Scientist and Co-Director
The Arthur and Sonia Labatt Brain Tumour
  Research Centre
Hospital for Sick Children
Hudson Chair in Neuro-Oncology
University of Toronto
Toronto, Ontario, Canada

Herbert B. Newton, MD, FAAN
Professor of Neurology, Neurosurgery, and Oncology
Esther Dardinger Endowed Chair in Neuro-Oncology
Department of Neurosurgery
Dardinger Neuro-Oncology Center
The Ohio State University Medical Center
James Cancer Hospital
Columbus, Ohio

Michael A. Vogelbaum, MD, PhD, FACS
The Robert and Kathryn Lamborn Chair for
  Neuro-Oncology
Associate Director of Neurosurgical Oncology
Department of Neurosurgery
Brain Tumor and Neuro-Oncology Center
Cleveland Clinic
Cleveland, Ohio

ASSOCIATE EDITORS

Melissa L. Bondy, PhD, Judith A. Schwartzbaum, PhD, and
Margaret R. Wrensch, MPH, PhD

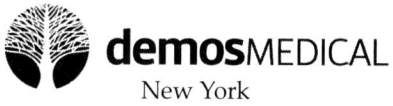

New York

Acquisitions Editor: Richard Winters
Cover Design: Joe Tenerelli
Compositor: NewGen Imaging
Printer: Bang Printing

Visit our website at www.demosmedpub.com

© 2011 Demos Medical Publishing, LLC. All rights reserved. This book is protected by copyright. No part of it may be reproduced, stored in a retrieval system, or transmitted in any form or by any means, electronic, mechanical, photocopying, recording, or otherwise, without the prior written permission of the publisher.

Medicine is an ever-changing science. Research and clinical experience are continually expanding our knowledge, in particular our understanding of proper treatment and drug therapy. The authors, editors, and publisher have made every effort to ensure that all information in this book is in accordance with the state of knowledge at the time of production of the book. Nevertheless, the authors, editors, and publisher are not responsible for errors or omissions or for any consequences from application of the information in this book and make no warranty, express or implied, with respect to the contents of the publication. Every reader should examine carefully the package inserts accompanying each drug and should carefully check whether the dosage schedules mentioned therein or the contraindications stated by the manufacturer differ from the statements made in this book. Such examination is particularly important with drugs that are either rarely used or have been newly released on the market.

Library of Congress Cataloging-in-Publication Data
Principles and practice of neuro-oncology : a multidisciplinary approach / editors, Minesh P. Mehta . . . [et al.] ;
associate editors, Melissa L. Bondy . . . [et al.].
   p. ; cm.
Includes bibliographical references and index.
ISBN 978-1-933864-78-5
1. Brain—Cancer. I. Mehta, Minesh P.
 [DNLM: 1. Brain Neoplasms. 2. Brain Neoplasms—therapy. WL 358 P957 2011]
RC280.B7P75 2011
616.99′481—dc22   2010022345

Special discounts on bulk quantities of Demos Medical Publishing books are available to corporations, professional associations, pharmaceutical companies, health care organizations, and other qualifying groups. For details, please contact:
Special Sales Department
Demos Medical Publishing
11 W. 42nd Street, 15th Floor
New York, NY 10036
Phone: 800–532–8663 or 212–683–0072
Fax: 212–941–7842
E-mail: rsantana@demosmedpub.com

Made in the United States of America

10 11 12 13 14   5 4 3 2 1

Contents

Preface ix
Acknowledgments xi
Contributors xiii

PART I: EPIDEMIOLOGY

Margaret R. Wrensch, Judith A. Schwartzbaum, and Melissa L. Bondy, Editors

Gliomas

1. Epidemiology and Etiology of Glioma: An Overview   *1*
   James L. Fisher, Judith A. Schwartzbaum, and Margaret R. Wrensch

2. Descriptive Epidemiology of Glioma   *4*
   Bridget J. McCarthy

3. Familial Factors and Inherited Susceptibility to Glioma   *14*
   Beatrice Melin and Melissa L. Bondy

4. Chemical Exposures Mediated Through Occupation, Environment and Lifestyle, and Brain Tumor Risk   *18*
   Dora Il'yasova, Faith G. Davis, Rose Lai, Therese A. Dolecek, and Siegal Sadetzki

5. Exposure to Ionizing Radiation and Glioma Risk   *26*
   Siegal Sadetzki and Lori Mandelzweig

6. Radiofrequency Fields and Glioma Risk   *31*
   Maria Feychting and Anders Ahlbom

7. Allergies and Glioma Risk   *39*
   Judith A. Schwartzbaum, Linda M. Karavodin, Margaret R. Wrensch, and Joseph Leo Wiemels

8. Glioma Survival and Prognosis   *47*
   Jeffrey S. Chang, Margaret R. Wrensch, Terri Rice, and James L. Fisher

Childhood Brain Tumors

9. Epidemiology of Childhood Brain Tumors   *57*
   Tarik Tihan, John K. Wiencke, Pedram Razavi, and Roberta McKean-Cowdin

10. Meningioma Genetics   *71*
    Yi Lu and Elizabeth B. Claus

PART II: MOLECULAR BIOLOGY

Abhijit Guha, Editor

11. Molecular Neuro-Oncology: Why is it Essential?   *79*
    Abhijit Guha

12. Brain Tumor Initiating Cells: History, New Advances, Therapeutic Promises, and Pitfalls   *81*
    Sameer Agnihotri, Diana Munoz, and Abhijit Guha

13. Molecular Pathogenesis of Glioma: Overview and Therapeutic Implications   *88*
    Ingeborg Fischer, Erik Sulman, and Ken Aldape

14. Molecular Heterogeneity and Tumor Microenvironment   *100*
    Daniel J. Brat and Sydney M. Evans

15. Molecular Regulators of Glioma Invasion   *112*
    Candece L. Gladson, Wei Michael Liu, and Michael E. Berens

16. Molecular Basis of Glioma Neovascularization and Its Therapeutic Applications   *122*
    Jean-Pierre Gagner, John G. Golfinos, Jerome J. Graber, and David Zagzag

17. Mouse Models of Central Nervous System Tumors   *145*
    Part 1 Transgenic Mouse Models of Central Nervous System Tumors   *145*
    Sameer Agnihotri and Abhijit Guha
    Part 2 Transplantation Mouse Models of Central Nervous System Tumors   *153*
    C. David James and Tomoko Ozawa

18. Pathology and Genetics of Meningiomas   *158*
    Hussein Alahmadi and Sidney E. Croul

19. Histopathology and Molecular Pathogenesis of Schwannomas   *167*
    Fabio Pereira Nunes, Scott R. Plotkin, and Anat O. Stemmer-Rachamimov

20. Histopathology and Molecular Pathogenesis of Pituitary Adenomas 174
    Siobhan C. Loeper, Shereen Ezzat, and Sylvia L. Asa

21. Histopathology and Molecular Pathogenesis of Neurofibromas and Malignant Peripheral Nerve Sheath Tumors 185
    Tim-Rasmus Kiehl and Kathleen Joy Khu

Pediatric Brain Tumors

22. The 'Cell of Origin' for Common Pediatric Brain Tumors 195
    Livia Garzia, Jessica Dawn Kessler, Robert J. Wechsler-Reya, and Michael David Taylor

23. Histopathological Features of Common Pediatric Brain Tumors 204
    Hisham AlKhalidi and Cynthia E. Hawkins

24. Molecular Genetics of Medulloblastoma and High-Grade Astrocytomas in Children 215
    Arnold B. Etame, Christian Smith, Uri Tabori, and James T. Rutka

25. Molecular Pathogenesis of Neuroblastomas 225
    Loretta M. S. Lau and Meredith S. Irwin

26. Pediatric Brain Tumor Syndromes and Murine Models 239
    Andrew B. Foy and Cynthia Wetmore

27. Predisposition Syndromes: Neurofibromatosis 1, Neurofibromatosis 2, and Tuberous Sclerosis Complex 249
    Rebecca J. Gutmann and David H. Gutmann

PART III: CLINICAL PRESENTATION AND SUPPORTIVE CARE

Herbert B. Newton, Editor

28. Presentation and Clinical Features of Supratentorial Gliomas in Adults 257
    Herbert B. Newton

29. Presentation and Clinical Features of Brain Metastases 262
    Deborah T. Blumenthal and Felix Bokstein

30. Presentation and Clinical Features of Medulloblastoma 267
    Roger J. Packer, Kevin C. DeBraganca, and Nadia Kadom

31. Presentation and Clinical Features of Pediatric Gliomas 273
    Ali I. Raja and Ian F. Pollack

32. Presentation and Clinical Features of Brainstem Tumors 278
    Paul Graham Fisher

33. Presentation and Clinical Features of Tumors of the Skull Base and Cranial Nerves 282
    Mario Ammirati and Hekmat Khodr Zarzour

34. Presentation and Clinical Features of Tumors of the Pituitary and Sellar Region 291
    Edward R. Laws, John A. Jane, Jr., Jay Jagannathan, and Laurence Katznelson

35. Presentation and Clinical Features of Spinal Cord Tumors 297
    Herbert H. Engelhard, III, Edward Andrew Michals, and John Lee Villano

Supportive Care and Quality of Life

36. Supportive Care in Neuro-Oncology 304
    Herbert B. Newton

37. Ethical Issues in Neuro-Oncology 311
    Herbert B. Newton

38. Role of Support Groups and Caregivers in Neuro-Oncology 316
    Sarah R. G. Gupta

39. Neurocognitive Function and Quality of Life 320
    Christina A. Meyers

40. Neuropsychological Sequelae of Adult Brain Tumors 326
    Martin Klein

41. Neuropsychological Sequelae Associated with Pediatric Brain Tumors: What We've Learned Over the Past 40 Years 334
    Sarah C. Carpentieri

42. Rehabilitation of Central Nervous System Tumors 342
    Subhadra L. Nori

43. Palliative Care in Neuro-Oncology 349
    Nina D. Wagner-Johnston and Stuart A. Grossman

Imaging

44. Imaging of Brain Tumors 353
    Yair Safriel and Volker Wilhelm Walter Stieber

PART IV: NEUROANATOMY AND NEUROSURGERY

Michael A. Vogelbaum, Editor

Anatomy

45. Functional Neuroanatomy 371
    Sameer A. Sheth, Bradley R. Buchbinder, and Fred G. Barker, II

46. Skull Base Anatomy, Pathology, and Approaches: An Overview 385
    Burak Sade and Joung H. Lee

Technology and Specialized Techniques

47. Surgical Navigation 392
    Gene H. Barnett

48. Stereotactic Brain Biopsy **400**
    S. Bulent Omay and Michael A. Vogelbaum

49. Intraoperative Anatomical Imaging **407**
    Salvatore M. Zavarella and Michael Schulder

50. Intraoperative Molecular Imaging **421**
    Walter Stummer and Jörg-Christian Tonn

51. Intraoperative Functional Mapping **428**
    R. Mark Richardson and Mitchel S. Berger

52. Endoscopy **435**
    Johnathan A. Engh, Amin B. Kassam, Daniel M. Prevedello, and Paul A. Gardner

Procedures

53. Transsphenoidal **445**
    Ashok R. Asthagiri, Adam S. Kanter, Edward H. Oldfield, and John A. Jane, Jr.

54. Spinal Neoplasms **453**
    Patrick C. Hsieh, John H. Chi, Ali Bydon, and Ziya L. Gokaslan

55. Spinal Cord Tumors **465**
    Sean J. Nagel, Kene T. Ugokwe, Paul Kim, and Edward C. Benzel

56. Low-Grade Gliomas **477**
    Michael L. Di Luna, Joachim M. Baehring, and Joseph M. Piepmeier

57. Pineal Gland Tumors **485**
    Gaetan Moise, Alfred T. Ogden, and Jeffrey N. Bruce

58. Intraventricular Tumors **496**
    Shakeel A. Chowdhry, Jonathan P. Miller, and Alan R. Cohen

59. Insular Tumors **505**
    Adam Wu and Frederick F. Lang

60. Pediatric Tumor Surgery **518**
    Shobhan Vachhrajani, Michael Ellis, and James T. Rutka

61. Brachial Plexus Tumors **534**
    Robert J. Spinner, Kimon Bekelis, and Kimberly K. Amrami

PART V: MEDICAL ONCOLOGY

Susan M. Chang, Editor

62. General Principles **547**
    Karine Michaud

63. Medical Management of Supratentorial Gliomas in Adults **556**
    Jennifer L. Clarke, Douglas Edward Ney, Charles C. Shyu, and Andrew B. Lassman

64. Medical Management for Pediatric Gliomas **579**
    Sabine Mueller

65. Medical Management of Primitive Neuroectodermal Tumors **589**
    Sabine Mueller and Susan M. Chang

66. Intracranial Meningiomas **599**
    Frank S. Lieberman

67. Medical Management for Brainstem Tumors **608**
    Sabine Mueller

68. Chemotherapy for Tumors of the Skull Base and Cranial Nerves **615**
    Jennifer L. Clarke and Andrew B. Lassman

69. Tumors of the Pituitary and Sellar Region **623**
    Lewis S. Blevins, Jr. and Jessica Koch Devin

70. Medical Treatment of Spinal Cord Tumors **633**
    Karine Michaud

71. Brain Metastases and Leptomeningeal Disease **638**
    Michelle E. Melisko

72. Primary Central Nervous System Lymphoma **650**
    Cigall Kadoch and James L. Rubenstein

73. Medical Treatment of Primary Central Nervous System Germ Cell Tumors **661**
    Raymond Liu

74. Medical Management for Choroid Plexus Tumors **664**
    Sabine Mueller and Susan M. Chang

Targeted Therapies

75. General Principles of Targeted Therapies **666**
    Nicholas Butowski

76. General Principles of Angiogenesis **669**
    Nicholas Butowski

77. Inhibitors of Signal Transduction Pathways in Malignant Glioma Therapy **676**
    Andrew D. Norden and Patrick Y. Wen

78. Biologics **692**
    Sith Sathornsumetee, John Howard Sampson, and David A. Reardon

79. Other Therapies **704**
    Daniela A. Bota and David A. Reardon

80. Alternative Therapies **710**
    Raymond Liu

PART VI: RADIATION THERAPY

Minesh P. Mehta, Editor

81. Introduction to Radiation Therapy **719**
    Tod W. Speer and Deepak Khuntia

Supratentorial Gliomas

82. Radiation for Glioblastoma **744**
    Samuel T. Chao and John H. Suh

83. Anaplastic Glioma **752**
    Malika L. Siker and Minesh P. Mehta

84. Low-Grade Glioma Radiation Therapy   760
    Nadia N. Issa Laack and Paul D. Brown

85. Ganglioglioma   769
    John C. Breneman

86. Optic Pathway Glioma   771
    Bernadine R. Donahue

87. The Current Role for Radiation Therapy in Pediatric Grade II-IV (Non-JPA) Gliomas   775
    Sameer Keole and Daniel J. Indelicato

88. Medulloblastoma and Primitive Neuroectodermal Tumors   781
    John C. Breneman

89. Adult and Pediatric Pilocytic Astrocytoma   795
    Bernadine R. Donahue

Posterior Fossa Tumors

90. Ependymoma (Intracranial)   799
    Lisa Hazard and C. Leland Rogers

91. Vestibular Schwannoma   808
    Bethany M. Anderson and Minesh P. Mehta

92. Hemangioblastoma and Hemangiopericytoma   818
    Malika L. Siker and Minesh P. Mehta

93. Radiation Therapy for Intracranial Meningiomas   820
    C. Leland Rogers

94. Adult and Pediatric Brainstem Glioma   842
    Carolyn R. Freeman

95. Tumors of the Base of Skull   846
    Kiran Devisetty, Robert S. Malyapa, and William M. Mendenhall

Tumors of the Pituitary and Sellar Region

96. Pituitary Tumors and Craniopharyngioma   861
    Tim J. Kruser, Vinai Gondi, and Minesh P. Mehta

97. Primary Central Nervous System Germ Cell Tumors, Pineal Tumors, and Other Tumors of the Pineal and Sellar Regions   874
    Kristin A. Bradley

98. Primary Central Nervous System Lymphoma   880
    Christopher J. Schultz and Joseph Bovi

Others

99. Neurocytoma   892
    Sayana Rachel Thomas and Deepak Khuntia

100. Radiation Therapy of Primary Spinal Cord Tumors   894
    Volker Wilhelm Walter Stieber

101. Metastatic Disease   902
    Carsten Nieder and Dirk Rades

Index   923

Preface

The field of neuro-oncology has experienced rapid growth in the last decade, characterized by robust advances in epidemiology, molecular biology, imaging, histopathologic harmonization, neurosurgical techniques, quality of life and cognitive functions, and therapeutic changes in terms of combined modality treatments, advanced radiation techniques, the advent of new drugs, especially targeted agents, and the tantalizing early promise of personalized therapeutic approaches. As dramatic as these changes are, we are merely at the cusp of an exponential explosion in knowledge in the field of neuro-oncology. This dramatic advance in our knowledge-base makes it almost impossible for any one person to keep pace, thereby underscoring the need for a comprehensive text incorporating these various elements in one common reference source.

This book is designed specifically with a multidisciplinary focus, as neuro-oncology today is a superb example of the intersection of various specialties for the optimum management of a patient with a brain tumor. The text is specifically designed for step-wise progression in the data and knowledge regarding various types of brain tumors, starting with epidemiology, progressing through with an understanding of etiologic factors, histopathogenesis, molecular biology, clinical presentation, imaging characteristics, and a comprehensive set of chapters on therapeutic options. Pulling together such a broad range of topics required expertise from various specialties, and this resulted in the creation of a truly multidisciplinary text.

It is our sincere hope that this text will be useful for both the basic scientist and the clinician, and will be actively utilized by people at all levels of training from students, to residents, to physicians and neuroscientists. The young trainee will find the large number of illustrations and the logical text a useful learning resource, whereas for the more experienced, this text will serve as an important reference source. It is our ultimate desire that whatever the joy or benefit this book provides, it actually translates to better patient management, for it is ultimately with the patient in mind that this work was undertaken.

Minesh P. Mehta, MD, FASTRO

Acknowledgments

The production of this text served up a major challenge in integration, juggling the needs and schedules of over 100 authors, and continually updating data and text as new publications rapidly came out in press. Through this process, my coeditors, Susan Chang, Abhijit Guha, Herbert Newton, and Michael Vogelbaum, as well as my associate editors, Melissa Bondy, Judith Schwartzbaum, and Margaret Wrensch rose to the challenge at every occasion and always co-ordinated their efforts with all of the individual chapter authors to deliver a superb product. I am highly indebted to all of them, for this book would not be possible otherwise. One of the coeditors battled through a personal health crisis of immense magnitude, and without batting an eyelid, and with superb grace and aplomb, continued through with the rigors of therapy, and still succeeded in delivering on a promise; one cannot ask for a better or more diligent colleague and friend. Malika Siker, my editorial assistant worked long hard hours through nights and weekends, while managing the rigors of residency training and motherhood, and I owe her a special debt of gratitude. My personal assistant Pat Lee was always there to restore my confidence that the book would see the light of day, and her organizational skills and patience were an enormous asset in this journey! Of course, a major "thank you" is owed to the staff of Demos Medical Publishing for their professionalism and support.

At a personal level, I wish to thank my patients for providing me the spark and incentive to continue with a project of this magnitude! Every time my energy would sap, I would think of the young man laboring through chemotherapy, the mother receiving radiation, the young child recovering from surgery, and the strength in their eyes, and the willpower behind their external façade provided me with the reinvigoration that I needed to go on! Finally, I owe my children, Tej and Sanjli, a big thank you for allowing me to miss all those parent-teacher conferences, tennis practices, musical performances, and for forgiving me all of the promises I failed to keep while working on this book.

Contributors

Sameer Agnihotri, BSc (Hons)
Graduate Student
Medical Biophysics
The Arthur and Sonia Labatt Brain Tumour Research Centre
Hospital for Sick Children
University of Toronto
Toronto, Ontario, Canada

Anders Ahlbom, PhD
Professor of Epidemiology
Institute of Environmental Medicine
Karolinska Institute
Stockholm, Sweden

Hussein Alahmadi, MD
Neurosurgery Resident
Division of Neurosurgery
University of Toronto
Toronto, Ontario, Canada

Ken Aldape, MD
Professor
Department of Pathology
The University of Texas MD Anderson Cancer Center
Houston, Texas

Hisham AlKhalidi, MBBS, FRCPC
Assistant Professor and Consultant
Department of Pathology
King Saud University
King Khalid University Hospital
Riyadh, Saudi Arabia

Mario Ammirati, MD, MBA
Professor of Neurosurgery and Radiation Oncology
Director of Skull Base Surgery and Stereotactic
  Radiosurgery
Director of Dardinger Microneurosurgery Skull Base Laboratory
Department of Neurological Surgery
The Ohio State University
Columbus, Ohio

Kimberly K. Amrami, MD
Professor
Department of Radiology
Mayo Clinic
Rochester, Minnesota

Bethany M. Anderson, MD
Assistant Professor
Department of Human Oncology
University of Wisconsin
Madison, Wisconsin

Sylvia L. Asa, MD, PhD
Pathologist-in-Chief
Medical Director, Laboratory Medicine Program
Department of Pathology
Senior Scientist
Ontario Cancer Institute
University Health Network
Toronto, Ontario, Canada

Ashok R. Asthagiri, MD
Staff Clinician
Surgical Neurology Branch
National Institute of Neurological Disorders
National Institutes of Health
Bethesda, Maryland

Joachim M. Baehring, MD, DSc
Associate Professor
Department of Neurology, Medicine, and Neurosurgery
Yale University School of Medicine
New Haven, Connecticut

Fred G. Barker, II, MD
Associate Visiting Neurosurgeon
Department of Neurosurgery
Massachusetts General Hospital
Associate Professor of Surgery (Neurosurgery)
Department of Surgery
Harvard Medical School
Boston, Massachusetts

Gene H. Barnett, MD, MBA, FACS
Professor of Surgery
Director, Brain Tumor and Neuro-Oncology Center
Department of Neurosurgery
Cleveland Clinic
Cleveland, Ohio

Kimon Bekelis, MD
Resident
Department of Neurologic Surgery
Dartmouth-Hitchcock Medical Center
Lebanon, New Hampshire

Edward C. Benzel, MD
Chairman
Department of Neurosurgery
Neurological Institute
Cleveland Clinic
Cleveland, Ohio

Michael E. Berens, PhD
Director and Senior Investigator
Department of Cancer and Cell Biology
The Translational Genomics Research Institute
Phoenix, Arizona
Associate Director
Van Andel Research Institute
Grand Rapids, Michigan

Mitchel S. Berger, MD
Kathleen M. Plant Distinguished Professor
Chairman
Department of Neurological Surgery
Director
Brain Tumor Research Center
University of California, San Francisco
San Francisco, California

Lewis S. Blevins, Jr., MD
Professor of Clinical Medicine and Neurological Surgery
Department of Neurological Surgery
University of California, San Francisco
San Francisco, California

Deborah T. Blumenthal, MD
Co-Director of Neuro-Oncology Service
Oncology Division
Tel-Aviv Sourasky Medical Center
Tel-Aviv, Israel
Adjunct Associate Professor of Neuro-Oncology
Division of Oncology
Department of Internal Medicine
The Huntsman Cancer Institute
University of Utah
Salt Lake City, Utah

Felix Bokstein, MD
Co-Director of Neuro-Oncology Service
Oncology Division
Tel-Aviv Sourasky Medical Center
Tel-Aviv, Israel

Melissa L. Bondy, PhD
Professor
Department of Epidemiology
Division of Cancer Prevention
The University of Texas MD Anderson Cancer Center
Houston, Texas

Daniela A. Bota, MD, PhD
Assistant Neurology Professor
Medical Co-Director
University of California Irvine Comprehensive
   Brain Tumor Program
Department of Neurology
University of California, Irvine Medical Center
Orange, California

Joseph Bovi, MD
Assistant Professor
Department of Radiation Oncology
Medical College of Wisconsin
Milwaukee, Wisconsin

Kristin A. Bradley, MD
Associate Professor
Department of Human Oncology
University of Wisconsin School of Medicine and Public Health
Madison, Wisconsin

Daniel J. Brat, MD, PhD
Professor and Vice Chair, Translational Programs
Department of Pathology and Laboratory Medicine
Emory University School of Medicine
Atlanta, Georgia

John C. Breneman, MD
Charles M. Barrett Professor of Radiation
   Oncology and Neurosurgery
Department of Radiation Oncology
University of Cincinnati
Cincinnati Children's Hospital Medical Center
Cincinnati, Ohio

Paul D. Brown, MD
Professor
Department of Radiation Oncology
The University of Texas MD Anderson Cancer Center
Houston, Texas

Jeffrey N. Bruce, MD
Edgar M. Housepian Professor
Vice-Chairman
Department of Neurological Surgery
Columbia University College of Physicians and Surgeons
New York, New York

Bradley R. Buchbinder, MD
Associate Radiologist
Department of Radiology
Division of Neuroradiology
Massachusetts General Hospital
Instructor in Radiology
Department of Radiology
Harvard Medical School
Boston, Massachusetts

Nicholas Butowski, MD
Associate Professor
Department of Neurological Surgery
University of California, San Francisco
San Francisco, California

Ali Bydon, MD
Assistant Professor
Department of Neurosurgery
Johns Hopkins University School of Medicine
Baltimore, Maryland

Sarah C. Carpentieri, PhD
Pediatric Neuropsychologist, Clinical Psychologist, and
   Research Consultant
Carpentieri and Associates
Houston, Texas

Jeffrey S. Chang, MD, PhD, MPH
Assistant Investigator
National Institute of Cancer Research
National Health Research Institutes
Tainan, Taiwan

Susan M. Chang, MD
Professor
Vice Chair, Neurological Surgery
Director, Division of Neuro-Oncology
University of California, San Francisco
San Francisco, California

Samuel T. Chao, MD
Assistant Professor
Department of Radiation Oncology
Cleveland Clinic
Cleveland, Ohio

John H. Chi, MD, MPH
Instructor
Department of Neurosurgery
Harvard Medical School
Brigham and Women's Hospital
Boston, Massachusetts

Shakeel A. Chowdhry, MD
Resident Physician
Department of Neurosurgery
Fellow, Endovascular Neurosurgery
University Hospitals Case Medical Center
Case Western Reserve University
Cleveland, Ohio

Jennifer L. Clarke, MD, MPH
Fellow
Department of Neurology
Memorial Sloan-Kettering Cancer Center
New York, New York
Assistant Clinical Professor of Neurology and
  Neurological Surgery
Department of Neurological Surgery
University of California, San Francisco
San Francisco, California

Elizabeth B. Claus, MD, PhD
Professor
Yale University School of Medicine
New Haven, Connecticut
Attending Neurosurgeon
Department of Neurosurgery
Brigham and Women's Hospital
Boston, Massachusetts

Alan R. Cohen, MD, FACS, FAAP
Surgeon-in Chief and Chief of Pediatric
  Neurological Surgery
Rainbow Babies and Children's Hospital
Reinberger Chair in Pediatric Neurological Surgery
Professor of Neurological Surgery and Pediatrics
Neurosurgery Residency Program Director
Case Western Reserve University School of Medicine
Cleveland, Ohio

Sidney E. Croul, MD, FRCPC
Professor and Head of Neuropathology
University Health Network
Member
The Arthur and Sonia Labatt Brain Tumour Research Centre
University of Toronto
Toronto, Ontario, Canada

Faith G. Davis, PhD
Professor
Department of Epidemiology and Biostatistics
University of Illinois at Chicago
Chicago, Illinois

Kevin C. DeBraganca, MD
Instructor
Department of Pediatrics and Neurology
Memorial Sloan-Kettering Cancer Center
New York, New York

Jessica Koch Devin, MD, MSCI
Endocrinology
Heritage Medical Associates
Nashville, Tennessee

Kiran Devisetty, MD
Assistant Professor
Department of Radiation Oncology
Medical College of Wisconsin
Milwaukee, Wisconsin

Michael L. Di Luna, MD
Assistant Professor
Neurosurgery
Yale University School of Medicine
New Haven, Connecticut

Therese A. Dolecek, PhD
Research Associate Professor
Department of Epidemiology
Institute for Health Research and Policy
University of Illinois at Chicago
Chicago, Illinois

Bernadine R. Donahue, MD
Clinical Director
Department of Radiation Oncology
Maimonides Cancer Center
Brooklyn, New York
Clinical Associate Professor
Department of Radiation Oncology
New York University School of Medicine
New York, New York

Michael Ellis, MD
Resident
Department of Neurosurgery
University of Toronto
Toronto, Ontario, Canada

Herbert H. Engelhard, III, MD, PhD
Associate Professor
Chief of Neuro-Oncology Section
Department of Neurosurgery
University of Illinois at Chicago
Chicago, Illinois

Johnathan A. Engh, MD
Assistant Professor
Department of Neurological Surgery
University of Pittsburgh Medical Center
Pittsburgh, Pennsylvania

Arnold B. Etame, MD
Neurosurgery Research Fellow
The Arthur and Sonia Labatt Brain Tumour Research Centre
Hospital for Sick Children
Toronto, Ontario, Canada

Sydney M. Evans, VMD, MS
Professor and Director of Faculty Affairs
Department of Radiation Oncology
University of Pennsylvania School of Medicine
Philadelphia, Pennsylvania

Shereen Ezzat, MD
Head of Endocrine Oncology
Princess Margaret Hospital
Senior Scientist
Ontario Cancer Institute
University Health Network
Professor
Department of Medicine
University of Toronto
Toronto, Ontario, Canada

Maria Feychting, PhD
Professor of Epidemiology
Institute of Environmental Medicine
Karolinska Institute
Stockholm, Sweden

Ingeborg Fischer, MD
Physician
Institute for Neuropathology
University of Zurich
Zurich, Switzerland

James L. Fisher, PhD
Research Scientist
Comprehensive Cancer Center
The Ohio State University
Columbus, Ohio

Paul Graham Fisher, MD
Professor
Department of Neurology, Pediatrics,
   Neurosurgery, and Human Biology
Stanford University
Palo Alto, California

Andrew B. Foy, MD
Clinical Fellow
Division of Neurosurgery
Children's Memorial Hospital
Chicago, Illinois

Carolyn R. Freeman, MBBS, FRCPC
Professor of Radiation Oncology and Pediatrics
McGill University
Head of Department of Radiation Oncology
McGill University Health Centre
Montreal, Canada

Jean-Pierre Gagner, MD, PhD
Assistant Professor of Surgery
Department of Surgery
New York University Langone Medical Center
New York, New York

Paul A. Gardner, MD
Assistant Professor
Department of Neurological Surgery
University of Pittsburgh Medical Center
Pittsburgh, Pennsylvania

Livia Garzia, PhD
Postdoctoral Fellow
The Arthur and Sonia Labatt Brain
   Tumour Research Centre
Hospital for Sick Children
Toronto, Ontario, Canada

Candece L. Gladson, MD
Professor of Molecular Medicine
Cleveland Clinic Lerner College of Medicine
Case Western Reserve University
Department of Cancer Biology
Cleveland Clinic
Brain Tumor and Neuro-Oncology Center
Cleveland, Ohio

Ziya L. Gokaslan, MD
Professor and Vice Chairman
Department of Neurosurgery
Johns Hopkins University School of Medicine
Baltimore, Maryland

John G. Golfinos, MD
Chairman
Department of Neurosurgery
Associate Professor of Neurosurgery
   and Otolaryngology
Department of Neurosurgery and Otolaryngology
New York University Langone Medical Center
New York, New York

Vinai Gondi, MD
Resident
Department of Human Oncology
University of Wisconsin School of Medicine
   and Public Health
Madison, Wisconsin

Jerome J. Graber, MD, MPH
Resident
Department of Neurology
New York University Langone Medical Center
Fellow
Department of Neurology
Memorial Sloan-Kettering Cancer Center
New York, New York

Stuart A. Grossman, MD
Professor of Oncology, Medicine, and Neurosurgery
Johns Hopkins School of Medicine
Baltimore, Maryland

Abhijit Guha, MSc, MD, FRCSC, FACS
Professor of Surgery (Neurosurgery)
Toronto Western Hospital
Senior Scientist and Co-Director
The Arthur and Sonia Labatt Brain Tumour Research Centre
Hospital for Sick Children
Hudson Chair in Neuro-Oncology
University of Toronto
Toronto, Ontario, Canada

Sarah R. G. Gupta, LICSW
Former Director of Support Services
National Brain Tumor Society
Boston, Massachusetts

David H. Gutmann, MS, MD, PhD
Donald O. Schnuck Family Professor
Department of Neurology
Washington University School of Medicine
St. Louis, Missouri

Rebecca J. Gutmann
Department of Neurology
Washington University School of Medicine
St. Louis, Missouri

Cynthia E. Hawkins, MD, PhD, FRCPC
Neuropathologist
Department of Paediatric Laboratory Medicine
Hospital for Sick Children
Associate Professor
Department of Laboratory Medicine and Pathobiology
University of Toronto
Toronto, Ontario, Canada

Lisa Hazard, MD
Associate Professor
Department of Radiation Oncology
University of Arizona
Tucson, Arizona

Patrick C. Hsieh, MD
Assistant Professor
Department of Neurological Surgery
University of Southern California Keck School of Medicine
Los Angeles, California

Dora Il'yasova, PhD
Assistant Professor
Department of Community and Family Medicine/Preston
    Robert Tisch Brain Tumor Center
Duke University School of Medicine
Durham, North Carolina

Daniel J. Indelicato, MD
Assistant Professor
Department of Radiation Oncology
University of Florida Proton Therapy Institute
University of Florida College of Medicine
Jacksonville, Florida

Meredith S. Irwin, MD
Associate Professor
Department of Pediatrics, Division of Hematology-Oncology
Hospital for Sick Children
Toronto, Ontario, Canada

Nadia N. Issa Laack, MD, MS
Assistant Professor
Department of Radiation Oncology
Mayo Clinic
Rochester, Minnesota

Jay Jagannathan, MD
Assistant Professor
Department of Neurosurgery
Wayne State University
Detroit, Michigan

C. David James, PhD
Professor of Neurological Surgery
Berthold and Belle N. Guggenhime Endowed Chair
Principal Investigator, Brain Tumor Research Center
Department of Neurological Surgery
University of California, San Francisco
San Francisco, California

John A. Jane, Jr., MD
Associate Professor
Department of Neurosurgery
University of Virginia
Charlottesville, Virginia

Cigall Kadoch, BA
Student and Research Associate
Division of Hematology/Oncology
University of California, San Francisco
San Francisco, California

Nadia Kadom, MD
Pediatric Neuroradiologist
Diagnostic Imaging and Radiology
Children's National Medical Center
Washington, DC

Adam S. Kanter, MD
Assistant Professor of Neurological Surgery
Department of Neurosurgery
University of Pittsburgh Medical Center
Pittsburgh, Philadelphia

Linda M. Karavodin, PhD
Principal Consultant
Karavodin Preclinical Consulting
Encinitas, California

Amin B. Kassam, MD
Medical Director, Neuroscience Institute
Department of Neurosurgery
St. John's Health Center
Santa Monica, California

Laurence Katznelson, MD
Professor
Department of Endocrinology/Neurosurgery
Stanford University
Stanford, California

Sameer Keole, MD
Adjunct Assistant Professor
Department of Radiation Oncology
Oklahoma University Health Science Center
Radiation Medicine Associates
Oklahoma City, Oklahoma

Jessica Dawn Kessler, PhD
Post-Doctoral Fellow
Verna and Marrs McLean Department of
 Biochemistry and Molecular Biology
Baylor College of Medicine
Houston, Texas

Kathleen Joy Khu, MD
Clinical Fellow in Neurosurgical Oncology
Neurosurgery
Toronto Western Hospital
University Health Network
Toronto, Ontario, Canada

Deepak Khuntia, MD
Associate Professor
Department of Human Oncology
University of Wisconsin
Madison, Wisconsin

Tim-Rasmus Kiehl, MD
Pathologist
Department of Pathology
University Health Network
Laboratory Medicine and Pathobiology
University of Toronto
Toronto, Ontario, Canada

Paul Kim, MD
Fellow
Department of Neurosurgery
Neurological Institute
Cleveland Clinic
Cleveland, Ohio

Martin Klein, PhD
Associate Professor
Clinical Neuropsychologist
Department of Medical Psychology
VU University Medical Center
Amsterdam, The Netherlands

Tim J. Kruser, MD
Resident
Department of Human Oncology
University of Wisconsin Carbone Cancer Center
Madison, Wisconsin

Rose Lai, MD
Assistant Professor
Department of Neurology
New York-Presbyterian Hospital
Columbia University
New York, New York

Frederick F. Lang, MD
Professor and Director of Clinical Research
Department of Neurosurgery
The University of Texas MD Anderson Cancer Center
Houston, Texas

Andrew B. Lassman, MD
Assistant Attending Neurologist
Department of Neurology
Memorial Hospital for Cancer and Allied Diseases
Assistant Member
Memorial Sloan-Kettering Cancer Center
New York, New York

Loretta M. S. Lau, MBBS, MMEd, PhD, FRACP
Paediatric Oncologist
Department of Oncology
The Children's Hospital at Westmead
Sydney Medical School
University of Sydney
Sydney, New South Wales, Australia

Edward R. Laws, MD, FACS
Professor
Department of Neurosurgery
Brigham and Women's Hospital
Harvard University
Boston, Massachusetts

Joung H. Lee, MD
Professor and Head, Section of Skull Base Surgery
Brain Tumor and Neuro-Oncology Center
Cleveland Clinic
Cleveland, Ohio

Frank S. Lieberman, MD
Director, Adult Neuro-Oncology Program
University of Pittsburgh Cancer Institute
University of Pittsburgh School of Medicine
Pittsburgh, Pennsylvania

Raymond Liu, MD
Associate Physician
Internal Medicine, Hematology-Oncology
The Permanente Medical Group
Kaiser Permanente
San Francisco, California

Wei Michael Liu, MD, PhD
Research Fellow
Department of Cancer Biology
Lerner Research Institute
Cleveland Clinic
Cleveland, Ohio

Siobhan C. Loeper, MD
Department of Nephrology, Endocrinology
 and Diabetes
University Hospital Hamburg-Eppendorf
Hamburg, Germany

Yi Lu, MD, PhD
Resident
Department of Neurosurgery
Brigham and Women's Hospital
Boston, Massachusetts

Robert S. Malyapa, MD, PhD
Assistant Professor
Department of Radiation Oncology
University of Florida Proton Therapy Institute
Jacksonville, Florida

Lori Mandelzweig, MPH, PhD
The Cancer and Radiation Epidemiology Unit
The Gertner Institute for Epidemiology and
 Health Policy Research
Chaim Sheba Medical Center, Tel-Hashomer
Ramat-Gan, Israel

Bridget J. McCarthy, PhD
Research Associate Professor
Department of Epidemiology/Biostatistics
University of Illinois at Chicago Cancer Center
University of Illinois at Chicago
Chicago, Illinois

Roberta McKean-Cowdin, PhD
Assistant Professor
Preventive Medicine
University of Southern California Keck School of Medicine
Los Angeles, California

Minesh P. Mehta, MD, FASTRO
Professor
Department of Human Oncology
University of Wisconsin
Madison, Wisconsin

Beatrice Melin, MD, PhD
Department of Oncology, Radiation Science
University Hospital
Umea, Sweden

Michelle E. Melisko, MD
Assistant Clinical Professor of Medicine
Division of Hematology and Oncology
University of California San Francisco
San Francisco, California

William M. Mendenhall, MD
Professor
Department of Radiation Oncology
University of Florida
Gainesville, Florida

Christina A. Meyers, PhD
Professor and Chief, Section of Neuropsychology
Department of Neuro-Oncology
The University of Texas MD Anderson Cancer Center
Houston, Texas

Edward Andrew Michals, MD
Director of Diagnostic Neuroradiology
Assistant Professor of Radiology
Diagnostic Radiology
University of Illinois at Chicago Medical Center
Chicago, Illinois

Karine Michaud, MD
Department of Neurosurgery
Centre hospitalier universitaire affilié l'Enfant-Jésus
Quebec, Canada

Jonathan P. Miller, MD
Director
Functional and Restorative Neurosurgery
Assistant Professor
Department of Neurological Surgery
Case Western Reserve University School of Medicine
Cleveland, Ohio

Gaetan Moise, MD
Resident
Department of Neurological Surgery
New York-Presbyterian Hospital
New York, New York

Sabine Mueller, MD, PhD
Assistant Professor
Departments of Pediatrics and Neurology
University of San Francisco
San Francisco, California

Diana Munoz, BSc (Hons)
Graduate Student
Department of Medical Biophysics
The Arthur and Sonia Labatt Brain Tumour Research Centre
Hospital for Sick Children
University of Toronto
Toronto, Ontario, Canada

Sean J. Nagel, MD
Resident
Department of Neurosurgery
Neurological Institute
Cleveland Clinic
Cleveland, Ohio

Herbert B. Newton, MD, FAAN
Professor of Neurology, Neurosurgery, and Oncology
Esther Dardinger Endowed Chair in Neuro-Oncology
Department of Neurosurgery
Dardinger Neuro-Oncology Center
The Ohio State University Medical Center
James Cancer Hospital
Columbus, Ohio

Douglas Edward Ney, MD
Fellow
Department of Neurology
Memorial Sloan-Kettering Cancer Center
New York, New York
Assistant Professor
Department of Neurology and Neurosurgery
University of Colorado School of Medicine
Aurora, Colorado

Carsten Nieder, MD
Professor
Department of Oncology and Palliative Medicine
Nordland Hospital
Bodø, Norway
Professor
Faculty of Health Sciences, Institute of Clinical Medicine
University of Tromsø
Tromsø, Norway

Andrew D. Norden, MD, MPH
Associate Neurologist
Division of Cancer Neurology
Department of Neurology
Brigham and Women's Hospital
Boston, Massachusetts

Subhadra L. Nori, MD
Regional Director
Department of Rehabilitation Medicine
Elmhurst Hospital Center
Elmhurst, New York
Regional Director
Department of Rehabilitation Medicine
Queens Hospital Center
Jamaica, New York
Assistant Professor, Rehabilitation Medicine
Mount Sinai School of Medicine
New York, New York

Fabio Pereira Nunes, MD
Instructor
Department of Neurology
Massachusetts General Hospital
Harvard Medical School
Boston, Massachusetts

Alfred T. Ogden, MD
Assistant Professor
Department of Neurological Surgery
Columbia University
New York, New York

Edward H. Oldfield, MD
Professor of Neurosurgery and Internal Medicine
Department of Neurosurgery
University of Virginia Health System
Charlottesville, Virginia

S. Bulent Omay, MD
Resident in Neurosurgery
Department of Neurosurgery
Yale University School of Medicine
New Haven, Connecticut

Tomoko Ozawa, MD, PhD
Research Specialist
Department of Neurological Surgery
University of California, San Francisco
San Francisco, California

Roger J. Packer, MD
Senior Vice-President, Neuroscience and Behavioral Medicine
Director, Brain Tumor Institute
Director, Gilbert Neurofibromatosis Institute
Center for Neuroscience and Behavioral Medicine
Children's National Medical Center
Professor
Department of Neurology and Pediatrics
The George Washington University
Washington, DC

Joseph M. Piepmeier, MD
Nixdorff/German Professor of Neurosurgery
Department of Neurosurgery
Yale University
New Haven, Connecticut

Scott R. Plotkin, MD, PhD
Assistant Professor of Neurology
Harvard Medical School
Director of Neurofibromatosis Clinic
Massachusetts General Hospital
Boston, Massachusetts

Ian F. Pollack, MD
Walter Dandy Professor
Department of Neurosurgery
University of Pittsburgh School of Medicine
Pittsburgh, Pennsylvania

Daniel M. Prevedello, MD
Assistant Professor
Department of Neurological Surgery
Director, Minimally Invasive Cranial Surgery Program
The Ohio State University
Columbus, Ohio

Dirk Rades, MD
Professor
Department of Radiation Oncology
University of Lubeck
Lubeck, Germany

Ali I. Raja, MD
Neurosurgeon
Department of Arkansas Neuroscience Institute
Little Rock, Arkansas

Pedram Razavi, MD, PhD
Research Associate
Preventive Medicine
University of Southern California
   Keck School of Medicine
Los Angeles, California

David A. Reardon, MD
Associate Deputy Director
The Preston Robert Tisch Brain Tumor Center
Associate Professor
Department of Surgery and Pediatrics
Duke University Medical Center
Durham, North Carolina

Terri Rice, MPH
Study Coordinator
Department of Neurological Surgery
University of California, San Francisco
San Francisco, California

R. Mark Richardson, MD, PhD
Resident, Neurological Surgery
University of California, San Francisco
San Francisco, California

C. Leland Rogers, MD
Department of Radiation Oncology
Gamma West Cancer Services
Salt Lake City, Utah

James L. Rubenstein, MD, PhD
Associate Professor of Medicine in Residence
Department of Hematology/Oncology
University of California, San Francisco
San Francisco, California

James T. Rutka, MD, PhD, FRCSC
Professor and Chairman
Department of Neurosurgery
University of Toronto
Toronto, Canada

Burak Sade, MD
Clinical Associate
Brain Tumor and Neuro-Oncology Center
Department of Neurosurgery
Cleveland Clinic
Cleveland, Ohio

Siegal Sadetzki, MD, MPH
Head
The Cancer and Radiation Epidemiology Unit
The Gertner Institute for Epidemiology and
    Health Policy Research
Chaim Sheba Medical Center, Tel-Hashomer
Ramat-Gan, Israel
Professor
Department of Epidemiology and Preventive Medicine
Sackler School of Medicine
Tel-Aviv University
Tel-Aviv, Israel

Yair Safriel, MD, MBBCh
Lead Neuroradiologist
Mease Dunedin Hospital
Assistant Clinical Professor
University of South Florida
Clearwater, Florida

John Howard Sampson, MD, PhD, MHSc
Robert H. and Gloria Wilkins Distinguished
    Professor of Surgery (Neurosurgery)
Professor of Pathology, Immunology, and Radiation Oncology
Department of Surgery
Duke University Medical Center
Durham, North Carolina

Sith Sathornsumetee, MD
Deputy Director, Adult Brain Tumor Program
Department of Medicine (Neurology)
Siriraj Cancer Center, Mahidol University
Bangkok, Thailand

Michael Schulder, MD
Professor and Vice Chairman
Department of Neurosurgery
Hofstra University School of Medicine
North Shore LIJ Health
Manhasset, New York

Christopher J. Schultz, MD
Professor
Department of Radiation Oncology
Medical College of Wisconsin
Milwaukee, Wisconsin

Judith A. Schwartzbaum, PhD
Associate Professor
Division of Epidemiology
College of Public Health
The Ohio State University
Columbus, Ohio

Sameer A. Sheth, MD, PhD
Resident
Department of Neurosurgery
Massachusetts General Hospital
Boston, Massachusetts

Charles C. Shyu, MD
Fellow
Department of Neurology
Memorial Sloan-Kettering Cancer Center
New York, New York
Neurologist
Christie Clinic
Champaign, Illinois

Malika L. Siker, MD
Resident Physician
Department of Radiation Oncology
Medical College of Wisconsin
Milwaukee, Wisconsin

Christian Smith, PhD
Research Associate
The Arthur and Sonia Labatt Brain Tumour Research Center
Hospital for Sick Children
University of Toronto
Toronto, Ontario, Canada

Tod W. Speer, MD
Clinical Assistant Professor
Department of Human Oncology
University of Wisconsin
Wausau, Wisconsin

Robert J. Spinner, MD
Professor
Department of Neurologic Surgery, Orthopedics, and Anatomy
Mayo Clinic
Rochester, Minnesota

Anat O. Stemmer-Rachamimov, MD
Assistant Professor
Department of Pathology
Massachusetts General Hospital
Massachusetts Eye and Ear Infirmary
Harvard Medical School
Boston, Massachusetts

Volker Wilhelm Walter Stieber, MD
Medical Director of Stereotactic Radiation Oncology
Department of Radiation Oncology
Derrick L. Davis Forsyth Regional Cancer Center
Winston-Salem, North Carolina

Walter Stummer, MD
Professor
Department of Neurosurgery
Universitätsklinikum Muenster
Muenster, Germany

John H. Suh, MD
Chairman
Department of Radiation Oncology
Cleveland Clinic
Cleveland, Ohio

Erik Sulman, MD
Assistant Professor
Radiation Oncology
The University of Texas MD Anderson Cancer Center
Houston, Texas

Uri Tabori, MD
Assistant Professor
Department of Neuro-Oncology
University of Toronto
Toronto, Ontario, Canada

Michael David Taylor, MD, PhD
Pediatric Neurosurgeon, Associate Professor
Division of Neurosurgery
The Arthur and Sonia Labatt Brain Tumour Research Center
Hospital for Sick Children
University of Toronto
Toronto, Ontario, Canada

Sayana Rachel Thomas, MD
Resident Physician
Department of Human Oncology
University of Wisconsin
Madison, Wisconsin

Tarik Tihan, MD, PhD
Professor of Pathology
Department of Pathology
University of California, San Francisco
San Francisco, California

Jörg-Christian Tonn, MD
Professor
Department of Neurosurgery
Ludwig Maximilians University
Munich, Germany

Kene T. Ugokwe, MD
Resident
Department of Neurosurgery
Neurological Institute
Cleveland Clinic
Cleveland, Ohio

Shobhan Vachhrajani, MD
Post-Doctoral Research Fellow
Department of Neurosurgery
University of Toronto
Toronto, Ontario, Canada

John Lee Villano, MD, PhD
Associate Professor of Medicine
College of Medicine
University of Illinois at Chicago
Chicago, Illinois

Michael A. Vogelbaum, MD, PhD, FACS
The Robert and Kathryn Lamborn Chair for Neuro-Oncology
Associate Director of Neurosurgical Oncology
Department of Neurosurgery
Brain Tumor and Neuro-Oncology Center
Cleveland Clinic
Cleveland, Ohio

Nina D. Wagner-Johnston, MD
Department of Internal Medicine
Division of Medical Oncology
Washington University School of Medicine
St. Louis, Missouri

Robert J. Wechsler-Reya, PhD
Associate Professor
Department of Pharmacology and Cancer Biology
Duke University Medical Center
Durham, North Carolina

Patrick Y. Wen, MD
Director
Center for Neuro-Oncology
Dana-Farber/Brigham and Women's Cancer Center
Professor of Neurology
Harvard Medical School
Boston, Massachusetts

Cynthia Wetmore, MD, PhD
Associate Member
Department of Oncology and Neuro-Oncology
St. Jude Children's Research Hospital
Memphis, Tennessee

Joseph Leo Wiemels, PhD
Associate Professor
Department of Epidemiology and Biostatistics
University of California, San Francisco
San Francisco, California

John K. Wiencke, PhD
Professor in Residence
Department of Neurosurgery
University of California, San Francisco
San Francisco, California

Margaret R. Wrensch, MPH, PhD
Professor
Department of Neurological Surgery
University of California, San Francisco
San Francisco, California

Adam Wu, MD
Fellow
Department of Neurosurgery
The University of Texas MD Anderson Cancer Center
Houston, Texas

David Zagzag, MD, PhD
Associate Professor of Pathology and Neurosurgery
Departments of Pathology and Neurosurgery
New York University Langone Medical Center
New York, New York

Hekmat Khodr Zarzour, MD
Clinical Fellow
Endovascular Neurosurgery/Interventional Neuroradiology
Department of Neurosurgery
Brigham and Women's Hospital
Boston, Massachusetts

Salvatore M. Zavarella, DO
Resident
Department of Neurosurgery
Hofstra University School of Medicine
North Shore LIJ Health
Manhasset, New York

Principles and Practice of Neuro-Oncology

PART I: EPIDEMIOLOGY

1 Epidemiology and Etiology of Glioma: An Overview

James L. Fisher, Judith A. Schwartzbaum, and Margaret R. Wrensch

In the following eight chapters, we summarize the descriptive and analytic epidemiologic research on glioma, a relatively rare tumor of neuroepithelial tissue and its precursors with an average annual incidence of 4.9 per 100,000 [1,2]. A salient descriptive feature of glioma is that the most common histologic type in adults, glioblastoma, is characterized by an extremely low survival probability, with only 3% of patients surviving more than 5 years from the time of diagnosis [1,2]. Another key feature of glioma epidemiology is that these tumors are generally more common in men than women [1,2]. Although only approximately 1% of gliomas can be directly attributed to inherited susceptibility, relatively little is known about environmental factors, other than exposure to ionizing radiation, that alter the risk of developing this tumor. Progress in identifying risk factors was impeded in the past because studies did not have sufficient numbers of observations to exclude the effects of statistical variation on the results. However, thanks to national and international collaboration, studies are now large enough to identify environmental and developmental factors and even to evaluate genetic interactions with these factors. The consistent inverse association between allergies and glioma has been the focus of epidemiologic, laboratory, and clinical studies on the potential role of the immune system in glioma etiology and growth. Finally, epidemiologists have recently turned their attention to identifying factors that may predict for improved survival.

As Bridget McCarthy points out in Chapter 2, glioma incidence has increased over time from the 1950's to the early 1990's [1,2]. However, much of the increase was probably due to the introduction of new diagnostic imaging technologies during the late 1970s and 1980s. In particular, computed tomography and magnetic resonance imaging of adults with new onset seizures helped identify several previously unidentified tumors. Since the 1980s, the incidence of glioma has stabilized [1,2]. Although there have been some changes in trends of some glial subgroups, these may be due to changing diagnostic criteria. Survival time for some glioma subtypes also has increased over the past 30 years [1–5]; however, these increases may be a result of improved ascertainment of indolent glioma rather than improved clinical management.

Glioma is thought to develop through the progressive accumulation of genetic and/or epigenetic alterations that permit cells to evade normal regulatory mechanisms and/or escape destruction by the immune system [2,3,6]. In chapter 3, Malmer and Bondy present evidence for inherited susceptibility to glioma. Studies have demonstrated increased risk of brain tumors among close relatives of glioma patients. Diseases or syndromes associated with mutations in highly penetrant genes (including neurofibromatosis types 1 and 2, tuberous sclerosis, retinoblastoma, Li-Fraumeni cancer family syndrome, and Turcot's syndrome) are known to increase glioma risk [4,7]. However, in a study of 500 glioma patients, less than 1% had a known hereditary syndrome [8]. Two recent genome-wide association studies discovered and confirmed that inherited variation in five regions—chromosome 5p15.33 (*TERT*), 9p21.3 (*CDKN2B*), 8q24, 11q23 (*PHLDB1*), and 20q13.3 (*RTEL1*)—influence glioma risk [9,10]. These findings open unique and novel research opportunities for more complete understanding of the etiology of this devastating disease.

Chemicals capable of inducing brain tumors in laboratory animals have been identified and are referred to as neurocarcinogens. In Chapter 4, Il'yasova et al review evidence for the influence of neurocarcinogens on human brain tumor risk. There is vast but inconclusive literature on the relationship of occupational exposure to carcinogenic substances and brain tumor risk. No single study has had sufficient numbers of cases to yield definitive conclusions and exposures vary so much over time and place that meta-analyses also have not yielded conclusive results. In addition, there is no consistent evidence that other sources of neurocarcinogens such as tobacco smoke or foods with neurocarcinogenic precursors alter glioma risk [2,4]. In addition to small study sample sizes, possible explanations for inconsistent findings include invalid or imprecise exposure measures (resulting from use of self-reports of exposure), inherited or developmental variation in metabolic and DNA repair pathways that modify the effect of environmental factors on brain tumor risk, and unaccounted-for protective environmental exposures or conditions. Exposure levels generally encountered for these compounds may be too low to measurably affect brain tumor risk.

Ionizing radiation is the only environmental factor found to be consistently associated with an increased risk of developing gliomas and/or other brain tumors. Sadetzki and Mandelzweig review the literature pertaining to ionizing radiation in chapter 5. Exposure to ionizing radiation occurred when the atomic bomb was exploded on Japan and continues to occur as the result of nuclear weapons testing, therapeutic and diagnostic medical procedures, occupational exposures, and natural sources. Results from prospective studies of people exposed to ionizing radiation are consistent and strong, suggesting a linear dose-response association between ionizing radiation exposure and glioma risk; however, results from case-control studies vary somewhat, perhaps due to underreporting of exposure, imprecise estimates of age at first exposure, or due to low prevalence of exposure to high doses of ionizing radiation. Future studies should consider the potential for interaction between ionizing radiation and age at exposure or genetic variation that may mediate exposure.

Due in large part to public concern over the potential health effects of mobile phone use, much recent research has focused on radiofrequency fields and glioma risk. In chapter 6, Feychting and Ahlbom report that results from epidemiologic studies suggest no consistent evidence for an effect of short-term mobile phone use on glioma risk [11–22]; however, there are limited data and inconsistent results pertaining to long-term use [12–16,19,20,22]. Although there is some evidence of increased glioma risk as the result of mobile phone use on the same side of the head as the phone was used [13,14,16,19,20], the decreased risk on the opposite side of the head indicate that these findings are probably due to recall bias. To avoid differential misclassification of exposure, information about mobile phone use is best collected prior to glioma diagnosis; that is, a cohort study is preferred and results from cohort studies, in this instance, are superior to those from case-control studies not nested in cohorts. The number of long-term mobile phone users is rapidly increasing and it will soon be possible to determine whether or not mobile phone use for a period longer than 15 years poses a threat. Although there have been a relatively large number of epidemiologic studies of mobile phone use and glioma risk, this line of inquiry has only recently evolved to construct more refined hypotheses and more sophisticated exposure assessment techniques that may be required to understand the potential role, if any, of mobile phone use in glioma etiology.

Perhaps the most intriguing factors emerging from epidemiologic studies of glioma over the past decade are the strong and consistent inverse associations between allergy, asthma, and immunoglobulin E and glioma risk. In chapter 7, Schwartzbaum et al review the evidence for a protective effect of allergy-related immune responses and inherited immunologic factors and discuss competing explanations for these findings. In addition, they argue that the effects of immunosuppressive regulatory T-cells and their associated cytokines, transforming growth factor-β and interleukin-10, provide a conceptual and mechanistic framework to explain an indirect relationship between allergies and antiglioma immune reactions. Finally, they point out that the unique architecture of the brain does not totally exclude gliomas from immune system interaction, although immune responses in the brain may be attenuated compared with those found in other organs. In addition, there is now evidence for infiltration of T and B-cells into the brains of brain tumor patients and the enhancement of such responses might form the basis of future glioma therapies.

Chang et al review the literature related to glioma survival and prognosis in chapter 8. The mechanisms for the strong, consistent inverse association between age and survival are poorly understood and deserve further exploration. Recent efforts to identify additional prognostic factors have focused on inherited genetic variation, tumor molecular markers, and serologic factors. For oligodendroglioma, it is now well established that the combined tumor loss of 1p and 19q confers a more favorable prognosis [23]. In addition, preliminary results from expression array studies of glioma, albeit limited by small sample sizes, have suggested that abnormal expression of some specific genes predicts survival. Although several studies of inherited variation in relation to glioma survival are suggestive, too few studies have been conducted to assess consistency and strength of association. Finally, evidence for the importance of immunologic factors in glioma progression and patient survival is accumulating, but more studies are needed to confirm the findings. Continued analyses of the immune status of patients diagnosed with glioma may help us to better understand the complex relationship between immune response, gliomagenesis, and prognosis.

REFERENCES

1. CBTRUS. *Statistical Report: Primary Brain Tumors in the United States, 2000–2004*. Hinsdale, IL: CBTRUS; 2008.
2. Fisher JL, Schwartzbaum J, Wrensch M, Wiemels JL. Epidemiology of brain tumors. *Neurol Clin.* 2007;25:867–890.
3. Schwartzbaum JA, Fisher JL, Aldape KD, Wrensch M. Epidemiology and molecular pathology of glioma. *Nat Clin Pract Neurol.* 2006;2:494–503.
4. Wrensch M, Minn Y, Chew T, Bondy M, Berger MS. Epidemiology of primary brain tumors: current concepts and review of the literature. *Neuro Oncol.* 2002;4:278–299.
5. Surveillance, Epidemiology, and End Results (SEER) Program (www.seer.cancer.gov) SEER*Stat Database: Incidence—SEER 13 Regs Public-Use, Nov 2005 Sub (1992–2003), National Cancer Institute, DCCPS, Surveillance Research Program, Cancer Statistics Branch, released April 2006, based on the November 2005 submission; 2006.
6. Wrensch M, Fisher JL, Schwartzbaum JA, Bondy M, Berger M, Aldape KD. The molecular epidemiology of gliomas in adults. *Neurosurg Focus.* 2005;19:E5.
7. Bondy M, Wiencke J, Wrensch M, Kyritsis AP. Genetics of primary brain tumors: a review. *J Neurooncol.* 1994;18:69–81.
8. Wrensch M, Lee M, Miike R, et al. Familial and personal medical history of cancer and nervous system conditions among adults with glioma and controls. *Am J Epidemiol.* 1997;145:581–593.
9. Wrensch M, Jenkins RB, Chang JS, et al. Variants in the CDKN2B and RTEL1 regions are associated with high-grade glioma susceptibility. *Nat Genet.* 2009;41:905–908.
10. Shete S, Hosking FJ, Robertson LB, et al. Genome-wide association study identifies five susceptibility loci for glioma. *Nat Genet.* 2009;41:899–904.

11. Auvinen A, Hietanen M, Luukkonen R, Koskela R-S. Brain tumors and salivary gland cancers among cellular telephone users. *Epidemiology* (Cambridge Mass). 2002;13:356–359.
12. Christensen HC, Schuz J, Kosteljanetz M, et al. Cellular telephones and risk for brain tumors: a population-based, incident case-control study. *Neurology*. 2005;64:1189–1195.
13. Hardell L, Carlberg M, Hansson Mild K. Case-control study on cellular and cordless telephones and the risk for acoustic neuroma or meningioma in patients diagnosed 2000–2003. *Neuroepidemiology*. 2005;25:120–128.
14. Hardell L, Mild KH, Carlberg M. Case-control study on the use of cellular and cordless phones and the risk for malignant brain tumours. *Int J Radiat Biol*. 2002;78:931–936.
15. Hardell L, Nasman A, Pahlson A, Hallquist A, Hansson Mild K. Use of cellular telephones and the risk for brain tumours: a case-control study. *Int J Oncol*. 1999;15:113–116.
16. Hepworth SJ, Schoemaker MJ, Muir KR, Swerdlow AJ, van Tongeren MJA, McKinney PA. Mobile phone use and risk of glioma in adults: case-control study. *BMJ* (Clinical Research ed). 2006;332:883–887.
17. Inskip PD, Tarone RE, Hatch EE, et al. Cellular-telephone use and brain tumors. *N Engl J Med*. 2001;344:79–86.
18. Johansen C, Boice JJ, McLaughlin J, Olsen J. Cellular telephones and cancer—a nationwide cohort study in Denmark. *J Natl Cancer Inst*. 2001;93:203–207.
19. Lahkola A, Auvinen A, Raitanen J, et al. Mobile phone use and risk of glioma in 5 North European countries. *Int J Cancer*. 2007;120:1769–1775.
20. Lonn S, Ahlbom A, Hall P, Feychting M, Feychting M. Long-term mobile phone use and brain tumor risk. *Am J Epidemiol*. 2005;161:526–535.
21. Muscat JE, Malkin MG, Thompson S, et al. Handheld cellular telephone use and risk of brain cancer. *JAMA*. 2000;284:3001–3007.
22. Schuz J, Bohler E, Berg G, et al. Cellular phones, cordless phones, and the risks of glioma and meningioma (Interphone Study Group, Germany). *Am J Epidemiol*. 2006;163:512–520.
23. Aldape K, Burger PC, Perry A. Clinicopathologic aspects of 1p/19q loss and the diagnosis of oligodendroglioma. *Arch Pathol Lab Med*. 2007;131:242–251.

2 Descriptive Epidemiology of Glioma

Bridget J. McCarthy

INTRODUCTION

Definitions and Classification Systems

Glioma is a class of neuroepithelial tumors that includes multiple histological types. As such, it is difficult to summarize the descriptive epidemiology of glioma because its definition depends on which histological subtypes are included. The histological subtypes that comprise glioma have changed over time and may vary among investigators. Early classification schemes for defining glioma included astrocytic, oligodendroglial, and ependymal tumors, as well as medulloblastoma, ganglioneuroma, pinealoma, and neuroepithelioma [1]. In later classification schemes, this broad group of tumors was renamed tumors of neuroepithelial tissue (Table 2.1) and was expanded to include additional histological types [2–7]. A summary of some of the methodological issues and suggestions for standardization of reporting was presented by Counsell and Grant [8].

The *International Classification of Diseases for Oncology, Third Edition* (ICD-O-3) is the standard classification system for cancer registries worldwide [9]. In *ICD-O-3*, the broad group "glioma" (938_–948_) consists of malignant glioma, not otherwise specified (NOS), ependymoma, subependymoma, oligodendroglial tumors, astrocytic tumors, mixed glioma, choroid plexus tumors, medulloblastoma, primitive neuroectodermal tumors, and dysembryoplastic neuroepithelial tumors (Table 2.1). In addition, each of these groups includes more specific histological subtypes. In *Histological Groups for Comparative Studies*, histologies included in the definition of "glioma" are the astrocytic, oligodendroglial, ependymal, and mixed tumors, as well as gliomas of uncertain origin (Table 2.1) [10]. Choroid plexus tumors and medulloblastoma are excluded from "glioma," and are included in the categories "other neuroepithelial tumors" and "embryonal tumors," respectively. As the grouping scheme for *Histological Groups for Comparative Studies* was written before *ICD-O-3* was published, desmoplastic infantile astrocytoma (9412/1), dysembryoplastic neuroepithelial tumor (9413/0), and chordoid glioma (9444/1) were not available as histological entities for categorization by cancer registries, and were not included in the definition of glioma [11]. The Central Brain Tumor Registry of the United States (CBTRUS) uses a definition of "glioma" that is similar to that found in *Histological Groups for Comparative Studies*, including astrocytic, oligodendroglial, ependymal, mixed tumors and the three histologies listed earlier (9412, 9413, and 9444) [7]. For childhood glioma, the International Classification of Childhood Cancer (ICCC) includes ependymoma and choroid plexus tumors, astrocytoma, and other glioma (Table 2.1) [12]. Despite these classification schemes, the definition of glioma continues to vary. Therefore, when known, we present the histological inclusion criteria described in the following text.

Most glioma subtypes are assigned a behavior code of malignant (/3), in ICD-O-3, whereas a few are considered nonmalignant [benign (/0) or uncertain (/1) behavior], including subependymoma (9383/1), subependymal giant cell astrocytoma (9384/1), choroid plexus papilloma (9390/0,1), myxopapillary ependymoma (9394/1), desmoplastic infantile astrocytoma (9412/1), dysembryoplastic neuroepithelial tumor (9413/0), gliofibroma (9442/1), and chordoid glioma (9444/1). Nonmalignant brain tumors are collected by some, but not all, cancer registries throughout the world. Beginning in 2004, the collection of all primary brain tumors was mandated by law (Benign Brain Tumor Cancer Registry Amendment Act, Public Law 107–260) in the United States. Although the behavior code for pilocytic astrocytomas was revised from malignant (/3) to uncertain (/1) in *ICD-O-3*, in the United States, pilocytic astrocytomas are still collected as malignant tumors to provide consistency with previous data reports [9].

Inclusion of differing primary sites may result in rates that are not comparable; for example, one registry may only include intracranial tumors, whereas another may collect spinal cord tumors as well. However, although misclassification may occur between histological subtypes (such as oligodendroglioma, mixed tumors, and astrocytoma), classification of a tumor as glioma is usually correct [13–16]. Standardization of rates to differing population standards (e.g., US 2000 Standard Population, World Standard Population [WSP], or the European Standard Population [ESP]) results in an additional source of variance.

Despite these classification and reporting differences among registries and population-based studies, demographic characteristics, incidence rates, and survival probabilities of "glioma" show similarities worldwide. In this chapter, we present basic clinical and demographic characteristics, incidence rates, and survival probabilities in population-based studies published after 2000. When possible,

Table 2.1 Categorization of Brain and CNS Glioma and Tumors of Neuroepithelial Tissue

	Histologies	ICD-O Version	Histology Codes
Glioma			
International Classification of Diseases for Oncology, Third Edition (ICD-O-3) [9]	Astrocytic tumors Oligodendroglial & mixed tumors Ependymal tumors Choroid plexus tumors Medulloblastoma Other glial tumors	3	9380–9480
Histological Groups for Comparative Studies [10]	Astrocytic tumors Ependymal tumors Oligodendroglial tumors and mixed gliomas Gliomas of uncertain origin	2	9384, 9400–9411, 9420–9421, 9424, 9440–9442 9383, 9391–9394 9382, 9450–9451 9380–9381, 9423, 9430, 9460, 9480
International Classification of Childhood Cancer (ICCC) [12]	Ependymoma and choroid plexus tumors Astrocytoma Other gliomas	3	9383, 9390–9394 [9380 in site code C72.3], 9381, 9400–9441 [9380 in site codes C70.0–72.2, 72.4–72.9], 9382, 9384, 9442–9460
Tumors of neuroepithelial tissue			
Histological Typing of Tumours of the CNS [2]	Astrocytic tumors Oligodendroglial tumors Ependymal tumors Mixed gliomas Choroid plexus tumors Gliomas of uncertain origin Neuronal/mixed neuronal–glial Pineal parenchymal tumors Embryonal tumors	1	9384, 9400–9411, 9420–9421, 9424, 9440–9442 9450–9451 9383, 9391–9394 9382 9390 9381, 9430, 9443 8690, 9490/0, 9505–9506, 9522–9523 9361–9362 9392, 9470–9473, 9490/1, 9500–9501
WHO 2000 Classification [3,4]	Astrocytic tumors Oligodendroglial tumors Ependymal tumors Oligoastrocytic tumors Choroid plexus tumors Gliomas of uncertain origin Neuronal/mixed neuronal–glial Pineal parenchymal tumors Embryonal tumors Neuroblastic tumors	3	9384, 9400–9411, 9420–9421, 9424, 9440–9442 9450–9451 9383, 9391–9394 9382 9390 9430, 9381, 9444 8680, 9412–9413, 9492–9493, 9505–9506 9361–9362 9392, 9470–9474, 9490, 9500–9501, 9508 9500, 9522–9523
Central Brain Tumor Registry of the United States[a] [7]	Astrocytic tumors Oligodendroglial tumors Ependymal tumors Oligoastrocytic tumors Malignant glioma, NOS Choroid plexus tumors Other neuroepithelial tumors Neuronal/mixed neuronal–glial Pineal parenchymal tumors Embryonal tumors	3	9383–9384, 9400–9411, 9420–9421, 9424, 9440–9442/3 9450–9451, 9460 9391–9394 9382 9380 9390 9381, 9423, 9430, 9444 8680–8682, 8690, 8693, 9412–9413, 9442/1, 9490–9493, 9500, 9505–9506, 9522–9523 9360–9362 8963, 9363–9364, 9470–9474, 9501–9503, 9508
WHO 2007 proposed classification [6]	Astrocytic tumors Oligodendroglial tumors Ependymal tumors Oligoastrocytic tumors Choroid plexus tumors Other neuroepithelial tumors Neuronal/mixed neuronal–glial Pineal parenchymal tumors Embryonal tumors	4[b]	9381, 9384, 9400–9411, 9420–9421, 9424, 9425[b], 9440–9442 9450–9451 9383, 9391–9394 9382 9390 9430, 9431[b], 9444 8680, 9412–9413, 9492–9493, 9505–9506, 9509 9361–9362, 9395[b] 9392, 9470–9471, 9473–9474, 9490, 9500–9501, 9508

[a] CBTRUS groupings are based on actual tumor histologies included in population-based cancer registry data and are classified into categories upon the recommendation of a consulting neuropathologist.

[b] Codes proposed for the 4th edition of ICD-O; subject to change until published.

incidence rates age-adjusted to the WSP are reported to allow comparability among studies. Tables summarizing "glioma" incidence rates from earlier studies are presented by Counsell and Grant [8], Elia-Pasquet et al [17], Christensen et al [18], and Ohgaki and Kleihues [19].

CLINICAL AND DEMOGRAPHIC CHARACTERISTICS

Frequency of Primary Gliomas

In the United States, 36% of all primary brain and central nervous system (CNS) tumors are classified as glioma (9380–9384, 9391–9460, 9480), whereas 81% of all malignant brain and CNS tumors are labeled malignant glioma [7]. In children aged 0 to 14 years, a higher percentage (56%) of all primary brain and CNS tumors are defined as glioma, whereas somewhat fewer (relative to adults) primary malignant brain tumors (76%) are so classified. This variation is attributable to nonmalignant histologies, meningioma and nerve sheath tumors, being more common in adults than children, while malignant embryonal and germ cell tumors are more common in children than adults. Gliomas account for 45% of all primary brain tumors in adults and 50% in children and adults combined, although differences in reporting and classification may affect the proportion of tumors when compared with other studies [17,20]. Forty-seven percent of all intracranial tumors are tumors of neuroepithelial tissue [21]. In children (aged 0–14 years) in Sweden, 47% of all CNS tumors were astrocytoma/glioma, with 75% of these being low grade [22].

Distribution of Glioma by Site (Tumor Location) and Histological Type

The most common primary site for glioma in the CBTRUS data was the frontal lobe (24.5%), followed by other brain, NOS (20.6%), and the temporal lobe (19.6%), with 61% of glioma occurring in one of the four lobes of the brain (Figure 2.1) [7]. Similarly, in a study from four Nordic countries, the frontal and temporal lobes were the most common primary sites for adult intracerebral glioma [23]. In Finland, 86% of all intracranial glioma in adults were found in one of the four lobes of the brain, with frontal (40%) and temporal (29%) being the most frequent site [24]. In Denmark, 40% of glioma (9380–9460) were located in the cerebrum, NOS, 25% in the frontal lobe, and 15% each in the parietal and temporal lobes [18].

Glioblastoma was the most frequent histological subtype of glioma (51.2%) in the CBTRUS 2000–2004 data, with astrocytic tumors, including glioblastomas, accounting for 75% of all primary glioma. Oligodendroglial and ependymal tumors accounted for 8.4 and 5.8%, respectively (Figure 2.2) [7]. Other studies have also found that glioblastoma is the most common subtype of all primary CNS tumors, of primary malignant brain tumors, and of adults with intracranial glioma [17,20,23–29]. In Zurich, glioblastoma accounted for 69% of incident astrocytic and oligodendroglial glioma cases [30]. In a population-based study of spinal glioma from England and Wales, the most

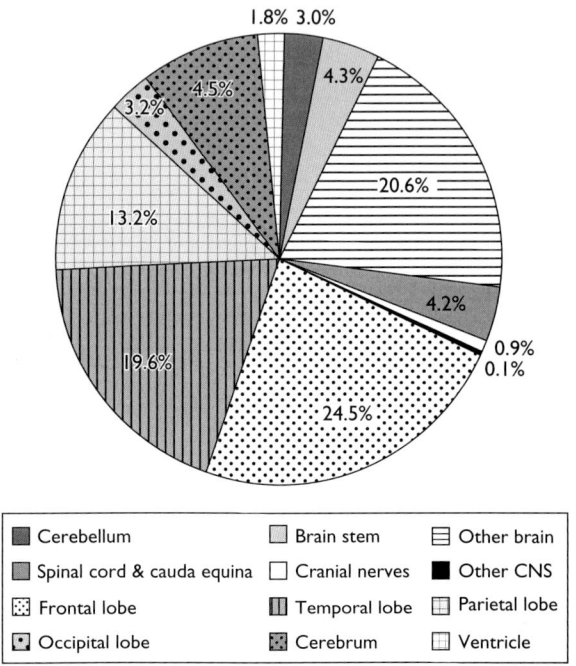

Figure 2.1 Distribution of all primary brain and CNS gliomas (9380–9384, 9391–9460, 9480) by site; CBTRUS 2000–2004. Reprinted with permission from CBTRUS [7].

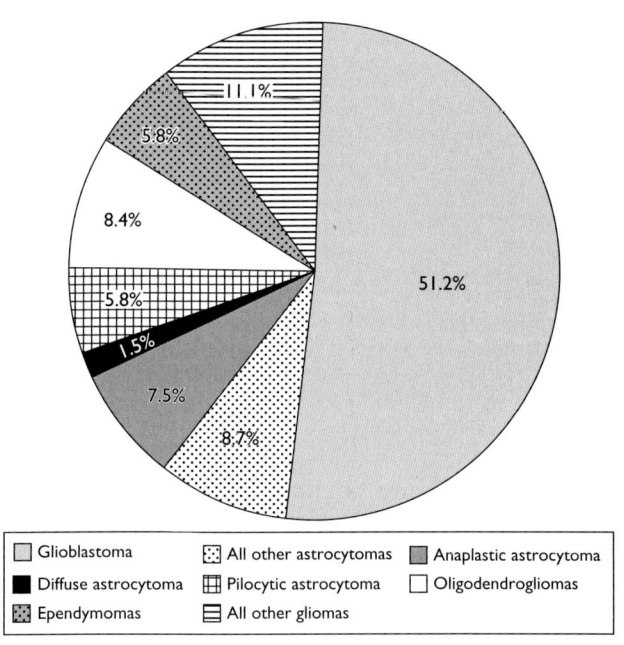

Figure 2.2 Distribution of all primary brain and CNS gliomas (9380–9384, 9391–9460, 9480) by histological subtype; CBTRUS 2000–2004. Reprinted with permission from CBTRUS [7].

common histologies were astrocytoma and ependymoma in both children (77% and 20%, respectively) and adults (60% and 37%, respectively) [31,32]. In children, astrocytic tumors were the most frequent neuroepithelial or brain tumor diagnosis, with most astrocytic tumors being pilocytic astrocytoma [22,25,29,33,34].

Frequency by Gender and Race

Gliomas are more frequent among males in most studies [7,20,23,25,33,35]. The frequency of gliomas was higher in whites than in other racial groups [7,26,27]. Whites had a higher frequency of glioblastoma and oligodendroglioma, whereas blacks had a higher frequency of astrocytoma, other glioma, NOS, and ependymoma [36]. Both white and black males were more commonly affected by glioma; further, a greater percentage of blacks were diagnosed at a younger age than whites [37].

INCIDENCE RATES

Overall Incidence Rates and By Ethnicity, and Age

Using data from the CBTRUS for cases diagnosed from 2000 to 2004, the incidence rate for all primary malignant and nonmalignant glioma (*ICD-O-3* histology codes: 9380–9384, 9391–9460, 9480) was 4.9/100,000 person-years (95% CI: 4.8–5.0), age-adjusted to the WSP [7]. Consistent with this result, the incidence rate for malignant glioma (9380–9384, 9391–9460, 9480), age-adjusted to the WSP, based on Surveillance, Epidemiology, and End Results (SEER) data from 17 US registries between 2000 and 2004 was 4.6/100,000 person-years (95% CI: 4.5–4.7) [38]. When both nonmalignant and malignant brain tumors were included, the SEER incidence rate for glioma was 4.7/100,000 person-years in 2004 (95% CI: 4.6–4.9), with an incidence rate of 4.5/100,000 person-years (95% CI: 4.4–4.7) for malignant glioma and 0.2/100,000 person-years (95%: 0.1–0.2; Figure 2.3) for nonmalignant glioma.

A summary of glioma and neuroepithelial tumor incidence rates from recent studies is presented in Table 2.2. Histological type is included, as is site, behavior, age group, and years of diagnosis. In addition, the standard population used for each study is noted. Incidence rates of glioma ranged from 2.1/100,000 in Japan to 7.0/100,000 in France, whereas incidence rates of tumors of neuroepithelial tissue ranged from 5.5/100,000 in the United States to 9.3/100,000 in Italy. Non-Hispanic whites had higher incidence rates of malignant glioma (5.5/100,000, 95% CI: 5.4–5.6), than blacks (2.7, 95% CI: 2.5–2.9), Hispanics (3.7, 95% CI: 3.6–3.9), or Asians (2.4, 95% CI: 2.3–2.6) in the United States (Figure 2.4). Incidence rates of both glial and neuroepithelial tumors were higher in children (aged 0–14 years), dipping in late adolescence (aged 15–19 years) and thereafter increasing with age (Figure 2.5).

Incidence Rates by Histological Type

Incidence rates by histological type for both the SEER and CBTRUS data are presented in Table 2.3. Glioblastomas had the highest incidence rates overall (range: 2.0–5.3/100,000 and in both males (range: 2.7–6.5/100,000) and females (range: 1.6–4.6/100,000) [7,17,19,23,24,26,28,41]. Incidence rates for glioblastomas were also higher in non-Latinos (2.5/100,000) than Latino whites (1.8) or blacks (1.5) [41]. The incidence of glioblastoma increased with age, peaking in the 70- to 79-year age group, and decreasing thereafter [7,41]. Incidence rates by age at diagnosis for glioblastoma

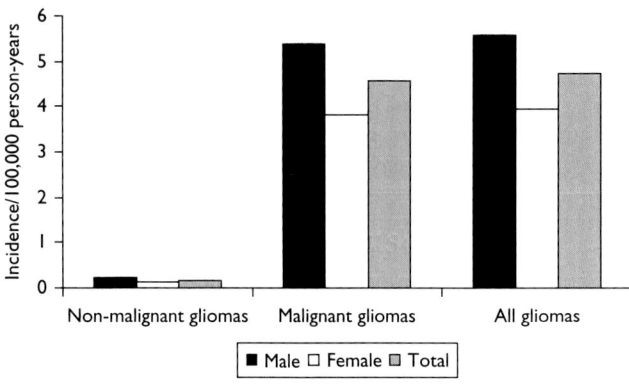

Figure 2.3 Incidence of all glioma, malignant glioma, and non-malignant glioma (9380–9384, 9391–9460, 9480) overall and by gender, age-adjusted to the World Standard Population; SEER 17 registries data from 2004 only.

and other selected glial histologies are presented in Figure 2.6. Incidence rates of both the oligodendroglial and mixed tumors peak in the 35- to 44-year age group. Malignant glioma NOS incidence rates peak in the 0- to 14-year age group, before dipping in late adolescence and then continuing to increase with age. The incidence rates for astrocytoma NOS and anaplastic astrocytoma increase with increasing age until they decline in the oldest age group. Ependymal tumors peak in childhood (0–14 years) and again in the 45- to 54-year age group. Incidence rate ratios for whites to blacks were 6.2 for glioblastoma, 3.5 for astrocytoma, and 4.3 for oligodendroglioma [27].

Incidence Rates by Gender

Higher incidence rates for glioma were observed among males (5.9/100,000, 95% CI: 5.7–6.2) than females (4.3/100,000, 95% CI: 4.1–4.5) in the SEER data (Figure 2.3), which is consistent with reports in the literature (Table 2.2). Male-to-female ratios of 1.4 to 1.5 were found for all primary glioma, whereas the male-to-female ratio was 1.26 for astrocytic and oligodendroglial glioma combined and 1.4 for supratentorial low-grade malignant glioma [7,17–19,30,42,43]. In Croatia, however, there was no significant difference in incidence rates between males and females for tumors of neuroepithelial tissue (male-to-female ratio = 1.1) [28]. By histology, there is some variability in the male-to-female ratio. In Zurich, Switzerland, most glioma histologies were more frequent in males than females, particularly the gemistocytic astrocytoma (3.5) and anaplastic oligodendroglioma (3.3). Oligodendroglioma, anaplastic astrocytoma, diffuse astrocytoma, and glioma NOS were about equally common among males and females, whereas anaplastic oligoastrocytoma and high-grade glioma were more common among females (male-to-female ratio = 0.6 and 0.7, respectively) [19,30]. Conversely, in the CBTRUS data, for all specific glial histologies, males were found to have higher or similar incidence compared to females [7]. In adults, glioblastoma was characterized by a male-to-female ratio of 1.6 [41]. In children under 15 years of age in Germany, oligodendroglioma occurred more often

Table 2.2 Incidence of Glioma and Tumors of Neuroepithelial Tissue in Recent Population-Based Studies

	Histology Codes	Years of Diagnosis/ Country	Standard Population	Nonmalignant Included?	Male Incidence/ 100,000	Female Incidence/ 100,000	All Incidence/ 100,000
Glioma							
CBTRUS [7]	ICD-O-3: 9380–9384,9391–9460,9480	2000–2004 US	WSP	Yes	5.76	4.17	4.92
SEER [38]	ICD-O-3: 9380–9384,9391–9460,9480	2000–2004 US	WSP	No	5.39	3.89	4.59
SEER [38]	ICD-O-3: 9380–9384,9391–9460,9480	2004 US	WSP	Yes	5.58	3.95	4.73
Ligant et al [25]	Kleihues et al [2]	1986–1996 Estonia	WSP	Yes	4.32 (Crude)	3.60 (Crude)	3.41
Kuratsu et al [39]	Kleihues et al [2]	1989–1998 Kumamoto, Japan	Pop. of Japan	Yes, Intracranial	NA	NA	2.13
Elia-Pasquet et al [17]	Astrocytomas, mixed tumors, glioblastomas, oligodendrogliomas	1999–2001 Gironde, France	Crude	Yes, Cerebral	8.5 (16+ years)	5.6 (16+ years)	7.0 (16+ years)
Christensen et al [18]	ICD-O: 9380–9460	1993–1997 Denmark	WSP	Yes	4.50	2.93	3.70
Ohgaki and Kleihues [19]	ICD-O-3: 9380, 9382, 9384, 9400–9401, 9411, 9420–9421, 9424, 9440–9442, 9450–9451	1980–1994 Zurich, Switzerland	ESP	Yes	NA	NA	5.27
Larjavaara et al [24]	ICD-O-3: 9380–9460	2000–2002 Finland	WSP	Yes, Intracranial	4.9 (20–69 years)	4.5 (20–69 years)	4.7 (20–69 years)
Tumors of neuroepithelial tissue							
CBTRUS [7]	CBTRUS, 2008 [7]	2000–2004 US	WSP	Yes	6.42	4.67	5.50
Pobereskin and Chadduck [21]	Astrocytoma, Ependymoma, Embryonal, Pineal, Oligodendroglioma	1992–1997 Devon & Cornwall	Pop. of England/ Wales	Yes, Intracranial	11.57	8.23	NA
Cordera et al [40]	Kleihues et al [2]	1992–1999 NW Italy	Pop. Of Italy	Yes, Intracranial	10.62	8.1	9.3
Dobec-Meic et al [28]	Kleihues et al [2]	1996–2004 Varazdin Co, Croatia	Crude	Yes; Intracranial	7.0 (18+ years)	6.3 (18+ years)	6.7 (18+ years)

Abbreviations: ESP, European Standard Population; NA, not available; WSP, World Standard Population.

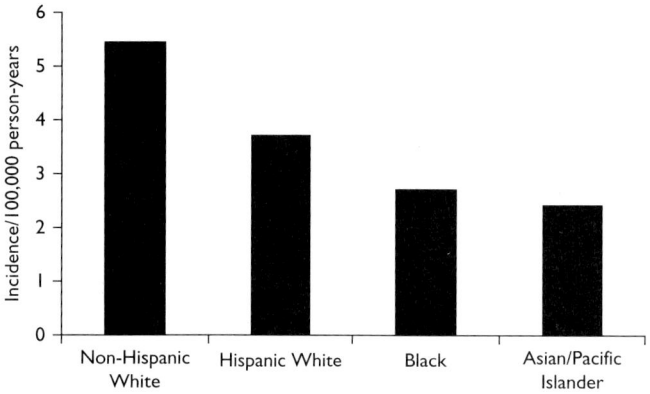

Figure 2.4 Incidence of malignant glioma (9380–9384, 9391–9460, 9480) by race/ethnicity, age-adjusted to the World Standard Population; SEER 17 registries data, 2000–2004.

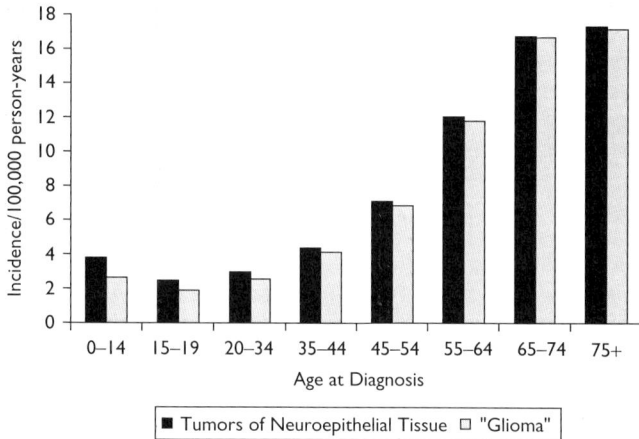

Figure 2.5 Incidence of tumors of neuroepithelial tissue and glioma (9380–9384, 9391–9460, 9480), age-adjusted to the World Standard Population; CBTRUS 2000–2004.

in males than in females (1.8), but ependymoma (1.1) and astrocytoma (1.1) occurred only slightly more often in males [44]. Similarly, pilocytic astrocytomas were found to be only slightly more common in males than females [7,45].

Incidence Rates in Childhood

In children, the incidence rates of glioma classified according to the ICCC were summarized by Kaatsch et al [12,44]. The incidence of astrocytic tumors ranged from 0.7 to 2.2/100,000, ependymoma from 0.2 to 0.5/100,000, and other glioma from 0 to 0.5/100,000. In the Netherlands for the years 1993–1999, the incidence of glioma was higher in females than males for those aged 0 to 14 years (1.8 vs 1.6/100,000) and 15 to 19 years (2.1 vs 1.3), but was lower in those aged 20 to 24 years (1.4 vs 2.3). The highest incidence of glioma was found in males 10 to 14 years of age and 20 to 24 years of age (2.3/100,000 for both), whereas the highest incidence in females was found for those 15 to 19 years of age (2.1/100,000) [46]. While glioblastomas are the most common glial histology overall and in adults, the glial histology with the highest incidence in children is pilocytic astrocytoma (Figure 2.7) [7]. Astrocytomas and malignant glioma NOS have the highest incidence in children aged 0 to 9 years, with a declining incidence through age 19, while the incidence of ependymomas is highest in children aged 0 to 4 years. Low-grade glioma (1.8/100,000) had a higher incidence in children aged 0 to 14 years than high-grade glioma (0.5/100,000) [22].

TRENDS IN INCIDENCE RATES

Incidence rates for tumors of neuroepithelial tissue leveled off after the 1980s in histologically confirmed tumors [33]. The incidence of all gliomas has significantly increased over time from the pre-1980s to the present (1951–1970 vs 1986–1996) [25], with a similar stabilization or leveling off of rates after the 1980s in Japan (1972–1992) [35], Italy (1986–1991 vs 1992–1999) [40], the Netherlands (1989–2003) [43], Denmark (1943–1997) [18], and in an analysis of four Nordic countries: Denmark, Finland, Norway and Sweden (1969–1998) [23]. In the United States, glioma incidence increased significantly from 1985 to 1999, but only in adults (AAPC: 0.8%, 95% CI: 0.2–1.3 in those 20–64 years and 2.2, 95% CI: 1.5–2.9 in those aged 65+) [47].

Trends in incidence rates differed according to histology. Increases in incidence rates have been noted for oligodendroglial and mixed tumor histologies at what appears to be the expense of astrocytomas, particularly astrocytoma NOS, in all age groups combined and in adults [26,42,48,49]. Using CBTRUS data from 1985 to 1999, the incidence of oligodendrogliomas (AAPC: 6.9%), anaplastic oligodendrogliomas (22.3%), and pilocytic astrocytomas (10.3%) increased, whereas astrocytoma, NOS decreased (–9.0%). Increases in incidence were limited to adults for glioblastoma (20–64 = 2.0%; 65+ = 3.2%) and to those aged 65 and above for anaplastic astrocytoma (6.7%) [47]. These findings confirmed results from earlier studies that had also reported that increasing incidence rates of anaplastic astrocytoma and glioblastoma were primarily observed among those in the oldest age groups [34,41,43,49,50]. Shifts in incidence rates within glial subgroups have occurred and may reflect changes in classification and reporting, as well as efforts to provide more specific diagnoses.

In children, increases in incidence rates of glioma were observed in boys aged 10 to 14 and 20 to 24 years, whereas in girls this increase was found only among those aged 15 to 19 years at diagnosis [46]. In children aged 0 to 14 years in Sweden, an increase (2.1%) in the incidence rates of low-grade glioma/astrocytoma between 1960 and 1998 was observed, although, similar to the increases seen in adults, these trends may be leveling off in recent years [22]. In the Netherlands, the incidence rates of all glioma, astrocytoma, and ependymoma demonstrated a decreasing trend between 1989 and 2003 in children, whereas the incidence rate of "gliomas of uncertain histology" rose [43]. Similarly, in Yorkshire, UK, for cases diagnosed between 1990 and 2001, no significant trends in specific glioma histologies were noted [34].

Table 2.3 Incidence by Gender and Histology for Primary Malignant Glioma Only (SEER 17 Registries Data, 2000–2004) and for All Primary Malignant and Nonmalignant Glioma (CBTRUS, 2000–2004)

	SEER (2000–2004)				CBTRUS (2000–2004)			
	Male		Female		Male		Female	
	Incidence	95% CI	Incidence	95% CI	Incidence	95% CI	Incidence	95% CI
Malignant glioma, NOS (9380)	0.37	0.35–0.40	0.37	0.34–0.40	0.41	0.38–0.44	0.38	0.35–0.40
Astrocytoma, NOS (9400)	0.47	0.44–0.50	0.36	0.34–0.39	0.42	0.39–0.45	0.33	0.30–0.35
Pilocytic astrocytoma (9421)	0.41	0.38–0.44	0.40	0.36–0.43	0.44	0.41–0.48	0.44	0.41–0.47
Fibrillary astrocytoma (9420)	0.08	0.07–0.10	0.06	0.05–0.07	0.08	0.07–0.10	0.07	0.06–0.08
Gemistocytic astrocytoma (9411)	0.06	0.05–0.07	0.03	0.02–0.04	0.04	0.03–0.05	0.03	0.02–0.04
Anaplastic astrocytoma (9401)	0.34	0.32–0.37	0.26	0.23–0.28	0.38	0.36–0.41	0.28	0.26–0.30
Glioblastoma, NOS (9440)	2.66	2.60–2.73	1.61	1.56–1.66	2.71	2.65–2.77	1.64	1.59–1.69
Mixed glioma (9382)	0.16	0.14–0.18	0.13	0.12–0.15	0.18	0.16–0.19	0.13	0.12–0.15
Oligodendroglioma (9450)	0.32	0.30–0.34	0.24	0.22–0.27	0.31	0.29–0.33	0.26	0.24–0.28
Anaplastic oligodendroglioma (9451)	0.13	0.11–0.14	0.10	0.09–0.12	0.15	0.13–0.16	0.12	0.11–0.14
Ependymoma/anaplastic ependymoma (9391–9394)	0.25	0.22–0.27	0.24	0.22–0.27	0.37	0.34–0.40	0.30	0.27–0.32
All glioma—Histological Groups for Comparative Studies (9380–9384, 9391–9460, 9480)	5.39	5.28–5.49	3.89	3.81–3.98	5.76	5.66–5.85	4.17	4.09–4.25

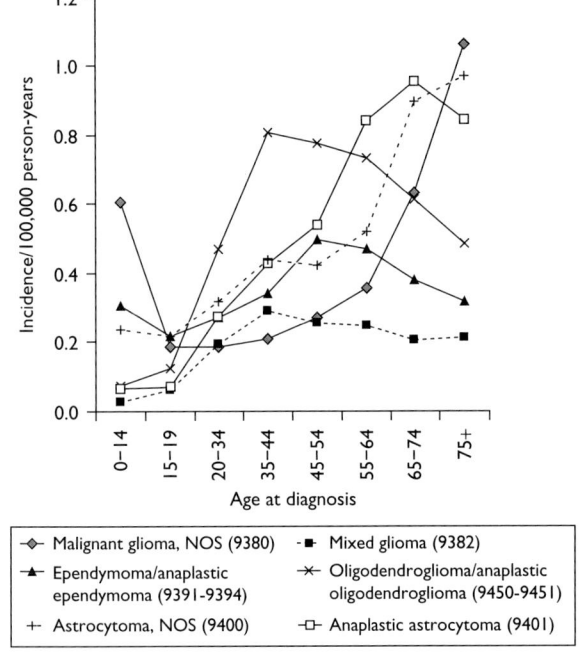

Figure 2.6 Incidence of selected glioma histologies by age at diagnosis, age-adjusted to the World Standard Population; CBTRUS 2000–2004.

SURVIVAL

One-, two- and five-year relative survival rates from the time of diagnosis for malignant glioma (9380–9384, 9391–9460, 9480) were 53.8%, 38.8%, and 31.7%, respectively (Figure 2.8A). Pilocytic astrocytoma had the highest 5-year survival rates: all pilocytic astrocytoma patients in Zurich, Switzerland, survived 5 years after diagnosis and 93.8% of American patients living in areas covered by the SEER Registry were also alive 5 years after diagnosis [19,30,38]. Other histologies with 5-year survival rates greater than 65% were oligodendroglioma and ependymoma (Figure 2.8A) [19,38]. In children, 5-year survival was 76% for astrocytoma and 57% for ependymoma [44]. Glioblastoma had the worst 5-year survival rates: 1.2% in Zurich, Switzerland, and 3.4% in the SEER data, with no improvement in survival after the 1980s (Figure 2.8B) [19,26,30,38,51]. Five-year survival for spinal gliomas was higher for adults with ependymoma (81.9%) and lower for those with astrocytoma (47.3%) compared with children (68.8% and 59.7%, respectively) [31,32].

In general, low-grade glioma had better 5-year survival probabilities than high-grade glioma in both children (76.3% vs 17.8%) and adults (75.0% vs 14.2%) [29]. Five-year survival for supratentorial low-grade glioma was 59.9%, with increased survival time associated with being female, white, diagnosed at a younger age, having an oligodendroglial tumor, or a later year of diagnosis [42]. Increased survival in adult glioma was also associated with younger age at diagnosis, female gender, and ependymal histology [52]. Median survival rates in adults with supratentorial low-grade glioma improved from 4.1 years between 1970 and 1981 to 9.2 years between 1982 and 1993, with increases seen in each histological subgroup [53]. Survival for adult glioma, overall, improved 16% between 1971–1975 and 1986–1990 [51].

Age is strongly inversely correlated with survival for all primary glioma with one exception. Children aged 0 to

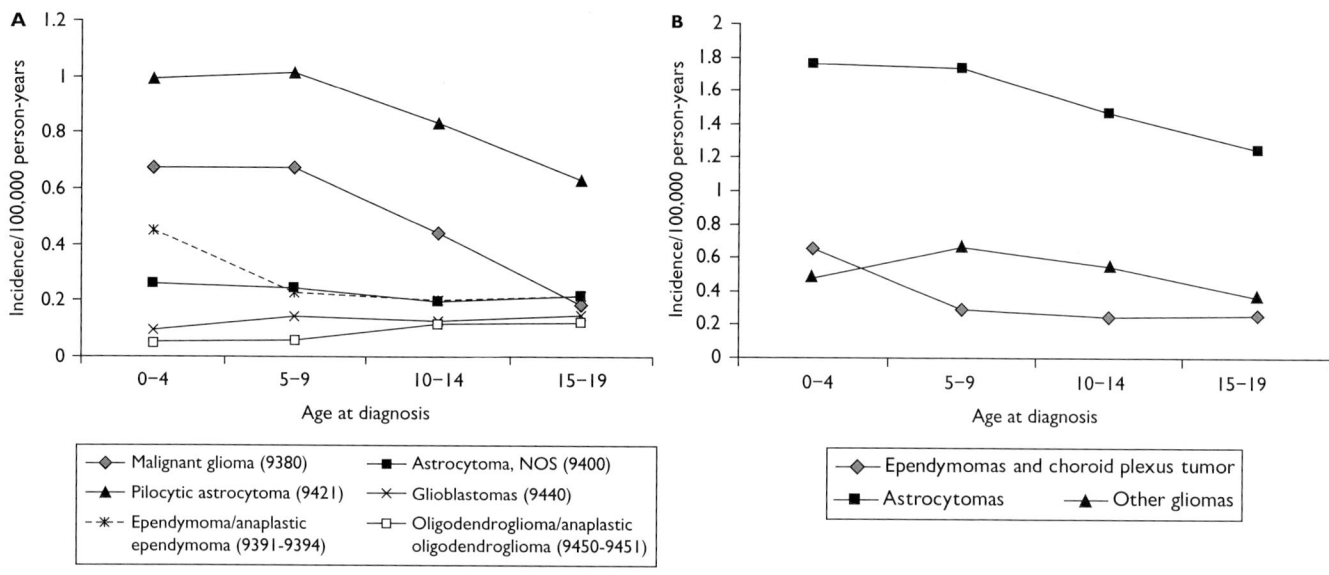

Figure 2.7 Childhood (aged < 20 years) incidence of **(A)** selected glioma histologies and **(B)** by ICCC classification by age at diagnosis, age-adjusted to the World Standard Population; CBTRUS 2000–2004.

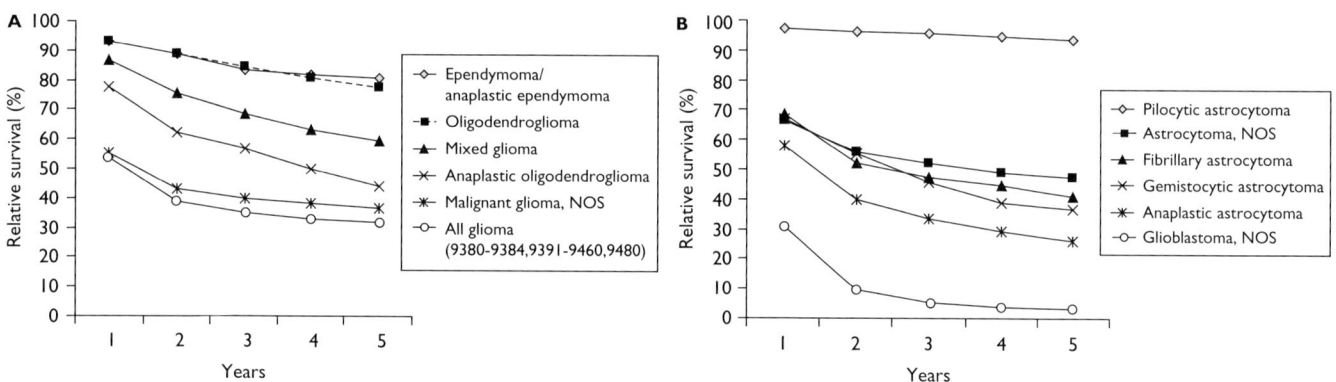

Figure 2.8 Relative survival for cases diagnosed with glioma, **(A)** overall and by selected histology and **(B)** for selected astrocytic tumors; SEER 13 registries, 1992–2004.

14 years had slightly worse survival than late adolescents aged 15 to 19 years (Figure 2.9) [38]. However, Feltbower et al [34] found that young adults (15–29 years) had significantly poorer survival than children (51.8% vs 83.4% 5-year survival for astrocytomas). In other studies, age has been a significant predictor of mortality for glioblastoma, low-grade diffuse glioma, adult glioma, malignant brain tumors, and supratentorial low-grade glioma [30,37,42,52,54].

Race-specific survival rates for glioma are not readily available; however, differences in survival by race for specific histologies and for all malignant brain tumors have been assessed. No survival differences were found between blacks and whites for glioblastoma, astrocytoma, or oligodendroglioma [27]. Using SEER data, blacks were found to have worse or similar survival than whites [36,42]. Further analysis of the SEER data showed that although no survival differences by race were apparent using a univariate model, adjusting for gender, age at diagnosis, surgery type, histology, site and SEER registry revealed a 13% increased risk of death among blacks [37]. Much of this increased risk of death occurred in blacks who underwent subtotal resections or surgery NOS. Conversely, using the same data, Deorah et al [26] found that whites had significantly worse survival compared to blacks. Careful adjustment for variables that differ by race or ethnicity will be important for future estimates of survival by race. In children, no significant differences among survival rates were found for low-grade astrocytoma, high-grade astrocytoma, or ependymoma between non-Hispanic whites, Hispanics, blacks, or Asians [55].

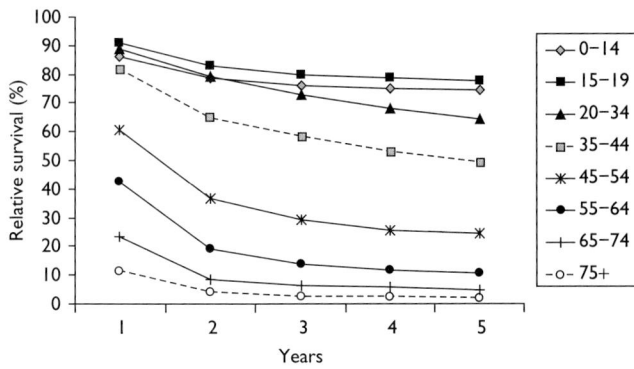

Figure 2.9 Relative survival for cases diagnosed with glioma (9380–9384, 9391–9460, 9480) by age at diagnosis; SEER 13 registries, 1992–2004.

CONCLUSIONS

- Comparisons of rates over time and among regions or countries can be difficult due to inconsistencies in classification schemes, variation in the definition of tumor behavior, and whether the definition of glioma is restricted to tumors that occur in the brain or elsewhere in the CNS. Differences in the ages and years of diagnosis included in the analyses and differences in the standard population used can also make comparison difficult.
- Glioma accounts for 36% to 50% of all primary brain tumors and 70% to 80% of all primary malignant brain tumors. Glioblastoma is the most common glioma histology accounting for approximately 50% of glioma. Glioma occurs most frequently in the cerebral lobes.
- Incidence rates of all primary glioma range from 2.1/100,000 to 7.0/100,000 in studies published after 1999 and are consistently higher among males than females and among whites compared with other racial/ethnic groups.
- The incidence of all glioma has stabilized since the 1980s, although trends within glial subgroups are apparent. Diagnoses of high-grade glioma have increased over time in the oldest age groups. Oligodendroglial and mixed tumor histologies have increased at the expense of less-specific histologies, such as astrocytoma NOS.
- People with low-grade glial tumors including pilocytic astrocytoma and oligodendroglioma have markedly better survival than those with higher grade glioma. People with the highest grade tumor, glioblastoma, have the poorest survival. In general, survival probabilities decrease with increasing age at diagnosis.

REFERENCES

1. van der Weil HJ. The biology of glioma. In: *Inheritance of Glioma: The Genetic Aspects of Cerebral Glioma and its Relation to Status Dysraphicus.* Amsterdam: Elsevier Publishing Company; 1960:31–55.
2. Kleihues P, Burger PC, Scheithauer BW, eds. *Histological Typing of Tumours of the Central Nervous System.* 2nd ed. Berlin, Germany: Springer-Verlag; 1993.
3. Kleihues P, Cavenee WK, eds. *World Health Organization Classification of Tumours: Pathology and Genetics of Tumours of the Nervous System.* Lyon, France: IARC Press; 2000.
4. Kleihues P, Louis DN, Scheithauer BW, et al. The WHO classification of tumours of the nervous system. *J Neuropathol Exp Neurol.* 2002;61:215–225.
5. van der Sanden GAC, Wesseling P, Schouten LJ, Teepen HLJM, Coebergh JWW. A uniform histological cluster scheme for ICD-O-coded primary central nervous system tumors. *Neuroepidemiology.* 1998;17:233–246.
6. Louis DN, Ohgaki H, Wiestler OD, et al. The 2007 WHO classification of tumours of the central nervous system. *Acta Neuropathol.* 2007;114:97–109.
7. CBTRUS. *Statistical Report: Primary Brain Tumors in the United States, 2000–2004.* Chicago, IL: Central Brain Tumor Registry of the United States; 2008.
8. Counsell CE, Grant R. Incidence studies of primary and secondary intracranial tumors: a systematic review of their methodology and results. *J Neurooncol* 1998;37:241–250.
9. Fritz A, Percy C, Jack A, et al, eds. *International Classification of Diseases for Oncology.* 3rd ed. Geneva, Switzerland: World Health Organization; 2000.
10. Parkin DM, Shanmugaratnam K, Sobin L, Ferlay J, Whelan SL. *Histological Groups for Comparative Studies. IARC Technical Report No. 31.* Lyon, France: International Agency for Research on Cancer; 1998.
11. Percy C, Van Holten V, Muir C, eds. *International Classification of Diseases for Oncology.* 2nd ed. Geneva, Switzerland: World Health Organization; 1990.
12. Steliarova-Foucher E, Stiller C, Lacour B, Kaatsch P. International classification of childhood cancer, third edition. *Cancer.* 2005;103:1457–1467.
13. Aldape K, Simmons ML, Davis RL, et al. Discrepancies in diagnoses of neuroepithelial neoplasms: the San Francisco Bay Area Adult Glioma Study. *Cancer.* 2000;88:2342–2349.
14. Bruner JM, Inouye L, Fuller GN, Langford LA. Diagnostic discrepancies and their clinical impact in a neuropathology referral practice. *Cancer.* 1997;79:796–803.
15. Castillo MS, Davis FG, Surawicz T, et al. Consistency of primary brain tumor diagnoses and codes in cancer surveillance systems. *Neuroepidemiology.* 2004;23:85–93.
16. Davis FG, Malmer BS, Aldape K, et al. Issues of diagnostic review in brain tumor studies: from the Brain Tumor Epidemiology Consortium (BTEC). *Cancer Epidemiol Biomarkers Prev.* 2008;17:484–489.
17. Elia-Pasquet S, Provost D, Jaffre A, et al. Incidence of central nervous system tumors in Gironde, France. *Neuroepidemiology.* 2004;23:110–117.
18. Christensen HC, Kosteljanetz M, Johansen C. Incidences of gliomas and meningiomas in Denmark, 1943 to 1997. *Neurosurgery.* 2003;52:1327–1334.
19. Ohgaki H, Kleihues P. Epidemiology and etiology of gliomas. *Acta Neuropathol.* 2005;109:93–108.
20. Buachet L, Rigau V, Mathieu-Daude H, et al. French brain tumor data bank: methodology and first results on 10,000 cases. *J Neurooncol.* 2007;84:189–199.
21. Pobereskin LH, Chadduck JB. Incidence of brain tumours in two English counties: a population-based study. *J Neurol Neurosurg Psychiatry.* 2000;69:464–471.
22. Dreifaldt AC, Carlberg M, Hardell L. Increasing incidence rates of childhood malignant diseases in Sweden during the period 1960–1998. *Eur J Cancer.* 2004;40:1351–1360.
23. Lonn S, Klaeboe L, Hall P, et al. Incidence trends of adult primary intracerebral tumors in four Nordic countries. *Int J Cancer.* 2004;108:450–455.
24. Larjavaara S, Mantyla R, Salminen T, et al. Incidence of gliomas by anatomic location. *Neuro Oncol.* 2007;9:319–325.
25. Liigant A, Asser T, Kulla A, Kaasik AE. Epidemiology of primary central nervous system tumors in Estonia. *Neuroepidemiology.* 2000;19:300–311.
26. Deorah S, Lynch CF, Sibenaller ZA, Ryken TC. Trends in brain cancer incidence and survival in the United States: Surveillance, Epidemiology, and End Results Program, 1973 to 2001. *Neurosurg Focus.* 2006;20:E1.

27. Robertson JT, Gunter BC, Somes GW. Racial differences in the incidence of gliomas: a retrospective study from Memphis, Tennessee. *Br J Neurosurg.* 2002;16:562–566.
28. Dobec-Meic B, Pikija S, Cvetko D, et al. Intracranial tumors in adult population of the Varazdin County (Croatia) 1996–2004: a population-based retrospective incidence study. *J Neurooncol.* 2006;78: 303–310.
29. Johannesen TB, Langmark F, Lote K. Cause of death and long-term survival in patients with neuro-epithelial brain tumours: a population-based study. *Eur J Cancer.* 2003;39:2355–2363.
30. Ohgaki H, Kleihues P. Population-based studies on incidence, survival rates, and genetic alterations in astrocytic and oligodendroglial gliomas. *J Neuropathol Exp Neurol.* 2005;64:479–489.
31. Tseng J-H, Tseng M-Y. Survival analysis of 81 children with primary spinal gliomas: a population-based study. *Pediatr Neurosurg.* 2006;42:347–353.
32. Tseng J-H, Tseng M-Y. Survival analysis of 459 adult patients with primary spinal cancer in England and Wales: a population-based study. *Surgical Neurology.* 2007;67:53–58.
33. Johannesen TB, Angell-Andersen E, Tretli S, Langmark F, Lote K. Trends in incidence of brain and central nervous system tumors in Norway, 1970–1999. *Neuroepidemiology.* 2004;23:101–109.
34. Feltbower RG, Picton S, Bridges LR, Crooks DA, Glaser AW, McKinney PA. Epidemiology of central nervous system tumours in children and young adults (0–29 years), Yorkshire, United Kingdom. *Pediatr Hematol Oncol.* 2004;21:647–660.
35. Kaneko S, Nomura K, Yoshimura T, Yamaguchi N. Trend of brain tumor incidence by histological subtypes in Japan: estimation from the Brain Tumor Registry of Japan, 1973–1993. *J Neurooncol.* 2002;60: 61–69.
36. Barnholtz-Sloan JS, Sloan AE, Schwartz AG. Relative survival rates and patterns of diagnosis analyzed by time period for individuals with primary malignant brain tumor, 1973–1997. *J Neurosurg.* 2003;99:458–466.
37. Barnholtz-Sloan JS, Sloan AE, Schwartz AG. Racial differences in survival after diagnosis with primary malignant brain tumor. *Cancer.* 2003;98:603–609.
38. Surveillance, Epidemiology, and End Results (SEER) Program. SEER*Stat Database: Incidence—SEER 17 Regs Limited-Use, Nov 2006 Sub (2000–2004)—Linked To County Attributes—Total U.S., 1969–2004 Counties, National Cancer Institute, DCCPS, Surveillance Research Program, Cancer Statistics Branch, released April 2007, based on the November 2006 submission. www.seer.cancer.gov. Accessed January 4, 2008.
39. Kuratsu J, Takeshima H, Ushio Y. Trends in the incidence of primary intracranial tumors in Kumamoto, Japan. *Int J Clin Oncol.* 2001;6:183–191.
40. Cordera S, Bottacchi E, D'Alessandro G, Machado D, De Gonda F, Corso G. Epidemiology of primary intracraneal tumours in NW Italy, a population-based study: stable incidence in the last two decades. *J Neurol.* 2002;249:281–284.
41. Chakrabarti I, Cockburn M, Cozen W, Wang Y-P, Preston-Martin S. A population-based description of glioblastoma multiforme in Los Angeles County, 1974–1999. *Cancer.* 2005;104:2798–2806.
42. Claus EB, Black PM. Survival rates and patterns of care for patients diagnosed with supratentorial low-grade gliomas. *Cancer.* 2006;106:1358–1363.
43. Houben MPWA, Aben KKH, Teepen JLJM, et al. Stable incidence of childhood and adult glioma in the Netherlands, 1989–2003. *Acta Oncologica.* 2006;45:272–279.
44. Kaatsch P, Rickert CH, Kuhl J, Schuz J, Michaelis J. Population-based epidemiologic data on brain tumors in German children. *Cancer* 2001;92:3155–3164.
45. Burkhard C, Di Patre P-L, Schuler D, et al. A population-based study of the incidence and survival rates in patients with pilocytic astrocytoma. *J Neurosurg.* 2003;98:1170–1174.
46. Reedijk AMJ, Janssen-Heijnen MLG, Louwman MWJ, Snepvangers Y, Hofhuis WJD, Coebergh JWW. Increasing incidence and improved survival of cancer in children and young adults in Southern Netherlands, 1973–1999. *Eur J Cancer.* 2005;41:760–769.
47. Hoffman S, Propp JM, McCarthy BJ. Temporal trends in incidence of primary brain tumors in the United States, 1985–1999. *Neuro-Oncol.* 2006;8:27–37.
48. McCarthy BJ, Propp JM, Davis FD, Burger PC. Time trends in oligodendroglial and astrocytic tumor incidence. *Neuroepidemiology.* 2008;30:34–44.
49. Hess KR, Broglio KR, Bondy ML. Adult glioma incidence trends in the United States, 1977–2000. *Cancer.* 2004;101:2293–2299.
50. McKinley BP, Michalek AM, Fenstermaker RA, Plunkett RJ. The impact of age and sex on the incidence of glial tumors in New York state from 1976 to 1995. *J Neurosurg.* 2000;93:932–939.
51. Paszat L, Laperriere N, Groome P, Schulze K, Mackillop W, Holowaty E. A population-based study of glioblastoma multiforme. *Int J Radiation Oncology Biol Phys.* 2001;51:100–107.
52. Tseng J-H, Tseng M-Y. Survival analysis for adult glioma in England and Wales. *J Formos Med Assoc.* 2005;104:341–348.
53. Johannesen TB, Langmark F, Lote K. Progress in long-term survival in adult patients with supratentorial low-grade gliomas: a population-based study of 993 patients in whom tumors were diagnosed between 1970 and 1993. *J Neurosurg.* 2003;99:854–862.
54. Okamoto Y, Di Patre P-L, Burkhard C, et al. Population-based study on incidence, survival rates, and genetic alterations of low-grade diffuse astrocytomas and oligodendrogliomas. *Acta Neuropathol* 2004;108:49–56.
55. Barnholtz-Sloan JS, Severson RK, Stanton B, Hamre M, Sloan AE. Pediatric brain tumors in Non-Hispanics, Hispanics, African Americans and Asians: differences in survival after diagnosis. *Cancer Causes Control.* 2005;16:587–592.

3 Familial Factors and Inherited Susceptibility to Glioma

Beatrice Melin and Melissa L. Bondy

There is increasing evidence of genetic susceptibility to glioma. In addition to known inherited syndromes that predispose to brain tumors, two recent genome-wide association studies discovered and confirmed that inherited variation in five regions (chromosome 5p15.33 (*TERT*), 9p21.3 (*CDKN2B*), 8q24, 11q23 (*PHLDB1*), and, 20q13.3 (*RTEL1*) influence glioma risk [1,2]. These findings open unique and novel research opportunities for more complete understanding of the etiology of this devastating disease. Several types of epidemiological study designs can be used to establish genetic susceptibility to a disease. These include the case series, cohort and case-control studies, segregation analysis to identify the mode of inheritance, and linkage studies to determine chromosomal regions and specific loci that explain the disorder. There has been evidence for genetic susceptibility to glioma from each of these study types. A summary of the evidence for familial aggregation of glioma and the link to inherited syndromes is presented in the following text.

FAMILIAL GLIOMA CASE REPORTS

Case series of glioma families have been published since the 1960s. One study reported 19 families: 6 families with 3 or more affected relatives, and 13 families with 2 affected family members [3]. There has been strong evidence of familial glioma and cancer susceptibility syndromes, especially with well-known entities such as the Li-Fraumeni syndrome (LFS) and neurofibromatosis type 1 (NF1) and type 2 (NF2). The other studies showing a familial association included siblings, which does not exclude the possibility that the associations could be due to common environmental factors [4]. A similar conclusion was drawn from another study of 72 consecutive families, where parents and children were affected in 33 families, siblings in 27 families, and spouses in 12 [5]. Since half of the cases were affected over a 5-year time period, it seemed possible that there could be an environmental cause to this familial aggregation. This latter study was not population-based, and therefore there could be an ascertainment bias [5].

CASE-CONTROL AND COHORT STUDIES OF FAMILIAL AGGREGATION OF GLIOMA

To determine whether there is a familial risk among close relatives of glioma patients, large sample sizes are needed in either a case-control or cohort study design. Most of the early studies did not find an increased risk of glioma or primary brain tumors (PBTs) among relatives [6–8] although one study did report an increased risk (odds ratio [OR] = 8.9) [9]. Small sample sizes probably account for the varying results.

During the past 10 years, several studies have shown a 2- to 3-fold increased incidence of brain tumors among close relatives of glioma patients. In a large population-based study from the Utah cancer registry data base, an increased risk for PBT cases was seen among first-degree relatives of PBT patients (relative risk [RR] = 1.96; 95% confidence interval [CI] =1.16–2.97) [10]. A 1997 case-control study calculated an increased RR for PBT of 2.3, 95% CI =1.0–5.8 [11]. More recent cohort studies have shown an increased risk of glioma but not other PBTs among first-degree relatives [12,13]. One larger cohort study found no increased risk of glioma among spouses of glioma patients [14]. Several studies reported an increased risk of malignant melanoma among close relatives of glioma patients [14–16]. In one family with individuals with glioma or melanoma, a *p16* deletion was detected in both [17]. In most glioma families, aside from the known hereditary syndromes described in the following text, the underlying genetic causes are unknown, but approximately 5% of all glioma cases have a family history of glioma among close relatives [18].

Segregation analysis also suggests an inherited etiology of glioma. A familial aggregation study of 250 childhood brain tumor patients supported multifactorial inheritance as causative, rather than random variation [19]. Segregation analyses of 600 adult glioma patient families revealed that a polygenic environment-interactive model best explained the pattern of occurrence of brain tumors [20]. Segregation analyses of 2141 first-degree relatives of 297 glioma families did not reject a multifactorial model, but an autosomal recessive model provided the best fit [18]. Certainly some glioma families likely have highly penetrant genes, and others may have low penetrant genes which interact with the environment. More work is required to delineate how genetic susceptibility affects risk.

In recent years, low penetrant but common genetic variants have been investigated using whole genome association studies and by pooling existing case-control studies in meta-analyses. As mentioned earlier, these approaches have led to the identification of novel susceptibility loci for glioma [1,2]. Only one linkage study has suggested a significant locus in familial glioma [21].

HEREDITARY SYNDROMES PREDISPOSING FOR PBTs

Some hereditary syndromes—such as Turcot and NF1 and NF2—pose a genetic predisposition to glioma [19], but Narod et al [22] estimated that it was a factor in only about 2% of brain tumors diagnosed in children in Great Britain. In a population-based study of 500 adults with glioma in San Francisco [11], less than 1% had a known hereditary syndrome—one had tuberous sclerosis and three had neurofibromatosis. While it is thought that genetic predisposition is influential in relatively few brain tumors (5–10%) [22], the proportion may be underestimated because some hereditary syndromes are not readily diagnosed and patients with a brain tumor are not routinely referred to a clinical geneticist. The well-known and identified syndromes associated with PBTs are listed in Table 3.1, adapted from the WHO classification book on nervous system tumors 2007 [23]. The clinical definitions of syndromes most commonly associated with glioma are more extensively presented in the following text.

Li-Fraumeni Syndrome

Li and Fraumeni described families where children developed sarcomas and young adults (45 years or younger) were diagnosed with breast and/or brain tumors. The authors proposed this as a new cancer-prone family syndrome. The LFS was later confirmed [24] when germline mutations were found in the *p53* gene located at chromosome 17p13 in some of the families. A population-based incidence rate of LFS does not exist, but it is rare. A database at the International Agency of Cancer Research (IARC, www.iarc.fr) contains some 170 LFS families. The *p53* germline mutations in these families are scattered along all 11 exons, even though some hotspots have been found for PBT patients: codon 175, 245, 248, and 273. The most common types of cancers in the LFS families are breast cancer (24%), brain tumors (12%), bone sarcomas (12.6%), and soft tissue sarcoma (11.6%) [25]. The clinical criteria for the LFS and for the Li–Fraumeni-like syndrome (LFL) [26] are listed in the following text. The LFL syndrome is more inclusive with slightly different criteria.

Li-Fraumeni Syndrome:

1. Occurrence of sarcoma at age 45 years or younger
2. At least one first-degree relative with any tumor diagnosed at age 45 years or younger
3. A first- or second-degree relative with any type of cancer diagnosed at age 45 years or younger or a sarcoma at any age.

Li–Fraumeni-Like Syndrome:

1. Three separate primary cancers, first diagnosed at age 45 or younger
2. Or a combination of
   (a) childhood cancer or LFS-associated neoplasm diagnosed at age 45 or younger
   (b) first- or second-degree relative with a LFS-associated tumor at any age
   (c) first- or second-degree relative with any cancer diagnosed at age 60 younger.

In some families with *p53* germline mutations, gliomas have been the main tumor in the family [27,28] without having any family members affected with sarcoma. Studies of LFS families have currently not shown that specific mutations predispose to gliomas, but certain mutations predispose to adrenocortical tumors in children [29]. However, families with missense mutations in the core DNA binding domain have a more severe phenotype with earlier age of onset and higher cancer incidence [26]. The glioma types in LFS are most often of astrocytic origin.

In LF-like families, *p53* mutations are not always identified [24], but new mutations are continually being discovered, including splice site mutations [30]. The tumor suppressor gene *hCHK2*, which closely regulates *p53*, has been shown to have germline mutations in one LFS family [31]. However, these data have been questioned because there are many homologues to the *hCHK2* gene which has since then been identified primarily as a low-penetrant breast cancer gene [32].

Genetic counseling is difficult in Li-Fraumeni families, because the occurrence of multiple tumor types makes it difficult to offer adequate surveillance. The practice of screening for breast tumors in these families starting in

Table 3.1 Inherited Syndromes Associated With PBTs

Hereditary Syndrome	Histopathology of PBT	Gene	Chromosomal Location	Estimated Incidence
NF1	Neurofibromas; neurofibrosarcomas; optic nerve glioma; astrocytoma	NF1	17q11	1:4000
Neurofibromatosis 2 (NF2)	Schwannoma; meningioma; glioma; ependymoma	NF2	22q12	1:40,000–1:25,000
Tuberous sclerosis	Subependymal giant cell astrocytoma	TSC1; TSC2	9q34; 16p13	1:5000
Retinoblastoma	Retinoblastoma; pineoblastoma; malignant glioma	RB1	13q14	1:20,000
Li-Fraumeni	Malignant glioma	TP53	17p13	Rare
Turcot syndrome	Medulloblastoma; glioma	APC; MMR	5q21	Rare

Abbreviation: NF1, neurofibromatosis 1; NF2, neurofibromatosis 2; PBT, primary brain tumor.

Adapted from Kleihues et al, 2007 [25].

early adolescence has been questioned. Breast tissue is presumably more sensitive to radiation-induced mutagenesis in these individuals as the germline mutation involves the DNA repair system. Mammography might therefore not be the most optimal screening method. Ultrasound or magnetic resonance imaging has been suggested as an alternative in these families.

Neurofibromatosis Type 1

NF1 is an autosomal dominant disease with an incidence of about 1:4000. Half of the cases are spontaneous germline mutations in the individual, and half have a family history of NF1. The syndrome is characterized by multiple neurofibromas, malignant peripheral nerve sheath tumors, optic nerve gliomas, and other astrocytomas.

The clinical criteria for NF1 are as follows [33] (patients must meet two of the following criteria to be identified with NF1):

1. Six or more cafe-au-lait patches, diameter at least 5 mm in prepubertal children and at least 15 mm in postpubertal individuals.
2. Two or more neurofibromas of any type or one plexiform neurofibroma.
3. Axillary and/or inguinal freckling.
4. Optic nerve glioma.
5. A distinct osseous lesion, such as dysplasia of the sphenoid wing, thinning of long bone cortex, with or without pseudoarthrosis.
6. A first-degree relative with NF1 according to the above criteria.

The frequency of brain tumors in NF1 patients is difficult to estimate, but about half of the children with optic glioma are diagnosed with NF1. An increased risk of brain tumors, apart from the optic nerve gliomas in NF1 patients, has been observed [34]. NF1 is 100% penetrant, but disease severity can differ widely within families. The *NF1* gene is large, including 60 exons located at chromosome 17q12 [35]. Genetic counseling can determine whether it is a new sporadic case (50%) or whether there is a family history, and the surveillance program for these patients includes annual clinical examination and visual field testing. Optic nerve gliomas are often of low grade and progress slowly. Some data purport that radiotherapy should be avoided in NF1-based optic nerve glioma as these patients might have a higher risk of radiotherapy-induced glioma in the radiation field with a median time to secondary neoplasia of 12 years [36].

Neurofibromatosis Type 2

NF2 is an autosomal dominant disorder with almost 100% penetrance by age 50. It is rare; with the incidence ranging from 1:40,000 to 1:25,000 [37,38]. NF2 patients have a predisposition for different types of PBTs such as schwannoma, meningioma, and glioma. Bilateral vestibular schwannoma are the characteristic and defining hallmark.

The clinical diagnostic criteria of NF2 are as follows:

1. Bilateral vestibular schwannomas
   or
2. A first-degree relative with NF2 and either
   (a) unilateral schwannoma or
   (b) two of the following: meningioma, schwannoma, glioma, posterior subcapsular lens opacity, or cerebral calcification
   or
3. Two of the following:
   (a) unilateral vestibular schwannoma
   (b) multiple meningioma
   (c) Either schwannoma, glioma, neurofibroma, posterior subcapsular lens opacity, or cerebral calcification.

The most common type of glioma associated with NF2 is spinal ependymoma, but astrocytomas may also occur [39]. Supratentorial gliomas are seen less frequently. The *NF2* gene is located on 22q12 and consists of 17 exons. Some studies indicate that the phenotype is worse with an earlier age at onset if the disease is maternally inherited [37]. A surveillance program for at-risk persons in families with NF2 includes magnetic resonance imaging, annual brainstem audiometry, and clinical examination. With surveillance programs, vestibular schwannoma can be diagnosed early, facilitating early therapeutic intervention and possible preservation of hearing.

Turcot Syndrome

Turcot syndrome was first described in 1959, and since then there have been several case reports [40,41]. It is rare and incidence numbers are not available, but it includes two major types. The first type is associated with glioma and hereditary nonpolyposis colorectal cancer with underlying germline mutations in the mismatch repair system in genes such as *hPMS*, *hMSH6 hMSH2*, or *hMLH1* (type 1). This subtype often has café au lait spots and may be misdiagnosed as neurofibromatosis. The second type displays familial adenomatous polyposis and medulloblastoma, with germline mutations in the adenomatous polyposis coli (*APC*) gene [41] (type 2).

Glioblastoma in Turcot syndrome occurs at a younger age (median age 26 years) than sporadic glioblastoma and, interestingly, patients with Turcot syndrome and glioblastoma have a longer median survival time of 27 months compared with 12 months among sporadic cases [42]. Defects in the mismatch repair genes can be investigated through microsatellite instability (MSI) in tumors, where some stable repetitive parts of the genome are examined. Gliomas, other than those occurring in Turcot syndrome are rarely MSI positive [43]. Nevertheless, four MSI positive tumors were found in 22 patients less than 45 years of age affected with glioblastoma [44]. Three patients later also developed colorectal cancer. Recently, patients with Turcot syndrome have been found to have compound heterozygote mutations in one or more of the mismatch repair genes [45]. Consanguinity is rather common, and population-based incidence numbers are not available. However, even among familial adenomatous polyposis and hereditary nonpolyposis colorectal cancer families medulloblastoma and glioma occur rarely.

REFERENCES

1. Shete S, Hosking FJ, Robertson LB, et al. Genome-wide association study identifies five susceptibility loci for glioma. *Nat Genet.* 2009;41:899–904.
2. Wrensch M, Jenkins RB, Chang JS, et al. Variants in the CDKN2B and RTEL1 regions are associated with high-grade glioma susceptibility. *Nat Genet.* 2009;41:905–908.
3. Ikizler Y, van Meyel DJ, Ramsay DA, et al. Gliomas in families. *Can J Neurol Sci.* 1992;19:492–497.
4. Vieregge P, Gerhard L, Nahser HC. Familial glioma: occurrence within the "familial cancer syndrome" and systemic malformations. *J Neurol.* 1987;234:220–232.
5. Grossman SA, Osman M, Hruban R, Piantadosi S. Central nervous system cancers in first-degree relatives and spouses. *Cancer Invest.* 1999;17:299–308.
6. Preston-Martin S, Mack W, Henderson BE. Risk factors for gliomas and meningiomas in males in Los Angeles County. *Cancer Res.* 1989;49:6137–6143.
7. Harvald B, Hauge M. On the heredity of glioblastoma. *J Natl Cancer Inst.* 1956;17:289–296.
8. Wrensch MR, Barger GR. Familial factors associated with malignant gliomas. *Genet Epidemiol* 1990;7:291–301.
9. Choi NW, Schuman LM, Gullen WH. Epidemiology of primary central nervous system neoplasms. II. Case-control study. *Am J Epidemiol* 1970;91:467–485.
10. Goldgar DE, Easton DF, Cannon-Albright LA, Skolnick MH. Systematic population-based assessment of cancer risk in first-degree relatives of cancer probands. *J Natl Cancer Inst.* 1994;86:1600–1608.
11. Wrensch M, Lee M, Miike R, et al. Familial and personal medical history of cancer and nervous system conditions among adults with glioma and controls. *Am J Epidemiol.* 1997;145:581–593.
12. Malmer B, Gronberg H, Bergenheim AT, Lenner P, Henriksson R. Familial aggregation of astrocytoma in northern Sweden: an epidemiological cohort study. *Int J Cancer.* 1999;81:366–370.
13. Hemminki K, Vaittinen P, Dong C, Easton D. Sibling risks in cancer: clues to recessive or X-linked genes? *Br J Cancer.* 2001;84:388–391.
14. Malmer B, Henriksson R, Gronberg H. Familial brain tumours-genetics or environment? A nationwide cohort study of cancer risk in spouses and first-degree relatives of brain tumour patients. *Int J Cancer.* 2003;106:260–263.
15. Paunu N, Pukkala E, Laippala P, et al. Cancer incidence in families with multiple glioma patients. *Int J Cancer.* 2002;97:819–822.
16. Scheurer ME, Etzel CJ, Liu M, et al. Aggregation of cancer in first-degree relatives of patients with glioma. *Cancer Epidemiol Biomarkers Prev.* 2007;16:2491–2495.
17. Tachibana I, Smith JS, Sato K, Hosek SM, Kimmel DW, Jenkins RB. Investigation of germline PTEN, p53, p16(INK4A)/p14(ARF), and CDK4 alterations in familial glioma. *Am J Med Genet.* 2000;92:136–141.
18. Malmer B, Iselius L, Holmberg E, Collins A, Henriksson R, Gronberg H. Genetic epidemiology of glioma. *Br J Cancer.* 2001;84:429–434.
19. Bondy M, Wiencke J, Wrensch M, Kyritsis AP. Genetics of primary brain tumors: a review. *J Neurooncol.* 1994;18:69–81.
20. de Andrade M, Barnholtz JS, Amos CI, Adatto P, Spencer C, Bondy ML. Segregation analysis of cancer in families of glioma patients. *Genet Epidemiol.* 2001;20:258–270.
21. Paunu N, Lahermo P, Onkamo P, et al. A novel low-penetrance locus for familial glioma at 15q23-q26.3. *Cancer Res.* 2002;62:3798–3802.
22. Narod SA, Lenoir GM. Are bilateral tumours hereditary? *Int J Epidemiol.* 1991;20:346–348.
23. Louis DN, Ohgaki H, Wiestler OD, et al. The 2007 WHO classification of tumours of the central nervous system. *Acta Neuropathol.* 2007;114:97–109.
24. Malkin D, Li FP, Strong LC, et al. Germ line p53 mutations in a familial syndrome of breast cancer, sarcomas, and other neoplasms. *Science.* 1990;250:1233–1238.
25. Kleihues P, Schauble B, zur Hausen A, Esteve J, Ohgaki H. Tumors associated with p53 germline mutations: a synopsis of 91 families. *Am J Pathol.* 1997;150:1–13.
26. Birch JM, Blair V, Kelsey AM, et al. Cancer phenotype correlates with constitutional TP53 genotype in families with the Li-Fraumeni syndrome. *Oncogene.* 1998;17:1061–1068.
27. Kyritsis AP, Bondy ML, Xiao M, et al. Germline p53 gene mutations in subsets of glioma patients. *J Natl Cancer Inst.* 1994;86:344–349.
28. Vital A, Loiseau H, Kantor G, et al. p53 protein expression in grade II astrocytomas: immunohistochemical study of 100 cases with long-term follow-up. *Pathol Res Pract.* 1998;194:831–836.
29. Ribeiro RC, Sandrini F, Figueiredo B, et al. An inherited p53 mutation that contributes in a tissue-specific manner to pediatric adrenal cortical carcinoma. *Proc Natl Acad Sci U S A.* 2001;98:9330–9335.
30. Verselis SJ, Rheinwald JG, Fraumeni JF Jr, Li FP. Novel p53 splice site mutations in three families with Li-Fraumeni syndrome. *Oncogene.* 2000;19:4230–4235.
31. Bell DW, Varley JM, Szydlo TE, et al. Heterozygous germ line hCHK2 mutations in Li-Fraumeni syndrome. *Science.* 1999;286:2528–2531.
32. Sodha N, Williams R, Mangion J, Bullock SL, Yuille MR, Eeles RA. Screening hCHK2 for mutations. *Science.* 2000;289:359.
33. Gutmann DH, Aylsworth A, Carey JC, et al. The diagnostic evaluation and multidisciplinary management of neurofibromatosis 1 and neurofibromatosis 2. *JAMA.* 1997;278:51–57.
34. Sorensen SA, Mulvihill JJ, Nielsen A. Long-term follow-up of von Recklinghausen neurofibromatosis. Survival and malignant neoplasms. *N Engl J Med.* 1986;314:1010–1015.
35. Seizinger BR, Rouleau GA, Ozelius LJ, et al. Genetic linkage of von Recklinghausen neurofibromatosis to the nerve growth factor receptor gene. *Cell.* 1987;49:589–594.
36. Sharif S, Ferner R, Birch JM, et al. Second primary tumors in neurofibromatosis 1 patients treated for optic glioma: substantial risks after radiotherapy. *J Clin Oncol.* 2006;24:2570–2575.
37. Evans DG, Huson SM, Donnai D, et al. A genetic study of type 2 neurofibromatosis in the United Kingdom. I. Prevalence, mutation rate, fitness, and confirmation of maternal transmission effect on severity. *J Med Genet.* 1992;29:841–846.
38. Evans DG, Watson C, King A, Wallace AJ, Baser ME. Multiple meningiomas: differential involvement of the NF2 gene in children and adults. *J Med Genet.* 2005;42:45–48.
39. Evans DG, Sainio M, Baser ME. Neurofibromatosis type 2. *J Med Genet.* 2000;37:897–904.
40. Turcot J, Despres JP, St Pierre F. Malignant tumors of the central nervous system associated with familial polyposis of the colon: report of two cases. *Dis Colon Rectum.* 1959;2:465–468.
41. Paraf F, Jothy S, Van Meir EG. Brain tumor-polyposis syndrome: two genetic diseases? *J Clin Oncol.* 1997;15:2744–2758.
42. Van Meir EG. "Turcot's syndrome": phenotype of brain tumors, survival and mode of inheritance. *Int J Cancer.* 1998;75:162–164.
43. Lundin DA, Blank A, Berger MS, Silber JR. Microsatellite instability is infrequent in sporadic adult gliomas. *Oncol Res.* 1998;10:421–428.
44. Leung SY, Chan TL, Chung LP, et al. Microsatellite instability and mutation of DNA mismatch repair genes in gliomas. *Am J Pathol.* 1998;153:1181–1188.
45. De Rosa M, Fasano C, Panariello L, et al. Evidence for a recessive inheritance of Turcot's syndrome caused by compound heterozygous mutations within the PMS2 gene. *Oncogene.* 2000;19:1719–1723.

4 Chemical Exposures Mediated Through Occupation, Environment and Lifestyle, and Brain Tumor Risk

Dora Il'yasova, Faith G. Davis, Rose Lai, Therese A. Dolecek, and Siegal Sadetzki

Occupational, environmental, and lifestyle exposures cause individuals to come in contact with known carcinogens, some of which induce brain tumors in animals and are therefore referred to as neurocarcinogens. An understanding of the relationships between these chemical exposures and risk of brain tumors would provide an opportunity for primary prevention of this devastating cancer. Data on human exposure to specific chemicals that cause brain tumors are sparse, although research in this area is emerging. In this chapter, we review the literature on chemical exposure through occupational, environmental, and other lifestyle experiences, including smoking, diet, and medication.

Occupational studies of brain tumors focus on workers exposed to neurocarcinogens identified in animal research (Table 4.1). The suspicion that chemical exposure, specifically in an occupational setting, can increase the risk of brain tumors in humans is not new. In 1982, the *Annals of the New York Academy of Sciences* devoted an issue to "Brain Tumors in the Chemical Industry" [1]. Occupational "exposure-risk" studies are initiated in response to apparent workplace hazards, the occurrence of brain tumor clusters, as extensions of animal studies of neurocarcinogens, or to study the effects of neurotoxins on brain tumor risk [2,3]. For example, a cluster of brain tumors in a petrochemical plant in Texas led to a longstanding investigation of whether polycyclic aromatic hydrocarbons (PAHs) can cause brain tumors [4–6]. However, current evidence that chemicals cause brain tumors in humans remains equivocal.

Environmental chemical exposure is usually addressed by studying highly exposed worker populations [7–9]. This review focuses on chemical exposure, specifically, to known and suspected animal neurocarcinogens, whether or not such exposure occurs in an occupational setting. As shown by Davis et al [2], a US survey of more than 30 industries showed that a substantial number of workers are exposed to known or suspected animal neurocarcinogens. Some of these chemicals can also be inhaled or are found in food or medication and can thus be ingested. In general, exposure to hazardous chemicals in occupational settings involves higher doses but smaller populations, whereas environmental and dietary exposures involve lower doses but larger populations. Often, occupational studies suffer from incomplete exposure assessment, because they do not take into account environmental and dietary exposures. However, such studies serve as a starting point to investigate the role of chemicals as causes of specific diseases. The major methodological weakness of most environmental and dietary exposure assessment is its low accuracy, because most of it is based on self-reporting. Taking these sources of bias into account, it is not surprising that, to-date, epidemiological studies on the relationship between exposure to chemicals and the risk of glioma have produced inconclusive results.

OCCUPATION

Evidence From Animal Studies Only

Several chemicals induce brain tumors in animals and have therefore been classified as animal neurocarcinogens. These include 1H-benzotriazole used to protect metals from corrosion [10], alkylating agents bromoethane and chloroethane used as chemical intermediates in various organic syntheses [11–13], and glycidol used as a stabilizer in the manufacture of vinyl polymers, an additive for oil and synthetic hydraulic fluids, and as a diluent in some epoxy resins [13–15]. Sills et al evaluated evidence for these compounds as neurocarcinogens and concluded with the following: for 1H-benzotriazole, bromoethane, and chloroethane, evidence is not strong, whereas for glycidol, there is clear evidence that it causes brain tumors in animals. Currently, no epidemiological data are available on the relationships between these compounds and the risk of brain tumors in humans.

Evidence From Epidemiological and Animal Studies

1,3-Butadiene and Isoprene

Isoprene and 1,3-butadiene are structurally related compounds. Isoprene is the monomer of natural rubber and naturally occurring terpenes and steroids, whereas 1,3-butadiene is a synthetic monomer used in the production of synthetic rubber. These compounds are found in many occupational settings including the production of rubber and petroleum-based products, transportation, waste treatment, as well as exposure to high levels of smoke,

Table 4.1 Occupations and Chemicals Implicated as Risk Factors for Brain Tumors[a]

CHEMICAL EXPOSURES
Known/Suspected Neurocarcinogens That Cause Gliomas in Animals

Industry/Occupation	1,3-Butadiene	3,3'-Dimethyl-benzidine Dihydrochloride	1H-Benzotriazole	Acrylamide	Acrylonitrile	PAHs[b]	Bromoethane	Chloroethane	CI Direct Blue	Ethylene Oxide	Glycidol	Isoprene	N-Nitroso Compounds
Acrylonitrile production					x								
Apparel and textile			x	x	x				x				
Chemical production	x	x	x	x			x	x	x	x	x		
Farmer										x			
Firefighter	x				x	x							
Health services		x	x	x			x	x	x	x			
Machine operators	x	x	x	x			x	x	x	x	x		
Pesticide applicator										x			
Petroleum products		x	x		x	x	x		x		x		
Rubber industry	x	x	x						x			x	x
Transport and material moving	x		x	x		x	x	x	x	x			

[a] This table excludes three compounds: diphenhydramine hydrochloride and furosemide are widely used drugs and are covered in the section related to medicine; occupational exposure to N2-fluorenylacetamide is not common. From ref. [2].

[b] Polycyclic aromatic hydrocarbons (PAHs), include benzo(a)pyrene and dimethylbenz(a)anthracene.

vehicle emissions, or gas/diesel fumes [16]. Nonoccupational exposure to 1,3-butadiene is virtually ubiquitous through smoke from cigarettes, fire, cooking with an open flame, etc [17,18]. 1,3-Butadiene is carcinogenic in both rats and mice [19–21] and is classified as a known human carcinogen by the Environmental Protection Agency [22] and the National Toxicology Program [23], whereas the International Association for Research on Cancer classified this compound as a probable human carcinogen [24]. There are more than 90 epidemiological investigations of the rubber industry and 9 of these studies are cohort studies that included brain tumors as an end point (5 of the 9 found excess risk in rubber workers). In addition, 4 of the 90 studies are case-control studies that included these tumors as an endpoint (3 of the 4 found excess risk). Such results may indicate an association between employment in the rubber industry and the risk of brain tumors, or they may reflect sampling variation between positive and negative studies. Suggesting this latter interpretation in a recent meta-analysis of 20 cohort studies, the summary estimate showed no association between employment in the rubber or tire industry and the risk of brain tumors [25].

Benzidine-Based Dyes: 3,3-Dimethoxybenzidine Dihydrochloride, 3,3'-Dimethylbenzidine Dihydrochloride, C.I. Direct Blue 15

Benzidine-based dyes are used as an intermediate in the production of bisazobiphenyl dyes for coloring textiles, paper, plastic, rubber, and leather as well as some polyurethane-based products [26]. Oral administration of these dyes cause various tumors in rats including astrocytoma [26]. However, Sills considered this evidence to be equivocal [13]. Epidemiological studies have found a connection between benzidine-based dyes and bladder cancer [26]. None of the occupational studies conducted among workers exposed to benzidine-based dyes reported an increased risk of brain tumors [27].

Acrylamide

Acrylamide has been used to manufacture water-soluble polymers (polyacrylamide) since the 1950s. High-level occupational exposure to acrylamide occurred in industrial accidents and, as documented, caused neurotoxicity [28]. No other effects have been documented by occupational studies on acrylamide [24,29,30]. In animal studies, chronic high-dose exposure to acrylamide was associated with increased incidence of several tumors including gliomas [31,32]. Currently, there is consensus that acrylamide and its metabolite glycidamide are genotoxic [28]. Recently, acrylamide has been found in fried and baked foods and coffee [33], expanding the question of this exposure beyond occupation to diet. Epidemiological studies have addressed dietary exposure to acrylamide in secondary analyses of case-control studies, with no convincing associations [24]. In addition to suffering from the common limitations of dietary assessment studies, these studies lack consensus on which foods constitutes significant sources of acrylamide and do not consider other occupational or environmental forms of exposure. Thus, the question whether dietary acrylamide is a risk factor for brain cancer (and all other cancers) remains unanswered.

Acrylonitrile

Acrylonitrile is an industrial chemical used in the manufacture of synthetic fibers, resins, plastics, elastomers, and rubber, and for use in various consumer goods. Primary routes of human exposure are dermal and inhalation [34]. Acrylonitrile causes tumors in various organs including the central nervous system. Meta-analysis of 12 epidemiological studies concluded that exposure to acrylonitrile is not associated with increased risk of brain tumors in humans [35]. Two cohort studies with the most detailed data on acrylonitrile exposure levels also have not found an association with brain tumors [36,37].

Ethylene Oxide

Ethylene oxide is widely used in chemical industries for the synthesis of several products [34,38] and as a sterilizing agent in the health care industry [2,34]. In rats, exposure to ethylene oxide increases the risk of brain tumors [34,39,40]. Several studies among health care professionals potentially exposed to ethylene oxide [2] found an increased risk of brain tumors, specifically among nurses and nursing assistants [41,42]. However, exposure to ethylene oxide in US hospitals has declined since 1984 [43]. Meta-analysis of 10 cohorts that include 29 800 workers and 2540 deaths concluded that occupational exposure to ethylene oxide is not associated with the increased risk of brain tumors [44]. Six years later, an update of this meta-analysis did not change this conclusion [38,45].

N-Nitroso Compounds

Humans are ubiquitously exposed to N-nitroso compounds: 75% of their exposure comes from diet, 25% from occupation, 2% from cigarette smoking, and 1% from other sources such as cosmetics, pharmaceuticals, and indoor and outdoor air [46,47]. In animals, only nitrosamides (e.g., methylnitrosourea and ethylnitrosourea) cause glioma with the highest potency associated with transplacental administration, that is, when a pregnant female is exposed to nitrosamides, her offspring develop brain tumors [47–49].

N-nitroso compounds are formed both in the environment (exogenous) and in the body (endogenous), complicating comprehensive exposure assessment of these compounds. In addition, other dietary components, such as vitamins, phenolic and sulfur compounds, inhibit formation of N-nitroso compounds [50], which further complicates exposure assessment, especially when performed using a dietary questionnaire. Epidemiological studies have assessed only partial exposure to N-nitroso compounds. For example, Ward et al evaluated exposure to nitrate and nitrite in drinking water and diet and found no association between such exposure and the risk of adult glioma [51]. Nor have a dozen dietary studies provided convincing evidence of an association between N-nitroso compound consumption and adult glioma [51–59]. However, most studies of childhood brain tumors (8 of 10 case-control studies) reviewed by Dietrich et al [60] found a positive association with maternal dietary intake of cured meats, a significant source of dietary N-nitroso compounds. These findings agree with the striking results from animal studies demonstrating extreme susceptibility of the fetal brain to chemical carcinogens [49,61,62]. Exposure to N-nitroso compounds also occurs in the rubber industry during the vulcanization processes [63]. Although specific exposure to N-nitroso compounds has not been evaluated among rubber industry workers, results of studies of these workers remain inconclusive (see section 1,3-Butadiene and Isoprene) [25,64].

Polycyclic Aromatic Hydrocarbons

PAHs are formed during incomplete combustion of coal, oil and gas, garbage, or other organic substances such as tobacco or charbroiled meat [65–67]. PAHs are a component of vehicle exhaust and are present in basic foods and drinking water. Human exposure to PAHs is widespread and unavoidable. Historically, a suspected cluster of brain tumors at a petrochemical plant in Texas City, Texas, generated a hypothesis that PAHs can cause brain tumors [4–6]. Maltoni showed that these compounds can cause brain tumors in animals [68].

Although exposure to PAHs is widespread, some occupations such as firefighting have particularly intensive exposure. A meta-analysis of 11 cohort and 5 case-control studies based on administrative records found no evidence of increased risk of brain tumors among firefighters [69]. However, when duration of employment was taken into account, firefighters with 30 or more years of employment had twice the risk of brain tumors [69]. Another well-studied example of occupational exposure to PAHs is among asphalt workers. A large international study among European asphalt workers found no convincing evidence that exposure to bitumen fume is associated with increased risk of any cancer [66]. Cordier et al report that paternal preconceptional exposure to PAH, from either tobacco smoke or occupational exposure, is associated with an increased risk for childhood brain tumors, especially astroglial tumors [70]. No effect was observed for maternal smoking or occupation before conception or during pregnancy. A previous study by the same group found that overall risk of brain tumors was elevated for fathers exposed to PAH. However, no dose-response relationship was found [71]. The data, therefore, remain inconclusive.

SMOKING

Although smoking is associated with increased cancer risk for a wide variety of tumors, a consistent relationship between smoking and development of glioma in adults does not exist [72]. The literature which addresses this association includes reports from 16 case-control and 5 cohort studies.

Among case-control studies that examined the relationship between ever-smoking cigarettes and glioma, seven reported ORs > 1, but were not statistically significant [55,73–78], two reported nonstatistically significant ORs < 1 [73,79], and one reported an OR of 1 [80]. Analyses presented separately by gender [54,56,81], and for current and former smokers [76,81–84], also provided risk estimates that did not reach statistical significance. Although some studies included dose-response analyses [74,76,78–81,85,86], only one reported a statistically significant trend for increased risk with increasing pack-years of plain (unfiltered) cigarettes ($p = 0.026$) [74]. The number of glioma cases included in the aforementioned studies ranged from 42 to 434.

Cohort studies that assessed the risk of glioma associated with smoking also demonstrated inconsistency among their findings, with very few reaching statistical significance. Two studies provided some indication of increased risk. Efird et al reported results from a cohort of 133 811 subscribers to the Kaiser Permanente Medical Care Program of Northern California. Assessment of the risk of glioma associated with smoking during a mean follow-up of 13.2 ± 6.7 years yielded relative risks of 1.4 (95% CI: 1.0–2.1) for ever versus never smokers ($p = 0.07$) and 1.6 (95%CI: 1.0–2.5) for current versus never smokers ($p = 0.06$) [87]. In addition, a dose-response relationship was observed among women (p for trend = 0.04). Consistent with this finding, a Canadian study of 89 709 women who had been recruited to participate in a National Breast Screening Study, also found a dose-response relationship between numbers of cigarettes per day (p for trend = 0.08), number of years smoking (p for trend = 0.06), and number of pack-years (p for trend = 0.07) and glioma [88].

A more recent study by Holick et al of three large US cohorts (Health Professionals Follow-up Study, Nurses' Health Study I, and Nurses' Health Study II), which included collection of smoking data during follow-up, in addition to baseline smoking data, did not confirm these trends [89]. Additional cohort studies that showed no increase in risk for glioma associated with smoking included a 6-year follow-up of a cohort of Seventh-day Adventists (RR: 0.82; 95% CI: 0.28–2.39) [90], and a 26-year follow-up of US veterans, for whom a relative risk of 1.1 (95% CI: 0.9–1.3) for mortality from brain cancer was observed among smokers relative to nonsmokers [91].

Although most of the aforementioned studies presented data on cigarette smoking only, a few studies also examined the risk of glioma associated with other tobacco products. All but one of these studies had either too little data on these substances to conduct an analysis [76,84], or did not find statistically significant associations with glioma [74,81]. When examining the risk associated with marijuana use at least once a month, adjusted for cigarette, cigar, and pipe smoking, as well as other possible confounders, Efird et al [87] reported a relative risk of 2.8 (1.3–6.2) ($p = 0.01$) for glioma.

One hypothesis that has been proposed to explain the lack of association between smoking and glioma observed in most studies is that the blood-brain barrier may limit the amount of carcinogens, such as N-nitroso compounds, reaching the brain tissue [81].

DIET

N-Nitroso Compound Exposure

Dietary studies of brain tumors have focused on foods and nutrients studied for other cancer sites and N-nitroso compounds. A number of dietary questionnaire and food composition database refinements were developed to improve N-nitroso compound exposure assessments for epidemiologic studies on cancer [58,92–95]. One study found that the incidence rate of gliomas was not related to cured meat consumption in men, although use of vitamin C tablets appeared protective [52]. Subsequent studies found that adults with glioma were more likely than controls to consume diets high in cured foods [56], and low in vitamin C–rich fruits and vegetables and to consume diets high in nitrites and low in vitamin C than were controls. These effects were more pronounced in men than in women. A population-based interview study in women with intracranial gliomas in Los Angeles County [55] found an increased risk associated with cured meat consumption, most notably bacon, and a decreased risk associated with vegetable consumption, including bell peppers. In addition, use of vitamin supplements appeared protective, and there was some suggestion that eating cured meats in combination with foods that inhibit endogenous nitrosation mitigates risk. Case-control studies conducted in Europe, Asia, and Australia suggest increased brain cancer risk from dietary intake of N-nitroso compounds. Consumption of processed meats increased the risk of gliomas and meningiomas in a German study [53]. In an Australian study, ingestion of high levels of bacon and corned meat [54] increased the risk of glial tumors in men, but the association was less evident in women. In another Australian study, N-nitroso compounds were not associated with glioma and meningioma [76]. In a Canadian study, spring water and wine intake increased the risk of brain tumors in adult males [74]. An increased risk of brain tumors among men who drank these two beverages is consistent with the N-nitroso compound hypothesis. Other reports and reviews extend the work over the past two decades on the role of N-nitroso compounds in brain and other cancers by contributing to biomarker development. First, improved food assays have been described by Mende et al [96] and Sen et al [97,98], who developed the methylnitrosourea equivalents (MNU) measure formed from foods under chemical conditions. Other advances include the direct measurement of endogenous formation of N-nitrosamides in the nonhuman stomach [99,100] and estimation of endogenous N-nitroso compounds from dietary precursors in the human stomach using a mathematical model [101], measurement of N-nitroso DNA adducts [102], and urinary N-nitroso excretion.

Vitamins and Antioxidants

Relatively few studies of brain tumors have focused on dietary components other than those related to NOC formation. Use of vitamin supplements has been found to reduce brain tumor risk in both adults [74,79] and in children. Risk may also be reduced by maternal prenatal vitamin use during pregnancy [103–105]. Antioxidants appear to be inversely associated with brain tumors through anti-inflammatory and oxidative stress reduction pathways. Oxidants can damage DNA and as this oxidative damage accumulates, cell repair mechanisms are impaired thus increasing risk of cancer. Antioxidants can either directly block the effects of oxidative DNA damage by removing or lowering the concentration of oxidants, minimize DNA or cellular damage, or enhance repair. Vitamin C is a known antioxidant acting as a scavenger of hydroxyl radicals that inhibits oxidative DNA lesions such as 8-hydroxydeoxyguanosine. Flavonoids inhibit low-density lipoprotein to lipoprotein oxidation, through downregulation of iNOS and COX-2 gene expression [106]. Carotenoids are lipophilic molecules with antioxidant properties implicated in scavenging peroxynitrite, modulating DNA repair [107], and possibly anti-inflammatory mechanisms. A few epidemiological studies have shown that antioxidant consumption from fruits and vegetables may be protective against adult glioma [55,56,58,108]. The primary mechanism centers on oxidative stress that induces a cellular redox imbalance, which has been found to be present in various cancer cells compared with normal cells; the redox imbalance may be related to oncogenic stimulation. DNA mutation is a critical step in carcinogenesis and elevated levels of oxidative DNA lesions (8-OH-G) have been noted in various tumors, strongly implicating such damage in the etiology of cancer. It appears that the DNA damage is predominantly linked with the initiation process. Both enzymatic (superoxide dismutase [Cu, Zn-SOD, Mn-SOD], catalase, glutathione peroxidase) and nonenzymatic antioxidants (Vitamin C, Vitamin E, carotenoids, thiol antioxidants [glutathione, thioredoxin, and lipoic acid], flavonoids, selenium, and others) may attenuate carcinogenesis. Most recently, a case-control study in Nebraska reported that increased intake of carotenoids reduces the risk of glioma by 50% and suggests that antioxidant as well as phytochemical nutrient intake is likely to play a protective role in adult glioma [58]. For carotenoid consumption, evidence of a protective effect on brain tumor risk has been consistent [108,109]. Carotenoids are lipophilic molecules with antioxidant properties implicated in scavenging peroxynitrite, modulating DNA repair [110], and possibly anti-inflammatory mechanisms [111].

Other Dietary Associations

Data on other dietary components are extremely limited. An inverse association between glioma and calcium consumption has been reported and hypothesized to function through inhibition of parathyroid hormone production in adults [112] and children [103,113]. Conflicting results with meat products, fresh fish, and poultry and use of salt with meat, fish, and vegetables require further clarification [55,57,114].

MEDICATIONS

COX-2 Inhibitors

There is a paucity of data on the use of common medications and their influence on brain tumor susceptibility. One actively investigated target is cyclooxygenase 2 (COX-2). COX-2 is an inducible isoform of COX, an enzyme that catalyzes the rate-limiting step in prostaglandin synthesis from arachidonic acid [115]. COX-2 is rapidly induced by cytokines, growth factors, tumor promotors, oncogenes, and carcinogens [116]. It enhances tumor cell motility and adhesion, and aberrant expression of COX-2 has been implicated in the pathogenesis of many cancer types, including malignant glioma [117]. To date, there is only one published study that evaluated the use of nonsteroidal anti-inflammatory drugs (NSAIDs), which are nonselective COX-2 inhibitors, in the risk of glioblastoma [118]. This population-based study was conducted in the San Francisco Bay Area. The authors recruited 236 glioblastoma cases and 401 frequency-matched controls. The use of NSAIDs was defined as having taken 600 or more pills within the past 10 years. Forty-one percent of interviews were completed by proxy. Analysis of the entire cohort showed an inverse association between NSAIDs use and risk of glioblastoma (OR = 0.76, 95% CI 0.5–1.1), suggestive of a protective effect of NSAIDs. When the analysis was restricted to self-reported cases, the results were consistent (OR = 0.53, 95% CI 0.3–0.8). The findings were also consistent for aspirin (OR = 0.51, 95% CI 0.3–0.8), ibuprofen (OR = 0.41, 95% CI 0.2–0.8), or naproxen (OR = 0.34, 95% CI 0.1–0.8). As glioblastoma patients may have used NSAIDs for recent onset of headache related to the development of their diseases, a sensitivity analysis was carried out by excluding those subjects who initiated NSAIDs use within the past 2 years. The result still showed that fewer subjects with glioblastoma than controls reported use of 600 or more NSAIDs (OR = 0.49, 95% CI 0.3–0.8). Results were also consistent for all types of NSAIDs. The study did not evaluate the use of selective COX-2 inhibitor, such as celecoxib; also, there were no data on dose-response relationships between NSAIDs and glioblastoma. Moreover, a possibility remains that drug evaluation in epidemiologic study would be confounded by their indication, that is, the underlying conditions for which the drugs were prescribed, and this study did not account for the reasons for which NSAIDs were used. In a pooled analysis that has only been published as an abstract, the San Francisco Bay cohort was combined with a separate cohort recruited in Harris County, Texas [119]. Overall, NSAIDs use was associated with a reduced risk of glioblastoma (OR = 0.69, 95% CI 0.51–0.94) but not other histological grades of glioma.

Antihistamines

In the same pooled analysis, the authors also investigated the use of antihistamine drugs and the risk of developing a glioma. The interest in this class of drugs is a result of consistent evidence showing that asthma and allergic conditions are inversely associated with the risk of glioma [120]. Histamine plays a major role in acute allergic inflammation because it is released from mast cells and basophils, and can be activated by immunologic and nonimmunologic stimuli such as allergens, IgE, and various cytokines [116,121]. Thus, antihistamine drugs possess antiallergic and anti-inflammatory properties, some of which may depend on histamine H_1-receptor blockade while others are receptor independent [122]. Antihistamine use was associated with an increased risk of anaplastic astrocytoma (AA, OR = 2.73, 95% CI 0.51–0.94) and low-grade glioma (LGG, OR = 1.86, 95% CI 1.11–3.11) but not GM [119]. More studies are necessary to confirm the relationships between LGG, AA and the use of antihistamine drugs, and the effect of these agents on the specific molecular pathogenesis of AA and LGG. Furthermore, the evidence for a positive association may be strengthened if a dose-response relationship can be shown. Also, the analysis of current versus past use of antihistamine may be helpful, as some have argued that only past history (childhood history) of allergic conditions causally reduces glioma risk. Their arguments are based on the immunosuppressive properties of glioma itself, and they claim that the subclinical tumor causes glioma patients to have fewer allergies than do controls proximate to the time of diagnosis.

Although the results of these studies are preliminary, they serve to stimulate further pharmacoepidemiological studies.

REFERENCES

1. Brain tumors in the chemical industry. *Ann N YAcad Sci.* 1982;381: 1–362.
2. Davis FG, Erdal S, Williams L, Bigner D. Work exposures to animal neurocarcinogens. *Int J Occup Environ Health.* 2006;12:16–23.
3. Maekawa A, Mitsumori K. Spontaneous occurrence and chemical induction of neurogenic tumors in rats. Influence of host factors and specificity of chemical structure. *CRC Crit Rev Toxicol.* 1990;20:287–310.
4. Alexander V, Leffingwell SS, Lloyd JW, Waxweiler RJ, Miller RL. Investigation of an apparent increased prevalence of brain tumors in a U.S. petrochemical plant. *Ann N Y Acad Sci.* 1982;381:97–107.
5. Alexander V, Leffingwell SS, Lloyd JW, Waxweiler RJ, Miller RL. Brain cancer in petrochemical workers: a case series report. *Am J Ind Med.* 1980;1:115–123.
6. Waxweiler RJ, Alexander V, Leffingwell SS, Haring M, Lloyd JW. Mortality from brain tumor and other causes in a cohort of petrochemical workers. *J Natl Cancer Inst.* 1983;70:75–81.
7. McLendon RE, Rosenblum MK, Bigner DD. Epidemiology of brain tumors: occupational studies. In: McLendon RE, Rosenblum MK, Bigner DD, eds. *Russell & Rubinstein's Pathology of Tumors of the Nervous System.* London: Hodder Arnold, 2006:29–32.
8. El-Zein R, Minn A, Wrensch M, Bondy ML. Epidemiology of brain tumors: industry and occupation. In: Levin VA, ed. *Cancer in the Nervous System.* New York: Oxford University Press; 2002:256–259.
9. Inskip PD, Linet MS, Heineman EF. Etiology of brain tumors in adults. *Epidemiol Rev.* 1995;17:382–414.
10. National Toxicology Program. Bioassay of 1H-benzotriazole for possible carcinogenecity. 1978;88:1–131
11. National Toxicology Program. Toxicology and carcinogenesis studies of bromoethane (ethyl bromide) (CAS No. 74–96-4) in F344/N rats and B6C3F1 mice (inhalation studies). 1989b;363:1–186..
12. National Toxicology Program. Toxicology and carcinogenesis studies of chloroethane (ethyl chloride) (CAS No. 75–00-3) in F344/N rats and B6C3F1 mice (inhalation studies). 1989;346:1–161.
13. Sills RC, Hailey JR, Neal J, Boorman GA, Haseman JK, Melnick RL. Examination of low-incidence brain tumor responses in F344 rats following chemical exposures in National Toxicology Program carcinogenicity studies. *Toxicol Pathol.* 1999;27:589–599.
14. U.S. Department of Labor OSHA. *Occupational Safety and Health Guideline for Glycidol.* Washington, DC: U.S. Department of Labor OSHA; 2007.
15. IARC. Glycidol. *IARC Monogr Eval Carcinog Risks Hum.* 2000;77:469–486.
16. Rice JM, Boffetta P. 1,3-Butadiene, isoprene and chloroprene: reviews by the IARC monographs programme, outstanding issues, and research priorities in epidemiology. *Chem Biol Interact.* 2001;135–136:11–26.
17. Sorsa M, Peltonen K, Anderson D, Demopoulos NA, Neumann HG, Osterman-Golkar S. Assessment of environmental and occupational exposures to butadiene as a model for risk estimation of petrochemical emissions. *Mutagenesis.* 1996;11:9–17.
18. U.S. EPA. *Cancer Risk from Outdoor Exposure to Air Toxics.* Vol. 1, Final Report. Research Triangle Park, NC: US Environmental Protection Agency; 1990.
19. National Toxicology Program. NTP toxicology and carcinogenesis studies of isoprene (CAS No. 78–79-5) in F344/N rats (Inhalation Studies). 1999;486:1–176
20. National Toxicology Program. NTP toxicology and carcinogenesis studies of 1,3-butadiene (CAS No. 106–99-0) in B6C3F1 mice (inhalation studies). 1984;288:1–111.
21. Huff JE, Melnick RL, Solleveld HA, Haseman JK, Powers M, Miller RA. Multiple organ carcinogenicity of 1,3-butadiene in B6C3F1 mice after 60 weeks of inhalation exposure. *Science.* 1985;227:548–549.
22. U.S. EPA. *Health Assessment of 1,3-Butadiene.* Washington, DC: U.S. EPA, Office of Research and Development, National Center for Environmental Assessment; 2002.
23. National Toxicology Program. *National Toxicology Program and U.S. Department of Health and Human Services, Ninth Report on Carcinogens: 1,3-Butadiene.* Research Triangle Park, NC: National Toxicology Program; 2000.
24. Rice JM. The carcinogenicity of acrylamide. *Mutat Res.* 2005;580: 3–20.
25. Borak J, Slade MD, Russi M. Risks of brain tumors in rubber workers: a metaanalysis. *J Occup Environ Med.* 2005;47:294–298.
26. Morgan DL, Dunnick JK, Goehl T, et al. Summary of the National Toxicology Program benzidine dye initiative. *Environ Health Perspect.* 1994;102:63–78.
27. Rosenman KD, Reilly MJ. Cancer mortality and incidence among a cohort of benzidine and dichlorobenzidine dye manufacturing workers. *Am J Ind Med.* 2004;46:505–512.
28. Exon JH. A review of the toxicology of acrylamide. *J Toxicol Environ Health B Crit Rev.* 2006;9:397–412.
29. Marsh GM, Youk AO, Buchanich JM, Kant IJ, Swaen G. Mortality patterns among workers exposed to acrylamide: updated follow up. *J Occup Environ Med.* 2007;49:82–95.
30. Swaen GM, Haidar S, Burns CJ, et al. Mortality study update of acrylamide workers. *Occup Environ Med.* 2007;64:396–401.
31. Johnson KA, Gorzinski SJ, Bodner KM, et al. Chronic toxicity and oncogenicity study on acrylamide incorporated in the drinking water of Fischer 344 rats. *Toxicol Appl Pharmacol.* 1986;85:154–68.
32. Friedman MA, Dulak LH, Stedham MA. A lifetime oncogenicity study in rats with acrylamide. *Fundam Appl Toxicol.* 1995;27:95–105.
33. Tareke E, Rydberg P, Karlsson P, Eriksson S, Tornqvist M. Analysis of acrylamide, a carcinogen formed in heated foodstuffs. *J Agric Food Chem.* 2002;50:4998–5006.
34. National Toxicology Program. *Eleventh Report on Carcinogens.* Research Triangle Park, NC: U.S. Department of Health and Human Services, Public Health Service, National Toxicology Program; 2004.
35. Collins JJ, Strother DE. CNS tumors and exposure to acrylonitrile: inconsistency between experimental and epidemiology studies. *Neuro Oncol.* 1999;1:221–230.
36. Blair A, Stewart PA, Zaebst DD, et al. Mortality of industrial workers exposed to acrylonitrile. *Scand J Work Environ Health.* 1998;24(suppl 2):25–41.
37. Swaen GM, Bloemen LJ, Twisk J, et al. Mortality update of workers exposed to acrylonitrile in The Netherlands. *J Occup Environ Med.* 2004;46:691–698.
38. Kolman A, Chovanec M, Osterman-Golkar S. Genotoxic effects of ethylene oxide, propylene oxide and epichlorohydrin in humans: update review (1990–2001). *Mutat Res.* 2002;512:173–194.
39. Garman RH, Snellings WM, Maronpot RR. Frequency, size and location of brain tumours in F-344 rats chronically exposed to ethylene oxide. *Food Chem Toxicol.* 1986;24:145–153.
40. Garman RH, Snellings WM, Maronpot RR. Brain tumors in F344 rats associated with chronic inhalation exposure to ethylene oxide. *Neurotoxicology.* 1985;6:117–137.
41. Aronson KJ, Howe GR, Carpenter M, Fair ME. Surveillance of potential associations between occupations and causes of death in Canada, 1965–91. *Occup Environ Med.* 1999;56:265–269.
42. Katz RM. Causes of death among registered nurses. *J Occup Med.* 1983;25:760–762.
43. LaMontagne A, Oakes J, Lopez-Turley R. Long-term ethylene oxide exposure trends in US hospitals: intervention needed to preserve gains made following 1984 OSHA standard. *Am J Public Health* 2004;94:1614–1619.
44. Shore RE, Gardner MJ, Pannett B. Ethylene oxide: an assessment of the epidemiological evidence on carcinogenicity. *Br J Ind Med.* 1993;50:971–997.
45. Teta MJ, Sielken RL Jr, Valdez-Flores C. Ethylene oxide cancer risk assessment based on epidemiological data: application of revised regulatory guidelines. *Risk Anal.* 1999;19:1135–1155.
46. Tricker AR. N-nitroso compounds and man: sources of exposure, endogenous formation and occurrence in body fluids. *Eur J Cancer Prev.* 1997;6:226–268.

47. Lijinsky W, Saavedra J, Kovatch R. Carcinogenesis in rats by nitrosodialkylureas containing methyl and ethyl groups given by gavage and in drinking water. *J Toxicol Environ Health.* 1989;28:27–38.
48. Lantos PL. Development of nitrosourea-induced brain tumours–with a special note on changes occurring during latency. *Food Chem Toxicol.* 1986;24:121–127.
49. Zook BC, Simmens SJ, Jones RV. Evaluation of ENU-induced gliomas in rats: nomenclature, immunochemistry, and malignancy. *Toxicol Pathol.* 2000;28:193–201.
50. Bartsch H, Ohshima H, Pignatelli B. Inhibitors of endogenous nitrosation. Mechanisms and implications in human cancer prevention. *Mutat Res.* 1988;202:307–324.
51. Ward MH, Heineman EF, McComb RD, Weisenburger DD. Drinking water and dietary sources of nitrate and nitrite and risk of glioma. *J Occup Environ Med.* 2005;47:1260–1267.
52. Preston-Martin S, Mack W. Gliomas and meningiomas in men in Los Angeles County: investigation of exposures to N-nitroso compounds. *IARC Sci Publ.* 1991;105:197–203.
53. Boeing H, Schlehofer B, Blettner M, Wahrendorf J. Dietary carcinogens and the risk for glioma and meningioma in Germany. *Int J Cancer.* 1993;53:561–565.
54. Giles GG, McNeil JJ, Donnan G, et al. Dietary factors and the risk of glioma in adults: results of a case-control study in Melbourne, Australia. *Int J Cancer.* 1994;59:357–362.
55. Blowers L, Preston-Martin S, Mack WJ. Dietary and other lifestyle factors of women with brain gliomas in Los Angeles County (California, USA). *Cancer Causes Control.* 1997;8:5–12.
56. Lee M, Wrensch M, Miike R. Dietary and tobacco risk factors for adult onset glioma in the San Francisco Bay Area (California, USA). *Cancer Causes Control.* 1997;8:13–24.
57. Kaplan S, Novikov I, Modan B. Nutritional factors in the etiology of brain tumors: potential role of nitrosamines, fat, and cholesterol. *Am J Epidemiol.* 1997;146:832–841.
58. Chen H, Ward MH, Tucker KL, et al. Diet and risk of adult glioma in eastern Nebraska, United States. *Cancer Causes Control.* 2002;13:647–655.
59. Huncharek M, Kupelnick B, Wheeler L. Dietary cured meat and the risk of adult glioma: a meta-analysis of nine observational studies. *J Environ Pathol Toxicol Oncol.* 2003;22:129–137.
60. Dietrich M, Block G, Pogoda JM, Buffler P, Hecht S, Preston-Martin S. A review: dietary and endogenously formed N-nitroso compounds and risk of childhood brain tumors. *Cancer Causes Control.* 2005;16:619–635.
61. Rice JM, Rehm S, Donovan PJ, Perantoni AO. Comparative transplacental carcinogenesis by directly acting and metabolism-dependent alkylating agents in rodents and nonhuman primates. *IARC Sci Publ.* 1989;96:17–34.
62. Zook BC, Simmens SJ. Neurogenic tumors in rats induced by ethylnitrosourea. *Exp Toxicol Pathol.* 2005;57:7–14.
63. Oury B, Limasset JC, Protois JC. Assessment of exposure to carcinogenic N-nitrosamines in the rubber industry. *Int Arch Occup Environ Health.* 1997;70:261–271.
64. Kogevinas M, Sala M, Boffetta P, Kazerouni N, Kromhout H, Hoar-Zahm S. Cancer risk in the rubber industry: a review of the recent epidemiological evidence. *Occup Environ Med.* 1998;55:1–12.
65. Boffetta P, Jourenkova N, Gustavsson P. Cancer risk from occupational and environmental exposure to polycyclic aromatic hydrocarbons. *Cancer Causes Control* 1997;8:444–472.
66. Boffetta P, Burstyn I, Partanen T, et al. Cancer mortality among European asphalt workers: an international epidemiological study. II. Exposure to bitumen fume and other agents. *Am J Ind Med* 2003;43:28–39.
67. IARC. *Polynuclear Aromatic Compounds, Part 1: Chemical, Environmental and Experimental Data.* Lyon, France: IARC Monogr Eval Carcinog Risk Chem Humans; 1983.
68. Maltoni C, Ciliberti A, Carretti D. Experimental contributions in identifying brain potential carcinogens in the petrochemical industry. *Ann N Y Acad Sci.* 1982;381:216–249.
69. Youakim S. Risk of cancer among firefighters: a quantitative review of selected malignancies. *Arch Environ Occup Health.* 2006;61:223–231.
70. Cordier S, Monfort C, Filippini G, et al. Parental exposure to polycyclic aromatic hydrocarbons and the risk of childhood brain tumors. The SEARCH International Childhood Brain Tumor Study. *Am J Epidemiol.* 2004;159:1109–1116.
71. Cordier S, Lefeuvre B, Filippini G, et al. Parental occupation, occupational exposure to solvents and polycyclic aromatic hydrocarbons and risk of childhood brain tumors (Italy, France, Spain). *Cancer Causes Control.* 1997;8:688–697.
72. U.S. Department of Health and Human Services. *The Health Consequences of Smoking: A Report of the Surgeon General.* Atlanta: U.S. Department of Health and Human Services, Centers for Disease Control and Prevention, National Center for Chronic Disease Prevention and Health Promotion, Office on Smoking and Health, 2004.
73. Ahlbom A, Navier IL, Norell S, Olin R, Spannare B. Nonoccupational risk indicators for astrocytomas in adults. *Am J Epidemiol.* 1986;124:334–337.
74. Burch JD, Craib KJ, Choi BC, Miller AB, Risch HA, Howe GR. An exploratory case-control study of brain tumors in adults. *J Natl Cancer Inst.* 1987;78:601–609.
75. Hu J, Johnson K, Mao Y, et al. Risk factors for glioma in adults: a case-control study in northeast China. *Cancer Detect Prev.* 1998;22:100–108.
76. Ryan P, Lee MW, North B, McMichael AJ. Risk factors for tumors of the brain and meninges: results from the Adelaide Adult Brain Tumor Study. *Int J Cancer.* 1992;51:20–27.
77. Zampieri P, Meneghini F, Grigoletto F, et al. Risk factors for cerebral glioma in adults: a case-control study in an Italian population. *J Neurooncol.* 1994;19:61–67.
78. Musicco M, Filippini G, Bordo BM, Melotto A, Morello G, Berrino F. Gliomas and occupational exposure to carcinogens: case-control study. *Am J Epidemiol.* 1982;116:782–790.
79. Preston-Martin S, Mack W, Henderson BE. Risk factors for gliomas and meningiomas in males in Los Angeles County. *Cancer Res.* 1989;49:6137–6143.
80. Hochberg F, Toniolo P, Cole P, Salcman M. Nonoccupational risk indicators of glioblastoma in adults. *J Neurooncol.* 1990;8:55–60.
81. Zheng T, Cantor KP, Zhang Y, Chiu BC, Lynch CF. Risk of brain glioma not associated with cigarette smoking or use of other tobacco products in Iowa. *Cancer Epidemiol Biomarkers Prev.* 2001;10:413–414.
82. Choi NW, Schuman LM, Gullen WH. Epidemiology of primary central nervous system neoplasms. II. Case-control study. *Am J Epidemiol.* 1970;91:467–485.
83. Brownson R, Reif J, Chang J, Davis J. An analysis of occupational risks for brain cancer. *Am J Public Health.* 1990;80:169–172.
84. Schlehofer B, Kunze S, Sachsenheimer W, Blettner M, Niehoff D, Wahrendorf J. Occupational risk factors for brain tumors: results from a population-based case-control study in Germany. *Cancer Causes Control.* 1990;1:209–215.
85. Hu J, La Vecchia C, Negri E, et al. Diet and brain cancer in adults: a case-control study in northeast China. *Int J Cancer.* 1999;81:20–23.
86. Hurley SF, McNeil JJ, Donnan GA, Forbes A, Salzberg M, Giles GG. Tobacco smoking and alcohol consumption as risk factors for glioma: a case-control study in Melbourne, Australia. *J Epidemiol Community Health.* 1996;50:442–446.
87. Efird JT, Friedman GD, Sidney S, et al. The risk for malignant primary adult-onset glioma in a large, multiethnic, managed-care cohort: cigarette smoking and other lifestyle behaviors. *J Neurooncol.* 2004;68:57–69.
88. Navarro-Silvera SA, Miller AB, Rohan TE. Cigarette smoking and risk of glioma: a prospective cohort study. *Int J Cancer.* 2006;118:1848–1851.
89. Holick CN, Giovannucci EL, Rosner B, Stampfer MJ, Michaud DS. Prospective study of cigarette smoking and adult glioma: dosage, duration, and latency. *Neuro-oncology.* 2007;9:326.
90. Mills PK, Preston-Martin S, Annegers JF, Beeson WL, Phillips RL, Fraser GE. Risk factors for tumors of the brain and cranial meninges in Seventh-day Adventists. *Neuroepidemiology.* 1989;8:266–275.
91. McLaughlin JK, Hrubec Z, Blot WJ, Fraumeni JF Jr. Smoking and cancer mortality among U.S. veterans: a 26-year follow-up. *Int J Cancer.* 1995;60:190–193.
92. Howe GR, Harrison L, Jain M. A short diet history for assessing dietary exposure to N-nitrosamines in epidemiologic studies. *Am J Epidemiol.* 1986;124:595–602.
93. Jakszyn P, Agudo A, Ibanez R, et al. Development of a food database of nitrosamines, heterocyclic amines, and polycyclic aromatic hydrocarbons. *J Nutr.* 2004;134:2011–2014.
94. Jakszyn P, Gonzalez CA. Nitrosamine and related food intake and gastric and oesophageal cancer risk: a systematic review of the epidemiological evidence. *World J Gastroenterol.* 2006;12:4296–4303.
95. Jakszyn P, Bingham S, Pera G, et al. Endogenous versus exogenous exposure to N-nitroso compounds and gastric cancer risk in the European Prospective Investigation into Cancer and Nutrition (EPIC-EURGAST) study. *Carcinogenesis.* 2006;27:1497.

96. Mende P, Spiegelhalder B, Preussmann R. Trace analysis of nitrosated foodstuffs for nitrosamides. *Food Chem Toxicol.* 1991;29:167–172.
97. Sen NP, Seaman SW, Burgess C, Baddoo PA, Weber D. Investigation on the possible formation of N-nitroso-N-methylurea by nitrosation of creatinine in model systems and in cured meats at gastric pH. *J Agric Food Chem.* 2000;48:5088–5096.
98. Sen NP, Seaman SW, Baddoo PA, Burgess C, Weber D. Formation of N-nitroso-N-methylurea in various samples of smoked/dried fish, fish sauce, seafoods, and ethnic fermented/pickled vegetables following incubation with nitrite under acidic conditions. *J Agric Food Chem.* 2001;49:2096–2103.
99. Maragos CM, Hotchkiss JH, Fubini SL. Quantitative estimates of N-nitrosotrimethylurea formation in the porcine stomach. *Carcinogenesis.* 1990;11:1587–1591.
100. Mirvish SS, Chu C. Chemical determination of methylnitrosourea and ethylnitrosourea in stomach contents of rats, after intubation of the alkylureas plus sodium nitrite. *J Natl Cancer Inst.* 1973;50:745–750.
101. Shephard SE, Schlatter C, Lutz WK. Assessment of the risk of formation of carcinogenic N-nitroso compounds from dietary precursors in the stomach. *Food Chem Toxicol.* 1987;25:91–108.
102. Gurney JG, Chen M, Skluzacek MC, et al. Null association between frequency of cured meat consumption and methylvaline and ethylvaline hemoglobin adduct levels: the N-nitroso brain cancer hypothesis. *Cancer Epidemiol Biomarkers Prev.* 2002;11:421–422.
103. Bunin GR, Kuijten RR, Buckley JD, Rorke LB, Meadows AT. Relation between maternal diet and subsequent primitive neuroectodermal brain tumors in young children. *N Engl J Med.* 1993;329:536–541.
104. Preston-Martin S, Pogoda JM, Mueller BA, Holly EA, Lijinsky W, Davis RL. Maternal consumption of cured meats and vitamins in relation to pediatric brain tumors. *Cancer Epidemiol Biomarkers Prev.* 1996;5:599–605.
105. Preston-Martin S, Pogoda JM, Mueller BA, et al. Results from an international case-control study of childhood brain tumors: the role of prenatal vitamin supplementation. *Environ Health Perspect.* 1998;106:887–892.
106. Raso GM, Meli R, Di Carlo G, Pacilio M, Di Carlo R. Inhibition of inducible nitric oxide synthase and cyclooxygenase-2 expression by flavonoids in macrophage J774A.1. *Life Sci.* 2001;68:921–931.
107. Astley SB, Hughes DA, Wright AJ, Elliott RM, Southon S. DNA damage and susceptibility to oxidative damage in lymphocytes: effects of carotenoids in vitro and in vivo. *Br J Nutr.* 2004;91:53–61.
108. Berleur MP, Cordier S. The role of chemical, physical, or viral exposures and health factors in neurocarcinogenesis: implications for epidemiologic studies of brain tumors. *Cancer Causes Control.* 1995;6:240–256.
109. Hara A, Okayasu I. Cyclooxygenase-2 and inducible nitric oxide synthase expression in human astrocytic gliomas: correlation with angiogenesis and prognostic significance. *Acta Neuropathol.* 2004;108:43–48.
110. Kritchevsky SB, Bush AJ, Pahor M, Gross MD. Serum carotenoids and markers of inflammation in nonsmokers. *Am J Epidemiol.* 2000;152:1065–1071.
111. Kamat JP, Devasagayam TP. Oxidative damage to mitochondria in normal and cancer tissues, and its modulation. *Toxicology.* 2000;155:73–82.
112. Tedeschi-Blok N, Schwartzbaum J, Lee M, Miike R, Wrensch M. Dietary calcium consumption and astrocytic glioma: the San Francisco Bay Area Adult Glioma Study, 1991–1995. *Nutr Cancer.* 2001;39:196–203.
113. Bunin GR, Kuijten RR, Boesel CP, Buckley JD, Meadows AT. Maternal diet and risk of astrocytic glioma in children: a report from the Childrens Cancer Group (United States and Canada). *Cancer Causes Control.* 1994;5:177–187.
114. Guo WD, Linet MS, Chow WH, Li JY, Blot WJ. Diet and serum markers in relation to primary brain tumor risk in China. *Nutr Cancer.* 1994;22:143–150.
115. Vane JR, Bakhle YS, Botting RM. Cyclooxygenases 1 and 2. *Annu Rev Pharmacol Toxicol.* 1998;38:97–120.
116. Walsh G. Anti-inflammatory properties of antihistamines: an update. Clin Exp Allergy Rev 2005;5:21–25.
117. Joki T, Heese O, Nikas DC, et al. Expression of cyclooxygenase 2 (COX-2) in human glioma and in vitro inhibition by a specific COX-2 inhibitor, NS-398. *Cancer Res.* 2000;60:4926–4931.
118. Sivak-Sears NR, Schwartzbaum JA, Miike R, Moghadassi M, Wrensch M. Case-control study of use of nonsteroidal anti-inflammatory drugs and glioblastoma multiforme. *Am J Epidemiol.* 2004;159:1131–1139.
119. Scheurer ME, Wrensch M, El-Zein RA, et al. Antihistamine and anti-inflammatory drug use associated differently for high-grade versus low-grade gliomas. AACRMTG 2006;2006:114–115.
120. Linos E, Raine T, Alonso A, Michaud D. Atopy and risk of brain tumors: a meta-analysis. *J Natl Cancer Inst.* 2007;99:1544–1550.
121. Bachert C. The role of histamine in allergic disease: re-appraisal of its inflammatory potential. *Allergy.* 2002;57:287–296.
122. Leurs R, Church MK, Taglialatela M. H1-antihistamines: inverse agonism, anti-inflammatory actions and cardiac effects. *Clin Exp Allergy.* 2002;32:489–498.

5 Exposure to Ionizing Radiation and Glioma Risk

Siegal Sadetzki and Lori Mandelzweig

INTRODUCTION

Ionizing radiation represents electromagnetic waves and particles that have sufficient energy to ionize atoms in the human body and thereby induce chemical changes with potential biological importance for cell function [1]. The main event, which initiates damage caused by radiation, is breaks in one or both strands of the DNA helix in cells, resulting in cell death, damage to chromosomes, or mutations [2]. Sources of exposure to ionizing radiation are both natural (e.g., cosmic rays, radon) and man made (mainly medical uses such as x-rays and nuclear medicine as well as accidents and nuclear power plants) [3].

The primary physical quantity of radiation dosimetry is the "absorbed dose," measured by the "gray" (Gy) unit, which equals $1\ \text{J kg}^{-1}$. The "equivalent dose" is the primary dosimetric quantity of radiation protection, which relates the absorbed dose to the effective biological damage of the radiation to the organ or tissue (measured by "sievert" [Sv]). The "effective dose" is a dosimetric quantity for the overall biological damage associated with exposure to radiation, which accounts for variations in equivalent dose among radiosensitive organs and tissues [1].

In diagnostic imaging procedures, effective doses are generally fairly low, ranging from 0.1 to 10 mSv. Exposures to therapeutic radiation for cancer are characterized by much higher doses, typically ranging from 20 to 60 Gy [3].

Evidence for the carcinogenic potential of ionizing radiation has been accumulating since the 1950s [4,5]. Sources of this evidence include studies of exposure to atomic bomb radiation in Japan [4,6], fallout and accidents from nuclear weapon testing [7,8], medical uses of ionizing radiation (including therapeutic radiation given for treatment of both cancer [9–11] and benign conditions [12–15] as well as diagnostic procedures [16–18]), occupational exposure [19–21], and environmental exposure from natural sources (e.g., radon) [22,23].

Although the association between ionizing radiation and brain tumors was discovered relatively late and is based on fewer studies, in comparison with other tumor sites, the role of ionizing radiation in brain tumor development is currently relatively well established [6,24–33].

CASE REPORTS

The idea that brain tumor development can be attributed to exposure to radiation was first raised on the basis of individual case reports. A recent review of the literature on radiation-induced gliomas reported 116 cases that developed after radiotherapy for cranial pathologies [34]. The most frequent reasons for radiotherapy, in descending order, were acute lymphoblastic leukemia (ALL), pituitary adenoma, and tinea capitis. The average radiation dose was 32 Gy, and the average latency period was 9.6 years. The authors described these patients as younger than those affected with spontaneous gliomas, with tumors originating in the previously irradiated area. Several cases of gliomas following radiosurgery (with maximum doses ranging from 27.5 to 40 Gy and the margin dose ranging from 11 to 20 Gy) have also been described by McIver [35].

PROSPECTIVE STUDIES

Tinea Capitis Cohorts

Prospective epidemiological studies of subjects who were treated during childhood for tinea capitis were the first to show increased risk for the development of brain tumors in irradiated compared with nonirradiated populations. One of the first and most conclusive sources of evidence for the association between ionizing radiation exposure and head and neck tumors comes from a follow-up study of Israeli subjects who underwent radiation therapy for tinea capitis during childhood in the 1950s [26]. The mean dose to the brain was 1.5 Gy (range: 1.0–6.0 Gy) [25,36]. The Israeli tinea capitis cohort includes 10,834 irradiated individuals with both matched population and sibling control groups. In a follow-up study conducted in 1980, a striking increased risk was found for meningioma RR = 9.5 (95% CI: 3.5–25.7), whereas a relative risk of 2.6 (95% CI: 0.8–8.6) was noted for gliomas [25]. With a median 40-year follow-up, the excess relative risks per gray (ERR/Gy) for the irradiated group were 4.63 (95% CI: 2.43–9.12) and 1.98 (95% CI: 0.73–4.69) for benign meningiomas and malignant brain tumors, respectively [32]. The ERR/Gy for malignant brain tumors decreased with increasing age at irradiation, from 3.56 for age < 5 to 0.47 for age ≥ 10, whereas no trend with age was observed for benign meningiomas; for both tumors, the risk remained elevated after a latent period of 30 years or more. For gliomas, the risk was not associated with gender or ethnic origin and was positively associated with dose; the linear dose response model described these data well. Analysis of excess absolute risk per 10,000 person-years yielded estimates of 0.31 and 0.48 per Gy/10,000 person-years for malignant brain tumors and benign meningiomas, respectively.

An additional cohort that was used to examine long-term effects of exposure to radiotherapy for treatment of tinea capitis is based on 2215 individuals exposed to brain doses of 175 cGy at the surface to 70 cGy at the base of the skull between 1940 and 1959 in New York [37–39]. The control group comprised 1395 individuals matched for age, sex, and race who were treated for tinea capitis during the same period using topical medications only. After a median follow-up of 39 years, 16 intracranial tumors (7 malignant brain tumors, 4 meningiomas, and 5 vestibular schwannoma) occurred in the irradiated group, compared with one vestibular schwannoma in the control group [12].

Hemangiomas Studies

Other follow-up studies of irradiated subjects include two Swedish cohorts of individuals who were exposed to radium (^{226}Ra) treatment for hemangiomas during infancy [40]. These subjects were exposed to low-dose ionizing radiation with a mean intracranial dose of 7 cGy. In a pooled analysis of these two cohorts, 83 intracranial tumors were observed in 26 949 people who had received radiotherapy, yielding a standardized incidence ratio (SIR) of 1.43 (95% CI: 1.14–1.78). Twenty of these tumors were meningiomas and 35 were gliomas, diagnosed on average 34 and 39 years, respectively, after the irradiation treatment. A linear dose-response model with dose-effect modification by age at first exposure fit the data best, indicating a higher risk for those exposed earlier in life. The estimated ERR/Gy for all the above-mentioned brain tumors using this model was 2.7 (95% CI: 1.0–5.6).

ALL Studies

Several reports of cohorts of children treated for ALL who were followed in order to determine the incidence of second neoplasms have also provided evidence of the effects of radiotherapy on the risk of brain tumors [9,10].

In a cohort study conducted in Nordic countries, 981 children treated for childhood leukemia were followed for 4.3 to 26.5 years for the development of second malignant neoplasms. Among those who had been treated with cranial radiation (58.4%), the number of brain tumors was close to 27 times greater (95% CI: 5.5–78.1) than expected, whereas no such tumors developed among those treated with chemotherapy [41]. The dose of radiation given to those who developed brain tumors was 24 Gy. Data from the Italian "Off Therapy Registry," which evaluated the incidence of second malignant tumors after the end of therapy for a first cancer in childhood, showed that among those who had been treated for ALL, 9 later developed malignant CNS tumors (SIR: 58.9; 95% CI: 26.8–111.8). All of these 9 cases had received prophylactic cranial radiotherapy (cumulative dose 2400 cGy in 7 patients and 1800 cGy and 3600 cGy, respectively, in the remaining 2) for treatment of childhood ALL [42]. Through the use of a database from the Berlin-Frankfurt-Munster study of treatment of children with ALL and the German Childhood Cancer Registry, Loning et al examined the rate of secondary neoplasms at a median 5.7-year follow-up (range: 1.5–18 years) of 5006 children. Among the 52 second neoplasms observed, 25% (n = 13) were CNS tumors, including 4 glioblastoma and 4 astrocytoma. All patients with secondary CNS tumors, except one with meningioma, had undergone cranial radiotherapy. Reported radiation doses were either 12 or ≥18 Gy. The estimated risk of developing a second neoplasm 15 years after diagnosis of ALL was significantly higher in those who had received radiation therapy in comparison with those who had not: 3.5% (95% CI: 1.5–5.5) versus 1.2% (95% CI: 0.2–2.3). A comparison of the observed incidence of CNS tumors in this study with the rate expected in the general population indicated a 19-fold increase of CNS neoplasms (95% CI: 9.8–29.4) [43].

Childhood Cancer Survivor Study

A report recently published from the Childhood Cancer Survivor Study, a collaborative effort of 26 institutions in the United States and Canada, presented data on subsequent primary neoplasms of the central nervous system among individuals who had survived childhood cancer for at least 5 years. Cases were matched with four controls by age, sex, and time since original cancer diagnosis [11]. Analysis of a cohort of 14 361 individuals identified subsequent primary CNS tumors among 116, the most frequent of which were meningiomas (n = 66) and gliomas (n = 40). Gliomas occurred in a median of 9 years from original diagnosis, while the median time to the development of meningioma was 17 years. Exposure to radiation therapy as treatment for the primary cancer was associated with statistically significant increased risks for the development of glioma (OR: 6.78; 95% CI: 1.54–29.7), meningioma (OR: 9.94; 95% CI: 2.17–45.6), and all CNS tumors combined (OR: 7.07; 95% CI: 2.76–18.1). Significant radiation dose-response relationships (p < 0.001) were observed for all CNS tumors combined as well as for gliomas individually. The ERR/Gy, equal to the slope of the linear dose-response function, was 0.33 (95% CI: 0.07–1.71) per Gy for glioma, 1.06 (95% CI: 0.21–8.15) per Gy for meningioma, and 0.69 (95% CI: 0.25–2.23) per Gy for all CNS tumors. For gliomas, the ERR/Gy was highest among children exposed when they were under the age of 5 years. The investigators concluded that exposure to radiation therapy is the most important risk factor for the development of a new CNS tumor in survivors of childhood cancer.

Atomic Bomb Survivor Study

The atomic bomb studies provide one of the most valuable sources of information about the long-term effects of exposure to ionizing radiation. Among the more recent publications based on these data was a quantitative study that examined the dose-response relationship, quantified radiation risks for specific histologic types of malignant and benign tumors, and evaluation of the role of modifying factors on dose response [6]. Based on 43 gliomas and 88 meningiomas, ERR/Sv of 0.6 (95% CI: −0.2–2.0) and 0.6 (95% CI: −0.01–1.8) were calculated for these tumors. A statistically significant dose-response was observed for all nervous system tumors combined, indicating that exposure to even moderate doses (<1 Sv) of radiation are associated with an elevated incidence of nervous system tumors. The linear dose-response model was shown to fit the data well for doses ranging from zero to two or more Sv.

Relative Risk Variance

Quantitative data on the association between ionizing radiation and brain tumor development have only been presented in four follow-up studies of the above-mentioned cohorts: Swedish infants with skin hemangioma [40], atomic bomb survivors in Hiroshima and Nagasaki [6], Israeli children treated for tinea capitis [32], and North American survivors of childhood cancer [11]. Comparison of these studies indicates some degree of discrepancy regarding risk estimates [32]. Although lower magnitudes of ERR/Sv associated with childhood exposure were observed in the atomic bomb studies (1.2 for all nervous system tumors excluding schwannoma) and studies of childhood leukemia treated with therapeutic radiation (1.06 for meningioma and 0.33 for gliomas), greater ERRs/Gy were reported in the Israeli tinea capitis cohort (4.63 for meningiomas and 1.98 for malignant brain tumors) and the Swedish cohorts of infants exposed to radiation treatment for hemangiomas (2.7 for all brain tumors combined). It is possible that the discrepancy in estimates may be partly attributed to differences in the age distributions of the cohorts [32]. Both the atomic bomb studies and the childhood cancer survivor cohort presented risk estimates for the age group of 20 years old and younger, whereas the age groups addressed in the tinea capitis and Swedish infant cohorts were 15 years and younger and infants, respectively [32]. The observation of higher risks in the younger cohorts is in-line with Soffer's suggestion that very young populations are more susceptible to the carcinogenic effect of ionizing radiation and are at greater risk of developing malignant tumors [44]. Other explanations that have been suggested include a higher genetic susceptibility to ionizing radiation in the Jewish population or a lower detection rate of brain tumors in the Japanese population [32,45].

Occupational Exposure

The majority of studies that have examined occupational exposure to ionizing radiation and risk of brain tumors have not reported evidence of an association [30]. Among the populations that have been studied are large cohorts of nuclear industry workers [19] as well as radiologists and x-ray technologists [21,46]. Although most of these studies found an increased risk for leukemia, particularly among workers in early periods, no excess risk for brain tumors was observed. However, a review of 14 cohort studies examining mortality estimated a statistically significant increased risk of about 15% for brain tumors among 140,000 white male workers exposed to ionizing radiation in US nuclear programs. This estimate was based on 300 cases of brain tumors during 3.8 million person-years of follow-up [47]. In a recent study of 90 305 radiology technologists in the United States who were followed between 1983 and 1998, 53 cases of brain cancer were found, yielding a SIR of 0.95 (95% CI: 0.75–1.16) [20].

CASE-CONTROL STUDIES

Although the risk of glioma associated with diagnostic medical exposure to ionizing radiation has been examined in several studies, the association remains unclear due to inconsistency in the results. Increased risks of glioma associated with x-ray of the head (OR: 5.49; 95% CI: 1.32–32) and with frequency of full-mouth dental x-ray examination (after age 25, p for trend 0.04) have been reported by Hu [48] and Preston-Martin [49], respectively. In contrast, significant decreased risk of glioma associated with exposure to diagnostic dental x-rays (RR: 0.42; 95% CI: 0.24–0.76; $p = 0.004$) [50], nondental diagnostic x-rays to the head and neck (OR: 0.7; 95% CI: 0.5–0.9), and any medical exposure to diagnostic ionizing radiation (OR: 0.63; 95% CI: 0.48–0.83) [51] have also been reported. In a study conducted by Wrensch et al, computed tomography and magnetic resonance imaging of the head, sources of ionizing and non-ionizing radiation, showed no association with glioma [52]. Additional case-control studies that examined the risk of glioma associated with diagnostic radiation yielded risk estimates that ranged from 0.4 to 2.67, but none reached statistical significance [53–55].

Regarding occupational exposure, in accordance with the lack of statistically significant findings in most of the prospective studies mentioned earlier, a recently published case-control study that used a Finnish job exposure matrix to assess exposure to radiation reported an odds ratio of 1.08 (95% CI: 0.55–2.12) for risk of glioma in the third tertile of exposure to ionizing radiation [56].

SUMMARY

In summary, evidence for a causal role of ionizing radiation in brain tumor development in general and glioma etiology in particular has been established. Indeed, it is the only environmental factor that has been conclusively shown to cause brain tumors. This association was consistently supported in cohort studies that examined groups of irradiated individuals. Case-control studies, however, have not been able to demonstrate this association consistently, possibly due to recall bias caused by underreporting of irradiation by cases or lack of accurate information on ages at exposure. Other explanations for null findings for an association of diagnostic radiation with adult glioma could include the low attributable risk for radiation exposure in adult brain tumors or the relatively low exposure doses from many (but not all) diagnostic procedures. The association has been quantified in only four cohort studies, all of which provide evidence of a linear dose-response association.

FUTURE DIRECTIONS FOR RESEARCH

Issues requiring further investigation include specification of the ages at which exposure to ionizing radiation is most likely to have harmful effects as well as the role of other factors that may influence the relationship, such as interactions between radiation and gender or other environmental or genetic factors. From a clinical perspective, determination of the extent to which exposure to low dose radiation, such as that used in diagnostic procedures, is associated with increased risk of glioma is of utmost importance, especially in light of the ever-increasing use of imaging procedures such as computed tomography. Furthermore, the precise effects of low-dose radiation exposure must be quantified so that safe levels of diagnostic radiation can be determined. Elucidation of these issues should be a goal of future research.

REFERENCES

1. IARC. *Monographs on the Evaluation of Carcinogenic Risks to Humans. Vol 75. Ionizing Radiation, Part I: x- and Gamma-Radiation, and Neutrons.* Lyon, France: IARC; 2000:35, 39. IARC publication no.: ISBN 92 832 1275 4.
2. United Nations Scientific Committee. *Sources and Effects of Ionizing Radiation. United Nations Scientific Committee on the Effects of Atomic Radiation, UNSCEAR 2000 Report to the General Assembly, with Scientific Annexes, Volume II: Effects.* New York: United Nations; 2000:77, 159. United Nations publication no.: 92-1-142239-6.
3. United Nations Scientific Committee. *Sources and Effects of Ionizing Radiation. United Nations Scientific Committee on the Effects of Atomic Radiation, UNSCEAR 2000 Report to the General Assembly, with Scientific Annexes, Volume I: Sources.* New York: United Nations; 2000:4–8, 333. United Nations publication no.: ISBN 92-1-142238-8.
4. Thompson DE, Mabuchi K, Ron E, et al. Cancer incidence in atomic bomb survivors. Part II: solid tumors, 1958–1987. *Radiat Res* 1994;137(21):17–6
5. Ron E. Cancer risks from medical radiation. *Health Phys.* 2003;85(1):47–59.
6. Preston DL, Ron E, Yonehara S, et al. Tumors of the nervous system and pituitary gland associated with atomic bomb radiation exposure. *J Natl Cancer Inst.* 2002;94(20):1555–1563.
7. Bauer S, Gusev BI, Pivina LM, Apsalikov KN, Grosche B. Radiation exposure due to local fallout from Soviet atmospheric nuclear weapons testing in Kazakhstan: solid cancer mortality in the Semipalatinsk historical cohort, 1960–1999. *Radiat Res.* 2005;164(4 pt 1):409–419.
8. Abylkassimova Z, Gusev B, Grosche B, Bauer S, Kreuzer M, Trott K. Nested case-control study of leukemia among a cohort of persons exposed to ionizing radiation from nuclear weapon tests in Kazakhstan (1949–1963). *Ann Epidemiol.* 2000;10(7):479.
9. Walter AW, Hancock ML, Pui CH, et al. Secondary brain tumors in children treated for acute lymphoblastic leukemia at St Jude Children's Research Hospital. *J Clin Oncol.* 1998;16(12):3761–3767.
10. Neglia JP, Meadows AT, Robison LL, et al. Second neoplasms after acute lymphoblastic leukemia in childhood. *N Engl J Med.* 1991;325(19):1330–1336.
11. Neglia JP, Robison LL, Stovall M, et al. New primary neoplasms of the central nervous system in survivors of childhood cancer: a report from the Childhood Cancer Survivor Study. *J Natl Cancer Inst.* 2006;98(21):1528–1537.
12. Shore RE, Moseson M, Harley N, Pasternack BS. Tumors and other diseases following childhood x-ray treatment for ringworm of the scalp (Tinea capitis). *Health Phys.* 2003;85(4):404–408.
13. Fürst CJ, Lundell M, Holm LE, Silfverswärd C. Cancer incidence after radiotherapy for skin hemangioma: a retrospective cohort study in Sweden. *J Natl Cancer Inst.* 1988;80(17):1387–1392.
14. Griem ML, Kleinerman RA, Boice JD Jr, Stovall M, Shefner D, Lubin JH. Cancer following radiotherapy for peptic ulcer. *J Natl Cancer Inst.* 1994;86(11):842–849.
15. Hildreth NG, Shore RE, Hempelmann LH, Rosenstein M. Risk of extrathyroid tumors following radiation treatment in infancy for thymic enlargement. *Radiat Res.* 1985;102(3):378–391.
16. Preston-Martin S, Paganini-Hill A, Henderson BE, Pike MC, Wood C. Case-control study of intracranial meningiomas in women in Los Angeles County, California. *J Natl Cancer Inst.* 1980;65(1):67–73.
17. Hoffman DA, Lonstein JE, Morin MM, Visscher W, Harris BS 3rd, Boice JD Jr. Breast cancer in women with scoliosis exposed to multiple diagnostic x rays. *J Natl Cancer Inst.* 1989;81(17):1307–1312.
18. Holm LE, Wiklund KE, Lundell GE, et al. Cancer risk in population examined with diagnostic doses of 131I. *J Natl Cancer Inst.* 1989;81(4):302–306.
19. Cardis E, Gilbert ES, Carpenter L, et al. Effects of low doses and low dose rates of external ionizing radiation: cancer mortality among nuclear industry workers in three countries. *Radiat Res.* 1995;142(2):117–132.
20. Sigurdson AJ, Doody MM, Rao RS, et al. Cancer incidence in the US radiologic technologists health study, 1983–1998. *Cancer.* 2003;97(12):3080–3089.
21. Wang JX, Inskip PD, Boice JD Jr, Li BX, Zhang JY, Fraumeni JF Jr. Cancer incidence among medical diagnostic X-ray workers in China, 1950 to 1985. *Int J Cancer.* 1990;45(5):889–895.
22. Darby S, Hill D, Deo H, et al. Residential radon and lung cancer–detailed results of a collaborative analysis of individual data on 7148 persons with lung cancer and 14,208 persons without lung cancer from 13 epidemiologic studies in Europe. *Scand J Work Environ Health.* 2006;32 (suppl 1):1–83.
23. Krewski D, Lubin JH, Zielinski JM, et al. A combined analysis of North American case-control studies of residential radon and lung cancer. *J Toxicol Environ Health Part A.* 2006;69(7):533–597.
24. Inskip PD, Linet MS, Heineman EF. Etiology of brain tumors in adults. *Epidemiol Rev.* 1995;17(2):382–414.
25. Ron E, Modan B, Boice JD Jr, et al. Tumors of the brain and nervous system after radiotherapy in childhood. *N Engl J Med.* 1988;319(16):1033–1039.
26. Modan B, Baidatz D, Mart H, Steinitz R, Levin SG. Radiation-induced head and neck tumours. *Lancet.* 1974;1(7852):277–279.
27. Longstreth WT Jr, Dennis LK, McGuire VM, Drangsholt MT, Koepsell TD. Epidemiology of intracranial meningioma. *Cancer.* 1993;72(3):639–648.
28. Bondy M, Ligon BL. Epidemiology and etiology of intracranial meningiomas: a review. *J Neurooncol.* 1996;29(3):197–205.
29. DeAngelis LM. Brain tumors. *N Engl J Med.* 2001;344(2):114–123.
30. Wrensch M, Minn Y, Chew T, Bondy M, Berger MS. Epidemiology of primary brain tumors: current concepts and review of the literature. *Neuro-oncology.* 2002;4(4):278–299.
31. Ohgaki H, Kleihues P. Epidemiology and etiology of gliomas. *Acta Neuropathol.* 2005;109(1):93–108.
32. Sadetzki S, Chetrit A, Freedman L, Stovall M, Modan B, Novikov I. Long-term follow-up for brain tumor development after childhood exposure to ionizing radiation for tinea capitis. *Radiat Res.* 2005;163(4):424–432.
33. Fisher JL, Schwartzbaum JA, Wrensch M, Wiemels JL. Epidemiology of brain tumors. *Neurol Clin.* 2007;25(4):867–90.
34. Salvati M, Frati A, Russo N, et al. Radiation-induced gliomas: report of 10 cases and review of the literature. *Surg Neurol.* 2003;60(1):60–67.
35. McIver JI, Pollock BE. Radiation-induced tumor after stereotactic radiosurgery and whole brain radiotherapy: case report and literature review. *J Neurooncol.* 2004;66(3):301–305.
36. Werner A, Modan B, Davidoff D. Doses to brain, skull and thyroid, following x-ray therapy for Tinea capitis. *Phys Med Biol.* 1968;13(2):247–258.
37. Albert RE, Omran AR, Brauer EW, et al. Follow-up study of patients treated by x-ray for tinea capitis. *Am J Public Health Nations Health.* 1966;56(12):2114–2120.
38. Schulz RJ, Albert RE. Follow-up study of patients treated by x-ray epilation for tinea capitis. III. Dose to organs of the head from the x-ray treatment of tinea capitis. *Arch Environ Health.* 1968;17(6):935–950.
39. Shore RE, Albert RE, Pasternack BS. Follow-up study of patients treated by X-ray epilation for tinea capitis. *Arch Environ Health* 1976;31:17–24.
40. Karlsson P, Holmberg E, Lundell M, Mattsson A, Holm LE, Wallgren A. Intracranial tumors after exposure to ionizing radiation during infancy: a pooled analysis of two Swedish cohorts of 28,008 infants with skin hemangioma. *Radiat Res.* 1998;150(3):357–364.

41. Nygaard R, Garwicz S, Haldorsen T, et al. Second malignant neoplasms in patients treated for childhood leukemia. A population-based cohort study from the Nordic countries. The Nordic Society of Pediatric Oncology and Hematology (NOPHO). *Acta Paediatr Scand.* 1991;80(12):1220–1228.
42. Rosso P, Terracini B, Fears TR, et al. Second malignant tumors after elective end of therapy for a first cancer in childhood: a multicenter study in Italy. *Int J Cancer.* 1994;59(4):451–456.
43. Löning L, Zimmermann M, Reiter A, et al. Secondary neoplasms subsequent to Berlin-Frankfurt-Münster therapy of acute lymphoblastic leukemia in childhood: significantly lower risk without cranial radiotherapy. *Blood.* 2000;95(9):2770–2775.
44. Soffer D, Gomori JM, Siegal T, Shalit MN. Intracranial meningiomas after high-dose irradiation. *Cancer.* 1989;63(8):1514–1519.
45. Ron E, Modan B. Thyroid and other neoplasms following childhood scalp irradiation. In: Boice JD and Fraumeni JF, eds. *Radiation Carcinogenesis Epidemiology and Biological Significance.* New York: Raven Press; 1984:139–151.
46. Doody MM, Mandel JS, Lubin JH, Boice JD Jr. Mortality among United States radiologic technologists, 1926–90. *Cancer Causes Control.* 1998;9(1):67–75.
47. Alexander V, DiMarco JH. Reappraisal of brain tumor risk among U.S. nuclear workers: a 10-year review. *Occup Med.* 2001;16(2):289–315.
48. Hu J, Johnson KC, Mao Y, et al. Risk factors for glioma in adults: a case-control study in northeast China. *Cancer Detect Prev.* 1998;22(2):100–108.
49. Preston-Martin S, Mack W, Henderson BE. Risk factors for gliomas and meningiomas in males in Los Angeles County. *Cancer Res.* 1989;49(21):6137–6143.
50. Ryan P, Lee MW, North B, McMichael AJ. Amalgam fillings, diagnostic dental x-rays and tumours of the brain and meninges. *Eur J Cancer B Oral Oncol.* 1992;28B(2):91–95.
51. Blettner M, Schlehofer B, Samkange-Zeeb F, Berg G, Schlaefer K, Schüz J. Medical exposure to ionising radiation and the risk of brain tumours: Interphone study group, Germany. *Eur J Cancer.* 2007;43(13):1990–1998.
52. Wrensch M, Miike R, Lee M, Neuhaus J. Are prior head injuries or diagnostic X-rays associated with glioma in adults? The effects of control selection bias. *Neuroepidemiology.* 2000;19(5):234–244.
53. Zampieri P, Meneghini F, Grigoletto F, et al. Risk factors for cerebral glioma in adults: a case-control study in an Italian population. *J Neurooncol.* 1994;19(1):61–67.
54. Hochberg F, Toniolo P, Cole P, Salcman M. Nonoccupational risk indicators of glioblastoma in adults. *J Neurooncol.* 1990;8(1):55–60.
55. Burch JD, Craib KJ, Choi BC, Miller AB, Risch HA, Howe GR. An exploratory case-control study of brain tumors in adults. *J Natl Cancer Inst.* 1987;78(4):601–609.
56. Karipidis KK, Benke G, Sim MR, Kauppinen T, Giles G. Occupational exposure to ionizing and non-ionizing radiation and risk of glioma. *Occup Med (Lond).* 2007;57(7):518–524.

6 Radiofrequency Fields and Glioma Risk

Maria Feychting and Anders Ahlbom

INTRODUCTION

Exposure to radiofrequency (RF) fields in the general population is a relatively recent phenomenon; this type of exposure has historically been limited to occupational settings or to the very low fields emitted by radio and television transmitters. With the introduction and widespread use of mobile phone technology, the number of people in the general population exposed to low-level RF fields has increased dramatically. The first mobile telecommunication devices were introduced in the beginning of the 1980s, the so-called bag phones, with the transmitting device and antenna carried in a "bag" and with a traditional telephone handset attached to the transmitter with a cord. The first handheld mobile phones were introduced during the latter half of the 1980s. These analog phones were used by a small proportion of the population. With the introduction of the second-generation mobile digital phones in 1993, use of mobile phones became increasingly popular. Nordic countries were among the earliest to adopt this new technology; in Sweden, for example, mobile phone use in the general population increased from a few percent in 1993 to more than 90% in 2006.

The rapid increase in mobile phone use has led to growing concern among the public about its potential harmful effects. Current exposure safety guidelines are based on acute effects from heating of tissue [1]. For exposure below guideline levels, there is no known mechanism by which RF fields might affect cancer risk. Nonetheless, if RF radiation had a carcinogenic effect, it would pose an important public health problem and excess numbers of intracranial tumors might result. In this chapter, we will review epidemiological evidence regarding potential effects on glioma risk from exposure to RF fields associated with mobile phone use that are below current guidelines and thus cannot cause substantial heating of tissue.

EXPOSURE ASSESSMENT

The primary source of low-level RF exposure today is mobile telephones. Currently, this technology uses frequencies from 450 to 2500 MHz, although the technology is constantly developing and therefore the frequency range may change in the future. The highest exposure occurs while talking on the phone itself. During telephone conversations, exposure is concentrated in the part of the head closest to the handset and the antenna, and it declines rapidly with distance to the antenna. Therefore, the use of hands-free equipment while talking on the phone reduces exposure to the head considerably, while usually increasing exposure of another part of the body that is near the phone's antenna, for example, if the phone is kept in a pocket or on a belt by the hip. Although exposure during mobile phone use is highly localized, mobile phone base stations give rise to whole-body exposure, though at levels at least a thousand times lower than localized exposure from the phone itself.

Radio and television transmitters that operate at frequencies between 200 and 900 MHz are also major sources of very low-level whole-body exposure in the general population. The third main source of exposure is occupational and includes, for example, work with RF polyvinyl chloride welding machines, plasma etching, and military or civil radar systems, each exposure source operating at different frequencies. Considering exposure to the head, most of the occupational exposure sources give rise to low-level far-field exposures.

Exposure misclassification occurs to a varying degree in all epidemiological studies. If misclassification of the exposure is unrelated to the disease, that is, the degree of exposure misclassification is similar for cases and others (nondifferential exposure misclassification), then the effect on the risk estimate will be a dilution toward unity. If the probability of exposure misclassification is related to the disease (differential exposure misclassification), the risk estimate can be reduced or elevated. If exposure information can be collected independently of the disease, for example, before disease onset or from historical records, the risk of differential exposure misclassification is minimized. In case-control studies, exposure information is often collected by asking study participants to complete a written questionnaire or interviewing them after disease occurrence. If cases and controls differ in their ability to remember their exposures, differential exposure misclassification may occur, that is, recall bias.

In epidemiological studies of mobile phone use, there are some examples where subscriber records kept by the mobile phone operators have been used as an independent source of exposure information. This approach has some limitations. It is usually not possible to get information about corporate subscriptions as these are not assigned to a specific person, but rather to a company. This means that people having corporate subscriptions will be regarded as unexposed, when in fact they may be among the heaviest users. Another problem is that the registered subscriber may not be the one actually using the phone, for example, when parents have subscriptions for their children who are too young to sign a subscriber contract themselves. These studies also lack information about the use of hands-free equipment, and on which side of the head the phone is usually held. These limitations may lead to a dilution of the risk estimates, should a true association exist. If the exposure is rare, as it was at the time when some of these studies were performed, the effect on the risk estimates will be negligible.

The most common exposure assessment method in epidemiological studies of mobile phone users has been self-report of mobile phone use either by requesting written responses to a questionnaire or interviewing patients some time after the occurrence of the disease. This approach may be subject to both nondifferential exposure misclassification and recall bias, and it may be especially problematic in studies of brain tumors, because the disease itself may affect the patient's ability to remember correctly. A validation study of healthy volunteers [2] conducted as part of a large international study of head and neck tumors in relation to mobile phone use (the Interphone study [3]) compared mobile phone use registered by the operators or by a software modified phone during a 3- to 8-month period with mobile phone use reported by the individuals themselves 6 to 12 months later. There was substantial individual variation in recall of both the number and duration of calls. The number of calls was generally underestimated, whereas their duration was generally overestimated. For 58% of the subjects, reported duration of phone use differed from that registered by at least a factor of 2. Furthermore, the ratio of recalled to actual duration of calls increased with increasing duration of phone use. The same pattern was seen for the number of calls. Thus, nondifferential exposure misclassification may be substantial. There is, as yet, no exposure validation study published assessing potential recall bias, which requires information from both cases and controls. In several case-control studies, however, there are indications of recall bias when reporting side of use, with a tendency among cases to over-report use on the same side as the tumor, which is discussed in detail later.

SELECTION BIAS

Selection bias can occur if controls in a case-control study are not selected randomly from the study population and if the probability of being selected as a control is related to the studied exposure, either directly or indirectly, for example, through socioeconomic status. Selection bias might also occur if not all identified cases and controls participate in the study and if the probability of participation is related to the exposure. In several case-control studies of mobile phone use and brain tumors, there are indications that nonparticipation is related to the exposure; mobile phone users seem to have been more willing to participate than nonusers [4,5]. As nonparticipation is more common among controls, this may bias the risk estimates downward.

EPIDEMIOLOGICAL STUDIES OF MOBILE PHONE USE AND GLIOMA RISK

Health effects related to RF exposure from mobile telephony is a relatively new research area. Available epidemiological studies have primarily focused on brain tumors, although a few have included other types of tumors. This review will focus on glioma as the outcome, but some studies have not reported results for specific types of brain tumors, and for these studies, the results for all brain tumors combined will be presented. As mobile telephony is a relatively new phenomenon, many of the available studies have no or only limited power to study long-term effects, something that needs to be taken into consideration when evaluating the evidence.

The biomedical literature database PubMed (www.ncbi.nlm.nih.gov/pubmed) was used to identify epidemiological studies of mobile phone use and glioma risk, as well as reference lists of the retrieved publications. Whenever multiple publications were available from the same study, the original publication was included in the review, and additional publications were considered only if they provided crucial information not available in the original publication. Fifteen studies of mobile phone use and brain tumors have been published so far (not counting studies of acoustic neuroma) [5–20]. Ten of these studies provide information on longer duration mobile phone use, the longest defined as "more than 10 years of use." One study included information on exposure lasting 1 year at most [12,21], and it is not discussed further here. Table 6.1 shows the relative risk (RR) estimates for glioma after a short duration of mobile phone use and the number of exposed cases included in the analyses, whereas Table 6.2 shows results for long-term mobile phone use.

Short-term Mobile Phone Use

The majority of the studies have found no effect on glioma risk after a short duration of use, but there are two exceptions. A Finnish case-control study found an increased risk of glioma primarily related to use of analogue phones [6]. Information about the exposure was collected from registries kept by the mobile phone operators, and therefore there was no risk of recall bias. The exposure misclassification is likely to be considerable as the investigators had no access to information about corporate mobile phone users, who are likely to be among the heaviest mobile phone users. This type of error cannot, however, explain the increased glioma risk because there is no reason to believe that the exposure misclassification would differ between cases and controls. The risk increase was found after only 1 to 2 years subscription to analogue phone service and was based on a very small number of exposed cases (Table 6.1). This very short time between exposure and effect seems unlikely to be real; it probably takes a longer time for a

Table 6.1 Epidemiological Studies on Short-term Mobile Phone Use and Glioma[a]

Study[b]	No. Exposed Cases	OR (95% CI)	Duration of Mobile Phone Use/Type of Brain Tumor
Hardell et al [8,22]	78	1.0 (0.7–1.4)	>1 year/all brain tumors combined
Muscat et al [11]	28	1.1 (0.6–2.0)	2–3 years/primary brain tumor (ICD9 191)
Inskip et al [9]	51	0.9 (0.5–1.6)	0.5–3 years/glioma
Johansen et al., [10] cohort study	87	1.1 (0.9–1.3)	1–4 years/brain and nervous system
Auvinen et al [6]	11 + 7[c]	1.6 (0.8–2.9)	1–2 years/glioma
Hardell et al [23][d]	36	1.1 (0.7–1.8)	1–6 years/malignant (analogue)
	100	1.1 (0.8–1.4)	1–6 years/malignant (digital)
Hardell et al [15][d]	0	–	1–5 years/malignant (analogue)
	20	1.8 (0.9–3.5)	>5–10 years/malignant (analogue)
	100	1.6 (1.1–2.4)	1–5 years/malignant (digital)
	79	2.2 (1.4–3.4)	>5–10 years/malignant (digital)
Lönn et al [5]	112	0.8 (0.6–1.1)	1–4 years/glioma
Christensen et al [13]	43	0.7 (0.3–1.0)	1–4 years/glioma
Hepworth et al [24]	271	0.9 (0.7–1.1)	1–4 years/glioma
Schüz et al [19]	82	0.9 (0.6–1.2)	1–4 years/glioma
Schüz et al., [20] cohort study	266	1.0 (0.9–1.2)	1–4 years/brain and nervous system
Lahkola et al [18]	384	0.8 (0.6–0.9)	0.5–4 years/glioma
Klaeboe et al [17]	27	0.6 (0.4–1.1)	<2 years/glioma

[a] If a study does not report glioma separately, results are shown for all malignant brain tumors or all brain tumors combined.
[b] Studies are case-control studies unless otherwise specified.
[c] Numbers of cases were given for analogue and digital phones separately, but may overlap.
[d] Results were only given for use of analogue and digital phones separately.

Table 6.2 Epidemiological Studies on Long-term Mobile Phone Use and Glioma[a]

Study[b]	No. Exposed Cases	OR (95% CI)	Duration of Mobile Phone Use/Type of Brain Tumor
Hardell et al [8,22]	16	1.2 (0.6–2.6)	>10 years/all brain tumors combined
Hardell et al [23][c]	43	1.2 (0.8–1.8)	>6 years/malignant (analogue)
	12	1.7 (0.7–4.3)	>6 years/malignant (digital)
Hardell et al [15][c]	48	3.5 (2.0–6.4)	>10 years/malignant (analogue)
	19	3.6 (1.7–7.5)	>10 years/malignant (digital)
Lönn et al [5]	25	0.9 (0.5–1.5)	≥10 yrs/glioma
Christensen et al [13]	14	0.7 (0.3–1.6)	≥10 years/glioma
Hepworth et al [24]	66	0.9 (0.6–1.3)	≥10 years/glioma
Schüz et al [19]	12	2.2 (0.9–5.1)	≥10 years/glioma
Schüz et al., [20] cohort study	28	0.7 (0.4–0.9)	≥10 years/brain and nervous system
Lahkola et al [18]	143	0.9 (0.7–1.2)	≥10 years/glioma
Klaeboe et al [17]	70	0.8 (0.5–1.2)	≥6 years/glioma

[a] If a study does not report glioma separately, results are shown for all malignant brain tumors or all brain tumors combined.
[b] Studies are case-control studies unless otherwise specified.
[c] Results were only given for use of analogue and digital phones separately.

tumor to develop and be diagnosed. If mobile phone use truly has an effect on glioma risk after such a short duration, the incidence of glioma should have increased during recent years in countries where there has been a rapid increase in mobile phone use in the general population. There was, however, no evidence of such an increase in a study of glioma incidence in the Nordic countries, where mobile phone use in the general population started relatively early [25]. The Finnish study [6] did not provide information about long-term mobile phone use.

A Swedish case-control study reported by Hardell et al [15] in 2006 observed a 60% increased risk of a malignant brain tumor after less than 5 years of use of a digital mobile phone, based on 100 exposed cases. No cases and three controls had used an analogue phone during such a short time period, but for 5 to 10 years duration, there was approximately a twofold risk increase regardless of type of phone used. Information about mobile phone use was collected through postal questionnaires after disease occurrence.

The other 12 available studies showed no indication of increased risks of brain tumors in general or glioma in particular after short-term mobile phone use (Table 6.1). A Danish study used similar exposure assessment methods as the Finnish case-control study discussed earlier, but it was designed as a cohort study, originally published in 2001 [10], and later updated in 2006 [20]. No indications were found of increased risks after short-term mobile phone use for any tumor types. This study has the same limitation as the Finnish case-control study in terms of exposure misclassification, and a modest risk increase would probably remain undetected.

Two case-control studies from the United States reported no association between brain tumor risk and mobile phone use [9,11]. Specific analyses of the side on which the mobile phone usually was held did not change these findings. These studies are hospital based; cases were identified at certain hospitals, and controls were selected from other patients at the same hospitals. This type of design assumes that patients with other diseases can be viewed as a representative sample of the population from which the brain tumor cases came and correctly reflects the exposure distribution, that is, mobile phone use, in this population. The studies used rapid case ascertainment, which is a considerable strength; this is important in a study of malignant brain tumors where the poor prognosis of the disease may prevent many cases from participating in the study. A limitation is the short period of mobile phone use in both studies; very few subjects had used a mobile phone for more than 5 years. Therefore, these studies do not provide information about potential effects of long-term exposure.

Two earlier case-control studies by Hardell and coworkers [8,22,23] reported no overall increase in brain tumor risk related to mobile phone use among ever users of mobile phones or among short-term users. These studies also used a postal questionnaire to collect information about historical mobile phone use and potential confounding factors. The first study published in 1999 included 78 mobile phone users among brain tumor cases [8,22], the majority of whom had used a mobile phone less than 5 years. The second study from 2002 included a large number of cases with short-term use, [23] but no risk increase was indicated in this group.

A multicenter international case-control study of head and neck tumors in relation to mobile phone use, the Interphone study [3], was initiated in the late 1990s, and from 2005 the first national publications have become available [5,13,17–19,24]. All centers used a common core study protocol, and data were collected using computer-assisted personal interviews. Detailed questions were asked about historical mobile phone use, phone use laterality, use of hands-free devices, and potential confounding factors. None of the hitherto published Interphone studies found any risk increase after short-term mobile phone use; rather, they found somewhat reduced relative risk estimates. A study based on pooled data from five North European countries participating in Interphone included more than 1500 glioma cases [18], of whom 384 had started to use a mobile phone less than 5 years prior to diagnosis. The study includes data from the Swedish [5], Danish [13], Norwegian [17], Finnish, and UK-South Interphone studies. The UK-South Study is also included as part of the study by Hepworth et al [24] Short-term mobile phone use was associated with an odds ratio (OR) of 0.8 (95% confidence interval [CI]: 0.6–0.9). The reduced OR is likely to be at least partly explained by a control participation bias; results from a nonresponder questionnaire [4,5] indicate that controls who were mobile phone users were more likely to participate than nonusers, which would lead to a downward bias of the relative risk estimate.

Long-term Mobile Phone Use

For long-term mobile phone use, numbers of exposed subjects are considerably smaller, as this is a relatively new technology (Table 6.2). Most of the studies that have provided some information on long-term mobile phone use have presented results for at least 10 years of use, although two have chosen at least 6 years of use as the lower limit of long-term use [17,23].

As can be seen from Table 6.2, it is mainly the study published by Hardell et al [15] in 2006 that reports increased relative risk estimates associated with long-term mobile phone use. As discussed earlier, this study also reported increased risks for short- and medium-term use. The German part of the Interphone study found an indication of increased risk after at least 10 years of use, but this result was based on only 12 exposed cases, and is also compatible with no effect. The large study pooling data from the Nordic and South-East UK Interphone studies [18] included 143 glioma cases who had started to use a mobile phone at least 10 years prior to diagnosis and observed an OR of 0.9 (95% CI: 0.7–1.1).

The updated Danish cohort of mobile phone subscribers [20] identified 28 brain and nervous system tumors in the part of the cohort that had been subscribers during at least 10 years, RR = 0.7 (0.4–0.9). The risk reduction observed cannot be explained by selection bias, which has been put forward as at least a partial explanation for the reduced ORs observed in the Interphone case-control studies. One alternative explanation for the cohort study is that persons who were early mobile phone subscribers belong to a segment of the population that is likely to be healthier than the general population, a "healthy subscriber effect," equivalent to the healthy worker effect. It is, however, not obvious that brain tumor risk would be affected to such an extent by a healthy worker or healthy subscriber effect; there are few well-established risk factors for brain tumors, and all are minor. Furthermore, there is some evidence that glioma increases with higher socioeconomic status [26].

Laterality of Mobile Phone Use

RF fields decrease rapidly with distance to the source, and the exposure is highly localized; therefore, the exposure is concentrated to the side of the head where the mobile phone is held during a phone call, whereas on the opposite side of the head, the exposure level is virtually similar to the general environment. If exposure to RF fields during mobile phone use has a carcinogenic effect, one would expect the tumor risk to be highest in the area that receives the highest exposure. Several of the case-control studies have collected information about the preferred side of mobile phone use and have analyzed the data according to laterality of mobile phone use. Table 6.3 displays the results for long-term mobile phone use according to laterality. All studies found a higher OR for having a brain tumor on the side of the head where the mobile phone was usually held,

Table 6.3 Long-term Mobile Phone Use and Glioma Risk According to Laterality of Phone Use

Study	Ipsilateral[a] OR (95% CI)	Contralateral[b] OR (95% CI)	Overall OR
Hardell et al [23][c]	1.8 (1.0–3.4)	0.7 (0.4–1.6)	1.2 (0.8–1.8)
Hardell et al [15][c,d]	3.1 (1.6–6.2)	2.6 (1.3–5.4)	2.6 (1.5–4.3)
Lönn et al [5]	1.6 (0.8–3.4)	0.7 (0.3–1.5)	0.9 (0.5–1.5)
Hepworth et al [24][d]	1.2 (1.0–1.5)	0.8 (0.6–0.9)	0.9 (0.8–1.1)
Lahkola et al [18]	1.4 (1.0–1.9)	1.0 (0.7–1.4)	0.9 (0.7–1.2)

[a] Ipsilateral = use of the mobile phone on the same side of the head as the tumor.
[b] Contralateral = use of the mobile phone on the opposite side of the head.
[c] Results for analogue phones
[d] Overall results; results according to laterality were not given for long-term use.

which is what would be expected given the higher exposure on this side. However, most of the studies observed a reduced OR on the opposite side and no risk increase overall. One plausible explanation for this could be recall bias when reporting side of use; it is possible that cases, knowing the side of their tumor, are more inclined to report using the mobile phone most often on this side. Such a recall bias would result in an increased risk of tumors on the same side as the phone was used, and a decreased risk on the opposite side. A causal explanation seems unlikely; it is biologically implausible that mobile phone use would protect against brain tumors on the opposite side of the head. There are two exceptions from the pattern of increased risk on the same side and a decreased risk on the opposite side; the study by Hardell et al in 2006 [15] found an increased risk of malignant brain tumors regardless of side of use, and is the only study that also found an increased risk overall associated with long-term mobile phone use. The study by Lahkola et al [18] observed a pattern that would be expected if there is a causal association between RF exposure and glioma risk; at least 10 years after first mobile phone use, there was a slightly increased risk on the same side as the phone was held, and on the opposite side the OR was 1. It is noteworthy, however, that for shorter latency periods in the Lahkola study, a pattern indicating recall bias when reporting side of use was observed. Thus, for subjects who started to use a mobile phone less than 5 years prior to diagnosis, the OR for ipsilateral use was 1.1 (95% CI: 0.9–1.3), whereas the OR for contralateral use was 0.7 (95% CI: 0.6–0.9). The same results were also seen for subjects who started to use a mobile phone 5 to 9 years prior to diagnosis. Other studies have observed a similar pattern for short-term mobile phone use, for example, the study by Hardell et al in 2002 [23], where no overall risk increase was found, but where the OR for ipsilateral use of analogue phones for less than 6 years was 1.93 (95% CI: 0.96–3.88), and the corresponding result for contralateral use was 0.49 (95% CI: 0.20–1.21). Similar results were found for use of digital phones.

OCCUPATIONAL STUDIES

Occupational exposure to RF fields has been studied over more than 20 years, and most investigations have focused on the risk of brain tumors and hematological malignancies, for example, leukemia. A variety of occupations have been investigated, including a range of different exposure frequencies, but exposure assessment methods have generally been poor. None of the studies have made measurements of the RF exposure for the subjects included in the study, and often the exposure classification has been based on the job title alone with no actual knowledge about the exposure levels for the workers in the particular occupations. No or only limited control of confounding has been made, and several of the studies have a poor statistical power.

A Norwegian study of 37,945 male electrical workers found a relative risk estimate for brain tumors below unity, with wide confidence intervals [27], based on a categorization of occupational titles as probably exposed to RF fields. The finding was based on only three exposed cases. Exposed occupations were, for example, radio/telegraph operators and radio/television repairmen, but no field measurements were made. Potential confounding factors were not controlled, although the comparison was made with the economically active population to limit the influence of the healthy worker effect.

A study of Polish military personnel reported increased risks for brain tumors, as well as other cancer types [28,29]. This study has severe methodological limitations and an unconventional study design. The authors put much more effort into finding exposures among the cancer cases than among other personnel, using multiple sources of information for the cases, but not for the healthy persons in the cohort. The bias introduced by this kind of procedure will inevitably lead to findings of increased cancer risks, even if no such associations exist; and no weight can be given to these studies in an evaluation of the scientific evidence on potential carcinogenic effects of RF exposure.

A case-control study nested within a cohort of male US Air Force members was conducted by Grayson et al. [30]. Incident cases of brain tumors were identified among subjects serving in the US Air Force during the study period, 1970–1989, but no attempt was made to follow those who left the cohort. Occupational histories were obtained for cases and matched controls; these were categorized according to extremely low-frequency, RF, and ionizing radiation exposure. RF exposure was associated with an OR for brain tumors of 1.39 (95% CI: 1.01–1.90), whereas the corresponding result for ionizing radiation was 0.58 (95% CI: 0.22–1.52). Apart from age and race, no control of confounding was made. The study reported an increased risk brain tumors associated with military rank, which is consistent with other reports of increased risk associated with high socioeconomic status [26].

A cohort study of 40,581 radar technicians in the US Navy reported a risk reduction for brain tumor mortality when compared with the general population [31]. A reduced mortality overall and for many specific diagnostic categories is noticeable in the comparisons with the general population, indicating a possible healthy worker effect. An internal comparison within the cohort showed a reduced risk of brain tumors in the highest exposed group compared with the group with low exposure potential, RR = 0.65 (95% CI: 0.43–1.01). No potential confounding factors were controlled in the analyses, and there were indications that smoking was less common in the cohort compared with the general population.

A cohort study of 195,775 workers employed in the design, manufacture, and testing of wireless devices such as mobile phones [32] reported reduced risks of brain tumor mortality when compared with the general population, standardized mortality ratio (SMR) = 0.53 (95% CI: 0.21–1.09). In addition, a considerably reduced overall mortality was noted (SMR = 0.66), as well as reduced overall cancer mortality (SMR = 0.78). Thus, there seems to be a considerable healthy worker effect. It is not clear, however, why this would affect brain tumors to such an extent, as discussed earlier also in connection to the cohort study of mobile phone subscribers [10,20]. Internal comparisons within the cohort did not indicate any associations between the exposure and disease risk. Exposure was assessed on the basis of expert opinion; no personal measurements were available.

The German Interphone study reported results on the effect of occupational exposure to RF fields on brain tumor risk, including 366 glioma cases and 1494 controls [33]. Exposure assessment was based on interviews with detailed questions on specific job tasks involving RF exposure. No association between brain tumor risk and occupational RF exposure was observed; the OR in the highest exposure group was 1.2 (95% CI: 0.7–2.2) based on 22 exposed glioma cases. As no measurements of the RF fields were made, it is unclear how well the exposure categorization captures individual RF exposure.

An Australian case-control study of occupational RF exposure and glioma risk reported contradictory findings [34]. Participants filled out a work history booklet, with information about each occupation, industry, tasks, and equipment used. They were also interviewed and asked whether they had been exposed to RF fields. Three different estimates of the exposure was used: the self-report, an assessment made by an industrial hygienist, and a job-exposure matrix (JEM). Only 18 cases were classified as exposed in the analyses based on the JEM, and no increased risks could be shown. Results for self-reported RF exposure were below unity, and when expert assessment was used, the OR was increased, but both results had wide confidence intervals.

DISCUSSION

For glioma in particular or malignant brain tumors in general, the current evidence does not indicate any increased risks related to short-term mobile phone use. This conclusion is based on 14 studies including in total a large number of brain tumor patients who had used a mobile phone for a short period, that is, generally less than 5 years prior to diagnosis. The available studies are very consistent; with only few exceptions, they all show relative risk estimates below or close to unity. The reduced relative risk observed in several studies is probably caused by control nonparticipation bias, although it is unclear whether this explains the whole risk reduction. When these studies were conducted, there was a rapid increase in the prevalence of mobile phone use in the general population, that is, a large proportion of the population started to use mobile phones. If early symptoms from the tumor, prior to its diagnosis, affect the likelihood of cases becoming a new mobile phone user, this would also result in an apparent risk reduction.

For long-term mobile phone use, less data are available; eight studies provide information about at least 10 years since first mobile phone use, but several of these include a small number of cases with long-term exposure. The largest study has almost 150 exposed cases [18] and found a relative risk estimate slightly below 1. Only one study reported an increased risk that cannot be explained by random variation; an almost fourfold risk increase was observed, with the lowest confidence bounds around 2. This study, however, also reported increased risks related to short- and medium-term use, which makes the results difficult to interpret, as there is a considerable amount of data speaking against an increased risk after short-term exposure.

Several studies report an increased risk of tumors on the same side of the head as the mobile phone was used, which would be indicative of a causal effect, as the exposure is highest on this side and virtually nonexistent on the other side. The findings of a decreased risk on the opposite side, however, speak against a causal interpretation, and make it more likely that recall bias when reporting side of use may explain the increased risk for ipsilateral use.

It is also important to note that the available evidence only relates to mobile phone use with a maximum induction period of slightly longer than 10 years, with probably only a small proportion of subjects having up to 15 years of use. Thus, conclusions about longer term exposure cannot be drawn based on the data available today.

Other limitations of the available data relate to the exposure assessment; validation studies of self-reported mobile phone use have shown a considerable amount of exposure misclassification. If the misclassification is unrelated to the disease, this may hamper the possibility to detect a modestly increased risk, should one exist. If cases and controls differ in the way they report their exposure, this may lead to differential exposure misclassification. The way questions are phrased may influence the degree of misclassification, for example, if the questions leave room for the participants' own interpretation of who is defined as a mobile phone user, there is a possibility that cases and controls interpret this differently. This problem could be overcome by using an independent source of exposure information, for example, the records kept by the mobile phone operators. However, information from mobile phone operators must be supplemented with questionnaires providing information about who uses the mobile phone, whether the phone is used by more than one person, whether hands-free devices are used, on which side of the head the phone is used, and similar information not available in registries. The questionnaire information should ideally be collected prior to disease occurrence, to avoid the possibility that the disease influences the answers. Therefore, the best approach is probably to perform a prospective cohort study of mobile phone users, where information about mobile phone use is collected both from operators and the subjects themselves, but before the occurrence of the disease. A cohort study has the additional advantage that several different outcomes can be studied at the same time.

Considerable improvements of exposure assessment methods are to be expected in future studies, with consideration taken of factors related to the adaptive power control used in mobile telephony that makes mobile phones down-regulate the output power to lower levels when the user is close to a base station, thereby decreasing the exposure up to 1000 times [35]. Relevant variables are, for example, mobile phone use in urban or rural areas, use of the phone inside or outside, or when stationary or moving.

Occupational studies have been performed over the last 20 years, but these studies are limited to certain occupational groups, generally with no information about the actual exposure in the included occupations. Although some increased brain tumor risk has been found in a few studies, the majority of studies report relative risk estimates close to or below unity. The available studies have not, however, convincingly demonstrated that occupational RF exposure has no effect on brain tumor risk, mainly because of limitations in the exposure assessment which could lead to a dilution of risk estimates, should there be an increased risk. There is also evidence of the so-called healthy worker effect in several of the studies, demonstrating considerably reduced risk estimates in comparison with the general population. A working population is generally healthier than the total population, and certain occupations make specific demands on good health, for example, policemen, so that comparing disease distributions of these occupations with those in the general population would be invalid. It is, however, noteworthy that relative risk estimates in several of these occupational studies are well below what would have been expected for brain tumors as a result of the healthy worker effect. Very few risk factors have been identified for glioma or brain tumors in general, and these can explain only a very small proportion of brain tumor incidence.

Efforts are being made to improve knowledge about RF exposure levels in different occupations and in the general environment, through actual measurements, but these efforts are not yet available for use in epidemiological studies. Meters suitable for use in large-scale epidemiological studies have been developed and are likely to improve our knowledge of the exposure distribution in the population and will increase our knowledge about the most important sources of RF exposure in occupations and in the general environment.

In summary, there is currently no or only very limited evidence from epidemiological studies suggesting an increased risk of brain tumors after exposure to low-level RF fields, with an exposure duration of up to 10 to 15 years. For longer durations, there are currently no data available.

REFERENCES

1. ICNIRP. International Commission on Non-ionizing Radiation Protection. Guidelines for limiting exposure to time varying electric, magnetic and electromagnetic fields (up to 300 GHz). *Health Phys.* 1998;74:494–522.
2. Vrijheid M, Cardis E, Armstrong BK, et al. Validation of short term recall of mobile phone use for the Interphone study. *Occup Environ Med.* 2006;63(4):237–243.
3. Cardis E, Richardson L, Deltour I, et al. The INTERPHONE Study: design, epidemiological methods, and description of the study population. *Eur J Epidemiol.* 2007;22(9):647–664.
4. Lahkola A, Salminen T, Auvinen A. Selection bias due to differential participation in a case-control study of mobile phone use and brain tumors. *Ann Epidemiol.* 2005;15(5):321–325.
5. Lönn S, Ahlbom A, Hall P, Feychting M. Long-term mobile phone use and brain tumor risk. *Am J Epidemiol.* 2005;161(6):526–535.
6. Auvinen A, Hietanen M, Luukkonen R, Koskela RS. Brain tumors and salivary gland cancers among cellular telephone users. *Epidemiology.* 2002;13(3):356–359.
7. Hardell L, Hallquist A, Mild KH, Carlberg M, Pahlson A, Lilja A. Cellular and cordless telephones and the risk for brain tumours. *Eur J Cancer Prev.* 2002;11(4):377–386.
8. Hardell L, Nasman A, Pahlson A, Hallquist A, Mild KH. Use of cellular telephones and the risk for brain tumours: A case-control study. *Int J Oncol.* 1999;15(1):113–116.
9. Inskip PD, Tarone RE, Hatch EE, et al. Cellular-telephone use and brain tumors. *N Engl J Med.* 2001;344(2):79–86.
10. Johansen C, Boice J, Jr., McLaughlin J, Olsen J. Cellular telephones and cancer: A nationwide cohort study in Denmark. *J Natl Cancer Inst.* 2001;93(3):203–207.
11. Muscat JE, Malkin MG, Thompson S, et al. Handheld cellular telephone use and risk of brain cancer. *JAMA.* 2000;284(23):3001–3007.
12. Rothman KJ, Loughlin JE, Funch DP, Dreyer NA. Overall mortality of cellular telephone customers. *Epidemiology.* 1996;7(3):303–305.
13. Christensen HC, Schuz J, Kosteljanetz M, et al. Cellular telephones and risk for brain tumors: A population-based, incident case-control study. *Neurology.* 2005;64(7):1189–1195.
14. Hardell L, Carlberg M, Mild KH. Case-control study on cellular and cordless telephones and the risk for acoustic neuroma or meningioma in patients diagnosed 2000–2003. *Neuroepidemiology.* 2005;25(3):120–128.
15. Hardell L, Carlberg M, Mild KH. Case-control study of the association between the use of cellular and cordless telephones and malignant brain tumors diagnosed during 2000–2003. *Environ Res.* 2006;100(2):232–241.
16. Hours M, Bernard M, Montestrucq L, et al. [Cell Phones and Risk of brain and acoustic nerve tumours: the French INTERPHONE case-control study.] *Rev Epidemiol Santé Publique.* 2007;55(5):321–332.
17. Klaeboe L, Blaasaas KG, Tynes T. Use of mobile phones in Norway and risk of intracranial tumours. *Eur J Cancer Prev.* 2007;16(2):158–164.
18. Lahkola A, Auvinen A, Raitanen J, et al. Mobile phone use and risk of glioma in 5 North European countries. *Int J Cancer.* 2007;120(8):1769–1775.
19. Schüz J, Bohler E, Berg G, et al. Cellular phones, cordless phones, and the risks of glioma and meningioma (Interphone study group, Germany). *Am J Epidemiol.* 2006;163(6):512–520.
20. Schüz J, Jacobsen R, Olsen JH, Boice JD, Jr., McLaughlin JK, Johansen C. Cellular telephone use and cancer risk: update of a nationwide Danish cohort. *J Natl Cancer Inst.* 2006;98(23):1707–1713.
21. Dreyer NA, Loughlin JE, Rothman KJ. Cause-specific mortality in cellular telephone users. *JAMA.* 1999;282(19):1814–1816.
22. Hardell L, Mild KH, Pahlson A, Hallquist A. Ionizing radiation, cellular telephones and the risk for brain tumours. *Eur J Cancer Prev.* 2001;10(6):523–529.
23. Hardell L, Mild KH, Carlberg M. Case-control study on the use of cellular and cordless phones and the risk for malignant brain tumours. *Int J Radiat Biol.* 2002;78(10):931–936.
24. Hepworth SJ, Schoemaker MJ, Muir KR, Swerdlow AJ, van Tongeren MJ, McKinney PA. Mobile phone use and risk of glioma in adults: case-control study. *BMJ.* 2006;332(7546):883–887.
25. Lönn S, Klaeboe L, Hall P, et al. Incidence trends of adult primary intracerebral tumors in four Nordic countries. *Int J Cancer.* 2004;108(3):450–455.
26. Chakrabarti I, Cokburn M, Cozen W, Wang YP, Preston-Martin S. A population-based description of glioblastoma multiforme in Los Angeles County, 1974–1999. *Cancer.* 2005;104:2798–2806.
27. Tynes T, Andersen A, Langmark F. Incidence of cancer in Norwegian workers potentially exposed to electromagnetic fields. *Am J Epidemiol.* 1992;136(1):81–88.
28. Szmigielski S. Cancer morbidity in subjects occupationally exposed to high frequency (radiofrequency and microwave) electromagnetic radiation. *Sci Total Environ.* 1996;180(1):9–17.

29. Szmigielski S, Sobiczewska E, Kubacki R. Carcinogenic potency of microwave radiation: overview of the problem and results of epidemiological studies on Polish military personnel. *Eur J Oncol.* 2001;6:193–199.
30. Grayson JK. Radiation exposure, socioeconomic status, and brain tumor risk in the US Air Force: a nested case-control study. *Am J Epidemiol.* 1996;143:480–486.
31. Groves FD, Page WF, Gridley G, et al. Cancer in Korean war navy technicians: mortality survey after 40 years. *Am J Epidemiol.* 2002;155(9):810–818.
32. Morgan RW, Kelsh MA, Zhao K, Exuzides KA, Heringer S, Negrete W. Radiofrequency exposure and mortality from cancer of the brain and lymphatic/hematopoietic systems. *Epidemiology.* 2000;11(2):118–127.
33. Berg G, Spallek J, Schuz J, et al. Occupational exposure to radio frequency/microwave radiation and the risk of brain tumors: Interphone Study Group, Germany. *Am J Epidemiol.* 2006;164(6):538–548.
34. Karipidis KK, Benke G, Sim MR, et al. Occupational exposure to ionizing and non-ionizing radiation and risk of non-Hodgkin lymphoma. *Int Arch Occup Environ Health.* 2007;80(8):663–670.
35. Lönn S, Forssén UM, Vecchia P, Ahlbom A, Feychting M. Output power levels from mobile phones in relation to the geographic position of the user. *Occup Environ Med.* 2004;61:769–772.

7 Allergies and Glioma Risk

Judith A. Schwartzbaum, Linda M. Karavodin, Margaret R. Wrensch, and Joseph Leo Wiemels

INVERSE ASSOCIATION BETWEEN ALLERGIC CONDITIONS, IMMUNOGLOBULIN E, AND GLIOMA

Epidemiological research on the influence of immune factors on glioma etiology has focused primarily on the potential role of allergic conditions in tumor immunosurveillance and growth inhibition. Allergic conditions are initiated by immune responses to common environmental proteins (e.g., pollen, dust mites, mold, dander, and certain foods) and typically result in elevated allergen-specific immunoglobulin E (IgE) antibody levels accompanied by allergic symptoms (e.g., runny nose, stuffy nose, sneezing, nasal itching, or skin rashes). Nearly 50 years ago, Burnet [1] and Thomas [2] proposed that some component of the allergic pathway is responsible for destroying cancer cells or at least inhibiting their growth. Since 1990, results from 10 case-control [3–12] and 1 of 2 cohort studies [13] show that self-reported allergies are inversely related to glioma risk (Table 7.1). Linos et al [14] conducted a formal meta-analysis of a subset of these studies and concluded that the strong inverse association between self-reported allergies and glioma (odds ratio [OR]: 0.61, 95% confidence interval [CI]: 0.55–0.67) is probably not attributable to methodological bias alone.

Literature on allergic conditions and cancer risk recently reviewed by Wang and Diepgen [15], Merrill et al [16], and Turner et al [17] lends further support to the allergy–glioma relationship. Wang and Diepgen concluded that although allergic conditions appear to increase the risk of tumors at several sites, the literature suggests an overall inverse association between allergic disease and cancer risk. More cautiously, Merrill et al reported that the inverse association is cancer-site specific but probably present for tumors at nine sites in addition to the brain. The most conservative report among these, by Turner et al, found strong evidence for an inverse association between allergic conditions and only two tumors: glioma and pancreatic cancer. Although almost all the inverse associations found in the literature are based on self-reported allergy histories, Wiemels et al [18] provide evidence for the validity of these self-reports among glioma patients by measuring serum allergen-specific and total IgE levels. They found that among people with elevated IgE, the proportion reporting allergies was similar for both controls and glioma patients; this observation strongly suggests that self-reports of allergies are generally factual, as validated by IgE levels. Interestingly, late-onset allergies that are less likely to be IgE-related were also associated with reduced risk, indicating that the associations are not specific to IgE-mediated allergic reactions.

Additional support for a possible relationship between IgE levels and glioma growth was reported by Wrensch et al [19]. They found that glioma patients with clinically elevated IgE levels survive an average of 9 months longer than do patients with borderline or normal IgE levels. If confirmed in other studies, this result could be due to direct action of IgE on the tumor itself or elevated IgE levels may indicate a robust antiglioma immune response leading to longer survival.

Consistent with IgE as a mere indicator of rather than a contributor to antiglioma immunity, Prins and Liau [20] point out that circulating antibodies do not easily cross the intact blood–brain barrier and do not appear to track to the tumor even when the blood–brain barrier is disrupted. Nonetheless, it is possible that IgE-producing cells may play a role in antiglioma immunity when they are extravasated (i.e., leaked from vessels into surrounding tissue) into the brain. In addition, evidence for a direct effect of IgE in the brain includes the presence of a low-affinity IgE receptor, CD23, on astrocytes, but the frequency of finding this receptor on glioma cells is not known [19]. Furthermore, Karagiannis et al [21] report that this low-affinity receptor mediates ovarian cancer cell killing by phagocytosis [22], whereas the high-affinity IgE receptor, FcεRI, accomplishes the same end result using cytotoxicity. In addition, Matta et al [23] saw a relationship similar to that observed by Wrensch et al between elevated IgE levels and myeloma patient survival. Specifically, they found that myeloma patients, who had clinically elevated IgE levels, live an average of 3 years longer than do patients whose IgE levels are not clinically elevated.

Also suggesting a role for IgE in affecting immune response to cancer are findings from a randomized clinical trial of omalizumab, an IgE-blocking drug for the treatment of asthma. Study participants in the treatment group had an incidence rate of solid tumors 3.8 times (95% CI: 0.9–34.3) greater than did participants in the control group [24]

Table 7.1 Studies of Association between Self-Reported Allergies, Asthma, and Glioma

Investigators	Glioma Cases	% Proxy Interview	Allergy (OR, 95% CI)	Asthma (OR, 95% CI)
Wigertz et al [11]	1527	13.0	0.70 (0.61–0.80)	0.65 (0.51–0.82)
Schoemaker et al [9]	965	0.0	0.73 (0.59–0.90)	0.71 (0.54–0.92)
Schwartzbaum et al [10]	174	9.0	0.98 (0.62–1.57)	0.64 (0.33–1.25)
Schwartzbaum et al [13]	37	0	0.45 (0.19–1.07)	Not given
Schwartzbaum et al [13]	42	0	2.05 (0.92–4.60)	Not given
Brenner et al [3]	489	24.0	0.67 (0.52–0.86)	0.63 (0.43–0.92)
Wiemels et al [12]	407	33.5	0.47 (0.33–0.67)	0.57 (0.38–0.86)
Schlehofer et al [8]	1178	26.7	0.59 (0.49–0.71)	0.75 (0.55–1.03)
Cicuttini et al [4]	416	43.7	Not given	0.80 (0.50–1.20)
Schlehofer et al [7]	115	4.0	0.71 (0.5–1.0)	Not given
Ryan et al [6]	110	24.7	0.54 (0.33–0.89)	0.40 (0.14–1.15)
Hochberg et al [5]	160	20.0	0.60 (0.40–1.00)	Not given
Average (random effects model)			0.66 (0.60–0.73)	0.68 (0.60–0.77)

Refs. [9–11] include some of same study participants as do refs. [7] and [8]. Ref. 13 is based on results from analysis of two cohorts.

(no gliomas were diagnosed in the treatment group but one was found in the control group). The small number of trial participants with tumors (omalizumab group: $n=16$, control group: $n=5$) may not have allowed equal allocation of individuals with differing prior risks of cancer to the treatment and control groups. Furthermore, the CIs indicate that the findings are consistent with equal tumor incidence rates in both groups. In addition, a group of "experts," noting that many of the tumors occurred during the first 6 months of study participation, judged that the treatment was unlikely to have caused excess tumors [25]. Another interpretation of the findings is that IgE may restrict growth of tumors, a process that Dunn and Schreiber [26] refer to as the equilibrium phase of the interaction between cancer and the immune system. During the equilibrium phase, a tumor is held in check by the immune system. If IgE is involved in this process, then the observed clinical trial findings are exactly what one would predict. That is, withdrawal of a mediator of immune equilibrium (e.g., IgE) would result in relatively rapid appearance of tumors [24]. Further clarification of these findings may come from a cohort study of omalizumab users and nonusers [27] that is currently being planned. At present, there is not sufficient evidence to determine whether IgE plays a direct or passive role in antiglioma immunity.

Allergy-Related Cytokines

Interleukin (IL)-4 and IL-13 are cytokines (immunoregulatory proteins) secreted by T-helper type 2 (Th2) cells that play central roles in IgE synthesis and allergic conditions [28]. The IL-4 receptor alpha (IL-4Rα) not only serves as an IL-4 receptor but also forms a heterodimer with the IL-13 receptor and also serves as an IL-13 receptor. The use of the common receptor may explain the shared functions of these cytokines.

In addition to their role in allergic conditions, the IL-4 and IL-13 cytokines also inhibit growth of glioma cell lines. Although IL-4 is not expressed in the normal adult brain, it is strongly expressed during brain injury [29] where invading T-cells may be a source of this cytokine [30]. Barna et al [30] found that three normal astrocytic, two low-grade astrocytoma, and three out of four glioblastoma cell lines expressed IL-4Rα. However, IL-4 suppresses DNA synthesis and cell proliferation only in normal astrocytic and low-grade astrocytoma cell lines but not in glioblastoma cell lines. Their results suggest that IL-4 could play a role in the inhibition of glioblastomas that arise from astrocytomas but may not be involved in glioblastomas that arise from other pathways [31]. In further support of a role for IL-4 in glioma pathology, Faber et al [32] reported that IL-4 increases the number of T-cell precursors in glioblastoma patients. Saleh et al [33] attributed the growth-inhibiting properties of mouse IL-4 on implanted C6 glioma cell lines to its ability to promote eosinophil infiltration and to inhibit angiogenesis. Furthermore, Saleh et al [34] observed that when c6 gliomas in rats are engineered to produce in situ retroviral IL-4, they are rapidly eradicated.

IL-13, like IL-4, inhibits astrocyte and low-grade astrocytoma proliferation but does not alter glioblastoma cell proliferation. Liu et al [35] found that although glial cells do not produce IL-13, IL-13 receptors are present in normal astrocytic tissue and in high- and low-grade glioma.

Further evidence for a role of IL-13 in glioma development is provided by overexpression (relative to expression levels in normal brain) of IL-13Rα2 in approximately 44% glioblastoma [36]. These receptors are found on the cell membrane, in the cell, and in soluble form in the blood, and under certain conditions, they down-regulate IL-13 levels [28]. Their presence may therefore account for the failure of IL-13 to inhibit growth of glioblastoma cell lines [30]. In addition, if IL-13 inhibits glioma cell growth, it is possible that glioma cells expressing receptors that down-regulate IL-13 maintain a survival advantage. Consistent with this hypothesis, Ma et al [37] found that melanoma cells that secrete IL-13 but not IL-13Rα2 have reduced tumorigenicity in vivo.

In view of a possible role of IL-4 and IL-13 in both allergic conditions and glioma, Schwartzbaum et al [10] took advantage of random allocation of genetic variants to determine whether allergic conditions reduce glioma risk or whether gliomas suppress allergic conditions. These authors identified polymorphisms of the *IL-4Rα* and *IL-13* genes that increase the risk of allergic conditions. Although these germline genetic variants are not sensitive indicators of the presence of allergic conditions, they do provide a measure of allergic condition risk that is free of differential reporting between cases and controls such as that leading to recall bias that may occur when cases are asked to report their histories of allergy after glioma diagnosis. In addition, because germline genetic variants exist prior to glioma development, they cannot be affected by the presence of the tumor as can serum IgE levels. Schwartzbaum et al hypothesized that individuals with *IL-4Rα* or *IL-13* polymorphisms that increase allergic condition risk would decrease glioblastoma risk. Using data from a small case-control study (111 glioblastoma cases, 422 controls), they found results consistent with their hypothesis. Each of the two *IL-4Rα* and *IL-13* single-nucleotide polymorphisms (SNPs) associated with increased allergic condition risk were also related to decreased glioblastoma risk. Wiemels et al [38] confirmed their finding for one of the *IL-13* SNPs in a larger case-control study of glioma (456 glioma cases, 541 controls). Furthermore, they reported that this *IL-13* SNP was inversely associated with IgE levels among controls ($p=0.04$). However, unlike Schwartzbaum et al, they did not find associations between the *IL-4Rα* SNPs and glioma, but they did see a borderline association between an *IL-4Rα* haplotype and glioma (OR: 1.5; 95% CI:, 1.0–2.3). They also identified a rare *IL-4* haplotype that was associated with decreased glioma risk (OR: 0.23; 95% CI 0.07–0.83).

A larger study of the four *IL-4Rα* and *IL-13* genetic variants by Schwartzbaum et al [39] did not provide strong support for their original observations. Nonetheless, they found an *IL-4Rα* haplotype associated with glioblastoma (OR: 2.26; 95% CI: 1.13–4.52) and inversely related to self-report of hay fever or asthma among controls (OR: 0.39; 95% CI: 0.16–0.98). Although Wiemels et al also found suggestive evidence for an association between an *IL-4Rα* haplotype and glioma, when they restricted their haplotype to the same *IL-4Rα* SNPs that Schwartzbaum et al examined, they observed no evidence for an association with glioma (OR: 1.13; 95% CI: 0.83–1.53).

Immunosuppression

One reason for the failure of Wiemels et al and Schwartzbaum et al's reports to consistently observe inverse associations between the *IL-4* and *IL-13* SNPs and glioma may be that these cytokines have paradoxical effects on glioma growth depending on their interaction with as yet unknown factors. Consistent with this hypothesis is a substantial body of evidence that suggests that IL-13 blocks tumor immunosurveillance in the colon [40] and breast [41]. The mechanism by which immunosurveillance is inhibited may be the signaling of IL-13 through the IL-13Rα2 receptor, leading to production of the immunosuppressive cytokine transforming growth factor (TGF)-β1. However, this explanation does not account for the fact that overexpression of the IL-13Rα2 receptor in breast and pancreatic cancer is associated with tumor regression [42].

The tumor itself may also have mechanisms that inhibit the ability of the immune system to eradicate it. In recent in vitro studies of glioma, human glioma cell lines were found to secrete immunosuppressive cytokines that can selectively recruit regulatory T-cells into the tumor microenvironment [43]. In addition, Chahlavi et al [44] demonstrated that glioma cell lines mediate immunosuppression by promoting T-cell death through tumor-associated antigens and gangliosides. Two of the major immunosuppressive cytokines that are present both in the glioma mircoenvironment and peripheral blood of glioma patients, IL-10 and TGF-β, induce immune tolerance, thereby inhibiting allergy and asthma [45]. Elevated IgE concentrations may therefore indicate low levels of immunosuppression and the resulting improved ability to conduct antitumor immunosurveillance against incipient glioma. Alternatively, the relative absence of allergies in glioma patients may merely suggest that tumor-induced cytokines have suppressed the immune system.

Role of IL-10 in Allergic Conditions

The IL-10 cytokine suppresses both total and allergen-specific IgE and is therefore essential for tolerance to allergens [46,47]. Recent analyses of nonallergic individuals demonstrate that their T-cells respond to IL-10 and that the amount of IL-10 is reduced in allergic individuals [48]. For example, bee keepers who have been stung multiple times have T-cells that do not respond to venom antigens, owing to the strong production of IL-10. Furthermore, when peripheral blood cells from healthy nonallergic individuals are stimulated and expanded with aeroallergens, IL-10-producing allergen-activated T-cells are present at a higher frequency than they are in allergic individuals. The suppressor activity of these activated cells is reduced by neutralization of IL-10 or TGF-β. As observed in a large cohort of allergic and nonallergic children, higher levels of IL-10 are related to negative allergy skin tests [45]. Liu and Ziu [49] found a correlation of −0.46 ($p<0.01$) between serum IL-10 and total serum IgE in a group of 50 allergic rhinitis patients.

Role of IL-10 in Glioma

Although IL-10 is commonly regarded as an anti-inflammatory and immunosuppressive cytokine that favors tumor escape from immune surveillance, it is now clear that depending on the tissue location and concentration, IL-10 may display either pro or anti-inflammatory effects [50]. In the normal brain, both astrocytes and microglia induce IL-10 production in response to systemic inflammation [51]. In glioma, the induction of IL-10 is increased [52] as it is in lymphoma [53], leukemia [54], pancreatic [55], and ovarian cancer [56]. Akasaki et al [57] found that COX-2 induces overexpression of IL-10 in a glioma cell line. Using a rodent glioma model, Zhang et al [58] observed that expression of IL-10 was elevated in glioma-associated microglia. Consistent with these cell and animal findings, Kumar et al [59] found that anaplastic astrocytoma and glioblastoma patients have higher levels of serum IL-10 than do controls. More recently, Samaras et al [60] observed higher levels of IL-10 secretion from peripheral mononuclear cells of glioma patients than from the same cells of controls.

IL-10 and Glioma Survival Time

Although there is no direct evidence that IL-10 concentration is associated with glioma survival time, IL-10 is involved in regulatory T-cell expression, and regulatory T-cells are related to glioma survival time (see later). In addition, IL-10 is related to prognosis of several other cancers. Colon cancer patients whose elevated serum IL-10 levels returned to normal after surgery were less likely to have a tumor recurrence and more likely to respond to chemotherapy than were patients whose IL-10 levels remained elevated [61]. In addition, serum IL-10 levels are positively related to factors that predict poor prognoses in ovarian [62] and non–small cell lung cancer [63] and adult T-cell leukemia/lymphoma [54].

Role of TGF-β in Allergic Conditions

There Are three closely related mammalian TGF-β isoforms (TGF-β1, 2, and 3) [52], and each has diverse effects including potent immunoregulatory properties, making them essential for the maintenance of immunological self-tolerance [46,47]. Most human cells express TGF-β receptors and synthesize TGF-β, which accounts for the complex consequences of TGF-β release by cells. In contrast to its known T-cell suppressive activity, TGF-β may also be involved in the pathogenesis of asthma, particularly in the remodeling of injured lung tissue in humans.

Role of TGF-β in Glioma

TGF-β signaling maintains tissue homeostasis, especially in the regulation of inflammation, thus reducing cancer risk [50,64]. In particular, within the brain, TGF-β terminates glial proliferation in response to injury [65]. In contrast, glioma growth facilitates the induction of regulatory T-cells that secrete IL-10 and TGF-β and suppress T-cell responses, thus blocking antitumor immunity. In addition to its immunosuppressive role, TGF-β controls the cell cycle and has antimitogenic functions. Again, in the course of glioma development, the effect of TGF-β is changed and this cytokine becomes mitogenic. One pathway for this alteration is through induction of a demethylated platelet-derived growth factor-B (PDGF-B) gene [66]. Once activated, TGF-β and PDGF-B induce glioma proliferation. Many studies have demonstrated the synthesis of TGF-β by glioma cells [67], and it has also been shown that the more advanced the glioma, the higher the level of TGF-β production [66,68]. Recently, the effects of TGF-β on neural stem cell proliferation have become an area of intense research interest. Aigner and Bogdahn [69] found that TGF-β initially inhibits neural stem cell proliferation but may subsequently affect the transition from a neural to a cancer stem cell. Later in tumor progression, TGF-β acts as an oncogene; it further promotes tumor growth by promoting angiogenesis and suppressing the immune system. Its role in stem cell transformation is especially important in view of the present focus on the role of neural stem cells in glioma development. Nor is glioma the only tumor characterized by elevated expression of TGF-β. Gastric [70] and pancreatic cancer [71] patients have higher levels of serum TGF-β than do controls.

TGF-β and Glioma Survival Time

In contrast to IL-10, there is direct evidence that TGF-β is associated with glioma survival time. It has been shown that mice with transplanted glioma cells survive longer when TGF-β signaling is inhibited [72], and Liu et al [73] found that inhibition of TGF-β2 augments the effect of tumor vaccine and improves survival. In humans, two groups report that TGF-β activity is inversely related to survival time from glioma diagnosis [66,68]. In response to the animal and human results, there are ongoing clinical trials to determine whether inhibition of TGF-β2 lengthens survival time from diagnosis of recurrent high-grade malignant glioma [74].

Immunosuppressive Regulatory T-cells (e.g., Natural Killer T, Tregs, and Tr1 cells)

Both IL-10 and TGF-β work in concert with immunosuppressive regulatory T cells. For example, TGF-β has been implicated in the conversion of naive CD4+ CD25–T cells into immunosuppressive CD4+ CD25+ regulatory T-cells by the induction of FOXP3. Regulatory T-cells control the immune response to self and allow appropriate response to pathogens or tumors while at the same time limiting potential damage to normal tissue. The balance between protection from pathogens and protection of self is delicate and sometimes prone to error. For example, regulatory T cells may suppress cancer immunity or their absence may produce an attack on normal cells as in autoimmune disease. Peripheral blood collected from cancer patients (including glioma) is characterized by elevation in the relative proportion of regulatory T-cells [75–86]. This excess has been attributed to the antitumor immunity inhibiting role of these cells and has been extensively documented in glioma [87]. Learn et al [88] compared differences in T-cell gene expression profiles in individuals with and without glioma. They found that genes in glioma cases involved in T-cell receptor ligation were down-regulated, whereas genes associated with regulatory T-cells and their immunosuppressive cytokines were upregulated. Grauer et al [89] showed that regulatory T-cells gradually accumulate in murine gliomas and suppress antitumor immunity. El Andaloussi and Lesniak [90] confirmed this observation in humans, noting that FOXP3 expressing regulatory T-cells increase during human glioma progression and that this increase is correlated with tumor grade.

Regulatory T-Cells and Glioma Survival Time

El Andaloussi et al [91] found that mice with glioma lived longer after depletion of their CD4+ CD25+ regulatory T-cells. Fecci et al [92] showed that blocking CTLA-4 (constitutively expressed on regulatory T-cells) lengthened survival of tumor-bearing mice by 80%. In any case, there is evidence that the higher the proportion of regulatory T-cells, the poorer the survival among patients with hepatocellular carcinoma [93] and renal cell [94], colorectal [95], and ovarian cancer [96].

Paradoxical Role of IL-10 and TGF-β

Although IL-10 and TGF-β play an immunosuppressive role in late glioma development, their anti-inflammatory properties may prevent tumor growth early in the tumor's natural history. This hypothesis is consistent with previous epidemiological research showing that people who use nonsteroidal anti-inflammatory drugs may have a lower risk of glioma than those who do not [97]. Also playing an anti-inflammatory role in the normal brain are the IL-4 and IL-13 cytokines [98] that may also suppress glioma development by interfering with inflammation.

The Role of Antibodies Against Tumor Antigens

Antibody-producing cells are likely to play a role, if any, when they are extravasated (i.e., leak from vessel into surrounding tissue) into the brain. Those individuals with B-cells reactive to tumor antigens may also have enhanced humoral responses to other antigens such as allergens; in this scenario, allergy is a marker of a hyper-reactive immune system rather than itself producing an antiglioma reaction. The observation that the major B-cell chemoattractant, CXCL13, is highly expressed during brain infection [99] is compatible with a role for B-cells in the remission of brain cancers that sometimes occurs subsequent to a strong intracranial infection following glioma surgery [100]. The tracking of IgE or IgG levels throughout the course glioma therapy would shed light on the role of these antibodies and the potential involvement of B-cells.

Current epidemiologic investigations have focused on IgE because of the inverse association between allergy and gliomas. However, since typical reactions against autoimmune targets involve IgG rather than IgE, a serum antibody response to a brain tumor would be more likely to involve IgGs against specific antigens expressed by a tumor. Tumors can express "tumor antigens," which are often normal embryonically expressed self-proteins but are recognized as "foreign" by the adult immune system (e.g., MAGE proteins). Other tumor antigens are proteins normally expressed at low levels, or only transiently by normal cells, but in large amounts by a tumor (e.g., heat shock proteins and survivin). Proteins do not easily pass into or out of the central nervous system (CNS) as noted earlier; however, modest amounts are able to enter the systemic immune system via cervical lymphatic drainage [101]. Proteins elevated in gliomas include transcription factors, and survivin [102–105]. It is unclear whether antibodies to these proteins can act on brain tumors directly to produce cytotoxicity or whether B-cells can enter the CNS in sufficient numbers to express antibodies. The presence and activation of B-cells in brain tumors should in the future be studied in relationship to survival and etiology.

Interestingly, brain cancers express CXCR4 and its cognate ligand SDF-1/CXCL12, which are critical in the formation of neovasculature to support the tumor and correlate strongly with tumor invasiveness and inversely with survival [106,107]. This chemokine is a key regulator of the differentiation and migration of B-cells in the bone marrow, in infection, and is also expressed by astrocytes and is important for their differentiation [108,109]. This and other chemokines are largely responsible for the positioning of B-cells within a tissue [110]. Although SDF-1/CXCL12 are thought to be involved in the recruitment of precursors to endothelial cells (which are stem cells that originally derive from the bone marrow, as do B-cells), the cytokine axis may be involved in antiglioma immune reactions. SDF-1/CXCR4 is a major signal for B-cell extravasation in inflammatory processes [111]. B-cell recruitment is a major feature of infection-associated inflammation that has been associated with glioma cure in anecdotal reports [100]. A strong inflammatory process due to an infection in the brain will disrupt immune equilibrium and may allow for the concomitant rejection of the tumor especially as negative regulation by regulatory T–cells, and the tumor itself will be disrupted during infection clearance.

Reverse Causality

As previously noted, the relative absence of allergic conditions among glioma patients may precede or result from glioma. There is, however, some evidence for a role of glioma in the suppression of allergies. In a study of 1527 glioma cases and 3309 randomly selected controls, Wigertz et al [11] found that hay fever or eczema present at the time of diagnosis is associated with reduced glioma risk, while a history of hay fever or eczema is not. Schoemaker et al [9] observed similar results for eczema. Further evidence for the absence of a causal association between allergies and cancer comes from a cohort study of a group of patients initially tested for total serum IgE levels and subsequently linked to a population-based cancer registry [112]. These authors report no effect of IgE levels on cancer risk at all sites combined; however, their sample was not large enough to investigate IgE levels and glioma separately. Still stronger evidence against an inverse causal association between allergies and non-Hodgkin's lymphoma (NHL) is based on a recent case-control study showing reduced risk of NHL among people reporting a history of allergies or having elevated aeroallergen-specific IgE levels [113]. When the same authors also tested sera from a case-control study nested in a cohort, they found no overall case-control differences. However, the nested case-control data did show a decline in aeroallergen-specific IgE levels among cases 4 years before NHL diagnosis, which would be expected if the tumor itself were responsible for declining IgE levels. This temporal pattern may also apply to the association between IgE and glioma. A clear caveat to the case-control component of this study, however, is the fact that the IgE measurements were made during pregnancy. Pregnancy is associated with Th1-suppression and concomitant enhancement of humoral (antibody) responses, which can result in elevated IgE levels irrespective of history of allergy status. Grulich et al [114] pointed out this potential error in interpretation; the role of allergy in the etiology of NHL is incompletely studied. Nonetheless, because all women in the sample were pregnant, the effect of pregnancy on the immune system would not have confounded the association between IgE levels and case status. It is still possible (but unlikely) that pregnancy might exert a modifying effect on the IgE, NHL association. If pregnancy modifies the effect of IgE on NHL risk, then the association between IgE and NHL would differ depending on whether one was a pregnant woman, a nonpregnant woman, or a man. There is no evidence that suggests the presence of such an effect, but it is possible.

CONCLUSIONS

Initial anecdotal reports of protective effects of allergy and the therapeutic role of infections have become the focus of intense epidemiologic, laboratory, and clinical investigation with great potential for new brain cancer prevention and treatment modalities. By far, the strongest and most consistent observation provided from the field of epidemiology is the inverse association between allergy and glioma, which remains the most consistent association among any risk factor for glioma besides, arguably, ionizing radiation, gender, age, and ethnicity.

The evidence reviewed in this chapter clearly places a diverse set of manifestations of immune function as significant in the glioma process—including allergic phenotypes, the atopic marker IgE, polymorphisms in allergy-related cytokines, active and repressive subsets of CD4+ T-cells, autoantibodies against tumor antigens, and specific roles of cytokines expressed by tumors and by the immune system in response to tumors. Several themes have emerged. First, active immune responses of the TH2 variety may be protective against glioma [42], in contrast to traditional tumor immunology concepts in which TH1 reactions dominate. Second, regulatory T-cells and their associated cytokines TGF-β and IL-10 repress effective antiglioma reactions and may provide a conceptual and mechanistic framework to explain an indirect relationship between allergies and antiglioma immune reactions. Third, the unique architecture of the brain does not exclude glioma from immune interaction; clearly, the brain supports attenuated immune responses, along with infiltration of T- and B-cells, and the enhancement of such responses is likely to form the basis of future effective glioma therapies.

Observational epidemiology has yielded key insights, but future studies must include sound immunological principles and mechanistic concepts for continuation of progress in these areas. Such studies must also move away from the traditional case-control approach to respond to the greatest criticism: reverse causality (i.e., the disease has created the immune phenotype studied). Studies of genetic inheritance (i.e., SNPs) are not subject to reverse causality and will provide the next set of critical insights into the epidemiology of immunity and glioma, but they will not be able to assess properties of the immune system influenced by development and environment. Creative uses of cohort and interventional studies are thus likely to provide future progress in understanding the relationship of immune phenotypes to glioma.

REFERENCES

1. Burnet FM. Cancer: a biological approach. IV. Practical application. *BMJ*. 1957;1:844–847.
2. Thomas L. Discussion. In: Lawrence HS, ed. *Cellular and Humoral Aspects of the Hypersensitive States*. New York, NY: Hoeber-Harper; 1959:529–532.
3. Brenner AV, Linet MS, Fine HA, et al. History of allergies and autoimmune diseases and risk of brain tumors in adults. *Int J Cancer*. 2002;99:252–259.
4. Cicuttini FM, Hurley SF, Forbes A. Association of adult glioma with medical conditions, family, and reproductive history. *Int J Cancer* 1997;71:203–207.
5. Hochberg F, Toniolo P, Cole P, Salcman M. Nonoccupational risk indicators of glioblastoma in adults. *J Neurooncol*. 1990;8:55–60.
6. Ryan P, Lee MW, North B, McMichael AJ. Risk factors for tumors of the brain and meninges: results from the Adelaide Adult Brain Tumor Study. *Int J Cancer*. 1992;51:20–27.
7. Schlehofer B, Blettner M, Becker N, Martinsohn C, Wahrendorf J. Medical risk factors and the development of brain tumors. *Cancer*. 1992;69:2541–2547.
8. Schlehofer B, Blettner M, Preston-Martin S, et al. Role of medical history in brain tumour development. Results from the international adult brain tumour study. *Int J Cancer*. 1999;82:155–160.
9. Schoemaker MJ, Swerdlow AJ, Hepworth SJ, McKinney PA, van Tongeren M, Muir KR. History of allergies and risk of glioma in adults. *Int J Cancer*. 2006;119(9):2165–2172.
10. Schwartzbaum J, Ahlbom A, Malmer B, et al. Polymorphisms associated with asthma are inversely related to glioblastoma multiforme. *Cancer Res*. 2005;65:6459–6465.
11. Wigertz A, Lönn S, Schwartzbaum J, et al. Allergic conditions and brain tumor risk. *Am J Epidemiol*. 2007;166(8):941–950.
12. Wiemels JL, Wiencke JK, Sison JD, Miike R, McMillan A, Wrensch M. History of allergies among adults with glioma and controls. *Int J Cancer*. 2002;98:609–615.
13. Schwartzbaum J, Jonsson F, Ahlbom A, et al. Cohort studies of association between self-reported allergic conditions, immune-related diagnoses and glioma and meningioma risk. *Int J Cancer*. 2003;106:423–428.
14. Linos E, Raine T, Alonso A, Michaud D. Atopy and risk of brain tumors: a meta-analysis. *J Natl Cancer Inst*. 2007;99:1544–1550.
15. Wang H, Diepgen TL. Is atopy a protective or a risk factor for cancer? A review of epidemiological studies. *Allergy*. 2005;60:1098–1111.
16. Merrill RM, Isakson RT, Beck RE. The association between allergies and cancer: what is currently known? *Ann Allergy Asthma Immunol*. 2007;99:102–116; quiz 17–19, 50.
17. Turner MC, Chen Y, Krewski D, Ghadirian P. An overview of the association between allergy and cancer. *Int J Cancer*. 2006;118:3124–3132.
18. Wiemels JL, Wiencke JK, Patoka J, et al. Reduced immunoglobulin E and allergy among adults with glioma compared with controls. *Cancer Res*. 2004;64:8468–8473.
19. Wrensch M, Wiencke JK, Wiemels J, et al. Serum IgE, tumor epidermal growth factor receptor expression, and inherited polymorphisms associated with glioma survival. *Cancer Res*. 2006;66:4531–4541.
20. Prins RM, Liau LM. Immunology and immunotherapy in neurosurgical disease. *Neurosurgery*. 2003;53:144–152; discussion 52–53.
21. Karagiannis SN, Bracher MG, Beavil RL, et al. Role of IgE receptors in IgE antibody-dependent cytotoxicity and phagocytosis of ovarian tumor cells by human monocytic cells. *Cancer Immunol Immunother*. 2008;57(2):247–263.
22. Karagiannis SN, Bracher MG, Hunt J, et al. IgE-antibody-dependent immunotherapy of solid tumors: cytotoxic and phagocytic mechanisms of eradication of ovarian cancer cells. *J Immunol*. 2007;179:2832–2843.
23. Matta GM, Battaglio S, Dibello C, et al. Polyclonal immunoglobulin E levels are correlated with hemoglobin values and overall survival in patients with multiple myeloma. *Clin Cancer Res*. 2007;13:5348–5354.
24. Genentech. Briefing Document on Safety (BLASTN 1039760/0): omalizumab (Xolair) for treatment of allergic asthma; 2003.
25. Holgate ST, Djukanovic R, Casale T, Bousquet J. Anti-immunoglobulin E treatment with omalizumab in allergic diseases: an update on anti-inflammatory activity and clinical efficacy. *Clin Exp Allergy*. 2005;35:408–416.

26. Dunn GP, Old LJ, Schreiber RD. The immunobiology of cancer immunosurveillance and immunoediting. *Immunity.* 2004;21:137–148.
27. Omalizumab: new drug. Asthma: too many unknowns for an anti-IgE. *Prescrire Int.* 2007;16:179–182.
28. Tabata Y, Khurana Hershey GK. IL-13 receptor isoforms: breaking through the complexity. *Curr Allergy Asthma Rep.* 2007;7:338–345.
29. Liu H, Prayson RA, Estes ML, et al. In vivo expression of the interleukin 4 receptor alpha by astrocytes in epilepsy cerebral cortex. *Cytokine.* 2000;12:1656–1661.
30. Barna BP, Estes ML, Pettay J, Iwasaki K, Zhou P, Barnett GH. Human astrocyte growth regulation: interleukin-4 sensitivity and receptor expression. *J Neuroimmunol.* 1995;60:75–81.
31. Louis DN. A molecular genetic model of astrocytoma histopathology. *Brain Pathol.* 1997;7:755–764.
32. Faber C, Terao E, Morga E, Heuschling P. Interleukin-4 enhances the in vitro precursor cell recruitment for tumor-specific T lymphocytes in patients with glioblastoma. *J Immunother.* 2000;23:11–16.
33. Saleh M, Davis ID, Wilks AF. The paracrine role of tumor-derived mIL-4 on tumour-associated endothelium. *Int J Cancer.* 1997;72:664–672.
34. Saleh M, Wiegmans A, Malone Q, Stylli SS, Kaye AH. Effect of in situ retroviral interleukin-4 transfer on established intracranial tumors. *J Natl Cancer Inst.* 1999;91:438–445.
35. Liu H, Jacobs BS, Liu J, et al. Interleukin-13 sensitivity and receptor phenotypes of human glial cell lines: non-neoplastic glia and low-grade astrocytoma differ from malignant glioma. *Cancer Immunol Immunother* 2000;49:319–324.
36. Jarboe JS, Johnson KR, Choi Y, Lonser RR, Park JK. Expression of interleukin-13 receptor alpha2 in glioblastoma multiforme: implications for targeted therapies. *Cancer Res.* 2007;67:7983–7986.
37. Ma HL, Whitters MJ, Jacobson BA, Donaldson DD, Collins M, Dunussi-Joannopoulos K. Tumor cells secreting IL-13 but not IL-13Ralpha2 fusion protein have reduced tumorigenicity in vivo. *Int Immunol.* 2004;16:1009–1017.
38. Wiemels JL, Wiencke JK, Kelsey KT, et al. Allergy-related polymorphisms influence glioma status and serum IgE levels. *Cancer Epidemiol Biomarkers Prev.* 2007;16:1229.
39. Schwartzbaum J, Ahlbom A, Lönn S, et al. An international case-control study of IL-4Ralpha, IL-13 and cyclooxygenase-2 polymorphisms and glioblastoma risk. *Cancer Epidemiol Biomarkers Prev.* 2007;16(11):2448–2454.
40. Park JM, Terabe M, van den Broeke LT, Donaldson DD, Berzofsky JA. Unmasking immunosurveillance against a syngeneic colon cancer by elimination of CD4+ NKT regulatory cells and IL-13. *Int J Cancer.* 2005;114:80–87.
41. Park JM, Terabe M, Donaldson DD, Forni G, Berzofsky JA. Natural immunosurveillance against spontaneous, autochthonous breast cancers revealed and enhanced by blockade of IL-13-mediated negative regulation. *Cancer Immunol Immunother.* 2008;57:907–912.
42. Ellyard JI, Simson L, Parish CR. Th2-mediated anti-tumour immunity: friend or foe? *Tissue Antigens.* 2007;70:1–11.
43. Jordan JT, Sun W, Hussain SF, DeAngulo G, Prabhu SS, Heimberger AB. Preferential migration of regulatory T cells mediated by glioma-secreted chemokines can be blocked with chemotherapy. *Cancer Immunol Immunother.* 2008;57:123–131.
44. Chahlavi A, Rayman P, Richmond AL, et al. Glioblastomas induce T-lymphocyte death by two distinct pathways involving gangliosides and CD70. *Cancer Res.* 2005;65:5428–5438.
45. Umetsu DT, DeKruyff RH. The regulation of allergy and asthma. *Immunol Rev.* 2006;212:238–255.
46. Akdis M, Akdis CA. Mechanisms of allergen-specific immunotherapy. *J Allergy Clin Immunol.* 2007;119:780–791.
47. Taylor A, Verhagen J, Blaser K, Akdis M, Akdis CA. Mechanisms of immune suppression by interleukin-10 and transforming growth factor-beta: the role of T regulatory cells. *Immunology.* 2006;117:433–442.
48. Akdis M. Healthy immune response to allergens: T regulatory cells and more. *Curr Opin Immunol.* 2006;18:738–744.
49. Liu G, Zhu R. Serum IL-10 level in allergic rhinitis patients and its effect on serum total IgE. *J Huazhong Univ Sci Technolog Med Sci.* 2005;25:724–725.
50. Lin WW, Karin M. A cytokine-mediated link between innate immunity, inflammation, and cancer. *J Clin Invest.* 2007;117:1175–1183.
51. Wu Z, Zhang J, Nakanishi H. Leptomeningeal cells activate microglia and astrocytes to induce IL-10 production by releasing pro-inflammatory cytokines during systemic inflammation. *J Neuroimmunol.* 2005;167:90–98.
52. Gomez GG, Kruse CA. Mechanisms of malignant glioma immune resistance and sources of immunosuppression. *Gene Ther Mol Biol.* 2006;10:133–146.
53. Cortes J, Kurzrock R. Interleukin-10 in non-Hodgkin's lymphoma. *Leuk Lymphoma.* 1997;26:251–259.
54. Inagaki A, Ishida T, Ishii T, et al. Clinical significance of serum Th1-, Th2- and regulatory T cells-associated cytokines in adult T-cell leukemia/lymphoma: high interleukin-5 and -10 levels are significant unfavorable prognostic factors. *Int J Cancer.* 2006;118:3054–3061.
55. Poch B, Lotspeich E, Ramadani M, Gansauge S, Beger HG, Gansauge F. Systemic immune dysfunction in pancreatic cancer patients. *Langenbecks Arch Surg.* 2007;392:353–358.
56. Mustea A, Konsgen D, Braicu EI, et al. Expression of IL-10 in patients with ovarian carcinoma. *Anticancer Res.* 2006;26:1715–1718.
57. Akasaki Y, Liu G, Chung NH, Ehtesham M, Black KL, Yu JS. Induction of a CD4+ T regulatory type 1 response by cyclooxygenase-2-overexpressing glioma. *J Immunol.* 2004;173:4352–4359.
58. Zhang L, Handel MV, Schartner JM, et al. Regulation of IL-10 expression by upstream stimulating factor (USF-1) in glioma-associated microglia. *J Neuroimmunol.* 2007;184:188–197.
59. Kumar R, Kamdar D, Madden L, et al. Th1/Th2 cytokine imbalance in meningioma, anaplastic astrocytoma and glioblastoma multiforme patients. *Oncol Rep.* 2006;15:1513–1516.
60. Samaras V, Piperi C, Korkolopoulou P, et al. Application of the ELISPOT method for comparative analysis of interleukin (IL)-6 and IL-10 secretion in peripheral blood of patients with astroglial tumors. *Mol Cell Biochem.* 2007;304:343–351.
61. Evans C, Dalgleish AG, Kumar D. Review article: immune suppression and colorectal cancer. *Aliment Pharmacol Ther.* 2006;24:1163–1177.
62. Lambeck AJ, Crijns AP, Leffers N, et al. Serum cytokine profiling as a diagnostic and prognostic tool in ovarian cancer: a potential role for interleukin 7. *Clin Cancer Res.* 2007;13:2385–2391.
63. Zeni E, Mazzetti L, Miotto D, et al. Macrophage expression of interleukin-10 is a prognostic factor in nonsmall cell lung cancer. *Eur Respir J.* 2007;30:627–632.
64. Salazar-Onfray F, Lopez MN, Mendoza-Naranjo A. Paradoxical effects of cytokines in tumor immune surveillance and tumor immune escape. *Cytokine Growth Factor Rev.* 2007;18:171–182.
65. Golestaneh N, Mishra B. TGF-beta, neuronal stem cells and glioblastoma. *Oncogene.* 2005;24:5722–5730.
66. Bruna A, Darken RS, Rojo F, et al. High TGFbeta-Smad activity confers poor prognosis in glioma patients and promotes cell proliferation depending on the methylation of the PDGF-B gene. *Cancer Cell.* 2007;11:147–160.
67. Wick W, Naumann U, Weller M. Transforming growth factor-beta: a molecular target for the future therapy of glioblastoma. *Curr Pharm Des.* 2006;12:341–349.
68. Schneider T, Sailer M, Ansorge S, Firsching R, Reinhold D. Increased concentrations of transforming growth factor beta1 and beta2 in the plasma of patients with glioblastoma. *J Neurooncol.* 2006;79:61–65.
69. Aigner L, Bogdahn U. TGF-beta in neural stem cells and in tumors of the central nervous system. *Cell Tissue Res.* 2008;331(1):225–241.
70. Lin Y, Kikuchi S, Obata Y, Yagyu K. Serum levels of transforming growth factor beta1 are significantly correlated with venous invasion in patients with gastric cancer. *J Gastroenterol Hepatol.* 2006;21:432–437.
71. Lin Y, Kikuchi S, Tamakoshi A, et al. Serum transforming growth factor-beta1 levels and pancreatic cancer risk: a nested case-control study (Japan). *Cancer Causes Control.* 2006;17:1077–1082.
72. Tran TT, Uhl M, Ma JY, et al. Inhibiting TGF-beta signaling restores immune surveillance in the SMA-560 glioma model. *Neuro Oncol.* 2007;9:259–270.
73. Liu Y, Wang Q, Kleinschmidt-DeMasters BK, Franzusoff A, Ng KY, Lillehei KO. TGF-beta2 inhibition augments the effect of tumor vaccine and improves the survival of animals with pre-established brain tumors. *J Neurooncol.* 2007;81:149–162.
74. Hau P, Jachimczak P, Schlingensiepen R, et al. Inhibition of TGF-beta2 with AP 12009 in recurrent malignant gliomas: from preclinical to phase I/II studies. *Oligonucleotides.* 2007;17:201–212.
75. Baecher-Allan C, Anderson DE. Regulatory cells and human cancer. *Semin Cancer Biol.* 2006;16:98–105.

76. Baecher-Allan C, Anderson DE. Immune regulation in tumor-bearing hosts. *Curr Opin Immunol.* 2006;18:214–219.
77. Beyer M, Kochanek M, Giese T, et al. In vivo peripheral expansion of naive CD4+CD25high FOXP3+ regulatory T cells in patients with multiple myeloma. *Blood.* 2006;107(10):3940–3949.
78. Beyer M, Schultze JL. Regulatory T cells in cancer. *Blood.* 2006;108(3):804–811.
79. Gray CP, Arosio P, Hersey P. Association of increased levels of heavy-chain ferritin with increased CD4+ CD25+ regulatory T-cell levels in patients with melanoma. *Clin Cancer Res.* 2003;9:2551–2559.
80. Ichihara F, Kono K, Takahashi A, Kawaida H, Sugai H, Fujii H. Increased populations of regulatory T cells in peripheral blood and tumor-infiltrating lymphocytes in patients with gastric and esophageal cancers. *Clin Cancer Res.* 2003;9:4404–4408.
81. Liyanage UK, Moore TT, Joo HG, et al. Prevalence of regulatory T cells is increased in peripheral blood and tumor microenvironment of patients with pancreas or breast adenocarcinoma. *J Immunol.* 2002;169:2756–2761.
82. Sasada T, Kimura M, Yoshida Y, Kanai M, Takabayashi A. CD4+CD25+ regulatory T cells in patients with gastrointestinal malignancies: possible involvement of regulatory T cells in disease progression. *Cancer.* 2003;98:1089–1099.
83. Wang X, Zheng J, Liu J, et al. Increased population of CD4(+) CD25(high), regulatory T cells with their higher apoptotic and proliferating status in peripheral blood of acute myeloid leukemia patients. *Eur J Haematol.* 2005;75:468–476.
84. Wolf AM, Wolf D, Steurer M, Gastl G, Gunsilius E, Grubeck-Loebenstein B. Increase of regulatory T cells in the peripheral blood of cancer patients. *Clin Cancer Res.* 2003;9:606–612.
85. Woo EY, Yeh H, Chu CS, et al. Cutting edge: regulatory T cells from lung cancer patients directly inhibit autologous T cell proliferation. *J Immunol.* 2002;168:4272–4276.
86. Fecci PE, Mitchell DA, Whitesides JF, et al. Increased regulatory T-cell fraction amidst a diminished CD4 compartment explains cellular immune defects in patients with malignant glioma. *Cancer Res.* 2006;66:3294–3302.
87. Terabe M, Berzofsky JA. Immunoregulatory T cells in tumor immunity. *Curr Opin Immunol.* 2004;16:157–162.
88. Learn CA, Fecci PE, Schmittling RJ, et al. Profiling of CD4+, CD8+, and CD4+CD25+CD45RO+FoxP3+ T cells in patients with malignant glioma reveals differential expression of the immunologic transcriptome compared with T cells from healthy volunteers. *Clin Cancer Res.* 2006;12:7306–7315.
89. Grauer OM, Nierkens S, Bennink E, et al. CD4+FoxP3+ regulatory T cells gradually accumulate in gliomas during tumor growth and efficiently suppress antiglioma immune responses in vivo. *Int J Cancer.* 2007;121:95–105.
90. El Andaloussi A, Lesniak MS. An increase in CD4+CD25+FOXP3+ regulatory T cells in tumor-infiltrating lymphocytes of human glioblastoma multiforme. *Neuro Oncol.* 2006;8(3):234–243.
91. El Andaloussi A, Han Y, Lesniak MS. Prolongation of survival following depletion of CD4+CD25+ regulatory T cells in mice with experimental brain tumors. *J Neurosurg.* 2006;105:430–437.
92. Fecci PE, Ochiai H, Mitchell DA, et al. Systemic CTLA-4 blockade ameliorates glioma-induced changes to the CD4+ T cell compartment without affecting regulatory T-cell function. *Clin Cancer Res.* 2007;13:2158–2167.
93. Fu J, Xu D, Liu Z, et al. Increased regulatory T cells correlate with CD8 T-cell impairment and poor survival in hepatocellular carcinoma patients. *Gastroenterology.* 2007;132:2328–2339.
94. Griffiths RW, Elkord E, Gilham DE, et al. Frequency of regulatory T cells in renal cell carcinoma patients and investigation of correlation with survival. *Cancer Immunol Immunother.* 2007;56(11):1743–1753.
95. Ling KL, Pratap SE, Bates GJ, et al. Increased frequency of regulatory T cells in peripheral blood and tumour infiltrating lymphocytes in colorectal cancer patients. *Cancer Immun.* 2007;7:7.
96. Dietl J, Engel JB, Wischhusen J. The role of regulatory T cells in ovarian cancer. *Int J Gynecol Cancer.* 2007;17:764–770.
97. Sivak-Sears N, Schwartzbaum J, Miike R, Moghadassi M, Wrensch M. Case-control study of non-steroidal anti-inflammatory drug use and glioblastoma multiforme. *Am J of Epidemiol.* 2004;159:1131–1139.
98. Yang MS, Ji KA, Jeon SB, et al. Interleukin-13 enhances cyclooxygenase-2 expression in activated rat brain microglia: implications for death of activated microglia. *J Immunol.* 2006;177:1323–1329.
99. Gelderblom H, Londono D, Bai Y, et al. High production of CXCL13 in blood and brain during persistent infection with the relapsing fever spirochete Borrelia turicatae. *J Neuropathol Exp Neurol.* 2007;66:208–217.
100. Bowles AP, Jr., Perkins E. Long-term remission of malignant brain tumors after intracranial infection: a report of four cases. *Neurosurgery.* 1999;44:636–642; discussion 42–43.
101. Harling-Berg CJ, Park TJ, Knopf PM. Role of the cervical lymphatics in the Th2-type hierarchy of CNS immune regulation. *J Neuroimmunol.* 1999;101:111–127.
102. Matsushita H, Uenaka A, Ono T, et al. Identification of glioma-specific RFX4-E and -F isoforms and humoral immune response in patients. *Cancer Sci.* 2005;96:801–809.
103. Pallasch CP, Struss AK, Munnia A, et al. Autoantibodies against GLEA2 and PHF3 in glioblastoma: tumor-associated autoantibodies correlated with prolonged survival. *Int J Cancer.* 2005;117:456–459.
104. Söling A, Plugge EM, Schmitz M, et al. Autoantibodies to the inhibitor of apoptosis protein survivin in patients with brain tumors. *Int J Oncol.* 2007;30:123–128.
105. Ueda R, Yoshida K, Kawakami Y, Kawase T, Toda M. Immunohistochemical analysis of SOX6 expression in human brain tumors. *Brain Tumor Pathol.* 2004;21:117–120.
106. Ehtesham M, Winston JA, Kabos P, Thompson RC. CXCR4 expression mediates glioma cell invasiveness. *Oncogene.* 2006;25:2801–2806.
107. Salmaggi A, Gelati M, Pollo B, et al. CXCL12 expression is predictive of a shorter time to tumor progression in low-grade glioma: a single-institution study in 50 patients. *J Neurooncol.* 2005;74:287–293.
108. Lazarini F, Tham TN, Casanova P, Arenzana-Seisdedos F, Dubois-Dalcq M. Role of the alpha-chemokine stromal cell-derived factor (SDF-1) in the developing and mature central nervous system. *Glia.* 2003;42:139–148.
109. Oh JW, Van Wagoner NJ, Rose-John S, Benveniste EN. Role of IL-6 and the soluble IL-6 receptor in inhibition of VCAM-1 gene expression. *J Immunol.* 1998;161:4992–4999.
110. Stein JV, Nombela-Arrieta C. Chemokine control of lymphocyte trafficking: a general overview. *Immunology.* 2005;116:1–12.
111. Kunkel EJ, Butcher EC. Plasma-cell homing. *Nat Rev Immunol.* 2003;3:822–829.
112. Lindelof B, Granath F, Tengvall-Linder M, Ekbom A. Allergy and cancer. *Allergy.* 2005;60:1116–1120.
113. Melbye M, Smedby KE, Lehtinen T, et al. Atopy and risk of non-Hodgkin lymphoma. *J Natl Cancer Inst.* 2007;99:158–166.
114. Grulich AE, Vajdic CM, Riminton S, Hughes AM, Kricker A, Armstrong BK. Re: Atopy and risk of non-Hodgkin lymphoma. *J Natl Cancer Inst.* 2007;99:1417.

8 Glioma Survival and Prognosis

Jeffrey S. Chang, Margaret R. Wrensch, Terri Rice, and James L. Fisher

Clinical trials as well as population registry data collect information on glioma survival and prognosis. Although studies from clinical trial groups provide useful information on prognostic factors for cases whose pathology has been centrally reviewed, most patients do not enter clinical trials. Thus, the results might not be applicable to, or representative of, the general population of patients with glioma. Although survival estimates from population registry data represent all patients diagnosed with glioma, these are potentially less precise than those from clinical trials because of substantial variation in diagnostic criteria over time and geographic region [1,2]. Population registry data are also limited by the fact that many patients are diagnosed by pathologists who have not had specific neuropathology training [3] and registries do not generally have as complete treatment data as is available in clinical trials. Detailed and regularly updated population-based survival data for glioma and other primary brain tumors are available through the Central Brain Tumor Registry of the United States (www.cbtrus.org) [4].

Histologic type and grade, age, extent of resection, tumor location, radiation therapy, and some chemotherapy regimens have been consistently and convincingly linked to survival in both population registry and clinical trial data [4–12] Histologic grade is an especially strong predictor of survival. For example, only 9% of glioblastoma (GM, grade IV) patients but 83% of patients with grade II oligodendroglial tumors survive 2 years or more [4].

A key unsolved problem in neuro-oncology is the very strong and consistent inverse relationship of age with survival; for example, in glioblastoma, the 2-year survival rate is approximately 30% for patients younger than 45 years, but only 3% for those diagnosed after 65 years. The reasons for this variation, whether due to properties related to the tumor or the host, are not well understood. It has been observed that in older patients, response to radiation is worse [13]. In this regard, one contributing factor may be related to different frequencies of molecular or chromosomal aberrations among tumors from older patients compared with those from younger patients.

In addition to age, glioblastoma survival may be associated with Karnofsky Performance Scale score, extent of resection, location and resectability, degree of necrosis, enhancement on preoperative magnetic resonance imaging studies, volume of residual disease, therapeutic approach, pre- and postoperative tumor size, noncentral tumor location (defined as infiltration of splenium, basal ganglia, thalamus, or midbrain), patient deterioration, patient condition before radiation therapy, and presurgical serum albumin level [14–18].

However, studying glioma survival is complicated by the very narrow range of survival times experienced by the vast majority of patients with malignant glioma. It is difficult to identify prognostic factors when there is not much difference in survival time between long-term and short-term survivors.

For low-grade (I and II) gliomas diagnosed in US Surveillance, Epidemiology, and End Results areas from 1973 to 2001, Claus and Black [14] reported better survival for females, whites versus non-Whites, and patients undergoing surgery only versus those undergoing surgery and radiation, radiation only, or no treatment as the first course of treatment. This latter factor is highly confounding, as only the higher risk low-grade glioma patients fall in the surgery plus radiation, or radiation only, or observation only categories, whereas the lowest risk patients typically undergo only surgery.

Recent efforts to identify prognostic factors for glioblastoma and other glioma subtypes have focused on genetic factors and molecular markers, which are described in the following text.

STUDIES OF TUMOR MARKERS IN RELATION TO SURVIVAL

It is now well established that the combined loss of 1p and 19q confers a more favorable prognosis for oligodendrogliomas [19]. Although results are inconsistent, and effects may be modified by other factors, such as age, there is some evidence that the following are prognostic indicators for glioblastoma and possibly some other glioma subtypes: p53 mutation and expression [20–29], overexpression or amplification of epidermal growth factor receptor (EGFR) [20–24,29], mutations in, loss of, or epigenetic silencing of the *PTEN* gene, CDKN2A alterations and deletions [20,21,23], and MDM2 amplifications [20,23,28–30]. A subset of tumors with EGFR amplification shows an additional change in the *EGFR* gene resulting from partial loss of the extracellular ligand-binding domain, called EGFR vIII, which results in constitutively activated signaling through the EGFR pathway, without the requirement of receptor-ligand binding and consequential receptor-receptor dimerization. A recent study showed that conventional prognostic factors for glioblastoma did not accurately predict outcome in patients whose tumors were EGFR vIII positive, although these results need to be confirmed [31]. Also interestingly, this study showed that glioblastoma patients whose tumor was negative both for EGFR vIII and expression of YKL-40 had better than expected survival. EGFR expression in patients with anaplastic astrocytoma was associated with nearly 3-fold poorer survival [29]; these patients had comparable survival with patients histologically diagnosed with glioblastoma. A recent study also showed that co-over expression of *EGFR/IGFBP-2/HIF-2A* genes was more predictive of poor prognosis than overexpression of any one individual marker.

Age-dependent associations between glioblastoma survival and 1p and CDKN2A have also been demonstrated [21]. Immunohistochemical studies show that p53 protein expression probably decreases with advancing age [21,32], and the association between p53 expression and survival from glioblastoma lost when adjusted for age in multivariate analysis. Loss of heterozygosity on chromosome 10q has been associated with shorter duration of survival from glioblastoma [26,33], and combined loss of heterozygosity on 1p and 19q may afford a more favorable prognosis to glioblastoma patients [26].

Other glioma tumor markers linked to survival have included geminin-labeling index [34], expression of cleaved caspase-3 [35], and expression of survivin in both the nucleus and the cytoplasm [36].

A post hoc unplanned subset analysis from a prospective trial of newly diagnosed glioblastoma suggested that methylation of the *MGMT* promoter in glioblastoma tumor samples was a marker of improved outcome, as measured by 2-year survival rate [37]. Interestingly, *MGMT* methylation appeared to be much more strongly associated with survival among patients who received front-line temozolomide as compared to those who did not [38], raising the possibility that *MGMT* methylation may be a predictive marker of response to this alkylating agent.

Insights From Expression Array Studies of Gliomas

Although some *a priori* candidate genes have been validated in large-scale expression array studies [39,40], many new genes whose expression had not been previously linked to glioma survival have recently been identified. Abnormal expression in certain classes of genes predicts survival. For example, in one report, best, intermediate, and worst survival were associated with abnormal expression of neurogenesis genes, cell proliferation and mitosis genes, and extracellular and extracellular matrix genes, respectively [40]. Other important findings are that loss of chromosome 10 was accompanied by gene expression changes across the genome and copy number loss of 10 and gains of 7, 19, and 20 were highly correlated with one another [39]. These findings, although compelling, are nevertheless preliminary due to the relatively small sample sizes typical of expression array studies. Candidate markers identified in such genome-wide screens, however, represent promising leads for possible validation in larger studies. A recent array study of oligodendroglioma and oligoastrocytoma found that tumor gain of 8q may be a negative prognostic factor [41].

CONSTITUTIVE GENETIC POLYMORPHISMS AND GLIOMA SURVIVAL

Several studies have assessed the prognosis of glioma associated with constitutive genetic polymorphisms (Table 8.1). Previous studies, most of which did not carry out multivariate analysis, showed that the overexpression or amplification of EGFR is a prognostic factor for glioblastoma and other glioma subtypes [21,23,29]. Therefore, it is logical to assess the constitutive genetic polymorphisms of *EGFR* gene and its ligand, epidermal growth factor (*EGF*), as potential prognostic factors for glioma. Only one study to date has assessed glioma survival associated with EGFR polymorphisms and found that the replacement of the G allele by a T allele at position 216 increases the promoter activity by 30% [54], and is associated with a modest improvement in median survival [42]. Based on a small number of (GM) subjects (31 *de novo* and 11 secondary GMs), Bhowmick et al [43] observed a significant association between *EGF* 61 A/G (rs4444903) and GM survival, with a more favorable survival for those with AA genotype compared to those with GA or GG genotypes. This result was not confirmed by two subsequent studies [44,45], though one of those two studies reported a borderline association between *EGF* 61 A/G and recurrence of GM [45].

Two studies have assessed the association between *TP53*, a tumor suppressor gene, and glioma survival [46,47]. Idbaih et al [46] reported no significant association between *TP53* 72 Arg/Pro (rs1042522) and oligodendroglioma survival. Similarly, Limas-Ramos et al [47] also reported no association between *TP53* 72 Arg/Pro and the survival of all glioma patients or of either GM or oligodendroglioma patients. However, among 42 glioma patients treated with adjuvant therapy, those with Arg/Pro or Pro/Pro genotypes had a longer median survival compared to those with the Arg/Arg genotype. *CHEK2*, another tumor suppressor gene, has been examined for its association with glioma survival. Simon et al [48] studied *CHEK2* rs2017309 A/T among GM cases, and found that those with AA genotype had the worst survival compared to those with AT or TT genotype; however, this association was no longer significant after adjusting for other prognostic factors including age, Karnofsky Performance Score, and postoperative treatment.

Carcinogen-metabolizing genes not only detoxify cancer causing chemicals but also determine the rates at which chemotherapeutic agents are excreted from the human body and thus influence the efficacy of therapy. Okcu et al [49] observed that among 78 patients with grade 3 gliomas, those with combined *GSTP1 *A/*A* and GSTM1-null genotypes survived longer than the rest of the group. A subsequent study by Wrensch et al [29] was not able to confirm the result observed by Okcu et al and reported a significantly shorter glioma survival for those with GSTT1-null genotype.

Table 8.1 Studies of Constitutive Genetic Polymorphisms and Glioma Survival

Author, Year, Location, Reference Genetic Polymorphisms Evaluated	Subject Recruitment	Type of Specimen Genotyped	Kaplan Meier Results	Cox Proportional Hazard Results (unless indicated otherwise)	Comments
EGFR/EGF					
Carpentier et al, 2006, France [42] EGFR -216 G/T -191 C/A	188 histologically confirmed glioblastoma multiforme (GM) cases without previous history of glioma, age ≥18, had clinical data and follow-up data, had blood DNA sample, and gave informed consent were identified from one hospital from 1997 to 2006.	Peripheral blood	*Overall survival* EGFR-**216 G/T** TT: 18.3 months GT+ GG = 14.4 months ($p = 0.05$) EGFR-**191C/A** Results were not presented		1. Survival analysis was not adjusted for any covariates.
Bhowmick et al, 2004, USA [43] EGF 61 A/G (rs4444903)	42 consecutive unselected GM patients with fresh tissue sample identified at a hospital. 31 were de novo GM and 11 were secondary GM.	Tumor tissue	*Progression free survival* AA: 9.14 months GA+GG: 5.64 months ($p = 0.04$)		1. Genotyping was performed on tumor tissue which may have undergone genetic mutations. 2. Survival analysis was not adjusted for any covariates. 3. Small sample size.
Costa et al, 2007, Portugal [44] EGF 61 A/G (rs4444903)	197 consecutive glioma patients, including 79 GM and 66 oligodendroglioma cases newly diagnosed at two hospitals, with available tumor materials. These 197 cases represented 60% of the glioma patients diagnosed between January 1990 and December 2004.	Tumor tissue	*Overall survival* GM: $p = 0.37$ Oligodendroglioma: ($p = 0.46$)		1. Genotyping was performed on tumor tissue that may have undergone genetic mutations; however, in 20 glioma cases where peripheral blood DNA was available, genotypes of the tumor tissue DNA and peripheral blood DNA were 100% concordant. 2. Survival analysis was not adjusted for any covariates.
Vauleon et al, 2007, France [45] EGF 61 A/G (rs4444903)	209 GM patients (mean age 55.9, range 22–83, overall survival = 16.5 months) selected from a neuro-oncology database out of 849 patients treated for GM from 1998 to 2004 (mean age 56.2, range 17–83, overall survival = 15 months). Eligibility criteria included histologically confirmed GM, age ≥18 years, clinical and follow-up data available in the database, no previous history of glioma, informed consent obtained, and blood and tumor sample available.	Peripheral blood	*Progression free survival* AA: 8.6 months AG: 8.2 months GG: 9.55 months ($p = 0.05$) *Overall survival* AA: 19 months AG: 16.5 months GG: 16.1 months ($p = 0.45$)	*Hazard ratio* AA: 1.0 AG: 1.3 (0.9–1.8) GG: 1.2 (0.7–1.8) (Cox proportional hazard regression model was performed adjusting for age, type of surgery, and postoperative treatment.)	

Continued

Table 8.1 Continued

Author, Year, Location, Reference Genetic Polymorphisms Evaluated	Subject Recruitment	Type of Specimen Genotyped	Kaplan Meier Results	Cox Proportional Hazard Results (unless indicated otherwise)	Comments
Tumor suppressor gene Idbaih et al, 2007, France [46] TP53 72 Arg/Pro (rs1042522)	275 patients with primary oligodendroglial tumors diagnosed between January 1995 and November 2006, with available blood DNA and paraffin-embedded tumor block, were selected from the tumor database of one hospital.	Peripheral blood	*Overall survival* Arg/Arg: 96.3 months Arg/Pro: median survival not reached Pro/Pro: median survival not reached ($p = 0.86$)		1. Survival analysis was not adjusted for any covariates.
Lima-Ramos et al, 2007, Portugal [47] TP53 72 Arg/Pro (rs1042522)	171 patients with glioma were identified from two hospitals. All patients were from northwestern Portugal and of European-origin ethnic background with a mean age of 49.5 years and 52.6% were male.	Tumor tissue	*Overall survival* **All 117[a] glioma patients** Arg/Arg vs. Arg/Pro vs. Pro/Pro ($p = 0.97$) No significant association was observed for GM and oligodendroglioma (Data were not shown) **42 glioma patients treated with adjuvant therapy** 5-year analysis: Arg/Arg: 13 months Arg/Pro: 24 months Pro/Pro: 57 months ($p = 0.03$) No statistical difference was observed in the 10-year analysis.		1. Genotyping was performed on tumor tissue that may have undergone genetic mutations. 2. Survival analysis was not adjusted for any covariates. 3. Small sample size for analysis with 42 glioma patients treated with adjuvant therapy.
Simon et al, 2006, Germany [48] CHEK2 rs2017309 A/T	213 patients newly diagnosed with primary GM, with available blood or tumor tissue were identified in one hospital between September 1994 and March 2003.	145 patients had peripheral blood samples, and 68 had tumor tissues only.	*Overall survival* **All 213 GM cases** AA patients had the worst survival compared to AT or TT ($p = 0.03$) **28 GM cases with postoperative chemo and radiotherapy** AA: no patients AT: 10.5 months TT: 15.5 months ($p = 0.008$)	Multivariate analysis[b] indicated that age, KPS, and postoperative treatment but not CHEK2 allele status are significant prognostic factors.	1. Genotyping was performed on tumor tissue for 68/213 patients. 2. Small sample size for analysis with 28 GM patients with postoperative chemo and radiotherapy.

Study	Sample		Results	Limitations
Carcinogen-metabolizing gene				
Okcu et al, 2004, USA [49] GSTM1 null GSTT1 null GSTP1 105 Ile/Val (rs1695) 114 Ala/Val (rs1138272) *A: 105Ile114Ala *B: *C: 105Val114Ala *D: 105Val114Val 105Ile114Val	278 patients were selected from 1594 patients with primary malignant glioma consecutively diagnosed and treated at one cancer center. Eligibility criteria were age <65 years at diagnosis, had complete medical records and peripheral blood DNA sample, diagnosed <1 year before the registration date, and consented to participate in the study.	Peripheral blood	*Overall survival* GSTM1 Null: 19.8 months Not null: 22.7 months ($p > 0.05$) GSTT1 Null: 21.6 months Not null: 21.4 months ($p > 0.05$) GSTP1 *A/*A: 27.0 months Others: 18.3 months ($p > 0.05$)	*Hazard ratio*[c] **All cases** GSTM1 Not null: 1.0 Null: 0.99 (0.70–1.40) GSTT1 Not null: 1.0 Null: 1.2 (0.73–1.80) GSTP1 not *A/*A: 1.0 *A/*A: 1.34 (0.95–1.89) **High Grade**[d] GSTP1 *A/*A and GSTM1 null 1.0 GSTP1 not *A/*A and GSTM1 null 0.7 (0.2–2.6) GSTP1 *A/*A and GSTM1 not null 0.5 (0.2–2.0) GSTP1 not *A/*A and GSTM1 not null 0.8 (0.2–3.1) **Medium Graded** GSTP1 *A/*A and GSTM1 null 1.0 GSTP1 not *A/*A and GSTM1 null 0.8 (0.2–3.0) GSTP1 *A/*A and GSTM1 not null 1.0 (0.3–3.8) GSTP1 not *A/*A and GSTM1 not null 0.2 (0.04–1.3)	1. Sample size was small for assessing gene-histology interactions.
Wrensch et al, 2006, USA [29] GSTT1 null EPHX1 139 Arg/His (rs2234922)	471 patients with glioma diagnosed between August 1991 and April 1994 (series 1) and between May 1997 and August 1999 (series 2) who resided in six San Francisco Bay Area counties at the time of diagnosis.	Peripheral blood or buccal specimen	*Over all survival months* All GM AA GSTT1 Not null 20.5 13.2 22.9 Null 17.2 10.2 14.7 EPHX1 139 His/His 19.9 12.9 19.1 His/Arg 27.0 14.1 NA Arg/Arg 30.7 9.7 NA	*Hazard ratio*[e] (null vs. not null) GSTT1 All Glioma 1.64 (1.25–2.16) Glioblastoma 1.54 (1.08–2.20) Anap. Astro. 1.74 (0.71–4.31) EPHX1 139 His/Arg[f] All Glioma 0.82 (0.64–1.05) Glioblastoma 0.95 (0.70–1.30) Anap. Astro. 0.14 (0.04–0.49)	
Immune function				
Tang et al, 2005, USA [50] HLA-A HLA-B HLA-C HLA-DRB1	155 GM patients diagnosed between August 1991 and April 1994 (series 1) and between May 1997 and August 1999 (series 2) who resided in six San Francisco Bay Area counties at the time of diagnosis, were non-Hispanic white, and had sufficient blood for DNA extraction.	Peripheral blood		*Hazard ratio* Other HLA type: 1.00 (reference) HLA-A*32: 0.40 (0.20–0.79) HLA-B*55: 2.26 (1.23–4.15) (Cox proportional hazard regression model was performed adjusting for age and gender.)	

Continued

Table 8.1 Continued

Author, Year, Location, Reference Genetic Polymorphisms Evaluated	Subject Recruitment	Type of Specimen Genotyped	Kaplan Meier Results			Cox Proportional Hazard Results (unless indicated otherwise)	Comments
Wrensch et al., 2006, USA [29]	471 patients with glioma diagnosed between August 1991 and April 1994 (series 1) and between May 1997 and August 1999 (series 2) who resided in six San Francisco Bay Area counties at the time of diagnosis.	Peripheral blood or buccal specimen	*Overall survival months*			*Hazard ratio*[f]	
CCR5 delta32				All	GM	AA	CCR5 delta32
IL4R			CCR delta 32				All Glioma 0.72 (0.52–0.98)
75 Ile/Val (rs1805010)			Homo.	19.5	12.2	20.6	GM 0.62 (0.41–0.93)
400 Glu/Ala (rs1805011)			not delta				Anap. Astro. 0.66 (0.16–2.68)
431 Cys/Arg (rs1805012)			Hetero.	30.6	14.9	30.7	**IL4R 75 Ile/Val**
503 Ser/Pro (rs1805015)			Homo. delta	150.9	NA	NA	All Glioma 0.87 (0.74–1.02)
576 Gln/Arg (rs1801275)							GM 0.84 (0.68–1.03)
752 Ser/Ala (rs1805016)			**IL4R 75 Ile/Val**				Anap. Astro. 0.87 (0.55–1.37)
			Ile/Ile	20.4	10.7	25.3	**IL4R 400 Glu/Ala**
			Ile/Val	18.1	12.7	20.7	All Glioma 0.78 (0.63–0.97)
			Val/Val	24.6	15.8	30.5	GM 0.82 (0.63–1.06)
			IL4R 400 Glu/Ala				Anap. Astro. 0.55 (0.27–1.15)
			Glu/Glu	18.5	12.3	20.0	**IL4R 431 Cys/Arg**
			Glu/Ala	21.7	12.8	46.8	All Glioma 0.76 (0.59–0.98)
			Ala/Ala	30.1	10.6	NA	GM 0.78 (0.57–1.07)
			IL4R 431 Cys/Arg				Anap. Astro. 0.60 (0.27–1.34)
			Cys/Cys	18.2	11.7	20.0	**IL4R 503 Ser/Pro**
			Cys/Arg	24.5	13.2	46.8	All Glioma 0.84 (0.68–1.04)
			Arg/Arg	43.7	19.0	NA	GM 0.82 (0.64–1.07)
			IL4R 503 Ser/Pro				Anap. Astro. 0.46 (0.24–0.91)
			Ser/Ser	18.5	12.4	19.7	**IL4R 576 Gln/Arg**
			Ser/Pro	19.9	12.4	38.1	All Glioma 0.85 (0.70–1.02)
			Pro/Pro	85.2	19.0	NA	GM 0.80 (0.63–1.01)
			IL4R 576 Gln/Arg				Anap. Astro. 0.54 (0.31–0.93)
			Gln/Gln	18.5	11.3	19.7	**IL4R 752 Ser/Ala**
			Gln/Arg	19.9	13.2	38.1	All Glioma 1.02 (0.73–1.41)
			Arg/Arg	25.5	17.9	NA	GM 0.95 (0.63–1.43)
			IL4R 752 Ser/Ala				Anap. Astro. 0.43 (0.16–1.16)
			Ser/Ser	19.9	12.5	20.1	**Number of IL4R variants**
			Ser/Ala	17.4	12.8	36.2	All Glioma 0.95 (0.89–1.00)
							IL4R **haplotype** with variants in all positions except 752 Ser/Ala
							All Glioma 0.64 (0.47–0.87)
DNA repair Wrensch et al., 2006, USA [29]	471 patients with glioma diagnosed between August 1991 and April 1994 (series 1) and between May 1997 and August 1999 (series 2) who resided in six San Francisco Bay Area counties at the time of diagnosis.	Peripheral blood or buccal specimen	*Overall survival months*			*Hazard ratio*[e]	
ERCC1			ERCC1 **8092 C/A**	All	GM	AA	ERCC1 **8092 C/A**
8092 C/A			C/C	18.1	11.1	20.1	All Glioma 0.72 (0.60–0.86)
MGMT			A/C	20.1	13.5	38.1	GM 0.73 (0.59–0.91)
84 Leu/Phe (rs12917)			A/A	23.4	17.4	NA	Anap. Astro. 0.57 (0.27–1.21)
XRCC1			MGMT **84 Leu/Phe**				MGMT **84 Leu/Phe**
280 His/Arg (rs25489)			Leu/Leu	19.8	12.4	30.7	All Glioma 1.03 (0.82–1.31)
			Leu/Phe	19.2	12.6	19.1	GM 0.91 (0.65–1.27)
			Phe/Phe	NA	NA	17.9	Anap. Astro. 1.77 (1.05–2.96)
			XRCC1 **280 His/Arg**				XRCC1 **280 His/Arg**
			His/His	20.0	12.7	20	All Glioma 1.32 (0.94–1.87)
			His/Arg	15.2	11.0	NA	GM 1.47 (0.93–2.33)
							Anap. Astro. 0.88 (0.29–2.67)

Study	Sample	Source	Overall survival	Hazard ratio[g]	Limitations
Chromosome 19q Yang et al, 2005, USA [51] ERCC2 rs1052555 C/T CD3EAP (ASE-1) rs3212986 C/A GLTSCR1 rs1035938 C/T	141 glioma patients who underwent surgical resection between December 1987 and December 2001, and had enough tumor samples and donated a blood sample.	Peripheral blood	*Overall survival* GLTSCR1 TT: 77% and 68% survival at 2 and 5 years. CT/CC: 56% and 34% survival at 2 and 5 years. ($p = 0.02$) ERCC2 **C/T** Not significant (Data not shown) CD3EAP (ASE-1) **C/A** Not significant (Data not shown)	*Hazard ratio[g]* *Grade <4, age < 57 years:* GLTSCR1 **CT or CC**, ERCC2 **CC** 1.0 *Grade <4, age < 57 years:* GLTSCR1 **TT** 0.11 (0.02–0.85) *Grade = 4, age ≥ 48 years:* GLTSCR1 **TT** 8.67 (4.51–16.68)	1. Small sample size ($n = 20$) for patients with SS genotypes.
Telomerase hTERT gene Wang et al, 2006, USA [52] MNS16A, which is a polymorphic tandem repeat in the downstream region of the hTERT gene. MNS16 has four alleles and are classified as either short (S) or long (L).	A subset of 299 de novo GM patients were identified from 2113 glioma patients consecutively diagnosed at a cancer center from 1994 to 2003. The eligibility criteria included the availability of complete medical records and peripheral blood DNA. Only non-Hispanic white patients were included in the analysis.	Peripheral blood	*Overall survival* SS: 25.1 months SL: 14.7 months LL: 14.6 months ($p = 0.04$)	*Hazard ratio* SL or LL vs. SS: HR = 1.78 (1.11–2.85) (Cox proportional hazard regression model, adjusting for age at diagnosis, sex, extent of surgery, chemotherapy, and interval between registration and surgery treatments.)	
Carpentier et al, 2007, France [53] hTERT MNS16A S/L	352 glioma patients (205 glioblastoma and 147 anaplastic gliomas), age ≥18 years, had clinical and follow-up data, and blood DNA sample.	Peripheral blood	hTERT MNS16A S/L GM SS: 15.8 months SL: 15.3 months LL: 16.8 months ($p = 0.625$) Anaplastic gliomas SS: 30.6 months SL: 31.8 months LL: 36.7 months ($p = 0.975$)	MNS16A was not significant in the multivariate analysis for survival (Multivariate analysis for overall survival, adjusting for age and the extent of surgery [biopsy + partial removal vs. complete removal].)	1. Small sample sizes (GM $n = 25$; anaplastic glioma $n = 27$) for patients with SS genotypes.

Abbreviations: AA or Anap Astro., anaplastic astrocytoma; All, all gliomas; GM, glioblastoma; Hetero., heterozygous; Homo., homozygous.

[a] Only 117 of the 171 with available survival and treatment data were included in the survival analysis.

[b] Multivariate analysis was performed and adjusted for age, degree of resection, postoperative radiotherapy, postoperative chemotherapy, and postoperative Karnofsky Performance Scale (KPS) Score.

[c] Cox proportional hazard regression model was performed and adjusted for age, degree of resection, postoperative radiotherapy, postoperative chemotherapy, and postoperative Karnofsky Performance Scale (KPS) Score.

[d] High Grade includes GM and Gliosarcoma. Medium grade includes Anaplastic astrocytoma, Anaplastic oligodendroglioma, Anaplastic oligo/astro, and Anaplastic ependymoma.

[e] Cox proportional hazard regression model was performed adjusting for age, gender, ethnicity (White/non-White), series, and types of treatment received.

[f] Hazard ratio associated with one copy of the variant allele.

[g] Cox proportional hazard regression model and classification and regression tree (CART) was performed with all 7 SNPs adjusting for tumor type, gender, race/ethnicity, age, geographic region of residence, tumor grade, primary vs recurrent tumor, and initial place of diagnosis.

As discussed previously, one of the most consistent findings among studies of glioma is the inverse association between glioma and allergies [55–64]. Wrensch et al [29] reported that several single-nucleotide polymorphisms (SNPs) and one haplotype of *IL4R*, the gene that codes for the receptor of the key Th2 cytokine IL4, were significantly associated with glioma survival. Tang et al [50] studied human leukocyte antigen (HLA), which plays a key role in immune function, and found that HLA-A*32 was associated with longer survival whereas HLA-B*55 was associated with shorter survival in GM patients.

Epigenetic silencing of MGMT, a DNA repair gene, by methylation of its promoter was associated with better outcomes among glioblastoma patients treated with radiotherapy and the alkylating agent temozolomide [65]. Thus, constitutive genetic polymorphisms that affect the expression of DNA repair genes may also be prognostic for glioma survival. Of the three DNA repair SNPs [*ERCC1* 8092 C/A, *MGMT* 84 Leu/Phe (rs12917), and XRCC1 280 His/Arg (rs25489] studied by Wrensch et al, [29] only *ERCC1* 8092 C/A was significantly associated with glioma survival, with a better prognosis for those who carried A alleles.

The loss of chromosome 19q is commonly observed in gliomas [66] and the candidate genes located in that chromosomal region may be important for both the etiology and progression of glioma. Yang et al [51] studied the association between three SNPs of three genes located on chromosome 19q (*ERCC2* rs1052555, *ASE-1* rs3213986, and *GLTSCR1* rs1035938) and the survival of patients with oligodendroglioma and found using univariate analysis that only *GLTSCR1* rs1035938 is a significant prognostic factor. Further exploration of gene-environment interactions showed a joint influence between age, grade of the tumor, ERCC2 rs1052555 and *GLTSCR1* rs1035938 on oligodendroglioma survival [51].

Two studies have examined the influence of the telomerase *hTERT* gene on glioma survival [52,53]. Telomerase activity is detected more often among higher-grade gliomas [67], and the high level of hTERT expression has been shown to be predictive of worse survival [68]. MNS16A is a polymorphic tandem repeat in the downstream region of the *hTERT* gene and it has four alleles that are classified as either short (S) or long (L) [69]. The S allele of MNS16 was associated with increased hTERT mRNA expression [69]. Wang et al [52] reported that GM patients with either SL or LL genotypes had significantly shorter survival. This result was not confirmed by Carpentier et al [53] who found no difference in the survival of GM or anaplastic glioma patients by MNS16 polymorphisms. The numbers of patients with SS genotype were small ($n<30$) in both studies, which could have made their results statistically unreliable.

Although several studies have suggested the potential roles of constitutive genetic polymorphisms as prognostic factors for glioma survival, results from published studies are inconclusive for the following reasons: (a) all of the polymorphisms have only been examined by a few studies (three or fewer), thus, the evidence for replication is lacking; (b) most studies have a small sample size, and (c) some studies did not adjust for other prognostic factors in their survival analyses.

SEROLOGIC AND IMMUNOLOGIC FACTORS

In addition to tumor markers and constitutive genetic factors, investigators have begun to explore the role of serologic factors. A large population-based case-control study found that glioblastoma patients with elevated immunoglobulin (Ig)E lived 9 months longer, compared to those with lower or normal IgE levels [29]. As discussed in other chapters, there is consistent and compelling evidence of protection against glioma as the result of allergies and immune-related conditions. A recent report indicates that amplification of interleukin(IL)-6, a cytokine which may promote glioblastoma, is significantly associated with decreased glioblastoma survival [70]. Analyses of atopy, IgE, and cytokines in relation to glioma prognosis may help us to better understand the complex nature of immunological response to gliomagenesis, including secreted tumor-specific factors and host immune responses, and such investigations may also have important implications for immunological therapy of glioma. Future studies should also include the examination of T-cell activities such as that of T-regulatory cells, which have been associated with tissue graft acceptance as well as brain tumor prognosis [71,72].

SUMMARY

An increasing spectrum of methods for interrogating molecular changes in genes, methylation patterns, chromosome numbers, transcripts, and proteins in tumors is allowing a much greater understanding of the complexities of changes in glial tumors. New technologies allow rapid genotyping of hundreds of thousands of inherited variants. With developing bioinformatic and statistical tools, investigators are examining the associations of survival with inherited variants both individually and in the context of biologic pathways. Furthermore, researchers are exploring the effects of immune status of patients on prognosis. In addition to efforts of individual investigators and research groups, The Cancer Genome Atlas (TCGA) (www.cancergenome.com), organized by the National Cancer Institute and the National Human Genome Research Institute, is a comprehensive and coordinated effort to accelerate our understanding of the molecular basis of cancer through the application of genome analysis technologies, including large-scale genome sequencing. Gliomas are the first cancer to be studied through the TCGA and early results are available to glioma researchers through the internet. These and other resources should accelerate our understanding of the biologic mechanisms responsible for glioma and thereby lay the groundwork for preventive and therapeutic strategies.

ACKNOWLEDGMENTS

Some of this material has been previously published by the authors [73,74]. The work was supported by R01 CA52689, P50 CA97257, and Dr. Jeffrey S. Chang was also supported by the National Cancer Institute (R25 CA112355).

REFERENCES

1. Karak AK, Singh R, Tandon PN, Sarkar C. A comparative survival evaluation and assessment of interclassification concordance in adult supratentorial astrocytic tumors. *Pathol Oncol Res.* 2000;6:46–52.
2. Coons SW, Johnson PC, Scheithauer BW, Yates AJ, Pearl DK. Improving diagnostic accuracy and interobserver concordance in the classification and grading of primary gliomas. *Cancer.* 1997;79:1381–1393.
3. Aldape K, Simmons ML, Davis RL, et al. Discrepancies in diagnoses of neuroepithelial neoplasms: the San Francisco Bay Area Adult Glioma Study. *Cancer.* 2000;88:2342–2349.
4. CBTRUS. *Primary Brain Tumors in the United States, Statistical Report 1998–2002.* Chicago, IL: Central Brain Tumor Registry of the United States; 2005–2006.
5. Curran WJ Jr, Scott CB, Horton J, et al. Recursive partitioning analysis of prognostic factors in three Radiation Therapy Oncology Group malignant glioma trials. *J Natl Cancer Inst.* 1993;85:704–710.
6. Davis FG, Freels S, Grutsch J, Barlas S, Brem S. Survival rates in patients with primary malignant brain tumors stratified by patient age and tumor histological type: an analysis based on Surveillance, Epidemiology, and End Results (SEER) data, 1973–1991. *J Neurosurg.* 1998;88:1–10.
7. Davis FG, McCarthy B, Jukich P. The descriptive epidemiology of brain tumors. *Neuroimaging Clin N Am.* 1999;9:581–594.
8. Horn B, Heideman R, Geyer R, et al. A multi-institutional retrospective study of intracranial ependymoma in children: identification of risk factors. *J Pediatr Hematol Oncol.* 1999;21:203–211.
9. Lamborn KR, Chang SM, Prados MD. Prognostic factors for survival of patients with glioblastoma: recursive partitioning analysis. *Neuro Oncol.* 2004;6:227–235.
10. Levin V, Liebel S, Gutin P. Neoplasms of the central nervous system (section 2). In: DeVita VTJ, Hellman S, Rosenberg SA, eds. *Cancer: Principles and Practice of Oncology.* 6th ed. Philadelphia, PA: Lipincott, Williams and Wilkins; 2001:2100–2160.
11. Scott JN, Rewcastle NB, Brasher PM, et al. Long-term glioblastoma multiforme survivors: a population-based study. *Can J Neurol Sci.* 1998;25:197–201.
12. Scott JN, Rewcastle NB, Brasher PM, et al. Which glioblastoma multiforme patient will become a long-term survivor? A population-based study. *Ann Neurol.* 1999;46:183–188.
13. Barker FG II, Chang SM, Larson DA, et al. Age and radiation response in glioblastoma multiforme. *Neurosurgery.* 2001;49:1288–1297; discussion 97–98.
14. Claus EB, Black PM. Survival rates and patterns of care for patients diagnosed with supratentorial low-grade gliomas: data from the SEER program, 1973–2001. *Cancer.* 2006;106:1358–1363.
15. Jeremic B, Milicic B, Grujicic D, Dagovic A, Aleksandrovic J. Multivariate analysis of clinical prognostic factors in patients with glioblastoma multiforme treated with a combined modality approach. *J Cancer Res Clin Oncol.* 2003;129:477–484.
16. Lacroix M, Abi-Said D, Fourney DR, et al. A multivariate analysis of 416 patients with glioblastoma multiforme: prognosis, extent of resection, and survival. *J Neurosurg.* 2001;95:190–198.
17. Lutterbach J, Sauerbrei W, Guttenberger R. Multivariate analysis of prognostic factors in patients with glioblastoma. *Strahlenther Onkol.* 2003;179:8–15.
18. Schwartzbaum JA, Lal P, Evanoff W, et al. Presurgical serum albumin levels predict survival time from glioblastoma multiforme. *J Neurooncol.* 1999;43:35–41.
19. Aldape K, Burger PC, Perry A. Clinicopathologic aspects of 1p/19q loss and the diagnosis of oligodendroglioma. *Arch Pathol Lab Med.* 2007;131:242–251.
20. Backlund LM, Nilsson BR, Liu L, Ichimura K, Collins VP. Mutations in Rb1 pathway-related genes are associated with poor prognosis in anaplastic astrocytomas. *Br J Cancer.* 2005;93:124–130.
21. Batchelor TT, Betensky RA, Esposito JM, et al. Age-dependent prognostic effects of genetic alterations in glioblastoma. *Clin Cancer Res.* 2004;10:228–233.
22. Deb P, Sharma MC, Mahapatra AK, Agarwal D, Sarkar C. Glioblastoma multiforme with long term survival. *Neurol India.* 2005;53:329–332.
23. Houillier C, Lejeune J, Benouaich-Amiel A, et al. Prognostic impact of molecular markers in a series of 220 primary glioblastomas. *Cancer.* 2006;106:2218–2223.
24. Layfield LJ, Willmore C, Tripp S, Jones C, Jensen RL. Epidermal growth factor receptor gene amplification and protein expression in glioblastoma multiforme: prognostic significance and relationship to other prognostic factors. *Appl Immunohistochem Mol Morphol.* 2006;14:91–96.
25. McLendon RE, Herndon JE II, West B, et al. Survival analysis of presumptive prognostic markers among oligodendrogliomas. *Cancer.* 2005;104:1693–1699.
26. Schmidt MC, Antweiler S, Urban N, et al. Impact of genotype and morphology on the prognosis of glioblastoma. *J Neuropathol Exp Neurol.* 2002;61:321–328.
27. Stander M, Peraud A, Leroch B, Kreth FW. Prognostic impact of TP53 mutation status for adult patients with supratentorial World Health Organization Grade II astrocytoma or oligoastrocytoma: a long-term analysis. *Cancer.* 2004;101:1028–1035.
28. Ushio Y, Tada K, Shiraishi S, et al. Correlation of molecular genetic analysis of p53, MDM2, p16, PTEN, and EGFR and survival of patients with anaplastic astrocytoma and glioblastoma. *Front Biosci.* 2003;8:e281-e288.
29. Wrensch M, Wiencke JK, Wiemels J, et al. Serum IgE, tumor epidermal growth factor receptor expression, and inherited polymorphisms associated with glioma survival. *Cancer Res.* 2006;66:4531–4541.
30. Ranuncolo SM, Varela M, Morandi A, et al. Prognostic value of Mdm2, p53 and p16 in patients with astrocytomas. *J Neurooncol.* 2004;68:113–121.
31. Pelloski CE, Ballman KV, Furth AF, et al. Epidermal growth factor receptor variant III status defines clinically distinct subtypes of glioblastoma. *J Clin Oncol.* 2007;25:2288–2294.
32. Simmons ML, Lamborn KR, Takahashi M, et al. Analysis of complex relationships between age, p53, epidermal growth factor receptor, and survival in glioblastoma patients. *Cancer Res.* 2001;61:1122–1128.
33. Ohgaki H, Dessen P, Jourde B, et al. Genetic pathways to glioblastoma: a population-based study. *Cancer Res.* 2004;64:6892–6899.
34. Shrestha P, Saito T, Hama S, et al. Geminin: a good prognostic factor in high-grade astrocytic brain tumors. *Cancer.* 2007;109:949–956.
35. Kobayashi T, Masumoto J, Tada T, Nomiyama T, Hongo K, Nakayama J. Prognostic significance of the immunohistochemical staining of cleaved caspase-3, an activated form of caspase-3, in gliomas. *Clin Cancer Res.* 2007;13:3868–3874.
36. Saito T, Arifin MT, Hama S, et al. Survivin subcellular localization in high-grade astrocytomas: simultaneous expression in both nucleus and cytoplasm is negative prognostic marker. *J Neurooncol.* 2007;82:193–198.
37. Stupp R, Mason WP, van den Bent MJ, et al. Radiotherapy plus concomitant and adjuvant temozolomide for glioblastoma. *N Engl J Med.* 2005;352:987–996.
38. Hegi ME, Diserens AC, Gorlia T, et al. MGMT gene silencing and benefit from temozolomide in glioblastoma. *N Engl J Med.* 2005;352:997–1003.
39. Nigro JM, Misra A, Zhang L, et al. Integrated array-comparative genomic hybridization and expression array profiles identify clinically relevant molecular subtypes of glioblastoma. *Cancer Res.* 2005;65:1678–1686.
40. Freije WA, Castro-Vargas FE, Fang Z, et al. Gene expression profiling of gliomas strongly predicts survival. *Cancer Res.* 2004;64:6503–6510.
41. Kitange G, Misra A, Law M, et al. Chromosomal imbalances detected by array comparative genomic hybridization in human oligodendrogliomas and mixed oligoastrocytomas. *Genes Chromosomes Cancer.* 2005;42:68–77.
42. Carpentier C, Laigle-Donadey F, Marie Y, et al. Polymorphism in Sp1 recognition site of the EGF receptor gene promoter and risk of glioblastoma. *Neurology.* 2006;67:872–874.
43. Bhowmick DA, Zhuang Z, Wait SD, Weil RJ. A functional polymorphism in the EGF gene is found with increased frequency in glioblastoma multiforme patients and is associated with more aggressive disease. *Cancer Res.* 2004;64:1220–1223.
44. Costa BM, Ferreira P, Costa S, et al. Association between functional EGF+61 polymorphism and glioma risk. *Clin Cancer Res.* 2007;13:2621–2626.
45. Vauleon E, Auger N, Benouaich-Amiel A, et al. The 61 A/G EGF polymorphism is functional but is neither a prognostic marker nor a risk factor for glioblastoma. *Cancer Genet Cytogenet.* 2007;172:33–37.
46. Idbaih A, Boisselier B, Marie Y, et al. TP53 codon 72 polymorphism, p53 expression, and 1p/19q status in oligodendroglial tumors. *Cancer Genet Cytogenet.* 2007;177:103–107.

47. Lima-Ramos V, Pacheco-Figueiredo L, Costa S, et al. TP53 codon 72 polymorphism in susceptibility, overall survival, and adjuvant therapy response of gliomas. *Cancer Genet Cytogenet.* 2008;180:14–19.
48. Simon M, Ludwig M, Fimmers R, et al. Variant of the CHEK2 gene as a prognostic marker in glioblastoma multiforme. *Neurosurgery.* 2006;59:1078–1085; discussion 85.
49. Okcu MF, Selvan M, Wang LE, et al. Glutathione S-transferase polymorphisms and survival in primary malignant glioma. *Clin Cancer Res.* 2004;10:2618–2625.
50. Tang J, Shao W, Dorak MT, et al. Positive and negative associations of human leukocyte antigen variants with the onset and prognosis of adult glioblastoma multiforme. *Cancer Epidemiol Biomarkers Prev.* 2005;14:2040–2044.
51. Yang P, Kollmeyer TM, Buckner K, Bamlet W, Ballman KV, Jenkins RB. Polymorphisms in GLTSCR1 and ERCC2 are associated with the development of oligodendrogliomas. *Cancer.* 2005;103:2363–2372.
52. Wang L, Wei Q, Wang LE, et al. Survival prediction in patients with glioblastoma multiforme by human telomerase genetic variation. *J Clin Oncol.* 2006;24:1627–1632.
53. Carpentier C, Lejeune J, Gros F, et al. Association of telomerase gene hTERT polymorphism and malignant gliomas. *J Neurooncol.* 2007;84:249–253.
54. Liu W, Innocenti F, Wu MH, et al. A functional common polymorphism in a Sp1 recognition site of the epidermal growth factor receptor gene promoter. *Cancer Res.* 2005;65:46–53.
55. Hochberg F, Toniolo P, Cole P, Salcman M. Nonoccupational risk indicators of glioblastoma in adults. *J Neurooncol.* 1990;8:55–60.
56. Ryan P, Lee MW, North B, McMichael AJ. Risk factors for tumors of the brain and meninges: results from the Adelaide Adult Brain Tumor Study. *Int J Cancer.* 1992;51:20–27.
57. Schlehofer B, Blettner M, Becker N, Martinsohn C, Wahrendorf J. Medical risk factors and the development of brain tumors. *Cancer.* 1992;69:2541–2547.
58. Cicuttini FM, Hurley SF, Forbes A, et al. Association of adult glioma with medical conditions, family and reproductive history. *Int J Cancer.* 1997;71:203–207.
59. Schlehofer B, Blettner M, Preston-Martin S, et al. Role of medical history in brain tumour development. Results from the international adult brain tumour study. *Int J Cancer.* 1999;82:155–160.
60. Wiemels JL, Wiencke JK, Sison JD, Miike R, McMillan A, Wrensch M. History of allergies among adults with glioma and controls. *Int J Cancer.* 2002;98:609–615.
61. Brenner AV, Linet MS, Fine HA, et al. History of allergies and autoimmune diseases and risk of brain tumors in adults. *Int J Cancer.* 2002;99:252–259.
62. Schwartzbaum J, Jonsson F, Ahlbom A, et al. Cohort studies of association between self-reported allergic conditions, immune-related diagnoses and glioma and meningioma risk. *Int J Cancer.* 2003;106:423–428.
63. Schoemaker MJ, Swerdlow AJ, Hepworth SJ, McKinney PA, van Tongeren M, Muir KR. History of allergies and risk of glioma in adults. *Int J Cancer.* 2006;119:2165–2172.
64. Schwartzbaum J, Ahlbom A, Malmer B, et al. Polymorphisms associated with asthma are inversely related to glioblastoma multiforme. *Cancer Res.* 2005;65:6459–6465.
65. Hegi ME, Diserens AC, Godard S, et al. Clinical trial substantiates the predictive value of O-6-methylguanine-DNA methyltransferase promoter methylation in glioblastoma patients treated with temozolomide. *Clin Cancer Res.* 2004;10:1871–1874.
66. Schwartzbaum JA, Fisher JL, Aldape KD, Wrensch M. Epidemiology and molecular pathology of glioma. *Nat Clin Pract Neurol.* 2006;2:494–503; quiz 1 p following 16.
67. Le S, Zhu JJ, Anthony DC, Greider CW, Black PM. Telomerase activity in human gliomas. *Neurosurgery.* 1998;42:1120–1124; discussion 4–5.
68. Boldrini L, Pistolesi S, Gisfredi S, et al. Telomerase activity and hTERT mRNA expression in glial tumors. *Int J Oncol.* 2006;28:1555–1560.
69. Wang L, Soria JC, Chang YS, Lee HY, Wei Q, Mao L. Association of a functional tandem repeats in the downstream of human telomerase gene and lung cancer. *Oncogene.* 2003;22:7123–7129.
70. Tchirkov A, Khalil T, Chautard E, et al. Interleukin-6 gene amplification and shortened survival in glioblastoma patients. *Br J Cancer.* 2007;96:474–476.
71. Fecci PE, Mitchell DA, Whitesides JF, et al. Increased regulatory T-cell fraction amidst a diminished CD4 compartment explains cellular immune defects in patients with malignant glioma. *Cancer Res.* 2006;66:3294–3302.
72. Yong Z, Chang L, Mei YX, Yi L. Role and mechanisms of CD4+CD25+ regulatory T cells in the induction and maintenance of transplantation tolerance. *Transpl Immunol.* 2007;17:120–129.
73. Fisher JL, Schwartzbaum JA, Wrensch M, Wiemels JL. Epidemiology of brain tumors. *Neurol Clin.* 2007;25:867–890, vii.
74. Wrensch M, Fisher JL, Schwartzbaum JA, Bondy M, Berger M, Aldape KD. The molecular epidemiology of gliomas in adults. *Neurosurg Focus.* 2005;19:E5.

9 Epidemiology of Childhood Brain Tumors

Tarik Tihan, John K. Wiencke, Pedram Razavi, and Roberta McKean-Cowdin

INTRODUCTION

An estimated 20,000 new patients are diagnosed with malignant central nervous system (CNS) tumors in the United States every year. This number accounts for 2.0% of all newly diagnosed cancers. Furthermore, approximately 12,000 patients die with malignant CNS tumors, which constitutes 5% of all cancer deaths annually [1]. The combined incidence of benign and malignant CNS tumors is more than twice that of malignant tumors alone [2]. In 2007, 43,800 patients were diagnosed with CNS tumors in the United States, of which approximately 3750 were children between 0 and 19 years of age [2]. CNS tumors are the leading cause of cancer deaths among children and the second most common form of cancer diagnosed among children following leukemia. Five-year survival rates for children 0 to 14 years of age at diagnosis improved from 57% between 1975 and 1977 to 74% between 1996 and 2003 [1]. However, survival can vary significantly depending on tumor histology and location. Many survivors of childhood brain tumors suffer severe neurocognitive deficits [3] or multiple late health effects including second primary malignancies resulting from treatment [4]. Despite interest in the disease due to its severity with respect to both morbidity and mortality, the etiology of the majority of CNS tumors remains unknown. Inherited syndromes that predispose affected individuals to CNS tumor development appear to be present in less than 5% of patients. Some environmental agents such as ionizing radiation are clearly implicated in the etiology of CNS tumors in a limited number of cases. Numerous other physical, chemical, and infectious agents have been suspected but not established as etiologically relevant risk factors.

In this chapter, we focus on both benign and malignant CNS tumors. The review discusses the new World Health Organization (WHO) 2007 classification system of CNS tumors as well as the importance of incorporating a standard, reproducible classification system into the successful design of epidemiological studies of childhood brain tumors. The review also includes a description of the incidence pattern of childhood brain tumors over time, the current understanding of environmental risk factors for the disease, and the genetic characteristics of the disease including the molecular genetic characteristics, constitutive genetic variation, and epigenetic regulation.

DEFINITION AND CLASSIFICATION OF CHILDHOOD BRAIN TUMORS

Childhood brain tumors include more than 100 different histological types and subtypes, and exhibit remarkable heterogeneity both within and among tumors, making accurate pathological diagnosis critical. More than 90% of tumors can be adequately classified using the current 2007 WHO classification scheme. The current WHO classification for adult and childhood brain tumors is based purely on morphological criteria and the "cell of origin" paradigm. The WHO categories and histological types are largely reproducible and well accepted in the pediatric neuro-oncology community. According to this classification scheme, neoplasms can be graded based on a four-tiered grading system: grade I CNS tumors are often well-circumscribed, progressing slowly, and can be cured by resection; grade II tumors are typically infiltrative with low proliferation rate, but have a higher likelihood of local recurrence; grade III tumors are histologically malignant and generally require more aggressive treatment; grade IV tumors are highly malignant and usually fatal. In addition, WHO 2007 identifies entities, variants and tissue patterns, only the latter of which have limited or no apparent prognostic significance.

The current WHO classification scheme does not consider childhood tumors as different entities from adult tumors, and ignores the mounting data that childhood and adult tumors of the same histological type may have distinctly different etiological factors and pathogenetic mechanisms. Another important issue is the changing definition of entities in three revisions of the scheme in 1993, 2000, and in 2007. Although many definitions of tumor types remained fairly constant through this evolution, comparisons of cases collected during pre-1993, between 1993 and 2000, and post-2007 periods require special consideration, especially if the tumors are to be segregated in large categories containing more than one histological type. Other challenges in the classification scheme include the fact that the accuracy of pathological diagnosis is often dependent on the experience and expertise of the (neuro) pathologist.

Epidemiologists face the challenge of establishing and developing accurate case ascertainment protocols to increase the probability of identifying homogeneous tumor groups in multi-institutional studies. Improving comparability of diagnostic results from different centers would ease such a task, and allow better interpretation of the results with respect to etiological hypotheses. Because of the potential for environmental and developmental differences among tumor entities, and because earlier epidemiological research (when childhood brain tumors were lumped into large, nonspecific categories) has not identified many risk factors, it is reasonable to think about splitting the tumor types for future studies. This requires larger sample. This approach has been successful in other tumor types with much higher incidence, but it is distinctly challenging for childhood brain tumors. Such studies require a strong effort to consolidate working groups into larger, and possibly nationwide consortia to retain statistical power while maintaining uniformity of the data gathering, and then split histological types to see if the data may trigger new hypotheses and help us learn more about risk factors. To accomplish this task, a coordinated effort that allows easy comparison, merging of data, and collection of comprehensive information from all children with brain tumors will be necessary, and requires a novel approach to the organization and funding of such research.

While the histological diversity of childhood brain tumors should not be ignored, four simplistic and broad categories are presented here to provide an overview: neuroepithelial tumors, embryonal tumors, glioneuronal tumors, and others (including more than 50 types and variants).

Neuroepithelial Tumors

Neuroepithelial tumors constitute a large and heterogeneous group of neoplasms, and contain the two most common tumor types seen in children; *pilocytic astrocytoma (9421/1) and ependymoma (9391/3)*. While *pilocytic astrocytoma* is coded as a malignant neoplasm by SEER (code 9421/3) for purposes of ascertainment, it is clearly a biologically indolent neoplasm with high probability long-term (>20 years) overall survival. Pilocytic astrocytomas have been considered WHO grade I neoplasms in all three versions of the WHO classification schemes. A new addition to the WHO 2007 scheme is the *pilomyxoid astrocytoma (9425/3-provisional)*, a more aggressive variant that corresponds to WHO grade II tumor. This less common variant of pilocytic astrocytoma has been historically included in the pilocytic astrocytoma groups. Diagnoses such as "cerebellar astrocytoma," "juvenile astrocytoma," and the majority of "optic gliomas" in children are in fact pilocytic astrocytomas, but may not have been recorded as such in earlier studies.

One critically important bit of knowledge that has developed over the last two decades is the need to distinguish infiltrating gliomas from localized or circumscribed gliomas. While the latter is often an indolent tumor with limited potential for recurrence, the former represents a spectrum that can progress and transform into higher grade tumors. Thus, diffuse astrocytoma (9400/3), anaplastic astrocytoma (9401/3), and glioblastoma (9440/3) constitute a continuum. Infiltrating astrocytomas also include most of the tumors known as "pontine glioma" or "bithalamic glioma."

Ependymomas constitute another large group within the glioma family, and although they often grow as solid masses, they have the ability to spread through the leptomeninges, cerebrospinal spaces, and even infiltrate the parenchyma. There are a number of ependymoma variants and tissue patterns, and their exact epidemiological and clinical significance is unclear. It is also critically important to identify variants such as *subependymoma (9383/1)*, and *myxopapillary ependymoma (9394/1)*, since they appear to behave in a distinctly more indolent manner, while the *clear-cell ependymoma* (9391/3; same code as classical ependymoma) seems to be more aggressive. Age, location, histological type and grade all seem to be critical factors in the study of these neoplasms. A number of genetic alterations have been identified in ependymomas, and their relevance is still being investigated.

Choroid plexus neoplasms (9390), for which there are now three types—*papilloma (9390/0)*, *atypical papilloma (9390/1-provisional)*, and *carcinoma (9390/3)*—are rare but predominantly occur in childhood. The *atypical choroid plexus papilloma* is a new addition to WHO 2007 classification scheme. Another neuroepithelial tumor group, *oligodendroglioma (9450/3)* is distinctly rare in children. Even when an exceptional oligodendroglioma is recognized in a child, the biological, genetic, and clinical characteristics differ quite strikingly from its adult counterpart.

Many additional tumor types and variants exist within the neuroepithelial tumor category. A new addition to the WHO 2007 is the so-called *angiocentric glioma (9431/1-provisional)*, a tumor with a unique histological appearance, more common to children, and remains poorly characterized to date. *Pleomorphic xanthoastrocytoma (9424/3)*, a tumor often confused with glioblastoma, and *subependymal giant cell astrocytoma (9384/1)*, are other examples that predominate in the young age, the latter being associated with the Tuberous Sclerosis Complex. *Astroblastomas (9430/3)* and *chordoid gliomas (9444/1)* are enigmatic members of this neuroepithelial tumor category and can be seen during childhood, even though the latter is more common in adults.

Embryonal Tumors

The most critical entity in this group is *medulloblastoma (9470/3)*, and there is significant progress in our understanding of the biology, but not the epidemiology of such tumors. With the recognition of histological variants, came our recognition of unique genetic alterations correlating with these subgroups. Medulloblastomas constitute one of the three most common tumor types in children, and the genes altered in variants of medulloblastoma also participate in the development of the cerebellum.

An important discovery is the *atypical teratoid/rhabdoid tumor (9508/3)*, a rare tumor with a unique genetic signature. While the histological, radiological and genetic features of the patients afflicted with this tumor is known, there is no study that links these features with a possible etiological agent beyond that of the well-characterized mutation of the *hSNF5/INI-1* gene.

Glioneuronal Tumors

The greatest expansion and diversification in the WHO 2007 classification scheme has occurred in the category of glioneuronal tumors. *Ganglioglioma (9505/1)* is the most typical and most common form of this group. Such novel entities such as *papillary glioneuronal tumor (9509/1-provisional)*, *rosette-forming glioneuronal tumor of the 4th ventricle (9509/1-provisional)*, and *extraventricular neurocytoma (9506/1-provisional)*, all of which sound like morphological descriptions rather than a specific entity, have emerged with the WHO 2007 classification. Our understanding of these tumors is rudimentary at best.

Other Childhood Brain Tumor Types

Many other tumors including primary germ cell tumors such as *teratoma (9080/1)*, pineal tumors (9361,9362), and *Craniopharyngioma (9350/1)*, peripheral nerve sheath tumors such as *neurofibroma (9540/0)* and *meningioma (9530/0)*, mesenchymal tumors such as *rhabdomyosarcoma (8900/3)*, and so on, are often placed in the "other" category because of their rarity, and the difficulty of gathering sufficient numbers of cases for epidemiological studies.

DESCRIPTIVE EPIDEMIOLOGY

Distribution by Gender, Race/Ethnicity, and Age

Brain tumors are the most common solid tumor in children less than 19 years of age. Of all childhood brain tumors, 52% are astrocytomas, 9% are ependymomas, 15% are other gliomas, and 21% are primitive neuroectodermal tumors (PNETs) or medulloblastomas. The overall age-adjusted incidence rates reported by the Central Brain Tumor Registry of the United States (CBTRUS) for males and females less than 19 years of age are 12.07 and 10.97 per 100,000, respectively [5]. Incidence rates overall are higher for males than females, but the male-to-female ratio varies by histological type of tumor. For example, incidence rates by gender are similar for pilocytic astrocytomas and other astrocytomas, but PNET/medulloblastomas and ependymomas are more frequent in males [6]. Incidence rates for childhood brain tumors are significantly lower among African-American children than among white children [5]. Racial differences in incidence rates vary, from one histological type of brain tumor to another. For example, the rate of neuroepithelial tumors is lower among African-American children than among white children, but the reverse is true for meningiomas [5]. The different histological types of childhood brain tumors have characteristic age distributions. Astrocytomas have two incidence peaks at 5 and 13 years of age, while ependymoma incidence peaks at age 2 and is rare among children aged 5 to 14. PNET/medulloblastomas peak in incidence at age 4 years [7]. Differences in histology-specific incidence rates by gender, race, and age suggest that different genetic or environmental risk factors may contribute to subgroups of brain tumors.

Trends

From the early 1970s through the mid 1990s incidence rates of childhood brain tumors steadily increased in the United States (see Figure 9.1), leading to speculation that the rising rates of brain tumors were being driven by changes in the environment or changes in lifestyle factors. Age-adjusted incidence rates of childhood brain tumors increased by 2% per year from 1973 to 1990, but were approximately level from 1990 through 2004 (annual percent change was not statistically significantly different from zero) [8]. The reason for the dramatic increase in the 1970s and 1980s is a continuing matter of debate. A discussion of these trends in two reports, based on analyses of SEER incidence data and National Center for Health Statistics mortality data, found that the changing patterns of incidence and mortality were consistent with increasing use of better diagnostic equipment—in particular computed tomography (CT) and magnetic resonance imaging (MRI) [9,10]. Legler et al [9] found that from 1975 to 1995 incidence rates were significantly increasing only among children less than 15 years of age and adults 65 years of age and older. During this same time period, mortality declined for the youngest age group suggesting that more low-grade tumors (better prognoses) were being diagnosed or that existing tumors were being identified and treated more effectively. Smith et al argued that improvements in diagnostic procedures and changes

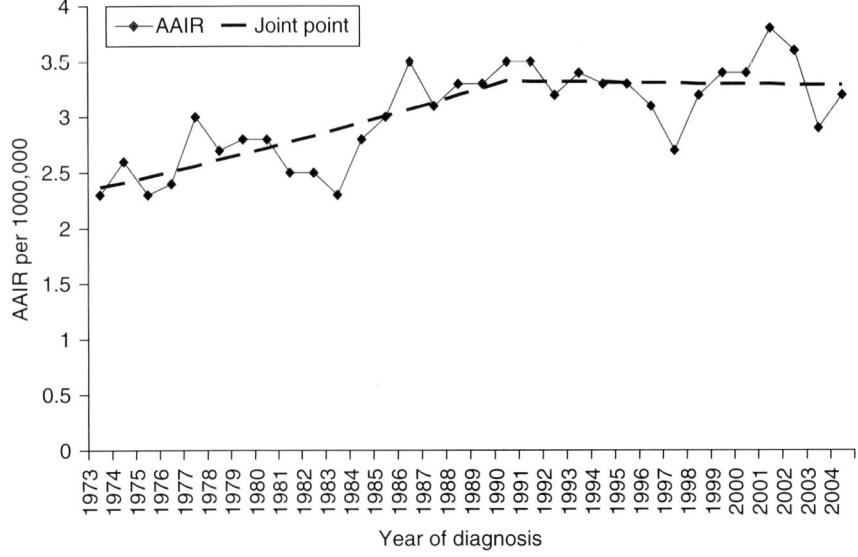

Figure 9.1 Age-adjusted incidence rate (AAIR) per 100,000 and best fit JoinPoint line for primary brain cancer by year of diagnosis for children 0 to 14 years of age, SEER, 1973 to 2004. *Age-adjusted to the 2000 US standard population.

in histological classification could explain the trends; these changes could result in the identification of new tumors or the classification of some tumors as malignant that previously would have been coded as benign [10]. Increasing rates were largely restricted to brain stem and low-grade cerebral tumors that could be explained by improvements in imaging equipment. Others have argued that large numbers of brain tumors in children would not have gone undetected [11–13]. The rise and stabilization of rates at a higher level could be consistent with a new environmental exposure causing new cases of brain tumors; however, no clear environmental factor to explain this pattern of change has been identified.

SUGGESTED CAUSES OF HUMAN CHILDHOOD BRAIN TUMORS

Environmental Risk Factors

This section reviews findings from epidemiological studies, which have investigated the association between various potential risk factors and childhood brain tumors. A summary of studies investigating these associations have been described in recent review articles [14]. Most studies of environmental factors have examined all brain tumors as a single entity, rather than by histological subtype. Results are described by histological groups when important differences were reported.

Ionizing Radiation

High-dose exposure to ionizing radiation is the only established environmental cause of brain tumors; the evidence supporting this association has been reviewed in detail in chapter 5 (Exposure to Ionizing Radiation and Glioma Risk). Briefly, several studies have shown an excess risk of brain tumors following exposure to high-dose therapeutic radiation (2500 cGy) for primary malignancies or benign conditions [15–17]. One of the strongest pieces of evidence supporting an association between therapeutic doses of ionizing radiation and brain tumor risk comes from an Israeli cohort study of adults irradiated as children for tinea capitis [18–21]. A significant excess of nervous system tumors also was found in atomic-bomb survivors, with those exposed during childhood having higher risks than survivors exposed as adults [22]. The relationship between brain tumors and low-dose diagnostic radiation is less certain [23–29]. A pooled analysis of two Swedish cohort studies found that exposure to low-level ionizing radiation during infancy was associated with an elevated risk of brain tumors and that risk was highest among children exposed before 5 months of age [30]. A more recent study of exposure to maternal prenatal pelvic x-rays found no association with pediatric brain cancer [31].

Nonionizing Radiation

Electromagnetic Fields

Electromagnetic fields (EMFs) from residential power lines and home electronics became a public health concern in the late 1970s when it was first reported that children living near high current power lines were potentially at increased risk of dying from leukemia and brain cancer [32]. This finding was controversial because extremely low-frequency EMFs (50–60 hertz) associated with power lines are not known to be genotoxic [33] or carcinogenic, however there is some evidence they may act as tumor promoters [34]. In the 1990s, numerous studies of electric and magnetic fields were completed to investigate the potential association with child and adult brain tumor risk, which have been described in several review articles [35–37]. While early studies of childhood brain tumors and residential EMFs exposure found significantly elevated risks based on power line wire-code configuration [32,38], these findings were not replicated in later studies using various exposure assessment methods including wire-code configuration [39,40], calculated magnetic fields [41–44], or direct measurements in the child's home [38,40,45,46]. Methodological limitations of studies have included the following: small sample sizes, in particular small numbers of subjects with high levels of exposure; challenges with retrospective exposure assessment; lack of a standardized reference interval for the evaluation of magnetic fields; and potential residual confounding due to unmeasured variables [47]. Other studies have looked for associations between electrical appliances used by the mother during pregnancy and childhood brain tumors; elevated risks were found for use of some individual electrical appliances, but findings were not consistent across studies [48,49]. Overall, the biological and epidemiological data do not support an association between residential EMF and childhood brain tumors, but the question remains open due to limitations in study design.

Occupational Exposures

Parental occupational exposure as a risk factor for childhood brain tumors has been investigated in numerous epidemiological studies [14,50–52]. High-risk jobs have been reported in most published studies, but few findings have been replicated more than once. Associations have been reported between childhood brain tumors and parental occupational exposures in both the pre-and postnatal periods [53–66], suggesting that multiple routes of exposure may be relevant, including exposure of the parents during the preconception period, transplacental exposures to the fetus, or direct exposure to the child from occupational chemicals or agents brought home by the parent on the clothing or skin. At least two studies reported increased risk of brain tumors for children whose fathers were employed as machinists [55,66,67], electrical workers [58,64,67], or in the aerospace and aircraft [56,61,62], agricultural [63], [67],or chemical industries [57,60,62,64]. While these job categories may suggest specific chemicals or agents for further investigation (eg, solvents, pesticides), none of the studies were able to recreate detailed exposure histories or had large enough numbers of individuals in a single employment group to implicate a specific exposure. One study specifically designed to examine polycyclic aromatic hydrocarbons (PAHs) found risk of PNETs was twice as high among fathers with occupational PAH exposure as those who were not exposed (odds ratio [OR] = 2.0; 95% confidence interval [CI]: 1.0–4.0) [68]. Similarly, a recent international case-control study found increased risk of all childhood brain tumors associated with paternal occupational exposure to PAH during the preconception period (OR = 1.3; 95% CI: 1.1–1.6) [69].

The inconsistency of findings across studies may be attributed in part to: the small sample sizes common to rare disease studies (leading to imprecise risk estimates), the different geographical areas (with different major industries) studied, the variation across studies in histological types of childhood brain tumors, differences in ages at diagnosis, or changes in industrial processes and agents over time. Studies of occupational job titles are further limited by the fact that occupation is acting as a surrogate for exposure to environmental agents, rather than an actual measurement of exposure.

Pesticides

Numerous epidemiological studies have investigated residential and occupational use of pesticides, insecticides, or herbicides as possible etiological factors for brain tumors [70]. Pesticides are designed to act on the nervous system and in some cases, may also be carcinogenic [71]. An occupational study of licensed pesticide applicators found an excess risk of adult brain cancer among licensed workers (SMR = 200) [72] and a case-control study found that occupational exposure to pesticides was associated with increased risk of adult gliomas (relative risk [RR] = 1.8; 95% CI: 0.6–5.1) [73]. Residential use of pesticides has been associated with risk of childhood brain tumors in one study [74], and specifically with maternal handling of flea and tick products during the child's pregnancy (OR = 1.7; 95% CI: 1.1–2.6) in another. Risk was strongest for children diagnosed under 5 years of age and a dose-response was found with number of pets treated [75]. Elevated but marginal associations were found for a case-control study of paternal occupational exposure to herbicides or fungicides (OR = 1.6; 95% CI: 1.0–2.6) and maternal exposure to insecticides (OR = 1.9; 95% CI: 1.1–3.3) with astrocytomas [76]. Associations of brain tumors with residential or occupational exposures to pesticides are suggestive, but additional work is needed to confirm the associations and evaluate the types of agents that may be neurocarcinogenic.

Nitroso Compounds

Although various chemical, physical and biological agents can cause nervous system tumors in experimental animals, N-nitroso compounds (NOCs), in particular the nitrosoureas, are by far the most specific and potent neurocarcinogens [77]. NOCs and their precursors are experimental carcinogens that have been investigated as potential causes of brain tumors in humans [77,78]. NOCs are divided into two major categories based on their chemical structure—nitrosamines and nitrosamides. Nitrosamines are carcinogenic in animal studies, but have never been shown to cause tumors in the nervous system [79]. Nitrosamides are direct acting agents that can cause DNA adducts and have been shown to be potent nervous system carcinogens in various species [80,81]. Ethylnitrosourea (ENU), a type of nitrosamide, has been shown to be a neurocarcinogen in rats, mice, rabbits, opossums, and monkeys through various routes of administration and when given in a single dose or through chronic low-dose exposure [82]. Transplacental exposure is the most potent route of exposure, as only one-fiftieth (1/50) of the dose of ENU required to induce tumors in adult animals is necessary to cause tumors in all fetal animals [83].

Population Exposure to NOC

The major sources of population exposure to NOCs in the United States are tobacco smoke, cosmetics, automobile interiors, cured meats, and some types of pesticides [78]. Only nitrosamines (not nitrosamides) have been widely measured in human environments and consumer products due to technical ability, even though many of these sources probably involve both nitrosamines and nitrosamides. Endogenous formation of NOCs in the stomach or bladder when both an amino compound and a nitrosating agent are present simultaneously is likely to be the primary source of human exposure to nitrosamides. Food is a major source of both highly concentrated nitrite solutions (eg, from cured meats) and amino compounds (eg, in fish and other foods, but also in many drugs). Another source of nitrite is reduction (eg, in the saliva) from nitrate which comes predominantly from vegetables in the diet; this source is likely to be a far less important contributor to the NOC formed endogenously because it is highly diluted (and, therefore, less readily reactive) and because vegetables also contain vitamins which inhibit the nitrosation reaction. Drinking water also contains nitrate (in the absence of vitamins), but this is a minor source unless levels are very high [84]. The level of NOC in the human body is also influenced by other factors such as presence of amino compounds, nitrosation inhibitors (eg, vitamins C or E), bacteria or other nitrosation catalysts, gastric pH, and other physiological factors. The active interaction of NOC precursors, inhibitors, and catalysts make this hypothesis a challenge to study.

Diet and Vitamin Supplementation

The majority of hypotheses regarding dietary factors and brain tumors have focused on cured meats, antioxidants, and inhibitors of nitrosation, including vitamins C and E. Eight of ten epidemiological studies which investigated the role of cured meats [48,85–93] during pregnancy found a significant positive association between the frequency of maternal cured meat intake by the mother and the risk of brain tumors. The individual foods most consistently found to be associated with increased risk were hot dogs and bacon. In a study of adults, serum levels of ascorbic acid (vitamin C) and alpha- and gamma-tocopherol (vitamin E) were both inversely related to glioblastoma risk [94]. Further, high intake of fruits and vegetables has been associated with lower risk of childhood brain tumors in several studies (maternal intake of fruits and vegetables during pregnancy) [93,95], and has also been reported in a number of studies of adult brain tumors [25,96]. Specifically, a case-control study of childhood PNET found significant protective trends with increasing levels of dietary vitamins A, C, β-carotene, and folate by the mother during pregnancy. In a related study of childhood astrocytoma, reduced risks were evident for dietary vitamins A and C, however these trends were not significant. An international case-control study from eight geographical areas in North America, Europe, and Israel suggested that maternal vitamin supplementation use for two trimesters may decrease the risk of brain tumors (OR 0.7, 95% CI: 0.5–0.9), with a lower risk with longer duration of use (p trend = 0.0007) [97]. A more recent study of maternal diet and PNET/medulloblastomas found an inverse association between fruit intake and risk, but no significant protective association for fruit juices, vegetables, or folate. There was no relationship of dietary β-carotene or folate with childhood astrocytoma. Although preliminary dietary results are promising, findings must be interpreted with caution because dietary histories were focused primarily on NOCs. Comprehensive dietary evaluations are necessary to evaluate the role of all possible dietary risk factors.

The apparent reduction in risk of brain tumors associated with fruits, vegetables, and vitamin intake may be interpreted as supportive of the NOC hypothesis due to the inhibition of the endogenous formation of NOCs in the presence of Vitamins C or E. The apparent protective effect also may be due to another mechanism such as the inhibition of free radical formation in the brain.

Prior Head Injury or Infection

Head Injury

Head injury may theoretically contribute to brain tumor risk by increasing cellular proliferation and inflammation [98]. Several case reports and series provide anecdotal evidence that prior head trauma is associated with brain tumor development. One report describes a case of malignant glioma occurring in the same spot where a man suffered a metal splinter injury 37 years earlier [99], most previous case reports of this sort have involved meningiomas [100]. An international case-control study of head injury and brain cancer risk found an increased risk, specifically for meningioma, among men who had a serious head injury 15 to 24 years before diagnosis [101]. Other investigators have found a weak relationship between injury and meningiomas [102]. Large studies from Sweden and Denmark have not found associations between head injury and risk [103,104]. Childhood brain tumors, which are predominantly neuroepithelial tumors, have sometimes been associated with birth trauma (eg, prolonged labor, forceps delivery, Caesarean section) [105]. Other studies have reported a slight increase in risk of childhood brain tumors among children who previously received medical treatment for a head injury, but found no association with birth trauma [105]. Because parents may be more likely to report a prior head injury for children with a brain tumor, it may be prudent to limit trauma histories to injuries of a certain minimum severity (such as those requiring medical attention or hospitalization) to minimize recall bias.

Infectious Agents

Several types of viruses cause brain tumors in experimental animals including: retro, papova, adeno, JC [106], BK, and simian immunodeficiency viruses (SV) [107]. In one of the earliest epidemiological studies of brain tumors, astrocytomas were associated with positive antibody titers to *Toxoplasma gondii* [108]; however more recent studies have failed to confirm this association [109]. It is believed that over 62% of the United States population have been exposed to SV40, a member of the *Polyomaviridae* family, through administration of contaminated polio vaccine between 1955 and 1963 [110–113]. Early animal studies showed that the virus was carcinogenic [114,115]. The tumorogenicity of JC and BK viruses has been well established through several *in vitro* and animal experimental studies [116–121], JC and BK viral DNA sequences have been isolated from a number of human CNS tumors including medulloblastoma, ependymoma, and gliomas [122–126]. A meta-analyses of studies measuring viral DNA or protein found that SV40 was significantly associated with brain tumors (OR = 3.9) and has specifically been found in brain tumors of infants and children [127].

Other studies have found associations between risk of maternal infections during pregnancy and childhood brain tumors. Bithell et al [128] found an increased risk of brain tumors among children of mothers who had chickenpox during their pregnancy. A case-control study of childhood brain tumors found that mothers with documented viral infections during pregnancy (eg, varicella, herpes zoster, rubella, mumps) were 11 times as likely to have a child with a brain tumor as mothers without infection [129]. Further, risk associated with likely exposure to viral infections from influenza or respiratory infection was double that of unexposed women [129].

Tobacco

Overall, the epidemiological data does not support an association between maternal smoking during pregnancy and risk of brain tumors, as described in a review [130] and meta-analyses [131,132]. However, a recent prospective study of 1.4 million Swedish births found an association between maternal smoking during pregnancy and risk of brain tumors (RR 1.24; 95% CI: 1.01–1.53) [133]. A meta-analysis of 10 studies found a small increase in risk (OR = 1.2; 95% CI: 1.1–-1.4) in relation to paternal smoking during pregnancy [131]. Paternal smoking also was associated with a 40% increase in risk of childhood astroglial tumors in a population-based case-control study [134].

Predisposing Genetic Syndromes and Familial Occurrence

Various hereditary syndromes have been associated with increased brain tumor risk including neurofibromatosis-1 and 2, Von Hippel-Lindau disease, Li-Fraumeni syndrome, tuberous sclerosis, and Gorlin's syndrome. However, these hereditary syndromes are rare and are likely to account for small numbers of cases in a population-based series of CNS neoplasia [135].

There are few studies of familial aggregation of CNS tumors. One study found that Connecticut children with CNS tumors were more likely to have relatives with nervous system tumors than control children, but this familial pattern was observed for fewer than 2% of the children with CNS tumors. Medulloblastoma and glioblastoma were over represented among children whose relatives had nervous system tumors [136]. Population-based studies that have studied predisposing genetic syndromes and familial aggregations suggest that the proportion of brain tumors attributable to highly penetrant, genetic traits is no more than 4% [137].

Molecular Genetic and Epigenetic Characteristics

Advances in molecular genetics is of growing importance for the correct classification of brain tumors, as well as the prediction of patient prognosis and treatment response. Details have been described in recent reviews [138–145]. As with other human malignancies, the pathogenesis of brain tumors is known to be associated with inactivation of tumor suppressor genes, and/or the activation of oncogenes [139], which may occur through several mechanisms including gene mutation, chromosomal loss, chromosomal amplification, or methylation. In the sections below we focus on several of the more common molecular genetic characteristics of brain tumors.

Chromosomal Loss

Molecular studies of adult gliomas indicate frequent loss of heterozygosity (LOH) at chromosomal regions 1p, 9p, 10q, 17p, 19q, and 22q [139,143] suggesting inactivation of tumor suppressor genes in these regions may contribute to the development of gliomas. In contrast, loss of these chromosomal regions in childhood gliomas is less frequent [144]. LOH 10q is one of the most frequent genetic alteration in gliomas, occurring in 40% to 50% of astrocytomas (grade II–III) [146] and 60% to 80% of glioblastomas [147–150]. Loss of one specific tumor suppressor gene on chromosome 10, PTEN, is associated with high-grade tumors in adults and has been observed in 15% to 40% of adult glioblastomas [142,151,152], but occurs infrequently in childhood brain tumors [153]. Mutations in PTEN can cause disruptions in cellular growth, migration, apoptosis, and interaction with the extracellular matrix [139].

Loss of chromosomal region 17p or mutations in the tumor suppressor gene *p53* located in that region is believed to play a major role in both the formation of low-grade adult glioma and in the transition of low-grade gliomas to malignant glioblastoma [139,142,154]. However few p53 mutations occur in children with gliomas, especially among children less than 3 years of age [155]. Reporting of p53 mutations in low-grade astrocytomas has varied in frequency across studies [156]. Loss of chromosome 17p is the most frequent molecular abnormality in childhood medulloblastomas, appearing in up to 50% of cases [157]. TP53 mutations are the earliest detectable change in gliomas [139] and have been observed in as many as 53% of low-grade and anaplastic astrocytomas (WHO grade II and III respectively) and 65% of glioblastomas [142]. Some studies suggest that there is no difference in survival between patients with or without a p53 mutation [158,159,] while others suggest there may be a survival benefit [160,161].

Chromosomal Gain

The epidermal growth factor receptor (EGFR), located on chromosome arm 7p, is a proto-oncogene amplified rarely in low-grade gliomas [162] and anaplastic oligodendrogliomas (<10%) [163] but in approximately 40% of primary glioblastomas [142]. EGRF overexpression is less common (<10%) among secondary glioblastomas and is also more common in primary glioblastomas (>60%) [142,164]. EGFR amplification is rarely seen in children (0–10%) [165]. This gene normally encodes a transmembrane receptor tyrosine kinase involved in cellular proliferation [166]. The prognostic value of EGFR is controversial. Some studies suggest that EGFR may contribute to radiotherapy resistance [167,168] and to overall poor prognosis; however, these differences may be due to confounding by age, because EGFR amplification is more common in older patients and survival significantly decreases with age [160]. EGFR amplification was not associated with survival in a recent meta-analysis [169]; however some studies suggest that EGFR is predictive of poor prognosis when present in younger patients [158,170,171] and others suggest that EGFR may be associated with better survival in children [165].

Other molecular changes in medulloblastomas may include inactivation of the *HIC-1* tumor suppressor gene through hypermethylation, amplification of *MYC*, overexpression of ErbB2, and mutations of the sonic hedgehog pathway (SHH) and the wingless (Wnt) pathway [144].

Epigenetic Alterations in Childhood Brain Tumors

Epigenetic mechanisms in cancer affect the expression of genes without attendant changes in the base pair composition of genomic DNA. Recent studies have highlighted the importance of epigenetic alterations in carcinogenesis and the fact that these changes can provide powerful new approaches for tumor classification in studies of disease etiology and for clinical diagnostic purposes [172]. In both adult and childhood tumors the disruption of gene expression through epigenetic mechanisms is common. Two fundamental aspects of these changes at the DNA level are the overall loss of methyl groups from genomic DNA [173] particularly in high-grade tumors [174] and the occurrence of focal DNA hypermethylation that can disrupt regulatory control regions of genes [175]. Hypermethylation of the 5′-regions of genes may block transcription factor binding and thereby suppress the transcription of genes leading to cancer. DNA methylation has been the focus of much epigenetic research but with the advent of new chromatin scanning technologies [176,177] the importance of protein modifications particularly those targeting nucleosomal histones has been brought to the forefront. Recent studies have linked alterations in DNA methylation with protein complexes that modify nucleosomal histone proteins [178]. Furthermore, important relationships have been shown to exist between these histone markings with epigenetic programs occurring in cancer stem cells and cancer progenitor cells [179–181]. Applying new epigenomic technologies and concepts linking stem cell and cancer biology is expected to greatly increase our understanding of the nature of epigenetic pathways in pediatric brain tumor pathogenesis.

The literature on methylation is extensive and focuses predominately on adult cancers as reviewed elsewhere [182–185]. Epigenetic mechanisms may be different in childhood brain tumors compared with adult brain tumors. For example, while aberrant DNA methylation and transcriptional silencing of p16IN4a, p15INK4b, p14ARF are very common in adult brain tumors [186–189] they are very uncommon in pediatric brain tumors [190–193]. Also most childhood brain tumors are of astrocytic origin and are low grade, in sharp contrast to adult glioma. Furthermore, previous studies have found few and in some case no genomic alterations such as TP53 mutation, a fact that points to epigenetic mechanisms.

Cyclin a1 is often methylated in astrocytoma including pediatric low-grade JPA [190,194]. In pediatric pilocytic astrocytoma some loci become undermethylated, for example, *MYOD1* [191] and mark epigenetic errors in gene regulation. The melanoma antigen family 1 gene [195] on the X chromosome, normally turned off in brain tissue, becomes unmethylated and transcriptionally active in pediatric astrocytoma [196]. Several neurogenesis genes were found to be remarkably down-regulated in JPA [197] and possess extensive CpG islands in their promoters (i.e., *BDNF, NEUROD2, NEUROD1*); *BDNF* is known to be methylated and transcriptionally regulated in this manner [198,199]. *OCT6* was found hypermethylated in 30% of both child and adult astrocytoma [190]. Several specific genes candidates were identified in pediatric ependymoma including *SCHIP-1, EB1*, and the chromatin remodeling protein *CBX7* [200]. Other well-known tumor suppressors and methylation targets occurring in CBTs include *RARβ2, CCND2, TMS1* [201,] *MGMT, & CDH1* [190,202]. HIC1 (hypermethylated in cancer) [203] was found to be completely methylated in 39% primary medulloblastoma and 60% high-grade glioma. MCT3 (monocarboxylate tansporter3) [204] transports lactate in choroid plexus epithelia, and functions in the blood-brain barrier and is silenced by DNA methylation in medulloblastoma. CYP1B1 metabolizes xenobiotics and estrogen and is expressed widely in the CNS and participates in the blood-brain barrier and is hypermethylated in medulloblastoma [202].

As one concept implies that childhood brain tumors arise from errors of differentiation in the developing CNS that may be influenced by environmental and genetic factors, it is worth emphasizing that epigenetic alterations may provide clues to etiological factors in pediatric brain tumors. This may arise by inappropriate silencing of critical genes as suggested above or by interference with normal epigenetic silencing that is an intrinsic part of the developmental program. Thus, epigenetic markers are also potentially etiologically relevant. For example, carcinogen exposures have been shown [205] to be related to gene methylation in tobacco related tumors [206,207]. Early smoking initiation (early teens) has been associated with *RASSF1* methylation in lung tumors [208]. One author suggested that RASSF1 methylation occurs in a significant proportion of all types of childhood cancers [209]. The RASSF1 protein interacts with DNA repair proteins and may regulate cell cycle progression. It is of interest that RASSF1 is frequently methylated in low-grade gliomas [190,210] that are common in children as well as pediatric neuroblastoma [211] and the childhood Wilm's kidney tumor [211,212]. Further study of DNA methylation and other epigenetic alterations may help to establish links between environmental exposures and the risk of developing a pediatric brain tumor.

Constitutive Genetic Variation

As only a small proportion of brain tumors are likely to be explained by inherited rare mutations, researchers have turned attention to polymorphisms and epigenetic mechanisms that might influence susceptibility to brain tumors. Genetic variation that affects carcinogen metabolism, oxidative metabolism, DNA repair, immune function, brain development pathways, and other pathways that have not yet been identified might plausibly confer genetic susceptibility to brain tumors. Only two epidemiological studies have reported on a limited number of polymorphisms in relation to brain tumor risk in children [213,214]. Because of the limited data available on childhood brain tumors, examples provided below include evidence from adult gliomas.

Carcinogen Metabolism Genes

Phase I and II metabolism genes are responsible for the activation and the detoxification of carcinogens. Phase I enzymes such as cytochrome p450 enzymes (CYP450s) can activate various chemicals to carcinogens, including benzene and PAHs [215,216]; while the phase II enzymes such as glutathione S-transferases (GSTs) facilitate the elimination of endogenous and exogenous sources of carcinogens [217]. Differential expression of metabolizing enzymes, as determined by genetic polymorphisms of the metabolizing genes, may determine the individual susceptibility to carcinogens. There has been no study of CYP450s and the risk of childhood brain tumors; among adults, one study showed that CYP2E1, the major CYP450 for the benzene metabolic pathway, may be associated with the risk of glioma [218]. One study of the association between GSTs and childhood brain tumors showed that GSTM1 and GSTP1 polymorphisms may be associated with high-grade pediatric astrocytomas [213].

Antioxidant Genes

Oxidative damage to DNA, which can result from normal metabolic processes, is hypothesized to be a contributing factor to many types of cancer [219]. Antioxidants, from both dietary (e.g., ascorbate, tocopherol, and carotenoids) and endogenous sources (physiological antioxidants and antioxidant enzymes), protect DNA from oxidative damage [220]. Genetic variation in antioxidant pathways may influence the efficiency of antioxidant enzymes, such as superoxide dismutase, catalase, glutathione peroxidase, and glutathione reductase and additionally modify the relationship between dietary antioxidants and brain tumor risk. Single nucleotide polymorphisms (SNPs) in genes associated with reduced antioxidant capacity also may be associated with hypermethylation [221,222].

Paraoxonase 1 (*PON1*), codes for the important organophosphate-detoxifying enzyme paraoxonase 1. The

T allele of the C-108T promoter polymorphism of *PON1* is associated with reduced *PON1* function, particularly among neonates [223]. A case-control study of childhood brain tumors observed an interaction between the -108T allele and reported home pesticide use, suggesting that OP insecticides confer risk of CBTs to those with low *PON1* function [214].

DNA Repair Genes

DNA repair genes, including those genes responsible for direct repair, base excision repair, nucleotide excision repair, mismatch repair, and double-strand break repair are important in guarding against DNA damage by various genotoxic chemicals [224]. Further, the DNA repair system is important during organogenesis; the development of the human brain is especially sensitive to the disruption of DNA repair pathways if some of the DNA repair genes are mutated [225]. Abnormalities of gene copy number of ERCC1 and ERCC2 have been observed in adult gliomas [226]. Among studies of adult brain tumors, polymorphisms of ERCC1 and ERCC2 have been associated with increased risk of glioma, especially oligoastrocytoma [227,228].

Immune Function Genes

Very little is known about the association between immune function and childhood brain tumors. Among adults, studies have consistently reported statistically inverse associations between gliomas and history of allergies and levels of serum IgE [229–231]. Two studies of adult gliomas and immune function genes (interleukin [IL-4RA], IL-13, ADAM33, and genes coding for human leukocyte antigen) found significant positive associations for some variants and negative associations for others [232,233].

Developmental Genes

The early embryonic neuroepithelium contains cells that have the potential to generate all the differentiated cells of the CNS [234,235]. The proper orchestration of signals for proliferation, differentiation, apoptosis, and cell migration are necessary for normal brain development and it is hypothesized that disruption of the balance of these signals may play a role in tumorigenesis [236]. The hypothesis of the association between the developmental genes and childhood brain tumors is supported by the fact that mutations in several developmental gene pathways are associated with familial syndromes characterized by increased brain tumor risk. For example, individuals with Gorlin syndrome have been found to have changes in the sonic hedgehog (Shh)/Patched1 (Ptc) pathway [237,238], individuals with Turcot syndrome frequently have mutations in the Wnt-signaling pathway [239–242]. Both genetic and epigenetic changes in developmental pathway genes may influence tumorigenesis. For example, Wnt pathway genes are mutated in some types of childhood brain tumors [157,243] and Wnt antagonists are often silenced by methylation in childhood and adult cancers [244,245].

FUTURE DIRECTIONS

The causes of most cases of brain tumors remain unexplained. Only ionizing radiation and a few, rare genetic syndromes are considered definitive risk factors for the disease. While somatic mutations of childhood brain tumors compared to adults have been well described, the role of epigenetic changes in childhood brain tumors is a more recent focus of research that continues to grow in importance. Recent studies have found that epigenetic changes are important contributors to carcinogenesis and may provide key information to tumor classification and to clinical diagnostics. The role of constitutional variation, or SNPs that may predispose a child to brain tumor development, deserves more research effort as few studies have investigated this important issue. A reason for the lack of genetic association studies, at least in part, is the high cost and time required to assemble large numbers of childhood cases and controls.

Environmental factors such as radiofrequency exposure from cell phones, and parental or childhood exposure to pesticides are all areas of recent public health interest and epidemiological research. Dietary factors, vitamin usage, parental occupational exposures, and tobacco use are other environmental and lifestyle exposures that may be of greater interest when considered in combination with refined tumor groupings and growing molecular and genetic data.

REFERENCES

1. SEER Cancer Statistics Review, 1975–2004. Bethesda: National Cancer Institute; 2006 based on November 2006 SEER data submission, posted to the SEER web site, 2007.
2. CBTRUS. *CBTRUS Fact Sheet*. Chicago, IL: CBTRUS; 2007.
3. Mulhern RK, Merchant TE, Gajjar A, Reddick WE, Kun LE. Late neurocognitive sequelae in survivors of brain tumours in childhood. *Lancet Oncol*. 2004;5(7):399–408.
4. Ron E. Childhood cancer–treatment at a cost. *J Natl Cancer Inst*. 2006;98(21):1510–1511.
5. CBTRUS. Statistical Report: Primary Brain Tumors in the United States, 1998–2002.: Central Brain Tumor Registry of the United States; 2005.
6. SEER Cancer Statistics Review, 1975–2002. National Cancer Institute, 2005. (Accessed at http://seer.cancer.gov/csr/1975_2004)
7. Gurney JG, Smith MA, Bunin GR. CNS and miscellaneous intracranial and intraspinal neoplasms. In: Ries LAG, Smith MA, Gurney JG, et al, eds. *Cancer Incidence and Survival among Children and Adolescents: United States SEER Program 1975–1995*. Bethesda: National Cancer Institute, SEER Program. NIH Pub. No. 99–4649; 1999.
8. Surveillance E, and End Results (SEER) Program (www.seer.cancer.gov). SEER*Stat Database: Incidence—SEER 9 Regs Public-Use, Nov 2005 Sub (1973–2003)—Linked to County Attributes—Total U.S., 1969–2003 Counties. In: National Cancer Institute, DCCPS, Surveillance Research Program, Cancer Statistics Branch; released April 2006, based on the Novermber 2005 submission.
9. Legler JM, Ries LA, Smith MA, et al. Cancer surveillance series [corrected]: brain and other central nervous system cancers: recent trends in incidence and mortality. *J Natl Cancer Inst*. 1999;91(16):1382–1390.
10. Smith MA, Freidlin B, Ries LA, Simon R. Trends in reported incidence of primary malignant brain tumors in children in the United States. *J Natl Cancer Inst*. 1998;90(17):1269–1277.
11. Kaiser J. No meeting of minds on childhood cancer. *Science*. 1999;286(5446):1832–1834.
12. Black WC. Increasing incidence of childhood primary malignant brain tumors–enigma or no-brainer? *J Natl Cancer Inst*. 1998;90(17):1249–1251.

13. Larsen NS. Brain tumor incidence rising; researchers ask why. *J Natl Cancer Inst.* 1993;85(13):1024–1025.
14. Baldwin RT, Preston-Martin S. Epidemiology of brain tumors in childhood–a review. *Toxicol Appl Pharmacol.* 2004;199(2):118–131.
15. Little MP, de Vathaire F, Shamsaldin A, et al. Risks of brain tumour following treatment for cancer in childhood: modification by genetic factors, radiotherapy and chemotherapy. *Int J Cancer.* 1998;78(3):269–275.
16. Shapiro S, Mealey J Jr, Sartorius C. Radiation-induced intracranial malignant gliomas. *J Neurosurg.* 1989;71(1):77–82.
17. Walter AW, Hancock ML, Pui CH, et al. Secondary brain tumors in children treated for acute lymphoblastic leukemia at St Jude Children's Research Hospital. *J Clin Oncol.* 1998;16(12):3761–3767.
18. Modan B, Baidatz D, Mart H, Steinitz R, Levin SG. Radiation-induced head and neck tumours. *Lancet.* 1974;1(7852):277–279.
19. Ron E, Modan B, Boice JD Jr, et al. Tumors of the brain and nervous system after radiotherapy in childhood. *N Engl J Med.* 1988;319(16):1033–1039.
20. Sadetzki S, Chetrit A, Freedman L, Stovall M, Modan B, Novikov I. Long-term follow-up for brain tumor development after childhood exposure to ionizing radiation for tinea capitis. *Radiat Res.* 2005;163(4):424–432.
21. Shore RE, Moseson M, Harley N, Pasternack BS. Tumors and other diseases following childhood x-ray treatment for ringworm of the scalp (Tinea capitis). *Health Phys.* 2003;85(4):404–408.
22. Preston DL, Ron E, Yonehara S, et al. Tumors of the nervous system and pituitary gland associated with atomic bomb radiation exposure. *J Natl Cancer Inst.* 2002;94(20):1555–1563.
23. Cardis E, Vrijheid M, Blettner M, et al. Risk of cancer after low doses of ionising radiation: retrospective cohort study in 15 countries. *BMJ.* 2005;331(7508):77.
24. Longstreth WT Jr, Phillips LE, Drangsholt M, et al. Dental X-rays and the risk of intracranial meningioma: a population-based case-control study. *Cancer.* 2004;100(5):1026–1034.
25. Preston-Martin S, Paganini-Hill A, Henderson BE, Pike MC, Wood C. Case-control study of intracranial meningiomas in women in Los Angeles County, California. *J Natl Cancer Inst.* 1980;65(1):67–73.
26. Preston-Martin S, Yu MC, Henderson BE, Roberts C. Risk factors for meningiomas in men in Los Angeles County. *J Natl Cancer Inst.* 1983;70(5):863–866.
27. Rodvall Y, Ahlbom A, Pershagen G, Nylander M, Spännare B. Dental radiography after age 25 years, amalgam fillings and tumours of the central nervous system. *Oral Oncol.* 1998;34(4):265–269.
28. Ryan P, Lee MW, North B, McMichael AJ. Amalgam fillings, diagnostic dental x-rays and tumours of the brain and meninges. *Eur J Cancer, B, Oral Oncol.* 1992;28B(2):91–95.
29. Blettner M, Schlehofer B, Samkange-Zeeb F, Berg G, Schlaefer K, Schüz J. Medical exposure to ionising radiation and the risk of brain tumours: Interphone study group, Germany. *Eur J Cancer.* 2007;43(13):1990–1998.
30. Karlsson P, Holmberg E, Lundell M, Mattsson A, Holm LE, Wallgren A. Intracranial tumors after exposure to ionizing radiation during infancy: a pooled analysis of two Swedish cohorts of 28,008 infants with skin hemangioma. *Radiat Res.* 1998;150(3):357–364.
31. Stålberg K, Haglund B, Axelsson O, Cnattingius S, Pfeifer S, Kieler H. Prenatal X-ray exposure and childhood brain tumours: a population-based case-control study on tumour subtypes. *Br J Cancer.* 2007;97(11):1583–1587.
32. Wertheimer N, Leeper E. Electrical wiring configurations and childhood cancer. *Am J Epidemiol.* 1979;109(3):273–284.
33. Otaka Y, Kitamura S, Furuta M, Shinohara A. Sex-linked recessive lethal test of Drosophila melanogaster after exposure to 50-Hz magnetic fields. *Bioelectromagnetics.* 1992;13(1):67–74.
34. McLean JR, Stuchly MA, Mitchel RE, et al. Cancer promotion in a mouse-skin model by a 60-Hz magnetic field: II. Tumor development and immune response. *Bioelectromagnetics.* 1991;12(5):273–287.
35. Kheifets LI. Electric and magnetic field exposure and brain cancer: a review. *Bioelectromagnetics.* 2001;suppl 5:S120-S131.
36. Ahlbom IC, Cardis E, Green A, Linet M, Savitz D, Swerdlow A; ICNIRP (International Commission for Non-Ionizing Radiation Protection) Standing Committee on Epidemiology. Review of the epidemiologic literature on EMF and Health. *Environ Health Perspect.* 2001;109 (suppl 6):911–933.
37. Gurney JG, van Wijngaarden E. Extremely low frequency electromagnetic fields (EMF) and brain cancer in adults and children: review and comment. *Neuro-oncology.* 1999;1(3):212–220.
38. Savitz DA, Wachtel H, Barnes FA, John EM, Tvrdik JG. Case-control study of childhood cancer and exposure to 60-Hz magnetic fields. *Am J Epidemiol.* 1988;128(1):21–38.
39. Gurney JG, Mueller BA, Davis S, Schwartz SM, Stevens RG, Kopecky KJ. Childhood brain tumor occurrence in relation to residential power line configurations, electric heating sources, and electric appliance use. *Am J Epidemiol.* 1996;143(2):120–128.
40. Preston-Martin S, Navidi W, Thomas D, Lee PJ, Bowman J, Pogoda J. Los Angeles study of residential magnetic fields and childhood brain tumors. *Am J Epidemiol.* 1996;143(2):105–119.
41. Tynes T, Haldorsen T. Electromagnetic fields and cancer in children residing near Norwegian high-voltage power lines. *Am J Epidemiol.* 1997;145(3):219–226.
42. Verkasalo PK, Pukkala E, Hongisto MY, et al. Risk of cancer in Finnish children living close to power lines. *BMJ.* 1993;307(6909):895–899.
43. Olsen JH, Nielsen A, Schulgen G. Residence near high voltage facilities and risk of cancer in children. *BMJ.* 1993;307(6909):891–895.
44. Feychting M, Ahlbom A. Magnetic fields and cancer in children residing near Swedish high-voltage power lines. *Am J Epidemiol.* 1993;138(7):467–481.
45. UK Childhood Cancer Study Investigators. Exposure to power-frequency magnetic fields and the risk of childhood cancer. *Lancet.* 1999;354(9194):1925–1931.
46. Skinner J, Mee TJ, Blackwell RP, et al.; United Kingdom Childhood Cancer Study Investigators. Exposure to power frequency electric fields and the risk of childhood cancer in the UK. *Br J Cancer.* 2002;87(11):1257–1266.
47. Linet MS, Hatch EE, Kleinerman RA, et al. Residential exposure to magnetic fields and acute lymphoblastic leukemia in children. *N Engl J Med.* 1997;337(1):1–7.
48. Kuijten RR, Bunin GR, Nass CC, Meadows AT. Gestational and familial risk factors for childhood astrocytoma: results of a case-control study. *Cancer Res.* 1990;50(9):2608–2612.
49. Savitz DA, John EM, Kleckner RC. Magnetic field exposure from electric appliances and childhood cancer. *Am J Epidemiol.* 1990;131(5):763–773.
50. Kuijten RR, Bunin GR. Risk factors for childhood brain tumors. *Cancer Epidemiol Biomarkers Prev.* 1993;2(3):277–288.
51. Savitz DA, Chen JH. Parental occupation and childhood cancer: review of epidemiologic studies. *Environ Health Perspect.* 1990;88:325–337.
52. Wrensch M, Minn Y, Chew T, Bondy M, Berger MS. Epidemiology of primary brain tumors: current concepts and review of the literature. *Neuro-oncology.* 2002;4(4):278–299.
53. Fabia J, Thuy TD. Occupation of father at time of birth of children dying of malignant diseases. *Br J Prev Soc Med.* 1974;28(2):98–100.
54. Feingold L, Savitz DA, John EM. Use of a job-exposure matrix to evaluate parental occupation and childhood cancer. *Cancer Causes Control.* 1992;3(2):161–169.
55. Gold EB, Diener MD, Szklo M. Parental occupations and cancer in children-a case-control study and review of the methodologic issues. *J Occup Med.* 1982;24(8):578–584.
56. Hicks N, Zack M, Caldwell GG, Fernbach DJ, Falletta JM. Childhood cancer and occupational radiation exposure in parents. *Cancer.* 1984;53(8):1637–1643.
57. Johnson CC, Annegers JF, Frankowski RF, Spitz MR, Buffler PA. Childhood nervous system tumors–an evaluation of the association with paternal occupational exposure to hydrocarbons. *Am J Epidemiol.* 1987;126(4):605–613.
58. Kuijten RR, Bunin GR, Nass CC, Meadows AT. Parental occupation and childhood astrocytoma: results of a case-control study. *Cancer Res.* 1992;52(4):782–786.
59. Kwa SL, Fine LJ. The association between parental occupation and childhood malignancy. *J Occup Med.* 1980;22(12):792–794.
60. Nasca PC, Baptiste MS, MacCubbin PA, et al. An epidemiologic case-control study of central nervous system tumors in children and parental occupational exposures. *Am J Epidemiol.* 1988;128(6):1256–1265.
61. Olshan AF, Breslow NE, Daling JR, Weiss NS, Leviton A. Childhood brain tumors and paternal occupation in the aerospace industry. *J Natl Cancer Inst.* 1986;77(1):17–19.
62. Peters FM, Preston-Martin S, Yu MC. Brain tumors in children and occupational exposure of parents. *Science.* 1981;213(4504):235–237.
63. Wilkins JR 3rd, Sinks T. Parental occupation and intracranial neoplasms of childhood: results of a case-control interview study. *Am J Epidemiol.* 1990;132(2):275–292.

64. McKean-Cowdin R, Preston-Martin S, Pogoda JM, Holly EA, Mueller BA, Davis RL. Parental occupation and childhood brain tumors: astroglial and primitive neuroectodermal tumors. *J Occup Environ Med*. 1998;40(4):332–340.
65. Cordier S, Mandereau L, Preston-Martin S, et al. Parental occupations and childhood brain tumors: results of an international case-control study. *Cancer Causes Control*. 2001;12(9):865–874.
66. Hemminki K, Saloniemi I, Salonen T, Partanen T, Vainio H. Childhood cancer and parental occupation in Finland. *J Epidemiol Community Health*. 1981;35(1):11–15.
67. Wilkins JR 3rd, Koutras RA. Paternal occupation and brain cancer in offspring: a mortality-based case-control study. *Am J Ind Med*. 1988;14(3):299–318.
68. Cordier S, Lefeuvre B, Filippini G, et al. Parental occupation, occupational exposure to solvents and polycyclic aromatic hydrocarbons and risk of childhood brain tumors (Italy, France, Spain). *Cancer Causes Control*. 1997;8(5):688–697.
69. Cordier S, Monfort C, Filippini G, et al. Parental exposure to polycyclic aromatic hydrocarbons and the risk of childhood brain tumors: The SEARCH International Childhood Brain Tumor Study. *Am J Epidemiol*. 2004;159(12):1109–1116.
70. Zahm SH, Ward MH. Pesticides and childhood cancer. *Environ Health Perspect*. 1998;106 (suppl 3):893–908.
71. Gurney JG, Smith MA, Olshan AF, Hecht SS, Kasum CM. Clues to the etiology of childhood brain cancer: N-nitroso compounds, polyomaviruses, and other factors of interest. *Cancer Invest*. 2001;19(6):630–640.
72. Blair A, Grauman DJ, Lubin JH, Fraumeni JF Jr. Lung cancer and other causes of death among licensed pesticide applicators. *J Natl Cancer Inst*. 1983;71(1):31–37.
73. Rodvall Y, Ahlbom A, Spännare B, Nise G. Glioma and occupational exposure in Sweden, a case-control study. *Occup Environ Med*. 1996;53(8):526–532.
74. Davis JR, Brownson RC, Garcia R, Bentz BJ, Turner A. Family pesticide use and childhood brain cancer. *Arch Environ Contam Toxicol*. 1993;24(1):87–92.
75. Pogoda JM, Preston-Martin S. Household pesticides and risk of pediatric brain tumors. *Environ Health Perspect*. 1997;105(11):1214–1220.
76. van Wijngaarden E, Stewart PA, Olshan AF, Savitz DA, Bunin GR. Parental occupational exposure to pesticides and childhood brain cancer. *Am J Epidemiol*. 2003;157(11):989–997.
77. Lijinsky W. *Chemistry and Biology of N-nitroso Compounds*. New York, NY: Cambridge University Press; 1992.
78. National Research Council Committee on Diet Nutrition and Cancer. *Diet Nutrition and Cancer*. Washington, DC: National Academy Press; 1982.
79. Sampson JH, Bigner DD. Experimental tumors and the evaluation of neurocarcinogens. In: Bigner DD, McLendon RE, Bruner JM, eds. *Russell and Rubinstein's Pathology of Tumors of the Nervous System* (6th ed.). New York: Oxford Univ. Press; 1998:167–230.
80. Magee PN, Montesano R, Preusmann R. N-nitroso compounds and related carcinogens. In: Searle ED, ed. *Chemical Carcinogens*. Washington, DC: American Chemical Society; 1976.
81. Bogovski P, Bogovski S. Animal Species in which N-nitroso compounds induce cancer. *Int J Cancer*. 1981;27(4):471–474.
82. Rice JM, Ward JM. Age dependence of susceptibility to carcinogenesis in the nervous system. *Ann N Y Acad Sci*. 1982;381:274–289.
83. Ivankovic S. Teratogenic and carcinogenic effects of some chemicals during perinatal life in rats, Syrian golden hamsters, and minipigs. *Natl Cancer Inst Monogr*. 1979;51:103–115.
84. Chilvers C, Inskip H, Caygill C, Bartholomew B, Fraser P, Hill M. A survey of dietary nitrate in well-water users. *Int J Epidemiol*. 1984;13(3):324–331.
85. Preston-Martin S, Mack W. Neoplasms of the nervous system. In: Fraumeni SDaJF Jr, ed. *Cancer Epidemiology and Prevention*. New York, NY: Oxford University Press; 1996:1231–1281.
86. Sarasua S, Savitz DA. Cured and broiled meat consumption in relation to childhood cancer: Denver, Colorado (United States). *Cancer Causes Control*. 1994;5(2):141–148.
87. Preston-Martin S, Yu MC, Benton B, Henderson BE. N-Nitroso compounds and childhood brain tumors: a case-control study. *Cancer Res*. 1982;42(12):5240–5245.
88. Bunin GR, Kuijten RR, Buckley JD, Rorke LB, Meadows AT. Relation between maternal diet and subsequent primitive neuroectodermal brain tumors in young children. *N Engl J Med*. 1993;329(8):536–541.
89. Bunin GR, Kuijten RR, Boesel CP, Buckley JD, Meadows AT. Maternal diet and risk of astrocytic glioma in children: a report from the Childrens Cancer Group (United States and Canada). *Cancer Causes Control*. 1994;5(2):177–187.
90. McCredie M, Maisonneuve P, Boyle P. Antenatal risk factors for malignant brain tumours in New South Wales children. *Int J Cancer*. 1994;56(1):6–10.
91. Lubin F, Farbstein H, Chetrit A, et al. The role of nutritional habits during gestation and child life in pediatric brain tumor etiology. *Int J Cancer*. 2000;86(1):139–143.
92. Preston-Martin S, Pogoda JM, Mueller BA, Holly EA, Lijinsky W, Davis RL. Maternal consumption of cured meats and vitamins in relation to pediatric brain tumors. *Cancer Epidemiol Biomarkers Prev*. 1996;5(8):599–605.
93. Cordier S, Iglesias MJ, Le Goaster C, Guyot MM, Mandereau L, Hemon D. Incidence and risk factors for childhood brain tumors in the Ile de France. *Int J Cancer*. 1994;59(6):776–782.
94. Schwartzbaum JA, Cornwell DG. Oxidant stress and glioblastoma multiforme risk: serum antioxidants, gamma-glutamyl transpeptidase, and ferritin. *Nutr Cancer*. 2000;38(1):40–49.
95. Bunin GR, Kushi LH, Gallagher PR, Rorke-Adams LB, McBride ML, Cnaan A. Maternal diet during pregnancy and its association with medulloblastoma in children: a children's oncology group study (United States). *Cancer Causes Control*. 2005;16(7):877–891.
96. Lee M, Wrensch M, Miike R. Dietary and tobacco risk factors for adult onset glioma in the San Francisco Bay Area (California, USA). *Cancer Causes Control*. 1997;8(1):13–24.
97. Preston-Martin S, Pogoda JM, Mueller BA, et al. Results from an international case-control study of childhood brain tumors: the role of prenatal vitamin supplementation. *Environ Health Perspect*. 1998;106(suppl 3):887–892.
98. Preston-Martin S, Pike MC, Ross RK, Jones PA, Henderson BE. Increased cell division as a cause of human cancer. *Cancer Res*. 1990;50(23):7415–7421.
99. Sabel M, Felsberg J, Messing-Jünger M, Neuen-Jacob E, Piek J. Glioblastoma multiforme at the site of metal splinter injury: a coincidence? Case report. *J Neurosurg*. 1999;91(6):1041–1044.
100. Walsh J, Gye R, Connelley TJ. Meningioma: a late complication of head injury. *Med J Aust*. 1969;1(18):906–908.
101. Preston-Martin S, Pogoda JM, Mueller BA, et al. Prenatal vitamin supplementation and risk of childhood brain tumors. *Int J Cancer Suppl*. 1998;11:17–22.
102. Longstreth WT Jr, Dennis LK, McGuire VM, Drangsholt MT, Koepsell TD. Epidemiology of intracranial meningioma. *Cancer*. 1993;72(3):639–648.
103. Inskip PD, Mellemkjaer L, Gridley G, Olsen JH. Incidence of intracranial tumors following hospitalization for head injuries (Denmark). *Cancer Causes Control*. 1998;9(1):109–116.
104. Nygren C, Adami J, Ye W, et al. Primary brain tumors following traumatic brain injury–a population-based cohort study in Sweden. *Cancer Causes Control*. 2001;12(8):733–737.
105. Gurney JG, Preston-Martin S, McDaniel AM, Mueller BA, Holly EA. Head injury as a risk factor for brain tumors in children: results from a multicenter case-control study. *Epidemiology*. 1996;7(5):485–489.
106. Khalili K. Human neurotropic JC virus and its association with brain tumors. *Dis Markers*. 2001;17(3):143–147.
107. Chrétien F, Boche D, Lorin de la Grandmaison G, et al. Progressive multifocal leukoencephalopathy and oligodendroglioma in a monkey co-infected by simian immunodeficiency virus and simian virus 40. *Acta Neuropathol*. 2000;100(3):332–336.
108. Schuman LM, Choi NW, Gullen WH. Relationship of central nervous system neoplasms to Toxoplasma gondii infection. *Am J Public Health Nations Health*. 1967;57(5):848–856.
109. Ryan P, Hurley SF, Johnson AM, et al. Tumours of the brain and presence of antibodies to Toxoplasma gondii. *Int J Epidemiol*. 1993;22(3):412–419.
110. Shah K, Nathanson N. Human exposure to SV40: review and comment. *Am J Epidemiol*. 1976;103(1):1–12.
111. Butel JS, Arrington AS, Wong C, Lednicky JA, Finegold MJ. Molecular evidence of simian virus 40 infections in children. *J Infect Dis*. 1999;180(3):884–887.
112. Shah KV, Rollison DE. Investigation of the SV40-human cancer association: look for the full signature of the virus. *Dis Markers*. 2001;17(3):159–161.

113. Pan American Health Organization. Proceedings of the Second International Conference on Live Poliovirus Vaccines. Pan American Health Organization, Washington, DC; 1960.
114. Eddy BE, Borman GS, Grubbs GE, Young RD. Identification of the oncogenic substance in rhesus monkey kidney cell culture as simian virus 40. *Virology*. 1962;17:65–75.
115. Girardi AJ, Sweet BH, Slotnick VB, Hilleman MR. Development of tumors in hamsters inoculated in the neonatal period with vacuolating virus, SV-40. *Proc Soc Exp Biol Med*. 1962;109:649–660.
116. Gordon L, McQuaid S, Cosby SL. Detection of herpes simplex virus (types 1 and 2) and human herpesvirus 6 DNA in human brain tissue by polymerase chain reaction. *Clin Diagn Virol*. 1996;6(1):33–40.
117. Franks RR, Rencic A, Gordon J, et al. Formation of undifferentiated mesenteric tumors in transgenic mice expressing human neurotropic polymavirus early protein. *Oncogene*. 1996;12(12):2573–2578.
118. Inskip PD, Linet MS, Heineman EF. Etiology of brain tumors in adults. *Epidemiol Rev*. 1995;17(2):382–414.
119. Small JA, Scangos GA, Cork L, Jay G, Khoury G. The early region of human papovavirus JC induces dysmyelination in transgenic mice. *Cell*. 1986;46(1):13–18.
120. Zu Rhein GM. Studies of JC virus-induced nervous system tumors in the Syrian hamster: a review. *Prog Clin Biol Res*. 1983;105:205–221.
121. Walker DL, Padgett BL, ZuRhein GM, Albert AE, Marsh RF. Human papovavirus (JC): induction of brain tumors in hamsters. *Science*. 1973;181(100):674–676.
122. Delbue S, Pagani E, Guerini FR, et al. Distribution, characterization and significance of polyomavirus genomic sequences in tumors of the brain and its covering. *J Med Virol*. 2005;77(3):447–454.
123. Arrington AS, Lednicky JA, Butel JS. Molecular characterization of SV40 DNA in multiple samples from a human mesothelioma. *Anticancer Res*. 2000;20(2A):879–884.
124. Boldorini R, Caldarelli-Stefano R, Monga G, et al. PCR detection of JC virus DNA in the brain tissue of a 9-year-old child with pleomorphic xanthoastrocytoma. *J Neurovirol*. 1998;4(2):242–245.
125. Krynska B, Del Valle L, Croul S, et al. Detection of human neurotropic JC virus DNA sequence and expression of the viral oncogenic protein in pediatric medulloblastomas. *Proc Natl Acad Sci USA*. 1999;96(20):11519–11524.
126. De Mattei M, Martini F, Corallini A, et al. High incidence of BK virus large-T-antigen-coding sequences in normal human tissues and tumors of different histotypes. *Int J Cancer*. 1995;61(6):756–760.
127. Vilchez RA, Kozinetz CA, Arrington AS, Madden CR, Butel JS. Simian virus 40 in human cancers. *Am J Med*. 2003;114(8):675–684.
128. Bithell JF, Draper GJ, Gorbach PD. Association between malignant disease in children and maternal virus infections during pregnancy. *Br J Prev Soc Med*. 1973;27(1):68.
129. Fear NT, Roman E, Ansell P, Bull D. Malignant neoplasms of the brain during childhood: the role of prenatal and neonatal factors (United Kingdom). *Cancer Causes Control*. 2001;12(5):443–449.
130. Norman MA, Holly EA, Preston-Martin S. Childhood brain tumors and exposure to tobacco smoke. *Cancer Epidemiol Biomarkers Prev*. 1996;5(2):85–91.
131. Boffetta P, Trédaniel J, Greco A. Risk of childhood cancer and adult lung cancer after childhood exposure to passive smoke: A meta-analysis. *Environ Health Perspect*. 2000;108(1):73–82.
132. Huncharek M, Kupelnick B, Klassen H. Maternal smoking during pregnancy and the risk of childhood brain tumors: a meta-analysis of 6566 subjects from twelve epidemiological studies. *J Neurooncol*. 2002;57(1):51–57.
133. Brooks DR, Mucci LA, Hatch EE, Cnattingius S. Maternal smoking during pregnancy and risk of brain tumors in the offspring. A prospective study of 1.4 million Swedish births. *Cancer Causes Control*. 2004;15(10):997–1005.
134. Cordier S, Monfort C, Filippini G, et al. Parental exposure to polycyclic aromatic hydrocarbons and the risk of childhood brain tumors: The SEARCH International Childhood Brain Tumor Study. *Am J Epidemiol*. 2004;159(12):1109–1116.
135. Preston-Martin S. Epidemiology of primary CNS neoplasms. *Neurol Clin*. 1996;14(2):273–290.
136. Farwell J, Flannery JT. Cancer in relatives of children with central-nervous-system neoplasms. *N Engl J Med*. 1984;311(12):749–753.
137. Bondy ML, Lustbader ED, Buffler PA, Schull WJ, Hardy RJ, Strong LC. Genetic epidemiology of childhood brain tumors. *Genet Epidemiol*. 1991;8(4):253–267.
138. Reifenberger G, Collins VP. Pathology and molecular genetics of astrocytic gliomas. *J Mol Med*. 2004;82(10):656–670.
139. Boudreau CR, Yang I, Liau LM. Gliomas: advances in molecular analysis and characterization. *Surg Neurol*. 2005;64(4):286–94; discussion 294.
140. Nutt CL. Molecular genetics of oligodendrogliomas: a model for improved clinical management in the field of neurooncology. *Neurosurg Focus*. 2005;19(5):E2.
141. Aldape KD, Okcu MF, Bondy ML, Wrensch M. Molecular epidemiology of glioblastoma. *Cancer J*. 2003;9(2):99–106.
142. Ohgaki H. Genetic pathways to glioblastomas. *Neuropathology*. 2005;25(1):1–7.
143. Bayani J, Pandita A, Squire JA. Molecular cytogenetic analysis in the study of brain tumors: findings and applications. *Neurosurg Focus*. 2005;19(5):E1.
144. Ullrich NJ, Pomeroy SL. Molecular genetics of pediatric central nervous system tumors. *Curr Oncol Rep*. 2006;8(6):423–429.
145. Pietsch T, Taylor MD, Rutka JT. Molecular pathogenesis of childhood brain tumors. *J Neurooncol*. 2004;70(2):203–215.
146. Roerig P, Nessling M, Radlwimmer B, et al. Molecular classification of human gliomas using matrix-based comparative genomic hybridization. *Int J Cancer*. 2005;117(1):95–103.
147. Rasheed BK, McLendon RE, Friedman HS, et al. Chromosome 10 deletion mapping in human gliomas: a common deletion region in 10q25. *Oncogene*. 1995;10(11):2243–2246.
148. Karlbom AE, James CD, Boethius J, et al. Loss of heterozygosity in malignant gliomas involves at least three distinct regions on chromosome 10. *Hum Genet*. 1993;92(2):169–174.
149. Ichimura K, Schmidt EE, Miyakawa A, Goike HM, Collins VP. Distinct patterns of deletion on 10p and 10q suggest involvement of multiple tumor suppressor genes in the development of astrocytic gliomas of different malignancy grades. *Genes Chromosomes Cancer*. 1998;22(1):9–15.
150. Ohgaki H, Schäuble B, zur Hausen A, von Ammon K, Kleihues P. Genetic alterations associated with the evolution and progression of astrocytic brain tumours. *Virchows Arch*. 1995;427(2):113–118.
151. Dahia PL. PTEN, a unique tumor suppressor gene. *Endocr Relat Cancer*. 2000;7(2):115–129.
152. Knobbe CB, Merlo A, Reifenberger G. Pten signaling in gliomas. *Neuro-oncology*. 2002;4(3):196–211.
153. Cheng Y, Ng HK, Zhang SF, et al. Genetic alterations in pediatric high-grade astrocytomas. *Hum Pathol*. 1999;30(11):1284–1290.
154. Wiencke JK, Aldape K, McMillan A, et al. Molecular features of adult glioma associated with patient race/ethnicity, age, and a polymorphism in O6-methylguanine-DNA-methyltransferase. *Cancer Epidemiol Biomarkers Prev*. 2005;14(7):1774–1783.
155. Pollack IF, Finkelstein SD, Burnham J, et al.; Children's Cancer Group. Age and TP53 mutation frequency in childhood malignant gliomas: results in a multi-institutional cohort. *Cancer Res*. 2001;61(20):7404–7407.
156. Ohgaki H, Kleihues P. Population-based studies on incidence, survival rates, and genetic alterations in astrocytic and oligodendroglial gliomas. *J Neuropathol Exp Neurol*. 2005;64(6):479–489.
157. Ellison D. Classifying the medulloblastoma: insights from morphology and molecular genetics. *Neuropathol Appl Neurobiol*. 2002;28(4):257–282.
158. Simmons ML, Lamborn KR, Takahashi M, et al. Analysis of complex relationships between age, p53, epidermal growth factor receptor, and survival in glioblastoma patients. *Cancer Res*. 2001;61(3):1122–1128.
159. Smith JS, Tachibana I, Passe SM, et al. PTEN mutation, EGFR amplification, and outcome in patients with anaplastic astrocytoma and glioblastoma multiforme. *J Natl Cancer Inst*. 2001;93(16):1246–1256.
160. Ohgaki H, Dessen P, Jourde B, et al. Genetic pathways to glioblastoma: a population-based study. *Cancer Res*. 2004;64(19):6892–6899.
161. Schmidt MC, Antweiler S, Urban N, et al. Impact of genotype and morphology on the prognosis of glioblastoma. *J Neuropathol Exp Neurol*. 2002;61(4):321–328.
162. Okamoto Y, Di Patre PL, Burkhard C, et al. Population-based study on incidence, survival rates, and genetic alterations of low-grade diffuse astrocytomas and oligodendrogliomas. *Acta Neuropathol*. 2004;108(1):49–56.
163. Reifenberger G, Louis DN. Oligodendroglioma: toward molecular definitions in diagnostic neuro-oncology. *J Neuropathol Exp Neurol*. 2003;62(2):111–126.

164. Okada Y, Hurwitz EE, Esposito JM, Brower MA, Nutt CL, Louis DN. Selection pressures of TP53 mutation and microenvironmental location influence epidermal growth factor receptor gene amplification in human glioblastomas. *Cancer Res.* 2003;63(2):413–416.
165. Sung T, Miller DC, Hayes RL, Alonso M, Yee H, Newcomb EW. Preferential inactivation of the p53 tumor suppressor pathway and lack of EGFR amplification distinguish de novo high grade pediatric astrocytomas from de novo adult astrocytomas. *Brain Pathol.* 2000;10(2):249–259.
166. Mendelsohn J, Baselga J. The EGF receptor family as targets for cancer therapy. *Oncogene.* 2000;19(56):6550–6565.
167. Barker FG 2nd, Simmons ML, Chang SM, et al. EGFR overexpression and radiation response in glioblastoma multiforme. *Int J Radiat Oncol Biol Phys.* 2001;51(2):410–418.
168. Chakravarti A, Chakladar A, Delaney MA, Latham DE, Loeffler JS. The epidermal growth factor receptor pathway mediates resistance to sequential administration of radiation and chemotherapy in primary human glioblastoma cells in a RAS-dependent manner. *Cancer Res.* 2002;62(15):4307–4315.
169. Huncharek M, Kupelnick B. Epidermal growth factor receptor gene amplification as a prognostic marker in glioblastoma multiforme: results of a meta-analysis.. *Oncol Res.* 2000;12(2):107–112.
170. Kleinschmidt-DeMasters BK, Lillehei KO, Varella-Garcia M. Glioblastomas in the older old. *Arch Pathol Lab Med.* 2005;129(5):624–631.
171. Muracciole X, Romain S, Dufour H, et al. PAI-1 and EGFR expression in adult glioma tumors: toward a molecular prognostic classification. *Int J Radiat Oncol Biol Phys.* 2002;52(3):592–598.
172. Jones PA, Baylin SB. The epigenomics of cancer. *Cell.* 2007;128(4):683–692.
173. Barresi V, Condorelli DF, Giuffrida Stella AM. GFAP gene methylation in different neural cell types from rat brain. *Int J Dev Neurosci.* 1999;17(8):821–828.
174. Zukiel R, Nowak S, Barciszewska AM, Gawronska I, Keith G, Barciszewska MZ. A simple epigenetic method for the diagnosis and classification of brain tumors. *Mol Cancer Res.* 2004;2(3):196–202.
175. Laird PW. Cancer epigenetics. *Hum Mol Genet.* 2005;14 Spec No 1:R65-R76.
176. Buck MJ, Lieb JD. ChIP-chip: considerations for the design, analysis, and application of genome-wide chromatin immunoprecipitation experiments. *Genomics.* 2004;83(3):349–360.
177. Mockler TC, Chan S, Sundaresan A, Chen H, Jacobsen SE, Ecker JR. Applications of DNA tiling arrays for whole-genome analysis. *Genomics.* 2005;85(1):1–15.
178. Stirzaker C, Song JZ, Davidson B, Clark SJ. Transcriptional gene silencing promotes DNA hypermethylation through a sequential change in chromatin modifications in cancer cells. *Cancer Res.* 2004;64(11):3871–3877.
179. Rajasekhar VK, Begemann M. Concise review: roles of polycomb group proteins in development and disease: a stem cell perspective. *Stem Cells.* 2007;25(10):2498–2510.
180. Ohm JE, Baylin SB. Stem cell chromatin patterns: an instructive mechanism for DNA hypermethylation? *Cell Cycle.* 2007;6(9):1040–1043.
181. Ohm JE, McGarvey KM, Yu X, et al. A stem cell-like chromatin pattern may predispose tumor suppressor genes to DNA hypermethylation and heritable silencing. *Nat Genet.* 2007;39(2):237–242.
182. Feinberg AP, Cui H, Ohlsson R. DNA methylation and genomic imprinting: insights from cancer into epigenetic mechanisms. *Semin Cancer Biol.* 2002;12(5):389–398.
183. Esteller M, Herman JG. Cancer as an epigenetic disease: DNA methylation and chromatin alterations in human tumours. *J Pathol.* 2002;196(1):1–7.
184. Jones PA. DNA methylation and cancer. *Oncogene.* 2002;21(35):5358–5360.
185. Jones PA, Baylin SB. The fundamental role of epigenetic events in cancer. *Nat Rev Genet.* 2002;3(6):415–428.
186. Costello JF, Berger MS, Huang HS, Cavenee WK. Silencing of p16/CDKN2 expression in human gliomas by methylation and chromatin condensation. *Cancer Res.* 1996;56(10):2405–2410.
187. Ghimenti C, Fiano V, Chiadò-Piat L, Chiò A, Cavalla P, Schiffer D. Deregulation of the p14ARF/Mdm2/p53 pathway and G1/S transition in two glioblastoma sets. *J Neurooncol.* 2003;61(2):95–102.
188. Wolter M, Reifenberger J, Blaschke B, et al. Oligodendroglial tumors frequently demonstrate hypermethylation of the CDKN2A (MTS1, p16INK4a), p14ARF, and CDKN2B (MTS2, p15INK4b) tumor suppressor genes. *J Neuropathol Exp Neurol.* 2001;60(12):1170–1180.
189. Dong SM, Pang JC, Poon WS, et al. Concurrent hypermethylation of multiple genes is associated with grade of oligodendroglial tumors. *J Neuropathol Exp Neurol.* 2001;60(8):808–816.
190. Yu J, Zhang H, Gu J, et al. Methylation profiles of thirty four promoter-CpG islands and concordant methylation behaviours of sixteen genes that may contribute to carcinogenesis of astrocytoma. *BMC Cancer.* 2004;4:65.
191. Uhlmann K, Rohde K, Zeller C, et al. Distinct methylation profiles of glioma subtypes. *Int J Cancer.* 2003;106(1):52–59.
192. Lindsey JC, Lusher ME, Anderton JA, et al. Identification of tumour-specific epigenetic events in medulloblastoma development by hypermethylation profiling. *Carcinogenesis.* 2004;25(5):661–668.
193. Watanabe T, Huang H, Nakamura M, et al. Methylation of the p73 gene in gliomas. *Acta Neuropathol.* 2002;104(4):357–362.
194. Tokumaru Y, Yamashita K, Osada M, et al. Inverse correlation between cyclin A1 hypermethylation and p53 mutation in head and neck cancer identified by reversal of epigenetic silencing. *Cancer Res.* 2004;64(17):5982–5987.
195. Cadieux B, Ching TT, VandenBerg SR, Costello JF. Genome-wide hypomethylation in human glioblastomas associated with specific copy number alteration, methylenetetrahydrofolate reductase allele status, and increased proliferation. *Cancer Res.* 2006;66(17):8469–8476.
196. Bodey B, Siegel SE, Kaiser HE. MAGE-1, a cancer/testis-antigen, expression in childhood astrocytomas as an indicator of tumor progression. *In Vivo.* 2002;16(6):583–588.
197. Wong KK, Chang YM, Tsang YT, et al. Expression analysis of juvenile pilocytic astrocytomas by oligonucleotide microarray reveals two potential subgroups. *Cancer Res.* 2005;65(1):76–84.
198. Martinowich K, Hattori D, Wu H, et al. DNA methylation-related chromatin remodeling in activity-dependent BDNF gene regulation. *Science.* 2003;302(5646):890–893.
199. Wade PA. Dynamic regulation of DNA methylation coupled transcriptional repression: BDNF regulation by MeCP2. *Bioessays.* 2004;26(3):217–220.
200. Suarez-Merino B, Hubank M, Revesz T, et al. Microarray analysis of pediatric ependymoma identifies a cluster of 112 candidate genes including four transcripts at 22q12.1-q13.3. *Neuro-oncology.* 2005;7(1):20–31.
201. Alaminos M, Davalos V, Cheung NK, Gerald WL, Esteller M. Clustering of gene hypermethylation associated with clinical risk groups in neuroblastoma. *J Natl Cancer Inst.* 2004;96(16):1208–1219.
202. Frühwald MC, O'Dorisio MS, Rush LJ, et al. Gene amplification in PNETs/medulloblastomas: mapping of a novel amplified gene within the MYCN amplicon. *J Med Genet.* 2000;37(7):501–509.
203. Ehrbrecht A, Müller U, Wolter M, et al. Comprehensive genomic analysis of desmoplastic medulloblastomas: identification of novel amplified genes and separate evaluation of the different histological components. *J Pathol.* 2006;208(4):554–563.
204. Nakamura M, Ishida E, Shimada K, et al. Frequent LOH on 22q12.3 and TIMP-3 inactivation occur in the progression to secondary glioblastomas. *Lab Invest.* 2005;85(2):165–175.
205. Wiencke JK, Thurston SW, Kelsey KT, et al. Early age at smoking initiation and tobacco carcinogen DNA damage in the lung. *J Natl Cancer Inst.* 1999;91(7):614–619.
206. Hirao T, Nelson HH, Ashok TD, et al. Tobacco smoke-induced DNA damage and an early age of smoking initiation induce chromosome loss at 3p21 in lung cancer. *Cancer Res.* 2001;61(2):612–615.
207. Kim DH, Nelson HH, Wiencke JK, et al. p16(INK4a) and histology-specific methylation of CpG islands by exposure to tobacco smoke in non-small cell lung cancer. *Cancer Res.* 2001;61(8):3419–3424.
208. Marsit CJ, Kim DH, Liu M, et al. Hypermethylation of RASSF1A and BLU tumor suppressor genes in non-small cell lung cancer: implications for tobacco smoking during adolescence. *Int J Cancer.* 2005;114(2):219–223.
209. Wong IH, Chan J, Wong J, Tam PK. Ubiquitous aberrant RASSF1A promoter methylation in childhood neoplasia. *Clin Cancer Res.* 2004;10(3):994–1002.
210. Gao Y, Guan M, Su B, Liu W, Xu M, Lu Y. Hypermethylation of the RASSF1A gene in gliomas. *Clin Chim Acta.* 2004;349(1–2):173–179.
211. Harada K, Toyooka S, Maitra A, et al. Aberrant promoter methylation and silencing of the RASSF1A gene in pediatric tumors and cell lines. *Oncogene.* 2002;21(27):4345–4349.

212. Wagner KJ, Cooper WN, Grundy RG, et al. Frequent RASSF1A tumour suppressor gene promoter methylation in Wilms' tumour and colorectal cancer. *Oncogene.* 2002;21(47):7277–7282.
213. Ezer R, Alonso M, Pereira E, et al. Identification of glutathione S-transferase (GST) polymorphisms in brain tumors and association with susceptibility to pediatric astrocytomas. *J Neurooncol.* 2002;59(2):123–134.
214. Searles Nielsen S, Mueller BA, De Roos AJ, Viernes HM, Farin FM, Checkoway H. Risk of brain tumors in children and susceptibility to organophosphorus insecticides: the potential role of paraoxonase (PON1). *Environ Health Perspect.* 2005;113(7):909–913.
215. Snyder R, Hedli CC. An overview of benzene metabolism. *Environ Health Perspect.* 1996;104(suppl 6):1165–1171.
216. Shimada T, Fujii-Kuriyama Y. Metabolic activation of polycyclic aromatic hydrocarbons to carcinogens by cytochromes P450 1A1 and 1B1. *Cancer Sci.* 2004;95(1):1–6.
217. Coles BF, Kadlubar FF. Detoxification of electrophilic compounds by glutathione S-transferase catalysis: determinants of individual response to chemical carcinogens and chemotherapeutic drugs? *Biofactors.* 2003;17(1–4):115–130.
218. De Roos AJ, Rothman N, Inskip PD, et al. Genetic polymorphisms in GSTM1, -P1, -T1, and CYP2E1 and the risk of adult brain tumors. *Cancer Epidemiol Biomarkers Prev.* 2003;12(1):14–22.
219. Ames BN, Shigenaga MK. Oxidants are a major contributor to aging. *Ann N Y Acad Sci.* 1992;663:85–96.
220. Ames BN, Shigenaga MK, Hagen TM. Oxidants, antioxidants, and the degenerative diseases of aging. *Proc Natl Acad Sci USA.* 1993;90(17):7915–7922.
221. Ingrosso D, Cimmino A, Perna AF, et al. Folate treatment and unbalanced methylation and changes of allelic expression induced by hyperhomocysteinaemia in patients with uraemia. *Lancet.* 2003;361(9370):1693–1699.
222. Valinluck V, Tsai HH, Rogstad DK, Burdzy A, Bird A, Sowers LC. Oxidative damage to methyl-CpG sequences inhibits the binding of the methyl-CpG binding domain (MBD) of methyl-CpG binding protein 2 (MeCP2). *Nucleic Acids Res.* 2004;32(14):4100–4108.
223. Chen J, Kumar M, Chan W, Berkowitz G, Wetmur JG. Increased influence of genetic variation on PON1 activity in neonates. *Environ Health Perspect.* 2003;111(11):1403–1409.
224. Yu Z, Chen J, Ford BN, Brackley ME, Glickman BW. Human DNA repair systems: an overview. *Environ Mol Mutagen.* 1999;33(1):3–20.
225. Vinson RK, Hales BF. DNA repair during organogenesis. *Mutat Res.* 2002;509(1–2):79–91.
226. Liang BC, Ross DA, Reed E. Genomic copy number changes of DNA repair genes ERCC1 and ERCC2 in human gliomas. *J Neurooncol.* 1995;26(1):17–23.
227. Chen P, Wiencke J, Aldape K, et al. Association of an ERCC1 polymorphism with adult-onset glioma. *Cancer Epidemiol Biomarkers Prev.* 2000;9(8):843–847.
228. Caggana M, Kilgallen J, Conroy JM, et al. Associations between ERCC2 polymorphisms and gliomas. *Cancer Epidemiol Biomarkers Prev.* 2001;10(4):355–360.
229. Wrensch M, Weinberg A, Wiencke J, et al. History of chickenpox and shingles and prevalence of antibodies to varicella-zoster virus and three other herpesviruses among adults with glioma and controls. *Am J Epidemiol.* 2005;161(10):929–938.
230. Schoemaker MJ, Swerdlow AJ, Hepworth SJ, McKinney PA, van Tongeren M, Muir KR. History of allergies and risk of glioma in adults. *Int J Cancer.* 2006;119(9):2165–2172.
231. Wiemels JL, Wiencke JK, Patoka J, et al. Reduced immunoglobulin E and allergy among adults with glioma compared with controls. *Cancer Res.* 2004;64(22):8468–8473.
232. Schwartzbaum J, Ahlbom A, Malmer B, et al. Polymorphisms associated with asthma are inversely related to glioblastoma multiforme. *Cancer Res.* 2005;65(14):6459–6465.
233. Tang J, Shao W, Dorak MT, et al. Positive and negative associations of human leukocyte antigen variants with the onset and prognosis of adult glioblastoma multiforme. *Cancer Epidemiol Biomarkers Prev.* 2005;14(8):2040–2044.
234. Lütolf S, Radtke F, Aguet M, Suter U, Taylor V. Notch1 is required for neuronal and glial differentiation in the cerebellum. *Development.* 2002;129(2):373–385.
235. Martí E, Bovolenta P. Sonic hedgehog in CNS development: one signal, multiple outputs. *Trends Neurosci.* 2002;25(2):89–96.
236. Jankowski JA, Bruton R, Shepherd N, Sanders DS. Cadherin and catenin biology represent a global mechanism for epithelial cancer progression. *MP, Mol Pathol.* 1997;50(6):289–290.
237. Hahn H, Wicking C, Zaphiropoulous PG, et al. Mutations of the human homolog of Drosophila patched in the nevoid basal cell carcinoma syndrome. *Cell.* 1996;85(6):841–851.
238. Johnson RL, Rothman AL, Xie J, et al. Human homolog of patched, a candidate gene for the basal cell nevus syndrome. *Science.* 1996;272(5268):1668–1671.
239. Jones SM, Phillips PC, Molloy PT, Lange BJ, Needle MN, Biegel JA. Congenital anomalies and genetic disorders in families of children with central nervous system tumours. *J Med Genet.* 1995;32(8):627–632.
240. Jones CT, Swingler RJ, Simpson SA, Brock DJ. Superoxide dismutase mutations in an unselected cohort of Scottish amyotrophic lateral sclerosis patients. *J Med Genet.* 1995;32(4):290–292.
241. Hung KL, Wu CM, Huang JS, How SW. Familial medulloblastoma in siblings: report in one family and review of the literature. *Surg Neurol.* 1990;33(5):341–346.
242. Hamilton SR, Liu B, Parsons RE, et al. The molecular basis of Turcot's syndrome. *N Engl J Med.* 1995;332(13):839–847.
243. Wechsler-Reya RJ. Analysis of gene expression in the normal and malignant cerebellum. *Recent Prog Horm Res.* 2003;58:227–248.
244. Roman-Gomez J, Jimenez-Velasco A, Agirre X, et al. Transcriptional silencing of the Dickkopfs-3 (Dkk-3) gene by CpG hypermethylation in acute lymphoblastic leukaemia. *Br J Cancer.* 2004;91(4):707–713.
245. Nozaki M, Tada M, Kobayashi H, et al. Roles of the functional loss of p53 and other genes in astrocytoma tumorigenesis and progression. *Neuro-oncology.* 1999;1(2):124–137.

10 Meningioma Genetics

Yi Lu and Elizabeth B. Claus

Meningioma is one of the most common tumors of the central nervous system [1]. Interest in meningiomas has continued ever since Harvey Cushing coined the term "meningioma" to describe this class of largely benign neoplasms that arise in the meninges of the brain and spinal cord. Little is understood in terms of the initiation, growth, and progression of meningiomas into more malignant lesions.

MENINGIOMA EPIDEMIOLOGY

The prevalence of meningioma is estimated to be approximately 97.5/100,000 in the United States with more than 150,000 individuals currently diagnosed with this tumor. Data from the Central Brain Tumor Registry of the United States reveal an age-adjusted incidence rate (per 100,000 person years) of 5.04 and 2.46 for women and men, respectively [1,2]. The incidence of meningioma increases with age. Women are affected two times more often than men. Although generally considered benign (World Health Organization [WHO] grade I), approximately 8% of meningiomas display aggressive features such as increased cellularity, high nuclear to cytoplasmic ratio, increased mitotic activity, patternless growth, and foci of necrosis and are classified as atypical meningioma (WHO grade II). Approximately 2% to 3% of meningiomas exhibit frank malignant histological signs and are classified as anaplastic or malignant meningiomas (WHO grade III). Atypical and anaplastic meningiomas account for significant morbidity and mortality. It is estimated that 3% to 20% of grade I meningiomas recur, compared to 30% to 40% of grade II and 50% to 80% grade III cases [3]. Interestingly, a recent report indicated that atypical and anaplastic meningiomas occur less frequently in the cranial base and spinal locations [4].

FAMILY HISTORY OF MENINGIOMA

Few studies have examined the relationship between a personal diagnosis of meningioma and a family history of meningioma although evidence that such a history is associated with risk does exist [5,6]. Using data from the Swedish Family-Cancer Database, Hemminki et al reported a statistically significant association between meningioma diagnosis and a parental history of meningioma (standardized incidence ratio: 2.5, 95% confidence interval [CI]: 1.3–4.3) [5]. A recently published hospital-based study [6] found that the risk of meningioma was increased among persons reporting a benign brain tumor (odds ratio [OR]: 4.5, 95% CI: 1.2–15.0). Population-based surveys suggest that highly penetrant but relatively rare inherited genes may exist for meningioma susceptibility, although it appears at present that these genes may be primarily seen in families with neurofibromatosis 2 (NF2). Collections of families with multiple family members diagnosed with meningioma and who do not appear to carry inherited mutations in NF2 are relatively rarely identified [7] despite the fact that up to 1% of the adult population may harbor such a diagnosis [8], indicating a wide spectrum of phenotypic expression. At present no family-based linkage studies of meningioma have been reported. Recently, data from Israel provide evidence for genetic predisposition to radiation-associated meningioma [7], highlighting the role of inherited genetic factors in meningioma risk modification. Thus it is likely, as for many neoplasms, that meningioma development and growth is a function of the effects of many genes that are relatively prevalent but not highly penetrant and that interact with environmental exposures to confer risk.

ASSOCIATION WITH BREAST CANCER

An association between breast cancer and meningioma has been examined in several studies [6,9–11]. A number of explanations have been proposed for this association including the presence of common risk factors including endogenous and exogenous hormones [12] as well as shared genetic predisposition, including variants in DNA repair polymorphisms [13]. A review of the literature as well as an analysis of the association between breast cancer and meningioma using the western Washington State cancer registry data is provided by Custer et al [9]. The relative risks observed across existing studies range between 1.5 and 2.0 with the majority statistically significant. Most of these studies have been conducted with tumor registry data and have relatively small sample sizes. Furthermore, none have been able to examine the association while controlling for risk factors that are likely to be shared by the two tumors, such as pregnancy and menstrual variables and exogenous hormone use. A hospital-based case-control study conducted by the National Cancer Institute between 1994 and 1998 [6] reported that family history of breast cancer was associated with an elevated meningioma risk among study subjects aged 18 to 49 years (OR: 3.9, 95% CI: 1.4–11.0) and a decreased risk among older subjects (OR: 0.2, 95% CI: 0.1–0.7), but again, sample sizes were small.

Investigators are only beginning to examine the prevalence of specific breast cancer associated genes within meningioma tumor samples. Although a small study of patients with sporadic meningioma showed no evidence of mutations in two breast cancer susceptibility genes, BRCA1 and BRCA2 [10], intriguing new data gathered from an analysis of five of the case-control series from the Interphone Study report suggest that variation in the breast cancer susceptibility gene 1 (BRCA1)-interacting protein 1 (BRIP1) is associated with meningioma risk [13]. Future studies will be needed to replicate this finding as well as define the functional significance of this variant.

MOLECULAR GENETICS

The overall genetic classification of meningiomas remains limited despite the fact that meningiomas were among the first solid neoplasms studied by cytogenetic analyses. Loss of chromosome 22 was reported in meningioma as early as 1967 and is seen in up to 70% of cases. Most meningiomas with loss on this chromosome have mutations in the NF2 gene located on the retained copy of 22q. Mutation or loss of this gene appears to represent an early genetic event in the development of many meningiomas as it is frequently the predominant genetic abnormality in grade I but not grade II (atypical) and III (anaplastic) meningiomas [14]. NF2 inactivation has been implicated to different extents in various subtypes of meningiomas. Inactivation of NF2 has been reported to be more highly associated with the fibroblastic relative to meningothelial subtype [14] and may also be associated with tumor progesterone status [15]. Hanssen et al [16] performed a comprehensive genetic and epigenetic analysis of sporadic meningiomas and reported that chromosome 22 monosomy was found in 47% of cases. Biallelic inactivation of NF2 was noticed in 36% of meningiomas, with 52% of cases of fibroblastic subtype showing biallelic inactivation compared to only 18% of cases of meningothelial subtypes. In addition, macromutation of chromosome 22q was more highly associated with fibroblastic (86%) subtypes compared to meningothelial (39%) subtypes [16].

The molecular mechanism by which merlin, the NF2 gene product, is involved in the initiation of meningiomas is still unknown. Merlin, a member of the protein 4.1 family of membrane-associated proteins, lacks any apparent catalytic or DNA-binding domain and displays significant homology to members of the Ezrin-Radixin-Moesin family of cytoskeleton linker proteins. It localizes underneath the plasma membrane at cell–cell junctions and other actin-rich sites. Recent studies indicate that merlin mediates contact inhibition of proliferation by blocking recruitment of Rac to the plasma membrane. In addition to neurofibromatosis, schwannomas, and meningiomas, NF2 has also been implicated in asbestos-induced malignant mesotheliomas, melanomas, and some other solid tumors [3]. Understanding the role of merlin in meningioma tumorigenesis should be of interest in future meningioma research [17].

In addition to NF2, several other genes are implicated in meningioma initiation. Gutmann et al identified another protein 4.1 gene, DAL-1/4.1B located on chromosome 18p11.3; it was involved in both the initiation of non–small cell lung carcinomas and meningiomas [18,19]. In addition, a DAL-1-binding protein TSLC1 (tumor suppressor in lung cancer 1) was found to be deficient in most meningiomas. TSLC1 encodes an immunoglobulin superfamily cell-adhesion molecule that binds to DAL-1. It was noticed that 48% of benign meningiomas, 69% of atypical meningiomas, and 85% of anaplastic meningiomas lack TSLC1 expression [20].

After chromosome 22, the genes most frequently found to have alterations in sporadic meningioma specimens are located on chromosomes 1p and 14q, particularly in atypical meningiomas and on 9p in anaplastic meningiomas [21]. FISH studies showed monosomy 1p in 70% of atypical and almost 100% of anaplastic meningioma, indicating a correlation between loss of 1p and meningioma progression [22]. Several genes have been implicated in the clinical effect of loss of 1p on meningiomas. Tissue nonspecific alkaline phosphatase (ALPL) gene is mapped to chromosome 1p36, a chromosome region that is frequently deleted in high-grade meningiomas; its enzymic activity was found to be completely absent in the meningioma samples with loss of chromosome 1p [23]. Another tumor suppressor gene mapped to 1p36 is p73, the protein product of which shows structural and functional similarities to p53. It has been noted that the promoter region of p73 undergoes methylation in most high-grade meningiomas but not in low-grade meningiomas [24]. A recently reported significant association between the DNA repair gene RAD54L 2290 C/T polymorphism and meningioma risk is of great interest given its location on 1p and its role in the DNA repair pathway [25].

Alteration in chromosome 14 has also been associated with meningioma progression; however, genes responsible for meningioma progression on chromosome 14 are not clearly identified. Recently, NDRG2 was identified on 14q11.2 as a potential meningioma-associated tumor suppressor gene. It was found that NDRG2 was consistently downregulated in anaplastic meningiomas and some atypical meningiomas and that the loss of NDRG2 expression was significantly associated with hypermethylation of the NDRG2 promotor that leads to decreased NDRG2 transcription [26].

Analyses of genetic aberrations in meningioma indicate that losses of chromosome 9p occur in approximately one third of cases and represent the third most frequently reported aberration in meningioma. Loss of 9q in meningioma is associated with loss of both wild-type copies of two genes associated with cell cycle control, CDKN2A (9p21) as well as CDKN2B (9p21) and this change is associated with progression to anaplastic meningiomas. Inactivation of the G(1)/S-phase cell cycle checkpoint seems to be an important aberration in anaplastic meningiomas [27].

These findings are of note in light of reports from Sadetzki et al of a variation in risk of meningioma associated with p16, given radiation exposure status [28]. Amplification of 17q has also been noted in anaplastic meningiomas; however, a clear association between this amplification and TP53 mutations has not yet been shown [29]. Recently, the *S6kinase* gene on chromosome 17q23 was associated with amplification of chromosome 17 in anaplastic meningiomas [30]. Using these alterations and their associations with stage, Weber et al [31] constructed a model of meningioma progression (Figure 10.1).

GENETIC POLYMORPHISMS

There are few studies involving meningioma risk and genetic polymorphisms; however the numbers are growing [13,28,32–37]. Results of these studies are presented in Table 10.1 with statistically significant (at $p = 0.05$) values presented in boldface. Because hormones and ionizing radiation have been consistently implicated in meningioma pathogenesis, the focus of these studies has been on genes that are involved in steroid biosynthesis, breakdown or metabolism as well as variants in DNA repair and cell cycle genes, either alone or accumulated across genes in a pathway. To date, little evidence exists for a relationship between variants drawn from genes in hormones (although few genes have been examined and the sample sizes are small) but a number of investigators have reported interesting results between variants in genes involved in DNA repair and cell cycle control pathways relative to meningioma risk [7,13,28,34–36]. In the most recent and largest study to date of genetic polymorphisms and meningioma risk, investigators from the Interphone Study examined 1127 tagging single nucleotide polymorphisms (SNPs) selected to capture common variation in 136 DNA repair genes as well as an additional 388 putative functional SNPs in a combined case-control series of 631 cases and 637 controls drawn from five case-control series from the Interphone Study [13]. The group reported a novel association between meningioma risk and the SNP rs496851, which maps to intron 4 of the gene that encodes BRIP1 (mapped at 17q22).

Several research groups have focused on the association between meningioma risk and genetic polymorphisms in another gene on chromosome 17, that is, the tumor suppressor gene, TP53 on 17p [34–36]. Using data from Sweden [34] and the Interphone Study [35], Malmer et al studied three polymorphisms in TP53 and found that overall there was no associated increased risk of meningioma for any of the individual polymorphisms or for the CC-CG-CC polymorphism combination. A second group based at the National Cancer Institute used data from a hospital-based case-control series conducted within the United States [36] and examined one of the same TP53 polymorphisms as did the Swedish group (rs1042522), obtaining similarly null results (Table 10.1). Interestingly enough, in the Swedish data, when restricting the analysis to those individuals with a family history of cancer, the association between the CC-CG-CC polymorphism TP53 combination and meningioma risk was increased 5.69-fold (95%CI: 1.81–17.96).

A number of additional genes from within the cell cycle control and DNA repair pathways have been studied [28,34–36] and are presented in Table 10.1. Malmer et al examined five polymorphisms in the ataxia-telangiectasia mutant gene (*ATM*), which regulates cellular response to DNA damage [35]. The group reported that the 1–1–1–2–1 ATM haplotype combination was significantly increased in meningioma cases compared to controls whereas the 2–1-2–1-1 haplotype was significantly decreased. Several additional SNPs were examined in an updated analysis of these data and again suggest an association between the *ATM* gene and meningioma risk [13]. Further genes from these pathways that have been implicated in meningioma risk include *CASP8* [36], *Ki-ras*, and *ERCC2* [28].

Several groups have examined the role of genes involved in the metabolism of a number of compounds including solvents and aromatic hydrocarbons and meningioma risk [32,33,39–42]. Examined polymorphisms include several in glutathione-S-transferase (GSTM1, -P1, -T1) and cytochrome P450 polypeptide 2E1 (CYP2E1); GSTM1 and GSTT1 code for cytosolic enzymes that are involved in the metabolism of xenobiotics or products of oxidative stress including a number of environmental carcinogens such as the polycyclic aromatic hydrocarbons present in diet and tobacco smoke. CYP2E1 is involved in the oxidation of various compounds including steroids, fatty acids, and xenobiotics. Data from several of the larger studies [32,33,39] are presented in Table 10.1. As can be seen by a review of these data (and as presented in a meta-analysis in 2005) [41], results do not consistently seem to indicate a strong relationship between GST or other metabolism genes and meningioma risk.

INTERACTION WITH THE ENVIRONMENT

Researchers from the Tinea Capitis Study have long been involved in examining the association between genetic variants in genes from DNA repair and cell cycle control pathways both in isolation as well as in concert with information on exposure to ionizing radiation [7,28,43]. Ionizing radiation is one of the most established risk factors associated with meningioma. Typically, radiation-induced meningiomas occur at multiple locations, show more aggressive histological features, and may be associated with a less favorable clinical prognosis [44,45]. In Israel, between 1949 and 1959, >20,000 children were treated with radiotherapy for tinea capitis [43]. A follow-up study revealed

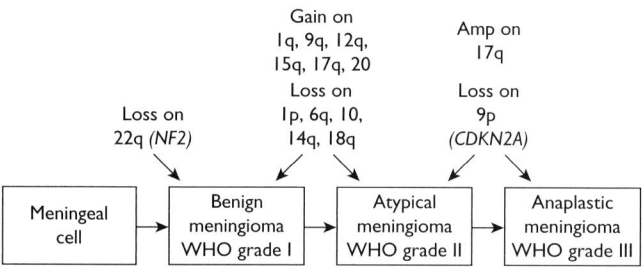

Figure 10.1 Weber's meningioma model. From Weber et al [31]. With permission from National Academy of Sciences, U.S.A., © 1997.

Table 10.1 Listing of SNPs Examined for Meningioma

Gene	SNP	Genotype	Odds Ratio	Significant Gene Environment Interaction
Meningioma susceptibility				
NF2	rs731647 [28]	AT	1.07 (0.59–1.96)	
		TT	1.36 (0.67–2.78)	
		TT+AT	1.16 (0.67–2.02)	
Breast cancer susceptibility				
BRIP1	rs4968451 [13]	Heterozygote	1.61 (1.26–2.06)	
		Homozygote	2.33 (1.25–4.34)	
Lead metabolism				
ALAD	rs1800435 [37]	ALAD2, lead−	1.1 (0.6–2.0)	With exposure to lead
		ALAD2, lead+	4.2 (1.7–10.4)	
Double-strand repair homologous				
RAD54L	2290C/T [38]	Ex18	3.4 (1.5–7.6)	
XRCC3	rs861539 [28]	CT	1.06 (0.58–1.94)	
		CC	1.18 (0.64–2.17)	
		TT+CT	1.13 (0.64–1.95)	
Double-strand repair nonhomologous				
XRCC5	rs828699 [28]	GT	1.22 (0.76–1.96)	
		TT	1.48 (0.86–2.57)	
		TT+GT	1.30 (0.84–2.03)	
Base excision repair				
XRCC1	rs1001581 [28]	TC	0.89 (0.58–1.37)	
		TT	0.91 (0.48–1.71)	
		CC+CT	0.89 (0.60–1.33)	
Cell cycle control and additional DNA repair				
Ki-ras	rs9266 [28]	CT	1.93 (1.14–3.31)	
		CC	1.49 (0.84–2.68)	
		CC+CT	1.76 (1.07–2.92)	
P16/CDKN2A	rs2811708 [28]	GT	0.75 (0.46–1.22)	With radiation
		TT	1.21 (0.56–2.67)	
		TT+TG	0.84 (0.54–1.31)	
CDKN2A	rs3731249 [36]	AG	0.7 (0.2–1.9)	
		AA	—	
		AG+AA	—	
Cyclin D1 (CCND1)	rs647451 [28]	CT	1.06 (0.62–1.81)	With radiation
		TT	1.38 (0.79–2.43)	
		TT+CT	1.18 (0.64–2.17)	
	rs678653 [36]	GC	0.6 (0.4–1.0)	
		CC	0.9 (0.5–1.6)	
		GC+CC	0.7 (0.5–1.0)	
	rs603965 [36]	AG	1.1 (0.7–1.7)	
		AA	1.5 (0.9–2.5)	
		AG+AA	1.2 (0.8–1.8)	
PTEN	rs1234214 [28]	AC	0.96 (0.60–1.54)	
		AA	1.18 (0.64–2.17)	
		AC+AA	1.02 (0.66–1.58)	
	rs701848 [36]	CT	0.8 (0.5–1.1)	
		CC	0.7 (0.4–1.3)	
		CT+CC	0.8 (0.5–1.1)	
E-cadherin	rs2010724 [28]	AG	1.34 (0.79–2.31)	
		AA	1.26 (0.73–2.21)	
		AA+AG	1.31 (0.80–2.16)	
TGFB1	rs2241715 [28]	GT	1.06 (0.62–1.81)	
		GG	1.35 (0.76–2.38)	
		GG+GT	1.17 (0.71–1.94)	
TGFBR2	rs877572 [28]	CG	0.75 (0.48–1.16)	
		GG	1.13 (0.62–2.08)	
		GG+CG	0.83 (0.54–1.26)	
ERCC2	rs1052559 [28]	AC	1.65 (0.96–2.89)	
		AA	1.71 (0.96–2.08)	
		AA+AC	1.68 (1.00–2.84)	
ATM	rs228599 [35]	TA	0.74 (0.58–0.94)	
		AA	0.70 (0.52–0.95)	

Continued

Table 10.1 Continued

Gene	SNP	Genotype	Odds Ratio	Significant Gene Environment Interaction
	rs3092992 [35]	AA	1.01 (0.70–1.45)	
		CC	2.54 (0.44–14.52)	
	rs664143 [35]	GA	0.75 (0.59–0.95)	
		AA	0.68 (0.50–0.92)	
	rs151964 [35]	AC	1.23 (0.98–1.54)	
		CC	1.41 (0.99–2.02)	
	rs3092993 [35]	CA	0.87 (0.68–1.120)	
		AA	1.19 (0.56–2.52)	
CASP8	rs13113 [36]	AT	0.8 (0.5–1.2)	
		AA	0.5 (0.3–0.9)	
		AT+AA	0.7 (0.5–1.1)	
	rs1045485 [36]	GC	1.4 (0.9–2.1)	
		CC	3.6 (1.0–13.1)	
		GC+CC	1.5 (1.0–2.3)	
CCNH	rs2266690 [36]	CT	1.2 (0.8–1.8)	
		CC	1.1 (0.4–3.2)	
		CT+CC	1.2 (0.8–1.8)	
CDKN1A	rs1801270 [36]	AC	0.8 (0.5–1.4)	
		AA	0.5 (0.1–3.3)	
		AC+AA	0.8 (0.5–1.4)	
CHEK1	rs506504 [36]	AG	0.8 (0.4–1.7)	
		AA	–	
		AG+AA	–	
CHEK2	rs2267130 [36]	AG	1.4 (0.9–2.2)	
		GG	1.2 (0.7–2.2)	
		AG+GG	1.3 (0.9–2.1)	
MDM2	rs769412 [36]	AG	1.4 (0.8–2.3)	
		GG	–	
		AG+GG	–	
P53	rs1042522 [36]	CG	1.1 (0.8–1.7)	
		CC	1.1 (0.5–2.3)	
		CG+CC	1.1 (0.8–1.7)	
	rs2287499 [34]	CG+GG	1.17 (0.75–1.83)	Interaction with family
	rs1042522 [34]	CG+GG	1.10 (0.74–1.61)	history and CC-CG-CC
	rs1625895 [34]	CT+TT	0.93 (0.58–1.49)	haplotype
	3-SNPs [34]	CC-CG-CC	5.69 (1.81–17.96)*	
Metabolic				
CYP1A1	I462V [33]	AG+GG	1.1 (0.6–2.1)	
	I462V [39]	AG+GG	1.31 (0.67–2.58)	
CYP1B1	V432L [33]	CG	1.0 (0.7–1.6)	
		GG	0.6 (0.3–1.0)	
CYP2E1	Rsa1 [32]		1.3 (0.6–2.6)	
	Ins96 [32]		0.8 (0.4–1.7)	
EPHX1	Y113H [33]	TC	0.7 (0.5–1.1)	
		CC	1.5 (0.8–2.9)	
GSTM3	*A/*B [33]	*A/*B	1.2 (0.8–1.9)	
		*B/*B	3.6 (1.3–9.8)	
	*A/*B [39]	*A/*B	1.24 (1.0–1.56)	
		*B/*B	1.02 (0.53–1.98)	
		*A/*B+*B/*B	1.22 (0.98–1.52)	
	63 [39]	AC	1.07 (0.86–1.33)	
		CC	0.84 (0.62–1.14)	
		AA+AC	0.81 (0.62–1.07)	
NQO1	P187S [33]	CT	0.8 (0.5–1.2)	
		TT	0.6 (0.2–2.0)	
	P187S [39]	CT+TT	1.21 (0.8–1.81)	
GSTP1	105 [32]	Val/Val	0.7 (0.4–1.5)	
	105 [39]	Val/Val	0.74 (0.57–1.15)	
	114 [32]	Ala/Val or Val/Val	0.9 (0.5–1.6)	
	114 [39]		1.07 (0.82–1.40)	
GSTM1	Null [32]		0.9 (0.6–1.3)	
	Null [39]		1.22 (0.85–1.75)	
GSTT1	Null [32]		1.5 (1.0–2.4)	
	Null [39]		0.98 (0.60–1.61)	

a relative risk of 9.5 of meningioma formation in the irradiated group compared with the nonirradiated controls. However, only a small subset of the irradiated subjects (<1%) developed meningioma, indicating the importance of the interplay between genes and the environment [43]. More recently, intriguing results involving the association between genetic variants, exposure to ionizing radiation, and meningioma risk have been presented using these same data [7,28]. This new analysis includes 150 meningioma patients irradiated for tinea capitis as children, 129 persons irradiated for tinea capitis as children who did not develop meningioma, 69 meningioma patients who had not been irradiated, and 92 population controls. SNPs from two genes in the cell cycle control pathway, *Ki-ras* (OR: 1.76, 95% CI: 1.07–2.92) and *ERCC2* (OR: 1.68, 95% CI: 1.00–2.68), were associated with meningioma risk. Furthermore, a significant association was found between radiation and cyclin D1 and p16 SNPs and meningioma risk ($p = 0.005$ and 0.057, respectively), suggesting these SNPs may be markers of genes that have an inverse effect on the risk of meningioma formation in irradiated and nonirradiated populations. The same group carried out a large-scale family study which confirmed that the irradiated family members of the initially identified patients with radiation-associated meningioma carry a significant increased risk for meningioma formation compared with control groups. This study confirmed the idea that genetic susceptibility increases the risk of radiation-associated meningioma formation [7,28].

The interplay between genes and the environment are again highlighted in work reported by Rajaraman et al [37] in which 151 patients with meningioma were genotyped for aminolevulinic acid dehydratase (ALAD), an enzyme that catalyzes the second step of heme synthesis and is strongly inhibited by lead. An increased risk of meningioma was seen in persons with occupational lead exposure with odds ratios ranging from 1.1 (95%CI: 0.3–4.5) for persons with low exposure to 12.8 (95% CI: 1.4–120.8) for persons with high exposure, potentially suggesting that lead may be implicated in meningioma risk in genetically susceptible persons. As the authors note, the sample size used to obtain these results is small; therefore, replications of these values are needed.

MICROARRAY ANALYSES

Few gene expression analyses exist utilizing meningioma specimens [46–48]; the ones that do examine expression by grade [48], anatomic location [47], and preparation [46]. More recently, meningioma gene expression has been examined by hormone receptor status [15]. A large number of investigators have examined both the prevalence and function of estrogen and progesterone receptors in meningioma, with these tumors in general showing a low expression level of estrogen receptors and a high level of progesterone receptors [45]. Although the specific role of both types of receptor as well as their isoforms remains unclear, there is growing evidence to support a role for progesterone receptors. A recent pilot study of 31 meningioma samples reported that gene expression appeared more strongly associated with PR status than with ER status [15]. Genes on the long arm of chromosome 22 and near the *NF2* gene (22q12) were most frequently noted to have expression variation, with significant upregulation in PR+ versus PR– lesions suggesting a higher rate of 22q loss in PR– lesions. Pathway analyses indicated that genes in collagen and extracellular matrix pathways were most likely to be differentially expressed by PR status. These data, although preliminary, are the first to examine gene expression for meningioma cases by hormone receptor status and indicate a stronger association with progesterone than with estrogen receptors. PR status is related to the expression of genes near the *NF2* gene, mutations which have been identified as the initial event in many meningiomas. These findings suggest that PR status may be a clinical marker for genetic subgroups of meningioma and warrant further examination in a larger data set [38].

CONCLUSION

Although the search for genes associated with meningioma risk is in its infancy, the data reviewed here provide intriguing preliminary results and suggest a number of research avenues to pursue. All of the results to date will require verification in additional, larger and collaborative data sets. To date, no genome-wide association study has been undertaken for meningioma although researchers from a number of groups including the Meningioma Consortium (Yale University, Brigham and Women's Hospital, Duke University, M.D. Anderson Cancer Center and the University of California at San Francisco), the Interphone Study, and the Tinea Capitis Study among others are working to collect such data. With the realization that most diseases are a product of a complex mixture of genes and the environment, it will only be through such collaborative efforts that advances in meningioma genetics will occur.

ACKNOWLEDGMENT

This work was supported by the Brain Science Foundation, the Meningioma Mommas and by NIH R01 grants CA109468 and CA109461.

REFERENCES

1. CBTRUS. *Statistical Report: Primary Brain Tumors in the United States, 1998–2002.* Hinsdale, IL: CBTRUS; 2005.
2. Claus EB, Bondy ML, Schildkraut JM, Wiemels J, Wrensch M, Black PM. Epidemiology of intra-cranial meningioma. *Neurosurgery.* 2005;57:1088–1095.
3. Perry A, Stafford SL, Scheithauer BW, Suman VJ, Lohse CM. Meningioma grading: an analysis of histologic parameters. *Am J Surg Pathol.* 1997;21:1455–1465.
4. Sade B, Chahlavi A, Krishnaney A, Nagel S, Choi E, Lee JH. World Health Organization Grades II and III meningiomas are rare in the cranial base and spine. *Neurosurgery.* 2007;61:1194–1198; discussion 1198.
5. Hemminki K, Li X. Familial risks in nervous system tumors. *Cancer Epidemiol Biomarkers Prev.* 2003;12:1137–1142.
6. Hill DA, Linet MS, Black PM, et al. Meningioma and schwannoma risk in adults in relation to family history of cancer. *Neuro Oncol.* 2004;6:274–280.

7. Flint-Richter P, Sadetzki S. Genetic predisposition for the development of radiation-associated meningioma: an epidemiological study. *Lancet Oncol.* 2007;8:403–410.
8. Vernooij MW, Ikram MA, Tanghe HL, et al. Incidental findings on brain MRI in the general population. *New Engl J Med.* 2007;357:1821–1828.
9. Custer BS, Koepsell TD, Mueller BA. The association between breast carcinoma and meningioma in women. *Cancer.* 2002;94:1626–1635.
10. Kirsch M, Zhu JJ, Black PM. Analysis of the BRCA1 and BRCA2 genes in sporadic meningiomas. *Genes Chromosomes Cancer.* 1997;20:53–59.
11. Malmer B, Tavelin B, Henriksson R, Gronberg H. Primary brain tumors as second primary: a novel association between meningioma and colorectal cancer. *Int J Cancer.* 2000;85:78–81.
12. Claus EB, Black PM, Bondy ML, et al. Exogenous hormone use and meningioma risk: what do we tell our patients? *Cancer.* 2007;110:471–476.
13. Bethke L, Murray A, Webb E, et al. Comprehensive analysis of DNA repair gene variants and risk of meningioma. *J Natl Cancer Inst.* 2008;100:270–276.
14. Buccoliero AM, Castiglione F, Degl'Innocenti DR, et al. NF2 gene expression in sporadic meningiomas: relation to grades or histotypes real time-PCR study. *Neuropathology.* 2007;27:36–42.
15. Claus EB, Park PJ, Carroll R, Chan J, Black PM. Specific genes expressed in association with progesterone receptors in meningioma. *Cancer Research.* 2008;68:314–322.
16. Hansson CM, Buckley PG, Grigelioniene G, et al. Comprehensive genetic and epigenetic analysis of sporadic meningioma for macromutations on 22q and micro-mutations within the NF2 locus. *BMC Genomics.* 2007;8:16.
17. Hirokawa Y, Tikoo A, Huynh J, et al. A clue to the therapy of neurofibromatosis type 2: NF2/merlin is a PAK1 inhibitor. *Cancer.* 2004;10:20–26.
18. Gutmann DH, Donahoe J, Perry A, et al. Loss of DAL-1, a protein 4.1-related tumor suppressor, is an important early event in the pathogenesis of meningiomas. *Hum Mol Genet.* 2000;9:1495–1500.
19. Kittiniyom K, Mastronardi M, Roemer M, et al. Allele-specific loss of heterozygosity at the DAL-1/4.1B (EPB41L3) tumor-suppressor gene locus in the absence of mutation. *Genes Chromosomes Cancer.* 2004;40:190–203.
20. Surace EI, Lusis E, Murakami Y, Scheithauer BW, Perry A, Gutmann DH. Loss of tumor suppressor in lung cancer-1 (TSLC1) expression in meningioma correlates with increased malignancy grade and reduced patient survival. *J Neuropathol Exp Neurol.* 2004;63:1015–1027.
21. Lopez-Gines C, Cerda-Nicolas M, Gil-Benso R, et al. Association of loss of 1p and alterations of chromosome 14 in meningioma progression. *Cancer Genet Cytogenet.* 2004;148:123–128.
22. Ketter R, Henn W, Niedermayer I, et al. Predictive value of progression-associated chromosomal aberrations for the prognosis of meningiomas: a retrospective study of 198 cases. *J Neurosurg.* 2001;95:601–607.
23. Muller P, Henn W, Niedermayer I, et al. Deletion of chromosome 1p and loss of expression of alkaline phosphatase indicate progression of meningiomas. *Clin Cancer Res.* 1999;5:3569–3577.
24. Nakane Y, Natsume A, Wakabayashi T, et al. Malignant transformation-related genes in meningiomas: allelic loss on 1p36 and methylation status of p73 and RASSF1A. *J Neurosurg.* 2007;107:398–404.
25. Mendiola M, Bello MJ, Alonso J, et al. Search for mutations of the hRAD54 gene in sporadic meningiomas with deletion at 1p32. *Mol Carcinog.* 1999;24:300–304.
26. Lusis EA, Watson MA, Chicoine MR, et al. Integrative genomic analysis identifies NDRG2 as a candidate tumor suppressor gene frequently inactivated in clinically aggressive meningioma. *Cancer Res.* 2005;65:7121–7126.
27. Bostrom J, Meyer-Puttlitz B, Wolter M, et al. Alterations of the tumor suppressor genes CDKN2A (p16(INK4a)), p14(ARF), CDKN2B (p15(INK4b)), and CDKN2C (p18(INK4c)) in atypical and anaplastic meningiomas. *Am J Pathol.* 2001;159:661–669.
28. Sadetzki S, Flint-Richter P, Starinsky S, et al. Genotyping of patients with sporadic and radiation-associated meningiomas. *Cancer Epidemiol Biomarkers Prev.* 2005;14:969–976.
29. Verheijen FM, Sprong M, Kloosterman JM, Blaauw G, Thijssen JH, Blankenstein MA. TP53 mutations in human meningiomas. *Int J Biol Markers.* 2002;17:42–48.
30. Surace EI, Lusis E, Haipek CA, Gutmann DH. Functional significance of S6K overexpression in meningioma progression. *Ann Neurol.* 2004;56:295–298.
31. Weber RG, Bostrom J, Wolter M, et al. Analysis of genomic alterations in benign, atypical, and anaplastic meningiomas: toward a genetic model of meningioma progression. *Proc Natl Acad Sci.* 1997;94:14719–14724.
32. De Roos AJ, Rothman N, Inskip PD, et al. Genetic polymorphisms in GSTM1, -P1, -T1, and CYP2E1 and the risk of adult brain tumors. *Cancer Epidemiol Biomarkers Prev.* 2003;12:14–22.
33. De Roos AJ, Rothman N, Brown M, et al. Variation in genes relevant to aromatic hydrocarbon metabolism and the risk of adult brain tumors. *Neuro Oncol.* 2006;8:145–155.
34. Malmer B, Feychting M, Lonn S, Ahlbom A, Henriksson R. p53 Genotypes and risk of glioma and meningioma. *Cancer Epidemiol Biomarkers Prev.* 2005;14:2220–2223.
35. Malmer BS, Feychting M, Lonn S, et al. Genetic variation in p53 and ATM haplotypes and risk of glioma and meningioma. *J Neurooncol.* 2007;82:229–237.
36. Rajaraman P, Wang SW, Rothman N, et al. Polymorphisms in apoptosis and cell cycle control genes and risk of brain tumors in adults. *Cancer Epidemiol Biomarkers Prev.* 2007;16:1655–1661.
37. Rajaraman P, Stewart PA, Samet JM, et al. Lead, genetic susceptibility, and risk of adult brain tumors. *Cancer Epidemiol Biomarkers Prev.* 2006;15:2514–2520.
38. Leone PE, Mendiola M, Alonso J, Paz-y-Mino C, Pestana A. Implications of a RAD54L polymorphism (2290C/T) in human meningiomas as a risk factor and/or a genetic marker. *BMC Cancer.* 2003;3:6.
39. Schwartzbaum JA, Ahlbom A, Lonn S, et al. An international case-control study of glutathione transferase and functionally related polymorphisms and risk of primary adult brain tumors. *Cancer Epidemiol Biomarkers Prev.* 2007;16:559–565.
40. Elexpuru-Camiruaga J, Buxton N, Kandula V, et al. Susceptibility to astrocytoma and meningioma: influence of allelism at glutathione S-transferase (GSTT1 and GSTM1) and cytochrome P-450 (CYP2D6) loci. *Cancer Research.* 1995;55:4237–4239.
41. Lai R, Crevier L, Thabane L. Genetic polymorphisms of glutathione S-transferases and the risk of adult brain tumors: a meta-analysis. *Cancer Epidemiol Biomarkers Prev.* 2005;14:1784–1790.
42. Pinarbasi H, Silig Y, Gurelik M. Genetic polymorphisms of GSTs and their association with primary brain tumor incidence. *Cancer Genet Cytogenet.* 2005;156:144–149.
43. Ron E, Modan B, Boice JD Jr, et al. Tumors of the brain and nervous system after radiotherapy in childhood. *N Engl J Med.* 1988;319:1033–1039.
44. Al-Mefty O, Topsakal C, Pravdenkova S, Sawyer JR, Harrison MJ. Radiation-induced meningiomas: clinical, pathological, cytokinetic, and cytogenetic characteristics. *J Neurosurg.* 2004;100:1002–1013.
45. Pravdenkova S, Al-Mefty O, Sawyer J, Husain M. Progesterone and estrogen receptors: opposing prognostic indicators in meningiomas. *J Neurosurg.* 2006;105:163–173.
46. Sasaki T, Hankins GR, Helm GR. Comparison of gene expression profiles between frozen original meningiomas and primary cultures of the meningiomas by GeneChip. *Neurosurgery.* 2003;52:892–899.
47. Sayagues JM, Tebernero MD, Maillo A, Trelles O, Espinosa AB, Sarasquete ME. Microarray-based analysis of spinal versus intracranial meningiomas: different clinical, biological, and genetic characteristics associated with distinct patterns of gene expression. *J Neuropathol Exp Neurol.* 2006;65:445–454.
48. Wrobel G, Roerig P, Kokocinski F, et al. Microarray-based gene expression profiling of benign, atypical, and anaplastic meningiomas identifies novel genes associated with meningioma progression. *Int J Cancer.* 2005;114:249–256

PART II: MOLECULAR BIOLOGY

11 Molecular Neuro-Oncology: Why is it Essential?

Abhijit Guha

Human nervous system tumors, like all cancers, arise from aberration(s) in the molecular controls of normal cellular developmental and biological processes. In essence cancer is a genetic disease, the understanding of which is critical toward improving our capability to diagnose, prognose, develop, and select specific biological targeted therapies. In conjunction with nontargeted surgical, radiation, and chemotherapy, it is hoped that rational biological therapies will improve the overall outcome of our patients. These molecular alterations that may arise at the level of DNA, RNA, or the proteins themselves are not singular but rather multiple in human nervous system tumors. Large-scale genomic studies, such as The Cancer Genome Atlas, and upcoming proteomic-based studies have already elucidated that there is much heterogeneity in the molecular profiles of nervous system tumors which are pathologically similar. This is even more pronounced between pediatric tumors and their adult counterparts, leading to some degree of separation of these topics in this section. Adding further complexity there is likely regional and temporal heterogeneity as the tumors adapt to different microenvironmental conditions and therapeutic interventions, as discussed in several chapters of this section. To make sense of the large current and emerging molecular data sets, like those available in adult malignant gliomas and pediatric medulloblastomas, grouping based on aberrant signaling pathways or prognosis has been undertaken. However, the ongoing challenge is to determine what are the key molecular alterations and their interactions that "drive" the origin or progression of the tumors versus those alterations that are secondary and "passengers." These require experimental paradigms using in vitro and in vivo model systems as discussed.

Some of the molecular alterations are germline, either inherited or acquired de-novo, and found in every cell of the body. These inherited syndromes, as discussed in several chapters of this section, underlie only a small percentage of human nervous system tumors, being more prevalent in pediatric tumors. The molecular understanding of these well-defined group of patients, which are part of predisposition syndromes, are important. Often, the key molecular alterations are similar in this largely pediatric group of nervous system tumors to their more common adult sporadically occurring counterparts. Furthermore, they form the basis of developing model systems, such as transgenic mice, to enhance our understanding of the large number of genetic alterations that are being deciphered in sporadic human nervous system tumors and also to provide platforms for therapeutic interventional studies.

The cell of origin of solid tumors, including nervous system tumors, has created much interest with the relatively recent Cancer Stem Cell (CSC) hypothesis. The well-known clonal evolution of cancer proposed by Nowell describes cancer to result from a stochastic accumulation of genetic alterations in differentiated cells. In contrast, the CSC hypothesis, much of which is based on our knowledge of hematological cancers, stipulates that the cell of origin has stem cell properties of self-renewal and differentiation capability, which acquires transforming genetic alterations in a hierarchical manner. The cell of origin in this case differs from differentiated tumor cells, which form the bulk of the solid tumor in terms of preferred biological niches and therapeutic sensitivity, thereby serving as a nidus for recurrence. Ongoing debate remains as to which of these model systems of the cell of origin is prevalent in both pediatric and adult nervous system tumors as discussed. It is likely that the answer is a composite of both theories, in keeping with the heterogeneity of transformed cells and their plasticity and adaptability to the tumor microenvironment.

Nervous system tumors include malignant and benign tumors of the central nervous system (CNS) and peripheral nervous system (PNS). In addition there are metastatic tumors to the CNS, which are increasing in frequency as their primary tumors are being detected earlier leading to better local control and increased patient longevity. The molecular biology of metastatic tumors is not addressed in this section as readers are referred to the large body of literature existing on this subject. In brief, it is of interest that the CNS or PNS microenvironment have several unique aspects of the "seed and soil" hypothesis of metastasis. For example, certain types of primaries such as melanomas have a propensity to involve the CNS. In contrast, other primaries such as prostate usually avoid the CNS parenchyma though they can metastasize to the skull and dura.

This section concentrates on primary malignant and benign nervous system tumors with their unique clinical presentation, pathology, molecular biology, and management. Emphasis is on the most common adult primary CNS tumors, the gliomas, especially the most malignant form known as glioblastoma multiforme. Invasion, angiogenesis, pathological and corresponding molecular heterogeneity are cardinal features, which makes this tumor subtype lethal even though some therapeutic progress has been made. Chapters dedicated to these key biological processes are a testament to these biological and thereby therapeutic roadblocks. Similarly, medulloblastomas and high-grade gliomas are the more common pediatric CNS tumors deserving of focused attention. In contrast to the malignant tumors mentioned earlier, benign CNS and PNS tumors are usually not invasive and more amenable to surgical or other focused therapies. However, due to their location in eloquent regions of the CNS or PNS they can cause significant morbidity and mortality with surgical treatment. Pathological and molecular understanding of these tumors, such as those of the pituitary region, meninges, peripheral, and cranial nerves are reviewed. Armed with this knowledge, additional biological therapies, such as those which have revolutionized management of most pituitary tumors, may emerge for these benign nervous system tumors.

In summary, the purpose of the chapters in this section is to give an overview of our current pathological and corresponding molecular knowledge of the variety of nervous system tumors. Readers are encouraged to utilize the references for additional detail. As evidenced, much controversy of fundamental questions about the origin and molecular biology of nervous system tumors remain. It is through collaborative efforts of clinicians, clinician-scientists, and basic scientists from a variety of backgrounds that the significant inroads into our knowledge of the molecular pathogenesis of nervous system tumors has been made to date and will be fostered in the future. This journey will be long, likely slow with many forks in the road, keeping with the complexity and diversity of these tumors. However, it is a journey that is essential toward our ultimate goals to improve the quality and quantity of our patients' lives.

12 Brain Tumor Initiating Cells: History, New Advances, Therapeutic Promises, and Pitfalls

Sameer Agnihotri, Diana Munoz, and Abhijit Guha

INTRODUCTION: STEM CELL HYPOTHESIS

Conventional approaches to the treatment and management of cancer have been to eliminate all tumor cells. This approach is primarily based on the *stochastic model* also known as the clonal evolution model in which all tumor cells have the potential to proliferate limitlessly, self-renew, and drive tumor growth [1,2]. However, treatments tailored to this model have resulted in minimal gains toward survival posttreatment in several cancers including glioblastoma multiforme (GBM) [3]. Current research has challenged the old paradigm of the stochastic model, as recent evidence suggests that a subset of cancer cells within a tumor are responsible for tumor initiation, maintenance, and resistance to therapy [4,5]. This new concept of a subset of cells within the tumor that has stem cell like properties, limitless expansion potential and can drive tumor formation, has been designated the cancer stem cell (CSC) hypothesis or *hierarchical model* (Figure 12.1).

In addition, bulk tumor cells that are derived from this stem cell like tumor cells have limited proliferating capacity, are partially differentiated cells, and cannot form tumors. The stem cell compartment of tumors have been termed cancer stem cells (CSCs), tumor-initiating cells (TICs), or tumor-propagating cells (TPCs) [6]. For simplicity, we will use the term TICs and brain tumor initiating cells (BTICs) to specifically refer to central nervous system (CNS) tumor formation. Additionally, we would like to clarify that our definition does not encompass the term cell of origin. This term refers to the original cell or group of cells that acquired neoplastic lesions to induce transformation. BTICs may be one possible candidate for the cell of origin.

TICs have been isolated from several cancers including brain tumors such as GBM and medulloblastomas (MB) [7–9]. These isolated BTICs constitute a tiny fraction of the total population of tumor cells and are characterized by several hallmark features in Table 12.1. BTICs are able to propagate in an undifferentiated manner and are able to recapitulate the tumor when injected in low numbers (10^3–10^4 versus 10^5–10^6 in nonpurified tumor cells) [7–10]. BTICs express markers including CD133, Nestin, SOX2, which are similar to normal neural stem cells and are isolated/derived using several means as summarized in Table 12.2 [4,7,11–14]. In this chapter, we will discuss sources of neural stem cells and BTICs and aberrant signaling pathways within these cells. We will further discuss how targeting BTICs may provide a new strategy for therapeutic targeting and outline potential limitations and pitfalls of the CSCs as therapeutic targets.

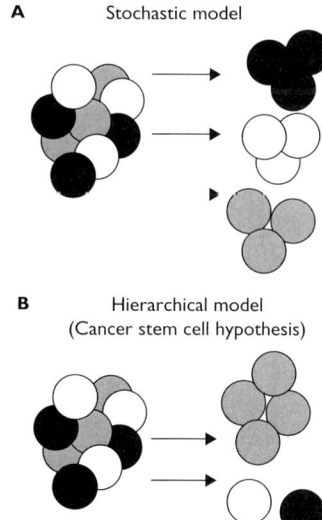

Figure 12.1 (A) The stochastic model predicts that any tumor cell, given the chance, will be able to form a new tumor. (B) The cancer stem cell model predicts that only a subset of cells (the gray cells in the figure) can generate a new tumor, whereas the other cells cannot.

Table 12.1 Hallmarks of Brain Tumor-Initiating Cells

Hallmark	Description
Self-renewal	Parent cell gives rise to two daughter cells, which retain all the stem cell-like properties of the parent cells
Multipotency	Potential to differentiate into different cell types and express markers of different lineages such as neurons, oligodendrocytes, and astrocytes
Proliferation	The ability to produce many progeny cells, which form primarily the bulk tumor

Table 12.2 Methods of Isolating BTICs

Method	Summary
Flow cytometry	Separating cells based on candidate stem cell surface markers into positive and negative fractions for the marker of interest [4,7,11]
Neurosphere assays	Growing tumor cells in neural basal cell medium with growth factors that enrich for neural stem cells [12,13]. Neurospheres can be passaged numerous times and display hallmarks from Table 12.1
Adherent stem cell cultures	Growing isolated BTICs on adherent laminin-coated plates to allow for increased purity and stability, uniform growth factor delivery, and reduce spontaneous differentiation [14]

DEFINITION AND SOURCES OF BTICS

The isolation of a subpopulation of stem-like cells from surgical specimens of malignant gliomas lent support to the CSC hypothesis [9]. The glioma stem cells or BTICs have features of normal neural stem cells such as self-renewal, multipotent differentiation, and the ability to recapitulate the tumor phenotype in vivo in small numbers. This discovery inferred that GBMs are composed of a heterogeneous collection of cancer cells with varying tumor initiation potential [9].

However, what is the origin of these BTICs remains controversial with several potential and not mutually exclusive hypotheses as schematized in Figure 12.2 and discussed later. BTICs can have different theoretical origins, which can be broadly grouped into three major underlying theories: (1) normal neuroglial stem cells (NSCs), which normally have tight regulation over their proliferative and differentiation potential, acquire mutations that render them tumorigenic and undergo transformation to BTICs [15,16]; (2) restricted neural or glial progenitors, which have limited self-renewal potential, acquire mutations that lead to the gain of unregulated transformed stem cell like properties; and (3) mature differentiated glia through acquisition of mutations dedifferentiate to acquire unregulated stem cell like properties.

The isolation of replication-competent, multipotent neural–glial progenitors from the postnatal brain [17,18] provided a hypothesis that these cells are the origin of BTICs in adults (Figure 12.2 [14,19]). These progenitor cells harboring stem cell properties of self-renewal and multipotent differentiation might represent a path of least resistance to transformation, since they already have activation of the genetic machinery for self-renewal. These multipotent neural progenitors are found in specialized neurogenic niches in adults such as the dentate gyrus and the subventricular zone (SVZ). The SVZ is an extensive germinal layer adjacent to the ependyma, containing astrocyte-like stem cells (also known as Type B cells in mice) [19]. These relative quiescent neural stem cells periodically give rise to lineage-restricted progenitors cells, which undergo limited mitosis before differentiating into mature cells [19]. A prevalent theory on the origin of BTICs asserts that they are a result of neural stem cell transformation, as there are several similarities between BTICs and neural stem cells. Both cells share multiple cell surface markers, exhibit a marked ability to migrate through the brain parenchyma, and are able to form neurospheres in vitro, but most importantly, pathways regulating normal stem cell self-renewal, proliferation, and survival may also be operative in BTICs.

In support of the neurogenic niche serving as the origin of BTICs is that gliomas are sometimes radiologically linked to the periventricular zone. However, this suggested link is often not present, though microscopic linkage not visualized on conventional imaging used to date with the periventricular zone cannot be ruled out. Additional support of the hypothesis is the observation that viral and chemical carcinogenesis preferentially induce tumors when inoculated adjacent to the SVZ rather than when introduced into nonproliferative regions such as the cortex [20,21]. More recently, further experimental models in mice have validated the paradigm that BTICs might arise from neural stem cell transformation. Alcantara et al. [22] developed a mouse model in which deletion of human astrocytoma-relevant tumor suppressors p53, Nf1, and PTEN was targeted to neural stem cells, through the use of an inducible Nestin-cre transgene, or alternatively using stereotactic viral delivery of Cre expressing adenovirus into the SVZ. This mice developed astrocytomas with a 100% penetrance, only when targeted to neural precursors cells but not differentiated glial cells [22].

A second hypothesis of the origin of BTICs is that they arise from restricted neural and glial progenitors (Figure 12.2 [2,5]), which have limited self-renewal potential. These cells will first need to acquire mutations that endow them with an increased self-renewal potential in order to experience additional mutations that would lead to transformation. Studies have shown that committed oligodendroglial progenitors can be induced through the modification of extracellular signals, to gain stem-like properties [23], resulting in the reactivation of the primitive neural epithelial marker Sox2 [23], which is prevalently expressed in human gliomas [24]. These results suggest that similar mechanisms might be operative in the transformation of restricted progenitors in the adult brain.

In contradiction to what is conceived as the CSC hypothesis, several studies have supported the idea that committed glial cells could be the precursors of BTICs, as depicted in Figure 12.2 [2–4]. Retroviral transduction of INK4a/Arf$^{-/-}$ mature astrocytes with a constitutively active mutant EGF receptor (EGFRvIII), prevalent in human GBMs, induces astrocyte dedifferentiation and GBM formation [25]. This phenomenon is also observed when GFAP$^+$ cells are infected with platelet-derived growth factor (PDGF) expressing retrovirus using the RCAS/tva system [24]. In addition, overexpression of the transcriptional factor c-myc in astrocytes results in the down-regulation of the astrocytic differentiation marker GFAP, and up-regulation of the astrocyte progenitor marker Nestin [11]. One of the most relevant pieces of evidence comes from the demonstration that adult fibroblast can be reprogrammed to a pluripotent stem cell state by transfection of a small number of transcription factors, the so-called induced pluripotent stem cell (IPS) [26]. In support, oncogenic stress and

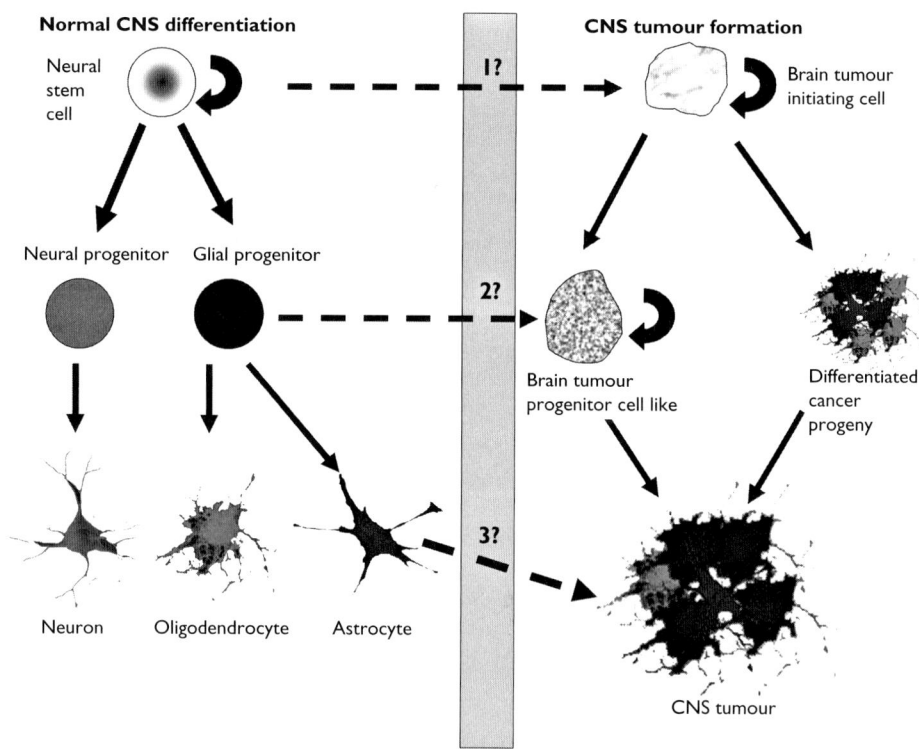

Figure 12.2 Normal central nervous system (CNS) differentiations and CNS tumor formation. During normal neuroglial stem cells (NSCs) differentiation, NSCs give rise to neural and glial progenitors, which give rise to differentiated cells such as neurons, oligodendrocytes, and astrocytes. BTICs have been theorized to come from terminally differentiated cells (1?) which acquire genetic mutations (?) which endow them with a proliferative advantage of a slow accumulation of critical mutations result in its transformation. Normal neural stem cells give rise to progenitors with limited proliferative and self-replicative capacity. BTICs have been theorized to form as a result of neural stem cells (2?) or neural progenitor transformation (3?). Curved arrow represents ability to self-renew.

induction of certain transcription factors have been shown to reprogram differentiated cells or restricted progenitor cells to a more pluripotent-like state [27–29]. Cumulatively, these and other experimental evidences suggest that permanently quiescent cells can be endowed stem cell like properties, arguing that a similar process might be relevant during brain tumor pathogenesis.

Lessons learned from other cancer systems also have raised questions in the applicability of the hierarchical model and BTICs in certain situations. In breast cancer, putative TICs shown to express CD24 or CD44 were genetically different within the same patient. This suggests that these cells, both of which express antigens associated with what is thought to be breast cancer TICs, actually originated from different subpopulations. This observation suggests that each subset of tumor cells undergoes differential transformations to gain growth advantages, in support of the stochastic model [30]. One study demonstrated that supplementing the long-term chemically used rat C6 glioma cell line with serum and certain growth conditions led to 100% of C6 cells able to proliferate, exhibit exponential growth without spontaneous differentiation, and the ability to self-renew. Once again this is more easily explained by the stochastic model and that the influence of microenvironment on conferring stem cell like properties to non-stem cell tumor cells can occur. In summary, the topic of the origin of BTICs remains controversial and may differ from one tumor type to another, between pediatric and adults, or even between the same tumor type in different patients. Currently there is experimental evidence in support or deference to several cell types of origin of BTICs, requiring an open mind in this area, with some of the reasons for this ongoing controversy discussed later.

However, the subject of the origin of BTICs is of great research and therapeutic interest, as the cancer causing genetic or epigenetic alterations may be quite different in the three cell populations outlined earlier in Figure 12.2.

CELL SURFACE MARKERS OF BTICS AND ABERRANT SIGNALING IN BTICS OF GBM

BTIC-Associated Markers

The concept of CSC originated from blood cancers where specific antigenic markers are well-defined and linked to the differentiation paradigm of hematopoietic lineage. However, this is not as clear in solid cancers such as gliomas as BTICs share many molecular markers once thought to be exclusively attributed to NSC, such as Nestin [31], CD133 [32], Musashi-1 [33], and SSEA-1 [34] (Table 12.3). Unfortunately, at this time no cell marker is absolute in identifying BTICs. However, two cell surface markers, Nestin and CD133 (Prominin-1), have been of particular interest in the study of brain tumor organization. It has been observed that these markers are associated with grade of malignancy and are likely prognostic markers for brain tumor patients [12,13].

The intermediate filament Nestin is expressed in all CNS lineage-restricted progenitors and in astrocytes [14]. Evidence suggests that Nestin expression is highly correlated with "stemness," whereas NSC progeny that takes on a more committed role results in a down-regulation of Nestin expression followed by up-regulation of more committed neuronal and astrocytic markers, such as GFAP [35]. Expression of Nestin has been reported in BTICs; however,

Table 12.3 Markers of BTICs

Marker	Summary
CD133	Used to isolate a subpopulation of tumorigenic cells from GBM operative specimens, capable of tumor initiation in vivo. Recent studies have reported its expression as a result of environmental stress, questioning its validity as a BTIC marker
Nestin	Expressed in all CNS lineage-restricted progenitors astrocytes and BTIC. However, the expression of this marker is variable and nonspecific to BTIC
Musashi-1	Expressed in normal NSC and BTIC. Its expression has been correlated with tumor grade and proliferative activity. Its role as a BTIC-specific marker is nonconclusive
SSEA-1	A neural stem progenitor marker shown to be expressed in GBM cells that fulfill the functional criteria of BTIC. Proposed to be a better BTIC marker in combination with CD133

its expression is variable and nonspecific for BTICs and also present in proliferating reactive astrocytes [31].

The neuronal stem cell marker CD133 (Prominin-1 in mice) has received particular interest, as its expression has been associated with both, tumor initiation capacity and radioresistance [9,36]. Initial reports indicated that as few as 100 CD133+ cells collected from GBM surgical specimens could form xenograft tumors in immunocompromised mice that recapitulated the phenotype of the tumor from which they were isolated [9]. This is in sharp contrast to the 10^6 CD133- cells required for the same phenotype [9]. Although there has been overwhelming evidence that supports this issue, more recent investigations have called into question the reliability of CD133 as a marker of BTICs. Griguer et al. [37] reported that alternations in mitochondrial function among glioma cells induce CD133 expression. Conversely, replacement of dysfunctional mitochondrial genes can reverse CD133 expression [37]. These results suggest that CD133 expression in gliomas is triggered as a response to environmental stress, questioning the reliability of CD133 as a BTIC marker.

Other markers that are shared by normal NSC and BTIC include the RNA-binding proteins, Musashi-1, which in normal stem cells is thought to repress the translation of mRNAs believed to be involved in the process of differentiation [5]. Increasing evidence points toward the involvement of Musashi-1 in the process of tumorigenesis, as its expression has been reported in neurospheres derived form GBM operative specimens, and its expression is highly correlated to the grade of malignancy and proliferative activity in gliomas [38]. However, its role as a specific BTIC marker remains questionable. More recently, Son et al. [34] identified the stage-specific embryonic antigen-1 (SSEA-1 also known as CD15/LeX) to be expressed in GBM cells that fulfill the functional criteria of BTICs. SSEA-1 cells are highly tumorigenic, can give rise to both SSEA-1+ and SSEA-1- populations, and have self-renewal and multilineage differentiation potential. However, further validation that will identify SSEA-1 as a specific marker of BTIC is still pending.

As inferred earlier, none of the makers by themselves seem to specifically identify a BTIC, a formidable impediment for research undertaken in this area. Research in thoroughly understanding neuroglial development and lineage differentiation with their associated regulatory controls (discussed later) and antigenic markers are ongoing and hopefully will shed further light into the characterization of origin of BTICs. As noted, there may not be a singular origin of BTICs and hence multiple markers may exist to define a BTIC and it may be only pertinent in that patient or a subgroup of patients. Of course these markers will also likely differ between different gliomas or other CNS tumor subtypes and also between pediatric and adults brain tumors, which we know are clinically and genetically different, even though pathologically may bear similarities to their adult counterparts.

Aberrant Signaling Pathways Associated with BTICs

Multiple signaling pathways have been implicated to be disrupted in BTICs. Interestingly they include those that serve to regulate the self-renewal, proliferation, and survival properties of normal stem cells. This include the hedgehog family of regulatory pathways that mediate the proliferation of progenitor cells through the activation of the transcription factor Gli, which promote cell cycle entry and DNA repair [39] In the adult CNS, Gli1 is expressed by neural progenitors in germinal regions such as the SVZ and the dentate gyrus, where it is thought to play a role in the maintenance of this stem cell population [40] Like the hedgehog pathway, the notch pathway has been linked to the biology of normal NCS as well as BTIC. Notch has been shown to be involved in the maintenance of "stemness," as its loss leads to enhance differentiation and reduce proliferation of neural progenitors in the SVZ in vivo. Both Gli and Notch are expressed in GBMs [41,42] and it is thought that these pathways may mediate the initiation and maintenance of these tumors, as they do for neural stem cells.

Mitogens and their respective tyrosine kinase receptors such as EGFR and PDGFR have been studied extensively in gliomas, as they are aberrantly expressed and activated in most adult high-grade gliomas [43] Both the PDGF and EGF receptors are expressed in progenitor populations in the SVZ. Overexpression of their ligand leads to reduced differentiation, followed by an increase in proliferation, leading to hyperplasias with some features of gliomas [44,45], suggestive of their role in glial progenitor differentiation and proliferation.

PTEN loss and AKT activation were shown to correlate with the aggressiveness and resistant phenotypes associated with BTICs [46]. Increased AKT through loss of PTEN leads to an increase in BTICs in mouse gliomas. In mouse meduloblastomas, combination of AKT pathway inhibitors with radiotherapy significantly decreases the survival of the stem-like pool [46]. Besides signaling pathways and their direct downstream effectors, transcription factors such as BMI-1 have also been shown to play a role in stem cell self-renewal by repressing the gene products of $p16_{INK4A}/p19_{ARF}$[43]. BMI-1 is expressed in human GBM tumors and is highly enriched in CD133+ cells. Stable BMI-1 knockdown using short hairpin RNA-expressing lentivirus resulted in inhibition of clonogenic potential in vitro and of brain tumor formation in vivo [47,60], suggesting its role in the regulation of BTICs self-renewal and proliferation.

THERAPEUTIC PROMISE OF TARGETING THE BTIC POPULATION

Traditional characterization of GBMs based on proliferation, apoptosis, angiogenesis, and invasion has been based on the bulk tumor, with of course recurrence. However, in light of the BTIC hypothesis, current and ongoing investigations suggest that the BTIC population may be an attractive and effective target to eliminate the tumor on a longer basis. Conventional nontargeted modalities of glioma treatment, chemotherapy, and radiation have demonstrated that the BTIC population are intrinsically resistant, providing a plausible explanation for recurrence [48,49]. For example, tumor cells expressing the CD133$^+$ candidate BTIC marker are significantly resistant to radiation compared with CD133$^-$ tumor cells. In terms of potential mechanisms, the CD133$^+$ glioma pool exhibited elevated levels of the DNA repair proteins CHK1 and CHK2 compared with their CD133$^-$ counterparts [33]. Therefore, targeted therapies to CHK1 and CHK2 may be an effective strategy to overcome radioresistance in the BTIC pool and make the entire glioma more sensitive. In addition to radioresistance, elevated levels of drug transporters ABCG2 and ABCA3 have been shown to promote temozolomide resistance in BTICs [49,50].

A novel approach for targeting BTICs may be promoting differentiation of these cells to limit their replication and self-renewal properties. Upregulation of the bone morphogenic proteins (BMPs) such as BMP4 has been shown to induce differentiation of BTICs, limit their self-renewal ability, and drastically reduce proliferation [51]. The vascular niche that promotes and allows BTICs to grow has also become a potential target. Use of the anti-VEGF antibody, bevacizumab has been shown to reduce the CD133$^+$ BTIC population in vitro and in vivo, illustrating that disruption of the BTIC niche may be an effective therapeutic strategy [52,53].

Recent advances into the CSC hypothesis and BTICs have allowed for a new paradigm in terms of treating brain tumor patients. By selectively targeting the cells that promote resistance and propagate the tumor, it might allow for treatment with effective and promising results. However, these are all at preclinical stage, though of high interest and hence worthy of further study, as discussed in the following. Novel-associated toxicities may also arise from targeting the BTIC niche in terms of neuroglial repair and most importantly neuroglial development especially in the pediatric population.

CURRENT LIMITATIONS TO THERAPEUTIC TARGETING OF BTICS

Although targeting the BTIC population may seem like a viable and attractive option, there still are unanswered questions as to how effective targeting BTICs truly are. First, many of the drugs used to treat GBMs and target BTICs namely BCNU, cisplatin, and cytarabine have shown to be toxic to normal stem cells of the SVZ and the dentate gyrus of the hippocampus at clinically relevant doses [54]. Therefore, direct targeting of BTICs with these compounds may also be harmful to normal NSCs. Second, although differentiation of BTICs may be another avenue of treatment, the complete picture is still unknown. For example, although BMP4 can promote reduction of the BTIC population as mentioned earlier, in certain subset of GBM patients, BMPs can paradoxically induce tumor proliferation and increase tumorigenicity [55].

Problems with xenotransplantation experiments can also limit the use of the BTIC and the CSC model. In most cases, only a small population of TICs have been shown to result in tumor growth when implanted into immunodeficient animals [56,57]. Using this system, TICs with certain phenotypes and markers have been shown to be more likely grown into a tumor (CD34$^+$CD38$^-$ in leukemia, CD44$^+$CD24$^-$ in breast, CD133$^+$ in brain), compared with cells negative for these markers. However, the environment of NOD-SCID mice removes many of the tumor cell–immune cell interactions and introduces tumor cells to a foreign milieu. How this environment of NOD-SCID mice contributes to tumorigenesis remains largely unanswered. Using NOD-SCID interleukin-2 receptor gamma chain null mice (more immunocompromised than traditional NOD-SCID mice), one group found 27% of melanoma cells could form a tumor with a single cell transplant [58]. Again this observation supports the stochastic theory of tumor formation, since a large population of tumor cells have the ability to form tumor. Last, as discussed there is the significant difficulty with BTIC/CSC markers. Several studies have shown that the CD133$^+$ compartment of BTICs form tumor compared with no tumor growth from CD133$^-$ GBM cell implants in NOD-SCID mice [9]. However, subsequent studies found that not only can CD133$^-$ GBM cells form tumors in immunodeficient mice, but they can also give rise to CD133$^+$ cells [59]. Identification of BTICs currently relies on several markers; however, each marker has limitations and it is highly likely that BTIC express several different markers under varying conditions. This provides great difficulty in isolating a truly pure population of BTICs from the tumor bulk to evaluate not only its genetic makeup, but also preferential sensitive therapies that may be tested in the clinic.

CONCLUSION

The concept of BTICs and CSCs is exciting and may provide new therapeutic targets for effective longer-term treatment. However, it remains an unproven hypothesis especially in solid cancers where lineage determination and associated markers are not as well-known, compared with blood cancers. It is an area of high interest with required ongoing research with an open mind. It is safe to argue that within a GBM lies a population of cells that exhibit BTIC properties, in addition to bulk differentiated tumor cells and cells that are more progenitor-like. However, the tumor microenvironment can influence the BTICs and differentiated tumor cells to become more plastic, stem cell like, or more differentiated. Selectively targeting the BTIC population, although hypothetically attractive, may not be an effective strategy. This is due to several reasons inducing toxicity to NSCs and the ability of bulk tumor cells to acquire stem cell like properties. Likely, targeting of all types of cells using combinatorial strategies would be most effective, without undue expectations that ablation of BTICs will lead to total ablation of the tumor as depicted by the simplified dandelion root and leaves analogy often used to promote the CSC hypothesis. Advancing our knowledge of the BTIC/CSC hypothesis and answering some of these outstanding questions may shed light and allow us to exploit this feature of GBM and other brain tumors, with hopeful incremental advantage to our patients.

REFERENCES

1. Tysnes BB, Bjerkvig R. Cancer initiation and progression: involvement of stem cells and the microenvironment. *Biochim Biophys Acta.* 2007;1775(2):283–297.
2. Heppner GH, Miller FR. The cellular basis of tumor progression. *Int Rev Cytol.* 1998;177:1–56.
3. Kleihues P, Sobin LH. World Health Organization classification of tumors. *Cancer.* 2000;88(12):2887.
4. Jordan CT, Guzman ML, Noble M. Cancer stem cells. *N Engl J Med.* 2006;355(12):1253–1261.
5. Bao S, Wu Q, Sathornsumetee S, et al. Stem cell-like glioma cells promote tumor angiogenesis through vascular endothelial growth factor. *Cancer Res.* 2006;66(16):7843–7848.
6. Hadjipanayis CG, Van Meir EG. Brain cancer propagating cells: biology, genetics and targeted therapies. *Trends Mol Med.* 2009;15(11):519–530.
7. Galli R, Binda E, Orfanelli U, et al. Isolation and characterization of tumorigenic, stem-like neural precursors from human glioblastoma. *Cancer Res.* 2004;64(19):7011–7021.
8. Taylor MD, Poppleton H, Fuller C, et al. Radial glia cells are candidate stem cells of ependymoma. *Cancer Cell.* 2005;8(4):323–335.
9. Singh SK, Hawkins C, Clarke ID, et al. Identification of human brain tumour initiating cells. *Nature.* 2004;432(7015):396–401.
10. Clarke MF, Dick JE, Dirks PB, et al. Cancer stem cells–perspectives on current status and future directions: AACR Workshop on cancer stem cells. *Cancer Res.* 2006;66(19):9339–9344.
11. Lassman AB, Dai C, Fuller GN, Vickers AJ, Holland EC. Overexpression of c-MYC promotes an undifferentiated phenotype in cultured astrocytes and allows elevated Ras and Akt signaling to induce gliomas from GFAP-expressing cells in mice. *Neuron Glia Biol.* 2004;1(2):157–163.
12. Thon N, Damianoff K, Hegermann J, et al. Presence of pluripotent CD133+ cells correlates with malignancy of gliomas. *Mol Cell Neurosci.* 2010;43(1):51–59.
13. Strojnik T, Røsland GV, Sakariassen PO, Kavalar R, Lah T. Neural stem cell markers, nestin and musashi proteins, in the progression of human glioma: correlation of nestin with prognosis of patient survival. *Surg Neurol.* 2007;68(2):133–43; discussion 143.
14. Morshead CM, Reynolds BA, Craig CG, et al. Neural stem cells in the adult mammalian forebrain: a relatively quiescent subpopulation of subependymal cells. *Neuron.* 1994;13(5):1071–1082.
15. Dirks PB. Brain tumor stem cells: bringing order to the chaos of brain cancer. *J Clin Oncol.* 2008;26(17):2916–2924.
16. Stiles CD, Rowitch DH. Glioma stem cells: a midterm exam. *Neuron.* 2008;58(6):832–846.
17. Sanai N, Tramontin AD, Quiñones-Hinojosa A, et al. Unique astrocyte ribbon in adult human brain contains neural stem cells but lacks chain migration. *Nature.* 2004;427(6976):740–744.
18. Eriksson PS, Perfilieva E, Björk-Eriksson T, et al. Neurogenesis in the adult human hippocampus. *Nat Med.* 1998;4(11):1313–1317.
19. Doetsch F. The glial identity of neural stem cells. *Nat Neurosci.* 2003;6(11):1127–1134.
20. Vick NA, Lin MJ, Bigner DD. The role of the subependymal plate in glial tumorigenesis. *Acta Neuropathol.* 1977;40(1):63–71.
21. Hopewell JW. The subependymal plate and the genesis of gliomas. *J Pathol.* 1975;117(2):101–103.
22. Alcantara Llaguno S, Chen J, Kwon CH, et al. Malignant astrocytomas originate from neural stem/progenitor cells in a somatic tumor suppressor mouse model. *Cancer Cell.* 2009;15(1):45–56.
23. Kondo T, Raff M. Oligodendrocyte precursor cells reprogrammed to become multipotential CNS stem cells. *Science.* 2000;289(5485):1754–1757.
24. Dai C, Celestino JC, Okada Y, Louis DN, Fuller GN, Holland EC. PDGF autocrine stimulation dedifferentiates cultured astrocytes and induces oligodendrogliomas and oligoastrocytomas from neural progenitors and astrocytes in vivo. *Genes Dev.* 2001;15(15):1913–1925.
25. Bachoo RM, Maher EA, Ligon KL, et al. Epidermal growth factor receptor and Ink4a/Arf: convergent mechanisms governing terminal differentiation and transformation along the neural stem cell to astrocyte axis. *Cancer Cell.* 2002;1(3):269–277.
26. Nakagawa M, Koyanagi M, Tanabe K, et al. Generation of induced pluripotent stem cells without Myc from mouse and human fibroblasts. *Nat Biotechnol.* 2008;26(1):101–106.
27. Rapp UR, Ceteci F, Schreck R. Oncogene-induced plasticity and cancer stem cells. *Cell Cycle.* 2008;7(1):45–51.
28. Kim JB, Greber B, Araúzo-Bravo MJ, et al. Direct reprogramming of human neural stem cells by OCT4. *Nature.* 2009;461(7264):649–643.
29. Zheng X, Shen G, Yang X, Liu W. Most C6 cells are cancer stem cells: evidence from clonal and population analyses. *Cancer Res.* 2007;67(8):3691–3697.
30. Shipitsin M, Campbell LL, Argani P, et al. Molecular definition of breast tumor heterogeneity. *Cancer Cell.* 2007;11(3):259–273.
31. Dahlstrand J, Collins VP, Lendahl U. Expression of the class VI intermediate filament nestin in human central nervous system tumors. *Cancer Res.* 1992;52(19):5334–5341.
32. Singh SK, Clarke ID, Hide T, Dirks PB. Cancer stem cells in nervous system tumors. *Oncogene.* 2004;23(43):7267–7273.
33. Bao S, Wu Q, McLendon RE, et al. Glioma stem cells promote radioresistance by preferential activation of the DNA damage response. *Nature.* 2006;444(7120):756–760.
34. Son MJ, Woolard K, Nam DH, Lee J, Fine HA. SSEA-1 is an enrichment marker for tumor-initiating cells in human glioblastoma. *Cell Stem Cell.* 2009;4(5):440–452.
35. Vescovi AL, Reynolds BA, Fraser DD, Weiss S. bFGF regulates the proliferative fate of unipotent (neuronal) and bipotent (neuronal/astroglial) EGF-generated CNS progenitor cells. *Neuron.* 1993;11(5):951–966.
36. Diehn M, Cho RW, Lobo NA, et al. Association of reactive oxygen species levels and radioresistance in cancer stem cells. *Nature.* 2009;458(7239):780–783.
37. Griguer CE, Oliva CR, Gobin E, et al. CD133 is a marker of bioenergetic stress in human glioma. *PLoS ONE.* 2008;3(11):e3655.
38. Toda M, Iizuka Y, Yu W, et al. Expression of the neural RNA-binding protein Musashi1 in human gliomas. *Glia.* 2001;34(1):1–7.
39. Sasaki H, Nishizaki Y, Hui C, Nakafuku M, Kondoh H. Regulation of Gli2 and Gli3 activities by an amino-terminal repression domain: implication of Gli2 and Gli3 as primary mediators of Shh signaling. *Development.* 1999;126(17):3915–3924.
40. Machold R, Hayashi S, Rutlin M, et al. Sonic hedgehog is required for progenitor cell maintenance in telencephalic stem cell niches. *Neuron.* 2003;39(6):937–950.
41. Hallahan AR, Pritchard JI, Hansen S, et al. The SmoA1 mouse model reveals that notch signaling is critical for the growth and survival of sonic hedgehog-induced medulloblastomas. *Cancer Res.* 2004;64(21):7794–7800.
42. Dahmane N, Sánchez P, Gitton Y, et al. The Sonic Hedgehog-Gli pathway regulates dorsal brain growth and tumorigenesis. *Development.* 2001;128(24):5201–5212.
43. Kesari S, Ramakrishna N, Sauvageot C, Stiles CD, Wen PY. Targeted molecular therapy of malignant gliomas. *Curr Oncol Rep.* 2006;8(1):58–70.
44. Doetsch F, Petreanu L, Caille I, Garcia-Verdugo JM, Alvarez-Buylla A. EGF converts transit-amplifying neurogenic precursors in the adult brain into multipotent stem cells. *Neuron.* 2002;36(6):1021–1034.
45. Jackson EL, Garcia-Verdugo JM, Gil-Perotin S, et al. PDGFR alpha-positive B cells are neural stem cells in the adult SVZ that form glioma-like growths in response to increased PDGF signaling. *Neuron.* 2006;51(2):187–199.

46. Bleau AM, Hambardzumyan D, Ozawa T, et al. PTEN/PI3K/Akt pathway regulates the side population phenotype and ABCG2 activity in glioma tumor stem-like cells. *Cell Stem Cell*. 2009;4(3):226–235.
47. Abdouh M, Facchino S, Chatoo W, Balasingam V, Ferreira J, Bernier G. BMI1 sustains human glioblastoma multiforme stem cell renewal. *J Neurosci*. 2009;29(28):8884–8896.
48. Rich JN. Cancer stem cells in radiation resistance. *Cancer Res*. 2007;67(19):8980–8984.
49. Liu G, Yuan X, Zeng Z, et al. Analysis of gene expression and chemoresistance of CD133+ cancer stem cells in glioblastoma. *Mol Cancer*. 2006;5:67.
50. Hirschmann-Jax C, Foster AE, Wulf GG, et al. A distinct "side population" of cells with high drug efflux capacity in human tumor cells. *Proc Natl Acad Sci USA*. 2004;101(39):14228–14233.
51. Piccirillo SG, Vescovi AL. Bone morphogenetic proteins regulate tumorigenicity in human glioblastoma stem cells. *Ernst Schering Found Symp Proc*. 2006;(5):59–81.
52. Keith B, Simon MC. Hypoxia-inducible factors, stem cells, and cancer. *Cell*. 2007;129(3):465–472.
53. Calabrese C, Poppleton H, Kocak M, et al. A perivascular niche for brain tumor stem cells. *Cancer Cell*. 2007;11(1):69–82.
54. Dietrich J, Han R, Yang Y, Mayer-Pröschel M, Noble M. CNS progenitor cells and oligodendrocytes are targets of chemotherapeutic agents *in vitro* and in vivo. *J Biol*. 2006;5(7):22.
55. Lee J, Son MJ, Woolard K, et al. Epigenetic-mediated dysfunction of the bone morphogenetic protein pathway inhibits differentiation of glioblastoma-initiating cells. *Cancer Cell*. 2008;13(1):69–80.
56. Al-Hajj M, Wicha MS, Benito-Hernandez A, Morrison SJ, Clarke MF. Prospective identification of tumorigenic breast cancer cells. *Proc Natl Acad Sci USA*. 2003;100(7):3983–3988.
57. Ricci-Vitiani L, Lombardi DG, Pilozzi E, et al. Identification and expansion of human colon-cancer-initiating cells. *Nature*. 2007;445(7123):111–115.
58. Quintana E, Shackleton M, Sabel MS, Fullen DR, Johnson TM, Morrison SJ. Efficient tumour formation by single human melanoma cells. *Nature*. 2008;456(7222):593–598.
59. Wang J, Sakariassen PØ, Tsinkalovsky O, et al. CD133 negative glioma cells form tumors in nude rats and give rise to CD133 positive cells. *Int J Cancer*. 2008;122(4):761–768.
60. Molofsky AV, Pardal R, Iwashita T, Park IK, Clarke MF, Morrison SJ. Bmi-1 dependence distinguishes neural stem cell self-renewal from progenitor proliferation. *Nature*. 2003;425(6961):962–967.

13 Molecular Pathogenesis of Glioma: Overview and Therapeutic Implications

Ingeborg Fischer, Erik Sulman, and Ken Aldape

INTRODUCTION

Diffuse gliomas in adults continue to have a dismal prognosis with the current standard of treatment, including maximal surgical resection, radiotherapy, and chemotherapy. The molecular pathogenesis of adult glioma is complex involving the loss of function of tumor suppressor genes and activation of oncogenes that are involved in a network of widely interconnected signaling pathways. Although currently available therapeutic modalities, including radiotherapy and alkylating agents, are nonspecific, a better understanding of the molecular pathogenesis of glioma may lead to a rational development of targeted therapies and discovery of predictive biomarkers. Despite the heterogeneity of gliomas, common mechanisms driving the malignant phenotype can be found. New treatments have emerged to target proliferation, angiogenesis, and invasion with the goal to increase specific treatment efficacy. This chapter gives an overview of the current knowledge about the pathogenesis of adult diffuse gliomas, emphasizing new targeted treatment approaches.

GLIOMA CLASSIFICATION

Diffuse adult gliomas include astrocytic, oligodendroglial, and mixed oligoastrocytic tumors according to the current World Health Organization Classification, which is based on the morphologic appearance and the presumed cell of origin. Patients with oligodendroglioma have a better prognosis than patients with astrocytoma, with survival rates of 78% at 5 years for oligodendroglioma, 70% at 5 years for oligoastrocytoma, and 65% at 5 years for fibrillary astrocytoma [1]. Although some genetic alterations such as TP53 mutations and loss of the phosphatase and tensin homolog (PTEN) protein are much more common in astrocytomas than in oligodendrogliomas, the determinants of the malignant phenotype in oligodendroglial and astrocytic tumors overlap to some extent [2]. Oligodendroglial and astrocytic tumors alike overexpress growth factors and angiogenic factors and have loss of function of important regulatory proteins of the cell cycle. The characteristics of the malignant glioma phenotype will therefore be discussed in general terms.

CELLS OF ORIGIN

Although the hypothesis was for many years that gliomas arise from differentiated oligodendrocytes or astrocytes, more recently, the discovery of brain tumor stem cells has put this hypothesis into question [3,4]. These cells make up a small percentage of malignant gliomas and are characterized by the potential for self-renewal and tumorigenesis. These brain tumor stem cells are generated by a carcinogenic insult to neural stem cells, which are more susceptible to oncogenic transformation than do more differentiated glial precursors [5–7]. If gliomas arise from undifferentiated stem cells that are not committed to either astrocytic or oligodendroglial lineage, the nature of the tumorigenic events presumably determines the phenotype and therefore the type of tumor. In mouse models, chronic platelet-derived growth factor (PDGF) signaling in glial progenitors leads to the formation of oligodendrogliomas, whereas chronic combined Ras and Akt give rise to astrocytomas [8].

PATHWAYS OF MALIGNANT PROGRESSION

Astrocytoma

Diffusely infiltrating gliomas have an inherent tendency to progress. The substrate of such progression is the accumulation of genetic abnormalities over time [9–12]. In gliomas, alternative pathways of tumor development and progression are implicated in oligodendrogliomas, astrocytomas, and primary and secondary glioblastoma (Figure 13.1). The affected tumor suppressor and oncogenes contribute to the development of the hallmarks of cancer: increased proliferation through self-sufficiency in growth signals and evasion of apoptosis, angiogenesis, and tissue invasion [13].

Although there is a functional redundancy of mechanisms, certain tumorigenic events (such as TP53 mutations and epidermal growth factor receptor [EGFR] amplification) are mutually exclusive in any individual glioma [14].

Certain genetic alterations typically occur early or late in the course of tumor progression. For example, TP53 mutations and overexpression of PDGF ligands and platelet-derived growth factor receptors (PDGFR) in low-grade

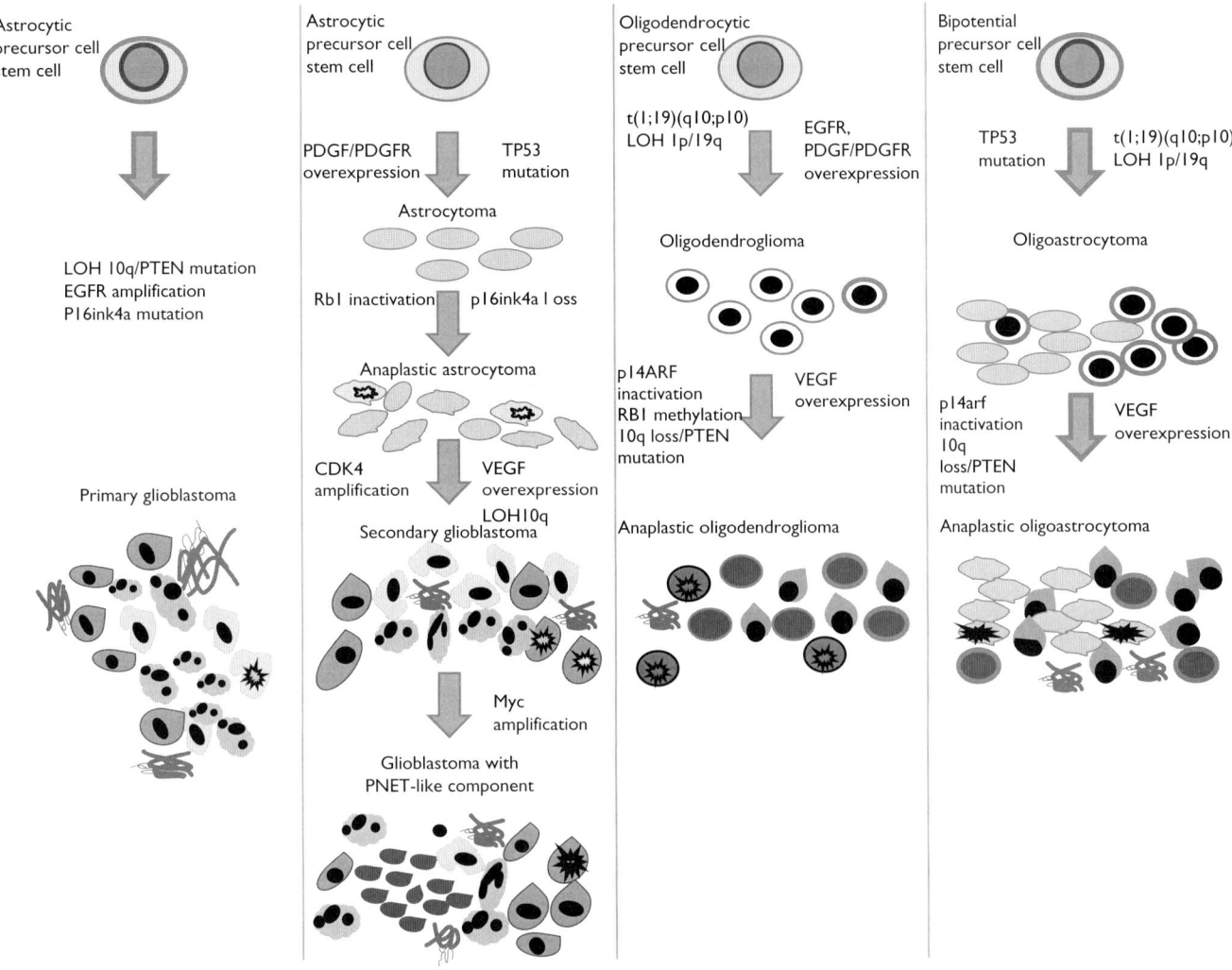

Figure 13.1 Glioma development and progression. Tumors originate from neural stem cells or glial precursor cells transformed through genetic alterations which accumulate during malignant progression.

astrocytomas are followed by accumulation of genetic alterations of cell cycle regulatory pathways, including deletion or mutations of cyclin-dependent kinase (CDK) inhibitor p16INK4A/CDKN2A or the retinoblastoma susceptibility locus 1 (pRB1) with the progression to anaplastic astrocytoma, followed by amplification or overexpression of CDK4 and LOH 10q in malignant progression of secondary glioblastomas [15–18].

In contrast, primary glioblastomas are believed to be characterized by frequent amplification of EGFR and infrequent TP53 mutations [2,11,14].

These two alternative pathways to glioblastoma represent an initial step toward molecularly based classification of high-grade gliomas. This model of alternative pathways will be further defined and perhaps expanded to include additional pathways. A recent example of further definition is the discovery that secondary glioblastomas in some instances acquire genotypic and phenotypic characteristics of primitive neuroectodermal tumors as described by Perry et al [19].

Oligodendroglioma

Oligodendrogliomas typically occur in the cerebral hemispheres of young adults and have a more favorable prognosis than do astrocytic tumors of the same grade [20]. Their molecular-genetic hallmark is deletion of the chromosomal arms 1p and 19q, which is present in up to 80% of cases and strongly associated with "classic" oligodendroglioma morphology. It is often due to an unbalanced translocation t(1;19)(q10;p10) [21].

The 1p/19q deletion is of both prognostic and predictive significance: a landmark study of 35 patients with anaplastic oligodendroglioma demonstrated that those patients whose tumors exhibited 1p/19q loss had a therapeutic response and longer survival times than patients whose tumors lacked this change [22]. Since that time, it has been suggested that oligodendrogliomas are inherently more responsive to treatment compared with other diffuse gliomas [20,23]. Putative tumor suppressor genes have not been identified on these chromosomal arms; therefore, the link between molecular pathogenesis of oligodendrogliomas and the therapeutic implication is still missing in this case. Nonetheless, the assessment of 1p/19q status in oligodendroglial tumors is currently a widely performed molecular-genetic test in neuro-oncologic practice [24,25].

Other mechanisms of tumor development and progression are identical to those seen in astrocytic tumors, including dysregulation of cell cycle proteins [15] and their inhibitors, loss of PTEN [26], and upregulation of angiogenic factors [27,28] with the progression to anaplastic oligodendroglioma.

Oligoastrocytoma

The molecular and genetic alteration underlying the tumorigenesis and progression of mixed oligoastrocytomas resemble those of either astrocytic or oligodendroglial tumors. Tumors that have 1p/19q deletions do not have TP53 mutations and vice versa, indicating that even if morphologically ambiguous, oligoastrocytomas genetically resemble either pure oligodendrogliomas or astrocytoma.

HALLMARKS OF MALIGNANT GLIOMAS

As outlined above, the pathogenesis of gliomas may be viewed as a series of genetic alterations that drive the progressive transformation of the normal cell of origin into their malignant derivatives. Observations made in animal models and human gliomas provide evidence that each of the genetic changes successively occurring in gliomas confers another type of growth advantage for the tumor cells.

Such genetic changes lead to functional alterations in the homeostasis of the tumor cells, which may be grouped into six different categories, which are also referred to as the hallmarks of cancer: self-sufficiency in growth signals, insensitivity to growth inhibitory signals, evasion of apoptosis, unlimited replicative potential, angiogenesis, and tissue invasion [13]. These characteristics apply to malignant glioma as to other forms of cancer, and they represent important targets for novel therapeutic approaches. A summary of novel treatments aimed at the components of the malignant phenotype is given in Figure 13.2.

Self-Sufficiency in Growth Signals

Mitogenic growth signals enable tumor cells to change from a quiescent state into a proliferative state. They are transmitted into the cell by transmembrane receptors that bind diffusible growth factors, extracellular matrix (ECM) components, and cell-to-cell adhesion or interaction molecules. Glioma cells (over)express both growth factors and corresponding receptors, for example PDGF, PDGFR, transforming growth factor (TGF)-β, and EGFR, allowing for paracrine and autocrine growth stimulation [29,30]. In addition, growth-stimulating signaling independently of ligand binding can occur in tyrosine kinase receptors as a result of a mutation (e.g., EGFRvIII, see the following).

PDGF/PDGFR

Coexpression of PDGF and PDGFR exists in gliomas of all grades and is held to be an early oncogenic event, even though expression directly increases with glioma grade [31]. PDGF promotes not only growth but also angiogenesis through an autocrine loop [31,32]. Imatinib mesylate (Gleevec; Novartis), a kinase inhibitor of PDGFR, c-Kit, and bcr-abl, has demonstrated a progression-free survival at 6 years of 32% in patients who had immunohistochemical expression of PDGFR [33]. Thus, detection of the target protein may be helpful in predicting response to agents directed to this target, but definitive evidence awaits clinical trials [34].

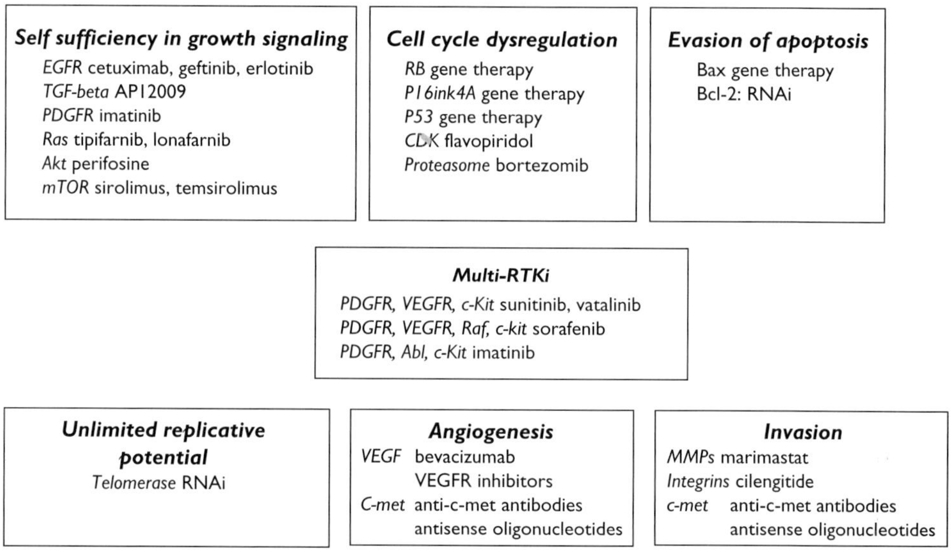

Figure 13.2 The hallmarks of cancer in glioma. Therapeutic approaches can specifically target individual or multiple aspects of the malignant phenotype.

Self sufficiency in growth signaling
EGFR cetuximab, geftinib, erlotinib
TGF-beta AP12009
PDGFR imatinib
Ras tipifarnib, lonafarnib
Akt perifosine
mTOR sirolimus, temsirolimus

Cell cycle dysregulation
RB gene therapy
P16ink4A gene therapy
P53 gene therapy
CDK flavopiridol
Proteasome bortezomib

Evasion of apoptosis
Bax gene therapy
Bcl-2: RNAi

Multi-RTKi
PDGFR, VEGFR, c-Kit sunitinib, vatalinib
PDGFR, VEGFR, Raf, c-kit sorafenib
PDGFR, Abl, c-Kit imatinib

Unlimited replicative potential
Telomerase RNAi

Angiogenesis
VEGF bevacizumab
VEGFR inhibitors
C-met anti-c-met antibodies
antisense oligonucleotides

Invasion
MMPs marimastat
Integrins cilengitide
c-met anti-c-met antibodies
antisense oligonucleotides

EGFR

EGFR is the most frequently amplified gene in glioblastoma [12,16,17]. EGFR amplification is associated with EGFR overexpression [35]. EGFRvIII is a truncated variant of EGFR found in 20% to 50% of glioblastomas with EGFR amplification. It results in a deletion in exons 2 to 7 of the EGFR mRNA, thereby removing the extracellular ligand-binding domain of the receptor [36,37]. Thus, EGFRvIII is constitutively activated, signaling through the PI3 kinase, RAS, and map kinase pathways, independently of its ligand. The increased activity of EGFR promotes tumor growth through many different mechanisms, promoting survival, invasion, and angiogenesis. For example, the antiapoptotic effect is mediated by the activation of Bcl-xl [38] and the increased invasiveness by upregulating the expression of matrix metalloproteinases (MMP) [39]. In accordance with these effects, EGFRvIII positivity in GBM has been linked to a more aggressive clinical phenotype with shorter overall survival times [40].

Because EGFRvIII does not occur on normal cells, it is a promising therapeutic target [41].

EGFR-targeted therapies include the monoclonal antibodies to EGFR (cetuximab, Erbitux, Bristol-Meyers Squibb) and EGFR kinase inhibitors, gefitinib (Iressa, ZD1839; AstraZeneca, Wilmington, DE) and erlotinib (Tarceva, OSI-774; Genentech, South San Francisco, CA). Cetuximab binds to EGFR and blocks activation of the receptor, resulting in G1 phase arrest, and promoting apoptosis and inhibiting angiogenesis in glioma cell lines and tumor xenografts [42]. In glioblastomas, clinical response to treatment with cetuximab has been reported in several cases [43]. Phase I and II clinical trials are ongoing. Gefitinib and erlotinib resulted in radiographic response, but no survival benefit in clinical trials for malignant gliomas. However, attempts at correlation of treatment response with molecular characteristics of gliomas produced notable result in retrospective evaluation of tumor tissues from patients enrolled in clinical trials: coexpression of normal PTEN and mutant EGFRvIII and combined low levels of AKT and overexpression of EGFR have been suggested as predictors of radiographic response [44–46], but these findings await confirmation in other trials.

TGF-β

TGF-β is a polypeptide growth factor that binds to its serine threonine kinase receptor TGF-βR. TGF-βR phosphorylates the Smad transcription factors that regulate the transcription of TGF-β responsive genes. In normal cells, TGF-β promotes apoptosis and differentiation and blocks cell proliferation. In neoplastic cells, inactivation of TGF-β through mutation of the receptor or downstream Smad proteins results in uncontrolled proliferation. Glioma coexpress both TGF-β and its receptors in an autocrine loop. The expression levels of TGF-β increase with tumor grade. However, the TGF-β receptors are not mutated in high-grade gliomas, suggesting a downstream signaling disruption [47,48]. TGF-β also promotes invasion by inducing the expression of MMP-2 [49]. Therapeutic exploitation of the TGF-β pathway has been attempted with antisense oligonucleotide AP12009, which has been tested in clinical trials on malignant gliomas with promising results; even complete regression of tumors was reported in 2 of 27 patients [50].

Mitogenic Signaling Pathways

Growth factor receptors activate intracellular effector molecules that are part of a downstream signaling cascade. Gliomas are often associated with either activation of these effector molecules or inactivating mutations of the negative regulators of these, such as PTEN in the PI3K pathway.

RAS-RAF-MEK-MAPK

The MAPK pathway is activated through integrins or receptor tyrosine kinase (RTK) that bind growth factors such as TGF-β. RTK activation results in receptor dimerization and downstream activation of Ras and phosphorylation of MAPK, which phosphorylates nuclear transcription factors that induce the expression of genes promoting cell cycle progression, for example cyclin D1. Although Ras is often activated in gliomas, it does not usually carry any mutations. Rather, Ras activity in gliomas is determined by inappropriate RTK or integrin activation [51–53]. The rate-limiting step of maturation of Ras is farnesylation and therefore farnesyltransferase inhibitors, including tipifarnib (Zarnestra, R115777; Johnson & Johnson, Brunswick, NJ) and lonafarnib (Sarasar, SCH66336; Schering-Plough, Kenilworth, NJ) are promising therapeutic agents [54].

PI3K/PTEN/AKT/mTOR

The PI3K pathway is an important mediator of cell growth and proliferation. Its activation is frequent and associated with poor prognosis in patients with glioma [55]. In many cases, loss of PTEN, a major tumor suppressor that is inactivated in up to 50% of high-grade gliomas by mutations or epigenetic mechanisms, results in uncontrolled PI3K signaling and AKT activation [17,56–58]. Akt activation detected by immunohistochemistry increases with tumor grade with 85% of GBM having activated Akt [59]. Downstream from Akt, the serine/threonine kinase mTOR regulates protein translation involving the initiation factor 4E-binding protein-1 (4E-BP1) and the ribosomal S6 kinase (p70s6K). Approaches to block this signaling cascade include the Akt inhibitor perifosine (Keryx Biopharmaceuticals, New York, NY), and the mTOR inhibitors Rapamycin (sirolimus; Wyeth, Madison, NJ) and its synthesized analogs, temsirolimus (CCI-779, Wyeth) and everolimus (RAD001, Novartis), which have been evaluated in clinical trials [60,61]. In a phase II clinical trial of temsirolimus on 65 patients with GBM, a radiographic response to treatment was observed in 36% of patients [60].

Insensitivity to Antigrowth Signals

Continuous rapid growth of tumor cells is fostered through different basic mechanisms: the physiological control of cell divisions is disrupted through inactivation of "brakes" on the cell cycle; tumor cells become resistant to physiologic cell death mechanisms (apoptosis and autophagy) and are "immortalized" through telomerase activity.

Cell Cycle Dysregulation

Rb Pathway

A central effector of the antiproliferative signaling is the retinoblastoma protein (pRb). It blocks proliferation by sequestering the transcription factor E2F, which is necessary for the progression from the G1 to S phase. Disruption of the retinoblastoma protein pathway liberates E2Fs and thus allows cell proliferation. The retinoblastoma pathway can be disrupted in different ways. Functional pRb may be lost through mutation of its gene, which occurs in 25% of high-grade gliomas. The Rb protein can be inactivated by Cyclin D1 and CDK4 and CDK6 complexes through hyperphosphorylation [53]. Amplification of the *CDK*4 and *CDK*6 genes also result in functional inactivation of RB in high-grade gliomas [62,63]. In addition, Rb activity is lost through the inactivation of a critical negative regulator of both CDK4 and CDK6, p16^{Ink4a} [64].

Disruptions of the Rb pathway are frequent in high-grade gliomas and tend to involve only one component of the pathway in any given tumor [65]. Therapeutic potential lies in the restoration of the function of the Rb pathway in gliomas through gene therapy approaches and small molecules that modulate the expression of the Rb pathway components. The results from preclinical trials are encouraging. In preclinical models, complementary DNA of the Rb gene transfected into glioma cell lines arrested growth of cells in G1 phase of the cell cycle [66]. A variant of the Rb gene delivered to glioma xenograft in mice through an adenoviral vector resulted in prolonged survival of glioma-bearing animals [67]. Similar gene therapy approaches have targeted dysregulation of CDKs and their inhibitors: transfer of p16ink4A to glioma cells resulted in demonstrated growth inhibition in vitro and in vivo [68–70].

Flavopiridol, a semisynthetic flavonoid derived from a plant alkaloid, is a small-molecule inhibitor of CDKs, which also induces G1 arrest and inhibits glioma growth in mouse xenograft models [71]. Because cyclins and CDK inhibitors are subject to proteosomal degradation, the cell cycle regulation can also be modified through proteasome inhibitors such as bortezomib (Velcade, Millenium Pharmaceuticals Inc.). This proteasome inhibitor induces expression of p21 and p27, decreases the levels of CDK2, CDK4, and E2F4, and leads to apoptosis in vitro glioma cell lines [72]. Phase I clinical trials for patients with recurrent malignant gliomas are ongoing.

p53 Pathway

The p53 protein plays a role in cell cycle control, DNA damage response, cell death, and differentiation. Its regulatory function in the cell cycle consists of a control function at the G1 to S phase transition point, which is effected through its downstream transcriptional target *CDNK1A*; which encodes the protein for the CDK2 inhibitor p21. The proapoptotic effect of p53 is mediated by its upregulation of proapoptotic proteins such as BAX (see "resistance to apoptotic signals"). The p53 protein itself is tightly regulated. The MDM2 gene binds to p53 protein, inhibiting its ability to activate transcription. In a negative feedback loop, the MDM2 gene is induced by the wild-type p53. MDM2 also promotes the degradation of the p53 protein. The p14arf gene (part of the CDKN2A complex gene) encodes the p14 protein, which inhibits MDM2-mediated p53 inhibition [73]. Therefore, loss of p53 function may be a consequence of altered function of TP53, MDM2, or p14ARF. More recently, the *MDM2*-related gene, *MDM4*, which inhibits *p53* transcription and enhances the ubiquitin ligase activity of MDM2, has been found to be amplified in a small subset of GBM with neither *TP53* mutation nor *MDM2* amplification [74].

Molecular therapeutic approaches directed at loss of p53 function in gliomas attempt to restore p53 function, mainly through delivery of the p53 gene [75]. In a phase I clinical trial of adenovirus-mediated gene transfer for recurrent gliomas, treatment was well tolerated by patients, and progression-free survival was 13 weeks and OS 43 weeks [76]. A limitation of this treatment approach has been poor diffusion of the vector into the affected brain tissue.

Evasion of Apoptosis

Among the central regulators of apoptosis are the members of the BCL-2 family of proteins, which includes both proapoptotic (Bax, Bak, Bid, and Bim) and antiapoptotic (Bcl-2, Bcl-X, and Bcl-W) proteins. These lead to death signaling through cytochrome c release from mitochondria, setting off a proteolytic cascade of caspase activation resulting in cell death. For example, the p53 protein elicits apoptosis by upregulating the expression of proapoptotic Bax in response to DNA damage; Bax in turn stimulates mitochondria to release cytochrome c. Resistance to apoptosis is most often acquired in gliomas by loss of a proapoptotic regulator through a mutation involving the *p53* tumor suppressor gene.

In addition, the PI3 kinase-AKT/PKB pathway is frequently activated through increased EGFR signaling or loss of the PTEN tumor suppressor in high-grade gliomas also transmits antiapoptotic signals [55] and therefore contributes to resistance to radiotherapy [77].

Apoptotic pathways are redundant in normal and neoplastic tissues. Restoration of the apoptotic pathways could be a goal of gene therapy; however, the crosstalk between parallel apoptotic signaling pathways in tumor cells may pose a therapeutic challenge.

As described above, a potential mechanism of restoring normal apoptotic properties in gliomas is restoration of p53 function. Adenoviral delivery of the proapoptotic Bax protein has been shown to cause apoptosis of glioma cells in vitro [78]. In addition, antisense techniques inhibiting the transcription and translation of antiapoptotic proteins as BCL-2 and BCL-xl hold promise [79,80]. Because survival signals are also transmitted through the EGFR and PDGFR pathways via Akt, which phosphorylates and deactivates Bax-9 and caspase-3 and inhibits cytochrome release from mitochondria, small-molecule inhibitors of Akt such as LY-294002 and perifosine may also induce apoptosis in gliomas [81,82].

Decrease of Autophagy

Autophagy is a physiologic cellular stress response and a mechanism of cell death that, in contrast to apoptosis, is not mediated through activation of caspases. The process is characterized by the formation of autophagic vacuoles that fuse with lysosomes to degrade cellular organelles such as the Golgi apparatus, polyribosomes, and endoplasmatic reticulum [83–86].. Triggers of autophagy include hypoxia, withdrawal of growth signals, toxins, and chemotherapeutic agents [86–89]. There is a significant overlap between autophagy and apoptosis, and in some instances, both cell death mechanisms may be observed in the same cell [90]. It is thus not surprising that the intracellular regulators are similar: the *PI3K/PTEN/AKT/mTOR* signaling pathway blocks autophagy and the p53 protein increases autophagy via regulation of mTOR [87,91–93]. In a large series of brain tumors, the expression of the proautophagic protein Beclin 1 was inversely correlated with tumor grade [94], and in gliomas, inhibition of mTOR signaling increases autophagy in vitro [95]. Temozolomide, an alkylating agent that led to a significant increase in the overall survival of patients with glioblastoma in an European Organisation for Research and Treatment of Cancer (EORTC) study [96], exerts part of its cytotoxic effect on glioma cells by causing autophagy [97]. The PDGFR inhibitor imatinib also has proapoptotic activity as demonstrated in chronic myelogenous leukemia in vitro [98]. Future therapeutic potential lies in the application of such proautophagic drugs to gliomas. Apart from the cytotoxic agents already applied to malignant gliomas in clinical trials, potential candidate bioactive substances have recently been identified through imaging-based screening. These include six Food and Drug Administration–approved drugs used in the treatment of cardiovascular disease and mental illness [99].

Unlimited Replicative Potential

Human chromosomes have repetitive DNA sequences at their ends, the telomeres, which are shortened with each cell division. This mechanism is the substrate of aging (senescence) on a cellular level. When the telomere length decreases below a critical level, the cell stops dividing. Telomere maintenance can be provided through telomerase, which adds hexanucleotide repeats onto the ends of telomeric DNA. In normal somatic cells, telomerase is not expressed. In contrast, most human neoplasms have telomerase expression [100]. In gliomas, telomerase expression increases with malignancy grade, and its pathogenetic importance has been demonstrated by the expression of telomerase in normal astrocytes being able to initiate the tumorigenic process by circumventing cellular senescence [101].

In orthotopic glioblastoma xenografts, telomerase inhibition with RNA interference methods results in decreased tumor growth [102].

Angiogenesis

Angiogenesis, the formation of new blood vessels from preexisting ones, is a key step in malignant progression of gliomas [103,104]. Angiogenesis is controlled through many angiogenic and antiangiogenic factors. High-grade gliomas have the ability to tip the angiogenic-antiangiogenic balance and induce vascular proliferation through a multitude of mediating substances, including vascular endothelial growth factor (VEGF), acidic and basic fibroblast growth factor, hepatocyte growth factor (HGF), and SDF-1 [32,105]. Of these, VEGF is perhaps the best studied.

The expression of VEGF is in part mediated by the transcription factor hypoxia-inducible factor -1, which is itself activated through hypoxia or upregulated expression of intracellular signaling pathways induced by growth factors such as epidermal growth factor, TGF-α, PDGF-A, and IGF-1 and -2 [32,106–108]. Its inhibition has found its way into clinical application in the form of (Avastin; Genentech, South San Francisco, CA) a humanized neutralizing monoclonal antibody to VEGF, which demonstrated a 63% radiographic response to treatment in a phase 2 clinical trial in malignant gliomas in combination with irinotecan. The 6-month progression-free survival in this study was 38%, and the 6-month overall survival probability was 72% [109,110]. A different strategy to inhibit VEGF-mediated angiogenesis is to block the tyrosine kinase activity of the VEGF receptors [111]. These tyrosine kinase inhibitors often have intrinsic activity against more than one receptor and are thus referred to as "multireceptor tyrosine kinase inhibitors." The advantage lies in the ability to block multiple signaling pathways active in the tumor. For example, the multireceptor tyrosine kinase inhibitors Sunitinib and Vatalanib block VEGF receptor, PDGFR, and c-kit signaling. Sorafenib unites activity against VEGF receptor, PDGFR, Raf, and c-kit. Phase I/II clinical trials of treatment of patients with high-grade gliomas are ongoing.

Another important mediator of angiogenesis in glioma is HGF and its tyrosine kinase receptor c-met. Its expression levels correlate with tumor grade and poor prognosis [112–115]. In orthotopic mouse models, a monoclonal antibody against c-met reduces tumor growth through antiangiogenic, antiproliferative, and proapoptotic mechanisms [116].

Invasion

Perhaps the most important hallmark of gliomas is their invasiveness. They diffusely infiltrate the surrounding brain tissue, making a complete resection impossible to achieve. For invasion to occur, tumor cells must be able to attach to the ECM, break down ECM components, and move by extension of membrane protrusion and reorganization of the cytoskeleton.

The ECM serves as a scaffold that also engages in signaling processes with invading glioma cells. In the brain parenchyma, the main constituent proteins are hyaluron and glycosaminoglycan and in the perivascular space, where glioma cells migrate preferentially, fibronectin, laminin, collagen, and vitronectin [117]. Tumor cells form attachments to these components, which is necessary for migration. The most important group of adhesion molecules is the integrin family of transmembrane proteins that mediate attachment to ECM components. The expression of integrin proteins has been shown to correlate with migration and invasion in gliomas [118]. Furthermore, integrins are important for migration of endothelial cells, thus fostering angiogenesis. Cilengitide (EMD121974; EMD Pharmaceuticals, Durham, NC), an inhibitor of avb3 and avb5 integrins, suppresses brain tumor growth through induction of apoptosis in vascular endothelial and brain tumor cells by blocking their interaction with the matrix proteins vitronectin and tenascin [118,119]. This drug is currently being tested in clinical trials.

Because the ECM is also a physiological barrier to cell migration, glioma cells can breakdown the ECM by secreting proteases such as matrix metalloproteases and urokinase plasminogen activator (uPA) [120]. The expression of MMPs and uPa increases with glioma grade and is inversely correlated with prognosis [121–123]. MMPs can be blocked by inhibitors such as marimastat, which has been tested in clinical trials on patients with glioma.

The motility of glioma cells is mediated, among other factors, through HGF and EGFR signaling. HGF interacts with its receptor c-met on glioma cells to promote not only tumor cell motility but also cell proliferation and angiogenesis in vivo, as discussed in the section on "angiogenesis." Inhibition of HGF has been shown to inhibit glioma motility [124].

EGFR signaling also contributes to invasion. Glioblastomas with constitutively active EGFRvIII receptors are more invasive in vitro than those with wild-type EGFR [39]. Downstream signaling molecules, most prominently phosphorylated Akt [125,126,] are also implicated in invasion, demonstrating that the PI3k-Akt pathway is instrumental not only to growth and inhibition of apoptosis but also for tumor invasion.

EXPRESSION PROFILING OF HUMAN GLIOMAS

Of all the brain tumor types, by far the largest numbers of profiled tumors have been gliomas (mainly astrocytic and oligodendroglial tumors), largely because of the greater availability of specimens as well as the research interest in discovery because of the poor outcome of high-grade gliomas. By using first-generation Affymetrix chips, 45 astrocytic tumors (19 grade I, 5 grade II, and 21 grade IV) and six normal brain specimens were profiled on approximately 6800 probes [127]. A unique profile of 360 genes was identified that distinguishes pilocytic (grade I) tumors from GBM (grade IV). Five genes upregulated in GBM, but not previously known to play a role in the tumor, were validated by quantitative real-time polymerase chain reaction and immunohistochemical staining of clinical tissue specimens. Some of these genes, such as *FOXM1*, have been subsequently reported by others to play functional roles in glioma tumorigenesis and progression [128–131]. The complexity and robustness of the microarray data obtained has improved based on improving technology, such that not only is nearly every known and predicted gene represented on a single, current-generation microarray, but gene splice variants can also be profiled using arrays containing oligonucleotides from potentially spiced exons. Such "exon" arrays have been used for glioma profiling [132,133].. Interesting, glioma-specific alternative splicing was a rare event in one study, with only 14 genes identified with tumor-specific splice variants [132].

A number of investigations have attempted to identify individual genes or signaling pathways from microarray data that are prognostic in malignant gliomas [134–143]. By using a group of only 19 gliomas, the chitinase-3-like-1 gene (*CHI3L1*), which encodes for the glycoprotein YKL-40, was found to be upregulated compared with normal brain, and its expression correlated to tumor grade [134]. By using a larger set of 34 GBMs, *CHI3L1* again emerged as a significant gene, and its expression correlated with decreased overall survival and in vitro radioresistance [137]. Subsequent studies have validated the role of *CHI3L1* as a biomarker and suggested a functional role for YKL-40 in tumor progression [144–146]. The EGFR and hypoxia-inducible factor-2α pathway have been implicated in high-grade pediatric astrocytomas based on microarray analysis [135]. An examination of genes overexpressed in GBMs identified a gene signature that differentiated long-term from typical survivors [136]. One of the genes in the signature, fatty acid–binding protein-7, was prognostic in an independent set of 105 patients. The ephrin receptor *EPHA2* gene was found to be a prognostic marker based on a novel integrative analysis of comparative genomic hybridization and mRNA microarray data [138]. Other studies have attempted to combine genomic structural information with expression profiling data to best identify prognostic genes, and this type of integrative approach represents the future of biomarker discovery [137,138,147].

Similar to the earliest studies mentioned previously [127], a number of groups have taken the approach of attempting to predict tumor classification (e.g., pathologic grade) based on expression profiling [131,148–155]. For example, analysis of 35 gliomas using Affymetrix U95A GeneChips identified a 170-gene signature that accurately classified tumors based on grade. Another group attempted to develop a molecular classifier based on microarray data, which could be used to help classify gliomas with "nonclassic" histologies [153]. Twenty-one tumors were used to build a gene classifier that was then applied to an additional 29 tumors with ambiguous histology (GBM vs. AO). Survival prediction based on the classifier was superior to that based on histologic diagnosis.

Specific studies have focused on oligodendroglioma array analysis [156–163]. In one report, a gene signature of approximately 1100 probes was capable of classifying based on grade (World Health Organization grade II vs. III) [156]. Because response to treatment in these tumors is related to deletion of human chromosome 1p/19q [22], several of the studies have attempted to identify unique expression profiles based on the 1p/19q status [157,160–162]. Expression of unique genes or gene signatures have been identified to correlate with 1p/19q deletion, such a neuron-related genes [159,162] or candidate tumor suppressor genes [161]. The concept of functional gene signatures that may be independent of histologic grade, but that reflect the underlying tumor biology, has been developed by a number of groups.

MOLECULAR SUBTYPES OF INFILTRATING GLIOMAS

Expression profiling followed by clustering of infiltrating gliomas (using both k-means and hierarchical methods) has led to the concept of molecular subtypes defined by genes overexpressed within each group. A group from the University of California, Los Angeles (UCLA) identified several subtypes, in a set of 84 tumors, which they termed *extracellular matrix*, mitosis, neurogenesis, and synaptic transmission [164]. An independent study then found subtypes with some similarities found by the UCLA group, specifically a "mesenchymal" group (corresponding to the ECM) proneural (corresponding to neural development) and "proliferative" (corresponding to mitosis) [165]. The subtype termed as "synaptic transmission" by the UCLA group was not found, and it is possible that this group represents cases with a high degree of normal/non-neoplastic brain within the sample. Subsequently, a group from the United Kingdom, in an independent study, highlighted the mesenchymal/angiogenic subtype (called "angio" by the authors) as clinically aggressive and characteristic of grade IV tumors [166]. This picture is still evolving, and the specific genes that describe each subtype are not identical among the various studies. However, a preliminary conclusion that can be reached is that a subset of gliomas exist that overexpress genes associated with mesenchyme and angiogenesis. This subgroup is composed almost solely of GBMs and are particular aggressive and generally resistant to therapy. A second group exists that may correspond to the "proneural" subtype. This group is overrepresented with lower-grade gliomas. Some GBMs also are included in this group, and these tend to be more responsive to therapy. This concept has also been extended to oligodendroglioma, which has been reported as having a proneural phenotype [159,162]. Although future work will clarify the robustness of these molecular subtypes, the concept of mesenchymal versus proneural gliomas does seems supported by several independent studies and represents a paradigm for future biologic investigations. Whether or not specific therapies are more or less effective within each molecular subgroup will no doubt be examined in future clinical trials.

Non-mRNA Based Markers

A recently emerging field of cancer research revolves around the role of micro-RNAs (miRNAs) in tumorigenesis. These small noncoding RNAs regulate gene expression on transcriptional and posttranscriptional levels and can function as oncogenes and tumor suppressor genes (therefore referred to as "oncomirs"). Many miRNAs are located in fragile regions of the human genome, which are disrupted in various types of cancer [167,168].. In glioblastoma, miRNA profiling experiments demonstrated that a specific signature of miRNA expression exists in comparison to normal tissue [169]. The miR-21 located on chromosome 17 is expressed at up to a 100-fold rate in glioblastomas. In vitro studies demonstrated that this miRNA has an antiapoptotic effect, which can be reversed by anti-miRNA oligonucleotides ("antagomirs") [170]. These anti-miRNA oligonucleotides hold promise for the treatment of gliomas in the future.

Additional non-mRNA-based platforms hold promise for molecular subtyping of gliomas, including epigenetic changes, which have only begun to be systematically explored in glioma. Large-scale projects, including The Cancer Genome Atlas, offers multidimensional profiling of a defined set of tumors. This approach will allow the integration of epigenetic, DNA, mRNA, and noncoding RNA platforms that will identify new pathways that may lead to an increased understanding of the biology.

SUMMARY AND FUTURE PERSPECTIVE

With the rapid development of molecular tools to identify the biological basis for glioma development and progression, much knowledge has been accumulated in the past years that will be translated into daily clinical practice by therapy targeting determinants of the malignant phenotype. Combining and integrating molecular analysis with clinical trials that combine cytotoxic therapies with targeted agents present the most realistic approach to improving outcomes for patients whose tumors exhibit biologically distinct molecular subtypes.

REFERENCES

1. Okamoto Y, Di Patre PL, Burkhard C, et al. Population-based study on incidence, survival rates, and genetic alterations of low-grade diffuse astrocytomas and oligodendrogliomas. *Acta Neuropathol.* 2004;108:49–56.
2. Ohgaki H, Kleihues P. Population-based studies on incidence, survival rates, and genetic alterations in astrocytic and oligodendroglial gliomas. *J Neuropathol Exp Neurol.* 2005;64:479–489.
3. Galli R, Binda E, Orfanelli U, et al. Isolation and characterization of tumorigenic, stem-like neural precursors from human glioblastoma. *Cancer Res.* 2004;64:7011–7021.
4. Singh SK, Clarke ID, Terasaki M, et al. Identification of a cancer stem cell in human brain tumors. *Cancer Res.* 2003;63:5821–5828.
5. Holland EC, Celestino J, Dai C, Schaefer L, Sawaya RE, Fuller GN. Combined activation of Ras and Akt in neural progenitors induces glioblastoma formation in mice. *Nat Genet.* 2000;25:55–57.
6. Sanai N, Alvarez-Buylla A, Berger MS. Neural stem cells and the origin of gliomas. *N Engl J Med.* 2005;353:811–822.
7. Vescovi AL, Galli R, Reynolds BA. Brain tumour stem cells. *Nat Rev Cancer.* 2006;6:425–436.
8. Dai C, Lyustikman Y, Shih A, et al. The characteristics of astrocytomas and oligodendrogliomas are caused by two distinct and interchangeable signaling formats. *Neoplasia.* 2005;7:397–406.
9. Lang FF, Miller DC, Koslow M, Newcomb EW. Pathways leading to glioblastoma multiforme: a molecular analysis of genetic alterations in 65 astrocytic tumors. *J Neurosurg.* 1994;81:427–436.
10. von Deimling A, Louis DN, von Ammon K, Petersen I, Wiestler OD, Seizinger BR. Evidence for a tumor suppressor gene on chromosome 19q associated with human astrocytomas, oligodendrogliomas, and mixed gliomas. *Cancer Res.* 1992;52:4277–4279.
11. von Deimling A, Louis DN, Wiestler OD. Molecular pathways in the formation of gliomas. *Glia.* 1995;15:328–338.
12. von Deimling A, von Ammon K, Schoenfeld D, Wiestler OD, Seizinger BR, Louis DN. Subsets of glioblastoma multiforme defined by molecular genetic analysis. *Brain Pathol.* 1993;3:19–26.
13. Hanahan D, Weinberg RA. The hallmarks of cancer. *Cell.* 2000;100:57–70.
14. Houillier C, Lejeune J, Benouaich-Amiel A, et al. Prognostic impact of molecular markers in a series of 220 primary glioblastomas. *Cancer.* 2006;106:2218–2223.
15. Wolter M, Reifenberger J, Blaschke B, et al. Oligodendroglial tumors frequently demonstrate hypermethylation of the CDKN2A (MTS1, p16INK4a), p14ARF, and CDKN2B (MTS2, p15INK4b) tumor suppressor genes. *J Neuropathol Exp Neurol.* 2001;60:1170–1180.
16. Ohgaki H, Kleihues P. Genetic pathways to primary and secondary glioblastoma. *Am J Pathol.* 2007;170:1445–1453.
17. Ohgaki H, Dessen P, Jourde B, et al. Genetic pathways to glioblastoma: a population-based study. *Cancer Res.* 2004;64:6892–6899.

18. Ohgaki H. Genetic pathways to glioblastomas. *Neuropathology*. 2005;25:1–7.
19. Perry A, Miller R, Guirati M, et al. Malignant gliomas with neuroblastic (PNET-like) components (GBM-PNET): a clinicopathologic and genetic study of 28 cases. *Neuro Oncol*. 2007;9:543.
20. van den Bent MJ. Anaplastic oligodendroglioma and oligoastrocytoma. *Neurol Clin*. 2007;25:1089–1109, ix–x.
21. Griffin CA, Burger P, Morsberger L, et al. Identification of der(1;19)(q10;p10) in five oligodendrogliomas suggests mechanism of concurrent 1p and 19q loss. *J Neuropathol Exp Neurol*. 2006;65:988–994.
22. Cairncross JG, Ueki K, Zlatescu MC, et al. Specific genetic predictors of chemotherapeutic response and survival in patients with anaplastic oligodendrogliomas. *J Natl Cancer Inst*. 1998;90:1473–1479.
23. Kros JM, Gorlia T, Kouwenhoven MC, et al. Panel review of anaplastic oligodendroglioma from European Organization For Research and Treatment of Cancer Trial 26951: assessment of consensus in diagnosis, influence of 1p/19q loss, and correlations with outcome. *J Neuropathol Exp Neurol*. 2007;66:545–551.
24. Jeuken JW, von Deimling A, Wesseling P. Molecular pathogenesis of oligodendroglial tumors. *J Neurooncol*. 2004;70:161–181.
25. Aldape K, Burger PC, Perry A. Clinicopathologic aspects of 1p/19q loss and the diagnosis of oligodendroglioma. *Arch Pathol Lab Med*. 2007;131:242–251.
26. Sasaki H, Zlatescu MC, Betensky RA, Ino Y, Cairncross JG, Louis DN. PTEN is a target of chromosome 10q loss in anaplastic oligodendrogliomas and PTEN alterations are associated with poor prognosis. *Am J Pathol*. 2001;159:359–367.
27. Chan AS, Leung SY, Wong MP, et al. Expression of vascular endothelial growth factor and its receptors in the anaplastic progression of astrocytoma, oligodendroglioma, and ependymoma. *Am J Surg Pathol*. 1998;22:816–826.
28. Christov C, Adle-Biassette H, Le Guerinel C, Natchev S, Gherardi RK. Immunohistochemical detection of vascular endothelial growth factor (VEGF) in the vasculature of oligodendrogliomas. *Neuropathol Appl Neurobiol*. 1998;24:29–35.
29. Maher PA. Nuclear translocation of fibroblast growth factor (FGF) receptors in response to FGF-2. *J Cell Biol*. 1996;134:529–536.
30. Guha A, Dashner K, Black PM, Wagner JA, Stiles CD. Expression of PDGF and PDGF receptors in human astrocytoma operation specimens supports the existence of an autocrine loop. *Int J Cancer*. 1995;60:168–173.
31. Hermanson M, Funa K, Hartman M, et al. Platelet-derived growth factor and its receptors in human glioma tissue: expression of messenger RNA and protein suggests the presence of autocrine and paracrine loops. *Cancer Res*. 1992;52:3213–3219.
32. Dunn IF, Heese O, Black PM. Growth factors in glioma angiogenesis: FGFs, PDGF, EGF, and TGFs. *J Neurooncol*. 2000;50:121–137.
33. Savage DG, Antman KH. Imatinib mesylate—a new oral targeted therapy. *N Engl J Med*. 2002;346:683–693.
34. Haberler C, Gelpi E, Marosi C, et al. Immunohistochemical analysis of platelet-derived growth factor receptor-alpha, -beta, c-kit, c-abl, and arg proteins in glioblastoma: possible implications for patient selection for imatinib mesylate therapy. *J Neurooncol*. 2006;76:105–109.
35. Tripp SR, Willmore-Payne C, Layfield LJ. Relationship between EGFR overexpression and gene amplification status in central nervous system gliomas. *Anal Quant Cytol Histol*. 2005;27:71–78.
36. Frederick L, Eley G, Wang XY, James CD. Analysis of genomic rearrangements associated with EGRFvIII expression suggests involvement of Alu repeat elements. *Neuro Oncol*. 2000;2:159–163.
37. Ekstrand AJ, Longo N, Hamid ML, et al. Functional characterization of an EGF receptor with a truncated extracellular domain expressed in glioblastomas with EGFR gene amplification. *Oncogene*. 1994;9:2313–2320.
38. Nagane M, Levitzki A, Gazit A, Cavenee WK, Huang HJ. Drug resistance of human glioblastoma cells conferred by a tumor-specific mutant epidermal growth factor receptor through modulation of Bcl-XL and caspase-3-like proteases. *Proc Natl Acad Sci USA*. 1998;95:5724–5729.
39. Lal A, Glazer CA, Martinson HM, et al. Mutant epidermal growth factor receptor up-regulates molecular effectors of tumor invasion. *Cancer Res*. 2002;62:3335–3339.
40. Pelloski CE, Ballman KV, Furth AF, et al. Epidermal growth factor receptor variant III status defines clinically distinct subtypes of glioblastoma. *J Clin Oncol*. 2007;25:2288–2294.
41. Jungbluth AA, Stockert E, Huang HJ, et al. A monoclonal antibody recognizing human cancers with amplification/overexpression of the human epidermal growth factor receptor. *Proc Natl Acad Sci USA*. 2003;100:639–644.
42. Eller JL, Longo SL, Hicklin DJ, Canute GW. Activity of anti-epidermal growth factor receptor monoclonal antibody C225 against glioblastoma multiforme. *Neurosurgery*. 2002;51:1005–1013; discussion 13–14.
43. Belda-Iniesta C, Carpeno Jde C, Saenz EC, Gutierrez M, Perona R, Baron MG. Long term responses with cetuximab therapy in glioblastoma multiforme. *Cancer Biol Ther*. 2006;5:912–914.
44. Mellinghoff IK, Wang MY, Vivanco I, et al. Molecular determinants of the response of glioblastomas to EGFR kinase inhibitors. *N Engl J Med*. 2005;353:2012–2024.
45. Haas-Kogan DA, Prados MD, Tihan T, et al. Epidermal growth factor receptor, protein kinase B/Akt, and glioma response to erlotinib. *J Natl Cancer Inst*. 2005;97:880–887.
46. Haas-Kogan DA, Prados MD, Lamborn KR, Tihan T, Berger MS, Stokoe D. Biomarkers to predict response to epidermal growth factor receptor inhibitors. *Cell Cycle*. 2005;4:1369–1372.
47. Yamada N, Kato M, Yamashita H, et al. Enhanced expression of transforming growth factor-beta and its type-I and type-II receptors in human glioblastoma. *Int J Cancer*. 1995;62:386–392.
48. Platten M, Wick W, Weller M. Malignant glioma biology: role for TGF-beta in growth, motility, angiogenesis, and immune escape. *Micros Res Tech*. 2001;52:401–410.
49. Wick W, Platten M, Weller M. Glioma cell invasion: regulation of metalloproteinase activity by TGF-beta. *J Neurooncol*. 2001;53:177–185.
50. Schlingensiepen KH, Schlingensiepen R, Steinbrecher A, et al. Targeted tumor therapy with the TGF-beta2 antisense compound AP 12009. *Cytokine Growth Factor Rev*. 2006;17:129–139.
51. Knobbe CB, Reifenberger J, Reifenberger G. Mutation analysis of the Ras pathway genes NRAS, HRAS, KRAS and BRAF in glioblastomas. *Acta Neuropathol*. 2004;108:467–470.
52. Jeuken J, van den Broecke C, Gijsen S, Boots-Sprenger S, Wesseling P. RAS/RAF pathway activation in gliomas: the result of copy number gains rather than activating mutations. *Acta Neuropathol*. 2007;114:121–133.
53. Aktas H, Cai H, Cooper GM. Ras links growth factor signaling to the cell cycle machinery via regulation of cyclin D1 and the Cdk inhibitor p27KIP1. *Mol Cell Biol*. 1997;17:3850–3857.
54. Cloughesy TF, Kuhn J, Robins HI, et al. Phase I trial of tipifarnib in patients with recurrent malignant glioma taking enzyme-inducing antiepileptic drugs: a North American Brain Tumor Consortium Study. *J Clin Oncol*. 2005;23:6647–6656.
55. Chakravarti A, Zhai G, Suzuki Y, et al. The prognostic significance of phosphatidylinositol 3-kinase pathway activation in human gliomas. *J Clin Oncol*. 2004;22:1926–1933.
56. Tohma Y, Gratas C, Biernat W, et al. PTEN (MMAC1) mutations are frequent in primary glioblastomas (de novo) but not in secondary glioblastomas. *J Neuropathol Exp Neurol*. 1998;57:684–689.
57. Knobbe CB, Reifenberger G. Genetic alterations and aberrant expression of genes related to the phosphatidyl-inositol-3′-kinase/protein kinase B (Akt) signal transduction pathway in glioblastomas. *Brain Pathol*. 2003;13:507–518.
58. Knobbe CB, Merlo A, Reifenberger G. Pten signaling in gliomas. *Neuro Oncol*. 2002;4:196–211.
59. Wang H, Zhang W, Huang HJ, Liao WS, Fuller GN. Analysis of the activation status of Akt, NFkappaB, and Stat3 in human diffuse gliomas. *Lab Invest*. 2004;84:941–951.
60. Galanis E, Buckner JC, Maurer MJ, et al. Phase II trial of temsirolimus (CCI-779) in recurrent glioblastoma multiforme: a North Central Cancer Treatment Group Study. *J Clin Oncol*. 2005;23:5294–5304.
61. Fan QW, Knight ZA, Goldenberg DD, et al. A dual PI3 kinase/mTOR inhibitor reveals emergent efficacy in glioma. *Cancer Cell*. 2006;9:341–349.
62. Reifenberger G, Reifenberger J, Ichimura K, Meltzer PS, Collins VP. Amplification of multiple genes from chromosomal region 12q13–14 in human malignant gliomas: preliminary mapping of the amplicons shows preferential involvement of CDK4, SAS, and MDM2. *Cancer Res*. 1994;54:4299–4303.
63. Reifenberger G, Ichimura K, Reifenberger J, Elkahloun AG, Meltzer PS, Collins VP. Refined mapping of 12q13-q15 amplicons in human malignant gliomas suggests CDK4/SAS and MDM2 as independent amplification targets. *Cancer Res*. 1996;56:5141–5145.

64. Serrano M, Hannon GJ, Beach D. A new regulatory motif in cell-cycle control causing specific inhibition of cyclin D/CDK4. *Nature*. 1993;366:704–707.
65. Ueki K, Ono Y, Henson JW, Efird JT, von Deimling A, Louis DN. CDKN2/p16 or RB alterations occur in the majority of glioblastomas and are inversely correlated. *Cancer Res*. 1996;56:150–153.
66. Fueyo J, Gomez-Manzano C, Alemany R, et al. A mutant oncolytic adenovirus targeting the Rb pathway produces anti-glioma effect in vivo. *Oncogene*. 2000;19:2–12.
67. McNeish IA, Bell SJ, Lemoine NR. Gene therapy progress and prospects: cancer gene therapy using tumour suppressor genes. *Gene Ther*. 2004;11:497–503.
68. Simon M, Simon C, Koster G, Hans VH, Schramm J. Conditional expression of the tumor suppressor p16 in a heterotopic glioblastoma model results in loss of pRB expression. *J Neurooncol*. 2002;60:1–12.
69. Komata T, Kanzawa T, Takeuchi H, et al. Antitumour effect of cyclin-dependent kinase inhibitors (p16(INK4A), p18(INK4C), p19(INK4D), p21(WAF1/CIP1) and p27(KIP1)) on malignant glioma cells. *Br J Cancer*. 2003;88:1277–1280.
70. Hung KS, Hong CY, Lee J, et al. Expression of p16(INK4A) induces dominant suppression of glioblastoma growth in situ through necrosis and cell cycle arrest. *Biochem Biophys Res Commun*. 2000;269:718–725.
71. Newcomb EW, Tamasdan C, Entzminger Y, et al. Flavopiridol inhibits the growth of GL261 gliomas in vivo: implications for malignant glioma therapy. *Cell Cycle*. 2004;3:230–234.
72. Yin D, Zhou H, Kumagai T, et al. Proteasome inhibitor PS-341 causes cell growth arrest and apoptosis in human glioblastoma multiforme (GBM). *Oncogene*. 2005;24:344–354.
73. Honda R, Tanaka H, Yasuda H. Oncoprotein MDM2 is a ubiquitin ligase E3 for tumor suppressor p53. *FEBS Lett*. 1997;420:25–27.
74. Riemenschneider MJ, Buschges R, Wolter M, et al. Amplification and overexpression of the MDM4 (MDMX) gene from 1q32 in a subset of malignant gliomas without TP53 mutation or MDM2 amplification. *Cancer Res*. 1999;59:6091–6096.
75. Hupp TR, Lane DP, Ball KL. Strategies for manipulating the p53 pathway in the treatment of human cancer. *Biochem J*. 2000;352(pt 1):1–17.
76. Lang FF, Bruner JM, Fuller GN, et al. Phase I trial of adenovirus-mediated p53 gene therapy for recurrent glioma: biological and clinical results. *J Clin Oncol*. 2003;21:2508–2518.
77. Chakravarti A, Dicker A, Mehta M. The contribution of epidermal growth factor receptor (EGFR) signaling pathway to radioresistance in human gliomas: a review of preclinical and correlative clinical data. *Int J Radiat Oncol Biol Phys*. 2004;58:927–931.
78. Shinoura N, Saito K, Yoshida Y, et al. Adenovirus-mediated transfer of bax with caspase-8 controlled by myelin basic protein promoter exerts an enhanced cytotoxic effect in gliomas. *Cancer Gene Ther*. 2000;7:739–748.
79. Zangemeister-Wittke U, Leech SH, Olie RA, et al. A novel bispecific antisense oligonucleotide inhibiting both bcl-2 and bcl-xL expression efficiently induces apoptosis in tumor cells. *Clin Cancer Res*. 2000;6:2547–2555.
80. Waxman DJ, Schwartz PS. Harnessing apoptosis for improved anticancer gene therapy. *Cancer Res*. 2003;63:8563–8572.
81. Kondapaka SB, Singh SS, Dasmahapatra GP, Sausville EA, Roy KK. Perifosine, a novel alkylphospholipid, inhibits protein kinase B activation. *Mol Cancer Ther*. 2003;2:1093–1103.
82. Marte BM, Downward J. PKB/Akt: connecting phosphoinositide 3-kinase to cell survival and beyond. *Trends Biochem Sci*. 1997;22:355–358.
83. Gozuacik D, Kimchi A. Autophagy as a cell death and tumor suppressor mechanism. *Oncogene*. 2004;23:2891–2906.
84. Kondo Y, Kanzawa T, Sawaya R, Kondo S. The role of autophagy in cancer development and response to therapy. *Nat Rev Cancer*. 2005;5:726–734.
85. Lefranc F, Facchini V, Kiss R. Proautophagic drugs: a novel means to combat apoptosis-resistant cancers, with a special emphasis on glioblastomas. *Oncologist*. 2007;12:1395–1403.
86. Lum JJ, Bauer DE, Kong M, et al. Growth factor regulation of autophagy and cell survival in the absence of apoptosis. *Cell*. 2005;120:237–248.
87. Guertin DA, Sabatini DM. An expanding role for mTOR in cancer. *Trends Mol Med*. 2005;11:353–361.
88. Kondo Y, Kondo S. Autophagy and cancer therapy. *Autophagy*. 2006;2:85–90.
89. Lockshin RA, Zakeri Z. Apoptosis, autophagy, and more. *Int J Biochem Cell Biol*. 2004;36:2405–2419.
90. Maiuri MC, Zalckvar E, Kimchi A, Kroemer G. Self-eating and self-killing: crosstalk between autophagy and apoptosis. *Nat Rev Mol Cell Biol*. 2007;8:741–752.
91. Feng Z, Zhang H, Levine AJ, Jin S. The coordinate regulation of the p53 and mTOR pathways in cells. *Proc Natl Acad Sci USA*. 2005;102:8204–8209.
92. Jin S. p53, autophagy and tumor suppression. *Autophagy*. 2005;1:171–173.
93. Sarbassov DD, Ali SM, Sabatini DM. Growing roles for the mTOR pathway. *Curr Opin Cell Biol*. 2005;17:596–603.
94. Miracco C, Cosci E, Oliveri G, et al. Protein and mRNA expression of autophagy gene Beclin 1 in human brain tumours. *Int J Oncol*. 2007;30:429–436.
95. Iwamaru A, Kondo Y, Iwado E, et al. Silencing mammalian target of rapamycin signaling by small interfering RNA enhances rapamycin-induced autophagy in malignant glioma cells. *Oncogene*. 2007;26:1840–1851.
96. Stupp R, Mason WP, van den Bent MJ, et al. Radiotherapy plus concomitant and adjuvant temozolomide for glioblastoma. *N Engl J Med*. 2005;352:987–996.
97. Kanzawa T, Germano IM, Komata T, Ito H, Kondo Y, Kondo S. Role of autophagy in temozolomide-induced cytotoxicity for malignant glioma cells. *Cell Death Differ*. 2004;11:448–457.
98. Ertmer A, Huber V, Gilch S, et al. The anticancer drug imatinib induces cellular autophagy. *Leukemia*. 2007;21:936–942.
99. Zhang L, Yu J, Pan H, et al. Small molecule regulators of autophagy identified by an image-based high-throughput screen. *Proc Natl Acad Sci USA*. 2007;104:19023–19028.
100. Falchetti ML, Larocca LM, Pallini R. Telomerase in brain tumors. *Childs Nerv Syst*. 2002;18:112–117.
101. Sonoda Y, Ozawa T, Hirose Y, et al. Formation of intracranial tumors by genetically modified human astrocytes defines four pathways critical in the development of human anaplastic astrocytoma. *Cancer Res*. 2001;61:4956–4960.
102. Falchetti ML, Fiorenzo P, Mongiardi MP, et al. Telomerase inhibition impairs tumor growth in glioblastoma xenografts. *Neurol Res*. 2006;28:532–537.
103. Brat DJ, Castellano-Sanchez AA, Hunter SB, et al. Pseudopalisades in glioblastoma are hypoxic, express extracellular matrix proteases, and are formed by an actively migrating cell population. *Cancer Res*. 2004;64:920–927.
104. Cheng SY, Huang HJ, Nagane M, et al. Suppression of glioblastoma angiogenicity and tumorigenicity by inhibition of endogenous expression of vascular endothelial growth factor. *Proc Natl Acad Sci USA*. 1996;93:8502–8507.
105. Fischer I, Gagner JP, Law M, Newcomb EW, Zagzag D. Angiogenesis in gliomas: biology and molecular pathophysiology. *Brain Pathol*. 2005;15:297–310.
106. Feldkamp MM, Lau N, Rak J, Kerbel RS, Guha A. Normoxic and hypoxic regulation of vascular endothelial growth factor (VEGF) by astrocytoma cells is mediated by Ras. *Int J Cancer*. 1999;81:118–124.
107. Maity A, Pore N, Lee J, Solomon D, O'Rourke DM. Epidermal growth factor receptor transcriptionally up-regulates vascular endothelial growth factor expression in human glioblastoma cells via a pathway involving phosphatidylinositol 3'-kinase and distinct from that induced by hypoxia. *Cancer Res*. 2000;60:5879–5886.
108. Zundel W, Schindler C, Haas-Kogan D, et al. Loss of PTEN facilitates HIF-1-mediated gene expression. *Genes Dev*. 2000;14:391–396.
109. Vredenburgh JJ, Desjardins A, Herndon JE 2nd, et al. Bevacizumab plus irinotecan in recurrent glioblastoma multiforme. *J Clin Oncol*. 2007;25:4722–4729.
110. Vredenburgh JJ, Desjardins A, Herndon JE 2nd, et al. Phase II trial of bevacizumab and irinotecan in recurrent malignant glioma. *Clin Cancer Res*. 2007;13:1253–1259.
111. Kubo K, Shimizu T, Ohyama S, et al. Novel potent orally active selective VEGFR-2 tyrosine kinase inhibitors: synthesis, structure-activity relationships, and antitumor activities of N-phenyl-N'-{4-(4-quinolyloxy)phenyl} ureas. *J Med Chem*. 2005;48:1359–1366.
112. Abounader R, Laterra J. Scatter factor/hepatocyte growth factor in brain tumor growth and angiogenesis. *Neuro Oncol*. 2005;7:436–451.
113. Lamszus K, Laterra J, Westphal M, Rosen EM. Scatter factor/hepatocyte growth factor (SF/HGF) content and function in human gliomas. *Int J Dev Neurosci*. 1999;17:517–530.

114. Laterra J, Nam M, Rosen E, et al. Scatter factor/hepatocyte growth factor gene transfer enhances glioma growth and angiogenesis in vivo. *Lab Invest.* 1997;76:565–577.
115. Rosen EM, Lamszus K, Laterra J, Polverini PJ, Rubin JS, Goldberg ID. HGF/SF in angiogenesis. *Ciba Found Symp.* 1997;212:215–226; discussion 27–29.
116. Martens T, Schmidt NO, Eckerich C, et al. A novel one-armed anti-c-Met antibody inhibits glioblastoma growth in vivo. *Clin Cancer Res.* 2006;12:6144–6152.
117. Gladson CL. The extracellular matrix of gliomas: modulation of cell function. *J Neuropathol Exp Neurol.* 1999;58:1029–1040.
118. Tonn JC, Wunderlich S, Kerkau S, Klein CE, Roosen K. Invasive behaviour of human gliomas is mediated by interindividually different integrin patterns. *Anticancer Res.* 1998;18:2599–2605.
119. Taga T, Suzuki A, Gonzalez-Gomez I, et al. alpha v-Integrin antagonist EMD 121974 induces apoptosis in brain tumor cells growing on vitronectin and tenascin. *Int J Cancer.* 2002;98:690–697.
120. Rao JS. Molecular mechanisms of glioma invasiveness: the role of proteases. *Nat Rev Cancer.* 2003;3:489–501.
121. Wang M, Wang T, Liu S, Yoshida D, Teramoto A. The expression of matrix metalloproteinase-2 and -9 in human gliomas of different pathological grades. *Brain Tumor Pathol.* 2003;20:65–72.
122. Demuth T, Berens ME. Molecular mechanisms of glioma cell migration and invasion. *J Neurooncol.* 2004;70:217–228.
123. Yamamoto M, Sawaya R, Mohanam S, et al. Expression and localization of urokinase-type plasminogen activator in human astrocytomas in vivo. *Cancer Res.* 1994;54:3656–3661.
124. Yamamoto S, Wakimoto H, Aoyagi M, Hirakawa K, Hamada H. Modulation of motility and proliferation of glioma cells by hepatocyte growth factor. *Jpn J Cancer Res.* 1997;88:564–577.
125. Joy AM, Beaudry CE, Tran NL, et al. Migrating glioma cells activate the PI3-K pathway and display decreased susceptibility to apoptosis. *J Cell Sci.* 2003;116:4409–4417.
126. Koul D, Shen R, Bergh S, et al. Inhibition of Akt survival pathway by a small-molecule inhibitor in human glioblastoma. *Mol Cancer Ther.* 2006;5:637–644.
127. Rickman DS, Bobek MP, Misek DE, et al. Distinctive molecular profiles of high-grade and low-grade gliomas based on oligonucleotide microarray analysis. *Cancer Res.* 2001;61:6885–6891.
128. Dai B, Kang SH, Gong W, et al. Aberrant FoxM1B expression increases matrix metalloproteinase-2 transcription and enhances the invasion of glioma cells. *Oncogene.* 2007;26:6212–6219.
129. Liu M, Dai B, Kang SH, et al. FoxM1B is overexpressed in human glioblastomas and critically regulates the tumorigenicity of glioma cells. *Cancer Res.* 2006;66:3593–3602.
130. Teh MT, Wong ST, Neill GW, Ghali LR, Philpott MP, Quinn AG. FOXM1 is a downstream target of Gli1 in basal cell carcinomas. *Cancer Res.* 2002;62:4773–4780.
131. van den Boom J, Wolter M, Kuick R, et al. Characterization of gene expression profiles associated with glioma progression using oligonucleotide-based microarray analysis and real-time reverse transcription-polymerase chain reaction. *Am J Pathol.* 2003;163:1033–1043.
132. Cheung HC, Baggerly KA, Tsavachidis S, et al. Global analysis of aberrant pre-mRNA splicing in glioblastoma using exon expression arrays. *BMC Genomics.* 2008;9:216.
133. French PJ, Peeters J, Horsman S, et al. Identification of differentially regulated splice variants and novel exons in glial brain tumors using exon expression arrays. *Cancer Res.* 2007;67:5635–5642.
134. Tanwar MK, Gilbert MR, Holland EC. Gene expression microarray analysis reveals YKL-40 to be a potential serum marker for malignant character in human glioma. *Cancer Res.* 2002;62:4364–4368.
135. Khatua S, Peterson KM, Brown KM, et al. Overexpression of the EGFR/FKBP12/HIF-2alpha pathway identified in childhood astrocytomas by angiogenesis gene profiling. *Cancer Res.* 2003;63:1865–1870.
136. Liang Y, Diehn M, Watson N, et al. Gene expression profiling reveals molecularly and clinically distinct subtypes of glioblastoma multiforme. *Proc Natl Acad Sci USA.* 2005;102:5814–5819.
137. Nigro JM, Misra A, Zhang L, et al. Integrated array-comparative genomic hybridization and expression array profiles identify clinically relevant molecular subtypes of glioblastoma. *Cancer Res.* 2005;65:1678–1686.
138. Liu F, Park PJ, Lai W, et al. A genome-wide screen reveals functional gene clusters in the cancer genome and identifies EphA2 as a mitogen in glioblastoma. *Cancer Res.* 2006;66:10815–10823.
139. Faury D, Nantel A, Dunn SE, et al. Molecular profiling identifies prognostic subgroups of pediatric glioblastoma and shows increased YB-1 expression in tumors. *J Clin Oncol.* 2007;25:1196–1208.
140. McDonald KL, O'Sullivan MG, Parkinson JF, et al. IQGAP1 and IGFBP2: valuable biomarkers for determining prognosis in glioma patients. *J Neuropathol Exp Neurol.* 2007;66:405–417.
141. Reddy SP, Britto R, Vinnakota K, et al. Novel glioblastoma markers with diagnostic and prognostic value identified through transcriptome analysis. *Clin Cancer Res.* 2008;14:2978–2987.
142. Ruano Y, Mollejo M, Camacho FI, et al. Identification of survival-related genes of the phosphatidylinositol 3′-kinase signaling pathway in glioblastoma multiforme. *Cancer.* 2008;112:1575–1584.
143. Scrideli CA, Carlotti CG Jr, Okamoto OK, et al. Gene expression profile analysis of primary glioblastomas and non-neoplastic brain tissue: identification of potential target genes by oligonucleotide microarray and real-time quantitative PCR. *J Neurooncol.* 2008;88:281–291.
144. Nutt CL, Betensky RA, Brower MA, Batchelor TT, Louis DN, Stemmer-Rachamimov AO. YKL-40 is a differential diagnostic marker for histologic subtypes of high-grade gliomas. *Clin Cancer Res.* 2005;11:2258–2264.
145. Pelloski CE, Mahajan A, Maor M, et al. YKL-40 expression is associated with poorer response to radiation and shorter overall survival in glioblastoma. *Clin Cancer Res.* 2005;11:3326–3334.
146. Pelloski CE, Lin E, Zhang L, et al. Prognostic associations of activated mitogen-activated protein kinase and Akt pathways in glioblastoma. *Clin Cancer Res.* 2006;12:3935–3941.
147. Persson O, Krogh M, Saal LH, et al. Microarray analysis of gliomas reveals chromosomal position-associated gene expression patterns and identifies potential immunotherapy targets. *J Neurooncol.* 2007;85:11–24.
148. Bozinov O, Kohler S, Samans B, et al. Candidate genes for the progression of malignant gliomas identified by microarray analysis. *Neurosurg Rev.* 2008;31:83–89; discussion 9–90.
149. Czernicki T, Zegarska J, Paczek L, et al. Gene expression profile as a prognostic factor in high-grade gliomas. *Int J Oncol.* 2007;30:55–64.
150. Godard S, Getz G, Delorenzi M, et al. Classification of human astrocytic gliomas on the basis of gene expression: a correlated group of genes with angiogenic activity emerges as a strong predictor of subtypes. *Cancer Res.* 2003;63:6613–6625.
151. Kim S, Dougherty ER, Shmulevich I, et al. Identification of combination gene sets for glioma classification. *Mol Cancer Ther.* 2002;1:1229–1236.
152. Margareto J, Leis O, Larrarte E, Idoate MA, Carrasco A, Lafuente JV. Gene expression profiling of human gliomas reveals differences between GBM and LGA related to energy metabolism and notch signaling pathways. *J Mol Neurosci.* 2007;32:53–63.
153. Nutt CL, Mani DR, Betensky RA, et al. Gene expression-based classification of malignant gliomas correlates better with survival than histological classification. *Cancer Res.* 2003;63:1602–1607.
154. Pomeroy SL, Tamayo P, Gaasenbeek M, et al. Prediction of central nervous system embryonal tumour outcome based on gene expression. *Nature.* 2002;415:436–442.
155. Shai R, Shi T, Kremen TJ, et al. Gene expression profiling identifies molecular subtypes of gliomas. *Oncogene.* 2003;22:4918–4923.
156. Watson MA, Perry A, Budhraja V, Hicks C, Shannon WD, Rich KM. Gene expression profiling with oligonucleotide microarrays distinguishes World Health Organization grade of oligodendrogliomas. *Cancer Res.* 2001;61:1825–1829.
157. Mukasa A, Ueki K, Matsumoto S, et al. Distinction in gene expression profiles of oligodendrogliomas with and without allelic loss of 1p. *Oncogene.* 2002;21:3961–3968.
158. Huang H, Okamoto Y, Yokoo H, et al. Gene expression profiling and subgroup identification of oligodendrogliomas. *Oncogene.* 2004;23:6012–6022.
159. Mukasa A, Ueki K, Ge X, et al. Selective expression of a subset of neuronal genes in oligodendroglioma with chromosome 1p loss. *Brain Pathol.* 2004;14:34–42.
160. French PJ, Swagemakers SM, Nagel JH, et al. Gene expression profiles associated with treatment response in oligodendrogliomas. *Cancer Res.* 2005;65:11335–11344.
161. Tews B, Felsberg J, Hartmann C, et al. Identification of novel oligodendroglioma-associated candidate tumor suppressor genes in 1p36 and 19q13 using microarray-based expression profiling. *Int J Cancer.* 2006;119:792–800.

162. Ducray F, Idbaih A, de Reynies A, et al. Anaplastic oligodendrogliomas with 1p19q codeletion have a proneural gene expression profile. *Mol Cancer.* 2008;7:41.
163. Hagerstrand D, Smits A, Eriksson A, et al. Gene expression analyses of grade II gliomas and identification of rPTPbeta/zeta as a candidate oligodendroglioma marker. *Neuro Oncol.* 2008;10:2–9.
164. Freije WA, Castro-Vargas FE, Fang Z, et al. Gene expression profiling of gliomas strongly predicts survival. *Cancer Res.* 2004;64:6503–6510.
165. Phillips HS, Kharbanda S, Chen R, et al. Molecular subclasses of high-grade glioma predict prognosis, delineate a pattern of disease progression, and resemble stages in neurogenesis. *Cancer Cell.* 2006;9:157–173.
166. Petalidis LP, Oulas A, Backlund M, et al. Improved grading and survival prediction of human astrocytic brain tumors by artificial neural network analysis of gene expression microarray data. *Mol Cancer Ther.* 2008;7:1013–1024.
167. Esquela-Kerscher A, Slack FJ. Oncomirs—microRNAs with a role in cancer. *Nat Rev Cancer.* 2006;6:259–269.
168. Chen CZ. MicroRNAs as oncogenes and tumor suppressors. *N Engl J Med.* 2005;353:1768–1771.
169. Ciafre SA, Galardi S, Mangiola A, et al. Extensive modulation of a set of microRNAs in primary glioblastoma. *Biochem Biophys Res Commun.* 2005;334:1351–1358.
170. Chan JA, Krichevsky AM, Kosik KS. MicroRNA-21 is an antiapoptotic factor in human glioblastoma cells. *Cancer Res.* 2005;65:6029–6033.

14 Molecular Heterogeneity and Tumor Microenvironment

Daniel J. Brat and Sydney M. Evans

INTRODUCTION

Human brain tumors are a heterogeneous group that display variable clinical behavior, histology, grade, location, proliferation, and invasiveness. In the past three decades, it has become apparent that individual tumors of the same histologic class and grade vary in their cellular and genetic composition [1–3]. A topic that has been less thoroughly investigated, but is likely to be equally important to future gains in biologic understanding, diagnosis, and therapy, is the role of cellular and molecular heterogeneity, including the tumor microenvironment, within a given patient's brain tumor. This chapter reviews the topic of cellular and molecular heterogeneity in relation to the microenvironment in human brain tumors with an emphasis on the infiltrating astrocytic neoplasms, including glioblastoma (GBM).

GROWTH PATTERNS OF ASTROCYTIC NEOPLASMS

The neuroimaging and pathologic features of diffusely infiltrating astrocytomas show a general pattern of increasing complexity and heterogeneity with advancing tumor grade. The World Health Organization uses a three-tiered grading system that includes infiltrative astrocytoma, grade II, anaplastic astrocytoma, grade III, and GBM, grade IV [4]. By magnetic resonance (MR) imaging, grade II and III astrocytomas show hyperintense T2-weighted signal abnormalities, reflecting both tumor cell infiltration into brain tissue and its consequence, vasogenic edema (Figure 14.1A). These lower-grade tumors expand the involved brain but usually have minimal or no contrast enhancement, suggesting an intact blood-brain barrier and an absence of tumor necrosis [5–8]. Histologic sections of grade II-III tumors support the MR imaging findings: neoplastic cells are found diffusely infiltrating between neuronal and glial processes, leading to architectural distortion and edema [9,10]. As astrocytomas advance through the pathologic spectrum from the lower end of grade II to the upper end of grade III, both the degree of nuclear anaplasia and the proliferative capacity increase resulting in a progressively more hypercellular tumor with a more aggressive biologic potential [11].

A defining feature of these tumors is the ability of individual tumor cells to infiltrate the central nervous system (CNS) parenchyma. Thus, all tumors will contain normal CNS structures, the content of which will depend on location. If the tumor involves primarily white matter, there will be axons with their myelin sheaths, oligodendroglia, microglia, vascular elements, including endothelial cells and pericytes, and dormant perivascular macrophages present within the neoplasm (Figure 14.2A). Tumors that infiltrate gray matter structures will contain, in addition to these features, a wide spectrum of incorporated neurons of variable size, shape, and function (Figure 14.2B). Thus, by neuroimaging and histologic criteria, grade II and III glial neoplasms are relatively homogeneous and vary mostly by their cellular density, histologic differentiation, and incorporated cellular elements.

Tumor dynamics and morphology fundamentally change in the transition to GBM and display considerably greater spatial diversity. MR images frequently reveal a central, contrast-enhancing component ("ring-enhancing mass") associated with a larger T2-weighted signal abnormality in the tumor's periphery (Figure 14.1B) [5,8]. The center of the ring-enhancing component consists of frank tumor necrosis and mostly includes cellular and proteinaceous debris. Studies using special imaging techniques, including MR spectroscopy, have shown that this area is highly acidic, and measurements of oxygen demonstrate low levels [12,13]. The histopathologic features that correspond to the ring-enhancing rim of GBM include (a) microscopic foci of necrosis, usually with evidence of surrounding cellular pseudopalisades ("pseudopalisading necrosis") and (b) microvascular hyperplasia, a form of angiogenesis that is morphologically recognized as endothelial proliferation within newly sprouted vessels (Figure 14.3) [2,4,11,14–19]. Recent studies have also demonstrated that intravascular thrombosis is a highly specific morphologic finding in GBM specimens and that this feature is commonly found near necrotic foci [20]. In peripheral regions of the GBM, distant from the contrast-enhancing region, there is diffuse infiltration of brain parenchyma that corresponds to T2 hyperintensity on MR imaging. In general, cell density decreases with increasing distance from the center of the neoplasm, and the leading infiltrative edge is characterized by invasion of individual cells. Curiously, foci of vascular hyperplasia are often

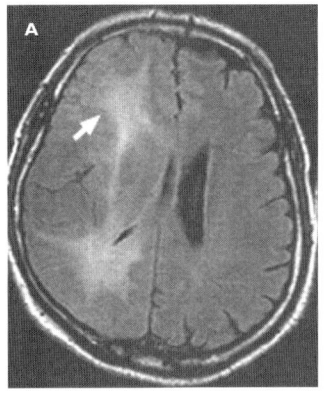
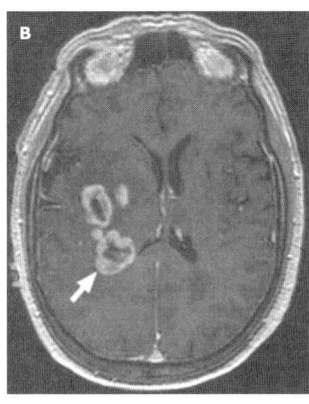

Figure 14.1 Anaplastic astrocytoma (AA; WHO grade III) and glioblastoma (GBM; WHO grade IV) have distinct growth patterns as demonstrated on magnetic resonance imaging (MRI). **(A)** Axial MRI of AA shows expansion of the involved brain and increased signal intensity on FLAIR imaging, reflecting the vasogenic edema that arises in response to infiltrating tumor cells. **(B)** Axial post-contrast MRI of GBM demonstrates a central contrast-enhancing component (arrow) that contains a necrotic center and an enhancing rim, which develops within the setting of a diffusely infiltrative astrocytoma.

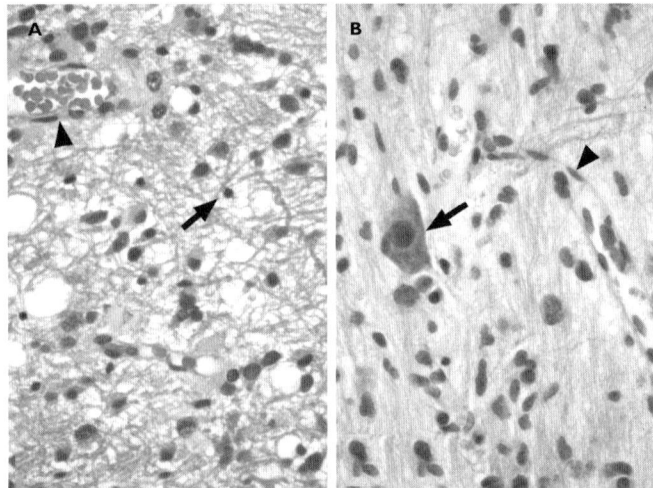

Figure 14.2 The microenvironment of infiltrating astrocytomas includes normal CNS structures that depend on tumor location. **(A)** The microenvironment of infiltrating tumors in the white matter includes axonal processes and myelin sheaths, oligodendrocytes (arrow), endothelial cells (arrowhead), astrocytes, and microglia. **(B)** Tumors that infiltrate the cortex or deep gray structures will also have a variety of neuronal cell bodies (arrow) and a prominent vasculature (arrowhead) within their immediate environment. *See color insert.*

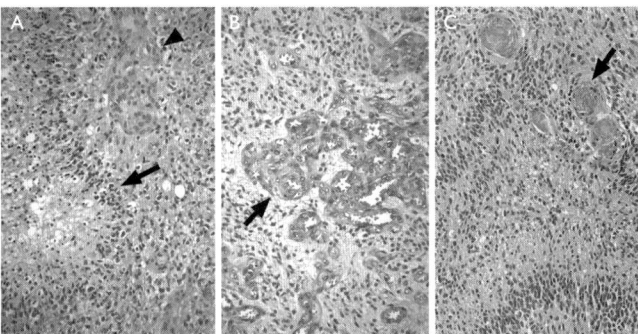

Figure 14.3 Pathologic features that define the microenvironment of glioblastoma. **(A)** Pseudopalisades (arrow) are characterized by a high cellular density of tumor cells that accumulate around a central zone of necrosis. (A,B) Microvascular hyperplasia (**B**, arrow) is a florid form of angiogenesis that can be noted in regions adjacent to necrosis but is also seen peripherally at the tumor's leading edge. **(C)** Intravascular thrombosis is present in nearly all GBMs and is usually identified adjacent to necrosis or within pseudopalisading cells associated with necrosis. *See color insert.*

present near the leading edge, distant from the central necrosis and hypoxia.

A current model of astrocytoma progression that incorporates the specific morphologic findings in GBM as compared with anaplastic astrocytoma suggests that vascular occlusion associated with intravascular thrombosis occurs as a first step in the center of the neoplasm [21,22].. The hypoxia and necrosis that develop in these regions lead to the secretion of hypoxia-inducible proangiogenic factors such as vascular endothelial growth factor (VEGF) and interleukin (IL)-8 causing microvascular proliferation and accelerated outward expansion of tumor cells toward a new vasculature [23].

One of the defining features of GBM is the presence of pseudopalisading tumor cells around necrosis. At early stages, these high-density collections of cells with associated necrosis can be found scattered throughout the tumor (Figure 14.3). As tumors progress, pseudopalisades enlarge and coalesce, giving rise to increasing expanses of coagulative necrosis [24]. Although cells in pseudopalisading regions are higher in density than in adjacent tumor, they are less proliferative and show increased levels of apoptosis. These observations suggest that accumulation of pseudopalisading cells is neither due to clonal expansion nor due to a survival advantage (Figure 14.4) [24–26]. It is possible that pseudopalisades represent a wave of actively migrating tumor cells that are moving away from an area of central hypoxia. This hypothesis is supported by the observations that [1] these cells dramatically upregulate hypoxia-inducible factor-1 (HIF-1), a nuclear transcription factor that orchestrates the cell's adaptive response to low oxygen, and [27] hypoxic GBM cells are more migratory than normoxic cells (Figure 14.4) [18,24,28,29]. Gene expression studies performed on microdissected pseudopalisading cells from human GBMs have demonstrated a pattern of upregulated transcripts that indicate a response to a hypoxic microenvironment. Some of the key adaptive response genes that are upregulated are those related to glycolysis, angiogenesis, and cell cycle control [30]. Moreover, hypoxic pseudopalisades also express increased levels of extracellular matrix proteases associated with invasion, including MMP-2 and uPAR [9,24,31–34].

VASCULAR HETEROGENEITY IN GBM

Normal CNS blood vessels are unique in that they allow only limited diffusion although their walls due to a highly

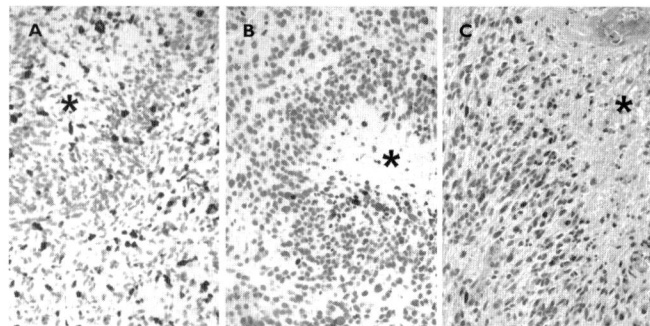

Figure 14.4 Heterogeneity of pseudopalisades and adjacent brain tumor. **(A)** Although the cells of the pseudopalisade around necrosis (*) have a higher cellular density than adjacent tumor cells, they have lower proliferation index as determined by immunohistochemistry for MIB-1 (nuclear stain). **(B)** Apoptotic cells are more frequent in pseudopalisading cells as determined by staining for cleaved caspase 3. **(C)** Cells adjacent to necrosis (*) express a high level of HIF-1α. See color insert.

restrictive blood-brain barrier, which is formed primarily by endothelial tight junctions in addition to astrocytic foot plates, extracellular matrix, and endothelial-pericytic interactions [35]. Vascular alterations that arise in the progression of glial neoplasms add to their complex topography and play a critical role in the growth, detection, and therapy of this process. The vasculature of increasing grades of astrocytomas has been compared with that of normal brain (both quantitatively and qualitatively) by analyzing vascular density and area, vessel diameter, microvascular proliferation, and endothelial cell hyperplasia [36,37]. Wesseling et al performed elegant studies on seven adult GBMs and detailed the vessel number, area, perimeter, and diameter in a variety of regions and compared these data to that of lower-grade astrocytomas and normal brain tissue [38,39]. Vascular parameters were not radically different between normal brain and grade II/III infiltrative astrocytomas, consistent with the concept that tumor cells in these neoplasms are infiltrating the normal brain structures and "co-opting" the host's native blood vessels [40,41]. In response to this process, it has been proposed that the vascular endothelial cells eventually undergo a number of changes that include hypertrophy, discohesion, and even apoptosis. It has been suggested that this damage may be initiated by the effects of angiopoietin-2 (Ang-2) on endothelial cells as a Tie-2 receptor antagonist [11].

In the transition from grade III to IV (GBM), blood vessels first become leaky, as evidenced by contrast enhancement on MR imaging. Specifically, increased vascular permeability to intravenous contrast agents (eg, gadolinium; Gd) and proteins that bind them (ie, albumin) result in their leakage from the blood stream into the extracelluar space of the brain parenchyma (Figure 14.1) [5,8]. When these damaged vessels are studied by electron microscopy, they appear fenestrated, show detachment of pericytes, and exhibit extracellular matrix alterations [35]. All factors that contribute to the increased permeability that initiates blood-brain barrier breakdown have not been defined, but VEGF (also known as VPF, vascular permeability factor) secretion by neoplastic cells has been implicated [42,43].

As opposed to grade II and III astrocytomas, GBM vasculature is distinct from normal brain, with increases in number, area, and perimeter of blood vessels [38,39]. However, there are also regions in these tumors, most often near the infiltrative peripheral edge, where the vascular density is quantitatively similar to that of normal cerebral white matter, emphasizing the high degree of regional heterogeneity. Microvascular hyperplasia, a defining morphologic feature of GBM, is most often noted in regions immediately adjacent to pseudopalisades and is hypothesized to be directly related to the development of hypoxia and necrosis [14,22]. Because necrosis and hypoxia are located in the GBM's core as well as near the contrast-enhancing rim, hypoxia-induced angiogenesis (in part due to VEGF secretion) occurs adjacent to this region, favoring neoplastic growth outward (Figures 14.2 and 14.4) [11,14,18]. In its most florid form, angiogenesis takes the shape of "glomeruloid bodies," a feature that is most characteristic of GBM, but is also an independent marker of poor prognosis in other forms of cancer [44]. This exuberant angiogenic response attempts to lay down a new vasculature for rapid neoplastic expansion, yet the function of these distorted vessels in oxygen and nutrient delivery has not been established.

VEGF is one of the most critical proangiogenic factors produced by pseudopalisades in GBMs. Pseudopalisading cells have been shown to express high levels of hypoxia-inducible transcription factors, including HIF-1, which is primarily controlled by tissue pO_2; a detailed understanding of the precise extent and distribution of hypoxia in GBM pseudopalisades remains unknown. Nonetheless, the *VEGF* gene contains a hypoxia-responsive element within its promoter that binds HIF-1, thereby activating transcription; VEGF is known to be an important mediator of GBM biology [23,28,45,46]. Once expressed and secreted, extracellular VEGF binds to its high-affinity receptors, VEGFR-1 and VEGFR-2, which are upregulated on endothelial cells of high-grade gliomas but are not present in normal brain [45]. Receptor activation then leads to angiogenesis in regions adjacent to pseudopalisades and eventually leads to a vascular density in GBMs that is among the highest of all human neoplasms (Figure 14.3).

A second proangiogenic factor that is highly upregulated in GBMs is IL-8 (CXCL8) [47]. Much like VEGF, hypoxia/anoxia strongly stimulates IL-8 expression, and it is also found at highest levels in GBM pseudopalisades [48,49]. IL-8 has a more punctate distribution than VEGF within pseudopalisades, and it remains unclear whether tumor cells or scattered infiltrating macrophages are most responsible for the majority of its expression. Hypoxic upregulation of IL-8 is HIF independent because there are no hypoxia-responsive elements within its promoter. Rather, the IL-8 promoter contains binding sites for other transcription factors, including NF-κB, AP-1, and C-EBP/NF-IL-6. AP-1 seems to mediate much of IL-8s upregulation by hypoxia/anoxia [50]. The IL-8 receptors that could potentially contribute to IL-8-mediated tumorigenic and angiogenic responses in GBM include CXCR1 and CXCR2, both of which are G-protein coupled.

HYPOXIC AND METABOLIC HETEROGENEITY IN GBM

Hypoxia is a well-known property of malignant neoplasms. In gliomas, only GBMs have a substantial degree of hypoxia [51,52]. This pathophysiologic property results from a diverse set of abnormalities, including abnormal vessel distribution and morphology, regions of decreased blood oxygen carrying capacity, and regions of high cellular respiration rates. The description of hypoxic heterogeneity (both in terms of level and pattern) within individual tumors depends on the technique used and the endpoint of "hypoxia" that is measured (see below). Methods for measuring hypoxia can be direct or indirect and invasive or noninvasive. For direct measurement of hypoxia, invasive techniques using needle electrodes have been reported most widely, but the decreased availability of the instrumentation has led to increased use of indirect methods. These include biopsy-based techniques using antibody-based detection of injected chemicals that bind to hypoxic cells (EF5, pimonidazole) or immunohistochemical detection of endogenous molecules that are upregulated under hypoxic conditions (ie, HIF, CA9, and Glut1). Less invasive indirect techniques include the use of positron emission tomography (PET) methods for detection of the radionucleotide-conjugated forms of the same or similar injected agents used for biopsy-based methods (18F-EF5, F-Miso, etc).

Needle electrodes were the first method that demonstrated hypoxia to be an important feature of human tumors; microelectrode measurements in human brain tumors were first reported in 1994 by Cruickshank and Rampling [53–55]. This measurement involves the insertion of an 8-cm, 26-gauge needle into the tumor using a ratcheting motion, usually over a length of 0.6 mm. The ratcheting motion decreases pressure on the electrode tip, eliminating this as a potential artifact. Three to five "passes" are typically performed, resulting in the collection of tens to hundreds of measurements. Depending on the number of passes, the spatial distribution of these measurements may be limited; some authors suggest that volumes that include as few as 50 cells can be sampled, whereas others contend that the tens of thousands of cells are required for optimal measurement [56]. It should be noted that the tissue sampled during the electrode passage may include normal tissue, necrotic cells, blood vessels, and interstitial and other fluids in addition to tumor cells. Nonetheless, valuable information on intratumoral heterogeneity can be obtained by examining the tumor histograms. Unfortunately, most studies to date have collected summary statistics on groups of patients to describe intertumoral heterogeneity, but have not addressed the question of intratumoral heterogeneity. In 1999, Collingridge et al used the needle electrode technique to study human brain tumors and included a small subset of patients with high-grade tumors (n = 3) [57]. Unfortunately, in this and other articles on this subject, only a single patient's histogram was shown as an example, and the remaining data were grouped (to demonstrate intertumoral heterogeneity). Among individual patients studied, the median values, but not the range or standard error, are reported. In the Collingridge study, it was reported that 15%, 59% and 80% of the oxygen values measured in these three high-grade gliomas were <2.5 mm Hg (0.3% oxygen), with the medians at 30.2, 2.1, and 0.9 mm, respectively [57]. Lally et al and Evans et al also measured the pO_2 in a series of brain tumors, including GBMs, and grouped pO_2 measurements were presented, but measurements of intratumoral heterogeneity were not [52,58].

Use of exogenously administered agents that bind intracellularly in hypoxic cells can provide the most tangible information on intratumoral heterogeneity because detection of these agents with immunohistochemistry can be evaluated on a cellular level. Currently, the two clinically relevant agents are EF5 and pimonidazole. These drugs are 2-nitroimidazoles and are reduced and covalently bound within cells at rates that are related to oxygen levels. Pimonidazole is reported to bind in cells at or below 10 mm Hg (eg, it has binary binding characteristics), but this has not been confirmed in a recent in vitro study in which antibody concentration has been shown to substantially affect the pO_2 dependence of binding [59,60]. EF5 has been shown to bind to cells over a range of pO_2 values, with increasing binding associated with decreasing pO_2, independent of antibody concentration [59]. The maximum sensitivity of the EF5 assay is between 0.01% and 5%, which is optimal for detection of oxygen levels in tumors [60]. Because of the continuous nature of the assay and the ability to convert the binding levels to pO_2, EF5 binding is particularly relevant for the analysis of intratumoral heterogeneity [51,60,61]. EF5 can also be synthesized for PET imaging, and the spatial distribution of hypoxia can be investigated in vivo (Figure 14.5). Importantly, the spatial sensitivity of the immunohistochemical assays is at the cellular level (10–20 μm), whereas the best resolution currently available for PET scanner is in the range of 3- to 4 mm. Clearly, the type of data on intratumoral heterogeneity garnered from these two methods (even though they are based on the same molecule, EF5) will determine their optimal use in patient care situations.

2-Nitroimidazoles bind to intracellular protein thiols, and importantly, EF5 binding is independent of other tissue properties (pH, glucose, etc) and inversely proportional to pO_2. For biopsy-based studies in humans, 21 mg/kg EF5 is given intravenously approximately 24 hours preoperatively. Biopsied tissue samples are frozen sand tissue sections are subsequently stained with fluorescent-labeled monoclonal antibodies.[1] Because of the technical development of quantitative immunofluorescence of EF5, the amount of binding can be quantified and reported as pO_2; pO_2 maps have been generated and published [51,61]. However, it should be emphasized that this technique relies on biopsied tissue and introduces potential sampling limitations. Studies on sampling limitations in canine tumors using an alternative hypoxia marker determined that four tissue samples provide adequate data to generalize findings to the whole tumor [62,63]. By using these data as guidelines, studies of intratumoral heterogeneity in human brain tumors have been performed (Figure 14.5). For each tumor, three endpoints are reported: the average of the highest binding (CF95 value[2]), the CF95 of the brightest slide, and the median EF5 value of all the slides evaluated (CF50). A number of observations can be made (Figure 14.6) as follows: [1] there is substantial intertumoral heterogeneity of hypoxia in gliomas [27], hypoxia is

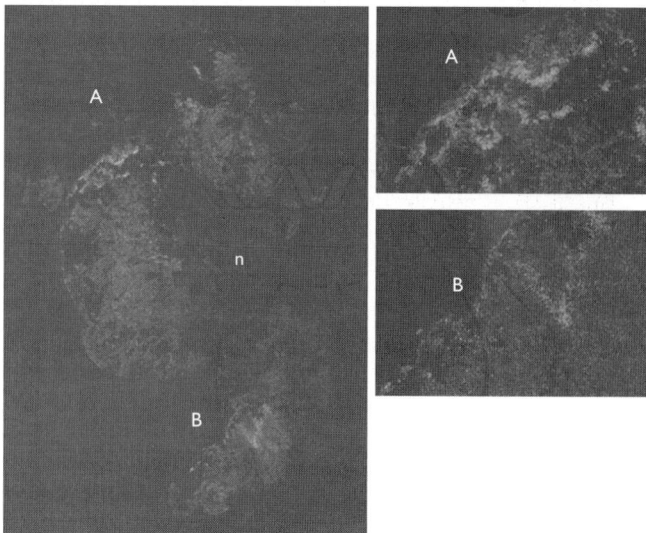

Figure 14.5 Intratumoral heterogeneity in a human glioblastoma. This image demonstrates the patterns, distributions, and levels of hypoxia (as measured by EF5 binding) in a human GBM. On the left is a tissue section (approximately 4 × 6 mm) from a GBM. A large portion of the central region is necrotic (n, macroscopic necrosis), but regions of viable oxic cells (green) are seen, even adjacent to this area. Two large areas of hypoxia (red regions A, B; also shown in detail (10×) on the right) are seen surrounding microscopic necrosis. Both regions are moderately hypoxic (pO$_2$ ≈ 0.5% oxygen). *See color insert*.

only present in high-grade glial neoplasms [64], GBMs are dominated by mild hypoxia, and a substantial percentage of the cells are oxic, and [65] regions of moderate to severe hypoxia can be identified in the majority of the GBMs. In several studies of three different human tumor types (sarcomas, high-grade gliomas, and head and neck cancer), the presence of moderate to severe hypoxia was the endpoint that best predicted patient outcome [52]. The predominance of mildly hypoxic or oxic cells in GBMs has substantial ramifications for therapies in which moderately or severely hypoxic cells are targeted because these cells are a relatively minor component of the whole tumor. In the cases in which chemotherapy is used, the distance of these relatively few but critical hypoxia cells from blood vessels may be an important determinant of patient outcome.

In addition to the presence of hypoxia in GBMs, an important consideration is the distribution of hypoxia and necrosis that often (although not always) accompanies it. Observations that there is an inverse relationship between the extent of necrosis and prognosis led Sawaya and coworkers to hypothesize that procoagulation and antiapoptotic mechanisms could prevent the completion of tumor necrosis factor (TNF)-induced apoptosis and promote necrosis as the final mode of cell death [17]. Studies using EF5 demonstrate that when binding is present adjacent to necrosis, the level of hypoxia is highest for that particular tumor [66]. GBMs (and other tumors) are often referred to as having "central necrosis," a concept that is supported by appearance of these tumors on imaging, particularly contrast-enhanced MR imaging [67]. The appearance of central necrosis is emphasized by the multi-mm spatial resolution of the imaging techniques, especially when compared with immunohistochemistry-based assays. Although a central region of macroscopic necrotic tissue may be present, it is extremely important to realize that regions of microscopic necrosis and hypoxia occur in all regions of GBMs, including the periphery. Microscopic regions of moderate to severe hypoxia, with or without necrosis, occur over distances of 100s of microns because it is on this scale that oxygen metabolism occurs. The location of hypoxic cells in the tumor periphery is likely to have substantial implications for prognosis. This is especially the case in tumors in which complete resections are not possible because hypoxic cells be biologically aggressive and produce proinvasion cytokines. Another interesting, but under-investigated, area of study is the spatial relationship between hypoxia and proliferation (Ki67 staining). We have found that GBM cells do proliferate in hypoxic regions (data not shown), yet the relationship between the presence of tissue hypoxia and its effects on tumor proliferation [66] and patient outcome remain unsettled.

PROTON MAGNETIC RESONANCE SPECTROSCOPY IMAGING OF TUMOR METABOLITES

Proton magnetic resonance spectroscopy (1H MRS) is often used to assess the presence, relative level, and distribution of organic compounds in brain tumors. It is a rapid (and therefore clinically relevant) method but is spatially limited; metabolite information is obtained in a 4- to 8-cc region [68]. As a result, detailed information on intratumoral heterogeneity is limited. Nonetheless, there have been numerous studies using multivoxel 1H MRS wherein a two-dimensional grid is superimposed over the Gd-enhanced T1-weighted MR imaging scan of the tumor, and the spectra from each region are displayed. In this way, spectra emanating from enhancing regions can be evaluated separately from necrotic or normal tissue. However, because of the voxel size, some overlap inevitably occurs. Various molecules can be assessed, but most studies emphasize portions of the spectra (peaks) corresponding to choline (Cho; alterations in phospholipid membrane turnover and cell density), creatine (Cre; cellular energetics), N-acetylaspartate (NAA; neuron and axon density), lactate (Lac, anaerobic metabolism), lipid (cellular breakdown), and alanine (cellular metabolic pathways) [69]. The work by Preul et al suggests that such measurements have the potential to discriminate between types of brain lesions [70]. In an elegant and technically challenging study, Croteau et al [71] paired image-guided biopsies with semiquantitative evaluations of tumor invasion. In a multivoxel 1H MRS study of 31 low- and high-grade glioma, they found that aggressive histologic phenotypes were correlated with choline-containing molecules. Unfortunately, only aggregate data for all patients were presented. However, one example demonstrated how regions of Gd signal enhancement can have substantially different metabolic spectra. Similarly, Nelson presented an example of a minimally enhancing GBM and demonstrated

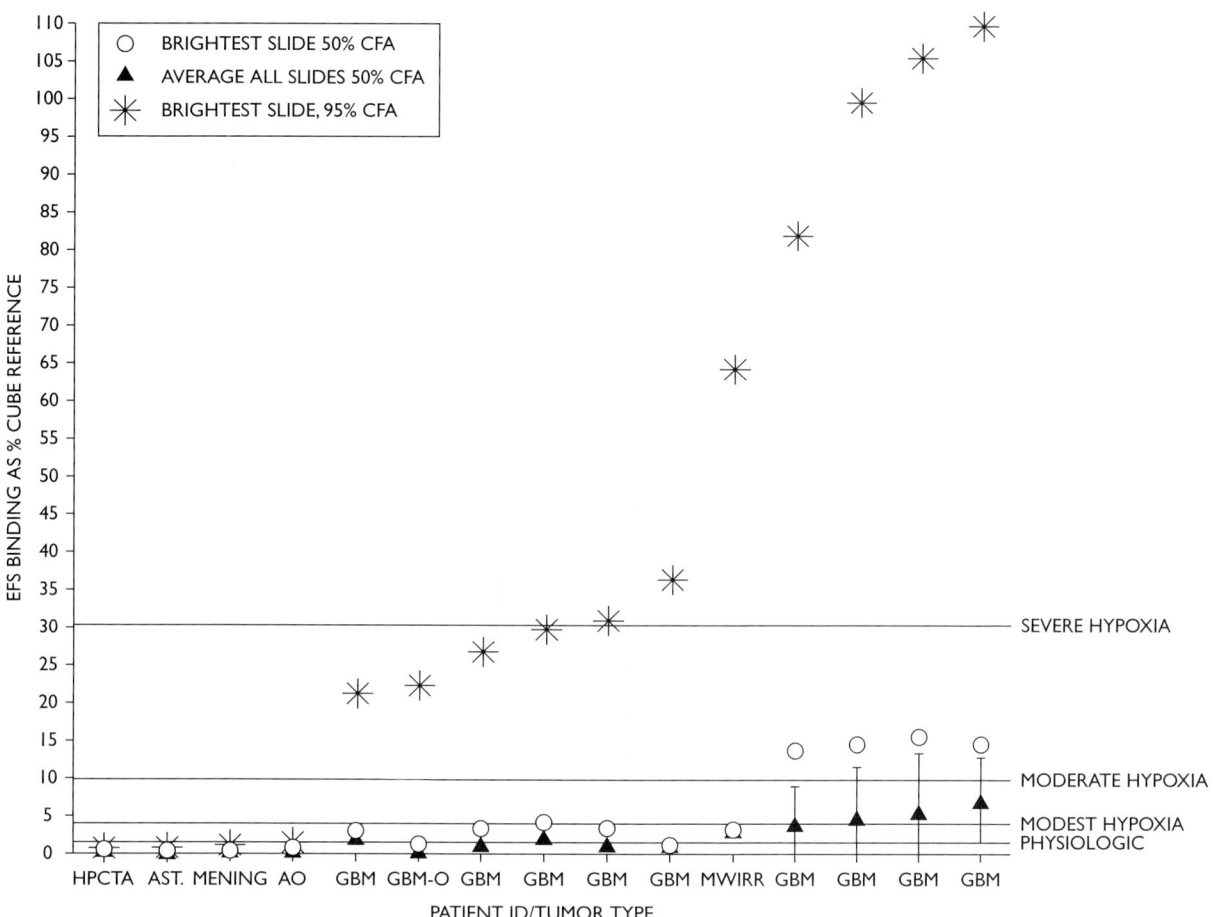

Figure 14.6 Intratumoral heterogeneity of EF5 binding in human brain tumors. De novo nonglioma (HPCTA—hemangiopericytoma, Mening—meningioma) and glial tumors are presented. WHO grade 2 (O = oligodendroglioma, A = astrocytoma, OA = oligoastrocytoma), grade 3 (AO = anaplastic oligoastrocytoma, AA = anaplastic astrocytoma), and grade 4 tumors (GBM—glioblastoma) and recurrent GBM (r-GBM) are illustrated; one high-grade tumor occurred in a previously irradiated site (Glioma-PIS). EF5 binding is presented as percentage of maximum binding (cube reference binding), and the physiologic descriptions are shown. As previously published, severe hypoxia: ≥30% binding, ≈≤0.1% oxygen = 0.76 mm Hg; Moderate hypoxia: 10–30% binding ≈0.5% oxygen = 3.8 mm Hg; mild hypoxia: 3–10% binding ≈2.5% oxygen =19 mmHg; oxia: <3% binding ≈>10% oxygen = 76 mm Hg. All of the WHO grade 2 tumors are oxic, and at least one of the grade 3 tumors contains regions of hypoxia. There is substantial heterogeneity in the maximum EF5 binding, yet the median level of pO_2 in all tumors is oxic.

heterogeneity, especially in lactate and lipid peaks [68]. This article evaluated whether regions of Gd enhancement corresponded to regions of abnormal metabolic signature. Although details of the spatial location were not provided, "a large variation in the maximum CNI (voxel with the most abnormal metabolic signature)" was reported. The article concluded that Gd enhancement does not usually correspond to the regions with the highest choline, supporting the hypothesis that 1H MRS is useful in the assessment of intratumoral heterogeneity.

CELLULAR HETEROGENEITY

Differentiation Patterns

On cytologic and histologic preparations, the majority of infiltrative astrocytomas (grades II and IV) are dominated by a "fibrillary" morphology, composed of tumor cells with elongated, delicate astrocytic processes. However, there is substantial histomorphologic diversity among astrocytomas and a stunning heterogeneity of differentiation patterns can be noted within individual human specimens. Descriptors such as gemistocytic, small cell, protoplasmic, sarcomatous, epithelioid, granular cell, and giant cell have been applied to specific variants [4,11]. In many instances, a single neoplasm will contain distinct regions of these differentiation patterns. The best understood mixed glioma is the oligoastrocytoma, which contains regions of both oligodendroglial and astrocytic differentiation. In grade II, III, or IV tumors, the presence of an oligodendroglial component is associated with a better prognosis [72].

Gemistocytic astrocytomas are composed of cells with abundant glassy pink cytoplasm and prominent stout cellular processes, whereas granular cell astrocytomas are populated by large, round tumor cells packed with eosinophilic granules that correspond at the ultrastructural level to autophagic vacuoles [73]. Both these cell variants seem to have more aggressive clinical behavior, even after adjusting for grade. The giant cell GBM is a distinct clinicopathologic entity, presenting clinically as a peripheral, cerebral hemispheric mass that is better circumscribed than other GBMs [74]; their slightly more favorable prognosis may be related to greater resectability [15]. Tumor cells in this variant are extremely large, misshapen, multinucleated with bizarre nuclei and contain a well-developed reticulin network. At the opposite end of the cytomorphologic spectrum, small-cell GBMs are composed of a monotonous, dense population of modest-sized, highly infiltrative tumor cells [75]. These lesions present more often in the elderly and have a rapid clinical progression. Gliosarcoma is a biphasic tumor consisting of malignant mesenchymal and glial components that are typically firmer and more discrete because of the high reticulin and collagen content in the sarcomatous component [76,77]. There does not seem to be any prognostic difference between gliosarcoma and typical GBM. The publications that describe these morphologic subtypes of astrocytomas usually restrict cases to tumors that are nearly homogeneous for a given morphology. However, it is much more common to have multiple morphologies present at least focally within an individual astrocytoma, leading to a histologically heterogeneous neoplasm.

Stem Cells/Glioma Progenitor Cells

Recent investigations have supported the hypothesis that a tumor stem cell (also referred to as glioma progenitor or tumor-initiating cells) population exists in human brain tumors, including gliomas [64,65,78,79]. This model suggests that a small subpopulation of neoplastic stem cells gives rise to a larger population of differentiated daughter cells that account for most of the biologic properties of the tumors. Progenitor cells that express CD133 (prominin) on their cell surface display tumor stem cell properties, including growth as neurospheres in culture, self-renewal, and differentiation along neural and glial lineages [79]. CD133$^+$ tumor cells are much more highly angiogenic and tumorigenic than the more numerous CD133$^-$ cells and are more radiation resistant, presumably due to differential ability to repair DNA [64]. These CD133$^+$ cells are believed to occupy a specialized "niche," yet its morphologic and spatial features have not been defined. Most of the original investigations of tumor stem cells were performed on cell suspensions produced from resected human GBM specimens and subjected to flow cytometry. As a result, little information was provided with regard to the spatial distribution of these cells within the tumor. The CD133$^+$ compartment of tumor specimens has only recently begun to be investigated by immunohistochemistry [80]. In grade II astrocytomas, CD133 immunoreactivity either was completely absent or was scattered in <1% of cells. The majority (62%) of grade III astrocytomas contained some CD133$^+$ cells, and these were noted either individually or in small clusters. Nearly, all GBMs (96%) showed CD133$^+$ cells, which were also EGFRvIII positive, confirming that they were tumor cells. Stem cell properties of gliomas seem to have an effect on patient outcome; a recent study has demonstrated that the "self-renewal" gene expression pattern, which includes HOX genes and prominin, was associated with treatment resistance and shorter survival [81].

In addition to tumor stem cells, endogenous (nonneoplastic) neural stem cells (NSCs) of the mature brain are thought to impact glioma biology. NSC in the adult mammalian brain function in neurogenesis and may be important in responses to brain injury. These cells have a striking tropism for brain tumors; even when NSCs are injected systemically or intrathecally, they find their way into the tumor mass [27]. Mechanisms responsible for this effect have not been totally elucidated, but VEGF secretion from tumor cells may have a trophic effect [82]. Studies of NSC using mice that express a green fluorescent protein under the regulation of the nestin promoter (a marker of NSC) demonstrated that green fluorescent protein-expressing cells from the subventricular zone, the primary site of NSCs, consistently invade into a xenografted brain tumor [83]. Interestingly, this effect occurred most robustly in younger mice. The influx of NSC was associated with smaller tumors (slower tumor growth) and improved survival. Thus, not only do gliomas seem to attract NSC but this cell population also seems to be antitumorigenic.

Proliferative/Apoptotic Heterogeneity

Proliferation within glioblastomas can be determined by counting mitotic cells on hematoxylin and eosin-stained slides or by using immunohistochemical stains to determine the percentage of tumor cells that are actively in the cell cycle. The most reliable and technically feasible method is the Ki-67/MIB-1 antibody. This antibody identifies an antigen present in the nuclei of cells in the G1, S, G2, and M phases of the cell cycle but is not expressed in the resting phase, G0. Investigations have demonstrated a significant positive correlation between Ki-67/MIB-1 indices (percentage of positive staining tumor cell nuclei) and histologic grade and have shown that higher Ki-67/MIB-1 proliferation indices are associated with shorter survivals [84]. However, within the population of GBMs, the relationship between proliferation and patient outcome is less clear [85]. Regional heterogeneity of proliferation within astrocytic neoplasms has been found to increase with increasing histologic grade [86]. There was also a tendency for more highly proliferative cells to cluster together, suggesting that they had arisen from clonal expansion. It might be expected that the proliferative activity of a neoplastic region would correspond to increasing cell density. In a comprehensive analysis of 54 supratentorial astrocytic tumors, grades II, III, and IV, the Ki67/MIB-1 expression was highly correlated with cellular density (measured using automated image analysis) [87]. Both cell density and proliferation correlated positively with histologic grade. The pseudopalisading cells around necrosis in GBM are a hypercellular collection of neoplastic cells and therefore might also be expected to be more highly proliferative than other cells within the neoplasm. However, MIB-1 analyses have shown that pseudopalisading cells are actually less proliferative than nonpseudopalisading cells within the same neoplasms, suggesting that they accumulate by mechanisms unrelated to proliferation [24].

It might also be expected that apoptosis, the programmed death of individual cells, would vary from region to region within a complex neoplasm such as GBM. Apoptosis is initiated through mechanisms that include death receptor (DR) ligation by members of the TNF family, including TNF-related apoptosis-inducing ligand/DR5 and FasL (CD95L)/Fas (CD95). Both Fas and FasL levels are higher in astrocytomas than in normal brain and correlate positively with tumor grade [88–90]. However, the overall levels of apoptosis have been shown to be low in malignant gliomas, and this type of cell death accounts for a small proportion when compared with coagulative-type necrosis. Moreover, apoptotic rates have not been found to be an independent risk factor for prognosis [91,92]. Most Fas expression in GBM is within pseudopalisading cells around necrosis, and physical interactions between tumor cells expressing Fas and FasL may promote apoptosis [26]. These observations are supported by a study of cleaved caspase 3 expression, an immunohistochemical marker of apoptosis, the level of apoptosis in pseudopalisading cells was found to be 6–20 times higher than that in the adjacent neoplastic cells [24].

GENETIC HETEROGENEITY

The genetic alterations associated with the development of gliomas have been well documented over the past three decades; some of the better studied alterations include *TP53* and *PTEN* mutations, epidermal growth factor receptor (EGFR) and *MDM2* amplifications, *CDKN2A(p16)* and *ARF(p14)* deletions, and loss of heterozygosity at 17p, 10q, 9p, 1p, and 19q. Many correlative studies have demonstrated relationships between tumor histology and grade with specific genetic alterations [11]. For example, nearly all gemistocytic astrocytomas have *TP53* mutations, whereas small-cell GBMs are defined by a high frequency of *EGFR* amplification [75,93]. Within a given neoplasm, there may be a heterogeneity of genetic alterations associated with clonal evolution, distinct morphologies, high-grade progression, or biologic properties. The research that has defined genetic heterogeneity has focused on either global gains and losses within distinct tumor regions (ie, by comparative genomic hybridization) or specific mutations, deletions, and amplifications (ie, *TP53* mutations or *EGFR* amplifications) within heterogeneous components.

The concept that malignant gliomas may have a heterogeneous genetic makeup was suggested by their high variable nuclear morphology, chromatin patterns, and DNA content. Flow cytometric analysis of human glioma specimens demonstrated that the ploidy of gliomas varies considerably within a given tumor, both in terms of its pattern and the percentage of aneuploid cells [94]. The prognostic significance of such nuclear heterogeneity has been studied in GBMs; Ki67-positive cells were larger and more regular in shape than those that were not Ki67 positive, indicating that nuclear heterogeneity may, at least in part, reflect the cell cycle [94]. Those tumors consisting of a high degree of intratumoral variation of nuclear shapes and sizes were associated with a poor prognosis. However, the finding of large cells by itself (without a high degree of nuclear heterogeneity) was not associated with a shorter survival. A similar morphologic analysis of the pseudopalisading cells revealed that the nuclei of these cells were more densely packed than adjacent cells, but the nuclear morphologic parameters of shape and size were not significantly different from adjacent astrocytoma cells [95]. The global genomic heterogeneity that may correspond to this variation in nuclear appearance has been studied using comparative genomic hybridization. Multiple distinct regions of 10 GBMs were evaluated for numerical chromosome gains and losses. The results not only demonstrated the presence of some chromosomal gains and losses that were common in all areas of a tumor but also identified region-specific aberrations. Some previously unreported alterations that were homogeneously distributed included gains on chromosome 4q, 5q, 12q, 13q, and 7 and losses on 22. Heterogeneity was noted for amplifications of chromosome 7p, the location of the *EGFR* gene, which was noted in only a single region of two tumors [96].

One of the most fundamental questions in defining genetic heterogeneity is whether brain tumors that have two distinct morphologic components have a single, shared genetic fingerprint or whether the two are distinct. The gliosarcoma, a biphasic tumor that displays both mesenchymal and glial differentiation, has been investigated as a model to answer this question. Two reported studies on this subject have demonstrated that patterns of *PTEN* mutation, *TP53* mutation, *CDKN2A* deletion, and *MDM2* and *CDK4* amplification were identical in the glial and mesenchymal components, suggesting a monoclonal origin for these morphologically distinct tumor regions [76,77]. Similarly, Walker et al investigated 13 gliomas that showed a high degree of morphologic heterogeneity, defined as having at least two distinct differentiation patterns (including oligodendroglioma, fibrillary astrocytoma, gemistocytic differentiation, low grade, high grade, or sarcomatous patterns) [97]. Analysis of microsatellite markers on chromosomes 1p, 19q, 17p, 10p, and 10q showed predominantly the same allelic loss pattern in the different regions of the gliomas. In particular, it was noted that those tumors with both oligodendroglioma and astrocytoma elements showed the same pattern of 1p and 19q deletion in each of the morphologically distinct regions. Other investigations have confirmed that 1p and 19q deletions are shared in both components of the majority of oligoastrocytomas [98–100]. However, a small subset of mixed tumors are defined molecularly by *TP53* mutations rather than 1p/19q codeletion, suggesting that some oligoastrocytomas are genetically similar to astrocytomas. In these less common cases, *TP53* mutations have been described in both the astrocytic and oligodendroglioma components or exclusively in the astrocytic component, but not exclusively in the oligodendroglial component. The most consistent additional genetic changes in oligoastrocytomas are loss of heterozygosity of 10q, 9p, and 13q, which occur in both elements of the mixed tumors, and these changes have been associated with tumor progression to a higher grade [97,98].

TP53 mutations are relatively common in low-grade, infiltrating astrocytomas (50–60%) and GBMs that arise from their progression (secondary GBMs). In many instances, *TP53* mutation is accompanied by allelic loss of the second *TP53* gene, leading to a complete loss of p53 function. One study evaluated mutations of *TP53* and allelic losses at 17p13.1, 9p21, and 10q23–25 in microdissected high- and low-grade elements of human GBM specimens. The majority of allelic losses in the high-grade components was also present in the low-grade components. However, compared with morphologically similar grade II and III astrocytomas, the low-grade elements of GBMs had higher frequencies of 10 loss, but fewer mutations of *TP53* [101].

In some instances, the evolution of *TP53* mutations and the subsequent alterations in protein function within a given tumor can be much more complex. Ren et al reported that in 11 gliomas (35 total samples analyzed), seven had alterations of TP53 and often this was characterized by more than one type of mutation [102]. For example, five tumors carried by two distinct *TP53* mutations, and these were most frequently noted in histologically distinct regions of the tumor (eg, low- and high-grade components). These findings suggest that *TP53* mutations arise in a polyclonal fashion rather than from monoclonal expansion after a single oncogenic mutation. Not all *TP53* mutations give rise to a transcriptionally inactive protein and therefore *TP53* mutations are not all functionally equal. A prime example of multiple *TP53* mutations evolving in a single astrocytoma was described by Fulci et al [103]. In this patient, born with a germline *TP53* mutation at codon 283, the gene produced a protein with partial functional activity. This same allele acquired a second mutation at codon 267 leading to complete protein inactivation. The second allele was later mutated at codon 258, and this mutation was also associated with complete loss of protein function. This example clearly demonstrates that the pattern of genomic alteration of *TP53* and the resulting dynamics of p53 functional loss can be complex, both spatially and temporally within a given neoplasm.

As a general principle, it would be expected that the mutations of *TP53* noted in grade II astrocytomas would be preserved in higher-grade tumors that arise from them. In one study, 12 of 22 primary grade II gliomas bore *TP53* mutations [104]. In all tumors, the identical *TP53* mutation was identified in the high-grade (grade III or IV) recurrences. It was consistently noted that the p53 protein expression was present in a significantly higher fraction of cells in the high-grade recurrences.

The *EGFR* gene is amplified in 40% to 50% of primary GBMs and occurs in the form of extrachromosomal double minutes, which can range from 10 to >100 copies per nucleus. The distribution and heterogeneity of the amplification event have been investigated using a number of approaches. One investigation used a set of six GBMs that had been shown to contain *TP53* mutations [105]. Although *TP53* mutations had been thought to be mutually exclusive with *EGFR* amplifications in GBMs, this report identified rare, scattered cells with amplified *EGFR* within four of these GBMs. The authors concluded that there is no selective pressure to maintain the amplified *EGFR* in these *TP53*-mutated tumors. In this same study, the spatial heterogeneity of *EGFR* amplification was investigated in four GBMs. The frequency of *EGFR* amplification was found to be much higher in tumor cells near the leading edge (>90% amplified) than at the center of the tumors (<20%), a distribution suggesting that the amplification event may be associated with infiltration. The distribution of *EGFR* amplification and its relation to biologic function have also been studied from the perspective of morphologically distinct regions within GBMs [106]. Semiquantitative polymerase chain reaction analysis of EGFR expression was compared with nuclear morphology and Ki-67 proliferation indices. A positive correlation between EGFR expression and Ki-67 was found, but nuclei with the highest degree of EGFR expression had more regular shapes.

Amplification of the *EGFR* gene is often accompanied by rearrangement or deletion. The most common mutant is *EGFRvIII*, which occurs in 50% of amplified tumors. EGFRvIII expression results in a constitutively active cell surface protein that lacks a functional ligand-binding domain. In most instances of amplification, both the wild type and mutant forms of the gene and protein product coexist, giving rise to intratumoral molecular heterogeneity [107]. In one immunohistochemical study of EGFR and EGFRvIII distribution, tumor cells showing EGFRvIII expression were found scattered diffusely through the tumor, suggesting that they may arise secondarily from the wild-type amplified cells. Thus, although it is assumed that EGFRvIII drives neoplastic properties in vivo, the precise functional relationship and clinical significance between wild-type and mutant tumor cells within the GBM remains unclear.

GBM heterogeneity has also been investigated by gene expression analysis of specific histologic regions [30]. The pseudopalisading neoplastic cells around necrosis are highly specific to GBM and account for substantial topographic diversity. The hypothesis was proposed that the genes expressed in these tumor cells might provide both insight into their biologic function and be prognostically significant. By using three frozen GBM specimens, the gene expression profile of 18 microdissected samples of pseudopalisades was compared with adjacent nonpseudopalisading cells. A total of 314 upregulated and 385 downregulated genes were identified in pseudopalisading cells. Pathway analysis of the specific gene families that were differentially regulated in this population revealed a pattern that indicated a hypoxic environment, high levels of glycolysis, and abnormal cell cycle regulation. Aldolase A, pyruvate kinase, phosphoglycerate kinase, glyceraldehyde-3-phosphate dehydrogenase, and GLUT1, a glucose transporter, were glycolytic genes that were upregulated in pseudopalisades. Other genes that were specifically upregulated in this population were *HIG2* (hypoxia-inducible protein-2), *POFUT2* (protein-o-fucosyltransferase 2), *PTDSR* (phosphatidylserine receptor), *PLOD2* (procollagen hydroxylase 2), *ATF5* (activating transcription factor 5), and *HK2* (hexokinase 2), whereas *OLIG2* (oligodendrocyte transcription factor 2) was most specifically expressed in nonpseudopalisading cells. The genes upregulated in pseudopalisading cells were tested for prognostic significance in a larger series of patients with GBM. PUFUT2 was found to be associated with a shorter survival [30].

CONCLUSION

It is clear that there is substantial intratumoral heterogeneity within specific brain tumors and that the tumor microenvironment plays a critical role in their biologic behavior. A classical example is GBM, in which enormous topographic diversity is present in nearly every tumor; this diversity includes regions with necrosis, severe hypoxia, varying differentiation patterns, diffuse infiltration into gray or white matter, florid angiogenesis, and as yet ill-defined biologic niches with normal stem cells and tumor initiating cells. Both the genetic and gene expression patterns vary within each neoplasm, and sometimes, but not always, these correlate with histologic grade and level of differentiation. The future of neuro-oncology research will certainly include a heightened understanding of the heterogeneity of these complex neoplasms. For example, it has been suggested that the failure of EGFR inhibitors to prolong survival of patients with GBM is due to the high degree of diversity of other tyrosine kinase receptors with overlapping function that are expressed on the surface of glial neoplasms [108]. The ability to predict responsiveness to therapy will need to take into account such molecular variability.

Finally, new biologic concepts are emerging from the study of tumor stem cells that may change the way we practice neuro-oncology [64,79]. The identification and characterization of these cell types in GBM specimens as a part of routine pathologic diagnosis may prove critical in prescribing therapy. Such techniques are still in their developmental stages, but they undoubtedly hold tremendous potential for improving the diagnostic stratification of glial neoplasms based on biologically meaningful data.

NOTES

[1] EF5 studies can be performed on paraffin embedded tissues as well; peroxidase-based staining is also possible.
[2] CF95 = 20 would mean that 95% of the EF5 values in the image are at or below 20% of maximum binding.

REFERENCES

1. CBTRUS. *Statistical report: primary brain tumors in the United States 1995–1999*. Chicago, IL: Central Brain Tumor Registry of the United States; 2002.
2. Kleihues P, Burger PC, Collins VP, Newcomb EW, Ohgaki H, Cavenee WK. *Pathology and Genetics of Tumours of the Nervous Systems*. Lyon, France: International Agency for Research on Cancer; 2000.
3. Ohgaki H, Kleihues P. Epidemiology and etiology of gliomas. *Acta Neuropathol (Berl)*. 2005;109:93–108.
4. Louis DN, Ohgaki H, Wiestler OD, Cavenee WK. *WHO Classification of Tumours of the Central Nervous System*. Lyon, France: International Agency for Research on Cancer; 2007.
5. Henson JW, Gaviani P, Gonzalez RG. MRI in treatment of adult gliomas. *Lancet Oncol*. 2005;6:167–175.
6. Mandonnet E, Delattre JY, Tanguy ML, et al. Continuous growth of mean tumor diameter in a subset of grade II gliomas. *Ann Neurol*. 2003;53:524–528.
7. Swanson KR, Bridge C, Murray JD, Alvord EC Jr. Virtual and real brain tumors: using mathematical modeling to quantify glioma growth and invasion. *J Neurol Sci*. 2003;216:1–10.
8. Zhu XP, Li KL, Kamaly-Asl ID, et al. Quantification of endothelial permeability, leakage space, and blood volume in brain tumors using combined T1 and T2* contrast-enhanced dynamic MR imaging. *J Magn Reson Imaging*. 2000;11:575–585.
9. Bellail AC, Hunter SB, Brat DJ, Tan C, Van Meir EG. Microregional extracellular matrix heterogeneity in brain modulates glioma cell invasion. *Int J Biochem Cell Biol*. 2004;36:1046–1069.
10. Gupta M, Djalilvand A, Brat DJ. Clarifying the diffuse gliomas: an update on the morphologic features and markers that discriminate oligodendroglioma from astrocytoma. *Am J Clin Pathol*. 2005;124:755–768.
11. Brat DJ, Castellano-Sanchez A, Kaur B, Van Meir EG. Genetic and biologic progression in astrocytomas and their relation to angiogenic dysregulation. *Adv Anat Pathol*. 2002;9:24–36.
12. Pirzkall A, McKnight TR, Graves EE, et al. MR-spectroscopy guided target delineation for high-grade gliomas. *Int J Radiat Oncol Biol Phys*. 2001;50:915–928.
13. Rampling R, Cruickshank G, Lewis AD, Fitzsimmons SA, Workman P. Direct measurement of pO2 distribution and bioreductive enzymes in human malignant brain tumors. *Int J Radiat Oncol Biol Phys*. 1994;29:427–431.
14. Brat DJ, Van Meir EG. Glomeruloid microvascular proliferation orchestrated by VPF/VEGF: a new world of angiogenesis research. *Am J Pathol*. 2001;158:789–796.
15. Burger PC, Green SB. Patient age, histologic features, and length of survival in patients with glioblastoma multiforme. *Cancer*. 1987;59:1617–1625.
16. Nelson JS, Tsukada Y, Schoenfeld D, Fulling K, Lamarche J, Peress N. Necrosis as a prognostic criterion in malignant supratentorial, astrocytic gliomas. *Cancer*. 1983;52:550–554.
17. Raza SM, Lang FF, Aggarwal BB, Fuller GN, Wildrick DM, Sawaya R. Necrosis and glioblastoma: a friend or a foe? A review and a hypothesis. *Neurosurgery*. 2002;51:2–12; discussion 12–13.
18. Brat DJ, Mapstone TB. Malignant glioma physiology: cellular response to hypoxia and its role in tumor progression. *Ann Intern Med*. 2003;138:659–668.
19. Daumas-Duport C, Scheithauer B, O'Fallon J, Kelly P. Grading of astrocytomas. A simple and reproducible method. *Cancer*. 1988;62:2152–2165.
20. Tehrani M, Friedman T, Olson JJ, Brat DJ. Intravascular thrombosis in central nervous system malignancies: a potential role in astrocytoma progression. *Brain Pathol*. 2008;18:164–171.
21. Brat DJ, Van Meir EG. Vaso-occlusive and prothrombotic mechanisms associated with tumor hypoxia, necrosis, and accelerated growth in glioblastoma. *Lab Invest*. 2004;84:397–405.
22. Rong Y, Durden DL, Van Meir EG, Brat DJ. 'Pseudopalisading' necrosis in glioblastoma: a familiar morphologic feature that links vascular pathology, hypoxia, and angiogenesis. *J Neuropathol Exp Neurol*. 2006;65:529–539.
23. Plate KH, Breier G, Weich HA, Risau W. Vascular endothelial growth factor is a potential tumour angiogenesis factor in human gliomas in vivo. *Nature*. 1992;59:845–848.
24. Brat DJ, Castellano-Sanchez AA, Hunter SB, et al. Pseudopalisades in glioblastoma are hypoxic, express extracellular matrix proteases, and are formed by an actively migrating cell population. *Cancer Res*. 2004;64:920–927.
25. Schiffer D, Cavalla P, Migheli A, et al. Apoptosis and cell proliferation in human neuroepithelial tumors. *Neurosci Lett*. 1995;195:81–84.
26. Tachibana O, Lampe J, Kleihues P, Ohgaki H. Preferential expression of Fas/APO1 (CD95) and apoptotic cell death in perinecrotic cells of glioblastoma multiforme. *Acta Neuropathol (Berl)*. 1996;92:431–434.
27. Aboody KS, Brown A, Rainov NG, et al. Neural stem cells display extensive tropism for pathology in adult brain: evidence from intracranial gliomas. *Proc Natl Acad Sci U S A*. 2000;97:12846–12851.
28. Semenza GL. Hypoxia-inducible factor 1: oxygen homeostasis and disease pathophysiology. *Trends Mol Med*. 2001;7:345–350.
29. Zagzag D, Zhong H, Scalzitti JM, Laughner E, Simons JW, Semenza GL. Expression of hypoxia-inducible factor 1alpha in brain tumors: association with angiogenesis, invasion, and progression. *Cancer*. 2000;88:2606–2618.
30. Dong S, Nutt CL, Betensky RA, Stemmer, et al. Histology-based expression profiling yields novel prognostic markers in human glioblastoma. *J Neuropathol Exp Neurol*. 2005;64:948–955.
31. Graham CH, Forsdike J, Fitzgerald CJ, Macdonald-Goodfellow S. Hypoxia-mediated stimulation of carcinoma cell invasiveness via upregulation of urokinase receptor expression. *Int J Cancer*. 1999;80:617–623.
32. Mori T, Abe T, Wakabayashi Y, et al. Up-regulation of urokinase-type plasminogen activator and its receptor correlates with enhanced invasion activity of human glioma cells mediated by transforming growth factor-alpha or basic fibroblast growth factor. *J Neurooncol*. 2000;46:115–123.

33. Pennacchietti S, Michieli P, Galluzzo M, Mazzone M, Giordano S, Comoglio PM. Hypoxia promotes invasive growth by transcriptional activation of the met protooncogene. *Cancer Cell.* 2003;3:347–361.
34. Yamamoto M, Mohanam S, Sawaya R, et al. Differential expression of membrane-type matrix metalloproteinase and its correlation with gelatinase A activation in human malignant brain tumors in vivo and in vitro. *Cancer Res.* 1996;56:384–392.
35. Dinda AK, Sarkar C, Roy S, et al. A transmission and scanning electron microscopic study of tumoral and peritumoral microblood vessels in human gliomas. *J Neurooncol.* 1993;16:149–158.
36. Brem S, Cotran R, Folkman J. Tumor angiogenesis: a quantitative method for histologic grading. *J Natl Cancer Inst.* 1972;48:347–356.
37. Sharma S, Sharma MC, Gupta DK, Sarkar C. Angiogenic patterns and their quantitation in high grade astrocytic tumors. *J Neurooncol.* 2006;79:19–30.
38. Wesseling P, van der Laak JA, de Leeuw H, Ruiter DJ, Burger PC. Computer-assisted analysis of the microvasculature in untreated glioblastomas. *J Neurooncol.* 1995;24:83–85.
39. Wesseling P, van der Laak JA, Link M, Teepen HL, Ruiter DJ. Quantitative analysis of microvascular changes in diffuse astrocytic neoplasms with increasing grade of malignancy. *Hum Pathol.* 1998;29:352–358.
40. Holash J, Maisonpierre PC, Compton D, et al. Vessel cooption, regression, and growth in tumors mediated by angiopoietins and VEGF. *Science.* 1999;284:1994–1998.
41. Zagzag D, Amirnovin R, Greco MA, et al. Vascular apoptosis and involution in gliomas precede neovascularization: a novel concept for glioma growth and angiogenesis. *Lab Invest.* 2000;80:837–849.
42. Fischer S, Clauss M, Wiesnet M, Renz D, Schaper W, Karliczek GF. Hypoxia induces permeability in brain microvessel endothelial cells via VEGF and NO. *Am J Physiol.* 1999;276:C812–820.
43. Senger DR, Galli SJ, Dvorak AM, Perruzzi CA, Harvey VS, Dvorak HF. Tumor cells secrete a vascular permeability factor that promotes accumulation of ascites fluid. *Science.* 1983;219:983–985.
44. Straume O, Chappuis PO, Salvesen HB, et al. Prognostic importance of glomeruloid microvascular proliferation indicates an aggressive angiogenic phenotype in human cancers. *Cancer Res.* 2002;62:6808–6811.
45. Plate KH. Mechanisms of angiogenesis in the brain. *J Neuropathol Exp Neurol.* 1999;58:313–320.
46. Shweiki D, Itin A, Soffer D, Keshet E. Vascular endothelial growth factor induced by hypoxia may mediate hypoxia-initiated angiogenesis. *Nature.* 1992;359:843–845.
47. Brat DJ, Bellail AC, Van Meir EG. The role of interleukin-8 and its receptors in gliomagenesis and tumoral angiogenesis. *Neuro Oncol.* 2005;7:122–133.
48. Desbaillets I, Diserens AC, de Tribolet N, Hamou MF, Van Meir EG. Regulation of interleukin-8 expression by reduced oxygen pressure in human glioblastoma. *Oncogene.* 1999;18:1447–1456.
49. Desbaillets I, Diserens AC, Tribolet N, Hamou MF, Van Meir EG. Upregulation of interleukin 8 by oxygen-deprived cells in glioblastoma suggests a role in leukocyte activation, chemotaxis, and angiogenesis. *J Exp Med.* 1997;186:1201–1212.
50. Garkavtsev I, Kozin SV, Chernova O, et al. The candidate tumour suppressor protein ING4 regulates brain tumour growth and angiogenesis. *Nature.* 2004;428:328–332.
51. Evans SM, Judy KD, Dunphy I, et al. Hypoxia is important in the biology and aggression of human glial brain tumors. *Clin Cancer Res.* 2004;10:8177–8184.
52. Evans SM, Judy KD, Dunphy I, et al. Comparative measurements of hypoxia in human brain tumors using needle electrodes and EF5 binding. *Cancer Res.* 2004;64:1886–1892.
53. Cruickshank GS, Rampling R. Peri-tumoural hypoxia in human brain: preoperative measurement of the tissue oxygen tension around malignant brain tumours. *Acta Neurochir Suppl (Wien).* 1994;60:375–377.
54. Cruickshank GS, Rampling RP, Cowans W. Direct measurement of the pO_2 distribution in human malignant brain tumours. *Adv Exp Med Biol.* 1994;345:465–470.
55. Hockel M, Knoop C, Schlenger K, et al. Intratumoral pO_2 predicts survival in advanced cancer of the uterine cervix. *Radiother Oncol.* 1993;26:45–50.
56. Jenkins WT, Evans SM, Koch CJ. Hypoxia and necrosis in rat 9L glioma and Morris 7777 hepatoma tumors: comparative measurements using EF5 binding and the Eppendorf needle electrode. *Int J Radiat Oncol Biol Phys.* 2000;46:1005–1017.
57. Collingridge DR, Piepmeier JM, Rockwell S, Knisely JP. Polarographic measurements of oxygen tension in human glioma and surrounding peritumoural brain tissue. *Radiother Oncol.* 1999;53:127–131.
58. Lally BE, Rockwell S, Fischer DB, Collingridge DR, Piepmeier JM, Knisely JP. The interactions of polarographic measurements of oxygen tension and histological grade in human glioma. *Cancer J.* 2006;12:461–466.
59. Koch CJ. Importance of antibody concentration in the assessment of cellular hypoxia by flow cytometry: EF5 and pimonidazole. *Radiat Res.* 2008;169:677–688.
60. Koch CJ, Evans SM, Lord EM. Oxygen dependence of cellular uptake of EF5 [2-(2-nitro-1H-imidazol-1-yl)-N-(2,2,3,3,3-pentafluoropropyl) acetamide]: analysis of drug adducts by fluorescent antibodies vs bound radioactivity. *Br J Cancer.* 1995;72:869–874.
61. Evans SM, Hahn S, Pook DR, et al. Detection of hypoxia in human squamous cell carcinoma by EF5 binding. *Cancer Res.* 2000;60:2018–2024.
62. Cline JM, Rosner GL, Raleigh JA, Thrall DE. Quantification of CCI-103F labeling heterogeneity in canine solid tumors. *Int J Radiat Oncol Biol Phys.* 1997;37:655–662.
63. Thrall DE, Rosner GL, Azuma C, McEntee MC, Raleigh JA. Hypoxia marker labeling in tumor biopsies: quantification of labeling variation and criteria for biopsy sectioning. *Radiother Oncol.* 1997;44:171–176.
64. Bao S, Wu Q, McLendon RE, Hao Y, et al. Glioma stem cells promote radioresistance by preferential activation of the DNA damage response. *Nature.* 2006;444:756–760.
65. Bao S, Wu Q, Sathornsumetee S, Hao Y, et al. Stem cell-like glioma cells promote tumor angiogenesis through vascular endothelial growth factor. *Cancer Res.* 2006;66:7843–7848.
66. Evans SM, Hahn SM, Magarelli DP, Koch CJ. Hypoxic heterogeneity in human tumors: EF5 binding, vasculature, necrosis, and proliferation. *Am J Clin Oncol.* 2001;24:467–472.
67. Sutherland RM, McCredie JA, Inch WR. Growth of multicell spheroids in tissue culture as a model of nodular carcinomas. *J Natl Cancer Inst.* 1971;46:113–120.
68. Nelson SJ. Multivoxel magnetic resonance spectroscopy of brain tumors. *Mol Cancer Ther.* 2003;2:497–507.
69. Gill SS, Thomas DG, Van Bruggen N, et al. Proton MR spectroscopy of intracranial tumours: in vivo and in vitro studies. *J Comput Assist Tomogr.* 1990;14:497–504.
70. Preul MC, Caramanos Z, Collins DL, et al. Accurate, noninvasive diagnosis of human brain tumors by using proton magnetic resonance spectroscopy. *Nat Med.* 1996;2:323–325.
71. Croteau D, Scarpace L, Hearshen D, et al. Correlation between magnetic resonance spectroscopy imaging and image-guided biopsies: semiquantitative and qualitative histopathological analyses of patients with untreated glioma. *Neurosurgery.* 2001;49:823–829.
72. Perry A. Oligodendroglial neoplasms: current concepts, misconceptions, and folklore. *Adv Anat Pathol.* 2001;8:183–199.
73. Brat DJ, Scheithauer BW, Medina-Flores R, Rosenblum MK, Burger PC. Infiltrative astrocytomas with granular cell features (granular cell astrocytomas): a study of histopathologic features, grading, and outcome. *Am J Surg Pathol.* 2002;26:750–757.
74. Peraud A, Watanabe K, Schwechheimer K, Yonekawa Y, Kleihues P, Ohgaki H. Genetic profile of the giant cell glioblastoma. *Lab Invest.* 1999;79:123–129.
75. Perry A, Aldape KD, George DH, Burger PC. Small cell astrocytoma: an aggressive variant that is clinicopathologically and genetically distinct from anaplastic oligodendroglioma. *Cancer.* 2004;101:2318–2326.
76. Biernat W, Aguzzi A, Sure U, Grant JW, Kleihues P, Hegi ME. Identical mutations of the p53 tumor suppressor gene in the gliomatous and the sarcomatous components of gliosarcomas suggest a common origin from glial cells. *J Neuropathol Exp Neurol.* 1995;54:651–656.
77. Reis RM, Konu-Leblebicioglu D, Lopes JM, Kleihues P, Ohgaki H. Genetic profile of gliosarcomas. *Am J Pathol.* 2000;156:425–432.
78. Dirks PB. Brain tumor stem cells: bringing order to the chaos of brain cancer. *J Clin Oncol.* 2008;26:2916–2924.
79. Singh SK, Hawkins C, Clarke ID, et al. Identification of human brain tumour initiating cells. *Nature.* 2004;432:396–401.
80. Zeppernick F, Ahmadi R, Campos B, et al. Stem cell marker CD133 affects clinical outcome in glioma patients. *Clin Cancer Res.* 2008;14:123–129.
81. Murat A, Migliavacca E, Gorlia T, et al. Stem cell-related "self-renewal" signature and high epidermal growth factor receptor expression associated with resistance to concomitant chemoradiotherapy in glioblastoma. *J Clin Oncol.* 2008;26:3015–3024.

82. Schmidt NO, Przylecki W, Yang W, et al. Brain tumor tropism of transplanted human neural stem cells is induced by vascular endothelial growth factor. *Neoplasia.* 2005;7:623–629.
83. Glass R, Synowitz M, Kronenberg G, et al. Glioblastoma-induced attraction of endogenous neural precursor cells is associated with improved survival. *J Neurosci.* 2005;25:2637–2646.
84. Torp SH. Diagnostic and prognostic role of Ki67 immunostaining in human astrocytomas using four different antibodies. *Clin Neuropathol.* 2002;21:252–257.
85. Bouvier-Labit C, Chinot O, Ochi C, Gambarelli D, Dufour H, Figarella-Branger D. Prognostic significance of Ki67, p53 and epidermal growth factor receptor immunostaining in human glioblastomas. *Neuropathol Appl Neurobiol.* 1998;24:381–388.
86. Coons SW, Johnson PC. Regional heterogeneity in the proliferative activity of human gliomas as measured by the Ki-67 labeling index. *J Neuropathol Exp Neurol.* 1993;52:609–618.
87. Kiss R, Dewitte O, Decaestecker C, et al. The combined determination of proliferative activity and cell density in the prognosis of adult patients with supratentorial high-grade astrocytic tumors. *Am J Clin Pathol.* 1997;107:321–331.
88. Gratas C, Tohma Y, Barnas C, Taniere P, Hainaut P, Ohgaki H. Up-regulation of Fas (APO-1/CD95) ligand and down-regulation of Fas expression in human esophageal cancer. *Cancer Res.* 1998;58:2057–2062.
89. Gratas C, Tohma Y, Van Meir EG, et al. Fas ligand expression in glioblastoma cell lines and primary astrocytic brain tumors. *Brain Pathol.* 1997;7:863–869.
90. Tohma Y, Gratas C, Van Meir EG, et al. Necrogenesis and Fas/APO-1 (CD95) expression in primary (de novo) and secondary glioblastomas. *J Neuropathol Exp Neurol.* 1998;57:239–245.
91. Migheli A, Cavalla P, Marino S, Schiffer D. A study of apoptosis in normal and pathologic nervous tissue after in situ end-labeling of DNA strand breaks. *J Neuropathol Exp Neurol.* 1994;53:606–616.
92. Coons SW, Johnson PC. Regional heterogeneity in the DNA content of human gliomas. *Cancer.* 1993;72:3052–3060.
93. Watanabe K, Tachibana O, Yonekawa Y, Kleihues P, Ohgaki H. Role of gemistocytes in astrocytoma progression. *Lab Invest.* 1997;76:277–284.
94. Nafe R, Franz K, Schlote W, Schneider B. Morphology of tumor cell nuclei is significantly related with survival time of patients with glioblastomas. *Clin Cancer Res.* 2005;11:2141–2148.
95. Nafe R, Franz K, Schlote W, Schneider B. The morphology of perinecrotic tumor cell nuclei in glioblastomas shows a significant relationship with survival time. *Oncol Rep.* 2006;16:555–562.
96. Brunner C, Jung V, Henn W, Zang KD, Urbschat S. Comparative genomic hybridization reveals recurrent enhancements on chromosome 20 and in one case combined amplification sites on 15q24q26 and 20p11p12 in glioblastomas. *Cancer Genet Cytogenet.* 2000;121:124–127.
97. Walker C, du Plessis DG, Joyce KA, et al. Phenotype versus genotype in gliomas displaying inter- or intratumoral histological heterogeneity. *Clin Cancer Res.* 2003;9:4841–4851.
98. Dong ZQ, Pang JC, Tong CY, Zhou LF, Ng HK. Clonality of oligoastrocytomas. *Hum Pathol.* 2002;33:528–535.
99. Kraus JA, Koopmann J, Kaskel P, et al. Shared allelic losses on chromosomes 1p and 19q suggest a common origin of oligodendroglioma and oligoastrocytoma. *J Neuropathol Exp Neurol.* 1995;54:91–95.
100. Qu M, Olofsson T, Sigurdardottir S, et al. Genetically distinct astrocytic and oligodendroglial components in oligoastrocytomas. *Acta Neuropathol.* 2007;113:129–136.
101. Cheng Y, Ng HK, Ding M, Zhang SF, Pang JC, Lo KW. Molecular analysis of microdissected de novo glioblastomas and paired astrocytic tumors. *J Neuropathol Exp Neurol.* 1999;58:120–128.
102. Ren ZP, Olofsson T, Qu M, et al. Molecular genetic analysis of p53 intratumoral heterogeneity in human astrocytic brain tumors. *J Neuropathol Exp Neurol.* 2007;66:944–954.
103. Fulci G, Ishii N, Maurici D, et al. Initiation of human astrocytoma by clonal evolution of cells with progressive loss of p53 functions in a patient with a 283H TP53 germ-line mutation: evidence for a precursor lesion. *Cancer Res.* 2002;62:2897–2905.
104. Reifenberger J, Ring GU, Gies U, et al. Analysis of p53 mutation and epidermal growth factor receptor amplification in recurrent gliomas with malignant progression. *J Neuropathol Exp Neurol.* 1996;55:822–831.
105. Okada Y, Hurwitz EE, Esposito JM, Brower MA, Nutt CL, Louis DN. Selection pressures of TP53 mutation and microenvironmental location influence epidermal growth factor receptor gene amplification in human glioblastomas. *Cancer Res.* 2003;63:413–416.
106. Nafe R, Glienke W, Burgemeister R, et al. Regional heterogeneity of EGFR gene amplification and nuclear morphology in glioblastomas. An investigation using laser microdissection and pressure catapulting. *Anal Quant Cytol Histol* 2004;26:65–76.
107. Nishikawa R, Ji XD, Harmon RC, et al. A mutant epidermal growth factor receptor common in human glioma confers enhanced tumorigenicity. *Proc Natl Acad Sci U S A.* 1994;91:7727–7731.
108. Stommel JM, Kimmelman AC, Ying H, et al. Coactivation of receptor tyrosine kinases affects the response of tumor cells to targeted therapies. *Science.* 2007;318:287–290.

15 Molecular Regulators of Glioma Invasion

Candece L. Gladson, Wei Michael Liu, and Michael E. Berens

THE PROCESS OF INVASION

In general, tumor cell invasion requires that multiple cellular events occur in a coordinated manner. These events can be summarized as remodeling of the extracellular matrix (ECM) by the secretion of proteases that degrade the ECM, the synthesis and secretion of new ECM components including growth factors, and the expression of cell surface receptors that promote or mediate tumor cell attachment and migration on the remodeled ECM (reviewed in ref. [1].). Current dogma suggests that the process of invasion requires altered expression of proteases, growth factors, growth factor receptors, and cell adhesion receptors, in addition to altered expression of ECM glycoproteins and proteoglycans [2]. The coordination of these events most likely involves temporal regulation as some of the processes occur sequentially, and it has been noted that although tumor cells are capable of moving and proliferating, they do not undergo both of these processes at the same time [3].

The coordination of the events associated with invasion is most likely also context-dependent as the molecular compositions of the different structures in the brain differ considerably; for example, the basement membrane of blood vessels differs considerably from the white matter tracts. The context may also be particularly important in determining the invasive behavior of glioma cells in vivo. In glioma tumors (WHO grades II–IV), tumor cells are described as invasive based on the observation of single tumor cells or groups of tumor cells at some distance from the main tumor mass [4]. Typically, glioma invasion is thought of as a steady advance of tumor cells along a localized front at the periphery of the tumor; however, malignant glioma cells also can "jump ahead" of the peripheral edge of the tumor creating distant sites of tumor invasion in the brain (or local brain metastases). This "jumping ahead" by glioma cells can be thought of as a field effect, which are considered to be local effects of glioma cells on the adjacent brain, for example, the mass effect of the tumor on the adjacent brain or, at a cellular level, the satellitosis of glioma cells about neurons that results in the death of the neurons and the utilization of vascular structures by glioma cells for invasion purposes (termed the secondary structures of Scherrer) [4]. It also is theoretically possible that the "jumping ahead" or invasion of the tumor cells to distant sites in the brain is due to the ability of glioma cells to attach and migrate on the vascular ECM structures (endothelial cell basement membrane and pial-glial membrane) without remodeling of these ECM structures.

In this chapter, we delineate some of the changes that occur in the ECM and on the surface of the tumor cells of malignant gliomas and discuss what is known currently regarding their coordination and the mechanism(s) by which they facilitate tumor cell migration and invasion.

MECHANISMS OF GLIOMA INVASION

Changes in the ECM

ECM molecules help to regulate cell migration and invasion through their interaction with specific cell surface receptors [5,6]. The ECM is altered in high-grade gliomas, such as glioblastoma, when compared to the ECM of the normal brain (also known as the neuropil). Alterations in the ECM of high-grade gliomas occur due to the synthesis of new ECM molecules by the tumor cells and activated stromal cells, increased expression of existing ECM molecules, as well as leakage of serum proteins across a disrupted blood-brain barrier. In glioblastoma tumors, there is upregulated or elevated expression of a number of glycoproteins and upregulated expression of certain proteoglycans (for examples, see Table 15.1). Some molecules are expressed in the ECM of both the normal brain and high-grade gliomas, such as osteopontin and thrombospondin (TSP)-1 [7,8], and other ECM molecules are down-regulated in high-grade gliomas, such as TSP-2 [9]. Certain components of the blood vessel basement membrane (e.g., collagen and laminin-9) are expressed in both the normal brain and high-grade gliomas [10,11,14]. An important constituent of the ECM of both the normal brain and glioma tumors is the glycosaminoglycan, hyaluronic acid, which is a major component of the ECM scaffold of the normal brain and interacts with other molecules, such as brevican [26–30]. Most recently, interest has focused on the expression of a family of carbohydrate-binding proteins known as galectins that can be found in the ECM as well as in the cell cytoplasm. Galectin-1 and galectin-3 are expressed in the normal brain, and galectin-1 expression is elevated in glioma tumors [12,13]. Synthesis of new ECM molecules by the tumor cells and activated stromal cells, increased expression of existing ECM molecules, as well as leakage

Table 15.1 Examples of Alterations in the Expression of Glycoproteins and Proteoglycans in Glioblastoma Tumors as Compared to Normal Brain

Cell Association or Localization	Localization in Normal Brain		Localization in Glioblastoma		Function(s) Promoted	Receptor/Binding Partner	Reference
	Vascular	Neural or Glial Cell	Vascular	Tumor Cell			
ECM Molecules							
Glycoproteins							
Fibronectin	+	wk+	++	wk+	Proliferation & Migration[a]	Integrin a5β1	[11]
ED-B-Fibronectin	−	−	++	−	Unclear	Integrin a5β1	[15]
Vitronectin	−	−	+	+	Survival & Proliferation, Less Promotion of Migration	Integrins avβ3, avβ5, avβ1, avβ8, etc.	[14]
Sparc (osteonectin)	−	Unclear	+	+	Migration & Invasion	Unclear	[16–19]
Osteopontin	−	+	+	+	Migration	Integrins avβ3, avβ5, and a5β1	[7]
Thrombospondin-1	+	wk+	++	wk+	Antiangiogenic	Integrins avß3 and a5β1	[8]
IGFBP7	−	−	+	−	Unclear	Unclear	[19,20]
YKL-40	Unclear	Unclear	+	+	Migration & Proangiogenic	Unclear	[21]
Laminin-8 (α4β1γ1)	−	(weak +)	++	focal +	Migration	Integrin a2β1	[22,23]
Laminin-5 (α3β3γ2)	Unclear	Unclear	+ (mRNA)	+ (mRNA)	Migration	Integrin a2β1	[22,23]
Tenascin-C	−	−	+	+ (Perivascular)	Migration	β1 and av integrins	[24,25]
Proteoglycans							
Brevican (BEHAB)	−	+	Unclear	++	Unclear	Unclear	[26]
Cleavage Product of Brevican (by ADAMTS-5)	Unclear	+	Unclear	++	Invasion	Unclear	[27–30]
NG2	wk+	(+ in cerebellum)	++	−	Proangiogenic	Angiostatin in the ECM	[31]
Perlecan (cleavage product-endorepellin)	−	−	++	−	Antiangiogenic (Endorepellin)	Integrin a2β1	[32]

[a] Cell migration is typically defined as cell motility that does not require protease digestion of the ECM. The assays used to measure cell migration include scratch/wounded monolayer assays, radial migration assays, and migration in a Boyden chamber under haptotactic or chemotactic conditions [3,7,25,32–36]. Cell invasion is typically defined as cell motility that occurs in a three-dimensional environment and requires the secretion of proteases that focally digest the ECM [1].

Invasion assays are usually conducted using two-well Boyden Chambers containing a filter coated with Matrigel or normal brain homogenate [7,16,30,37]. Slices of normal brain in organotypic culture also are used to assay migration or invasion depending on the conditions (time and buffer) and method of analysis [37]. +, protein expression; wk+, weak and focal expression; −, no detectable protein expression; IGFB-P7, insulin-like growth factor-binding protein; ECM, extracellular matrix.

of serum proteins across a disrupted blood-brain barrier all occur in glioma tumors.

Current thinking suggests that tumor cell synthesis of ECM molecules that promote cell attachment or motility allows tumors to create a pathway for invasion [1]. For example, expression of galectin-1 and sparc is increased in malignant glioma tumors, and both molecules promote glioma cell migration and invasion in vitro. Sparc appears to promote glioma cell migration through its activation of focal adhesion kinase (FAK) and integrin-linked kinase [38], its activation of the urokinase/urokinase receptor (uPA/uPAR) pathway [39], and its activation of HSP27 [40]. It also has been shown that sparc promotes invasion in vivo in a mouse xenograft model of glioma [17].

Several ECM molecules that are newly expressed or upregulated in high-grade gliomas, such as the glycoproteins tenascin-C, the ED-B-isoform of fibronectin, laminin-8, IGFBP-7, TSP-1, and perlecan, as well as the elevated expression of the proteoglycan NG2, are localized nearly exclusively or predominantly to neovessels or to a perivascular location. This suggests that the vascular cells and associated cells (endothelial cells, pericytes, smooth muscle cells, and associated astrocytes) are induced by the tumor cells or by the activated stromal cells to express an altered repertoire of ECM molecules. This altered repertoire of ECM molecules at the neovessels can be part of a host antitumor/antiangiogenesis response, can promote further neovascularization, or can promote glioma cell migration on the remodeled vascular basement membrane. For example, there is upregulation of laminin-8 (a promigratory ECM molecule) in the basement membrane of blood vessels in malignant gliomas [10,41,42], and the ability of laminin-8 to promote angiogenesis is supported by both in vitro and in vivo data. It is thought that laminin-8 promotes angiogenesis through its promotion of endothelial cell migration [41]. It does not appear to promote migration of malignant glioma cells [42].

The expression of TSP-1 also is increased in the neovasculature in glioblastoma tumors [8], but TSP-1 is likely part of a host antitumor/antiangiogenesis response.

Some ECM molecules are more promigratory than others, for example, laminin has a greater promigratory effect than vitronectin on glioma cells [43]. This is likely due to

Table 15.2 Examples of Integrin Expression in Malignant Gliomas

Integrin	Elevated mRNA Expression	Ligands	Function	Reference
β1				
a2β1	not tested	COL	β1 mAb blocks glioma migration on all the purified ligands in the column to the readers left	[41–46]
a3β1	not tested	COL, LM, FN		
a5β1	not tested	FN;		
a6β1	not tested	LM		
β3				
avβ3	+	VN; OPN, TN, Degraded COL	Promotes migration and invasion toward normal brain homogenate, and towards the purified ligands listed in the column to the readers left.	[7,14,45–48]
av				
avβ5	+	FN, VN, OPN	Promotes migration and invasion toward normal brain homogenate, and toward the purified ligands listed in the column to the readers left.	[7,14,45–48]

+, elevated mRNA expression when compared to normal brain tissue; COL, collagen; FIB, fibrinogen; FN, fibronectin; LN, laminin; OPN, osteopontin; TN, tenascin; VN, vitronectin.

the differences in the reorganization of the cytoskeleton promoted by these two ECM molecules [6,43]. Ultimately, successful glioma cell invasion requires tumor cell proliferation as well as migratory and invasive behavior. ECM molecules that promote a more adherent phenotype with actin stress fiber formation, such as those seen in glioma cells adherent to vitronectin [7], are likely conducive to cell proliferation, whereas ECM molecules that promote a less organized actin cytoskeleton with filopodia or lamellipodia, such as laminin and osteopontin [7,41], are conducive to cell motility.

Changes in Expression of Cell Surface Receptors

Changes in the expression of multiple different classes of cell surface receptors (e.g., integrins, growth factor receptors, and the Eph/Ephrin family) have been described in malignant gliomas (see Tables 15.2 and 15.3).

Integrins are heterodimeric (aß) transmembrane-spanning receptors that largely recognize ECM molecules as ligands and mediate both outside-to-in and inside-to-out directional signaling across the cell membrane (from the ECM to the actin cytoskeleton and vice versa) [5,6]. Directed cell migration requires a sequence of events in which the cell extends protrusions at the front of the cell and retracts the tail at the rear, forms focal adhesions with the ECM via integrin receptors at the front of the cell (this stabilizes the forward protrusions), and then uses these adhesions to pull the cell body forward [6]. The focal adhesions that relocalize to the rear of the cell as the cells move forward are disassembled. Analyses of biopsy specimens indicate that multiple integrin receptors are expressed on glioblastoma cells, such as integrins a3ß1, a2ß1, avß3, and avß5, and in some instances integrin expression is upregulated (see Table 15.2) [7,47,48,53,54]. The promotion of motility requires an optimal level of integrin expression on the cell; very high levels of an integrin can promote a stationary phenotype and inhibit cell migration [5]. In malignant gliomas, integrin signaling that promotes migration could theoretically be amplified by the elevated expression of ECM molecules; for example, the upregulation of laminin-8 in the vascular basement membrane likely primes the endothelial cell for signaling by integrin a3ß1 [10,41,42].

As shown in Tables 15.1 and 15.2, several of the integrins that have been shown to be expressed on glioblastoma cells in biopsies recognize as ligands some of the above described upregulated ECM molecules.

Integrin receptors cooperate or coordinate with growth factor receptors to promote cell migration, as well as proliferation and angiogenesis, and this is exemplified by the cooperation of integrin avß3 with the platelet-derived growth factor receptor (PDGFr) ß, vascular endothelial growth factor receptor (VEGFR), or Insulin-like growth factor receptor (IGFR), and the coordination of integrin a6ß1 with the VEGFR [6,55–58]. The importance of integrin receptor coordination with growth factor receptors is supported by the observation that overexpression of the integrin ß3 subunit decreased tumor growth in an immunodeficient rat model of human glioma; however, when the integrin ß3 subunit

Table 15.3 Examples of Growth Factor Receptor Expression in Malignant Gliomas

Growth Factor Receptor	Elevated Expression on Glioma Cells	Function(s) Promoted	Reference
EGFR[a]	+	Migration and Proliferation	[34,49]
PDGFr	+	Migration	[50]
FGFR4	+	Unclear	[51]
c-met	+	Migration	[52]

[a] EGFR is amplified in ~40% of glioblastoma tumors; and the vIII variant (constitutively active) is frequently expressed [49].

was overexpressed with a cooperating growth factor, such as VEGF, glioma growth was restored [59].

Certain growth factor receptors are upregulated on glioma cells in vivo. These include the PDGFr (α and β), the epidermal growth factor receptor (EGFR), the c-met, and the fibroblast growth factor receptor 4 (FGFR-4); see Table 15.3). In most instances, the receptor and its growth factor are upregulated in the tumor. For example, the expression of hepatocyte growth factor (HGF)/scatter factor (SF) and its receptor (c-met) is elevated in malignant glioma cells in biopsies [52], suggesting that an autocrine or paracrine mechanism exists for HGF/SF promotion of malignant glioma cell migration and invasion.

CD44 is a cell adhesion receptor that recognizes hyaluronic acid and osteopontin as ligands [60]. CD44 promotes glioma cell migration and invasion in vitro [61–63]. In some cells, CD44 cooperates with a specific integrin to promote cell migration [64]. Another family of cell adhesion receptors, the cadherin family, is known to mediate homophilic cell-cell adhesion, and in glioblastoma cells, there appears to be altered organization of the cadherin-catenin pathway [65]. E-cadherin is not expressed in astrocytic gliomas (WHO Grades II, III, or IV) [66], and N-cadherin protein expression levels are similar in glioblastoma and normal brain samples [67,68].

Lastly, the Eph family of cell adhesion receptors also plays an important role in glioma cell migration and invasion. The Eph receptors are tyrosine kinases that recognize the ephrins as ligands with the receptors and ligands being divided into A and B subfamilies [69]. This receptor ligand family induces bidirectional signaling between interacting cells. Typically, the Eph-B receptors bind transmembrane Ephrin-B ligands and their cytoplasmic tail engages in signaling activities, and the Eph-A receptors bind glycosylphosphatidylinositol-anchored Ephrin-A ligands (some exceptions to this rule exist) [69]. Both in vitro and animal studies suggest that the Eph-B2 receptor and ephrin-B3 ligand promote glioma cell migration and invasion [70,71]. In malignant glioma tissue, the expression of Eph-A2 and Eph-A7 is elevated [70,72].

Taken together, the available data suggest that specific cell surface receptors from different classes cooperate or coordinate their signaling in a manner that is temporally dependent and context-dependent during the promotion of malignant glioma cell invasion in vivo.

Changes in Protease/Protease Receptor Expression

Current dogma suggests that cell invasion requires that the cells focally digest the surrounding ECM and create an invasion pathway [1]. Proteases involved in invasion are typically localized to the surface of cells through their receptor or binding partner(s) (reviewed in ref. [1,2,73,74]). This cell surface localization restricts the enzymatic activity to a defined region of the cell membrane, for example, the serine protease uPA, which binds to its cell surface receptor uPAR on tumor cells, thus localizing uPA-mediated digestion of molecules to a defined region of the cell membrane [73]. Furthermore, uPAR associates with specific integrin receptors, which further localizes the enzymatic function of uPA on the cell membrane. uPA acts proteolytically to digest a number of ECM molecules, such as fibronectin. Studies utilizing malignant glioma cell lines indicate that uPAR promotes cell migration and invasion in vitro and it has been shown to promote invasion in vivo in mouse models of malignant glioma [73]. Furthermore, in glioblastoma tumor samples, both uPA and uPAR mRNA and proteins are upregulated on the tumor cells (reviewed in ref. 73, 75).

Another family of proteases that are important for glioma invasion are the matrix metalloproteinases (MMPs) (reviewed in ref. [74]). MMP-2 and -9 in particular have been shown to promote malignant glioma invasion in vitro and in vivo in mouse models of glioma, and downregulation of either protease inhibits glioma invasion. The expression of both MMP-2 and -9 is elevated in malignant glioma tumors in vivo [74]. The function of these proteases also is likely localized to defined regions of the cell membrane through a binding partner; for example, pro-MMP-2 is activated by binding to cell surface integrin $\alpha v\beta 3$ [76]. Also, MMP-2 activation can be promoted by the tissue inhibitor of metalloproteinase (TIMP)-2 in glioma cells [77]. MMPs proteolytically degrade some of the above discussed ECM molecules, including galectin and perlecan, and thereby alter the function of these ECM molecules [78,79]. In addition, uPA activates pro-MMPs by proteolytic cleavage. Conversely, ECM molecules help to regulate the expression and function of the MMPs; for example, sparc upregulates the expression of a transmembrane MMP, MT1-MMP, and increases the activity of MMP-2 [78]. This suggests that the tumor cell synthesis of sparc increases tumor cell invasion in part by increasing proteolytic degradation of the ECM and is an example of the coordination that occurs during glioma invasion.

Other proteases involved in glioma invasion include the cathepsins, the ADAMTS family of metalloproteases [29,30,73], and the hyalurolytic enzymes that degrade hyaluronan [80]. Expression of the ADAMTS-5 protease, a member of the ADAMTS family, is increased in malignant gliomas [29], and it is thought to be important in malignant gliomas as it cleaves brevican resulting in a brevican fragment that promotes glioma invasion [30,81].

Role of Cytoplasmic Kinases

A number of cytoplasmic tyrosine kinases serve as common downstream effectors of the above classes of cell surface receptors. This use of common downstream signaling effectors by different classes of cell surface receptors may underlie the cooperation of these different classes of cell surface receptors in promoting cell migration and invasion.

The FAK/proline-rich tyrosine kinase (Pyk2 or RAFTK) family was identified in 1992 when FAK was found to be a constitutively phosphorylated protein in viral-Src-transformed cells (reviewed in ref. [82]). FAK is rapidly activated (phosphorylated) when cells attach to an ECM ligand via integrin receptors, and FAK colocalizes with integrin receptors to sites of cell-matrix adhesions in adherent cells (reviewed in ref. [83]). FAK is also activated when cells are stimulated with multiple different growth factors [84]. Pyk2 is highly homologous to FAK in its domain structure, but it is activated (phosphorylated) by different stimuli, for example, by increases in cytoplasmic Ca^{2+} [85]. The FAK/Pyk2 family of cytoplasmic tyrosine kinases can promote cell migration and invasion. One relatively well-defined mechanism by which this occurs requires both the kinase and scaffolding functions of FAK and Pyk2 and involves their association with cellular Src and members of the Crk-associated substrate (CAS) family of adaptor molecules [86]. CAS family members bind activated FAK or Pyk2, followed by cellular Src phosphorylation of the substrate domain of the bound CAS family member, recruitment of another adaptor molecule from the Crk family, and activation of a small GTPase (i.e., Rac1 or Cdc42) that signal(s) actin polymerization, membrane protrusion, and cell polarity (see Figure 15.1; reviewed in refs. [83,87,88]). The small GTPase, Rho, also modulates cell migration in glioma cells; in rat glioma cells, the Rho effector mDia1 controls cell polarity by promoting the localization of Cdc42 to the front of the cell and controls focal adhesion turnover at the rear of the cell that is mediated by cellular Src [88].

The expression and activity of FAK are elevated in anaplastic astrocytoma biopsy samples as compared to the nonneoplastic brain when analyzed by western blotting [89], and FAK expression is increased in glioblastoma tumors when analyzed by immunohistochemistry [33–35,90]. In glioblastoma tumors, FAK localizes to cells expressing EGFR or PDGFr [91]. In support of a role for FAK in promoting the migration and invasion of malignant glioma cells in vitro, investigators using different cell lines have shown that inhibition of FAK function blocks EGF-stimulated migration on fibronectin and PDGF-stimulated migration on vitronectin and osteopontin, as well as invasion through Matrigel and homogenates of normal brain [33,34,92]. The expression of Pyk2 also is elevated in glioblastoma tumor biopsy samples as compared to the normal brain when analyzed by immunohistochemistry [90,93]. In support of a role for Pyk2 in promoting malignant glioma cell migration and invasion in vitro, investigators have shown that Pyk2 promotes migration of several malignant glioma cell lines adherent to laminin, although, in these conditions, FAK did not appear to play a promigratory role [94]. Recent in vivo data in a xenograft model of malignant glioma indicated the downregulation of Pyk2 or of FAK-inhibited glioma invasion; the downregulation of Pyk2 appeared to inhibit glioma invasion to a greater extent, although the downregulation of Pyk2 or of FAK prolonged survival similarly [95]. Thus, both FAK and Pyk2 participate in promoting malignant glioma cell migration and invasion, and the participating family member is likely context-dependent.

Members of the Src family of cytoplasmic tyrosine kinases also participate in the regulation of cell migration and invasion [96]. Similar to FAK, cellular Src is rapidly activated when integrin receptors bind their ligand in the ECM. Src family members signal through their tyrosine phosphorylation of substrates, and this phosphorylation is promoted by cellular Src association with substrates through its SH2 and SH3 domains. In the adult human brain and in anaplastic astrocytoma and glioblastoma tumor samples, the predominant Src family members are Fyn, Lyn, and c-Src based on western blotting of tissue biopsies; very low levels of Yes and Lck were also detected [97]. Furthermore, kinase assays and western blotting showed that the activity of Lyn kinase is significantly elevated in glioblastoma tumor biopsy samples as compared to the normal brain or nonneoplastic brain. This was not due solely to increased levels of Lyn message and protein, which suggests that increased expression of cell surface receptors that activate cellular Src (such as integrins and growth factor receptors) is likely responsible at least in part for the increase in Lyn kinase activity [97]. Importantly, Lyn kinase has been shown to be necessary for the migration of malignant glioma cells mediated through cooperation of integrin avß3 and the PDGFrß [55].

Adaptor Molecules

The CAS family of adaptor molecules (p130CAS, HEF1, and Sin/Efs) act downstream of FAK or Pyk2 and cellular Src to promote cell migration (reviewed in refs. [83,87]). Regarding CAS family member expression, p130CAS is thought to be expressed ubiquitously [98], HEF1 is expressed in the developing hindbrain [99–101], and Sin/Efs is expressed in embryonic and adult brain tissue [102,103]. The CAS family members may be activated (phosphorylated) by different cellular stimuli in a cell- and context-dependent manner [92,104]. For example, HEF1 is activated in PDGF-stimulated malignant glioma cells adherent to vitronectin or osteopontin and promotes cell migration and invasion in vitro [92], whereas p130CAS is activated in malignant glioma cells adherent to fibronectin and promotes cell migration in vitro [104–106].

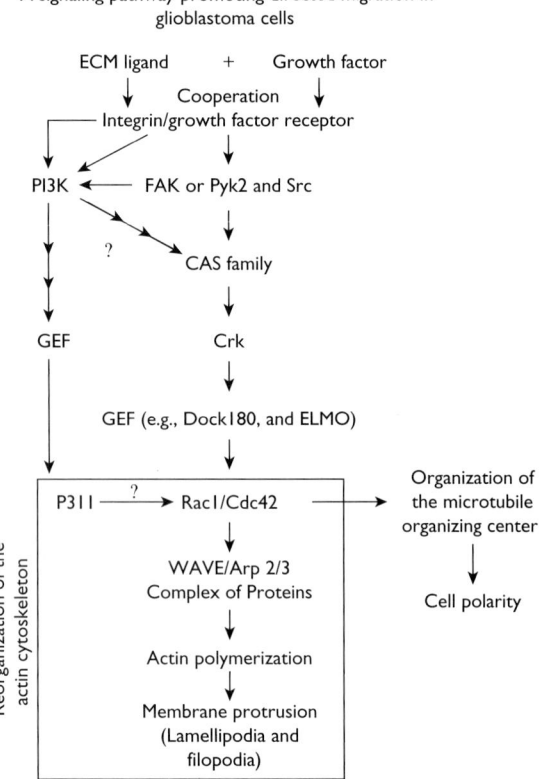

Figure 15.1 A signaling pathway promoting directed migration in glioblastoma cells.

Members of another family of adaptor/scaffolding molecules, the Crk family, also promote cell migration and invasion [87]. The *crk* gene is translated into Crk I and II proteins by alternative splicing [107]. Studies of Crk mRNA levels in tissue samples indicate that Crk II is expressed in the normal brain and glioblastoma tumor tissue, whereas Crk I is upregulated in glioblastoma tumor tissue [107]. Crk proteins bind through their SH2 domain to the phosphorylated substrate domain of CAS family members and through their SH3 domain to guanine exchange factors (GEFs), such as Dock 180, that activate or promote the GTP-bound form of Rac1 or Cdc42 (reviewed in refs. [83,87]).

Phosphatidylinositol-3-Hydroxyl Kinase, PTEN, and Protein Kinase C

Several other kinases have been implicated in glioma cell migration and invasion. A number of studies indicate that phosphatidylinositol-3-hydroxyl kinase (PI3K) promotes glioma cell migration and invasion in vitro [104,108,109]. In non-glioma cells, PI3K can promote migration through its activation of Vav1, a GEF that activates a small GTPase promoting actin polymerization and membrane protrusion [110]. Also in non-glioma cells, PI3K can phosphorylate p130 CAS promoting migration [111]. The phosphatase, PTEN, also regulates migration, as re-expression of PTEN in malignant glioma cells lacking a functional PTEN resulted in an inhibition of cell migration in vitro [104,105]. In addition, protein kinase C promotes migration of glioma cells [112].

QUESTIONS REMAINING/FUTURES STUDIES AND THERAPEUTIC IMPLICATIONS

Although our understanding of the regulation of glioma cell invasion is still in its infancy, the current knowledge of the molecular events that regulate glioma cell invasion and how these processes are coordinated has already suggested several potential targets and therapeutic strategies. In terms of therapeutic targeting of the ECM molecules in malignant glioma tumors or their use in localization, Phase I and II clinical trials in glioblastoma patients with a radiolabeled monoclonal antibody directed toward tenascin-C have shown promising results [113,114]. The targeting of newly expressed ECM molecules may prove to be a very important therapeutic approach. Expression of the ECM molecule YKL-40 in glioblastoma tumors correlates with a poor response to radiation therapy [19,115]. This suggests that the reduction of YKL-40 expression in these tumors could improve the response to radiation. As targeting of an ECM molecule could enhance its turnover (reduce its half-life) in the ECM, knowledge of the half-life of the molecule in the ECM and the mechanisms involved in its turnover would assist in the development of therapeutic strategies. The ECM molecules TSP-1 and TSP-2 are internalized by the scavenger receptor low-density lipoprotein receptor-related protein 1 (LRP1) and targeted for lysosomal degradation [116] (reviewed in ref. [117]). TSP-1 and TSP-2 also bind MMP-2 and the complex of TSP-1/MMP-2 or TSP-2/MMP-2 is internalized by LRP1, suggesting the antiangiogenic molecules TSP-1 and TSP-2 can reduce invasion by clearing MMP-2 [117,118]. Evidence supporting a role for TSP-2 in clearing MMP-2 in these tumors has been obtained by propagation of malignant glioma cells in a TSP-2-null mouse, which resulted in increased angiogenesis and tumor growth, likely due to the increased levels of MMP-2 found at the tumor vessels [119]. It is possible that other unidentified ECM molecules are upregulated in high-grade gliomas, and their identification could prove useful for diagnostic or prognostic purposes.

Although the mechanism(s) by which different classes of cell surface receptors cooperate or coordinate in promoting glioma cell invasion may prove to be excellent therapeutic targets or assist in directed targeting, these mechanisms must be better defined. It will be necessary to determine whether the cooperation of two different cell surface receptors is due either to a direct interaction or to a colocalization to a membrane structure and whether there is a hierarchy of receptor function. It has been shown in glioma cells that the function of integrin avß3 requires engagement of integrin a5ß1 [120], and this could be important in glioblastomas as integrin avß3 is upregulated on glioblastoma tumor cells in biopsy samples [14,47,48,53,54]. Determining the regulators of integrin expression in glioblastoma tumors is also important, for example, some evidence suggests that an aberrant constitutive activation of nuclear factor kappaB may regulate integrin expression in glioblastoma tumors [121,122]. Targeting cell signaling pathways with small molecule inhibitors of various kinases (such as EGFR) that are known to participate in the invasion process has also received considerable attention, and the results are promising [123] (reviewed in ref. [124]). Identification of other cell membrane molecules that affect receptor function may provide additional targets [125]. An enlarging family of membrane proteins known as tetraspanins regulate integrin function [126], but little is known as to their expression or function in malignant gliomas. Another exciting approach that is evolving is the targeting of myosin in migrating/invading glioma cells [127].

Basic research in three areas of unique interest should prove to be especially informative, that is, the role of stromal cells (astrocytes, microglia, and vascular cells) in the process of invasion, the role of tumor cells expressing markers of stem cells or progenitor cells in the process of invasion, and the delineation of the differences in gene and protein expression profiles in the invading glioma cells as compared to the glioma cells in the main tumor mass. The literature indicates that certain stromal cells, such as microglia and astrocytes, are activated and respond to glioma tumors by proliferating and migrating to the tumor and by altering the repertoire of proteins they express [11,128,129]. The importance of the stromal or bystander cell response in gliomas was highlighted recently by the work of Assanah et al [130]. that demonstrated that large numbers of stromal or bystander cells are recruited to the tumor and contribute significantly to the tumor mass in a rat model of glioblastoma. Thus, further experimentation is needed to identify the factors or environmental conditions resulting in the activation or recruitment of stromal cells to gliomas and how these stromal or bystander cells are potentially co-opted to contribute to glioma cell invasion or survival or proliferation. Recent studies from several groups have suggested that tumor cells expressing markers of stem or progenitor cells are the highly invasive cells in human gliomas [131] (reviewed in refs. [132,133]). This suggests that the difficulties glioma biologists have faced in modeling human glioma invasion in vivo can be overcome by utilizing tumor cells that express stem or progenitor cell markers. This approach could be particularly informative as we know very little regarding the function of glioma cells expressing such markers [132]. Recent work indicates that there are significant alterations in gene expression in the invading glioma cells as compared to those in the main tumor mass, such as increased expression of the P311 polypeptide that promotes cell migration (see Figure 15.1), as well as increased expression of the fibroblast growth factor-inducible 14 molecule and p38 MAP kinase [134–137]. Expansion of this work will likely lead to the identification of genes that could be targeted therapeutically as well as further insights into the molecular mechanisms by which the invasive behavior is regulated.

REFERENCES

1. Brinckerhoff CE, Matrisian LM. Matrix metalloproteinases: a tail of a frog that became a prince. *Nat Rev Mol Cell Biol.* 2002;3(3):207–214.
2. Borg TK. It's the matrix! ECM, proteases, and cancer. *Am J Pathol.* 2004;164(4):1141–1142.
3. Berens ME, Giese A. "... those left behind." Biology and oncology of invasive glioma cells. *Neoplasia.* 1999;1(3):208–219.
4. Burger PC, Vogel FS, Green SB, Strike TA. Glioblastoma multiforme and anaplastic astrocytoma. Pathologic criteria and prognostic implications. *Cancer.* 1985;56(5):106–111.
5. Hynes RO. Integrins: versatility, modulation, and signaling in cell adhesion. *Cell.* 1992;69:11–25.
6. Berrier AL, Yamada KM. Cell-matrix adhesion. *J Cell Physiol.* 2007;213(3):565–573.
7. Ding Q, Stewart J Jr, Prince CW, et al. Promotion of malignant astrocytoma cell migration by osteopontin expressed in the normal brain: differences in integrin signaling during cell adhesion to osteopontin versus vitronectin. *Cancer Res.* 2002;62(18):5336–5343.
8. Pijuan-Thompson V, Grammer JR, Stewart J, et al. Retinoic acid alters the mechanism of attachment of malignant astrocytoma and neuroblastoma cells to thrombospondin-1. *Exp Cell Res.* 1999;249(1):86–101.
9. Kazuno M, Tokunaga T, Oshika Y, et al. Thrombospondin-2 (TSP2) expression is inversely correlated with vascularity in glioma. *Eur J Cancer.* 1999;35(3):502–506.
10. Ljubimova JY, Fujita M, Khazenzon NM, et al. Association between laminin-8 and glial tumor grade, recurrence, and patient survival. *Cancer.* 2004;101(3):604–612.
11. Novak U, Kaye AH. Extracellular matrix and the brain: components and function. *J Clin Neurosci.* 2000;7(4):280–290.
12. Stillman BN, Mischel PS, Baum LG. New roles for galectins in brain tumors—from prognostic markers to therapeutic targets. *Brain Pathol.* 2005;15(2):124–132.
13. Rorive S, Belot N, Decaestecker C, et al. Galectin-1 is highly expressed in human gliomas with relevance for modulation of invasion of tumor astrocytes into the brain parenchyma. *Glia.* 2001;33(3):241–255.
14. Gladson CL, Cheresh DA. Glioblastoma expression of vitronectin and the $\alpha v \beta 3$ integrin: adhesion mechanism for transformed glial cells. *J Clin Invest.* 1991;88:1924–1932.
15. Castellani P, Viale G, Dorcaratto A, et al. The fibronectin isoform containing the ED-B oncofetal domain: a marker of angiogenesis. *Int J Cancer.* 1994;59(5):612–618.
16. Golembieski WA, Ge S, Nelson K, Mikkelsen T, Rempel SA. Increased SPARC expression promotes U87 glioblastoma invasion in vitro. *Int J Dev Neurosci.* 1999;17(5–6):463–472.
17. Schultz C, Lemke N, Ge S, Golembieski WA, Rempel SA. Secreted protein acidic and rich in cysteine promotes glioma invasion and delays tumor growth in vivo. *Cancer Res.* 2002;62(21):6270–6277.
18. Rempel SA, Golembieski WA, Ge S, et al. SPARC: a signal of astrocytic neoplastic transformation and reactive response in human primary and xenograft gliomas. *J Neuropathol Exp Neurol.* 1998;57(12):1112–1121.
19. Pen A, Moreno MJ, Martin J, Stanimirovic DB. Molecular markers of extracellular matrix remodeling in glioblastoma vessels: microarray study of laser-captured glioblastoma vessels. *Glia* 2007;55(6):559–572.
20. Holtkamp N, Ziegenhagen N, Malzer E, Hartmann C, Giese A, von DA. Characterization of the amplicon on chromosomal segment 4q12 in glioblastoma multiforme. *Neuro Oncol.* 2007;9(3):291–297.
21. Nutt CL, Betensky RA, Brower MA, Batchelor TT, Louis DN, Stemmer-Rachamimov AO. YKL-40 is a differential diagnostic marker for histologic subtypes of high-grade gliomas. *Clin Cancer Res.* 2005;11(6):2258–2264.
22. Ljubimova JY, Fujita M, Khazenzon NM, Ljubimov AV, Black KL. Changes in laminin isoforms associated with brain tumor invasion and angiogenesis. *Front Biosci.* 2006;11:81–88.
23. Fukushima Y, Ohnishi T, Arita N, Hayakawa T, Sekiguchi K. Integrin alpha3beta1-mediated interaction with laminin-5 stimulates adhesion, migration and invasion of malignant glioma cells. *Int J Cancer.* 1998; 76(1):63–72.
24. Zagzag D, Friedlander DR, Dosik J, et al. Tenascin-C expression by angiogenic vessels in human astrocytomas and by human brain endothelial cells in vitro. *Cancer Res.* 1996;56(1):182–189.
25. ZagZag D, Shiff B, Jallo GI, et al. Tenascin-C promotes microvascular cell migration and phosphorylation of focal adhesion kinase. *Cancer Res.* 2002;62(9):2660–2668.
26. Jaworski DM, Kelly GM, Piepmeier JM, Hockfield S. BEHAB (brain enriched hyaluronan binding) is expressed in surgical samples of glioma and in intracranial grafts of invasive glioma cell lines. *Cancer Res.* 1996;56(10):2293–2298.
27. Viapiano MS, Bi WL, Piepmeier J, Hockfield S, Matthews RT. Novel tumor-specific isoforms of BEHAB/brevican identified in human malignant gliomas. *Cancer Res.* 2005;65(15):6726–6733.
28. Viapiano MS, Matthews RT, Hockfield S. A novel membrane-associated glycovariant of BEHAB/brevican is up-regulated during rat brain development and in a rat model of invasive glioma. *J Biol Chem.* 2003;278(35):33239–33247.
29. Nakada M, Miyamori H, Kita D, et al. Human glioblastomas overexpress ADAMTS-5 that degrades brevican. *Acta Neuropathol.* 2005;110(3):239–246.
30. Viapiano MS, Hockfield S, Matthews RT. BEHAB/brevican requires ADAMTS-mediated proteolytic cleavage to promote glioma invasion. *J Neurooncol.* 2008;88(3):261–272.
31. Schrappe M, Klier FG, Spiro RC, Waltz TA, Reisfeld RA, Gladson CL. Correlation of chondroitin sulfate proteoglycan expression on proliferating brain capillary endothelial cells with the malignant phenotype of astroglial cells. *Cancer Res.* 1991;51:4986–4993.
32. Mongiat M, Sweeney SM, San Antonio JD, Fu J, Iozzo RV. Endorepellin, a novel inhibitor of angiogenesis derived from the C terminus of perlecan. *J Biol Chem.* 2003;278(6):4238–4249.
33. Wang D, Grammer JR, Cobbs CS, et al. p125 focal adhesion kinase promotes malignant astrocytoma cell proliferation in vivo. *J Cell Sci.* 2000;113(pt 23):4221–4230.
34. Jones G, Machado J Jr, Merlo A. Loss of focal adhesion kinase (FAK) inhibits epidermal growth factor receptor-dependent migration and induces aggregation of NH2-terminal FAK in the nuclei of apoptotic glioblastoma cells. *Cancer Res.* 2001;61:4978–4981.
35. Jones G, Machado J Jr, Tolnay M, Merlo A. PTEN-independent induction of caspase-mediated cell death and reduced invasion by the focal adhesion targeting domain (FAT) in human astrocytic brain tumors which highly express focal adhesion kinase (FAK). *Cancer Res.* 2001;61:5688–5691.
36. Berens ME, Beaudry C. Radial monolayer cell migration assay. *Methods Mol Med.* 2004;88:219–224.
37. Valster A, Tran NL, Nakada M, Berens ME, Chan AY, Symons M. Cell migration and invasion assays. *Methods.* 2005;37(2):208–215.
38. Shi Q, Bao S, Song L, et al. Targeting SPARC expression decreases glioma cellular survival and invasion associated with reduced activities of FAK and ILK kinases. *Oncogene.* 2007;26(28):4084–4094.
39. Kunigal S, Gondi CS, Gujrati M, et al. SPARC-induced migration of glioblastoma cell lines via uPA-uPAR signaling and activation of small GTPase RhoA. *Int J Oncol.* 2006;29(6):1349–1357.

40. Golembieski WA, Thomas SL, Schultz CR, et al. HSP27 mediates SPARC-induced changes in glioma morphology, migration, and invasion. *Glia*. 2008;56(10):1061–1075.
41. Fujiwara H, Kikkawa Y, Sanzen N, Sekiguchi K. Purification and characterization of human laminin-8. Laminin-8 stimulates cell adhesion and migration through alpha3beta1 and alpha6beta1 integrins. *J Biol Chem*. 2001;276(20):17550–17558.
42. Kawataki T, Yamane T, Naganuma H, et al. Laminin isoforms and their integrin receptors in glioma cell migration and invasiveness: evidence for a role of alpha5-laminin(s) and alpha3beta1 integrin. *Exp Cell Res*. 2007;313(18):3819–3831.
43. Giese A, Rief MD, Loo MA, Berens ME. Determinants of human astrocytoma migration. *Cancer Res*. 1994;54:3897–3904.
44. Paulus W, Baur I, Beutler AS, Reeves SA. Diffuse brain invasion of glioma cells requires beta 1 integrins. *Lab Invest*. 1996;75(6):819–826.
45. Friedlander DR, ZagZag D, Shiff B, et al. Migration of brain tumor cells on extracellular matrix proteins in vitro correlates with tumor type and grade and involves alphaV and beta1 integrins. *Cancer Res*. 1996;56(8):1939–1947.
46. Deryugina EI, Bourdon MA. Tenascin mediates human glioma cell migration and modulates cell migration on fibronectin. *J Cell Sci*. 1996;109(pt 3):643–652.
47. Paulus W, Baur I, Schuppan D, Roggendorf W. Characterization of integrin receptors in normal and neoplastic human brain. *Am J Pathol*. 1993;143(1):154–163.
48. Gladson CL, Wilcox JN, Sanders L, Gillespie GY, Cheresh DA. Cerebral microenvironment influences expression of the vitronectin gene in astrocytic tumors. *J Cell Sci*. 1995;108(pt 3):947–956.
49. Wong AJ, Bigner SH, Bigner DD, Kinzler KW, Hamilton SR, Vogelstein B. Increased expression of the epidermal growth factor receptor gene in malignant gliomas is invariably associated with gene amplification. *Proc Natl Acad Sci U S A*. 1987;84(19):6899–6903.
50. Hermanson M, Funa K, Koopmann J, et al. Association of loss of heterozygosity on chromosome 17p with high platelet-derived growth factor alpha receptor expression in human malignant gliomas. *Cancer Res*. 1996;56(1):164–171.
51. Yamada SM, Yamada S, Hayashi Y, Takahashi H, Teramoto A, Matsumoto K. Fibroblast growth factor receptor (FGFR) 4 correlated with the malignancy of human astrocytomas. *Neurol Res*. 2002;24(3):244–248.
52. Koochekpour S, Jeffers M, Rulong S, et al. Met and hepatocyte growth factor/scatter factor expression in human gliomas. *Cancer Res*. 1997;57(23):5391–5398.
53. Gingras MC, Roussel E, Bruner JM, Branch CD, Moser RP. Comparison of cell adhesion molecule expression between glioblastoma multiforme and autologous normal brain tissue. *J Neuroimmunol*. 1995;57(1–2):143–153.
54. Bello L, Francolini M, Marthyn P, et al. Alpha(v)beta3 and alpha(v)beta5 integrin expression in glioma periphery. *Neurosurgery*. 2001;49(2):380–389.
55. Ding Q, Stewart JE Jr, Olman MA, Klobe MR, Gladson CL. The pattern of enhancement of Src kinase activity on platelet-derived growth factor stimulation of glioblastoma cells is affected by the integrin engaged. *J Biol Chem*. 2003;278:39882–39891.
56. Borges E, Jan Y, Ruoslahti E. Platelet derived growth factor receptor β and vascular endothelial growth factor receptor 2 bind to the β3 integrin through its extracellular domain. *J Biol Chem*. 2000;275:39867–39873.
57. Alam N, Goel HL, Zarif MJ, et al. The integrin-growth factor receptor duet. *J Cell Physiol*. 2007;213(3):649–653.
58. Lee TH, Seng S, Li H, Kennel SJ, Avraham HK, Avraham S. Integrin regulation by vascular endothelial growth factor in human brain microvascular endothelial cells: role of alpha6beta1 integrin in angiogenesis. *J Biol Chem*. 2006;281(52):40450–40460.
59. Kanamori M, Vanden B Sr, Bergers G, Berger MS, Pieper RO. Integrin beta3 overexpression suppresses tumor growth in a human model of gliomagenesis: implications for the role of beta3 overexpression in glioblastoma multiforme. *Cancer Res*. 2004;64(8):2751–2758.
60. Weber GF, Ashkar S, Glimcher MJ, Cantor H. Receptor-ligand interaction between CD44 and osteopontin (Eta-1). *Science*. 1996;271(5248):509–512.
61. Radotra B, McCormick D. Glioma invasion in vitro is mediated by CD44-hyaluronan interactions. *J Pathol*. 1997;181(4):434–438.
62. Koochekpour S, Pilkington GJ, Merzak A. Hyaluronic acid/CD44H interaction induces cell detachment and stimulates migration and invasion of human glioma cells in vitro. *Int J Cancer*. 1995;63(3):450–454.
63. Merzak A, Koocheckpour S, Pilkington GJ. CD44 mediates human glioma cell adhesion and invasion in vitro. *Cancer Res*. 1994;54(15):3988–3992.
64. Fujisaki T, Tanaka Y, Fujii K, et al. CD44 stimulation induces integrin-mediated adhesion of colon cancer cell lines to endothelial cells by up-regulation of integrins and c-Met and activation of integrins. *Cancer Res*. 1999;59(17):4427–4434.
65. Perego C, Vanoni C, Massari S, et al. Invasive behaviour of glioblastoma cell lines is associated with altered organisation of the cadherin-catenin adhesion system. *J Cell Sci*. 2002;115(pt 16):3331–3340.
66. Utsuki S, Sato Y, Oka H, Tsuchiya B, Suzuki S, Fujii K. Relationship between the expression of E-, N-cadherins and beta-catenin and tumor grade in astrocytomas. *J Neurooncol*. 2002;57(3):187–192.
67. Shinoura N, Paradies NE, Warnick RE, et al. Expression of N-cadherin and alpha-catenin in astrocytomas and glioblastomas. *Br J Cancer*. 1995;72(3):627–633.
68. Asano K, Duntsch CD, Zhou Q, et al. Correlation of N-cadherin expression in high grade gliomas with tissue invasion. *J Neurooncol*. 2004;70(1):3–15.
69. Pasquale EB. Eph receptor signalling casts a wide net on cell behaviour. *Nat Rev Mol Cell Biol*. 2005;6(6):462–475.
70. Nakada M, Niska JA, Tran NL, McDonough WS, Berens ME. EphB2/R-Ras signaling regulates glioma cell adhesion, growth, and invasion. *Am J Pathol*. 2005;167(2):565–576.
71. Nakada M, Drake KL, Nakada S, Niska JA, Berens ME. Ephrin-B3 ligand promotes glioma invasion through activation of Rac1. *Cancer Res*. 2006;66(17):8492–8500.
72. Wang LF, Fokas E, Juricko J, et al. Increased expression of EphA7 correlates with adverse outcome in primary and recurrent glioblastoma multiforme patients. *BMC Cancer*. 2008;8:79.
73. Lakka S, Rao J. Role and regulation of proteases in human gliomas. In: Lendeckel U, Hooper N, eds. *Proteases in the Brain*. New York, NY: Springer; 2005:151–177.
74. Lakka S, Rao J. Role and regulation of matrix metalloproteases in brain tumors. In: Gottschall P, ed. *MMPs in the Central Nervous System*. London: Imperial College Press; 2005:263–278.
75. Gladson CL, Pijuan-Thompson V, Olman MA, Gillespie GY, Yacoub IZ. Up-regulation of urokinase and urokinase receptor genes in malignant astrocytoma. *Am J Path*. 1995;146:1150–1160.
76. Brooks PC, Strombland S, Sanders LC, et al. Localization of matrix metalloproteinase MMP-2 to the surface of invasive cells by interaction with integrin avβ3. *Cell*. 1996;85:683–693.
77. Lu KV, Jong KA, Rajasekaran AK, Cloughesy TF, Mischel PS. Upregulation of tissue inhibitor of metalloproteinases (TIMP)-2 promotes matrix metalloproteinase (MMP)-2 activation and cell invasion in a human glioblastoma cell line. *Lab Invest*. 2004;84(1):8–20.
78. McClung HM, Thomas SL, Osenkowski P, et al. SPARC upregulates MT1-MMP expression, MMP-2 activation, and the secretion and cleavage of galectin-3 in U87MG glioma cells. *Neurosci Lett*. 2007;419(2):172–177.
79. Gonzalez EM, Reed CC, Bix G, et al. BMP-1/Tolloid-like metalloproteases process endorepellin, the angiostatic C-terminal fragment of perlecan. *J Biol Chem*. 2005;280(8):7080–7087.
80. Novak U, Stylli SS, Kaye AH, Lepperdinger G. Hyaluronidase-2 overexpression accelerates intracerebral but not subcutaneous tumor formation of murine astrocytoma cells. *Cancer Res*. 1999;59(24):6246–6250.
81. Matthews RT, Gary SC, Zerillo C, et al. Brain-enriched hyaluronan binding (BEHAB)/brevican cleavage in a glioma cell line is mediated by a disintegrin and metalloproteinase with thrombospondin motifs (ADAMTS) family member. *J Biol Chem*. 2000;275(30):22695–22703.
82. Parsons JT. Focal adhesion kinase: the first ten years. *J Cell Sci*. 2003;116(pt 8):1409–1416.
83. Cox BD, Natarajan M, Stettner MR, Gladson CL. New concepts regarding focal adhesion kinase promotion of cell migration and proliferation. *J Cell Biochem*. 2006;99(1):35–52.
84. Sieg DJ, Hauck CR, Ilick D, et al. FAK integrates growth-factor and integrin signals to promote cell migration. *Nat Cell Biol*. 2000;2:249–256.
85. Lev S, Moreno H, Martinez R, et al. Protein tyrosine kinase PYK2 involved in Ca(2+)-induced regulation of ion channel and MAP kinase functions. *Nature*. 1995;376(6543):737–745.

86. Hsia DA, Mitra SK, Hauck CR, et al. Differential regulation of cell motility and invasion by FAK. *J Cell Biol.* 2003;160(5):753–767.
87. Schlaepfer DD, Mitra SK, Ilic D. Control of motile and invasive cell phenotypes by focal adhesion kinase. *Biochim Biophys Acta.* 2004;1692(2–3):77–102.
88. Yamana N, Arakawa Y, Nishino T, et al. The Rho-mDia1 pathway regulates cell polarity and focal adhesion turnover in migrating cells through mobilizing Apc and c-Src. *Mol Cell Biol.* 2006;26(18):6844–6858.
89. Hecker TP, Grammer JR, Gillespie GY, Stewart J Jr, Gladson CL. Focal adhesion kinase enhances signaling through the Shc/extracellular signal-regulated kinase pathway in anaplastic astrocytoma tumor biopsy samples. *Cancer Res.* 2002;62(9):2699–2707.
90. Gutenberg A, Bruck W, Buchfelder M, Ludwig HC. Expression of tyrosine kinases FAK and Pyk2 in 331 human astrocytomas. *Acta Neuropathol.* 2004;108(3):224–230.
91. Riemenschneider MJ, Mueller W, Betensky RA, Mohapatra G, Louis DN. In situ analysis of integrin and growth factor receptor signaling pathways in human glioblastomas suggests overlapping relationships with focal adhesion kinase activation. *Am J Pathol.* 2005;167(5):1379–1387.
92. Natarajan M, Stewart JE, Golemis EA, et al. HEF1 is a necessary and specific downstream effector of FAK that promotes the migration of glioblastoma cells. *Oncogene.* 2006;25(12):1721–1732.
93. Lipinski CA, Tran NL, Menashi E, et al. The tyrosine kinase pyk2 promotes migration and invasion of glioma cells. *Neoplasia.* 2005;7(5):435–445.
94. Lipinski CA, Tran NL, Bay C, et al. Differential role of proline-rich tyrosine kinase 2 and focal adhesion kinase in determining glioblastoma migration and proliferation. *Mol Cancer Res.* 2003;1:323–332.
95. Lipinski CA, Tran NL, Viso C, et al. Extended survival of Pyk2 or FAK deficient orthotopic glioma xenografts. *J Neurooncol.* 2008;90(2):181–189.
96. Thomas SM, Brugge JS. Cellular functions regulated by Src family kinases. *Annu Rev Cell Dev Biol.* 1997;13:513–609.
97. Stettner MR, Wang W, Nabors LB, et al. Lyn kinase activity is the predominant cellular SRC kinase activity in glioblastoma tumor cells. *Cancer Res.* 2005;65(13):5535–5543.
98. Sakai R, Iwamatsu A, Hirano N, et al. A novel signaling molecule, p130 forms stable complex in vivo with v-Crk and c-Src in a tyrosine phosphorylation-dependent manner. *EMBO J.* 1994;13:3748–3756.
99. Law SF, Estojak J, Wang B, Mysliwiec T, Kruh G, Golemis EA. Human enhancer of filamentation 1, a novel p130 cas-like docking protein, associated with focal adhesion kinase and induces pseudohyphal growth in Saccharomyces cerevisiae. *Mol Cell Biol.* 1996;16:3327–3337.
100. Minegishi M, Tachibana K, Sato T, Iwata S, Nojima Y, Morimoto C. Structure and function of Cas-L, a 105-kD Ckr-associated substrate-related protein that is involved in beta 1 integrin-mediated signaling in lymphocytes. *J Exp Med.* 1996;184:1365–1375.
101. Merrill RA, See AW, Wertheim ML, Clagett-Dame M. Crk-associated substrate (Cas) family member, NEDD9, is regulated in human neuroblastoma cells and in the embryonic hindbrain by all-trans retinoic acid. *Dev Dyn.* 2004;231(3):564–575.
102. Ishino M, Ohba T, Sasaki H, Sasaki T. Molecular cloning of a cDNA endocing a phosphoprotein, Efs, which contains a Src homology 3 domain and associates with Fyn. *Oncogene.* 1995;11:2331–2338.
103. Alexandropoulos K, Donlin LT, Xing L, Regelmann AG. Sin: good or bad? A T lymphocyte perspective. *Immunol Rev.* 2003;192:181–195.
104. Tamura M, Gu J, Takino T, Yamada KM. Tumor suppressor PTEN inhibition of cell invasion, migration, and growth: differential involvement of focal adhesion kinase and p130Cas. *Cancer Res.* 1999;59(2):442–449.
105. Tamura M, Gu J, Tran H, Yamada KM. PTEN Gene and Integrin Signaling in Cancer. *J Natl Cancer Inst.* 1999;91(21):1820–1828.
106. Gu J, Tamura M, Pankov R, et al. Shc and FAK differentially regulate cell motility and directionality modulated by PTEN. *J Cell Biol.* 1999;146(2):389–403.
107. Takino T, Nakada M, Miyamori H, Yamashita J, Yamada KM, Sato H. CrkI adapter protein modulates cell migration and invasion in glioblastoma. *Cancer Res.* 2003;63(9):2335–2337.
108. Ling J, Liu Z, Wang D, Gladson CL. Malignant astrocytoma cell attachment and migration to various matrix proteins is differentially sensitive to phosphoinositide 3-OH kinase inhibitors. *J Cell Biochem.* 1999;73(4):533–544.
109. Wei Q, Clarke L, Scheidenhelm DK, et al. High-grade glioma formation results from postnatal PTEN loss or mutant epidermal growth factor receptor expression in a transgenic mouse glioma model. *Cancer Res.* 2006;66(15):7429–7437.
110. Whetton AD, Lu Y, Pierce A, Carney L, Spooncer E. Lysophospholipids synergistically promote primitive hematopoietic cell chemotaxis via a mechanism involving Vav 1. *Blood.* 2003;102(8):2798–2802.
111. Ojaniemi M, Vuori K. Epidermal growth factor modulates tyrosine phosphorylation of p130Cas. Involvement of phosphatidylinositol 3′-kinase and actin cytoskeleton. *J Biol Chem.* 1997;272(41):25993–25998.
112. Besson A, Davy A, Robbins SM, Yong VW. Differential activation of ERKs to focal adhesions by PKC epsilon is required for PMA-induced adhesion and migration of human glioma cells. *Oncogene.* 2001;20(50):7398–7407.
113. Bigner DD, Brown MT, Friedman AH, et al. Iodine-131-labeled antitenascin monoclonal antibody 81C6 treatment of patients with recurrent malignant gliomas: phase I trial results. *J Clin Oncol.* 1998;16(6):2202–2212.
114. Reardon DA, Akabani G, Coleman RE, et al. Phase II trial of murine (131)I-labeled antitenascin monoclonal antibody 81C6 administered into surgically created resection cavities of patients with newly diagnosed malignant gliomas. *J Clin Oncol.* 2002;20(5):1389–1397.
115. Pelloski CE, Mahajan A, Maor M, et al. YKL-40 expression is associated with poorer response to radiation and shorter overall survival in glioblastoma. *Clin Cancer Res.* 2005;11(9):3326–3334.
116. Chen H, Strickland DK, Mosher DF. Metabolism of thrombospondin 2. Binding and degradation by 3t3 cells and glycosaminoglycan-variant Chinese hamster ovary cells. *J Biol Chem.* 1996;271(27):15993–15999.
117. Armstrong L, Bornstein P. Thrombospondin 1 and 2 function as inhibitors of angiogenesis. *Matrix Biol.* 2003;22:63–71.
118. Bein K, Simons M. Thrombospondin type 1 repeats interact with matrix metalloproteinase-2. Regulation of metalloproteinase activity. *J Biol Chem.* 2000;275:32167–32173.
119. Fears CY, Grammer JR, Stewart JE Jr, et al. Low-density lipoprotein receptor-related protein contributes to the antiangiogenic activity of thrombospondin-2 in a murine glioma model. *Cancer Res.* 2005;65(20):9338–9346.
120. Pijuan-Thompson V, Gladson CL. Ligation of integrin a5ß1 is required for internalization of vitronectin by integrin avß3. *J Biol Chem.* 1997;272(5):2736–2743.
121. Raychaudhuri B, Han Y, Lu T, Vogelbaum MA. Aberrant constitutive activation of nuclear factor kappaB in glioblastoma multiforme drives invasive phenotype. *J Neurooncol.* 2007;85(1):39–47.
122. Ritchie CK, Giordano A, Khalili K. Integrin involvement in glioblastoma multiforme: possible regulation by NF-kappaB. *J Cell Physiol.* 2000;184(2):214–221.
123. Wang MY, Lu KV, Zhu S, et al. Mammalian target of rapamycin inhibition promotes response to epidermal growth factor receptor kinase inhibitors in PTEN-deficient and PTEN-intact glioblastoma cells. *Cancer Res.* 2006;66(16):7864–7869.
124. Mellinghoff IK, Cloughesy TF, Mischel PS. PTEN-mediated resistance to epidermal growth factor receptor kinase inhibitors. *Clin Cancer Res.* 2007;13(2 pt 1):378–381.
125. Hoelzinger DB, Demuth T, Berens ME. Autocrine factors that sustain glioma invasion and paracrine biology in the brain microenvironment. *J Natl Cancer Inst.* 2007;99(21):1583–1593.
126. Liu WM, Zhang XA. KAI1/CD82, a tumor metastasis suppressor. *Cancer Lett.* 2006;240(2):183–194.
127. Beadle C, Assanah MC, Monzo P, Vallee R, Rosenfeld SS, Canoll P. The Role of myosin II in glioma invasion of the brain. *Mol Biol Cell.* 2008;19(8):3357–3368.
128. Markovic DS, Glass R, Synowitz M, Rooijen N, Kettenmann H. Microglia stimulate the invasiveness of glioma cells by increasing the activity of metalloprotease-2. *J Neuropathol Exp Neurol.* 2005;64(9):754–762.
129. Le DM, Besson A, Fogg DK, et al. Exploitation of astrocytes by glioma cells to facilitate invasiveness: a mechanism involving matrix metalloproteinase-2 and the urokinase-type plasminogen activator-plasmin cascade. *J Neurosci.* 2003;23(10):4034–4043.
130. Assanah M, Lochhead R, Ogden A, Bruce J, Goldman J, Canoll P. Glial progenitors in adult white matter are driven to form malignant gliomas by platelet-derived growth factor-expressing retroviruses. *J Neurosci.* 2006;26(25):6781–6790.

131. Lee J, Kotliarova S, Kotliarov Y, et al. Tumor stem cells derived from glioblastomas cultured in bFGF and EGF more closely mirror the phenotype and genotype of primary tumors than do serum-cultured cell lines. *Cancer Cell.* 2006;9(5):391–403.
132. Dirks PB. Cancer: stem cells and brain tumours. *Nature.* 2006;444(7120):687–688.
133. Gilbertson RJ, Rich JN. Making a tumour's bed: glioblastoma stem cells and the vascular niche. *Nat Rev Cancer.* 2007;7(10):733–736.
134. Mariani L, McDonough WS, Hoelzinger DB, et al. Identification and validation of P311 as a glioblastoma invasion gene using laser capture microdissection. *Cancer Res.* 2001;61(10):4190–4196.
135. Tran NL, McDonough WS, Savitch BA, et al. Increased fibroblast growth factor-inducible 14 expression levels promote glioma cell invasion via Rac1 and nuclear factor-kappaB and correlate with poor patient outcome. *Cancer Res.* 2006;66(19):9535–9542.
136. Demuth T, Reavie LB, Rennert JL, et al. MAP-ing glioma invasion: mitogen-activated protein kinase kinase 3 and p38 drive glioma invasion and progression and predict patient survival. *Mol Cancer Ther.* 2007;6(4):1212–1222.
137. McDonough WS, Tran NL, Berens ME. Regulation of glioma cell migration by serine-phosphorylated P311. *Neoplasia.* 2005;7(9):862–872.

16 Molecular Basis of Glioma Neovascularization and Its Therapeutic Applications

Jean-Pierre Gagner, John G. Golfinos, Jerome J. Graber, and David Zagzag

INTRODUCTION

> The glial cells [of glioblastoma multiforme] vary greatly, but there is one constant finding in these tumors and that is the endothelial and adventitial hyperplasia of the vessels which is practically always present.... I think it is quite possible that often the vessel change is primary and the polymorphism of neoplastic cells secondary to the consequent rapid alteration in blood supply. On the other hand, the vessel change is not wholly responsible for the growth, for the neoplastic cells themselves metastasize through the spinal fluid.
>
> *Dr. Wilder Penfield in 1935 [1].*

Early observations and histological analyses of brain tumors drew attention to the impressive number of blood vessels in a tumor mass, most commonly seen in the more malignant tumors like glioblastoma multiforme (GBM). They also raised fundamental questions about their biological significance, for example, whether these vascular structures were "being part and parcel of the neoplastic process?" [1]. Possibly some of the greatest advances in the biology of cancer came many years later with the demonstration that solid tumors are endowed with angiogenic capability and that their growth, invasion, and metastasis depend on the formation of new blood vessels [2–4]. Judah Folkman introduced the concept that tumors probably secrete diffusible angiogenic molecules that could stimulate the growth of new blood vessels toward the tumor and that the resulting tumor neovascularization could conceivably be prevented or interrupted by angiogenesis inhibitors. Through various mechanisms, acquisition of this angiogenic capability can be seen as an expression of progression from neoplastic transformation to tumor growth and metastasis and is considered one of the functional hallmarks of most, if not all, cancer development [5]. Promotion and regulation of new blood vessel formation are essential not only for cancer but for organ growth and repair and for numerous ischemic, inflammatory, infectious, and immune disorders [6–8]. The process of blood vessel growth and tissue vascularization encompasses primarily two distinct mechanisms: *angiogenesis*, the proliferation and migration of mature, differentiated endothelial cells resulting in sprouting and remodeling of capillaries from preexisting vessels, and *vasculogenesis*, the de novo assembly of capillaries from undifferentiated endothelial precursors and other hematopoietic progenitors, not only in the embryo but also probably in adults [6–8]. Although neovascularization of glioma tumors (Figure 16.1) [9–18] has been demonstrated to occur via angiogenesis [15,19], recent experimental evidence suggests that vasculogenesis may play an important role in this process and involve the mobilization and recruitment of bone marrow-derived proangiogenic cells to the tumor vascular bed as well [20–22].

Preceded by the intense research on the biological significance and the mechanisms of tumor neovascularization, we are assisting in the development and application of new antiangiogenic therapies in the clinical setting in combination with standard treatments for patients with gliomas [23–26]. However, several challenging issues, such as assessing tumor neovascularization and its therapeutic response in patients and counteracting tumor escape from antiangiogenic therapies, currently limit the benefit of this new therapeutic approach. In this chapter, we summarize the current understanding of the molecular and cellular mechanisms of neovascularization in gliomas and the lessons from clinical studies using antiangiogenic therapies in patients with gliomas. We also discuss the challenges and potential directions of these efforts.

ANGIOGENESIS IN GLIOMAS

Molecular Pathology of Gliomas

The World Health Organization (WHO) classification distinguishes low-grade (I–II) from high-grade (III–IV) gliomas based on histopathological features that include high vascular density, "glomeruloid" microvascular proliferation, pseudopalisading cells, and necrosis, which have also been identified as independent prognostic indicators [27,28]. Vascular proliferation in brain tumors correlates with the contrast enhancement and peritumoral edematous changes seen on gadolinium-enhanced magnetic resonance imaging (MRI) and predicts biological aggressiveness of the tumors, time to progression, and patient survival [23,28]. GBM (WHO Grade IV) can either evolve from a lower-grade precursor tumor (secondary GBM) over a variable time interval of several years or present as a high-grade lesion from the outset, so-called de novo

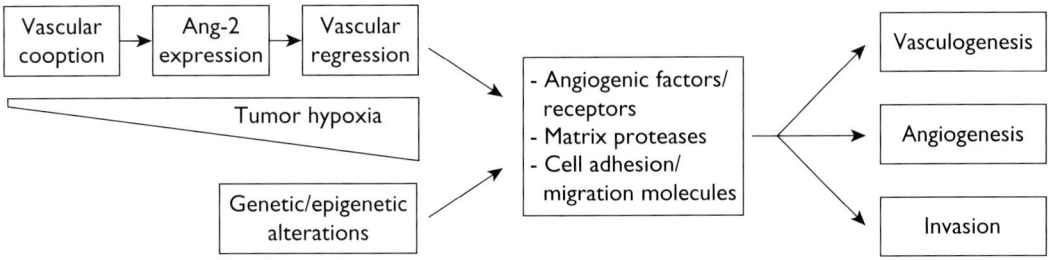

Figure 16.1 Molecular mechanisms by which tumor hypoxia and genetic/epigenetic alterations promote tumor neovascularization, invasion, and growth. In gliomas, as tumor cells first accumulate around existing vasculature (see Figure 16.2), the endothelial cells of the co-opted blood vessels express angiopoietin-2 (Ang-2), which leads to the destabilization of the blood vessel wall, vascular regression, and necrosis [9,10]. Tumor cells respond to decreased tissue O_2 level by increasing hypoxia-inducible factor (HIF)-1 transcriptional activity, which induces adaptive changes in gene expression patterns (e.g., increased vascular endothelial growth factor [VEGF] and its receptors [VEGFR]) that result in enhanced tumor angiogenesis, vasculogenesis, invasion, and survival [11–14]. In addition, genetic alterations, such as gain-of-function mutations in oncogenes (e.g., epidermal growth factor receptor [EGFR]), loss-of-function mutations in tumor-suppressor genes (e.g., phosphatase and tensin homologue [PTEN], p53), and chromosomal alterations accumulate in tumor cells that lead to O_2-independent increase in HIF-1 activity associated with similar changes in gene expression patterns [15,16]. Severe intratumoral hypoxia itself can induce genetic instability that can result in genetic and chromosomal alterations [17,18]. These adaptive responses have been associated with tumor growth advantage, increased malignancy, as well as treatment resistance and failure [12,13].

or primary GBM. Molecular genetic studies suggest that GBMs are composed of multiple molecular genetic subsets [28–30]. Notwithstanding the diversity of genetic changes leading to the GBM phenotype, the vascular changes that evolve in this disease, presumably favoring further growth, are morphologically indistinguishable. Underlying genetic changes in GBM may tilt the balance in favor of an angiogenic phenotype by upregulation of proangiogenic factors and downregulation of endogenous angiogenic inhibitors [15,19,31]. Increased vascularity and endothelial cell proliferation in GBMs are also driven by hypoxia-induced expression of proangiogenic cytokines, such as vascular endothelial growth factor (VEGF).

In vivo experimental models with orthotopic gliomas (C6 and GL261 cells) provided evidence for the sequential progression of glioma angiogenesis in which co-option, the adoption of preexisting vessels by migrating tumor cells, precedes true angiogenesis. As illustrated in Figure 16.2, glioma cells first accumulate around existing vasculature (stage I). In response, the endothelial cells of the co-opted blood vessels express angiopoietin-2 (Ang-2) [9,10,32]. This leads to the destabilization of the blood vessel wall associated with decreased pericyte coverage. In stage II, perivascular proliferation takes place. In stage III, these blood vessels become apoptotic and undergo involution with vascular collapse and loss of neighboring tumor cells [9,10,32]. In addition, a procoagulant state associated with vascular thrombosis may contribute to the necrosis observed in GBMs [33,34]. In stage IV, angiogenic sprouting and remodeling adjacent to the necrotic area is triggered in response to increased tumor hypoxia and expression of hypoxia-inducible factor (HIF)-1α and VEGF in pseudopalisading tumor cells around the areas of necrosis, a process that rescues the remaining tumor cells [9,11]. These results suggest that the sequence of events leading to angiogenesis begins with Ang-2 expression in co-opted vessels, followed by vascular regression leading to hypoxia, which results in HIF-1α activation, VEGF synthesis and secretion in pseudopalisading tumor cells and angiogenesis. Based on this experimental model, it appears that human astrocytomas first acquire their blood supply by co-opting existing normal brain blood vessels without initiating angiogenesis necessarily. They instead grow along blood vessels. When Grade III gliomas progress into GBM, they become hypoxic and necrotic, partly due to vessel regression and increased tumor cell proliferation. These conditions, in turn, induce formation of new blood vessels that results in the growth of the tumors [2–4].

Angiogenesis and its Regulation by Tumor Hypoxia and Metabolism

Angiogenesis is the process of new vessel sprouting from existing vessels, a normal part of embryonic development and wound healing, as well as malignancies, which depends on the balance of various factors that influence endothelial and supporting cell survival and activity [6–8]. This process depends on the disassembly of an existing endothelium and its supporting pericytes and extracellular matrix (ECM), followed by endothelial cell proliferation and the reassembly of a new vascular wall and ECM. However, most solid tumors are subjected to low oxygen or hypoxic environments because of a combination of rapid growth, high oxygen consumption, and inadequate blood supply. Cellular sensing of oxygen tension drives the coordinated expression of the signals necessary for angiogenesis to occur, largely mediated by hydroxylation of the transcription factor HIF α-subunit by the hydroxylase factor-inhibiting HIF (FIH-1) and prolyl hydroxylase domain (PHD) enzymes [12,13,35].

The HIF-1 transcriptional complex is a heterodimer composed of two basic helix loop helix-Per/ARNT/Sim

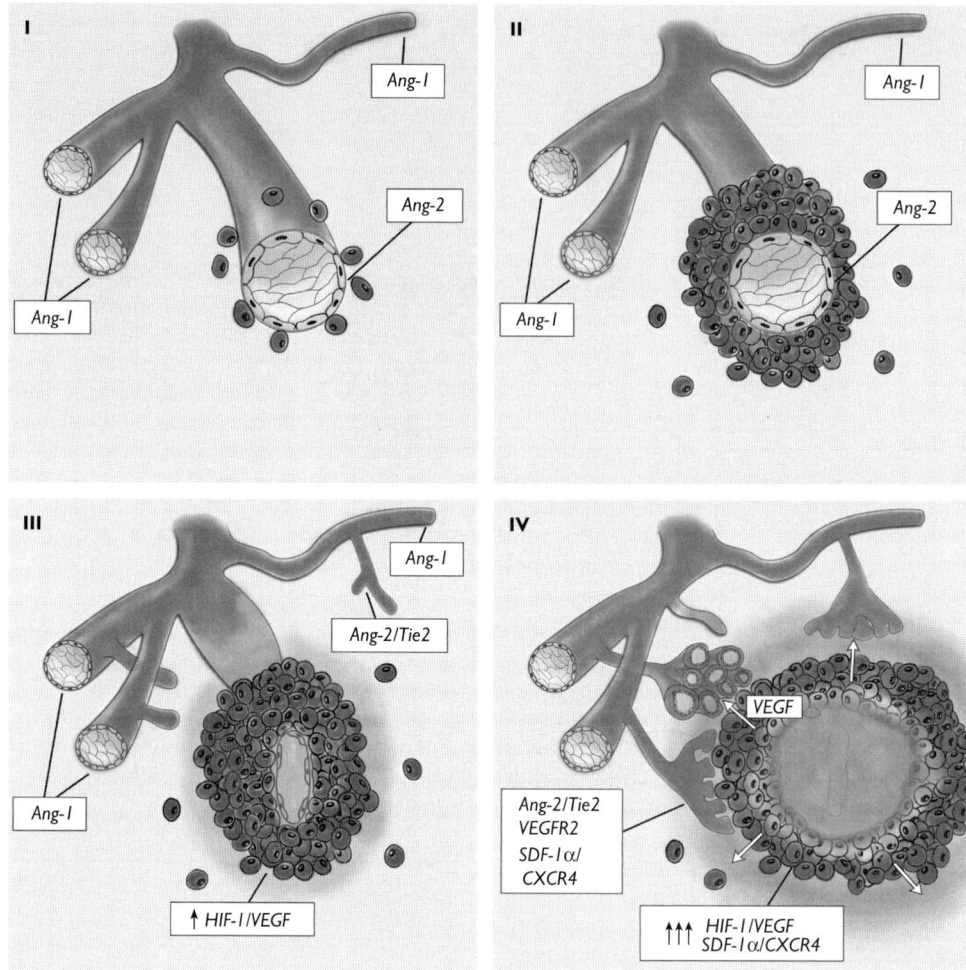

Figure 16.2 Distinct stages of glioma neovascularization in a murine model. Stage I (day 7 post-tumor implantation): *Perivascular organization* in which tumor cells aggregate around some native cerebral vessels, thereby inducing angiopoietin-2 (Ang-2) expression in vascular endothelial cells. Quiescent vessel endothelium expresses Ang-1. Stage II (day 14): *Tumor proliferation* phase during which tumor cells actively proliferate around existing viable blood vessels. Stage III (day 21): *Vascular involution* resulting in degeneration of blood vessels. This leads to focal thrombosis, necrosis, and hypoxia, which in turn promotes hypoxia-inducible factor (HIF-1)-regulated gene expression and early vascular sprouting, associated with expression of Ang-2 and Tie-2, the Ang receptor. Stage IV (day 28): *Angiogenesis* occurs as blood vessels grow toward and vascularize the tumor cells around necrotic areas. These pseudopalisading cells show stabilization of HIF-1α and release vascular endothelial growth factor (VEGF) and stromal cell-derived factor (SDF)-1α, leading to the induction of angiogenesis in neighboring blood vessels. These vessels express Ang-2 and SDF-1α. See color insert.

domain subunits, HIF-1α and HIF-1β (also termed aryl hydrocarbon nuclear translocator [ARNT]) [12,13]. Three HIF-α isoforms have been described, with the best characterized being HIF-1α and HIF-2α [36,37]. Although the β-subunit of HIF-1 is constitutively expressed, the α-subunit is subject to complex regulatory mechanisms at the transcriptional, posttranscriptional and posttranslational level [38–40]. In the presence of adequate oxygen levels, hydroxylation of HIF-1α at an asparagyl residue catalyzed by FIH-1 inhibits its transcriptional activity by preventing the recruitment of coactivator p300/CBP (cAMP-response element-binding protein [CREB]-binding protein). Also, hydroxylation of HIF-1α at prolyl residues by PHD isozymes allows for binding of the von Hippel-Lindau protein (pVHL), which mediates ubiquitination of HIF-1α and subsequent proteasomal degradation. However, when oxygen levels are inadequate for cellular growth, these hydroxylases are inactive, resulting in accumulation of the constitutively expressed HIF-1α protein. On phosphorylation by extracellular signal-related protein kinase (ERK)-1/2, the alpha subunit is translocated to the nucleus, where it dimerizes with the β-subunit, recruits p300/CBP, binds to hypoxia-response elements (HREs) in the promoter region of a wide array of HIF-1-regulated target genes, and initiates their transcription [12,41,42]. Additional hypoxia-responsive transcription factors integrate with HIF-1 or HIF-2 in their response to angiogenic stimuli [43] including activator protein-1 [44], early growth response gene-1 [45], and v-ets erythroblastosis virus E26 oncogene homolog 1 (ETS-1) [46,47]. Nuclear factor κB transcriptional activity [48] may involve posttranslational hydroxylation of inhibitor of κB proteins by oxygen-dependent FIH-1 [49]. Finally, posttranscriptional and posttranslational regulation of HIF-1α has also been described, including c-myc-mediated repression of HIF-1α mRNA translation through induction of miR-17–92 microRNA (miRNA) cluster [50] and acetylation, phosphorylation, and SUMOylation of HIF-1α protein [51].

These gene products promote numerous aspects of tumor progression, including angiogenesis, cellular metabolism and mitochondrial function, proliferation and survival, and ECM function and motility [12,15,41]. In particular, we and others have noted a correlation between increased HIF-1 expression and advanced disease stage, increased angiogenesis, and poor prognosis [11,52]. Moreover, the expression of HIF-2α is upregulated in GBMs both at the mRNA and protein levels [36,37]. As a result, HIF-1/2, its signaling pathways, and gene products have become targets for the development of cancer antiangiogenic therapy [12,13,53].

In contrast to normal cells, cancer cells, including gliomas, exhibit a high glycolytic rate even under aerobic conditions sufficient to maintain mitochondrial function (Warburg effect) [54,55]. As illustrated in Figure 16.3, HIF-1 has been implicated in regulating many of the genes responsible for the metabolic difference [13,41]; its activation by tumor hypoxia and/or nonhypoxic oncogenic events (discussed under Angiogenesis and Genetic/Epigenetic Alterations) leads to the metabolic reprogramming of tumor cells [83,84]. In addition, non–HIF-1-dependent mechanisms contribute to the angiogenic response at the posttranscriptional, translational, and posttranslational levels [78,80,85,86]. Recent findings underscore the clinical significance of the regulation of angiogenesis by cellular metabolism. For example, mutations in the isocitrate dehydrogenase (IDH) genes, IDH1 (cytoplasmic) and IDH2 (mitochondrial), are implicated in the pathogenesis of malignant gliomas [59,60]. HIF-1-regulated glucose transporter-1 is an independent prognostic indicator in patients with gliomas [56]. Glioma stem cells have been linked to hypoxic environments [87,88], and neural stem cells preferentially migrate to sites with oxygen deprivation [89]. Finally, tumor hypoxia has also been implicated in the mechanisms of evasion of solid tumors to antiangiogenic therapy [90–92], in addition to its known association with resistance to both radiotherapy and chemotherapy.

Angiopoietins and VEGFs

Among the proangiogenic factors produced by gliomas, the most important in tumor progression include the Angs and VEGFs [15,19,31]. The receptor tyrosine kinase with immunoglobulin and epidermal growth factor homology domain 2 (Tie2) and its ligands, the Angs, play an essential role in vascular development and glioma-associated angiogenesis [15,93,94]. The Angs constitute a family of angiogenic factors that include Ang-1 and Ang-2 that bind competitively to Tie2 [9]. While the binding of Ang-1 to Tie2 promotes survival of endothelial cells and stabilizes their interactions with vascular pericytes, the binding of Ang-2 to Tie2 antagonizes Ang-1 binding and destabilizes endothelial cells from the vessel wall, a necessary step for new vessel sprouting [93]. Ang-2 induces vascular regression in the absence of VEGF [9]. Ang-2 expression is induced in the endothelium of co-opted tumor vessels prior to their regression [9,10,32,95]. Tie2 expression is increased in the vasculature of gliomas, its levels correlate with increasing tumor grade, and its inhibition results in decreased tumor growth in animal models [96–98]. Ang-2 expression also promotes glioma cell invasiveness [9,32,93,99]. In response to hypoxia, Ang-2 is induced through HIF-1 binding to an HRE in the first intron of the Ang-2 gene [100]. Conversely, Ang-2 reduced VEGF expression by modulating HIF-1α levels, demonstrating the intrinsic coordination among these factors in angiogenesis [101].

Central nervous system (CNS) tumors stimulate angiogenesis through processes driven primarily by the potent angiogenic factor VEGF [15,19,31,102]. The VEGF family consists of five members: VEGF-A (referred to here as VEGF), VEGF-B, VEGF-C, VEGF-D, and placental growth factor (PlGF). VEGF and its receptors (VEGFR) are increased in malignant gliomas and their expression displays a temporal and spatial relationship with angiogenesis and correlates with tumor grade [103–105]. VEGF also increases vascular permeability, leading to increased interstitial fluid pressure and vasogenic edema [106,107]. Of the several spliced forms of VEGF, $VEGF_{165}$ is predominant in GBMs [108]. VEGF mRNA is highly expressed in the hypoxic pseudopalisading cells around areas of necrosis, one of the hallmarks of GBM pathology [109,110]. Tumor cells are the major source of VEGF, but endothelial cells also express VEGF to a lesser extent [110]. Increased VEGF levels also appear to stimulate migration of glioma cells by inducing stromal cell-derived factor (SDF)-1α expression [14]. Similarly, PlGF is upregulated in GBMs, correlates with tumor grade and acts synergistically with VEGF in increasing tumor vascularization [111–113].

There are three cognate VEGF receptor tyrosine kinases, VEGFR-1/FLT-1, VEGFR-2/Flk-1/KDR, and VEGFR-3 [102,114–116], and two VEGFR coreceptors, the neuropilins (NRP)-1 and NRP-2 [117–119]. Inhibition of VEGF binding to VEGFR or its intracellular signaling pathways reduces angiogenesis in animal models of glioma [120–122]. The effect of VEGF signaling including increased vascular permeability and proliferation, differentiation, survival, and migration of endothelial cells depends on the receptor subtype [102,114–116]. For example, angiogenesis is mainly mediated through VEGFR-2, which activates the phosphatidylinositol 3-kinase (PI3K)/Akt and Ras-mitogen-activated protein kinase (MEK)-1/2 pathways, leading to proliferation and activation of several integrins stimulating cell adhesion and migration. VEGFR-1 acts as a positive regulator of angiogenesis by inducing endothelial cell protease and growth factor expression [102,123–125].

NRP receptors are also expressed in malignant gliomas. NRP-1 is expressed on endothelial cells and on tumor cells [126], and its expression correlates with glioma grade [117–119]. Although NRP-1 enhances the binding of VEGF to VEGFR-2 [127], it may also regulate endothelial

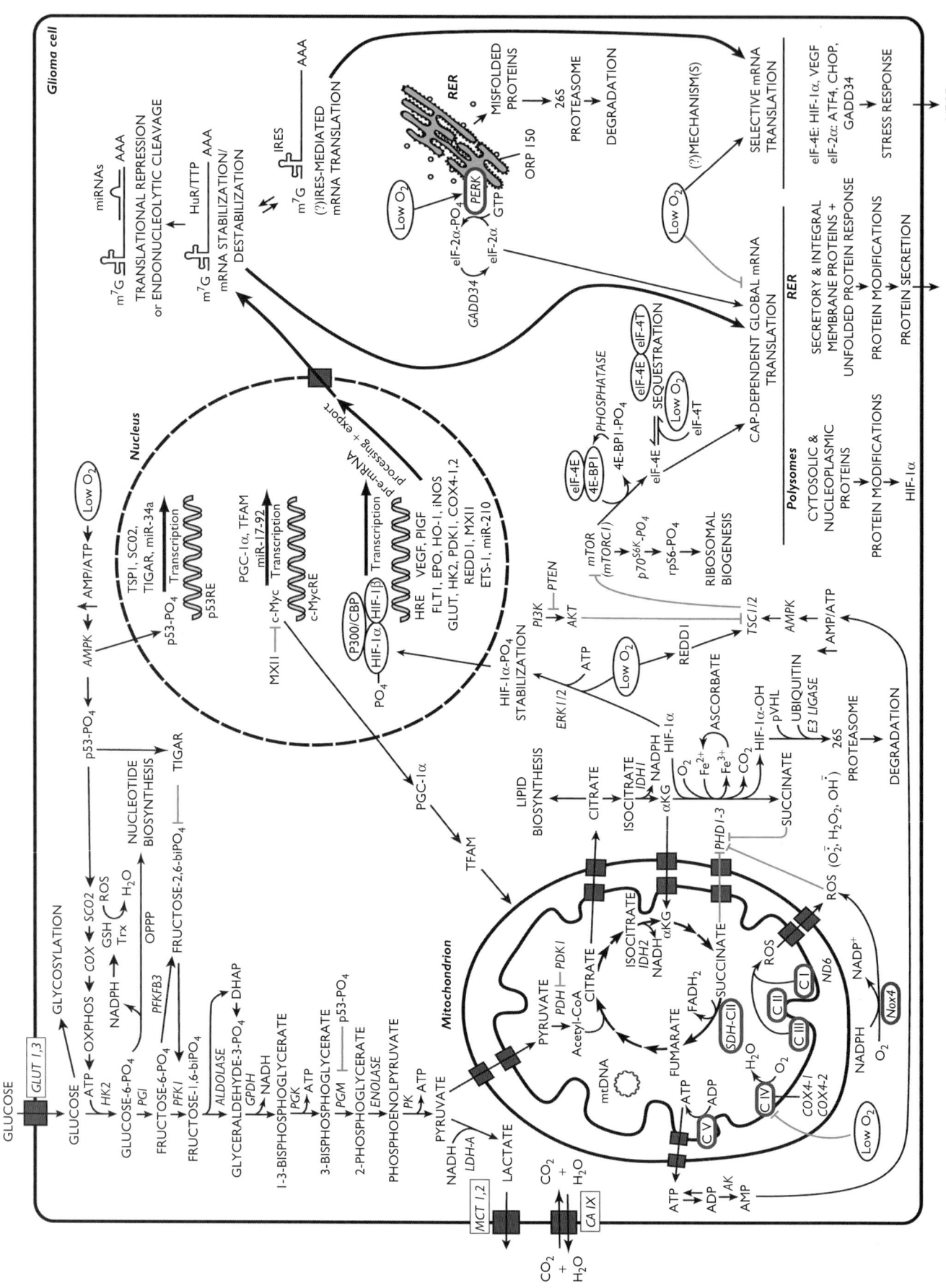

Figure 16.3 Tumor hypoxia selectively suppresses cellular energy metabolism and biosynthetic machinery through hypoxia-inducible factor (HIF)-dependent and independent mechanisms. In contrast to normal cells, cancer cells including glioma avidly consume glucose to produce pyruvate and lactate, even in conditions of adequate oxygenation (Warburg effect). HIF-1 has been implicated in regulating many of the genes responsible for the metabolic difference [13,41,56]; its activation by tumor hypoxia and/or nonhypoxic oncogenic events leads to an increase in some metabolic pathways (glucose uptake, glycolysis, lactate secretion) and a decrease in others (mitochondrial functions owing to HIF-1-dependent pyruvate dehydrogenase kinase-I [PDKI] induction, decreased mitochondrial biogenesis through MAX interactor 1 [MXII] induction [which antagonizes c-myc activity], and switched cytochrome oxidase subunit 4 isoform 1 [COX4–1] to the high-efficiency COX4–2 isoform to minimize reactive oxygen species [ROS] production). In normoxic conditions, O_2-dependent hydroxylation of HIF-1α subunits by prolyl hydroxylase domain (PHD) proteins-1 to 3 or by factor-inhibiting HIF (FIH)-1 (not shown) targets HIF-1α to degradation by the ubiquitin-proteasome system or inhibits its transcriptional activity, respectively. These hydroxylase activities are regulated by Krebs cycle metabolites (α-ketoglutarate, succinate, fumarate) [57] and by ROS produced by O_2-dependent nicotinamide adenine dinucleotide phosphate (NADPH) oxidase (Nox). Overexpression of Nox 4 [58] and mutations in isocitrate dehydrogenase (IDH) 1 and 2 [59,60] and mitochondrial complex I NADH dehydrogenase subunit 6 (ND6) [61] may occur in gliomas, possibly altering their regional hypoxic response [62]. In response to energy depletion (elevated AMP:ATP ratio) secondary to hypoxia, AMP-activated protein kinase (AMPK) inhibits mammalian target of rapamycin (mTOR) activity, thereby reducing eukaryotic translation initiation factor eIF-4E availability and cap-dependent global mRNA translation [63–65]. In addition, AMPK activates p53-dependent modulation of glycolysis and respiration by stimulating synthesis of cytochrome c oxidase-2 (SCO2) and Tp53-inducible glycolysis and apoptosis regulator [TIGAR], thereby enhancing the elimination of ROS by the NADPH-generating oxidative phase of the pentose phosphate pathway (OPPP) [66–68]. Mitochondrial biogenesis, which is controlled by c-myc-regulated mitochondrial transcription factor A (TFAM), is enhanced in glioma because of the formation of an alternately transcribed inhibitor of c-myc (MXII–0) [69,70]. HIF-1-regulated mRNA transcripts may also be regulated posttranscriptionally by mRNA-binding proteins (stability factor HuR, decay factor TTP) [38,71,72] and by microRNAs [50,73–75]. Responses to hypoxia also include the endoplasmic reticulum (ER) unfolded protein response (UPR) through activation of pancreatic ER kinase (PKR)-like ER kinase (PERK), which phosphorylates eIF-2α, also causing inhibition of cap-dependent global mRNA translation [76–79]. However, mRNAs such as HIF-1α, vascular endothelial growth factor (VEGF), and activating transcription factor 4 (ATF4) are selectively translated through incompletely characterized mechanisms, possibly involving utilization of mRNA internal ribosomal entry sites (IRESs) [78,80]. Finally, ER-resident chaperone molecule 150 kDa O_2-regulated protein (ORP-150) participates in VEGF protein folding prior to secretion [81,82]. These metabolic pathways have been implicated in tumor angiogenesis, but not all of them have been studied in gliomas. In this diagram, gene products regulated by HIF-1 are indicated in BLUE, and genetic or chromosomal abnormalities in RED. Inhibitory effect of a product is indicated by a BLUNT ENDED RED LINE.

Abbreviations: AAA, polyadenylate tail; AcetylCoA, acetyl coenzyme A; AK, adenylate kinase; αKG, α-ketoglutarate; AMP, adenosine-5′-monophosphate; ATP, adenosine-5′-triphosphate; C1 - CV, respiratory chain complexes I to V; CA IX, carbonic anhydrase IX; CHOP, CCAAT/enhancer-binding protein homologous protein; c-mycRE, c-myc-response element; COX4–1,2, cytochrome c oxidase subunit 4 isoform 1,2; DHAP, dihydroxyacetone phosphate; 4E-BP1, eukaryotic translation initiation factor 4E (eIF-4E)-binding protein 1; eIF-2α/4E/4T, eukaryotic translation initiation factor-2α/4E/4T; EPO, erythropoietin; ERK1/2, extracellular signal-regulated protein kinase-1/2; ETS-1, v-ets erythroblastosis virus E26 oncogene homolog 1; FLT-1, fms-related tyrosine kinase 1/VEGF receptor 1; GADD34, growth arrest and DNA-damage-inducible gene 34; GPDH, glyceraldehyde 3-phosphate dehydrogenase; GSH, glutathione; GTP, guanosine-5′-triphosphate; HK2, hexokinase-2; HRE, hypoxia-response element; HuR, human antigen R; IRES, internal ribosome entry site; LDH-A, lactate dehydrogenase-A; m7G, N7-methylguanosine; MCT-1,2, monocarboxylate transporter-1,2; miRNA, microRNA; mtDNA, mitochondrial DNA; mTOR(C1), mammalian target of rapamycin (complex 1); MXII, MAX interactor 1; NAD(P), nicotinamide adenine dinucleotide (phosphate); OPPP, oxidative phase of pentose phosphate pathway; ORP-150, 150 kDa oxygen-regulated protein; OXPHOS, oxidative phosphorylation; p53RE, p53-response element; p70S6K, 70 kDa ribosomal protein S6 kinase; P300/CBP, cAMP-response element-binding protein (CREB) binding protein; PDH, pyruvate dehydrogenase; PDK1, pyruvate dehydrogenase kinase-1; PERK, pancreatic ER kinase (PKR)-like ER kinase; PFK1, phosphofructokinase-1; PFKFB3, 6-phosphofructo-2-kinase/fructose-2,6-bisphosphatase-3; PGI, phosphoglucose isomerase; PGK, phosphoglycerate kinase; PGM, phosphoglycerate mutase; PHD1–3, HIF-1α prolyl hydroxylase domain proteins-1 to 3; PK, pyruvate kinase; pVHL, protein von Hippel-Lindau; REDD1, regulated in development and DNA damage responses-1; RER, rough endoplasmic reticulum; rpS6, ribosomal protein S6; SCO2, synthesis of cytochrome c oxidase-2; TFAM, mitochondrial transcription factor A; TIGAR, Tp53-inducible glycolysis and apoptosis regulator; Trx, thioredoxin; TSC1/2, tuberous sclerosis complex-1/2; TSP-1, thrombospondin-1; TTP, tristetraprolin. See color insert.

cell migration and attachment independently of VEGFR-2 [128,129].

As we discussed earlier, under hypoxic conditions, the expression of VEGF is enhanced largely through the transcription factor HIF-1 [12,13]. However, other transcription factors regulate VEGF, including the ETS-1 proto-oncogene and signal transducer and activator of transcription (STAT-3) [130–132]. HIF-1-independent upregulation of VEGF by the transcriptional coactivator peroxisome proliferator-activated receptor γ coactivator (PGC)-1α has recently been demonstrated [133]. In addition, genetic alterations seen in gliomas, for example, epidermal growth factor receptor (EGFR) amplification and phosphatase and tensin homologue (PTEN) mutation, lead to enhanced VEGF expression [29,134–136].

Other Endogenous Angiogenic Factors

A number of other factors stimulate VEGF expression and angiogenesis in gliomas [15,19,137,138] such as epidermal growth factor (EGF), basic fibroblast growth factor (bFGF) [139], platelet-derived growth factors (PDGFs) [140,141], tumor necrosis factor-α [142], interleukin-6 [132], insulin [143], tissue factor [144], thrombin [145], stem cell factor [146], and delta-like 4 ligand [147,148]. Although several angiogenic factors (e.g., VEGF, Ang-1/2) directly stimulate angiogenesis via binding to receptors on vascular cells (endothelial, pericyte), others act indirectly by triggering tumor cells (e.g., EGF) or other cell types (Ang on Tie 2-expressing monocytes [TEMs], discussed under Vasculogenesis in Gliomas) to release angiogenic factors onto vascular cells.

Scatter Factor/Hepatocyte Growth Factor, and c-Met

Expression of scatter factor (SF), also known as hepatocyte growth factor (HGF), and its tyrosine kinase receptor c-Met play an important role not only in embryogenesis and development but also in angiogenesis and glioma growth [149–151]. SF/HGF directly or indirectly stimulates angiogenesis by regulating cell adhesion, migration, survival, and proliferation. Enhanced SF/HGF expression correlates with glioma tumor grade [152]. In animal models of glioma, SF/HGF increases tumor growth and angiogenesis by enabling degradation of the existing ECM matrix via matrix metalloprotease and urokinase production, stimulating endothelial cell migration and proliferation and promoting tubule formation [153,154]. SF/HGF is expressed in tumor blood vessels, upregulates VEGF and its receptor, and downregulates antiangiogenic thrombospondin-1 (TSP-1) [154,155]. SF/HGF has also been shown to be capable of inducing angiogenesis even in the setting of VEGF inhibition [156]. Blockade of SF/HGF or c-Met activity in animal models reduced glioma growth, inhibited angiogenesis, and prolonged survival [152,157–159]. Factors known to enhance VEGF function, including NRP-1 and transforming growth factor-β, have also been shown to enhance SF/HGF expression and activity [160,161]. The SF/HGF c-Met is part of a signaling complex acting in cooperation with other receptor tyrosine kinases in gliomas [162]. Hypoxia-induced c-met expression also plays a role in glioma invasiveness [163].

SDF-1α/CXCR4

SDF-1α, also known as CXCL12, is a ligand of the CXC chemokine receptor-4 (CXCR4) [164,165]. Both SDF-1α and CXCR4 are expressed in hypoxic tissues, an expression, at least in part, mediated by HIF-1 [166–168]. SDF-1α acts as a chemoattractant for endothelial cells, induces endothelial cell proliferation in vitro, and promotes capillary branching in vivo [169,170]. CXCR4 is normally expressed at low levels in resting endothelial cells but is increased in response to VEGF stimulation [14,168,171]. Immunoreactivity for SDF-1α is intense in tumor-associated vessels in GBMs [14,168,172]. The SDF-1α/CXCR4 ligand receptor system also activates signaling pathways known to induce glioma invasiveness [14]. For instance, treatment of glioma cells with SDF-1α enhanced phosphorylation of focal adhesion kinase, Akt, and ERK-1/2, which have been implicated in glioma cell migration [14,173–175].

In addition, experimental evidence suggests that SDF-1α contributes to the recruitment of CXCR4$^+$ bone marrow-derived cells to sites of neovascularization (discussed under Vasculogenesis in Gliomas) associated with hypoxic/ischemic and neoplastic processes [167,176].

Endogenous Antiangiogenic Factors

Several endogenous inhibitors of angiogenesis demonstrated in gliomas act through multiple protein-protein or protein-proteoglycan interactions (e.g., angiostatin, endostatin), specific receptor binding (e.g., interferons), or downregulation of VEGF or other proangiogenic molecules [15,177–179]. These include angiostatin, endostatin, TSP-1 and -2, tissue inhibitor of metalloprotease (TIMP)-1 and -4, and pigment endothelial-derived factor. Their expression variably correlates with glioma grade [178–181].

Angiogenesis and Genetic/Epigenetic Alterations

Genetic Alterations

Malignant transformation in gliomas results from the sequential accumulation of genetic and chromosomal alterations and the deregulation of some of these growth factor signaling pathways [28–30,136,182–184]. Some of these anomalies may promote angiogenesis independently of hypoxia [31,185]. Gain of function of the oncogenes EGF, PDGF, and their receptors (EGFR amplification, EGFR variant III mutation, PDGFR overexpression) and loss of function of tumor-suppressor genes (mutations of p53 and PTEN, etc.) have been linked to glioma neovascularization [136,186]. Also, the loss of heterozygosity of chromosome arms 1p, 10p, 10q, 19q, and 22q has been associated with deletion of the PTEN locus and/or loss of other gene loci encoding proangiogenic and/or antiangiogenic factors or their receptors [15,23,31,185]. These genetic alterations may combine with hypoxia to drive chromosome instability [17,18] promoting continual selective growth advantage for the tumor cells. The frequency and association of these genetic anomalies differ according to pathological grade and the subtype (primary or secondary GBM). These genetic aberrations result in chronic activation of HIF-1 through stimulation of the intracellular PI3K-Akt or Ras-MEK-1/2 pathways [30,135,187,188].

Additional genetic alterations in cancer cells, including gliomas, can deregulate the expression of HIF-1α protein [31,185]. Although rare in gliomas, loss of function of the pVHL gene results in diminished ubiquitination and proteasomal degradation of HIF-1α, leading to chronic overexpression of HIF-1-inducible gene products and abnormal vascular proliferations [12,189]. Loss of function of genes encoding subunits of succinate dehydrogenase or fumarate hydratase also impedes PHD isozyme activity and HIF-1α proteasomal degradation [59,60]. Gliomas also show mutation in mitochondrial complex I NADH dehydrogenase subunit 6 [ND6] associated with defective response to hypoxia [61,62].

Epigenetic Alterations

Epigenetics are defined, in broad terms, as heritable changes to the expression of genes without affecting the DNA sequence itself [190,191]. DNA methylation and histone modifications are two classical means to regulate gene expression, but miRNAs and microvesicles or exosomes have also recently been documented to govern phenotypic expression in normal as well as cancer cells [190,191]. For example, genes encoding PTEN, TSP-1, and TIMPs are inactivated by methylation in 28% to 71% of gliomas [192,193]. Hypermethylation of CpG islands in the O^6-methylguanine DNA methyltransferase gene initiates defects in DNA repair in glioma cells [192,193]. Histone modifications at the VEGFR-1 promoter region mediate the angiogenic activity of the HIF-2α/ETS-1 transcription factors [194].

miRNAs, an emerging class of highly conserved, noncoding 19 to 24 nucleotide single-stranded RNAs, regulate gene expression by sequence-specific base pairing in the 3′-untranslated regions of target mRNAs [195]. miRNAs, which normally suppress expression of target transcripts, may become activators of expression during stress [73]. A variety of miRNAs have been identified in gliomas and medulloblastomas [196,197]. Some have been shown to regulate various aspects of angiogenesis [85,86,198,199]. Proangiogenic miRNAs include miR-17–92 cluster, miR-27b, miR-126, miR-130a, miR-210, miR-296, miR-378, and Let-7f. Other miRNAs with antiangiogenic properties include miR-15, miR-16, miR-20a/b, miR-125a, miR-221, and miR-222. In particular, the expression of miR-296 induced by angiogenic growth factors (VEGF, EGF) regulates the overexpression of VEGFR-2 and PDGFR-β in glioma-associated endothelial cells [198]. This positive-feedback loop is mediated by miR-296 directly inhibiting mRNA for HGF-regulated tyrosine kinase substrate, thereby allowing the accumulation of VEGFR-2 and PDGFR-β proteins by attenuating their degradation. Inhibition of miR-296 with antagomirs reduces angiogenesis in tumor xenografts in vivo. Manipulation of miRNAs implicated in the neovascularization of gliomas may demonstrate potential therapeutic applications.

Finally, tumor cells can release vesicular structures, defined as microvesicles or exosomes, carrying a large array of cellular content that can promote the horizontal propagation of oncogenes and their associated transforming phenotype among subsets of normal and cancer cells [200]. Glioblastoma tumor cells have been shown to release microvesicles containing mRNAs, miRNAs, angiogenic proteins [201] as well as oncogenic proteins such as EGFRvIII [202] that are taken up by normal host cells, such as brain microvascular endothelial cells, or other tumor cells, and alter their phenotypic or angiogenic properties.

"Glioma Stem Cells" and Tumor Neovascularization

Although the genetic and signaling pathways involved in the progression of malignant gliomas have been relatively well characterized, the cellular origins of these tumors are unknown. Experimental evidence suggests that glioma stem cells can be isolated from human brain tumors [203–207]. Glioma stem cells may be operationally defined as "a tumor subpopulation that can self-renew in culture, perpetuate a tumor in orthotopic transplant *in vivo*, and generate diversified neuron-like and glia-like postmitotic progeny *in vivo* and *in vitro*" [207]. Such cells growing as neurospheres in culture and expressing prominin-1 (CD133) and nestin were isolated from human brain tumors including GBMs. Although typically a minor subset of the total cells within gliomas, they are generally the most tumorigenic component of the tumor [207]. Moreover, these cells were able to promote angiogenesis, at least in part, through the release of VEGF and SDF-1α [208–211]. Glioma stem cells may contribute to the resistance of malignant gliomas to chemotherapy and radiotherapy [205,206,212]. Like normal neural stem cells, glioma stem cells occupy and support a specialized vascular niche for their function [213–216]. This vascular niche may be a hypoxic environment as HIF-2α has been shown to be upregulated together with VEGF in perivascular immature stem cells of neuroblastomas [217]. However, recent reports question the identity of glioma stem cells [88,218].

Cancer stem cells can enter into a long-term dormant state before progressing, which begs the question of how tumors progress [219–221]. Examining glioblastomas and other cancer types, a genome-wide transcriptional analysis of the molecular mechanisms underlying the switch of dormant tumors identified the angiogenesis process (e.g., TSP, ephrin receptor A5) as the most significantly affected functional gene category [222].

VASCULOGENESIS IN GLIOMAS

Comparison of Angiogenesis and Vasculogenesis

Tumor vasculature is derived not only from endothelial cell sprouting and co-option of preexisting vessels, as we have seen, but can also be acquired from postnatal vasculogenesis [6,7,15,19]. Comparison of these major mechanisms reveals that the main difference relates to the source of the endothelial cells (Table 16.1) [223–229]. Angiogenesis occurs as mature, differentiated endothelial cells, pericyte,

Table 16.1 Vasculogenesis and Angiogenesis in CNS Ontogeny and Oncogeny

	Vasculogenesis	Angiogenesis
Source of endothelial precursor cells	Hemangioblast (embryo) or HSC (adult)	ECs of existing vessels
Embryonic development	In situ differentiation of ECs from angioblasts, which share an origin (mesoderm hemangioblast) with hematopoietic progenitors	Sprouting and remodeling of new EC-lined vessels from preexisting vessels to expand the vascular network
Adult life/tumor	Mobilization, recruitment, and differentiation of BM-derived proangiogenic cells (EPCs, PPCs TEMs, etc.) into nascent blood vessels	Sprouting and remodeling of new EC-lined vessels from preexisting vessels to expand the vascular network
Example	De novo formation of blood vessels	Branching and remodeling of existing blood vessels
Mechanism sequence	In embryo 1. Establishment of nascent endothelial tubes from endothelial precursors (angioblast) induced by VEGF 2. Formation of primitive vascular network from array of nascent endothelial tubes 3. Assembly of the vessel wall (pericytes, smooth muscle cells, or astrocytes [in CNS blood-brain barrier]) In adult life/tumor 1. Self-repopulating HSCs develop into EPCs and other proangiogenic cells in the BM 2. Proliferation and mobilization of these progenitor cells in response to tissue-derived plasma angiogenic stimuli 3. Recruitment and differentiation of these progenitor cells into mature cells that may integrate in nascent vessels	Common mechanism 1. New capillaries originate from small venules or other capillaries 2. Local degradation of basement membrane and extracellular matrix on the side of parental vessels closest to angiogenic stimuli, by secretion and activation of proteases 3. Migration of ECs toward angiogenic cues to form sprouts 4. Local proliferation of ECs within capillary sprouts 5. Generation of capillary lumen (tube formation) 6. Resynthesis of basement membrane and matrix 7. Recruitment of mural cells (pericytes, smooth muscle cells, or astrocytes [in CNS blood-brain barrier])
Molecular regulation		
1. Vascular compartment	Cytokines/receptors (VEGF/VEGFR, SDF-1α/CXCR4, etc.) Proteases (e.g., EPC cathepsin L activity) Adhesion/migration molecules (integrins, cadherins, etc.)	Cytokines/receptors (VEGF/VEGFR, SDF-1α/CXCR4, etc.) Proteases (MMPs, cathepsins, serine proteases, etc.) Adhesion/migration molecules (integrins, cadherins, etc.)
2. BM compartment	Cytokines/receptors (VEGF/VEGFR, SDF-1α/CXCR4, etc.) Proteases (e.g., MMP-9 releases sKitL, which leads to mobilization of EPCs and hematopoietic cells from BM) Adhesion/migration molecules (integrins, cadherins, etc.)	Not determined

During embryonic development, vasculogenesis and angiogenesis occur sequentially in the process of blood vessel formation: establishment of the initial vascular network contributes to its subsequent remodeling and expansion [223–225]. Although angiogenesis contributes to wound healing and other processes in adults, the in vivo contribution of vasculogenesis to postnatal neovascularization remains an area of intense debate, owing to the lack of definitive markers of endothelial progenitors [224,226,227]. The interactions of angiogenic molecular mechanisms seen in embryonic development and physiological neovascularization may also occur in solid tumors; however, the tumor cells themselves, and host endothelial, stromal, and inflammatory cells (when present), provide sources of angiogenic stimuli, and the resulting vessels' architecture and function are abnormal [4,19,228]. Tumors may also acquire new blood supply through a third mechanism, the co-option of normal capillaries, while infiltrating along blood vessels [9,10,19,229]. Abbreviations: BM, bone marrow; CNS, central nervous system; CXCR4, CXC chemokine receptor-4; EC, endothelial cell; EPC, endothelial progenitor cell; HSC, hematopoietic stem cell; MMP, matrix metalloprotease; PPC, pericytic progenitor cell; SDF-1α, stromal cell-derived factor-1α; sKitL, soluble kit ligand; TEM, Tie2-expressing monocyte; VEGFR(R), vascular endothelial growth factor (receptor).

and other vessel wall cells break free from their basement membrane and proliferate as well as migrate to form sprouts from parental vessels. In contrast, vasculogenesis involves bone marrow-derived endothelial progenitor cells (EPCs) and other proangiogenic cells which circulate to sites of neovascularization, where they differentiate in situ into mature endothelial cells or other perivascular cells, respectively. Growth factors (e.g., VEGF) and cytokines (e.g., SDF-1α) released in response to tumor tissue hypoxia and/or genetic alterations act to promote mobilization, proliferation, and differentiation of these proangiogenic cells [19,21]. The same factors may stimulate local endothelial cell processes during angiogenesis. Considerable overlap also exists between these two mechanisms with regard to the matrix proteases, cell adhesion, and motility molecules involved [228–231].

Evidence of Circulating Endothelial Lineage Cells in Glioma Neovascularization

Accumulating evidence suggests that subsets of bone marrow-derived pro-angiogenic cells circulate in the blood and home to sites of physiological and pathological neovascularization (Figure 16.4)[20–22,226,227,232–239]. Although some of these blood cells are relatively rare (e.g., EPCs), interference with the recruitment of endothelial and hematopoietic precursor cells was shown to impair tumor neovascularization and growth in tumor models (227,240).

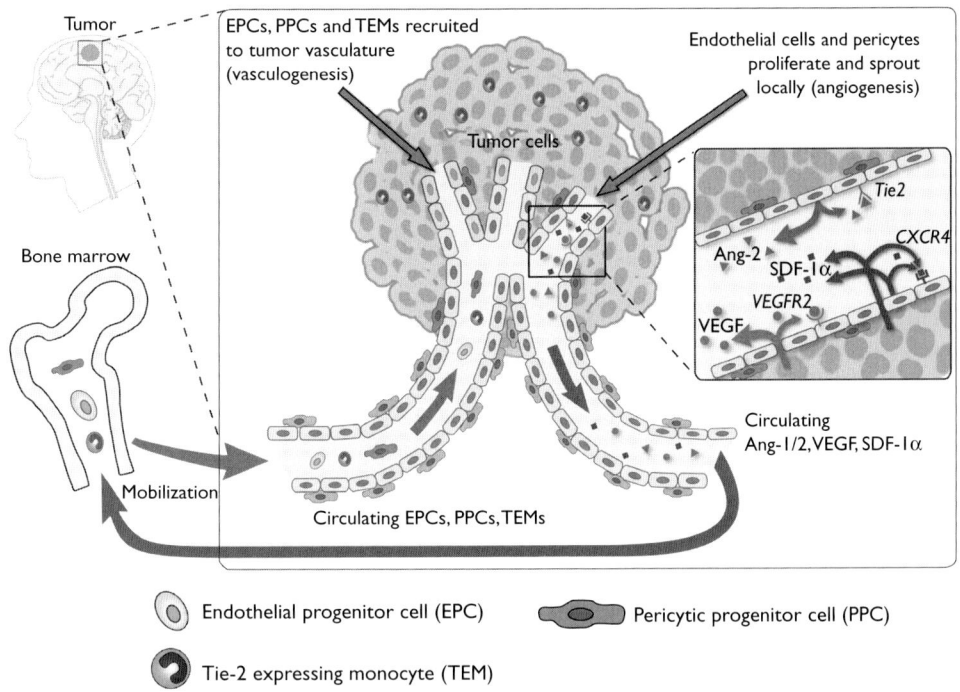

Figure 16.4 Mobilization and recruitment of bone marrow-derived proangiogenic cells to the site of tumor neovascularization. Experimental evidence, particularly in murine models, suggests that solid tumors can produce and release cytokines, such as angiopoietin-2 (Ang-2), vascular endothelial growth factor (VEGF), stromal cell-derived factor (SDF)-1α, and platelet-derived growth factor (PDGF) into the systemic circulation, that can mobilize various populations of proangiogenic cells from the bone marrow [20–22]. Following entry in tumor tissues, these cell populations exert different roles in neovascularization. Among them, the endothelial and pericyte progenitor cells (EPCs, PPCs) may be incorporated into the growing vasculature of the tumor where they differentiate and mature in situ [20,21,232]. These cells may also secrete angiogenic factors locally [227]. On the other hand, recruited Tie2-expressing monocytes (TEMs) and other bone marrow-derived myeloid cells localize in the perivascular space and secrete a panel of angiogenic factors, including VEGF, that stimulate angiogenesis locally in a paracrine manner [22,233]. Antigen expression profile and other methods are currently used to identify these cell types, but their exact identity, differentiation, and function are the subject of debate because of the considerable overlap of expression of these cellular markers [20,22,226,234,235]. Illustrated in this diagram are EPCs (that express VEGFR2$^+$CD45^{dim}(CXCR4$^+$)CD117$^+$ in mice, VEGFR2$^+$CD45^{dim}(CXCR4$^+$)CD34$^+$CD133$^+$ in humans) [176,226,234–236], PPCs (PDGFRβ$^+$Sca-1$^+$CD11b$^+$ in mice, PDGFRβ$^+$CD11b$^+$ in humans) [20,237,238], and TEMs (Tie2$^+$CD45$^+$CD11b$^+$Gr-1$^{dim/-}$ in mice, Tie2$^+$CD45$^+$CD11b$^+$CD14^{dim}CD16$^+$ in humans) [22,233,239]. In addition, mature endothelial cells may also be shed into the peripheral blood as circulating endothelial cells (not illustrated) that lack CD117/CD133 expression [226]. See *color insert*.

The molecular identity and differentiation lineage of EPCs is under debate; however, these cells are generally defined by their expression of progenitor (CD34, CD133) and endothelial (CD31, VEGFR2) markers in humans [226,241–243], which was confirmed by oligonucleotide microarray analysis of cultured EPCs from human umbilical cord blood [244]. Elevated levels of circulating EPCs have been reported in patients with neoplastic conditions [243,245,246], including gliomas [247] relative to control subjects. These were associated with concomitant tissue hypoxia [167,248], increased serum levels of SDF-1α, bFGF, or VEGF [121,249], and recruitment of EPCs into intratumoral capillaries [246,249]. Blood EPC levels also increased in patients with tumor progression after interruption of anti-VEGF receptor therapy [121,250]. Using MRI microimaging, locally implanted magnetically labeled CD133$^+$ cells were shown to migrate to the periphery of glioma tumor at the site of active neovascularization [251]. Interestingly, EPCs express CXCR4 and VEGFR-2 and migrate toward gradients of SDF-1α or VEGF [249,252–255]. Expression of the Ang-2/Tie2 receptor, which is essential for the progression of murine and human gliomas [10,94,97], has also been linked to the recruitment of EPCs in tumors, including gliomas [256–259].

Studies of vasculogenesis in mice bearing brain tumors and other tumor types have produced discordant findings [232,237,253,260], raising doubts as to the contribution of marrow-derived EPCs or periendothelial cells to brain tumor neovascularization. Importantly, different experimental tumors and strains of mice have been shown to vary in their levels of circulating EPCs, which may help to account for those differences [227,253,261]. Thus, the role EPCs play in the neovascularization of brain tumors remains incompletely elucidated.

Evidence of Other Circulating Proangiogenic Cells in Glioma Neovascularization

Different populations of marrow-derived pro-angiogenic cells appear to have specific roles temporally and spatially in promoting vasculogenesis in tumors (Figure 16.4). Of those, EPCs and pericyte progenitor cells (PPCs) may incorporate into the nascent vessel wall, where they differentiate into mature endothelial cells (as discussed above) and pericytes, the perivascular support cells, respectively [20,227,237,238,262]. Other subsets of marrow-derived cells incorporate perivascularly and may contribute to neovascularization primarily in a paracrine manner by secreting various angiogenic factors, such as VEGF, and/or proteolytic enzymes, such as MMPs [21,22,226]. These cells include CD11b+ TEMs [22,233,263], VEGFR1+CD11b+CXCR4+ hemangiocytes [176,254], and CD11b+Gr-1+ neutrophils and myeloid suppressor cells [21,264]. Among myeloid cells, the newly discovered TEMs represent a subset of tumor-infiltrating CD11b+ cells characterized by the expression of Tie2 as well as F4/80, Sca-1, and CD45 [22,233,239,265]. In mice, the circulating Tie2+CD45+ hematopoietic cells are mostly CD11b+Gr-1$^{low/-}$, whereas in humans they express CD14, CD16, and CD11c [239,265]. The surface marker profile of mouse and human TEMs is distinct from the classic inflammatory monocytes and so-called resident monocytes [265,266]. Importantly, the vast majority of the circulating Tie2+ cells lack expression of EPC antigens such as VEGFR-2, CD133, CD146, and CD34 [22,267]. TEMs are important promoters of tumor vasculogenesis and were found in several mouse tumor models, including human GBM explants in the mouse brain, and spontaneous pancreatic tumors developing in RIP1-Tag2 transgenic mice [237]. They have also been detected in human blood and tumor tissues [22,265,266,268]. Labeled monocytes/macrophages were shown to target brain tumors, a process that could be monitored noninvasively using MRI [269]. Hypoxia upregulates Tie2 expression on TEMs and, together with Ang-2, down-regulates their antitumoral functions [239,267]. Like EPCs, TEMs may express CXCR4 [237]. Interestingly, the tumor-homing capacity of TEMs and other marrow-derived tumor-infiltrating progenitor cells may provide the means for selective drug delivery, such as interferon-α [270] or suicide genes [271,272], and produce effective, targeted inhibition of tumor angiogenesis.

Potential Molecular and Cellular Biomarkers of Glioma Neovascularization and Antiangiogenic Response

The dependence of tumor growth, progression, and metastasis on new blood vessel formation makes tumor neovascularization a pivotal target of therapy [2,19,23,31]. Considering that the mechanisms of action of these new antiangiogenic therapies are preferentially cytostatic rather than directly cytotoxic [23–25,31], biomarkers previously used for chemotherapeutic agents (e.g., maximum tolerated dose, tumor shrinkage) do not seem to be adequate for monitoring antiangiogenic drugs [273–275]. Also, the efficacy of antiangiogenic treatment may depend on many factors, such as tumor stage, heterogeneity and perfusion of tumor vasculature, and response profile of neoplastic cells [19,275,276]. Choosing an optimal biological dose, which is probably lower than the maximum tolerated dose and dose-limiting toxicity, is sought for the development of these agents. Although patients with colorectal, lung, and breast cancer, for example, experienced prolonged survival or progression-free survival from antiangiogenic therapies, it is often by achieving partial tumor stabilization or regression and transient remission of their disease before the patient tumors develop resistance typically after a few months of receiving therapy [19,277]. Surrogate biomarkers would have the potential to better identify patients to treat and optimize drug dosage and schedule, improve the therapeutic index, inform early clinical benefit, assess the development of acquired resistance, and guide potential alternative therapy [273–275].

Parallel to the progress of clinical trials of angiogenesis inhibitors, objective measures of antiangiogenic activity are currently being investigated, but none have been clinically validated thus far [30,273–275]. When tumor tissue biopsy or resection specimen can be obtained, tumor histology including microvascular density counts and antigenic and gene expression profiles for tumor angiogenic factors and receptors may be informative for initial patient selection and the choice of antiangiogenic drug dosage and schedule [23,274]. In contrast to tissue markers, dynamic biomarkers are relatively noninvasive and better suited for repeated measurements needed to monitor the response to antiangiogenic therapy. Although tumor and/or circulating VEGF concentrations have been associated with tumor progression and/or poor prognosis, these data do not appear to be predictive of response to anti-VEGF therapy [274,278]. Current methods of VEGF quantification exhibit several limitations, for example, VEGF released from nontumor sources (platelets, leukocytes) can contribute significant proportions of circulating VEGF [274]. However, truncated forms of the VEGFR-2 receptor (sVEGFR-2) and the vascular cell adhesion molecule (sVCAM-1) appear to correlate with antiangiogenic inhibitor treatments [278,279]. Also, circulating levels of SDF-1α and bFGF appear to predict disease relapse in patients with GBM receiving the VEGFR/PDGFR/Kit tyrosine kinase inhibitor cediranib [121]. The concentration of circulating endothelial cells and/or progenitors also correlated with anti-VEGF treatment [19,31,250,278]. Alternatively, several imaging techniques, such as dynamic contrast-enhanced MRI, positron emission tomography, dynamic computerized tomography (CT), and functional ultrasound, are valuable in determining tumor blood volume and vascular permeability [19,23,280–283]. These preliminary studies need confirmation and validation in larger prospective clinical trials.

ANTIANGIOGENIC THERAPIES IN PATIENTS WITH GLIOMAS

Rationale, Patient Selection, and Outcome Measure

Because of the dependence of low- to high-grade gliomas on new vessel formation for their growth and progression, it has been thought that malignant gliomas would be highly susceptible to antiangiogenic therapy [15,19,23,31]. Unlike conventional high-dose chemotherapy, antiangiogenic agents target endothelial cells lining the vasculature that nourish tumor growth [23,283,284]. Endothelial cells are easily accessible for antiangiogenic drugs administered intravenously, as opposed to chemotherapeutic drugs that have to overcome physical barriers (blood-brain barrier, stromal cells and matrix, interstitial fluid) before reaching the tumor cells. Because VEGF is expressed in glioma from early stages of growth and stimulates endothelial cell proliferation, survival, and migration as well as vascular permeability, agents interfering with VEGF signaling have been developed [26,285]. Also targeted are oncogenic receptors and signaling pathways in glioma cells that lead to the overexpression of proangiogenic factors, such as VEGF, and new vessel formation [25,26,286]. Other vascular cells (e.g., pericytes, smooth muscle cells, circulating marrow-derived proangiogenic cells) constitute additional potential targets for antiangiogenic therapy [239,287]. Potential mechanisms of action of anti-VEGF therapies have been characterized and include (a) inhibition of new vessel growth, (b) regression of newly formed tumor vasculature, (c) alteration of vascular function and tumor blood flow (normalization), and (d) possibly direct effects on tumor cells [277,285,288,289]. The potential pleiotropic effects of these therapies occur because VEGF receptors are expressed not only on tumor-associated endothelial cells but also on subsets of hematopoietic cells, stromal cells, and malignant cells in some human cancers.

The selection of patients most likely to respond to antiangiogenic agents remains a major challenge [273,290,291]. Successful precedents of individualized molecular therapy based on biomarkers include the use of trastuzumab in HER-2 overexpressing breast cancer, cetuximab in EGFR expressing colorectal cancer, and imatinib in c-Kit expressing gastrointestinal stromal tumor [290,291]. In contrast, antiangiogenic drugs have mostly been studied in patient populations selected based on clinical criteria rather than on molecular profiles as no biomarkers that reflect the efficacy of these agents have been validated in clinical practice [23,273,290,291]. For instance, despite considerable evidence for the association of intratumoral and/or plasma VEGF levels with tumor progression and/or poor prognosis, pretreatment VEGF levels do not appear to be predictive of response to antiangiogenic therapy [278,290].

Because of the presumed cytostatic mechanism of action of antiangiogenic agents, their efficacy is most appropriately assessed through survival end points rather than the objective-response end points that have traditionally been used with cytotoxic agents [277,292,293]. For instance, the vascular effects of antiangiogenic therapy pose problems for evaluating brain tumor response based on contrast-enhanced MRI, which are now being reexamined [294–297]. Nevertheless, bevacizumab has been shown to increase the response rates with chemotherapy in almost all tumor types studied in Phase III trials [284].

Clinical Trials of Antiangiogenic Therapies in Patients with Glioma

The early promise of antiangiogenesis treatment in solid tumors was quickly adopted for the treatment of malignant gliomas for obvious reasons. Malignant gliomas, as we have seen, are hotbeds of neovascularization. High hopes were held for antiangiogenesis strategies. The following clinical vignette illustrates the promise and limitations of this therapeutic approach in malignant glioma (Figure 16.5).

Clinical Vignette

An otherwise healthy 30-year-old school teacher presented after a first-time generalized tonic-clonic seizure (Panel A). MRI revealed a left motor strip nonenhancing T2 intense lesion. She underwent a partial resection with motor mapping to spare her right hand function (Panel B1). Pathology of the lesion revealed a WHO II mixed glioma that was not immunopositive for p53. She returned to teaching and did well for 4 years until progression of the T2 signal abnormality prompted treatment. She received proton beam radiation therapy and was again well, with occasional focal motor seizures until 5 years after her first surgery. MRI now began to reveal patchy contrast enhancement in the lesion, which was interpreted as a possible radiation effect. One year later, the lesion progressed with vigorous contrast enhancement. She now had a right hemiparesis and Karnofsky performance score declined to 60 (Panel B2). Six years after her first surgery, she underwent a second surgery with gross total resection of the contrast-enhancing tumor in the motor strip. Pathology was now interpreted as a high-grade mixed glioma with 50% of tumor cells immunopositive for p53. She was now treated with bevacizumab (Avastin, 10 mg/kg iv q2weeks) and temozolomide (Temodar, 75 mg/m^2 po qd) as well as radiation boost (36 Gy) to the involved area, with a dramatic near-complete response (Panel B3). Four months after resection, MRI revealed no contrast enhancement, no mass effect, and minimal T2 signal abnormality. Two months later, she deteriorated rapidly, with a complete aphasia and lethargy. MRI now revealed diffuse areas of contrast enhancement and T2 signal in both cerebral hemispheres whereas the original resection bed remained quiescent (Panel B4). Stereotactic biopsy of a left frontal pole lesion, far removed from the initial resection bed, showed high-grade mixed glioma, now with 100% of the tumor cells staining for p53.

Bevacizumab has been used for recurrent malignant glioma as both a single agent and in combination with cytotoxic chemotherapies, most commonly irinotecan [298–300]. Our group observed radiographic responses in 73.6% of cases after treatment with bevacizumab in combination with either irinotecan or carboplatin. These sometimes dramatic radiographic responses have been well characterized and are thought to relate to normalization of tumor vasculature by VEGF blockade [121,288]. Some authors have argued that the apparent therapeutic effect of bevacizumab and VEGF blockade is really just a radiological effect from stabilization of the blood-brain barrier [301]. However, the reported 6-month progression-free survival of 43% for patients with glioblastoma [298,299] argues for a real therapeutic effect. Similarly, the MRI results often include loss of mass effect and brain shift in addition to simple loss of contrast enhancement (Figure 16.5).

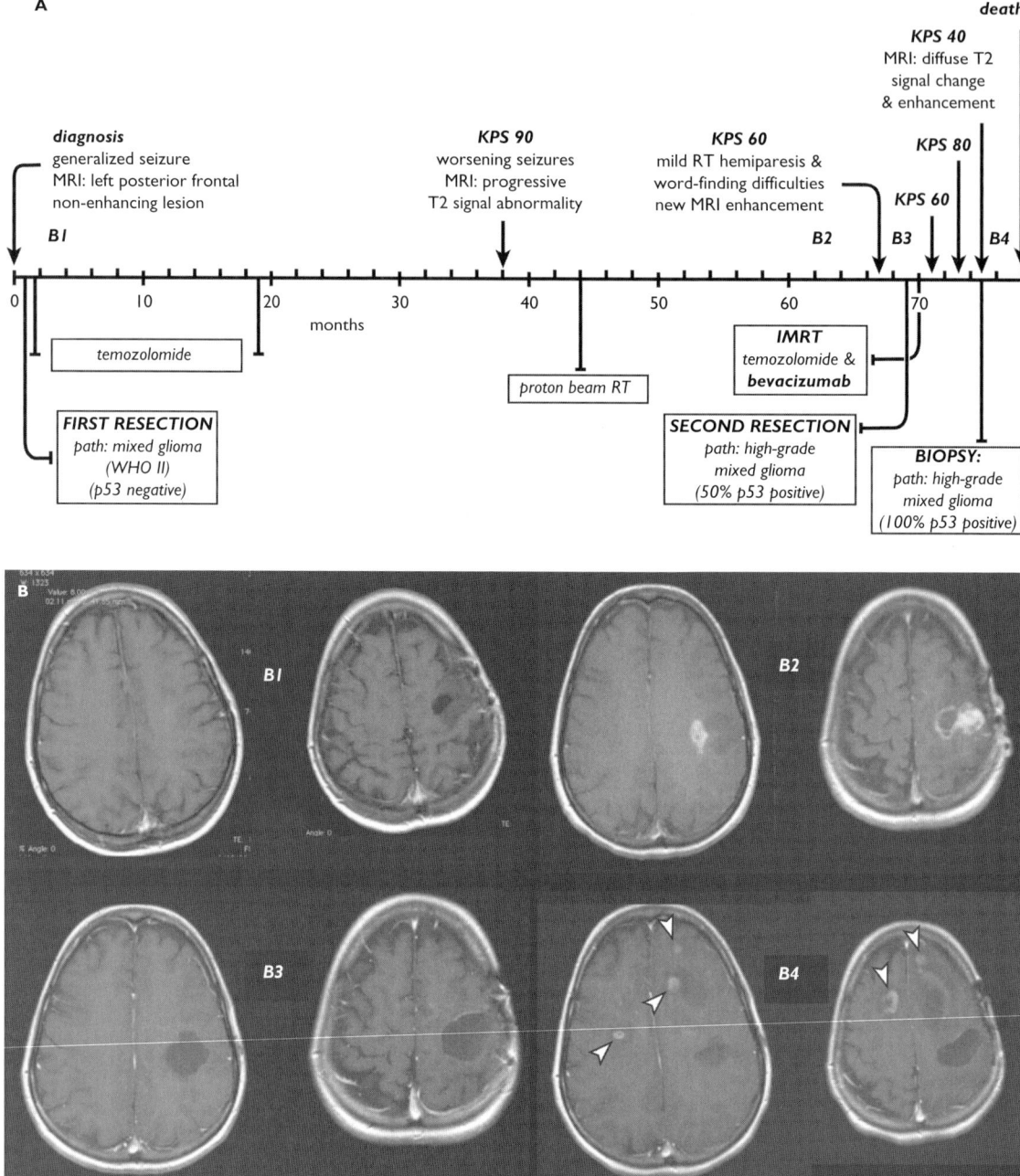

Figure 16.5 Case illustration of antiangiogenic therapy in a young female with glioma progression. Clinical timeline (Panel A). Bevacizumab was started 70 months following initial diagnosis with a World Health Organization (WHO) II mixed glioma and less than 1 month following her second resection and tumor progression to a high-grade tumor. T1 weighted axial magnetic resonance imaging (MRI) demonstrating left posterior frontal tumor resection cavity (after gross total resection of WHO II mixed glioma [Panel B1]). The patient presented with seizures and underwent 19 months of adjuvant chemotherapy with temozolomide. Three years later, local tumor recurrence was treated with proton beam radiotherapy without resection. More than 5 years after initial diagnosis, surveillance MRI revealed a local recurrence (Panel B2). The patient underwent resection, and pathology revealed tumor progression to WHO Grade III mixed glioma. Following resection and adjuvant bevacizumab, temozolomide, and intensity-modulated radiation therapy (IMRT), the patient was without evidence of recurrence for 8 months (Panel B3). However, almost 7 years after initial diagnosis, the patient developed multifocal disease progression (white arrow heads) following treatment with bevacizumab (Panel B4).

The promising results in recurrent glioblastoma and the relatively low incidence of serious complications have also led to consideration of antiangiogenesis therapy as a frontline treatment. A recently completed Phase I trial of 15 patients treated with radiation, temozolomide, and bevacizumab showed that 13 patients were able to successfully complete the treatment regimen [302]. There were four Grade III-IV nonhematological toxicities (malignant hypertension, ulceration, thromboembolism) (see later). The 1-year progression-free survival was 59.3% in this cohort of high-grade gliomas.

Although VEGF is the best characterized proangiogenic factor, several other ligands, receptors, and signaling pathways deregulated in glioma and associated endothelial cells contribute directly or indirectly to the process of glioma neovascularization [15,19,31]. As illustrated in Figure 16.6 [11,23–25,122,135,185,298–300,303–322], a variety of molecularly targeted approaches [23,284,285], such as neutralizing monoclonal antibodies against angiogenic factors and their receptors, competitive decoy angiogenic factor receptors, competitive receptor kinase inhibitors, and signaling pathway inhibitors, often in combination with chemoradiotherapy, have been explored in clinical studies. Based on comparative analyses of Phase II trials completed to date [24,25,307,323], minimal efficacy has been demonstrated for single agents tested in patients with brain tumors. However, the combinations of bevacizumab and irinotecan (Camptostar) or bevacizumab and temozolomide (Temodar) have emerged as the most promising new treatments for malignant glioma [298,300,302,304]. A 6-month progression-free survival of 40% to 50% exceeds that of any previously assessed treatment of this malignant neoplasm. Also, these treatment combinations reduced peritumoral edema in many patients, which likely improved their quality of life. Similar studies are being pursued, with some success in pediatric patients bearing brain tumors [324–326] as well as in patients with metastatic tumors (especially melanoma and breast cancer) to the brain [327–329].

Mechanisms of Resistance to Antiangiogenic Therapies in Patients with Glioma

The early enthusiasm for bevacizumab and other antiangiogenic agents in high-grade glioma has been somewhat tempered by the unusual patterns of failure seen in these patients, that is, initial response followed by dissemination of disease in a mode reminiscent of gliomatosis [301]. As with the patient in our clinical vignette (Figure 16.5), recurrence in bevacizumab-treated patients can occur as diffuse and distant invasive disease in perhaps as many as 50% of cases [26,302]. The mechanisms for this apparent increased invasiveness remain unclear [6,277,330]. Based on emerging data, two modes of resistance have been proposed [331]: *acquired evasive resistance*, in which initial objective responses are circumvented and followed by growth and progression, like in our clinical vignette's patient (Figure 16.5), and *intrinsic resistance*, in which no discernable benefit is ever achieved. Accordingly, evasion of antiangiogenic therapy (*acquired resistance*) is seen to occur through (a) upregulation of alternative proangiogenic signaling circuits, such as bFGF, SDF-1α, and PDGF [121,332–334]; (b) recruitment of vascular progenitor cells and proangiogenic monocytes from the bone marrow, such as EPCs and CD11b$^+$Gr-1$^+$ myeloid cells [121,264,335]; (c) increased and tight pericyte coverage of tumor vasculature [336]; or (d) increased capabilities for perivascular invasion and co-option without angiogenesis [120,300,337,338]. Worsening hypoxia in tumors that undergo antiangiogenic therapy because of vessel regression may contribute to this escape mechanism. Alternatively, the tumor may be indifferent to antiangiogenic therapy (*intrinsic resistance*) because of (a) preexisting multiplicity of redundant proangiogenic signals, such as concomitantly activated receptor tyrosine kinases [164], (b) preexisting inflammatory cell-mediated vascular protection, such as marrow-derived endothelial, pericytic, and myeloid cells [264], (c) characteristic hypovascularity and indifference toward angiogenesis inhibitors, such as expression of multidrug resistance genes in glioma-associated endothelial cells [339], or (d) invasive co-option of normal vessels without requisite angiogenesis [9,229,331,340]. In those instances where compensatory or intrinsic mechanisms could facilitate glioma cells to infiltrate within the adjacent normal brain tissue where they may co-opt the existing vasculature, antiangiogenic therapy alone would not be adequate in eradicating those cells [23,338].

The future therefore may bring increased use of multiagent therapy with VEGF blockade accompanied by simultaneous blockade of other proangiogenic or promigratory pathways with the overarching goal of decreasing glioma cell invasiveness. Furthermore, the marked cellular and genetic heterogeneity of glioma cells, the redundancy and crosstalk among molecular pathways in tumors, as well as the lack of benefit from single antiangiogenic agents in clinical trials argue for the need of combined blockade of functionally linked and relevant multiple targets, such as angiogenic and oncogenic signaling pathways [286] or angiogenic and invasion mechanisms [341].

Complications of Angiogenic Factors and Antiangiogenic Therapies in Patients with Glioma

Deep venous thrombosis and pulmonary embolism are frequent complications in the course of cancer, particularly in patients with brain tumors [342]. Their risk of developing such complications correlates with the plasma level of coagulation factors as well as that of VEGF [342]. Multiple and complex interactions between tumor cells, endothelial cells, circulating plasma proteins, and angiogenic factors can affect both angiogenesis and blood coagulation [343–345]. Tissue Factor (TF) exposed after endothelium disruption during tumor growth and thrombin (factor IIa) promote angiogenesis by both coagulation-dependent and -independent pathways [343]. TF initiates the clotting cascade but also upregulates the expression of VEGF and activates the protease-activated receptor (PAR)-2 on tumor cells. Conversely, VEGF induces vascular permeability to plasma coagulation factors [34]. Furthermore, thrombin activates PAR-1/-4, which stimulates angiogenic factors, such as Ang-2. Following bevacizumab administration, the protective function of VEGF on endothelial cells would be diminished, which may result in endothelial cell damage and bleeding (see below). In a meta-analysis of patients

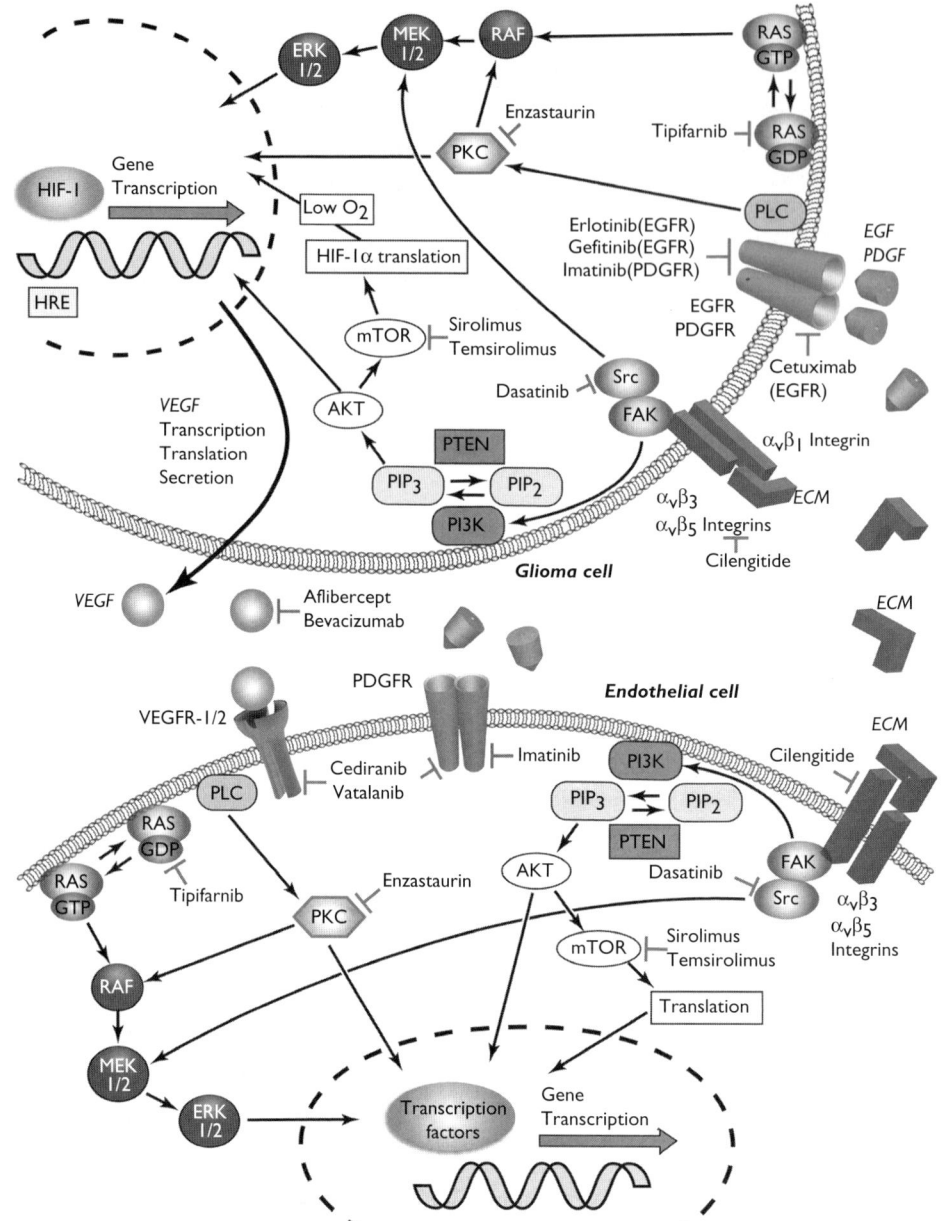

Figure 16.6 Molecular signaling pathways targeted by antiangiogenic drugs in clinical trials for malignant gliomas. During malignant transformation, common deregulation of growth factor signaling pathways involving epidermal growth factor receptor (EGFR amplification/EGFR variant III mutation) and platelet-derived growth factor receptor (PDGFR overexpression) lead to enhanced hypoxia-inducible factor (HIF)-1-regulated expression of vascular endothelial growth factor (VEGF) and other effector molecules in glioma cells (illustrated on top) that induce signaling pathways that result in cell survival, proliferation and migration, increased tube formation, and vascular permeability in tumor endothelium (at the bottom) [11,135,185]. These aberrations have become important potential targets of antiangiogenic therapy for malignant gliomas [23–25,303]. In published clinical trials, a variety of therapeutic approaches have been evaluated, most commonly monoclonal antibodies, receptor decoys, low-molecular-weight receptor kinase inhibitors, and signaling pathway inhibitors, often in combination with chemoradiotherapy. These include neutralizing anti-VEGF antibody *bevacizumab* (Avastin) [298–300,302,304]; VEGFR/PDGFR/Kit tyrosine kinase inhibitors *cediranib* (Recentin, AZD2171) [26,121] and *vatalanib* (PTK787/ZK222584) [24,25]; neutralizing anti-EGFR antibody *cetuximab* (Erbitux) [305]; EGFR tyrosine kinase inhibitors *erlotinib* (Tarceva) and *gefitinib* (Iressa) [306–308]; and PDGFR/Kit/Bcr-Abl tyrosine kinase inhibitor *imatinib mesylate* (Gleevec) [309,310]. In addition, common signal transduction pathways activated by these growth factors have been targeted: the Ras-mitogen-activated protein kinase (MEK)-1/2 pathway using the farnesyltransferase inhibitor *tipifarnib* (Zarnestra) [311], the phosphatidylinositol 3-kinase (PI3K)-Akt-mammalian target of rapamycin (mTOR) pathway using the mTOR inhibitors *temsirolimus* (CCI-779) [312–315] and *sirolimus* (Rapamycin) [314], the protein kinase C (PKC)-β2 pathway using the inhibitor *enzastaurin* (LY317615) [24]. (Of note, constitutive activation of PI3K pathways is frequently observed in gliomas associated with the loss of tumor-suppressor gene phosphatase and tensin homologue (PTEN) [135,315].) Also evaluated were the αvβ3/αvβ5 integrin inhibitor *cilengitide* (EMD121974) [316–318] and the 26S proteasome inhibitor *bortezomib* (Velcade) (not shown) [76,319]. Other potential therapeutic targets include VEGFR by means of the soluble VEGF receptor decoy *aflibercept* (VEGF Trap) [122] and the focal adhesion kinase (FAK)/src pathway using the Src/PDGFR/Bcr-Abl inhibitor *dasatinib* (BMS-354825), for example [320–322]. Abbreviations: Akt, protein kinase B; ECM, extracellular matrix; ERK-1/2, extracellular signal-regulated protein kinase-1/2; HRE, hypoxia-response element; MEK-1/2, mitogen-activated protein (MAP) kinase and extracellular signal-regulated protein kinase-1/2 kinase; PIP2, phosphatidylinositol [4,5] bisphosphate; PIP3, phosphatidylinositol [3–5] trisphosphate; PLC, phospholipase C; Raf, protein product of c-raf; Ras-GTP, protein product of c-ras - guanosine-5′-triphosphate; src, protein product of c-src. *See color insert.*

with a variety of advanced solid tumors (excluding brain tumors), the use of bevacizumab was significantly associated with an increased risk of developing venous thromboembolism [346]. Nevertheless, a study of the safety of anticoagulation combined with bevacizumab therapy in patients with glioma concluded that anticoagulation did not lead to any major hemorrhages and did not appear to be a contraindication for starting bevacizumab [347].

Contrary to initial expectations, anti-VEGF antibody and VEGFR-2 kinase inhibitors have caused toxicities in patients with cancer [301,348–350]. The distinct profile of adverse effects attributed to bevacizumab reflects its interference in VEGF's physiological functions in many organs [351,352], including hypertension, thromboembolic events, bleeding complications, gastrointestinal perforation, impaired wound healing, proteinuria, hypothyroidism, myelosuppression, and neurotoxicity. For example, bevacizumab-induced hypertension may be secondary to decreased VEGF-regulated nitric oxide and prostacylin production, which results in endothelial dysfunction, microvascular density rarefaction, increased peripheral resistance, and disrupted balance of endogenous vasoconstrictor endothelium-1 [350,352,353]. These are usually manageable by conventional medical approaches. In terms of neurotoxicity, reversible posterior leukoencephalopathy syndrome (RPLS) has been described, which consists of increased vascular permeability in the posterior circulation of the brain, associated clinically with headache, altered mental status, seizures, cortical blindness, and posterior subcortical white matter changes on CT and MRI. While most commonly associated with hypertension, a number of chemotherapeutic and immunotherapeutic agents have been associated with RPLS. Cases of RPLS have been reported in patients receiving bevacizumab as a single agent or in combination with other chemotherapy for systemic cancers and glioma [354,355]. Isolated brainstem symptoms that resolved after cessation of bevacizumab and antihypertensive therapy have also been reported [355,356]. Both hypertensive and vascular permeability side effects of bevacizumab are postulated to play a role in these rare cases.

CONCLUDING REMARKS

Much has been learned about CNS tumors since the times of Dr. Penfield, but the intricacies of their biology continue to amaze and challenge. In recent years, new fields of research have uncovered glioma cancer stem cells and the perivascular niche, cancer cell metabolism under hypoxia, miRNAs, tumor-shed microvesicles and intercellular communication, and marrow-derived proangiogenic cells and postnatal vasculogenesis, for example.

Although the demonstration that tumor neovascularization could be prevented or interrupted by antiangiogenic therapies and result in tangible benefits for patients with malignant gliomas is eagerly awaited, the quest is ongoing. Several questions remain unanswered. These include (a) the appropriate strategies for selection of patients, (b) the design of antiangiogenic agents and optimal treatment regimens, (c) the study design and proper end points for preclinical and clinical studies using these agents, (d) the monitoring of patients' responses to antiangiogenic therapies, (e) the biological consequences of sustained suppression of angiogenesis on tumor biology and normal tissue homeostasis, and (f) the synergy between antiangiogenic therapy and chemoradiotherapy. New questions have emerged, such as (a) the mechanisms of tumor escape from antiangiogenic therapies and (b) the development of antiinvasion drugs and other therapeutic approaches to counteract resistance to antiangiogenic therapies. As these challenging and limiting issues are resolved, we hope to achieve improved response and benefit from antiangiogenic drugs as components of standard-of-care therapy in neuro-oncology.

ACKNOWLEDGMENTS

This work was supported by grants from the National Institutes of Health (R01 CA100426), the Goldhirsh Foundation, and the Making Headway Foundation, Inc (DZ), and by the Alice M. and Thomas J. Tisch Foundation (JGG) and the S. Arthur Localio Laboratory (JPG). We express our gratitude to Amanda Najjar for her editorial assistance, Yevgeniy Lukyanov, MD, and Julio Garcia for their illustration work and Robert J. Bollo, MD, for the clinical vignette material. The authors declare no competing financial interests.

REFERENCES

1. Elvidge A, Penfield W, Cone W. The gliomas of the central nervous system. A study of two hundred and ten verified cases. *Res Publ Assoc Res Nerv Ment Dis*. 1935;16:107–181; discussion 175–178.
2. Zetter BR. The scientific contributions of M. Judah Folkman to cancer research. *Nat Rev Cancer*. 2008;8:647–654.
3. Folkman J. Tumor angiogenesis: therapeutic implications. *N Engl J Med*. 1971;285:1182–1186.
4. Folkman J. How is blood vessel growth regulated in normal and neoplastic tissue? G.H.A. Clowes Memorial Award Lecture. *Cancer Res*. 1986;46:467–473.
5. Hanahan D, Weinberg RA. The hallmarks of cancer. *Cell*. 2000;100:57–70.
6. Carmeliet P. Angiogenesis in life, disease and medicine. *Nature*. 2005;438:932–936.
7. Adams RH, Alitalo K. Molecular regulation of angiogenesis and lymphagenesis. *Nat Rev Mol Cell Biol*. 2007;8:464–478.
8. Ribatti D, Nico B, Crivellato E. Morphological and molecular aspects of physiological vascular morphogenesis. *Angiogenesis*. 2009;12:101–111.
9. Holash J, Maisonpierre PC, Compton D, et al. Vessel cooption, regression, and growth in tumors mediated by angiopoietins and VEGF. *Science*. 1999;284:1994–1998.
10. Zagzag D, Hooper A, Friedlander DR, et al. In situ expression of angiopoietins in astrocytomas identifies angiopoietin-2 as an early marker of tumor angiogenesis. *Exp Neurol*. 1999;159:391–400.
11. Zagzag D, Zhong H, Scalzitti JM, Laughner E, Simons JW, Semenza GL. Expression of hypoxia-inducible factor 1α in brain tumors: association with angiogenesis, invasion, and progression. *Cancer*. 2000;88:2606–2618.
12. Semenza GL. Targeting HIF-1 for cancer therapy. *Nat Rev Cancer*. 2003;3:721–732.
13. Semenza GL. Hypoxia-inducible factor 1 and cancer pathogenesis. *IUBMB Life*. 2008;60:591–597.
14. Zagzag D, Esencay M, Mendez O, et al. Hypoxia- and vascular endothelial growth factor-induced stromal cell-derived factor-1α/CXCR4 expression in glioblastomas. One plausible explanation of Scherer's structures. *Am J Pathol*. 2008;178:545–560.
15. Fischer I, Gagner JP, Law M, Newcomb EW, Zagzag D. Angiogenesis in gliomas: biology and molecular pathophysiology. *Brain Pathol*. 2005;15:297–310.

16. Puputti M, Tynninen O, Sihto H, et al. Amplification of KIT, PDGFRA, VEGFR2, and EGFR in gliomas. *Mol Cancer Res.* 2006;4:927–934.
17. Weinmann M, Belka C, Plasswilm L. Tumour hypoxia: impact on biology, prognosis and treatment of solid malignant tumours. *Onkologie.* 2004;27:83–90.
18. Reynolds TY, Rockwell S, Glazer PM. Genetic instability induced by the tumor micro-environment. *Cancer Res.* 1996;56:5754–5757.
19. Jain RK, di Tomaso E, Duda DG, Loeffler JS, Sorensen AG, Batchelor TT. Angiogenesis in brain tumours. *Nat Rev Neurosci.* 2007;8:610–622.
20. Lamagna C, Bergers G. The bone marrow constitutes a reservoir of pericyte progenitors. *J Leukoc Biol.* 2006;80:677–681.
21. Kerbel RS. Tumor angiogenesis. *N Engl J Med.* 2008;358:2039–2049.
22. Murdoch C, Muthana M, Coffelt SB, Lewis CE. The role of myeloid cells in the promotion of tumour angiogenesis. *Nat Rev Cancer.* 2008;8:618–631.
23. Gagner JP, Law M, Fischer I, Newcomb EW, Zagzag D. Angiogenesis in gliomas: imaging and experimental therapeutics. *Brain Pathol.* 2005;15:342–363.
24. Omuro AM, Faivre S, Raymond E. Lessons learned in the development of targeted therapy for malignant gliomas. *Mol Cancer Ther.* 2007;6:1909–1919.
25. Sathornsumetee S, Reardon DA, Desjardins A, Quinn JA, Vredenburgh JJ, Rich JN. Molecularly targeted therapy for malignant glioma. *Cancer.* 2007;110:13–24.
26. Norden AD, Drappatz J, Wen PY. Novel anti-angiogenic therapies for malignant gliomas. *Lancet Neurol.* 2008;7:1152–1160.
27. Daumas-Duport C, Koziak M, Miquel C, Nataf F, Jouvet A, Varlet P. [Reappraisal of the Sainte-Anne Hospital classification of oligodendrogliomas in view of retrospective studies]. *Neurochirurgie.* 2005;51:247–253.
28. Kleihues P, Burger PC, Aldape KD, et al. Glioblastoma. In: Louis DN, Ohgaki H, Wiestler OD, Cavenee WK, eds. *WHO Classification of Tumours of the Central Nervous System.* 4th ed. Lyon, France, International Agency for Research on Cancer; 2007:33–49.
29. Louis DN. Molecular pathology of malignant gliomas. *Annu Rev Pathol.* 2006;1:97–117.
30. Wen PY, Kesari S. Malignant gliomas in adults. *N Engl J Med.* 2008;359:492–507.
31. Jouanneau E. Angiogenesis and gliomas: current issues and development of surrogate markers. *Neurosurgery.* 2008;62:31–50; discussion 50–52.
32. Zagzag D, Amirnovin R, Greco MA, et al. Vascular apoptosis and involution in gliomas precedes neovascularization: a novel concept for glioma growth and angiogenesis. *Lab Invest.* 2000;80:837–849.
33. Brat DJ, Castellano-Sanchez AA, Hunter SB, et al. Pseudopalisades in glioblastoma are hypoxic, express extracellular matrix proteases, and are formed by an actively migrating cell population. *Cancer Res.* 2004;64:920–927.
34. Rong Y, Post DE, Pieper RO, Durden DL, van Meir EG, Brat DJ. PTEN and hypoxia regulate tissue factor expression and plasma coagulation by glioblastoma. *Cancer Res.* 2005;65:1406–1413.
35. Aragonés J, Fraisl P, Baes M, Carmeliet P. Oxygen sensors at the crossroad of metabolism. *Cell Metab.* 2009;9:11–22.
36. Khatua S, Peterson KM, Brown KM, et al. Overexpression of the EGFR/FKBP12/HIF-2alpha pathway identified in childhood astrocytomas by angiogenesis gene profiling. *Cancer Res.* 2003;63:1865–1870.
37. Acker T, Diez-Juan A, Aragones J, et al. Genetic evidence for a tumor suppressor role of HIF-2alpha. *Cancer Cell.* 2005;8:131–141.
38. Galbán S, Kuwano Y, Pullmann R Jr, et al. RNA-binding proteins HuR and PTB promote the translation of hypoxia-inducible factor 1alpha. *Mol Cell Biol.* 2008;28:93–107.
39. Kenneth NS, Rocha S. Regulation of gene expression by hypoxia. *Biochem J.* 2008;414:19–29.
40. Yee Koh M, Spivak-Kroizman TR, Powis G. HIF-1 regulation: not so easy come, easy go. *Trends Biochem Sci.* 2008;33:526–534.
41. Semenza GL. Oxygen-dependent regulation of mitochondrial respiration by hypoxia-inducible factor 1. *Biochem J.* 2007;405:1–9.
42. Kaluz S, Kaluzová M, Stanbridge EJ. Regulation of gene expression by hypoxia: integration of the HIF-transduced hypoxic signal at the hypoxia-responsive element. *Clin Chim Acta.* 2008;395:6–13.
43. Cummins EP, Taylor CT. Hypoxia-responsive transcription factors. *Pflugers Arch.* 2005;450:363–371.
44. Laderoute KR. The interaction between HIF-1 and AP-1 transcription factors in response to low oxygen. *Semin Cell Dev Biol.* 2005;16:502–513.
45. Rong Y, Hu F, Huang R, et al. Early growth response gene-1 regulates hypoxia-induced expression of tissue factor in glioblastoma multiforme through hypoxia-inducible factor-1-independent mechanisms. *Cancer Res.* 2006;66:7067–7074.
46. Elvert G, Kappel A, Heidenreich R, et al. Cooperative interaction of hypoxia-inducible factor-2alpha (HIF-2alpha) and Ets-1 in the transcriptional activation of vascular endothelial growth factor receptor-2 (Flk-1). *J Biol Chem.* 2003;278:7520–7530.
47. Hahne JC, Okuducu AF, Sahin A, Fafeur V, Kiriakidis S, Wernert N. The transcription factor ETS-1: its role in tumour development and strategies for its inhibition. *Mini Rev Med Chem.* 2008;8:1095–1105.
48. Li L, Gondi CS, Dinh DH, Olivero WC, Gujrati M, Rao JS. Transfection with anti-p65 intrabody suppresses invasion and angiogenesis in glioma cells by blocking nuclear factor-kappaB transcriptional activity. *Clin Cancer Res.* 2007;13:2178–2190.
49. Cockman ME, Lancaster DE, Stolze IP, et al. Posttranslational hydroxylation of ankyrin repeats in IkappaB proteins by the hypoxia-inducible factor (HIF) asparaginyl hydroxylase, factor inhibiting HIF (FIH). *Proc Natl Acad Sci USA.* 2006;103:14767–14772.
50. Taguchi A, Yanagisawa K, Tanaka M, et al. Identification of hypoxia-inducible factor-1 alpha as a novel target for miR-17–92 microRNA cluster. *Cancer Res.* 2008;68:5540–5545.
51. Brahimi-Horn C, Mazure N, Pouysségur J. Signalling via the hypoxia-inducible factor-1α requires multiple posttranslational modifications. *Cell Signal.* 2005;17:1–9.
52. Birner P, Gatterbauer B, Oberhuber G, et al. Expression of hypoxia-inducible factor-1 alpha in oligodendrogliomas: its impact on prognosis and on neoangiogenesis. *Cancer.* 2001;92:165–171.
53. Brahimi-Horn MC, Pouysségur J. Harnessing the hypoxia-inducible factor in cancer and ischemic disease. *Biochem Pharmacol.* 2007;73:450–457.
54. Bartrons R, Caro J. Hypoxia, glucose metabolism and the Warburg's effect. *J Bioenerg Biomembr.* 2007;39:223–229.
55. Denko NC. Hypoxia, HIF1 and glucose metabolism in the solid tumour. *Nat Rev Cancer.* 2008;8:705–713.
56. Flynn JR, Wang L, Gillespie DL, et al. Hypoxia-regulated protein expression, patient characteristics, and preoperative imaging as predictors of survival in adults with glioblastoma multiforme. *Cancer.* 2008;113:1032–1042.
57. Hewitson KS, Liénard BM, McDonough MA, et al. Structural and mechanistic studies on the inhibition of the hypoxia-inducible transcription factor hydroxylases by tricarboxylic acid cycle intermediates. *J Biol Chem.* 2007;282:3293–3301.
58. Shono T, Yokoyama N, Uesaka T, et al. Enhanced expression of NADPH oxidase Nox4 in human gliomas and its roles in cell proliferation and survival. *Int J Cancer.* 2008;123:787–792.
59. Thompson CB. Metabolic enzymes as oncogenes or tumor suppressors. *N Engl J Med.* 2009;360:813–815.
60. Yan H, Parsons DW, Jin G, et al. IDH1 and IDH2 mutations in gliomas. *N Engl J Med.* 2009;360:765–773.
61. DeHaan C, Habibi-Nazhad B, Yan E, Salloum N, Parliament M, Allalunis-Turner J. Mutation in mitochondrial complex I ND6 subunit is associated with defective response to hypoxia in human glioma cells. *Mol Cancer.* 2004;3:19.
62. Santandreu FM, Brell M, Gene AH, et al. Differences in mitochondrial function and antioxidant systems between regions of human glioma. *Cell Physiol Biochem.* 2008;22:757–768.
63. Neurath KM, Keough MP, Mikkelsen T, Claffey KP. AMP-dependent protein kinase alpha 2 isoform promotes hypoxia-induced VEGF expression in human glioblastoma. *Glia.* 2006;53:733–743.
64. Riemenschneider MJ, Betensky RA, Pasedag SM, Louis DN. AKT activation in human glioblastomas enhances proliferation via TSC2 and S6 kinase signaling. *Cancer Res.* 2006;66:5618–5623.
65. Ermoian RP, Kaprealian T, Lamborn KR, et al. Signal transduction molecules in gliomas of all grades. *J Neurooncol.* 2009;91:19–26.
66. Thoreen CC, Sabatini DM. AMPK and p53 help cells through lean times. *Cell Metab.* 2005;1:287–288.
67. Corcoran CA, Huang Y, Sheikh MS. The regulation of energy generating metabolic pathways by p53. *Cancer Biol Ther.* 2006;5:1610–1613.
68. Teodoro JG, Evans SK, Green MR. Inhibition of tumor angiogenesis by p53: a new role for the guardian of the genome. *J Mol Med.* 2007;85:1175–1186.
69. Engstrom LD, Youkilis AS, Gorelick JL, et al. Mxi1-0, an alternatively transcribed Mxi1 isoform, is overexpressed in glioblastomas. *Neoplasia.* 2004;6:660–673.

70. Löfstedt T, Fredlund E, Noguera R, et al. HIF-1alpha induces MXI1 by alternate promoter usage in human neuroblastoma cells. *Exp Cell Res.* 2009;315:1924–1936.
71. Ido K, Nakagawa T, Sakuma T, Takeuchi H, Sato K, Kubota T. Expression of vascular endothelial growth factor-A and mRNA stability factor HuR in human astrocytic tumors. *Neuropathology.* 2008;28:604–611.
72. Suswam E, Li Y, Zhang X, et al. Tristetraprolin down-regulates interleukin-8 and vascular endothelial growth factor in malignant glioma cells. *Cancer Res.* 2008;68:674–682.
73. Leung AK, Sharp PA. MicroRNAs: a safeguard against turmoil? *Cell.* 2007;130:581–585.
74. Chang TC, Wentzel EA, Kent OA, et al. Transactivation of miR-34a by p53 broadly influences gene expression and promotes apoptosis. *Mol Cell.* 2007;26:745–752.
75. Fasanaro P, D'Alessandra Y, Di Stefano V, et al. MicroRNA-210 modulates endothelial cell response to hypoxia and inhibits the receptor tyrosine kinase ligand Ephrin-A3. *J Biol Chem.* 2008;283:15878–15883.
76. Wouters BG, Koritzinsky M. Hypoxia signaling through mTOR and the unfolded protein response in cancer. *Nat Rev Cancer.* 2008;8:851–864.
77. Koumenis C, Wouters BG. "Translating" tumor hypoxia: unfolded protein response (UPR)-dependent and UPR-independent pathways. *Mol Cancer Res.* 2006;4:423–436.
78. Young RM, Wang SJ, Gordan JD, Ji X, Liebhaber SA, Simon MC. Hypoxia-mediated selective mRNA translation by an internal ribosome entry site-independent mechanism. *J Biol Chem.* 2008;283: 16309–16319.
79. Bi M, Naczki C, Koritzinsky M, et al. ER stress-regulated translation increases tolerance to extreme hypoxia and promotes tumor growth. *EMBO J.* 2005;24:3470–3481.
80. Holcik M, Sonenberg N. Translational control in stress and apoptosis. *Nat Rev Cell Biol.* 2005;6:318–327.
81. Ozawa K, Tsukamoto Y, Hori O, et al. Regulation of tumor angiogenesis by oxygen-regulated protein 150, an inducible endoplasmic reticulum chaperone. *Cancer Res.* 2001;61:4206–4213.
82. Abcouwer SF, Marjon PL, Loper RK, Vander Jagt DL. Response of VEGF expression to amino acid deprivation and inducers of endoplasmic reticulum stress. *Invest Ophthalmol Vis Sci.* 2002;43:2791–2798.
83. DeBerardinis RJ, Lum JJ, Hatzivassiliou G, Thompson CB. The biology of cancer: metabolic reprogramming fuels cell growth and proliferation. *Cell Metab.* 2008;7:11–20.
84. Fraisl P, Mazzone M, Schmidt T, Carmeliet P. Regulation of angiogenesis by oxygen and metabolism. *Dev Cell.* 2009;16:167–179.
85. Kulshreshtha R, Davuluri RV, Calin GA, Ivan M. A microRNA component of the hypoxic response. *Cell Death Differ.* 2008;15:667–671.
86. Urbich C, Kuehbacher A, Dimmeler S. Role of microRNAs in vascular diseases, inflammation, and angiogenesis. *Cardiovasc Res.* 2008;79:581–588.
87. Das B, Tsuchida R, Malkin D, Koren G, Baruchel S, Yeger H. Hypoxia enhances tumor stemness by increasing the invasive and tumorigenic side population fraction. *Stem Cells.* 2008;26:1818–1830.
88. Griguer CE, Oliva CR, Gobin E, et al. CD133 is a marker of bioenergetic stress in human glioma. *PLoS ONE.* 2008;3:e3655.
89. Zhao D, Najbauer J, Garcia E, et al. Neural stem cell tropism to glioma: critical role of tumor hypoxia. *Mol Cancer Res.* 2008;6:1819–1829.
90. Toffoli S, Michiels C. Intermittent hypoxia is a key regulator of cancer cell and endothelial cell interplay in tumours. *FEBS J.* 2008;275:2991–3002.
91. Loges S, Mazzone M, Hohensinner P, Carmeliet P. Silencing or fueling metastasis with VEGF inhibitors: antiangiogenesis revisited. *Cancer Cell.* 2009;15:167–170.
92. Pàez-Ribes M, Allen E, Hudock J, et al. Antiangiogenic therapy elicits malignant progression of tumors to increased local invasion and distant metastasis. *Cancer Cell.* 2009;15:220–231.
93. Reiss T, Machein MR, Plate KH. The role of angiopoietins during angiogenesis in gliomas. *Brain Pathol.* 2005;15:311–377.
94. Martin V, Lie D, Fueyo J, Gomez-Manzano C. Tie2: a journey from normal angiogenesis to cancer and beyond. *Histol Histopathol.* 2008;23:773–780.
95. Stratmann A, Risau W, Plate KH. Cell type-specific expression of angiopoietin-1 and angiopoietin-2 suggests a role in glioblastoma angiogenesis. *Am J Pathol.* 1998;153:1459–1466.
96. Ding H, Roncari L, Wu X, et al. Expression and hypoxic regulation of angiopoietins in human astrocytomas. *Neuro Oncol.* 2001;3:1–10.
97. Zadeh G, Qian B, Okhowat A, Sabha N, Kontos CD, Guha A. Targeting the Tie2/Tek receptor in astrocytomas. *Am J Pathol.* 2004;164:467–476.
98. Lee OH, Xu J, Fueyo J, et al. Expression of the receptor tyrosine kinase Tie2 in neoplastic glial cells is associated with integrin beta-1-dependent adhesion to the extracellular matrix. *Mol Cancer Res.* 2006;4:915–926.
99. Hu B, Jarzynka MJ, Guo P, Imanishi Y, Schlaepfer DD, Cheng SY. Angiopoietin 2 induces glioma cell invasion by stimulating matrix metalloprotease 2 expression through the alphavbeta1 integrin and focal adhesion kinase signaling pathway. *Cancer Res.* 2006;66: 775–783.
100. Simon MP, Tournaire R, Pouyssegur J. The angiopoietin-2 gene of endothelial cells is up-regulated in hypoxia by a HIF binding site located in its first intron and by the central factors GATA-2 and Ets-1. *J Cell Physiol.* 2008;217:809–818.
101. Lee OH, Xu J, Fueyo J, et al. Angiopoietin-2 decreases vascular endothelial growth factor expression by modulating HIF-1 alpha levels in gliomas. *Oncogene.* 2008;27:1310–1314.
102. Ferrara N, Gerber HP, LeCouter J. The biology of VEGF and its receptors. *Nat Med.* 2003;9:669–676.
103. Machein MR, Plate KH. VEGF in brain tumors. *J Neurooncol.* 2000;50:109–120.
104. Sonoda Y, Kanamori M, Deen DF, Cheng SY, Berger MS, Pieper RO. Overexpression of vascular endothelial growth factor isoforms drives oxygenation and growth but not progression to glioblastoma multiforme in a human model of gliomagenesis. *Cancer Res.* 2003;63:1962–1968.
105. Tse V, Xu L, Yung YC, et al. The temporal-spatial expression of VEGF, angiopoietins-1 and 2, and Tie-2 during tumor angiogenesis and their functional correlation with tumor neovascular architecture. *Neurol Res.* 2003;25:729–738.
106. Kaal EC, Vecht CJ. The management of brain edema in brain tumors. *Curr Opin Oncol.* 2004;16:593–600.
107. Nagy JA, Benjamin L, Zeng H, Dvorak AM, Dvorak HF. Vascular permeability, vascular hyperpermeability and angiogenesis. *Angiogenesis.* 2008;11:109–119.
108. Robinson CJ, Stringer SE. The splice variants of vascular endothelial growth factor (VEGF) and their receptors. *J Cell Sci.* 2001;114:853–865.
109. Shweiki D, Itin A, Soffer D, Keshet E. Vascular endothelial growth factor induced by hypoxia may mediate hypoxia-initiated angiogenesis. *Nature.* 1992;359:843–845.
110. Zagzag D, Capo V. Angiogenesis in the central nervous system: a role for vascular endothelial growth factor/vascular permeability factor and tenascin-C. Common molecular effectors in cerebral neoplastic and non-neoplastic "angiogenic diseases." *Histol Histopathol.* 2002;17:301–321.
111. Carmeliet P, Moons L, Luttun A, et al. Synergism between vascular endothelial growth factor and placental growth factor contributes to angiogenesis and plasma extravasation in pathological conditions. *Nat Med.* 2001;7:575–583.
112. Autiero M, Waltenberger J, Communi D, et al. Role of PlGF in the intra- and intermolecular cross talk between the VEGF receptors Flt1 and Flk1. *Nat Med.* 2003;9:936–943.
113. Luttun A, Autiero M, Tjwa M, Carmeliet P. Genetic dissection of tumor angiogenesis: are PlGF and VEGFR-1 novel anti-cancer targets? *Biochim Biophys Acta.* 2004;1654:79–94.
114. Hicklin DJ, Ellis LM. Role of vascular endothelial growth factor pathway in tumor growth and angiogenesis. *J Clin Oncol.* 2005;23: 1011–1027.
115. Kowanetz M, Ferrara N. Vascular endothelial growth factor signaling pathways: therapeutic perspective. *Clin Cancer Res.* 2006;12:5018–5022.
116. Roskoski R Jr. Vascular endothelial growth factor (VEGF) signaling in tumor progression. *Crit Rev Oncol Hematol.* 2007;62:179–213.
117. Ding H, Wu X, Roncari L, et al. Expression and regulation of neuropilin-1 in human astrocytomas. *Int J Cancer.* 2000;88:584–592.
118. Broholm H, Laursen H. Vascular endothelial growth factor (VEGF) receptor neuropilin-1's distribution in astrocytic tumors. *APMIS.* 2004;112:257–263.
119. Osada H, Tokunaga T, Nishi M, et al. Overexpression of the neuropilin (NRP1) gene correlated with poor prognosis in human glioma. *AntiCancer Res.* 2004;24:547–552.
120. Kunkel P, Ulbricht U, Bohlen P, et al. Inhibition of glioma angiogenesis and growth in vivo by systemic treatment with a monoclonal

antibody against vascular endothelial growth factor receptor-2. *Cancer Res.* 2001;61:6624–6628.
121. Batchelor TT, Sorensen AG, di Tomaso E, et al. AZD2171, a pan-VEGF receptor tyrosine kinase inhibitor, normalizes tumor vasculature and alleviates edema in glioblastoma patients. *Cancer Cell.* 2007;11:83–95.
122. Gomez-Manzano C, Holash J, Fueyo J, et al. VEGF Trap induces antiglioma effect at different stages of disease. *Neuro Oncol.* 2008;10:940–945.
123. Heidenreich R, Machein M, Nicolaus A, et al. Inhibition of solid tumor growth by gene transfer of VEGF receptor-1 mutants. *Int J Cancer.* 2005;111:348–357.
124. Shibuya M. Vascular endothelial growth factor receptor-1 (VEGFR-1/Flt-1): a dual regulator for angiogenesis. *Angiogenesis.* 2006;9:225–230.
125. Fischer C, Mazzone M, Jonckx B, Carmeliet P. FLT1 and its ligands VEGFB and PlGF: drug targets for anti-angiogenic therapy? *Nat Rev Cancer.* 2008;8:942–956.
126. Ellis LM. The role of neuropilins in cancer. *Mol Cancer Ther.* 2006;5:1099–1107.
127. Soker S, Miao HQ, Nomi M, Takashima S, Klagsbrun M. VEGF165 mediates formation of complexes containing VEGFR-2 and neuropilin-1 that enhance VEGF165-receptor binding. *J Cell Biochem.* 2002;85:357–368.
128. Wang L, Zeng H, Wang P, Soker S, Mukhopadhyay D. Neuropilin-1-mediated vascular permeability factor/vascular endothelial growth factor-dependent endothelial cell migration. *J Biol Chem.* 2003;278:48848–48860.
129. Murga M, Fernandez-Capetillo O, Tosato G. Neuropilin-1 regulates attachment in human endothelial cells independently of vascular endothelial growth factor receptor-2. *Blood.* 2005;105:1992–1999.
130. Valter MM, Hugel A, Huang HJ, et al. Expression of the Ets-1 transcription factor in human astrocytomas is associated with Fms-like tyrosine kinase-1 (Flt-1)/vascular endothelial growth factor receptor-1 synthesis and neoangiogenesis. *Cancer Res.* 1999;59:5608–5614.
131. Sahin A, Velten M, Pietsch T, et al. Inaction of ETS 1 transcription factor by a specific decoy strategy reduces rat C6 glioma cell proliferation and MMP-9 expression. *Int J Mol Med.* 2005;15:771–776.
132. Loeffler S, Fayard B, Weis J, Weissenberger J. Interleukin-6 induces transcriptional activation of vascular endothelial growth factor (VEGF) in astrocytes in vivo and regulates VEGF promoter activity in glioblastoma cells via direct interaction between STAT3 and Sp1. *Int J Cancer.* 2005;115:202–213.
133. Arany Z, Foo SY, Ma Y, et al. HIF-independent regulation of VEGF and angiogenesis by the transcriptional coactivator PGC-1alpha. *Nature.* 2008;451:1008–1012.
134. Pore N, Liu S, Haas-Kogan DA, O'Rourke DM, Maity A. PTEN mutation and epidermal growth factor receptor activation regulate vascular endothelial growth factor (VEGF) mRNA expression in human glioblastoma cells by transactivating the proximal VEGF promoter. *Cancer Res.* 2003;63:236–241.
135. Furnari FB, Fenton T, Bachoo RM, et al. Malignant astrocytic glioma: genetics, biology, and paths to treatment. *Genes Dev.* 2007;21:2683–2710.
136. Endersby R, Baker SJ. PTEN signaling in brain: neuropathology and tumorigenesis. *Oncogene.* 2008;27:5416–5430.
137. Zagzag D. Angiogenic growth factors in neural embryogenesis and neoplasia. *Am J Pathol.* 1995;146:293–309.
138. Dunn IF, Heese O, Black PM. Growth factors in glioma angiogenesis: FGFs, PDGF, EGF, and TGFs. *J Neurooncol* 2000;50:121–137.
139. Zagzag D, Miller DC, Sato Y, Rifkin DB, Burstein DE. Immunohistochemical localization of basic fibroblast growth factor in astrocytomas. *Cancer Res.*1990;50:7393–7398.
140. Guo P, Hu B, Gu W, et al. Platelet-derived growth factor-B enhances glioma angiogenesis by stimulating vascular endothelial growth factor expression in tumor endothelia and by promoting pericyte recruitment. *Am J Pathol.* 2003;162:1083–1093.
141. Shih AH, Holland EC. Platelet-derived growth factor (PDGF) and glial tumorigenesis. *Cancer Lett.* 2006;232:139–147.
142. Nabors LB, Suswam E, Huang Y, Yang X, Johnson MJ, King PH. Tumor necrosis factor alpha induces angiogenic factor upregulation in malignant glioma cells: a role for RNA stabilization and HuR. *Cancer Res.* 2003;63:4181–4187.
143. Zelzer E, Levy Y, Kahana C, Shilo BZ, Rubinstein M, Cohen B. Insulin induces transcription of target genes through the hypoxia-inducible factor HIF-1 alpha/ARNT. *EMBO J.* 1998;17:5085–5094.
144. Takano S, Tsuboi K, Tomono Y, et al. Tissue factor, osteopontin, alpha-v-beta3 integrin expression in microvasculature of gliomas associated with vascular endothelial growth factor expression. *Br J Cancer.* 2000;82:1967–1973.
145. Yamahata H, Takeshima H, Kuratsu J, et al. The role of thrombin in the neo-vascularization of malignant gliomas: an intrinsic modulator for the up-regulation of vascular endothelial growth factor. *Int J Oncol.* 2002;20:921–928.
146. Sun L, Hui AM, Su Q, et al. Neuronal and glioma-derived stem cell factor induces angiogenesis within the brain. *Cancer Cell.* 2006;9:287–300.
147. Noguera-Troise I, Daly C, Papadopoulos NJ, et al. Blockade of Dll4 inhibits tumour growth by promoting non-productive angiogenesis. *Nature.* 2006;444:1032–1037.
148. Li JL, Sainson RC, Shi W, et al. Delta-like 4 Notch ligand regulates tumor angiogenesis, improves tumor vascular function, and promotes tumor growth in vivo. *Cancer Res.* 2007;67:11244–11253.
149. Arrieta O, Gracia E, Guevara P, et al. Hepatocyte growth factor is associated with poor prognosis of malignant gliomas and is a predictor for recurrence of meningioma. *Cancer.* 2002;94:3210–3218.
150. Zhang YW, Su Y, Volpert OV, Vande Woude GF. Hepatocyte growth factor/scatter factor mediates angiogenesis through positive VEGF and negative thrombospondin 1 regulation. *Proc Natl Acad Sci U S A.* 2003;100:12718–12723.
151. Comoglio PM, Giordan S, Trusolino L. Drug development of MET inhibitors: targeting oncogene addiction and expedience. *Nat Rev Drug Discov.* 2008;7:504–506.
152. Abounader R, Laterra J. Scatter factor/hepatocyte growth factor in brain tumor growth and angiogenesis. *Neuro Oncol.* 2005;7:436–451.
153. Lamszus K, Schmidt NO, Jin L, et al. Scatter factor promotes motility of human glioma and neuro-microvascular endothelial cells. *Int J Cancer.* 1998;75:19–28.
154. Schmidt NO, Westphal M, Hagel C, et al. Levels of vascular endothelial growth factor, hepatocyte growth factor/scatter factor and basic fibroblast growth factor in human gliomas and their relationship to angiogenesis. *Int J Cancer.* 1999;84:10–18.
155. Moriyama T, Kataoka H, Hamasuna R, et al. Up-regulation of vascular endothelial growth factor induced by hepatocyte growth factor/scatter factor stimulation in human glioma cells. *Biochem Biophys Res Commun.* 1998;249:73–77.
156. Sengupta S, Gherardi E, Sellers LA, Wood JM, Sasisekharan R, Fan TP. Hepatocyte growth factor/scatter factor can induce angiogenesis independently of vascular endothelial growth factor. *Arterioscler Thromb Vasc Biol.* 2003;23:69–75.
157. Martens T, Schmidt NO, Eckerich C, et al. A novel one-armed anti-c-met antibody inhibits glioblastoma growth in vivo. *Clin Cancer Res.* 2006;12:6144–6152.
158. Sattler M, Salgia R. c-Met and hepatocyte growth factor: potential as novel targets in cancer therapy. *Curr Oncol Rep.* 2007;9:102–108.
159. Tseng JR, Kang KW, Dandekar M, et al. Preclinical efficacy of the c-Met inhibitor CE-355621 in a U87 MG mouse xenograft model evaluated by 18F-FDG small-animal PET. *J Nucl Med.* 2008;49:129–134.
160. Hu B, Guo P, Bar-Joseph I, et al. Neuropilin-1 promotes human glioma progression through potentiating the activity of the HGF/SF autocrine pathway. *Oncogene.* 2007;26:5577–5586.
161. Chu S, Ma Y, Zhang H, et al. Hepatocyte growth factor production is stimulated by gangliosides and TGF-β isoforms in human glioma cells. *J Neurooncol.* 2007;35:33–38.
162. Stommel JM, Kimmelman AC, Ying H, et al. Coactivation of receptor tyrosine kinases affects the response of tumor cells to targeted therapies. *Science.* 2007;318:287–290.
163. Eckerich C, Zapf S, Fillbrandt R, Loges S, Westphal M, Lamszus K. Hypoxia can induce c-Met expression in glioma cells and enhance SF/HGF-induced cell migration. *Int J Cancer.* 2007;121:276–283.
164. Strieter RM, Belperio JA, Phillips RJ, Keane MP. CXC chemokines in angiogenesis of cancer. *Semin Cancer Biol.* 2004;4:195–200.
165. Li M, Ransohoff RM. The roles of chemokine CXCL12 in embryonic and brain tumor angiogenesis. *Semin Cancer Biol.* 2009;19:111–115.
166. Rempel SA, Dudas S, Ge S, Gutierrez JA. Identification and localization of the cytokine SDF1 and its receptor, CXC chemokine receptor

4, to regions of necrosis and angiogenesis in human glioblastoma. *Clin Cancer Res.* 2000;6:102–111.
167. Ceradini DJ, Gurtner GC. Homing to hypoxia: HIF-1 as a mediator of progenitor cell recruitment to injured tissue. *Trends Cardiovasc Med.* 2005;15:57–63.
168. Zagzag D, Lukyanov Y, Lan Li, et al. Hypoxia-inducible factor 1 and VEGF upregulate CXCR4 in glioblastoma: implications for angiogenesis and glioma cell invasion. *Lab Invest.* 2006;86:1221–1232.
169. Salvucci O, Yao L, Villalba S, Sajewicz A, Pittaluga S, Tosato G. Regulation of endothelial cell branching morphogenesis by endogenous chemokine stromal-derived factor-1. *Blood.* 2002;99:2703–2711.
170. Salmaggi A, Gelati M, Pollo B, et al. CXCL12 in malignant glial tumors: a possible role in angiogenesis and cross-talk between endothelial and tumoral cells. *J Neurooncol.* 2004;67:305–317.
171. Salcedo R, Wasserman K, Young HA, et al. Vascular endothelial growth factor and basic fibroblast growth factor induce expression of CXCR4 on human endothelial cells: in vivo neovascularization induced by stromal-derived factor-1alpha. *Am J Pathol.* 1999;154:1125–1135.
172. Rubin JB, Kung AL, Klein RS, et al. A small-molecule antagonist of CXCR4 inhibits intracranial growth of primary brain tumors. *Proc Natl Acad Sci USA.* 2003;100:13513–13518.
173. Lakka SS, Jasti SL, Gondi C, et al. Downregulation of MMP-9 in ERK-mutated stable transfectants inhibits glioma invasion in vitro. *Oncogene.* 2002;21:5601–5608.
174. Chandrasekar N, Mohanam S, Gujrati M, Olivero WC, Dinh DH, Rao JS. Downregulation of uPA inhibits migration and PI3k/Akt signaling in glioblastoma cells. *Oncogene.* 2003;22:392–400.
175. Cox BD, Natarajan M, Stettner MR, Gladson CL. New concepts regarding focal adhesion kinase promotion of cell migration and proliferation. *J Cell Biochem.* 2006;99:35–52.
176. Petit I, Jin D, Rafii S. The SDF-1-CXCR4 signaling pathway: a molecular hub modulating neo-angiogenesis. *Trends Immunol.* 2007;28:299–307.
177. Nyberg P, Xie L, Kalluri R. Endogenous inhibitors of angiogenesis. *Cancer Res.* 2005;65:3967–3979.
178. Rege TA, Fears CY, Gladson CL. Endogenous inhibitors of angiogenesis in malignant gliomas: nature's antiangiogenic therapy. *Neuro Oncol.* 2005;7:106–121.
179. Anderson JC, McFarland BC, Gladson CL. New molecular targets in the angiogenic vessels of glioblastoma tumors. *Expert Rev Mol Med.* 2008;10:e23.
180. Kazuno M, Tokunaga T, Oshika Y, et al. Thrombospondin-2 (TSP2) expression is inversely correlated with vascularity in glioma. *Eur J Cancer.* 1999;35:502–506.
181. Wang D, Anderson JC, Gladson CL. The role of the extracellular matrix in malignant glioma tumors. *Brain Pathol.* 2005;15:318–326.
182. Ohgaki H, Dessen P, Jourde B, et al. Genetic pathways to glioblastoma: a population-based study. *Cancer Res.* 2004;64:6892–6899.
183. Okamoto Y, Di Patre PL, Burkhard C, et al. Population-based study on incidence, survival rates, and genetic alterations of low-grade diffuse astrocytomas and oligodendrogliomas. *Acta Neuropathol (Berl)* 2004;108:49–56.
184. Cancer Genome Atlas Research Network. Comprehensive genomic characterization defines human glioblastoma genes and core pathways. *Nature* 2008;455:1061–1068.
185. Hirota K, Semenza GL. Regulation of angiogenesis by hypoxia-inducible factor 1. *Crit Rev Oncol Hematol.* 2006;59:15–26.
186. Zheng H, Ying H, Yan H, et al. Pten and p53 converge on c-myc to control differentiation, self-renewal, and transformation of normal and neoplastic stem cells in glioblastoma. *Cold Spring Harb Symp Quant Biol.* 2008;73:427–437.
187. Guha A. Ras activation in astrocytomas and neurofibromas. *Can J Neurol Sci.* 1998;25:267–281.
188. Mizukami Y, Kohgo Y, Chung DC. Hypoxia-inducible factor-1 independent pathways in tumor angiogenesis. *Clin Cancer Res.* 2007;13:5670–5674.
189. Zagzag D, Krishnamachary B, Yee H, et al. Stromal cell-derived factor-1 alpha and CXCR4 expression in hemangioblastoma and clear cell-renal cell carcinoma: von Hippel-Lindau loss-of-function induces expression of a ligand and its receptor. *Cancer Res.* 2005;65:6178–6188.
190. Esteller M. Epigenetics in cancer. *N Engl J Med.* 2008;358:1148–1159.
191. Delcuve GP, Rastegar M, Davie JR. Epigenetic control. *J Cell Physiol.* 2009;219:243–250.
192. Burgess R, Jenkins R, Zhang Z. Epigenetic changes in gliomas. *Cancer Biol Ther.* 2008;7:1326–1334.
193. Hesson LB, Krex D, Latif F. Epigenetic markers in human gliomas: prospects for therapeutic intervention. *Expert Rev Neurother.* 2008;8:1475–1496.
194. Dutta D, Ray S, Vivian JL, Paul S. Activation of the VEGFR1 chromatin domain: an angiogenic signal-ETS1/HIF-2alpha regulatory axis. *J Biol Chem.* 2008;283:25404–25413.
195. Esquela-Kerscher A, Slack FJ. Oncomirs-microRNAs with a role in cancer. *Nat Rev Cancer.* 2006;6:259–269.
196. Nicoloso MS, Calin GA. MicroRNA involvement in brain tumors: from bench to bedside. *Brain Pathol.* 2008;18:122–129.
197. Ferretti E, DeSmaele E, Po A, et al. MicroRNA profiling in human medulloblastoma. *Int J Cancer.* 2009;124:568–577.
198. Würdinger T, Tannous BA, Saydam O, et al. miR-296 regulates growth factor receptor overexpression in angiogenic endothelial cells. *Cancer Cell.* 2008;14:382–393.
199. Fish JE, Srivastava D. MicroRNAs: opening a new vein in angiogenesis research. *Sci Signal.* 2009;1:pe1.
200. Iero M, Valenti R, Huber V, et al. Tumour-released exosomes and their implications in cancer immunity. *Cell Death Differ.* 2008;15:80–88.
201. Skog J, Würdinger T, van Rijn S, et al. Glioblastoma microvesicles transport RNA and proteins that promote tumour growth and provide diagnostic biomarkers. *Nat Cell Biol.* 2008;10:1470–1476.
202. Al-Nedawi K, Meehan B, Micallef J, et al. Intercellular transfer of the oncogenic receptor EGFRvIII by microvesicles derived from tumour cells. *Nat Cell Biol.* 2008;10:619–624.
203. Singh SK, Clarke ID, Terasaki M, et al. Identification of a cancer stem cell in human brain tumors. *Cancer Res.* 2003;63:5821–5828.
204. Singh SK, Hawkins C, Clarke ID, et al. Identification of human brain tumour initiating cells. *Nature.* 2004;432:396–401.
205. Liu G, Yuan X, Zeng Z, et al. Analysis of gene expression and chemoresistance of CD133+ cancer stem cells in glioblastoma. *Mol Cancer.* 2006;5:67–78.
206. Bao S, Wu Q, McLendon RE, et al. Glioma stem cells promote radioresistance by preferential activation of the DNA damage response. *Nature.* 2006;444:756–760.
207. Stiles CD, Rowitch DH. Glioma stem cells: a midterm exam. *Neuron.* 2008;58:832–846.
208. Bao S, Wu Q, Sathornsumetee S, et al. Stem cell-like glioma cells promote tumor angiogenesis through vascular endothelial growth factor. *Cancer Res.* 2006;66:7843–7848.
209. Salmaggi A, Boiardi A, Gelati M, et al. Glioblastoma-derived tumorospheres identify a population of tumor stem-like cells with angiogenic potential and enhanced multidrug resistance phenotype. *Glia.* 2006;54:850–860.
210. Oka N, Soeda A, Inagaki A, et al. VEGF promotes tumorigenesis and angiogenesis of human glioblastoma stem cells. *Biochem Biophys Res Commun.* 2007;360:553–559.
211. Yao XH, Ping YF, Chen JH, et al. Glioblastoma stem cells produce vascular endothelial growth factor by activation of a G-protein coupled formylpeptide receptor FPR. *J Pathol.* 2008;215:369–376.
212. Dean M, Fojo T, Bates S. Tumour stem cells and drug resistance. *Nat Rev Cancer.* 2005;5:275–284.
213. Calabrese C, Poppleton H, Kocak M, et al. A perivascular niche for brain tumor stem cells. *Cancer Cell.* 2007;11:69–82.
214. Folkins C, Man S, Xu P, Shaked Y, Hicklin DJ, Kerbel RS. Anticancer therapies combining antiangiogenic and tumor cell cytotoxic effects reduce the tumor stem-like cell fraction in glioma xenograft tumors. *Cancer Res.* 2007;67:3560–3564.
215. Christensen K, Schroder HD, Kristensen BW. CD133 identifies perivascular niches in grade II-IV astrocytomas. *J Neurooncol.* 2008;90:157–170.
216. Veeravagu A, Bababeygy SR, Kalani MY, Hou LC, Tse V. The cancer stem cell-vascular niche complex in brain tumor formation. *Stem Cells Dev.* 2008;17:859–867.
217. Pietras A, Gisselsson D, Ora I, et al. High levels of HIF-2α highlight an immature neural crest-like neuroblastoma cell cohort located in a perivascular niche. *J Pathol.* 2008;214:482–488.
218. Shmelkov SV, Butler JM, Hooper AT, et al. CD133 expression is not restricted to stem cells, and both CD133+ and CD133- metastatic colon cancer cells initiate tumors. *J Clin Invest.* 2008;118:2111–2120.

219. Aguirre-Ghiso JA. Models, mechanisms and clinical evidence for cancer dormancy. *Nat Rev Cancer.* 2007;7:834–846.
220. Naumov GN, Folkman J, Straume O, Akslen LA. Tumor-vascular interactions and tumor dormancy. *APMIS.* 2008;116:569–585.
221. Trumpp A, Wiestler OD. Mechanisms of disease: cancer stem cells--targeting the evil twin. *Nat Clin Pract Oncol.* 2008;5:337–347.
222. Almog N, Ma L, Raychowdhury R, et al. Transcriptional switch of dormant tumors to fast-growing angiogenic phenotype. *Cancer Res.* 2009;69:836–844.
223. Cogle CR, Scott EW. The hemangioblast: cradle to clinic. *Exp Hematol.* 2004;32:885–890.
224. Fischer C, Schneider M, Carmeliet P. Principles and therapeutic implications of angiogenesis, vasculogenesis and arteriogenesis. *Handb Exp Pharmacol.* 2006;176:157–212.
225. Ribatti D. Genetic and epigenetic mechanisms in the early development of the vascular system. *J Anat.* 2006;208:139–152.
226. Bertolini F, Shaked Y, Mancuso P, Kerbel RS. The multifaceted circulating endothelial cell in cancer: towards marker and target identification. *Nat Rev Cancer.* 2006;6:835–845.
227. Gao D, Nolan D, McDonnell K, et al. Bone marrow-derived endothelial progenitor cells contribute to the angiogenic switch in tumor growth and metastatic progression. *Biochim Biophys Acta.* 2009;1796:33–40.
228. van Hinsbergh VW, Engelse MA, Quax PH. Pericellular proteases in angiogenesis and vasculogenesis. *Arterioscler Thromb Vasc Biol.* 2006;26:716–728.
229. Farin A, Suzuki SO, Weiker M, Goldman JE, Bruce JN, Canoll P. Transplanted glioma cells migrate and proliferate on host brain vasculature: a dynamic analysis. *Glia.* 2006;53:799–808.
230. Ahn GO, Brown JM. Matrix metalloproteinase-9 is required for tumor vasculogenesis but not for angiogenesis: role of bone marrow-derived myelomonocytic cells. *Cancer Cell.* 2008;13:193–205.
231. Avraamides CJ, Garmy-Susini B, Varner JA. Integrins in angiogenesis and lymphangiogenesis. *Nat Rev Cancer.* 2008;8:604–617.
232. Aghi M, Chiocca EA. Contribution of bone marrow-derived cells to blood vessels in ischemic tissues and tumors. *Mol Ther.* 2005;12:994–1005.
233. De Palma M, Venneri MA, Galli R, et al. Tie2 identifies a hematopoietic lineage of proangiogenic monocytes require for tumor vessel formation and a mesenchymal population of pericyte progenitors. *Cancer Cell.* 2005;8:211–226.
234. Gagner JP, Shamamian P. Antigen expression profile in circulating endothelial progenitor cells. *Nat Rev Cancer.* 2007;7:68.
235. Zerbini G, Lorenzi M, Palini A, Kerbel RS. Tumor angiogenesis. *N Engl J Med.* 2008; 359:763–764.
236. Beaudry P, Force J, Naumov GN, et al. Differential effects of vascular endothelial growth factor receptor-2 inhibitor ZD6474 on circulating endothelial progenitors and mature circulating endothelial cells: implications for use as a surrogate marker of antiangiogenic activity. *Clin Cancer Res.* 2005;11:3514–3522.
237. Du R, Lu KV, Petritsch C, et al. HIF1alpha induces the recruitment of bone marrow-derived vascular modulatory cells to regulate tumor angiogenesis and invasion. *Cancer Cell.* 2008;13:206–220.
238. Bababeygy SR, Cheshier SH, Hou LC, Higgins DM, Weissman IL, Tse VC. Hematopoietic stem cell-derived pericytic cells in brain tumor angio-architecture. *Stem Cells Dev.* 2008;17:11–18.
239. De Palma M, Murdoch C, Venneri MA, Naldini L, Lewis CE. Tie2-expressing monocytes: regulation of tumor angiogenesis and therapeutic implications. *Trends Immunol.* 2007;28:519–524.
240. Lyden D, Hattori K, Dias S, et al. Impaired recruitment of bone-marrow-derived endothelial and hematopoietic precursor cells blocks tumor angiogenesis and growth. *Nat Med.* 2001;7:1194–1201.
241. Ribatti D, Nico B, Crivellato E, Vacca A. Endothelial progenitor cells in health and disease. *Histol Histopathol.* 2005;20:1351–1358.
242. Schatteman G. Are circulating CD133+ cells biomarkers of vascular disease? *Arterioscler Thromb Vasc Biol.* 2005;25:270–271.
243. Dome B, Timar J, Ladanyi A, et al. Circulating endothelial cells, bone marrow-derived endothelial progenitor cells and proangiogenic hematopoietic cells in cancer: from biology to therapy. *Crit Rev Oncol Hematol.* 2009;69:108–124.
244. Furuhata S, Ando K, Oki M, et al. Gene expression profiles of endothelial progenitor cells by oligonucleotide microarray analysis. *Mol Cell Biochem.* 2007;298:125–138.
245. Fürstenberger G, von Moos R, Lucas R, et al. Circulating endothelial cells and angiogenic serum factors during neoadjuvant chemotherapy of primary breast cancer. *Br J Cancer.* 2006;94:524–531.
246. Döme B, Timar J, Dobos J, et al. Identification and clinical significance of circulating endothelial progenitor cells in human non-small cell lung cancer. *Cancer Res.* 2006; 66:7341–7347.
247. Zheng PP, Hop WC, Luider TM, Sillevis Smitt PA, Kros JM. Increased levels of circulating endothelial progenitor cells and circulating endothelial nitric oxide synthase in patients with gliomas. *Ann Neurol.* 2007;62:40–48.
248. Raida M, Weiss T, Leo C, et al. Circulating endothelial progenitor cells are inversely correlated with the median oxygen tension in the tumor tissue of patients with cervical cancer. *Oncol Rep.* 2006;16: 597–601.
249. Li B, Sharpe EE, Maupin AB, et al. VEGF and PLGF promote adult vasculogenesis by enhancing EPC recruitment and vessel formation at the site of tumor neovascularization. *FASEB J.* 2006;20:664–676.
250. Willett CG, Duda DG, di Tomaso E, et al. Complete pathological response to bevacizumab and chemoradiation in advanced rectal cancer. *Nat Clin Pract Oncol.* 2007;4:316–321.
251. Arbab AS, Pandit SD, Anderson SA, et al. Magnetic resonance imaging and confocal microscopy studies of magnetically labeled endothelial progenitor cells trafficking to sites of tumor angiogenesis. *Stem Cells.* 2006;24:671–678.
252. Moore XL, Lu J, Sun L, Zhu CJ, Tan P, Wong MC. Endothelial progenitor cells' "homing" specificity to brain tumors. *Gene Ther.* 2004;11:811–818.
253. Aghi M, Cohen KS, Klein RJ, Scadden DT, Chiocca EA. Tumor stromal-derived factor-1 recruits vascular progenitors to mitotic neovasculature, where microenvironment influences their differentiated phenotypes. *Cancer Res.* 2006;66:9054–9064.
254. Jin DK, Shido K, Kopp HG, et al. Cytokine-mediated deployment of SDF-1 induces revascularization through recruitment of CXCR4+ hemangiocytes. *Nat Med.* 2006;12:557–567.
255. Tabatabai G, Frank B, Möhle R, Weller M, Wick W. Irradiation and hypoxia promote homing of haematopoietic progenitor cells towards gliomas by TGF-beta-dependent HIF-1alpha-mediated induction of CXCL12. *Brain.* 2006;129:2426–2435.
256. Shaw JP, Basch R, Shamamian P. Hematopoietic stem cells and endothelial cell precursors express Tie-2, CD31 and CD45. *Blood Cells Mol Dis.* 2004;32:168–175.
257. Gill KA, Brindle NPJ. Angiopoietin-2 stimulates migration of endothelial progenitors and their interaction with endothelium. *Biochem Biophys Res Commu.* 2005;36:392–396.
258. Udani V, Santarelli J, Yung Y, et al. Differential expression of angiopoietin-1 and angiopoietin-2 may enhance recruitment of bone-marrow-derived endothelial precursor cells into brain tumors. *Neurol Res.* 2005;27:801–806.
259. Kim KL, Shin IS, Kim JM, et al. Interaction between Tie receptors modulates angiogenic activity of angiopoietin2 in endothelial progenitor cells. *Cardiovasc Res.* 2006;72:394–402.
260. Machein MR, Renninger S, de Lima-Hahn E, Plate KH. Minor contribution of bone marrow-derived endothelial progenitors to the vascularization of murine gliomas. *Brain Pathol.* 2003;13:582–597.
261. Shaked Y, Bertolini F, Man S, et al. Genetic heterogeneity of the vasculogenic phenotype parallels angiogenesis; Implications for cellular surrogate marker analysis of antiangiogenesis. *Cancer Cell* 2005;7:101–11.
262. Bexell D, Gunnarsson S, Tormin A, et al. Bone marrow multipotent mesenchymal stroma cells act as pericyte-like migratory vehicles in experimental gliomas. *Mol Ther.* 2009;17:183–190.
263. McLean K, Buckanovich RJ. Myeloid cells functioning in tumor vascularization as a novel therapeutic target. *Transl Res.* 2008;151:59–67.
264. Shojaei F, Wu X, Malik AK, et al. Tumor refractoriness to anti-VEGF treatment is mediated by CD11b+Gr1+ myeloid cells. *Nat Biotechnol.* 2007;25:911–920.
265. Venneri MA, De Palma M, Ponzoni M, et al. Identification of proangiogenic TIE2-expressing monocytes (TEMs) in human peripheral blood and cancer. *Blood.* 2007;109:5276–5285.
266. Lewis CE, Hughes R. Inflammation and breast cancer. Microenvironmental factors regulating macrophage function in breast tumours: hypoxia and angiopoietin-2. *Breast Cancer Res.* 2007;9:209–212.
267. Murdoch C, Tazzyman S, Webster S, Lewis CE. Expression of Tie-2 by human monocytes and their responses to angiopoietin-2. *J Immunol.* 2007;178:7405–7411.

268. Riccioni R, Diverio D, Mariani G, et al. Expression of Tie-2 and other receptors for endothelial growth factors in acute myeloid leukemias is associated with monocytic features of leukemic blasts. *Stem Cells.* 2007;25:1862–1871.
269. Valable S, Barbier EL, Bernaudin M, et al. In vivo MRI tracking of exogenous monocytes/macrophages targeting brain tumors in a rat model of glioma. *Neuroimage.* 2008;40:973–983.
270. De Palma M, Mazzieri R, Politi LS, et al. Tumor-targeted interferon-alpha delivery by Tie2-expressing monocytes inhibits tumor growth and metastasis. *Cancer Cell* 2008;14:299–311.
271. De Palma M, Venneri MA, Roca C, Naldini L. Targeting exogenous genes to tumor angiogenesis by transplantation of genetically modified hematopoietic stem cells. *Nat Med.* 2003;9:789–795.
272. Miletic H, Fischer YH, Giroglou T, et al. Normal brain cells contribute to the bystander effect in suicide gene therapy of malignant glioma. *Clin Cancer Res.* 2007;13:6761–6768.
273. Jubb AM, Oates AJ, Holden S, Koeppen H. Predicting benefit from anti-angiogenic agents in malignancy. *Nat Rev Cancer.* 2006;6:626–635.
274. Longo R, Gasparini G. Anti-VEGF therapy: the search for clinical biomarkers. *Expert Rev Mol Diagn.* 2008;8:301–314.
275. Sessa C, Guibal A, Del Conte G, Rüegg C. Biomarkers of angiogenesis for the development of antiangiogenic therapies in oncology: tools or decorations? *Nat Clin Pract Oncol.* 2008;5:378–391.
276. Eberhard A, Kahlert S, Goede V, Hemmerlein B, Plate KH, Augustin HG. Heterogeneity of angiogenesis and blood vessel maturation in human tumors: implications for antiangiogenic tumor therapies. *Cancer Res.* 2000;60:1388–1393.
277. Ellis LM, Hicklin DJ. Pathways mediating resistance to vascular endothelial growth factor-targeted therapy. *Clin Cancer Res.* 2008;14:6371–6375.
278. Bertolini F, Mancuso P, Shaked Y, Kerbel RS. Molecular and cellular biomarkers for angiogenesis in clinical oncology. *Drug Discov Today.* 2007;12:806–812.
279. Denduluri N, Yang SX, Berman AW, et al. Circulating biomarkers of bevacizumab activity in patients with breast cancer. *Cancer Biol Ther.* 2008;7:15–20.
280. Perini R, Choe R, Yodh AG, Sehgal C, Divgi CR, Rosen MA. Noninvasive assessment of tumor neovasculature: techniques and clinical applications. *Cancer Metastasis Rev.* 2008;27:615–630.
281. Sathornsumetee S, Cao Y, Marcello JE, et al. Tumor angiogenic and hypoxic profiles predict radiographic response and survival in malignant astrocytoma patients treated with bevacizumab and irinotecan. *J Clin Oncol.* 2008;26:271–278.
282. Veeravagu A, Hou LC, Hsu AR, et al. The temporal correlation of dynamic contrast-enhanced magnetic resonance imaging with tumor angiogenesis in a murine glioblastoma model. *Neurol Res.* 2008;30:952–959.
283. Cao Y. Molecular mechanisms and therapeutic development of angiogenesis inhibitors. *Adv Cancer Res.* 2008;100:113–131.
284. Ellis LM, Hicklin DJ. VEGF-targeted therapy: mechanisms of antitumour activity *Nat Rev Cancer.* 2008;8:579–591.
285. Ferrara N, Kerbel RS. Angiogenesis as a therapeutic target. *Nature.* 2005;438:967–974.
286. Tortora G, Ciardiello F, Gasparini G. Combined targeting of EGFR-dependent and VEGF-dependent pathways: rationale, preclinical studies and clinical applications. *Nat Clin Pract Oncol.* 2008;5:521–530.
287. Bergers G, Song S, Meyer-Morse N, Bergsland E, Hanahan D. Benefits of targeting both pericytes and endothelial cells in the tumor vasculature with kinase inhibitors. *J Clin Invest.* 2003;111:1287–1295.
288. Jain RK. Normalization of tumor vasculature: an emerging concept in antiangiogenic therapy. *Science.* 2005;307:58–62.
289. Duda DG, Batchelor TT, Willett CG, Jain RK. VEGF-targeted cancer therapy strategies: current progress, hurdles and future prospects. *Trends Mol Med.* 2007;13:223–230.
290. Longo R, Gasparini G. Challenges for patient selection with VEGF inhibitors. *Cancer Chemother Pharmacol.* 2007;60:151–170.
291. Le Tourneau C, Vidal L, Siu LL. Progress and challenges in the identification of biomarkers for EGFR and VEGFR targeting anticancer agents. *Drug Resist Updat.* 2008;11:99–109.
292. Kitzen JJEM, de Jonge MJA, Verweij J. How to define treatment success or failure if tumours do not shrink. Consequences for trial design. In: Teicher BA, Ellis LM, eds. *Antiangiogenic Agents in Cancer Therapy.* 2nd ed. Totowa, NJ: Humana Press; 2008:657–674.
293. Norden AD, Young GS, Setayesh K, et al. Bevacizumab for recurrent malignant gliomas: efficacy, toxicity, and patterns of recurrence. *Neurology.* 2008;70:779–787.
294. Ananthnarayan S, Bahng J, Roring J, et al. Time course of imaging changes of GBM during extended bevacizumab treatment. *J Neurooncol.* 2008;88:339–347.
295. Brandsma D, Stalpers L, Taal W, Sminia P, van den Bent MJ. Clinical features, mechanisms, and management of pseudoprogression in malignant gliomas. *Lancet Oncol.* 2008;9:453–461.
296. Sorensen AG, Batchelor TT, Wen PY, Zhang WT, Jain RK. Response criteria for glioma. *Nat Clin Pract Oncol.* 2008;5:634–644.
297. Varallyay CG, Muldoon LL, Gahramanov S, et al. Dynamic MRI using iron oxide nanoparticles to assess early vascular effects of antiangiogenic versus corticosteroid treatment in a glioma model. *J Cereb Blood Flow Metab.* 2009;29:853–860.
298. Vredenburgh JJ, Desjardins A, Herndon JE 2nd, et al. Bevacizumab plus irinotecan in recurrent glioblastoma multiforme. *J Clin Oncol.* 2007;25:4722–4729.
299. Desjardins A, Reardon DA, Herndon JE 2nd, et al. Bevacizumab plus irinotecan in recurrent WHO grade 3 malignant gliomas. *Clin Cancer Res* 2008;14:7068–7073.
300. Narayana A, Kelly P, Golfinos J, et al. Antiangiogenic therapy using bevacizumab in recurrent high-grade glioma: impact on local control and patient survival. *J Neurosurg.* 2009;110:173–180.
301. Dietrich J, Norden AD, Wen PY. Emerging antiangiogenic treatments for gliomas - efficacy and safety issues. *Curr Opin Neurol.* 2008;21:736–744.
302. Narayana A, Golfinos JG, Fischer I, et al. Feasibility of using bevacizumab with radiation therapy and temozolomide in newly diagnosed high-grade glioma. *Int J Radiat Oncol Biol Phys.* 2008;72:383–389.
303. Norden AD, Drappatz J, Wen PY. Antiangiogenic therapy in malignant gliomas. *Curr Opin Oncol.* 2008;20:652–661.
304. de Groot JF, Yung WK. Bevacizumab and irinotecan in the treatment of recurrent malignant gliomas. *Cancer J.* 2008;14:279–285.
305. Belda-Iniesta C, Carpeño Jde C, et al. Long term responses with cetuximab therapy in glioblastoma multiforme. *Cancer Biol Ther.* 2006;5:912–914.
306. Rich JN, Reardon DA, Peery T, et al. Phase II trial of gefitinib in recurrent glioblastoma. *J Clin Oncol.* 2004;22:133–142.
307. Prados MD, Chang SM, Butowski N, et al. Phase II study of erlotinib plus temozolomide during and after radiation therapy in patients with newly diagnosed glioblastoma multiforme or gliosarcoma. *J Clin Oncol.* 2009;27:579–584.
308. Brandes AA, Franceschi E, Tosoni A, Hegi ME, Stupp R. Epidermal growth factor receptor inhibitors in neuro-oncology: hopes and disappointments. *Clin Cancer Res.* 2008;14:957–960.
309. Wen PY, Yung WK, Lamborn KR, et al. Phase I/II study of imatinib mesylate for recurrent malignant gliomas: North American Brain Tumor Consortium Study 99–08. *Clin Cancer Res.* 2006;12: 4899–4907.
310. Raymond E, Brandes AA, Dittrich C, et al. European Organisation for Research and Treatment of Cancer Brain Tumor Group Study. Phase II study of imatinib in patients with recurrent gliomas of various histologies: a European Organisation for Research and Treatment of Cancer Brain Tumor Group Study. *J Clin Oncol.* 2008;26:4659–4665.
311. Cloughesy TF, Wen PY, Robins HI, et al. Phase II trial of tipifarnib in patients with recurrent malignant glioma either receiving or not receiving enzyme-inducing antiepileptic drugs: a North American Brain Tumor Consortium Study. *J Clin Oncol.* 2006;24:3651–3656.
312. Chang SM, Wen P, Cloughesy T, et al. North American Brain Tumor Consortium and the National Cancer Institute. Phase II study of CCI-779 in patients with recurrent glioblastoma multiforme. *Invest New Drugs* 2005;23:357–361.
313. Galanis E, Buckner JC, Maurer MJ, et al. North Central Cancer Treatment Group. Phase II trial of temsirolimus (CCI-779) in recurrent glioblastoma multiforme: a North Central Cancer Treatment Group Study. *J Clin Oncol* 2005;23:5294–304.
314. Reardon DA, Quinn JA, Vredenburgh JJ, et al. Phase 1 trial of gefitinib plus sirolimus in adults with recurrent malignant glioma. *Clin Cancer Res.* 2006;12:860–868.
315. Castellino RC, Durden DL. Mechanisms of disease: the PI3K-Akt-PTEN signaling node--an intercept point for the control of angiogenesis in brain tumors. *Nat Clin Pract Neurol.* 2007;3:682–693.
316. Natarajan M, Hecker TP, Gladson CL. FAK signaling in anaplastic astrocytoma and glioblastoma tumors. *Cancer J.* 2003;9:126–133.

317. Oliveira-Ferrer L, Hauschild J, Fiedler W, et al. Cilengitide induces cellular detachment and apoptosis in endothelial and glioma cells mediated by inhibition of FAK/src/AKT pathway. *J Exp Clin Cancer Res*. 2008;27:86.
318. Reardon DA, Fink KL, Mikkelsen T, et al. Randomized phase II study of cilengitide, an integrin-targeting arginine-glycine-aspartic acid peptide, in recurrent glioblastoma multiforme. *J Clin Oncol*. 2008;26:5610–5617.
319. Kubicek GJ, Werner-Wasik M, Machtay M, et al. Phase I trial using proteasome inhibitor bortezomib and concurrent temozolomide and radiotherapy for central nervous system malignancies. *Int J Radiat Oncol Biol Phys*. 2009;74:433–439.
320. Mitra SK, Schlaepfer DD. Integrin-regulated FAK-Src signaling in normal and cancer cells. *Curr Opin Cell Biol*. 2006;18:516–523.
321. Coluccia AM, Cirulli T, Neri P, et al. Validation of PDGFRbeta and c-Src tyrosine kinases as tumor/vessel targets in patients with multiple myeloma: preclinical efficacy of the novel, orally available inhibitor dasatinib. *Blood*. 2008;112:1346–1356.
322. Du J, Bernasconi P, Clauser KR, et al. Bead-based profiling of tyrosine kinase phosphorylation identifies SRC as a potential target for glioblastoma therapy. *Nat Biotechnol*. 2009;27:77–83.
323. Chang SM, Lamborn KR, Kuhn JG, et al. Neurooncology clinical trial design for targeted therapies: lessons learned from the North American Brain Tumor Consortium. *Neuro Oncol*. 2008;10:631–642.
324. Kieran MW. Anti-angiogenic therapy in pediatric neuro-oncology. *J Neurooncol*. 2005;75:327–334.
325. Grizzi F, Weber C, Di Ieva A. Antiangiogenic strategies in medulloblastoma: reality or mystery. *Pediatr Res*. 2008;63:584–590.
326. Rössler J, Taylor M, Geoerger B, et al. Angiogenesis as a target in neuroblastoma. *Eur J Cancer*. 2008;44:1645–1656.
327. Orlando L, Cardillo A, Ghisini R, et al. Trastuzumab in combination with metronomic cyclophosphamide and methotrexate in patients with HER-2 positive metastatic breast cancer. *BMC Cancer*. 2006;6:225–232.
328. Palmieri D, Chambers AF, Felding-Habermann B, Huang S, Steeg PS. The biology of metastasis to a sanctuary site. *Clin Cancer Res*. 2007;13:1656–1662.
329. González-Cao M, Viteri S, Díaz-Lagares A, et al. Preliminary results of the combination of bevacizumab and weekly paclitaxel in advanced melanoma. *Oncology*. 2008;74:12–16.
330. Dempke WC, Heinemann V. Resistance to EGF-R (erbB-1) and VEGF-R modulating agents. *Eur J Cancer*. 2009;45:1117–1128.
331. Bergers G, Hanahan D. Modes of resistance to anti-angiogenic therapy. *Nat Rev Cancer*. 2008;8:592–603.
332. Fernando NT, Koch M, Rothrock C et al. Tumor escape from endogenous, extracellular matrix-associated angiogenesis inhibitors by up-regulation of multiple proangiogenic factors. *Clin Cancer Res*. 2008;14:1529–1539.
333. Saidi A, Javerzat S, Bellahcène A, et al. Experimental anti-angiogenesis causes upregulation of genes associated with poor survival in glioblastoma. *Int J Cancer*. 2008;122:2187–2198.
334. Crawford Y, Kasman I, Yu L, et al. PDGF-C mediates the angiogenic and tumorigenic properties of fibroblasts associated with tumors refractory to anti-VEGF treatment. *Cancer Cell*. 2009;15:21–34.
335. Shojaei F, Zhong C, Wu X, Yu L, Ferrara N. Role of myeloid cells in tumor angiogenesis and growth. *Trends Cell Biol*. 2008;18:372–378.
336. Erber R, Thurnher A, Katsen AD, et al. Combined inhibition of VEGF and PDGF signaling enforces tumor vessel regression by interfering with pericyte-mediated endothelial cell survival mechanisms. *FASEB J*. 2004;18:338–340.
337. Rubenstein JL, Kim J, Ozawa T, et al. Anti-VEGF antibody treatment of glioblastoma prolongs survival but results in increased vascular cooption. *Neoplasia*. 2000;2:306–314.
338. Lamszus K, Kunkel P, Westphal M. Invasion as limitation to anti-angiogenic glioma therapy. *Acta Neurochir Suppl*. 2003;88:169–177.
339. Lu C, Shervington A. Chemoresistance in gliomas. *Mol Cell Biochem*. 2008;312:71–80.
340. Friedl P, Wolf K. Tumour-cell invasion and migration: diversity and escape mechanisms. *Nat Rev Cancer*. 2003;3:362–374.
341. Chi A, Norden AD, Wen PY. Inhibition of angiogenesis and invasion in malignant gliomas. *Expert Rev Anticancer Ther*. 2007;7:1537–1560.
342. Sciacca FL, Ciusani E, Silvani A, et al. Genetic and plasma markers of venous thromboembolism in patients with high grade glioma. *Clin Cancer Res*. 2004;10:1312–1317.
343. Elice F, Jacoub J, Rickles FR, Falanga A, Rodeghiero F. Hemostatic complications of angiogenesis inhibitors in cancer patients. *Am J Hematol*. 2008;83:862–870.
344. Milsom C, Yu J, May L, Magnus N, Rak J. Diverse roles of tissue factor-expressing cell subsets in tumor progression. *Semin Thromb Hemost*. 2008;34:170–181.
345. Rak J, Milsom C, Yu J. Tissue factor in cancer. *Curr Opin Hematol*. 2008;15:522–528.
346. Nalluri SR, Chu D, Keresztes R, Zhu X, Wu S. Risk of venous thromboembolism with the angiogenesis inhibitor bevacizumab in cancer patients: a meta-analysis. *JAMA*. 2008;300:2277–2285.
347. Nghiemphu PL, Green RM, Pope WB, Lai A, Cloughesy TF. Safety of anticoagulation use and bevacizumab in patients with glioma. *Neuro Oncol*. 2008;10:355–360.
348. Kamba T, McDonald DM. Mechanisms of adverse effects of anti-VEGF therapy for cancer. *Br J Cancer*. 2007;96:1788–1795.
349. Verheul HM, Pinedo HM. Possible molecular mechanisms involved in the toxicity of angiogenesis inhibition. *Nat Rev Cancer*. 2007;7:475–485.
350. Roodhart JM, Langenberg MH, Witteveen E, Voest EE. The molecular basis of class side effects due to treatment with inhibitors of the VEGF/VEGFR pathway. *Curr Clin Pharmacol*. 2008;3:132–143.
351. Carmeliet P. Blood vessels and nerves: common signals, pathways and diseases. *Nat Rev Genet*. 2003;4:710–720.
352. Daher IM, Yeh ET. Vascular complications of selected cancer therapies. *Nat Clin Pract Cardiovasc Med*. 2008;5:797–805.
353. Mourad JJ, des Guetz G, Debbabi H, Levy BI. Blood pressure rise following angiogenesis inhibition by bevacizumab. A crucial role for microcirculation. *Ann Oncol*. 2008;19:927–934.
354. Glusker P, Recht L, Lane B. Reversible posterior leukoencephalopathy syndrome and bevacizumab. *N Engl J Med*. 2006;354:980–982.
355. Vaughn C, Zhang L, Schiff D. Reversible posterior leukoencephalopathy syndrome in cancer. *Curr Oncol Rep*. 2008;10:86–91.
356. El Maalouf G, Mitry E, Lacout A, et al. Isolated brainstem involvement in posterior reversible leukoencephalopathy induced by bevacizumab. *J Neurol*. 2008;255:295–296.

17 Mouse Models of Central Nervous System Tumors

Part I: Transgenic Mouse Models of Central Nervous System Tumors

Sameer Agnihotri and Abhijit Guha

INTRODUCTION

The most common primary central nervous system (CNS) tumors are gliomas, where other than a few subtypes such as oligodendrogliomas, the survival has remained unchanged despite advances in surgical, chemotherapy and radiation therapy, especially for the most malignant and common glioma: glioblastoma multiforme (GBM). Recent novel therapies such as immunotherapy and gene therapy have shown some promise in existing preclinical models but have failed to demonstrate therapeutic benefit in patients. The reasons for such failures include our incomplete understanding of the molecular pathogenesis of these tumors and testing of novel biological therapies in less than ideal preclinical models, which for the most part have included xenografts established in mice from glioma cell lines or patient explants. These xenografts fail to resemble human gliomas especially with respect to the inherent invasive nature of gliomas and their vascularity and molecular heterogeneity, all of which are the main biological hurdles that have led to their resistance to the multitude of attempted therapies.

Schwannomas and neurofibromas are the most common peripheral nerve tumors and unlike gliomas are usually localized noninvasive benign tumors that are potentially surgically respectable when indicated. However, because of their location, such as in cranial nerves, their multiplicity or chance of malignant conversion when they are in the context of cancer predisposition syndromes such as neurofibromatosis-1 (NF-1: neurofibromas and other CNS tumors) or neurofibromatosis-2 (NF-2: multiple schwannomas and other CNS tumors), significant morbidity and mortality can arise with surgical therapy. Hence, increased molecular understanding and appropriate preclinical models to test biological therapies in these peripheral nerve tumors are also desirable.

Transgenic mouse models offer an opportunity to develop and use an easily replenished, reproducible, manipulated spontaneous, and more appropriate preclinical model of human cancers that we can use to add to our molecular knowledge and to test promising therapies. The recent completion of the human and mouse genomes has revealed a high homology (>95%) between the two genomes. Taking advantage of this resource, several techniques to manipulate the mouse genome have been developed to suppress the expression of candidate tumor suppressor genes or overexpress putative gain of function genes. In this outline, these techniques and how they have been used to develop mouse models for gliomas and peripheral nerve tumors in the context of NF-1 and NF-2 will be discussed in further detail.

TECHNIQUES FOR MOUSE TRANSGENESIS

Homologous Recombination

Homologous recombination was a breakthrough that rapidly progressed the use of mouse models because it allowed for an unprecedented manipulation of the mouse genome (Figure 17.1). The mouse genome could be effectively manipulated by targeted insertion of a replacement allele, leading to deletion of a relevant gene of interest. It takes advantage of flanking homologous regions around the targeted allele that can undergo normal homologous recombination during meiosis. Creation of a targeting vector containing these homologous regions flanking the replacement and nonfunctional allele, with appropriate selection conditions (ie, neomycin and puromycin), can allow for the selection of cells harboring the appropriate homologous recombination event (Figure 17.1). The reader is referred to review articles for further details of this extremely useful technology [1,2]. This technique has been further refined, using Cre recombinase and other transgenic technologies, to allow more cell/tissue-specific and regional-targeted deletions of an allele.

Pronuclear Injection

Microinjection has been extensively used to introduce foreign DNA into the male pronuclei of fertilized

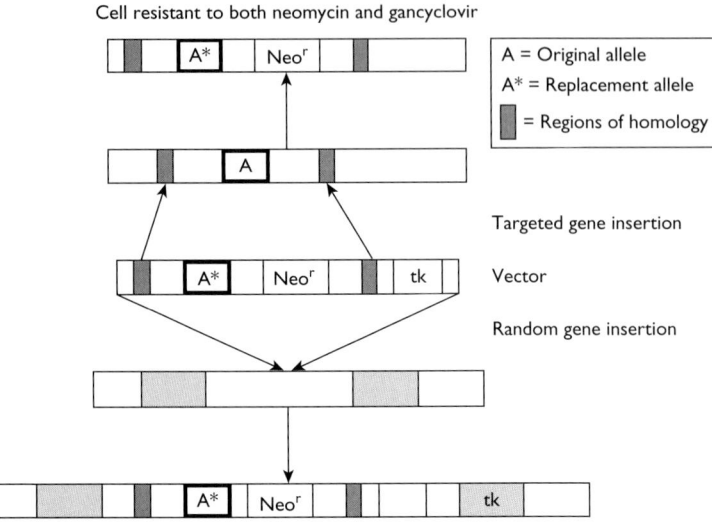

Figure 17.1 Homologous recombination used to target and knockout specific genes. This technique has been used to knockout globally a variety of tumor suppressor genes. Recent use of Cre-loxP technology can be combined with homologous recombination to knockout genes in a cell-specific manner, a useful adjunct when global knockout is embryonic lethal.

mammalian eggs, which are then implanted into a foster mother for the remainder of embryonic development (Figure 17.2). One of the major drawbacks of this method is the high frequency of multiple-copy integration of a transgene into the host genome, which can result in variation or sometimes even inhibition of the transgene expression. In comparison, embryonic stem (ES) cell-mediated transgenesis provides a higher frequency of low-copy number or even single-copy transgene integration. A few models of gliomas have been developed using pronuclear injection technology with relevant oncogenes [3–5].

ES Cell-Mediated Transgenesis

ES cells are derived from early embryos (blastocyst stage) and can be maintained in culture under the proper growth conditions as undifferentiated, pluripotent cells (Figure 17.3). ES cells can be manipulated to alter their genetic composition by introducing foreign gene of interest under ubiquitous or cell/tissue-specific promoters using various transfection techniques and selected with antibiotics and selectable markers such as LacZ. Then, the ES cells are injected into the host blastocyst, followed by aggregation as a morula stage embryo into a pseudopregnant mouse. The resulting pups are chimeras consisting of transfected ES cell lineage cells and those cells derived from nontransfected wild-type ES cells in the host blastocyst. Because of this chimeric representation in all tissue types, many transgenes, which if ubiquitously expressed would be lethal, do not cause lethality unlike pronuclear injections. Depending on the effects of the transgene on viability and fertility, the chimeric pups can go on to germline transmission, allowing development of established mouse lines carrying the altered gene(s). This technique has been used in the creation of astrocytomas and oligodendrogliomas in transgenic mouse models by our group and several others [6,7].

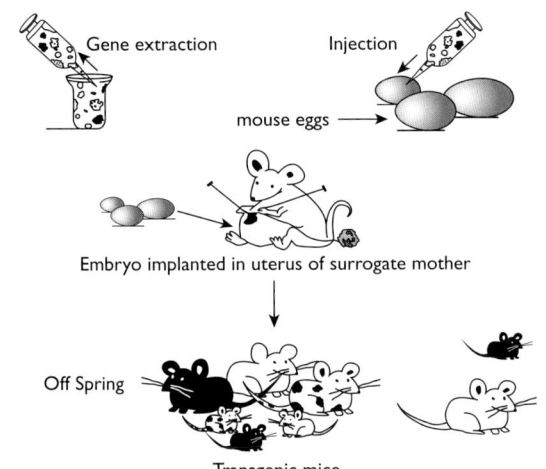

Figure 17.2 Pronuclear injection technique to develop transgenic mice. Nuclei of fertilized eggs are injected with genes of interest, with random and multiple integration sites, and subsequently reimplanted in surrogate mothers. Transgenic offspring harboring the transgene in every cell type is obtained with the potential of germline transmission.

Cell/Tissue-Specific Transgenesis

This is one of the most popular and powerful techniques for producing mouse models in which the altered gene is expressed or deleted in the cells/tissues of interest and not in all cell types (Figure 17.4). Advantages of this system include bypassing a potential embryonic lethal phenotype or lack of germline transmission because only a specific cell type will be affected. Second, targeting cell types/tissue at different time points can also be investigated for studying the role of specific gene(s) during development or disease progression. These systems depend on the use of a bacteriophage-derived recombinase enzyme, such as Cre or Flp recombinase, to specifically excise out a portion of a

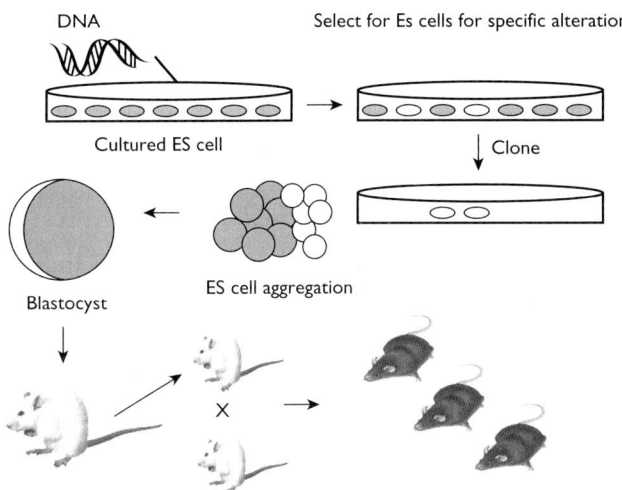

Figure 17.3 Embryonic stem cell transgenesis DNA vector carrying gene of interest is transfected into cultured mouse ES cells. In our case, we used a retrovirus carrying the ^{V12}Ha-Ras gene under the control of the astrocyte-specific human GFAP promoter and a neomycin selection marker expression cassette. Selection of ES cells with the transgene of interest is first accomplished by selecting for neomycin-resistant clones. Thereafter, NeoR ES clones are tested for their ability to express the transgene by in vitro differentiation to astrocytes. This process confirms activation of the GFAP promoter expression and specificity. Positive ES cells undergo aggregations and are transferred to a pseudopregnant female mouse to create chimeric embryos (striped mouse in picture). The chimeric mice are bred to normal mice and those mice having incorporated the transgene in their germ line will generate transgenic offspring.

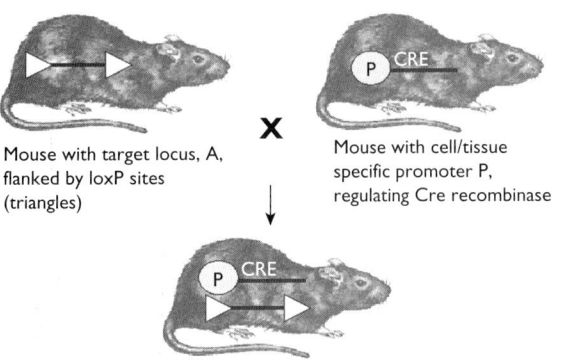

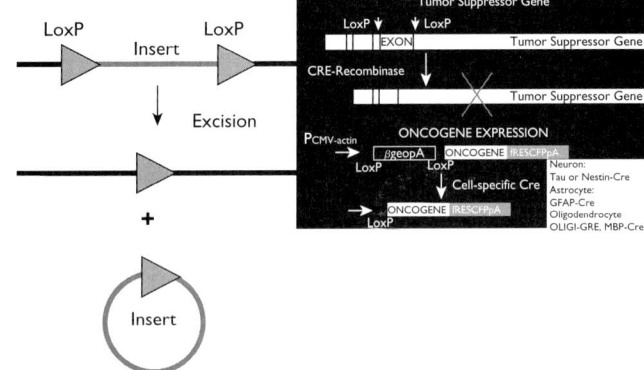

Figure 17.4 Cre-loxP system. Mouse with the gene of interest flanked by loxP recognition sites (top). The loxP sites can flank a critical coding exon, which if excised would lead to a nonfunctioning protein such as a tumor suppressor gene (bottom). It can also flank a stop codon (such as β-geopA bottom), which after excision would allow expression of an oncogene. Cre recombinase, to excise out the loxP flanked regions, can be delivered by cell- or tissue-specific promoters such as GFAP. These can be in the form of other transgenic mice, adenoviral or other gene delivery techniques.

gene that is flanked by specific nucleotide sequences recognized by these recombinases. The loxP recombination site is 34 bp long and consists of two 13-bp palindromes separated by an asymmetric 8-bp core sequence. A consensus loxP sequence is the following: ATAACTTCGTATA (13 bp) ATGTATGC (8-bp core) TATACGAAGTTAT(13-bp palindrome to first 13 bp) [8]. Flp recombinase is used to a lesser extent but is similar in principle and recognizes a unique 34-bp sequence from Cre recombinase. The targeted region of a gene, which is crucial for its transcription or function, is flanked by recombinase recognition nucleotide sequence sites (ie, loxP recognized by Cre recombinase or FRT recognized by Flp recombinase), that are placed in a way that gene function is not compromised when the respective recombinase is absent (Figure 17.4). In the presence of the recombinase, which is both necessary and sufficient for catalyzing recombination between the recognition sites, the intervening DNA segment is deleted. The Cre-loxP recombinase system is at present the most widely used system in mammals. By using specific cell/tissue-type promoters and expressing recombinase in the desired cells/tissues, targeted manipulation of the gene of interest in only those cells/tissues can be undertaken, thereby avoiding embryonic or other developmental defects due to more global alterations of an important gene. For example, one can excise out the flanked portion of a gene to delete it or remove a stop sequence to express a gene in astrocytes, by expressing Cre recombinase under the astroglial-specific GFAP promoter. In addition, recent technology allows for inducible expression of the recombinase under regulation of agents such as tamoxifen or tetracycline in the adult mouse, if expressing or deleting a particular gene even restricted to a specific cell/tissue such as astrocytes leads to embryonic lethal (e.g., by severely interfering with brain development).

Somatic Gene Transfer Using RCAS-tva System

This system uses an avian leukemia retrovirus vector (RCAS) carrying the transgene, which binds to its specific cell surface tva receptor, resulting in incorporation and random integration of the retrovirus in the genome of the cell, with subsequent expression of the transgene (Figure 17.5). The transgene is expressed from a spliced message under control of the constitutive retroviral LTR promoter, with the retroviral genes spliced out to prevent viral replication in mammalian cells. The specificity arises from cell type-specific promoters used to create transgenic

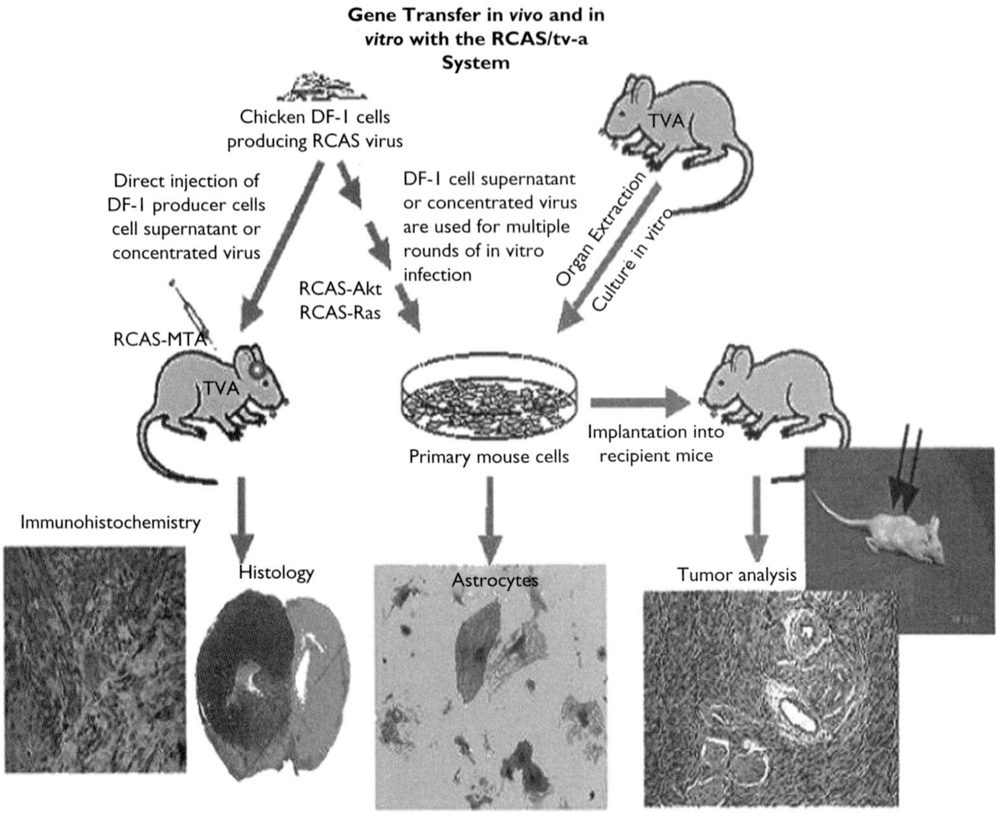

Figure 17.5 RCAS-tva system. The tva receptor is specific for recognizing and incorporating the RCAS retrovirus. Cell- or tissue-specific transgenic tva mice (such as GFAP-tva) are made and can be mated with other genetically modified mice (such as Ink4A/Arf null mice). The RCAS retrovirus, with the transgene of interest, can be inoculated into the adult tva mice, either alone or in combination, to yield focal gliomas, as undertaken by Holland et al [11].

mice, where expression of the tva is only in the cells in which that promoter is active. Hence, only these cells in the adult transgenic tva mouse can be transfected with the intracranially injected RCAS vector carrying the transgene. For example, the GFAP-tva or Nestin-tva mice have been used to express relevant transgenes in differentiated GFAP-positive and progenitor Nestin-positive glial precursor cells in several models of gliomas [9–14].

ANIMAL MODELS OF CNS TUMORS

Specific Mouse Glioma Models

Strategies Using Transgenic and Knockout Mice

Molecular progression of gliomas, like most solid tumors, involves accumulation of genetic aberrations, which results in the inactivation of tumor suppressor genes (PTEN, p53, p16, p19, and Rb) or activation of oncogenic pathways (p21-Ras, PI3-Kinase, epidermal growth factor receptor [EGFR], CDK4, and MDM2) [15] (Table 17.1). Most of the current strategies for creating transgenic mouse models is based on manipulating the mouse genome, using some of the techniques discussed above, to overexpress and/or loose expression of these relevant molecular alterations that have been deciphered from human tumor data (Table 17.2).

For example, there are transgenic mouse glioma models that target the Rb or p53 cell cycle regulatory pathways. Astrocyte-specific inactivation of pRb and pRb-related proteins, p107 and p130 [4], by expression of a single copy of the viral T121 oncogene driven by the GFAP promoter, led to gliomas that are pathologically similar to grade III anaplastic astrocytomas. One hundred percent of GFAP:T121 transgenic mice developed these high-grade astrocytomas at approximately 6 months of age, a latency that was shortened with the addition of a single null PTEN allele. This supported the critical role of the pRb-regulated pathways in astrocytoma formation and loss of PTEN in astrocytoma progression (Table 17.3).

The relevance of the p53-regulated cell cycle pathways, which also involves p19 and MDM2, has also been demonstrated in mouse models. p53 null mice by themselves do not develop gliomas, although they develop and die of a variety of other non-CNS tumors. However, a combined deletion of *Nf-1* (neurofibromatosis-1 gene that encodes for neurofibromin, an inactivator of the important mitogenic

Table 17.1 Genetic Aberration in Human Astrocytomas

Gain of Function	Loss of Function

Aberrant receptors:
    EGFR/ EGFRvIII
    PDGFR
	Cell cycle pathway gene:
	    p53, p19
	    Rb, p16

Aberrant signaling pathway:
    p21-Ras
    PI3-Kinase
    Src
	In-activators of signaling pathway:
	    PTEN inhibits PI3-Kinase
	    NF-1 inhibits p21-Ras

Aberrant cyclin activators CDK4	
Aberrant in-activators of p53 MDM2	

Table 17.2 Transgenic or Knockout Mouse Glioma Models

Tumour Type	Transgene	Knockout	Cell of Origin	References
Astrocytomas	v-Src		GFAP	Weissenberger et al., 1997
Astrocytomas	V^{12}Ha-ras		GFAP	Ding, Guha et al., 2001
Oligodendroglioma Mixed Oligo-astrocytma	V^{12}Ha-ras & EGFRvIII		GFAP	Ding, Guha et al., 2003
High-grade astrocytomas	T121	pRb (−/−), PTEN(+/−)	GFAP	Xiao, vanDyke et al., 2002
Oligodendroglioma	v-erbB	Ink4a-ARF (−/−)	S-100	Weiss, Israel et al., 2003
GBM (strain specific)		Nf1;Trp53 (cis KO)	All cells	Reilly, Jacks et al., 2000
		p53 (+/−), NF-1 (−/−)		Zhu, Paragda, 2002
Astrocytomas			GFAP	
Oligodendrogliomas		P19 (−/−)	All cells	Kamijo, Sherr et al., 1999

Table 17.3 Mouse Models of Gliomas: Virus Infection

Tumor Type	Signal Transduction Abnormality	Cell Cycle Arrest Disruption	Cell Of Origin/ Affected Cells	References
GBM (Mixed gliomas)	PDGF (v-sis)	Ink4a-ARF (−/−)	Mixed population (nestin+, GFAP+)	Uhrborm et al., 1998, Dai et al., 2001
GBM	K-ras & Akt	Ink4a-ARF (−/−)	GFAP+ Nestin+	Holland et al., 2000 L. Uhrbom et al, 2002
Mixed gliomas	EGFRvIII	P53 +/−, Cdk4+	Nestin+	Holland et al, 1998
Mixed gliomas	MTAg		GFAP+	Holland et al., 2000

p21-Ras signaling pathway) and *p53* [16,17] results in generating malignant gliomas. Loss of neurofibromin by itself results in astrogliosis but not glioma formation; however, when p53 expression is first lost and then followed by loss of neurofibromin, malignant astrocytomas develop [16]. The importance of aberrations in the p53 pathway early in gliomagenesis is also demonstrated by the small incidence of gliomas in mice deficient for p19, a protein involved in regulating the stability of p53 through its negative regulation of MDM2 [18].

Overexpression of relevant oncogenic aberrations such as receptors or downstream signaling pathways has also been used in developing mouse glioma models. These have been either alone or in combination with mice harboring specific knockouts of relevant cell cycle regulatory proteins. For example, the S-100 glial precursor promoter-regulated *v-erbB* (an activated member of the EGFR family) transgenic mice develop oligodendrogliomas, which is potentiated in terms of shorter latency and increased malignancy when undertaken in mice deficient for both p16 and p19 (Ink4a/ARF null mice) [5]. Because wild-type EGFR and mutant EGFRvIII are the most common gain of function alterations in malignant human astrocytomas, our group has recently created mice expressing these proteins under regulation of the GFAP promoter [7]. Mice with GFAP-regulated expression of EGFR and EGFRvIII, both did not result in gliomas, suggesting that, similar to human gliomas, these are not initiation factors. However, when these mice were mated with a mouse that is prone to develop gliomas, such as the GFAP-regulated activated p21-Ras mouse described below, the EGFRvIII but not the EGFR mice potentiated glioma formation. In addition, expression of EGFRvIII also altered the glioma subtype, with the double transgenic mice (activated p21-Ras + EGFRvIII) developing oligodendrogliomas and mixed oligoastrocytomas, compared with the mainly astrocytic lineage tumors in the single transgenic activated p21-Ras mouse described in further detail below.

There are several examples of aberrant expression of relevant downstream signaling pathways, in mouse glioma modeling. These include astrocytomas of varying grades resulting from GFAP-regulated expression of v-src [3]. Our laboratory has used our initial observation of aberrant activation of the p21-Ras signaling pathway in astrocytomas to develop glioma models using ES transgenesis [6,7]. GFAP-regulated oncogenic/activated p21-Ras led to multifocal astrocytomas of varying grades in a p21-Ras activity dose-dependent manner. Mice with extremely high levels of p21-Ras activity in the brain died as chimeras with GBM-like tumors. Moderate levels of p21-Ras activation led to germline transmission, with mice that are born normally but start to develop and die of their multifocal astrocytomas of varying grades commencing at approximately 12 to 14 weeks. Of interest, expression of activated p21-Ras in adult astrocytes leads to senescence; therefore, the developmental expression of p21-Ras in early glial progenitor cells is of importance. Furthermore, expression of activated p21-Ras in the early glial progenitors leads to genetic instability, but we believe that does not suffice alone for transformation, because the astrocytomas occur after a period of development postbirth. When the GBM-like tumors are examined in these mice, additional genetic alterations such as those found in human GBMs (overexpression of EGFR, CDK4, and MDM2; decreased expression of p16, p19, p53, and PTEN) [15] are present, which we hypothesize are facilitated by the genetic instability created by activated p21-Ras. As described above, experiments involving mating these p21-Ras mice to other genetically defined mice such as EGFRvIII have already commenced and are continuing, with the potential of these mouse models serving not only as useful preclinical reagents but also to increase our understanding of the in vivo interactions of these molecular alterations in the pathogenesis of gliomas.

Strategies Using Viral and Transgenic Mice

The models described above, for the most part, involve modulating the mouse genome commencing at an early embryonic stage. This has the potential advantage of generating a renewable resource of genetically defined mice that develop gliomas at a certain frequency and hence can be used for a variety of experiments. However, cancer is mainly an adult somatic disease arising from a clone of cells that have become transformed because of accumulation of genetic alterations. Viral-transduced expression of relevant gain of function alterations, in combination with transgenic mouse technology, allows one to model such somatic alterations at a later stage in life, although it does not lead to germline colonies.

Although the link between a viral etiology and human gliomas is weak, retroviruses that have been engineered to express relevant gain of function genes have been used to create glioma models in mice and other mammals [9–14]. This includes members of the Rous sarcoma virus family and simian sarcoma virus, whose transforming properties are a result of overexpression of the viral oncogene *v-sis*, the cellular counterpart of which is c-sis or platelet derived growth factor (PDGF)-B [19]. Overexpression of PDGF and activation of PDGF receptors are well recognized in gliomagenesis [9,12,19]. Retroviruses carrying *v-sis* (PDGF-B), when injected into normal mice, have yielded astrocytic tumors with varying glioma types when injected in Ink4a/ARF null mice [9]. The frequency of gliomas using this retroviral strategy was between 40% and 80%, with the most frequent histology being high-grade gliomas that have characteristics similar to GBMs.

One of the best examples of coupling retroviruses to express somatically defined gain of function genes in varying cell lineages and genetic backgrounds to model gliomas is the RCAS-*tva* system, detailed previously [9–14] (Figure 17.3). This system develops focal gliomas, the subtype and grade of which varies with the injected retroviral-transduced gene (ie, PDGF-B, EGFRvIII, activated p21-Ras, and activated Akt), the lineage of the cell expressing the *tva* receptor (GFAP, Nestin), and underlying genetic cell cycle alterations in the mice (deficient for Ink4a/ARF, p53, etc). For example, retroviral-transduced expression of *v-sis* or PDGF-B in GFAP-*tva* mice developed oligodendroglioma or mixed oligoastrocytoma in 40% of the mice, with 60% developing similar gliomas in Nestin-*tva* mice [10]. When these experiments were undertaken in Ink4a/ARF null mice, the gliomas formed with a shorter latency and were of higher grade. Another example with the RCAS-*tva* system is experiments with retroviral transduction of activated p21-Ras and Akt, representing the two most implicated aberrant signaling pathways in gliomas, as previously discussed. Neither of these activated signaling molecules by itself formed gliomas, but when expressed together in more primitive Nestin-positive precursor glial cells, astrocytomas developed. Furthermore, activated p21-Ras by itself could give rise to astrocytomas if transduced in Nestin-positive cells in Ink4a/ARF null mice. This is consistent with the results we obtained and described above with ES transgenesis of activated p21-Ras [6]. Activated p21-Ras is transforming only if expressed in early glial lineage cells, with the transformed astrocytes deficient in the gene products encoded by the Ink4a/ARF locus (p16 and p19) and expressing Nestin. Similar results with EGFRvIII have also been obtained by our ES transgenesis model [7] and those with the RCAS-*tva* system [13]. In both, expression of EGFRvIII by itself is not transforming because it is a progression not an initiation factor. In the RCAS-*tva* system, retroviral transduction of both EGFRvIII and CDK4 in mice deficient for p53, was required for formation of mixed gliomas.

Recently, The Cancer Genome Atlas initiative involved integrative analysis of DNA copy number variation, gene expression, and DNA methylation aberrations in 206 glioblastomas [20]. This study provided new insights into the roles of ERBB2, NF-1, and TP53 as p53 mutations were discovered to be more widespread in primary GBMs than previously thought. Furthermore, novel NF-1 point mutations were discovered helping support the case for NF-1 being a critical GBM tumor suppressor gene. The p53 mutation observations were further investigated in mouse models in which co-loss of p53 and Pten in murine neural stem cells resulted in the formation of a penetrant acute-onset high-grade glioma with a pathological and molecular profile resembling primary GBMs. In addition to The Cancer Genome Atlas study, another group sequenced more than 20 661 protein-coding genes in GBM operative samples and human xenograft models [21]. P53 once again was observed to have a high mutation rate in primary GBMs. Interestingly, isocitrate dehydrogenase-1 (IDH1), an enzyme involved in the oxidative carboxylation of isocitrate to α-ketoglutarate, resulting in the production of nicotinamide adenine dinucleotide phosphate, was found to be mutated in 12% of all GBMs [21–23], with >80% mutation in secondary GBMs. Of the five IDH genes, IDH1 and IDH2 were found to be mutated and that point mutations were consistently observed in the substrate-binding site at residue R132 and R172, respectively. Interestingly, no insertion or deletion mutations (InDels) were identified at the IDH1 locus, suggesting a critical role for the point mutation. A recent study has shown that cancer-associated IDH1 mutations result in a new ability of the enzyme to catalyse the nicotinamide adenine dinucleotide phosphate-dependent reduction of α-ketoglutarate to R(−)-2-hydroxyglutarate (2HG), a metabolite that increases in patients with GBM [24]. Finally, IDH1 mutations were seen in a younger population of patients with GBM, and patients with IDH1 mutations had better overall survival compared with patients with wild type intact [21]. Mouse models would truly provide an invaluable insight into the role of this gene in gliomagenesis, and these studies show how high-throughput tumor profiling coupled with mouse models can be an excellent combination of tools.

Specific Mouse Models of Peripheral Nerve Tumors

Neurofibromatosis 1

After cloning the *Nf-1* gene on chromosome 17q, knockout technology was used by two groups to delete the *Nf-1* gene in all cell types, resulting in identical phenotypes [25,26]. In both, the *Nf-1* (–/–) null mice were embryonically lethal, with major cardiovascular developmental disorders, in support of the critical function of neurofibromin in development. The heterozygous *Nf-1* (+/–) mice were born normally but died of non-neuroectodermal tumors slightly earlier than their matched control littermates. Chimeric mice generated from *Nf-1* (–/–) and *Nf-1* (+/+) ES cells were embryonically viable, as per discussion previously of one of the potential benefits of this technology [6,7]. Expectant neurofibromas did form in these chimeric mice, from derivatives of the *Nf-1* (–/–) ES cells, proving that loss of neurofibromin expression in Schwann cells was indeed causal toward developing neurofibromas in patients with NF-1. The embryonic lethality was also overcome with cell-specific deletion of *Nf-1*, using the previously described Cre-loxP system. For example, the normal NF-1/*flox* mouse can be used to specifically delete neurofibromin in astrocytes, by breeding the NF-1/*flox* mouse to GFAP:Cre mouse. From this kind of manipulation, much has been learned about development of astrocytomas in the context of NF-1. Astrocyte-specific deletion of neurofibromin only led to increased number of astrocytes but not ones that were transformed. However, if neurofibromin was deleted in the presence of existing p53 null astrocytes, then astrocytomas of varying grades formed [16]. Similar strategies have been used to examine the biological consequences due to loss of neurofibromin in other cell types. For example, by mating the NF-1/*flox* mouse with endothelial cell-specific Cre recombinase–expressing transgenic mice (Tie2:Cre), insights into the crucial effects of loss of neurofibromin on vascular development have been deciphered [27]. Finally, mouse models have also given insights into the molecular basis of progression of benign neurofibromas to malignant peripheral nerve sheath tumors (MPNST). Taking advantage of the fact that in mice the *Nf-1*, *p53*, and *Nf-2* loci are on the same chromosome and relatively close together, transgenic mice in which both *Nf-1l* and *p53* could be deleted were generated [16]. These mice developed MPNST, which is in keeping with the loss of p53 in a large subset of human MPNST, and suggests that a second hit with p53 loss is involved in this malignant conversion of neurofibromas.

Neurofibromatosis 2

Similar to *NF-1*, cloning the *Nf-2* gene on chromosome 22q soon led to it being knocked out in mice. The *Nf-2* (–/–) null mice died in embryo similar to *Nf-1* null mice, with the heterozygotes developing osteosarcomas and other tumors but not the expectant schwannomas [28,29]. The Cre-loxP system was used to overcome this embryonic lethality when *Nf-2* was deleted globally, with Schwann cell-specific Cre recombinase expression leading to development of schwannomas [30]. Meningiomas, which are highly prevalent in patients with NF-2 also formed, with meninges-specific excision of the *Nf-2* gene using adenoviral delivered Cre into the CSF of NF-2/*flox* mice [31].

Potential Use of Transgenic Mouse Models

The ability to manipulate the mouse genome with a variety of technologies, such as those discussed above, has opened the doors for many research and potential preclinical applications. The marked similarity between the mouse and human genome, with syntenic regions mapped between the two species, has allowed us to target specific genes that are causal for human diseases such as gliomas and peripheral nerve tumors in mice. In addition to allowing us to study the temporal, spatial, and cellular interactions between these known genetic alterations toward causing the human disease, transgenic mouse models also serve as agents to decipher novel genetic alterations that may not have been recognized from human samples. These can then be tested in human samples and, if indicated, incorporated in subsequent models.

Characterization and better understanding of the molecular and pathological progression of tumors, such as those in the nervous system, is another use of transgenic mouse models, which cannot be readily undertaken in humans. Understanding interactions of tumor cells with other cellular elements such as the vascular system, immunological system, extracellular matrix, and other stromal cells, is another area of research that is facilitated by transgenic mouse models. Having a spontaneous orthotopic occurring model in an immunocompetent mammal, of course lends itself well to preclinical trials of established and novel biological therapies. To augment this vital translational use of transgenic mouse modeling of human diseases, a variety of readouts, such as small animal imaging, are also being developed to follow the efficacy of the therapeutic interventions being tested. Although much progress has been made in development of better human disease models using transgenic and other technologies, one must remember that significant epigenetic differences between mice and humans do exist, and the ultimate test of therapies will still rely on properly designed clinical trials. However, with better models of human diseases such as those being developed for nervous system tumors using transgenic technologies, the chance of promising preclinical therapies translating to efficacy in clinical trials should be much improved in the future.

REFERENCES

1. Babinet C, Cohen-Tannoudji M. Genome engineering via homologous recombination in mouse embryonic stem (ES) cells: an amazingly versatile tool for the study of mammalian biology. *An Acad Bras Cienc*. 2001;73(3):365–383.
2. Vasquez KM, Marburger K, Intody Z, Wilson JH. Manipulating the mammalian genome by homologous recombination. *Proc Natl Acad Sci U S A*. 2001;98(15):8403–8410.
3. Weissenberger J, Steinbach JP, Malin G, Spada S, Rulicke T, Aguzzi A. Development and malignant progression of astrocytomas in GFAP-v-src transgenic mice. *Oncogene*. 1997;14(17):2005–2013.
4. Xiao A, Wu H, Pandolfi PP, Louis DN, van Dyke T. Astrocyte inactivation of the pRb pathway predisposes mice to malignant astrocytoma development that is accelerated by PTEN mutation. *Cancer Cell*. 2002;1(2):157–168.

5. Weiss WA, Burns MJ, Hackett C, et al. Genetic determinants of malignancy in a mouse model for oligodendroglioma. *Cancer Res.* 2003;63(7):1589–1595.
6. Ding H, Roncari L, Shannon P, et al. Astrocyte-specific expression of activated p21-ras results in malignant astrocytoma formation in a transgenic mouse model of human gliomas. *Cancer Res.* 2001;61(9):3826–3836.
7. Ding H, Shannon P, Lau N, et al. Oligodendrogliomas result from the expression of an activated mutant epidermal growth factor receptor in a RAS transgenic mouse astrocytoma model. *Cancer Res.* 2003;63(5):1106–1113.
8. Hoess RH, Ziese M, Sternberg N. P1 site-specific recombination: nucleotide sequence of the recombining sites. *Proc Natl Acad Sci U S A.* 1982;79(11):3398–3402.
9. Uhrbom L, Hesselager G, Nister M, Westermark B. Induction of brain tumors in mice using a recombinant platelet-derived growth factor B-chain retrovirus. *Cancer Res.* 1998;58(23):5275–5279.
10. Dai C, Celestino JC, Okada Y, Louis DN, Fuller GN, Holland EC. PDGF autocrine stimulation dedifferentiates cultured astrocytes and induces oligodendrogliomas and oligoastrocytomas from neural progenitors and astrocytes in vivo. *Genes Dev.* 2001;15(15):1913–1925.
11. Holland EC, Li Y, Celestino J, et al. Astrocytes give rise to oligodendrogliomas and astrocytomas after gene transfer of polyoma virus middle T antigen in vivo. *Am J Pathol.* 2000;157(3):1031–1037.
12. Uhrbom L, Dai C, Celestino JC, Rosenblum MK, Fuller GN, Holland EC. Ink4a-Arf loss cooperates with KRas activation in astrocytes and neural progenitors to generate glioblastomas of various morphologies depending on activated Akt. *Cancer Res.* 2002;62(19):5551–5558.
13. Holland EC, Hively WP, DePinho RA, Varmus HE. A constitutively active epidermal growth factor receptor cooperates with disruption of G1 cell-cycle arrest pathways to induce glioma-like lesions in mice. *Genes Dev.* 1998;12(23):3675–3685.
14. Holland EC, Celestino J, Dai C, Schaefer L, Sawaya RE, Fuller GN. Combined activation of Ras and Akt in neural progenitors induces glioblastoma formation in mice. *Nat Genet.* 2000;25(1):55–57.
15. Holland EC. Gliomagenesis: genetic alterations and mouse models. *Nat Rev Genet.* 2001;2(2):120–129.
16. Reilly KM, Loisel DA, Bronson RT, McLaughlin ME, Jacks T. Nf1;Trp53 mutant mice develop glioblastoma with evidence of strain-specific effects. *Nat Genet.* 2000;26(1):109–113.
17. Kamijo T, Bodner S, van de KE, Randle DH, Sherr CJ. Tumor spectrum in ARF-deficient mice. *Cancer Res.* 1999;59(9):2217–2222.
18. King D, Yang G, Thompson MA, Hiebert SW. Loss of neurofibromatosis-1 and p19(ARF) cooperate to induce a multiple tumor phenotype. *Oncogene.* 2002;21(32):4978–4982.
19. Potapova O, Fakhrai H, Baird S, Mercola D. Platelet-derived growth factor-B/v-sis confers a tumorigenic and metastatic phenotype to human T98G glioblastoma cells. *Cancer Res.* 1996;56(2):280–286.
20. McLendon R, Friedman A, Bigner D, et al. Comprehensive genomic characterization defines human glioblastoma genes and core pathways. *Nature.* 2008;455(7216):1061–1068.
21. Jones S, Zhang X, Parsons DW, et al. Core signaling pathways in human pancreatic cancers revealed by global genomic analyses. *Science.* 2008;321(5897):1801–1806.
22. Geisbrecht BV, Gould SJ. The human PICD gene encodes a cytoplasmic and peroxisomal NADP(+)-dependent isocitrate dehydrogenase. *J Biol Chem.* 1999;274(43):30527–30533.
23. Xu X, Zhao J, Xu Z, et al. Structures of human cytosolic NADP-dependent isocitrate dehydrogenase reveal a novel self-regulatory mechanism of activity. *J Biol Chem.* 2004;279(32):33946–33957.
24. Dang L, White DW, Gross S, et al. Cancer-associated IDH1 mutations produce 2-hydroxyglutarate. *Nature.* 2009;462(7274):739–744.
25. Jacks T, Shih TS, Schmitt EM, Bronson RT, Bernards A, Weinberg RA. Tumour predisposition in mice heterozygous for a targeted mutation in Nf1. *Nat Genet.* 1994;7(3):353–361.
26. Brannan CI, Perkins AS, Vogel KS, et al. Targeted disruption of the neurofibromatosis type-1 gene leads to developmental abnormalities in heart and various neural crest-derived tissues. *Genes Dev.* 1994;8(9):1019–1029.
27. Forde A, Constien R, Grone HJ, Hammerling G, Arnold B. Temporal Cre-mediated recombination exclusively in endothelial cells using Tie2 regulatory elements. *Genesis.* 2002;33(4):191–197.
28. McClatchey AI, Saotome I, Mercer K, et al. Mice heterozygous for a mutation at the Nf2 tumor suppressor locus develop a range of highly metastatic tumors. *Genes Dev.* 1998;12(8):1121–1133.
29. McClatchey AI, Saotome I, Ramesh V, Gusella JF, Jacks T. The Nf2 tumor suppressor gene product is essential for extraembryonic development immediately prior to gastrulation. *Genes Dev.* 1997;11(10):1253–1265.
30. Giovannini M, Robanus-Maandag E, van der Valk M, et al. Conditional biallelic Nf2 mutation in the mouse promotes manifestations of human neurofibromatosis type 2. *Genes Dev.* 2000;14(13):1617–1630.
31. Kalamarides M, Niwa-Kawakita M, Leblois H, et al. Nf2 gene inactivation in arachnoidal cells is rate-limiting for meningioma development in the mouse. *Genes Dev.* 2002;16(9):1060–1065.

Mouse Models of Central Nervous System Tumors

Part 2: Transplantation Mouse Models of Central Nervous System Tumors

C. David James and Tomoko Ozawa

INTRODUCTION

Transplantation models for studying central nervous system (CNS) cancer have been an essential part of neuro-oncology research for more than 40 years [1,2]. To many, the method that is associated with the propagation of brain tumors in animals, in nearly all cases involving rodents, is represented by the collection of cells from culture flasks, followed by use of the collected cells for subcutaneous injection and tumor establishment in mice. Indeed, this represents the most commonly used method, but one which is having proportionately less use in current neuro-oncology research. Over the past 10 years, there has been increasing diversity and sophistication of approach in the use of transplantation models, some of which is reviewed below, accompanied by discussion of conventional methods.

IMMUNOCOMPETENT HOSTS

Chemically Induced Tumor Cells

The use of chemically induced rodent brain tumors, converted to permanent cell lines, for establishing syngeneic tumors in corresponding strains of rodents, represents one of the most accepted and utilitarian transplant systems in neuro-oncology research. Among these, the 9L and C6 glioma cell lines, derived from the Fisher and Wistar rats, respectively [3,4], that had been subjected to repetitive treatment with N-nitrosomethylurea (MNU), have seen the greatest extent of use and continue to be a common choice for studies in which immunocompetent hosts are of importance. However, it is important to note that the C6 line was developed in outbred Wistar rats, and as a result, these cells are not truly syngeneic to any strain of rodent and are capable of inducing an alloimmune response when used for in vivo study. Aside from the 9L Fisher rat combination, additional rodent tumor models with syngeneic hosts include the F98 and RG2 lines that were derived from Fisher rats treated with ethylnitrosourea [5] and the CNS-1 line derived from Lewis rats treated with MNU [6]. Each of these cell lines is conveniently maintained in vitro using conventional, serum-supplemented media and are highly reliable with respect to their successful engraftment as well as their in vivo growth kinetics. Major concerns for the use of these cell lines have been their rodent origin and their initiation through chemical treatment that has called into question the accuracy with which they represent their human cancer counterparts. However, analysis of rodent glioma cell lines and their tumors has revealed gene alterations consistent with genetic signature lesions associated with human gliomas [7–9], and their immunohistochemical characterization has additionally demonstrated shared features with corresponding human tumors [6,10].

Published studies involving the use of chemically induced rodent tumors show a strong orientation toward application in therapeutic testing, especially for therapies dependent on or associated with host immune response. This is not to indicate, however, the use of rodent glioma cell lines to the exclusion of mechanistic studies involving the role of specific genes and proteins in tumor biology. For example, it is evident that RNA interference has spurred increased interest in C6 and 9L for addressing protein functional properties, through the development of cell line derivatives that are used for comparing the effects of short- or long-term suppression of gene expression [11,12]. Nonetheless, and despite such research activity, it is anticipated that the syngeneic, rodent glioma tumor models will continue to see predominant application in evaluating experimental therapies.

Transgenic Models

Although seldom used in the context of transplant model systems, many of the genetically modified mouse tumor models developed over the past decade may well be adaptable for use in rodent transplantation research. Examples supporting the feasibility of this approach are few in number but are nonetheless intriguing in suggesting the potential for genetically modified mouse tumors for significantly expanding the number of syngeneic and allogeneic models that are currently available. A recent report indicating the application of this concept used GFAP promoter-regulated v-src-transformed astrocytes for establishing orthotopic tumors in syngeneic B6C3F1 mice [13]. In addition to the use of spontaneously arising tumors, nontransformed CNS tissue can be harvested from genetically modified mice and further modified, ex vivo, to produce fully transformed cancer cells for use in a syngeneic transplant model context [14].

By using genetically modified mouse tumor cells in a conventional transplant/engraftment paradigm, mouse modelers of human cancer could potentially address one of the major shortcomings of genetically modified mouse models: the difficulty in adapting spontaneous CNS tumor models for therapeutic testing. Transplantation of these tumors, either in syngeneic animal hosts or as allografts (e.g., in athymic mice), would expand their use for therapeutic testing, which has been a major goal of the mouse model community of investigators [15].

HUMAN TUMOR XENOGRAFT MODELS

Cell Culture–Based Methods

The establishment of xenografts from permanent human tumor cell lines represents one of the most widely used procedures in cancer research. With respect to human gliomas, several series of permanent cell lines have been developed and have seen extensive use for in vivo and in vitro study. The first such series was established by Westermark and coworkers at the Uppsala University [16], and the use of the corresponding "U" series of glioblastoma multiformes (GBM), especially the U87 line, abstract references for which number more than 1000, has significantly influenced our current and collective understanding of glioblastoma. Other widely distributed and used series of GBM cell lines include the "D" series from Duke University [17], the "SF" series from the University of California, San Francisco [18], and the "LN" series from the University of Lausanne [19]. Aside from adult GBM, medulloblastoma is the only other type of CNS tumor for which a series of cell lines has been developed, suggesting that: (a) grade IV malignancy may be a requirement for permanent CNS tumor cell line establishment and (b) tumor incidence is important for developing a cell line series for a specific tumor (i.e., GBM and medulloblastoma are the most common grade IV malignancy CNS tumors of adults and children, respectively).

It is important to note that there are members from each series of established GBM cell lines that are nontumorigenic in immunocompromised rodents [20]; therefore, careful review of existing literature is required before selection for anticipated in vivo experimentation. In addition to lack of tumorigenicity for some of these cell lines, their lengthy in vitro propagation, using conventional cell culture conditions, has undoubtedly contributed to alterations in other biological properties that are manifested in human tumors. This is perhaps most evident with respect to the orthotopic (intracranial) growth pattern of tumorigenic cell lines, which is often well circumscribed [21,22] rather than diffusely infiltrative, as is often the case in patients.

Because of the changes in tumor cell properties that result from extended in vitro propagation, when using conventional serum-supplemented medias, alternative approaches have been described in recent years for promoting the maintenance of tumor-initiating cells, in vitro, that recapitulate intracranial growth patterns in immunocompromised rodents, and that are more representative of those seen in patients [23]. The so-called "stem cell," "neurosphere," or "neuroprogenitor" medias that are most often supplemented with epidermal and fibroblast growth factors rather than serum, and that are used in association with culture conditions that promote the maintenance of unattached cellular aggregates [24] rather than attached cell monolayers, have gained a broad acceptance and use in neuro-oncology research. An example of the growth pattern associated with orthotopic tumor propagation of a GBM neurosphere culture is shown in Figure 17.6.

Xenograft-Based Tumor Propagation

Although less commonly used than cell culture methods of propagation, the sustained growth of GBM surgical specimens as subcutaneous xenografts has been described by a few groups [25,26]. At least one advantage of this approach is readily apparent: any specimen maintained as a xenograft is, by definition, tumorigenic and therefore useful in association with in vivo studies. Less obvious, but nonetheless apparent in association with information reported by multiple groups, is that subcutaneous tumor tissue, or cells dispersed from resected subcutaneous tumors, produce highly infiltrative tumors on intracranial injection in immunocompromised mice [27]. Moreover, GBM propagation as a subcutaneous xenograft promotes retention of tumor epidermal growth factor receptor (EGFR) amplification [26,28], a key genetic alteration observed in approximately one-third of the patients with GBMs. In fact, xenografts established from human tumors have been shown to faithfully maintain all genetic

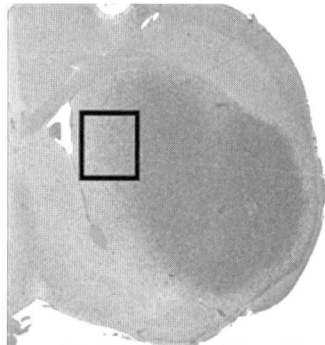

Figure 17.6 Intracranial xenograft tumor established from human GBM neurosphere culture. Growth is as a highly cellular mass with infiltrating cells at the tumor margin (black rectangle). *See color insert.*

signature alterations identified in corresponding human tumors [25,26].

Disadvantages to the xenograft-based approach for tumor propagation include the need for an appropriate facility to house animals and to perform animal procedures, the need for appropriately trained animal technical staff, and the increased difficulty, relative to working with cell cultures, in manipulating and modifying tumor cells to investigate gene/protein function (ie, the development of isogenic derivatives). In addition, there is decreased convenience regarding the timing of experiments because the availability of tumor cells is dependent on having ready access to specific- and appropriately sized subcutaneous tumors. Through additional studies addressing the benefits and shortcomings of tumor cell propagation in growth factor supplemented media versus propagation as subcutaneous xenografts, it is anticipated that a clearer picture will emerge regarding the most appropriate circumstances for using either method.

Orthotopic (Intracranial) Versus Heterotopic (Subcutaneous) Tumor Cell Growth

Xenograft-enabled research, as well as research associated with the use of syngeneic rodent tumor models, has been and will undoubtedly continue to be primarily oriented toward therapeutic testing. Routinely used methods for assessing tumor response to treatment with experimental therapies have been largely based on the following approaches, used either singularly or in different combinations:

- Determination of control versus treatment group volume differences through caliper-based measurements of subcutaneous tumors.
- Determination of control versus treatment group differences in tumor size at arbitrary, albeit identical, time points in animals sacrificed subsequent to orthotopic tumor implantation.
- Determination of control versus treatment group differences in survival time in animals receiving orthotopic tumor implants.

For CNS tumors, the basis for concern over the first approach is primarily associated with the assumption that subcutaneous tumor response is indicative of intracranial tumor response. Because of the different growth patterns of heterotopic versus orthotopic tumors [27], one would more likely anticipate different therapeutic responses between circumscribed (subcutaneous) and infiltrative (intracranial) growths, with therapeutic response of the latter type being more subject to properties of the normal tissue within which the tumor cells have invaded.

Because the procedure for stereotactic intracranial implantation of tissue culture–derived brain tumor cells has been significantly refined since its initial description [29], the success rate of orthotopic tumor establishment is high, with minimal procedure-related animal death. Consequently, one might anticipate its near-obligate use among neuro-oncology researchers. However, a major shortcoming associated with this approach, as indicated by the latter two points listed above, is that an investigator is only allowed a single observation per experimental animal.

EFFECT OF BIOLUMINESCENCE IMAGING

It is reasonable to speculate that much of the resistance to the use of orthotopic brain tumor transplantation approaches has stemmed from the inability to continuously monitor intracranial tumor growth and response to therapeutic testing. However, in recent years, bioluminescence imaging (BLI) has provided researchers with the ability to perform noninvasive, longitudinal studies for continuous monitoring of tumor biological processes, such as growth rate, during initial establishment and response to therapy [30]. In contrast to survival as an indication of agent activity, BLI is not limited to a single observation per animal used in an experiment.

Although other small animal imaging modalities are being used in neuro-oncology research, including magnetic resonance imaging and micro-positron emission tomography, none currently compare with BLI with respect to combined considerations of cost, speed, and sensitivity. In addition to noninvasive serial monitoring of tumor growth and response to therapy, BLI improves animal treatment group randomization because randomization is based on actual tumor burden as indicated by BLI. Furthermore, BLI facilitates more relevant timing of treatment initiation by allowing investigators to determine when injected tumor cells have achieved log-phase growth (Figure 17.7). In many cancer therapy-tumor response experiments, treatments are initiated shortly after intracranial tumor cell injection such that efficacy evaluations are conducted under conditions that favor interpretation of significant antitumor activity, thereby contributing to

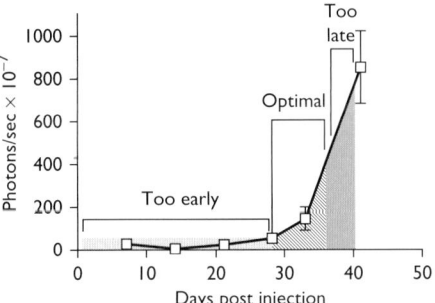

Figure 17.7 Results from bioluminescence monitoring of intracranial U87 xenograft growth, with a graph showing mean luminescence of 3 mice subsequent to injection of 500,000 luciferase-modified cells in each (standard error of mean indicated at each time point). Note that progressive growth of the tumor is not evident until day 28 imaging, with exponential growth evident at day 33 imaging. Initiation of therapy before tumor establishment and progressive growth at day 28 (dark gray area) would yield results less meaningful for assessing efficacy, and clinical translation, than would initiation of therapy after day 28 (light gray area). Optimal therapy administration, for efficacy evaluation, is after indication of progressive growth, but prior to a level of tumor burden that is too extensive for therapeutic response to be evident.

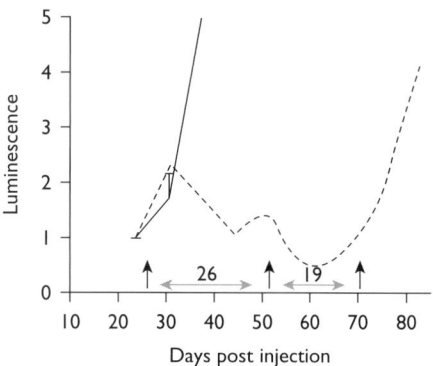

Figure 17.8 Intracranial xenograft bioluminescence signal variation associated with repeated 100 mg/kg temozolomide treatments at days 25, 51, and 70 (indicated by arrows); solid black line represents the luminescence plot for an untreated mouse and shows rapid, exponential tumor growth beyond day 22 posttumor cell injection. Monitoring tumor regrowth of the TMZ-treated mouse provides the opportunity to test novel therapies in an animal model that mimics the clinical scenario of cancer relapse. For this example, note the decreasing benefit of temozolomide therapy, that is indicated by the decreasing length of time for antiproliferative effect when comparing first vs. second treatment (26 vs. 19 days, respectively). The third treatment, at day 70, has essentially no anti-tumor effect. By comparing molecular characteristics of tumors obtained from untreated versus once-treated versus twice-treated animals, candidate genes and corresponding proteins associated with acquired resistance to therapy can be identified.

unrealistic expectations for human clinical trial results due to successful pre-clinical outcomes.

A related and additional application of BLI is for conducting experiments to test the efficacy of salvage therapies against recurrent tumor. Continuous bioluminescence monitoring permits the determination of intracranial tumor regrowth after initial therapeutic response (Figure 17.8) and provides opportunity to treat mice in a context analogous to that of a patient whose cancer has relapsed. Because most novel therapies are initially tested in a setting of recurrent cancer, this approach provides a therapy evaluation paradigm that should, in principle, more closely resemble the clinical scenario in which the therapy would first be evaluated in patients. In addition to creating a salvage therapy evaluation context, this approach is also useful for studying the molecular biology associated with cancer acquisition of resistance to therapy, by comparing molecular profiles of untreated tumors versus once-treated tumor versus tumors subjected to multiple cycles of therapy (Figure 17.8).

HUMAN TUMOR PANELS AND HIGH-THROUGHPUT PRECLINICAL TESTING

By combining GBM panels, maintained either as cell cultures or as subcutaneous grafts, with BLI, the concept of conducting high-throughput and relevant preclinical testing of experimental therapies, against multiple molecular subtypes of GBM, is making progress toward becoming reality. Recent demonstrations in support of a panel approach for investigating therapeutic efficacy have included the analysis of a large series of GBM xenografts for radiation sensitivity [31], as well as for response to the EGFR kinase inhibitor erlotinib [32]. Given the large number of existing therapeutics, the steady supply of novel therapeutics from the industry, and the importance of testing therapies in combinations, it is clear that there are more therapeutic options to evaluate than there are patients to support evaluations through clinical trial activity. Consequently, the need for high-throughput and relevant animal model preclinical testing is essential. It seems likely that advances in our approaches to propagating GBM, combined with advances in monitoring orthotopic growth of GBM in animal models, will help address this need.

REFERENCES

1. Krigman MR, Manuelidis EE. Distribution of fluorescent tracers in heterologously transplanted intracerebral tumors. *Cancer Res.* 1964;24:1749–1759.
2. Norrell HA Jr, Wilson CB. Heterologous transplantation of human glial tumors. *Surg Forum.* 1966;17:431–432.
3. Benda P, Someda K, Messer J, Sweet WH. Morphological and immunochemical studies of rat glial tumors and clonal strains propagated in culture. *J Neurosurg.* 1971;34:310–323.
4. Schmidek HH, Nielsen SL, Schiller AL, Messer J. Morphological studies of rat brain tumors induced by N-nitrosomethylurea. *J Neurosurg.* 1971;34:335–340.
5. Ko L, Koestner A, Wechsler W. Morphological characterization of nitrosourea-induced glioma cell lines and clones. *Acta Neuropathol.* 1980;51:23–31.
6. Kruse CA, Molleston MC, Parks EP, et al. A rat glioma model, CNS-1, with invasive characteristics similar to those of human gliomas: a comparison to 9L gliosarcoma. *J Neurooncol.* 1994;22:191–200.
7. Asai A, Miyagi Y, Sugiyama A, et al. Negative effects of wild-type p53 and s-Myc on cellular growth and tumorigenicity of glioma cells. Implication of the tumor suppressor genes for gene therapy. *J Neurooncol.* 1994;19:259–268.
8. Schlegel J, Piontek G, Kersting M, et al. The p16/Cdkn2a/Ink4a gene is frequently deleted in nitrosourea-induced rat glial tumors. *Pathobiology.* 1999;67:202–206.
9. Park CM, Park MJ, Kwak HJ, et al. Ionizing radiation enhances matrix metalloproteinase-2 secretion and invasion of glioma cells through Src/epidermal growth factor receptor-mediated p38/Akt and phosphatidylinositol 3-kinase/Akt signaling pathways. *Cancer Res.* 2006;66:8511–8519.
10. Chekhonin VP, Baklaushev VP, Yusubalieva GM, et al. Modeling and immunohistochemical analysis of C6 glioma in vivo. *Bull Exp Biol Med.* 2007;143:501–509.
11. Santra M, Zhang X, Santra S, et al. Ectopic doublecortin gene expression suppresses the malignant phenotype in glioblastoma cells. *Cancer Res.* 2006;66:11726–11735.
12. Bates DC, Sin WC, Aftab Q, Naus CC. Connexin43 enhances glioma invasion by a mechanism involving the carboxy terminus. *Glia.* 2007;55:1554–1564.
13. Smilowitz HM, Weissenberger J, Weis J, et al. Orthotopic transplantation of v-src-expressing glioma cell lines into immunocompetent mice: establishment of a new transplantable in vivo model for malignant glioma. *J Neurosurg.* 2007;106:652–659.
14. Bachoo RM, Maher EA, Ligon KL, et al. Epidermal growth factor receptor and Ink4a/Arf: convergent mechanisms governing terminal differentiation and transformation along the neural stem cell to astrocyte axis. *Cancer Cell.* 2002;1:269–277.
15. Fomchenko EI, Holland EC. Mouse models of brain tumors and their applications in preclinical trials. *Clin Cancer Res.* 2006;12:5288–5297.
16. Beckman G, Beckman L, Ponten J, Westermark B. G-6-PD and PGM phenotypes of 16 continuous human tumor cell lines. Evidence

against cross-contamination and contamination by HeLa cells. *Hum Hered.* 1971;21:238–241.
17. Bigner DD, Bigner SH, Pontén J, et al. Heterogeneity of Genotypic and phenotypic characteristics of fifteen permanent cell lines derived from human gliomas. *J Neuropathol Exp Neurol.* 1981;40:201–229.
18. Rutka JT, Giblin JR, Dougherty DY, et al. Establishment and characterization of five cell lines derived from human malignant gliomas. *Acta Neuropathol.* 1987;75:92–103.
19. de Muralt B, de Tribolet N, Diserens AC, et al. Phenotyping of 60 cultured human gliomas and 34 other neuroectodermal tumors by means of monoclonal antibodies against glioma, melanoma and HLA-DR antigens. *Eur J Cancer Clin Oncol.* 1985;21:207–16.
20. Ishii N, Maier D, Merlo A, et al. Frequent co-alterations of TP53, p16/CDKN2A, p14ARF, PTEN tumor suppressor genes in human glioma cell lines. *Brain Pathol.* 1999;9:469–479.
21. Bullard DE, Schold SC Jr, Bigner SH, Bigner DD. Growth and chemotherapeutic response in athymic mice of tumors arising from human glioma-derived cell lines. *J Neuropathol Exp Neurol.* 1981;40:410–427.
22. Finkelstein SD, Black P, Nowak TP, Hand CM, Christensen S, Finch PW. Histological characteristics and expression of acidic and basic fibroblast growth factor genes in intracerebral xenogeneic transplants of human glioma cells. *Neurosurgery.* 1994;34:136–143.
23. Lee J, Kotliarova S, Kotliarov Y, et al. Tumor stem cells derived from glioblastomas cultured in bFGF and EGF more closely mirror the phenotype and genotype of primary tumors than do serum-cultured cell lines. *Cancer Cell.* 2006;9:391–403.
24. Engebraaten O, Hjortland GO, Hirschberg H, Fodstad O. Growth of precultured human glioma specimens in nude rat brain. *J Neurosurg.* 1999;90:125–32.
25. Leuraud P, Taillandier T, Aguirre-Cruz L. Correlation between genetic alterations and growth of human malignant glioma xenografted in nude mice. *Br J Cancer.* 2003;89:2327–2332.
26. Pandita A, Aldape KD, Zadeh G, et al. Contrasting in vivo and in vitro fates of glioblastoma cell subpopulations with amplified EGFR. *Genes Chromosomes Cancer.* 2004;39:29–36.
27. Giannini C, Sarkaria JN, Saito A, et al. Patient tumor EGFR and PDGFRA gene amplifications retained in an invasive intracranial xenograft model of glioblastoma multiforme. *Neuro Oncol.* 2005;7:164–176.
28. Bigner SH, Humphrey PA, Wong AJ, et al. Characterization of the epidermal growth factor receptor in human glioma cell lines and xenografts. *Cancer Res.* 1990;50:8017–8022.
29. Barker M, Hoshino T, Gurcay O, et al. Development of an animal brain tumor model and its response therapy with 1,3-bis (2-chloroethyl)-1-nitrosourea. *Cancer Res.* 1973;33: 976–986.
30. Gross S, Piwnica-Worms D. Spying on cancer: molecular imaging in vivo with genetically encoded reporters. *Cancer Cell.* 2005;7:5–15.
31. Sarkaria JN, Carlson BL, Schroeder MA, et al. Use of an orthotopic xenograft model for assessing the effect of epidermal growth factor receptor amplification on glioblastoma radiation response. *Clin Cancer Res.* 2006;12:2264–2271.
32. Sarkaria JN, Yang L, Grogan PT, et al. Identification of molecular characteristics correlated with glioblastoma sensitivity to EGFR kinase inhibition through use of an intracranial xenograft test panel. *Mol Cancer Ther.* 2007;6:1167–1174.

18 Pathology and Genetics of Meningiomas

Hussein Alahmadi and Sidney E. Croul

GRADING

The majority of meningiomas are World Health Organization (WHO) grade I, based on their benign histology and the potential for cure by surgical excision. A minority are WHO grade II, atypical, or WHO grade III, anaplastic. Grade II and III meningiomas show a greater tendency to recur and metastasize than do grade I tumors [1].

LOCATION

Meningiomas are usually dural-based tumors and are often found adjacent to venous sinuses and dural infoldings. This accounts for some of the common sites of origin falx cerebri, olfactory grooves, optic nerves, sphenoid wings, petrous ridge, tentorium cerebelli, sella turcica, and spinal dura. Occasional intraventricular meningiomas are probably caused by arachnoid rests entrapped in the ventricular system during development [2,3]. Rare meningiomas occur outside the central nervous system, particularly in the lung, again as a consequence of developmental arachnoid rests [4]. Metastatic tumors, which occur in 0.1% of tumors, can be found in the lung, as well as liver and bone [5].

INCIDENCE

Meningiomas are the most common primary intracranial tumors. They comprise 32% of histologically confirmed primary brain tumors in the Central Brain Tumor Registry of the United States [6]. In a population-based study, the prevalence of asymptomatic meningiomas was 0.9% (1.1% in women and 0.7% in men) [7]. The incidence of meningiomas rises steadily over the lifespan from a low of less than 1 per 100,000 person-years in the first two decades to 30 per 100,000 person-years by the ninth decade [6]. Benign meningiomas (WHO grade I) are diagnosed twice as frequently in women compared with men [6]. This female predominance is not replicated in atypical (WHO grade II) or anaplastic (WHO grade III) meningiomas [8,9]. Although large North American studies show no compelling evidence for a difference in incidence of grade I meningiomas between populations of different racial backgrounds [6], studies of smaller populations such as Polynesians [10] suggest that risk factors may segregate among some ethnic groups.

PATHOLOGY

Macroscopic

Meningiomas tend to be rubbery and firm. A gritty consistency on section is often indicative of calcific psammoma bodies. They are usually attached to the dura and often have a central mass of tumor that gradually tapers out into a thin tail. Compression of the underlying brain is usual (Figure 18.1A and 18.1B). Invasion of the dura, overlying bone and skin, and adjacent structures such as the orbital contents is common as well (Figure 18.2A and 18.2B). Bony invasion is often associated with hyperostosis, readily seen on standard x-rays and computed tomography scans. Invasion of the brain is the exception. Even in the case of malignant meningiomas, brain invasion tends to be limited to a few millimeters below the pial surface. Adjacent vessels are frequently ensheathed by meningothelial tumors, but the walls of these vessels are rarely breached (Figure 18.2B) [1].

Microscopic

The similarities between arachnoid villi and these tumors led Cushing and Eisenhardt [11] to coin the term *meningioma* in their 1938 monograph. Hyperplastic clusters of normal arachnoid cap cells are often histologically identical to microscopic fields of grade I meningiomas (Figure 18.3A and 18.3B). They have pale round nuclei with evenly dispersed chromatin and

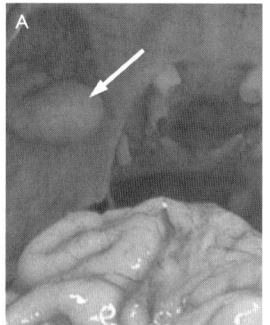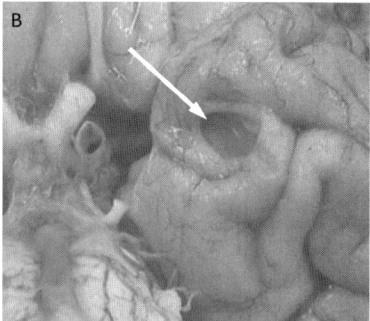

Figure 18.1 An incidental middle fossa meningioma found at autopsy (**A**) compresses but does not invade the inferior surface of the temporal lobe (**B**). *See color insert.*

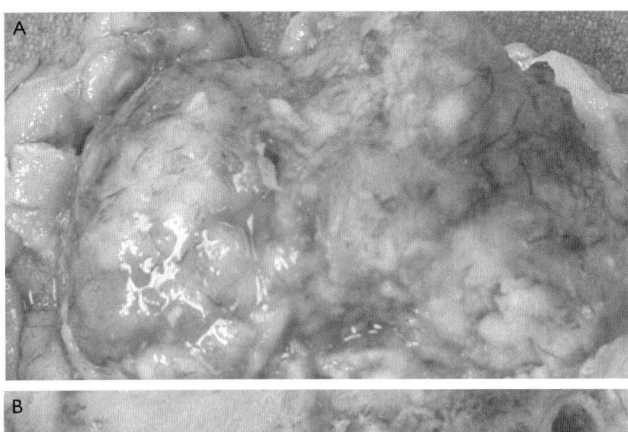

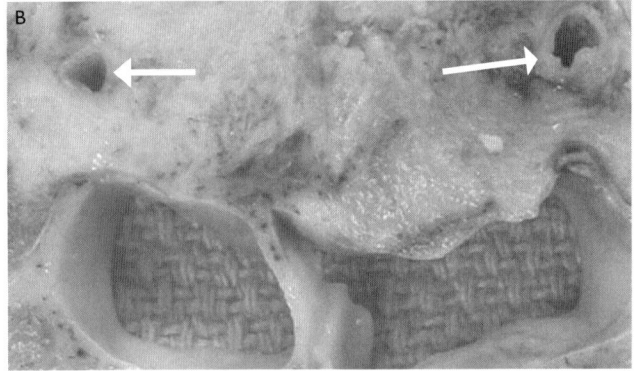

Figure 18.2 A histologically benign olfactory groove meningioma **(A)** encases the cavernous sinuses **(B, arrows)**, invades the skull, and grows into the sinuses. See color insert.

occasional clear cytoplasmic invaginations. Borders between cells are indistinct because of interdigitation of adjacent cell membranes, which may give the cells a syncytial appearance. Groups of cells form whorls, the centers of which may become mineralized, forming psammoma bodies.

Since Cushing and Eisenhardt's delineation of nine major types and 22 subtypes of meningiomas [11], the classification has gone through several modifications. The current WHO scheme ([1]; Table 18.1) recognizes 15 types. Of these, nine are WHO grade I. They differ in their histological patterns but have nearly equal biological behavior. Meningothelial tumors are more syncytial in appearance (Figure 18.4A), fibroblastic meningiomas have elongated fascicular cells (Figure 18.4B), and transitional meningiomas contain elements of both types (Figure 18.4C). Psammomatous meningiomas (Figure 18.4D) are rich in those lamellar calcifications and angiomatous meningiomas in small vessels (Figure 18.4E). Microcystic meningiomas are notable for a loose, vacuolated background (Figure 18.4F). The chronic inflammatory infiltrate of lymphoplasmacyte-rich tumors can obscure the meningothelial features, making diagnosis difficult. They are a rare and a somewhat controversial entity. The argument has been made that these tumors actually represent primary inflammatory processes that have been misdiagnosed. Metaplastic meningiomas demonstrate focal mesenchymal elements such as bone, cartilage, and fat (Figure 18.4G). Secretory meningiomas have brightly eosinophilic intracellular inclusions, which have been called pseudopsammoma

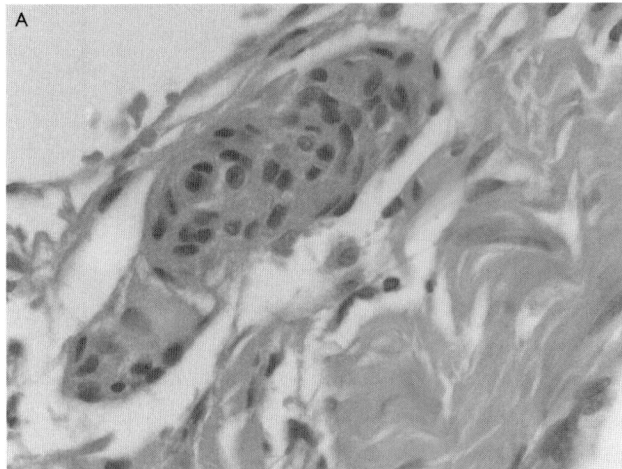

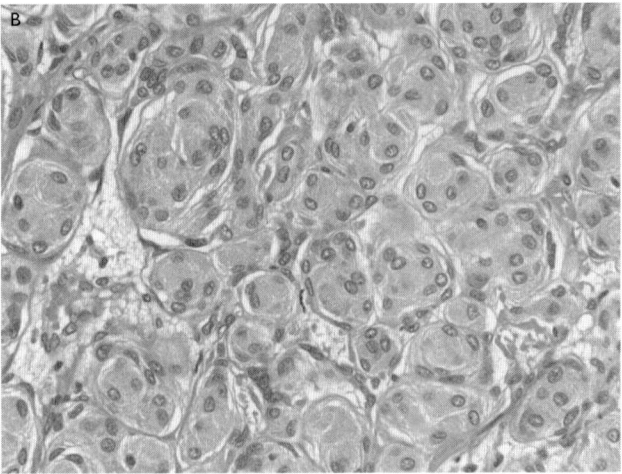

Figure 18.3 Arachnoid cap cells **(A)** and the whorls of a meningothelial meningioma **(B)** share both architecture and cytology. See color insert.

Table 18.1 The 2007 WHO Classification of Meningiomasa Recognizes 15 Types of Which 9 are Grade I, 3 Grade II, and 3 Grade III

Grade I
   Meningothelial
   Fibrous (Fibroblastic)
   Transitional (Mixed)
   Psammomatous
   Angiomatous
   Microcystic
   Secretory
   Lymphoplasmacyte—rich
   Metaplastic

Grade II
   Chordoid
   Clear cell
   Atypical

Grade III
   Papillary
   Rhabdoid
   Anaplastic

From ref. [1].

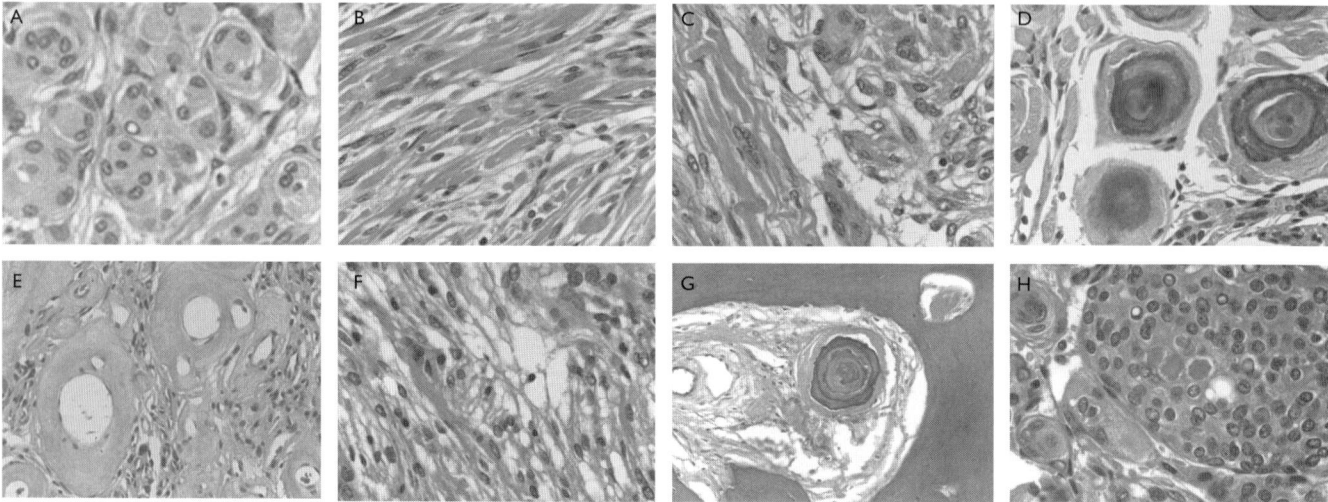

Figure 18.4 WHO grade I histological subtypes include meningothelial meningiomas **(A)**, fibroblastic meningiomas **(B)**, and transitional meningiomas with elements of both meningothelial and fibroblastic tumors **(C)**. Psammomatous meningiomas **(D)** have calcifications, angiomatous meningiomas have small vessels **(E)**, and microcystic meningiomas have a vacuolated background **(F)**. Metaplastic meningiomas demonstrate focal mesenchymal elements such as the bone seen here **(G)**. Secretory meningiomas demonstrate eosinophilic intracellular inclusions **(H)**. *See color insert.*

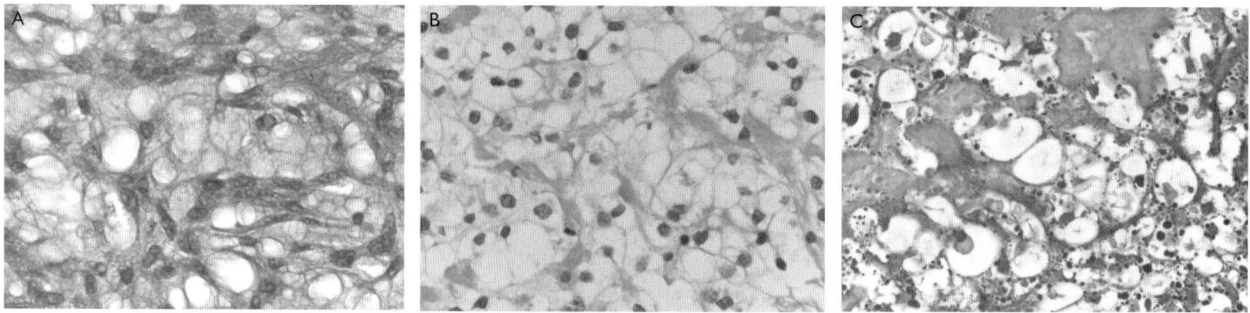

Figure 18.5 Both chordoid **(A)** and clear cell meningiomas **(B, C)** are WHO grade II/atypical. The chordoid tumors feature a myxoid background with vacuolated cells, whereas in the clear cell variant, the cytoplasm of the tumor cells is glycogen rich, accounting for the stunning PAS positivity **(C)**. *See color insert.*

bodies. They differ biologically from the other eight WHO grade I tumors in that they are more associated with edema of surrounding central nervous system tissues [12,13].

Three subtypes of meningioma are classified as WHO grade II/atypical tumors because of their high rates of recurrence after resection. Chordoid meningiomas [14–16] are named for their resemblance to chordomas. These tumors feature zones with a myxoid background in which there are trabeculae of eosinophilic cells with vacuolated cytoplasm (Figure 18.5A). These are intermixed with other zones displaying more typical meningothelial features. Clear cell meningiomas [17,18] feature cells with glycogen-rich cytoplasm (Figure 18.5B and 18.5C) and often lack many of the common secondary structures of meningiomas, particularly the distinctive whorled pattern. Meningiomas without the features of these three subtypes can also be classified as grade II if they exhibit four mitotic figures per 10 high-power fields (Figure 18.6A), microscopic evidence of brain invasion (Figure 18.6B), or three of following features: patternless growth, hypercellularity, foci of small cells with high nuclear:cytoplasmic ratio, prominent nucleoli, or foci of necrosis (Figure 18.7A to 18.7D; [19]).

Meningiomas classified as WHO grade III/anaplastic or malignant pursue a more aggressive clinical course. Median survival for these tumors is less than 2 years [20]. Papillary meningiomas are characterized by a perivascular pseudopapillary growth pattern (Figure 18.8A and 18.8B). They tend to occur in young patients, demonstrate brain invasion, recur frequently, and can metastasize both within the subarachnoid space and outside the nervous system [21]. Rhabdoid meningiomas are named for their intracytoplasmic eosinophilic masses of intermediate filaments similar to those found in rhabdoid tumors from other organs, particularly the kidney (Figure 18.8C). Most rhabdoid meningiomas have high proliferative indices and other histological features of malignancy [22]. As in the case of atypical meningiomas, tumors need not demonstrate papillary or rhabdoid features to be classified as

18 • *Pathology and Genetics of Meningiomas* 161

anaplastic. The findings of either cytological malignancy or 20 or more mitotic figures per 10 high-power fields are sufficient to warrant the diagnosis [20].

Immunohistochemistry and Electron Microscopy

Most meningiomas demonstrate expression of epithelial membrane antigen by immunohistochemistry (Figure 18.9A; [23]). Secretory meningiomas show positivity for carcinoembryonic antigen (Figure 18.9B). The intracytoplasmic masses of rhabdoid meningiomas are positive for vimentin (Figure 18.9C). Electron microscopy can occasionally be of value in the diagnosis of meningothelial tumors. Large numbers of intermediate filaments, interdigitated membranes, and desmosomal junctions are characteristic of meningiomas.

MIB1/Ki67 immunohistochemistry is currently used by many pathologists to assess the proliferation index of meningiomas. Although absolute values vary between laboratories, the percentage of positive cells tends to be lowest in grade I and highest in grade III tumors. A MIB1/Ki67 index of 5% to 10% in the absence of histological features of a grade II tumor is a predictor for early tumor recurrence (Figure 18.10A and 18.10B). Two thirds of meningiomas express progesterone receptors (Figure 18.10C). Progesterone receptor negativity, although not a risk factor by itself, tends to occur more frequently in higher-grade meningiomas and may be an indicator of poor prognosis when combined with increased proliferation index and higher grade. Progesterone receptor–negative tumors also tend to be larger than those that express progesterone receptors [24–26].

GENETICS

Background

The contribution of inheritance to the occurrence of meningiomas has been recognized since the clinical association of multiple meningiomas and meningioangiomatosis with neurofibromatosis was made almost a century ago [27,28]. Family groups with increased incidence of meningiomas but without the stigmata of neurofibromatosis have also been described [29]. Meningiomas may also occur in the context of other inherited diseases such as Gorlin and Cowden syndromes [30,31].

Although the current WHO classification system defines the grade of meningothelial tumors solely on histological criteria, the genetic profile of meningiomas provides further predictive information. The majority of this work has grown out of cytogenetic studies and is therefore presented here in the context of chromosomal aberrations and telomeric stability.

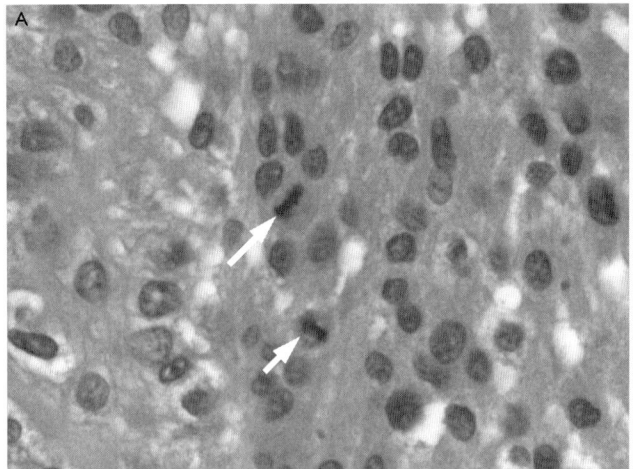
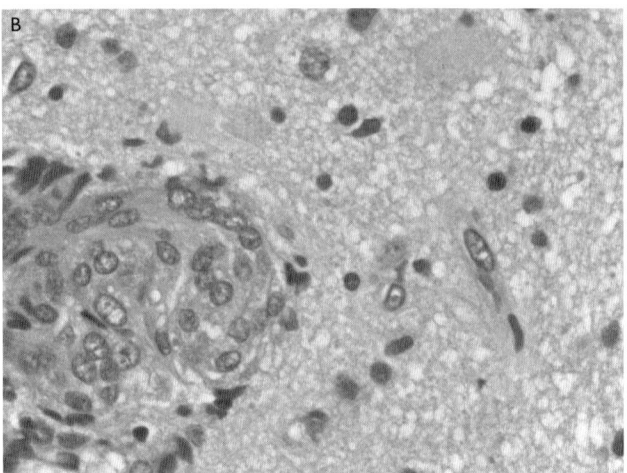

Figure 18.6 In the absence of chordoid or clear cell morphologies, either four mitoses/10 high-power fields (**arrows, A**) or brain invasion by tumor (**B**) is sufficient to make the diagnosis of atypical meningioma. *See color insert.*

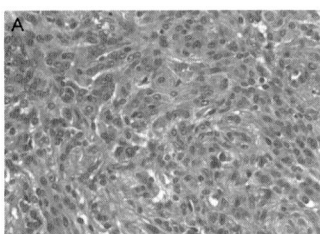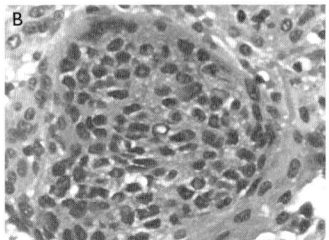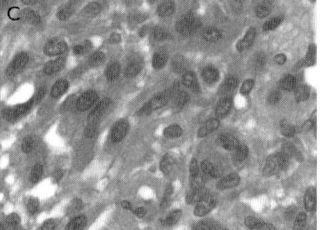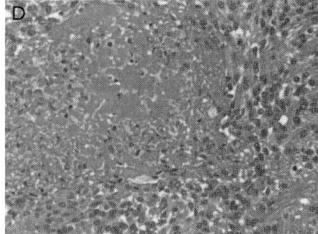

Figure 18.7 Tumors demonstrating three of the following: patternless growth (**A**), hypercellularity, foci of small cells with high nuclear:cytoplasmic ratio (**B**), prominent nucleoli (**C**), or foci of necrosis (**D**) are also considered grade II/ atypical. *See color insert.*

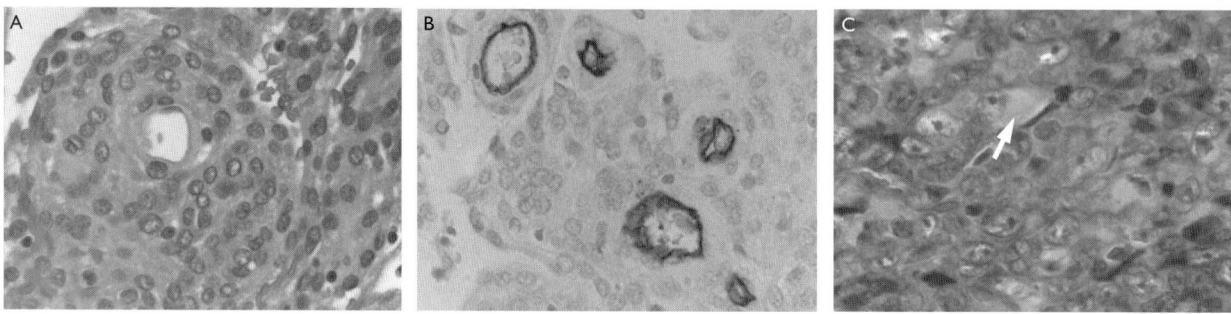

Figure 18.8 The perivascular growth pattern of papillary meningiomas can be seen with hematoxylin and eosin staining **(A)** but is even clearer with immunohistochemistry for CD34 **(B)** which clarifies the structure of the vascular cores. The intracytoplasmic inclusions of rhabdoid meningiomas **(C arrow)** are brightly eosinophilic. See color insert.

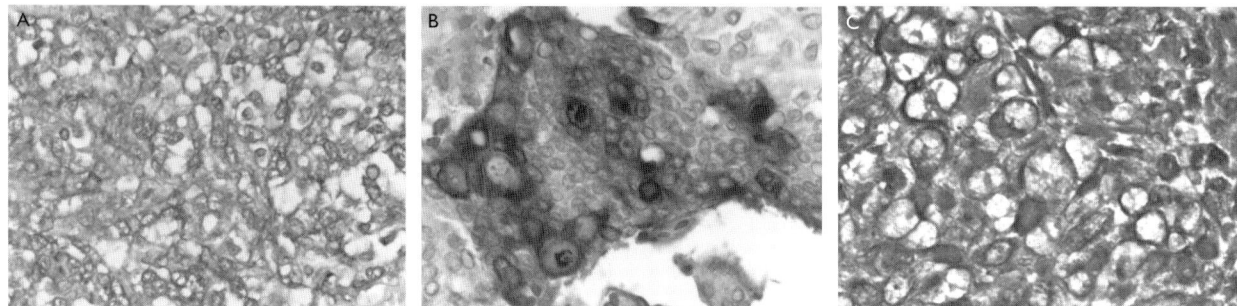

Figure 18.9 Epithelial membrane antigen immunohistochemistry stains most meningiomas **(A)**, whereas carcinoembryonic antigen is positive in secretory meningiomas **(B)** and vimentin marks the intracytoplasmic filamentous accumulations of rhabdoid meningiomas **(C)**. See color insert.

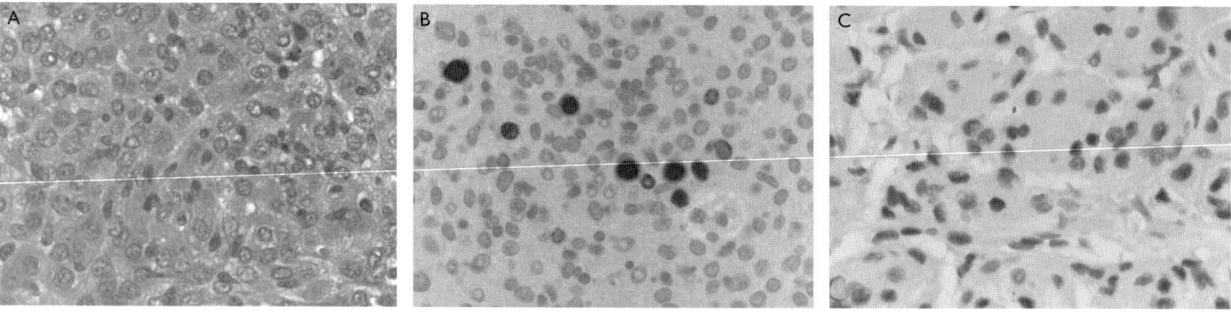

Figure 18.10 Meningiomas that are WHO grade I by standard morphological criteria **(A)** but have proliferation indices of 5% to 10% by MIB-1 staining **(B)** have an increased risk of early recurrence. Progesterone receptor expression can be demonstrated by immunohistochemistry in most meningiomas **(C)**. See color insert.

Chromosomal aberrations

Chromosome 22q

Loss of the long arm of chromosome 22, which is usually associated with inactivation of the NF2 gene, is the most common genetic abnormality found in meningiomas (Figure 18.11A; [32,33,34]). NF2, which codes for the merlin (schwannomin) protein, is a tumor suppressor because its inactivation by mutation, methylation of the 5′ region, or proteolysis results in the phenotype of peripheral neurofibromas and multiple meningiomas [34,35]. Sporadic merlin (schwannomin) inactivation is most common in fibroblastic and transitional meningiomas but uncommon in meningothelial and secretory meningiomas [35,36]. Although NF2 inactivation has been documented in all grades of meningiomas, there is a high frequency of additional complex genetic abnormalities in the higher-grade tumors. This has led to the hypothesis that NF2 inactivation initiates low-grade tumors followed by the additional genetic events that are responsible for the progression to high-grade tumors [34].

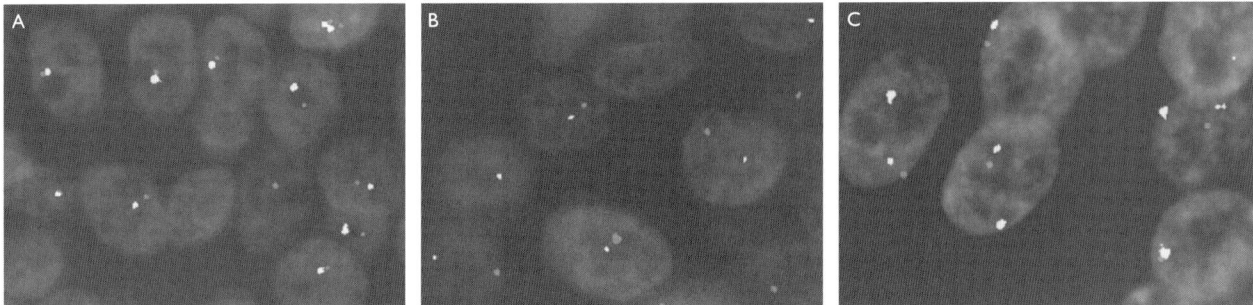

Figure 18.11 Fluorescent in situ hybridization (FISH) is used to detect chromosomal abnormalities in meningiomas. 22q deletion is demonstrated with a probe for NF2 (22q12) in red and another for BCR (22q11.2) in green. The presence of only one of each in most nuclei is consistent with either monosomy of chromosome 22 or a large 22q deletion **(A)**. Loss of both 1p and 14q is demonstrated with a probe for 1p32 labeled in green and another for 14q32 labeled in red. Again, most cells have one green and one red, consistent with deletions of both chromosomal regions **(B)**. Hemizygous deletion of 9p21 is shown with CEP9 (centromere enumerating probe for chromosome 9) in green (2 signals in most nuclei) and the p16 (CDKN2A) gene region (9p21) in red (1 signal in most cells) **(C)**. Courtesy of Arie Perry, MD, Department of Pathology, University of California at San Francisco. See color insert.

Chromosome 1p

Loss of heterozygosity for chromosome 1p is associated with increases in both grade and recurrence rate of meningiomas (Figure 18.11B). The rate of 1p loss increases from a low of 25% in WHO grade I to a high of 85% in grade III meningiomas [37]. Meningiomas with loss of 1p have also been reported to be those with the highest risk of recurrence [9]. The critical region of chromosomal loss has been narrowed to the 1p32, 1p34, and 1p36 loci [38–43]. Although several genes within these regions, including p18, CDKN2C, p73, GADD45A, and EPB41, have been examined for mutations and polymorphisms, none has been detected [37,44–46]. A few studies have demonstrated promoter methylation of p73 [47,48] and RASSF1A [48], implying that downregulation of these genes may play a role in meningioma progression. At the same time, more maps of these loci have generated further lists of candidate genes [40,43], the analyses of which have yet to be reported.

Chromosome 14q

Loss of 14q is associated with grade II and III meningiomas ([38,49–53]; Figure 18.11B). The 14q loss may also be a predictor of early recurrence in grade I meningiomas and poorer outcome in grade III meningiomas [53–55]. A candidate tumor suppressor gene, NDRG2, located at 14q11.2, has been identified. Decreased expression of its transcripts and protein product has been demonstrated in lower-grade meningiomas with aggressive clinical behavior [56].

Chromosome 9p

The frequency of deletions in 9p21 (Figure 18.11C) is increased proportionally with increases in grade of meningiomas [37,57] and may be an independent predictor of poor outcome in anaplastic meningiomas [57]. Several tumor suppressor genes are located on 9p, including CDKN2a, a regulator of the G1/S-phase transition, CDKN2b, which is involved in cell cycle G1 progression, and p14ARF, a regulator of p53 activity. The role that these genes may play in 9p-related meningioma progression remains unclear. Although in one study [37], homozygous deletions of all three genes were found in a small percentage of grade II and approximately half of grade III meningiomas, another study [58] has reported only promoter methylation not consistently related to changes in gene expression.

Chromosome 10

Abnormalities of chromosome 10 are also correlated with meningioma progression from grade I to grades II and III. These include loss of heterozygosity [38,59,60], trisomy [61], and homozygous deletion [51,62] of 10q. One recent study [63], which applied both high-density single-nucleotide polymorphism arrays and multicolor fluorescence in situ hybridization to single atypical meningioma, reported both loss of heterozygosity at 10q21.1 and a reciprocal translocation involving 10q22: t(10;16)(q2;q12.1).

Chromosome 17

Abnormalities of 17q have also been associated with higher-grade meningiomas. Both fluorescent and chromogenic in situ hybridization [61,64] showed gains in chromosome 17. Restriction fragment length polymorphism has demonstrated loss at 17p in malignant meningiomas [65]. Comparative genomic hybridization has narrowed this region of interest to 17q22–23 [66].

Telomere Stability

Telomere shortening with progressive cell division is involved in the normal regulation of cell division and senescence. Conversely, maintenance of telomere length by the reverse transcriptase telomerase is a common feature of human tumors. Several studies have examined measures of telomere stability in meningiomas. Telomerase activity is detectable in few grade I meningiomas but in most grade II and II tumors [67–73].

Radiation

The only proven environmental risk factor for meningiomas is ionizing radiation. Evidence for this comes from patients with tinea capitis treated with low-dose radiotherapy before the introduction of griseofulvin in the 1960s [74,75], children and teenagers who received full mouth dental x-rays with doses of 1 to 2.8 Gy or more [76], survivors of the Hiroshima and Nagasaki atomic bombs [77,78], and more recent studies of children receiving high-dose radiation therapy for cancer [79]. Although the relative risk in the patients who received low-dose radiotherapy was 9.5 times higher than the general population, less than 1% of patients treated developed meningiomas [75]. Radiation-induced meningiomas are more often multiple and have higher recurrence rates than standard meningiomas [80–82]. Most of these tumors are pathologically WHO grade I. One or two of the histological findings associated with grade II tumors (small cell change, nuclear enlargement, hypercellularity, and sheeting) may be found in a greater percentage of the radiation-induced tumors than in standard meningiomas [80,82]. Although it is not clear whether a significant proportion of radiation-induced meningiomas are WHO grades II or III at initial presentation, progression in grade is certainly seen in the recurrent tumors [82].

It has been suggested that radiation induces meningiomas in individuals with genetic predispositions to radiation-induced tumorigenesis. Support for this notion comes from an epidemiological analysis that found an 11% prevalence of meningiomas in first-degree relatives of irradiated patients with meningiomas compared with less than 1% prevalence of meningiomas in first-degree relatives of irradiated patients without meningiomas [83]. In addition, the patients who developed meningioma after irradiation had a higher incidence of other radiation-induced cancers in their siblings.

Cytogenetic analyses show that the most frequent chromosomal loss in radiation-induced meningiomas occurs at 1p followed by 22. Losses of 6q, 7p, 9p, 18q, and 19q and gains of 8 and 12 have also been reported but with less consistency [82,84–89]. The increased frequency of chromosome 1p over 22 losses may help explain the more aggressive phenotype of radiation-induced meningiomas. It also brings into question whether these tumors depend on oncogenic pathways that are different from those that have been characterized in meningiomas not associated with radiation. In regards to NF2, the results of studies are variable. Although some report a paucity of NF2 mutations and normal merlin expression in radiation-induced meningiomas [88,90], others report underexpression of NF2 transcripts in meningiomas regardless of a history of radiation exposure [82].

REFERENCES

1. Louis DN, Ohgaki H, Wiestler OD, Cavenee WK. *WHO Classification of Tumours of the Central Nervous System*. 4th ed. Lyon, France: International Agency for Research on Cancer; 2007.
2. Burger PC, Scheithauer BW, Vogel FS. *Surgical Pathology of the Nervous System and its Coverings* New York, NY: Churchill Livingstone; 2002.
3. Bhatoe HS, Singh P, Dutta V. Intraventricular meningiomas: a clinicopathological study and review. *Neurosurg Focus*. 2006;20:E9.
4. Incarbone M, Ceresoli GL, Di Tommaso L, et al. Primary pulmonary meningioma: report of a case and review of the literature. *Lung Cancer*. 2008;62:401–407.
5. Drummond KJ, Bittar RG, Fearnside MR. Metastatic atypical meningioma: case report and review of the literature. *J Clin Neurosci*. 2000;7:69–72.
6. Central Brain Tumor Registry of the United States. *Statistical Report: Primary Brain Tumors in the United States, 2000–2004*. Illinois: Central Brain Tumor Registry of the United States; 2008.
7. Vernooij MW, Ikram MA, Tanghe HL, et al. Incidental findings on brain MRI in the general population. *N Engl J Med*. 2007;357:1821–1828.
8. Simon M, Boström JP, Hartmann C. Molecular genetics of meningiomas: from basic research to potential clinical applications. *Neurosurgery*. 2007;60:787–798; discussion 787–798.
9. Ketter R, Henn W, Niedermayer I, et al. Predictive value of progression-associated chromosomal aberrations for the prognosis of meningiomas: a retrospective study of 198 cases. *J Neurosurg*. 2001;95:601–607.
10. Olson S, Law A. Meningiomas and the Polynesian population. *ANZ J Surg*. 2005;75:705–709.
11. Cushing H, Eisenhardt L. *Meningiomas, Their Classification, Regional Behavior, Life History, and Surgical Results*. Springfield, IL: Charles C Thomas; 1938.
12. Regelsberger J, Hagel C, Emami P, Ries T, Heese O, Westphal M. Secretory meningiomas: a benign subgroup causing life-threatening complications. *Neuro Oncol*. 2009;11:819–824.
13. Jagadha V, Deck JH. Massive cerebral edema associated with meningioma. *Can J Neurol Sci*. 1987;14:55–58.
14. Kepes JJ, Chen WY, Connors MH, Vogel FS. "Chordoid" meningeal tumors in young individuals with peritumoral lymphoplasmacellular infiltrates causing systemic manifestations of the Castleman syndrome. A report of seven cases. *Cancer*. 1988 15;62:391–406.
15. Zuppan CW, Liwnicz BH, Weeks DA. Meningioma with chordoid features. *Ultrastruct Pathol*. 1994;18:29–32.
16. Couce ME, Aker FV, Scheithauer BW. Chordoid meningioma: a clinicopathologic study of 42 cases. *Am J Surg Pathol*. 2000;24:899–905. Erratum in: *Am J Surg Pathol*. 2000;24:1316–1317.
17. Kubota T, Sato K, Kabuto M, et al. Clear cell (glycogen-rich) meningioma with special reference to spherical collagen deposits. *Noshuyo Byori*. 1995;12:53–60.
18. Zorludemir S, Scheithauer BW, Hirose T, Van Houten C, Miller G, Meyer FB. Clear cell meningioma. A clinicopathologic study of a potentially aggressive variant of meningioma. *Am J Surg Pathol*. 1995;19:493–505.
19. Perry A, Stafford SL, Scheithauer BW, Suman VJ, Lohse CM. Meningioma grading: an analysis of histologic parameters. *Am J Surg Pathol*. 1997;21:1455–1465.
20. Perry A, Scheithauer BW, Stafford SL, Lohse CM, Wollan PC. "Malignancy" in meningiomas: a clinicopathologic study of 116 patients, with grading implications. *Cancer*. 1999;85:2046–2056.
21. Ludwin SK, Rubinstein LJ, Russell DS. Papillary meningioma: a malignant variant of meningioma. *Cancer*. 1975;36:1363–1373.
22. Kepes JJ, Moral LA, Wilkinson SB, Abdullah A, Llena JF. Rhabdoid transformation of tumor cells in meningiomas: a histologic indication of increased proliferative activity: report of four cases. *Am J Surg Pathol*. 1998;22:231–238.
23. Winek RR, Scheithauer BW, Wick MR. Meningioma, meningeal hemangiopericytoma (angioblastic meningioma), peripheral hemangiopericytoma, and acoustic schwannoma. A comparative immunohistochemical study. *Am J Surg Pathol*. 1989;13:251–261.
24. Hsu DW, Efird JT, Hedley-Whyte ET.MIB-1 (Ki-67) index and transforming growth factor-alpha (TGF alpha) immunoreactivity are significant prognostic predictors for meningiomas. *Neuropathol Appl Neurobiol*. 1998;24:441–452.

25. Perry A, Stafford SL, Scheithauer BW, Suman VJ, Lohse CM. The prognostic significance of MIB-1, p53, and DNA flow cytometry in completely resected primary meningiomas. *Cancer.* 1998;82:2262–2269.
26. Roser F, Nakamura M, Bellinzona M, Rosahl SK, Ostertag H, Samii M. The prognostic value of progesterone receptor status in meningiomas. *J Clin Pathol.* 2004;57:1033–1037.
27. Bassoe P, Nuzum F. Report of a case of central and peripheral neurofibromatosis. *J Nerv Ment Dis.* 1915;42:785–796.
28. Omeis I, Hillard VH, Braun A, Benzil DL, Murali R, Harter DH. Meningioangiomatosis associated with neurofibromatosis: report of 2 cases in a single family and review of the literature. *Surg Neurol.* 2006;65:595–603.
29. Maxwell M, Shih SD, Galanopoulos T, Hedley-Whyte ET, Cosgrove GR. Familial meningioma: analysis of expression of neurofibromatosis 2 protein Merlin. Report of two cases. *J Neurosurg.* 1998;88:562–569.
30. Gorlin RJ. Nevoid basal-cell carcinoma syndrome. *Medicine (Baltimore).* 1987;66:98–113.
31. Rimbau J, Isamat F. Dysplastic gangliocytoma of the cerebellum (Lhermitte-Duclos disease) and its relation to the multiple hamartoma syndrome (Cowden disease). *J Neurooncol.* 1994;18:191–197.
32. Leuraud P, Dezamis E, Aguirre-Cruz L, et al. Prognostic value of allelic losses and telomerase activity in meningiomas. *J Neurosurg.* 2004;100:303–309.
33. Lee JY, Finkelstein S, Hamilton RL, Rekha R, King JT Jr, Omalu B. Loss of heterozygosity analysis of benign, atypical, and anaplastic meningiomas. *Neurosurgery.* 2004;55:1163–1173.
34. Seizinger BR, de la Monte S, Atkins L, Gusella JF, Martuza RL. Molecular genetic approach to human meningioma: loss of genes on chromosome 22. *Proc Natl Acad Sci USA.* 1987;84:5419–5423.
35. Wellenreuther R, Kraus JA, Lenartz D, et al. Analysis of the neurofibromatosis 2 gene reveals molecular variants of meningioma. *Am J Pathol.* 1995;146:827–832.
36. Hartmann C, Sieberns J, Gehlhaar C, Simon M, Paulus W, von Deimling A. NF2 mutations in secretory and other rare variants of meningiomas. *Brain Pathol.* 2006;16:15–19.
37. Boström J, Meyer-Puttlitz B, Wolter M, et al. Alterations of the tumor suppressor genes CDKN2A (p16(INK4a)), p14(ARF), CDKN2B (p15(INK4b)), and CDKN2C (p18(INK4c)) in atypical and anaplastic meningiomas. *Am J Pathol.* 2001;159:661–669.
38. Simon M, von Deimling A, Larson JJ, et al. Allelic losses on chromosomes 14, 10, and 1 in atypical and malignant meningiomas: a genetic model of meningioma progression. *Cancer Res.* 1995;55:4696–4701.
39. Sulman EP, Dumanski JP, White PS, et al. Identification of a consistent region of allelic loss on 1p32 in meningiomas: correlation with increased morbidity. *Cancer Res.* 1998;58:3226–3230.
40. Sulman EP, White PS, Brodeur GM. Genomic annotation of the meningioma tumor suppressor locus on chromosome 1p34. *Oncogene.* 2004;23:1014–1020.
41. Bello MJ, de Campos JM, Vaquero J, Kusak ME, Sarasa JL, Rey JA. High-resolution analysis of chromosome arm 1p alterations in meningioma. *Cancer Genet Cytogenet.* 2000;120:30–36.
42. Murakami M, Hashimoto N, Takahashi Y, Hosokawa Y, Inazawa J, Mineura K. A consistent region of deletion on 1p36 in meningiomas: identification and relation to malignant progression. *Cancer Genet Cytogenet.* 2003;140:99–106.
43. Buckley PG, Jarbo C, Menzel U, et al. Comprehensive DNA copy number profiling of meningioma using a chromosome 1 tiling path microarray identifies novel candidate tumor suppressor loci. *Cancer Res.* 2005;65:2653–2661.
44. Leuraud P, Marie Y, Robin E, et al. Frequent loss of 1p32 region but no mutation of the p18 tumor suppressor gene in meningiomas. *J Neurooncol.* 2000;50:207–213.
45. Lomas J, Bello MJ, Arjona D, et al. Analysis of p73 gene in meningiomas with deletion at 1p. *Cancer Genet Cytogenet.* 2001;129:88–91.
46. Piaskowski S, Rieske P, Szybka M, et al. GADD45A and EPB41 as tumor suppressor genes in meningioma pathogenesis. *Cancer Genet Cytogenet.* 2005;162:63–67.
47. Lomas J, Amiñoso C, Gonzalez-Gomez P, et al. Methylation status of TP73 in meningiomas. *Cancer Genet Cytogenet.* 2004;148:148–151.
48. Nakane Y, Natsume A, Wakabayashi T, et al. Malignant transformation-related genes in meningiomas: allelic loss on 1p36 and methylation status of p73 and RASSF1A. *J Neurosurg.* 2007;107:398–404.
49. Menon AG, Rutter JL, von Sattel JP, et al. Frequent loss of chromosome 14 in atypical and malignant meningioma: identification of a putative 'tumor progression' locus. *Oncogene.* 1997;14:611–616.
50. Tse JY, Ng HK, Lau KM, Lo KW, Poon WS, Huang DP. Loss of heterozygosity of chromosome 14q in low- and high-grade meningiomas. *Hum Pathol.* 1997;28:779–785.
51. Lamszus K, Kluwe L, Matschke J, Meissner H, Laas R, Westphal M. Allelic losses at 1p, 9q, 10q, 14q, and 22q in the progression of aggressive meningiomas and undifferentiated meningeal sarcomas. *Cancer Genet Cytogenet.* 1999;110:103–110.
52. Leone PE, Bello MJ, de Campos JM, et al. NF2 gene mutations and allelic status of 1p, 14q and 22q in sporadic meningiomas. *Oncogene.* 1999;18:2231–2239.
53. Cai DX, Banerjee R, Scheithauer BW, Lohse CM, Kleinschmidt-Demasters BK, Perry A. Chromosome 1p and 14q FISH analysis in clinicopathologic subsets of meningioma: diagnostic and prognostic implications. *J Neuropathol Exp Neurol.* 2001;60:628–636.
54. Tabernero MD, Espinosa AB, Maíllo A, et al. Characterization of chromosome 14 abnormalities by interphase in situ hybridization and comparative genomic hybridization in 124 meningiomas: correlation with clinical, histopathologic, and prognostic features. *Am J Clin Pathol.* 2005;123:744–751.
55. Maillo A, Orfao A, Espinosa AB, et al. Early recurrences in histologically benign/grade I meningiomas are associated with large tumors and coexistence of monosomy 14 and del(1p36) in the ancestral tumor cell clone. *Neuro Oncol.* 2007;9:438–446.
56. Lusis EA, Watson MA, Chicoine MR, et al. Integrative genomic analysis identifies NDRG2 as a candidate tumor suppressor gene frequently inactivated in clinically aggressive meningioma. *Cancer Res.* 2005;65:7121–7126.
57. Perry A, Banerjee R, Lohse CM, Kleinschmidt-DeMasters BK, Scheithauer BW. A role for chromosome 9p21 deletions in the malignant progression of meningiomas and the prognosis of anaplastic meningiomas. *Brain Pathol.* 2002;12:183–190.
58. Tse JY, Ng HK, Lo KW, et al. Analysis of cell cycle regulators: p16INK4A, pRb, and CDK4 in low- and high-grade meningiomas. *Hum Pathol.* 1998;29:1200–1207.
59. Rempel SA, Schwechheimer K, Davis RL, Cavenee WK, Rosenblum ML. Loss of heterozygosity for loci on chromosome 10 is associated with morphologically malignant meningioma progression. *Cancer Res.* 1993;53(10 suppl):2386–2392.
60. Mihaila D, Gutiérrez JA, Rosenblum ML, Newsham IF, Bögler O, Rempel SA; NABTT CNS Consortium. Meningiomas: analysis of loss of heterozygosity on chromosome 10 in tumor progression and the delineation of four regions of chromosomal deletion in common with other cancers. *Clin Cancer Res.* 2003;9:4435–4442.
61. Scholz M, Gottschalk J, Striepecke E, Firsching R, Harders A, Füzesi L. Intratumorous heterogeneity of chromosome 10 and 17 in meningiomas using non-radioactive in situ hybridization. *J Neurosurg Sci.* 1996;40:17–23.
62. Ozaki S, Nishizaki T, Ito H, Sasaki K. Comparative genomic hybridization analysis of genetic alterations associated with malignant progression of meningioma. *J Neurooncol.* 1999;41:167–174.
63. Krupp W, Holland H, Koschny R, et al. Genome-wide genetic characterization of an atypical meningioma by single-nucleotide polymorphism array-based mapping and classical cytogenetics. *Cancer Genet Cytogenet.* 2008;184:87–93.
64. Kasai H, Kawamoto K. Cytogenical analysis of brain tumors by FISH (fluorescence in situ hybridization) and FCM (flow cytometry). *Noshuyo Byori.* 1995;12:75–82.
65. Kim JH, Lee SH, Rhee CH, Park SY, Lee JH. Loss of heterozygosity on chromosome 22q and 17p correlates with aggressiveness of meningiomas. *J Neurooncol.* 1998;40:101–106.
66. Büschges R, Ichimura K, Weber RG, Reifenberger G, Collins VP. Allelic gain and amplification on the long arm of chromosome 17 in anaplastic meningiomas. *Brain Pathol.* 2002;12:145–153.
67. Langford LA, Piatyszek MA, Xu R, Schold SC Jr, Wright WE, Shay JW. Telomerase activity in ordinary meningiomas predicts poor outcome. *Hum Pathol.* 1997;28:416–420.
68. Hiraga S, Ohnishi T, Izumoto S, et al. Telomerase activity and alterations in telomere length in human brain tumors. *Cancer Res.* 1998;58:2117–2125.
69. Carroll T, Maltby E, Brock I, Royds J, Timperley W, Jellinek D. Meningiomas, dicentric chromosomes, gliomas, and telomerase activity. *J Pathol.* 1999;188:395–399.
70. Chen HJ, Liang CL, Lu K, Lin JW, Cho CL. Implication of telomerase activity and alternations of telomere length in the histologic characteristics of intracranial meningiomas. *Cancer.* 2000;89:2092–2098.

71. Boldrini L, Pistolesi S, Gisfredi S, et al. Telomerase in intracranial meningiomas. *Int J Mol Med*. 2003;12:943–947.
72. Maes L, Kalala JP, Cornelissen R, de Ridder L. Telomerase activity and hTERT protein expression in meningiomas: an analysis in vivo versus in vitro. *Anticancer Res*. 2006;26:2295–2300.
73. Maes L, Van Neste L, Van Damme K, et al. Relation between telomerase activity, hTERT and telomere length for intracranial tumours. *Oncol Rep*. 2007;18:1571–1576.
74. Modan B, Baidatz D, Mart H, Steinitz R, Levin SG. Radiation-induced head and neck tumours. *Lancet*. 1974;1:277–279.
75. Ron E, Modan B, Boice JD Jr, Alfandary E, Stovall M, Chetrit A, Katz L. Tumors of the brain and nervous system after radiotherapy in childhood. *N Engl J Med*. 1988;319:1033–1039.
76. Preston-Martin S, Paganini-Hill A, Henderson BE, Pike MC, Wood C. Case-control study of intracranial meningiomas in women in Los Angeles County, California. *J Natl Cancer Inst*. 1980;65:67–73.
77. Shibata S, Sadamori N, Mine M, Sekine I. Intracranial meningiomas among Nagasaki atomic bomb survivors. *Lancet*. 1994;344:1770.
78. Shintani T, Hayakawa N, Hoshi M, et al. High incidence of meningioma among Hiroshima atomic bomb survivors. *J Radiat Res (Tokyo)*. 1999;40:49–57.
79. Musa BS, Pople IK, Cummins BH. Intracranial meningiomas following irradiation—a growing problem? *Br J Neurosurg*. 1995;9:629–637.
80. Rubinstein AB, Shalit MN, Cohen ML, Zandbank U, Reichenthal E. Radiation-induced cerebral meningioma: a recognizable entity. *J Neurosurg*. 1984;61:966–971.
81. Soffer D, Pittaluga S, Feiner M, Beller AJ. Intracranial meningiomas following low-dose irradiation to the head. *J Neurosurg*. 1983;59:1048–1053.
82. Lillehei KO, Donson AM, Kleinschmidt-DeMasters BK. Radiation-induced meningiomas: clinical, cytogenetic, and microarray features. *Acta Neuropathol*. 2008;116:289–301.
83. Flint-Richter P, Sadetzki S. Genetic predisposition for the development of radiation-associated meningioma: an epidemiological study. *Lancet Oncol*. 2007;8:403–410.
84. Al-Mefty O, Topsakal C, Pravdenkova S, Sawyer JR, Harrison MJ. Radiation-induced meningiomas: clinical, pathological, cytokinetic, and cytogenetic characteristics. *J Neurosurg*. 2004;100:1002–1013.
85. Pagni CA, Canavero S, Fiocchi F, Ponzio G. Chromosome 22 monosomy in a radiation-induced meningioma. *Ital J Neurol Sci*. 1993;14:377–379.
86. Rajcan-Separovic E, Maguire J, Loukianova T, Nisha M, Kalousek D. Loss of 1p and 7p in radiation-induced meningiomas identified by comparative genomic hybridization. *Cancer Genet Cytogenet*. 2003;144:6–11.
87. Rienstein S, Loven D, Israeli O, et al. Comparative genomic hybridization analysis of radiation-associated and sporadic meningiomas. *Cancer Genet Cytogenet*. 2001;131:135–140.
88. Shoshan Y, Chernova O, Juen SS, et al. Radiation-induced meningioma: a distinct molecular genetic pattern? *J Neuropathol Exp Neurol*. 2000;59:614–620.
89. Zattara-Cannoni H, Roll P, Figarella-Branger D, et al. Cytogenetic study of six cases of radiation-induced meningiomas. *Cancer Genet Cytogenet*. 2001;126:81–84.
90. Joachim T, Ram Z, Rappaport ZH, et al. Comparative analysis of the NF2, TP53, PTEN, KRAS, NRAS and HRAS genes in sporadic and radiation-induced human meningiomas. *Int J Cancer*. 2001;94:218–221.

19 Histopathology and Molecular Pathogenesis of Schwannomas

Fabio Pereira Nunes, Scott R. Plotkin, and Anat O. Stemmer-Rachamimov

CLINICAL FEATURES

Schwannomas (also known as neurinomas or neurilemmomas) are benign tumors uniformly composed of differentiated neoplastic Schwann cells and correspond to WHO (World Health Organization) Grade I tumors.

Schwannomas may arise from nerve roots (cranial or spinal), from small myelinated peripheral nerve fibers (cutaneous, subcutaneous, and visceral) or rarely within the parenchyma of the brain or spinal cord [1,2].

Schwannomas are common and account for approximately 8% of all primary intracranial tumors and 29% of primary spinal tumors [3,4]. The incidence in the general population is highest in the fourth to sixth decades and both sexes are equally affected. Most schwannomas (90%) are single tumors (sporadic) [5]. Multiple schwannomas (syndromic) are seen in the setting of neurofibromatosis 2 (NF2) and schwannomatosis. Pigmented schwannomas are a component of Carney complex.

SITES

The most common intracranial site for a schwannoma is the eighth cranial nerve; specifically its vestibular division. These tumors are more correctly referred to as vestibular schwannomas, rather than acoustic neuromas. The latter is an erroneous term as the tumors arise from the vestibular (not acoustic) branch of the eighth cranial nerve and are schwannomas (tumors), not neuromas (reactive proliferation of Schwann cells).

Vestibular schwannomas constitute 80% of all intracranial schwannomas [6] and typically present as slowly progressive unilateral sesorineural hearing loss. Large tumors may extend from the internal auditory canal to the cerebellopontine angle, with compression of the cerebellum and brainstem. Schwannomas arising from other cranial nerves may occur, especially in the context of NF2 or schwannomatosis, with the fifth cranial nerve most frequently affected [7,8].

In the spinal cord, schwannomas have a predilection for sensory spinal roots, especially at the lumbosacral region and cauda equina. The tumors are intradural and extramedullary, often extending from the spinal root in the intravertebral foramen with a dumbbell configuration. The tumors may be asymptomatic, or cause local pain and myelopathy due to compression.

Schwannomas arising from peripheral nerves have a predilection for the flexor surfaces of the upper and lower extremities [9]. Visceral schwannomas are rare and mostly involve the gastrointestinal tract [10–12]. Schwannomas may also present as large, encapsulated tumors in soft tissue of the retroperitoneum or mediastinum [9] (Figure 19.1).

Cutaneous and subcutaneous schwannomas arise from small peripheral nerves and may appear as discrete, firm nodules or as diffuse dermal lesions (Figure 19.2). Cutaneous and subcutaneous schwannomas are an early manifestation of NF2. Histologically, cutaneous schwannomas often have a plexiform growth pattern [13].

Intraparenchymal schwannomas are rare. In the brain, most are in the cerebral hemispheres or cerebellum. Most intracerebral tumors occur in the pediatric and young adult groups (30 years or younger) [2,14–17].

NEUROIMAGING

Schwannomas appear as well-delineated, isodense, round/oval masses that are bright on heavily weighted T2 sequences. Cystic changes and hemorrhages may occur with resulting heterogeneous patterns on T1- and T2-weighted images. Schwannomas are usually not calcified and show homogeneous enhancement following gadolinium administration.

MULTIPLE SCHWANNOMA SYNDROMES

Multiple schwannomas are associated with an underlying genetic predisposition and are seen in the setting of NF2 and schwannomatosis. Psammomatous pigmented schwannomas are associated with Carney syndrome and may be multiple.

The hallmark lesion in NF2 is the vestibular schwannoma. Nonvestibular schwannomas are also common. In addition to multiple schwannomas, NF2 patients have increased risk of meningiomas and ependymomas as well as of other, nonneoplastic manifestations including meningioangiomatosis, glial hamartia, peripheral polyneuropathy, posterior subcapsular cataracts, and a variety of retinal abnormalities [18,19]. The disease is autosomal dominant, with full penetrance, so the genetic risk to offspring is 50%. However, half of the patients have no family

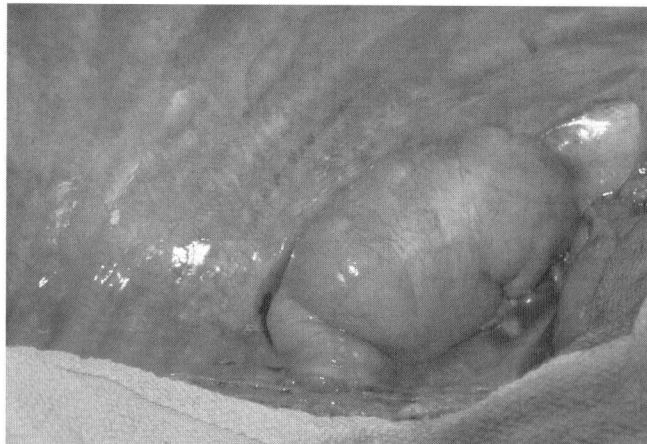

Figure 19.1 Retroperitoneal schwannoma. A large retroperitoneal schwannoma in an NF2 patient. *See color insert.*

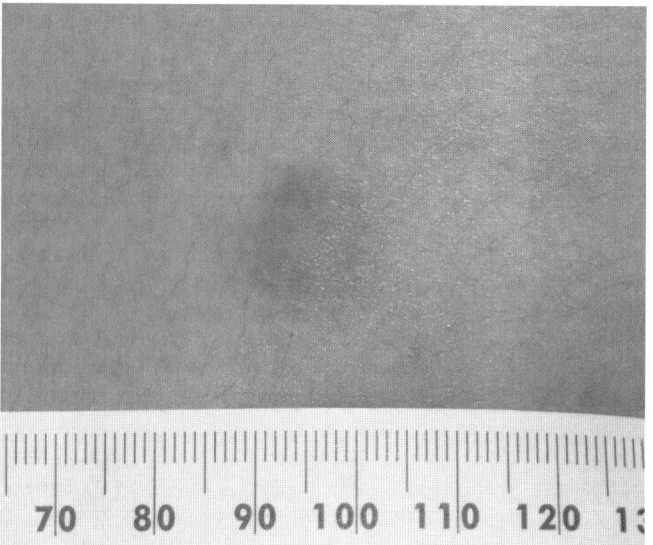

Figure 19.2 Cutaneous schwannoma. Cutaneous schwannomas often appear as discrete nodules under a mildly hyperpigmented skin. Cutaneous schwannomas are common in NF2. *See color insert.*

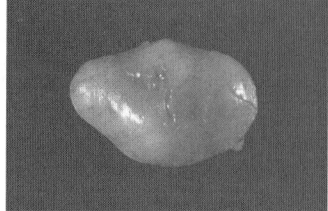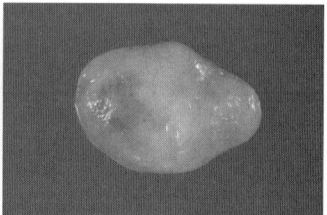

Figure 19.3 Schwannoma, gross appearance. Schwannomas are discrete, encapsulated tumors with smooth external surface (right). Cut surface may show areas of yellow (lipid rich) and red/brown (hemorrhages) discoloration (left). *See color insert.*

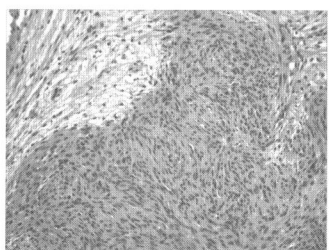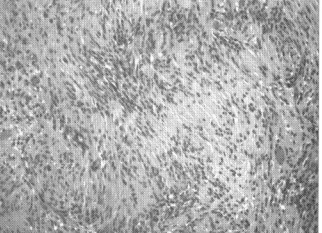

Figure 19.4 Schwannoma, histology. Typical features in schwannoma include a biphasic pattern of compact (Antoni A) and loose (Antoni B) areas (right) and nuclear palisades with formation of Verocay bodies (left). *See color insert.*

history of NF2 and represent founders. The median age of onset of NF2 is the first to third decade, earlier than that of sporadic tumors in the general population [7,20,21].

Multiple schwannomas are also associated with schwannomatosis in which patients develop multiple schwannomas (in peripheral or cranial nerves) with the absence of vestibular schwannomas (an important distinctive characteristic from NF2) [22]. Schwannomatosis patients have a unique propensity to develop severe chronic pain associated with their tumors [23]. There may be an association of schwannomatosis with meningiomas but not with other tumors or nonneoplastic manifestations [24]. Only 15% of schwannomatosis cases are familial and segmental forms are common (33%). Recent studies have implicated the gene *SMARCB1/INI1* in familial and sporadic forms of schwannomatosis [25–31].

Carney syndrome is an inherited autosomal dominant, multiple neoplasia disorder, characterized by skin lesions (lenigines and nevi), variety of nonendocrine tumors (most important are cardiac myxomas), endocrine overreactivity (secondary to hyperplasia and adenomas of various glands), and tumors of the peripheral nerves (schwannomas). The schwannomas associated with Carney syndrome are pigmented and psammomatous and are unique in their propensity for malignant transformation (10% of the cases) [32,33].

PATHOLOGY

Macroscopy

Schwannomas are typically soft, globoid, and well-circumscribed tumors. The distinct borders are due to a thick capsule consisting of epineurium and collagen. The nerve of origin may be identified in the periphery of the tumors. The cut surface is tan and may show areas of yellow discoloration (lipid-laden macrophages) and foci of cystic degeneration or hemorrhages (Figure 19.3).

Histology

Schwannomas are composed of a homogeneous cell population of neoplastic Schwann cells. Tumor cells are spindled with large elongated nuclei that have tapered ends. The hallmark histological feature of conventional or classical schwannomas is a biphasic pattern of growth with alternating compact (Antoni A) and loose (Antoni B) areas (Figure 19.4). In the compact (Antoni A) areas, the cells are arranged in fascicles and may form the typical Verocay bodies, a pattern of two parallel rows of stacked nuclear palisades around a central anuclear zone (Figure 19.4). Antoni A areas and Verocay bodies are prominent in spinal schwannomas.

The loose Antoni B areas are often hypocellular with microcystic or myxoid matrix that may mimic the matrix observed in neurofibromas. However, in contrast to schwannomas, the cellular composition of neurofibromas is heterogeneous and includes perineural cells, Schwann cells, and fibroblasts. Immunostaining for S100 highlights the Schwann cells component in the lesions and may aid in the differential diagnosis of Antoni B areas of schwannomas (diffuse staining) from neurofibroma (focal staining). However, the histological distinction between "Schwann cell-rich" neurofibromas and schwannomas with prominent myxoid change may in some cases be very difficult. Problematic tumors that cannot be classified are coined "hybrid lesions" [34].

Clusters of large vessels with tortuous, thick, hyalinized walls are often present in schwannomas and may at times be so prominent as to resemble vascular malformations. Clusters of dilated sinusoidal vessels in "back-to-back" arrangement may mimic cavernous hemangiomas. There are often adjacent hemosiderin-laden macrophages or hemorrhages associated with these vessels. Thrombosis, necrosis, granulation tissue, and aggregates of lipid-laden macrophages are also common.

Some schwannomas exhibit prominent cytological atypia with scattered large, hyperchromatic, and pleomorphic nuclei (ancient change) [35]. Importantly, these changes do not represent malignant transformation, but rather degenerative changes (Figure 19.5). Malignant transformation in conventional schwannomas is exceedingly rare and the tumor often assumes an epithelioid appearance [36].

Epithelial structures, glands, and small squamous islands have been described in schwannomas and are thought to represent epithelial differentiation in the tumor (glandular schwannomas) [37].

Analysis of the histological features of NF-associated schwannomas and sporadic/solitary schwannomas has identified unique histological features associated with each schwannoma clinical subtype. Sporadic/solitary vestibular schwannomas frequently have prominent vascular malformations, thrombosis, and inflammation while lobular, "grape-like" appearance, due to distinct, round/oval lobules within the tumor is common in NF2-associated tumors [38]. In addition, entrapped nerve axons are common in NF2-related tumors but not in sporadic/solitary tumors [39,40]. Interestingly, tumors from schwannomatosis patients often display a prominent myxoid stroma and an intraneural growth pattern. These features may account for high rate of misdiagnosis of these tumors as neurofibromas [23].

Plexiform Schwannoma

Plexiform schwannomas grow along the nerve, expanding it to produce a rope-like mass, similar to the appearance of nerves involved by a plexiform neurofibroma. The distinction between plexiform schwannomas and plexiform neurofibromas is important as only plexiform neurofibromas have the propensity to undergo malignant degeneration.

Plexiform schwannomas are often superficial, cutaneous, or subcutaneous tumors that have the histological appearance of multiple expanded nerve fascicles with otherwise the typical histological features of a conventional schwannomas (Antoni A areas, Verocay bodies) (Figure 19.6). Plexiform schwannomas are associated with NF2 and with schwannomatosis but may also occur as sporadic tumors. Plexiform schwannomas are not associated with NF1 [41,42].

Cellular Schwannoma

Cellular schwannomas are hypercellular variants of schwannomas, often exhibiting mitotic activity. Cellular schwannomas are often composed predominantly or exclusively of compact (Antoni A) areas and lack Verocay bodies. The tumors may display cytological atypia and small areas of necrosis. In spite of these worrisome histological

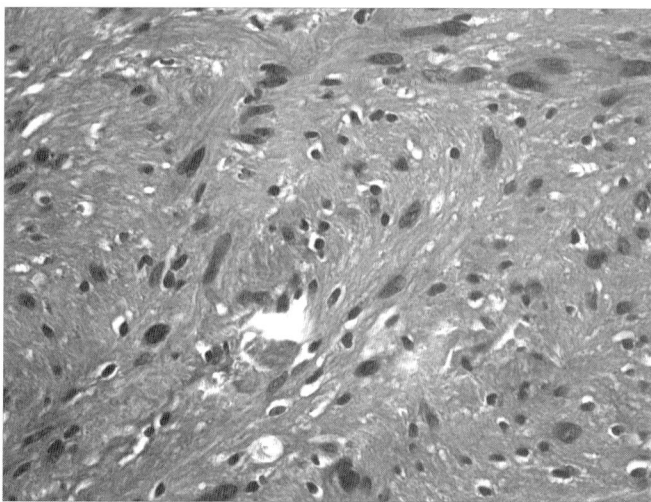

Figure 19.5 Schwannoma, histology. Large, hyperchromatic and atypical nuclei are often encountered in conventional schwannomas and are not indicative of malignant transformation. *See color insert.*

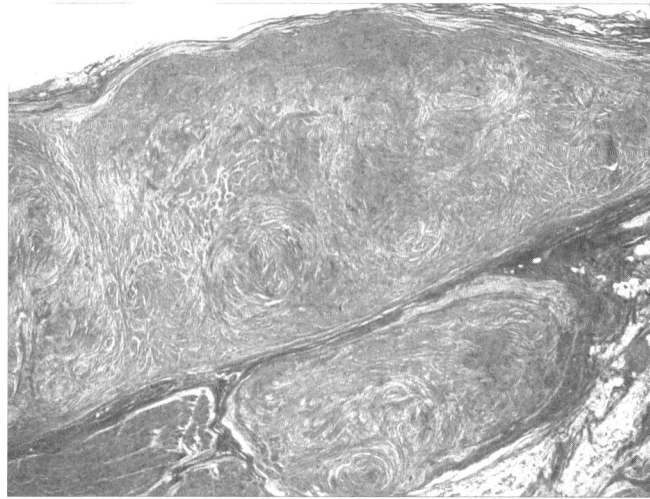

Figure 19.6 Plexiform schwannoma, histology. Expansion of multiple peripheral nerves by a plexiform schwannoma in an NF2 patient. Plexiform schwannomas may mimic the gross appearance of plexiform neurofibromas. *See color insert.*

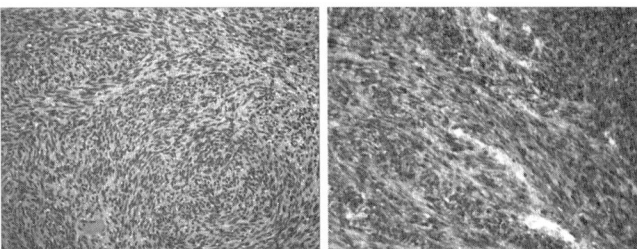

Figure 19.7 Cellular schwannoma, histology. Cellular schwannomas are cellular and mitotically active. Biphasic pattern and Verocay bodies are often absent (right). Diagnosis is confirmed by diffuse S100 immunostaining of the tumor (left). *See color insert.*

features, cellular schwannomas carry the same prognosis as conventional schwannomas and do not follow a malignant clinical course. Cellular schwannomas are more commonly encountered in the spine, retroperitoneum, and mediastinum and must not be confused with malignant peripheral nerve sheath tumors, sarcoma, or meningioma. Cellular schwannomas are diffusely S100 immunopositive [43–45] (Figure 19.7).

Melanotic Schwannomas

Melanotic schwannomas are rare tumors composed of neoplastic Schwann cells that contain melanin and are reactive to melanin markers. The mean age of presentation is at 35 years (a decade earlier than conventional schwannomas) and the tumors appear as pigmented, well-circumscribed masses. Approximately half of melanotic schwannomas are of the psammomatous type, defined by the presence of concentrically laminated, periodic acid-Schiff–positive bodies. Approximately half of psammomatous melanotic schwannomas are associated with Carney complex and may undergo malignant degeneration [46,47]. Nonpsammomatous (conventional) melanotic schwannomas have a benign course, similar to other conventional schwannomas.

Electron Microscopy

Ultrastructural examination of schwannomas shows a tumor composed exclusively of neoplastic Schwann cells. The cells have long, narrow cytoplasmic processes, lined by a continuous basal lamina. Long-spacing collagen in the stroma or encircled by Schwann cell processes may be seen.

MOLECULAR BIOLOGY

NF2 Gene

Inactivation of the *NF2* gene is the most important genetic event in schwannoma formation. Inactivating mutations of *NF2* gene have been found in sporadic schwannomas, NF2-associated schwannomas, and schwannomatosis-associated schwannomas.

NF2 was simultaneously cloned by two independent groups in 1993 [48,49] and is located on chromosome 22q12. The gene is composed of 17 exons with alternative splicing of exon 16. Both isoforms can be found in tissues [50,51].

The *NF2* gene product is a 595 aminoacid protein (590 for isoform 2) and belongs to the 4.1 protein family, which includes moesin, ezrin, radixin, and DAL-1. The NF2 protein is referred to as merlin (moesin, ezrin, radixin like protein) [49] or schwannomin, based on its role on schwannoma formation [48]. Merlin has an ERM domain that shows a conserved homology with other members of the 4.1 protein family, a unique α-helix domain and a C-terminal domain that lacks the actin-binding site seen in other 4.1 protein family members.

Merlin is ubiquitously expressed, and forms inter- and intramolecular associations that regulate protein function [52–56]. Merlin is active when the N- and C-terminal domains are connected forming a closed conformation. An open conformation of merlin leads to inactivation of the protein and a tumor-permissive state. Interestingly, isoform 2 of merlin cannot form a closed conformation and has been shown to lack tumor-suppressor function [55,56].

Merlin's activation and tumor-suppressor function is regulated by protein phosphorylation at position Ser518 [57,58]. Merlin phosphorylation can be accomplished by p21-activated kinases and cyclic adenosine monophosphate–dependent protein kinase A [58–60].

The mechanism by which merlin suppresses tumor growth is not clear and is most likely related to complex interactions with components of the cellular cytoskeleton and cellular growth activators [61].

NF2 Inactivation in Schwannomas

The mechanism of *NF2* inactivation in schwannomas has been recently summarized in comprehensive databases. The majority of reported cases are vestibular tumors, with only few studies of nonvestibular schwannomas [62–64].

The NF2 Gene in Sporadic Schwannomas

Inactivation of the *NF2* gene is found in 78% to 86% of sporadic schwannomas. If *NF2* loss of heterozygosity is also considered, at least one allele of *NF2* is inactivated in up to 92% of sporadic schwannomas, confirming that *NF2* is the main genetic event involved in sporadic schwannoma formation [65,66].

NF2 mutations can occur in exons 1 to 15, while no mutations occur in the alternatively spliced exons 16 and 17. Truncating mutations are seen in over three quarters of the tumors, with frameshift mutations accounting for about 60% [62–64]. Interestingly, frameshift mutations in sporadic schwannomas get more frequent with increase in the patients' age, suggesting an increased rate of mutagenesis or reduced efficiency in DNA repair in older patients [67].

Few genotype-phenotype studies have been published in sporadic schwannomas. A recent study found a correlation between presence of frameshift and missense mutations in the tumors and a higher rate of tumor growth and cell proliferation index when compared with tumors carrying splice site mutations [68].

The NF2 Gene in Neurofibromatosis 2

The spectrum of NF2 germline mutations is significantly different than the mutations observed in sporadic schwannomas, with nonsense germline mutations occurring in 40% of NF2 patients and frameshift mutations seen in only 27%. Nonsense mutations in the NF2 gene occur frequently in methylated CpG islands on codons 169 (exon 2), 586 (exon 6), 784 (exon 8), and 1021 (exon 11) [62–64]. These nonsense mutations are caused by deamination of a methylated cytosine into a thymine, leading to a change from an arginine (CGA) to a stop codon (TGA). This difference of mutation type observed in somatic mutations in solitary, sporadic schwannomas and germline mutations in NF2 patients may be secondary to different mechanisms of mutagenesis; more frequent nonsense mutations during meiosis in early embryogenic development or more frequent frameshift mutations postzygotically during mitosis.

Patients with truncating NF2 germline mutations have been associated with a more severe phenotype, while presence of missense or large gene deletions have been found to cause a milder phenotype. Splice site mutations are associated with phenotype variability in patients [69–72].

The NF2 Gene in Schwannomatosis

Schwannomatosis is a recently described form of neurofibromatosis in which patients develop multiple nonvestibular schwannomas, often associated with severe, chronic pain [73–77]. Schwannomatosis is thought to be as common as NF2 [5] Only 15% of schwannomatosis cases are familial and many patients have segmental presentation [23,77].

Germline mutations in the NF2 gene have been excluded as the cause of familial schwannomatosis. However, somatic inactivation of NF2 gene is common in schwannomas resected from schwannomatosis patients. Furthermore, multiple tumors from the same individual often harbor independent NF2 mutations, suggesting molecular instability of the NF2 gene in the neoplastic Schwann cells [78].

The SMARCB1/INI1 Gene

SMARCB1/INI1 is located at 22q11.2, in the schwannomatosis candidate region identified by linkage analysis [78]. SMARCB1/INI1 encodes a member of the SWI/SNF multiprotein complex involved in transcription and chromatin-remodeling [79,80]. Biallelic inactivation of SMARCB1/INI1 has previously been shown in malignant rhabdoid tumors and in atypical teratoid rhabdoid tumors [79,81,82]. Germline mutations of SMARCB1/INI1 are associated with increased predisposition to rhabdoid tumors in familial clusters [83,84].

SMARCB1/INI1 Gene in Schwannomas

In 2007, a germline SMRCB1/INI1 mutation was identified from a father and a daughter with familial schwannomatosis [25]. Subsequent studies in multiple cohorts found germline SMARCB1/INI1 mutations in familial schwannomatosis kindred (33%–60%) and sporadic schwannomatosis (7%) patients, confirming the role of SMARCB1/INI1 in schwannomas. In addition, biallelic inactivation of SMARCB1/INI1 was found in tumors. These findings suggest a "four hit" mechanism with comutation of NF2 and SMARCB1/INI1 in some schwannomatosis tumors [26,27,29].

Furthermore, a comprehensive immunohistochemistry analysis of INI1 protein expression in a large series of schwannomas showed a mosaic pattern of staining (suggestive of inactivation of SMARCB1/INI1) in more than 90% of familial schwannomatosis tumors and half of sporadic schwannomatosis tumors. Surprisingly, a mosaic pattern of INI1 immunostaining was also observed in 83% of NF2-associated schwannomas, implicating the SMARCB1/INI1 gene in tumorigenesis in NF2. In contrast, INI1 was diffusely expressed in over 90% of the single, sporadic tumors, suggesting a distinct pathogenesis for sporadic tumors [85].

Further work is needed to determine the extent of SMARCB1/INI1 involvement in sporadic and familial schwannomatosis and the mechanism by which SMARCB1/INI1 causes NF2 instability.

REFERENCES

1. Herregodts P, Vloeberghs M, Schmedding E, Goossens A, Stadnik T, D'Haens J. Solitary dorsal intramedullary schwannoma. Case report. *J Neurosurg.* 1991;74:816–820.
2. Cruz-Sanchez F, Cervos-Navarro J, Kashihara M, Ferszt R. Intracerebral neurinomas in a case of von Recklinghausen's disease (neurofibromatosis). *Clin Neuropathol.* 1987;6:174–178.
3. Chandler CL, Ramsden RT. Acoustic schwannoma. *Br J Hosp Med.* 1993;49:335–343.
4. Russell DSaR, LJ. *Pathology of Tumors of the Nervous System*. London: Edward Arnold; 1989.
5. Antinheimo J, Sankila R, Carpen O, Pukkala E, Sainio M, Jaaskelainen J. Population-based analysis of sporadic and type 2 neurofibromatosis-associated meningiomas and schwannomas. *Neurology.* 2000;54:71–76.
6. Consensus Development Panel. National Institutes of Health consensus development conference statement on acoustic neuroma. *Arch Neurol.* 1994;51(2):201–207.
7. Evans DG, Huson SM, Donnai D, et al. A clinical study of type 2 neurofibromatosis. *Q J Med.* 1992;84:603–618.
8. Parry DM, Eldridge R, Kaiser-Kupfer MI, Bouzas EA, Pikus A, Patronas N. Neurofibromatosis 2 (NF2): clinical characteristics of 63 affected individuals and clinical evidence for heterogeneity. *Am J Med Genet.* 1994;52:450–461.
9. Enzinger FM, Weiss SW. *Benign Tumors of Peripheral Nerves. Soft Tissue Tumors*. China: Mosby-Year Book; 2008:853 869.
10. Prevot S, Bienvenu L, Vaillant JC, de Saint-Maur PP. Benign schwannoma of the digestive tract: a clinicopathologic and immunohistochemical study of five cases, including a case of esophageal tumor. *Am J Surg Pathol.* 1999;23:431–436.
11. Nabeya Y, Watanabe Y, Tohnosu N, et al. Diffuse schwannoma involving the entire large bowel with huge extramural development: report of a case. *Surg Today.* 1999;29:637–641.
12. Sarlomo-Rikala M, Miettinen M. Gastric schwannoma—a clinicopathological analysis of six cases. *Histopathology.* 1995;27:355–360.
13. Mautner VF, Lindenau M, Baser ME, Kluwe L, Gottschalk J. Skin abnormalities in neurofibromatosis 2. *Arch Dermatol.* 1997;133:1539–15343.
14. Casadei GP, Komori T, Scheithauer BW, Miller GM, Parisi JE, Kelly PJ. Intracranial parenchymal schwannoma. A clinicopathological and neuroimaging study of nine cases. *J Neurosurg.* 1993;79:217–222.
15. Ezura M, Ikeda H, Ogawa A, Yoshimoto T. Intracerebral schwannoma: case report. *Neurosurgery.* 1992;30:97–100.
16. Frim DM, Ogilvy CS, Vonsattal JP, Chapman PH. Is intracerebral schwannoma a developmental tumor of children and young adults? Case report and review. *Pediatr Neurosurg.* 1992;18:190–194.

17. Bhatoe HS, Srinivasan K, Dubey AK. Intracerebral schwannoma. *Neurol India.* 2003;51:125–127.
18. Stemmer-Rachamimov A, Wiestler OD, Louis DN. Neurofibromatosis type 2. In: Cavenee WK, ed. *WHO Classification of Tumours of the Central Nervous System.* Lyon, France: IARC Press; 2007:210–214.
19. Mautner VF, Hazim W, Pohlmann K, Berger R, Kluwe L, Haase W. Ophthalmologic spectrum of neurofibromatosis type 2 in childhood. *Klin Monatsbl Augenheilkd.* 1996;208:58–62.
20. Martuza RL, Eldridge R. Neurofibromatosis 2 (bilateral acoustic neurofibromatosis). *N Engl J Med.* 1988;318:684–688.
21. Baser ME, Evans DGR, Gutmann DH. Neurofibromatosis 2. *Curr Opin Neurol.* 2003;16:27–33.
22. Wolkenstein P, Benchikhi H, Zeller J, Wechsler J, Revuz J. Schwannomatosis: a clinical entity distinct from neurofibromatosis type 2. *Dermatology.* 1997;195:228–231.
23. MacCollin M, Chiocca EA, Evans DG, et al. Diagnostic criteria for schwannomatosis. *Neurology.* 2005;64:1838–1845.
24. Garretto NS, Monteverde D, Giocoli H, et al. Schwannomatosis: report of a new case. *Arq Neuropsiquiatr.* 1992;50:539–542.
25. Hulsebos TJ, Plomp AS, Wolterman RA, Robanus-Maandag EC, Baas F, Wesseling P. Germline mutation of INI1/SMARCB1 in familial schwannomatosis. *Am J Hum Genet.* 2007;80:805–810.
26. Sestini R, Bacci C, Provenzano A, Genuardi M, Papi L. Evidence of a four-hit mechanism involving SMARCB1 and NF2 in schwannomatosis-associated schwannomas. *Hum Mutat.* 2008;29:227–231.
27. Hadfield KD, Newman WG, Bowers NL, et al. Molecular characterisation of SMARCB1 and NF2 in familial and sporadic schwannomatosis. *J Med Genet.* 2008;45:332–339.
28. Gutmann DH, Giovannini M. Mouse models of neurofibromatosis 1 and 2. *Neoplasia.* 2002;4:279–290.
29. Boyd C, Smith MJ, Kluwe L, Balogh A, Maccollin M, Plotkin SR. Alterations in the SMARCB1 (INI1) tumor suppressor gene in familial schwannomatosis. *Clin Genet.* 2008;74:358–366.
30. Dereure O. Molecular characterisation of SMARCB1 and NF2 in familial and sporadic schwannomatosis: An evolving paradigm. *Ann Dermatol Venereol.* 2008;135:888–889.
31. Swensen JJ, Keyser J, Coffin CM, Biegel JA, Viskochil DH, Williams MS. Familial occurrence of schwannomas and malignant rhabdoid tumour associated with a duplication in SMARCB1. *J Med Genet.* 2009;46:68–72.
32. Martin-Reay DG, Shattuck MC, Guthrie FW Jr. Psammomatous melanotic schwannoma: an additional component of Carney's complex. Report of a case. *Am J Clin Pathol.* 1991;95:484–489.
33. Handley J, Carson D, Sloan J, et al. Multiple lentigines, myxoid tumours and endocrine overactivity; four cases of Carney's complex. *Br J Dermatol.* 1992;126:367–371.
34. Feany MB, Anthony DC, Fletcher CD. Nerve sheath tumours with hybrid features of neurofibroma and schwannoma: a conceptual challenge. *Histopathology.* 1998;32:405–410.
35. Dahl I. Ancient neurilemmoma (schwannoma). *Acta Pathol Microbiol Scand [A].* 1977;85:812–818.
36. Woodruff JM, Selig AM, Crowley K, Allen PW. Schwannoma (neurilemoma) with malignant transformation. A rare, distinctive peripheral nerve tumor. *Am J Surg Pathol.* 1994;18:882–895.
37. Brooks JJ, Draffen RM. Benign glandular schwannoma. *Arch Pathol Lab Med.* 1992;116:192–195.
38. Sobel RA. Vestibular (acoustic) schwannomas: histological features in neurofibromatosis 2 and in unilateral cases. *J Neuropathol Exp Neurol.* 1993;52:106–113.
39. Jaaskelainen J, Paetau A, Pyykko I, Blomstedt G, Palva T, Troupp H. Interface between the facial nerve and large acoustic neurinomas. Immunohistochemical study of the cleavage plane in NF2 and non-NF2 cases. *J Neurosurg.* 1994;80:541–547.
40. Hamada Y, Iwaki T, Fukui M, Tateishi J. A comparative study of embedded nerve tissue in six NF2-associated schwannomas and 17 nonassociated NF2 schwannomas. *Surg Neurol.* 1997;48:395–400.
41. Megahed M. Plexiform schwannoma. *Am J Dermatopathol.* 1994;16:288–293.
42. Fletcher CD, Davies SE. Benign plexiform (multinodular) schwannoma: a rare tumour unassociated with neurofibromatosis. *Histopathology.* 1986;10:971–980.
43. Casadei GP, Scheithauer BW, Hirose T, Manfrini M, Van Houton C, Wood MB. Cellular schwannoma. A clinicopathologic, DNA flow cytometric, and proliferation marker study of 70 patients. *Cancer.* 1995;75:1109–1119.
44. Woodruff JM, Godwin TA, Erlandson RA, Susin M, Martini N. Cellular schwannoma: a variety of schwannoma sometimes mistaken for a malignant tumor. *Am J Surg Pathol.* 1981;5:733–744.
45. White W, Shiu MH, Rosenblum MK, Erlandson RA, Woodruff JM. Cellular schwannoma. A clinicopathologic study of 57 patients and 58 tumors. *Cancer.* 1990;66:1266–1275.
46. Myers JL, Bernreuter W, Dunham W. Melanotic schwannoma. Clinicopathologic, immunohistochemical, and ultrastructural features of a rare primary bone tumor. *Am J Clin Pathol.* 1990;93:424–429.
47. Carney JA. Psammomatous melanotic schwannoma. A distinctive, heritable tumor with special associations, including cardiac myxoma and the Cushing syndrome. *Am J Surg Pathol.* 1990;14:206–222.
48. Rouleau GA, Merel P, Lutchman M, et al. Alteration in a new gene encoding a putative membrane-organizing protein causes neurofibromatosis type 2. *Nature.* 1993;363:515–521.
49. Trofatter JA, MacCollin MM, Rutter JL, et al. A novel moesin-, ezrin-, radixin-like gene is a candidate for the neurofibromatosis 2 tumor suppressor. *Cell.* 1993;75:826.
50. Bianchi AB, Hara T, Ramesh V, et al. Mutations in transcript isoforms of the neurofibromatosis 2 gene in multiple human tumour types. *Nat Genet.* 1994;6:185–192.
51. Pykett MJ, Murphy M, Harnish PR, George DL. The neurofibromatosis 2 (NF2) tumor suppressor gene encodes multiple alternatively spliced transcripts. *Hum Mol Genet.* 1994;3:559–564.
52. den Bakker MA, Vissers KJ, Molijn AC, Kros JM, Zwarthoff EC, van der Kwast TH. Expression of the neurofibromatosis type 2 gene in human tissues. *J Histochem Cytochem.* 1999;47:1471–1480.
53. Stemmer-Rachamimov AO, Gonzalez-Agosti C, Xu L, et al. Expression of NF2-encoded merlin and related ERM family proteins in the human central nervous system. *J Neuropathol Exp Neurol.* 1997;56:735–742.
54. Schipper H, Papp T, Johnen G, et al. Mutational analysis of the nf2 tumour suppressor gene in three subtypes of primary human malignant mesotheliomas. *Int J Oncol.* 2003;22:1009–1017.
55. Sherman L, Xu HM, Geist RT, et al. Interdomain binding mediates tumor growth suppression by the NF2 gene product. *Oncogene.* 1997;15:2505–2509.
56. Gutmann DH, Hirbe AC, Haipek CA. Functional analysis of neurofibromatosis 2 (NF2) missense mutations. *Hum Mol Genet.* 2001;10:1519–1529.
57. Xiao GH, Beeser A, Chernoff J, Testa JR. p21-activated kinase links Rac/Cdc42 signaling to merlin. *J Biol Chem.* 2002;277:883–886.
58. Kissil JL, Wilker EW, Johnson KC, Eckman MS, Yaffe MB, Jacks T. Merlin, the product of the Nf2 tumor suppressor gene, is an inhibitor of the p21-activated kinase, Pak1. *Mol Cell.* 2003;12:841–849.
59. Gronholm M, Vossebein L, Carlson CR, et al. Merlin links to the cAMP neuronal signaling pathway by anchoring the RIbeta subunit of protein kinase A. *J Biol Chem.* 2003;278:41167–41172.
60. Alfthan K, Heiska L, Gronholm M, Renkema GH, Carpen O. Cyclic AMP-dependent protein kinase phosphorylates merlin at serine 518 independently of p21-activated kinase and promotes merlin-ezrin heterodimerization. *J Biol Chem.* 2004;279:18559–18566.
61. Scoles DR. The merlin interacting proteins reveal multiple targets for NF2 therapy. *Biochim Biophys Acta.* 2008;1785:32–54.
62. Baser M. The distribution of constitutional and somatic mutations in neurofibromatosis 2 gene. *Hum Mutat.* 2006;27:297–306.
63. Nunes F, Ahronowitz I, MacCollin M. Molecular biology of neurofibromatosis 2 and related conditions. *Recent Res Dev Mol Cell Biol.* 2004:171–196.
64. Ahronowitz I, Xin W, Kiely R, Sims K, MacCollin M, Nunes FP. Mutational spectrum of the NF2 gene: a meta-analysis of 12 years of research and diagnostic laboratory findings. *Hum Mutat.* 2007;28:1–12.
65. Jacoby LB, MacCollin M, Louis DN, et al. Exon scanning for mutation of the NF2 gene in schwannomas. *Hum Mol Genet.* 1994;3:413–419.
66. Jacoby LB, MacCollin M, Barone R, Ramesh V, Gusella JF. Frequency and distribution of NF2 mutations in schwannomas. *Genes Chromosomes Cancer.* 1996;17:45–55.
67. Evans DG, Maher ER, Baser ME. Age related shift in the mutation spectra of germline and somatic NF2 mutations: hypothetical role of DNA repair mechanisms. *J Med Genet.* 2005;42:630–632.
68. Bassoe P, Nuzum F. Report of a case of central and peripheral neurofibromatosis. *J Nerv Ment Dis.* 1915;42:785–796.
69. Kluwe L, Mautner VF. A missense mutation in the NF2 gene results in moderate and mild clinical phenotypes of neurofibromatosis type 2. *Hum Genet.* 1996;97:224–227.

70. Kluwe L, MacCollin M, Tatagiba M, et al. Phenotypic variability associated with 14 splice-site mutations in the NF2 gene. *Am J Med Genet.* 1998;77:228–233.
71. Ruttledge MH, Andermann AA, Phelan CM, et al. Type of mutation in the neurofibromatosis type 2 gene (NF2) frequently determines severity of disease. *Am J Hum Genet.* 1996;59:331–342.
72. Evans DG, Trueman L, Wallace A, Collins S, Strachan T. Genotype/phenotype correlations in type 2 neurofibromatosis (NF2): evidence for more severe disease associated with truncating mutations. *J Med Genet.* 1998;35:450–455.
73. MacCollin M, Woodfin W, Kronn D, Short MP. Schwannomatosis: a clinical and pathologic study. *Neurology.* 1996;46:1072–1079.
74. Jacoby LB, Jones D, Davis K, et al. Molecular analysis of the NF2 tumor-suppressor gene in schwannomatosis. *Am J Hum Genet.* 1997;61:1293–1302.
75. Seppala MT, Sainio MA, Haltia MJ, Kinnunen JJ, Setala KH, Jaaskelainen JE. Multiple schwannomas: schwannomatosis or neurofibromatosis type 2? *J Neurosurg.* 1998;89:36–41.
76. Jacoby LB, MacCollin M, Parry DM, et al. Allelic expression of the NF2 gene in neurofibromatosis 2 and schwannomatosis. *Neurogenetics.* 1999;2:101–108.
77. Kaufman DL, Heinrich BS, Willett C, et al. Somatic instability of the NF2 gene in schwannomatosis. *Arch Neurol.* 2003;60:1317–1320.
78. MacCollin M, Willett C, Heinrich B, et al. Familial schwannomatosis: exclusion of the NF2 locus as the germline event. *Neurology.* 2003;60:1968–1974.
79. Biegel JA, Kalpana G, Knudsen ES, et al. The role of INI1 and the SWI/SNF complex in the development of rhabdoid tumors: meeting summary from the workshop on childhood atypical teratoid/rhabdoid tumors. *Cancer Res.* 2002;62:323–328.
80. Muchardt C, Yaniv M. The mammalian SWI/SNF complex and the control of cell growth. *Semin Cell Dev Biol.* 1999;10:189–195.
81. Versteege I, Sevenet N, Lange J, et al. Truncating mutations of hSNF5/INI1 in aggressive paediatric cancer. *Nature.* 1998;394:203–206.
82. Biegel JA, Zhou JY, Rorke LB, Stenstrom C, Wainwright LM, Fogelgren B. Germ-line and acquired mutations of INI1 in atypical teratoid and rhabdoid tumors. *Cancer Res.* 1999;59:74–79.
83. Biegel JA, Fogelgren B, Wainwright LM, Zhou JY, Bevan H, Rorke LB. Germline INI1 mutation in a patient with a central nervous system atypical teratoid tumor and renal rhabdoid tumor. *Genes Chromosomes Cancer.* 2000;28:31–37.
84. Fujisawa H, Takabatake Y, Fukusato T, Tachibana O, Tsuchiya Y, Yamashita J. Molecular analysis of the rhabdoid predisposition syndrome in a child: a novel germline hSNF5/INI1 mutation and absence of c-myc amplification. *J Neurooncol.* 2003;63:257–262.
85. Patil S, Perry A, Maccollin M, et al. Immunohistochemical analysis supports a role for INI1/SMARCB1 in hereditary forms of schwannomas, but not in solitary, sporadic schwannomas. *Brain Pathol.* 2008;18:517–519.

20 Histopathology and Molecular Pathogenesis of Pituitary Adenomas

Siobhan C. Loeper, Shereen Ezzat, and Sylvia L. Asa

INTRODUCTION

Tumors of the pituitary gland are common intracranial neoplasms derived from adenohypophysial cells of the anterior pituitary lobe. Their clinical manifestations are either local compressive or mass effects or symptoms of hormonal hyper- or hyposecretion. The histomorphological and immunohistochemical characterizations of pituitary adenomas are necessary to classify the different subtypes and are important for patient management. The molecular pathogenesis of pituitary tumor formation and progression differs significantly from that of other tumor types, as mutations in "classic" tumor suppressor genes (TSG) or oncogenes are rarely identified. Dysregulation of hormones, growth factors, and their receptors contribute to cell proliferation in the pituitary, but their function in tumor initiation and progression is not clear. Changes of the epigenome are increasingly recognized as a common feature of pituitary adenomas, but again their exact contribution to tumor initiation and progression still remains to be elucidated.

Definition

Pituitary adenomas are nonmetastasizing neoplasms arising from the adenohypophysis—the epithelial component of the gland that consists of the anterior and intermediate lobes as well as the pars tuberalis and comprises six different cell types (Figure 20.1) [1,2].

Most of the tumors are localized in the sella turcica, yet ectopic adenomas can occur, most frequently in the sphenoid sinuses or in the suprasellar region. The tumors exhibit a wide range of hormonal as well as proliferative behaviors. While some tumors produce excess hormones and give rise to clinical syndromes, such as acromegaly or Cushing disease with significant morbidity and mortality, other adenomas are hormonally inactive. If these adenomas are small and have a slow growth rate, they are not usually detected clinically and are discovered either as a radiographic "incidentaloma" or at postmortem examination. If they grow more rapidly, pituitary tumors can give rise to symptoms associated with an intracranial mass, such as visual field disturbances, hypopituitarism, or signs of local invasion into the cavernous sinuses or the brain parenchyma. Pituitary carcinomas, which metastasize to distant sites in the central nervous system or other locations throughout the body, are very rare.

Epidemiology

Pituitary adenomas clearly represent an important clinical entity; it is estimated that they account for 10% of all intracranial neoplasms and 25% of surgically resected intracranial tumors [3,4].

The peak incidence of pituitary tumors occurs between the ages of 30 and 60 years and they are equally distributed among the sexes in autopsy series [5,6]. In epidemiologic studies, which primarily report clinically apparent pituitary adenomas, they occur with a prevalence of 19 cases/100 000 population in Italy [7], 28 cases/100 000 in the United Kingdom [8], and 94 cases/100 000 in Belgium [9]. A meta-analysis of postmortem and radiologic data estimated the prevalence of mostly clinically silent pituitary adenomas to be much higher: the overall prevalence was 17%, and the prevalence across postmortem studies was 14% compared with 23% in radiographic studies [10]. The majority of these clinically silent tumors represent nonfunctioning adenomas of gonadotroph differentiation or prolactinomas that have not caused clinical symptoms [8,11]. Prolactinomas are also the most common type of clinically apparent adenoma in surgical series from the United States and Canada (30–40%), followed by clinically nonfunctional adenomas (25–30%) and growth hormone (GH) or adrenocorticotropic hormone (ACTH)-producing adenomas (10–15%) while thyrotropin (TSH)-secreting adenomas are exceedingly rare [12,13].

Pituitary adenomas occur in a familial setting in 5% of the cases and five different gene mutations have been identified to date (see Table 20.1). Approximately half of the familial pituitary adenomas are due to loss of function of the TSG *MEN1* coding for the nuclear protein MENIN in the multiple endocrine neoplasia type 1 syndrome [14,15]. Prolactinomas and somatotrophinomas are the commonest pituitary tumor subtypes in this disorder and are found in 30% to 40% of affected patients. Patients with Carney complex due to genetic defects in one of the regulatory subunits of protein kinase A (*PRKAR1A; protein kinase A I α-regulatory subunit*) [16,17], with the multiple endocrine neoplasia type 4 due to mutations in the *cyclin-dependent kinase inhibitor 1B (CDKN1B)* gene (encoding p27kip1) [18,19], and with McCune-Albright syndrome due to somatic mutations in the adenylate cyclase-stimulating

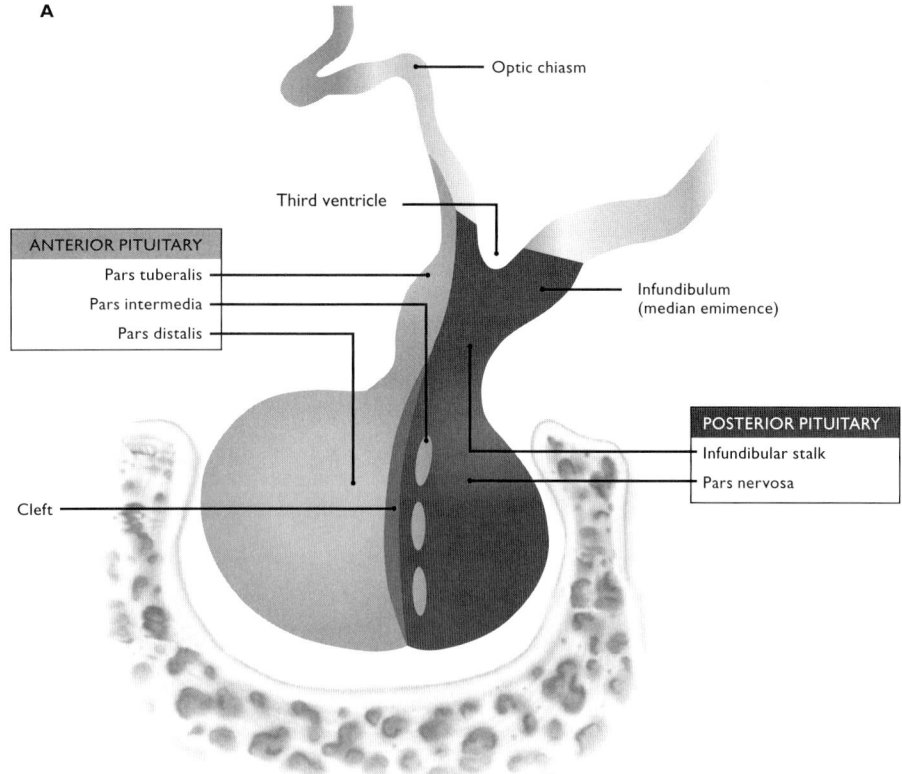

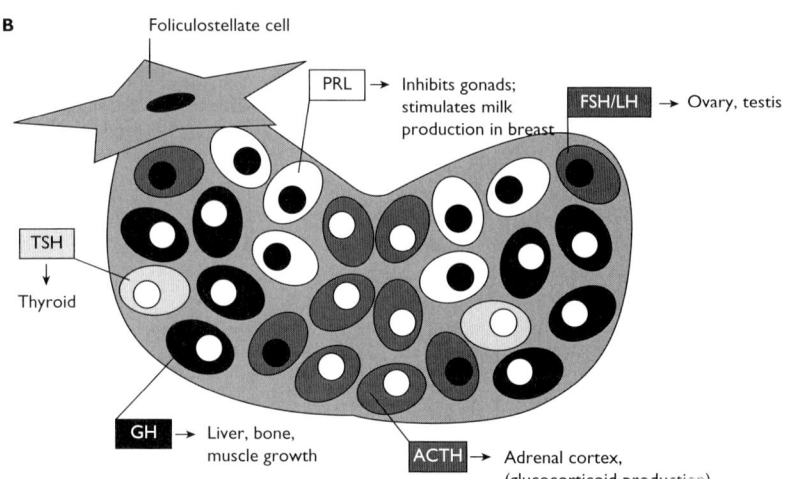

Figure. 20.1 Pituitary adenomas are non-metastasizing neoplasms arising from the adenohypophysis—the epithelial component of the gland which consists of the anterior and intermediate lobes as well as the pars tuberalis (**A**) and comprises six different cell types (**B**).

G α-protein (*guanine-nucleotide activating α subunit adenylate cyclase-stimulating G α-protein* complex locus, *GNAS*) account only for a small percentage of familial pituitary adenomas [20–22]. Recently mutations in the *aryl hydrocarbon receptor interacting protein* gene (*AIP*) were reported in association with familial acromegaly kindreds and in 15% of familial isolated pituitary adenoma kindreds with all subtypes of pituitary adenomas [23,24]. It is important to note that these gene mutations are rare in sporadic pituitary adenomas.

Classification

There are several classification schemes for pituitary adenomas [25].

Clinically, pituitary adenomas are classified as hormonally active, functioning adenomas associated with the specific hormone excess syndrome and as nonfunctioning, silent adenomas.

Based on size and invasiveness, pituitary adenomas are also classified anatomically/radiologically as microadenomas (tumors less than 1 cm) and macroadenomas (larger than 1 cm). Micro- and macroadenomas can both invade surrounding structures, for example, bone, dura, sinuses. Invasiveness appears to correlate to some extent with tumor type and size. Thyrotroph and silent corticotroph adenomas as well as the unusual plurihormonal subtype 3 adenoma are more commonly invasive and macroadenomas are more often invasive than microadenomas [26].

Table 20.1 Familial Syndromes Involving Pituitary Adenomas

Syndrome	Gene	Molecular Pathology	Clinical Features
MEN1	MEN1 (Ch11q13)	Decreased expression/function of the tumor suppressor gene product MENIN	Parathyroid, enteropancreatic, anterior pituitary (all subtypes but mostly nonfunctioning, PRL or GH cell adenoma) tumors, lipomas, angiofibromas
MEN4	CDKN1B (Ch12p13)	Decreased expression of cell cycle inhibitor p27	2 patients; parathyroid tumors, carcinoid tumor, renal and testicular cancer, GH or ACTH cell adenoma
CNC	PPKR1A (Ch17q22–24) ? Ch2p16	Decreased PKA regulatory subunit α expression/ function results in increased PKA signaling	Skin and cardiac myxomas, spotty skin pigmentation, schwannomas, GH or GH-PRL cell adenoma
MAS	GNAS1 (Ch20q13.2 mosaic)	Activating gsp mutation results in reduced GTPase activity, increased adenyl cyclase activity and constitutive cAMP elevation	Polyostotic fibrous dysplasia, pigmented skin patches, precocious puberty, GH or ACTH cell adenoma
FIPA	AIP (Ch11q13.32) ? Other genes	? Altered interaction with aryl-hydrocarbon receptor; abnormal functioning of phosphodiesterase	Pituitary adenomas: all subtypes 15% of all FIPA cases; 50% of familial acromegaly cases

Abbreviations: AIP, aryl-hydrocarbon receptor-interacting protein; ACTH, adenocorticotropic hormone; cAMP, cyclic adenosine monophosphate; CDKN1B, cyclin-dependent kinase inhibitor 1B; CNC, Carney complex syndrome; FIPA, familial isolated pituitary adenoma; GH, growth hormone; GNAS1, guanine-nucleotide activating α subunit adenylate cyclase-stimulating G α-protein; GTPase, guanine triphosphatase; MAS, McCune-Albright syndrome; MEN 1/4, multiple endocrine neoplasia type 1/4 syndrome; PKA, protein kinase A; PPKR1A, protein kinase A regulatory subunit α; PRL, prolactin.

Incorporating clinical information on the specific hormone excess and pathological information on the hormone content of the tumors using immunohistochemistry permits maximal structure-function correlation and a valuable clinicopathological classification described in Table 20.2 [27].

The histological classification, based on histochemical stains, divides adenomas into those that are acidophilic, basophilic, and chromophobic. This classification is of limited value and has largely been abandoned.

The immunohistochemical classification categorizes pituitary adenomas based primarily on hormone content with additional information provided by immunoreactivity for transcription factors and keratins as shown in Tables 20.2 and 20.3 [27].

The transcription factors utilized for the immunohistochemical classification are part of a complex network of temporally and spatially differentially expressed factors that govern the cytodifferentiation of adenohypophyseal cells. Three major pathways in cell lineage development from precursor cells have been identified in the pituitary as shown in Figure 20.2 [25,28]. The proopiomelanocortin expressing corticotrophs are the first cells to differentiate in the human fetal pituitary. By stimulation of proopiomelanocortin expression, the T-box-transcription factor Tpit/Tbox19 promotes terminal differentiation of corticotrophs in concert with the biocoid transcription factor Pitx1 and the basic helix-loop-helix transcription factor NeuroD1 [29–32]. Loss of Tpit function is associated with neonatal onset isolated ACTH deficiency [33].

The second line of differentiation in the fetal human gland is determined by the POU-domain containing transcription

Table 20.2 Clinicopathological Classification of Pituitary Adenomas

Clinically Functioning Adenomas	Clinically Silent Adenomas
Adenomas causing GH excess Somatotroph adenomas Mammosomatotroph adenomas	Silent somatotroph adenomas
Adenomas causing hyperprolactinemia Lactotroph adenomas Lactotroph adenomas with GH	Silent lactotroph adenomas
Adenomas causing TSH excess Thyrotroph adenomas	Silent thyrotroph adenomas
Adenomas causing ACTH excess Corticotroph adenomas	Silent corticotroph adenomas
Adenomas causing gonadotropin excess Gonadotroph adenomas	Silent gonadotroph adenomas
Plurihormonal adenomas	Hormone negative adenomas

Abbreviations: ACTH adrenocorticotropic hormone; GH: growth hormone; TSH: thyroid-stimulating hormone (thyrotropin).

Adapted from Asa SL, 2008 [27].

factor Pit-1 (in concert with the transcription factor Prop-1). Pit-1 is essential for the terminal differentiation and expansion of the somatotroph, lactotroph, and thyrotroph cell lineages as well as for repressing gonadotroph cell fate [34–36]. Furthermore, Pit-1 is necessary for the transcriptional regulation of genes encoding the hormone products of these cell types, including GH, prolactin (PRL), and TSH (reviewed in ref. [37]). Mutations in the Pit-1 gene result in hypopituitarism in humans with hypoplasia of somatotrophs, lactotrophs, and thyrotrophs [38,39]. Pit-1 initiates GH expression

Table 20.3 Immunohistochemical Classification of Pituitary Adenoma

Tumor	Transcription Factor	Hormone(s)	CAM 5.2
GH-producing adenomas	Pit-1		
Somatotroph adenomas		GH	
Densely granulated somatotroph adenomas		GH, α-SU	
Sparsely granulated somatotroph adenomas		GH	Fibrous bodies
Mammosomatotroph adenomas	Pit-1, ER	GH, PRL, α-SU	
Mixed somatotroph-lactotroph adenomas		GH, PRL, α-SU	
Plurihormonal GH-producing adenomas	Pit-1, ER, TEF, GATA-2	GH, PRL, α-SU, β-TSH	
PRL-producing adenomas	Pit-1, ER		
Lactotroph adenomas		PRL	
Densely granulated lactotroph adenomas		PRL (Golgi)	
Sparsely granulated lactotroph adenomas		PRL (diffuse)	
Acidophilic stem cell adenomas		PRL, GH	Fibrous bodies
TSH-producing adenomas	Pit-1, TEF, GATA-2		
Thyreotroph adenomas		α-SU, β-TSH	
ACTH-producing adenomas	Tpit		
Densely granulated coricotroph adenomas		ACTH	
Sparsely granulated coricotroph adenomas		ACTH	
Crooke cell adenomas		ACTH	Dense bands
Gonadotropin-producing adenomas	SF-1, ER, GATA-2		
Gonadotroph adenomas		α-SU, β-FSH, β-LH	
Plurihormonal adenomas	? Multiple		
Silent subtype 3 adenomas		Multiple	
Unusual plurihormonal adenomas		Multiple	
Hormone negative adenomas	None	None	
Null cell adenomas			

Abbreviations: α-SU, α-subunit; ACTH, adrenocorticotropic hormone; ER, estrogen receptor; FSH, follicle-stimulating hormone; GH, growth hormone; LH, luteinizing hormone; Pit-1, pituitary transcription factor 1; PRL, prolactin; SF-1, steroidogenic factor 1; TEF, thyrotroph embryonic factor; TSH, thyroid-stimulating hormone (thyrotropin). Adapted from Asa SL, 2008 [27].

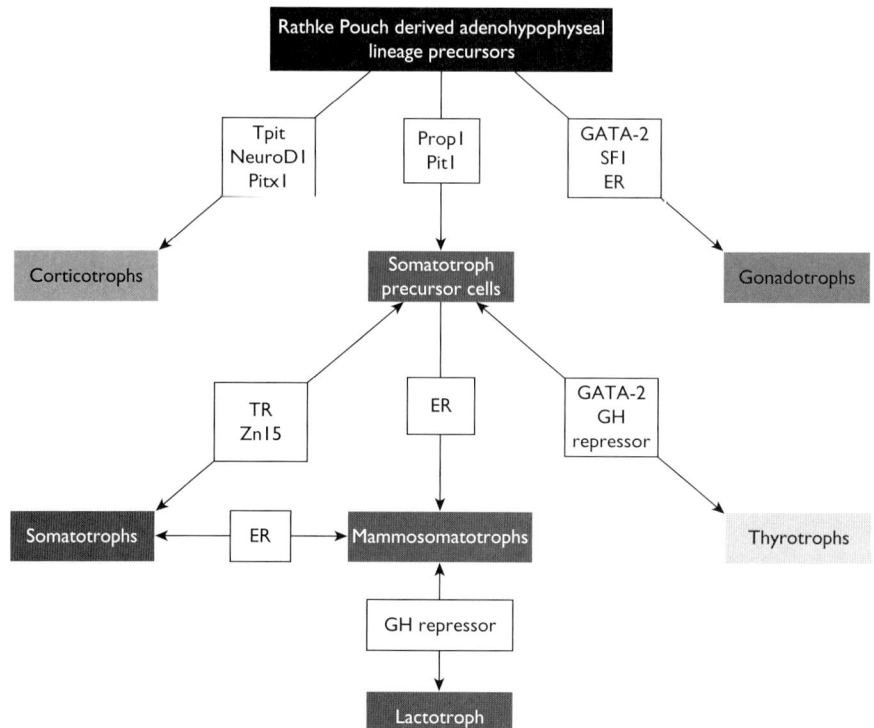

Figure 20.2 Three major pathways in cell lineage development from precursor cells have been identified in the pituitary.

and somatotroph differentiation while additional transcription factors are necessary for the differentiation of lactotrophs and thyrotrophs. Expression of the estrogen receptor allows the expression of GH and PRL in a bihormonal population of mammosomatotrophs [40]. The development of mature lactotrophs is dependent on the presence of a putative GH repressor [41]. Some of the Pit-1-expressing cells develop into thyrotrophs in the presence of a putative GH repressor and the zinc-finger transcription factor GATA-2 [35]. In physiologic states somatotrophs, mammosomatotrophs, and lactotrophs transdifferentiate in what is thought to be a reversible fashion [42]. In animal models, even the transdifferentiation of somatotrophs into thyrotrophs has been shown in severe hypothyroidism [43]. These findings suggest a fluidity of all four cell types that express Pit-1.

The third line of cytodifferentiation is that of the gonadotrophs whose hormone production is dependent on steroidogenic factor-1 and GATA-2 in the presence of estrogen receptor [35,44].

Finally, ultrastructural classification based on electron microscopy allows recognition of specific subcellular characteristics of pituitary adenomas, especially the differentiation of densely or sparsely granulated lactotroph and somatotroph adenomas; however, other immunohistochemical markers, such as keratins, have largely obviated the need for this additional technology. Only in the analysis of unusual plurihormonal adenomas does electron microscopy continue to play an important role in determining cytodifferentiation and structure-function correlations.

HISTOPATHOLOGY

The majority of pituitary adenomas are composed of monomorphic proliferations of cells with uniform round nuclei, delicate stippled chromatin, and moderate quantities of cytoplasm. In contrast to hyperplasia, pituitary adenomas are characterized by complete disruption of the reticulin fiber network as demonstrated with the reticulin stain. Mitoses are seldom in most adenomas. Ki-67 antigen (clone MIB-1) labeling indices are usually less than 3%. Some adenomas, though, have atypical morphological features suggestive of aggressive behavior such as invasive growth, elevated mitotic and Ki-67 labeling indices, as well as extensive nuclear p53 reactivity and are described as "atypical" adenomas. Distant metastasis are required for classification of pituitary carcinoma, as histomorphologically the primary tumor cannot be distinguished from an adenoma.

Clinically Functioning Adenomas
GH-Producing Adenomas

Somatotroph adenomas, which cause two clinically related phenotypes, acromegaly and gigantism depending on the age of onset, are subclassified histomorphologically into five distinct variants (see Table 20.3). These distinctions, especially densely versus sparsely granulated somatotroph adenoma, can affect medical therapy, as the pathophysiology of the lesions determines their response to the current therapies: somatostatin analogues versus GH-antagonists and possibly dopamine agonists [45,46]. In this regard, it is of interest that Gsα mutations have only been shown in densely granulated adenomas providing an intracellular target for somatostatin inhibition in this tumor subtype. In contrast, sparsely granulated adenomas demonstrate heterozygous mutations in the GH-receptor implicated in the formation of fibrous bodies. This mutation results in disruption of GH autoregulation rendering GH-receptor antagonism a more appropriate therapeutic option less likely to be associated with treatment-induced tumor activation [47].

GH-producing adenomas exhibit nuclear Pit-1 reactivity and variable cytoplasmic GH positivity. Mammosomatotroph adenomas stain for PRL as well in the same cell while mixed somatotroph-lactotroph adenomas stain for GH and PRL in different cell populations; the unusual plurihormonal adenomas contain β-TSH in addition to GH and PRL. All of the densely granulated adenomas, including mammosomatotrophs, mixed GH-PRL-producing adenomas, and plurihormonal adenomas, are acidophilic and stain for α-subunit. The sparsely granulated adenoma is chromophobic and immunoreactivity for GH is often weak or negative. It often shows a more aggressive phenotype compared to the densely granulated adenoma and varying degrees of cellular und nuclear pleomorphism are seen. The CAM 5.2 antibody against keratin 7 and 8 is used to identify the hallmark feature of the sparsely granulated adenomas: fibrous bodies, perinuclear keratin globules that are composed of an admixture of intermediate filaments, and smooth endoplasmic reticulum located in the Golgi region and indenting the nuclei. In contrast, densely granulated adenomas show diffuse perinuclear cytoplasmatic keratin staining.

PRL-Producing Adenomas

Lactotroph adenomas causing hyperprolactinemia can be subclassified into three different variants. Sparsely granulated adenomas are chromophobic and exhibit abundant cytoplasm with characteristic juxtanuclear PRL immunoreactivity (Golgi-pattern). These adenomas are usually highly responsive to dopamine-agonist-treatment and therefore frequently display major histomorphological changes induced by therapy: the lesions then are composed of small cells in a fibrous stroma, resembling inflammation, plasmacytoma, or lymphoma. The diagnosis is confirmed by strong nuclear Pit-1 immunoreactivity and at least focal PRL positivity. The rare densely granulated lactotroph adenomas are composed of acidophilic cells with strong and diffuse cytoplasmic positivity for PRL. The unusual acidophilic stem cell adenoma (which some authors also consider to be a subtype of GH-producing adenoma) is characterized by Pit-1 nuclear staining, variable PRL and GH reactivity, oncocytic cytoplasm with abundant spherulated and often dilated giant mitochondria, and fibrous bodies identified with the CAM 5.2. immunostain.

TSH-Producing Adenomas

The rare thyrotroph adenomas causing secondary hyperthyroidism are usually highly infiltrative macroadenomas with stromal fibrosis and marked nuclear atypia. The tumors are composed of chromophobic cells and exhibit a sinusoidal growth pattern. Immunohistochemically, they express Pit-1, α-subunit and β-TSH. The adenomas are sometimes plurihormonal with positive staining for GH and PRL as well.

ACTH-Producing Adenomas

Most ACTH-producing adenomas that cause Cushing syndrome are small microadenomas, measuring 4 to 6 mm. The classical microadenoma is a densely granulated adenoma composed of strongly basophilic cells that stain with periodic acid-Schiff (PAS). Immunohistochemically, the cells demonstrate expression of ACTH and strong reactivity with the CAM 5.2 antibody. The surrounding nonneoplastic corticotrophs typically demonstrate Crooke hyaline change due to accumulation of cytokeratin positive intermediate filaments in the cytoplasm, a morphological marker of feedback suppression. Some adenomas, usually macroadenomas, are chromophobic and only weakly PAS- and ACTH-positive. Staining for treponema pallidum immobilization test is often useful in this setting to establish the diagnosis.

A rare variant of corticotroph adenoma is the Crooke cell adenoma, in which the adenomatous cells exhibit the features of suppressed corticotrophs. The morphology of these lesions is quite atypical with prominent nuclear pleomorphism and large cells with only focal positivity with PAS and ACTH immunohistochemistry and a dense ring of keratin (identified with CAM 5.2) that fills the tumor cell cytoplasm. They have a higher rate of recurrence than other corticotroph adenomas.

Clinically Nonfunctioning Adenomas

The diagnosis of a clinically nonfunctioning adenoma requires an adequate classification for prognostication. The majority of clinically nonfunctioning adenomas are gonadotroph adenomas. Occasionally clinically silent adenomas are positive for Pit-1 and GH, PRL, or β-TSH; these lesions should be classified as adenomas of the appropriate type as indicated previously, with the additional qualification of "silent" adenoma. Silent corticotroph adenoma subtype 1 and subtype 2 as well as the silent (plurihormonal) subtype 3 and the null cell adenoma are rare tumors but behave more aggressively and recur more frequently than the other silent adenomas.

Gonadotropin-Producing Adenomas

These tumors rarely present with clinical or biochemical evidence of hormone excess. Nevertheless, they produce follicle-stimulating and/or luteinizing hormone and they express the transcription factors steroidogenic factor-1, GATA-2, and estrogen receptor that prove gonadotroph differentiation. Several histological patterns are observed but the majority of adenomas consist of uniform, tall, polar cells forming a sinusoidal pattern with characteristic pseudorosettes around vessels and of polygonal cells that comprise the bulk of the lesion. In general, gonadotropin-producing adenomas are chromophobic and PAS negative. Gonadotroph adenoma cells express α-subunit, β-follicle-stimulating hormone subunit and less frequently β-luteinizing hormone subunit in scattered patterns and to a variable degree.

Clinically Silent ACTH-Producing Adenomas

Clinically silent ACTH-producing adenomas are usually large, invasive tumors that may be either basophilic and densely granulated with strong PAS positivity (corticotroph adenoma subtype 1) or chromophobic and sparsely granulated with weak PAS reactivity (corticotroph adenoma subtype 2). There is no associated Crooke's hyaline change in the surrounding nontumorous corticotrophs. These tumors are considered to arise from cells that fail to process the ACTH precursor, proopiomelanocortin, into the biologically active 1–39 ACTH. They stain for Tpit and ACTH and show strong immunoreactivity for CAM 5.2. These adenomas are generally much more aggressive than other silent adenomas and recurrence is very common.

Null Cell Adenoma

The rare tumor that is completely negative for all hormones and transcription factors is classified as null cell adenoma. These tumors are often macroadenomas, invade the cavernous sinuses, and extend upwards into the suprasellar area or downward into the nasal cavity. Null cell adenomas may be poorly differentiated or may exhibit some ultrastructural features of gonadotroph adenomas. They are classically composed of chromophobic cells but oncocytic change is common, resulting in focal to extensive acidophilia; they have a diffuse architectural growth pattern and elongated small cells may form pseudorosettes around markedly dilated capillaries.

Plurihormonality

Plurihormonal adenomas are unusual tumors that show immunoreactivities for more than one pituitary hormone, in patterns that are not explained by normal cytogenesis. The application of highly specific monoclonal antibodies and the understanding of cell differentiation have clarified many of the controversies, for example, reports of adenomas expressing GH or PRL with gonadotropins are now recognized to reflect nonspecific cross-reactivity of the β-follicle-stimulating hormone or β-luteinizing hormone antibodies with the α-subunit, which is positive in many cells of the Pit-1-lineage [48]. Most lesions respect the lines of differentiation attributable to the three transcription factor-induced cell lineages. Even the rare silent subtype 3 adenomas are usually positive for Pit-1, PRL, GH, and β-TSH with other reported reactivities likely reflecting α-subunit cross-reactivity. It is important to classify this adenoma subtype correctly, as it is often highly invasive with parasellar extension and/or invasion of the base of the skull; it exhibits rapid growth and a high recurrence rate. Histologically, these tumors are chromophobic or slightly acidophilic and PAS negative. They are composed of spindle-shaped cells, and intense stromal fibrosis as well as high vascularity are characteristic [49]. For correct diagnosis, ultrastructural confirmation is often necessary to document the presence of nuclear spheridia [50].

Very rarely, tumors express hormones and transcription factors suggestive of "translineage" differentiation as in the case of corticotroph adenomas expressing GH or of somatotroph adenomas expressing ACTH. These tumors express the transcription factors Pit-1 as well as Neuro-D1 suggesting translineage differentiation [51].

Pituitary Carcinomas

Pituitary carcinoma, by definition a lesion that exhibits distant cerebrospinal and/or systemic metastasis, is a very rare tumor. The majority of reported cases secrete ACTH or PRL [52]. The prognosis of patients with pituitary carcinoma is poor with a few exceptions [53]. It cannot be defined by morphological characteristics of the primary tumor or by proliferative index, as it does not differ from an invasive atypical macroadenoma.

Prognosis

In the World Health Organization classification of 2004, a Ki67/MIB-1 labeling index of more than 3% of adenoma nuclei and an elevated mitotic index are the main criteria for atypical adenoma [2]. Nonetheless, the evaluation of proliferative activity using markers such as cyclins, proliferating cell nuclear antigen, antiapoptotic Bcl-2, DNA topoisomerase IIα, and Ki-67/MIB-1 has not demonstrated a consistent correlation with tumor invasiveness or recurrence [54–56]. Other markers such as Cyclooxygenase-2 expression [57], Galectin-3 expression [58], or the reduced expression of the cell cycle inhibitory proteins p16 [59], p27 [60], or p53 [61] are also not helpful in this setting. Therefore, the best predictive marker remains the tumor classification based on hormone content and cell structure.

MOLECULAR PATHOGENESIS

Pituitary tumorigenesis involves both intrinsic pituitary-cell alterations as well as changes in endocrine and paracrine regulatory factors. The exact nature of the intrinsic pituitary-cell defect still has to be established; mutations in oncogenes and TSG, which have been identified in other human malignancies, are restricted to a very small subset of pituitary neoplasms. Gene mutations associated with hereditary pituitary tumors are also rare in sporadic adenomas. Various hypophysiotropic hormones and growth factors govern pituitary cell proliferation. There is an ongoing dispute if these hormones/growth factors stimulate pituitary hyperplasia thus making the cells susceptible to genetic changes or if genetic changes occur first and the hormones and growth factors act as promoters of cell growth in genetically transformed cells. Epigenetic changes are increasingly recognized in pituitary adenomas and clearly have functional consequences in pituitary tumor evolution.

Clonality

Several studies examining X-chromosome inactivation have shown that pituitary adenomas are monoclonal [62,63]. This finding is used to support the idea that pituitary tumors are caused by intrinsic pituitary-cell defects leading to the expansion of a single cell clone resulting in tumor formation. Loss of heterozygosity analysis of a small number of corticotroph adenomas demonstrated oligoclonality/polyclonality in 30% of the analyzed adenomas [64,65]. According to recent reviews, which argue against the monoclonal nature of pituitary adenomas, this documented multiclonality would favor a scenario of pituitary tumor development in which the initiating event is hyperplasia (due to intrapituitary growth factors or extrinsic hormone stimulation) rendering different cells susceptible to different genetic alterations resulting in distinct clones within a tumor [66,67]. This theory may apply in rare corticotroph adenomas but has not been substantiated in any other adenoma type.

Oncogene Activation in Pituitary Tumors

Several reports have excluded involvement of classic proto-oncogenes, including ras [68], c-myc [69], c-fos [69], and c-erbB-2 [70], in pituitary tumors. H-ras mutation [71] has been described in a single aggressive prolactinomas and in metastases of pituitary carcinomas and might play a role in the very rare malignant transformation of pituitary tumors. The association between gain-of-function mutations in the Gsα-subunit of heterotrimeric G-proteins and the development of somatotroph adenomas remains the most important oncogene-associated mechanism yet identified in pituitary adenomas. Gsα point mutations have been demonstrated in approximately 40% of GH-secreting pituitary tumors but in less than 10% of other pituitary tumor subtypes [21]. These mutations inhibit Gsα guanine triphosphatase activity, resulting in GH-releasing hormone receptor ligand-independent constitutive activation of cyclic adenosine monophosphate, which results in GH-transcriptional activation and somatotroph proliferation via a cyclic adenosine monophosphate response element-binding protein in the GH promoter (for review see [72]). Another putative oncogene, the pituitary tumor-transforming gene (PTTG) regulates chromosome separation by inhibition of a group of proteins called separins and, when disrupted, predisposes to aneuploidy through inappropriate timing of chromosomal segregation [73]. PTTG is present at very low levels in normal pituitary tissue and is overexpressed in many pituitary adenomas without demonstrating activating mutations or promoter insertions (for review see [74]). Overexpression correlates with pituitary tumor invasiveness in vivo and with increased hyperplasia in vitro, but the mechanism involved in this proposed oncogenic function is still obscure [75,76]. Recently, high mobility group A2 was shown to be overexpressed and amplified in human prolactinomas and overexpression in transgenic mice induced pituitary tumor formation [77]. A very interesting mechanism for the oncogenic function was proposed in that high mobility group A2 binds to phosphorylated retinoblastoma (Rb) leading to displacement of histone deacetylase 1 from the pRB/E2F1 complex, resulting in enhanced acetylation of both E2F1 and DNA-associated histones causing activation of E2F1 and DNA transcription initiation (for review see [78]).

TSG Inactivation in Pituitary Tumors

TSG act to prevent uncontrolled cell growth and can be inactivated by heterozygous deletion of one of the two alleles encoding the TSG (so-called loss of heterozygosity) or by homozygous loss of both the alleles. Epigenetic events such as promoter cytosine preceding guanine (CpG)-island methylation constitute a third mechanism reducing TSG protein expression.

Allelic losses on chromosomes 10q26, 11q13, and 13q12–14 occur in up to 30% of pituitary adenomas and correlate with increasingly invasive behavior [79]. The putative TSG involved have not been identified.

Although p53 is commonly mutated in human tumors, no mutations have been identified in pituitary adenomas [80]. In mice, loss of Rb and of p27, a member of the cyclin-dependent kinase inhibitor family, results in adenoma formation of the intermediate lobe [81,82]. In humans, mutations in both genes have been excluded, but both proteins are underexpressed or absent in a variable percentage of pituitary adenomas [83,84]. Homozygous mutations of p16, another member of the cyclin-dependent kinase inhibitor family, occur infrequently in human pituitary tumors. However, p16 expression is silenced in 70% of nonfunctioning pituitary adenomas and 10% of somatotroph adenomas by methylation; the significance of these changes for adenoma formation is still under debate [85].

Hormones and Their Receptors

Pituitary gene expression and hormone secretion are regulated by several stimulatory and inhibitory polypeptides and steroid hormones released from the hypothalamus or peripheral endocrine organs that may promote pituitary tumor development (for review please refer to [1,86]). Evidence supporting a hormonal etiology includes paradoxical pituitary hormone responsiveness to exogenous hormonal stimulation of pituitary adenomas, the development of pituitary adenomas in the rare event of stimulatory hypothalamic hormone excess or reduced feedback suppression by target gland hormones, and local production of hypothalamic hormones in the anterior pituitary. In favor are also different animal models with hypothalamic dysregulation, which develop pituitary adenomas (mostly preceded by hyperplasia which is uncommon in humans), for example, transgenic animals overexpressing GH-releasing hormone or Dopamine 2-receptor deficient mice [1]. Arguments against a hormonal etiology, however, are the rarity of hyperplastic changes associated with adenomas in humans, the lack of true adenomatous change in the pituitary even after sustained exposure to hypothalamic hormone stimulation, for example, true for GH-releasing hormone, corticotropin-releasing hormone, gonadotropin-releasing hormone, thyrotropin-releasing hormoneexposure, and the low frequency of recurrence after successful tumor resection. Furthermore, the releasing-hormone receptors are rarely constitutively activated by mutations. Mutations of inhibitory hormone receptors such as somatostatin and dopamine have also not been identified in humans.

Growth and Angiogenic Factors and Their Receptors

The pituitary is the site of synthesis and the target of several proteins that modulate hormone production and are believed to regulate in part pituitary-cell growth and angiogenesis. Angiogenesis has emerged as a key component of the tumor phenotype although the role of angiogenesis in pituitary tumor formation is unresolved. As for hypothalamic and steroid hormones, much evidence supports a permissive role for growth and angiogenic factors in pituitary tumor pathogenesis. The factors implicated in pituitary tumorigenesis include fibroblast growth factors (FGF) and their receptors, particularly FGF-2 (bFGF), FGF-4, and ptd-FGFR4 (pituitary tumor-derived FGFR4) [87,88], the epidermal growth factor family including epidermal growth factor, the epidermal growth factor receptor [89], and transforming growth factor-α [90] as well as the transforming growth factor-β family including activin, inhibin, and bone morphogenic factor-4 (for review see [1,25,91]). The expression of hypoxia-inducible factor 1α, which is an important transcription factor involved in the adaptive response to hypoxia and matrix metalloproteinases, a family of proteins involved in angiogenesis and tissue breakdown as part of invasion and metastases, has also been identified in pituitary tumors [92–94].

Hereditary Syndromes

Several hereditary syndromes (see Table 20.1) are associated with pituitary tumors, although with the exception of Gsα mutations in McCune-Albright syndrome, the molecular events in the hereditary syndromes appear distinct from those implicated in sporadic pituitary tumors.

Epigenetic Changes

Epigenetics describes the mechanisms that result in heritable alterations in gene expression profiles without an accompanying change in DNA sequence. Three main types of epigenetic inheritance—DNA methylation of CpG islands, genomic imprinting, and histone modifications—have been described and these changes are interrelated. Epigenetically regulated gene dysregulation is a common feature associated with human pituitary tumorigenesis (for review see [95]).

The TSG Rb is only rarely mutated in pituitary tumors that are deficient of the protein but is silenced frequently through CpG island methylation [96]. Similarly methylation and silencing of p16 in pituitary tumors occurs at high frequency and seems to be an early event in pituitary tumorigenesis [85,97]. Expression of GADD45γ, a member of a growth arrest and DNA damage-(GADD-) inducible gene family, is reduced in pituitary tumors through CPG island promoter methylation [98]. The Ras-association domain 1A gene (*RASSF1A*) is frequently inactivated in pituitary adenomas by promoter hypermethylation [99]. In addition, MEG3, a human homolog of mouse maternally imprinted Gtl2 gene, is also down-regulated in human nonfunctioning pituitary tumors through promoter hypermethylation [100]. Decreased expression of the FGFR2-IIIb isoform in a significant proportion of primary pituitary tumors is associated with DNA methylation of the promoter-associated CpG island [101,102]. In tumors with reduced expression of FGFR2, the expression of the normally silent cancer-testis antigen, melanoma-associated antigen A3 gene (*MAGE-A3*) gene is apparent and is associated, in contrast to normal pituitary, with hypomethylation of CpG islands [103]. The imprinted gene neuronatin (*NNAT*) is abundantly expressed in normal pituitary, while pituitary adenomas irrespective of subtype predominantly do not express NNAT, which is in line with the hypermethylation of the associated CpG island [104]. The zinc-finger transcription factor Ikaros (Ik) and its isoforms modulate chromatin accessibility through associations with members of the nucleosome remodeling and deacetylase complex including histone deacetylase complexes. Ik is expressed in normal pituitary while the dominant negative (dn) isoform of this protein, Ik6, is expressed in nearly half of all primary pituitary tumors [105]. Altered Ik expression is implicated in altered regulation of the FGFR4 gene that gives rise to ptd-FGFR4 [106,107]. The dominant negative Ik6 isoform results in neoplastic growth in mouse genetic studies and is associated with enhanced protection against apoptosis and with up-regulation of the antiapototic factor Bcl-Xl through selective acetylation of histone 3 sites [108].

REFERENCES

1. Asa SL, Ezzat S. The pathogenesis of pituitary tumours. *Nat Rev Cancer.* 2002;2:836–849.
2. DeLellis RA, Lloyd RV, Heitz PU, Eng C. *Pathology and Genetics of Tumors of Endocrine Organs, World Health Organization Classification of Tumors.* Lyon, France: IARC Press; 2004:9–45.
3. Kovacs K, Horvath E. Tumors of the pituitary gland. In: Hartmann WH, Sobin LH. *Atlas of Tumor Pathology.* 2nd series, Fascicle 21. Washington, DC: Armed Forces Institute of Pathology; 1986.
4. Scheithauer BW. Surgical pathology of the pituitary: the adenomas. Part I. *Pathol Annu.* 1984;19:317–374.
5. Faglia G. Epidemiology and pathogenesis of pituitary adenomas. *Acta Endocrinol.* 1993;129(suppl 1):1–5.
6. Molitch ME. Pituitary incidentalomas. *Endocrinol Metab Clin North Am.* 1997;26:725–740.
7. Ambrosi B, Faglia G. Epidemiology of pituitary tumors. In: Faglia G, Beck-Peccoz P, Ambrosi B, Travaglini P, Spada A, eds. *Pituitary Adenomas: New Trends in Basic and Clinical Research.* Amsterdam, The Netherlands: Elsevier; 1991:159–168.
8. Davis JR, Farrell WE, Clayton RN. Pituitary tumours. *Reproduction.* 2001;121:363–371.
9. Daly A, Rixhon M, Adam C, Dempegioti A, Tichomirowa MA, Beckers A. High prevalence of pituitary adenomas: a cross sectional study in the Province of Liege, Belgium. *J Clin Endocrinol Metab.* 2006;91:4769–4775.
10. Ezzat S, Asa SL, Couldwell WT, et al. The prevalence of pituitary adenomas: a systematic review. *Cancer.* 2004;101:613–619.
11. McComb DJ, Ryan N, Horvath E, Kovacs K. Subclinical adenomas of the human pituitary. New light on old problems. *Arch Pathol Lab Med.* 1983;107:488–491.
12. Mindermann T, Wilson CB. Age-related and gender-related occurrence of pituitary adenomas. *Clin Endocrinol.* 1994;41:359–364.
13. Burrow GN, Wortzman G, Rewcastle NB, Holgate RC, Kovacs K. Microadenomas of the pituitary and abnormal sellar tomograms in an unselected autopsy series. *N Engl J Med.* 1981;304:156–158.
14. Chandrasekharappa SC, Guru SC, Manickam P, et al. Positional cloning of the gene for multiple endocrine neoplasia-type 1. *Science.* 1997;276:404–407.
15. Daly AF, Tichomirow MA, Beckers A. Update on familial pituitary tumors: from multiple endocrine neoplasia type 1 to familial isolated pituitary adenoma. *Horm Res.* 2009;71(suppl 1):105–111.
16. Casey M, Mah C, Merliss AD, et al. Identification of a novel genetic locus for familial cardiac myxomas and Carney complex. *Circulation.* 1998;98:2560–2566.
17. Boikos SA, Stratakis CA. Carney complex: the first 20 years. *Curr Opin Oncol.* 2007;19:24–29.
18. Pellegata NS, Quintanilla-Martinez L, Siggelkow H, et al. Germline mutations in p27Kip1 cause a multiple endocrine neoplasia syndrome in rats and humans. *Proc Natl Acad Sci USA.* 2006;103:15558–15563.
19. Georgitsi M, Raitila A, Karhu A, et al. Germline CDKN1B/p27Kip1 mutation in multiple endocrine neoplasia. *J Clin Endocrinol Metab.* 2007;92:3321–3325.
20. Landis CA, Masters SB, Spada A, Pace AM, Bourne HR, Vallar L. GTPase inhibiting mutations activate the chain of Gs and stimulate adenylyl cyclase in human pituitary tumours. *Nature.* 1989;340:692–696.
21. Lyons J, Landis CA, Harsch G, et al. Two G protein oncogenes in human endocrine tumors. *Science.* 1990;249:655–659.
22. Lumbroso S, Paris F, Sultan C. Activating Gs-alpha mutations: analysis of 113 patients with signs of McCune-Albright syndrome—a European collaborative study. *J Clin Endocr Metab.* 2004;89:2107–2113.
23. Vierimaa O, Georgitsi M, Lehtonen R, et al. Pituitary adenoma predisposition caused by germline mutations in the AIP gene. *Science.* 2006;312:1228–1230.
24. Daly AF, Vanbellinghen JF, Khoo SK, et al. Aryl hydrocarbon receptor-interacting protein gene mutations in familial isolated pituitary adenomas: analysis in 73 families. *J Clin Endocrinol Metab.* 2007;92:1891–1896.
25. Asa SL, Ezzat S. The cytogenesis and pathogenesis of pituitary adenomas. *Endocr Rev.* 1998;19:798–827.
26. Sautner D, Saeger W. Invasiveness of pituitary adenomas. *Pathol Res Pract.* 1991;187:632–636.
27. Asa SL. Practical pituitary pathology. *Arch Pathol Lab Med.* 2008;132:1231–1240.
28. Asa SL, Ezzat S. Molecular basis of pituitary development and cytogenesis. *Front Horm Res.* 2004;32:1–19.
29. Liu J, Lin C, Gleiberman A, et al. Tbx19, a tissue-selective regulator of POMC gene expression. *Proc Natl Acad Sci USA.* 2001;98:8674–8679.
30. Lamolet B, Pulichino AM, Lamonerie T, et al. A pituitary cell-restricted T box factor, Tpit, activates POMC transcription in cooperation with Pitx homeoproteins. *Cell.* 2001;104:849–859.
31. Lamonerie T, Tremblay JJ, Lanctot C, Therrien M, GauthierY, Drouin J. Ptx1, a bicoid-related homeo box transcription factor involved in transcription of the pro-opiomelanocortin gene. *Genes Dev.* 1996;10:1284–1295.
32. Poulin G, Turgeon B, Drouin J. NeuroD1/beta2 contributes to cell-specific transcription of the proopiomelanocortin gene. *Mol Cell Biol.* 1997;17:6673–6682.
33. Pulichino AM, Vallette-Kasic S, Couture C, et al. Human and mouse TPIT gene mutations cause early onset pituitary ACTH deficiency. *Genes Dev.* 2003;17:711–716.
34. Camper SA, Saunders TL, Katz RW, Reeves RH. The Pit-1 transcription factor gene is a candidate for the murine Snell dwarf mutation. *Genomics.* 1990;8:586–590.
35. Dasen JS, O'Connell SM, Flynn SE, et al. Reciprocal interactions of Pit1 and GATA2 mediate signaling gradient induced determination of pituitary cell types. *Cell.* 1999;97:587–598.

36. Li S, Crenshaw EB, Rawson EJ, Simmons DM, Swanson LW, Rosenfeld MG. Dwarf locus mutants lacking three pituitary cell types result from mutations in the POU-domain gene pit-1. *Nature.* 1990;347:528–533.
37. Andersen B, Rosenfeld MG. POU domain factors in the neuroendocrine system: lessons from developmental biology provide insights into human disease. *Endocr Rev.* 2001;22:2–35.
38. Pfäffle RW, DiMattia GE, Parks JS, et al. Mutation of the POU-specific domain of Pit-1 and hypopituitarism without pituitary hypoplasia. *Science.* 1992;257:1118–1121.
39. Tatsumi K, Miyai K, Notomi T, et al. Cretinism with combined hormone deficiency caused by a mutation in the PIT1 gene. *Nat Genet.* 1992;1:56–58.
40. Day RN, Koike S, Sakai M, Muramatsu M, Maurer RA. Both Pit-1 and the estrogen receptor are required for estrogen responsiveness of the rat prolactin gene. *Mol Endocrinol.* 1990;4:1964–1971.
41. Scully KM, Jacobson EM, Jepsen K, et al. Allosteric effects of Pit-1 DNA sites on long-term repression in cell type specification. *Science.* 2000;290:1127–1131.
42. Frawley LS, Boockfor FR. Mammosomatotropes: presence and functions in normal and neoplastic pituitary tissue. *Endocr Rev.* 1991;12:337–355.
43. Horvath E, Lloyd RV, Kovacs K. Propylthiouracil-induced hypothyroidism results in reversible transdifferentiation of somatotrophs into thyroidectomy cells: a morphologic study of the rat pituitary including immunoelectron microscopy. *Lab Invest.* 1990;63:511–520.
44. Asa SL, Bamberger A-M, Cao B, Wong M, Parker KL, Ezzat S. The transcription activator steroidogenic factor-1 is preferentially expressed in the human pituitary gonadotroph. *J Clin Endocrinol Metab.* 1996;81:2165–2170.
45. Ezzat S, Kontogeorgos G, Redelmeier DA, Horvath E, Harris AG, Kovacs K. In vivo responsiveness of morphological variants of growth hormone-producing pituitary adenomas to octreotide. *Eur J Endocrinol.* 1995;133:686–690.
46. Bhayana S, Booth GL, Asa SL, Kovacs K, Ezzat S. The implication of somatotroph adenoma phenotype to somatostatin analog responsiveness in acromegaly. *J Clin Endocrinol Metab.* 2005;90:6290–6295.
47. Asa SL, Digiovanni R, Jiang J, et al. A growth hormone receptor mutation impairs growth hormone autofeedback signaling in pituitary tumors. *Cancer Res.* 2007;67:7505–7511.
48. Labat-Moleur F, Trouillas J, Seret-Begue D, Kujas M, Delisle MB, Ronin C. Evaluation of 29 monoclonal and polyclonal antibodies used in the diagnosis of pituitary adenomas: a collaborative study from pathologists of the Club Francais de l'Hypophyse. *Pathol Res Pract.* 1991;187:534–538.
49. Horvath E, Kovacs K, Killinger DW, Smyth HS, Platts ME, Singer W. Silent corticotropic adenomas of the human pituitary gland: a histologic, immunocytologic, and ultrastructural study. *Am J Pathol.* 1980;98:617–638.
50. Horvath E, Kovacs K, Smyth HS, Cusimano M, Singer W. Silent adenoma subtype 3 of the pituitary–immunohistochemical and ultrastructural classification: a review of 29 cases. *Ultrastruct Pathol.* 2005;29:511–524.
51. Tahara S, Kurotani R, Ishii Y, Sanno N, Teramoto A, Osamura RY. A case of Cushing's disease caused by pituitary adenoma producing adrenocorticotropic hormone and growth hormone concomitantly: aberrant expression of transcription factors NeuroD1 and Pit-1 as a proposed mechanism. *Mod Pathol.* 2002;15:1102–1105.
52. Ragel BT, Couldwell WT. Pituitary carcinoma: a review of the literature. *Neurosurg Fokus.* 2004;16:E7.
53. Pernicone PJ, Scheithauer BW, Sebo TJ, et al. Pituitary carcinoma: a clinicopathologic study of 15 cases. *Cancer.* 1997;79:804–812.
54. Amar AP, Hinton DR, Krieger MD, Weiss MH. Invasive pituitary adenomas: significance of proliferation parameters. *Pituitary.* 1999;2:117–122.
55. Thapar K, Kovacs K, Scheithauer BW, et al. Proliferative activity and invasiveness among pituitary adenomas and carcinomas: an analysis using the MIB-1 antibody. *Neurosurgery.* 1996;38:99–106.
56. Vidal S, Kovacs K, Horvath E, et al. Topoisomerase II alpha expression in pituitary adenomas and carcinomas: relationship to tumor behavior. *Mod Pathol.* 2002;15:1205–1212.
57. Vidal S, Kovacs K, Bell D, Horvath E, Scheithauer BW, Lloyd RV. Cyclooxygenase-2 expression in human pituitary tumors. *Cancer.* 2003;97:2814–2821.
58. Riss D, Jin L, Qian X, et al. Differential expression of galectin-3 in pituitary tumors. *Cancer Res.* 2003;63:2251–2255.
59. Simpson DJ, Bicknell JE, McNicol AM, Clayton RN, Farrell WE. Hypermethylation of the p16/CDKN2A/MTSI gene and loss of protein expression is associated with nonfunctional pituitary adenomas but not somatotrophinomas. *Genes Chromosomes Cancer.* 2003;37:225–236
60. Korbonits M, Chahal HS, Kaltsas G, et al. Expression of phosphorylated p27(Kip1) protein and Jun activation domain-binding protein 1 in human pituitary tumors. *J Clin Endocrinol Metab.* 2002;87:2635–2643.
61. Schreiber S, Saeger W, Lüdecke DK. Proliferation markers in different types of clinically non-secreting pituitary adenomas. *Pituitary.* 1999;1:213–220.
62. Herman V, Fagin J, Gonsky R, Kovacs K, Melmed S. Clonal origin of pituitary adenomas. *J Clin Endocrinol Metab.* 1990;71:1427–1433.
63. Alexander JM, Biller BM, Bikkal H, Zervas NT, Arnold A, Klibanski A. Clinically nonfunctioning pituitary tumors are monoclonal in origin. *J Clin Invest.* 1990;86:336–340.
64. Schulte HM, Oldfield EH, Allolio B, Katz DA, Berkman RA, Ali IU. Clonal composition of pituitary adenomas in patients with Cushing's disease: determination by X-chromosome inactivation analysis. *J Clin Endocrinol Metab.* 1991;73:1302–1308.
65. Biller BM, Alexander JM, Zervas NT, Hedley-Whyte ET, Arnold A, Klibanski A. Clonal origins of adrenocorticotropin-secreting pituitary tissue in Cushing's disease. *J Clin Endocrinol Metab.* 1992;75:1303–1309.
66. Levy A. Molecular and trophic mechanisms of tumorigenesis. *Endocrinol Metab Clin N Am.* 2008;37:23–50.
67. Clayton RN, Farrell WE. Pituitary tumour clonality revisited. *Front Horm Res.* 2004;32:186–204.
68. Herman V, Drazin NZ, Gonsky R, Melmed S. Molecular screening of pituitary adenomas for gene mutations and rearrangements. *J Cin Endocrinol Metab.* 1993;77:50–55.
69. Woloschak M, Roberts JL, Post K. c-myc, c-fos, and c-myb gene expression in human pituitary adenomas. *J Clin Endocrinol Metab.* 1994;79:253–257.
70. Ezzat S, Zheng L, Smyth HS, Asa SL. The c-erbB-2/neu proto-oncogene in human pituitary tumours. *Clin Endocrinol.* 1997;46:599–606.
71. Pei L, Melmed S, Scheithauer B, Kovacs K, Prager D. H-ras mutations in human pituitary carcinoma metastases. *J Clin Endocrinol Metab.* 1994;78:842–846.
72. Lania A, Mantovani G, Spada A. G protein mutations in endocrine diseases. *Eur J Endocrinol.* 2001;145:543–559.
73. Zou H, McGarry TJ, Bernal T, Kirschner MW. Identification of a vertebrate sister-chromatid separation inhibitor involved in transformation and tumorigenesis. *Science.* 1999;285:418–422.
74. Salehi F, Kovacs K, Scheithauer BW, Lloyd RV, Cusimano M. Pituitary tumor-transforming gene in endocrine and other neoplasms: a review and update. *Endocr Relat Cancer.* 2008;15:721–743.
75. Abbud RA, Takumi I, Barker EM, et al. Early multipotential pituitary focal hyperplasia in the alpha-subunit of glycoprotein hormone-driven pituitary tumor-transforming gene transgenic mice. *Mol Endocrinol.* 2005;19:1383–1391.
76. Zhang X, Horwitz GA, Heaney AP, et al. Pituitary tumor transforming gene (PTTG) expression in pituitary adenomas. *J Clin Endocrinol Metab.* 1999;84:761–767.
77. Fedele M, Battista S, Kenyon L, et al. Overexpression of the HMGA2 gene in transgenic mice leads to the onset of pituitary adenomas. *Oncogene.* 2002;21:3190–3198.
78. Fedele M, Pierantoni GM, Visone R, Fusco A. Critical Role of HMGA2 gene in pituitary adenomas. *Cell Cycle.* 2006;5:2045–2048.
79. Bates AS, Farrell WE, Bicknell EJ, et al. Allelic deletion in pituitary adenomas reflects aggressive biological activity and has potential value as a prognostic marker. *J Clin Endocrinol Metab.* 1997;82:818–824.
80. Levy A, Hall L, Yeudall WA, Lightman SL. p53 gene mutations in pituitary adenomas: rare events. *Clin Endocrinol.* 1994;41:809–814.
81. Jacks T, Fazeli A, Schmitt EM, Bronson RT, Goodell MA, Weinberg RA. Effects of an Rb mutation in the mouse. *Nature.* 1992;359:295–300.
82. Kiyokawa H, Kineman RD, Manova-Todorova KO, et al. Enhanced growth of mice lacking the cyclin-dependent kinase inhibitor function of p27(Kip1). *Cell.* 1996;85:721–732.
83. Cryns VL, Alexander JM, Klibanski A, Arnold A. The retinoblastoma gene in human pituitary tumors. *J Clin Endocrinol Metab.* 1993;77:644–646.
84. Lidhar K, Korbonits M, Jordan S, et al. Low expression of the cell cycle inhibitor p27Kip1 in normal corticotroph cells, corticotroph tumors, and malignant pituitary tumors. *J Clin Endocrinol Metab.* 1999;84:3823–3830.

85. Simpson DJ, Magnay J, Bicknell JE, McNichol AM, Clayton RN, Farrell WE. Hypomethylation of the p16/CDKN2A/MTS1 gene and loss of protein expression is associated with nonfunctional pituitary adenomas but not somatotrophinomas. *Genes Chromosomes Cancer.* 1999;24:328–336.
86. Melmed S. Mechanisms for pituitary tumorigenesis: the plastic pituitary. *J Clin Invest.* 2003;112:737–740.
87. Ezzat S, Smyth HS, Ramyar L, Asa SL. Heterogenous in vivo and in vitro expression of basic fibroblast growth factor by human pituitary adenomas. *J Clin Endocrinol Metab.* 1995;80:878–884.
88. Ezzat S, Zheng L, Zhu XF, Wu GE, Asa SL. Targeted expression of a human pituitary tumor-derived isoform of FGF receptor-4 recapitulates pituitary tumorigenesis. *J Clin Invest.* 2002;109:69–78.
89. LeRiche VK, Asa SL, Ezzat S. Epidermal growth factor and its receptor (EGF-R) in human pituitary adenomas: EGF-R correlates with tumor aggressiveness. *J Clin Endocrinol Metab.* 1996;81:656–662.
90. Ezzat S, Walpola IA, Ramyar L, Smyth HS, Asa SL. Membrane-anchored expression of transforming growth factor-alpha in human pituitary adenoma cells. *J Clin Endocrinol Metab.* 1995;80:534–539.
91. Heaney AP. Pituitary tumour pathogenesis. *Br Med Bull.* 2006;75:81–97.
92. Yoshida D, Kim K, Yamazaki M, Teramoto A. Expression of hypoxia-inducible factor alpha and cathespin D in pituitary adenomas. *Endocr Pathol.* 2005;16:123–131.
93. Turner HE, Nagy Zs, Esiri MM, Harris AL, Wass JAH. Role of matrix metalloproteinase 9 in pituitary tumor behavior. *J Clin Endocrinol Metab.* 2000;85:2931–2935.
94. Liu W, Matsumoto Y, Okada M et al. Matrix metalloproteinase 2 and 9 expression correlated with cavernous sinus invasion of pituitary adenomas. *J Med Invest.* 2005;52:151–158.
95. Ezzat S. Epigenetic control in pituitary tumors. *Endocr J.* 2008;55:951–957.
96. Simpson DJ, Hibberts NA, McNicol AM, Clayton RN, Farrell WE. Loss of pRb expression in pituitary adenomas is associated with methylation of the RB1 CpG island. *Cancer Res.* 2000;60:1211–1216.
97. Woloschak M, Yu A, Post KD. Frequent inactivation of the p16 gene in human pituitary tumors by gene methylation. *Mol Carcinog.* 1997;19:221–224.
98. Bahar A, Bicknell JE, Simpson DJ, Clayton RN, Farrell WE. Loss of expression of the growth inhibitory gene GADD45gamma, in human pituitary adenomas, is associated with CpG island methylation. *Oncogene.* 2004;23:936–944.
99. Qian ZR, Sano T, Yoshimoto K, et al. Inactivation of RASSF1A tumor suppressor gene by aberrant promoter hypermethylation in human pituitary adenomas. *Lab Invest.* 2005;85:464–473.
100. Zhao J, Dahle D, Zhou Y, Zhang X, Klibanski A. Hypermethylation of the promoter region is associated with the loss of MEG3 gene expression in human pituitary tumors. *J Clin Endocrinol Metab.* 2005;90:2179–2186.
101. Abbass SAA, Asa SL, Ezzat S. Altered expression of fibroblast growth factor receptors in human pituitary adenomas. *J Clin Endocrinol Metab.* 1997;82:1160–1166.
102. Zhu X, Lee K, Asa SL, Ezzat S. Epigenetic silencing through DNA and histone 20 methylation of fibroblast growth factor receptor 2 in neoplastic pituitary cells. *Am J Pathol.* 2007;170:1618–1628
103. Zhu X, Asa SL, Ezzat S. Fibroblast growth factor 2 and estrogen control the balance of histone 3 modifications targeting MAGE-A3 in pituitary neoplasia. *Clin Cancer Res.* 2008;14:1984–1996.
104. Dudley KJ, Revill K, Whitby P, Clayton RN, Farrell WE. Genome wide analysis in a murine Dnmt1 knockdown model identifies epigenetically silenced genes in primary human pituitary tumors. *Mol Cancer Res.* 2008;6:1567–1574.
105. Ezzat S, Yu S, Asa SL. Ikaros isoforms in human pituitary tumors: distinct localization, histone acetylation, and activation of the 5′ fibroblast growth factor receptor-4 promoter. *Am J Pathol.* 2003;163:1177–1184.
106. Yu S, Asa SL, Ezzat S. Fibroblast growth factor receptor 4 is a target for the zinc-finger transcription factor Ikaros in the pituitary. *Mol Endocrinol.* 2002;16:1069–1078.
107. Yu S, Asa SL, Weigel RJ, Ezzat S. Pituitary tumor AP-2alpha recognizes a cryptic promoter in intron 4 of fibroblast growth factor receptor 4. *J Biol Chem.* 2003;278:19597–19602.
108. Ezzat S, Zhu X, Loeper S, Fischer S, Asa SL. Tumor-derived Ikaros 6 acetylates the Bcl-XL promoter to up-regulate a survival signal in pituitary cells. *Mol Endocrinol.* 2006;20:2976–2986.

21 Histopathology and Molecular Pathogenesis of Neurofibromas and Malignant Peripheral Nerve Sheath Tumors

Tim-Rasmus Kiehl and Kathleen Joy Khu

BACKGROUND ON NEUROFIBROMAS AND MALIGNANT PERIPHERAL NERVE SHEATH TUMORS

Neurofibromas are benign nerve sheath tumors that may occur sporadically or, in 50% of cases, in association with the neurofibromatosis 1 (NF1) syndrome. Different types of neurofibroma can be distinguished in terms of their growth pattern and infiltrative behavior, among them dermal neurofibroma (DNF) and plexiform neurofibroma (PNF) [1,2]. DNF, although often disfiguring and painful, generally remains clinically asymptomatic and does not tend to progress to higher-grade malignancies. In contrast, PNF leads to higher morbidity and may exhibit a tendency for malignant transformation in 10% to 15% of cases [3–5].

NF1, also known as von Recklinghausen disease, is one of the most common human cancer predisposition syndromes, occurring in 1 per 3500 to 4000 individuals [6]. It is transmitted in an autosomal dominant fashion with virtually 100% penetrance by the age 10 years [7]. Men and women are affected in roughly equal proportions. All individuals with NF1 are born with one functional and one nonfunctional (mutated) copy of the NF1 gene in every cell in their body [8]. The presence of two or more neurofibromas of any type or one or more PNFs is one of the diagnostic criteria of NF1 [4]. Patients with NF1 have a lifetime risk of approximately 10% for developing a malignant peripheral nerve sheath tumor (MPNST) [9]. The majority of patients with NF1 have multiple benign DNFs but only about 30% to 50% of them develop one or more PNFs. These often grow along major nerve tracts where they may involve multiple fascicles and nerve branches. When such PNFs grow sufficiently large, their growth rates and developmental patterns tend to become somewhat unpredictable. Patients with a deep-seated PNF are up to 20 times more likely to eventually develop an MPNST compared with individuals with NF1 without such tumors [10]. The risk for an MPNST is low for a patient with NF1, ranging from 5% to 13% [11,12]. Clinical parameters that may indicate the possibility of transformation to MPNST include pain and neurological deficits, rapid growth, and invasion of adjacent structures. Surgery reduces metastasis and prolongs survival [13], especially if tumor-free margins are obtained. Radiotherapy is usually the next treatment modality, although tumor resistance to radiotherapy and chemotherapy is often seen. Current imaging modalities such as computed tomography still lack the sensitivity to reliably detect this malignant transformation. The diagnostic potential of 18-fluorodeoxyglucose-positron emission tomography/computed tomography for this application is currently under investigation [14–18].

MOLECULAR PATHOGENESIS OF NEUROFIBROMAS

The NF1 gene is located on chromosome 17q11.2 and comprises 60 exons spanning 350 kb of genomic DNA. It codes for the protein neurofibromin, which is expressed in all tissues but is most abundant in neurons, astrocytes, oligodendrocytes, Schwann cells, adrenal medullary cells, white blood cells, as well as gonadal tissue [19]. Neurofibromin functions as a tumor suppressor or negative growth regulator [8].

Neurofibromas arise from Schwann cells that have undergone biallelic inactivation of the NF1 gene [20–22]. Consistent with Knudson's two-hit hypothesis of tumor suppressor gene inactivation [23,24], one NF1 allele carries a genetic alteration in all cells of a patient with NF1 (germline), and loss of the second NF1 allele (somatic) then results in functional loss of neurofibromin. Both copies of the NF1 gene are mutated in NF1 tumors, but contrary to the classical "two-hit" hypothesis, most of these never become malignant [7].

Loss of heterozygosity (LOH) or inactivation of both NF1 genes can occur by means of several mechanisms. Genetic testing for NF1 is complicated by the fact that more than 250 different NF1 germline mutations have been reported thus far. These include large deletions (>700 kb where the entire NF1 gene is deleted), microdeletions, single base pair substitutions, duplications, insertions, splicing errors, and translocations [25,26]. Mutations may also occur as a result of nondisjunction, loss of an entire chromosome 17, or somatic recombination [7].

Most of these mutations result in premature truncation of the gene product, which in turn results in an inactive protein and reduced amounts of active, functional neurofibromin [7,25].

Genetic differences between DNFs, PNFs, and MPNSTs have been detected. Pandita et al [27] analyzed DNA from transformed tumor cells and reported that chromosomal losses were more prevalent in benign tumors, compared with mainly gains in MPNSTs.

Aside from changes at the DNA level, it has been found that alterations at the mRNA level also play a role in NF1 gene expression. Levy et al [19] found that 30 genes were significantly upregulated in PNFs compared with DNFs and that none were downregulated. The upregulated genes mainly encoded transcription factors and growth factors, as well as secreted proteins, cytokines, and their receptors. This points to a role of defects in paracrine and autocrine signaling in the genesis of PNFs [19]. "mRNA editing" is a posttranscriptional alteration of mRNA coding that can occur either as "insertion" or as "base modification" editing [25]. NF1 mRNA isolated from benign and malignant tumors showed higher levels of mRNA editing compared with mRNA from tissues of individuals without NF1 [25]. This may be another mode of inactivation of both NF1 alleles that works by modification of their transcripts without a mutation in the NF1 gene and could account for some of the cases in which LOH was not detectable at the DNA level in some tumor tissues.

The specifics of NF1 mRNA processing could also play a role in determining the type of tumor that develops. Benign cutaneous neurofibromas show the least amount of mRNA editing in their NF1 mRNA, PNFs have an intermediate amount, and MPNSTs have the greatest amount of mRNA editing [26].

Neurofibromin functions as a tumor suppressor via various mechanisms. The functional part of neurofibromin is a guanosine triphospatase-activating protein that helps maintain the proto-oncogene RAS in an inactive form. This is achieved by accelerating the conversion of GTP-RAS to GDP-RAS. RAS functions as part of a signal transduction pathway that is activated by growth factors and their receptors, including receptor tyrosine kinases such as epidermal growth factor (EGF), nerve growth factor, and platelet-derived growth factor (PDGF), via guanine nucleotide exchange factors [3]. RAS also signals via the Raf/MEK/ERK mitogen-activated protein kinase and P13K/Akt/mammalian target of rapamycin pathways [28]. These two pathways are aberrantly activated when there is loss of neurofibromin in tumor cells. Activation contributes to the malignant transformation of mammalian cells and is associated with uncontrolled cell proliferation and resistance to apoptosis [28]. Ultimately, loss of neurofibromin results in increased levels of activated GTP-RAS, leading to dysregulated cell growth and tumorigenesis [29].

The significant role of RAS in the pathogenesis of neurofibromas was investigated by several authors [26,30]. It was found that neurofibromin was not expressed in NF1 tumors and that levels of activated RAS-GTP in NF1 PNFs and MPNSTs were 5 and 15 times higher, respectively, compared with non-NF1 schwannomas [30]. Cell lines derived from tumors of patients with NF1 can have undetectable levels of neurofibromin, decreased neurofibromin guanosine triphospatase-activating protein -like activity, and increased levels of activated RAS [26].

In addition to regulating RAS, neurofibromin also positively regulates cyclic adenosine monophosphate levels [8,29,31]. Increased cyclic adenosine monophosphate levels are associated with reduced cell growth, possibly through interference with multiple mitogenic signaling pathways [8].

The Schwann cell has been identified as the progenitor cell of neurofibroma formation because LOH was found specifically in involved Schwann cells but not in other cellular components of a neurofibroma, such as fibroblasts [7,29]. In addition, the transformed Schwann cells have other unique in vitro characteristics that may contribute to tumorigenesis, such as a higher potential to be severely compromised by mutations compared with other cells. They express less NF1 mRNA than fibroblasts and translation of mRNA into protein is slow and inefficient. They have increased active RAS and RAS-GTP. They have an altered morphology, delayed senescence, lack of density-limited growth, and a propensity to form proliferative cell aggregates rich in extracellular matrix spontaneously. They promote angiogenesis and invade basement membranes. They also show a loss of negative autocrine growth control. All of these features contribute to the growth advantage of Schwann cells in a neurofibroma [7].

The tumor bulk and growth of a neurofibroma is not solely attributed to the proliferative features of the transformed Schwann cells. Neurofibromas also contain fibroblasts, perineural cells, axons, and mast cells embedded in an extracellular matrix [32]. In patients with NF1, these supporting cells are heterozygous (NF1+/−); thus, half of the normal activity of the neurofibromin protein is lost. The single active NF1 allele may not generate enough functional protein to maintain an appropriate biological function, which may confer a growth advantage. Such haploinsufficiency of NF1 in the microenvironment of neurofibromas contributes to its tumorigenicity [7]. Haploinsufficiency of NF1 has also been associated with increased mast cell proliferation, survival, and colony formation, and enhanced RAS mitogen-activated protein kinase C activity [29].

The other heterozygous components in the cellular microenvironment contribute to tumor formation in various ways. NF1+/− fibroblasts demonstrate abnormal responses to cytokines, increased collagen deposition, and increased proliferation [7]. One study suggests that mouse fibroblasts with one functioning NF1 allele (NF1+/−) show abnormal wound healing and continued fibroblast proliferation in vivo [6]. These fibroblasts may contribute to the development of a neurofibroma by responding aberrantly to proliferative signals imparted by "neoplastic" Schwann cells [6].

Mast cells also play a role in tumor initiation, progression, and angiogenesis. NF1+/− mast cells show increased infiltration into preneoplastic peripheral nerves [7], and mouse NF1+/− mast cells exhibit abnormal growth properties and dysregulated RAS signaling [6]. Neurofibromin-deficient Schwann cells secrete five times the normal amount of kit ligand, a growth factor that serves as a chemoattractant for mast cells [7]. This demonstrates that the loss of NF1 in Schwann cells results in increased growth factor production. This initiates an autocrine or paracrine loop, which is important for tumorigenesis to progress [7]. In addition, heterozygous inactivation of NF1+/− promotes rapid migration of mast cells on alpha-4B1 integrins (mast cell surface proteins) in response to the kit ligand [7], facilitating attachment to endothelial cells and promoting angiogenesis. Other cells such as NF1 heterozygous bone marrow cells may also contribute to tumor formation [33], reflecting the influence of tumor microenvironment.

Certain epigenetic factors have been found to contribute to neurofibroma formation and growth. These include increased expression of growth factors and their receptors, including EGF, PDGF, and vascular endothelial growth factor (VEGF) [6]. Other Schwann cell mitogens that promote tumorigenesis include hepatocyte growth factor, basic fibroblast growth factor, insulin growth factor-1, and pigment epithelium-derived growth factor [7]. Transforming growth factor-β1 and nerve growth factor have also been implicated [25]. The angioinvasive properties of the neoplastic Schwann cells in a neurofibroma may result from increased production of proteins that breakdown the extracellular matrix, such as matrix metalloproteinases (MMPs), which are increased in neurofibromas [6,31]. In addition to promoting growth, some proteins such as EGF receptor (EGFR) serve as a survival factor by avoiding apoptosis [7]. The presence of supporting cells and growth factors demonstrate the critical role of the microenvironment in the pathogenesis of neurofibromas.

Future Directions

An improved understanding of the cellular and molecular pathogenesis of neurofibromas has made it possible to develop treatment strategies that specifically target the molecular abnormalities in NF1. Various agents, including antihistamines (ketotifen), maturation enhancers (cis-retinoic acid), and antiangiogenic drugs (interferon-α, thalidomide) have been tried in the past, with only limited success [12]. Targets for future treatment include the RAS signal transduction pathway and the many growth factors involved in the tumorigenesis of neurofibroma.

Because RAS plays a crucial role in cell proliferation, one potential therapy involves the inactivation of RAS by preventing it from undergoing secondary posttranslational modifications, such as farnesylation. Inhibition of the enzyme involved in this process via farnesyltransferase inhibitors prevents the activation of the RAS signaling pathway [25]. One such drug, tipifarnib, is currently undergoing phase II clinical trials [6–8].

Other means of targeting the RAS effector pathway include inhibitors that target downstream effectors such as MEK, which reverts many aspects of cellular transformation, and P13K, which induces apoptosis [7,28]. Another treatment option is the use of gene therapy vectors with functional NF1 GD proteins or with dominant negative RAS, which blocks RAS activity [7]. Other RAS inhibitors such as antisense RNA may have a promising role [4].

Another agent that is under phase II trial is pirfenidone, a broad-spectrum antifibrotic drug that modulates actions of cytokines such as PDGF, fibroblast growth factor, EGF, transforming growth factor, and intracellular adhesion molecules. Inhibition of these cytokines decreases proliferation and collagen matrix synthesis in fibroblasts [6–8].

Other agents that target growth receptors are being studied for use in neurofibromas. These include imatinib mesylate, which inhibits PDGF and c-kit receptors [7], and AZD2171, an inhibitor of the VEGF receptor [8].

HISTOPATHOLOGY OF NEUROFIBROMA

The macroscopic appearance of solitary neurofibromas is variable and depends on location, the size of the nerve involved, and whether a single nerve or a deep nerve bundle or trunk is affected. Tumors growing along a nerve often have a fusiform shape (Figures 21.1A, B). Deeply situated tumors tend to be larger at the time of diagnosis. Preexisting structures, such as dorsal root ganglia, may be incorporated into the tumor. Neurofibromas may lack a distinct capsule, especially when originating from a small nerve. The cut surface often has a yellow-white or grey-tan, gelatinous appearance. The consistency is often soft or only moderately firm. PNFs, usually found in the context of NF1, may show a convoluted appearance (Figure 21.1C) when they occur in trunks of a nerve plexus. The complete surgical resection of such lesions may be difficult.

Microscopically, neurofibromas are characterized by the variable presence of wavy strands of collagen (Figure 21.1D), often without much architectural patterning. The collagenous fibers have been described as resembling "shredded carrots" (Figure 21.1E). A loose matrix of mucopolysaccharides is often present. The diffusely infiltrating growth of a neurofibroma may lead to the incorporation of adjacent preexisting structures, for example soft tissue elements and blood vessels. In a DNF, skin adnexal structures may be incorporated into the tumor. Architecturally, neurofibromas can easily be distinguished from schwannomas because they lack nuclear palisades and biphasic patterns [34]. Higher magnification demonstrates that neurofibromas are proliferations of neoplastic Schwann cells as the predominant cellular element (Figure 21.1E). Cells are mostly spindle shaped with small amounts of cytoplasm. Nuclei have a wavy and elongated or less commonly ovoid shape. They are generally significantly smaller than the nuclei of schwannomas. Some tumors may show multinucleated floret-like giant cells [35]. The chromatin is bland to slightly hyperchromatic, and nucleoli are small and indistinct. In addition to the neoplastic Schwann cells, there are other components derived from the peripheral nerve, such as fibroblasts and perineurial cells (Figure 21.1E). Occasional mast cells may be seen in the stroma [36,37], a feature that is also shared with schwannomas. Residual axons are present to varying degrees in a neurofibroma and tend to be less numerous in larger tumors. As in other neuroectodermal tumors [38,39], pigmentation (melanin) may sometimes be seen [40]. This *pigmented neurofibroma*, also known as melanotic neurofibroma, represents less than 1% of all neurofibromas. Such tumors contain neuromelanin granules, which can be highlighted with a melanin stain. Other frequently positive markers in these tumors are Melan-A, microphthalmia-associated transcription factor

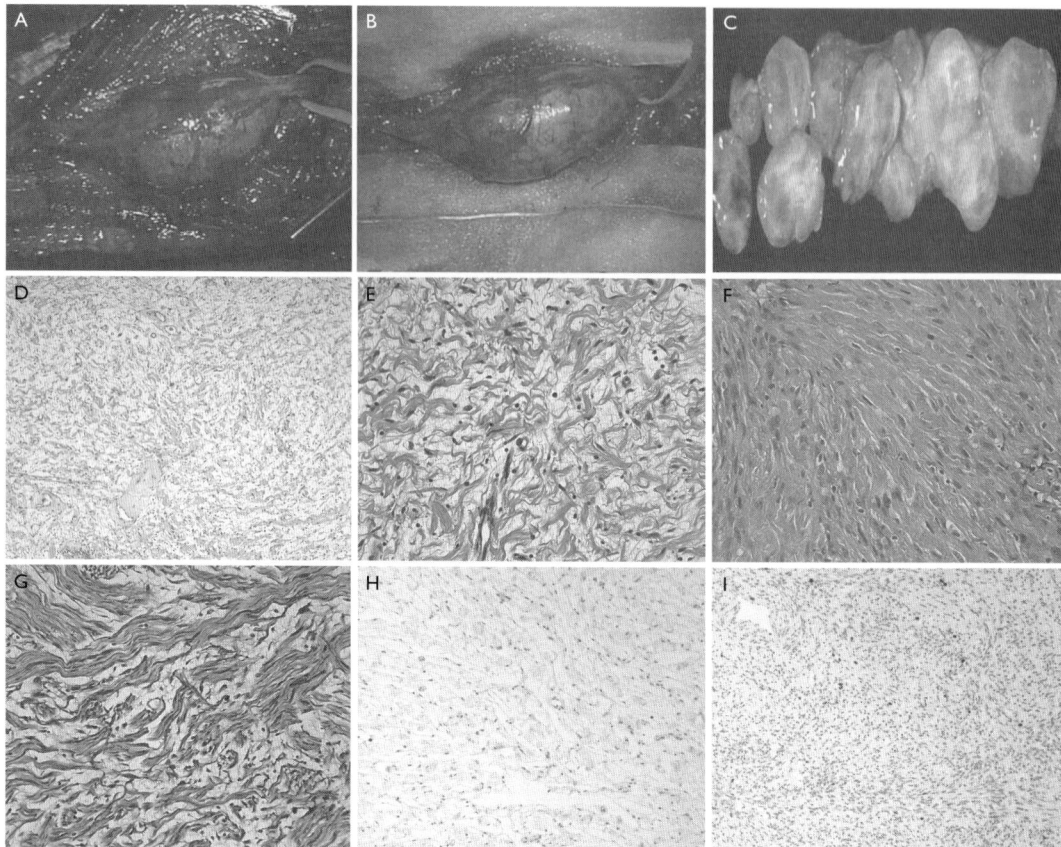

Figure 21.1 Neurofibromas often have a fusiform shape **(A, B)** because they tend to grow along a nerve. The cut surface often has a yellow-white or grey-tan, gelatinous appearance **(C)**. The consistency is often soft or only moderately firm. Microscopically, neurofibromas show wavy strands of collagen **(D)**, often without much architectural patterning. Higher magnification demonstrates that neurofibromas are proliferations of neoplastic Schwann cells as the predominant cellular element **(E)**, but also contain fibroblasts and perineurial cells. The collagenous fibers are sometimes described as resembling "shredded carrots." In an atypical neurofibroma **(F)**, there is increased cellularity and nuclear atypia. Neurofibromas are nearly always positive for S-100 **(G)**. The MIB-1 (KI-67) proliferation index is low in neurofibromas, labeling only 1% to 2% of nuclei **(H)**, but may reach 5% to 15 % in atypical neurofibromas **(I)**. See color insert.

(MITF), and variably HMB45 [41,42]. Among the diagnostic considerations are melanocytic tumors, melanotic schwannoma, and pigmented dermatofibrosarcoma protuberans (DFSP, Bednar tumor) [43].

The term *atypical neurofibroma* (Figure 21.1F) denotes those rare cases in which increased cellularity and nuclear atypia occur. This type of tumor is often symptomatic, showing both active cell growth and increased glucose uptake on 18-fluorodeoxyglucose-positron emission tomography [44,45]. Atypical neurofibroma is characterized by increased nuclear atypia, for example nuclear enlargement and hyperchromasia. In other words, this entity exhibits some features observed in both benign neurofibromas and low-grade MPNST [46]. Bizarre nuclei may be present. Mitotic activity is only mildly increased or may even be absent. Atypia can be a focal finding, involving only a portion of the tumor. As with regular neurofibromas, the primary differential diagnosis is schwannoma. In contrast, *cellular neurofibroma* does not have this degree of nuclear atypia but shows hypercellularity as a dominant feature [34,47]. Occasional mitotic figures may be present. There is no necrosis, which is an important feature to distinguish it from MPNST. Immunohistochemistry in cellular neurofibroma may show an increased MIB-1 (KI-67) proliferation index and an increased staining for p53. Among the principal differential diagnostic considerations are cellular schwannoma and MPNST. In superficial, especially cutaneous locations, an important differential diagnosis is DFSP, characterized by a storiform pattern and locally infiltrative behavior. Finally, *cellular neurofibroma with atypia* [45] has both increased nuclear atypia and small numbers of mitoses. It must be distinguished from MPNST. Histological signs of a transformation to MPNST include increased mitotic activity, nuclear pleomorphism, and regional necrosis. The tumor can also easily be mistaken for different types of soft tissue sarcoma, both histologically and cytologically. Immunohistochemistry may show loss of reactivity to S-100. P53 immunoreactivity seems to be similarly low as in neurofibroma [45].

The role of the *intraoperative consultation* in a neurofibroma case is twofold: (a) to exclude another type of peripheral nerve tumor, such as a schwannoma and (b) to detect features that may suggest the presence of atypia or malignancy. Nuclear atypia can be difficult to assess on a frozen sample because of distortion and other artifacts of freezing. Changes in personnel and specimen handling may introduce further variables. Therefore, a cytological preparation (smear) is often useful because it only minimally delays the diagnosis and provides excellent detail on nuclear features.

Immunohistochemistry may be required to distinguish neurofibromas from other neoplasms of the peripheral nerve. Neurofibromas are nearly always positive for S-100 (Figure 21.1G), although the staining intensity may vary and is less vigorous than in schwannomas. Intratumoral axons, individually and in bundles, can be demonstrated by immunohistochemistry for neurofilament or neuron-specific enolase. Axons are easier to demonstrate in smaller tumors and become more "diluted" in larger tumors. In schwannomas, axons are usually present in bundles, but more diffuse entrapment also occurs. Neurofibromas are generally fairly reactive to vimentin. Most neurofibromas contain certain numbers of cells that are positive for epithelial membrane antigen (EMA) [48,49]. These are perineurial cells, which are residual structures of the original perineurium. In large tumors, they are often strongly diluted, with only a few of these EMA-positive cells present, typically in the periphery of the lesion. This pattern helps to distinguish the tumor from a perineurioma, which has strong and ubiquitous EMA reactivity. As mentioned above, in superficial locations, a diagnosis of DFSP may be considered when the lesion is highly cellular. DFSPs are strongly positive for CD34 but negative for S-100. In contrast, neurofibromas only show CD34 expression in blood vessels and in small numbers of amoeboid dendritic cells that are also positive for factor XIIIa [50–52]. The MIB-1 (KI-67) cellular proliferation index in neurofibromas is low, labeling only approximately 1% to 2% of nuclei (Figure 21.1H) but reaches 5% to 15% in atypical neurofibromas (Figure 21.1I).

The principal *differential diagnostic* considerations for neurofibroma include schwannoma and other spindle-cell neoplasms associated with the peripheral nerve. The clinical importance of the distinction between neurofibroma and schwannoma lies in the association of neurofibroma with NF1 and the risk of progression to MPNST. Often, clinical parameters (e.g., stigmata of NF1) will help with the diagnosis. In some rare cases, further investigations may be required. Grossly, a neurofibroma is more likely to have a soft consistency, in contrast to a schwannoma, which is often firm. Immunoreactivity for S-100 is a feature that is shared with schwannomas and therefore cannot be used as a distinguishing criterion. The MIB-1 (KI-67) proliferation index can be similar in both tumors. However, the growth pattern of these two entities is often different: while neurofibromas tend to grow diffusely, leading to fusiform expansion of the nerve, schwannomas are more likely to exhibit extrafascicular growth.

Electron microscopy of a neurofibroma is only rarely indicated for diagnostic purposes. It reveals the various cellular components, for example Schwann cells, perineurial cells, fibroblasts, and occasional mast cells. Also present are axons, frequent basement membranes as well as a stroma that is rich in collagen fibers. Mucinous material may be visible on EM.

BACKGROUND ON MPNSTS

MPNSTs have also been referred to as neurogenic sarcoma, malignant schwannoma, and neurofibrosarcoma. They account for 3% to 10% of all soft tissue sarcomas, and approximately half of them arise from NF1-associated PNFs [1,53]. Individuals with NF1 have a 7% to 13% lifetime risk for developing MPNSTs [9]. This tumor may arise from a preexisting plexiform or subcutaneous neurofibroma but not from a cutaneous neurofibroma or DNF [54]. Clinical findings of an increase in tumor size, new neurological deficits, and pain should alert to the possibility of transformation from a benign PNF to MPNST. Despite recent advancements in imaging techniques [14], the radiologic diagnosis of PNF versus MPNST remains somewhat challenging. Several similarities between neurofibromas and MPNSTs exist, and MPNSTs often arise from a preexisting neurofibroma. First, the cell of origin is also the transformed Schwann cell. Both types of tumor are also characterized by their cellular heterogeneity. Both are a mixture of the primary transformed NF1−/− cells and various untransformed components of NF1+/− cells, significantly complicating the investigations. Similar to neurofibromas, MPNSTs contain large numbers of stromal cells, fibroblasts, vascular elements, and mast cells [55–57].

MOLECULAR PATHOGENESIS OF MPNSTS

The genetic alterations leading to the initiation and malignant transformation of MPNSTs are still largely unknown. A shared feature of neurofibromas and MPNSTs at the genetic level is the frequent LOH of the NF1 gene, resulting in decreased levels of neurofibromin [25,56]. This was observed in both NF1-related and sporadic MPNSTs [58]. In addition to the lack of neurofibromin, NF1-associated MPNSTs also have increased levels of activated RAS GTP compared with neurofibromas [25,32]. Feldkamp et al [30] measured the RAS activity in tumor tissue and found that the levels of activated RAS-GTP in NF1 MPNSTs and NF1 PNFs were 15 and 5 times higher, respectively, than in non-NF1 schwannomas. This supports the view that the RAS signaling pathway is crucial in the tumorigenesis of MPNSTs.

Aside from increased RAS levels secondary to a mutation in the NF1 gene, additional genetic abnormalities are necessary for the malignant transformation of a neurofibroma into an MPNST. These may involve inactivation of key cell cycle regulators such as p53, p27-kip1, and p16 [6,32,58]. MPNSTs have been found to harbor mutations in another tumor suppressor gene, p53, in addition to inactivation of the NF1 gene [26]. In support of this hypothesis, mutations in both NF1 and p53 in mice gave rise to the development of MPNSTs [26,32]. The loss of the p53 gene has been observed in many NF1 MPNSTs but not in benign neurofibromas, resulting in abnormalities in DNA damage-induced cell cycle arrest and apoptosis [7].

LOH in the CDKN2A gene, also known as INK4A gene, has also been observed in MPNSTs. This gene encodes two tumor suppressor genes, p16^{INK4A} and p14^{ARF} [7,56]. Loss of p16^{INK4A} leads to a failure to inactivate the cyclin D/cdk4 complex that promotes retinoblastoma proliferation, which in turn results in a release of inhibition of E2F, increasing cellular proliferation [7]. On the other hand, loss of p14^{ARF} protein stabilizes and activates p53 pathways by inhibiting the Mdm-2-induced p53 degradation and transactivational silencing [7]. Another cell cycle regulator, p27^{Kip1}, has also been implicated [56]. Overall, increased mitogenic activity resulting from a combination of neurofibromin loss and defective cell cycle control and tumor surveillance may be involved in malignant transformation.

Chromosomal imbalances in MPNSTs may contribute to malignant transformation. Pandita et al [27] found chromosomal gains in the DNA of transformed MPNST cells. Gains in chromosomes 7, 8q, 15q, and 17q have been reported, as have chromosomal losses and amplifications [7]. Levy et al [59] found that the expression of 28 of 489 genes was significantly different between MPNSTs and PNFs. The altered genes were mainly involved in cell proliferation, senescence, apoptosis, and extracellular matrix remodeling. Meanwhile, the other genes were involved in the RAS and Hedgehog-Gli signaling pathways. These results suggest that the Hedgehog-Gli pathway may be involved in the malignant transformation of PNFs [58].

There is increased gene expression and protein upregulation of certain cell growth mediators in MPNSTs, especially EGFR [25,31,56]. Activation of EGFR by the EGF mitogen results in the inactivation of RAS and other small signaling proteins [56]. Other upregulated proteins include MMP-13, PDGF-α, hepatocyte growth factor, pigment epithelium-derived growth factor, VEGF, and EGF [6,7,25]. These growth factors stimulate cell proliferation or survival, support invasion, and stimulate angiogenesis.

Certain molecules have been implicated in invasion and metastasis in MPNSTs. One such molecule is CD44, a cell surface glycoprotein that plays a role in cell-cell adhesion, cell migration, growth factor signaling, and metastasis [31,54]. It has been found that high levels of CD44 expression in MPNST cells contribute to their invasive behavior [31]. Increased levels of another molecule, brain lipid-binding protein, have been found in mouse and human MPNSTs [31].

Several molecular risk factors characterize the development of MPNSTs. A particular microdeletion in the NF1 gene has been identified as a risk factor [54,60], with the lifetime risk for MPNST in patients with NF1 microdeletion twice that of the general NF1 population [60]. Levy et al [19] described a gene expression profile, which identified PNFs most likely to undergo malignant transformation. This profile is based on the following genes: MMP9, FLT4/VEGFR3, TNFRSF10B/TRAILR2, SHH, and GLI1 [19].

Future Directions

Biologically targeted therapies for MPNSTs are basically similar to those of PNFs because the two share several common elements in their pathogenesis. Farnesyltransferase inhibitors prevent the anchoring of RAS to the cell membrane, thereby blocking its activation. This drug has been found to inhibit the growth of an NF1 MPNST cell line in vitro [7]. Agents that block the downstream signaling pathways of RAS activation also show promise. In a recently completed study, a MEK inhibitor, ARRY-509, and a mammalian target of rapamycin inhibitor, rapamycin, have been found to significantly inhibit the growth of NF1 MPNST in vivo [9]. MMP inhibitors with a high selectivity for MMP9 could also be considered [19].

HISTOPATHOLOGY OF MPNST

The pathological diagnosis of MPNST remains challenging, due in part to issues of heterogeneity and paucity of clearly defined histological criteria. The macroscopic appearance of MPNSTs is highly variable. These tumors arise from a peripheral nerve, which is almost always the trunk of a large nerve or plexus of the extremities or the neck. They are typically fusiform, oval, or multilobulated masses that average 5 cm in diameter [61]. They can be enveloped by a thin fibrous capsule, although this is more likely to be a pseudocapsule of infiltrated adjacent tissue. Often, no apparent capsule can be demonstrated, and surrounding tissues, such as fat, are rather diffusely infiltrated (Figure 21.2A). Peripheral nerves can often be seen entering and exiting the lesion. When situated near central nervous system (CNS) tissue, such as in spinal intradural locations, there may be invasion of CNS parenchyma [62]. The cut surface is white to yellow and may show areas of hemorrhage and necrosis. The consistency is also variable and may show soft and firm regions.

MPNSTs are histologically heterogenous, and therefore, multiple samplings are required because some regions may retain their benign PNF characteristics, whereas other regions may show varying grades of malignancy and dedifferentiation. Microscopically, these neoplasms have highly variable features. Their cellularity tends to be even higher than in cellular neurofibroma. In addition, characteristic low-power tissue patterns are present. In high-grade tumors, these include well-delineated areas of "geographic" necrosis (Figure 21.2B), which occur in more than 70% of MPNSTs. This pattern can resemble the necrosis seen in many glioblastomas, although nuclear palisading around necrosis is rare. MPNSTs often have large, monomorphic sheets of cells. A herringbone-type pattern of interlacing fascicles and sheets is often seen (Figure 21.2C), resembling fibrosarcoma. Loose and paucicellular areas may occur and may represent regions that retain the morphology of the original lower-grade lesion [63]. At higher magnification, cells are often spindle shaped and have variable amounts of eosinophilic cytoplasm (Figure 21.2D). They have elongated hyperchromatic nuclei that are often many times larger than those of a typical neurofibroma. In addition, large numbers of small, round, and hyperchromatic nuclei may be present. Mitotic activity is often brisk (Figure 21.2E).

Grading is performed on the basis of cellularity, presence of necrosis, nuclear pleomorphism, and mitotic activity. Most MPNSTs are of high histological grade. Only

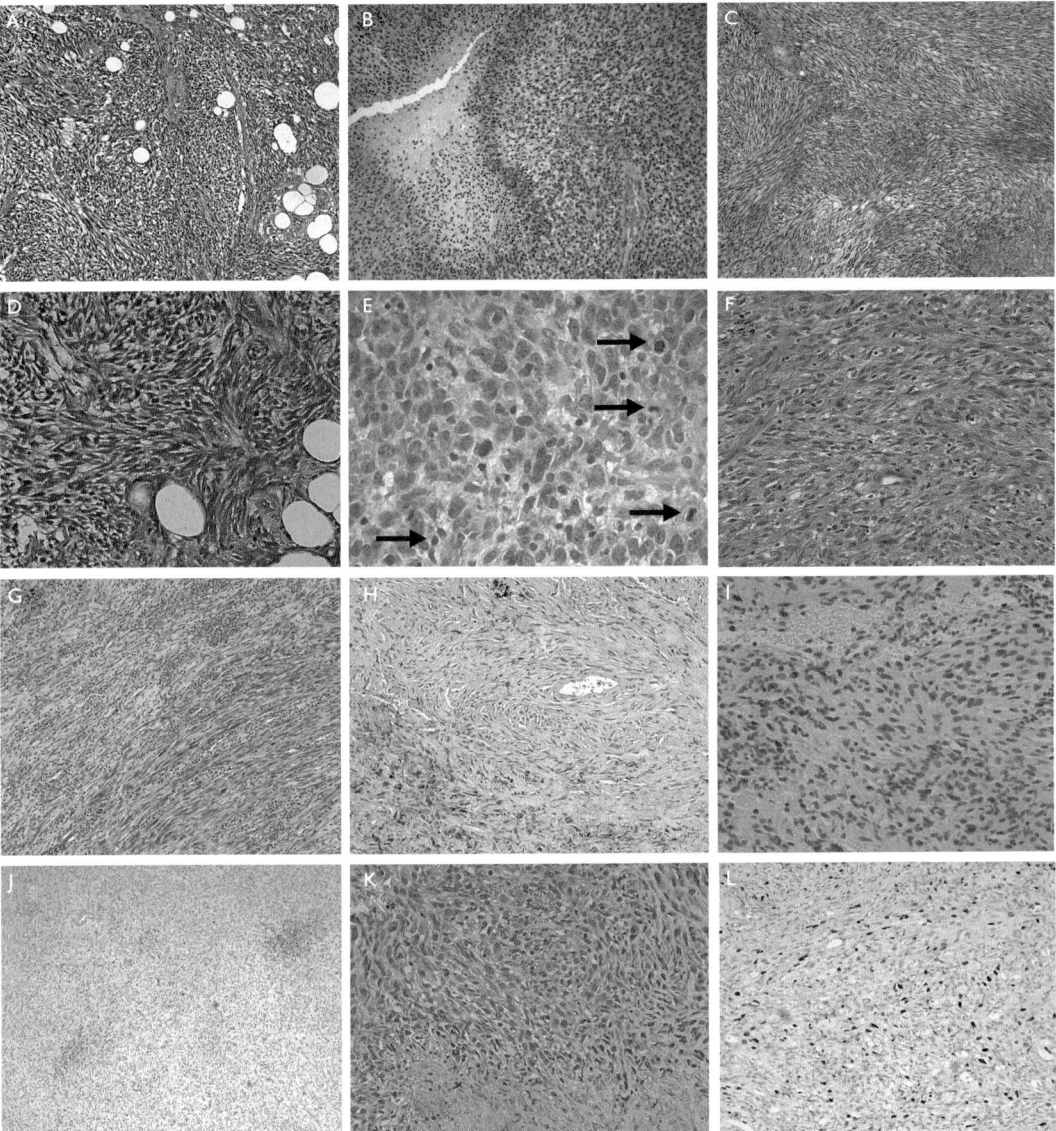

Figure 21.2 MPNST can often diffusely invade surrounding tissues so that adjacent structures such as adipose tissue become incorporated into the tumor (**A**). Cellularity is high, and there are often well-delineated areas of "geographic" necrosis (**B**). A herringbone-type pattern of interlacing fascicles and sheets may be seen (**C**), resembling fibrosarcoma. At higher magnification, cells are often spindle-shaped and have variable amounts of eosinophilic cytoplasm (**D**). They have large, hyperchromatic nuclei and brisk mitotic activity (**E**). In low-grade MPNST, there is no necrosis, cellularity tends to be lower, and nuclei are smaller (**F**). One of several variant histological types is the so-called "MPNST with mesenchymal differentiation," here shown with immunoreactivity to smooth muscle actin (SMA; **G**). Reactivity for S-100 is inversely correlated with tumor grade and can be only focal in high-grade MPNSTs (**H**). Immunoreactivity for p53 is common in MPNST (**I**). Intratumoral lymphocytes can give the appearance of increased cellularity and can be highlighted with a CD45 stain (**J**). Vimentin is usually positive (**K**). The KI-67 (MIB-1) proliferation index is markedly increased in high-grade MPNST, easily labeling 20% to 50% of nuclei (**L**). *See color insert.*

a minority of about 10% can be classified as low-grade MPNST [64]. In the World Health Organization system, tumors with necrosis are classified as grade IV, whereas tumors without necrosis are grade III [64]. In well-differentiated tumors, the spectrum overlaps with cellular neurofibroma. Low-grade MPNSTs are relatively less cellular, show less nuclear hyperchromasia, and have a reduced number of mitoses [61] (Figure 21.2F).

Several histological *variant forms* of MPNST have been recognized, with approximately 15% to 20% of MPNSTs showing some degree of divergent differentiation [65]. The most common among these are rhabdomyoblastic and other heterologous mesenchymal elements. These rare tumors are referred to as malignant triton tumor (MTT) or "MPNST with mesenchymal differentiation." This tumor was first described in a patient with NF1 [66]. About two thirds of MTT cases occur in NF1 [67]. Histologically in MTT, rhabdomyoblasts are mixed in among the more typical cells of a high-grade MPNST. By immunohistochemistry, they may be positive for markers of muscle differentiation, such as myoglobin, myogenin, and smooth muscle actin (Figure 21.2G). Other mesenchymal elements, such as osteosarcomatous or chondrosarcomatous differentiation, may rarely be seen in MPNST. Another variant is epithelioid MPNST, which makes up approximately 5% of MPNSTs. It has a nodular growth pattern and is composed of plump, polygonal epithelial-like cells. It may resemble carcinoma or melanoma and has to be distinguished from these. Another subtype is the MPNST with glandular differentiation, characterized by well-differentiated gland-forming epithelium and mucin secretion. The important distinction of this tumor from metastatic adenocarcinoma may be complicated by the fact that the glands may be cytokeratin immunopositive [68].

The *intraoperative consultation* plays an important role in the management of MPNSTs because its results can significantly affect the extent of surgical resection. In situations in which the resection of the affected nerve is of little or no clinical significance, wide local excision may be attempted. The often large size of an MPNST necessitates the preparation of multiple samples from different areas for frozen section. Some of the samples may show features of an earlier tumor stage, for example PNF. The presence of palisading of cells around areas of necrosis is helpful in distinguishing high-grade MPNST from lower-grade lesions such as cellular neurofibroma or a large cellular schwannoma. A cytological preparation (smear) can demonstrate the spindle-shaped cytomorphology and the presence of mitoses in cases in which no necrosis is present.

The *ultrastructural examination* is not typically helpful in the diagnosis of MPNST because of the poor differentiation level of this tumor. Rarely, a degree of neuroendocrine differentiation [69] or perineurial differentiation [70] can be demonstrated by electron microscopy.

Immunohistochemistry plays an important role in the workup of these tumors. Reactivity for S-100 is only seen in approximately 50% to 70% of MPNSTs and is inversely correlated with tumor grade: high-grade MPNSTs can show only focal staining [71,72] (Figure 21.2H). Immunoreactivity for p53 is common in MPNST, whereas it is unusual in neurofibroma [73] (Figure 21.2I). CD57 (Leu7) expression is variably present [74]. Frequently there are collections of lymphocytes, which can give the appearance of increased cellularity. They can be highlighted with a CD45 stain (Figure 21.2J). Vimentin is usually positive (Figure 21.2K). EMA is only occasionally seen in the standard variety of MPNSTs but is more common in the subtype with glandular differentiation, which may also express keratin and carcino-embryonic antigen (CEA) [68]. The KI-67 (MIB-1) proliferation index is markedly increased in high-grade MPNST, easily labeling 20% to 50% of nuclei (Figure 21.2L). The results are much less conclusive for low-grade MPNST, where the proliferation index can be so low as to overlap with findings in neurofibromas [14].

The *differential diagnosis* of MPNST is complex because of the rather variable histomorphology. The most important considerations are other highly cellular neoplasms that originate from peripheral nerve. In the absence of areas of necrosis and with a low mitotic activity, consideration should be given to cellular neurofibroma instead of low-grade MPNST. No standardized criteria for the distinction of high-grade MPNST from various types of soft tissue sarcomas currently exist. Fibrosarcomas often have a "herringbone" pattern at low power, which is sometimes seen in MPNST. However, cytologically fibrosarcoma can resemble MPNST closely. Fibrosarcomas are also typically negative for S-100. Leiomyosarcoma may resemble MPNST but is usually immunopositive for muscle-specific markers such as smooth muscle actin or desmin and negative for S-100. In locations near the vertebral column, synovial sarcoma can be considered, which would be positive for EMA or cytokeratin. Biphasic synovial sarcoma may be confused with glandular MPNST or metastatic adenocarcinoma. Molecular studies for the characteristic translocation t(x;18)(p11.2;q11.2) will help with the diagnosis [75]. The morphological features of hemangiopericytoma (HPC) can sometimes be similar to those of an MPNST and include high cellularity and mitotic activity. However, areas of necrosis are uncommon in HPC. Nuclear pleomorphism can be much lower in HPC than in MPNST. HPC is also often highly vascular. Morphological clues such as the characteristic "staghorn" branching vasculature in HPC should help in making the distinction. Immunohistochemistry for HPC is almost never positive for S-100 but often reactive for CD34. The morphology of malignant melanoma can be highly variable and can be confused with the epithelioid variant of MPNST in particular. Immunohistochemistry for HMB45 and Melan-A may help with the diagnosis, whereas S-100 is less useful. Epithelioid MPNST may also be confused with various forms of metastatic carcinoma. In locations near CNS tissue, high-grade glioma (glioblastoma) may be considered, which can be morphologically indistinguishable from MPNST but would frequently have strong glial fibrillary acidic protein (GFAP) reactivity.

REFERENCES

1. Bhattacharyya AK, Perrin R, Guha A. Peripheral nerve tumors: management strategies and molecular insights. *J Neurooncol*. 2004;69:335–349.
2. Huson SM, Compston DA, Clark P, Harper PS. A genetic study of von Recklinghausen neurofibromatosis in south east Wales I: prevalence, fitness, mutation rate, and effect of parental transmission on severity. *J Med Genet*. 1989;26:704–711.
3. Lynch TM, Gutmann DH. Neurofibromatosis 1. *Neurol Clin*. 2002, 20:841–865.
4. Korf BR. Clinical features and pathobiology of neurofibromatosis 1. *J Child Neurol*. 2002;17:573–577; discussion 602–604, 646–651.
5. Friedman JM. Neurofibromatosis 1: clinical manifestations and diagnostic criteria. *J Child Neurol*. 2002;17:548–554.
6. Packer RJ, Gutmann DH, Rubenstein A, et al. Plexiform neurofibromas in NF1: toward biologic-based therapy. *Neurology*. 2002;58:1461–1470.
7. Gottfried ON, Viskochil DH, Fults DW, Couldwell WT. Molecular, genetic, and cellular pathogenesis of neurofibromas and surgical implications. *Neurosurgery*. 2006;58:1–16.
8. Williams VC, Lucas J, Babcock MA, Gutmann DH, Korf B, Maria BL. Neurofibromatosis type 1 revisited. *Pediatrics*. 2009;123:124–133.
9. Evans DG, Baser ME, McGaughran J, Sharif S, Howard E, Moran A. Malignant peripheral nerve sheath tumours in neurofibromatosis 1. *J Med Genet*. 2002;39:311–314.

10. Tucker T, Wolkenstein P, Revuz J, Zeller J, Friedman JM. Association between benign and malignant peripheral nerve sheath tumors in NF1. *Neurology*. 2005;65:205–211.
11. Hosoi K. Multiple neurofibromatosis (von Recklinghausen disease) with special reference to malignant transformation. *Arch Surg*. 1931;22:265–281.
12. Sørensen SA, Mulvihill JJ, Nielsen A. Long-term follow-up of von Recklinghausen neurofibromatosis. Survival and malignant neoplasms. *N Engl J Med*. 1986;314:1010–1015.
13. Wong WW, Hirose T, Scheithauer BW, Schild SE, Gunderson LL. Malignant peripheral nerve sheath tumor: analysis of treatment outcome. *Int J Radiat Oncol Biol Phys*. 1998;42:351–360.
14. Karabatsou K, Kiehl TR, Wilson DM, Hendler A, Guha A. Potential role of 18fluorodeoxyglucose-positron emission tomography/computed tomography in differentiating benign neurofibroma from malignant peripheral nerve sheath tumor associated with neurofibromatosis 1. *Neurosurgery*. 2009;65(4 Suppl):160–170.
15. Delbeke D. Oncological applications of FDG PET imaging: brain tumors, colorectal cancer lymphoma and melanoma. *J Nucl Med*. 1999;4:591–603.
16. Di Chiro G, DeLaPaz RL, Brooks RA, et al. Glucose utilization of cerebral gliomas measured by [18F] fluorodeoxyglucose and positron emission tomography. *Neurology*. 1982;32:1323–1329.
17. Lucas JD, O'Doherty MJ, Cronin BF, et al. Prospective evaluation of soft tissue masses and sarcomas using fluorodeoxyglucose positron emission tomography. *Br J Surg*. 1999;86:550–556.
18. Nieweg OE, Pruim J, van Ginkel RJ, et al. Fluorine-18-fluorodeoxyglucose PET imaging of soft-tissue sarcoma. *J Nucl Med*. 1996;37:257–261.
19. Levy P, Bieche I, Leroy K, et al. Molecular profiles of neurofibromatosis type 1-associated plexiform neurofibromas: identification of a gene expression signature of poor prognosis. *Clin Cancer Res*. 2004;10:3763–3771.
20. Kluwe L, Friedrich R, Mautner VF. Loss of NF1 allele in Schwann cells but not in fibroblasts derived from an NF1-associated neurofibroma. *Genes Chromosomes Cancer*. 1999;24:283–285.
21. Seizinger BR, Rouleau GA, Ozelius LJ, et al. Genetic linkage of von Recklinghausen neurofibromatosis to the nerve growth factor receptor gene. *Cell*. 1987;49:589–594.
22. Serra E, Rosenbaum T, Winner U, et al. Schwann cells harbor the somatic NF1 mutation in neurofibromas: evidence of two different Schwann cell subpopulations. *Hum Mol Genet*.2000;9: 3055–3064.
23. Nordling C. A new theory on cancer-inducing mechanism. *Br J Cancer*. 1953;7:68–72.
24. Knudson AG. Mutation and cancer: statistical study of retinoblastoma. *Proc Natl Acad Sci USA*. 1971;68: 820–823.
25. Lakkis MM, Tennekoon GI. Neurofibromatosis type 1: general overview. *J Neurosci Res*. 2000;62:755–763.
26. Reed N, Gutmann DH. Tumorigenesis in neurofibromatosis: new insights and potential therapies. *Trends Mol Med*. 2001;7:157–162.
27. Pandita A, Bereskin L, Mukherjee J, Karim Z, Shannon P, Guha A. Construction of a high-resolution genetic alteration map of early and progressive changes in transformed cells in neurofibromas using laser capture microdissection and arrayCGH, submitted to Neoplasia.
28. Bhola P, Banerjee S, Mukherjee J, et al. Preclinical in vivo evaluation of rapamycin in human malignant peripheral nerve sheath explant xenograft. *Int J Cancer*. 2010;126:563–571.
29. Yohay KH. The genetic and molecular pathogenesis of NF1 and NF2. *Semin Pediatr Neurol*. 2006;13:21–26.
30. Feldkamp MM, Angelov L, Guha A. Neurofibromatosis type 1 peripheral nerve tumors: aberrant activation of the Ras pathway. *Surg Neurol*. 1999;51:211–218.
31. Arun D, Gutmann DH. Recent advances in neurofibromatosis type 1. *Curr Opin Neurol*. 2004;17:101–105.
32. Ferner RE, O'Doherty MJ. Neurofibroma and schwannoma. *Curr Opin Neurol*. 2002;15:679–684.
33. Radovanovic I, Guha A. Neurogenetics and the molecular biology of human brain tumors. In: Kaye AH, Laws ER, eds. *Brain Tumors*. 3rd ed. In press.
34. Enzinger FM, Weiss SW. Benign and malignant tumors of peripheral nerves. In: Enzinger FM, Weiss SW, eds. *Soft Tissue Tumors*. 3rd ed. St. Louis, MO: Mosby-Year Book; 1995:829–863.
35. Magro G, Amico P, Vecchio GM, et al. Multinucleated floret-like giant cells in sporadic and NF1-associated neurofibromas: a clinicopathologic study of 94 cases. *Virchows Arch*. 2010;456:71–76.
36. Johnson MD, Kamso-Pratt J, Federspiel CF, Whetsell WO Jr. Mast cell and lymphoreticular infiltrates in neurofibromas. Comparison with nerve sheath tumors. *Arch Pathol Lab Med*. 1989;113:1263–1270.
37. Pineda A. Mast cells—their presence and ultrastructural characteristics in peripheral nerve tumors. *Arch Neurol*. 1965;13:372–382.
38. Bednar B. Storiform neurofibromas of the skin, pigmented and non-pigmented. *Cancer*. 1957;10:368–376.
39. Bird CC, Willis RA. The histogenesis of pigmented neurofibromas. *J Pathol*. 1969;97:631–637.
40. Williamson DM, Suggit RI. Pigmented neurofibroma. *Br J Dermatol*. 1977;97:685–688.
41. Fetsch JF, Michal M, Miettinen M. Pigmented (melanotic) neurofibroma: a clinicopathologic and immunohistochemical analysis of 19 lesions from 17 patients. *Am J Surg Pathol*. 2000;24:331–343.
42. Motoi T, Ishida T, Kawato A, Motoi N, Fukayama M. Pigmented neurofibroma: review of Japanese patients with an analysis of melanogenesis demonstrating coexpression of c-met protooncogene and microphthalmia-associated transcription factor. *Hum Pathol*. 2005;36:871–877.
43. Dupree WB, Langloss JM, Weiss SW. Pigmented dermatofibrosarcoma protuberans (Bednar tumor). A pathologic, ultrastructural, and immunohistochemical study. *Am J Surg Pathol*. 1985;9:630–639.
44. Ferner RE, Gutmann DH. International consensus statement on malignant peripheral nerve sheath tumors in neurofibromatosis. *Cancer Res*. 2002;62:1573–1577.
45. Woodruff JM, Horten BC, Erlandson RA. Pathology of peripheral nerves and paragangliomas. In: Silverberg SG, ed. *Principles and Practice of Surgical Pathology*. New York: Wiley; 1983:1509–1515.
46. Brems H, Beert E, de Ravel T, Legius E. Mechanisms in the pathogenesis of malignant tumours in neurofibromatosis type 1. *Lancet Oncol*. 2009;10:508–515.
47. Coffin CM, Dehner LP. Cellular peripheral neural tumors (neurofibromas) in children and adolescents: a clinicopathological and immunohistochemical study. *Pediatr Pathol*. 1990;10:351–361.
48. Theaker JM, Fletcher CD. Epithelial membrane antigen expression by the perineurial cell: further studies of peripheral nerve lesions. *Histopathology*. 1989;14:581–592.
49. Scheithauer BW, Woodruff JM, Erlandson RA. *Tumors of the Peripheral Nervous System*. Washington DC: Armed Forces Institute of Pathology; 1999.
50. Khalifa MA, Montgomery EA, Ismiil N, Azumi N. What are the CD34+ cells in benign peripheral nerve sheath tumors? Double immunostaining study of CD34 and S-100 protein. *Am J Clin Pathol*. 2000;114:123–126.
51. Takata M, Imai T, Hirone T. Factor-XIIIa-positive cells in normal peripheral nerves and cutaneous neurofibromas of type-1 neurofibromatosis. *Am J Dermatopathol*. 1994;16:37–43.
52. Weiss SW, Nickoloff BJ. CD-34 is expressed by a distinctive cell population in peripheral nerve, nerve sheath tumors, and related lesions. *Am J Surg Pathol*. 1993;17:1039–1045.
53. McCarron KF, Goldblum JR. Plexiform neurofibroma with and without associated malignant peripheral nerve sheath tumor: a clinicopathologic and immunohistochemical analysis of 54 cases. *Mod Pathol*. 1998;11:612–617.
54. Ferner RE. Neurofibromatosis 1 and neurofibromatosis 2: a twenty first century perspective. *Lancet Neurol*. 2007;6:340–351.
55. Lynch TM, Gutmann DH. Neurofibromatosis 1. *Neurol Clin*. 2002;20:841–865.
56. Dasgupta B, Gutmann DH: Neurofibromatosis 1. Closing the GAP between mice and men. *Curr Opin Genet Dev*. 2003;13:20–27.
57. Feldkamp MM, Gutmann DH, Guha A. Neurofibromatosis type 1: piecing the puzzle together. *Can J Neurol Sci*. 1998;25:181–191.
58. Frahm S, Mautner VF, Brems H, et al. Genetic and phenotypic characterization of tumor cells derived from malignant peripheral nerve sheath tumors of neurofibromatosis type 1 patients. *Neurobiol Dis*. 2004;16:85–91.
59. Levy P, Vidaud D, Leroy K, et al. Molecular profiling of malignant peripheral nerve sheath tumors associated with neurofibromatosis type 1, based on large-scale real-time RT-PCR. *Mol Cancer*. 2004;3:20.
60. De Raedt T, Brems H, Wolkenstein P, et al. Elevated risk for MPNST in NF1 microdeletion patients. *Am J Hum Genet*. 2003;72:1288–1292.

61. Ducatman BS, Scheithauer BW, Piepgras DG, Reiman HM, Ilstrup DM. Malignant peripheral nerve sheath tumors. A clinicopathologic study of 120 cases. *Cancer*. 1986;57:2006–2021.
62. Deinsberger W, Kästner S, Schachenmayr W, Böker DK. Malignant peripheral nerve sheath tumour infiltrating the spinal cord. *Acta Neurochir (Wien)*. 2000;142:1071–1072.
63. Spurlock G, Knight SJ, Thomas N, Kiehl TR, Guha A, Upadhyaya M. Molecular evolution of a neurofibroma to malignant peripheral nerve sheath tumour (MPNST) in an NF1 patient: correlation between histopathological, clinical, and molecular findings. *J Cancer Res Clin Oncol*. 2010 Mar 15 (Epub ahead of print).
64. Louis DN, Ohgaki H, Wiestler OD, Cavenee WK, eds. *WHO Classification of Tumours of the Central Nervous System*. 4th ed. Geneva, Switzerland: World Health Organization; 2007.
65. Ducatman BS, Scheithauer BW. Malignant peripheral nerve sheath tumors with divergent differentiation. *Cancer*. 1984;54:1049–1057.
66. Masson P. *Recklinghausen's Neurofibromatosis. Sensory Neuromas and Motor Neuromas*. New York: International Press; 1932:2.
67. Brooks JS, Freeman M, Enterline HT. Malignant "Triton" tumors. Natural history and immunohistochemistry of nine new cases with literature review. *Cancer*. 1985;55:2543–2549.
68. Woodruff JM, Christensen WN. Glandular peripheral nerve sheath tumors. *Cancer*. 1993;72:3618–3628.
69. Christensen WN, Strong EW, Bains MS, Woodruff JM. Neuroendocrine differentiation in the glandular peripheral nerve sheath tumor. Pathologic distinction from the biphasic synovial sarcoma with glands. *Am J Surg Pathol*. 1988;12:417–426.
70. Hirose T, Scheithauer BW, Sano T. Perineurial malignant peripheral nerve sheath tumor (MPNST): a clinicopathologic, immunohistochemical, and ultrastructural study of seven cases. *Am J Surg Pathol*. 1998;22:1368–1378.
71. Daimaru Y, Hashimoto H, Enjoji M. Malignant peripheral nerve-sheath tumors (malignant schwannomas). An immunohistochemical study of 29 cases. *Am J Surg Pathol*. 1985;9:434–444.
72. Weiss SW, Langloss JM, Enzinger FM. Value of S-100 protein in the diagnosis of soft tissue tumors with particular reference to benign and malignant Schwann cell tumors. *Lab Invest*. 1983;49:299–308.
73. Halling KC, Scheithauer BW, Halling AC, et al. p53 expression in neurofibroma and malignant peripheral nerve sheath tumor. An immunohistochemical study of sporadic and NF1-associated tumors. *Am J Clin Pathol*. 1996;106:282–288.
74. Zhou H, Coffin CM, Perkins SL, Tripp SR, Liew M, Viskochil DH. Malignant peripheral nerve sheath tumor: a comparison of grade, immunophenotype, and cell cycle/growth activation marker expression in sporadic and neurofibromatosis 1-related lesions. *Am J Surg Pathol*. 2003;27:1337–1345.
75. Coindre JM, Pelmus M, Hostein I, Lussan C, Bui BN, Guillou L. Should molecular testing be required for diagnosing synovial sarcoma? A prospective study of 204 cases. *Cancer*. 2003;98:2700–2707.

22 The 'Cell of Origin' for Common Pediatric Brain Tumors

Livia Garzia, Jessica Dawn Kessler, Robert J. Wechsler-Reya, and Michael David Taylor

Current dogma states that most cancers, including pediatric brain tumors, arise from a single transformed normal cell. Efforts to determine the cell of origin for the various histological subtypes of pediatric brain tumors have shown some recent success building on a very long history. Very early efforts to classify brain tumors noted the similarity between cell types in the developing human brain and the various histological types of brain tumors. The extent to which oncology recapitulates ontogeny is thought to be particularly marked among pediatric brain tumors. Identification of the cell of origin of pediatric brain tumors is thought to be of benefit as it will improve our pathological classification system and help us understand the biology of the various histologies, more effectively model specific histologies in other organisms, and ultimately develop novel and more effective therapeutics strategies. Recent advances in understanding the normal development of the nervous system, particularly in the area of stem cell biology, have lead to an explosion of data on the cell of origin for many pediatric brain tumors.

In the early 1960s, Altman et al [1,2] demonstrated that neurogenesis in the mammalian brain extends beyond the embryonic and early postnatal period, as new neurons are continuously added in specific regions of the brain. But it was not until the early 1990s it was demonstrated that neurons are generated from neural stem cells (NSCs), which can be taken from the adult brain and propagated in culture supplemented with epidermal growth factor and fibroblast growth factor. These tissue culture conditions promote the formation of spherical aggregates termed "neurospheres," which have the potential to both self-renew and differentiate into cells of all 3 major neural lineages: neurons, oligodendrocytes, and astrocytes [3] (Figure 22.1). Only a subpopulation of cells within a neurosphere are true NSCs. Although it has been suggested that some brain tumors may arise through dedifferentiation of more mature, differentiated cells [4], the preponderance of the current literature suggests that brain tumors arise from less differentiated cell populations such as stem cells or progenitors (Figure 22.2). Among the earliest lines of evidence that brain tumors may arise from transformation of NSCs or progenitor cells came from studies in the early 1970s, in which inoculation with avian sarcoma viruses resulted in intracranial tumors [5,6]. The observation that brain tumors retain an undifferentiated phenotype, being mostly composed of densely packed proliferating cells is supportive of a nondifferentiated cell of origin [7].

More recently, other types of evidence have also suggested that brain tumors may arise from transformation of NSCs or progenitor cells. Microarray experiments have shown that human medulloblastomas share similar gene expression patterns with cells of the normal developing brain. At molecular level, developmental signaling pathways such as Sonic Hedgehog (Shh), Notch, and Wnt, which are key regulators of stem cell and progenitor growth and differentiation, have been shown to be mutated or activated in brain tumors [8–10]. These findings highlight the similarities in the mechanisms that normal stem cells and cancer cells employ for self-renewal. Our model of the brain tumor cell of origin has evolved as researchers have defined the expression patterns of molecular markers of pluripotency or differentiation. Glial fibrillary acidic protein (GFAP) has been traditionally defined as one of the markers of terminal differentiation in the astrocyte lineage [11,12]. However, when its promoter was used to drive expression of avian retrovirus receptors, allowing (through infection with avian retroviruses) restricted expression of oncogenes such as *Kras* and *Akt*, no tumor formation was seen. When the same strategy was applied using the Nestin promoter, tumors formed in 7 of 27 mice. The authors concluded that GFAP-expressing cells represented terminally differentiated astrocytes and that undifferentiated (Nestin positive) neural or glial progenitors were more likely to act as the cell of origin for glioblastoma [13]. More recently these conclusions have been challenged in a spontaneously occurring animal model of low- and high-grade astrocytoma based on the expression of an activated form of p21-ras, the oncogene expression was driven by the GFAP promoter in a transgenic mouse. In this model, GFAP positive cells are still "competent" to give rise to tumors after an initiating event [14,15]. Further research on the expression of GFAP in the adult mammalian brain showed that astrocytes globally indeed possess NSC attributes during embryonic and early postnatal development [16,17]. These attributes disappear near the end of the second postnatal week, except for subventricular zone (SVZ) astrocytes, which continue to form neurospheres even when derived from adult animals.

Although recent findings support the hypothesis that the cell of origin of brain tumors is a NSC or progenitor cell, the alternative interpretation—that mature cells can

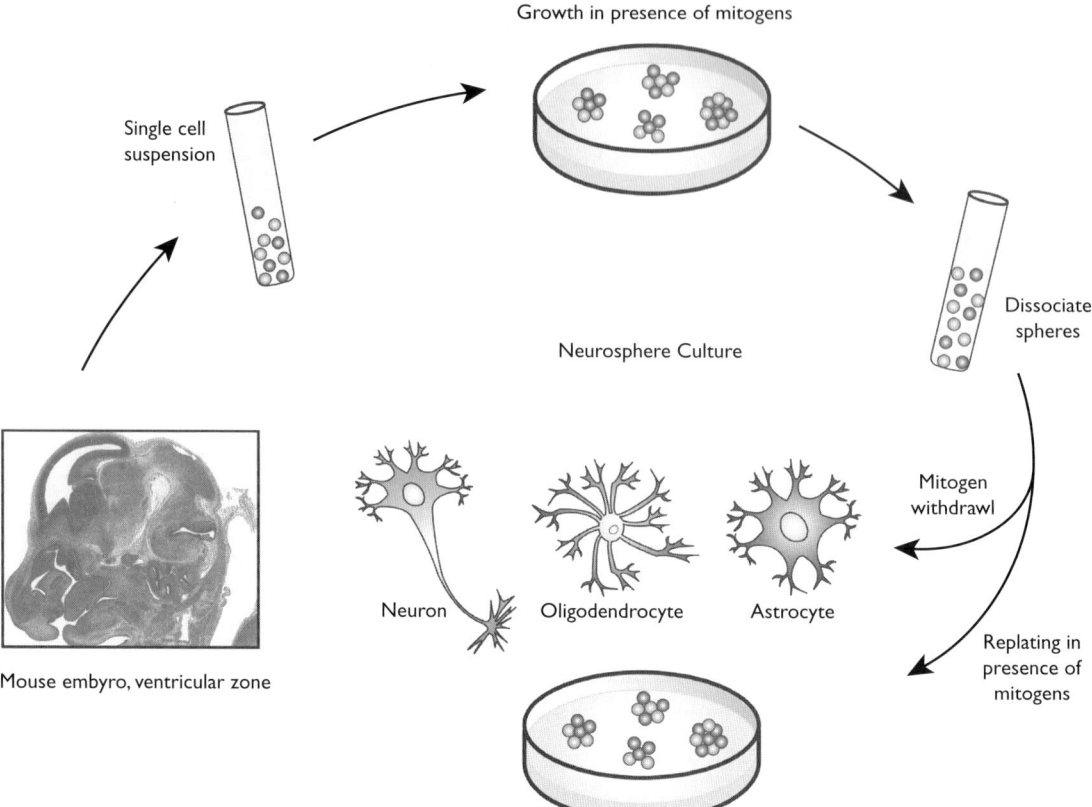

Figure 22.1 The neurosphere culture. The subventricular zone of an embryo of 14 to 15 days is removed and enzymatically digested to give a single cell suspension. The cells are then cultured in presence of growth factors as βFGF and EGF. In these conditions, the cells maintain their pluripotency only if deprived of mitogens differentiate producing mature neurons, oligodendrocytes, and astrocytes.

be induced to dedifferentiate by initiating events—has recently been reexplored in the context of retinoblastoma. Dedifferentiation and transdifferentiation are phenomena well known in the mammalian retina: Müller glia cells (the equivalent of radial glia cells [RGCs] in the eye) in the central retina of adult mammals proliferate in response to neurotoxin-induced damage and generate new retinal neurons, highlighting the regenerative potential of the adult mammalian retina. Work by Dyer and colleagues have demonstrated that mouse retinoblastoma can arise from differentiated horizontal interneurons, shaking the traditional view that cell cycle arrest must precede differentiation. In early stages of the disease, retinoblastoma presents a much more differentiated phenotype compared with end-stage tumors, with tumor cells expressing markers characteristic of horizontal interneurons that extend processes and form synapses [18,19]. In spite of these exciting findings, NSCs and progenitors remain stronger candidates for the cell of origin for brain tumors: as they are already endowed with the capacity for proliferation, survival and migration, they are likely to require fewer mutations to achieve malignancy.

Ultimately, whether the transforming events that result in brain tumors occur in NSCs or in more differentiated cells must be determined for each type of tumor. Indeed, it is quite possible that more than one type of cell has the potential to act as a cell of origin, even for a single histological type of brain tumor.

ORIGINS OF MEDULLOBLASTOMA

The link between normal development and tumorigenesis is particularly relevant for pediatric malignancies compromised of primitive neuroepithelial cells, such as medulloblastoma. Medulloblastoma is an aggressive tumor of the cerebellum that is the most common malignant pediatric brain tumor [20]. Although it occurs predominantly in children, approximately 30% of cases present in adulthood [21]. Current treatment for medulloblastoma involves a combination of surgical resection, chemotherapy, and radiotherapy. These therapies have markedly improved prognosis: more than 90% of standard risk patients and more than 60% of high risk patients survive more than 5 years after diagnosis [20]. Although these statistics are encouraging, patients who undergo these treatments often develop severe and lasting side effects including cognitive and motor deficits, endocrine disorders, and a high incidence of secondary tumors later in life. Understanding the cellular and molecular origins of medulloblastoma is a critical first step in the development of better approaches to diagnosis and treatment of this disease.

The origins of medulloblastoma have been the subject of debate since the tumor was first described by Percival Bailey and Harvey Cushing in 1925 [22,23]. In their seminal work, they described the histopathology of medulloblastoma and demonstrated the presence of both neuronal and glial cells

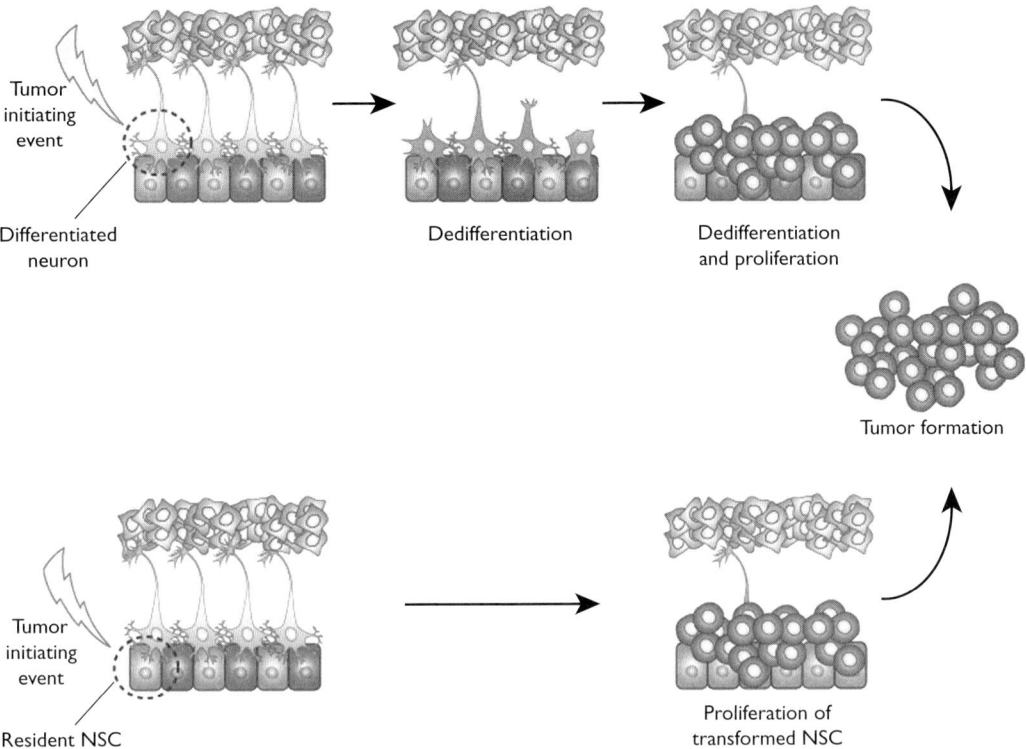

Figure 22.2 Two potential models for tumor initiation. Differentiated neurons or resident NSCs can be both hosts for tumor-initiating events. In the first case, a de-differentiation step is necessary to allow for the acquisition of a malignant phenotype. Resident NSCs already posses a cell machinery permissive to transformation.

within the tumors. Based on these observations, they postulated that the tumor originated from a primitive cell (a "medulloblast") that was capable of giving rise to multiple cell types. In contrast, the neuropathologist Pio del Rio Hortega, noting the predominantly neuronal nature of these tumors, referred to them as "cerebellar neuroblastomas" and suggested that they arose from progenitors that were restricted to the neuronal lineage [24]. In retrospect, these differing views likely resulted from the diversity of the cells within a given tumor and from the distinct characteristics of the tumors that were classified as medulloblastomas.

Although medulloblastoma was initially viewed as a single disease, advances in histochemical and immunological staining have increased our appreciation of the heterogeneity of the tumor. Today, the World Health Organization (WHO) recognizes several distinct subtypes of medulloblastoma. Among these, the most common are classic medulloblastomas, which consist of sheets of small, round, undifferentiated cells [25,26]. These tumors are more common in children and are associated with a relatively poor prognosis. Nodular/desmoplastic medulloblastomas, in contrast, contain "pale islands" of differentiated cells surrounded by areas of highly proliferative cells. These tumors account for one-quarter to one-third of all cases, occur more commonly in adulthood, and tend to have a better prognosis than the classic type [27]. Finally, large-cell/anaplastic medulloblastomas consist of large, heterogeneous cells with prominent nucleoli and abundant cytoplasm [28,29]. These tumors represent a minority of cases, but recur and metastasize more frequently than other types of medulloblastoma, and are associated with a much poorer prognosis.

The diversity of medulloblastoma subtypes raises the possibility that there is not a single cell of origin, but rather, distinct cells of origin for distinct subtypes of the disease. In that context, it is worth considering the different classes of progenitors in the cerebellum, each of which could represent a cell of origin for one or more types of medulloblastoma. The developing cerebellum contains two spatially distinct germinal zones [30]. The first is the ventricular zone (VZ), which contains multipotent NSCs that give rise to the majority of the cell types in the cerebellum. VZ stem cells are thought to differentiate into more restricted progenitors that migrate radially outward from the ventricle and in turn give rise to Purkinje, Golgi, basket and stellate neurons as well as astrocytes and oligodendrocytes. The VZ itself exists only in the embryonic cerebellum, but recent studies have suggested that multipotent stem cells can also be found in the cerebellar white matter at postnatal stages, and even in adulthood [31,32]. Assuming medulloblastomas originate from cells that have at least some capacity to generate neurons, stem cells in the VZ and white matter, and their progeny that commit to neuronal lineages, could all represent cells of origin for the disease.

Although most of the cell types in the cerebellum arise from the VZ, the most abundant cell type—the granule neuron—is generated in a distinct germinal zone on the surface of the cerebellum, called the external granule layer

(EGL). The EGL is comprised of highly proliferative granule neuron precursors (GNPs) that are restricted to the granule lineage [30]. These cells proliferate on the surface of the cerebellum from mid-embryogenesis until about 3 weeks after birth (in rodents), at which point all GNPs have differentiated and migrated away from the surface into the internal granule layer. The abundance of GNPs and the observation that some tumors can be found on the surface of the cerebellum [33,34] have lent support to the notion that at least a subset of medulloblastomas may arise from GNPs.

Considering the multitude of possible cells of origin for medulloblastoma, determining which cell types actually give rise to the disease has been a challenge. Historically, the cell of origin has been inferred from expression of cell surface and intracellular markers by tumor cells. For example, based on the abundant expression of neuronal markers such as β-III tubulin, microtubule-associated protein 2 (Map2), synaptophysin, and NeuN [35–37] most investigators believe that medulloblastomas arise from cells that are capable of giving rise to neurons. The fact that some tumors (particularly those of the nodular/desmoplastic subtype) express the low-affinity neurotrophin receptor p75, TrkC, Zic1, and Math1—genes normally found in the developing EGL—has led some investigators to suggest that these tumors arise from GNPs [38–41]. In contrast, tumors that express markers associated with stem cells (Nestin, CD133) [42–44] or with nongranule neurons (Calbindin, Neurogenin) [45,46] have been suggested to arise from multipotent progenitors, such as those in the VZ or white matter.

Although these data are consistent with the notion that different medulloblastoma subtypes arise from distinct stem/progenitor cell populations, there are caveats to using marker expression to identify the cell of origin. First, since oncogenic mutations can dramatically alter expression of genes and proteins within tumor cells, the presence or absence of a particular marker might not reflect the cell of origin but the consequences of transformation. In addition, it is important to note that solid tumors do not consist solely of tumor cells. In the context of medulloblastoma, expression of glial markers within the tumor could suggest that tumor cells have undergone glial differentiation, or it could mean that nontransformed glial cells have invaded or become trapped within the tumor. Thus, expression of individual markers in a tumor, while suggestive of a cell of origin, must be interpreted with caution.

To overcome the dependence on individual markers, recent studies have turned to microarray analysis, which provides a more comprehensive profile of the genes expressed within a tumor. In one of the first such studies, Pomeroy et al demonstrated that classic and desmoplastic medulloblastomas exhibited significant differences in gene expression [8]. In particular, desmoplastic tumors had increased expression of targets of the Shh signaling pathway, including *PTCH*, *GLI*, and *MYCN*. In light of evidence that Shh is a potent mitogen for GNPs in the EGL [47,48], these data supported the hypothesis that desmoplastic tumors arise from GNPs. More recent studies have combined high-resolution gene expression profiling with mutational analysis as well as clinical and histological data [49,50]. These studies have classified medulloblastomas into five distinct subtypes based on shared genetic signatures. Two of these groups were associated with mutations in the Shh and Wnt pathways and exhibited increased expression of targets of these pathways; the others contained distinct mutational and expression profiles.

The use of gene expression analysis has allowed more precise classification of medulloblastoma and has provided important insight into the molecular biology of the disease. But whether these data have advanced our understanding of the cell of origin remains a matter of debate. As with individual markers, gene expression profiles may reflect the cell from which a tumor arises, or the consequences of activation of a particular signaling pathway, or both. Another drawback of both types of analysis is that they are performed on end-stage tumors, which have often accumulated numerous mutations and changed markedly from the normal cells that gave rise to them. Because of these issues, conclusive identification of the cell of origin for human medulloblastoma may be impossible. To address this problem, some researchers have turned to mouse models of the disease.

The past decade has seen the creation of a number of mouse models of medulloblastoma. One of the most widely studied model contains a mutation in the *patched* gene that results in activation of the Shh signaling pathway [51]. Homozygotes from this strain die during embryogenesis, but heterozygotes survive and 15% to 20% develop medulloblastoma. Crossing these mice with animals lacking the *p53* tumor suppressor gene results in a marked increase in tumor incidence, with 95% to 100% of animals developing medulloblastoma [52,53]. Mice expressing an activated form of the Shh signal-transducing molecule Smoothened also develop medulloblastoma with high penetrance [54,55]. Interestingly, animals with mutations in various cell cycle and DNA repair genes (together with homozygous loss of *p53*) also develop medulloblastoma, and in each of these strains, genomic loss of *patched* is observed [56–59], suggesting that the Shh pathway is a critical regulator of tumorigenesis in mice, as it is in a subset of patients with the disease. *patched* mutant mice and other mouse models have been used to study many aspects of medulloblastoma, including the early stages of the disease [60,61], the interactions between the Shh pathway and other oncogenes and tumor suppressors [52,57,62–64] and the efficacy of hedgehog antagonists for therapy [53,65]. However, since most of these animals carry the etiological mutations in all of their cells (or at least in multiple cell types in the cerebellum), they cannot be used to identify the cell of origin for the disease.

To gain insight into the cell of origin of such tumors, it would be helpful to target mutations to a particular cell type. This can be achieved using conditional knockout or transgenic mice, in which deletion of a tumor suppressor gene or activation of an oncogene is dependent on concomitant expression of the Cre recombinase. By crossing such animals with transgenic mice expressing Cre in different cell types, it is possible to determine whether a particular cell type is capable of giving rise to a tumor. We and others have recently used this approach to examine the cell of origin for medulloblastomas resulting from activation of the Shh pathway [66,67]. These studies revealed that deletion of *patched* or activation of Smoothened in GNPs resulted in tumor formation in 100% of mice, strongly supporting the notion that GNPs could represent cells of origin for Shh pathway–associated tumors. Interestingly, activation of Shh signaling in VZ stem cells also caused tumors with 100% penetrance; however, these tumors only formed once mutant cells had committed to the granule lineage. These results suggest that medulloblastoma can be initiated in either GNPs or stem cells, but that GNPs may provide a critical context for the oncogenic effects of Shh signaling.

These studies provide insight into the origin of Shh pathway–associated tumors, and provide an experimental paradigm for investigating the origin of other medulloblastoma subtypes. The success of this approach depends on identification of the genetic mutations that are required for tumor initiation, and on the availability of promoters that can target these mutations to the appropriate progenitors. With the increasing availability of gene expression and mutation data for human medulloblastoma [8,49,50,68], there are now numerous genes whose expression is known to be altered in distinct subtypes of the disease; which of these are important for tumor initiation or progression and which are merely consequences of transformation remains to be determined. Transgenic animals that can be used to target these mutations to specific cell types are also becoming more widely available [67,68]. However, in cases where no appropriate promoter can be found, it is also possible to isolate the relevant progenitors, use somatic delivery (e.g., retroviruses) to introduce oncogenes or delete tumor suppressors of interest, and then transplant these cells into naïve hosts to see if they generate tumors. This approach has been used successfully for other types of tumors [69–71], and is likely to be a viable approach for identifying the cell of origin for medulloblastoma as well.

In the long run, identifying the cell of origin for medulloblastoma may have important implications for both understanding and treatment of the disease. At a molecular level, comparing tumor cells to the appropriate population of normal cells can provide insight into the genes and proteins that are critical for tumor initiation and progression. Moreover, knowing the cell of origin can allow one to draw inferences about the behavior of tumor cells from the biology of their normal counterparts. As just one example, basic fibroblast growth factor is a potent mitogen for NSCs, but promotes cell cycle exit and differentiation of GNPs [32,72]. Given this, therapies based on basic fibroblast growth factor signaling might be effective for treating tumors that arise from GNPs, but would presumably not be appropriate for tumors derived from, or resembling, stem cells. Thus, identifying the cell of origin for particular subtypes of medulloblastoma may be critical for designing appropriate strategies.

ORIGINS OF EPENDYMOMA

Ependymomas are central nervous system (CNS) tumors originally thought to originate from the walls of the ventricular system. The ventricular system is lined by ependymal cells that face the lumen, and a SVZ lying beneath the ependymal layer. Ependymal cells are cuboidal/columnar with apical surfaces covered in a layer of cilia, which circulate cerebrospinal fluid around the CNS. Ependymal cells derive from RGCs, the primary progenitors in the embryonic VZ, that shortly after birth become postmitotic. In the developing brain, neural progenitors reside in the VZ as a pseudostratified epithelium in direct contact with the ventricles through an apical process. In the adult brain, primary neural progenitors instead reside in the SVZ, displaced in their contact with the ventricles by ependymal cells. In the adult the largest germinal center is the SVZ, which maintains a hierarchy of cells, with NSCs at the top differentiating into more dedicated neural progenitor cells that, shortly after birth, transform into astrocytes [16,73–76].

Ependymomas are found in the supratentorial region, the posterior fossa, and the spinal cord. Ependymomas originating from different anatomical regions are largely histologically indistinguishable, but the anatomic distinction between intracranial and spinal locations has an epidemiological and clinical correlate. In children, approximately 90% of ependymomas are intracranial, whereas in adults and adolescents, 75% of ependymomas arise within the spinal cord. Overall ependymomas are the third most common malignant pediatric brain tumor, with more than 50% of cases arising in children younger than 5 years of age [77–79].

Early cytogenetic works as well as comparative genomic hybridization studies indicated that ependymomas from different anatomical locations had specific chromosomal aberrations, suggesting that tumors from different locations were different molecular diseases [80–84].

If cancer arises from transformed stem cells, then subgroups of the same histological tumor type might be derived from distinct populations of progenitor cells in the tissue of origin. In the recent past, the availability of genome-wide expression analysis and high definition comparative genomic hybridization tools has generated a great deal of knowledge about the genetic alterations in end-stage tumors. One factor hindering interpretation of these studies is an absence of knowledge about the normal counterpart of ependymomas, the cell of origin of ependymoma.

We recently hypothesized that ependymomas from the supratentorial region, the posterior fossa (fourth ventricle), and the spinal cord are clinically heterogeneous because they arise from different populations of neural progenitor cells [9]. To test this, we compared a 103 ependymomas arising from different anatomical region and found that subsets of ependymoma exhibited distinct patterns of gene expression and region of chromosome gain and loss. The genes that distinguished the supratentorial, posterior fossa, and spinal ependymomas included regulators of neural precursor cell proliferation and differentiation that were expressed in the corresponding region of the CNS. Supratentorial tumors express markedly elevated levels of members of the EPHB-EPHRIN and NOTCH signaling pathways, key regulators of NSC self-renewal and migration. Conversely, spinal ependymomas express multiple homeobox family members, which are involved in the anteroposterior patterning of the hindbrain and spinal cord during embryonic development.

One possible explanation for the observed molecular signatures is that subsets of ependymoma either maintain or recapitulate the developmental expression profiles of anatomically restricted progenitor cells from which they are derived. Analysis of the expression pattern of the genes specific for the supratentorial and spinal ependymoma subgroups, through *in situ* hybridization techniques, showed that in the developing mouse the site of expression coincided precisely, in anatomical site and timing, with local populations of RGCs. Further experiments using RGC markers suggested that RGCs within the brain and spine are the cells of origin of supratentorial and spinal ependymomas, respectively.

Detailed knowledge of the cell of origin of ependymoma and other brain tumors has recently gained further clinical significance as a result of the increasing body of evidence supporting the cancer stem cell (CSC) hypothesis [85–87]. This hypothesis proposed that, much like during normal organogenesis, a hierarchy exists in tumors where CSC proliferate to give rise to tumor cells that have significantly less, or no proliferative potential (Figure 22.3). Accordingly to this hypothesis, only a relatively small fraction of the tumor cell bulk, the CSCs, is able to propagate the disease. The existence of CSCs may also be responsible for therapeutic failures due to their intrinsic resistance to chemotherapy and radiotherapy. CSCs share many of the molecular markers once thought to be exclusively attributed only to NSCs, two cell surface markers, Nestin and CD133 (prominin-1), have been used to prospectively isolate CSCs from ependymomas, as CD133+ve cells were able to propagate the tumors in immunocompromised mice whereas the CD133-ve fraction was not [9].

If the CSC theory proves true for ependymomas and other tumors, it would lead to a key switch in our approach to design treatment strategies; research will have to focus on the genes and pathways that are dysregulated in CSC compared with its normal counterpart, the cell of origin. The comparison between the two will lead to potentially new therapeutic approaches which can selectively target CSCs and spare NSCs, impairing the intracellular pathways CSC rely on for proliferation and migration.

ORIGINS OF ASTROCYTOMA

Pediatric astrocytoma is the most common childhood brain tumor, accounting for more than half of all primary CNS malignancies. Most patients are diagnosed in the first decade of life, with the peak age at 6 to 8 years [88]. Astrocytomas are mostly slow growing, low-grade (i.e., WHO grade I–II) tumors that arise in midline locations, such as the cerebellum and the diencephalon, including the visual pathway and hypothalamus. Malignant high-grade tumors (i.e., WHO grade III–IV) are generally found in the cerebral hemispheres or in the pons. Therapy usually comprises surgical resection when anatomically permissible, and which alone is sufficient to cure most low-grade astrocytomas. However, the prognosis remains poor for high-grade astrocytomas in spite of the addition of radiotherapy and chemotherapy. Recent findings seem to indicate that the difference between the clinicopathological entities of astrocytoma (i.e., WHO grades I–IV) reflect the genetic events acquired during the process of malignant transformation.

As with medulloblastoma and ependymoma there has been a lot of debate about the cell of origin of astrocytomas. In 1926, Bailey [22] proposed that astrocytic tumors arise from the abnormal maturation of progenitor cells of astrocytes. Astrocytoma in its histological appearance is a very heterogeneous disease, varying from the low cellularity,

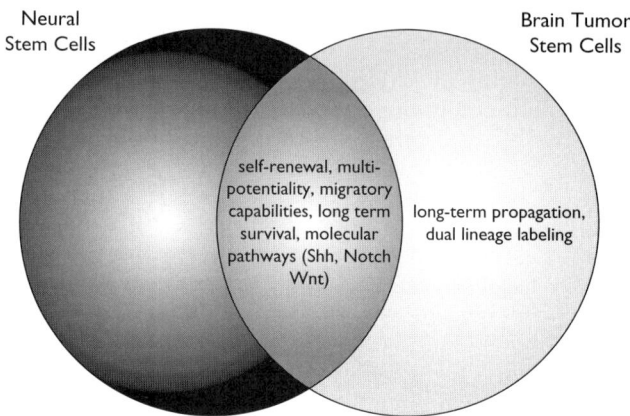

Figure 22.3 NSC versus BTSC; differences and similarities.

low proliferative and mitotic activity of pilocytic astrocytomas (WHO grade I) to the highly cellular, high proliferative and mitotic activity of the glioblastoma multiforme (GBM). GBM in some cases has been proposed to arise as a malignant progression from low-grade astrocytoma through anaplastic astrocytoma to secondary GBM, or else it may arise "de novo" as primary GBM. Both types of GBM are usually histologically indistinguishable. It is certainly feasible, indeed likely that different types of pediatric astrocytomas will arise from distinct cells of origin. Tumorigenesis is a multistep process; therefore it is reasonable that a given sequence of initiating events has to arise in the astrocytoma cell of origin to drive its transformation through low-grade astrocytomas to high grades of the disease. Recent evidence indicates that several loci are frequently amplified and/or overexpressed in astrocytomas, including genes such as *EGFR* (7p11-p12) [89–91], *GAC1*, *ELF3*, *MDM4*, and *REN1* (1q32) [92–94], *PDGFR-α* (4q11) [95], *MDM2*, and *CDK4* (12q13) [96,97]. Gene inactivation also plays a key role in astrocytoma; genes such as *RB1* [98], *INK4A* [99], *PTEN* [100], and *TP53* [101] exhibit sequence changes and/or loss of heterozygosity in a significant number of astrocytic tumors.

The hypothesis that malignant progression relies on sequential mutations in the same cell of origin has been accumulating evidence. For example, it has been shown that malignant progression and poor prognosis of low-grade astrocytic tumors are *TP53* dependent through clonal expansion of mutated cells [101]. By comparing alterations involved in low grade astrocytic tumors versus those found in GBM, it has been found that genes such as *MDM2* are preferentially subject to amplification/overexpression in malignant gliomas [102,103].

The discrepancies between the molecular alterations found in malignant versus low-grade glioma support the hypothesis that the former can arise as a *de novo* disease. Using human tumor tissues, it has not been possible to conclusively demonstrate which cell type gives rise to astrocytoma, and debate continues about whether astrocytomas arise from differentiated astrocytes, astroglial progenitor cells, or NSCs. Indeed, each of these may be true for different histologies, or between different patients. The major limitation resides in the fact that when working with human samples the only specimens available are from advanced

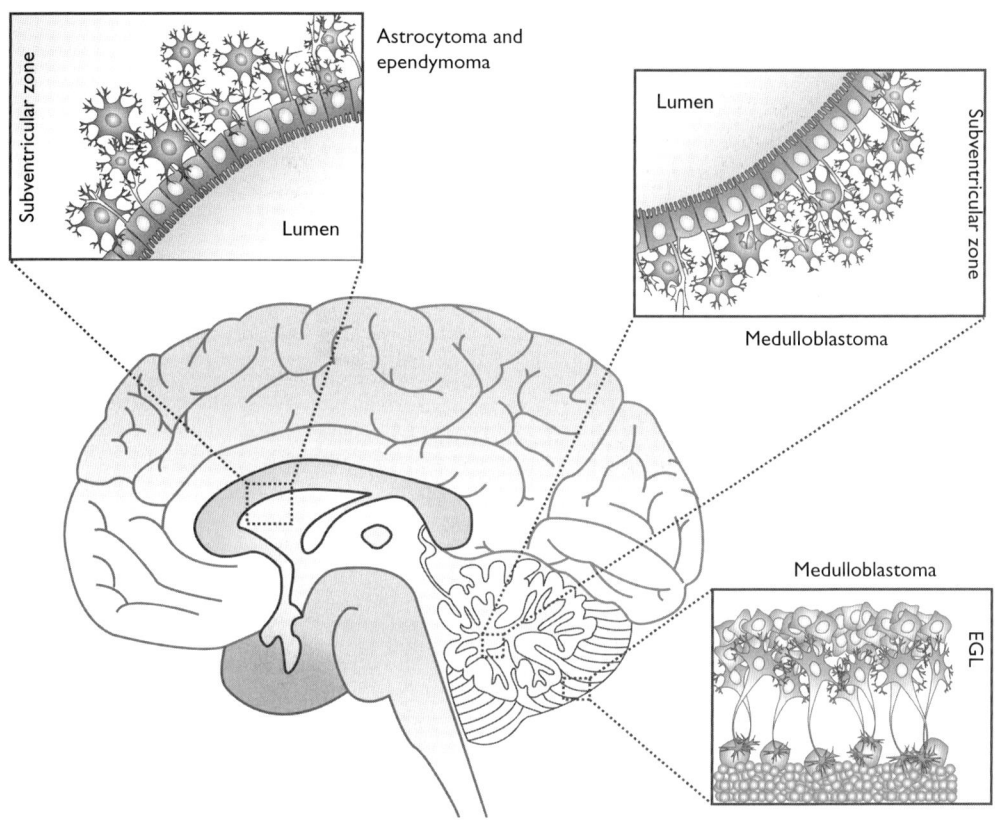

Figure 22.4 Anatomical sites of origin of pediatric brain tumors. Anatomical location where the potential cells of origin of pediatric brain tumors reside.

tumors. For this reason the cell of origin can merely be hypothesized from markers expressed in its progeny. This line of reasoning has been shown to be unreliable, especially in the case of astrocytomas. As discussed earlier in this chapter, GFAP, previously thought to be expressed in differentiated astrocytes, is also expressed in NSCs in the VZ [16,17,74]. Furthermore if a tumor cell expresses a marker of a particular lineage that does not necessarily imply that the tumor arose from cells of that lineage, because expression could have been acquired during tumor progression.

An alternative way to investigate the cell of origin of astrocytoma is to take advantage of genetically or virally engineered mouse models. As described above, oncogene expression driven by the GFAP or Nestin promoters can result in astrocytoma. However, Nestin-expressing cells tend to be more permissive than GFAP-expressing cells to initiating events, as both markers are expressed in the same compartment but with slightly different timing (Nestin expression begins earlier during development). Therefore, it seems plausible that the timing of the transforming events together with the cellular context plays a role in the gliomagenesis [13]. Most of the research in the current literature has been devoted to the study of adult onset astrocytomas. We await the extension of these findings to study the cell of origin of pediatric astrocytomas.

CONCLUSIONS

Recent advances in genomics, developmental biology, and mouse modeling have allowed us to learn a great deal more about the cell of origin for common pediatric brain tumors (Figure 22.4). Learning the cell of origin will feed back and provide increased insights into genomic, cell biology, developmental biology, and mouse-modeling experiments studying the etiology and pathogenesis of brain tumors. Ultimately, it is hoped that in-depth understanding of the specific cell of origin and the specific genetic/epigenetic transformative events will lead to more effective and less toxic therapies for pediatric patients with brain tumors.

REFERENCES

1. Altman J. Are new neurons formed in the brains of adult mammals? *Science*. 1962;135:1127–1128.
2. Altman J, Das GD. Autoradiographic and histological evidence of postnatal hippocampal neurogenesis in rats. *J Comp Neurol*. 1965;124(3):319–335.
3. Reynolds BA, Weiss S. Generation of neurons and astrocytes from isolated cells of the adult mammalian central nervous system. *Science*. 1992;255(5052):1707–1710.
4. Bachoo RM, Maher EA, Ligon KL, et al. Epidermal growth factor receptor and Ink4a/Arf: convergent mechanisms governing terminal differentiation and transformation along the neural stem cell to astrocyte axis. *Cancer Cell*. 2002;1(3):269–277.
5. Copeland DD, Vogel FS, Bigner DD. The induction of intracranial neoplasms by the inoculation of avian sarcoma virus in perinatal and adult rats. *J Neuropathol Exp Neurol*. 1975;34(4):340–358.
6. Copeland DD, Bigner DD. The role of the subependymal plate in avian sarcoma virus brain tumor induction: comparison of incipient tumors in neonatal and adult rats. *Acta Neuropathol*. 1977;38(1):1–6.
7. Rubinstein LJ. Presidential address. Cytogenesis and differentiation of primitive central neuroepithelial tumors. *J Neuropathol Exp Neurol*. 1972;31(1):7–26.
8. Pomeroy SL, Tamayo P, Gaasenbeek M, et al. Prediction of central nervous system embryonal tumour outcome based on gene expression. *Nature*. 2002;415(6870):436–442.

9. Taylor MD, Poppleton H, Fuller C, et al. Radial glia cells are candidate stem cells of ependymoma. *Cancer Cell.* 2005;8(4):323–335.
10. Northcott PA, Nakahara Y, Wu X, et al. Multiple recurrent genetic events converge on control of histone lysine methylation in medulloblastoma. *Nat Genet.* 2009;41(4):465–472.
11. Uyeda CT, Eng LF, Bignami A. Immunological study of the glial fibrillary acidic protein. *Brain Res.* 1972;37(1):81–89.
12. Bignami A, Dahl D. Astrocyte-specific protein and neuroglial differentiation. An immunofluorescence study with antibodies to the glial fibrillary acidic protein. *J Comp Neurol.* 1974;153(1):27–38.
13. Holland EC, Celestino J, Dai C, Schaefer L, Sawaya RE, Fuller GN. Combined activation of Ras and Akt in neural progenitors induces glioblastoma formation in mice. *Nat Genet.* 2000;25(1):55–57.
14. Ding H, Roncari L, Shannon P, et al. Astrocyte-specific expression of activated p21-ras results in malignant astrocytoma formation in a transgenic mouse model of human gliomas. *Cancer Res.* 2001;61(9):3826–3836.
15. Shannon P, Sabha N, Lau N, Kamnasaran D, Gutmann DH, Guha A. Pathological and molecular progression of astrocytomas in a GFAP:12 V-Ha-Ras mouse astrocytoma model. *Am J Pathol.* 2005;167(3):859–867.
16. Doetsch F, Caillé I, Lim DA, García-Verdugo JM, Alvarez-Buylla A. Subventricular zone astrocytes are neural stem cells in the adult mammalian brain. *Cell.* 1999;97(6):703–716.
17. Quiñones-Hinojosa A, Sanai N, Soriano-Navarro M, et al. Cellular composition and cytoarchitecture of the adult human subventricular zone: a niche of neural stem cells. *J Comp Neurol.* 2006;494(3):415–434.
18. Ajioka I, Martins RA, Bayazitov IT, et al. Differentiated horizontal interneurons clonally expand to form metastatic retinoblastoma in mice. *Cell.* 2007;131(2):378–390.
19. Johnson DA, Zhang J, Frase S, Wilson M, Rodriguez-Galindo C, Dyer MA. Neuronal differentiation and synaptogenesis in retinoblastoma. *Cancer Res.* 2007;67(6):2701–2711.
20. Crawford JR, MacDonald TJ, Packer RJ. Medulloblastoma in childhood: new biological advances. *Lancet Neurol.* 2007;6(12):1073–1085.
21. Cervoni L, Maleci A, Salvati M, Delfini R, Cantore G. Medulloblastoma in late adults: report of two cases and critical review of the literature. *J Neurooncol.* 1994;19(2):169–173.
22. Bailey P, Cushing H. *A Classification of the Tumors of the Glioma Group on a Histogenetic Basis With a Correlated Study of Prognosis.* Philadelphia: Lippincott; 1926.
23. Ferguson S, Lesniak MS. Percival Bailey and the classification of brain tumors. *Neurosurg Focus.* 2005;18(4):e7.
24. Katsetos CD, Del Valle L, Legido A, de Chadarévian JP, Perentes E, Mörk SJ. On the neuronal/neuroblastic nature of medulloblastomas: a tribute to Pio del Rio Hortega and Moises Polak. *Acta Neuropathol.* 2003;105(1):1–13.
25. Ellison D. Classifying the medulloblastoma: insights from morphology and molecular genetics. *Neuropathol Appl Neurobiol.* 2002;28(4):257–282.
26. Gilbertson RJ, Ellison DW. The origins of medulloblastoma subtypes. *Annu Rev Pathol.* 2008;3:341–365.
27. McManamy CS, Pears J, Weston CL, et al. Nodule formation and desmoplasia in medulloblastomas-defining the nodular/desmoplastic variant and its biological behavior. *Brain Pathol.* 2007;17(2):151–164.
28. Leonard JR, Cai DX, Rivet DJ, et al. Large cell/anaplastic medulloblastomas and medullomyoblastomas: clinicopathological and genetic features. *J Neurosurg.* 2001;95(1):82–88.
29. Eberhart CG, Burger PC. Anaplasia and grading in medulloblastomas. *Brain Pathol.* 2003;13(3):376–385.
30. Altman J, Bayer SA. *Development of the Cerebellar System: In Relation to its Evolution, Structure and Functions.* Boca Raton, FL: CRC Press; 1997.
31. Klein C, Butt SJ, Machold RP, Johnson JE, Fishell G. Cerebellum- and forebrain-derived stem cells possess intrinsic regional character. *Development.* 2005;132(20):4497–4508.
32. Lee A, Kessler JD, Read TA, et al. Isolation of neural stem cells from the postnatal cerebellum. *Nat Neurosci.* 2005;8(6):723–729.
33. Kadin ME, Rubinstein LJ, Nelson JS. Neonatal cerebellar medulloblastoma originating from the fetal external granular layer. *J Neuropathol Exp Neurol.* 1970;29(4):583–600.
34. Miyata H, Ikawa E, Ohama E. Medulloblastoma in an adult suggestive of external granule cells as its origin: a histological and immunohistochemical study. *Brain Tumor Pathol.* 1998;15(1):31–35.
35. Maraziotis T, Perentes E, Karamitopoulou E, et al. Neuron-associated class III beta-tubulin isotype, retinal S-antigen, synaptophysin, and glial fibrillary acidic protein in human medulloblastomas: a clinicopathological analysis of 36 cases. *Acta Neuropathol.* 1992;84(4):355–363.
36. Giordana MT, Cavalla P, Dutto A, Borsotti L, Chiò A, Schiffer D. Is medulloblastoma the same tumor in children and adults? *J Neurooncol.* 1997;35(2):169–176.
37. Eberhart CG, Kaufman WE, Tihan T, Burger PC. Apoptosis, neuronal maturation, and neurotrophin expression within medulloblastoma nodules. *J Neuropathol Exp Neurol.* 2001;60(5):462–469.
38. Yokota N, Aruga J, Takai S, et al. Predominant expression of human zic in cerebellar granule cell lineage and medulloblastoma. *Cancer Res.* 1996;56(2):377–383.
39. Pomeroy SL, Sutton ME, Goumnerova LC, Segal RA. Neurotrophins in cerebellar granule cell development and medulloblastoma. *J Neurooncol.* 1997;35(3):347–352.
40. Bühren J, Christoph AH, Buslei R, Albrecht S, Wiestler OD, Pietsch T. Expression of the neurotrophin receptor p75NTR in medulloblastomas is correlated with distinct histological and clinical features: evidence for a medulloblastoma subtype derived from the external granule cell layer. *J Neuropathol Exp Neurol.* 2000;59(3):229–240.
41. Salsano E, Pollo B, Eoli M, Giordana MT, Finocchiaro G. Expression of MATH1, a marker of cerebellar granule cell progenitors, identifies different medulloblastoma sub-types. *Neurosci Lett.* 2004;370(2-3):180–185.
42. Valtz NL, Hayes TE, Norregaard T, Liu SM, McKay RD. An embryonic origin for medulloblastoma. *New Biol.* 1991;3(4):364–371.
43. Hemmati HD, Nakano I, Lazareff JA, et al. Cancerous stem cells can arise from pediatric brain tumors. *Proc Natl Acad Sci USA.* 2003;100(25):15178–15183.
44. Singh SK, Clarke ID, Terasaki M, et al. Identification of a cancer stem cell in human brain tumors. *Cancer Res.* 2003;63(18):5821–5828.
45. Katsetos CD, Herman MM, Krishna L, et al. Calbindin-D28k in subsets of medulloblastomas and in the human medulloblastoma cell line D283 Med. *Arch Pathol Lab Med.* 1995;119(8):734–743.
46. Salsano E, Croci L, Maderna E, et al. Expression of the neurogenic basic helix-loop-helix transcription factor NEUROG1 identifies a subgroup of medulloblastomas not expressing ATOH1. *Neuro-oncology.* 2007;9(3):298–307.
47. Wallace VA. Purkinje-cell-derived Sonic hedgehog regulates granule neuron precursor cell proliferation in the developing mouse cerebellum. *Curr Biol.* 1999;9(8):445–448.
48. Wechsler-Reya RJ, Scott MP. Control of neuronal precursor proliferation in the cerebellum by Sonic Hedgehog. *Neuron.* 1999;22(1):103–114.
49. Thompson MC, Fuller C, Hogg TL, et al. Genomics identifies medulloblastoma subgroups that are enriched for specific genetic alterations. *J Clin Oncol.* 2006;24(12):1924–1931.
50. Kool M, Koster J, Bunt J, et al. Integrated genomics identifies five medulloblastoma subtypes with distinct genetic profiles, pathway signatures and clinicopathological features. *PLoS ONE.* 2008;3(8):e3088.
51. Goodrich LV, Milenkovic L, Higgins KM, Scott MP. Altered neural cell fates and medulloblastoma in mouse patched mutants. *Science.* 1997;277(5329):1109–1113.
52. Wetmore C, Eberhart DE, Curran T. Loss of p53 but not ARF accelerates medulloblastoma in mice heterozygous for patched. *Cancer Res.* 2001;61(2):513–516.
53. Romer JT, Kimura H, Magdaleno S, et al. Suppression of the Shh pathway using a small molecule inhibitor eliminates medulloblastoma in Ptc1(+/-)p53(-/-) mice. *Cancer Cell.* 2004;6(3):229–240.
54. Hallahan AR, Pritchard JI, Hansen S, et al. The SmoA1 mouse model reveals that notch signaling is critical for the growth and survival of sonic hedgehog-induced medulloblastomas. *Cancer Res.* 2004;64(21):7794–7800.
55. Hatton BA, Villavicencio EH, Tsuchiya KD, et al. The Smo/Smo model: hedgehog-induced medulloblastoma with 90% incidence and leptomeningeal spread. *Cancer Res.* 2008;68(6):1768–1776.
56. Lee Y, McKinnon PJ. DNA ligase IV suppresses medulloblastoma formation. *Cancer Res.* 2002;62(22):6395–6399.
57. Uziel T, Zindy F, Xie S, et al. The tumor suppressors Ink4c and p53 collaborate independently with Patched to suppress medulloblastoma formation. *Genes Dev.* 2005;19(22):2656–2667.
58. Yan CT, Kaushal D, Murphy M, et al. XRCC4 suppresses medulloblastomas with recurrent translocations in p53-deficient mice. *Proc Natl Acad Sci USA.* 2006;103(19):7378–7383.

59. Frappart PO, Lee Y, Russell HR, et al. Recurrent genomic alterations characterize medulloblastoma arising from DNA double-strand break repair deficiency. *Proc Natl Acad Sci USA*. 2009;106(6):1880–1885.
60. Oliver TG, Read TA, Kessler JD, et al. Loss of patched and disruption of granule cell development in a pre-neoplastic stage of medulloblastoma. *Development*. 2005;132(10):2425–2439.
61. Kessler JD, Hasegawa H, Brun SN, et al. N-myc alters the fate of pre-neoplastic cells in a mouse model of medulloblastoma. *Genes Dev*. 2009;23(2):157–170.
62. Pogoriler J, Millen K, Utset M, Du W. Loss of cyclin D1 impairs cerebellar development and suppresses medulloblastoma formation. *Development*. 2006;133(19):3929–3937.
63. Briggs KJ, Corcoran-Schwartz IM, Zhang W, et al. Cooperation between the Hic1 and Ptch1 tumor suppressors in medulloblastoma. *Genes Dev*. 2008;22(6):770–785.
64. Lelievre V, Seksenyan A, Nobuta H, et al. Disruption of the PACAP gene promotes medulloblastoma in ptc1 mutant mice. *Dev Biol*. 2008;313(1):359–370.
65. Berman DM, Karhadkar SS, Hallahan AR, et al. Medulloblastoma growth inhibition by hedgehog pathway blockade. *Science*. 2002;297(5586):1559–1561.
66. Schüller U, Heine VM, Mao J, et al. Acquisition of granule neuron precursor identity is a critical determinant of progenitor cell competence to form Shh-induced medulloblastoma. *Cancer Cell*. 2008;14(2):123–134.
67. Yang ZJ, Ellis T, Markant SL, et al. Medulloblastoma can be initiated by deletion of Patched in lineage-restricted progenitors or stem cells. *Cancer Cell*. 2008;14(2):135–145.
68. Schüller U, Kho AT, Zhao Q, Ma Q, Rowitch DH. Cerebellar 'transcriptome' reveals cell-type and stage-specific expression during postnatal development and tumorigenesis. *Mol Cell Neurosci*. 2006;33(3):247–259.
69. Huntly BJ, Shigematsu H, Deguchi K, et al. MOZ-TIF2, but not BCR-ABL, confers properties of leukemic stem cells to committed murine hematopoietic progenitors. *Cancer Cell*. 2004;6(6):587–596.
70. Zender L, Xue W, Cordón-Cardo C, et al. Generation and analysis of genetically defined liver carcinomas derived from bipotential liver progenitors. *Cold Spring Harb Symp Quant Biol*. 2005;70:251–261.
71. Krivtsov AV, Twomey D, Feng Z, et al. Transformation from committed progenitor to leukaemia stem cell initiated by MLL-AF9. *Nature*. 2006;442(7104):818–822.
72. Fogarty MP, Emmenegger BA, Grasfeder LL, Oliver TG, Wechsler-Reya RJ. Fibroblast growth factor blocks Sonic hedgehog signaling in neuronal precursors and tumor cells. *Proc Natl Acad Sci USA*. 2007;104(8):2973–2978.
73. Voigt T. Development of glial cells in the cerebral wall of ferrets: direct tracing of their transformation from radial glia into astrocytes. *J Comp Neurol*. 1989;289(1):74–88.
74. Doetsch F, García-Verdugo JM, Alvarez-Buylla A. Cellular composition and three-dimensional organization of the subventricular germinal zone in the adult mammalian brain. *J Neurosci*. 1997;17(13):5046–5061.
75. Spassky N, Merkle FT, Flames N, Tramontin AD, García-Verdugo JM, Alvarez-Buylla A. Adult ependymal cells are postmitotic and are derived from radial glial cells during embryogenesis. *J Neurosci*. 2005;25(1):10–18.
76. Mirzadeh Z, Merkle FT, Soriano-Navarro M, Garcia-Verdugo JM, Alvarez-Buylla A. Neural stem cells confer unique pinwheel architecture to the ventricular surface in neurogenic regions of the adult brain. *Cell Stem Cell*. 2008;3(3):265–278.
77. Duffner PK, Krischer JP, Sanford RA, et al. Prognostic factors in infants and very young children with intracranial ependymomas. *Pediatr Neurosurg*. 1998;28(4):215–222.
78. Schwartz TH, Kim S, Glick RS, et al. Supratentorial ependymomas in adult patients. *Neurosurgery*. 1999;44(4):721–731.
79. Grill J, Le Deley MC, Gambarelli D, et al. Postoperative chemotherapy without irradiation for ependymoma in children under 5 years of age: a multicenter trial of the French Society of Pediatric Oncology. *J Clin Oncol*. 2001;19(5):1288–1296.
80. Ebert C, von Haken M, Meyer-Puttlitz B, et al. Molecular genetic analysis of ependymal tumors. NF2 mutations and chromosome 22q loss occur preferentially in intramedullary spinal ependymomas. *Am J Pathol*. 1999;155(2):627–632.
81. Hirose Y, Aldape K, Bollen A, et al. Chromosomal abnormalities subdivide ependymal tumors into clinically relevant groups. *Am J Pathol*. 2001;158(3):1137–1143.
82. Carter M, Nicholson J, Ross F, et al. Genetic abnormalities detected in ependymomas by comparative genomic hybridisation. *Br J Cancer*. 2002;86(6):929–939.
83. Dyer S, Prebble E, Davison V, et al. Genomic imbalances in pediatric intracranial ependymomas define clinically relevant groups. *Am J Pathol*. 2002;161(6):2133–2141.
84. Jeuken JW, Sprenger SH, Gilhuis J, Teepen HL, Grotenhuis AJ, Wesseling P. Correlation between localization, age, and chromosomal imbalances in ependymal tumours as detected by CGH. *J Pathol*. 2002;197(2):238–244.
85. Bonnet D, Dick JE. Human acute myeloid leukemia is organized as a hierarchy that originates from a primitive hematopoietic cell. *Nat Med*. 1997;3(7):730–737.
86. Singh SK, Hawkins C, Clarke ID, et al. Identification of human brain tumour initiating cells. *Nature*. 2004;432(7015):396–401.
87. Clarke MF, Fuller M. Stem cells and cancer: two faces of eve. *Cell*. 2006;124(6):1111–1115.
88. Kaderali Z, Lamberti-Pasculli M, Rutka JT. The changing epidemiology of paediatric brain tumours: a review from the Hospital for Sick Children. *Childs Nerv Syst*. 2009;25(7):787–793.
89. Libermann TA, Nusbaum HR, Razon N, et al. Amplification, enhanced expression and possible rearrangement of EGF receptor gene in primary human brain tumours of glial origin. *Nature*. 1985;313(5998):144–147.
90. Ekstrand AJ, James CD, Cavenee WK, Seliger B, Pettersson RF, Collins VP. Genes for epidermal growth factor receptor, transforming growth factor alpha, and epidermal growth factor and their expression in human gliomas in vivo. *Cancer Res*. 1991;51(8):2164–2172.
91. Arjona D, Bello MJ, Alonso ME, et al. Molecular analysis of the EGFR gene in astrocytic gliomas: mRNA expression, quantitative-PCR analysis of non-homogeneous gene amplification and DNA sequence alterations. *Neuropathol Appl Neurobiol*. 2005;31(4):384–394.
92. Riemenschneider MJ, Büschges R, Wolter M, et al. Amplification and overexpression of the MDM4 (MDMX) gene from 1q32 in a subset of malignant gliomas without TP53 mutation or MDM2 amplification. *Cancer Res*. 1999;59(24):6091–6096.
93. Riemenschneider MJ, Knobbe CB, Reifenberger G. Refined mapping of 1q32 amplicons in malignant gliomas confirms MDM4 as the main amplification target. *Int J Cancer*. 2003;104(6):752–757.
94. Arjona D, Bello MJ, Alonso ME, et al. Real-time quantitative PCR analysis of regions involved in gene amplification reveals gene overdose in low-grade astrocytic gliomas. *Diagn Mol Pathol*. 2005;14(4):224–229.
95. Hermanson M, Funa K, Koopmann J, et al. Association of loss of heterozygosity on chromosome 17p with high platelet-derived growth factor alpha receptor expression in human malignant gliomas. *Cancer Res*. 1996;56(1):164–171.
96. Reifenberger G, Reifenberger J, Ichimura K, Meltzer PS, Collins VP. Amplification of multiple genes from chromosomal region 12q13–14 in human malignant gliomas: preliminary mapping of the amplicons shows preferential involvement of CDK4, SAS, and MDM2. *Cancer Res*. 1994;54(16):4299–4303.
97. Reifenberger G, Ichimura K, Reifenberger J, Elkahloun AG, Meltzer PS, Collins VP. Refined mapping of 12q13-q15 amplicons in human malignant gliomas suggests CDK4/SAS and MDM2 as independent amplification targets. *Cancer Res*. 1996;56(22):5141–5145.
98. Simpson DJ, Hibberts NA, McNicol AM, Clayton RN, Farrell WE. Loss of pRb expression in pituitary adenomas is associated with methylation of the RB1 CpG island. *Cancer Res*. 2000;60(5):1211–1216.
99. Nakamura M, Watanabe T, Klangby U, et al. p14ARF deletion and methylation in genetic pathways to glioblastomas. *Brain Pathol*. 2001;11(2):159–168.
100. Li J, Yen C, Liaw D, et al. PTEN, a putative protein tyrosine phosphatase gene mutated in human brain, breast, and prostate cancer. *Science*. 1997;275(5308):1943–1947.
101. Ishii N, Tada M, Hamou MF, et al. Cells with TP53 mutations in low grade astrocytic tumors evolve clonally to malignancy and are an unfavorable prognostic factor. *Oncogene*. 1999;18(43):5870–5878.
102. Collins VP. Gene amplification in human gliomas. *Glia*. 1995;15(3):289–296.
103. Momand J, Jung D, Wilczynski S, Niland J. The MDM2 gene amplification database. *Nucleic Acids Res*. 1998;26(15):3453–3459.

23 Histopathological Features of Common Pediatric Brain Tumors

Hisham AlKhalidi and Cynthia E. Hawkins

INTRODUCTION

Central nervous system (CNS) tumors are the most common solid tumors in the pediatric population and are the leading cause of cancer-related death in this age group. In childhood, most of these tumors originate from neural elements within the brain. They constitute a diagnostically challenging group of divergent diseases that frequently share similar histopathological features. Ancillary studies, including immunohistochemistry, electron microscopy, cytogenetics, or molecular studies, may help in defining the tumor; however, in some cases they do not fit neatly into a diagnostic category.

In this chapter, we provide the reader with a brief overview of the main diagnostic histopathological features of the common pediatric CNS tumors. In addition, we describe a few examples of relatively rare entities that are more frequent in the pediatric population and/or may overlap morphologically with the more common ones. There are excellent texts available that we encourage the readers to consult for a more detailed review of neuropathology of brain tumors [1–3].

NEUROEPITHELIAL TUMORS

Astrocytic Tumors

Pilocytic Astrocytoma

Pilocytic astrocytoma [4] (WHO grade I) is the most common glioma in the pediatric population. They occur most commonly in the cerebellum followed by the hypothalamic/optic pathways. Grossly, they are typically well demarcated and may contain areas of calcification. They can form small nodules in a cystic cavity, giving them a similar gross appearance to ganglioglioma, hemangioblastoma, and pleomorphic xanthoastrocytoma (PXA).

On microscopic examination, pilocytic astrocytoma classically demonstrates a biphasic morphological pattern (Figure 23.1A). One is a cellular component formed by parallel fascicles of bipolar hair-like (piloid) cells (Figure 23.1B) in a fibrillary background that is rich in Rosenthal fibers. These fibers (Figure 23.1C) are brightly eosinophilic intracytoplasmic masses that are characteristic of, but not specific to, pilocytic astrocytoma (Table 23.1).

The second pattern consists of loose, hypocellular, microcystic areas. Here, the cells exhibit small, round nuclei and fine processes in which eosinophilic granular bodies (EGBs) are commonly found (Figure 23.1D). EGBs are globular, brightly eosinophilic aggregates within the cellular processes.

The presence of microscopic foci of infiltration in the surrounding brain tissue, or in the subarachnoid space, occasional mitotic figures, isolated foci of necrosis, or microvascular proliferation, does not indicate malignancy. In addition, degenerative changes can occur and may lead to misdiagnosis of a malignant glioma. These degenerative changes include nuclear atypia and pleomorphism that is associated with smudgy chromatin and nuclear pseudoinclusions. Another example of a degenerative change is the "pennies-on-a-plate" pattern, a term used to describe degenerative multinucleated giant cells (Figure 23.1E). On the other hand, nonneoplastic, reactive gliosis can look similar to a pilocytic astrocytoma. A classical example is the rim of a craniopharyngioma or a hemangioma where the surrounding brain tissue creates a dense gliotic background filled with Rosenthal fibers. A biopsy from such areas may be misinterpreted as a pilocytic astrocytoma.

Pilomyxoid Astrocytoma

This tumor is not as common as pilocytic astrocytoma, but they share some gross and microscopic features. The term "pilomyxoid astrocytoma" was introduced in 1999 by Tihan et al [5], who distinguished the entity from pilocytic astrocytoma with which it was previously grouped. Pilomyxoid astrocytoma recurs more frequently after resection and spreads within the subarachnoid space more often than pilocytic astrocytomas do. On this basis, pilomyxoid astrocytoma has been recognized as a distinct entity and given a WHO grade of II in the most recent WHO classification [3]. It typically arises in the hypothalamic/chiasmatic region.

Grossly, pilomyxoid astrocytoma is a well-circumscribed, solid, gelatinous, or cystic lesion that is difficult to distinguish macroscopically from pilocytic astrocytoma. Microscopic examination (Figure 23.2A) shows that pilomyxoid astrocytoma is monophasic. The matrix is predominantly myxoid, a feature that can be highlighted with Alcian blue staining (Figure 23.2B). Embedded within the myxoid matrix are bland bipolar cells that have a tendency

Table 23.1 Common Central Nervous System Tumors With Rosenthal Fibers

Pilocytic astrocytoma
Ganglioglioma
Pleomorphic xanthoastrocytoma

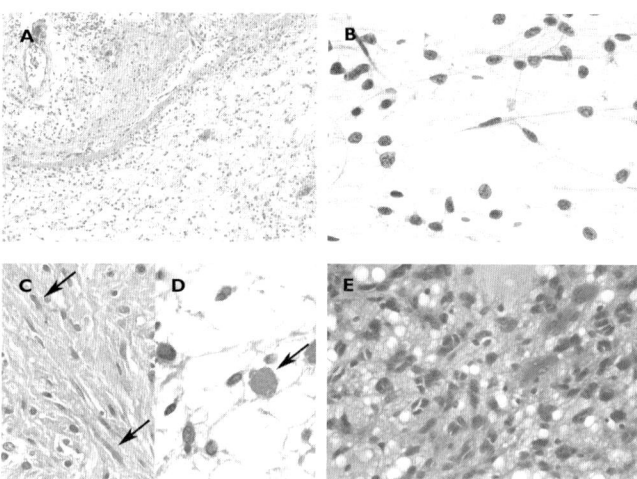

Figure 23.1 (A) Pilocytic astrocytoma showing a biphasic architecture, with both a loose, hypocellular pattern (lower right half) and a compact cellular pattern (upper left half). H&E, original magnification ×100. (B) A smear of a pilocytic astrocytoma showing bipolar hair-like processes that characterize the piloid cell. H&E, original magnification ×400. (C) Rosenthal fibers (arrows) scattered within the compact piloid component of a pilocytic astrocytoma. H&E, original magnification ×400. (D) Eosinophilic granular body (arrow) within a loose area in a pilocytic astrocytoma. H&E, original magnification ×600. (E) Pilocytic astrocytoma with scattered tumor cells showing degenerative changes, which include hyperchromatic and mild-to-moderate pleomorphic nuclei and multinucleation. H&E, original magnification ×400. *See color insert.*

to form an angiocentric pattern (Figure 23.2C). This tumor rarely exhibits protoplasmic cells, EGBs, or calcifications. Rosenthal fibers are not found, however.

Angiocentric Glioma

This is a recently described entity [6] that has been added to the WHO 2007 classification [3]. It usually occurs superficially in the frontoparietal or temporal lobes or in the hippocampal region. This benign (WHO grade I) and variably infiltrative tumor is histopathologically characterized by monomorphous bipolar cells with a prominent angiocentric growth pattern (Figure 23.3A). As for most astrocytic neoplasms, this tumor is usually positive for glial fibrillary acidic protein (GFAP) but, in addition, it shows an intracytoplasmic, dot-like pattern of staining with epithelial membrane antigen (EMA) (Figure 23.3B). The latter feature, in addition to the perivascular rosetting pattern, has led to the suggestion that this tumor may be related to ependymal tumors [7].

Diffuse Astrocytoma

Diffuse astrocytoma (WHO grade II) can occur anywhere in the CNS. In the pediatric population, diffuse astrocytoma rarely transforms to a higher grade, a phenomenon that is typical in the adult population. Grossly this tumor forms an ill-defined and occasionally cystic mass that causes enlargement and distortion of the involved anatomical structure.

Microscopically, diffuse astrocytoma is cellular and forms sheets of spindle cells within a fibrillar background (Figure 23.4A). Its infiltrative nature is often evinced by the finding of entrapped neurons (Figure 23.4B) and the formation of secondary structures of Scherer. These structures are descriptive patterns of perineuronal, perivascular, subpial, and subependymal aggregates of neoplastic cells. The nuclei of the neoplastic astrocytic cells are usually different from reactive astrocytes; they are more angular, hyperchromatic, and mildly pleomorphic. GFAP is the main immunohistochemical stain that highlights the neoplastic astrocytic cells and corresponds to intracytoplasmic intermediate filaments seen ultrastructurally.

Other morphological variants of the same tumor and grade are the protoplasmic and the gemistocytic variants. The former is a rare hypocellular, mucoid, and microcystic lesion that is predominantly composed of cells with small nuclei, low content of glial filaments, and scant GFAP expression. The gemistocytic variant shows a predominant population of cells with abundant eosinophilic cytoplasm, nuclei that are displaced to the periphery, and strong, consistent GFAP expression.

Anaplastic Astrocytoma

Compared to the diffuse astrocytomas, anaplastic astrocytoma (WHO grade III) is a high-grade astrocytic tumor that shows increased cellularity and more nuclear pleomorphism and hyperchromasia than WHO grade II diffuse astrocytomas. In children, an increased mitotic count is a particularly important feature to distinguish these malignant neoplasms from low-grade mimics such as pilocytic astrocytoma (Figure 23.4C). Though the finding of pyknotic nuclei is still consistent with this category, geographic areas of necrosis or microvascular proliferation are usually indicative of glioblastoma (GBM).

Glioblastoma

GBM is a malignant and aggressive astrocytic tumor (WHO grade IV). Grossly, it usually shows necrosis, hemorrhage, peritumoral edema, and occasional pseudocapsule formation, in addition to a yellowish discoloration from myelin breakdown (Figure 23.5A). Microscopically, GBM can exhibit variable architectural patterns and cellular morphologies. These include multinucleated giant cells, small cells, granular cells, and lipidized cells. The two main histopathological features that are mandatory for the diagnosis of GBM are (1) coagulative necrosis, typically with pseudopalisading of tumor cells (Figure 23.5B), and (2) microvascular proliferation (Figure 23.5C). Nodular primitive neuroectodermal components may be seen in GBMs,

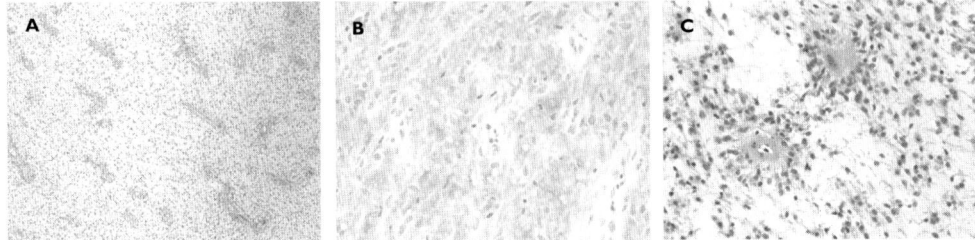

Figure 23.2 **(A)** Pilomyxoid astrocytoma showing a monophasic architecture. There is an impression of the angiocentric pattern at this low power, which is better seen at higher power (C). H&E, original magnification ×40. **(B)** Alcian blue highlights the prominent myxoid background of pilomyxoid astrocytoma. Original magnification ×200. **(C)** Angiocentric pattern of pilomyxoid astrocytoma. H&E, original magnification ×200. See color insert.

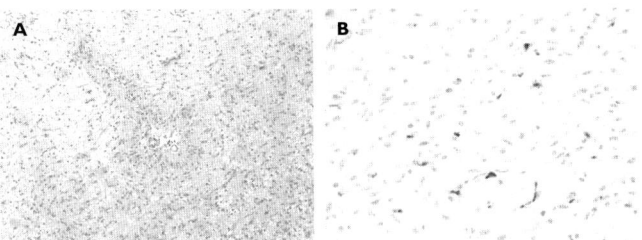

Figure 23.3 **(A)** Angiocentric glioma showing elongated astrocytic tumor cells. The angiocentric pattern is noted centrally. H&E, original magnification ×100. **(B)** A dot-like staining pattern with epithelial membrane antigen (EMA) immunohistochemistry is a characteristic feature of angiocentric glioma. Original magnification ×400. See color insert.

but these mixed tumors are still considered to fall within the malignant-glioma category [8].

Pleomorphic Xanthoastrocytoma

PXA (WHO grade II) is a relatively rare astrocytic tumor with unique morphologic features. It is a supratentorial lesion that commonly involves the leptomeninges and the cerebral cortex of children and young adults. On average, 50% of PXAs occur in the temporal lobe [9].

A cyst with a nodule in its cavity is a frequent gross and radiological finding. Microscopically, PXA is composed of highly pleomorphic, fibrillary astrocytes, some of which are lipidized (Figures 23.6A and 23.6B); large, bizarre, multinucleated cells are an additional feature. Reticulin characteristically highlights the background (Figure 23.6C). EGBs, chronic inflammation, and hemorrhage are common associated features.

Because of the potentially worrisome nuclear pleomorphism, it is important to consider this tumor in the differential diagnosis of malignant astrocytic tumors such as anaplastic astrocytoma or GBM. PXA usually has few mitoses, unless the tumor has "anaplastic features." It has been proposed that a mitotic count of 5 or more per 10 high-power fields is indicative of anaplasia, but the presence of necrosis alone was not found to be an independent predictor of survival [9]. The neoplastic cells in

PXA are positive for S100 and variably positive for GFAP (Figure 23.6D) and CD34 [10]. PXAs may focally express a neuronal phenotype, and there are multiple reports of distinct, coincident PXA and ganglioglioma in the same tumor. A neuroepithelial precursor cell type common to both astrocytic and neuronal lineages has been suggested as a source for such composite tumors [11].

Embryonal Tumors

Medulloblastoma

Medulloblastoma is the most common malignant, pediatric brain tumor and is given a WHO grade of IV. It characteristically occurs in the cerebellum and the fourth ventricle roof areas, where it forms a well-circumscribed, soft, grey mass (Figure 23.7A). It has a tendency to infiltrate the leptomeninges and metastasize via the CSF pathways. It can be divided into classic medulloblastoma, desmoplastic/nodular medulloblastoma, medulloblastoma with extensive nodularity, anaplastic medulloblastoma, and large cell medulloblastoma.

Classic Medulloblastoma

Classic medulloblastomas are formed by sheets of small round blue cells with a high nucleus-to-cytoplasmic ratio and sit within a finely fibrillary background. Homer-Wright rosettes (Figure 23.7B) and rarely differentiating ganglion-euronal elements may be seen. Medulloblastomas usually exhibit a high mitotic rate, numerous apoptotic bodies, and small areas of necrosis. The tumor cells are positive with neuronal immunohistochemical markers such as synaptophysin, NeuN, anti-Hu, and neuron-specific enolase, in addition to focal positivity with glial markers like GFAP.

Medulloblastoma Variants

Medulloblastoma can exhibit different morphological patterns that do not have clinical implications, such as medulloblastomas with melanotic or myogenic differentiation. Medulloblastoma with extensive nodularity is a rare variant, usually seen in infants, with a favorable prognosis (Figure 23.7C) [12]. In this variant, a lobular architecture

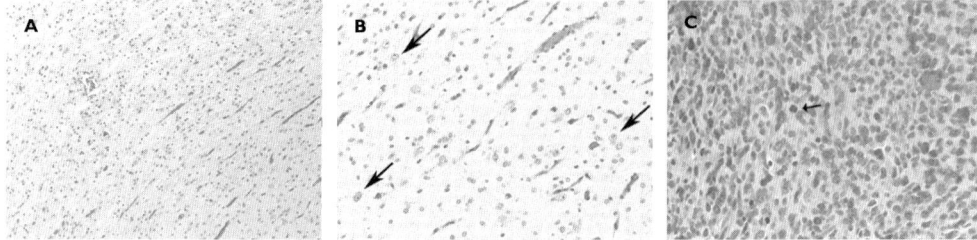

Figure 23.4 **(A)** At low power, diffuse astrocytoma can be recognized as areas of hypercellularity within the brain. H&E, original magnification ×100. **(B)** On higher power, entrapped neurons (arrows) can be seen demonstrating the infiltrative nature of the tumor. H&E, original magnification ×200. **(C)** Anaplastic astrocytoma showing markedly increased cellularity, nuclear pleomorphism, and mitosis (arrow). H&E, original magnification ×200. *See color insert.*

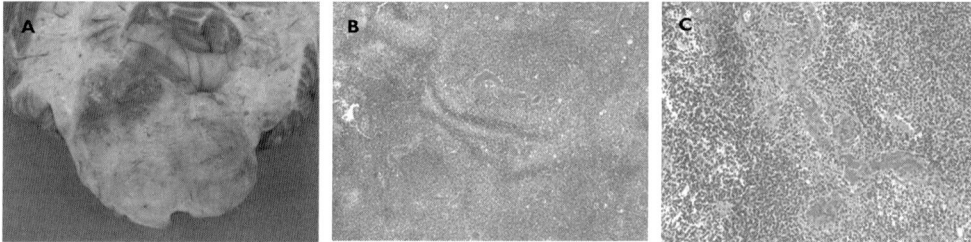

Figure 23.5 **(A)** Grossly, glioblastoma causes enlargement and distortion of the involved brain tissue. It is usually necrotic, hemorrhagic, and exhibits yellowish discoloration. Microscopically, the classical palisading of the neoplastic cells around areas of necrosis **(B)** and vascular endothelial proliferation **(C)** is seen. H&E, original magnification ×40 (B) and ×100 **(C)**. *See color insert.*

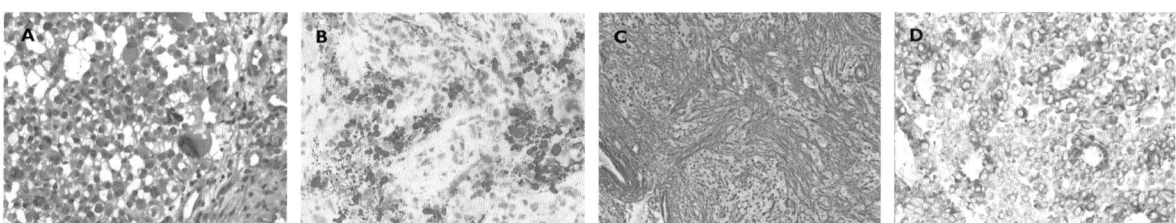

Figure 23.6 **(A)** PXA showing pleomorphic fibrillary astrocytes, including large, bizarre cells. H&E, original magnification ×200. **(B)** Oil red-O stain highlighting the intracellular lipid components in PXA. Original magnification ×200. **(C)** PXA typically exhibits an extensive reticulin network. Reticulin, original magnification ×40. **(D)** GFAP immunostain confirming the glial nature of the neoplastic cells in PXA. Original magnification ×200. *See color insert.*

predominates with large, elongated, reticulin-free zones that contain small, round, neurocytic cells in a fibrillary background. The internodular component of reticulin-rich areas that is commonly seen in desmoplastic medulloblastoma is largely reduced. Desmoplastic medulloblastoma is a more common variant. Grossly, it has a firm consistency. Microscopically, zones of pale, reticulin-poor tumor surrounded by cellular, reticulin-rich, and highly proliferative areas are seen (Figures 23.7D and 23.7E). The prognostic significance of this variant is less clear.

Other well-recognized medulloblastoma variants that are associated with a poorer prognosis are "anaplastic" and "large cell," which may coexist in the same tumor [13–16].

The concept of anaplasia grading in medulloblastoma has expanded this poor prognostic category to include tumors with moderate or severe anaplasia but without the classic large-cell morphology. However, drawing the borders between anaplastic and nonanaplastic tumors can be difficult, and questions about the prognostic significance of such classification have also been raised [17]. Anaplastic medulloblastoma is classically described to show marked nuclear pleomorphism, molding, high mitotic count, prominent necrosis, and apoptosis (Figure 23.7F). Large-cell medulloblastoma has noncohesive, monomorphic, and large cells with abundant eosinophilic cytoplasm (Figure 23.7G). The nuclei are round with open chromatin and prominent nucleoli.

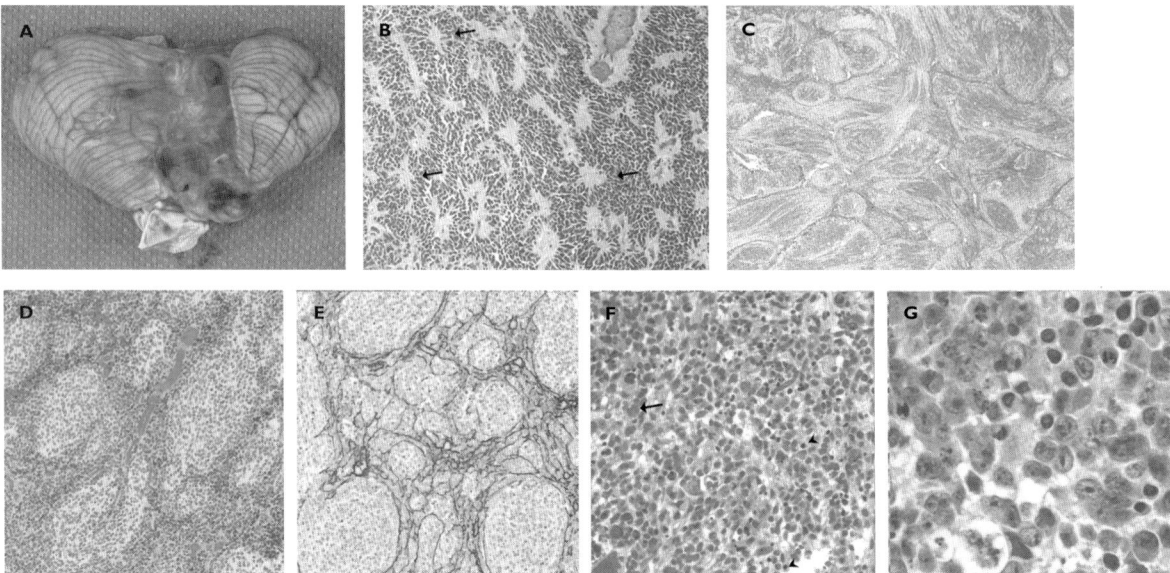

Figure 23.7 (A) Macroscopic appearance of a cerebellar medulloblastoma. (B) Small, round, blue cells arranged in rows and exhibiting Homer-Wright rosettes (arrows) in medulloblastoma. H&E, original magnification ×100. (C) Markedly prominent nodular pattern created by small, round, blue cells lying in a background of neuropil in medulloblastoma with extensive nodularity. H&E, original magnification ×40. (D) Desmoplastic medulloblastoma showing pale nodular areas in-between more cellular internodular regions. H&E, original magnification ×100. (E) Reticulin rich internodular regions in desmoplastic medulloblastoma. Reticulin, original magnification ×100. (F) Anaplastic medulloblastoma showing markedly pleomorphic cells, cell wrapping (arrow) and prominent apoptosis (arrowheads). H&E, original magnification ×200. (G) Large cell medulloblastoma showing large anaplastic cells with prominent nucleoli and vesicular chromatin. Note the prominent apoptosis. H&E, original magnification ×400. *See color insert.*

Supratentorial Primitive Neuroectodermal Tumor

Supratentorial primitive neuroectodermal tumors (sPNETs) (WHO grade IV) usually affect the cerebral hemispheres in children and adolescents. Compared to the morphologically similar medulloblastoma, sPNET is less frequent, has a worse survival, and a different genetic profile. This tumor is mostly deep seated and often has cystic components. The gross distinction from the surrounding brain tissue can be difficult. Microscopically, it exhibits sheets of poorly differentiated small, round blue cells with hyperchromatic nuclei and a high nucleus-to-cytoplasmic ratio (Figure 23.8A). Homer-Wright rosettes are found with variable frequency. Areas of necrosis, abundant mitoses, and apoptosis can be seen. Immunohistochemistry may demonstrate areas of divergent differentiation, including neuronal and glial lineages, or, more rarely, mesenchymal lineages. Differentiated neurons can also be present, in which case the term "ganglioneuroblastoma" may be used.

Other Embryonal Neoplasms

Similar and very rare primitive embryonal tumors include those with predominant neural-tube formation termed "medulloepithelioma" (Figure 23.8B) and "ependymoblastoma" for tumors with predominant ependymoblastic rosettes (Figure 23.8C). A newly described variant

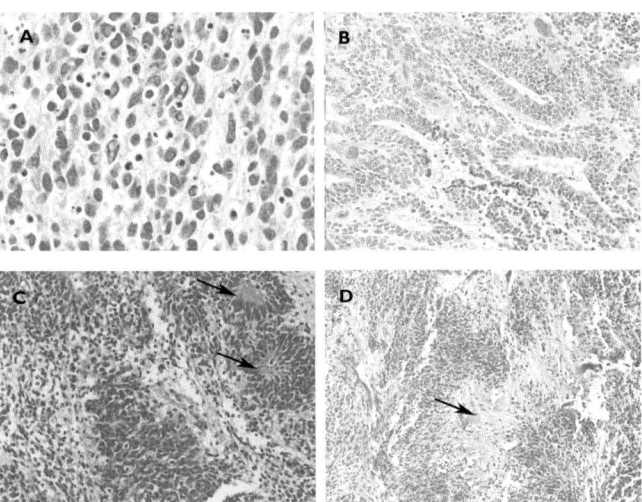

Figure 23.8 (A) sPNET showing a cellular neoplasm with hyperchromatic, anaplastic nuclei and numerous apoptotic bodies. H&E, original magnification ×200. (B) Medulloepithelioma showing the characteristic tubular structures mimicking the primitive neural tube. H&E, original magnification ×200. (C) Ependymoblastoma showing ependymoblastic, multilayered rosette formation (arrows) within sheets of round blue cells. H&E, original magnification ×200. (D) Embryonal tumor with abundant neuropil and true rosettes demonstrating the biphasic architecture with hypercellular regions abutting hypocellular fibrillar regions. H&E, original magnification ×100. *See color insert.*

is "embryonal tumor with abundant neuropil and true rosettes" (Figure 23.8D) that has an extremely poor outcome [18].

Atypical Teratoid/Rhabdoid Tumor

Atypical teratoid/rhabdoid tumor (ATRT) is a high-grade and primitive tumor that can occur in the cerebral hemispheres, the cerebellar hemispheres, the cerebellopontine angles, or the brain stem. It commonly affects children below the age of 3 years. Like other embryonal tumors, ATRT creates a soft-pink mass with foci of necrosis (Figure 23.9A). This tumor has the capacity to show widely divergent differentiation along epithelial, mesenchymal, neuronal, or glial lineages. The word "rhabdoid" refers to the characteristic cells that are not mandatory, however, for the diagnosis. These are large pleomorphic cells with clear margins and abundant eosinophilic cytoplasm that has filamentous inclusions and vacuoles displacing an eccentric round nucleus with a prominent nucleolus (Figure 23.9B). Bizarre, multinucleated giant cells, small cells, or epithelioid cells with granular components may be seen. Necrotic areas are common. Mitoses are usually abundant and the Mib-1 proliferative index is typically very high (up to 80%). Immunohistochemical studies may show tumor-cell positivity for vimentin, EMA, smooth-muscle actin, as well as focally for GFAP, cytokeratin, neurofilament, and synaptophysin. They are typically negative for desmin. By definition, the tumor cells are immunonegative for INI-1 (Figure 23.9C) [19,20] and show 22q11.2 deletions involving the hSNF5/INI1 gene. This feature is very useful in distinguishing ATRT from sPNET, choroid plexus carcinoma (CPC), and medulloblastoma that it may mimic.

Ependymomas

Ependymal tumors comprise a group of tumors with variable biological and morphological patterns and include ependymoma, anaplastic ependymoma, myxopapillary ependymoma, and subependymoma. The two most common entities in the pediatric population are ependymoma (WHO grade II) and its anaplastic variant (WHO grade III). In the pediatric population, though ependymomas most commonly occur in the fourth ventricle, they can be also seen throughout the neuraxis. They commonly show a solid, fibrillary pattern with the formation of perivascular pseudorosettes (Figure 23.10A). The latter structures are zones of fibrillary eosinophilic process, free of nuclei, and abutting blood vessels. It is less common, however, for this tumor to show true ependymal rosettes (Figure 23.10B). The cells usually have bland uniform nuclei with granular chromatin. The neoplastic cells usually show positive reactivity with GFAP, vimentin, and S100. They are occasionally positive with cytokeratin, in addition to EMA, where a characteristic intracytoplasmic dot-like pattern is described. Ultrastructural examination is often important in distinguishing the ependymal versus astrocytic lineage of the neoplastic cells. The finding of abnormal cilia, intracytoplasmic lumens with microvilli, and long junctional complexes point to an ependymal lineage (Figure 23.10C). Morphological variants of ependymoma include cellular, clear-cell, papillary and tanycytic ependymomas.

The WHO grade III version of ependymoma is anaplastic ependymoma. Grossly, it tends to remain well demarcated (Figure 23.11A); however, frankly invasive foci can also be seen. Reproducible criteria for distinguishing grade III from grade II ependymoma have been somewhat elusive. Although some authors report prognostic significance of some histologic features [21,22], others have not found a correlation [23–27]. A more recent study that included an extensive review shows histological grade using the WHO criteria does not correlate with overall survival, but it is still an independent prognostic factor for event-free survival [28]. The authors of this study used the WHO criteria and their review and experience to define more objective criteria for the grading of posterior fossa ependymomas. In their study, two of the following features were needed for the diagnosis of a grade III ependymoma [28]: bona fide vascular endothelial proliferation with endothelial layering (Figure 23.11B), mitotic rate greater than 10 per 10 high-power fields, palisading necrosis, and marked hypercellularity with nuclear pleomorphism and/or hyperchromasia. It is only hoped that adoption of these criteria will lead to more consistent grading of these tumors.

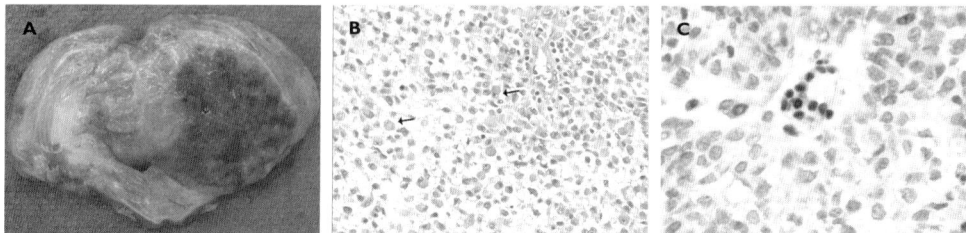

Figure 23.9 (A) A large destructive, hemorrhagic and necrotic mass occupying most of a cerebellar hemisphere that was found to be ATRT. (B) ATRT showing sheets of large pleomorphic cells, some of which exhibits globular cytoplasmic eosinophilic material that push the nucleus to the cell edges (arrows). Note the prominent nucleoli within vesicular nuclei. H&E, original magnification ×100. (C) In ATRT, the tumor cells are negative for INI-1. Also present are scattered lymphocytes and a vessel (center of the picture) that show normal, positive, nuclear staining for INI-1. Original magnification ×200. See color insert.

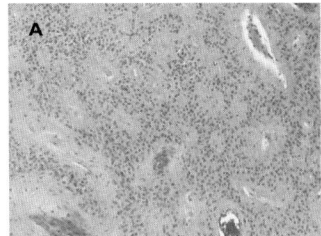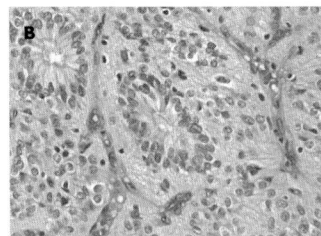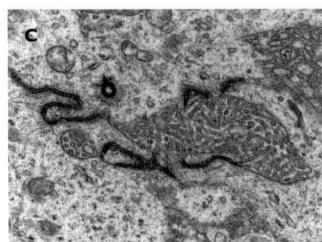

Figure 23.10 **(A)** Ependymoma showing small, bland cells within a fibrillary background. Note the perivascular nuclear-free zones that are a typical, low-power appearance of ependymoma. H&E, original magnification ×100. **(B)** True ependymal rosettes with the formation of lumens are sometimes found in ependymoma. H&E, original magnification ×200. **(C)** Ultrastructural features of an ependymoma showing microvilli in lumina and long intracellular junctions. See color insert.

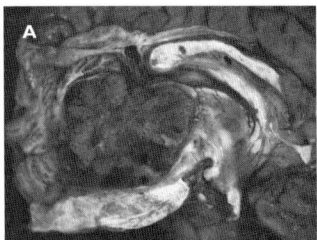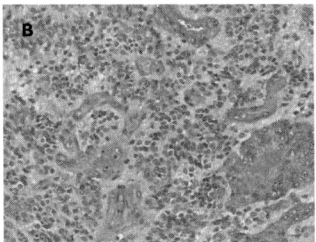

Figure 23.11 **(A)** Gross appearance of an anaplastic ependymoma showing a soft, fleshy, and well-demarcated mass protruding into the lumen of the fourth ventricle. **(B)** Anaplastic ependymoma showing increased cellularity and abundant vascular-endothelial proliferation. See color insert.

Choroid Plexus Papilloma and Carcinoma

Choroid plexus papilloma (CPP, WHO grade I) constitutes 2% to 4% of pediatric CNS tumors. CPC (WHO grade III) is 5 times less common. Both occur in areas where choroid plexus is normally found [29], mainly in the lateral ventricles [30], and to a lesser degree, in the fourth ventricle (the commonest location in adults). Grossly, CPP forms a cauliflower-like and well-delineated mass that is larger than the normal choroid plexus. Microscopically, it exhibits a normal choroid plexus-like histology with true fibrovascular cores (Figure 23.12A), with the tumor cells typically resting on a basement membrane (Figure 23.12B)—a feature that is helpful in distinguishing it from papillary ependymoma. However, the lining epithelial cells are mildly atypical and appear more crowded and piled-up when compared with normal papillae (Figure 23.12C). CPP tumor cells can exhibit a wide variety of cellular changes, including oncocytic change, mucinous degeneration, and melanization. Immunohistochemical studies show that the lining epithelium is positive for cytokeratin, transthyretin, vimentin, CK7, and focally for GFAP and EMA. They are usually negative for CK20 [31].

CPC usually demonstrates more hemorrhage, necrosis, and invasiveness than CPP. Brain invasion is common (Figure 23.13A). Microscopically, sheets of frankly anaplastic, highly cellular tumor with areas of necrosis and frequent mitoses (Figure 23.13B) are commonly associated with foci that are still reminiscent of a papilloma. Otherwise, the papillary structures are usually blurred by more solid patterns. The neoplastic cells are usually immunopositive for EMA, cytokeratin, and S100. CPCs can create poorly differentiated patterns that may be confused with embryonal tumors like ATRT.

Atypical CPP is a new entity that has been added to the 2007 WHO classification. It is essentially similar to CPP but with an increased mitotic activity. Two or more mitoses per 10 random high-power fields are required for the diagnosis of this atypical entity. In addition, two out of four features are commonly seen. These include cellularity, nuclear pleomorphism, blurring of the papillary pattern, and necrosis [32].

Neuronal and Mixed Neuroglial Tumors

Ganglioglioma

Ganglioglioma usually forms a well-defined mass that can exhibit cystic features with little mass effect and has a temporal-lobe predilection. This tumor typically exhibits variable degrees of two distinct neoplastic cell populations: (1) glial, and (2) neuronal/gangliocytic (Figure 23.14A). When the tumor is composed solely of neuronal/gangliocytic components, it is referred to as "gangliocytoma, WHO grade I." When a neoplastic glial component is recognized, the term "ganglioglioma" is used and is graded on the basis of the glial component; a pilocytic-like glial component is given a WHO grade of I, whereas an anaplastic glial component leads to a WHO grade III designation. Criteria for grade II ganglioglioma have been suggested; however, this is not currently an official WHO category [33].

Microscopically, the neurons appear like ganglion cells, with large nuclei, prominent nucleoli, and abundant cytoplasm where Nissl basophilic material is present (Figure 23.14B). A "neoplastic or atypical ganglion cell" is a descriptor used for the ganglion cells that show abnormal clustering, pleomorphism, bi- or multinucleation, or exhibit large, bizarre nuclei. EGBs are typically present, and Rosenthal fibers can also be seen. Calcifications and

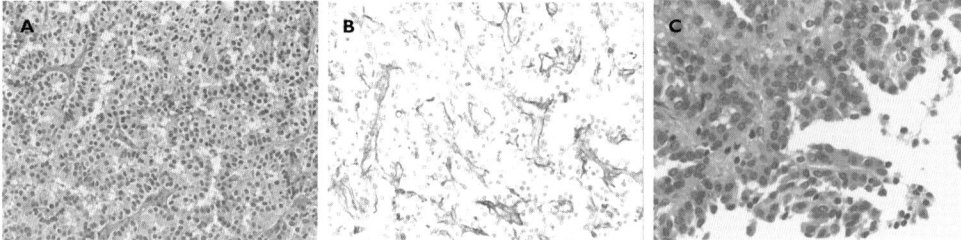

Figure 23.12 **(A)** Choroid-plexus papilloma showing the papillary architecture where the papillae are formed by fibrovascular stroma with overlying columnar epithelium. H&E, original magnification ×200. **(B)** Immunohistochemical staining for laminin highlighting the basement membrane in CPP. Original magnification ×200. **(C)** The epithelial cells lining the papillae are slightly crowded and exhibit minor atypical changes such as mild nuclear pleomorphism and hyperchromasia. H&E, original magnification ×400. *See color insert.*

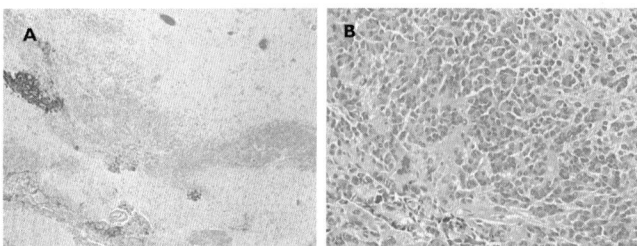

Figure 23.13 **(A)** Choroid plexus carcinoma showing sheets of anaplastic tumor cells that are invading adjacent brain tissue. Melanization of some of the tumor cells can be seen. H&E, original magnification ×40. **(B)** A higher-power view of the tumor showing nuclear atypia, blurring of the papillary pattern, and increased cell density compared with CPP. H&E, original magnification ×200. *See color insert.*

perivascular inflammation within a prominent capillary network are common features. Mitotic figures are rare in low-grade gangliogliomas but are present in the anaplastic version.

The neuronal/gangliocytic cells are highlighted by immunohistochemistry for NeuN, synaptophysin, or chromogranin. The glial component is highlighted by GFAP. Ultrastructural examination may be used to confirm the presence of both a glial and neuronal/gangliocytic component. The former shows glial processes with intracytoplasmic dense fascicles of intermediate filaments, whereas the latter shows microtubules, electron-dense neurosecretory vesicles, and neuritic-type processes (Figure 23.14C).

Developmental abnormalities such as cortical dysplasia should be considered in the differential diagnosis of gangliocytoma or low-grade ganglioglioma. Cortical dysplasia may also be seen in association with these tumors. It has been suggested that distinguishing anaplastic ganglioglioma from anaplastic astrocytoma is important as gross, total resection is suggested to be curative in the former [34].

Desmoplastic Infantile Astrocytoma/Ganglioglioma

Desmoplastic infantile astrocytoma/ganglioglioma (DIA/G) is a unique and rare pediatric tumor (WHO grade I) [35]. It usually affects the supratentorial compartment of children who are aged less than 18 months. Grossly, it is large, well-demarcated, superficial, and typically cystic, with involvement of multiple lobes and an attachment to the overlying dura. DIA has low cellularity within a remarkably desmoplastic stroma within which fascicles, storiform, or whorled patterns of spindled, strongly GFAP-immunopositive astrocytes are embedded (Figures 23.15A, 23.15B, 23.15C). A cortical component without desmoplasia may be observed. This component is usually nodular and often formed by small astrocytes with oval nuclei and eosinophilic cytoplasm. If a population of abnormal, binucleated ganglion cells is present then the tumor is labeled "DIG." The ganglion cells can be difficult to detect without the use of immunohistochemical markers such synaptophysin. DIA/G usually has only rare mitoses, no necrosis, and no microvascular proliferation. However, the presence of one or more of these latter features is not indicative of a high-grade tumor as the significance of such findings remains to be established [36,37]. Areas similar to a poorly differentiated embryonal tumor with high mitotic index can be found; however, these also should not be considered as a high-grade feature as their prognostic significance in the context of DIA/G is not clear.

Dysembryoplastic neuroepithelial tumor

Dysembryoplastic neuroepithelial tumor (DNET) is a low-grade cortically based tumor (WHO grade I) that has a predilection for the temporal and frontal lobes. It should not demonstrate mass effect on the surrounding brain tissue. Grossly, it is a well-defined neoplasm that affects the cerebral cortex and can exhibit multinodular, cystic, and/or gelatinous features. Different patterns have been described whose prognostic significance is unclear. These are "typical," "complex," and "nonspecific" [38]. In the simple form, the main constituent is the classic glioneuronal element. This is made up of bland oligodendroglial-like cells that flank axons, highlighted with immunostaining for synaptophysin or neurofilament, which run perpendicular to the cortical surface (Figure 23.16A). There is a mucinous background where floating mature neurons are

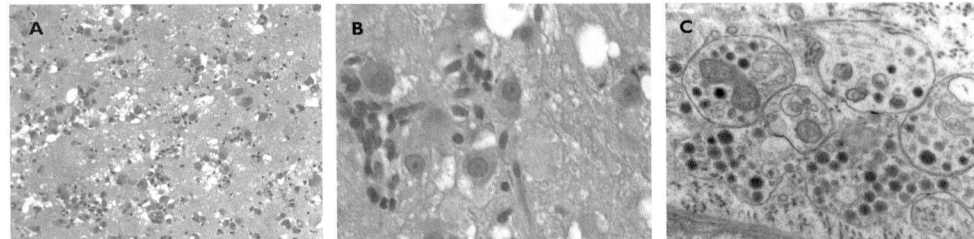

Figure 23.14 **(A)** Ganglioglioma showing scattered ganglion cells within a rich fibrillary background. H&E, original magnification ×40. **(B)** Ganglion cells are large cells with prominent nucleoli and abundant eosinophilic cytoplasm; some contain basophilic Nissl substance in the periphery of the cytoplasm. H&E, original magnification ×400. **(C)** Ultrastructurally, electron-dense neurosecretory vesicles can be seen in the cytoplasm of the tumor cells. *See color insert.*

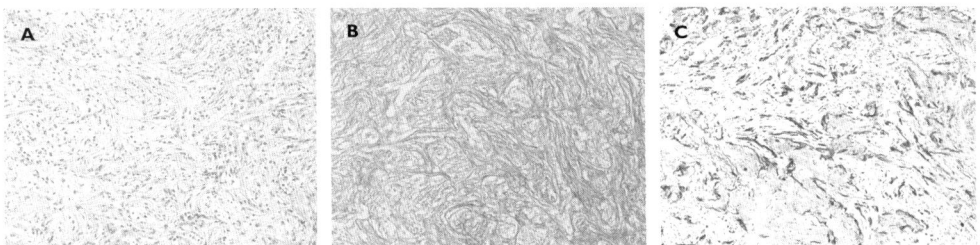

Figure 23.15 **(A)** Desmoplastic infantile ganglioglioma/astroctyoma showing fascicles of spindled astrocytes within a desmoplastic stroma that is highlighted with reticulin staining **(B)**. **(C)** Immunohistochemical staining is positive for GFAP. All pictures original magnification ×100. *See color insert.*

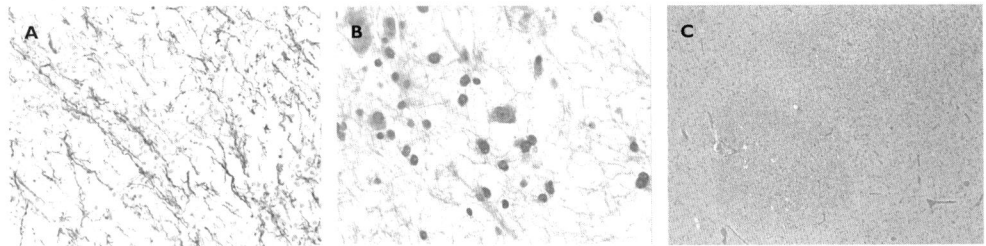

Figure 23.16 **(A)** DNET showing the typical glioneuronal component. The axons are highlighted with immunohistochemical staining for neurofilament. Original magnification ×200. **(B)** Within the hypocellular myxoid areas of DNET, scattered, floating neurons are present. H&E, original magnification ×400. **(C)** Tumor nodules within the cortex in a case of complex DNET. H&E, original magnification ×40. *See color insert.*

present. The floating neuronal component is composed of large cells with large bland nuclei and prominent nucleoli (Figure 23.16B). Atypical ganglion cells should not be seen. Adjacent foci of cortical dysplasia are usually present [38]. Rarely, microvascular proliferation, mitoses, or necrosis can be seen in DNET and shouldn't change the grade by themselves. The oligodendroglial-like cells show positive immunohistochemical reactivity with S100, MAP2, and olig2. In addition, a subpopulation of cells may be positive for neuronal markers such as NeuN or synaptophysin. GFAP stains the glial components.

"Complex" is a term that is used when the tumor has glial nodules in addition to the specific glioneuronal element (Figure 23.16C). More diffuse glial components can also be seen. These often mimic a low-grade glioma but may also show some atypical features like nuclear atypia, occasional mitoses, microvasular-like proliferation, or ischemic necrosis [3]. In addition to the complex form, a controversial concept of a "nonspecific" variant exists that is essentially based on clinicopathological correlation. The lesion in this latter variant is formed by glial elements in the absence of glioneuronal elements. The required clinical criteria for lesions that would otherwise be categorized as low-grade gliomas to be put under the "nonspecific" DNET variant include partial seizures, age <20 years, absence of neurological deficits, stable cortical topography, and absence of mass effects unless they relate to a cyst.

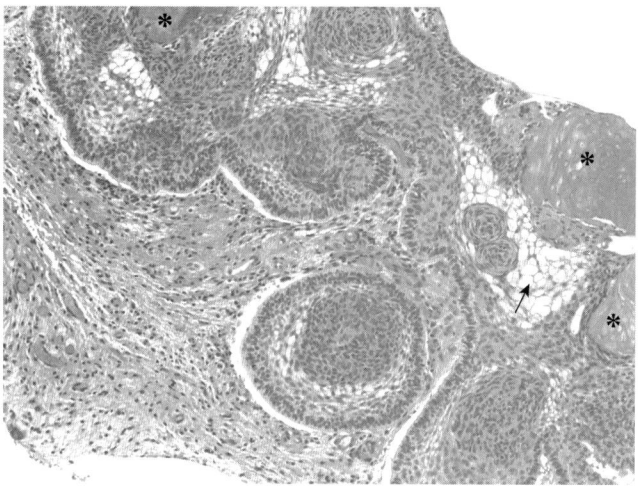

Figure 23.17 Craniopharyngioma showing palisaded epithelial cells, the loose stellate reticulum (arrow) and wet keratin (*). H&E, original magnification ×100. *See color insert.*

Nonneuroepithelial Tumors

Craniopharyngioma

Craniopharyngioma (WHO grade I) usually affects the suprasellar region where it is thought to arise from Rathke's pouch remnants. It has two variants: adamantinomatous and papillary. The former is most common in the pediatric population where it accounts for 5 to 10% of intracranial tumors, making it the most common form of nonneuroepithelial neoplasm [39]. It usually has solid, firm, and cystic components with contents that resemble motor oil due to the nature of the mixture of blood, proteins, and cholesterol crystals. The tumor exhibits poor circumscription and has nests and trabeculae of epithelial-cell sheets in a fibrous stroma. The epithelium demonstrates a characteristic morphology where the peripheral cells show nuclear palisading, whereas the central cells form a loose "stellate reticulum" (Figure 23.17). Also present are characteristic areas of "wet keratin" that frequently calcify. The presence of one of the latter two features (the stellate reticulum or the wet keratin) is diagnostic of craniopharyngioma [2]. In addition, cystic changes, xanthogranulomatous reaction, and cholesterol clefts are frequent findings in a craniopharyngioma. Variable degrees of necrosis can be seen, which does not indicate a malignant nature. Craniopharyngioma can be associated with a rim of reactive brain tissue where Rosenthal fibers are prominent. The latter can be confused with low-grade astrocytic neoplasms, particularly on frozen section.

REFERENCES

1. Burger PC, Scheithauer BW. *Tumors of the central nervous system.* Washington, DC: American Registry of Pathology in collaboration with the Armed Forces Institute of Pathology; 2007.
2. Burger PC, Scheithauer BW, Vogel FS. *Surgical Pathology of the Nervous System and its Coverings.* New York: Churchill Livingstone; 2002.
3. Louis DN. *WHO Classification of Tumours of the Central Nervous System.* Lyon: International Agency for Research on Cancer; 2007.
4. Hayostek CJ, Shaw EG, Scheithauer B, et al. Astrocytomas of the cerebellum. A comparative clinicopathologic study of pilocytic and diffuse astrocytomas. *Cancer.* 1993;72(3):856–869.
5. Tihan T, Fisher PG, Kepner JL, et al. Pediatric astrocytomas with monomorphous pilomyxoid features and a less favorable outcome. *J Neuropathol Exp Neurol.* 1999;58(10):1061–1068.
6. Wang M, Tihan T, Rojiani AM, et al. Monomorphous angiocentric glioma: a distinctive epileptogenic neoplasm with features of infiltrating astrocytoma and ependymoma. *J Neuropathol Exp Neurol.* 2005;64(10):875–881.
7. Lehman NL. Central nervous system tumors with ependymal features: a broadened spectrum of primarily ependymal differentiation? *J Neuropathol Exp Neurol.* 2008;67(3):177–188.
8. Perry A, Miller CR, Gujrati M, et al. Malignant gliomas with primitive neuroectodermal tumor-like components: a clinicopathologic and genetic study of 53 cases. *Brain Pathol.* 2009;19(1):81–90.
9. Giannini C, Scheithauer BW, Burger PC, et al. Pleomorphic xanthoastrocytoma: what do we really know about it? *Cancer.* 1999;85(9):2033–2045.
10. Reifenberger G, Kaulich K, Wiestler OD, Blumcke I. Expression of the CD34 antigen in pleomorphic xanthoastrocytomas. *Acta Neuropathol.* 2003;105(4):358–364.
11. Yeh DJ, Hessler RB, Stevens EA, Lee MR. Composite pleomorphic xanthoastrocytoma-ganglioglioma presenting as a suprasellar mass: case report. *Neurosurgery.* 2003;52(6):1465–1468; discussion 8–9.
12. Giangaspero F, Perilongo G, Fondelli MP, et al. Medulloblastoma with extensive nodularity: a variant with favorable prognosis. *J Neurosurg.* 1999;91(6):971–977.
13. Brown HG, Kepner JL, Perlman EJ, et al. "Large cell/anaplastic" medulloblastomas: a Pediatric Oncology Group Study. *J Neuropathol Exp Neurol.* 2000;59(10):857–865.
14. Eberhart CG, Kepner JL, Goldthwaite PT, et al. Histopathologic grading of medulloblastomas: a Pediatric Oncology Group Study. *Cancer.* 2002;94(2):552–560.
15. Giangaspero F, Wellek S, Masuoka J, Gessi M, Kleihues P, Ohgaki H. Stratification of medulloblastoma on the basis of histopathological grading. *Acta Neuropathol.* 2006;112(1):5–12.
16. Lamont JM, McManamy CS, Pearson AD, Clifford SC, Ellison DW. Combined histopathological and molecular cytogenetic stratification of medulloblastoma patients. *Clin Cancer Res.* 2004;10(16):5482–5493.
17. Min HS, Lee YJ, Park K, Cho BK, Park SH. Medulloblastoma: histopathologic and molecular markers of anaplasia and biologic behavior. *Acta Neuropathol.* 2006;112(1):13–20.
18. Eberhart CG, Brat DJ, Cohen KJ, Burger PC. Pediatric neuroblastic brain tumors containing abundant neuropil and true rosettes. *Pediatr Dev Pathol.* 2000;3(4):346–352.
19. Biegel JA, Fogelgren B, Zhou JY, et al. Mutations of the INI1 rhabdoid tumor suppressor gene in medulloblastomas and primitive neuroectodermal tumors of the central nervous system. *Clini Cancer Res.* 2000;6(7):2759–2763.
20. Judkins AR, Mauger J, Ht A, Rorke LB, Biegel JA. Immunohistochemical analysis of hSNF5/INI1 in pediatric CNS neoplasms. *Am J Surg Pathol.* 2004;28(5):644–650.
21. Figarella-Branger D, Civatte M, Bouvier-Labit C, et al. Prognostic factors in intracranial ependymomas in children. *J Neurosurg.* 2000;93(4):605–613.
22. Merchant TE, Jenkins JJ, Burger PC, et al. Influence of tumor grade on time to progression after irradiation for localized ependymoma in children. *Int J of Radiat Oncol Biol Phys.* 2002;53(1):52–57.
23. Agaoglu FY, Ayan I, Dizdar Y, Kebudi R, Gorgun O, Darendeliler E. Ependymal tumors in childhood. *Pediatr Blood Cancer.* 2005;45(3):298–303.
24. Bouffet E, Perilongo G, Canete A, Massimino M. Intracranial ependymomas in children: a critical review of prognostic factors and a plea for cooperation. *Med Pediatr Oncol.* 1998;30(6):319–329; discussion 29–31.
25. Foreman NK, Love S, Thorne R. Intracranial ependymomas: analysis of prognostic factors in a population-based series. *Pediatr Neurosurg.* 1996;24(3):119–125.
26. Jaing TH, Wang HS, Tsay PK, et al. Multivariate analysis of clinical prognostic factors in children with intracranial ependymomas. *J Neurooncol.* 2004;68(3):255–261.
27. Robertson PL, Zeltzer PM, Boyett JM, et al. Survival and prognostic factors following radiation therapy and chemotherapy for ependymomas in children: a report of the Children's Cancer Group. *J Neurosurg.* 1998;88(4):695–703.

28. Tihan T, Zhou T, Holmes E, Burger PC, Ozuysal S, Rushing EJ. The prognostic value of histological grading of posterior fossa ependymomas in children: a Children's Oncology Group study and a review of prognostic factors. *Mod Pathol.* 2008;21(2):165–177.
29. Rickert CH, Paulus W. Epidemiology of central nervous system tumors in childhood and adolescence based on the new WHO classification. *Childs Nerv Syst.* 2001;17(9):503–511.
30. Wolff JE, Sajedi M, Brant R, Coppes MJ, Egeler RM. Choroid plexus tumours. *Br J Cancer.* 2002;87(10):1086–1091.
31. Gyure KA, Morrison AL. Cytokeratin 7 and 20 expression in choroid plexus tumors: utility in differentiating these neoplasms from metastatic carcinomas. *Mod Pathol.* 2000;13(6):638–643.
32. Jeibmann A, Hasselblatt M, Gerss J, et al. Prognostic implications of atypical histologic features in choroid plexus papilloma. *J Neuropathol Exp Neurol.* 2006;65(11):1069–1073.
33. Luyken C, Blumcke I, Fimmers R, Urbach H, Wiestler OD, Schramm J. Supratentorial gangliogliomas: histopathologic grading and tumor recurrence in 184 patients with a median follow-up of 8 years. *Cancer.* 2004;101(1):146–155.
34. Varlet P, Soni D, Miquel C, et al. New variants of malignant glioneuronal tumors: a clinicopathological study of 40 cases. *Neurosurgery.* 2004;55(6):1377–1391; discussion 91–92.
35. Pommepuy I, Delage-Corre M, Moreau JJ, Labrousse F. A report of a desmoplastic ganglioglioma in a 12-year-old girl with review of the literature. *J Neurooncol.* 2006;76(3):271–275.
36. De Munnynck K, Van Gool S, Van Calenbergh F, et al. Desmoplastic infantile ganglioglioma: a potentially malignant tumor? *Am J Surg Pathol.* 2002;26(11):1515–1522.
37. Setty SN, Miller DC, Camras L, Charbel F, Schmidt ML. Desmoplastic infantile astrocytoma with metastases at presentation. *Mod Pathol.* 1997;10(9):945–951.
38. Daumas-Duport C, Varlet P, Bacha S, Beuvon F, Cervera-Pierot P, Chodkiewicz JP. Dysembryoplastic neuroepithelial tumors: nonspecific histological forms—a study of 40 cases. *J Neurooncol.* 1999;41(3):267–280.
39. Adamson TE, Wiestler OD, Kleihues P, Yasargil MG. Correlation of clinical and pathological features in surgically treated craniopharyngiomas. *J Neurosurg.* 1990;73(1):12–17.

24 Molecular Genetics of Medulloblastoma and High-Grade Astrocytomas in Children

Arnold B. Etame, Christian Smith, Uri Tabori, and James T. Rutka

INTRODUCTION

Brain tumors represent the most common solid tumor in children, with a peak incidence of 4 in 100,000 person years in the United States [1]. Most children present with the disease between the ages of 3 and 7. Supratentorial tumors are usually seen in older children, whereas infratentorial tumors are more common in the younger age group. Medulloblastomas and malignant gliomas are the most common malignant brain tumors in children. Recent advances in microneurosurgical techniques, radiation therapy, and chemotherapy have led to significant improvement in survival for children with medulloblastoma. However, this has come at the expense of neurocognitive function [2]. It is now well recognized that craniospinal irradiation is the primary cause of cognitive dysfunction in children treated for medulloblastoma [2]. Similarly, high-dose conventional chemotherapy has its toxic limitations [2]. In spite of these advances for medulloblastoma, children with high-grade gliomas continue to have a dismal prognosis with 2-year progression-free survival at less than 20% [3]. As a result, there has been an increased emphasis on identifying critical molecular pathways that belie tumor behavior and differential response to therapy. Recent advances in molecular techniques have provided some insights into the molecular mechanisms of tumor initiation, propagation, and progression. Ultimately, these molecular advances should pave the way for development of therapies that are more specific and less toxic. In this chapter, we examine the molecular genetics of diffuse intrinsic pontine glioma, supratentorial high-grade astrocytomas and medulloblastoma, as well as the potential role of molecularly directed translational therapies.

DIFFUSE PONTINE BRAINSTEM GLIOMA

Brief Clinical Overview

Diffuse intrinsic pontine glioma (DIPG) accounts for approximately 80% of pediatric brainstem tumors. The median survival after presentation is less than 1 year, and the long-term survival remains less than 10% [4]. The vast majority of patients present between the ages of 5 and 10. Diagnosis is typically ascertained radiographically; hence, surgical biopsies are rarely performed. A radiographic view of DIPG is depicted in Figure 24.1. DIPG can demonstrate histopathologic features consistent with either grade III or even grade IV gliomas. The disease is not amenable to surgery due to its very diffuse and infiltrative nature. Radiation therapy is the treatment modality of choice. Whereas radiation leads to clinical and radiological responsiveness, the vast majority of children experience early progression of disease [4]. Neither high-dose chemotherapy protocols [5], using myeloablation with autologous stem-cell rescue [6], nor high-dose hyperfractionated radiotherapy [7] have prolonged survival.

Molecular Genetics

The dismal outcome of DIPG has generated an impetus toward identifying critical genetic alterations associated with tumor pathogenesis—see Table 24.1. As the disease is usually diagnosed by radiography, surgical specimens are extremely rare. As a result, there is a limitation to studying surgical specimens for molecular analysis and also ascertaining any statistically significant molecular patterns. It is, therefore, not surprising that there is a paucity of data in the literature pertaining to the molecular genetics of DIPG.

However, molecular analysis on DIPG shows a predilection toward p53 mutation when compared to gliomas of other locations [8,9]. In addition, there appears to be a correlation with loss of heterozygosity (LOH) on chromosome 17p. In one analysis of 7 gliomas, LOH 17p was demonstrated in 4 patients [9]. All patients with LOH on 17p had a concurrent p53 mutation. In the same study, LOH on chromosome 10 was also noted in 4 patients, 3 of whom had a concurrent LOH on 17p.

Another genetic alteration noted in DIPG involves the overexpression and amplification of the epidermal growth factor receptor (EGFR). The extent of EGFR expression has been correlated with tumor grade [10]. From this respect, DIPG may share similar genetic alterations to adult glioblastoma multiforme (GBM).

Recently, Lee et al [11]. performed a genetic analysis of DIPGs using high-resolution single-nucleotide polymorphism (SNP) arrays and using whole genome-amplified DNA. In this study, SNP analysis led to the observation that the platelet-derived growth factor (PDGF), sonic hedgehog (SHH), and wingless (Wnt) signaling pathways

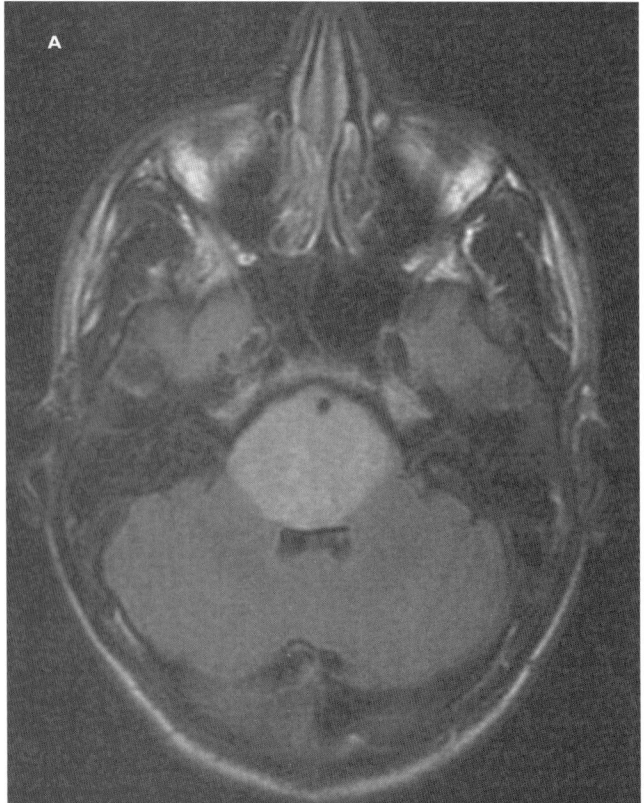

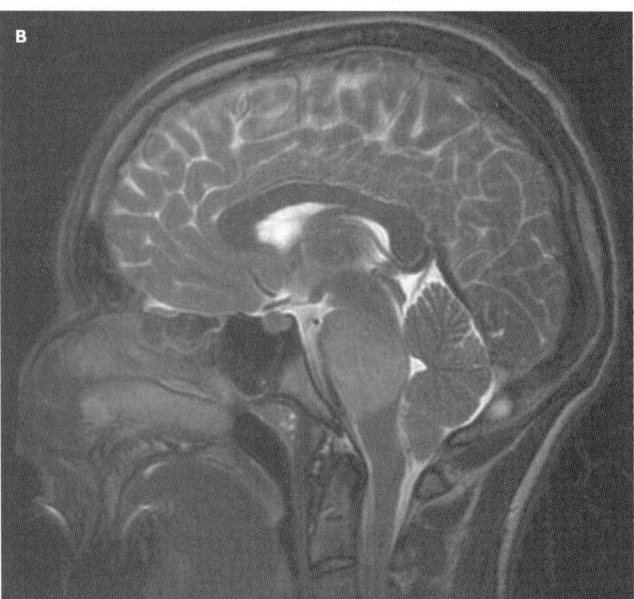

Figure 24.1 Brainstem glioma. **(A)** Axial T1-FLAIR MR in 6-year-old autistic child, one of identical twins, who presented with a brief history of headache, head tilt, and VI nerve palsy. MR image shows high signal region occupying the pons. Note the basilar artery, which is surrounded by tumor. **(B)** Sagittal T2 TSE-weighted MR in the same patient demonstrates a high signal expansile lesion within the pons.

were affected in several tumors examined [11]. It is hoped that future studies will complete the genomic map for DIPG and that this will lead to targets that can be validated across several centers.

Table 24.1 Key Genetic Alterations in Diffuse Intrinsic Pontine Gliomas

Chromosomal deletions
  LOH 17p
  LOH 10P
Tumor-suppressor mutations
  p53
Aberrant receptor signaling
  EGRF

Translational Therapies

The increased EGFR signaling in DIPG, and the correlation of EGFR expression with DIPG grade, has made this pathway an ideal target. The anti-EGFR monoclonal antibody, nimotuzumab, was recently evaluated in patients with relapsing DIPG. In a clinical trial of 22 patients, 10 demonstrated stable disease and partial remission when treated with nimotuzumab [5]. Another area of exploration is the employment of antiangiogenic agents as radio sensitizers, as has been applied in adult patients [1]. As DIPGs share similar genetic alterations with adult GBM, future directives would entail applying adult-directed molecular-pathway therapies to similar pathways in children. In the interim, DIPG remains a uniformly fatal entity.

HIGH-GRADE ASTROCYTOMAS

Brief Clinical Overview

In general, astrocytomas represent 40% of all pediatric brain tumors. World Health Organization (WHO) classifies four grades of astrocytomas: grades I and II, representing the low-grade tumors, and grade III and IV, representing high-grade tumors. The most common pediatric astrocytoma is the juvenile pilocytic astrocytoma (JPA) that is a grade I tumor. Most JPA patients are cured through complete surgical resection. Grade II astrocytomas can be classified as either fibrillary, gemistocytic, and protoplasmic on the basis of histology. Grade III and IV tumors represent the anaplastic astrocytoma and the GBM, respectively. A radiographic view of a high-grade astrocytoma is depicted in Figure 24.2. Patients with grade III and IV lesions have a much poorer prognosis than those with low-grade astrocytomas, in spite of aggressive multimodal therapy, including radiation, surgical resection, and chemotherapy. Children with GBM have the worst outcome within the spectrum [12]. In contrast to adults, high-grade tumors are relatively rare in children. Furthermore, pediatric high-grade astrocytomas have a slightly better prognosis compared to adult astrocytoma [13].

Molecular Genetics

Chromosomal Alterations

Cytogenetics studies demonstrated distinct cytogenetic alterations in children with high-grade astrocytomas relative to adults with similar tumors—see Table 24.2 and Figure 24.3. Extensive data from the study of adult high-grade astrocytomas suggest two possible pathways for tumor pathogenesis [14,15]. In the first pathway, loss of

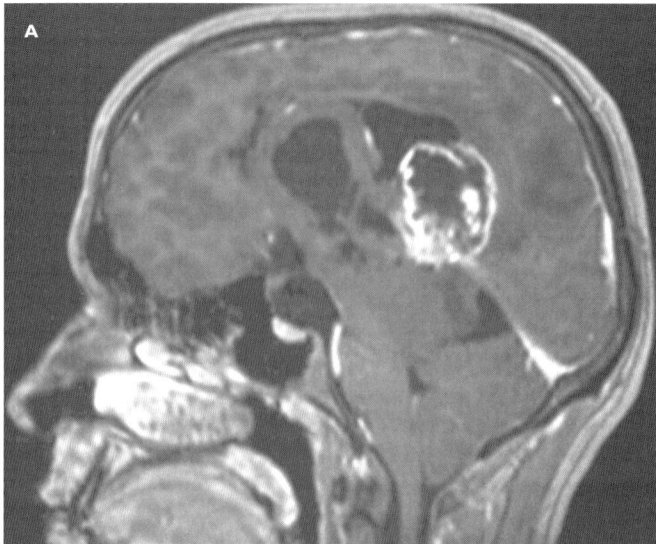

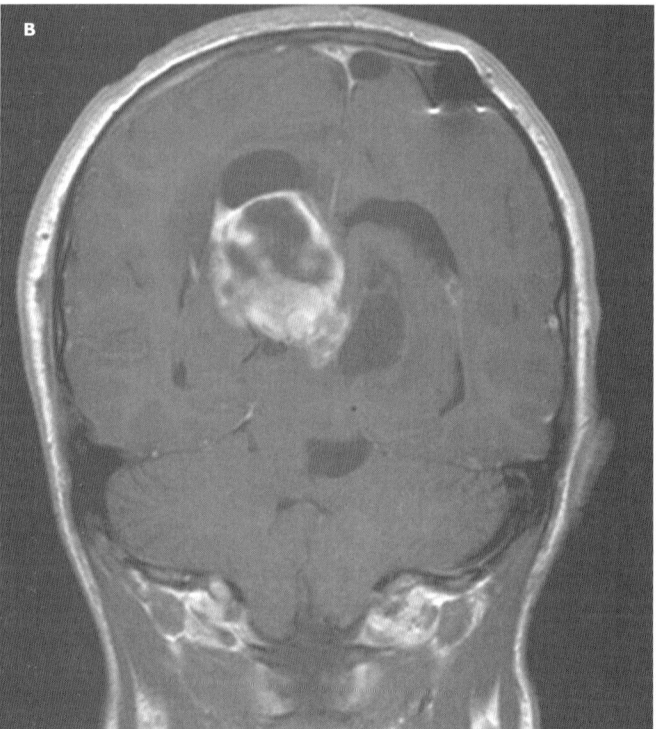

Figure 24.2 High-grade glioma. **(A)** Sagittal T1-weighted MR with gadolinium in 14-year-old man with a heterogeneous ring enhancing posterior thalamic mass. Note the anterior displacement of the corpus callosum as well as effacement of the ventricles. **(B)** Axial T1-weighted MR with contrast showing lesion in the right thalamus with some involvement of the left thalamus.

Table 24.2 Key Genetic Alterations in Pediatric High-Grade Astrocytomas

Chromosomal deletions in AA
6q, 9q, 12q, 22q
Chromosomal gains in AA
5q
Chromosomal deletions in pediatric GBM
8q, 17p
Chromosomal gains in pediatric GBM
1q, 3q, 16p

Abreviations: AA, anaplastic astrocytoma; GBM, glioblastoma multiforme.

this has been observed in 63% of GBM [14]. These GBMs are considered *de novo* or primary GBMs. Furthermore, concomitant LOH of 10 and amplification of a mutant EGRF(EGFR/c-erbB1) has been estimated to occur in approximately 45% of adult GBMs, suggesting that the increased tyrosine kinase activity from increased activation of the EGFR pathway appears to be a crucial component in the *de novo* formation of GBMs [18–20].

Other interesting chromosomal findings that have been associated with adult GBM include duplication of chromosome 7, loss of 9p, monosomy 10, deletion of 22q, and double-minute chromosomes [21]. Genes associated with some of the chromosomal alterations have been further elucidated. Schmidt et al [22] associated the 9p deletion with loss of *CDKN2/p16*. Similarly, some patients with loss of 10q have deletions of *MMAC1/PTEN*[23,24] or *DMBT1* [25]. Such findings are relatively rare in children, suggesting that, in children, such pediatric astrocytomas occur via distinct molecular paradigms and pathways when compared to their adult counterparts.

The most common chromosomal alterations in pediatric high-grade gliomas include loss of chromosome 16p, 17p, 19p, 19q, and 22 [26]. Gain of chromosome 5q as well as losses of chromosome 6q, 9q, 12q, and 22q are characteristic findings in pediatric anaplastic astrocytomas [27]. Pediatric GBMs are often rare tumors and demonstrate loss of chromosome 8q and 17p, as well as gain of chromosome 1q, 3q, and 16p [27]. The reported frequency of LOH of 17p in pediatric astrocytomas appears to be considerably lower when compared to adult high-grade astrocytomas. When Litofsky et al [28], examined 21 pediatric astrocytomas for LOH of 17p, only 5 tumors demonstrated the delection. Another series with a similar number of pediatric patients reported the mutation in only 1 patient whose tumor was a GBM [29].

Mutations in DNA mismatch repair have been shown to be a key factor in tumorigenesis, especially with respect to colorectal cancer [30]. Such defects result in accumulation of mutated DNAs of varying length, a condition termed "microsatellite instability." Approximately, 25% of pediatric high-grade astrocytomas are characterized with microsatellite instability, in contrast to adult high-grade gliomas where this phenotype is extremely rare or even absent [31].

Nakamura et al [32] studied 44 pediatric gliomas using LOH analysis, mutational analysis for p53 and PTEN,

chromosome 17p leads to the transformation of a diffuse astrocytoma into an anaplastic astrocytoma or a GBM. GBMs resulting from this pathway are often referred to as secondary GBMs. LOH of 17p is seen in 40% of anaplastic astrocytomas and 30% of GBM [15–17]. Other subsequent alterations include LOH on chromosomes 9p, 19p, and 22. The second pathway involves transformation of glial cell into a GBM secondary to LOH on chromosome 10, and

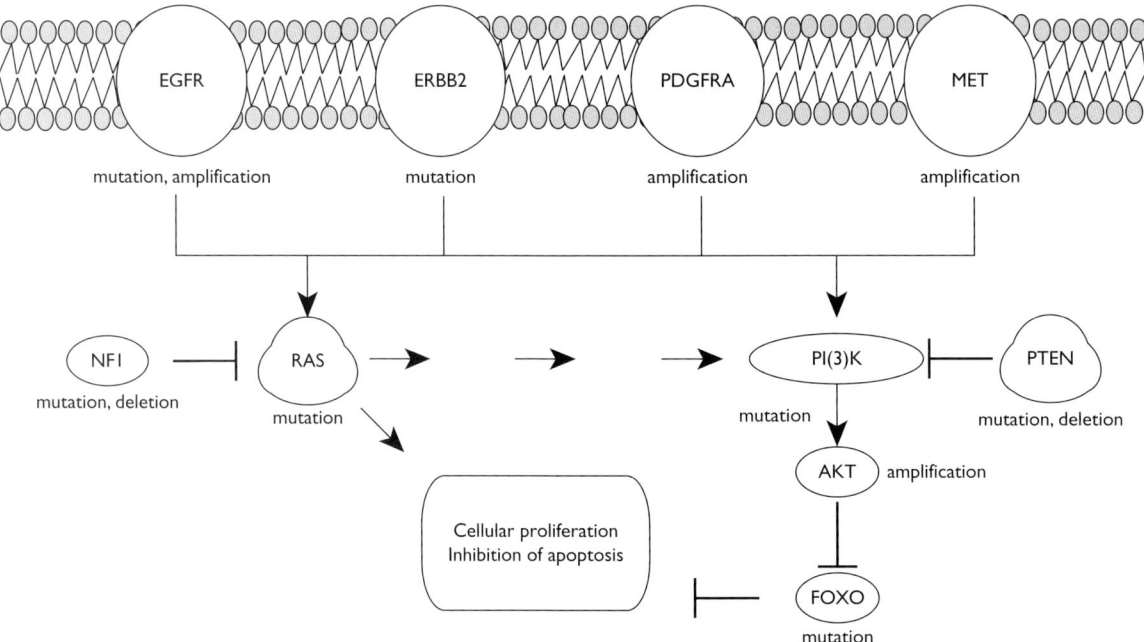

Figure 24.3 The activated RAS pathway in high-grade astrocytomas is illustrated. Arrows highlighted in *red* are activated, whereas those in *black* are suppressed. The net effect is cellular proliferation and inhibition of apoptosis. *See color insert.*

and EGFR and PDGFR-α amplification techniques. They showed a higher frequency of p53 mutations in children older than 6, a relatively infrequent rate of PTEN mutations, infrequent LOH on 1p/19q, and rare amplification of EGFR or PDGFR-α [32]. Their results suggest that there are several differences in children compared to adults in the genetic pathways, which in turn lead to the formation of *de novo* astrocytic tumors.

Faury et al [33] used 19K spotted cDNA arrays against 14 pediatric and 7 adult GBMs to detect differences in gene expression between these two age groups. They identified at least two subsets of pediatric GBMs: One subset was associated with the Ras and Akt pathway in which children had a poor prognosis, and the other was associated with astroglial precursor cells in which children had a better prognosis. It is interesting that, in both subsets, overexpression of Y-box-protein-1 was observed, which may help to drive oncogenesis [33]. Traditionally, the availability of fresh tumor specimens was a major rate-limiting step in many gene-profiling experiments. However, the same group showed in a follow-up study that formalin-fixed paraffin embedded pediatric GBMs could serve as a reasonable alternative [34]. Here, RNA was extracted after scrape or laser-capture microdissection and amplified by reverse-transcription polymerase chain reaction. The investigators showed that they could reproduce the results obtained from fresh frozen pediatric GBMs using this strategy, thus opening the door to the analysis of a large number of pediatric GBMs [34].

Wong et al [35] used SNP-arrays on 14 high-grade, and 14 low-grade pediatric gliomas to show that most low-grade gliomas, as expected, had virtually no detectable alterations. However, the high-grade gliomas demonstrated amplification of EGFR or PDGFR-α on one allele, but LOH on the other. This may represent a new molecular mechanism underlying progression in pediatric gliomas [35].

Recent advances in DNA-sequencing platforms and their utility in genomic analyses have resulted in a number of coordinated efforts focused on comprehensive characterization of the GBM genome. The Cancer Genome Atlas, published by the National Cancer Institute and the National Human Genome Research Institute, recently published its findings in 206 adult GBMs, integrating DNA copy number, gene expression, and DNA methylation profiles [36]. PCR-directed exon resequencing was performed for 601 selected genes in 91 of the tumors. This approach of integrating multidimensional genomic data from GBMs revealed the consistent deregulation of p53, RB, and PI(3) kinase-signaling pathways in the majority of tumors and established a connection between *MGMT* promoter methylation and a hypermutator phenotype in some cases [36]. In a similar study, 22 adult GBMs were comprehensively profiled by exon resequencing of 20 661 protein-coding genes, which were analyzed for copy-number aberrations, using SNP arrays, and gene expression, studied by combining SAGE (Serial Analysis of Gene Expression) with next-generation sequencing [37]. This report identified recurrent mutations in *IDH1* in 12% of GBM patients, mostly in young patients and those with secondary GBMs, and showed that patients harboring *IDH1* mutations had increased overall survival. The high-throughput afforded by next-generation sequencing has recently enabled several significant breakthroughs in genomics. It can be anticipated that many of these novel sequencing-based methods will be routinely applied in cancer genomics, including the study of pediatric brain tumors in the near future.

Translational Therapies

The development of translational therapies for high-grade astrocytomas in children is fraught with challenges. Primarily, there is very limited information relating to the molecular genetics of malignant pediatric astrocytomas as compared to similar tumors in adults. Furthermore, although there is extensive body of knowledge regarding genetic and molecular abnormalities found in adult high-grade astrocytomas, the current data on pediatric high-grade astrocytomas suggest that pediatric astrocytomas are molecularly distinct from their adult counterparts. Hence, novel strategies employed in adult tumors may not be applicable in pediatric patients.

Nonetheless, with failure in current treatment modalities, there is an impetus toward developing molecular therapies that target the tyrosine kinase activity [38], as well as tumor angiogensis [39]. The use of bevacizumab, an antiangiogenic agent in combination with irinotecan (CPT-11), a topoisomerase I inhibitor, appears promising as observed in a Phase 2 trial involving adults, where there was a meaningful improvement in 6-month progression-free survival, as well as overall survival [40]. Attempts are currently underway by the Pediatric Brain Tumor Consortium in ascertaining whether the these findings can be replicated in children with malignant astrocytomas and diffuse/intrinsic brainstem astrocytomas.

MEDULLOBLASTOMA

Brief Clinical Overview

Medulloblastoma is the most common pediatric malignant brain tumor. This tumor belongs to the family of primitive neuroectodermal tumors (PNETs). A PNET arising from the cerebellum is termed a "medulloblastoma." Medulloblastomas are generally very invasive tumors with a predilection for children, with a peak age of diagnosis of 7 years. Based on the World Health Organization classification, medulloblastomas are grade IV tumors with five distinct histologic variants: (a) classical medulloblastoma, (b) desmoplastic medulloblastoma, (c) large-cell anaplastic medulloblastoma, (d) the melanotic medulloblastoma, and (e) the medullomyoblastoma [41]. Patients with medulloblastomas are stratified as standard risk or high risk, on the basis of age, extent of resection, and the presence of metastasis at the time of diagnosis. Standard-risk patients have a more favorable prognosis. High-risk patients are those who are younger than 3 years of age, or who have more than 1.5 cm^2 of residual tumor following surgery or who have disseminated disease at diagnosis [42]. Multimodality treatment, including maximum surgical resection, craniospinal radiation, and adjuvant chemotherapy is standard care [42–45]. Craniospinal radiation is not typically recommended for children under the age of 3 years, in order to minimize long-term neurologically sequelae [46,47]. The 5-year survival for the standard-risk group is estimated at 80%, whereas the high-risk patients have a 5-year survival of approximately 40% to 70%[2]. A radiographic view of medulloblastoma is depicted in Figure 24.4. Current multimodality treatment with surgery, radiation therapy, and chemotherapy are limited by the highly invasive nature of these tumors, as well as severe toxicities of conventional chemotherapy. As a result, there has been a tremendous focus on studying molecular pathways associated with these tumors, with a hope of developing molecularly directed therapies with less adverse effects than what is currently available.

Molecular Genetics of Medulloblastomas

There has been a significant expansion of our understanding of the molecular genetics of medulloblastomas over the past decade. Information acquired from elucidating distinct signaling pathways associated with tumorigenesis suggests that medulloblastomas are genetically heterogeneous tumors. Although most medulloblastomas are sporadic, there exists a subset that occurs in conjunction with familial cancer syndromes such as Turcot, Gorlin, and Li-Fraumeni syndromes. Molecular analysis of familial cancer syndromes has provided valuable insights into the molecular pathogenesis of medulloblastomas. Implicated pathways such as the Hedgehog (Hh), Wnt, and Notch are critical for both embryonic development, as well as cerebellar development [48–53]. Hence, medulloblastomas could well represent the aftermath of a dysregulated pattern of normal neuroembryogenesis [52]. Familiar cancer syndromes as well as aberrancies of signaling pathways are discussed in what follows. The key genetic pathways are summarized in Tables 24.3 and 24.4.

Familiar Cancer Syndromes Associated With Medulloblastoma

Turcot Syndrome

Patients with Turcot syndrome often present with colorectal cancer and a malignant brain tumor. The colorectal cancers in Turcot can either present as hereditary nonpolyposis (HNP) or as familial adenomatous polyposis (FAP) colon cancers. The molecular basis of HNP involves a germline mutation in DNA mismatch-repair genes, and such patients typically develop GBM. On the other hand, patients with FAP will typically have a medulloblastoma as part of the Turcot complex. A germline mutation of the tumor-suppressor gene, *APC*, is responsible for FAP. *APC* normally regulates β-catenin, which is a downstream activator of Wnt signaling pathway [54–57].

Gorlin Syndrome

Patients with Gorlin syndrome have basal-cell carcinomas of the skin, in conjunction with multiple malformations and tumors, including, but not limited to, ovarian fibromas and medulloblastomas. A germline mutation in the *PTCH* gene is frequently seen in most of these patients. It is interesting that the *PCTH* gene encodes a critical plasma-membrane protein receptor within the Hh signaling pathway [58].

Li-Fraumeni Syndrome

Patients with Li-Fraumeni syndrome have a predilection to multiple cancers, including medulloblastomas [59]. The

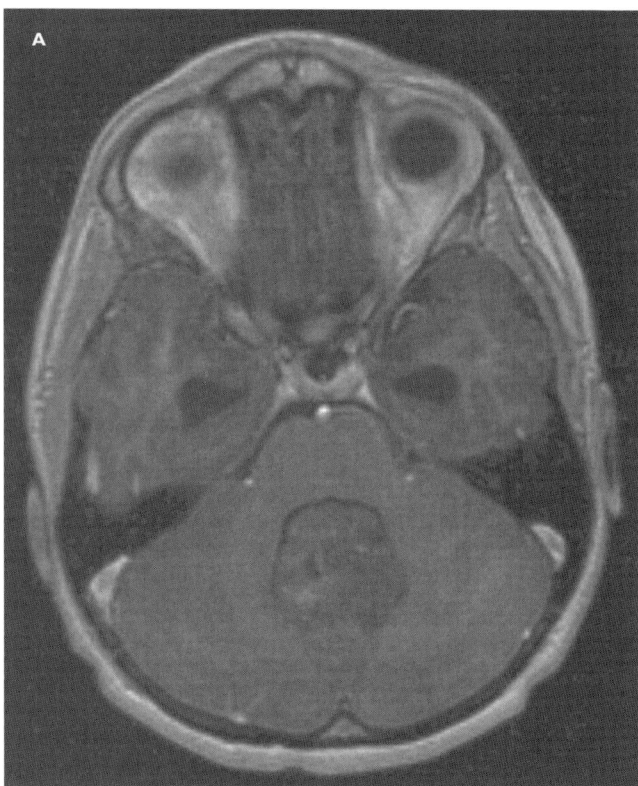
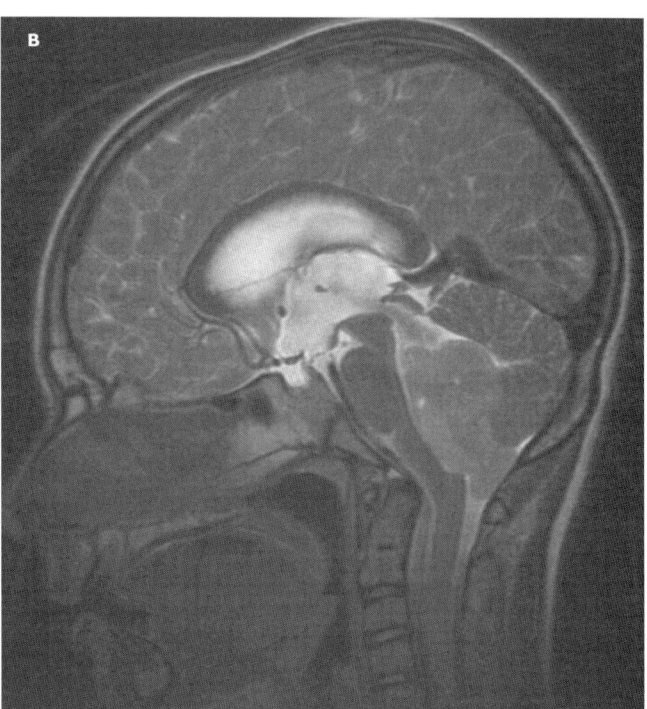

Figure 24.4 Medulloblastoma. **(A)** Axial T1-weighted gadolinium enhanced MR in 4-year-old man with 1-month history of nausea, vomiting, and ataxia. The MR shows a minimally enhancing lesion occupying the region of the fourth ventricle. **(B)** Sagittal T2 TSE MR image showing tumor extending from the fourth ventricle into the cerebellum. The tumor extends below the foramen magnum.

Table 24.3 Genetic Diseases with a Predisposition to Development of Medulloblastomas

Disease	Gene
Turcot syndrome	APC (5q21)
Gorlin syndrome	PTCH (9q22)
Li-Fraumeni syndrome	TP53 (17Q13)

Table 24.4 Key Aberrant Signaling Pathways in Medulloblastomas

Pathway	Mutated Genes
Hedgehog pathway	PTCH, SMOH, SUFU
Wnt pathway	AXIN 1, APC, β-catenin
Notch pathway	NOTCH 1, NOTCH 2
Growth factor pathway	HER2, HER4, IGFR

underlying molecular defect is a mutation of the tumor-suppressor gene, *p53*.

Chromosomal Alterations

The most commonly reported cytogenetic abnormality in 30 to 40% medulloblastomas is the isochromosome 17q that has been reported in more than 30 to 40% of tumors [21,23,43,60]. In addition, chromosomal gains in 4, 7, 8, 9, and 18, as well as losses in 1, 2, 8, 10, 11, 16, and 19, have been reported [43,61]. The significance of these chromosomal abnormalities with respect to prognosis is yet to be determined. The main poor prognostic factor in medulloblastoma is amplification of the *MYC* oncogene [62,63].

Signaling Pathways in Medulloblastoma

Sonic Hedgehog Pathway

Aberrant activity of the SHH signaling pathway has been implicated in the pathogenesis of medulloblastomas [48]. This pathway is involved in normal cerebellar development. There are three Hedgehog proteins in mammals: (1) SHH, (2) Indian hedgehog, and (3) desert hedgehog [49]. The SHH proteins have the most relevance to medulloblastoma pathogenesis because they play a very active role in the development of the cerebellum [50]. SHH is a potent mitogen for progenitor cells of the granular cell layer of the cerebellum. The activities of the SHH signaling pathway are controlled by the *PCTH* gene that is a negative regulator. It is interesting, however, that inactivating mutations of the *PTCH* gene occur in approximately 8% of sporadic medulloblastomas [52,64]. Patients with Gorlin syndrome have a mutation in *PTCH* and present with medulloblastomas in addition to other tumors. In mice, it has been demonstrated that medulloblastoma formation can occur with deletion of one of the PTCH alleles[65,66]. Furthermore, there appears to be a correlation between LOH of the PTCH locus at 9q22.3q32, and medulloblastomas [58,67]. In general, mutations of genes within the SHH pathway occur in approximately 25% of medulloblastomas [68]. Additional low-frequency activating mutations of the Hh pathway seen in medulloblastomas include mutations of the SMOH gene[69] and SUFU gene [70]. Medulloblastomas resulting from aberrant SHH signaling, and SUFU mutations in particular, correlate histologically with the desmoplastic subtype of medulloblastoma [71,72]. A simplified schematic of this pathway is depicted in Figure 24.5.

Wnt/B-Catenin Pathway

The role of the Wnt pathway in medulloblastoma pathogenesis has been extensively studied. It is estimated that this pathway is aberrant in approximately 15% of sporadic medulloblastomas [73–78]. The pathway is normally involved in cellular regulation and differentiation during embryological development [79]. In this pathway, the interaction of Wnt proteins and associated receptors leads to the nuclear translocation and accumulation of β-catenin. A polymeric multisubunit protein complex composed of axin 1, the APC protein, and glycogen synthase kinase 3-β negatively regulates the intracellular levels of β-catenin. Nuclear translocation of β-catenin leads to activation of mitogenic and oncogenic transcription factors such as C-MYC, cyclin D, MMP-7, and CD44 [51]. Hence, inactivating mutations in APC, axin 1, and glycogen synthase kinase 3-β can result in increased β-catenin-mediated transcription of oncogenes. APC mutations have been found in 4% of medulloblastomas [74]. Deletions of the AXIN 1 gene have also been reported [75]. Furthermore, mutations of β-catenin leading to activation of the Wnt signaling pathway occur in 10% of sporadic medulloblastomas [73]. Increased nuclear expression of β-catenin has been demonstrated in 18 to 25% of medulloblastomas, using immunohistochemical techniques [76]. It is interesting to note that increased β-catenin activation correlates with a favorable prognosis in children with medulloblastomas [80]. A simplified schematic of this pathway is depicted in Figure 24.5.

The Notch Pathway

This is a developmental pathway involved in cellular differentiation as well as cell-fate determination [81]. The pathway that includes five ligands and four distinct notch receptors was initially associated with acute lymphoblastic leukemia [82]. The exact role of the Notch pathway in the tumorigenesis of medulloblastomas has not been fully elucidated. However, recent gene-profiling and hybridization studies have demonstrated amplification, as well as overexpression of Notch 2 in approximately 15% of cases [63,83]. Moreover, inhibition of the Notch pathway by receptor function by γ-secretase, a known inhibitor of notch signaling, resulted in growth inhibition of medulloblastoma cells [63]. A simplified schematic of this pathway is depicted in Figure 24.5.

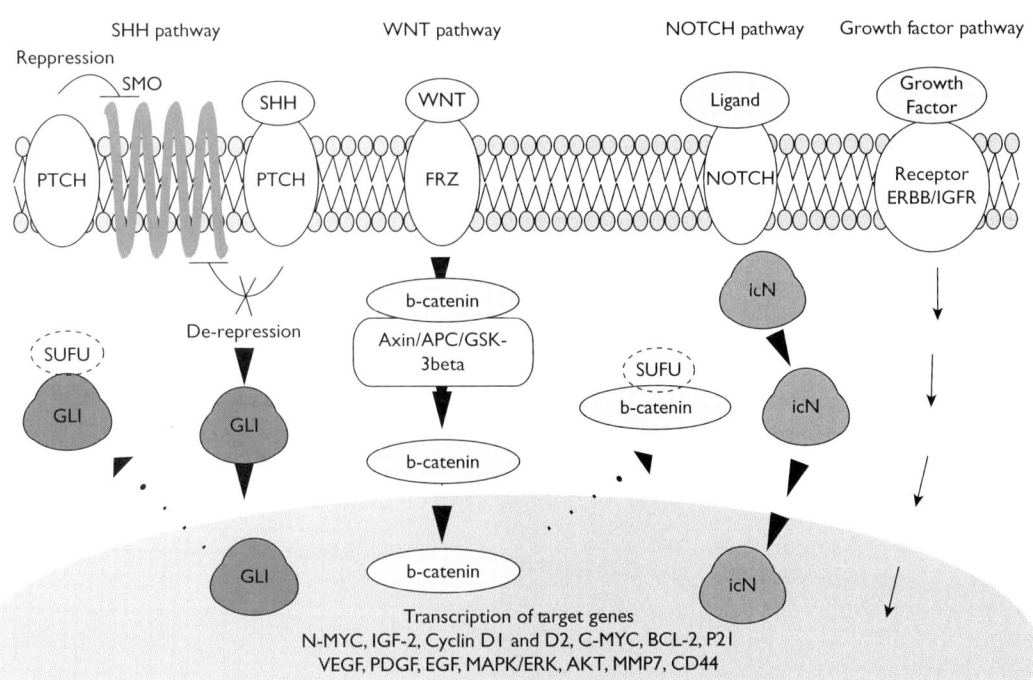

Figure 24.5 Medulloblastoma Pathways. Simplified schematic representation of critical pathways involved in medulloblastoma formation. Illustrated are the different embryonic signaling pathways (Hh, Wnt, and Notch), growth factor pathways, associated ligands, membrane receptors, transcriptions factors, and downstream activation of target genes.

Other Signaling Pathways

Several signaling pathways involved with cellular proliferation have been found to be upregulated in medulloblastomas. A member of the epidermal growth factor family of receptor tyrosine kinases, ErbB2(Her2) is overexpressed in medulloblastomas, and portends a poor prognosis if coexpressed with ErbB4(Her4) [84]. Upregulation of proliferation factors such as protein kinase B (Akt) [85,86], extracellular signal-regulated kinase (Erk) [85,86], as well as insulin-like growth factor receptor [87], has also been described in medulloblastomas.

Epigenetics and Medulloblastoma

Epigenetic silencing of tumor-suppressor genes through aberrant methylation of cytosine-guanine dinucleotides, so-called CpG islands, within promoter regions has been postulated as a potential mechanism of medulloblastoma formation. Extensive hypermethylation of the tumor-suppressor gene, *RASSF1A* [88,89], as well as complete methylation of the *HIC1* tumor suppressor [90,91], have been well documented in medulloblastomas. Furthermore, other tumor-suppressor and apoptotic genes such as *CASP8, MGMT, GSTP1, p14, p15, p16, p18, TIMP3, S100A6, S100A10,* and *DNAJDI*, have been implicated [92–94]. Recently, Kongkham et al [95] identified a novel, putative, tumor-suppressor gene, *SPINT2*, as being epigenetically silenced in medulloblastomas.

Association With the T-antigen of the JC Virus

Medulloblastomas have been associated with the oncogenic T-antigen in both neonatal hamsters and transgenic mice models. The T-antigen inactivates tumor-suppressor proteins of the p53 and pRb pathways leading to oncogenesis [96]. In one study, more than 80% of neonatal hamsters developed medulloblastomas as well as other PNETs following intracerebral inoculation with the JC virus [96,97]. Similarly, transgenic mice expressing the T-antigen from the JC virus have been shown to develop medulloblastomas [96,97] These findings, in conjunction with immunohistochemical correlation of T-antigen levels and expressions of p53 and pRb proteins in medulloblastomas[97] suggest a possible role for JC virus in the tumorigenesis of medulloblastomas.

Translational Therapies

Increased focus on the molecular biology of medulloblastomas has led to a better understanding of molecular mechanisms involved in both tumor development as well as tumor progression. This new knowledge should ultimately translate into therapies that are molecularly specific. Clinical studies have shown that expression of the epidermal growth factor, ERBB2, confers a negative prognosis with a 50% reduction in 5-year survival [3,98]. As overexpression of ERBB2 in medulloblastoma serves as a marker for medulloblastoma invasiveness, inhibitors of ERBB2, such as OSI-774, have been introduced into clinical trial by the Children's Oncology Group and the Pediatric Brain Tumor Consortium [10].

Inhibitors of the SHH pathway in medulloblastomas have equally gained momentum. In particular, cyclopamine, a steroid alkaloid has been shown to inactivate the pathway by binding to SMO and, in turn, leading to downregulation of the pathway [99]. The end result is cell-cycle arrest. The drug has been demonstrated to promote tumor regression in murine allografts *in vivo* as well as apoptosis of medulloblastoma cells [99,100]. This drug remains in preclinical trials.

Small-molecule inhibitors generated from binding assays provide another avenue for targeting the SHH pathway in medulloblastomas [48,99–102]. One of these antagonists of the SHH pathway targets SMO with high affinity and exhibits dose-dependent inhibition of cell proliferation, as well as promotes apoptosis [103,104]. The drug remains in preclinical trials.

The feasibility of employing valproic acid, a histone deacetylase inhibitor that is used to inhibit cell growth and induce apoptosis in medulloblastoma cell lines, has been assessed. HDAC plays a role in gene expression by modulating the interaction of genomic DNA with histone proteins. Valproic acid has been shown to suppress tumor growth both in medulloblastoma cell lines and xenograft models [105,106]. Further studies are warranted to establish the safety and the efficacy of valproic acid in medulloblastoma.

CONCLUSION

The technological revolution in molecular biology over the past decade has contributed to our understanding of the molecular pathogenesis of malignant gliomas and medulloblastomas. Studies on the limited molecular data that are now available show that these tumors appear to have distinct alterations when compared to similar tumors in the adult population. In most cases, the prognosis remains guarded, despite advances in surgical techniques, chemotherapy regimens, and radiotherapy protocols. Several critical molecular pathways have been implicated. Ultimately, further elucidation of these critical pathways would allow for molecularly derived and molecular-specific therapies, which may have the potential to improve outcome.

REFERENCES

1. Gottardo NG, Gajjar A. Chemotherapy for malignant brain tumors of childhood. *J Child Neurol.* 2008;23:1149–1159.
2. Gajjar A, Chintagumpala M, Ashley D, et al. Risk-adapted craniospinal radiotherapy followed by high-dose chemotherapy and stem-cell rescue in children with newly diagnosed medulloblastoma (St Jude Medulloblastoma-96): long-term results from a prospective, multicentre trial. *Lancet Oncol.* 2006;7:813–820.
3. Broniscer A, Gajjar A. Supratentorial high-grade astrocytoma and diffuse brainstem glioma: two challenges for the pediatric oncologist. *Oncologist.* 2004;9:197–206.
4. Hargrave D, Bartels U, Bouffet E. Diffuse brainstem glioma in children: critical review of clinical trials. *Lancet Oncol.* 2006;7:241–248.
5. Massimino M, Gandola L, Spreafico F, et al. No salvage using high-dose chemotherapy plus/minus reirradiation for relapsing previously irradiated medulloblastoma. *Int J Radiat Oncol Biol Phys.* 2009;73:1358–1363.
6. Dunkel IJ, Garvin JH Jr, Goldman S, et al. High dose chemotherapy with autologous bone marrow rescue for children with diffuse

pontine brain stem tumors. Children's Cancer Group. *J Neurooncol.* 1998;37:67–73.
7. Packer RJ, Allen JC, Goldwein JL, et al. Hyperfractionated radiotherapy for children with brainstem gliomas: a pilot study using 7,200 cGy. *Ann Neurol.* 1990;27:167–173.
8. Cheng Y, Ng HK, Zhang SF, et al. Genetic alterations in pediatric high-grade astrocytomas. *Hum Pathol.* 1999;30:1284–1290.
9. Louis DN, Rubio MP, Correa KM, Gusella JF, von Deimling A. Molecular genetics of pediatric brain stem gliomas. Application of PCR techniques to small and archival brain tumor specimens. *J Neuropathol Exp Neurol.* 1993;52:507–515.
10. Gilbertson RJ, Hill DA, Hernan R, et al. ERBB1 is amplified and over-expressed in high-grade diffusely infiltrative pediatric brain stem glioma. *Clin Cancer Res.* 2003;9:3620–3624.
11. Lee E, Monsalves E, Solomon L, Bartels U, Hawkins C. Genetic analysis of pediatric brain stem gliomas by high-resolution single-nucleotide polymorphism arrays using whole-genome amplified DNA. Society of Neuro-Oncology Annual Meeting, Las Vegas, NV, 2008; Abstract GE-11.
12. Geyer JR, Finlay JL, Boyett JM, et al. Survival of infants with malignant astrocytomas. A Report from the Childrens Cancer Group. *Cancer.* 1995;75:1045–1050.
13. Tamber MS, Rutka JT. Pediatric supratentorial high-grade gliomas. *Neurosurg Focus.* 2003;14:e1.
14. von Deimling A, von Ammon K, Schoenfeld D, Wiestler OD, Seizinger BR, Louis DN. Subsets of glioblastoma multiforme defined by molecular genetic analysis. *Brain Pathol.* 1993;3:19–26.
15. el-Azouzi M, Chung RY, Farmer GE, et al. Loss of distinct regions on the short arm of chromosome 17 associated with tumorigenesis of human astrocytomas. *Proc Natl Acad Sci U S A.* 1989;86:7186–7190.
16. Fults D, Tippets RH, Thomas GA, Nakamura Y, White R. Loss of heterozygosity for loci on chromosome 17p in human malignant astrocytoma. *Cancer Res.* 1989;49:6572–6577.
17. James CD, Carlbom E, Nordenskjold M, Collins VP, Cavenee WK. Mitotic recombination of chromosome 17 in astrocytomas. *Proc Natl Acad Sci U S A.* 1989;86:2858–2862.
18. Burgart LJ, Robinson RA, Haddad SF, Moore SA. Oncogene abnormalities in astrocytomas: EGF-R gene alone appears to be more frequently amplified and rearranged compared with other protooncogenes. *Mod Pathol.* 1991;4:183–186.
19. Chaffanet M, Chauvin C, Laine M, et al. EGF receptor amplification and expression in human brain tumours. *Eur J Cancer.* 1992;28:11–17.
20. Kyritsis AP, Saya H. Epidemiology, cytogenetics, and molecular biology of brain tumors. *Curr Opin Oncol.* 1993;5:474–480.
21. Bigner SH, Mark J, Friedman HS, Biegel JA, Bigner DD. Structural chromosomal abnormalities in human medulloblastoma. *Cancer Genet Cytogenet.* 1988;30:91–101.
22. Schmidt EE, Ichimura K, Reifenberger G, Collins VP. CDKN2 (p16/MTS1) gene deletion or CDK4 amplification occurs in the majority of glioblastomas. *Cancer Res.* 1994;54:6321–6324.
23. Biegel JA. Genetics of pediatric central nervous system tumors. *J Pediatr Hematol Oncol.* 1997;19:492–501.
24. Steck PA, Pershouse MA, Jasser SA, et al. Identification of a candidate tumour suppressor gene, MMAC1, at chromosome 10q23.3 that is mutated in multiple advanced cancers. *Nat Genet.* 1997;15:356–362.
25. Mollenhauer J, Wiemann S, Scheurlen W, et al. DMBT1, a new member of the SRCR superfamily, on chromosome 10q25.3–26.1 is deleted in malignant brain tumours. *Nat Genet.* 1997;17:32–39.
26. Warr T, Ward S, Burrows J, et al. Identification of extensive genomic loss and gain by comparative genomic hybridisation in malignant astrocytoma in children and young adults. *Genes Chromosomes Cancer.* 2001;31:15–22.
27. Rickert CH, Strater R, Kaatsch P, et al. Pediatric high-grade astrocytomas show chromosomal imbalances distinct from adult cases. *Am J Pathol.* 2001;158:1525–1532.
28. Litofsky NS, Hinton D, Raffel C. The lack of a role for p53 in astrocytomas in pediatric patients. *Neurosurgery.* 1994;34:967–972; discussion 72–73.
29. Lang FF, Miller DC, Koslow M, Newcomb EW. Pathways leading to glioblastoma multiforme: a molecular analysis of genetic alterations in 65 astrocytic tumors. *J Neurosurg.* 1994;81:427–436.
30. Boland CR, Sato J, Saito K, et al. Genetic instability and chromosomal aberrations in colorectal cancer: a review of the current models. *Cancer Detect Prev.* 1998;22:377–382.
31. Alonso M, Hamelin R, Kim M, et al. Microsatellite instability occurs in distinct subtypes of pediatric but not adult central nervous system tumors. *Cancer Res.* 2001;61:2124–2128.
32. Nakamura M, Shimada K, Ishida E, et al. Molecular pathogenesis of pediatric astrocytic tumors. *Neuro Oncol.* 2007;9:113–123.
33. Faury D, Nantel A, Dunn SE, et al. Molecular profiling identifies prognostic subgroups of pediatric glioblastoma and shows increased YB-1 expression in tumors. *J Clin Oncol.* 2007;25:1196–1208.
34. Haque T, Faury D, Albrecht S, et al. Gene expression profiling from formalin-fixed paraffin-embedded tumors of pediatric glioblastoma. *Clin Cancer Res.* 2007;13:6284–6292.
35. Wong KK, Tsang YT, Chang YM, et al. Genome-wide allelic imbalance analysis of pediatric gliomas by single nucleotide polymorphic allele array. *Cancer Res.* 2006;66:11172–11178.
36. Comprehensive genomic characterization defines human glioblastoma genes and core pathways. *Nature.* 2008;455:1061–1068.
37. Parsons DW, Jones S, Zhang X, et al. An integrated genomic analysis of human glioblastoma multiforme. *Science.* 2008;321:1807–1812.
38. Khanna C, Helman LJ. Molecular approaches in pediatric oncology. *Annu Rev Med.* 2006;57:83–97.
39. Kerbel RS. Antiangiogenic therapy: a universal chemosensitization strategy for cancer? *Science.* 2006;312:1171–1175.
40. Vredenburgh JJ, Desjardins A, Herndon JE II, et al. Phase II trial of bevacizumab and irinotecan in recurrent malignant glioma. *Clin Cancer Res.* 2007;13:1253–1259.
41. Giangaspero F EC, Haapasalo H, et al. Medulloblastoma. Medulloblastoma. In: Louis D M N, Ohgaki H, Wiestler O D, et al., eds. *WHO classification of tumors of the central nervous system.* 4th edn. Lyon: IARC Press, 2007:132–140.
42. Packer RJ, Rood BR, MacDonald TJ. Medulloblastoma: present concepts of stratification into risk groups. *Pediatr Neurosurg.* 2003;39:60–67.
43. Crawford JR, MacDonald TJ, Packer RJ. Medulloblastoma in childhood: new biological advances. *Lancet Neurol.* 2007;6:1073–1085.
44. Mazzola CA, Pollack IF. Medulloblastoma. *Curr Treat Options Neurol.* 2003;5:189–198.
45. Packer RJ, Cogen P, Vezina G, Rorke LB. Medulloblastoma: clinical and biologic aspects. *Neuro Oncol.* 1999;1:232–250.
46. Geyer JR, Sposto R, Jennings M, et al. Multiagent chemotherapy and deferred radiotherapy in infants with malignant brain tumors: a report from the Children's Cancer Group. *J Clin Oncol.* 2005;23:7621–7631.
47. Grill J, Sainte-Rose C, Jouvet A, et al. Treatment of medulloblastoma with postoperative chemotherapy alone: an SFOP prospective trial in young children. *Lancet Oncol.* 2005;6:573–580.
48. Dellovade T, Romer JT, Curran T, Rubin LL. The hedgehog pathway and neurological disorders. *Annu Rev Neurosci.* 2006;29:539–563.
49. Fuccillo M, Joyner AL, Fishell G. Morphogen to mitogen: the multiple roles of hedgehog signalling in vertebrate neural development. *Nat Rev Neurosci.* 2006;7:772–783.
50. Ingham PW, Placzek M. Orchestrating ontogenesis: variations on a theme by sonic hedgehog. *Nat Rev Genet.* 2006;7:841–850.
51. Johnson ML, Rajamannan N. Diseases of Wnt signaling. *Rev Endocr Metab Disord.* 2006;7:41–49.
52. Marino S. Medulloblastoma: developmental mechanisms out of control. *Trends Mol Med.* 2005;11:17–22.
53. Reya T, Clevers H. Wnt signalling in stem cells and cancer. *Nature.* 2005;434:843–850.
54. Hamada H, Kurimoto M, Endo S, Ogiichi T, Akai T, Takaku A. Turcot's syndrome presenting with medulloblastoma and familiar adenomatous polyposis: a case report and review of the literature. *Acta Neurochir (Wien).* 1998;140:631–632.
55. Hamilton SR, Liu B, Parsons RE, et al. The molecular basis of Turcot's syndrome. *N Engl J Med.* 1995;332:839–847.
56. Paraf F, Jothy S, Van Meir EG. Brain tumor-polyposis syndrome: two genetic diseases? *J Clin Oncol.* 1997;15:2744–2758.
57. Van Meir EG. "Turcot's syndrome": phenotype of brain tumors, survival and mode of inheritance. *Int J Cancer.* 1998;75:162–164.
58. Zurawel RH, Allen C, Wechsler-Reya R, Scott MP, Raffel C. Evidence that haploinsufficiency of Ptch leads to medulloblastoma in mice. *Genes Chromosomes Cancer.* 2000;28:77–81.
59. Malmer B, Feychting M, Lonn S, Ahlbom A, Henriksson R. p53 Genotypes and risk of glioma and meningioma. *Cancer Epidemiol Biomarkers Prev.* 2005;14:2220–2223.
60. Griffin CA, Hawkins AL, Packer RJ, Rorke LB, Emanuel BS. Chromosome abnormalities in pediatric brain tumors. *Cancer Res.* 1988;48:175–180.

61. Rickert CH, Paulus W. Chromosomal imbalances detected by comparative genomic hybridisation in atypical teratoid/rhabdoid tumours. *Childs Nerv Syst.* 2004;20:221–224.
62. Lamont JM, McManamy CS, Pearson AD, Clifford SC, Ellison DW. Combined histopathological and molecular cytogenetic stratification of medulloblastoma patients. *Clin Cancer Res.* 2004;10:5482–5493.
63. Eberhart CG, Kratz J, Wang Y, et al. Histopathological and molecular prognostic markers in medulloblastoma: c-myc, N-myc, TrkC, and anaplasia. *J Neuropathol Exp Neurol.* 2004;63:441–449.
64. Fogarty MP, Kessler JD, Wechsler-Reya RJ. Morphing into cancer: the role of developmental signaling pathways in brain tumor formation. *J Neurobiol.* 2005;64:458–475.
65. Corcoran RB, Scott MP. A mouse model for medulloblastoma and basal cell nevus syndrome. *J Neurooncol.* 2001;53:307–318.
66. Kim JY, Nelson AL, Algon SA, et al. Medulloblastoma tumorigenesis diverges from cerebellar granule cell differentiation in patched heterozygous mice. *Dev Biol.* 2003;263:50–66.
67. Raffel C, Jenkins RB, Frederick L, et al. Sporadic medulloblastomas contain PTCH mutations. *Cancer Res.* 1997;57:842–845.
68. Carlotti CG Jr, Smith C, Rutka JT. The molecular genetics of medulloblastoma: an assessment of new therapeutic targets. *Neurosurg Rev.* 2008;31:359–368; discussion 68–69.
69. Reifenberger J, Wolter M, Weber RG, et al. Missense mutations in SMOH in sporadic basal cell carcinomas of the skin and primitive neuroectodermal tumors of the central nervous system. *Cancer Res.* 1998;58:1798–1803.
70. Taylor MD, Liu L, Raffel C, et al. Mutations in SUFU predispose to medulloblastoma. *Nat Genet.* 2002;31:306–310.
71. Pomeroy SL, Tamayo P, Gaasenbeek M, et al. Prediction of central nervous system embryonal tumour outcome based on gene expression. *Nature.* 2002;415:436–442.
72. Thompson MC, Fuller C, Hogg TL, et al. Genomics identifies medulloblastoma subgroups that are enriched for specific genetic alterations. *J Clin Oncol.* 2006;24:1924–1931.
73. Zurawel RH, Chiappa SA, Allen C, Raffel C. Sporadic medulloblastomas contain oncogenic beta-catenin mutations. *Cancer Res.* 1998;58:896–899.
74. Huang H, Mahler-Araujo BM, Sankila A, et al. APC mutations in sporadic medulloblastomas. *Am J Pathol.* 2000;156:433–437.
75. Dahmen RP, Koch A, Denkhaus D, et al. Deletions of AXIN1, a component of the WNT/wingless pathway, in sporadic medulloblastomas. *Cancer Res.* 2001;61:7039–7043.
76. Eberhart CG, Tihan T, Burger PC. Nuclear localization and mutation of beta-catenin in medulloblastomas. *J Neuropathol Exp Neurol.* 2000;59:333–337.
77. Baeza N, Masuoka J, Kleihues P, Ohgaki H. AXIN1 mutations but not deletions in cerebellar medulloblastomas. *Oncogene.* 2003;22:632–636.
78. Yokota N, Nishizawa S, Ohta S, et al. Role of Wnt pathway in medulloblastoma oncogenesis. *Int J Cancer.* 2002;101:198–201.
79. Gajjar A, Hernan R, Kocak M, et al. Clinical, histopathologic, and molecular markers of prognosis: toward a new disease risk stratification system for medulloblastoma. *J Clin Oncol.* 2004;22:984–993.
80. Ellison DW, Onilude OE, Lindsey JC, et al. beta-Catenin status predicts a favorable outcome in childhood medulloblastoma: the United Kingdom Children's Cancer Study Group Brain Tumour Committee. *J Clin Oncol.* 2005;23:7951–7957.
81. Eberhart CG. In search of the medulloblast: neural stem cells and embryonal brain tumors. *Neurosurg Clin N Am.* 2007;18:59–69, viii-ix.
82. Sjolund J, Manetopoulos C, Stockhausen MT, Axelson H. The Notch pathway in cancer: differentiation gone awry. *Eur J Cancer.* 2005;41:2620–2629.
83. Yokota N, Mainprize TG, Taylor MD, et al. Identification of differentially expressed and developmentally regulated genes in medulloblastoma using suppression subtraction hybridization. *Oncogene.* 2004;23:3444–3453.
84. Gilbertson RJ, Perry RH, Kelly PJ, Pearson AD, Lunec J. Prognostic significance of HER2 and HER4 coexpression in childhood medulloblastoma. *Cancer Res.* 1997;57:3272–3280.
85. Hartmann W, Digon-Sontgerath B, Koch A, et al. Phosphatidylinositol 3'-kinase/AKT signaling is activated in medulloblastoma cell proliferation and is associated with reduced expression of PTEN. *Clin Cancer Res.* 2006;12:3019–3027.
86. Wlodarski P, Grajkowska W, Lojek M, Rainko K, Jozwiak J. Activation of Akt and Erk pathways in medulloblastoma. *Folia Neuropathol.* 2006;44:214–220.
87. Del Valle L, Enam S, Lassak A, et al. Insulin-like growth factor I receptor activity in human medulloblastomas. *Clin Cancer Res.* 2002;8:1822–1830.
88. Lindsey JC, Lusher ME, Anderton JA, et al. Identification of tumour-specific epigenetic events in medulloblastoma development by hypermethylation profiling. *Carcinogenesis.* 2004;25:661–668.
89. Lusher ME, Lindsey JC, Latif F, Pearson AD, Ellison DW, Clifford SC. Biallelic epigenetic inactivation of the RASSF1A tumor suppressor gene in medulloblastoma development. *Cancer Res.* 2002;62:5906–5911.
90. Rood BR, Zhang H, Weitman DM, Cogen PH. Hypermethylation of HIC-1 and 17p allelic loss in medulloblastoma. *Cancer Res.* 2002;62:3794–3797.
91. Waha A, Koch A, Meyer-Puttlitz B, et al. Epigenetic silencing of the HIC-1 gene in human medulloblastomas. *J Neuropathol Exp Neurol.* 2003;62:1192–1201.
92. Lindsey JC, Anderton JA, Lusher ME, Clifford SC. Epigenetic events in medulloblastoma development. *Neurosurg Focus.* 2005;19:E10.
93. Lindsey JC, Lusher ME, Anderton JA, Gilbertson RJ, Ellison DW, Clifford SC. Epigenetic deregulation of multiple S100 gene family members by differential hypomethylation and hypermethylation events in medulloblastoma. *Br J Cancer.* 2007;97:267–274.
94. Uziel T, Zindy F, Sherr CJ, Roussel MF. The CDK inhibitor p18Ink4c is a tumor suppressor in medulloblastoma. *Cell Cycle.* 2006;5:363–365.
95. Kongkham PN, Northcott PA, Ra YS, et al. An epigenetic genome-wide screen identifies SPINT2 as a novel tumor suppressor gene in pediatric medulloblastoma. *Cancer Res.* 2008;68:9945–9953.
96. Caracciolo V, Reiss K, Khalili K, De Falco G, Giordano A. Role of the interaction between large T antigen and Rb family members in the oncogenicity of JC virus. *Oncogene.* 2006;25:5294–5301.
97. Del Valle L, Baehring J, Lorenzana C, Giordano A, Khalili K, Croul S. Expression of a human polyomavirus oncoprotein and tumour suppressor proteins in medulloblastomas. *Mol Pathol.* 2001;54:331–337.
98. Bal MM, Das Radotra B, Srinivasan R, Sharma SC. Does c-erbB-2 expression have a role in medulloblastoma prognosis? *Indian J Pathol Microbiol.* 2006;49:535–539.
99. Berman DM, Karhadkar SS, Hallahan AR, et al. Medulloblastoma growth inhibition by hedgehog pathway blockade. *Science.* 2002;297:1559–1561.
100. Romer J, Curran T. Targeting medulloblastoma: small-molecule inhibitors of the sonic hedgehog pathway as potential cancer therapeutics. *Cancer Res.* 2005;65:4975–4978.
101. Kiselyov AS. Targeting the hedgehog signaling pathway with small molecules. *Anticancer Agents Med Chem.* 2006;6:445–449.
102. Lauth M, Toftgard R. The hedgehog pathway as a drug target in cancer therapy. *Curr Opin Investig Drugs.* 2007;8:457–461.
103. Romer JT, Kimura H, Magdaleno S, et al. Suppression of the Shh pathway using a small molecule inhibitor eliminates medulloblastoma in Ptc1(+/-)p53(-/-) mice. *Cancer Cell.* 2004;6:229–240.
104. Sasai K, Romer JT, Lee Y, et al. Shh pathway activity is down-regulated in cultured medulloblastoma cells: implications for preclinical studies. *Cancer Res.* 2006;66:4215–4222.
105. Shu Q, Antalffy B, Su JM, et al. Valproic acid prolongs survival time of severe combined immunodeficient mice bearing intracerebellar orthotopic medulloblastoma xenografts. *Clin Cancer Res.* 2006;12:4687–4694.
106. Li XN, Shu Q, Su JM, Perlaky L, Blaney SM, Lau CC. Valproic acid induces growth arrest, apoptosis, and senescence in medulloblastomas by increasing histone hyperacetylation and regulating expression of p21Cip1, CDK4, and CMYC. *Mol Cancer Ther.* 2005;4:1912–1922.

25 Molecular Pathogenesis of Neuroblastomas

Loretta M. S. Lau and Meredith S. Irwin

INTRODUCTION

Neuroblastoma is the most common extracranial pediatric solid tumor and contributes to 15% of all cancer-related deaths in children. It accounts for 7% to 10% of all childhood cancers, with an annual incidence of 10 per million children under the age of 15 years [1]. Neuroblastoma is a tumor derived from primordial neural-crest cells that ultimately populate the sympathetic ganglia and the adrenal medulla. As tumors can arise from any site along the sympathetic nervous system chain, there is a broad spectrum of clinical presentations. In older children with metastatic neuroblastoma, the disease can be very aggressive; however, in a subset of infants neuroblastoma has the remarkable ability to regress spontaneously or mature into a benign ganglioneuroma. Recent advances in the understanding of the biology and genetics of neuroblastoma have provided considerable insight into the mechanisms underlying the biological heterogeneity, which contributes to the diverse natural history and clinical behavior of neuroblastoma. The identification of specific genetic changes and biological features associated with prognostic significance has resulted in the ability to classify these tumors into prognostic subsets with distinct clinical behavior and deliver risk-adapted therapies [2].

CLINICAL PRESENTATION

Neuroblastoma occurs predominantly in young children with a median age of 18 months at the time of diagnosis. The annual incidence of neuroblastoma decreases from 64 per million during the first year of life to 29 per million in second year of life and gradually declines to 1 per million for the 10 to 14 years age group . The clinical presentation is highly variable due to different locations of primary tumors, the propensity to metastasize to distant sites, and the potential for paraneoplastic syndromes. The majority of neuroblastomas arise in the adrenal glands. Other primary sites include the paraspinal sympathetic ganglia in the neck and thorax, the retroperitoneal paraganglia, and the visceral ganglia. Abdominal tumors often present with constipation, pain, and, rarely, obstruction. Cervical and upper-thoracic tumors can be associated with respiratory distress and Horner's syndrome manifesting as unilateral ptosis, miosis, and enophthalmos [3]. Paraspinal tumors can extend into the neural foramina of the vertebral bodies through to the contralateral side forming a "dumb-bell" tumor and can cause nerve roots or spinal cord compression [4]. More than 50% of the patients present with metastatic disease at diagnosis. Neuroblastomas metastasize via both the lymphatic and hematogenous route to regional and distant lymph nodes, bone, bone marrow, liver, and skin, and, at times, to the brain and lungs. Periorbital infiltration by tumor can produce the characteristic "raccoon eye" with periorbital ecchymosis and proptosis. Opsoclonus-myoclonus syndrome is a paraneoplastic syndrome observed in 4% of neuroblastoma patients, who suffer from myoclonic jerks, random eye movements, and cerebellar ataxia [5]. Though these patients generally have excellent survival, a significant proportion have long-term neurocognitive deficits [6]. A small number of patients may be affected by hypertension due to tumor compression of the renal artery leading to stimulation of the renin-angiotensin system or due to excessive secretion of catecholamines [7]. On rare occasions, neuroblastomas can produce vasoactive intestinal peptide causing intractable secretory diarrhea [8].

DISEASE STAGING

In order to stage patients uniformly and to facilitate comparisons of results from clinical trials and biological studies worldwide, the International Neuroblastoma Staging System (INSS) was established in 1991 [9] and has been widely adopted (Table 25.1). Stage 1 and 2A are localized tumors with complete and incomplete gross resection, respectively. Stage 2B is a localized tumor with ipsilateral lymph-node involvement. Stage 3 represents unresectable unilateral tumor infiltrating across the midline or localized unilateral tumor with contralateral regional lymph-node involvement. Stage 4 neuroblastoma includes all metastatic disease, except for stage 4S disease that is limited to infants aged less than 1 year with localized primary tumor (stage 1 or 2) and dissemination confined to skin, liver, or bone marrow (<10% infiltration). Disease evaluation includes computed tomography or magnetic resonance imaging of the primary tumor (Figure 25.1) and urine catecholamine screen for elevated homovanilic acid and vanillylmandelic acid. Metastatic disease is assessed by bone-marrow examination and imaging with bone scan and meta-iodobenzylguanidine scintigraphy (Figure 25.2),

Table 25.1 International Neuroblastoma Staging System

1	Localized tumor with completer gross excision, with or without microscopic residual disease; representative ipsilateral lymph node negative for tumor microscopically (nodes attached to and removed with the primary tumor could be positive)
2A	Localized tumor with incomplete gross excision; representative, ipsilateral, nonadherent lymph nodes negative for tumor microscopically
2B	Localized tumor with or without complete gross excision; with ipsilateral, nonadherent lymph nodes positive for tumor. Enlarged contralateral lymph nodes should be negative microscopically
3	Unresectable unilateral tumor infiltrating across the midline, with or without regional lymph-node involvement, or localized unilateral tumor with contralateral regional lymph-node involvement, or midline tumor with bilateral extension by infiltration (unresectable) or by lymph-node involvement
4	Any primary tumor with dissemination to distant lymph node, bone, bone marrow, liver, skin, or other organs (except as defined by stage 4S)
4S	Localized primary tumor in infants aged less than 1 year (as defined for Stages 1, 2A, or 2B) with dissemination limited to skin, liver, or bone marrow (<10% malignant cells)

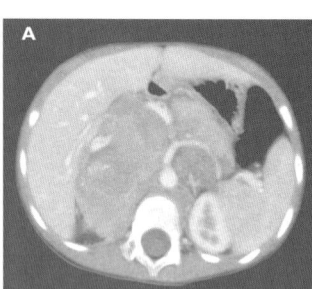
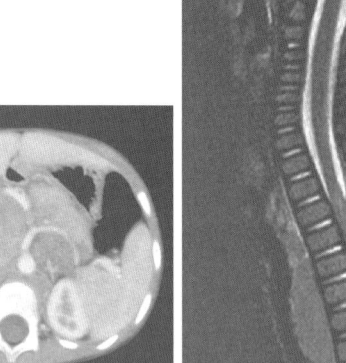

Figure 25.1 CT scan images of neuroblastoma tumors. (A) Contrast-enhanced CT demonstrates right-sided retroperitoneal mass that encases the aorta and vena cava. Small areas of calcification are present at the periphery. (B) MRI demonstrates large heterogenous paravertebral tumor extending from lower T2 vertebrae through T10. It extends into the spinal canal resulting in cord compression.

a tracer that selectively concentrates in neuroblastoma and pheochromocytoma tumors. A final diagnosis is confirmed by biopsy of the primary mass (Figure 25.3) or elevated catecholamines in the setting of a bone-marrow aspirate demonstrating neuroblasts.

Approximately 40% of neuroblastoma patients present with localized disease (INSS stage 1 to 3). Some patients can be adequately treated with surgery alone, and others may require adjuvant chemotherapy, depending on the stage and biology of the tumor. The prognosis of localized neuroblastoma is generally good with a survival rate between 70% and 90% [10,11]. Unfortunately, more than 50% of the children present with aggressive and disseminated (stage 4) disease at diagnosis. Patients with high-risk neuroblastoma (stage 4 disease and localized disease with specific poor prognostic biological markers) require multimodal treatment, including very intensive chemotherapy, radiotherapy, and stem-cell transplantation, which carry significant toxicities and long-term complications. Despite very good initial responses to chemotherapy in 80% of high-risk patients, more than 50% will relapse with a dismal outcome. Less than one-third of children with high-risk neuroblastoma can be cured [12,13]. Patients are now stratified into risk categories on the basis of clinical as well as molecular and genetic characteristics. The specific risk categories (low, intermediate, and high) are discussed in a later section and included in Table 25.2.

MOLECULAR PATHOGENESIS

Although neuroblastoma is one of the most extensively studied human cancers from the genetic point of view, the key specific events leading to the pathogenesis of neuroblastoma remain elusive. In many adult cancers, malignant transformation is often a consequence of stepwise progression of multiple "hits" or genetic alterations, best exemplified by the transformation of adenomas to adenocarcinomas in the colon [14]. In some pediatric malignancies, only a few or even a single initiation event may result in tumor development. Examples of these initiation events are specific translocations with subsequent oncogene activation in the majority of Ewings sarcoma with t(11:22) EWS:FLI translocation and in Philadelphia-positive leukemia-harboring t(9:22) BCR:ABL translocation. Other examples include gene deletions or mutations leading to loss of tumor-suppressor function such as in retinoblastoma carrying *Rb* mutations and in Wilm's Tumor with loss of heterozygosity (LOH) at *WT-1* [15]. By contrast, the genetic changes in neuroblastoma are complex and heterogeneous; thus far, no single genetic abnormality common to the majority of neuroblastoma has been identified, despite persistent research efforts. There is increasing evidence that neuroblastoma is the result of multiple genetic and molecular changes and the combination of specific alterations may explain the tumor heterogeneity. The numerous identified genetic loci, specific candidate genes, and their protein products are discussed in the following section.

Neuroblastoma Predisposition

Familial neuroblastoma is rare (~1%) and follows an autosomal dominant pattern with incomplete penetrance [16,17]. In contrast to sporadic cases, patients with familial neuroblastoma present at an earlier age and often have bilateral adrenal or multifocal primary tumors. Disease heterogeneity within a pedigree suggests that tumor phenotype is likely affected by acquired secondary genetic abnormalities, consistent with Knudson's two-hit hypothesis [18,19]. Constitutional chromosomal abnormalities involving chromosome 1p36 and 11q14–23, two loci deleted in a large number of sporadic tumors, have only been reported in a few neuroblastoma patients [20,21]. No

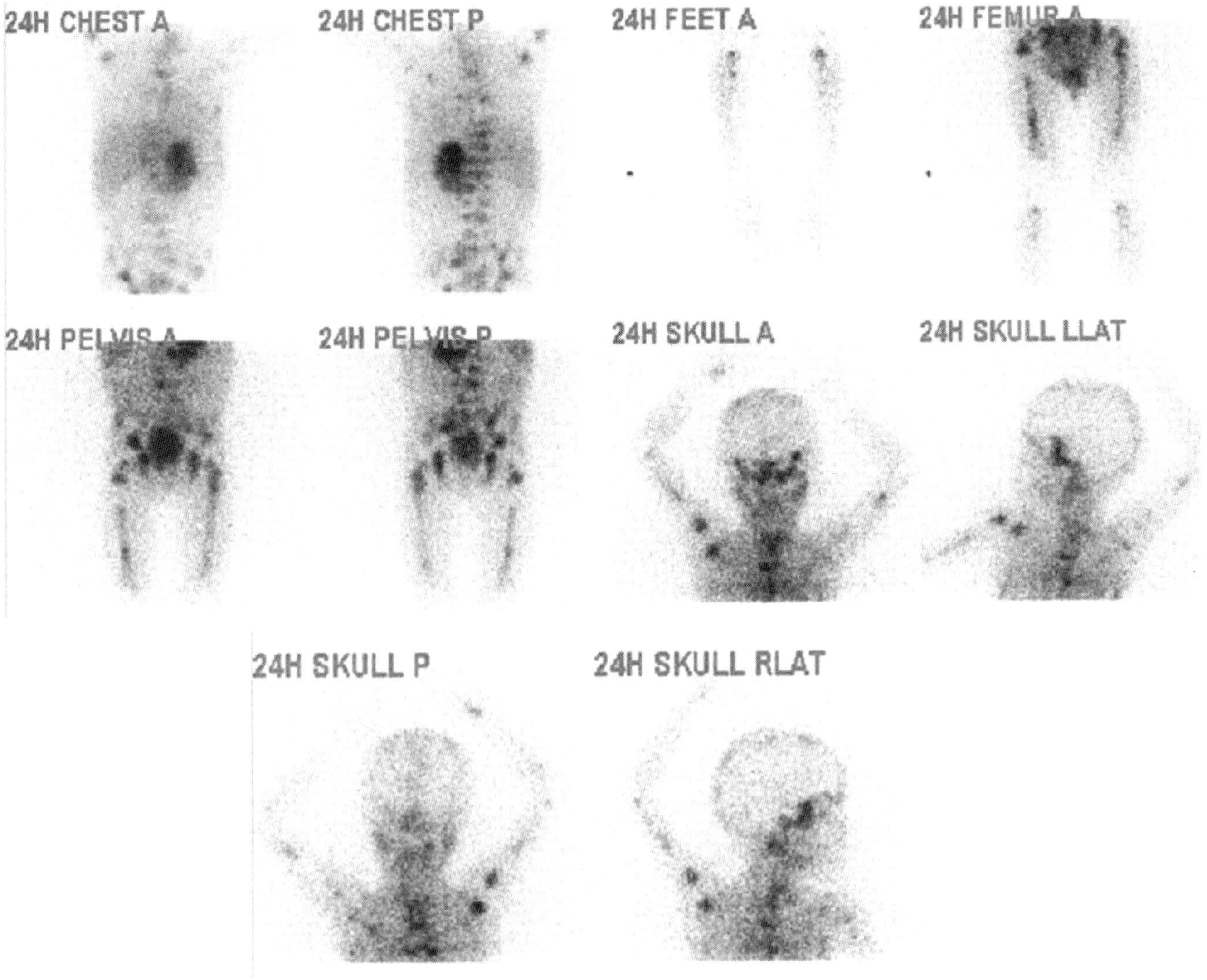

Figure 25.2 Meta-iodobenzylguanidine (MIBG) scan. MIBG images of patient with numerous metastases, including areas of the femur, vertebrae, and skull. Images, courtesy of Dr. Martin Charron, Diagnostic Imaging and Nuclear Medicine, Hospital for Sick Children, Toronto, Ontario, Canada.

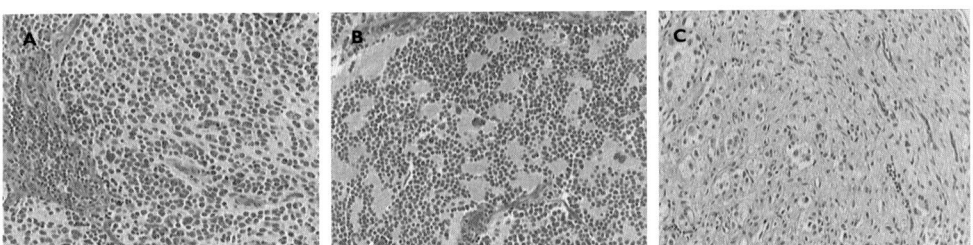

Figure 25.3 Histopathology of neuroblastoma tumors. (A) Neuroblastoma that is categorized as undifferentiated and stroma poor with a high MKI (mitosis–karryorhexis index), (B) Neuroblastoma that is poorly differentiated with a lower MKI and classic rosette formation of tumor cells. (C) Ganglioneuroblastoma with significant areas of well-differentiated larger cells, stroma rich, and dense neuropil. Images, courtesy of Dr. Paul Thorner, Department of Laboratory Medicine and Pathology, Hospital for Sick Children. See color insert.

Table 25.2 Children's Oncology Group (COG) Risk Stratification Schema

	Age	MYCN	Ploidy	Histology	Other	Risk Group
1						Low
2A/2B		Not amplified			>50% resection	Low
		Not amplified			<50% resection	Intermediate
		Not amplified			Biopsy only	Intermediate
		Amplified				High
3	<547 days	Not amplified				Intermediate
	<547 days	Not amplified		Favorable		Intermediate
		Amplified				High
	<547 days	Not amplified		Unfavorable		High
4	<365 days	Amplified				High
	<365 days	Not amplified				Intermediate
	365–547 days	Amplified				High
	365–547 days		DI = 1			High
	365–547 days			Unfavorable		High
	365–547 days	Not amplified	DI >1	Favorable		Intermediate
	<547 days					High
4S	<365 days	Not amplified	DI >1	Favorable	Asymptomatic	Low
	<365 days	Not amplified	DI = 1			Intermediate
	<365 days	Missing	Missing	Missing		Intermediate
	<365 days	Not amplified			Symptomatic	Intermediate
	<365 days	Not amplified		Unfavorable		Intermediate
	<365 days	Amplified				High

constitutional chromosomal rearrangements are consistently present in either sporadic or familial neuroblastoma. Genetic-linkage analysis of neuroblastoma predisposition suggests that chromosome 16p12–13 is one candidate locus [22]. An increased incidence of neuroblastoma has also been described in patients with neurofibromatosis [23] and Hirschsprung disease and/or central hypoventilation (Ondine's curse) [19,24], all of which are disorders of neural crest-derived cells. Recently, germline mutations of paired-like homeobox 2B (PHOX2B) have been detected in these patients with hereditary neuroblastoma, who also demonstrate other abnormalities of neural-crest development [25,26]. PHOX2B is a homeobox gene that regulates neurogenesis and is mutated in congenital central hypoventilation syndrome [27,28], suggesting that PHOX2B may play a role in tumor initiation in a subset of neuroblastoma. The majority of primary tumors express high levels of PHOX2B mRNA [29]. Overexpression of the PHOX2B protein in neuroblastoma cells inhibits proliferation and enhances differentiation in response to retinoic acid. To date, PHOX2B mutations have not been identified in sporadic tumors. Recently, four independent groups identified genomic amplification of chromosome 2p23–24 in a subset of families with hereditary neuroblastoma [30–33]. Amplification and activating mutations of the tyrosine kinase anaplastic lymphoma kinase (ALK) were identified in both familial and sporadic cases of neuroblastoma. The implications of ALK mutations in prognosis and the development of therapeutics are discussed in the section on "Oncogenes". Familial neuroblastoma predisposition is likely due to more than one causal gene, and tumor initiation involves multiple genetic alterations. Nevertheless, clinical testing for PHOX2B and ALK mutations will be available soon. The identification of familial neuroblastoma predisposition genes will not only benefit affected families but also contribute to our better understanding of the initiation of sporadic neuroblastoma.

Chromosomal Abnormalities

Chromosomal abnormalities in neuroblastoma tumors were originally detected by conventional cytogenetic studies, which could be hampered by low mitotic index during metaphase. Allelic loss and fluorescence in-situ hybridization (FISH) analyses provide specific information on the targeted genetic regions, but other genomic regions are not examined. Comparative genomic hybridization (CGH) has the advantages of detecting imbalances of whole genomic regions in a large number of samples but cannot identify balanced translocations. More recently, high-throughput assays to detect copy-number variation (CNV) and single-nucleotide polymorphisms (SNPs) have led to discovery of new genetic loci not previously implicated in neuroblastoma. Combinations of these techniques will continue to be utilized to study chromosomal aberrations in an effort to identify better prognostic markers and novel therapeutic targets for neuroblastoma. Furthermore, recent efforts now also include analysis of genomic DNA associations that may predispose to the development of neuroblastoma.

Deletion or Allelic Loss at 1p and 11q

Utilizing DNA polymorphism approaches and CGH, LOH of chromosome 1p36 and 11q23 have been found to be the most common genetic abnormalities in neuroblastoma, with an overall incidence of 25% to 35% [34,35] and 35% to 45% [36,37], respectively; 1p LOH, as detected by PCR and FISH (Figure 25.4), is strongly associated with MYCN amplification and other high-risk disease features [37]. Though 90% of MYCN-amplified tumors have 1p deletion, 1p LOH is only present in 20% of MYCN nonamplified tumors [38]. By contrast, 11q LOH is uncommon in MYCN-amplified tumors, even though it remains highly correlated with other high-risk factors [37]. Current evidence suggests that 1p and 11q

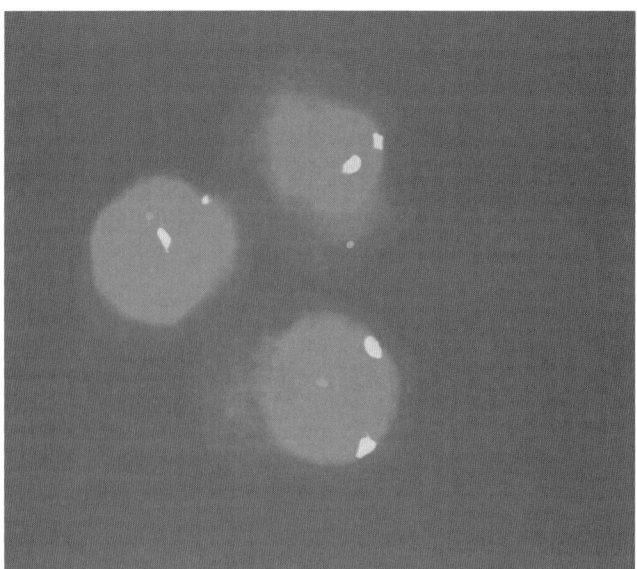

Figure 25.4 1p deletion in neuroblastoma detected by FISH (Fluourescence In situ hybridization). Tumor-cell nuclei are stained in blue (DAPI staining). Loss of 1p chromosome is demonstrated by staining of a single 1p allele in each cell (with a probe labeled with red fluorescence). By contrast, two 1q alleles are detected with the 1q probe labeled with light-blue fluorescence. Images provided by the Dr. Mary Shago, Cytogenetics Laboratory, Hospital for Sick Children, Toronto, Ontario. See *color insert*.

LOH are both independent markers of inferior event-free survival in patients without *MYCN* amplification [37,39]. Current therapeutic studies for patients with nonmetastatic disease will prospectively examine the independent role of *1p* and *11q* LOH in prognosis and risk stratification.

Most 1p deletion studies have localized the smallest region of overlap (SRO) to the short arm of chromosome 1 at 1p36. However, attempts to further narrow the exact site of 1p36 SRO by different groups have resulted in identification of several discrete regions [40]. In most cases, distal 1p (1p36.2–3) is deleted, but the breakpoints are variable. As evidence suggests that there is more than one site of consistent deletion on distal 1p in neuroblastoma, researchers have speculated about the presence of one or more putative neuroblastoma-suppressor gene in this region. Of note, the 1p deletions of *MYCN*-amplified neuroblastomas are generally large, including a region from 1p35–1p36.1 to the telomere, whereas 1p deletions of *MYCN* single-copy tumors commonly have a smaller SRO confined to 1p36.3 [41]. In addition, there is evidence of preferential deletion of the maternally inherited copy of chromosome 1 in *MYCN* nonamplified tumors, indicating that the 1p36.3 suppressor locus may be subject to genomic imprinting [38]. This has led to further speculation of an imprinted locus within distal 1p that is inactivated in *MYCN* single-copy tumors and a more proximal nonimprinted tumor suppressor in *MYCN*-amplified tumors. To date, several tumor-suppressor loci have been identified, but no single genetic abnormality is universal in neuroblastoma. Nevertheless, many investigators are actively pursuing the identification of specific genes that map to 1p36 and 11q23 that may encode putative neuroblastoma tumor-suppressor proteins. It seems likely that the combination of alterations (complete inactivation, haploinsufficiency) of one or more different contiguous genes at these two loci may influence the development of neuroblastoma. The candidate proteins at these loci, in which there is evidence for a role in neuroblastoma, are discussed in the "Tumor Suppressor Gene" section.

Chromosome 17q Gain

Chromosome 17q gain is detected in more than 50% of all neuroblastoma and is by far the most common cytogenetic changes that occurs in neuroblastoma [42,43]; 17q is often translocated to various chromosomal partners resulting in unbalanced translocations and 17q gain. The most frequent partner site for these translocations is 1p, followed by 11q [44]; 17q gain from unbalanced translocation is frequently associated with other adverse prognostic factors, including advanced-stage disease and near-diploid tumors. *MYCN* amplification and/or 1p deletion are found in 75% of tumors with 17q gain [42], and 17q gain has also been reported to be a predictor of adverse outcome [42,45,46]. Its prognostic significance in relation to other genetic factors warrants validation in large prospective clinical trials. How 17q gain contributes to the malignant phenotype of neuroblastoma remains to be elucidated. Unbalanced translocation not only results in 17q gain but also loss of material on the partner chromosome, raising the possibility of the lost of putative tumor-suppressor genes on 1p and 11q. Overexpression of genes on 17q such as *PMM1D* [47], *NM23* [47], and *BIRC5* (Survivin) [48] have been proposed to confer tumor cells survival advantages and malignant phenotype. Further studies identifying genes located close to the 17q breakpoints may also shed light on the role of unbalanced translocation on neuroblastoma initiation.

Chromosome 6 Polymorphism

In contrast to the abnormalities in chromosomes 1p, 11q, and 17q found in the genomic DNA of primary tumors, genome-wide associations are now being analyzed in the germline in blood samples of neuroblastoma patients. In one recent study, Maris and colleagues genotyped blood from more than 1,000 patients and confirmed findings in three independent neuroblastoma patient cohorts [49]. They detected an association between neuroblastoma and the common minor alleles of three SNPs on chromosome 6p22. Homozygosity of the allele was significantly linked with the development of neuroblastoma as well as more common development of metastatic disease, MYCN amplification and disease relapse. Two predicted genes of unknown function FLJ22536 and FLJ44180 map to this region. Further studies are needed to determine whether one of these two genes or both are involved in neuroblastoma pathogenesis or metastasis. Additional SNPs and CNVs in germline DNA are likely to be identified, and some of the genes involved may be important in neuroblastoma predisposition or may modify the tumor phenotype.

ONCOGENE AMPLIFICATION AND ACTIVATION

Overexpression of specific genes that are involved in the regulation of cell proliferation confers survival advantage to cancer cells. Amplification is one of the mechanisms by which cancer cells overexpress genes that possess oncogenic properties. This can manifest as a few additional copies to thousands of copies of the gene per cell. How neuroblastoma and other cancer cells amplify large regions of DNA is still not clear.

MYCN Amplification

Amplification of the *MYCN* gene is the most prominent genomic abnormality in neuroblastoma and is prototypic for recurrent amplification of a protooncogene in human cancers. *MYCN* amplification, detected by FISH (Figure 25.5), is present in about 20% of neuroblastoma tumors and confers a very poor prognosis [2]. However, the specific mechanisms by which *MYCN* amplification contributes to the aggressive tumor phenotype remains enigmatic. *MYCN*, a member of the *MYC* gene family, maps to chromosome 2p24. The amplified *MYCN* DNA can be found in extrachromosomal chromatin bodies known as double minutes or can be integrated into chromosomal positions distinct from 2p24 to form homogeneously staining regions (HSRs) [50,51]. The specific mechanism by which MYCN is amplified (eg, double minutes vs HSRs) has not been linked with prognosis [52]. The size of the *MYCN* amplicon (unit of amplified DNA) ranges from 350kb to 1 Mb, of which the *MYCN* gene takes up only 7 kb [53,54]. Although flanking genes can be coamplified with *MYCN*, *MYCN* has emerged as the gene that is most consistently amplified in this locus [53,55]. Genes that have been shown to be coamplified with *MYCN* in neuroblastoma include *ODC* (orthinine decarboxylase), *RRM2* (ribonucleotide reductase), *Syndecan-1*, and *DDX1* [56]. In addition, as mentioned in the following, high levels of ALK have been detected in tumors with amplification of 2p23–24 [32]. The *DDX1* gene coamplifies with *MYCN* in 50% of MYCN-amplified neuroblastomas [57]; however, *DDX1* amplification without concomitant *MYCN* amplification has not been observed. *DDX1* belongs to the DEAD-box protein family that regulates RNA metabolism [58] and which, potentially, can enhance the oncogenicity of *MYCN*.

Like its homologue MYC-C that is involved in various hematologic malignancies, the MYCN oncoprotein is a nuclear transcription factor that can bind to the promoters and activate or repress genes involved in a variety of oncogenic cellular processes, which include cell-cycle progression [59], transcriptional regulation [60], genomic stability [61], and apoptosis [62]. MYC activity is regulated by the formation of heterodimers with the MAX protein. However, despite persistent research effort, the effector genes of MYCN that are crucial for neuroblastoma tumorigenesis are yet to be identified. Recently, Slack et al [63,64] identified *MDM2* as a direct transcriptional target of MYCN and demonstrated that MYCN-induced centromere amplification and genomic instability was mediated through MDM2 in neuroblastoma [65]. MDM2 is not only the key negative regulator of the tumor-suppressor p53 but it also functions as an oncoprotein, independent of p53 [66,67]. Through a naturally occurring SNP309, MDM2 has also been shown to affect genetic susceptibility to cancers [68]. Hence, MYCN and MDM2 may cooperate to induce malignant transformation, and further research into the MYCN/MDM2 pathway may provide insight into the pathogenesis of MYCN-driven tumors.

Different experimental models have shown that enhanced *MYCN* expression leads to malignant transformation and cell-cycle progression [69,72] This includes a transgenic mouse model whereby targeted overexpression of the human *MYCN* cDNA to the murine neural crest elicits development of neuroblastoma [73,74]. Furthermore, MYCN expression may affect response to chemotherapies in vitro [75]. Hence, elevated levels of *MYCN* expression were thought to play an essential role in the clinically aggressive phenotype of *MYCN*-amplified tumors. However, in contrast to *MYCN* gene amplification, *MYCN* expression does not always correlate with poor outcome. In a subset of *MYCN* nonamplified neuroblastoma that expresses high levels of *MYCN* mRNA or MYCN protein, *MYCN* overexpression does not correlate with inferior survival [76,77]. The prognostic significance of *MYCN* expression appears to be dependent on the subset of patients being analyzed [78,79]. Neuroblastoma is biologically heterogeneous. It is plausible that while loss of *MYCN* transcriptional regulation may contribute to the aggressive phenotype in some patients, factors other than *MYCN* expression may play an important role in tumorigenesis in other patients. For example, approximately 50% of the patients older than

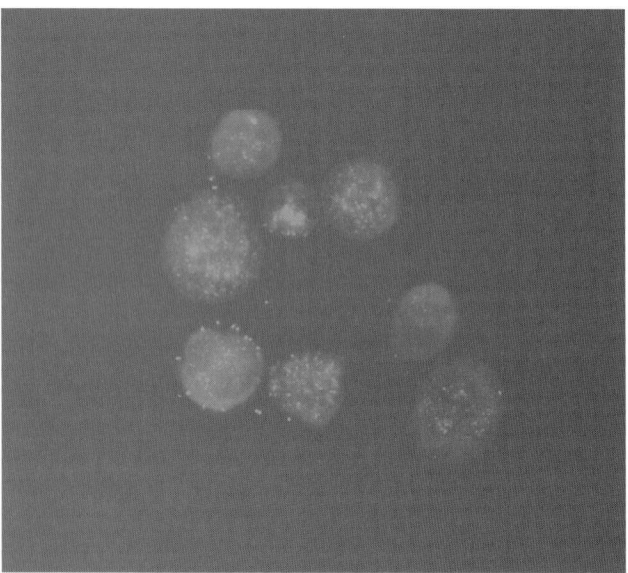

Figure 25.5 N-myc amplification. FISH using a probe to N-myc (labeled with red fluorescence) demonstrates high levels of N-myc in nuclei of tumor cells (nuclei are stained in blue). Amplification of N-myc is defined as greater than 10 copies of N-myc genes detected per cell as per the INRG (International Neuroblastoma Risk Group) guidelines. Images provided by the Dr. Mary Shago, Cytogenetics Laboratory, Hospital for Sick Children, Toronto, Ontario. *See color insert.*

1 year of age, with advanced-stage disease, lack *MYCN* amplification, yet their outcome is poor. *MYCN* may also have distinct regulatory roles on the expression of downstream target genes that can promote or repress tumor progression in different subsets of patients.

Amplification and Mutation of ALK Oncogene

Amplification of other gene loci that are nonsyntenic with the *MYCN* locus at chromosome 2p24 can occur concurrently with *MYCN* amplification. These include the *MYCL* gene at 1p32 [80] and the *MDM2* gene at 12q12–14 [81,82]. Most gene amplifications in neuroblastoma are found to be concomitant with *MYCN* amplification. However, recent data using a variety of techniques, including whole genome-scanning, demonstrates independent amplification of a region of chromosome 2p23–4 that encodes ALK. ALK abnormalities had previously been detected in anaplastic large-cell lymphomas (translocations) as well as some lung cancers [83] and rare tumors, including inflammatory myofibroblastic tumors. Notably, amplification of *ALK* has been detected in neuroblastomas without amplification of the *MYCN* loci [30–33]. ALK mutations have also been detected in some neuroblastomas. Most mutations map to the tyrosine kinase domain of ALK and result in constitutive phosphorylation. Early studies suggest an incidence of ALK abnormalities (combination of amplification and mutations) in approximately 12% of neuroblastomas. Thus far, it is unclear whether ALK mutations are more common in tumors in certain stages and/or whether ALK status is associated with prognosis. Furthermore, studies are underway to determine which ALK mutations are driver, rather than passenger, mutations in the pathogenesis of neuroblastoma. Knockdown of ALK in neuroblastoma cell lines and xenografts results in decreased tumor growth. Furthermore, pharmacologic inhibitors of ALK have shown promising early activity in preclinical studies [33]; however, whether these drugs will have efficacy only in tumors with abnormal ALK expression or activity has not been fully determined. Nevertheless, due to the promising preclinical data and the presence of ALK abnormalities in several malignancies, in addition to neuroblastoma in children, adults Phase I studies are currently underway.

RAS Activation

Activating mutations in the proto-oncogenes, H-RAS, K-RAS, and N-RAS, have been identified in a wide variety of human cancers. N-RAS was initially identified as the transforming gene of a human neuroblastoma cell line. Furthermore, activated RAS cooperates with the MYCN gene to promote tumorigenesis [84] and stabilizes the MYC proteins through posttranslational modifications [85]. However, subsequent studies have shown that activating mutations of the RAS genes [86,87] and alterations of Ras-MAPK/PI3K signaling are rare in neuroblastoma [88] and, therefore, do not support the role of RAS in neuroblastoma. In fact, key oncogenes and their associated pathways frequently targeted for activation or inactivation in human cancers are rarely mutated in neuroblastomas.

Tumor-Suppressor Inactivation

p53

p53 is the most extensively studied tumor-suppressor gene. It plays a critical role in cellular responses during DNA damage and is a key regulator of cell-cycle control and apoptosis [89]. Though *p53* is mutated in 50% of all human cancers, it is rarely mutated in *de novo* neuroblastoma [90] and only rarely detected in the inherited cancer predisposition, Li-Fraumeni syndrome, characterized by germline *p53* mutations [91]. Mechanisms inactivating wild-type p53, including *MDM2* amplification [81], p53 cytoplasmic sequestration in undifferentiated neuroblastoma [92,93], and H-TWIST overexpression [94], have been proposed. However, *p53* mutations have been observed in cell lines derived from patients at relapses [82,95] and are thought to contribute to chemoresistance in recurrent disease. In vitro and xenograft data demonstrate that specific inactivation of p53 in neuroblastoma cells results in resistance to commonly used chemotherapeutic agents [96].

p73

p73 is a *p53* homologue and maps to chromosome 1p36.33, a region of frequent LOH in neuroblastoma [97]. This raises the possibility that this region could harbor a neuroblastoma-suppressor gene and *p73* is a candidate gene for the imprinted distal 1p suppressor gene. However, mutations on the second allele of *p73* have only rarely been detected in neuroblastoma and other cancers [98]. Furthermore, studies of epigenetic alterations, such as methylation status, have not provided consistent evidence for p73 inactivation [99–101]. Thus, p73 does not fulfill Knudson's criteria for a canonical tumor suppressor gene. On the other hand, there is emerging evidence that the relative abundance of different p73 isoforms is an important determinant of tumorigenicity [102]. *p73* encodes multiple, functionally distinct isoforms as a result of alternative-promoter utilization and splicing. The N-terminus truncated Δ Np73 isoforms lack the transactivation domain and function as dominant negative inhibitors of p53 and the full-length proapoptotic TAp73 isoforms [102]. The truncated Δ *Np73* isoforms are found to be overexpressed in a variety of cancers, including neuroblastoma, in which high levels of Δ *Np73* expression is associated with poor outcome, independent of disease stage and MYCN amplification. In a study of 52 neuroblastoma patients, the overall survival declined from 80% to 0% in tumors with Δ *Np73* overexpression [103]; p73 has also been implicated in chemosensitivity and neuronal differentiation and survival. Hence, p73 may a role in neuroblastoma development in a far more complex model than that of a classical tumor-suppressor model. In addition to *p73*, other genes at 1p36 have been implicated in neuroblastoma.

CHD5

The chromatin helicase-binding domain 5 (*CHD5*) gene is one of the 20 genes initially localized to the 1p36 region most commonly deleted in neuroblastoma. Recent evidence demonstrates that the second allele of *CHD5* is often inactivated by methylation in neuroblastoma cell lines [104]. Furthermore, high levels of expression of CHD5 are associated with favorable prognosis. In addition, decreased expression of CHD5 in neuroblastoma xenografts as a result of CHD5 antisense treatment resulted in inhibition of tumor growth. CHD5 has been shown to control proliferation, apoptosis, and senescence via the p19Arf/ p53 pathway [105]. Mice with heterozygous inactivation of the region, including CHD5, develop spontaneous tumors, including lymphomas, squamous-cell carcinomas, and mesenchymal neoplasms.

KIFI Beta

Germline deletion of the kinesin KIF1β is a rare cause of familial neural-crest-derived malignancy and maps to the region of 1p36 frequently deleted in neuroblastoma. Rare missense loss of function mutations have been identified in the second allele for some patients with neuroblastoma as well as the related tumors, pheochromocytoma and medulloblastoma [106]. KIF1β plays a critical role in apoptosis of primary sympathetic neurons in the absence of nerve growth factor (NGF). Knockdown of KIF1β by short interfering RNA (siRNA) results in protection from apoptosis in primary neurons, and overproduction of KIF1β in neuroblastoma cells leads to enhanced cell death.

CDKN2A

The *CDKN2A* gene-encoding INK4A/p16 is an important cell-cycle regulatory gene and is frequently inactivated by deletion or mutation in various cancers. Although homozygous deletion of *CDKN2A* at chromosome 9p21 have been observed in a subset of neuroblastoma cell lines, deletion of this locus in primary neuroblastoma is uncommon [107,108]; therefore, it is not a potential tumor-suppressor candidate gene in a large number of neuroblastoma.

Abnormal Gene Expression

Neurotrophin Receptors

Advances in molecular embryology have identified neurotrophin receptors (TrkA, TrkB, and TrkC) as important players in the embryonic development and differentiation of neural-crest cells to sympathetic neurons [109]. Neuroblastoma cells are derived from sympathetic neuroblasts and have the propensity to undergo spontaneous or induced differentiation into ganglioneuroblastoma or ganglioneuroma. Hence, a similar mechanism involving neurotrophin receptor signaling may be involved in neuroblastomas [110]. The TrkA (NTRK1) tyrosine kinase transmembrane neurotrophin receptor is expressed in normal embryonic cells at the later stage of sympathetic/adrenal development. Binding of its ligand-NGF to TrkA signals the differentiation of immature sympathetic neurons into mature ganglion cells, whereas inhibition of TrkA activation results in apoptosis [111]. Similarly, primary-culture studies of neuroblastoma expressing TrkA have shown that exogenous NGF provokes differentiation and withdrawal of NGF induces apoptosis [112]. By contrast, a splice variant of TrkA (TrkAIII) promotes neuroblastoma tumor growth by inhibiting NGF/TrkA signaling [113]. In the clinical context, TrkA is a favorable prognostic factor [112,114]. This supports that the anti-oncogenic NGF/TrkA pathway is functional in TrkA-expressing neuroblastoma. In a subset of neuroblastoma, NGF/TrkA signaling is likely to mediate differentiation or regression, depending on the microenvironment. It is plausible that the spontaneous regression observed in TrkA-expressing neuroblastomas in infants results from the decline of NGF in the microenvironment, leading to apoptosis [115].

TrkB (NTRK2), a second neurotrophin receptor, is commonly associated with unfavorable neuroblastomas, particularly those with *MYCN* amplification [116]. TrkB is expressed in normal sympathetic neurons at an earlier embryonic stage than TrkA [117]. Hence, the expression of TrkB in *MYCN*-amplified tumor may represent arrest of differentiation of neural-crest cells prior to TrkA expression. TrkB signaling is generally intact in neuroblastoma cell lines and promotes survival and neurite outgrowth [116]. The coexpression of TrkB with it ligand brain-derived neurotrophic factor (BDNF) is thought to provide a survival advantage through an autocrine or paracrine loop, thereby promoting chemoresistance, angiogenesis, and metastasis [118,119]. Like TrkA, TrkC (NTRK3) is expressed in predominantly biologically favorable neuroblastomas [120]. Truncated isoforms of TrkB and TrkC lacking the catalytic tyrosine kinase domain are also expressed in favorable tumors. In conclusion, these neurotrophic receptors represent one of the key molecules that contribute to our understanding of neuroblastoma biology and could be potential therapeutic targets in the treatment of neuroblastoma. One trkB inhibitor K252a is in early clinical trials.

Multidrug Resistance Genes

The development of resistance to multiple and structurally and functionally distinct chemotherapeutic agents is implicated in treatment failure. Multidrug resistance is a prominent feature of *MYCN*-amplified and relapsed neuroblastomas. One of the underlying mechanisms for multidrug resistance (MDR) is enhancement of drug efflux. The P-glycoprotein encoded by the *MDR1* gene belongs to the ATP-binding cassette (ABC) transporters family and is known to efflux hydrophobic drugs. *MDR1* overexpression is a poor prognostic indicator in tumors lacking MYCN amplification [121]. A second ABC transporter, the *MRP1* (MDR-associated protein) gene, has also been demonstrated to confer poor survival after adjusting for the effect of MYCN amplification [122]. There is evidence that *MRP1* is a transcription target of the MYCN protein and response to cytotoxic agents is influenced by MYCN-mediated regulation of *MRP* expression [75]. More recently, *MRP4* overexpression has also been found to be a poor prognostic marker [123]. Identification and characterization of genes that mediate MDR provides insights into neuroblastoma biology and the drug resistant-phenotype and help define novel compounds that can modulate drug-efflux mechanisms.

Telomerase Activity

Telomeres are specialized structures that protect the ends of chromosomes and shorten progressively with each cell division due to end-replication problem. As telomeres reach a critically short length, normal cells enter senescence, whereas cancer cells achieve immortality by maintaining the length of telomeres through activation of the reverse-transcriptase telomerase [124]. In neuroblastoma, telomerase activity correlates with advanced disease stage, MYCN amplification, and poor outcome for both localized and metastatic disease [125–127]. In stage 4S disease, the lack of telomerase activity is associated with spontaneous regression [125,126]. Like stage 4S neuroblastoma, pediatric low-grade gliomas lacking telomerase undergo spontaneous regression and long telomere length is predictive of recurrence in low-grade gliomas [128]. Furthermore, in pediatric ependymoma, the enzymatic subunit of telomerase hTERT is a poor prognostic marker [129]. Although telomerase activity is associated with specific prognostic markers, the specific mechanisms by which telomerase may be involved in neuroblastoma pathogenesis is not known.

BCL-2

Apoptosis, programmed cell death, is a critical process during neuronal development [111], and the BCL-2 gene family consisting of both pro- and anti-apoptotic genes have been shown to play a role in neurogenesis [130,131]. Neuroblastoma has the highest frequency of spontaneous regression observed in human cancers and may represent the delayed activation of an intact apoptotic pathway. Conversely, the highly aggressive phenotype suggests defects in the apoptotic machinery. The antiapoptotic BCL-2 is highly expressed in most neuroblastoma cell lines and primary tumors [132], and the expression level is inversely related to the degree of differentiation and apoptotic fraction [133]. BCL-2 and BCL-X_L have been shown to inhibit chemotherapy-induced apoptosis in neuroblastoma [134,135] and may be amenable to drug targeting to overcome chemoresistance. Furthermore, in vitro cell death triggered by serum deprivation is attenuated by BCL-2 [136].

DNA Content

The DNA content of tumor cells can be determined by karyotyping, which may not always be successful in neuroblastoma. Total DNA content (DNA index) can be analyzed by flow cytometry, which, though easy to use, offers no specific information on chromosome rearrangements. The DNA content or ploidy of neuroblastomas can be categorized into near-diploid and hyperdiploid (or near-triploid). Near-diploid tumors are commonly unfavorable tumors, whereas hyperdiploid tumors are more likely to be favorable tumors. Tumor ploidy has been shown to offer prognostic information primarily in patients less than 1 year of age with advanced-stage disease [137]. The loss of its prognostic significance in older patients [138,139] is likely related to the structural rearrangements present in the near-diploid tumors of older patients, as opposed to the whole-chromosome gain without structural rearrangements in the hyperdiploid tumors of infants. However, recent prospective studies of patients with intermediate-risk neuroblastoma suggests that tumors with diploid DNA content are associated with a poorer outcome than those with hyperdiploidy; thus, DNA content is still used in the current risk stratification [138].

CANCER STEM CELLS

There is growing evidence to suggest that within a tumor there is a reservoir or subpopulation of cells that share some properties with normal stem cells and drive tumorigenesis [140]. These cells termed "tumor-initiating cells" (TIC) are the "cancer stem cells" that have been described in leukemia and, more recently, in many solid tumors, including central-nervous-system tumors [141]. Recently, using culture conditions favoring neural stem-cell growth neuroblastoma TICs have been isolated as neurospheres from primary tumors and bone-marrow metastases [142]. These cells were identified on the basis of their ability to self-renew, differentiate into cellular lineages observed in primary tumors, and form tumors following serial transplantation into immunocompromised mice in vivo. Unlike brain tumor stem cells that are characterized by the cell-surface marker CD133, the neuroblastoma TICs cannot be identified by a single marker. However, in contrast to more than 1 million cultured adherent neuroblastoma cells that are required to form a tumor in orthotopic murine neuroblastoma models, as few as 10 TIC cells will result in tumors in vivo. It is likely that the TIC cells represent the cells in a neuroblastoma that are responsible for disease relapse. Thus, these cells may be an important model for identifying and testing novel therapies. In addition, genetic studies on TICs may also shed light on the genes and signaling pathways involved in neuroblastoma tumor initiation. Furthermore, in the future, it may be possible to isolate TICs from an individual patient and examine the genetic and molecular profiles as well as sensitivity to therapies.

Genetic Model of Neuroblastoma Development

Tumor Initiation and Progression

On the basis of the different DNA content observed in neuroblastoma tumors, a genetic model of neuroblastoma initiation and progression has been proposed [40]. It is based on the hypothesis that all neuroblastomas have a common, yet to be identified, mutation; however, a commitment made shortly after tumor initiation leads to the development of two main types of tumor with different DNA content. The first type is characterized by mitotic dysfunction with whole-chromosome gains without structural rearrangements, resulting in a hyperdiploid/near-triploid karyotype. These tumors tend to have a benign behavior, express high levels of TrkA, and are responsive to differentiation and apoptosis stimuli and NGF in the microenvironment. *MYCN* amplification that occurs in a small percentage of these triploid tumors is a consequence of secondary hit acquired at a later stage of tumor development. The second type generally has a diploid/near-diploid DNA content and a fundamental defect in genomic stability, resulting in gross chromosomal aberrations. These tumors tend to be unfavorable, frequently demonstrate

17q gain, and do not express *TrkA*. They can be further subdivided into an aggressive subtype with *MYCN* amplification, *1p* LOH, and *TrkB* and *BDNF* expression. The other less aggressive subtype does not have *MYCN* amplification and is characterized by *11q* deletion and other chromosomal rearrangements. All of these genetic aberrations are acquired as "second-hit" changes. Genetic abnormalities responsible for the first hit during the very early evolutionary stage of tumor development remain elusive.

Spontaneous Regression

The hallmark of neuroblastoma is its biological diversity and its propensity to undergo spontaneous regression. However, specific clinical and biological features have been linked to tumors that undergo spontaneous regression. These tumors are usually characterized by age less than 12 months, triploid DNA content, and absence of *1p* deletion and *MYCN* amplification [143–145]. This peculiar phenomenon has been explained by two different mechanisms. One is the delayed onset of apoptosis, based on the assumption that the triploid genome is responsible for the delayed apoptosis and that tumor regression represents the activation of this naturally occurring programmed cell death [146,147]. As NGF plays an important role in neuronal death in the perinatal period [111,148], the interaction of growth factors and their receptors such as NGF and TrkA may be of crucial importance in the spontaneous regression process. The second mechanism represents an immunologic process based on the observations that normal human serum is cytotoxic to neuroblastoma cells and immune factors such as IgM and complements trigger apoptosis and tumor regression [149–151].

RISK STRATIFICATION

Substantial research efforts throughout the years have provided convincing evidence that the biological features of neuroblastoma are highly predictive of clinical behavior. Improvement in the outcome of patients with neuroblastoma over the past few decades is a result of the ability to stratify patients into prognostic subsets and thereby allows pediatric oncologists to deliver risk-adapted therapies. To standardize risk stratification in clinical trials and to enable accurate comparison of treatment outcomes worldwide, an International Neuroblastoma Risk Group (INRG) classification system was established in 2005, using age, stage, and *MYCN* status as the backbone of the schema. Other potential biological variables will also be introduced, depending on further statistical analyses. In addition, surgical risk-factor-scoring systems [152] will be prospectively incorporated into cooperative group studies.

Age at diagnosis and disease stage are considered to be the two most important clinical factors for predicting outcome in neuroblastoma. Survival is inversely related to age and stage of disease, with the exception of stage 4S disease [1]. Traditionally, the age cutoff in risk stratification schema had been set at 12 months. However, for tumors lacking MYCN amplification, intensive therapy yielded a better survival in patients aged 12 to 18 months [153–155]. With evidence suggesting a more appropriate age cutoff at 18 months of age, upcoming clinical trials of the Children's Oncology Group will assess the safety of therapy reduction in children aged between 12 and 18 months with INSS stage 3 or 4 disease and favorable biology. These patients, previously considered high-risk, are now included in the intermediate-risk group.

Tumor histology is another important prognostic variable. The degree of neuroblastic maturation toward ganglion cells has long been recognized to confer prognostic importance in neuroblastoma [156,157]. The International Neuroblastoma Pathology Classification System (INPC), a modification of the Shamada system, classifies tumors into favorable and unfavorable histology on the basis of the degree of neuroblastic differentiation, Schwannian stroma content, mitosis-karyorrhexis (MKI), and age at diagnosis [158]. More recently, the presence of nodular histology in a rare subset of patients has been correlated with poor survival [159].

The genetic composition of a tumor has played an increasingly important role in risk stratification in neuroblastoma. *MYCN* gene amplification is the most well-studied genetic variable. MYCN amplification is detected in about 20% of all primary tumors and is closely related to stage 4 disease, other genetic aberrations, treatment failure, and poor survival [137,160]. However, the usefulness of *MYCN* amplification in risk stratification lies in its capability to predict inferior outcome in patients with otherwise favorable diseases such as localized disease and disseminated disease in infants. For instance, in infants less than 1 year of age with metastatic disease, the 3-year event-free survival decreased from 93% to 10% for those with *MYCN*-nonamplified and *MYCN*-amplified tumors, respectively [161]. In addition, DNA index has been shown to independently predict outcome in patients less than 2 years of age with metastatic disease [138,139]. DNA ploidy is divided into two broad groups: (1) diploid/near-diploid, and (2) hyperdiploid/near-triploid; the former is associated with advanced-stage disease and the latter with lower-stage tumors. Hence, DNA ploidy has generally been used to separate stage 4S and stage 4 patients aged less than 12 months into different risk category among *MYCN*-nonamplified tumors. In addition, Trk expression [115] and chromosome 1p, 11q, and 17q abnormalities [37,42] have also been shown to correlate with clinical outcomes. Their clinical applicability in risk stratification will need to be confirmed in future clinical trials.

The Children's Oncology Group has stratified patients into low-, intermediate-, and high-risk groups on the basis of age at diagnosis, INSS stage, tumor histology, DNA index, and *MYCN* status. Patients treated in the low- and intermediate-risk groups have an event-free survival of close to 90%, whereas patients in the high-risk group have an event-free survival of less than 30%, despite intensive multimodal treatment [2]. In addition to improving survival, the major goals of continuing clinical trials are to prospectively validate updated risk stratification schemas and to integrate potential prognostic markers into future algorithms to further refine the risk-group classification system. Recently, the risk stratification schema has been revised to accommodate the modification of age cutoff to 18 months (Table 25.2). In addition, on the basis of data on the prognostic predictability of *1p* and *11q* LOH in tumors lacking *MYCN* amplification, upcoming clinical trials will stratify intermediate-risk patients by 1p and 11q allelic status and aim to establish the appropriate therapy on the basis of chromosomal aberrations involving 1p and 11q. Future studies will also validate the importance of newly identified genes involved in neuroblastoma such as ALK.

CONCLUSIONS

Knowledge of the biology and genetics of neuroblastoma has allowed identification of biological-based risk groups and the choice of more appropriate treatment. Neuroblastoma serves as model in which the genetic and biological analyses of the tumor cells have become conventional determinants of patient management. Understanding the fundamental genetic alterations responsible for the spontaneous regression, differentiation, or malignant transformation of neuroblastoma will provide insights into developing more effective and less toxic therapies, as well as the much-needed novel therapies to treat the aggressive tumors. However, thus far, other than MYCN amplification that occurs in only a subset of aggressive tumors, no other oncogene has been shown to be consistently activated in human neuroblastomas. Despite the discovery of MYCN amplification 20 years ago, the molecular mechanisms underlying MYCN amplification and the critical effector molecules downstream of MYCN that mediates MYCN-dependent transformation and progression have remained enigmatic. Furthermore, some of the major oncogenic pathways that are frequently deregulated in human cancers seem to be intact in neuroblastoma. Cytogenetic and molecular analyses have shown that several chromosomal regions are frequently deleted in neuroblastoma, suggesting the presence of one or more tumor-suppressor genes in these regions. Despite persistent effort, no tumor-suppressor loci have been identified. A better understanding of normal neuronal development of the sympathetic/adrenal system, neural stem cells, together with innovative techniques in genetic and molecular profiling of primary tumors, metastases and germline DNA (eg, by CNV and SNP arrays), will help pin-point the key mutational events responsible for tumor initiation and progression in neuroblastoma. The ultimate goal is to precisely prognosticate on the basis of both patient-specific and tumor-specific genetic variables and to provide effective and safe treatment by exploiting pathways leading to the specific phenotype of this heterogeneous pediatric tumor. Individualized prognostic assessment and treatment may eventually depend on an individual tumor's complex genetic and proteomic signaling pathways.

REFERENCES

1. Brodeur GM, Maris JM. Neuroblastoma. In: Pizzo PA, Poplack DG, eds. *Principals and Practice of Pediatric Oncology*. 5th ed. Philadelphia: J B Lippincott Company; 2006:993–970.
2. Maris JM, Hogarty MD, Bagatell R, Cohn SL. Neuroblastoma. *Lancet*. 2007;369:2106–2120.
3. Mahoney NR, Liu GT, Menacker SJ, Wilson MC, Hogarty MD, Maris JM. Pediatric horner syndrome: etiologies and roles of imaging and urine studies to detect neuroblastoma and other responsible mass lesions. *Am J Ophthalmol*. 2006;142:651–659.
4. De Bernardi B, Pianca C, Pistamiglio P, et al. Neuroblastoma with symptomatic spinal cord compression at diagnosis: treatment and results with 76 cases. *J Clin Oncol*. 2001;19:183–190.
5. Matthay KK, Blaes F, Hero B, et al. Opsoclonus myoclonus syndrome in neuroblastoma a report from a workshop on the dancing eyes syndrome at the advances in neuroblastoma meeting in Genoa, Italy, 2004. *Cancer Lett*. 2005;228:275–282.
6. Mitchell WG, Davalos-Gonzalez Y, Brumm VL, et al. Opsoclonus-ataxia caused by childhood neuroblastoma: developmental and neurologic sequelae. *Pediatrics*. 2002;109:86–98.
7. Weinblatt ME, Heisel MA, Siegel SE. Hypertension in children with neurogenic tumors. *Pediatrics*. 1983;71:947–951.
8. El Shafie M, Samuel D, Klippel CH, Robinson MG, Cullen BJ. Intractable diarrhea in children with VIP-secreting ganglioneuroblastomas. *J Pediatr Surg*. 1983;18:34–36.
9. Brodeur GM, Pritchard J, Berthold F, et al. Revisions of the international criteria for neuroblastoma diagnosis, staging, and response to treatment. *J Clin Oncol*. 1993;11:1466–1477.
10. Cheung NK, Kushner BH, LaQuaglia MP, et al. Survival from non-stage 4 neuroblastoma without cytotoxic therapy: an analysis of clinical and biological markers. *Eur J Cancer*. 1997;33:2117–2120.
11. Garaventa A, De Bernardi B, Pianca C, et al. Localized but unresectable neuroblastoma: treatment and outcome of 145 cases. Italian Cooperative Group for Neuroblastoma. *J Clin Oncol*. 1993;11:1770–1779.
12. Matthay KK, Villablanca JG, Seeger RC, et al. Treatment of high-risk neuroblastoma with intensive chemotherapy, radiotherapy, autologous bone marrow transplantation, and 13-cis-retinoic acid. Children's Cancer Group. *N Engl J Med*. 1999;341:1165–1173.
13. De Bernardi B, Nicolas B, Boni L, et al. Disseminated neuroblastoma in children older than one year at diagnosis: comparable results with three consecutive high-dose protocols adopted by the Italian Co-Operative Group for Neuroblastoma. *J Clin Oncol*. 2003;21:1592–1601.
14. Vogelstein B, Fearon ER, Hamilton SR, et al. Genetic alterations during colorectal-tumor development. *N Engl J Med*. 1988;319:525–532.
15. Rubnitz JE, Crist WM. Molecular genetics of childhood cancer: implications for pathogenesis, diagnosis, and treatment. *Pediatrics*. 1997;100:101–108.
16. Robertson CM, Tyrrell JC, Pritchard J. Familial neural crest tumours. *Eur J Pediatr*. 1991;150:789–792.
17. Kushner BH, Gilbert F, Helson L. Familial neuroblastoma. Case reports, literature review, and etiologic considerations. *Cancer*. 1986;57:1887–1893.
18. Knudson AG Jr, Strong LC. Mutation and cancer: neuroblastoma and pheochromocytoma. *Am J Hum Genet*. 1972;24:514–532.
19. Maris JM, Chatten J, Meadows AT, Biegel JA, Brodeur GM. Familial neuroblastoma: a three-generation pedigree and a further association with Hirschsprung disease. *Med Pediatr Oncol*. 1997;28:1–5.
20. Biegel JA, White PS, Marshall HN, et al. Constitutional 1p36 deletion in a child with neuroblastoma. *Am J Hum Genet*. 1993;52:176–182.
21. Mosse Y, Greshock J, King A, Khazi D, Weber BL, Maris JM. Identification and high-resolution mapping of a constitutional 11q deletion in an infant with multifocal neuroblastoma. *Lancet Oncol*. 2003;4:769–771.
22. Maris JM, Weiss MJ, Mosse Y, et al. Evidence for a hereditary neuroblastoma predisposition locus at chromosome 16p12–13. *Cancer Res*. 2002;62:6651–6658.
23. Kushner BH, Hajdu SI, Helson L. Synchronous neuroblastoma and von Recklinghausen's disease: a review of the literature. *J Clin Oncol*. 1985;3:117–120.
24. Bolande RP. Neurocristopathy: its growth and development in 20 years. *Pediatr Pathol Lab Med*. 1997;17:1–25.
25. Trochet D, Bourdeaut F, Janoueix-Lerosey I, et al. Germline mutations of the paired-like homeobox 2B (PHOX2B) gene in neuroblastoma. *Am J Hum Genet*. 2004;74:761–764.
26. Mosse YP, Laudenslager M, Khazi D, et al. Germline PHOX2B mutation in hereditary neuroblastoma. *Am J Hum Genet*. 2004;75:727–730.
27. Weese-Mayer DE, Berry-Kravis EM, Zhou L, et al. Idiopathic congenital central hypoventilation syndrome: analysis of genes

pertinent to early autonomic nervous system embryologic development and identification of mutations in PHOX2b. *Am J Med Genet A.* 2003;123:267–278.
28. Amiel J, Laudier B, Attie-Bitach T, et al. Polyalanine expansion and frameshift mutations of the paired-like homeobox gene PHOX2B in congenital central hypoventilation syndrome. *Nat Genet.* 2003;33:459–461.
29. Raabe EH, Laudenslager M, Winter C, et al. Prevalence and functional consequence of PHOX2B mutations in neuroblastoma. *Oncogene.* 2008;27:469–476.
30. Mosse YP, Laudenslager M, Longo L, et al. Identification of ALK as a major familial neuroblastoma predisposition gene. *Nature.* 2008;455:930–935.
31. Janoueix-Lerosey I, Lequin D, Brugieres L, et al. Somatic and germline activating mutations of the ALK kinase receptor in neuroblastoma. *Nature.* 2008;455:967–970.
32. Chen Y, Takita J, Choi YL, et al. Oncogenic mutations of ALK kinase in neuroblastoma. *Nature.* 2008;455:971–974.
33. George RE, Sanda T, Hanna M, et al. Activating mutations in ALK provide a therapeutic target in neuroblastoma. *Nature.* 2008;455:975–978.
34. White PS, Thompson PM, Gotoh T, et al. Definition and characterization of a region of 1p36.3 consistently deleted in neuroblastoma. *Oncogene.* 2005;24:2684–2694.
35. Martinsson T, Sjoberg RM, Hedborg F, Kogner P. Deletion of chromosome 1p loci and microsatellite instability in neuroblastomas analyzed with short-tandem repeat polymorphisms. *Cancer Res.* 1995;55:5681–5686.
36. Guo C, White PS, Weiss MJ, et al. Allelic deletion at 11q23 is common in MYCN single copy neuroblastomas. *Oncogene.* 1999;18:4948–4957.
37. Attiyeh EF, London WB, Mosse YP, et al. Chromosome 1p and 11q deletions and outcome in neuroblastoma. *N Engl J Med.* 2005;353:2243–2253.
38. Caron H, van Sluis P, van Hoeve M, et al. Allelic loss of chromosome 1p36 in neuroblastoma is of preferential maternal origin and correlates with N-myc amplification. *Nat Genet.* 1993;4:187–190.
39. Maris JM, Weiss MJ, Guo C, et al. Loss of heterozygosity at 1p36 independently predicts for disease progression but not decreased overall survival probability in neuroblastoma patients: a Children's Cancer Group study. *J Clin Oncol.* 2000;18:1888–1899.
40. Brodeur GM. Neuroblastoma: biological insights into a clinical enigma. *Nat Rev Cancer.* 2003;3:203–216.
41. Caron H, Peter M, van Sluis P, et al. Evidence for two tumour suppressor loci on chromosomal bands 1p35–36 involved in neuroblastoma: one probably imprinted, another associated with N-myc amplification. *Hum Mol Genet.* 1995;4:535–539.
42. Bown N, Cotterill S, Lastowska M, et al. Gain of chromosome arm 17q and adverse outcome in patients with neuroblastoma. *N Engl J Med.* 1999;340:1954–1961.
43. Plantaz D, Mohapatra G, Matthay KK, Pellarin M, Seeger RC, Feuerstein BG. Gain of chromosome 17 is the most frequent abnormality detected in neuroblastoma by comparative genomic hybridization. *Am J Pathol.* 1997;150:81–89.
44. Van Roy N, Laureys G, Cheng NC, et al. 1;17 translocations and other chromosome 17 rearrangements in human primary neuroblastoma tumors and cell lines. *Genes Chromosomes Cancer.* 1994;10:103–114.
45. Caron H, van Sluis P, de Kraker J, et al. Allelic loss of chromosome 1p as a predictor of unfavorable outcome in patients with neuroblastoma. *N Engl J Med.* 1996;334:225–230.
46. Lastowska M, Cotterill S, Pearson AD, et al. Gain of chromosome arm 17q predicts unfavourable outcome in neuroblastoma patients. U.K. Children's Cancer Study Group and the U.K. Cancer Cytogenetics Group. *Eur J Cancer.* 1997;33:1627–1633.
47. Godfried MB, Veenstra M, v Sluis P, et al. The N-myc and c-myc downstream pathways include the chromosome 17q genes nm23-H1 and nm23-H2. *Oncogene.* 2002;21:2097–2101.
48. Islam A, Kageyama H, Takada N, et al. High expression of Survivin, mapped to 17q25, is significantly associated with poor prognostic factors and promotes cell survival in human neuroblastoma. *Oncogene.* 2000;19:617–623.
49. Maris JM, Mosse YP, Bradfield JP, et al. Chromosome 6p22 locus associated with clinically aggressive neuroblastoma. *N Engl J Med.* 2008;358:2585–2593.
50. Corvi R, Amler LC, Savelyeva L, Gehring M, Schwab M. MYCN is retained in single copy at chromosome 2 band p23–24 during amplification in human neuroblastoma cells. *Proc Natl Acad Sci U S A.* 1994;91:5523–5527.
51. Schwab M, Varmus HE, Bishop JM, et al. Chromosome localization in normal human cells and neuroblastomas of a gene related to c-myc. *Nature.* 1984;308:288–291.
52. Moreau LA, McGrady P, London WB, et al. Does MYCN amplification manifested as homogeneously staining regions at diagnosis predict a worse outcome in children with neuroblastoma? A Children's Oncology Group study. *Clin Cancer Res* 2006;12:5693–5697.
53. Reiter JL, Brodeur GM. High-resolution mapping of a 130-kb core region of the MYCN amplicon in neuroblastomas. *Genomics.* 1996;32:97–103.
54. Schneider SS, Hiemstra JL, Zehnbauer BA, et al. Isolation and structural analysis of a 1.2-megabase N-myc amplicon from a human neuroblastoma. *Mol Cell Biol.* 1992;12:5563–5570.
55. Reiter JL, Brodeur GM. MYCN is the only highly expressed gene from the core amplified domain in human neuroblastomas. *Genes Chromosomes Canc.* 1998;23:134–140.
56. George RE, Kenyon RM, McGuckin AG, Malcolm AJ, Pearson AD, Lunec J. Investigation of co-amplification of the candidate genes ornithine decarboxylase, ribonucleotide reductase, syndecan-1 and a DEAD box gene, DDX1, with N-myc in neuroblastoma. United Kingdom Children's Cancer Study Group. *Oncogene.* 1996;12:1583–1587.
57. Squire JA, Thorner PS, Weitzman S, et al. Co-amplification of MYCN and a DEAD box gene (DDX1) in primary neuroblastoma. *Oncogene.* 1995;10:1417–1422.
58. Linder P, Lasko PF, Ashburner M, et al. Birth of the D-E-A-D box. *Nature.* 1989;337:121–122.
59. Nesbit CE, Tersak JM, Prochownik EV. MYC oncogenes and human neoplastic disease. *Oncogene.* 1999;18:3004–3016.
60. Alaminos M, Mora J, Cheung NK, et al. Genome-wide analysis of gene expression associated with MYCN in human neuroblastoma. *Cancer Res.* 2003;63:4538–4546.
61. Felsher DW, Bishop JM. Transient excess of MYC activity can elicit genomic instability and tumorigenesis. *Proc Natl Acad Sci U S A.* 1999;96:3940–3944.
62. Lutz W, Fulda S, Jeremias I, Debatin KM, Schwab M. MycN and IFNgamma cooperate in apoptosis of human neuroblastoma cells. *Oncogene.* 1998;17:339–346.
63. Slack A, Shohet JM. MDM2 as a critical effector of the MYCN oncogene in tumorigenesis. *Cell Cycle.* 2005;4:857–860.
64. Slack A, Chen Z, Tonelli R, et al. The p53 regulatory gene MDM2 is a direct transcriptional target of MYCN in neuroblastoma. *Proc Natl Acad Sci U S A.* 2005;102:731–736.
65. Slack AD, Chen Z, Ludwig AD, Hicks J, Shohet JM. MYCN-directed centrosome amplification requires MDM2-mediated suppression of p53 activity in neuroblastoma cells. *Cancer Res.* 2007;67:2448–2455.
66. Iwakuma T, Lozano G. MDM2, an introduction. *Mol Cancer Res.* 2003;1:993–1000.
67. Ganguli G, Wasylyk B. p53-independent functions of MDM2. *Mol Cancer Res.* 2003;1:1027–1035.
68. Bond GL, Hu W, Bond EE, et al. A single nucleotide polymorphism in the MDM2 promoter attenuates the p53 tumor suppressor pathway and accelerates tumor formation in humans. *Cell.* 2004;119:591–602.
69. Schwab M, Varmus HE, Bishop JM. Human N-myc gene contributes to neoplastic transformation of mammalian cells in culture. *Nature.* 1985;316:160–162.
70. Schweigerer L, Breit S, Wenzel A, Tsunamoto K, Ludwig R, Schwab M. Augmented MYCN expression advances the malignant phenotype of human neuroblastoma cells: evidence for induction of autocrine growth factor activity. *Cancer Res.* 1990;50:4411–4416.
71. Schmidt ML, Salwen HR, Manohar CF, Ikegaki N, Cohn SL. The biological effects of antisense N-myc expression in human neuroblastoma. *Cell Growth Differ.* 1994;5:171–178.
72. Peverali FA, Orioli D, Tonon L, et al. Retinoic acid-induced growth arrest and differentiation of neuroblastoma cells are counteracted by N-myc and enhanced by max overexpressions. *Oncogene.* 1996;12:457–462.
73. Weiss WA, Aldape K, Mohapatra G, Feuerstein BG, Bishop JM. Targeted expression of MYCN causes neuroblastoma in transgenic mice. *Embo J.* 1997;16:2985–2995.
74. Weiss WA, Godfrey T, Francisco C, Bishop JM. Genome-wide screen for allelic imbalance in a mouse model for neuroblastoma. *Cancer Res.* 2000;60:2483–2487.

75. Haber M, Bordow SB, Gilbert J, et al. Altered expression of the MYCN oncogene modulates MRP gene expression and response to cytotoxic drugs in neuroblastoma cells. *Oncogene.* 1999;18:2777–2782.
76. Cohn SL, London WB, Huang D, et al. MYCN expression is not prognostic of adverse outcome in advanced-stage neuroblastoma with nonamplified MYCN. *J Clin Oncol.* 2000;18:3604–3613.
77. Tang XX, Zhao H, Kung B, et al. The MYCN enigma: significance of MYCN expression in neuroblastoma. *Cancer Res.* 2006;66:2826–2833.
78. Chan HS, Gallie BL, DeBoer G, et al. MYCN protein expression as a predictor of neuroblastoma prognosis. *Clin Cancer Res.* 1997;3:1699–1706.
79. Bordow SB, Norris MD, Haber PS, Marshall GM, Haber M. Prognostic significance of MYCN oncogene expression in childhood neuroblastoma. *J Clin Oncol.* 1998;16:3286–3294.
80. Jinbo T, Iwamura Y, Kaneko M, Sawaguchi S. Coamplification of the L-myc and N-myc oncogenes in a neuroblastoma cell line. *Jpn J Cancer Res.* 1989;80:299–301.
81. Corvi R, Savelyeva L, Breit S, et al. Non-syntenic amplification of MDM2 and MYCN in human neuroblastoma. *Oncogene.* 1995;10:1081–1086.
82. Carr J, Bell E, Pearson AD, et al. Increased frequency of aberrations in the p53/MDM2/p14(ARF) pathway in neuroblastoma cell lines established at relapse. *Cancer Res.* 2006;66:2138–2145.
83. Soda M, Choi YL, Enomoto M, et al. Identification of the transforming EML4-ALK fusion gene in non-small-cell lung cancer. *Nature.* 2007;448:561–566.
84. Yaari S, Jacob-Hirsch J, Amariglio N, Haklai R, Rechavi G, Kloog Y. Disruption of cooperation between Ras and MycN in human neuroblastoma cells promotes growth arrest. *Clin Cancer Res.* 2005;11:4321–4330.
85. Sears R, Nuckolls F, Haura E, Taya Y, Tamai K, Nevins JR. Multiple Ras-dependent phosphorylation pathways regulate Myc protein stability. *Genes Dev.* 2000;14:2501–2514.
86. Ballas K, Lyons J, Janssen JW, Bartram CR. Incidence of ras gene mutations in neuroblastoma. *Eur J Pediatr.* 1988;147:313–314.
87. Ireland CM. Activated N-ras oncogenes in human neuroblastoma. *Cancer Res.* 1989;49:5530–5533.
88. Dam V, Morgan BT, Mazanek P, Hogarty MD. Mutations in PIK3CA are infrequent in neuroblastoma. *BMC Cancer.* 2006;6:177.
89. Vogelstein B, Lane D, Levine AJ. Surfing the p53 network. *Nature.* 2000;408:307–310.
90. Vogan K, Bernstein M, Leclerc JM, et al. Absence of p53 gene mutations in primary neuroblastomas. *Cancer Res.* 1993;53:5269–5273.
91. Rossbach HC, Baschinsky D, Wynn T, Obzut D, Sutcliffe M, Tebbi C. Composite adrenal anaplastic neuroblastoma and virilizing adrenocortical tumor with germline TP53 R248W mutation. *Pediatr Blood Cancer.* 2008;50:681–683.
92. Moll UM, Ostermeyer AG, Haladay R, Winkfield B, Frazier M, Zambetti G. Cytoplasmic sequestration of wild-type p53 protein impairs the G1 checkpoint after DNA damage. *Mol Cell Biol.* 1996;16:1126–1137.
93. Moll UM, LaQuaglia M, Benard J, Riou G. Wild-type p53 protein undergoes cytoplasmic sequestration in undifferentiated neuroblastomas but not in differentiated tumors. *Proc Natl Acad Sci U S A.* 1995;92:4407–4411.
94. Valsesia-Wittmann S, Magdeleine M, Dupasquier S, et al. Oncogenic cooperation between H-Twist and N-Myc overrides failsafe programs in cancer cells. *Cancer Cell.* 2004;6:625–630.
95. Tweddle DA, Malcolm AJ, Bown N, Pearson AD, Lunec J. Evidence for the development of p53 mutations after cytotoxic therapy in a neuroblastoma cell line. *Cancer Res.* 2001;61:8–13.
96. Xue C, Haber M, Flemming C, et al. p53 determines multidrug sensitivity of childhood neuroblastoma. *Cancer Res.* 2007;67:10351–10360.
97. Kovalev S, Marchenko N, Swendeman S, LaQuaglia M, Moll UM. Expression level, allelic origin, and mutation analysis of the p73 gene in neuroblastoma tumors and cell lines. *Cell Growth Differ.* 1998;9:897–903.
98. Irwin MS, Kaelin WG Jr. Role of the newer p53 family proteins in malignancy. *Apoptosis* 2001;6:17–29.
99. Ichimiya S, Nimura Y, Kageyama H, et al. Genetic analysis of p73 localized at chromosome 1p36.3 in primary neuroblastomas. *Med Pediatr Oncol.* 2001;36:42–44.
100. Barrois M, Eychenne MK, Terrier-Lacombe MJ, et al. Genomic and allelic expression status of the p73 gene in human neuroblastoma. *Med Pediatr Oncol.* 2001;36:45–47.
101. Norris MD, Gilbert J, Smith SA, et al. Expression of the putative tumour suppressor gene, p73, in neuroblastoma and other childhood tumours. *Med Pediatr Oncol.* 2001;36:48–51.
102. Moll UM, Slade N. p63 and p73: roles in development and tumor formation. *Mol Cancer Res.* 2004;2:371–386.
103. Casciano I, Mazzocco K, Boni L, et al. Expression of DeltaNp73 is a molecular marker for adverse outcome in neuroblastoma patients. *Cell Death Differ.* 2002;9:246–251.
104. Fujita T, Igarashi J, Okawa ER, et al. CHD5, a tumor suppressor gene deleted from 1p36.31 in neuroblastomas. *J Natl Cancer Inst.* 2008;100:940–949.
105. Bagchi A, Papazoglu C, Wu Y, et al. CHD5 is a tumor suppressor at human 1p36. *Cell.* 2007;128:459–475.
106. Schlisio S, Kenchappa RS, Vredeveld LC, et al. The kinesin KIF1beta acts downstream from EglN3 to induce apoptosis and is a potential 1p36 tumor suppressor. *Genes Dev.* 2008;22:884–893.
107. Thompson PM, Maris JM, Hogarty MD, et al. Homozygous deletion of CDKN2A (p16INK4a/p14ARF) but not within 1p36 or at other tumor suppressor loci in neuroblastoma. *Cancer Res.* 2001;61:679–686.
108. Beltinger CP, White PS, Sulman EP, Maris JM, Brodeur GM. No CDKN2 mutations in neuroblastomas. *Cancer Res.* 1995;55:2053–2055.
109. Bothwell M. Keeping track of neurotrophin receptors. *Cell.* 1991;65:915–918.
110. Nakagawara A. Trk receptor tyrosine kinases: a bridge between cancer and neural development. *Cancer Lett.* 2001;169:107–114.
111. Oppenheim RW. Cell death during development of the nervous system. *Annu Rev Neurosci.* 1991;14:453–501.
112. Nakagawara A, Arima-Nakagawara M, Scavarda NJ, Azar CG, Cantor AB, Brodeur GM. Association between high levels of expression of the TRK gene and favorable outcome in human neuroblastoma. *N Engl J Med.* 1993;328:847–854.
113. Tacconelli A, Farina AR, Cappabianca L, et al. TrkA alternative splicing: a regulated tumor-promoting switch in human neuroblastoma. *Cancer Cell.* 2004;6:347–360.
114. Suzuki T, Bogenmann E, Shimada H, Stram D, Seeger RC. Lack of high-affinity nerve growth factor receptors in aggressive neuroblastomas. *J Natl Cancer Inst.* 1993;85:377–384.
115. Nakagawara A. Molecular basis of spontaneous regression of neuroblastoma: role of neurotrophic signals and genetic abnormalities. *Hum Cell.* 1998;11:115–124.
116. Nakagawara A, Azar CG, Scavarda NJ, Brodeur GM. Expression and function of TRK-B and BDNF in human neuroblastomas. *Mol Cell Biol.* 1994;14:759–767.
117. Levi-Montalcini R. The nerve growth factor 35 years later. *Science.* 1987;237:1154–1162.
118. Acheson A, Conover JC, Fandl JP, et al. A BDNF autocrine loop in adult sensory neurons prevents cell death. *Nature.* 1995;374:450–453.
119. Matsumoto K, Wada RK, Yamashiro JM, Kaplan DR, Thiele CJ. Expression of brain-derived neurotrophic factor and p145TrkB affects survival, differentiation, and invasiveness of human neuroblastoma cells. *Cancer Res.* 1995;55:1798–1806.
120. Yamashiro DJ, Nakagawara A, Ikegaki N, Liu XG, Brodeur GM. Expression of TrkC in favorable human neuroblastomas. *Oncogene.* 1996;12:37–41.
121. Haber M, Bordow SB, Haber PS, Marshall GM, Stewart BW, Norris MD. The prognostic value of MDR1 gene expression in primary untreated neuroblastoma. *Eur J Cancer.* 1997;33:2031–2036.
122. Norris MD, Bordow SB, Marshall GM, Haber PS, Cohn SL, Haber M. Expression of the gene for multidrug-resistance-associated protein and outcome in patients with neuroblastoma. *N Engl J Med.* 1996;334:231–238.
123. Norris MD, Smith J, Tanabe K, et al. Expression of multidrug transporter MRP4/ABCC4 is a marker of poor prognosis in neuroblastoma and confers resistance to irinotecan in vitro. *Mol Cancer Ther.* 2005;4:547–553.
124. Neumann AA, Reddel RR. Telomere maintenance and cancer—look, no telomerase. *Nat Rev Cancer.* 2002;2:879–884.
125. Hiyama E, Hiyama K, Yokoyama T, Matsuura Y, Piatyszek MA, Shay JW. Correlating telomerase activity levels with human neuroblastoma outcomes. *Nat Med.* 1995;1:249–255.

126. Poremba C, Willenbring H, Hero B, et al. Telomerase activity distinguishes between neuroblastomas with good and poor prognosis. *Ann Oncol.* 1999;10:715–721.
127. Choi LM, Kim NW, Zuo JJ, et al. Telomerase activity by TRAP assay and telomerase RNA (hTR) expression are predictive of outcome in neuroblastoma. *Med Pediatr Oncol.* 2000;35:647–650.
128. Tabori U, Vukovic B, Zielenska M, et al. The role of telomere maintenance in the spontaneous growth arrest of pediatric low-grade gliomas. *Neoplasia.* 2006;8:136–142.
129. Tabori U, Ma J, Carter M, et al. Human telomere reverse transcriptase expression predicts progression and survival in pediatric intracranial ependymoma. *J Clin Oncol.* 2006;24:1522–1528.
130. Deckwerth TL, Elliott JL, Knudson CM, Johnson EM, Jr., Snider WD, Korsmeyer SJ. BAX is required for neuronal death after trophic factor deprivation and during development. *Neuron.* 1996;17:401–411.
131. Garcia I, Martinou I, Tsujimoto Y, Martinou JC. Prevention of programmed cell death of sympathetic neurons by the bcl-2 proto-oncogene. *Science.* 1992;258:302–304.
132. Castle VP, Heidelberger KP, Bromberg J, Ou X, Dole M, Nunez G. Expression of the apoptosis-suppressing protein bcl-2, in neuroblastoma is associated with unfavorable histology and N-myc amplification. *Am J Pathol.* 1993;143:1543–1550.
133. Oue T, Fukuzawa M, Kusafuka T, et al. In situ detection of DNA fragmentation and expression of bcl-2 in human neuroblastoma: relation to apoptosis and spontaneous regression. *J Pediatr Surg.* 1996;31:251–257.
134. Dole M, Nunez G, Merchant AK, et al. Bcl-2 inhibits chemotherapy-induced apoptosis in neuroblastoma. *Cancer Res.* 1994;54:3253–3259.
135. Dole MG, Jasty R, Cooper MJ, Thompson CB, Nunez G, Castle VP. Bcl-xL is expressed in neuroblastoma cells and modulates chemotherapy-induced apoptosis. *Cancer Res.* 1995;55:2576–2582.
136. Ushmorov A, Hogarty MD, Liu X, Knauss H, Debatin KM, Beltinger C. N-myc augments death and attenuates protective effects of Bcl-2 in trophically stressed neuroblastoma cells. *Oncogene.* 2008;27:3424–3434.
137. Look AT, Hayes FA, Shuster JJ, et al. Clinical relevance of tumor cell ploidy and N-myc gene amplification in childhood neuroblastoma: a Pediatric Oncology Group study. *J Clin Oncol.* 1991;9:581–591.
138. Bagatell R, Rumcheva P, London WB, et al. Outcomes of children with intermediate-risk neuroblastoma after treatment stratified by MYCN status and tumor cell ploidy. *J Clin Oncol.* 2005;23:8819–8827.
139. Bowman LC, Castleberry RP, Cantor A, et al. Genetic staging of unresectable or metastatic neuroblastoma in infants: a Pediatric Oncology Group study. *J Natl Cancer Inst.* 1997;89:373–380.
140. Clarke MF, Dick JE, Dirks PB, et al. Cancer stem cells--perspectives on current status and future directions: AACR Workshop on cancer stem cells. *Cancer Res.* 2006;66:9339–9344.
141. Singh SK, Hawkins C, Clarke ID, et al. Identification of human brain tumour initiating cells. *Nature.* 2004;432:396–401.
142. Hansford LM, McKee AE, Zhang L, et al. Neuroblastoma cells isolated from bone marrow metastases contain a naturally enriched tumor-initiating cell. *Cancer Res.* 2007;67:11234–11243.
143. Yamamoto K, Hanada R, Kikuchi A, et al. Spontaneous regression of localized neuroblastoma detected by mass screening. *J Clin Oncol.* 1998;16:1265–1269.
144. Evans AE, Chatten J, D'Angio GJ, Gerson JM, Robinson J, Schnaufer L. A review of 17 IV-S neuroblastoma patients at the children's hospital of philadelphia. *Cancer.* 1980;45:833–839.
145. Haas D, Ablin AR, Miller C, Zoger S, Matthay KK. Complete pathologic maturation and regression of stage IVS neuroblastoma without treatment. *Cancer.* 1988;62:818–825.
146. Pritchard J, Hickman JA. Why does stage 4s neuroblastoma regress spontaneously? *Lancet.* 1994;344:869–870.
147. Ikeda H, Hirato J, Akami M, et al. Massive apoptosis detected by in situ DNA nick end labeling in neuroblastoma. *Am J Surg Pathol.* 1996;20:649–655.
148. Hamburger V. History of the discovery of neuronal death in embryos. *J Neurobiol.* 1992;23:1116–1123.
149. Bolande RP, Mayer DC. The cytolysis of human neuroblastoma cells by a natural IgM 'antibody'-complement system in pregnancy serum. *Cancer Invest.* 1990;8:603–611.
150. David K, Ollert MW, Vollmert C, et al. Human natural immunoglobulin M antibodies induce apoptosis of human neuroblastoma cells by binding to a Mr 260,000 antigen. *Cancer Res.* 1999;59: 3768–3775.
151. Ollert MW, David K, Schmitt C, et al. Normal human serum contains a natural IgM antibody cytotoxic for human neuroblastoma cells. *Proc Natl Acad Sci U S A.* 1996;93:4498–4503.
152. Cecchetto G, Mosseri V, De Bernardi B, et al. Surgical risk factors in primary surgery for localized neuroblastoma: the LNESG1 study of the European International Society of Pediatric Oncology Neuroblastoma Group. *J Clin Oncol.* 2005;23:8483–8489.
153. London WB, Castleberry RP, Matthay KK, et al. Evidence for an age cutoff greater than 365 days for neuroblastoma risk group stratification in the Children's Oncology Group. *J Clin Oncol.* 2005;23:6459–6465.
154. Schmidt ML, Lal A, Seeger RC, et al. Favorable prognosis for patients 12 to 18 months of age with stage 4 nonamplified MYCN neuroblastoma: a Children's Cancer Group Study. *J Clin Oncol.* 2005;23:6474–6480.
155. George RE, London WB, Cohn SL, et al. Hyperdiploidy plus nonamplified MYCN confers a favorable prognosis in children 12 to 18 months old with disseminated neuroblastoma: a Pediatric Oncology Group study. *J Clin Oncol.* 2005;23:6466–6473.
156. Shimada H, Chatten J, Newton WA Jr, et al. Histopathologic prognostic factors in neuroblastic tumors: definition of subtypes of ganglioneuroblastoma and an age-linked classification of neuroblastomas. *J Natl Cancer Inst.* 1984;73:405–416.
157. Joshi VV, Cantor AB, Altshuler G, et al. Age-linked prognostic categorization based on a new histologic grading system of neuroblastomas. A clinicopathologic study of 211 cases from the Pediatric Oncology Group. *Cancer.* 1992;69:2197–2211.
158. Shimada H, Ambros IM, Dehner LP, et al. The International Neuroblastoma Pathology Classification (the Shimada system). *Cancer.* 1999;86:364–372.
159. Peuchmaur M, d'Amore ES, Joshi VV, et al. Revision of the International Neuroblastoma Pathology Classification: confirmation of favorable and unfavorable prognostic subsets in ganglioneuroblastoma, nodular. *Cancer.* 2003;98:2274–2281.
160. Tonini GP, Boni L, Pession A, et al. MYCN oncogene amplification in neuroblastoma is associated with worse prognosis, except in stage 4s: the Italian experience with 295 children. *J Clin Oncol.* 1997;15:85–93.
161. Schmidt ML, Lukens JN, Seeger RC, et al. Biologic factors determine prognosis in infants with stage IV neuroblastoma: a prospective Children's Cancer Group study. *J Clin Oncol.* 2000;18:1260–1268.

26 Pediatric Brain Tumor Syndromes and Murine Models

Andrew B. Foy and Cynthia Wetmore

Brain tumors are the most common solid tumors of childhood with an average overall 5-year survival of approximately 50% [1]. Treating brain tumors in children, whose nervous system continues to develop throughout the first decade of life, is a particular challenge [1–3]. There is very little information on the molecular pathogenesis of pediatric brain tumors and one of the obstacles to progress in treating brain tumors is a lack of understanding of the subtle differences in signal transduction that differentiate physiologic cell cycle progression and mitosis from neoplastic proliferation.

The molecular pathogenesis of pediatric brain tumors has been informed by developmental biology, as several pathways important to normal development are aberrantly expressed and are hypothesized to play a role in medulloblastoma, a malignant brain tumor with peak incidence between 2 and 7 years [4–6]. Medulloblastoma is also one of the most extensively studied brain tumors as the developing mouse cerebellum provides an excellent model system in which to study proliferation, migration, and differentiation of neural stem and precursor cells [7,8]. A substantial body of experimental evidence indicates that medulloblastoma can arise by transformation of granule cell precursors (GCPs), and recent evidence suggests that tumors may also arise from less well-differentiated stem-like cells of the cerebellum [4,9–12]. During embryogenesis, undifferentiated GCPs originate from the rhombic lip in the developing hindbrain. The GCPs migrate away from the rhombic lip to the developing cortical surface of the cerebellum where these proliferating GCPs form a secondary germinal zone called the external granular layer. In mice and humans, GCPs undergo a phase of rapid proliferation in the early postnatal period (2 weeks in the mouse, 9 months in the human) [13,14], which is supported by the morphogen and mitogen, Sonic hedgehog (Shh). Shh is produced by the Purkinje cells, released into the external granular layer, and supports the tremendous proliferative expansion of the GCPs [15], which then exit the cell cycle, differentiate, and migrate inward through the Purkinje cell layer to generate the internal granule cell layer of the mature cerebellum (see Figure 26.1 for schematic) [7,16,17]. Sustained signaling through the Shh pathway is associated with malignant transformation of neural progenitor cells and provides one of the most tenable models of medulloblastoma (discussed later in this chapter).

Several of the pathways that are crucial to normal nervous system development also appear to play a role

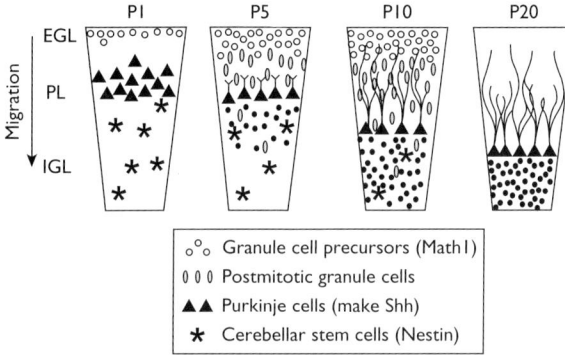

Figure 26.1 Diagram of postnatal development of murine cerebellum. Proliferating granule cell precursors (GCPs; designated as small circles) express Math1 while undergoing proliferative expansion in the external germinal layer (EGL). Proliferation is supported in part by Sonic hedgehog (Shh) produced by the Purkinje cells (designated by triangles). GCPs exit the cell cycle, persist in the inner EGL for approximately 24 hours, and begin to differentiate and lose Math1 expression (designated as ellipses) prior to migrating to their location in the mature cerebellum to comprise the inner granule cell layer (IGL). A population of nestin-expressing neural stem cells (NSCs) persists in the IGL of the mature cerebellum, though reduced in number. Modified from Wetmore [12].

in neoplastic proliferation. Within the last decade, a number of mouse models of brain tumors have become available [18,19] and many of these are based upon knowledge gained from cancer predisposition syndromes as well as through the analyses of sporadic tumor tissues. This chapter will discuss the most common cancer predisposition syndromes involving brain tumors (NF1 and tuberous sclerosis will be discussed in a separate chapter) and their respective murine models as well as a discussion of several additional genes thought to be important in the molecular pathogenesis of pediatric brain tumors.

VON-HIPPEL LINDAU

Clinical Features and Diagnostic Criteria

von-Hippel Lindau (VHL) is an autosomal dominant disorder caused by inactivating mutations in the VHL tumor suppressor gene. VHL is a multisystem disorder that predisposes affected individuals to develop a number of neoplasms including renal clear cell carcinoma, pheochromocytoma, pancreatic neuroendocrine tumors, and retinal and cerebellar hemangioblastomas [20]. VHL has an estimated incidence of 1 in 36,000 with more than 90% penetrance by age 65 [21,22].

Hemangioblastomas are benign and often cystic neoplasms that preferentially occur in the posterior fossa, retina, and spinal cord and affect 60% to 80% of all patients with VHL [23,24]. They are best diagnosed with contrast-enhanced T1 magnetic resonance imaging (MRI) and frequently show intense enhancement and an associated cyst. Angiography shows a strong persistent vascular blush. They are well-circumscribed masses that are highly vascular and grossly have a reddish hue. Histologically, these tumors are composed of neoplastic stromal cells and a dense vascular network.

The diagnosis of VHL is based primarily upon clinical findings. Patients with a family history and any of the tumors commonly associated with VHL are diagnosed with the disease. Those without family history and evidence of two central nervous system (S) hemangioblastomas or one S hemangioblastoma and one visceral tumor common to VHL patients also meet diagnostic criteria. Genetic testing for the VHL gene mutations often confirms a clinical diagnosis. Patients with a single S hemangioblastoma should be screened for VHL at the time of diagnosis with surveillance abdominal CT scan, complete neuroaxial MRI, opthalmological examination, and possibly genetic testing. Younger patients in particular with an isolated hemangioblastoma should be monitored for VHL [23].

Molecular Pathogenesis

VHL results from a germline mutation of *VHL*, a tumor suppressor gene on chromosome 3p25 [25]. Typically, patients inherit a single germline mutation of the gene, and tumor formation occurs only after inactivation of the single wild-type *VHL* gene in susceptible organs and tissues. De novo mutations can also occur in sporadic hemangioblastomas but are less common than in patients with VHL. The VHL protein targets the oxygen-sensing alpha subunit of hypoxia inducible factor-1 for proteosomal degradation and is involved in the intracellular adaptation to tissue hypoxia. Cells lacking the VHL protein have increased hypoxia inducible factor-1 leading to unregulated cellular growth and an increase in the production of angiogenic factors such as vascular endothelial growth factor [26].

Therapy and Prognosis

Surgical resection is the preferred treatment for symptomatic hemangioblastomas. The majority of hemangioblastomas of the S are amenable to surgical resection with acceptable surgical morbidity [27–29]. In cases of multiple S hemangioblastomas or persistent recurrence, stereotactic radiosurgery has been utilized. Patients with smaller lesions without cysts have had stabilization of tumor volume following stereotactic radiosurgery; however, large studies with long-term follow-up have not been reported [30,31].

Animal Models

VHL is essential for embryonic development and mouse embryos carrying homozygous deletion of the gene die during midgestation due to placental vascular dysgenesis [32]. Tissue specific conditional deletion and point mutations of *Vhlh* (murine *VHL*) have been accomplished and have given insight into the multiple roles of VHL protein within various tissues [33–35]. However, investigators have not been successful in modeling S hemangioblastomas as deletion of *Vhlh* in neuroepithelial cells results in embryonic death [34].

NEVOID BASAL CELL CARCINOMA SYNDROME

Clinical Features and Diagnostic Criteria

Nevoid basal cell carcinoma syndrome (NBCCS), also known as Gorlin syndrome, is an autosomal dominant genetic disorder characterized by a predisposition to develop basal cell carcinomas, medulloblastoma, pitting of the palms and soles, larger overall body size, and various skeletal and developmental anomalies [36–38]. NBCCS has an estimated incidence of approximately 1 in 50,000 to 150,000 [38,39] and has been mapped to chromosome 9q22.3–31 [39,40], an area now known to contain the *Patched* (*PTCH* in human; *Ptc* in mouse) gene [41,42], which encodes a repressive component of the Shh receptor [43,44].

In patients carrying a germline mutation of *PTCH*, the incidence of medulloblastoma increased from 2 per million in the general population to 4 per 100 in children less than 18 years of age [45,46]. Patients with NBCCS have a 3% to 5% lifetime risk of developing medulloblastoma and patients with NBCCS account for 1% to 2% of all cases of medulloblastoma [38,47]. As well, patients with NBCCS have a 5% lifetime risk of developing meningiomas, which are likely treatment related [37,48,49]. Patients with NBCCS typically develop medulloblastoma at an earlier age and frequently have the desmoplastic variant of medulloblastoma [50]. These tumors usually arise in the cerebellar vermis and fill the fourth ventricle. Children often present with evidence of ataxia or headache and vomiting due to raised intracranial pressure. Desmoplastic medulloblastoma has a more favorable survival rate and patients with NBCCS typically have a better overall survival rate than patients with sporadic medulloblastoma [51,52]. Diagnosis of NBCCS is made on the basis of clinical findings compatible with the disorder and DNA testing for the *PTCH* gene.

Molecular Pathogenesis

Cancer predisposition syndromes such as NBCCS have provided insight into mechanisms of tumorigenesis of medulloblastoma. However, it is also important to document whether similar potentially growth-promoting lesions are also detected in sporadic tumors. It has been demonstrated through a number of studies that a subset of human medulloblastomas express high levels of *PTCH* and *glioma-related oncogene (GLI1)* mRNA, indicating activation of the Shh pathway [50,53,54]. Additional developmental pathways that include aberrations in *Wnt* [2,55–59], *Notch* [59–63], and *Insulin-like growth factor 1 (IGF1)* [64–66] signaling are also found in human medulloblastoma but have not been found to play a role in syndromic brain tumors.

The Hedgehog (Hh) pathway was originally described in *Drosophila melanogaster* where, in the first few hours of embryogenesis, Hh guides the formation of body segmentation and, at later stages, controls cell fate specification and the pattern of expression of cuticle hairs [67,68]. In vertebrates, activation of the Shh pathway results in activation of *Gli1*, a member of a family of zinc-finger DNA binding proteins that function as transcriptional mediators of the Shh signaling cascade (see schematic diagram in Figure 26.2) [69–73]. Aberrant activation of the Shh pathway is known to contribute to tumorigenesis in the nervous system and other tissues [12,74–80].

PTCH encodes a 12-pass transmembrane receptor for the ligand *Shh*, a secreted morphogen essential for normal embryonic development and maintenance of progenitor cell populations [78,81–84]. *PTCH* associates with another transmembrane protein, *Smoothened* (*SMOH* in human; *Smo* in mouse), to repress the SMOH-mediated activation of *GLI1* and other Shh pathway target genes. Under normal conditions, in the absence of ligand, PTCH/Ptc represses the constitutive activity of SMOH/Smo, and Gli1 remains tethered in the cytoplasm to a microtubule-containing complex by Fused and Suppressor of fused. When Shh is present, Gli1 is released from Suppressor of fused, undergoes translocation to the nucleus, and results in the induction of target genes, including *Cyclin D, N-myc, Gli1*, and *Ptc* itself [69,71,72,85]. Mutation of other regulatory components of the Shh pathway have been found in sporadic human tumors, indicating the importance of this pathway to the etiology of this tumor [86,87].

Therapy and Prognosis

Treatment of patients with NBCCS and medulloblastoma is similar but less intense than for patients with sporadic medulloblastoma. Patients are treated with aggressive surgical resection, radiation, and chemotherapy. Medulloblastomas are classified into either a standard or high risk category. High risk patients are defined by any of the following criteria: age 3 or less, evidence of dissemination at diagnosis, or greater than 1.5 cm^2 of residual tumor after resection. Standard risk patients are usually treated with craniospinal radiation, involved field radiation to the posterior fossa, and chemotherapy consisting of cisplatin, lomustine, and vincristine. High risk patients are treated with chemotherapy and higher doses of involved field and craniospinal radiation [51,88]. Due to the significant morbidity associated with craniospinal radiation, particularly in younger patients, radiation therapy may be reserved in favor of surgical resection and chemotherapy in patients aged less than 3 [51,89].

Extensive craniospinal radiation therapy is avoided in NBCCS patients due to the sensitivity to ionizing radiation and propensity to develop basal cell nevi in the radiation field [90–92]. It has been known for some time that NBCCS patients [93–95] and mice [96,97] with activation of the Shh pathway have increased sensitivity to ionizing radiation, but only recently has the mechanism of this sensitivity been elucidated [98]. Patients that do receive radiation therapy should be evaluated on a yearly basis for the development of basal cell nevi and with a complete neurologic examination to screen for any focal findings that may suggest the presence of a secondary intracranial neoplasm [99–101].

Animal Models

Several groups have demonstrated that a subset of mice haploinsufficient for *Ptc* spontaneously develop medulloblastoma, a tumor of neural origin believed to arise from immature progenitor cells within the cerebellum [75,102]. Loss of *Ptc* reduces the inhibition of Smo, and Shh pathway is chronically activated, resulting in increased proliferation of GCPs and increased incidence of medulloblastoma. Haploinsufficiency of Ptc alone is not sufficient to promote tumorigenesis as only 15% of the *Ptc*$^{+/-}$ mice develop brain tumors by 10 months of age, suggesting additional genetic events contribute to malignant transformation of cerebellar precursor cells [75,102]. Many murine and human medulloblastomas continue to express the wild-type *PTCH/Ptc* allele, demonstrating that loss of heterozygosity of *PTCH/Ptc* may not be required for tumorigenesis [102–104]. However, the tumors appear to be accelerated by homozygous deletion of *Ptc* in cells already committed to the granule cell lineage [11,105]. A further refinement of murine models of human medulloblastoma came with the discovery that mice carrying activating mutations in *Smo*, an activating component of the

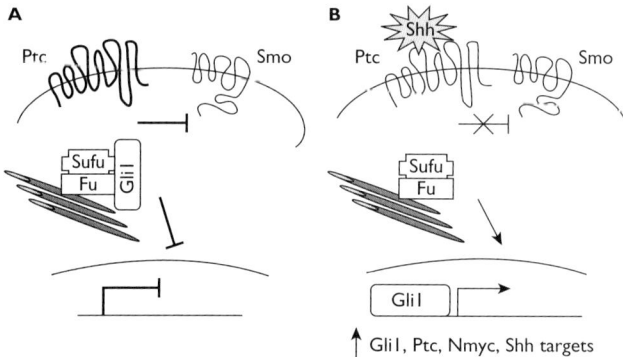

Figure 26.2 Shh signaling pathway. **(A)** *Ptc* encodes a 12-pass membrane protein that—in the absence of the ligand Shh—represses the constitutive activity of Smoothened (Smo). In the quiescent cell, Gli1 is tethered to a microtubule-containing complex by Fused (Fu) and Suppresser of fused (Sufu). **(B)** When Shh is bound to Ptc, repression of Smo is released, Gli1 dissociates from Sufu complex, enters the nucleus and initiates transcription of downstream target genes (e.g., *Gli1, N-myc, cyclin D, Ptc* itself, and others). Modified from Wetmore [12].

Shh receptor, develop an aggressive form of medulloblastoma with leptomeningeal spread, a relatively common clinical finding that carries an especially poor prognostic value in humans [62,106].

Other signaling pathways in addition to Hh contribute to the proliferation and transformation of cerebellar GCPs, including members of the IGF and Myc genes. IGF receptor and insulin receptor substrate 1 are activated and more highly expressed in tumor over nonmalignant cerebellar tissues [107]. Insulin receptor substrate 1 is stabilized by Shh pathway activation and is also required for Shh-induced proliferation of nonneoplastic GCPs [65]. Both c-Myc and N-myc are highly expressed in some medulloblastomas and each have been found to participate in Shh-induced proliferation of GCPs (N-Myc) [108] and in the transformation of cerebellar neural stem cells (c-Myc) [109]. Interestingly, intact N-myc and IGF2 signaling is required for tumorigenesis in mice with constitutive activation of Shh pathway as germline deletion of Igf2 [110] or N-myc [111] abrogates development of medulloblastoma in $Ptc^{+/-}$ mice or mice with activated Smo, respectively.

Germline absence of P53 results in increased genomic instability and dramatically accelerates tumor formation in some murine models of brain tumors. For example, Greater than 95% of $Ptc^{+/-}/P53^{-/-}$ mice develop tumors by 12 weeks of age compared to a 14% incidence of medulloblastomas in $Ptc^{+/-}$ mice by 10 months of age [112]. Cytogenetic analysis of medulloblastomas from $Ptc^{+/-}/P53^{-/-}$ mice demonstrated an increase in chromosomal aberrations compared to tumors from $Ptc^{+/-}$ mice, suggesting that the effect of p53 deficiency on tumor induction may be related to genomic instability and consequently acquisition of secondary mutations in growth control genes [112]. Despite the impact of p53 deficiency on medulloblastoma formation in genetically engineered mice, loss-of-function mutations in the P53 gene are not common in human medulloblastomas [113–116].

The $Ptc^{+/-}/P53^{-/-}$ murine model has been used to demonstrate that inhibition of Shh pathway with specific antagonists is an effective treatment for murine medulloblastoma in vivo, and has provided the preclinical data for a future phase 1 study [117]. However, Shh antagonists developed to date are not specific to the malignant Shh signal transduction and will likely also disrupt signaling in neural stem and progenitor sells in other tissues, which also rely upon Shh for their maintenance [118]. It has been reported that chronic activation of the Shh pathway through haploinsufficiency of Ptc is transduced in murine neural stem cells by a different constellation of Gli transcription factors than the acute activation by exposure to the ligand Shh [119]. Further refinement of signaling differences between normal vs. neoplastic and chronic vs. acute Shh pathway activation will be needed in order to develop molecular inhibitors that will spare the Hh activity that is essential to maintain progenitor cells of normal tissues.

Other models of medulloblastoma are based upon somatic rather than germline activation of Shh pathway and require transduction of progenitor cells during early postnatal development of the cerebellum and are beyond the scope of this chapter [120–122].

TURCOT SYNDROME

Clinical Features and Diagnostic Criteria

Turcot syndrome is the name given to a group of disorders that involves the development of primary S neoplasms in the setting of familial colorectal tumors. Originally described as a single disorder in 1959 [123], it is now recognized that mutation of several genes can give rise to the phenotype of familial colorectal cancer syndromes that are associated with nervous system tumors. There are two distinct subsets of this group of disorders. The first is familial adenonomatous polyposis (FAP), more recently termed brain tumor polyposis syndrome type 2, which involves the development of numerous small adenomas of the colon early in life and eventual transformation to colorectal carcinoma. Patients with FAP have mutations in the *adenomatous polyposis coli* (APC) gene. These patients are at risk of developing S tumors, most commonly medulloblastoma, astrocytoma and ependymoma. Medulloblastoma is particularly common, representing 60% to 80% of the S tumors seen in patients with FAP [124,125]. The relative risk of a person developing a brain tumor in the context of FAP is increased by greater than 20-fold [125].

The second disorder is hereditary nonpolyposis colorectal cancer (HNPCC), also known as brain tumor polyposis syndrome type 1. HNPCC differs from FAP in that fewer colon polyps are seen; however, there is a greater likelihood of developing colonic adenocarcinoma if the colon is not removed. HNPCC results from germline mutation of nucleotide mismatch repair genes *hMLH1*, *hMSH2*, *hMSH6*, and *hPMS2*. Patients with HNPCC are also at risk of developing S neoplasms, most commonly high-grade glioma [125]. Patients are typically diagnosed clinically when there is evidence of polyposis and a S neoplasm. Genetic testing can distinguish among mutations of the *APC* gene and mutations of the mismatch repair genes.

Molecular Pathogenesis

Turcot syndrome can result from several distinct genetic mechanisms. FAP is an autosomal dominant disorder that results from germline mutations of the *APC* gene on chromosome 5q21 [126]. *APC* participates in the phosphorylation of beta catenin, a primary effector of Wnt signaling. Phosphorylation of beta catenin marks it for destruction through proteosomal degradation. Loss of APC function results in activation of the Wnt signaling pathway through accumulation of beta-catenin, leading to unrestrained cell proliferation [127]. While increased Wnt pathway signaling is often found in sporadic cases of colorectal cancer and a subset of medulloblastomas [128,129], *APC* mutations are rarely found in sporadic tumors outside of the gastrointestinal tract [127]. This suggests that while dysregulation of the Wnt pathway may play a role in sporadic brain tumors, activation of this pathway more commonly occurs by a mechanism other than by mutation of *APC*.

HNPCC is an autosomal dominant disorder that results from germline mutation of one of the nucleotide mismatch repair genes [130]. Mutation of any of the mismatch repair genes can lead to HPNCC; however, the most common mutations are to the genes *hMSH2* and *hMLH1*. Patients with HPNCC show evidence of replication errors, or microsatellite instability, and have misalignment of the DNA strands. This has been shown to increase the risk of malignant transformation and increase the risk of developing high-grade gliomas [131].

Therapy and Prognosis

At present, there are no specific treatment recommendations for patients with Turcot syndrome that develop S tumors. However, ionizing radiation and other DNA damaging agents should be used with some caution as the risk for secondary malignancy is likely elevated in this population of patients. Two intriguing case studies have reported long-term (7 and 15 years) remission in Turcot syndrome patients with glioblastoma multiforme with retinoic acid therapy [132,133]. There are currently no guidelines for surveillance intracranial imaging in patients with FAP or HNPCC; however, patients should be monitored closely for the development of any neurologic symptoms. Frequent surveillance for the development of colonic adenocarcinoma and prophylactic colectomy has improved survival in patients with Turcot syndrome [134]. Patients with germline mutation of mismatch repair genes may have less benefit from the alkylating agents that are most commonly used to treat malignant gliomas such as carmustine (bis-chloroethyl nitrosourea or BU), lomustine (chloroethylnitrosourea), and temozolomide. The cytotoxicity of these agents relies upon an intact mismatch repair capability so that the tumor cells recognize and initiate apoptosis in response to mismatched nucleotide base pairing [135].

Animal Models

Mice carrying heterozygous mutation of the *Apc* gene are useful for modeling the intestinal neoplasia and some of the extra S challenges of Turcot syndrome [136,137]. However, *Apc* mutant mice do not develop spontaneous brain tumors even when bred onto mice heterozygous for *Ptc*, which are predisposed to develop medulloblastoma [112]. Interestingly, although patients carrying germline mutation of *APC* have an increased risk of developing medulloblastoma, loss of heterozygosity of the *APC* alleles are not consistently found in sporadic medulloblastomas [138,139], suggesting that loss or mutation of *APC* may not actively contribute to tumorigenesis within the nervous system.

LI-FRAUMENI

Clinical Features and Diagnostic Criteria

First described in 1969, Li-Fraumeni syndrome (LFS) is an autosomal dominant disorder characterized by increased susceptibility to a wide range of soft tissue, visceral, hematologic, and nervous system malignancies [140,141]. Sarcomas and early-onset breast carcinoma are the most frequent tumors seen in patients with LFS. Approximately 14% of patients with LFS develop S tumors, most commonly malignant gliomas, although medulloblastoma and supratentorial primitive neuroectodermal tumors have also been reported [142]. Brain tumors often occur at an early age in patients with LFS with an average age at diagnosis of 16 years.

LFS is diagnosed based on clinical criteria. LFS is diagnosed in patients younger than 45 years with a sarcoma as well as a first-degree relative younger than 45 years with any cancer and another first- or second-degree relative with any cancer younger than 45 years or a sarcoma at any age [143]. A version of Li-Fraumeni sydrome known as Li-Fraumeni-like syndrome (LFL) has also been described. LFL is diagnosed in patients with any childhood tumor or a sarcoma, brain tumor, or adrenocortical tumor before the age of 45 as well as a first- or second-degree relative with a typical LFS tumor at any age and another first- or second-degree relative with any tumor younger than 60 years [144].

Molecular Pathogenesis

The vast majority of patients with LFS harbor a germline mutation in the *P53* gene. Genetic analysis shows mutations of *P53* on chromosome 17p13 in 77% of LFS patients and 40% of LFL patients [145]. *P53* is a tumor suppressor gene encoding the protein p53, often referred to as the "guardian of the genome," which has diverse functions and is the most commonly mutated gene in human cancer [146]. p53 plays an essential role in tissue homeostasis by maintaining cell cycle checkpoints in response to cellular stress and DNA damage [147]. Cell cycle checkpoints are activated in response to various forms of cellular stress to block cell cycle progression and replication of potentially damaged DNA until the stress has been resolved. In normal cells, p53 protein levels are very low due to rapid degradation of p53 through interaction with the E3 ubiquitin protein ligase, Mdm2. However, under conditions of rapid proliferation, p53 is activated and contributes to the cellular phenotypes of cell cycle arrest (senescence), increased DNA repair, and apoptosis [148,149]. Loss of p53 function leads to poorly controlled cell cycle progression, resulting in inappropriate DNA replication and cell division [150]. Mutation of *P53* is found in up to 50% of all solid tumors and recent evidence has suggested that aberrations in the downstream pathway of p53 or amplification of critical regulators of p53 such as Mdm2 may play a role in tumor formation in patients with tumors that have wild-type *P53* [151,152]. Development of brain tumors is particularly common in patients with missense mutations of *P53* in the DNA binding loop and brain tumors developed earlier in patients with complete loss of the P53 protein or complete absence of P53 function [142]. A smaller number of patients harbor germline mutations of *CHEK2* on chromosome 22 although the role of this gene in LFS and LFL is still unclear [153]. *CHEK2* is another regulator of the G1-S cell cycle transition and participates in enforcing G1 arrest and the induction of apoptosis in cells exposed to genotoxic stress. Thus the loss of P53 or Chek2 function may result in premature replication of damaged DNA and/or mitosis, which contributes to malignant transformation.

Therapy and Prognosis

Treatment of brain tumors in LFS patients is no different than for patients with sporadic tumors; however, these patients have an increased sensitivity to ionizing radiation. Patients who have undergone radiation should be screened frequently for the development of secondary malignancies.

Animal Models

While *P53*-null mice rarely develop brain tumors, the loss of p53 results in the development of medulloblastoma in other strains of genetically engineered mice that do not otherwise develop spontaneous brain tumors. In addition to acceleration of medulloblastoma in mice deficient in *Ptc* (see previous discussion in NBCCS Animal Models section), mice lacking the gene encoding *poly (ADP-ribose) polymerase (Parp-1)*, a molecule that senses DNA strand breaks and participates in DNA damage response, develop spontaneous posterior fossa tumors when bred onto a background deficient in *P53* [154,155]. Compound loss of *P53* and the gene encoding *DNA ligase IV (Lig4)*, an enzyme that is critical for repairing double-strand DNA breaks, results in development of medulloblastoma-like lesions within the first month of life [156,157]. Interestingly, *Lig4-/-* mice die in early embryogenesis due to widespread neural apoptosis, yet normal neural development is rescued by the additional loss of *P53* [158].

Retinoblastoma *(Rb)*, the first tumor-suppressor gene cloned, is mutated in a variety of human tumors and plays a role in cell cycle entry and cell fate determination in several tissues [159,160]. Conditional compound deletion of *P53* and *Rb* from astrocytes in the developing brain results in aggressive posterior fossa tumors that also resemble medulloblastoma histologically [161]. While loss of several of these genes alone is not sufficient for tumorigenesis, when paired with compound loss of *P53* a dramatic increase in medulloblastoma formation is observed. These and other genetically engineered mouse models have demonstrated that mutation of several genes can give rise to tumors that phenotypically resemble primitive neuroectodermal tumors of the cerebellum.

COWDEN DISEASE

Clinical Features and Diagnostic Criteria

Cowden disease (CD) is an autosomal dominant disorder characterized by the development of benign hamartomas is many organ systems and an increased risk of breast, thyroid, and endometrial cancer. Cutaneous lesions are also common and tricholemmomas, a benign cutaneous tumor of the hair follicle, are considered to be pathognomonic for the disease. Neurologically, patients with CD frequently have megalencephaly, cognitive delay, and there is a strong association between Lhermitte-Duclos disease (LDD) and CD. The incidence of CD is estimated to be quite low at 1 in 200,000 to 1 in 250,000; however, the disease has variable and often subtle expression, which may lead to underestimation of the true incidence [162].

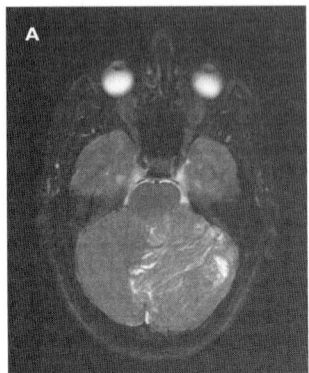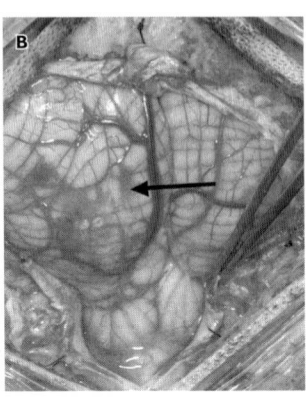

Figure 26.3 Appearance of cerebellum in Lhermitte-Duclos disease. **(A)** T2-weighted MR image showing the dramatic enlargement of the folia of left cerebellar hemisphere and the hallmark "tiger-stripe" appearance seen in Lhermitte-Duclos disease. **(B)** Intraoperative photograph showing the enlarged folia (arrow) of the left cerebellar folia. Photo courtesy of Dr. John Atkinson and Mayo Medical Photography.

The most notable neurologic manifestation of CD is LDD, also known as dysplastic gangliocytoma of the cerebellum. LDD is a hamaratomatous enlargement of the cerebellar hemisphere marked by the presence of hypertrophic ganglion cells, loss of the Purkinje layer, and increased myelination. The disease is slowly progressive and usually presents in early adulthood with mild ataxia or evidence of raised intracranial pressure from effacement of the fourth ventricle. MRI findings of LDD are distinct and the diagnosis can often be made based on MRI findings. On T2-weighted imaging, the enlarged cerebellar folia have a distinct "tiger-stripe" appearance and there is an absence of enhancement on gadolinium-enhanced images (Figure 26.3A and 26.3B)

Molecular Pathogenesis

The genetic basis of CD has been attributed to germline mutation of the Phosphatase and tensin homolog deleted on chromosome 10 *(PTEN)* gene located on chromosome 10q22–23 [163]. *PTEN* is a phosphatase that represses signal transduction in the PI3K/AKT/mTOR pathway and inactivating mutation of this protein leads to unrestrained activation of AKT signaling. The PI3K/AKT/mTOR pathway has diverse functions in cellular homeostais and loss of PTEN regulation leads to aberrant cell cycle progression, autocrine growth stimulation, migration, and cellular survival. *PTEN* is now recognized as a tumor suppressor gene [164–166] and mutations of *PTEN* have been found in a number of sporadic malignancies including glioblastoma multiforme [167–169]. Germline *PTEN* mutations, though, have a varied phenotype and clinical penetrance and a number of disorders are associated with *PTEN* mutation. Some of these disorders, like CD, are associated with an increased risk of malignancy, but others, such as Bannayan-Riley-Ruvalcaba syndrome, juvenile polyposis syndrome, and proteus syndrome, are not [164]. The relationship between specific mutations of the *PTEN* gene and clinical phenotype has not been fully determined.

Therapy and Prognosis

Treatment of LDD is usually reserved for patients that have symptomatic raised intracranial pressure or clinical evidence of brainstem compression. The mainstay of treatment involves suboccipital craniectomy and debulking of the affected cerebellar hemisphere. This treatment may worsen the ataxia but will alleviate the pressure on the fourth ventricle and brainstem and normalize the intracranial pressure. Ventricular shunting will alleviate the raised intracranial pressure but will not help progressive brainstem compression. Posterior fossa radiation has not been reported to be beneficial in the treatment of LDD.

Animal Models

Mice with germline deletion of PTEN show numerous histoarchitectural abnormalities within the nervous system due in part to shortened time for cell cycle progression and increased proliferation of neural stem cells [170], but not of cerebellar GCPs [171,172]. While cellular dysplasia was described, no invasive malignancies were found in the transgenic mouse brains after deletion of PTEN. However, on a background of compound deficiency for *P53* and *Neurofibromin-1*, heterozygous deletion of *Pten* resulted in accelerated development of grade III astrocytoma with a further evolution to grade IV astrocytomas with loss of the second *Pten* allele [173]. In addition, *PTEN* deficient astrocytes demonstrated increased proliferation in vitro, suggesting that there may be a developmental and/or cell-type specific result from *PTEN* loss [174].

MULTIPLE ENDOCRINCE NEOPLASIA

Clinical Features and Diagnostic Criteria

Multiple endocrince neoplasia (MEN) is a group of disorders characterized by the development of more than one endocrine tumor. MEN type 1 is characterized by the development of primary hyperparathyroidism due to parathyroid adenoma, entero-pancreatic tumors, adrenocortical tumors, and pituitary adenomas. Approximately 30% of patients with MEN-1 develop pituitary adenomas. Similar to sporadic cases of pituitary adenoma, the vast majority are either prolactin-secreting or nonfunctional tumors. Pituitary tumors in childhood are extremely rare, with an incidence of fewer than 1 per million children younger than 19 years and are often associated with an underlying genetic condition such as MEN [175]. Patients are diagnosed with MEN-1 based on clinical and radiographic evidence of tumors common to affected individuals. Genetic testing for the gene responsible for MEN-1 also aids in diagnosis. Patients with MEN-1 should have biochemical screening on a yearly basis.

Molecular Pathogenesis

Mutation in the gene *MEN-1* on chromosome 11q13, which produces the protein menin is responsible for the development of MEN-1 [176]. MEN-1 acts as a tumor suppressor gene. The exact mechanism of action is unclear, but loss of menin leads to cell cycle progression and increased cellular proliferation.

Therapy and Prognosis

Treatment of patients with MEN-1 and pituitary adenoma is the same as for patients with sporadic pituitary tumors. Prolactinomas are often successfully treated with dopamine agonists such as bromocriptine. Large nonfunctional tumors are frequently treated with endoscopic transsphenoidal tumor resection to decompress the optic chiasm.

Animal Models

There are no animal models that reproduce the molecular pathology of S manifestations of MEN.

REFERENCES

1. Packer RJ. Brain tumors in children. *Arch Neurol*. 1999;56(4):421–425.
2. Pietsch T, Taylor MD, Rutka JT. Molecular pathogenesis of childhood brain tumors. *J Neurooncol*. 2004;70(2):203–215.
3. Rutka JT, Kuo JS, Carter M, Ray A, Ueda S, Mainprize TG. Advances in the treatment of pediatric brain tumors. *Expert Rev Neurother*. 2004;4(5):879–893.
4. Wechsler-Reya R, Scott MP. The developmental biology of brain tumors. *Annu Rev Neurosci*. 2001;24:385–428.
5. Dyer MA. Mouse models of childhood cancer of the nervous system. *J Clin Pathol*. 2004;57(6):561–576.
6. Grimmer MR, Weiss WA. Childhood tumors of the nervous system as disorders of normal development. *Curr Opin Pediatr*. 2006;18(6):634–638.
7. Goldowitz D, Hamre K. The cells and molecules that make a cerebellum. *Trends Neurosci*. 1998;21(9):375–382.
8. Hatten ME, Alder J, Zimmerman K, Heintz N. Genes involved in cerebellar cell specification and differentiation. *Curr Opin Neurobiol*. 1997;7(1):40–47.
9. Oliver TG, Read TA, Kessler JD, et al. Loss of patched and disruption of granule cell development in a pre-neoplastic stage of medulloblastoma. *Development*. 2005;132(10):2425–2439.
10. Oliver TG, Wechsler-Reya RJ. Getting at the root and stem of brain tumors. *Neuron*. 2004;42(6):885–888.
11. Schuller U, Heine VM, Mao J, et al. Acquisition of granule neuron precursor identity is a critical determinant of progenitor cell competence to form Shh-induced medulloblastoma. *Cancer Cell*. 2008;14(2):123–134.
12. Wetmore C. Sonic hedgehog in normal and neoplastic proliferation: insight gained from human tumors and animal models *Curr Opin Genet Dev*. 2003;13(1):34–42.
13. Altman J, Bayer SA. *Development of the Cerebellar System in Relation to its Evolution, Structure and Functions*. Boca Raton, FL: CRC Press; 1997.
14. Altman J, Das GD. Autoradiographic and histological studies of postnatal neurogenesis. I. A longitudinal investigation of the kinetics, migration and transformation of cells incorporating tritiated thymidine in neonate rats, with special reference to postnatal neurogenesis in some brain regions. *J Comp Neurol*. 1966;126(3):337–389.
15. Wechsler-Reya RJ, Scott MP. Control of neuronal precursor proliferation in the cerebellum by Sonic Hedgehog. *Neuron*. 1999;22(1):103–114.
16. Hatten ME, Heintz N. Mechanisms of neural patterning and specification in the developing cerebellum. *Annu Rev Neurosci*. 1995;18:385–408.
17. Jacobson M. *Developmental Neurobiology*. 3rd ed. New York and London: Plenum Press; 1991.
18. Reilly KM, Jacks T. Genetically engineered mouse models of astrocytoma: GEMs in the rough? *Semin Cancer Biol*. 2001;11(3):177–191.
19. Reilly KM, Rubin JB, Gilbertson RJ, Garbow JR, Roussel MF, Gutmann DH. Rethinking brain tumors: the fourth Mouse Models of Human

Cancers Consortium nervous system tumors workshop. *Cancer Res.* 2008;68(14):5508–11.
20. Kaelin WG Jr. The von hippel-lindau tumor suppressor protein: an update. *Methods Enzymol.* 2007;435:371–383.
21. Maher ER, Iselius L, Yates JR, et al. Von Hippel-Lindau disease: a genetic study. *J Med Genet.* 1991;28(7):443–447.
22. Maher ER, Yates JR, Harries R, et al. Clinical features and natural history of von Hippel-Lindau disease. *Q J Med.* 1990;77(283):1151–1163.
23. Wanebo JE, Lonser RR, Glenn GM, Oldfield EH. The natural history of hemangioblastomas of the central nervous system in patients with von Hippel-Lindau disease. *J Neurosurg.* 2003;98(1):82–94.
24. Filling-Katz MR, Choyke PL, Oldfield E, et al. Central nervous system involvement in Von Hippel-Lindau disease. *Neurology.* 1991;41(1):41–46.
25. Seizinger BR, Rouleau GA, Ozelius LJ, et al. Von Hippel-Lindau disease maps to the region of chromosome 3 associated with renal cell carcinoma. *Nature.* 1988;332(6161):268–269.
26. Carmeliet P, Dor Y, Herbert JM, et al. Role of HIF-1alpha in hypoxia-mediated apoptosis, cell proliferation and tumour angiogenesis. *Nature.* 1998;394(6692):485–490.
27. Lonser RR, Weil RJ, Wanebo JE, DeVroom HL, Oldfield EH. Surgical management of spinal cord hemangioblastomas in patients with von Hippel-Lindau disease. *J Neurosurg.* 2003;98(1):106–116.
28. Weil RJ, Lonser RR, DeVroom HL, Wanebo JE, Oldfield EH. Surgical management of brainstem hemangioblastomas in patients with von Hippel-Lindau disease. *J Neurosurg.* 2003;98(1):95–105.
29. Jagannathan J, Lonser RR, Smith R, DeVroom HL, Oldfield EH. Surgical management of cerebellar hemangioblastomas in patients with von Hippel-Lindau disease. *J Neurosurg.* 2008;108(2):210–222.
30. Pan L, Wang EM, Wang BJ, et al. Gamma knife radiosurgery for hemangioblastomas. *Stereotact Funct* Neurosurg. 1998;70(suppl 1):179–186.
31. Patrice SJ, Sneed PK, Flickinger JC, et al. Radiosurgery for hemangioblastoma: results of a multiinstitutional experience. *Int J Radiat Oncol Biol Phys.* 1996;35(3):493–499.
32. Gnarra JR, Ward JM, Porter FD, et al. Defective placental vasculogenesis causes embryonic lethality in VHL-deficient mice. *Proc Natl Acad Sci U S A.* 1997;94(17):9102–9107.
33. Doedens A, Johnson RS. Transgenic models to understand hypoxia-inducible factor function. Methods Enzymol. 2007;435:87–105.
34. Haase VH. The VHL tumor suppressor in development and disease: functional studies in mice by conditional gene targeting. *Semin Cell Dev Biol.* 2005;16(4–5):564–574.
35. Rathmell WK, Hickey MM, Bezman NA, Chmielecki CA, Carraway NC, Simon MC. In vitro and in vivo models analyzing von Hippel-Lindau disease-specific mutations. *Cancer Res.* 2004;64(23):8595–8603.
36. Gorlin RJ, Sedano HO. The multiple nevoid basal cell carcinoma syndrome revisited. *Birth Defects* Orig Artic Ser. 1971;7(8):140–148.
37. Kimonis VE, Goldstein AM, Pastakia B, et al. Clinical manifestations in 105 persons with nevoid basal cell carcinoma syndrome. *Am J Med Genet.* 1997;69(3):299–308.
38. Shanley S, Ratcliffe J, Hockey A, et al. Nevoid basal cell carcinoma syndrome: review of 118 affected individuals. *Am J Med Genet.* 1994;50(3):282–290.
39. Farndon PA, Del Mastro RG, Evans DG, Kilpatrick MW. Location of gene for Gorlin syndrome. *Lancet.* 1992;339(8793):581–582.
40. Gailani MR, Bale SJ, Leffell DJ, et al. Developmental defects in Gorlin syndrome related to a putative tumor suppressor gene on chromosome 9. *Cell.* 1992;69(1):111–117.
41. Hahn H, Wicking C, Zaphiropoulous PG, et al. Mutations of the human homolog of Drosophila patched in the nevoid basal cell carcinoma syndrome. *Cell.* 1996;85(6):841–851.
42. Johnson RL, Rothman AL, Xie J, et al. Human homolog of patched, a candidate gene for the basal cell nevus syndrome. *Science.* 1996;272(5268):1668–1671.
43. Marigo V, Davey RA, Zuo Y, Cunningham JM, Tabin CJ. Biochemical evidence that patched is the Hedgehog receptor [see comments]. *Nature.* 1996;384(6605):176–179.
44. Marigo V, Tabin CJ. Regulation of patched by sonic hedgehog in the developing neural tube. *Proc Natl Acad Sci USA.* 1996;93(18):9346–9351.
45. Kleihues P, Cavenee WK. *World Health Organization Classification of Tumors: Pathology and Genetics of tumors of the Nervous System.* Lyon, France: IARCPress; 2000.

46. Wicking C, Bale AE. Molecular basis of the nevoid basal cell carcinoma syndrome. *Curr Opin* Pediatr. 1997;9(6):630–635.
47. Evans DG, Farndon PA, Burnell LD, Gattamaneni HR, Birch JM. The incidence of Gorlin syndrome in 173 consecutive cases of medulloblastoma. *Br J Cancer.* 1991;64(5):959–961.
48. Campbell RM, Mader RD, Dufresne RG Jr. Meningiomas after medulloblastoma irradiation treatment in a patient with basal cell nevus syndrome. *J Am Acad Dermatol.* 2005;53(5 suppl 1):S256-S259.
49. Pribila JT, Ronan SM, Trobe JD. Multiple intracranial meningiomas causing papilledema and visual loss in a patient with nevoid Basal cell carcinoma syndrome. *J Neuroophthalmol.* 2008;28(1):41–46.
50. Pomeroy SL, Tamayo P, Gaasenbeek M, et al. Prediction of central nervous system embryonal tumour outcome based on gene expression. *Nature.* 2002;415(6870):436–442.
51. Polkinghorn WR, Tarbell NJ. Medulloblastoma: tumorigenesis, current clinical paradigm, and efforts to improve risk stratification. *Nat Clin Pract Oncol.* 2007;4(5):295–304.
52. Weiss WA, Banerjee A. Can mouse models for brain tumors inform treatment in pediatric patients? *Semin Cancer Biol.* 2004;14(1):71–77.
53. Ehrbrecht A, Müller U, Wolter M, et al. Comprehensive genomic analysis of desmoplastic medulloblastomas: identification of novel amplified genes and separate evaluation of the different histological components. *J Pathol.* 2006;208(4):554–563.
54. Thompson MC, Fuller C, Hogg TL, et al. Genomics identifies medulloblastoma subgroups that are enriched for specific genetic alterations. *J Clin Oncol.* 2006;24(12):1924–1931.
55. Dahmen RP, Koch A, Denkhaus D, et al. Deletions of AXIN1, a component of the WNT/wingless pathway, in sporadic medulloblastomas. *Cancer Res.* 2001;61(19):7039–7043.
56. Baeza N, Masuoka J, Kleihues P, Ohgaki H. AXIN1 mutations but not deletions in cerebellar medulloblastomas. *Oncogene.* 2003;22(4):632–636.
57. Taylor MD, Zhang X, Liu L, et al. Failure of a medulloblastoma-derived mutant of SUFU to suppress WNT signaling. *Oncogene.* 2004;23(26):4577–4583.
58. Dakubo GD, Mazerolle CJ, Wallace VA. Expression of Notch and Wnt pathway components and activation of Notch signaling in medulloblastomas from heterozygous patched mice. *J Neurooncol.* 2006;79(3):221–227.
59. Fan X, Eberhart CG. Medulloblastoma stem cells. *J Clin Oncol.* 2008;26(17):2821–2827.
60. Fan X, Matsui W, Khaki L, et al. Notch pathway inhibition depletes stem-like cells and blocks engraftment in embryonal brain tumors. *Cancer Res.* 2006;66(15):7445–7452.
61. Sjölund J, Manetopoulos C, Stockhausen MT, Axelson H. The Notch pathway in cancer: differentiation gone awry. *Eur J Cancer.* 2005;41(17):2620–2629.
62. Hallahan AR, Pritchard JI, Hansen S, et al. The SmoA1 mouse model reveals that notch signaling is critical for the growth and survival of sonic hedgehog-induced medulloblastomas. *Cancer Res.* 2004;64(21):7794–7800.
63. Fan X, Mikolaenko I, Elhassan I, et al. Notch1 and notch2 have opposite effects on embryonal brain tumor growth. *Cancer Res.* 2004;64(21):7787–7793.
64. Hartmann W, Koch A, Brune H, et al. Insulin-like growth factor II is involved in the proliferation control of medulloblastoma and its cerebellar precursor cells. *Am J Pathol.* 2005;166(4):1153–1162.
65. Parathath SR, Mainwaring LA, Fernandez-L A, Campbell DO, Kenney AM. Insulin receptor substrate 1 is an effector of sonic hedgehog mitogenic signaling in cerebellar neural precursors. *Development.* 2008;135(19):3291–3300.
66. Rao G, Pedone CA, Del Valle L, Reiss K, Holland EC, Fults DW. Sonic hedgehog and insulin-like growth factor signaling synergize to induce medulloblastoma formation from nestin-expressing neural progenitors in mice. *Oncogene.* 2004;23(36):6156–6162.
67. Perrimon N. Hedgehog and beyond. *Cell.* 1995;80(4):517–520.
68. Perrimon N, Mahowald AP. Multiple functions of segment polarity genes in Drosophila. *Dev Biol.* 1987;119(2):587–600.
69. Marigo V, Johnson RL, Vortkamp A, Tabin CJ. Sonic hedgehog differentially regulates expression of GLI and GLI3 during limb development. *Dev Biol.* 1996;180(1):273–283.
70. Dahmane N, Lee J, Robins P, Heller P, Ruiz i Altaba A. Activation of the transcription factor Gli1 and the Sonic hedgehog signalling pathway in skin tumours. *Nature.* 1997;389(6653):876–881.

71. Hynes M, Stone DM, Dowd M, et al. Control of cell pattern in the neural tube by the zinc finger transcription factor and oncogene Gli-1. *Neuron.* 1997;19(1):15–26.
72. Lee J, Platt KA, Censullo P, Ruiz i Altaba A. Gli1 is a target of Sonic hedgehog that induces ventral neural tube development. *Development.* 1997;124(13):2537–2552.
73. Borycki AG, Mendham L, Emerson CP Jr. Control of somite patterning by Sonic hedgehog and its downstream signal response genes. *Development.* 1998;125(4):777–790.
74. Fan H, Oro AE, Scott MP, Khavari PA. Induction of basal cell carcinoma features in transgenic human skin expressing Sonic Hedgehog. *Nat Med.* 1997;3(7):788–792.
75. Goodrich LV, Milenkovic L, Higgins KM, Scott MP. Altered neural cell fates and medulloblastoma in mouse patched mutants. *Science.* 1997;277(5329):1109–1113.
76. Matise MP, Joyner AL. Gli genes in development and cancer. *Oncogene.* 1999;18(55):7852–7859.
77. Taipale J, Beachy PA. The Hedgehog and Wnt signalling pathways in cancer. *Nature.* 2001;411(6835):349–354.
78. Ruiz i Altaba A, Sanchez P, Dahmane N. Gli and hedgehog in cancer: tumours, embryos and stem cells. *Nat Rev Cancer.* 2002;2(5):361–372.
79. Berman DM, Karhadkar SS, Maitra A, et al. Widespread requirement for Hedgehog ligand stimulation in growth of digestive tract tumours. *Nature.* 2003;425(6960):846–851.
80. Liu S, Dontu G, Mantle ID, et al. Hedgehog signaling and Bmi-1 regulate self-renewal of normal and malignant human mammary stem cells. *Cancer Res.* 2006;66(12):6063–6071.
81. Lai K, Kaspar BK, Gage FH, Schaffer DV. Sonic hedgehog regulates adult neural progenitor proliferation *in vitro* and in vivo. *Nat Neurosci.* 2003;6(1):21–27.
82. Machold R, Hayashi S, Rutlin M, et al. Sonic hedgehog is required for progenitor cell maintenance in telencephalic stem cell niches. *Neuron.* 2003;39(6):937–950.
83. Palma V, Lim DA, Dahmane N, et al. Sonic hedgehog controls stem cell behavior in the postnatal and adult brain. *Development.* 2005;132(2):335–344.
84. Blank U, Karlsson G, Karlsson S. Signaling pathways governing stem-cell fate. *Blood.* 2008;111(2):492–503.
85. Ingham PW. Signalling by hedgehog family proteins in Drosophila and vertebrate development. *Curr Opin Genet Dev.* 1995;5(4):492–498.
86. Ng D, Stavrou T, Liu L, et al. Retrospective family study of childhood medulloblastoma. *Am J Med Genet A.* 2005;134(4):399–403.
87. Taylor MD, Liu L, Raffel C, et al. Mutations in SUFU predispose to medulloblastoma. *Nat Genet.* 2002;31(3):306–310.
88. Gajjar A, Chintagumpala M, Ashley D, et al. Risk-adapted craniospinal radiotherapy followed by high-dose chemotherapy and stem-cell rescue in children with newly diagnosed medulloblastoma (St Jude Medulloblastoma-96): long-term results from a prospective, multicentre trial. *Lancet Oncol.* 2006;7(10):813–820.
89. Mulhern RK, Palmer SL, Merchant TE, et al. Neurocognitive consequences of risk-adapted therapy for childhood medulloblastoma. *J Clin Oncol.* 2005;23(24):5511–5519.
90. Atahan IL, Yildiz F, Ozyar E, Uzal D, Zorlu F. Basal cell carcinomas developing in a case of medulloblastoma associated with Gorlin's syndrome. *Pediatr Hematol Oncol.* 1998;15(2):187–191.
91. O'Malley S, Weitman D, Olding M, Sekhar L. Multiple neoplasms following craniospinal irradiation for medulloblastoma in a patient with nevoid basal cell carcinoma syndrome. Case report. *J Neurosurg.* 1997;86(2):286–288.
92. Walter AW, Pivnick EK, Bale AE, Kun LE. Complications of the nevoid basal cell carcinoma syndrome: a case report. *J Pediatr Hematol Oncol.* 1997;19(3):258–262.
93. Bale AE. The nevoid basal cell carcinoma syndrome: genetics and mechanism of carcinogenesis. *Cancer Invest.* 1997;15(2):180–186.
94. Chan GL, Little JB. Cultured diploid fibroblasts from patients with the nevoid basal cell carcinoma syndrome are hypersensitive to killing by ionizing radiation. *Am J Pathol.* 1983;111(1):50–55.
95. Evans DG, Birch JM, Orton CI. Brain tumours and the occurrence of severe invasive basal cell carcinoma in first degree relatives with Gorlin syndrome. *Br J Neurosurg.* 1991;5(6):643–646.
96. Hahn H, Wojnowski L, Zimmer AM, Hall J, Miller G, Zimmer A. Rhabdomyosarcomas and radiation hypersensitivity in a mouse model of Gorlin syndrome. *Nat Med.* 1998;4(5):619–622.
97. Pazzaglia S, Mancuso M, Atkinson MJ, et al. High incidence of medulloblastoma following X-ray-irradiation of newborn Ptc1 heterozygous mice. *Oncogene.* 2002;21(49):7580–7584.
98. Leonard J, Ye, H, Wetmore, C, Karnitz, L. Sonic hedgehog signaling impairs ionizing radiation-induced checkpoint activation and induces genomic instability. *J Cell Biol.* 2008;183(3):385–391.
99. Choudry Q, Patel HC, Gurusinghe NT, Evans DG. Radiation-induced brain tumours in nevoid basal cell carcinoma syndrome: implications for treatment and surveillance. *Childs Nerv Syst.* 2007;23(1):133–136.
100. Stavrou T, Bromley CM, Nicholson HS, et al. Prognostic factors and secondary malignancies in childhood medulloblastoma. *J Pediatr Hematol Oncol.* 2001;23(7):431–436.
101. Büyükpamukçu M, Varan A, Yazici N, et al. Second malignant neoplasms following the treatment of brain tumors in children. *J Child Neurol.* 2006;21(5):433–436.
102. Wetmore C, Eberhart DE, Curran T. The normal patched allele is expressed in medulloblastomas from mice with heterozygous germline mutation of patched. *Cancer Res.* 2000;60(8):2239–2246.
103. Raffel C, Jenkins RB, Frederick L, et al. Sporadic medulloblastomas contain PTCH mutations. *Cancer Res.* 1997;57(5):842–845.
104. Vorechovský I, Tingby O, Hartman M, et al. Somatic mutations in the human homologue of Drosophila patched in primitive neuroectodermal tumours. *Oncogene.* 1997;15(3):361–366.
105. Yang ZJ, Ellis T, Markant SL, et al. Medulloblastoma can be initiated by deletion of Patched in lineage-restricted progenitors or stem cells. *Cancer Cell.* 2008;14(2):135–145.
106. Hatton BA, Villavicencio EH, Tsuchiya KD, et al. The Smo/Smo model: hedgehog-induced medulloblastoma with 90% incidence and leptomeningeal spread. *Cancer Res.* 2008;68(6):1768–1776.
107. Del Valle L, Enam S, Lassak A, et al. Insulin-like growth factor I receptor activity in human medulloblastomas. *Clin Cancer Res.* 2002;8(6):1822–1830.
108. Kenney AM, Cole MD, Rowitch DH. Nmyc upregulation by sonic hedgehog signaling promotes proliferation in developing cerebellar granule neuron precursors. *Development.* 2003;130(1):15–28.
109. Su X, Gopalakrishnan V, Stearns D, et al. Abnormal expression of REST/NRSF and Myc in neural stem/progenitor cells causes cerebellar tumors by blocking neuronal differentiation. *Mol Cell Biol.* 2006;26(5):1666–1678.
110. Hahn H, Wojnowski L, Specht K, et al. Patched target Igf2 is indispensable for the formation of medulloblastoma and rhabdomyosarcoma. *J Biol Chem.* 2000;275(37):28341–28344.
111. Hatton BA, Knoepfler PS, Kenney AM, et al. N-myc is an essential downstream effector of Shh signaling during both normal and neoplastic cerebellar growth. *Cancer Res.* 2006;66(17):8655–8661.
112. Wetmore C, Eberhart DE, Curran T. Loss of p53 but not ARF accelerates medulloblastoma in mice heterozygous for patched. *Cancer Res.* 2001;61(2):513–516.
113. Adesina AM, Nalbantoglu J, Cavenee WK. p53 gene mutation and mdm2 gene amplification are uncommon in medulloblastoma. *Cancer Res.* 1994;54(21):5649–5651.
114. Badiali M, Iolascon A, Loda M, et al. p53 gene mutations in medulloblastoma. Immunohistochemistry, gel shift analysis, and sequencing. *Diagn Mol Pathol.* 1993;2(1):23–28.
115. Biegel JA, Burk CD, Barr FG, Emanuel BS. Evidence for a 17p tumor related locus distinct from p53 in pediatric primitive neuroectodermal tumors. *Cancer Res.* 1992;52(12):3391–3395.
116. Saylors RL 3rd, Sidransky D, Friedman HS, et al. Infrequent p53 gene mutations in medulloblastomas. *Cancer Res.* 1991;51(17):4721–4723.
117. Romer JT, Kimura H, Magdaleno S, et al. Suppression of the Shh pathway using a small molecule inhibitor eliminates medulloblastoma in Ptc1(+/-)p53(-/-) mice. *Cancer Cell.* 2004;6(3):229–240.
118. Kimura H, Ng JM, Curran T. Transient inhibition of the Hedgehog pathway in young mice causes permanent defects in bone structure. *Cancer Cell.* 2008;13(3):249–260.
119. Galvin KE, Ye H, Wetmore C. Differential gene induction by genetic and ligand-mediated activation of the Sonic hedgehog pathway in neural stem cells. *Dev Biol.* 2007;308(2):331–342.
120. Fuller GN, Su X, Price RE, et al. Many human medulloblastoma tumors overexpress repressor element-1 silencing transcription (REST)/neuron-restrictive silencer factor, which can be functionally countered by REST-VP16. *Mol Cancer Ther.* 2005;4(3):343–349.
121. Fults DW. Modeling medulloblastoma with genetically engineered mice. *Neurosurg Focus.* 2005;19(5):E7.

122. Weiner HL, Bakst R, Hurlbert MS, et al. Induction of medulloblastomas in mice by sonic hedgehog, independent of Gli1. *Cancer Res.* 2002;62(22):6385–6389.
123. Turcot J, Despres JP, St Pierre F. Malignant tumors of the central nervous system associated with familial polyposis of the colon: report of two cases. *Dis Colon Rectum.* 1959;2:465–468.
124. Attard TM, Giglio P, Koppula S, Snyder C, Lynch HT. Brain tumors in individuals with familial adenomatous polyposis: a cancer registry experience and pooled case report analysis. *Cancer.* 2007;109(4):761–766.
125. Hamilton SR, Liu B, Parsons RE, et al. The molecular basis of Turcot's syndrome. *N Engl J Med.* 1995;332(13):839–847.
126. Groden J, Thliveris A, Samowitz W, et al. Identification and characterization of the familial adenomatous polyposis coli gene. *Cell.* 1991;66(3):589–600.
127. Polakis P. The many ways of Wnt in cancer. *Curr Opin Genet Dev.* 2007;17(1):45–51.
128. Gilbertson RJ, Ellison DW. The origins of medulloblastoma subtypes. *Annu Rev Pathol.* 2008;3:341–365.
129. Zurawel RH, Chiappa SA, Allen C, Raffel C. Sporadic medulloblastomas contain oncogenic beta-catenin mutations. *Cancer Res.* 1998;58(5):896–899.
130. Peltomäki P, Aaltonen LA, Sistonen P, et al. Genetic mapping of a locus predisposing to human colorectal cancer. *Science.* 1993;260(5109):810–812.
131. Leung SY, Chan TL, Chung LP, et al. Microsatellite instability and mutation of DNA mismatch repair genes in gliomas. *Am J Pathol.* 1998;153(4):1181–1188.
132. Gottschling S, Reinhard H, Pagenstecher C, et al. Hypothesis: Possible role of retinoic acid therapy in patients with biallelic mismatch repair gene defects. *Eur J Pediatr.* 2008;167(2):225–229.
133. Rutz HP, de Tribolet N, Calmes JM, Chapuis G. Long-time survival of a patient with glioblastoma and Turcot's syndrome. Case report. *J Neurosurg.* 1991;74(5):813–815.
134. Galiatsatos P, Foulkes WD. Familial adenomatous polyposis. *Am J Gastroenterol.* 2006;101(2):385–398.
135. Sarkaria JN, Kitange GJ, James CD, et al. Mechanisms of chemoresistance to alkylating agents in malignant glioma. *Clin Cancer Res.* 2008;14(10):2900–2908.
136. Dietrich WF, Lander ES, Smith JS, et al. Genetic identification of Mom-1, a major modifier locus affecting Min-induced intestinal neoplasia in the mouse. *Cell.* 1993;75(4):631–639.
137. Moser AR, Luongo C, Gould KA, Meley MK, Shoemaker AR, Dove WF. ApcMin: a mouse model for intestinal and mammary tumorigenesis. *Eur J Cancer.* 1995;31A(7–8):1061–1064.
138. Vortmeyer AO, Stavrou T, Selby D, et al. Deletion analysis of the adenomatous polyposis coli and PTCH gene loci in patients with sporadic and nevoid basal cell carcinoma syndrome-associated medulloblastoma. *Cancer.* 1999;85(12):2662–2667.
139. Yong WH, Raffel C, von Deimling A, Louis DN. The APC gene in Turcot's syndrome. *N Engl J Med.* 1995;333(8):524.
140. Li FP, Fraumeni JF Jr. Soft-tissue sarcomas, breast cancer, and other neoplasms. A familial syndrome? *Ann Intern Med.* 1969;71(4):747–752.
141. Li FP, Fraumeni JF Jr. Rhabdomyosarcoma in children: epidemiologic study and identification of a familial cancer syndrome. *J Natl Cancer Inst.* 1969;43(6):1365–1373.
142. Olivier M, Goldgar DE, Sodha N, et al. Li-Fraumeni and related syndromes: correlation between tumor type, family structure, and TP53 genotype. *Cancer Res.* 2003;63(20):6643–6650.
143. Li FP, Fraumeni JF Jr, Mulvihill JJ, et al. A cancer family syndrome in twenty-four kindreds. *Cancer Res.* 1988;48(18):5358–5362.
144. Birch JM, Hartley AL, Tricker KJ, et al. Prevalence and diversity of constitutional mutations in the p53 gene among 21 Li-Fraumeni families. *Cancer Res.* 1994;54(5):1298–1304.
145. Varley JM. Germline TP53 mutations and Li-Fraumeni syndrome. *Hum Mutat.* 2003;21(3):313–320.
146. Wang W, El-Deiry WS. Restoration of p53 to limit tumor growth. *Curr Opin Oncol.* 2008;20(1):90–96.
147. Hofseth LJ, Hussain SP, Harris CC. p53: 25 years after its discovery. *Trends Pharmacol Sci.* 2004;25(4):177–181.
148. Fridman JS, Lowe SW. Control of apoptosis by p53. *Oncogene.* 2003;22(56):9030–9040.
149. Oren M, Rotter V. Introduction: p53—the first twenty years. *Cell Mol Life Sci.* 1999;55(1):9–11.
150. Sherr CJ. Principles of tumor suppression. *Cell.* 2004;116(2):235–246.
151. Ohgaki H, Dessen P, Jourde B, et al. Genetic pathways to glioblastoma: a population-based study. *Cancer Res.* 2004;64(19):6892–6899.
152. Ohgaki H, Kleihues P. Genetic pathways to primary and secondary glioblastoma. *Am J Pathol.* 2007;170(5):1445–1453.
153. Sodha N, Houlston RS, Bullock S, et al. Increasing evidence that germline mutations in CHEK2 do not cause Li-Fraumeni syndrome. *Hum Mutat.* 2002;20(6):460–462.
154. Tong WM, Hande MP, Lansdorp PM, Wang ZQ. DNA strand break-sensing molecule poly(ADP-Ribose) polymerase cooperates with p53 in telomere function, chromosome stability, and tumor suppression. *Mol Cell Biol.* 2001;21(12):4046–4054.
155. Tong WM, Ohgaki H, Huang H, Granier C, Kleihues P, Wang ZQ. Null mutation of DNA strand break-binding molecule poly(ADP-ribose) polymerase causes medulloblastomas in p53(-/-) mice. *Am J Pathol.* 2003;162(1):343–352.
156. Lee Y, McKinnon PJ. DNA ligase IV suppresses medulloblastoma formation. *Cancer Res.* 2002;62(22):6395–6399.
157. Lee Y, Miller HL, Jensen P, et al. A molecular fingerprint for medulloblastoma. *Cancer Res.* 2003;63(17):5428–5437.
158. Lee Y, Barnes DE, Lindahl T, McKinnon PJ. Defective neurogenesis resulting from DNA ligase IV deficiency requires Atm. *Genes Dev.* 2000;14(20):2576–2580.
159. Jacks T, Fazeli A, Schmitt EM, Bronson RT, Goodell MA, Weinberg RA. Effects of an Rb mutation in the mouse. *Nature.* 1992;359(6393):295–300.
160. Weinberg RA. The molecular basis of retinoblastomas. *Ciba Found Symp.* 1989;142:99–105; discussion 106.
161. Marino S, Vooijs M, van Der Gulden H, Jonkers J, Berns A. Induction of medulloblastomas in p53-null mutant mice by somatic inactivation of Rb in the external granular layer cells of the cerebellum. *Genes Dev.* 2000;14(8):994–1004.
162. Nelen MR, Kremer H, Konings IB, et al. Novel PTEN mutations in patients with Cowden disease: absence of clear genotype-phenotype correlations. *Eur J Hum Genet.* 1999;7(3):267–273.
163. Nelen MR, Padberg GW, Peeters EA, et al. Localization of the gene for Cowden disease to chromosome 10q22–23. *Nat Genet.* 1996;13(1):114–116.
164. Gustafson S, Zbuk KM, Scacheri C, Eng C. Cowden syndrome. *Semin Oncol.* 2007;34(5):428–434.
165. Cully M, You H, Levine AJ, Mak TW. Beyond PTEN mutations: the PI3K pathway as an integrator of multiple inputs during tumorigenesis. *Nat Rev Cancer.* 2006;6(3):184–192.
166. Endersby R, Baker SJ. PTEN signaling in brain: neuropathology and tumorigenesis. *Oncogene.* 2008;27(41):5416–5430.
167. Li J, Yen C, Liaw D, et al. PTEN, a putative protein tyrosine phosphatase gene mutated in human brain, breast, and prostate cancer. *Science.* 1997;275(5308):1943–1947.
168. Okami K, Wu L, Riggins G, et al. Analysis of PTEN/MMAC1 alterations in aerodigestive tract tumors. *Cancer Res.* 1998;58(3):509–511.
169. Guanti G, Resta N, Simone C, et al. Involvement of PTEN mutations in the genetic pathways of colorectal cancerogenesis. *Hum Mol Genet.* 2000;9(2):283–287.
170. Groszer M, Erickson R, Scripture-Adams DD, et al. Negative regulation of neural stem/progenitor cell proliferation by the Pten tumor suppressor gene in vivo. *Science.* 2001;294(5549):2186–2189.
171. Backman SA, Stambolic V, Suzuki A, et al. Deletion of Pten in mouse brain causes seizures, ataxia and defects in soma size resembling Lhermitte-Duclos disease. *Nat Genet.* 2001;29(4):396–403.
172. Kwon CH, Zhu X, Zhang J, et al. Pten regulates neuronal soma size: a mouse model of Lhermitte-Duclos disease. *Nat Genet.* 2001;29(4):404–411.
173. Kwon CH, Zhao D, Chen J, et al. Pten haploinsufficiency accelerates formation of high-grade astrocytomas. *Cancer Res.* 2008;68(9):3286–3294.
174. Fraser MM, Zhu X, Kwon CH, Uhlmann EJ, Gutmann DH, Baker SJ. Pten loss causes hypertrophy and increased proliferation of astrocytes in vivo. *Cancer Res.* 2004;64(21):7773–7779.
175. Keil MF, Stratakis CA. Pituitary tumors in childhood: update of diagnosis, treatment and molecular genetics. *Expert Rev Neurother.* 2008;8(4):563–574.
176. Chandrasekharappa SC, Guru SC, Manickam P, et al. Positional cloning of the gene for multiple endocrine neoplasia-type 1. *Science.* 1997;276(5311):404–407.

27 Predisposition Syndromes: Neurofibromatosis 1, Neurofibromatosis 2, and Tuberous Sclerosis Complex

Rebecca J. Gutmann and David H. Gutmann

INTRODUCTION

Although the vast majority of nervous system tumors arise in a sporadic fashion, there are a number of inherited cancer syndromes that predispose affected individuals to the development of nervous system tumors. These inherited cancer syndromes are particularly important to recognize clinically, since at-risk individuals are likely to develop additional tumors and family members will require genetic counseling and screening. In addition, study of these genetic conditions has already provided key insights into the molecular and cellular pathogenesis of sporadic nervous system tumors. In this chapter, we will discuss three of the most common cancer predisposition syndromes (Table 27.1): neurofibromatosis-1 (NF1), neurofibromatosis-2 (NF2), and tuberous sclerosis complex (TSC).

The genetic basis for these inherited cancer syndromes was first recognized by Alfred Knudson for retinoblastoma in 1971 [1]. Because individuals with these conditions begin life with one mutated (nonfunctional) copy of a given tumor suppressor gene (TSG; eg, *NF1* gene), only one additional genetic change (inactivation of the one remaining functional copy) is required for a tumor to form in individuals with an inherited cancer syndrome. In the general population, the probability of both copies of a TSG becoming inactivated by mutation in a single cell is very small. However, in individuals with these cancer predisposition syndromes, tumors form at an increased frequency (Figure 27.1).

NEUROFIBROMATOSIS-1

NF1, also known as peripheral neurofibromatosis or von Recklinghausen disease, is the most common of the three inherited cancer syndromes. NF1 is found in all ethnic groups and populations worldwide, occurring with an incidence between 1 in 2500 and 1 in 3000 [2]. The diagnosis of NF1 requires the presence of at least two features from a list of seven diagnostic criteria (Table 27.2).

The most common and typically earliest sign of NF1 is the presence of hyperpigmented regions on the skin and the iris. *Café-au-lait* macules are hyperpigmented macules

Table 27.1 Inherited Brain Tumor Predisposition Syndromes

Syndrome	Gene	Nervous System Tumors
Gorlin syndrome	PTCH1 (9q22)	Medulloblastoma
Li-Fraumeni syndrome	TP53 (17p13)	Astrocytoma, primitive neuroectodermal tumors
Neurofibromatosis 1	NF1 (17q11)	Astrocytoma, optic glioma, neurofibroma
Neurofibromatosis 2	NF2 (22q12)	Schwannoma, meningioma, ependymoma
Tuberous sclerosis complex	TSC1 (9p34) TSC2 (16p13)	Subependymal giant cell astrocytoma
Turcot syndrome	APC (7p22)	Medulloblastoma
Von Hippel-Lindau	VHL (5q21)	Hemangioblastoma

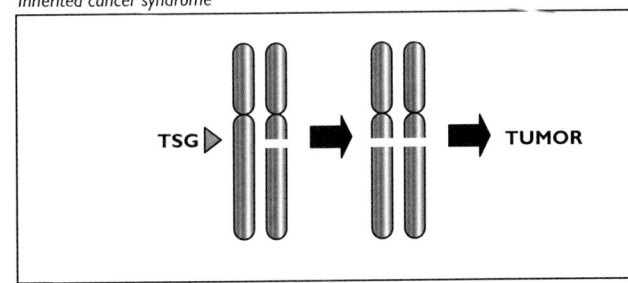

Figure 27.1 Genetic basis for inherited tumor syndromes. Tumor formation requires the inactivation of both copies of a specific tumor suppressor gene (TSG; eg, *NF1* gene) in any given cell (eg, Schwann cell). In individuals with an inherited cancer syndrome, children are born with one nonfunctional copy of a specific tumor suppressor gene. Tumor formation only requires one additional genetic event—inactivation of the remaining functional tumor suppressor.

Table 27.2 Diagnostic Criteria for Neurofibromatosis 1

Two or more of the following features are required:
1. Six or more café-au-lait spots with diameters greater than 0.5 mm before puberty or 1.5 cm after puberty
2. Two or more neurofibromas or single plexiform neurofibroma
3. Freckling in the axillary or inguinal regions
4. Optic pathway tumor
5. Lisch nodules (hamartomas of the iris)
6. A distinctive bony lesion: dysplasia of the sphenoid bone or dysplasia/thinning of long bone cortex
7. A first-degree relative diagnosed with NF1

that usually appear within the first year of life. Similarly, children with NF1 often have freckles in their axilla and inguinal creases, termed skinfold freckling. Lastly, hyperpigmented nodules on the iris (iris hamartomas or Lisch nodules) are nearly pathognomonic for NF1. These iris hamartomas do not interfere with vision, but are most reliably identified by an experienced ophthalmologist using a slit lamp.

The most common nervous system tumors in patients with NF1 involve the peripheral nervous system. These peripheral nerve tumors, termed neurofibromas, represent complex benign neoplasms composed of numerous distinct cell types. The neoplastic cell in the neurofibroma is the Schwann cell [3,4]; however, other cell types, including endothelial cells, mast cells, and fibroblasts, also contribute to tumorigenesis and growth. Neurofibromas typically become apparent in early adolescence and often herald the onset of puberty [5]. These characteristic discrete neurofibromas can develop anywhere on the body and do not transform into malignant tumors. Discrete neurofibromas involve a single nerve fascicle and may be located on the skin, underneath the skin, or deep within the body.

More diffuse neurofibromas involving greater than one nerve fascicle, termed plexiform neurofibromas, are found in 25% to 30% of all individuals with NF1 [6]. Plexiform neurofibromas may be associated with significant morbidity due to the involvement of associated structures, including the spinal cord (Figure 27.2), blood vessels, and bones. Unlike their discrete counterparts, plexiform neurofibromas can transform into malignant peripheral nerve sheath tumors (MPNSTs). MPNSTs are highly aggressive metastatic cancers with poor responses to both radiation and chemotherapy [7]. The lifetime risk of developing a MPNST in NF1 has been estimated as high as 10% [8].

The second most common tumor in individuals with NF1 is the optic pathway glioma (OPG), which is seen in 15% of children with NF1 [9]. OPGs in patients with NF1 are usually World Health Organization grade I pilocytic astrocytomas arising within the optic nerves, chiasm, postchiasmatic optic radiations, and hypothalamus (Figure 27.2). When they affect the hypothalamus, children with NF1 may present with diencephalic syndrome or precocious puberty [10]. OPGs in the context of NF1 are typically brain tumors of early childhood, most frequently affecting children between the ages of 2 and 6 years. Although visual impairment can develop, most NF1-associated OPGs run an indolent course and less than one third will require treatment [11]. Treatment is usually chemotherapy involving the combination of carboplatin and vincristine. There is a very limited role for surgery [12,], and radiation therapy should be avoided owing to the high rate of secondary brain tumors in this tumor-prone population [13].

In addition to OPGs, individuals with NF1 are prone to the development of brainstem gliomas [14] as well as high-grade gliomas in adulthood [15]. In these studies, the observed prevalence of brain tumors in patients with NF1 is between 10 and 100 times greater than expected, and this increased risk remains elevated at all ages.

Finally, individuals with NF1 also develop numerous other medical problems, including specific learning disabilities (visual-spatial learning problems and attention deficit disorder) [16,], vascular abnormalities (moya-moya disease and renal artery stenosis) [17,], bony abnormalities (sphenoid wing and long bone dysplasia), and other cancers (pheochromocytoma). Clinicians caring for children with NF1 may find hyperintensities on T2-weighted magnetic resonance imaging (MRI). These abnormalities are of unknown clinical significance, but can be confused with noncontrast-enhancing low-grade gliomas [18].

With the advent of positional cloning, the *NF1* gene was identified and found to encode a large cytoplasmic protein, termed neurofibromin [19]. Analysis of the predicted protein sequence of neurofibromin revealed that it shares sequence and functional similarity with a family of proteins known to negatively regulate the Ras proto-oncogene [20]. In many cell types, active Ras leads to increased cell growth and transformation, suggesting that neurofibromin, as a tumor suppressor, regulates cell growth by maintaining Ras in an inactive conformation. Subsequent work from a number of laboratories have shown that neurofibromin not only inhibits Ras activity but also promotes the generation of cyclic AMP [21,22,], a second messenger that can inhibit cell growth in some cell types. Moreover, further dissection of the neurofibromin growth control pathway revealed that neurofibromin negatively regulates mammalian target of rapamycin (mTOR) signaling [23,24]. The identification of Ras and mTOR as targets for neurofibromin function has led to the development of clinical trials using drugs that inhibit Ras and mTOR activity (Figure 27.3).

Over the past decade, several research groups have generated robust small animal models of specific NF1 clinical phenotypes. Genetically engineered mice have been developed to model NF1-associated plexiform neurofibromas [25,], MPNSTs [26,27,], bony abnormalities [28,], leukemia [29,], pheochromocytoma [30,], learning disabilities [31,], high-grade gliomas [32,], and optic gliomas [33–35.] Each of these models provides the opportunity to understand more about the molecular and cellular pathogenesis of the clinical features of NF1 as well as to evaluate new biologically targeted therapies (eg, rapamycin) prior to human clinical studies [36,37]. *Nf1* mouse models of plexiform neurofibroma and optic glioma have shown that the tumor microenvironment (stroma) is critical for tumor formation and growth [38–40.] With the identification of these growth regulatory signals from the tumor microenvironment, additional antitumor therapies that target stromal growth factors might emerge.

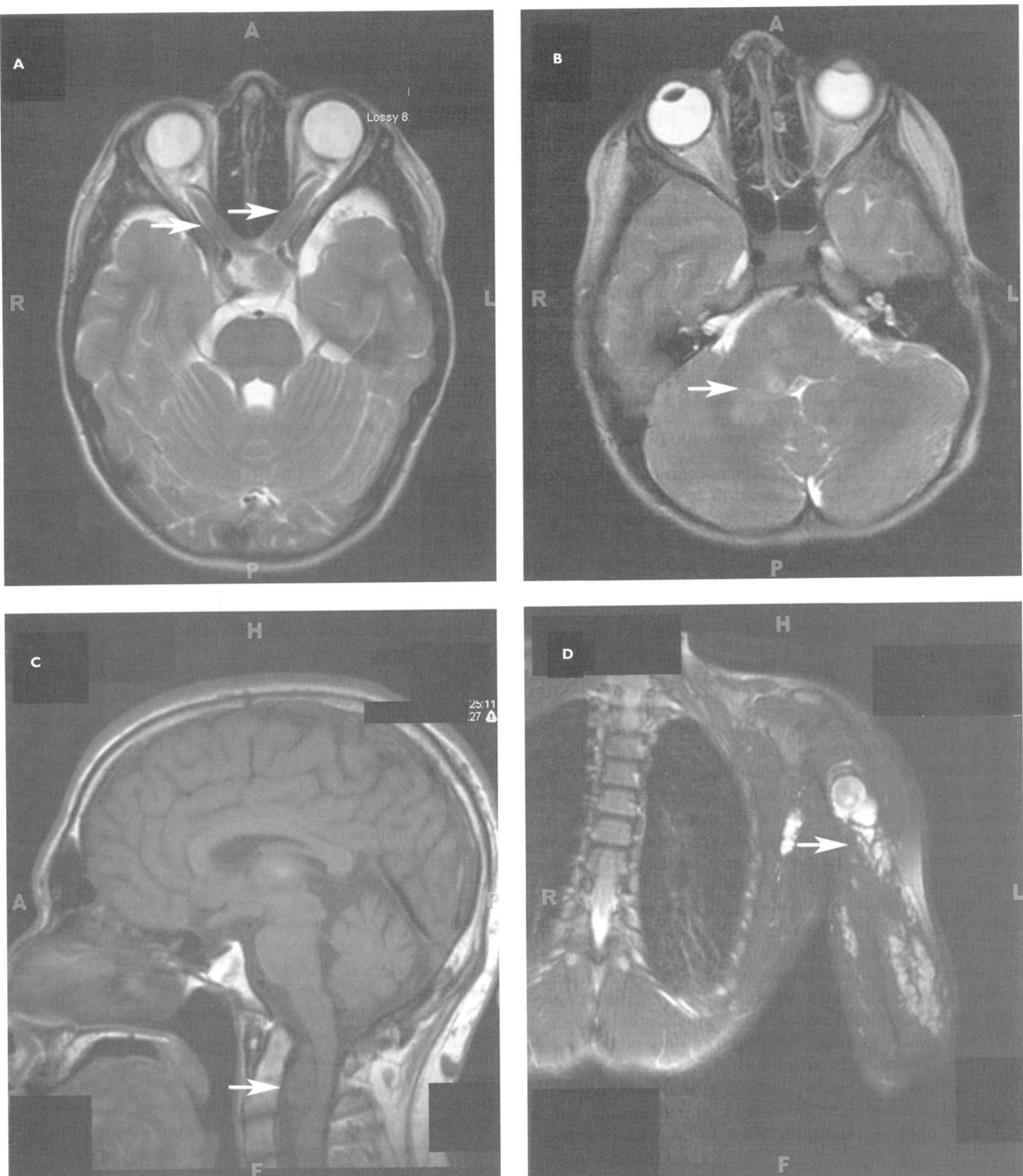

Figure 27.2 Nervous system tumors in neurofibromatosis 1. (**A**) Bilateral optic nerve gliomas are denoted by the arrows. (**B**) Brainstem glioma with extension into the cerebellar peduncles is denoted by the arrow. (**C**) Plexiform neurofibroma compressing the cervical spinal cord is denoted by the arrow. (**D**) Extensive plexiform neurofibroma involving the left upper arm.

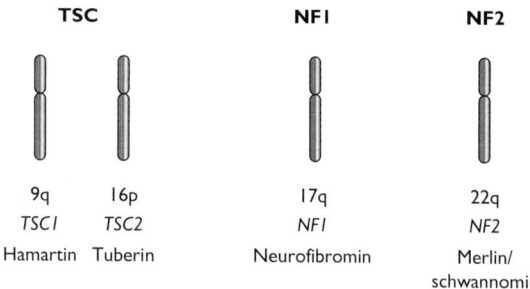

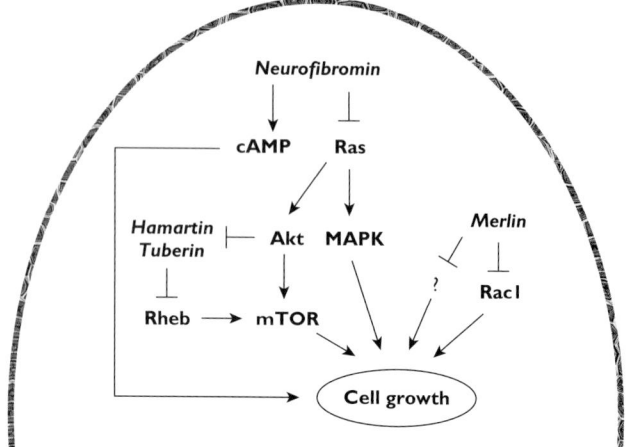

Figure 27.3 Molecular basis for inherited nervous system tumor disposition syndromes. The chromosomal location and protein names for the NF1, NF2, and TSC tumor suppressor syndromes are shown. Neurofibromin, tuberin/hamartin, and merlin/schwannomin each negatively regulate cell growth by controlling the activity of specific intracellular signaling proteins. Loss of function of neurofibromin, tuberin/hamartin, or merlin/schwannomin leads to deregulated intracellular signaling and increased cell growth.

NEUROFIBROMATOSIS 2

NF2, unlike NF1, is a condition where patients predominantly develop numerous nervous system tumors. It is far less common than NF1 and affects 1 in 25,000 individuals worldwide [41]. The diagnosis of NF2 is usually established in an adolescent or young adult who presents with hearing and balance problems attributable to compression of the eighth cranial (vestibular) nerve by schwannomas (Figure 27.4). The presence of bilateral vestibular schwannomas (VS) is pathognomonic for NF2 [42]; however, in the absence of this classic clinical picture, the diagnosis can be rendered using established diagnostic criteria (Table 27.3).

Schwannomas are the most common tumors seen in individuals with NF2 and can affect any nerve in the body. Unlike neurofibromas, schwannomas tend to grow eccentrically to the nerve and compress the nerve. These tumors are also simpler in composition and are usually composed of only neoplastic Schwann cells. Surgery is the mainstay of management, although efforts are currently focused on developing medical antitumoral therapies.

The second most common tumor is the meningioma, which tends to occur in multiple locations along the

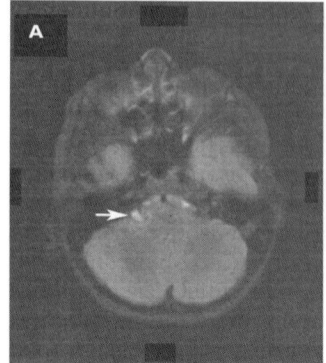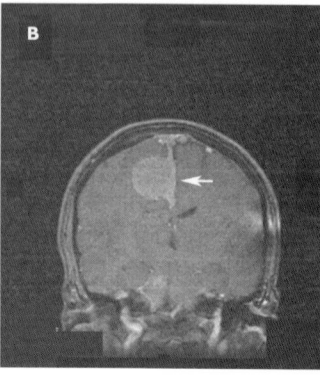

Figure 27.4 Nervous system tumors in neurofibromatosis 2. (**A**) Eighth cranial nerve schwannoma is denoted by the arrow. (**B**) A large meningioma is denoted by the arrow.

Table 27.3 Diagnostic Criteria for Neurofibromatosis 2

Definite NF2
1. Bilateral vestibular schwannomas (VS)
2. Family history of NF2 plus either
   a. Unilateral VS at <30 years or
   b. Any two of the following:
      i. Meningioma
      ii. Glioma (ependymoma)
      iii. Schwannoma
      iv. Juvenile posterior subcapsular lenticular opacities (cataract)

Probable NF2
1. Unilateral VS at <30 years plus at least any one of the following:
   a. Meningioma
   b. Glioma (ependymoma)
   c. Schwannoma
   d. Juvenile posterior subcapsular lenticular opacities (cataract)
2. Multiple meningiomas (two or more) plus unilateral VS at <30 years or
3. Any one of the following:
   a. Meningioma
   b. Glioma (ependymoma)
   c. Schwannoma
   d. Juvenile posterior subcapsular lenticular opacities (cataract)

leptomeninges (Figure 27.4). Individuals with NF2 are also prone to the development of ependymomas in the spinal cord. The management of both of these tumor types is largely surgical. Finally, retinal lesions and posterior sublenticular cataracts may be seen in the context of NF2.

As with NF1, the discovery of the *NF2* gene by two groups led to the identification of the *NF2* protein, termed merlin (or schwannomin) [43,44]. Analysis of the predicted protein sequence revealed that merlin belonged to a family of proteins that associate with cell membrane glycoproteins [45]. Although the exact function of merlin as a tumor suppressor has not been resolved (Figure 27.3), it most likely functions to transmit growth regulatory signals that emanate from the plasma membrane, including growth factor receptor and contact inhibition signaling [46–48.]

The two NF2-associated tumors that have been successfully modeled in genetically engineered mice are schwannomas and meningiomas. These mouse models of schwannoma and meningioma result from merlin loss in Schwann cells and leptomeningeal cells, respectively [49,50]. Interestingly, unlike NF1, tumor formation does not appear to require participating cells in the tumor microenvironment and may result from cell autonomous effects of *NF2* loss on Schwann cells and leptomeningeal cells.

TUBEROUS SCLEROSIS COMPLEX

TSC is relatively common, affecting between 1 in 7500 and 11 in 10,000 individuals [51]. While tumors are frequently found in children and adults with TSC, the most devastating problems are mental retardation and epilepsy [52]. Similar to NF1, children with TSC are frequently identified when they present with pigmentary abnormalities. Children with TSC harbor hypopigmented macules, detectable by direct visual inspection or using a Wood's lamp. The diagnosis of TSC is rendered using established diagnostic criteria [53] (Table 27.4).

Children with TSC most frequently present with mental retardation, autistic behaviors, and intractable epilepsy [54]. Neuroimaging often demonstrates the presence of subependymal nodules, which can progress to low-grade brain tumors, termed subependymal giant cell astrocytomas (SEGAs). These tumors can obstruct cerebrospinal fluid flow and lead to hydrocephalus. Other tumors not affecting the nervous system include renal cell carcinoma and pulmonary lymphoangiomatosis.

Unlike NF1 and NF2, there are two distinct genetic loci for TSC. Some families have germline mutations in the *TSC1* gene located on chromosome 9p while others harbor germline mutations in the *TSC2* gene on chromosome 16p [55,56]. Until the protein products of the *TSC1* and *TSC2* genes were identified, it was not clear how TSC could arise from dysfunction of either the *TSC1* or *TSC2* gene; however, biochemical studies have demonstrated that the *TSC1* protein, hamartin, forms a complex with the *TSC2* protein, tuberin [57]. It is this tuberin-hamartin complex that functions to negatively regulate cell growth. Further insights into the mechanism underlying hamartin-tuberin complex function derived from an analysis of the predicted protein sequence of tuberin. A small region of tuberin contains a Ras-like regulatory domain, similar to neurofibromin. Instead of inhibiting Ras, the tuberin-hamartin complex inhibits a different Ras-like protein, called Rheb (*R*as *h*omolog *e*xpressed in *b*rain). Rheb, when active, activates mTOR signaling and leads to increased cell growth [58]. Accordingly, loss of either hamartin or tuberin function renders the complex incapable of inhibiting Rheb activity and leads to increased mTOR signaling (Figure 27.3). As with NF1, current clinical trials are underway using rapamycin and rapamycin analogs to treat TSC-related tumors.

Current mouse models have yet to recapitulate the central nervous system tumors seen in individuals with TSC. However, two groups have generated genetically engineered mice that develop epilepsy [59,60]. These mice have been used to determine how seizures result from impaired astrocyte and neuronal function in TSC [61,62] as well as to evaluate conventional and novel therapies for TSC-associated epilepsy [63]. In these studies, defects in glutamate homeostasis were shown to partly contribute to the pathogenesis of neuronal hyperexcitability. Excitingly, rapamycin treatment dramatically reduced the seizure frequency in *TSC* genetically engineered mice.

SUMMARY

With the identification of the *NF1*, *NF2*, and *TSC* genes, it is possible that the next generation of therapies will target the specific biochemical abnormalities that result from neurofibromin, merlin, or tuberin-hamartin dysfunction. The availability of more targeted therapies coupled with the development of robust small-animal models for many of these important clinical abnormalities provides researchers an ideal situation to rapidly evaluate promising compounds prior to human clinical study. As we learn more about the molecular and cellular pathogenesis of these inherited cancer syndromes, it is highly likely that discoveries that were derived from studies of NF1, NF2, or TSC will lead to improved therapies for histologically similar brain tumors arising in the general population.

Table 27.4 Diagnostic Criteria for Tuberous Sclerosis Complex

Definite TSC: Either two major features or one major feature and two minor features
Probable TSC: One major and one minor feature
Possible TSC: Either one major or one minor feature

Major features
1. Facial angiofibromas or forehead plaque
2. Nontraumatic ungual or periungual fibroma
3. Three of more hypomelanotic macules
4. Shagreen patch
5. Multiple retinal nodular hamartomas
6. Cortical tuber
7. Subependymal nodule
8. Subependymal giant cell astrocytoma
9. Cardiac rhabdomyoma
10. Lymphangiomyomatosis
11. Renal angiomyolipoma

Minor features
1. Multiple dental enamel pits
2. Rectal hamartomas (polyp)
3. Bone cysts
4. Cerebral white matter radial lines
5. Gingival fibromas
6. Nonrenal hamartomas
7. Retinal achromic patch
8. Confetti skin lesions
9. Multiple renal cysts

REFERENCES

1. Knudson AG. Mutation and cancer: statistical study of retinoblastoma. *Proc Natl Acad Sci USA*. 1971;68(4):820–823.
2. Friedman JM. Epidemiology of neurofibromatosis type 1. *Am J Med Genet*. 1999;89(1):1–6.
3. Rutkowski JL, Wu K, Gutmann DH, Boyer PJ, Legius E. Genetic and cellular defects contributing to benign tumor formation in neurofibromatosis type 1. *Hum Mol Genet*. 2000;9(7):1059–1066.
4. Perry A, Roth KA, Banerjee R, Fuller CE, Gutmann DH. NF1 deletions in S-100 protein-positive and negative cells of sporadic and neurofibromatosis 1 (NF1)-associated plexiform neurofibromas and malignant peripheral nerve sheath tumors. *Am J Pathol*. 2001;159(1):57–61.
5. Korf BR. Plexiform neurofibromas. *Am J Med Genet*. 1999;89(1):31–37.
6. Waggoner DJ, Towbin J, Gottesman G, Gutmann DH. Clinic-based study of plexiform neurofibromas in neurofibromatosis 1. *Am J Med Genet*. 2000;92(2):132–135.

7. Ferner RE, Gutmann DH. International consensus statement on malignant peripheral nerve sheath tumors in neurofibromatosis. *Cancer Res.* 2002;62(5):1573–1577.
8. Evans DG, Baser ME, McGaughran J, Sharif S, Howard E, Moran A. Malignant peripheral nerve sheath tumours in neurofibromatosis 1. *J Med Genet.* 2002;39(5):311–314.
9. Listernick R, Charrow J, Greenwald M, Mets M. Natural history of optic pathway tumors in children with neurofibromatosis type 1: a longitudinal study. *J Pediatr.* 1994;125(1):63–66.
10. Habiby R, Silverman B, Listernick R, Charrow J. Precocious puberty in children with neurofibromatosis type 1. *J Pediatr.* 1995;126(3):364–367.
11. Listernick R, Ferner RE, Liu GT, Gutmann DH. Optic pathway gliomas in neurofibromatosis-1: controversies and recommendations. *Ann Neurol.* 2007;61(3):189–198.
12. Leonard JR, Perry A, Rubin JB, King AA, Chicoine MR, Gutmann DH. The role of surgical biopsy in the diagnosis of glioma in individuals with neurofibromatosis-1. *Neurology.* 2006;67(8):1509–1512.
13. Sharif S, Ferner R, Birch JM, et al. Second primary tumors in neurofibromatosis 1 patients treated for optic glioma: substantial risks after radiotherapy. *J Clin Oncol.* 2006;24(16):2570–2575.
14. Bilaniuk LT, Molloy PT, Zimmerman RA, et al. Neurofibromatosis type 1: brain stem tumours. *Neuroradiology.* 1997;39(9):642–653.
15. Gutmann DH, Rasmussen SA, Wolkenstein P, et al. Gliomas presenting after age 10 in individuals with neurofibromatosis type 1 (NF1). *Neurology.* 2002;59(5):759–761.
16. Hyman SL, Shores A, North KN. The nature and frequency of cognitive deficits in children with neurofibromatosis type 1. *Neurology.* 2005;65(7):1037–1044.
17. Friedman JM, Arbiser J, Epstein JA, et al. Cardiovascular disease in neurofibromatosis 1: report of the NF1 Cardiovascular Task Force. *Genet Med.* 2002;4(3):105–111.
18. Hyman SL, Gill DS, Shores EA, Steinberg A, North KN. T2 hyperintensities in children with neurofibromatosis type 1 and their relationship to cognitive functioning. *J Neurol Neurosurg Psychiatr.* 2007;78(10):1088–1091.
19. Gutmann DH, Collins FS. The neurofibromatosis type 1 gene and its protein product, neurofibromin. *Neuron* 1993;10(3):335–343.
20. Weiss B, Bollag G, Shannon K. Hyperactive Ras as a therapeutic target in neurofibromatosis type 1. *Am J Med Genet.* 1999;89(1):14–22.
21. Tong J, Hannan F, Zhu Y, Bernards A, Zhong Y. Neurofibromin regulates G protein-stimulated adenylyl cyclase activity. *Nat Neurosci.* 2002;5(2):95–96.
22. Dasgupta B, Dugan LL, Gutmann DH. The neurofibromatosis 1 gene product neurofibromin regulates pituitary adenylate cyclase-activating polypeptide-mediated signaling in astrocytes. *J Neurosci.* 2003;23(26):8949–8954.
23. Dasgupta B, Yi Y, Chen DY, Weber JD, Gutmann DH. Proteomic analysis reveals hyperactivation of the mammalian target of rapamycin pathway in neurofibromatosis 1-associated human and mouse brain tumors. *Cancer Res.* 2005;65(7):2755–2760.
24. Johannessen CM, Reczek EE, James MF, Brems H, Legius E, Cichowski K. The NF1 tumor suppressor critically regulates TSC2 and mTOR. *Proc Natl Acad Sci USA.* 2005;102(24):8573–8578.
25. Zhu Y, Ghosh P, Charnay P, Burns DK, Parada LF. Neurofibromas in NF1: Schwann cell origin and role of tumor environment. *Science.* 2002;296(5569):920–922.
26. Cichowski K, Shih TS, Schmitt E, et al. Mouse models of tumor development in neurofibromatosis type 1. *Science.* 1999;286(5447):2172–2176.
27. Vogel KS, Klesse LJ, Velasco-Miguel S, Meyers K, Rushing EJ, Parada LF. Mouse tumor model for neurofibromatosis type 1. *Science* 1999;286(5447):2176–2179.
28. Kolanczyk M, Kossler N, Kühnisch J, et al. Multiple roles for neurofibromin in skeletal development and growth. *Hum Mol Genet.* 2007;16(8):874–886.
29. Mahgoub N, Taylor BR, Le Beau MM, et al. Myeloid malignancies induced by alkylating agents in Nf1 mice. *Blood.* 1999;93(11):3617–3623.
30. Tischler AS, Shih TS, Williams BO, Jacks T. Characterization of pheochromocytomas in a mouse strain with a targeted disruptive mutation of the neurofibromatosis gene Nf1. *Endocr Pathol.* 1995;6(4):323–335.
31. Silva AJ, Frankland PW, Marowitz Z, et al. A mouse model for the learning and memory deficits associated with neurofibromatosis type I. *Nat Genet.* 1997;15(3):281–284.
32. Reilly KM, Loisel DA, Bronson RT, McLaughlin ME, Jacks T. Nf1;Trp53 mutant mice develop glioblastoma with evidence of strain-specific effects. *Nat Genet.* 2000;26(1):109–113.
33. Bajenaru ML, Hernandez MR, Perry A, et al. Optic nerve glioma in mice requires astrocyte Nf1 gene inactivation and Nf1 brain heterozygosity. *Cancer Res.* 2003;63(24):8573–8577.
34. Bajenaru ML, Garbow JR, Perry A, Hernandez MR, Gutmann DH. Natural history of neurofibromatosis 1-associated optic nerve glioma in mice. *Ann Neurol.* 2005;57(1):119–127.
35. Zhu Y, Harada T, Liu L, et al. Inactivation of NF1 in CNS causes increased glial progenitor proliferation and optic glioma formation. *Development.* 2005;132(24):5577–5588.
36. Gutmann DH, Hunter-Schaedle K, Shannon KM. Harnessing preclinical mouse models to inform human clinical cancer trials. *J Clin Invest.* 2006;116(4):847–852.
37. Hegedus B, Banerjee D, Yeh TH, et al. Preclinical cancer therapy in a mouse model of neurofibromatosis-1 optic glioma. *Cancer Res.* 2008;68(5):1520–1528.
38. Warrington NM, Woerner BM, Daginakatte GC, et al. Spatiotemporal differences in CXCL12 expression and cyclic AMP underlie the unique pattern of optic glioma growth in neurofibromatosis type 1. *Cancer Res.* 2007;67(18):8588–8595.
39. Daginakatte GC, Gutmann DH. Neurofibromatosis-1 (Nf1) heterozygous brain microglia elaborate paracrine factors that promote Nf1-deficient astrocyte and glioma growth. *Hum Mol Genet.* 2007;16(9):1098–1112.
40. Munchhof AM, Li F, White HA, et al. Neurofibroma-associated growth factors activate a distinct signaling network to alter the function of neurofibromin-deficient endothelial cells. *Hum Mol Genet.* 2006;15(11):1858–1869.
41. Evans DG, Sainio M, Baser ME. Neurofibromatosis type 2. *J Med Genet.* 2000;37(12):897–904.
42. MacCollin M, Chiocca EA, Evans DG, et al. Diagnostic criteria for schwannomatosis. *Neurology.* 2005;64(11):1838–1845.
43. Trofatter JA, MacCollin MM, Rutter JL, et al. A novel moesin-, ezrin-, radixin-like gene is a candidate for the neurofibromatosis 2 tumor suppressor. *Cell.* 1993;75(4):826.
44. Rouleau GA, Merel P, Lutchman M, et al. Alteration in a new gene encoding a putative membrane-organizing protein causes neurofibromatosis type 2. *Nature.* 1993;363(6429):515–521.
45. Sun CX, Robb VA, Gutmann DH. Protein 4.1 tumor suppressors: getting a FERM grip on growth regulation. *J Cell Sci.* 2002;115(pt 21):3991–4000.
46. Morrison H, Sherman LS, Legg J, et al. The NF2 tumor suppressor gene product, merlin, mediates contact inhibition of growth through interactions with CD44. *Genes Dev.* 2001;15(8):968–980.
47. Shaw RJ, Paez JG, Curto M, et al. The Nf2 tumor suppressor, merlin, functions in Rac-dependent signaling. *Dev Cell.* 2001;1(1):63–72.
48. Curto M, Cole BK, Lallemand D, Liu CH, McClatchey AI. Contact-dependent inhibition of EGFR signaling by Nf2/Merlin. *J Cell Biol.* 2007;177(5):893–903.
49. Giovannini M, Robanus-Maandag E, van der Valk M, et al. Conditional biallelic Nf2 mutation in the mouse promotes manifestations of human neurofibromatosis type 2. *Genes Dev.* 2000;14(13):1617–1630.
50. Kalamarides M, Niwa-Kawakita M, Leblois H, et al. Nf2 gene inactivation in arachnoidal cells is rate-limiting for meningioma development in the mouse. *Genes Dev.* 2002;16(9):1060–1065.
51. Gómez MR. History of the tuberous sclerosis complex. *Brain Dev.* 1995;17 (suppl):55–57.
52. Marcotte L, Crino PB. The neurobiology of the tuberous sclerosis complex. *Neuromolecular Med.* 2006;8(4):531–546.
53. Roach ES, Sparagana SP. Diagnosis of tuberous sclerosis complex. *J Child Neurol.* 2004;19(9):643–649.
54. Ess KC. The neurobiology of tuberous sclerosis complex. *Semin Pediatr Neurol.* 2006;13(1):37–42.
55. van Slegtenhorst M, de Hoogt R, Hermans C, et al. Identification of the tuberous sclerosis gene TSC1 on chromosome 9q34. *Science.* 1997;277(5327):805–808.
56. Identification and characterization of the tuberous sclerosis gene on chromosome 16. *Cell.* 1993;75:1305–15.
57. Crino PB, Nathanson KL, Henske EP. The tuberous sclerosis complex. *N Engl J Med.* 2006;355(13):1345–1356.

58. Kwiatkowski DJ, Manning BD. Tuberous sclerosis: a GAP at the crossroads of multiple signaling pathways. *Hum Mol Genet.* 2005;14 Spec No. 2:R251-R258.
59. Uhlmann EJ, Wong M, Baldwin RL, et al. Astrocyte-specific TSC1 conditional knockout mice exhibit abnormal neuronal organization and seizures. *Ann Neurol.* 2002;52(3):285–296.
60. Meikle L, Talos DM, Onda H, et al. A mouse model of tuberous sclerosis: neuronal loss of Tsc1 causes dysplastic and ectopic neurons, reduced myelination, seizure activity, and limited survival. *J Neurosci.* 2007;27(21):5546–5558.
61. Wong M, Ess KC, Uhlmann EJ, et al. Impaired glial glutamate transport in a mouse tuberous sclerosis epilepsy model. *Ann Neurol.* 2003;54(2):251–256.
62. Zeng LH, Ouyang Y, Gazit V, et al. Abnormal glutamate homeostasis and impaired synaptic plasticity and learning in a mouse model of tuberous sclerosis complex. *Neurobiol Dis.* 2007;28(2):184–196.
63. Zeng LH, Xu L, Gutmann DH, Wong M. Rapamycin prevents epilepsy in a mouse model of tuberous sclerosis complex. *Ann Neurol.* 2008;63(4):444–453.

PART III: CLINICAL PRESENTATION AND SUPPORTIVE CARE

28 Presentation and Clinical Features of Supratentorial Gliomas in Adults

Herbert B. Newton

Primary brain tumors represent approximately 2% of newly diagnosed malignancies each year in the United States, with an annual incidence across all age groups of 6 to 9 per 100,000 population [1,2]. This corresponds to about 17,000 to 20,000 pathologically verified new cases per year. Supratentorial gliomas are an important subgroup of primary brain tumors that can occur at any age and are quite variable in their degree of histological malignancy [3]. In adults, the most common age range for development of a supratentorial glioma is 45 to 55 years, with lower grade tumors tending to occur in younger patients, and malignant tumors more often affecting older patients. High-grade tumors such as glioblastoma multiforme and anaplastic astrocytoma are the most commonly diagnosed supratentorial gliomas. Lower grade tumors, including oligodendroglioma, astrocytoma, and ganglioglioma, are diagnosed at a much lower frequency.

The neurological presentation of supratentorial gliomas is quite variable [1,3]. They can elevate intracranial pressure (ICP), often causing generalized symptoms such as headache, nausea, and diplopia. Focal symptoms and signs can also develop depending on the location of the neoplasm and can affect eloquent areas of brain that mediate functions such as language, vision, or sensation. In benign tumors (e.g., pilocytic astrocytoma), the clinical course is slow and indolent, with symptoms developing over months to years. In more malignant tumors (e.g., glioblastoma) the onset of symptoms is more rapid, occurring over days, weeks, or a few months.

PRESENTING SIGNS AND SYMPTOMS

The most important feature of the clinical presentation in most patients with supratentorial gliomas is the *progressive nature* of the symptoms [1]. The evolving presentation is variable and depends on many factors, including the type of tumor and its method of growth (infiltrative versus expansile), the location of the tumor within the brain, the rapidity of growth, and the degree of associated edema and mass effect. Table 28.1 lists the common symptoms noted at presentation in a large series of adult patients with supratentorial gliomas. Individually, none of these symptoms is pathognomonic for an intracranial tumor. However, the clinical suspicion should increase if several of these symptoms occur together in the context of a *progressive* neurological illness. The symptoms (and signs) associated with an intracranial neoplasm can be divided into two groups: generalized, produced by disturbances of ICP regulation; and focal, produced by alteration of function of specialized regions of the brain due to tissue destruction and/or compression.

Neurological Symptoms

The most common generalized symptoms of intracranial neoplasms are headache, generalized seizure activity, cognitive and personality changes, nausea and emesis, diplopia, and alteration of consciousness [1,3]. These symptoms occur as the expanding tumor and associated edema raise ICP and compress localized nervous system structures. Compression of ventricular pathways by the tumor and associated edema may cause hydrocephalus, which will further augment elevated ICP.

Headache is the most common symptom produced by intracranial tumors, present in two-thirds of patients with gliomas. Headaches are probably caused by a combination of elevated ICP and traction on sensitive structures such as blood vessels and overlying dura mater. The headache usually occurs in the frontal or vertex region, but may be more diffuse. Headaches may be most severe in the morning because of elevated pCO_2 that develops during the hypoventilation of sleep, increasing cerebral blood volume and exacerbating peritumoral edema, and because of reduced cerebrospinal fluid drainage in the recumbent position. However, morning headache is not specific only to brain tumors, because patients with migraine can also develop this pattern. Brain tumor–related headache is usually of moderate to severe intensity and will often last for hours at a time. The intensity of pain may be increased by coughing, sneezing, straining, or other maneuvers that increase intrathoracic (and consequently intracranial) pressure. In most patients with intracranial neoplasms, the headaches are progressive in frequency and intensity and are more resistant to analgesics than prior non-tumor-related headaches. Nausea and emesis are present in one-third of patients with intracranial tumors and are not always correlated with headaches. They are caused by elevation of ICP and are also frequently most severe in the morning.

Table 28.1 Common Symptoms at Presentation of Patients with Supratentorial Gliomas

Symptom	All Gliomas (% Cases) N = 653
Headache	70
Seizure activity:	54
Partial motor	23
Generalized tonic-clonic	20
Partial complex	9
Absence	2
Cognitive/personality change	52
Focal weakness	43
Nausea/vomiting	31
Speech disturbance	27
Alteration of consciousness	25
Sensory abnormalities	14
Visual disturbances	8

Adapted from refs. 1 and 2.

Table 28.2 Common Neurologic Signs in Patients with Supratentorial Gliomas

Neurological Sign	All Gliomas (% Cases) N = 1251
Hemiparesis	57
Cranial nerve palsies	54
Papilledema	53
Cognitive changes/confusion	45
Depressed sensorium	37
Hemianesthesia	30
Hemianopsia	29
Dysphasia	25

Adapted from refs. 1 and 2.

Generalized seizures occur in the form of tonic-clonic or absence seizures in one-fifth of patients. Irritation and compression of neural tissues occurs as the tumor grows, producing epileptogenic activity that generalizes to the whole brain. Generalized seizures can often be the initial symptom of an intracranial neoplasm, which therefore should always be included in the differential diagnosis of a first seizure, especially in patients greater than 20 to 25 years of age.

Changes in cognition and personality may be caused by elevation of ICP, mass effect, and disruption of central pathways. Mild alterations of memory, concentration, and reasoning are commonly noticed by family members. Dulling of affect or loss of energy and initiative may also develop. Elevated ICP can also disturb the patient's level of consciousness, producing lethargy, drowsiness, irritability, or coma. The most common alteration is excessive daytime sleepiness or lethargy that is typically noted by a spouse or parent.

Complaints of double vision and other general visual disturbances may develop. Diplopia is caused by dysfunction of the sixth cranial nerve secondary to elevated ICP, as the nerve courses from the brainstem to the orbit. It is considered a false localizing sign, as it is not due to a direct effect of tumor on the nerve. It is often apparent to the patient before dysconjugation is noted by the physician.

Focal symptoms are helpful for localization of the tumor and occur because of destruction, compression, or irritation of specialized regions of the brain. Tumors near the cerebral cortex can induce focal motor or sensory seizures, most often affecting the contralateral face and arm. Todd's postictal paralysis, prolonged weakness of the limbs that develops after seizure activity, is more common with intracranial tumors than other conditions. Focal symptoms such as personality or cognitive changes (e.g., apathy, dulling of affect, jocularity, forgetfulness), limb weakness or loss of sensation, speech disturbances, visual field changes, gait disturbances (e.g., ataxia, imbalance), and limb incoordination occur frequently in patients with brain tumors and are commonly progressive.

Neurological Signs

The neurological examination is an important tool for analyzing the signs that develop in brain tumor patients. The common neurological signs from a series of adults with supratentorial gliomas are listed in Table 28.2. Hemiparesis, cranial nerve palsies, and papilledema are noted in most patients [1,3]. Hemiparetic weakness often involves the arm more than the leg and may be accompanied by an ipsilateral increase in tendon reflexes and a Babinski sign. Arm weakness is usually more severe in extensor than flexor muscles. The most common cranial nerve palsies are lower facial weakness (ipsilateral to the hemiparesis), caused by seventh nerve dysfunction and incomplete eye abduction, secondary to sixth nerve dysfunction. A detailed funduscopic examination is necessary when considering an intracranial neoplasm. Papilledema is seen as swelling of the optic nerve head with blurring of the disc margin and reduced venous pulsations; in more severe stages, retinal venous engorgement and hemorrhages may occur. Severe papilledema may produce central visual field defects because of enlargement of the blind spot. Hemianopic visual field defects are found on examination in almost one-third of patients. If the defect develops slowly, the patient may remain unaware of the deficit. Speech disturbances can manifest as difficulty with articulation (dysarthria) or as a deficit in language (dysphasia), with an impaired ability to express or understand speech. Further characterization of the symptoms and signs of an intracranial neoplasm will depend on the specific anatomical location of the tumor within the intracranial cavity. The clinical manifestations of tumors located in different supratentorial regions of the brain will be discussed in the following text.

NEOPLASMS OF THE CEREBRAL HEMISPHERES

Supratentorial gliomas of the cerebral hemispheres usually occur in adults between 35 and 55 years of age. The degree of neurological compromise will depend on the size of the tumor, the specific lobe (or lobes) of the brain affected, and whether the tumor is on the dominant or nondominant side of the brain [1,3]. In all right-handed and most left-handed patients, the left hemisphere is dominant for speech. Tumor growth within or near the pars opercularis of the dominant inferior frontal lobe (Broca area) results in a nonfluent "expressive" language deficit (dysphasia), with an impaired ability to articulate speech. The patient is often frustrated and states he can think of what he wants to say, but can't get the words out. Comprehension remains intact, whereas repetition is disturbed in most patients. In addition to expressive language function, the frontal lobes also mediate many aspects of personality and executive activities. Symptoms are more severe in bifrontal lesions, but can occur with unilateral tumors. Orbitofrontal neoplasms often cause disinhibited behavior, irritability, jocularity, and lack of social awareness. Dorsal midline tumors may cause abulia, with profoundly slowed initiation of thought, speech, and motor behavior. Tumors affecting the dorsolateral convexity region usually cause apathy, depressed mentation, impaired planning, and lack of motivation. Bifrontal inferomedial lesions (eg, "butterfly" gliomas) may present as a dementia resembling Alzheimer disease. Frontal lobe release signs may appear with any of these lesions, including the glabellar, snout, and palmomental reflexes. Compression or destruction of the precentral gyrus (primary motor cortex) will result in varying degrees of contralateral spastic hemiparesis. Parasagittal lesions can present similar to a myelopathy, with spastic paraparesis and impaired bowel and bladder function. Seizures are common with tumors of the frontal lobes. They can be generalized, focal, or partial complex. Focal seizures usually manifest as clonic activity affecting the contralateral face and arm, less commonly the leg. They can also cause speech arrest and, if the frontal eye field (premotor cortex) is irritated, contralateral conjugate deviation of the eyes and head. Partial complex seizures may occur with tumors in the prefrontal region, as manifested by altered level of consciousness and automatisms. In some patients with high-grade, infiltrative gliomas of the frontal lobes, the neurological examination may be normal.

Tumors developing within the parietal lobes most often disturb the postcentral gyrus (primary sensory cortex), causing contralateral sensory loss, astereognosis, and agraphesthesia. Posteriorly placed tumors on the dominant side may disturb Wernicke area, causing a fluent "receptive" language deficit with impaired repetition. These patients speak fluently, often with excessive "empty" speech, yet lack comprehension of spoken or written words. Most patients with receptive aphasia are unaware of their deficit and do not appear frustrated. Dominant side lesions near the angular gyrus may produce Gerstmann syndrome, with agraphia, acalculia, right/left disorientation, and finger agnosia. Nondominant parietal lesions may result in a neglect syndrome, as manifested in mild cases by contralateral extinction to sensory stimuli. In more severe cases, parietal lobe neglect can cause severe spatial disorientation, with complete inattention to the contralateral side of the body and environment. Parietal lesions may also cause apraxias, the inability to formulate and execute complex motor behaviors such as dressing or constructions, despite intact strength and coordination. Tumors of either parietal lobe can cause apraxia, but it is more common on the nondominant side. Disturbance of the deep parietal white matter can affect the optic radiations, causing a contralateral lower homonymous quadrantanopsia. Generalized and focal seizures can also develop from tumors within the parietal lobes. Focal seizures usually present as intermittent sensory phenomena on the contralateral side of the body.

Temporal lobe gliomas may be clinically silent if located anteriorly. Seizures are very common with medial and posterior neoplasms. They are often partial complex, associated with alteration of consciousness and motor automatisms, although generalized seizures can also occur. Large superomedial tumors may cause motor deficits by compressing the adjacent frontal lobe. Dominant side medially placed tumors may cause loss of verbal memory, whereas nondominant side lesions may affect visuo-spatial memory. Disturbance of deep white matter can cause a contralateral superior homonymous quadrantanopsia. Tumors affecting the uncus or parahippocampal gyrus may cause olfactory hallucinations (eg, metallic or unpleasant odors) and impaired memory. If the posterior aspect of the dominant superior temporal gyrus is affected, a fluent "receptive" dysphasia may develop, similar to Wernicke's.

Lesions affecting the occipital lobes usually cause a contralateral partial or complete homonymous hemianopsia. Dominant side occipital lobe tumors, in association with damage to the posterior corpus callosum, may present with the syndrome of "alexia without agraphia," in which the patient is unable to read, but still has intact spoken and written language skills. Seizures caused by tumors of the occipital region usually manifest as intermittent flashing lights or unformed images.

NEOPLASMS OF THE THALAMUS AND BASAL GANGLIA

Thalamic tumors cause headache, contralateral sensory loss, and contralateral weakness with pyramidal tract signs if the mass compresses the internal capsule [4]. The sensory loss may be subtle in some patients, but should be suspected if there is hyperpathia with a distinctive "burning" quality to it. On the dominant side, thalamic neoplasms may cause a nonfluent form of dysphasia, as well as behavioral changes that may resemble dementia. Less often, patients develop a nonspecific, persistent headache secondary to hydrocephalus and elevated ICP pressure. Other less frequent symptoms and signs include visual loss, impaired cognition, reduced level of alertness, and seizures.

Tumors that originate within the basal ganglia, or infiltrate there from nearby regions of brain (i.e., thalamus), have a similar presentation to primary thalamic gliomas. The most common symptoms and signs are headache, contralateral weakness with pyramidal tract signs, gait impairment, and impaired cognition. In addition, gliomas in this region may cause movement disorders, such as tremor and hemiballismus [5]. Tumors isolated to the basal ganglia do not typically have a prominent sensory component.

NEOPLASMS OF THE PINEAL REGION

A large variety of tumors can develop in this region (e.g., germinoma, pineoblastoma), including gliomas

[6]. Headache is common and results from elevated ICP, with or without associated hydrocephalus. Pineal tumors often cause hydrocephalus by compressing the aqueduct of Sylvius during its course through the midbrain. Compression of the nearby dorsal midbrain by tumor often causes Parinaud syndrome, which consists of paralysis of upgaze, retraction nystagmus, pupillary light-near dissociation, and impaired convergence. Further compression or infiltration of tumor into the brainstem or cerebellum will result in pyramidal tract signs, cranial nerve palsies, dysmetria, and ataxia. Rarely, endocrine abnormalities can be noted with pineal tumors, including diabetes insipidus.

RADIOLOGIC DIAGNOSIS

In a patient with a history and neurologic examination suspicious for a supratentorial glioma, neuroimaging is an essential tool for diagnosis. Magnetic resonance imaging (MRI), in combination with a paramagnetic contrast agent, has become the modality of choice for diagnosing intracranial neoplasms [7]. The tumor will appear as a region of altered signal with surrounding edema and mass effect (see Figure 28.1). Most malignant tumors enhance with contrast, due to an alteration of the blood-brain barrier within tumor vasculature. However, MRI can clearly demonstrate low-grade tumors and allows the differentiation of vascular masses from tumors. In addition, MR images can be formatted into axial, coronal, and sagittal sections, which can be very useful for detection of tumors in certain supratentorial locations, such as the medial temporal lobes or pineal region.

Despite the overall superiority of MRI for the diagnosis of supratentorial tumors, computed tomography (CT) remains an excellent diagnostic technique. After the addition of a contrast agent, CT can readily demonstrate the enhancing mass, surrounding edema, and mass effect associated with most tumors (see Figure 28.2).

COMMON DIAGNOSTIC DILEMMAS

As mentioned earlier, many of the common neurological signs and symptoms of patients with supratentorial gliomas are not specific to brain tumors. The progressive nature of these complaints will eventually differentiate them from their non-neoplastic counterparts. Headaches occur frequently in the general population. The vast majority of these headaches are not related to intracranial tumors. Acute and chronic tension headaches present with head and neck pain described as tight, pressing, squeezing, and band-like. They are often precipitated by fatigue, family crises, work deadlines, or other stressful situations. Tension headaches respond well to mild analgesics and, after cessation of the causative stimulus, usually improve. Migraine headaches are typically described as pounding or throbbing and are often associated with nausea, emesis, and photophobia. Cluster headaches occur in periodic cycles and are extremely painful. The pain usually affects one eye and is associated with ipsilateral scleral injection, tearing, rhinorrhea, and sinus congestion. Differentiating brain tumor–related headaches from other common headaches by history is very difficult. Patients previously free of headaches who now develop them should be evaluated carefully, especially if they are in an older age group. Patients with stable headache disorders that have a well-described pain pattern who then complain of a *new type* of headache, or of a progressive worsening of their headaches, need close observation and possibly neuroimaging. Normal neurological examination and absence of papilledema significantly lower the risk for presence of a brain neoplasm but do not rule it out. Disorders such as glaucoma and temporal arteritis should also be investigated using tonometry and an erythrocyte sedimentation rate, respectively. Other common conditions that might cause headaches should also be discussed, including hypertension, allergies, cervical degenerative joint disease, oral contraceptive usage, and

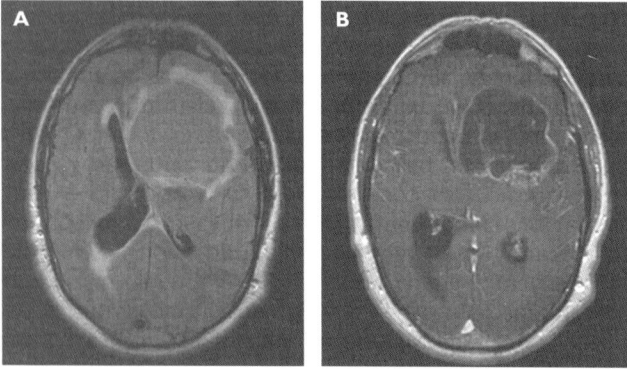

Figure 28.1 MRI scan of 59-year-old male with progressive headache, expressive language dysfunction, and dysnomia. (A) Axial FLAIR image demonstrating large, cystic, lesion within the left frontal lobe, with surrounding edema, mass effect, and midline shift. (B) Axial T1-weighted image after contrast injection with gadolinium-DTPA, demonstrating enhancement of the noncystic portions of the lesion. Resection proved this to be a glioblastoma.

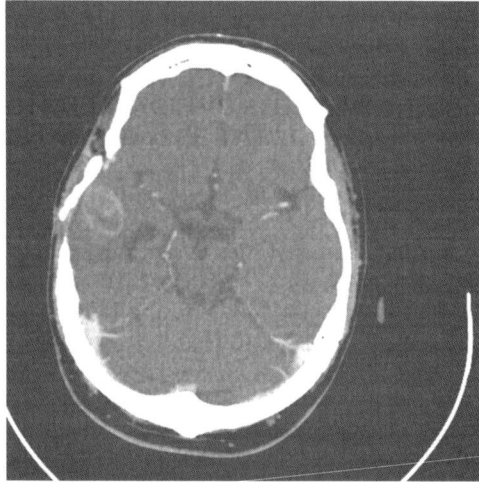

Figure 28.2 CT scan of a 27-year-old male with complaints of headache, left-sided weakness, leg stiffness, and gait imbalance. This axial contrast-enhanced image clearly shows an enhancing mass in the right temporal lobe. This proved to be a recurrent anaplastic ependymoma.

visual refractive errors. Nausea and emesis are common symptoms of numerous gastrointestinal ailments. When these symptoms occur as part of the presentation of a brain tumor, the clinician may significantly delay proper diagnosis and treatment if a central nervous system cause is not considered. Extensive gastrointestinal evaluations are occasionally performed early in the course of brain tumor patients when nausea and emesis can be prominent, and other symptoms may be more subtle (eg, spasticity, gait difficulty, weakness, and diplopia).

The clinical presentation of non-neoplastic disorders can, on occasion, be suggestive of an intracranial tumor. Focal symptoms and signs can be seen with multiple sclerosis, stroke, abscess, enlarging aneurysm, encephalitis, infectious or neoplastic meningitis, cerebral vasculitis, and others. A detailed history and neurological examination, enhanced MRI scan, and, if necessary, cerebrospinal fluid evaluation will usually differentiate these diseases from an intracranial neoplasm. On occasion, the CT or MRI findings may be equivocal, so that the diagnosis remains unclear. Cerebral abscess is the only entity which typically has a progressive course and ring-enhancing appearance that is similar to a brain neoplasm on contrast-enhanced CT or MRI. Biopsy is often necessary to clarify the diagnosis between intracranial tumor and abscess.

REFERENCES

1. Newton HB. Primary brain tumors: review of etiology, diagnosis, and treatment. *Am Fam Phys.* 1994;49:787–797.
2. Buckner JC, Brown PD, O'Neill BP, Meyer FB, Wetmore CJ, Uhm JH. Central nervous system tumors. *Mayo Clin Proc.* 2007;82:1271–1286.
3. Berger MS, Leibel SA, Bruner JM, Finlay JL, Levin VA. Primary central nervous system tumors of the supratentorial compartment. In: Levin VA, ed. *Cancer in the Nervous System.* New York: Churchill Livingstone; 1996:57–126.
4. Nishio S, Morioka T, Suzuki S, Takeshita I, Fukui M. Thalamic gliomas: a clinicopathologic analysis of 20 cases with reference to patient age. *Acta Neurochir (Wien).* 1997;139:336–342.
5. Krauss JK, Nobbe F, Wakhloo AK, Mohadier M, Vach W, Mundinger F. Movement disorders in astrocytomas of the basal ganglia and the thalamus. *J Neurol Neurosurg Psych.* 1992;55:1162–1167.
6. Blakeley JO, Grossman SA. Management of pineal region tumors. *Curr Treat Options Oncol.* 2006;7:505–516.
7. Jenkinson MD, Plessis DG, Walker C, Smith TS. Advanced MRI in the management of adult gliomas. *Br J Neurosurg.* 2007;21:550–561.

29 Presentation and Clinical Features of Brain Metastases

Deborah T. Blumenthal and Felix Bokstein

EPIDEMIOLOGY

Brain metastases occur in 15% to 40% of patients with a known synchronous or prior diagnosis of solid cancer [1,2]. The annual incidence of brain metastases in the United States may be as high as 170,000 cases. These numbers are increased compared with older data [3]. This increase may reflect better reporting, better detection with advanced imaging, or actual increased incidence of cases related to prolonged survival of patients being treated for their systemic neoplasm.

A newly presenting space-occupying brain lesion is much more likely to be a metastasis, even without a prior diagnosis of systemic neoplasm, than a primary glioma, which occurs at about one-tenth the frequency [2]. Autopsy studies were a primary source of epidemiological data for brain metastases in the past decades but are becoming more limited in their utility, as they are performed less often. Magnetic resonance imaging (MRI)–based studies are more representative of the incidence of brain metastases in the population at large. Data culled from various primary tumor–specific autopsy studies showed a 20% to 50% incidence of brain metastases in lung cancers (brain metastases occur less commonly in squamous type lung adenocarcinomas), approximately 20% incidence in breast cancers, 46% to 68% incidence in melanomas, 10% to 17% incidence in renal cell cancers, and 6% incidence in gastrointestinal cancers [4,5]. Although brain metastases may be diagnosed at the time of systemic disease discovery in up to one-third of cases, most brain metastases are seen in later stage, advanced cancer, or at the time of recurrence [6,7].

More than 10% of brain metastases are from an unknown primary origin, and 25% to 50% of these will remain unknown despite extensive diagnostic work-up [8,9]. Immunohistochemical stains, as described in Correlation To Systemic Disease section, combined with appropriate imaging, can identify a primary site in a substantial portion of cases.

Most brain metastases are located in the larger volume of the cerebral hemispheres (~80%), with 10% to 15% found in the cerebellum and less than 5% in the brainstem. There appears to be a higher incidence of pelvic and gastrointestinal primary sources in infratentorial metastases [9].

Although older reports cite a rate of 50% for solitary metastases, more cases are likely multiple. MRI is a superior modality for detecting smaller metastases and those in areas prone to volumetric artifacts. Thirty percent of patients with a single metastasis found on computed tomography will have multiple lesions on MRI. Hence, brain MRI with contrast is the examination of choice for diagnostic evaluation of suspected metastases (see Figure 29.1) [9,10].

In recent years, as systemic treatments have become more successful in prolonging longevity, the central nervous system has become a "reservoir" of disease, or a physiologically isolated site not broached by otherwise successful systemic biochemotherapy, wherein brain metastases develop. In addition, advanced methods of imaging and more frequent surveillance of the central nervous system in asymptomatic patients may be increasing the incidence of reported brain metastases.

Most brain metastases are of primary histologies of lung, breast, and melanoma neoplasms. Lung and breast remain the most commonly diagnosed systemic cancers, whereas other less frequent cancers such as melanoma, which represents less than 5% of all cancers, have a higher propensity for brain involvement [2]. Melanoma spreads to the central nervous system in approximately half of the cases of advanced disease [11]. Renal cell cancer and gastrointestinal cancers are the next most commonly seen primary cancers that metastasize to the brain.

CLINICAL PRESENTATION, DIAGNOSIS, AND IMAGING

The differential diagnosis for space-occupying intracranial lesions includes brain metastases, primary brain tumor, brain abscess, intracranial hemorrhage, demyelinating disease, and cerebral infarct. A landmark study, which established the important role of surgery for single, accessible brain metastases, showed that 11% of known cancer patients with a single brain lesion unexpectedly had diagnoses other than brain metastases when the lesion was biopsied or resected [12].

MRI is the established imaging mode of choice for diagnosis of brain metastases [13]. Classically, metastases appear rounded, with vivid uptake of contrast agent (Gd-DTPA, gadolinium). They may have a central cystic or necrotic component. Their borders tend to be defined, which can differentiate them radiographically from more infiltrative and diffuse primary glial tumors (see Figure 29.2). Vasogenic edema in the extracellular spaces of

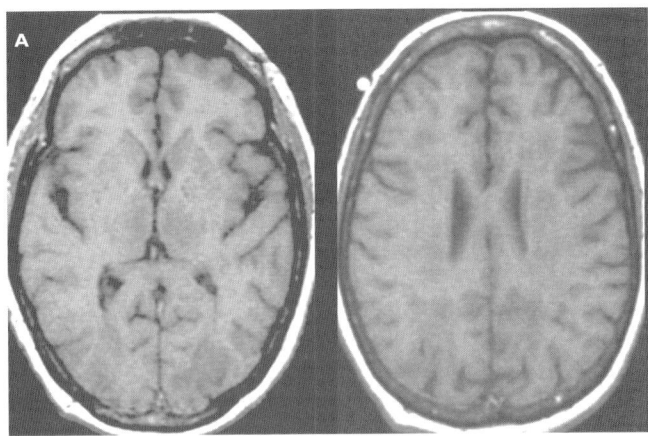
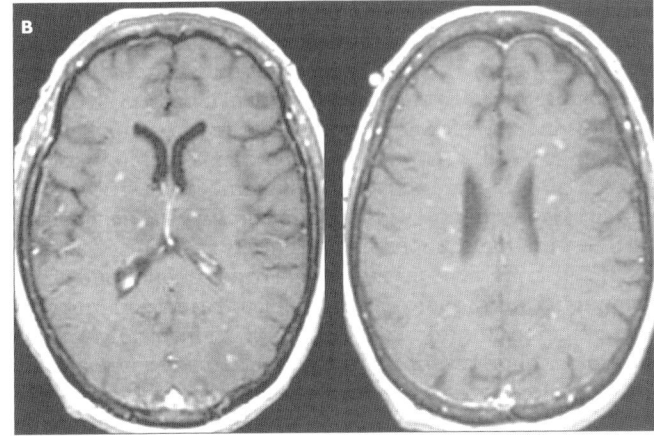

Figure 29.1 Patient with multiple miliary breast cancer metastases. **(A)** T1-weighted axial MRI without gadolinium. **(B)** T1-weighted axial MRI with gadolinium.

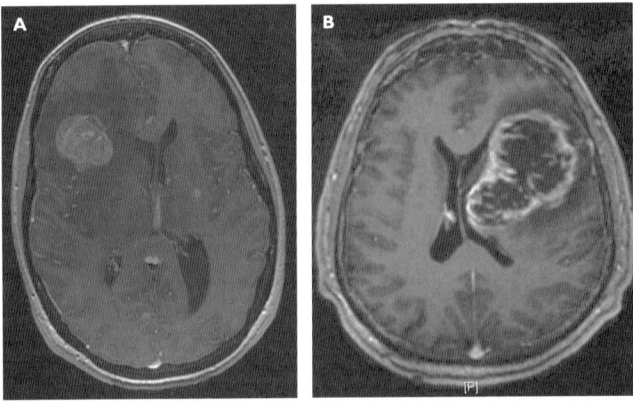

Figure 29.2 Axial T1-weighted gadolinium enhanced MRIs. **(A)** 33-year-old woman with NSCLC, large right frontal lesion, numerous miliary nodules. Note relatively rounded, enhancing lesion, with surrounding moderate edema and mass effect. Note two other small, enhancing lesions in left insula and right medial occipital lobes. **(B)** 59-year-old man presenting with cognitive changes and dysphasia. Note infiltrative left frontal mass emanating from the white matter, with irregular border, and heterogenous enhancement. Diagnosis: glioblastoma multiforme, primary brain tumor.

the white matter is typically present, and can be marked in some cases, not necessarily corresponding with the size of the inciting metastatic lesion. The severity of neurological symptoms associated with the lesions and edema depends not only upon their overall volume but also upon the location/compartment of the metastasis; posterior fossa lesions may be more symptomatic as they can lead to early hydrocephalus from fourth ventricle compression.

Brain metastases can present acutely, related to an associated event such as hemorrhage, seizure, or acute increase in intracranial pressure; or more progressively, related to gradual growth of tumor volume and associated edema; or development of hydrocephalus. The most common presenting symptom of brain metastases is headache; headaches are the presenting complaint in up to 50% of patients with brain metastatic involvement. However, more than 70% of known cancer patients who complain of headaches have causes other than brain metastases [14]. Focal presenting symptoms are related to the location of the metastasis relative to eloquent or symptomatic areas in the brain. Such symptoms include lateralized weakness, aphasia, hemisensory loss, or ataxia. Lesions related to increased pressure include headache and papilledema, nausea and vomiting, or mental status/level of consciousness changes. Seizures may be seen in about 10% of cases.

Between 2% and 7% of brain metastases may present with hemorrhage before any intervention. The most common hemorrhagic brain metastases are from lung origin, related to the largest denominator of brain metastases being of lung primary source (although only about 5% of brain metastases from lung have a hemorrhagic component) [15,16]. Choriocarcinoma and melanoma metastases to the brain have the highest relative incidence of hemorrhage. Up to 80% of melanoma brain metastases are associated with hemorrhage, although often the bleed is clinically asymptomatic (see Figure 29.3) [17]. There may be an increased risk of hemorrhage in larger metastases following treatment with radiosurgery within the month of treatment, although this remains speculative [18,19].

CORRELATION TO SYSTEMIC DISEASE; PATHOLOGICAL DIAGNOSIS-SPECIAL STAINS; PROGNOSTIC FACTORS

Close to half of newly diagnosed brain metastases are not readily associated with a primary systemic cancer of origin at time of diagnosis. Fifty to seventy percent of such cases will ultimately be identified as being from a lung source [20]. Specific immunohistochemical stains may be useful in identifying the likely organs of origin for adenocarcinoma brain metastases and can guide in choosing specific tests to locate the primary source of disease.

Cytokeratin 7 and thyroid transcription factor-1 positivity indicate a lung origin, whereas cytokeratin 20 positivity with negative cytokeratin 7 indicates a colorectal source. Melanoma is associated with positive staining of vimentin, S100, HMB-45, and negative cytokeratin [21].

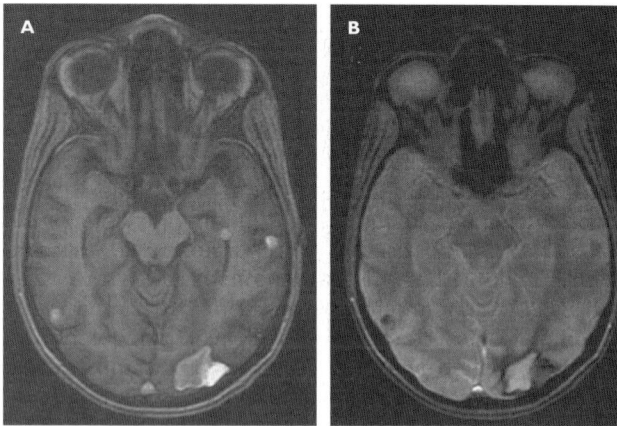

Figure 29.3 A 43-year-old woman with forehead melanoma resected 7 years earlier, presenting with headaches and subacute visual field disturbance. Axial MRI images: **(A)** T1-gadolinium enhanced sequence showing contrast-enhancing metastatic lesions. **(B)** T2 gradient echo sequence more clearly demonstrating hemorrhagic components of larger left occipital and smaller right posterior temporal lesions.

Breast cancer is associated with positive CA 15–3, cytokeratin 7, estrogen and progesterone receptor staining in some cases, and negative thyroid transcription factor-1, CA 125, and CA 19–9 [22,23].

Once a metastatic lesion is identified, the status of systemic disease (in known malignancies as well) needs to be established, as this has an effect on the overall prognosis and influences treatment decisions that need to be made regarding the brain disease.

Prediction of the biological behavior of a metastatic lesion may have an effect on the decision to treat with adjuvant modalities after resection, specifically, radiotherapy. A recent study of resected single metastases, which were followed without radiation after surgery, showed a propensity for early relapse (within 2 months of resection) for those lesions with a higher proliferative index. The same study also correlated a higher incidence of early brain metastasis relapse with synchronous metastases (those occurring before or within 2 months of systemic neoplasm diagnosis) compared with metachronous metastases [24]. A separate study of non–small cell lung cancer patients with brain metastases compared with non–small cell lung cancer without brain involvement correlated higher primary tumor Ki-67 index, lower caspase-3 expression, higher vascular endothelial growth factor-C (VEGF-C) expression, and lower E-cadherin with development of brain metastases.

The relevance of HER2/neu status in the prognosis of breast cancer patients with brain metastases is emerging. Some studies suggest a higher incidence of spread to the brain in those patients who initially respond to trastuzumab treatment [25].

A recent retrospective study of breast cancer patients with brain metastases showed that hormone-positive disease, younger age (<50 years), Karnofsky Performance Score >80, and favorably responsive systemic disease were factors associated with better survival on multivariate analysis. Median survival after diagnosis of brain metastases was 14.4 months. Brain metastases associated with breast cancer presented at a median of 38 months from systemic disease diagnosis (triple the median latency time seen for presentation of lung cancer brain metastases), and at a shorter period for hormone-negative patients. The HER2/neu status was neither associated with difference in survival in these patients nor with a shorter time to presentation of metastases after primary disease diagnosis [26].

Aside from treatment, which will be addressed in a later chapter and which has the greatest effect on prognosis, there are several clinical factors that have been repeatedly shown to be associated with improved survival. These include the status of systemic disease, the age of the patient, and the clinical (Karnofsky) performance score. A Radiation Therapy Oncology Group study validated these factors by recursive partitioning analysis (RPA) of 1200 patients with brain metastases (single or "oligometastases") treated on several prospective trials (see Table 29.1) [27,28]. Patients younger than 65 years with independent clinical function and controlled systemic disease had median survival of 7.1 months, compared with older patients with poorly controlled disease (4.2 months) and poorer clinical function (2.3 months). The RPA classification may be used as a guide in determining candidates for surgical or other treatment interventions. However, some patients, despite a poorer RPA score or presence of more than three metastatic lesions, may still benefit from palliative intervention to alleviate focal neurologic or pressure-related symptoms of a given metastatic lesion.

A large review of more than 1200 patients from the Netherlands confirmed the importance of three clinical prognostic factors: performance status, response to steroids, and evidence of active systemic disease. Serum lactate dehydrogenase level was also found to be significant on multivariate analysis. Treatment (steroids, neurosurgery, and radiation) was found to be the most influential modality correlating to improved outcome [29].

THEORIES OF SPREAD, MIGRATION, PROPENSITIES

Brain metastases are thought to arrive at the end organ via hematogenous routes. As such, most lesions are seen

Table 29.1 RTOG RPA Classification of Brain Metastases

RPA Class	Criteria	Median Survival (months)
1	KPS ≥ 70 Age < 65 years No extracranial metastases Controlled primary tumor	7.1
2	KPS ≥ 70 At least one of the following: Age > 65 years Uncontrolled primary tumor Systemic metastases	4.2
3	KPS < 70	2.3

Abbreviations: KPS, Karnofsky performance score; RPA, recursive partitioning analysis; RTOG, Radiation Therapy Oncology Group.

at grey-white junctions at the "watershed" end zones of the middle cerebral artery branches [9]. The vascular routes of entry to the brain include the carotid arteries, vertebrobasilar circulation, and venous plexuses (Batson venous plexus). Metastases may commonly reach the brain from the lung arterial circulation, primary lung sources, or from metastases traveling via the lung. About 80% of brain metastatic lesions are found in the cerebrum, 15% in the cerebellum, and about 5% in the brainstem, reflecting the distribution of the intracranial blood flow [3,9]. Some types of primary tumors show specific predilections to different parts of the brain, such as melanoma to the cerebral cortex and basal ganglia, or pelvic and abdominal tumors to the posterior fossa [9,30]. Formation of brain metastases is usually the result of interaction between metastasizing tumor cells and brain tissue microenvironment, whereas the processes of invasion, proliferation, and angiogenesis are strongly influenced by brain tissue–derived growth factors [31,32].

Vasogenic edema associated with brain metastases may be mediated by VEGF and nitric oxide. Migratory activity of metastatic cells and binding with tissue matrix integrins may be partly influenced by VEGF interactions with adhesion kinases and tyrosine kinase beta [33]. Nitric oxide synthase isoenzymes (NOS) may be induced in the metabolic hypoxic milieu at the site of brain metastasis. Certain NOS forms (NOS III) may be associated with less vasogenic edema. There may be a positive correlation between NOS expression, VEGF receptor, and the presence of microglia and macrophages, which may affect tumor migration [33].

Retroviral manipulation of osteosarcoma cell lines show Notch pathway gene expression to be associated with invasive and metastatic potential [34]. Microarray gene expression profile studies of cell lines derived from breast cancer metastases have shown the Notch signaling pathway to play an important role in migration and invasion [35].

Additional studies of breast cancer metastatic to brain models show significantly more expression of VEGF-A and interleukin 8 in culture supernatants than the original cell lines, and more VEGF-A RNA expression when cultured. Decreased cell survival is seen when these lines are treated with VEGF-receptor tyrosine kinase inhibitor, suggesting a potential target for therapy based on the VEGF-R mechanism [36].

SUPPORTIVE TREATMENT

Definitive treatment of brain metastases, which includes surgical resection, radiation therapy, radiosurgery, and chemotherapy, is addressed in separate chapters. Supportive therapies provide initial, maintenance, and often later stage palliation for patients, and can prolong survival.

Steroids can be helpful to acutely contain the clinical symptoms secondary to metastases and associated edema. However, steroids can cause multiple side effects that limit the quality of life for patients with brain metastases; they are not required for asymptomatic lesions. Once definitive treatment is initiated (surgery, radiosurgery, radiation) steroids can often be successfully weaned relatively quickly, before such unwanted side effects such as Cushingoid changes, proximal myopathy, mood lability, and insomnia occur [37]. Dexamethasone is usually the drug of choice because of its high potency and lack of prominent mineralocorticoid effects, with starting doses of 4 to 8 mg per day usually sufficient for rapid symptomatic improvement [38]. About 25% of patients develop steroid dependence and need longstanding steroid treatment for maintaining a reasonable level of neurological function.

The use of anti-epileptic medications should be judicious and employed only in the cases of symptomatic seizures, and not as a prophylactic measure. Prophylactic use does not seem to decrease the incidence of seizures, and puts the patient at risk for significant dermatological and other adverse effects associated with antiepileptic therapies [39–41.]

Patients with brain metastases may have prior thromboembolic events (related to hypercoagulable systemic state from their cancer) or may be at increased risk for such, due to hemiparesis and decreased mobility secondary to their tumor. The question of safety of use of anticoagulative medications often arises. There is no absolute contraindication for use of therapeutical or prophylactic anticoagulative treatment in patients with brain metastases; in fact, there is evidence of a higher rate of complications related to vena cava filters (recurrent thromboemboli or filter thromboses) than complications (hemorrhage) related to use of anticoagulants [42,43]. The potential risk of intracranial hemorrhage related to anticoagulation should be discussed with the patient but should not prevent treatment of thromboembolic disease when indicated.

SUMMARY

Brain metastases are the most common intracranial neoplasms and are becoming more prevalent with advances in systemic neoplastic treatment. The extent of systemic illness, functional score, and age of the patient should be taken into account to manage the metastases optimally. Appropriate systemic treatment, supportive and definitive, can significantly influence the prognosis of the patient with brain metastases. Better understanding of the mechanisms of migration and invasion of metastastic cells in the brain may provide us with future targeted therapies.

REFERENCES

1. Khuntia D, Brown P, Li J, Mehta MP. Whole-brain radiotherapy in the management of brain metastasis. *J Clin Oncol.* 2006;24(8):1295–1304.
2. Jemal A, Siegel R, Ward E, et al. Cancer statistics, 2008. *CA Cancer J Clin.* 2008;58(2):71–96.
3. Posner JB, Chernik NL. Intracranial metastases from systemic cancer. *Adv Neurol.* 1978;19:579–592.
4. Wang SY, Ye X, Ou W, Lin YB, Zhang BB, Yang H. Risk of cerebral metastases for postoperative locally advanced non-small-cell lung cancer. *Lung Cancer.* 2009;64(2):238–243.
5. Sawaya R, Bindal RK, Lang FF, Abi-Said D. Metastatic brain tumors. In: Kaye AH, Laws ER, eds. *Brain Tumors: An Encyclopedic Approach.* Edinburgh, UK: Churchill Livingstone; 2001:999–1026.
6. El Kamar FG, Posner JB. Brain metastases. *Semin Neurol.* 2004;24(4):347–362.

7. Schouten LJ, Rutten J, Huveneers HA, Twijnstra A. Incidence of brain metastases in a cohort of patients with carcinoma of the breast, colon, kidney, and lung and melanoma. *Cancer.* 2002;94(10):2698–2705.
8. Polyzoidis KS, Miliaras G, Pavlidis N. Brain metastasis of unknown primary: a diagnostic and therapeutic dilemma. *Cancer Treat Rev.* 2005;31(4):247–255.
9. Delattre JY, Krol G, Thaler HT, Posner JB. Distribution of brain metastases. *Arch Neurol.* 1988;45(7):741–744.
10. Schellinger PD, Meinck HM, Thron A. Diagnostic accuracy of MRI compared to CCT in patients with brain metastases. *J Neurooncol.* 1999;44(3):275–281.
11. Douglas JG, Margolin K. The treatment of brain metastases from malignant melanoma. *Semin Oncol.* 2002;29(5):518–524.
12. Patchell RA, Tibbs PA, Walsh JW, et al. A randomized trial of surgery in the treatment of single metastases to the brain. *N Engl J Med.* 1990;322(8):494–500.
13. Davis PC, Hudgins PA, Peterman SB, Hoffman JC Jr. Diagnosis of cerebral metastases: double-dose delayed CT vs contrast-enhanced MR imaging. *AJNR Am J Neuroradiol.* 1991;12(2):293–300.
14. Clouston PD, DeAngelis LM, Posner JB. The spectrum of neurological disease in patients with systemic cancer. *Ann Neurol.* 1992;31(3):268–273.
15. Graus F, Rogers LR, Posner JB. Cerebrovascular complications in patients with cancer. *Medicine (Baltimore).* 1985;64(1):16–35.
16. Salcman M. Intracranial hemorrhage caused by brain tumor. In: Kaufman HH, ed. *Intracerebral Hematomas.* New York, NY: Raven Press;1992:96–106.
17. Nutt SH, Patchell RA. Intracranial hemorrhage associated with primary and secondary tumors. *Neurosurg Clin N Am.*1992;3(3): 591–599.
18. Suzuki H, Toyoda S, Muramatsu M, Shimizu T, Kojima T, Taki W. Spontaneous haemorrhage into metastatic brain tumours after stereotactic radiosurgery using a linear accelerator. *J Neurol Neurosurg Psychiatry.* 2003;74(7):908–912.
19. Schrader B, Barth H, Lang EW, et al. Spontaneous intracranial haematomas caused by neoplasms. *Acta Neurochir (Wien).* 2000;142(9):979–985.
20. Debevec M. Management of patients with brain metastases of unknown origin. *Neoplasma.*1990;37(5):601–606.
21. Baisden BL, Askin FB, Lange JR, Westra WH. HMB-45 immunohistochemical staining of sentinel lymph nodes: a specific method for enhancing detection of micrometastases in patients with melanoma. *Am J Surg Pathol.* 2000;24(8):1140–1146.
22. Drlicek M, Bodenteich A, Urbanits S, Grisold W. Immunohistochemical panel of antibodies in the diagnosis of brain metastases of the unknown primary. *Pathol Res Pract.* 2004;200(10):727–734.
23. Perry A, Parisi JE, Kurtin PJ. Metastatic adenocarcinoma to the brain: an immunohistochemical approach. *Hum Pathol.* 1997;28(8):938–943.
24. Peev NA, Tonchev AB, Penkowa M, Kalevski SK, Haritonov DG, Chaldakov GN. Cell proliferation index predicts relapse of brain metastases in non-irradiated patients. *Acta Neurochir (Wien).* 2008;150(10):1043–1048; discussion 1048.
25. Shmueli E, Wigler N, Inbar M. Central nervous system progression among patients with metastatic breast cancer responding to trastuzumab treatment. *Eur J Cancer.* 2004;40(3):379–382.
26. Melisko ME, Moore DH, Sneed PK, De Franco J, Rugo HS. Brain metastases in breast cancer: clinical and pathologic characteristics associated with improvements in survival. *J Neurooncol.* 2008;88(3):359–365.
27. Gaspar L, Scott C, Rotman M, et al. Recursive partitioning analysis (RPA) of prognostic factors in three Radiation Therapy Oncology Group (RTOG) brain metastases trials. *Int J Radiat Oncol Biol Phys.* 1997;37(4):745–751.
28. Gaspar LE, Scott C, Murray K, Curran W. Validation of the RTOG recursive partitioning analysis (RPA) classification for brain metastases. *Int J Radiat Oncol Biol Phys.* 2000;47(4):1001–1006.
29. Lagerwaard FJ, Levendag PC, Nowak PJ, Eijkenboom WM, Hanssens PE, Schmitz PI. Identification of prognostic factors in patients with brain metastases: a review of 1292 patients. *Int J Radiat Oncol Biol Phys.* 1999;43(4):795–803.
30. Byrne TN, Cascino TL, Posner JB. Brain metastasis from melanoma. *J Neurooncol.* 1983;1(4):313–317.
31. Fidler IJ, Yano S, Zhang RD, Fujimaki T, Bucana CD. The seed and soil hypothesis: vascularisation and brain metastases. *Lancet Oncol.* 2002;3(1):53–57.
32. Nicolson GL, Menter DG, Herrmann JL, Yun Z, Cavanaugh P, Marchetti D. Brain metastasis: role of trophic, autocrine, and paracrine factors in tumor invasion and colonization of the central nervous system. *Curr Top Microbiol Immunol.* 1996;213 (pt 2): 89–115.
33. Ludwig HC, Ahkavan-Shigari R, Rausch S, et al. Oedema extension in cerebral metastasis and correlation with the expression of nitric oxide synthase isozymes (NOS I-III). *Anticancer Res.* 2000;20(1A):305–310.
34. Zhang P, Yang Y, Zweidler-McKay PA, Hughes DP. Critical role of notch signaling in osteosarcoma invasion and metastasis. *Clin Cancer Res.* 2008;14(10):2962–2969.
35. Nam DH, Jeon HM, Kim S, et al. Activation of notch signaling in a xenograft model of brain metastasis. *Clin Cancer Res.* 2008;14(13):4059–4066.
36. Kim LS, Huang S, Lu W, Lev DC, Price JE. Vascular endothelial growth factor expression promotes the growth of breast cancer brain metastases in nude mice. *Clin Exp Metastasis.* 2004;21(2): 107–118.
37. Hempen C, Weiss E, Hess CF. Dexamethasone treatment in patients with brain metastases and primary brain tumors: do the benefits outweigh the side-effects? *Support Care Cancer.* 2002;10(4): 322–328.
38. Vecht CJ, Hovestadt A, Verbiest HB, van Vliet JJ, van Putten WL. Dose-effect relationship of dexamethasone on Karnofsky performance in metastatic brain tumors: a randomized study of doses of 4, 8, and 16 mg per day. *Neurology.* 1994;44(4):675–680.
39. Forsyth PA, Weaver S, Fulton D, et al. Prophylactic anticonvulsants in patients with brain tumour. *Can J Neurol Sci.* 2003;30(2):106–112.
40. Glantz MJ, Cole BF, Friedberg MH, et al. A randomized, blinded, placebo-controlled trial of divalproex sodium prophylaxis in adults with newly diagnosed brain tumors. *Neurology.* 1996;46(4): 985–991.
41. Glantz MJ, Cole BF, Forsyth PA, et al. Practice parameter: anticonvulsant prophylaxis in patients with newly diagnosed brain tumors. Report of the Quality Standards Subcommittee of the American Academy of Neurology. *Neurology.* 2000;54(10):1886–1893.
42. Levin JM, Schiff D, Loeffler JS, Fine HA, Black PM, Wen PY. Complications of therapy for venous thromboembolic disease in patients with brain tumors. *Neurology.* 1993;43(6):1111–1114.
43. Schiff D, DeAngelis LM. Therapy of venous thromboembolism in patients with brain metastases. *Cancer.* 1994;73(2):493–498.

30 Presentation and Clinical Features of Medulloblastoma

Roger J. Packer, Kevin C. DeBraganca, and Nadia Kadom

INTRODUCTION

Medulloblastoma is the most common malignant brain tumor of childhood and the primary central nervous system tumor most likely to develop in the posterior fossa during the pediatric years [1,2]. Medulloblastoma may also, less frequently, occur in adults [1–3]. It is a malignant, invasive, embryonal tumor which is believed to arise from one of two germinal zones in the cerebellum, the external granular layer that lines the outside of the cerebellum, or the ventricular zone that forms the inner-most boundary of the cerebellum. Prognosis and clinical presentation depends on where in the cerebellum the tumor arises.

Because of its primitive nature, medulloblastomas can disseminate throughout the nervous system at the time of diagnosis or at relapse [2]. Dissemination to nonprimary central nervous system sites can occur, but is less frequent. Prognosis for medulloblastoma has improved over the past decades—especially in older children [4,5]. Treatment is highly dependent upon extent of disease at the time of diagnosis, although earlier diagnosis has not been shown to correlate with a lower rate of dissemination or higher likelihood of survival.

INCIDENCE

The annual incidence of medulloblastoma has been estimated to be 0.5 per 100,000 children younger than 15 years [6–8]. The tumor comprises approximately 25% of all childhood brain tumors. Most cases are diagnosed in patients between 3 and 10 years of age with a peak occurrence in children between 5 and 9 years of age [2,6–10]. Some studies have suggested a bimodal peak distribution in childhood, with maximal occurrences at 3 to 5 years of age and 8 to 9 years of age. The percentage of children younger than 3 years with medulloblastoma has varied between series. Approximately 20% of all medulloblastomas arise in children younger than 3, although this number may be overestimated because of the past inclusion of other types of embryonal tumors within the medulloblastoma grouping in very young children. Immunohistochemical and molecular genetic techniques have demonstrated that as many as one-quarter of all children younger than 3 years who were thought to have medulloblastoma, based on light microscopy finding, actually had atypical teratoid/rhabdoid tumors (AT/RTs) [6].

Medulloblastomas are more likely to occur in Caucasians as compared with other ethnic groups, as in most epidemiological series in the United States nearly 80% of all medulloblastomas occur in non-Hispanic white children [7–13]. This ethnic pattern is even more marked in cooperative group trials, as in the most recent large prospective COG study the ratio of Caucasian children entered on study as compared with blacks was nearly 15:1 and raises questions about disparity in access or utilization of health care [4]. However, within other ethnic groups, the relative ratio of medulloblastoma to other types of childhood brain tumors is similar to that which occurs in non-Hispanic white children [7–13].

Medulloblastoma comprises approximately 1% or less of all adult brain tumors [14]. It usually occurs in young adults, predominantly those between 21 and 40 years of age, but has also been reported in the elderly [15].

ETIOLOGY

The etiology for most patients with medulloblastoma is unknown [16,17]. Familial cases have been reported, but they are rare [18]. Medulloblastoma does arise with increased frequency in various syndromes—primarily the nevoid basal cell carcinoma syndrome and the familial adenomatous polyposis syndrome [19,20]. Histologically, five primary subtypes of medulloblastoma have been identified in the most recent World Health Organization Classification of Tumors of the Central Nervous System including classical medulloblastoma, desmoplastic/nodular medulloblastoma, medulloblastoma with extensive nodularity, anaplastic medulloblastoma, and large cell medulloblastoma. Patients with the nevoid basal cell carcinoma syndrome (also known as Gorlin syndrome) have been noted to have a higher likelihood of harboring desmoplastic lesions [20–22]. Abnormalities in the sonic hedgehog pathway, known to be present in Gorlin syndrome, have been identified with increased frequency in patients with desmoplastic tumors, as well as some patients with more classical lesions. Similarly, abnormalities in the WNT pathway, which is aberrant in the familial adenomatous polyposis syndrome (Turcot), have also been identified in up to 10% of patients with medulloblastoma [23]. Medulloblastomas have also been diagnosed in children with other syndromes such as the Rubenstein-Taybi and Fanconi syndromes [24–29]. However, whether this is a chance occurrence or related to an increased predisposition is unclear.

Environmental factors responsible for the development of medulloblastoma are essentially unknown [16,17]. Medulloblastomas do occur more frequently after exposure to cranial irradiation. A viral etiology for this tumor has never been proven, although there has been some suggestions of a relationship with the development of the tumor and exposure to the SV-40 virus [2]. More recent epidemiological studies refute this relationship. A seasonal variation for development of medulloblastoma has been identified with a peak occurrence in October [30,31]. Since the peak rate of cerebellar development is between 8 and 16 weeks of development, this would correspond to a possible exposure to a viral or other agent in late winter or early spring. In addition, an increased risk for medulloblastoma has been found in children born before term. The association between development of medulloblastoma and other environmental exposures such as pesticides, maternal diet, exposure to products containing N-nitroso compounds in utero, and father's occupation have been suggested, but not conclusively proven [16,17].

CLINICAL PRESENTATION

Medulloblastoma, which by definition is a tumor that arises in the posterior fossa, may cause signs and symptoms due to either obstruction of cerebrospinal fluid pathways or direct damage to cerebellar or other brainstem structures. Most children with medulloblastoma present with vomiting and headaches [2]. This is most likely due to obstruction of cerebrospinal fluid flow at the outlet of the third or fourth ventricle and secondary hydrocephalus, as 80% to 90% of patients with medulloblastoma will have radiographic evidence of hydrocephalus at the time of diagnosis. At the time of onset of symptoms, the diagnosis is usually in the 1 to 3-month range with the majority being diagnosed 45 to 60 days after onset of symptoms [7,9,12,31]. Patients with metastatic disease are more likely to be diagnosed earlier, possibly due to the greater biological aggressivity of their tumors.

Children with medulloblastoma often have various types of headaches. Early in the course of illness, they are often nonspecific, but later the headaches are those more classically associated with increased intracranial pressure, primarily occurring upon awakening and associated with vomiting. Some degree of unsteadiness, which is often initially ill-defined, occurs before diagnosis in between 50% and 80% of patients. Because of the tumors' midline location in most cases, this unsteadiness is more frequently truncal than lateralized. More lateralized masses, such as those associated with desmoplastic (external granular layer lineage) lesions, may have more lateralized cerebellar deficits [2,7,9,12,32]. Other clinical findings which can occur include head tilt, stiff neck, and weight loss. Ophthalmological signs are often poorly characterized in reports, but one ophthalmological deficit, including nystagmus or frank cranial nerve deficits, such as sixth nerve palsies, has been reported in as high as 90% of patients at the time of diagnosis [7,8,12,32]. Because of the associated hydrocephalus, between 60% and 80% of patients will have papilledema.

Occasionally, medulloblastomas will present with the acute onset of alteration of consciousness, including coma, although it is most common in young children [7,9,12,13,33]. Although this may be due to acute obstruction of cerebrospinal fluid flow, it has also been related to spontaneous hemorrhage within the tumor with resultant increase in the size of the posterior fossa mass, and possible direct brain stem compression.

Presentations in infants and young children are somewhat more subtle [7,9,12,13,34]. Children younger than 3 years are more likely to have large heads, unexplained intermittent lethargy, head tilt, and poorly characterized ophthalmological findings such as strabismus. Although the "setting sun" sign can be seen in children with medulloblastoma, which is the downward deviation of the eyes due to tectal pressure either secondary to tumor or hydrocephalus, it probably occurs in less than 5% of infants.

Presentation in adults does not differ dramatically from that which occurs in children. In most adult series, the time to diagnosis has been slightly longer [14,35,36]. However, by the time of diagnosis, most adults have developed headaches, nausea, and ataxia. Reports in both adults and children have suggested that cerebellopontine angle presentations for patients with medulloblastoma, with resultant sixth and seventh nerve and possibly eighth nerve paresis, are rare [14,35–37]. The occurrence of these findings is probably underestimated. In infants, a cerebellopontine angle presentation was considered to be somewhat more frequent; however, in retrospect, many of the children with such signs and symptoms may have had AT/RTs.

The other tumors which occur in the posterior fossa in childhood may mimic medulloblastomas, but usually present differently. Cerebellar gliomas, usually pilocytic astrocytomas, are more likely to develop in the cerebellar hemispheres and cause lateralized cerebellar deficits, such as unilateral dysmetria or ill-defined clumsiness early in illness. Cerebellar astrocytomas are more often diagnosed later after the onset of symptoms, 3 to 6 months in most series, and secondarily grow toward the midline. By the time of diagnosis, most (75–90%) patients will have obstructive hydrocephalus with resultant headaches and vomiting. Patients with midline, solid cerebellar glial tumors, which are somewhat more common in adults and may be more histologically aggressive, present with symptoms that are often difficult to distinguish from those occurring in patients with medulloblastomas, but the course of illness tends to be more protracted.

Brain stem gliomas, arising both in children and adults, usually cause multiple cranial nerve palsies, long-tract signs, cerebellar deficits, and sensory abnormalities early in disease and overshadow other findings, such as headaches. Because of the availability of magnetic resonance imaging (MRI), patients with brain stem gliomas are often diagnosed within 1 to 2 months of onset of symptoms and one-third or less will have hydrocephalus at diagnosis. Patients with tectal lesions often develop only headaches, due to third ventricular obstruction, by the time of diagnosis. Those with exophytic posterior medullary lesions may present insidiously with nausea and vomiting before the development of focal neurological findings.

Adults and children with posterior-fossa ependymomas often have more laterally placed lesions, causing cranial nerve and cerebellopontine dysfunction, with sixth, seventh, and eighth nerve palsies and unsteadiness. The onset of symptoms is usually a bit slower than is seen in patients with medulloblastoma, but clinical distinction is often difficult. By the time of diagnosis, well over 50% of patients will have headaches and hydrocephalus.

As stated previously, AT/RTs tend to occur in younger children, especially those younger than 2 years. They are often clinically indistinguishable from infant medulloblastomas, but seem to have a predilection for the cerebellopontine angle.

NEURORADIOGRAPHIC FINDINGS

The typical appearance of pediatric medulloblastoma is a midline posterior fossa mass arising from the inferior medullary velum of the vermis (see Figure 30.1A) [38,39]. High cellularity accounts for the relatively hyperdense appearance on computed tomography images (see Figure 30.2A) and relatively low signal intensity on T2-weighted MRI images (see Figure 30.3A), close to the signal intensity of normal cerebellar cortex [39]. The high cellularity also causes slightly restricted appearance of medulloblastoma on diffusion-weighted images and ADC maps (see Figure 30.4A, top and bottom). Contrast enhancement is usually present (see Figure 30.5A).

Less frequent aspects of pediatric medulloblastoma appearance include calcifications, hemorrhage (see Figure 30.2A), cysts, necrosis, peritumoral edema, and lack of contrast enhancement. Major differential considerations for medulloblastoma among pediatric posterior fossa tumors include teratoid/rhabdoid tumor (B, all figures) and ependymoma (C, all figures). The neuroradiographic differentiation of these tumors becomes especially difficult in large lesions because the origin of the mass is difficult to identify. The configuration and location of ependymoma can be similar to medulloblastoma, but ependymoma has bright signal on diffusion-weighted images without corresponding restriction on ADC maps (see Figure 30.4C), and tends to be calcified on computed tomography. Ependymomas have a greater propensity for contiguous spread, especially to the upper surface of the cervical cord. AT/RT is very similar to medulloblastoma in T1, T2, and diffusion signal behavior (B, all figures) and there is no distinguishing imaging feature [39]. The tumor is somewhat more necrotic and hemorrhagic than medulloblastoma. AT/RTs tend to locate near the cerebellopontine angle (see Figure 30.3B), a less common location for medulloblastoma and less frequently have hydrocephalus.

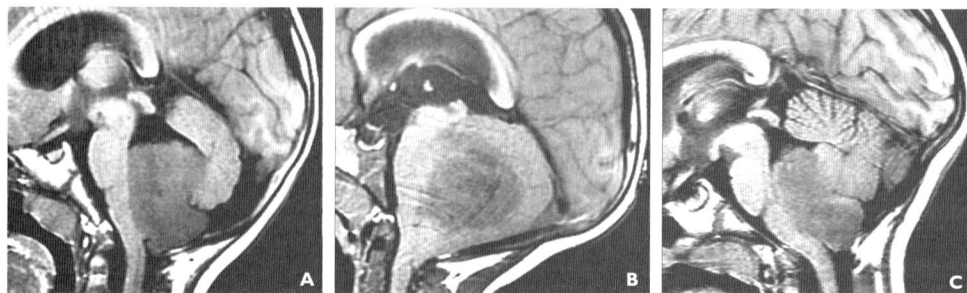

Figure 30.1 Sagittal noncontrast T1 MRI: medulloblastoma **(A)** compared to atypical teratoid/rhabdoid tumor **(B)** and ependymoma **(C)**. Note the similar extension within the 4th ventricle, especially in the medulloblastoma (A) and ependymoma (C). Note the difficulty of defining lesion origin in very large masses (B).

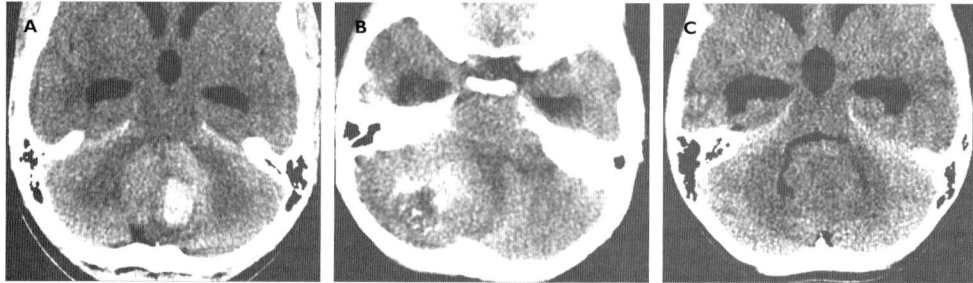

Figure 30.2 Axial noncontrast head CT: medulloblastoma **(A)** compared to atypical teratoid/rhabdoid tumor **(B)** and ependymoma **(C)**. There is a small hemorrhage in the medulloblastoma (A) but note the increased density of the underlying mass when compared to the ependymoma (C). Calcifications are more common with atypical teratoid/rhabdoid tumor (B) than with medulloblastoma.

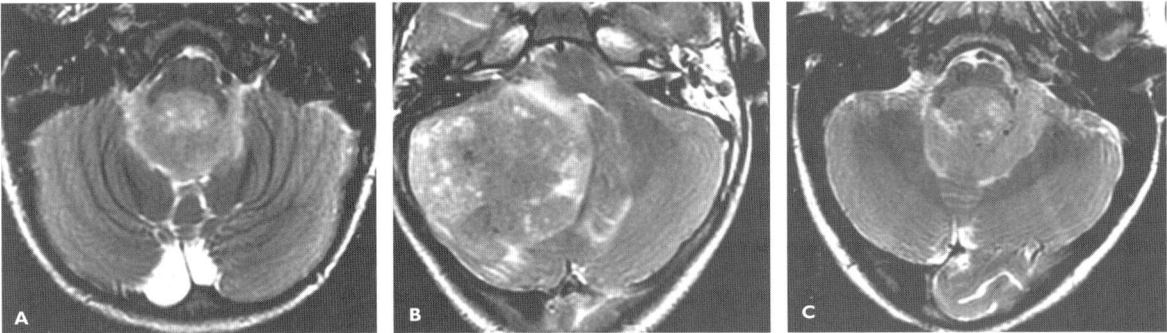

Figure 30.3 Axial T2 MRI: medulloblastoma **(A)** compared to atypical teratoid/rhabdoid tumor **(B)** and ependymoma **(C)**. Note the similar extension of tumor into the foramen of Luschkae in both medulloblastoma (A) and ependymoma (C). Note the similarity of T2 signal quality in all three lesions.

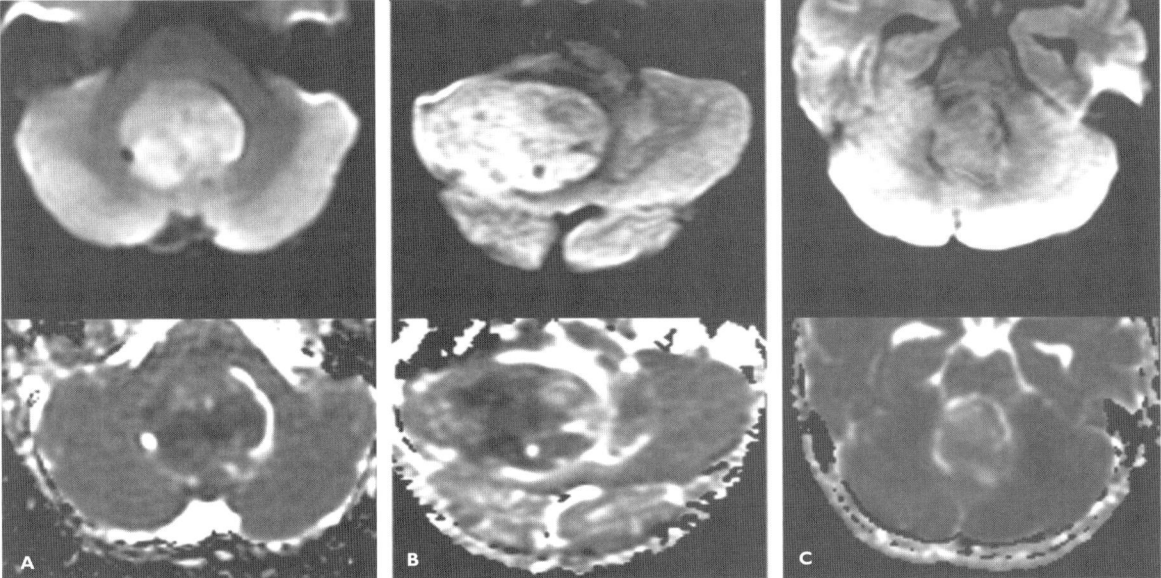

Figure 30.4 Axial diffusion-weighted images, DWI on the top and ADC map on the bottom: medulloblastoma **(A)** compared to atypical teratoid/rhabdoid tumor **(B)** and ependymoma **(C)**. Note the T2 restriction in medulloblastoma (A, bottom) versus T2 shine through in ependymoma (C, bottom). Note the similarity of medulloblastoma (A) and atypical teratoid/rhabdoid tumor (B).

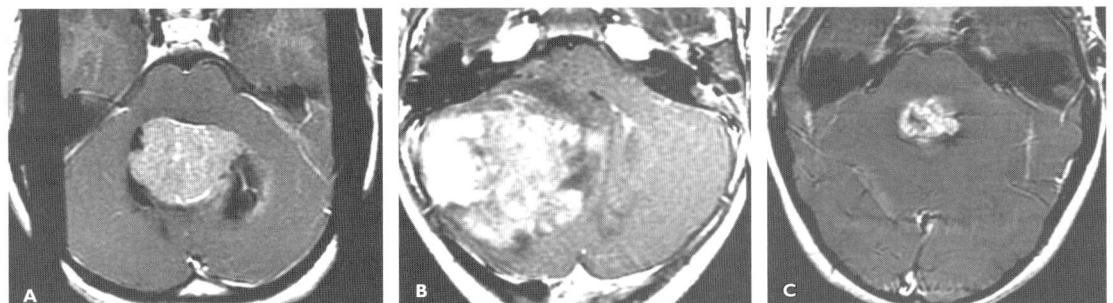

Figure 30.5 Axial postcontrast T1 MRI: medulloblastoma **(A)** compared to atypical teratoid/rhabdoid tumor **(B)** and ependymoma **(C)**. Note the more homogeneous enhancement pattern in the medulloblastoma A).

Complications of medulloblastoma include hydrocephalus from 4th ventricle obstruction and leptomeningeal metastasis. Detection of leptomeningeal metastasis is especially difficult in medulloblastoma cases where the primary lesion does not show contrast enhancement on MRI [4,39]. Meticulous screening of fluid attenuated inversion-recovery and diffusion-weighted sequences in the brain as well as high resolution T1 images of the spine are required for diagnosis.

DISSEMINATION

Dissemination along cerebrospinal fluid pathways, primarily to the surface of the spinal cord and less frequently to other regions of brain, is a major clinical finding in patients of all ages with medulloblastoma. It occurs in anywhere between 10% and 30% of patients at the time of diagnosis, occurring more frequently in infants and less frequently (probably less than 10%) in adults [2,4,5]. The true incidence of dissemination in adults is somewhat difficult to determine because in some series adult patients have not undergone an as extensive evaluation for disseminated disease as in pediatric studies.

Although dissemination outside the central nervous system into bone marrow, and less likely bone or lung, may occur, this occurs at diagnosis predominantly in infants or in patients with wide-spread disseminated central nervous system disease [2,4].

In spite of occurring in a substantial minority of patients with medulloblastoma, central nervous system dissemination at the time of diagnosis is usually asymptomatic. MRI of the entire brain and spine and cerebrospinal fluid lumbar cytological examination are complementary in the diagnosis of tumor dissemination. In most recent series, 10% to 15% of patients with disseminated disease will be missed if assessment is performed only by MRI scanning [2,4]. Although MRI is presently the gold standard for assessing dissemination, the uniformity of quality of such assessments is far from optimal. In recent multicenter international pediatric trials, upon central neuroradiographic review, nearly 10% of patients considered to have nondisseminated disease were found to have evidence of leptomeningeal disease, primarily spinal involvement, and another 10% to 15% were found to have studies that were inadequate for complete interpretation [4]. Determination of leptomeningeal dissemination is especially problematic in patients with predominantly nonenhancing medulloblastomas. The lack of detection of disseminated disease is a major clinical problem, as in series, those patients with incorrectly interpreted or inadequate studies had poorer overall survivals when treated with less-aggressive (reduced dose craniospinal radiotherapy) therapy regimens developed for children with non-disseminated disease [4].

STAGING

A major component of the management of children with medulloblastoma has been the stratification of patients into risk groups. Two major risk groups have been identified, based on clinical findings; patients with so-called "average-risk" disease, which include those with nondisseminated tumors that had been totally or near-totally resected, and those patients with "high-risk" or "poor-risk" disease who have tumors that are not totally resected and/or have evidence of dissemination on staging studies [2,4]. Other clinical parameters such as the signs and symptoms present at the time of diagnosis have not been shown to improve the accuracy of disease stratification. However, molecular genetic studies and possibly histological features have been shown to be predictive of outcome and may aid, if not supplant, the clinical and neuroradiographic stratification of patients into appropriate risk groups [2,5,20,40–42]. For infants, disease stratification based on extent of dissemination and extent of resectability is somewhat less useful, although those children with widely disseminated disease have a very poor prognosis. It is likely that biological (molecular genetic) differences in medulloblastoma subgroups underlie most clinical parameters used for stratification.

SUMMARY

Management of medulloblastoma has improved over the past decade, especially in older children. Clinical presentation for most patients is relatively stereotyped and most patients are diagnosed within 3 months of the onset of symptoms. Presentations for infants and adults with medulloblastoma may be somewhat different than those that occur in older children; however, patients of all ages share similar symptomatology. Although early diagnosis is important and may aid management, it has not been clearly related to improve the outcomes. The primary determinant of outcome for patients with medulloblastoma is the underlying biology of the disease.

REFERENCES

1. CBTRUS. *Statistical Report: Primary Brain Tumors in the United States, 1995–1999*. Hinsdale, IL: CBTRUS; 2002.
2. Packer RJ, Cogen P, Vezina G, Rorke LB. Medulloblastoma: clinical and biologic aspects. *Neuro Oncol*. 1999;7:232–250.
3. Herrlinger U, Steinbrecher A, Rieger J, et al. Adult medulloblastoma: prognostic factors and response to therapy at diagnosis and at relapse. *J Neurol*. 2005;252:291–299.
4. Packer RJ, Gajjar A, Vezina G, et al. Phase III Study of craniospinal radiation therapy followed by adjuvant chemotherapy for newly diagnosed average-risk medulloblastoma. *J Clin Oncol*. 2006;24(25):4202–4208.
5. Gajjar A, Hernan R, Kovak M, et al. Clinical, histopathologic, and molekular markers of prognosis: toward a new disease risk stratification system for medulloblastoma. *J Clin Oncol*. 2004;22(6):984–993.
6. McNeil DE, Cote TR, Clegg L, Rorke LB. Incidence and trends in pediatric malignancies medulloblastoma/primitive neuroectodermal tumor: a SEER update. *Med Pediatr Oncol*. 2002;39:190–194.
7. Monteith SJ, Heppner PA, Woodfield MJ, Law AJJ. Paediatric central nervous system tumours in a New Zealand population: a 10-year experience of epidemiology, management strategies and outcomes. *J Clin Neurosci*. 2006;13:722–729.
8. Suh YL, Koo H, Kim TS, et al. Tumors of the central nervous system in Korea: a multicenter study of 3221 cases. *J Neurooncol*. 2002;56:251–259.
9. Chan MY, Teo WY, Seow WT, Tan AM. Epidemiology, management and treatment outcome of medulloblastoma in Singapore. *Ann Acad Med Singapore*. 2007;36(5):314–318.

10. Dreifaldt AC, Carlberg M, Hardell L. Increasing incidence rates of childhood malignant diseases in Sweden during the period 1960–1998. *Eur J Cancer.* 2004;40:1351–1360.
11. Kadri H, Mawla AA, Murad L. Incidence of childhood brain tumors in Syria (1993–2002). *Pediatr Neurosurg.* 2005;41:173–177.
12. Alston RD, Newton R, Kelsey A, et al. Childhood medulloblastoma in northwest England 1954 to 1997: incidence and survival. *Develop Med & Child Neurol.* 2003;45:308–314.
13. Barnholtz-Sloan JS, Severson RK, Stanton B, et al. Pediatric brain tumors in non-Hispanics, Hispanics, African Americans and Asians: differences in survival after diagnosis. *Cancer Causes Control.* 2005;16:587–592.
14. Malheiros SMF, Franco CMR, Stavale JN, et al. Medulloblastoma in adults: a series from Brazil. *J Neurooncol.* 2002;60:247–253.
15. Yong RL, Kavanagh EC, Fenton D, et al. Midline cerebellar medulloblastoma in a seventy-one-year-old patient. *Can J Neurol Sci.* 2006;33:101–104.
16. Bunin GR, Gallagher PR, Rorke-Adams LB et al. Maternal supplement, micronutrient, and cured meat intake during pregnancy and risk of medulloblastoma during childhood: a children's oncology group study. *Cancer Epidemiol Biomarkers Prev.* 2006;15(9):1660–1667.
17. Bunin GR, Kushi LH, Gallagher PR, et al. Maternal diet during pregnancy and its association with medulloblastoma in children: a children's oncology group study (United States). *Cancer Causes Control.* 2005;16:877–891.
18. Razak ARA, Nasser Q, Morris P, et al. Medulloblastoma in two successive pregnancies. *J Neuro-Oncol.* 2005;73:89–90.
19. Fukushima Y, Oka H, Utsuki S, Iwamoto K, Fujii K. Nevoid basal cell carcinoma syndrome with medulloblastoma and meningioma. *Neurol Med Chir (Tokyo).* 2004;44:665–668.
20. Taylor MD, Mainprize TG, Rutka JT. Molecular insight into medulloblastoma and central nervous system primitive neuroectodermal tumor biology from hereditary syndromes: a review. *Neurosurgery.* 2000;47(4):888–901.
21. Amlashi SFA, Riffaud L, Brassier G, Morandi X. Nevoid baxal cell carcinoma syndrome: relation with desmoplastic medulloblastoma in infancy. A population-based study and review of the literature. *Cancer.* 2003;98(3):618–624.
22. Stavrou T, Bromley CM, Nicholson HS, et al. Prognostic factors and secondary malignancies in childhood medulloblastoma. *J Ped Hematol/Oncol.* 2001;23(7):431–436.
23. Attard TM, Giglio P, Kooppula S, et al. Brain tumors in individuals with familial adenomatous polyposis. A Cancer Registry Experience and Pooled Case Report Analysis. *Cancer.* 2007;109(4):761–766.
24. Taylor MD, Mainprize TG, Rutka JT, et al. Medulloblastoma in a child with Rubenstein-Taybi syndrome: case report and review of the literature. *Pediatr Neurosurg.* 2001;35:235–238.
25. Tischkowitz MD, Chisholm J, Gaze M, et al. Medulloblastoma as a first presentation of fanconi anemia. *Pediatr Hematol Oncol.* 2004;26(1):52–55.
26. Palmer L, Nordborg C, Steneryd K, et al. Large-cell medulloblastoma in Aicardi syndrome. Case report and literature review. *Neuropediatrics.* 2004;35:307–311.
27. Ozisik PA, Akalan N, Palaoglu S, Topcu M. Medulloblastoma in a child with the metabolic disease L-2-hydroxyglutaric aciduria. *Pediatr Neurosurg.* 2002;37:22–26.
28. Ng D, Stavrou T, Liu L, et al. Retrospective family study of childhood medulloblastoma. *Am J Med Genet.* 2005;134A:399–403.
29. Ruud E, Wesenberg F. Microcephalus, medulloblastoma and excessive toxicity from chemotherapy: an unusual presentation of Fanconi anaemia. *Acta Paediatr.* 2001;90:580–583.
30. Halperin EC, Miranda ML, Watson DM, George SL, Stanberry M. Medulloblastoma and birth date: evaluation of 3 U.S. datasets. *Arch Environ Health.* 2004;59(1):26–30.
31. Hoffman S, Schellinger KA, Propp JM, et al. Seasonal variation in incidence of pediatric medulloblastoma in the United States, 1995–2001. *Neuroepidemiology.* 2007;29:89–95.
32. Modha A, Vassilyadi M, George A, Kuehn S, Hsu E, Ventureyra EC. Medulloblastoma in children—the Ottawa experience. *Child's Nerv Syst.* 2000;16:341–350.
33. Elgamal EA, Richards PG, Patel UJ. Fatal haemorrhage in medulloblastoma following ventricular drainage. A case report and review of the literature. *Pediatr Neurosurg.* 2006;42:45–48.
34. Kumar R, Achari G, Banerjee D, Chhara DK. Uncommon presentation of medulloblastoma. *Child's Nerv Syst.* 2001;17:538–542.
35. Urberuaga A, Navajas A, Burgos J, Pijoan JI. A review of clinical and histological features of Spanish paediatric medulloblastomas during the last 21 years. *Childs Nerv Syst.* 2006;22:466–474.
36. Akay KM, Erdogan E, Izci Y, Kaya A, Timurkaynak E. Medulloblastoma of the cerebellopontine angle. *Neurol Med Chir (Tokyo).* 2003;43:555–558.
37. Jaiswal AK, Mahapatra AK, Sharma MC. Cerebellopontine angle medulloblastoma. *J clin Neurosci.* 2004;11(1):42–45.
38. Malheiros SMF, Carrete Jr H, Stavale JN, et al. MRI of medulloblastoma in adults. *Neuroradiology.* 2003;45:463–467.
39. Vézina LG, Booth T. Imaging of tumors of the pediatric central nervous system. In: Keating RF, Goodrich JT, Packer R, eds. *Tumors of the Pediatric Central Nervous System.* New York, NY: Thieme; 2001:27–43.
40. Koral K, Gargan L, Bowers DC, Gimi B, Timmons CF, et al. Imaging characteristics of atypical teratoid-rhabdoid tumor in children compared with medulloblastoma. *AJR Am J Roentgenol.* 2008;190(3):809–814.
41. Grotzer MA, von Hoff K, von Bueren AO, et al. Which clinical and biological tumor markers proved predictive in the prospective multicenter trial HIT ,91—Implications for investigating childhood medulloblastoma. *Klin Padiatr.* 2007;219:312–317.
42. Lopez-Aguilar E, Sepulveda-Vildosola AC, Rivera-Marquez H, et al. Clinical and molecular parameters for risk stratification in Mexican children with medulloblastoma. *Arch Med Res.* 2007;38:769–773.

31 Presentation and Clinical Features of Pediatric Gliomas

Ali I. Raja and Ian F. Pollack

INTRODUCTION

Neoplasms of the central nervous system are the most frequently encountered solid tumors in children[1,2]. These are estimated to occur at a rate of 3.6 per 100,000 population. Of these, 90.7% to 93.6% are intracranial tumors. Overall, infratentorial tumors are more common in the pediatric population. One exception to this rule is the age group below 3 years, in which supratentorial tumors occur more commonly. Approximately 60% of hemispheric tumors in children are low-grade astrocytomas (WHO grades I and II). Fifty percent of supratentorial midline tumors are also low-grade tumors of glial origin. Grade I or II astrocytomas constitute more than half of these tumors[1,2]. The remainder are mixed gliomas, oligodendrogliomas, gangliogliomas, and other less common lesions such as pleomorphic xanthoastrocytoma, dysembryoplastic neuroepithelial tumor, and desmoplastic infantile ganglioglioma [3–8]. High-grade malignant gliomas of the cerebral and cerebellar hemispheres, which are the most common intrinsic brain tumors in adults, account for a minority of gliomas in children. However, the majority of intrinsic brainstem gliomas in children are malignant [1].

A clear environmental or genetic mechanism for pathogenesis is not apparent for most gliomas. In a small percentage of patients, an underlying genetic syndrome predisposing to the development of gliomas has been identified. Some of these syndromes include neurofibromatosis type 1, tuberous sclerosis, and Turcot's syndrome. Neurofibromatosis type 1 is caused by a mutation in the neurofibromin gene on chromosome 17q11.2, which encodes a protein with GTPase-activating properties that modulates growth signaling [9,10]. The most common intracranial neoplasms in affected patients are visual pathway gliomas, but other glial neoplasms are also frequent[11]. Patients with tuberous sclerosis typically have seizures, mental retardation, and adenoma sebaceum (facial angiofibromas) in addition to cortical and subependymal hamartomas (tubers), angioleiomyomas of the kidney, and rhabdomyomas of the heart. Mutations in genes that influence mammalian target of rapamycin signaling are thought to be responsible for this syndrome[12]. Subependymal giant cell astrocytomas are the characteristic intracranial neoplasms in these patients.

CLASSIFICATION OF PEDIATRIC GLIOMAS

Tumors of glial origin in the pediatric population can be categorized in different ways. One classification is based on tumor location. This classification divides these tumors into gliomas of the cerebral hemisphere, diencephalon and visual pathway, brainstem, and cerebellum. Another scheme of classification for pediatric gliomas takes into account the histological grade, and includes high-grade (malignant) and low-grade gliomas. Low-grade gliomas are further subdivided into several groups, based on their histologic appearance [4]. These include astrocytic tumors (e.g., pilocytic and nonpilocytic astrocytomas, pleomorphic xanthoastrocytomas, and subependymal giant cell astrocytomas), oligodendroglial tumors, mixed gliomas, and benign neuroepithelial tumors, such as ganglioglioma, desmoplastic infantile ganglioglioma, and dysembryoplastic neuroepithelial tumor. Malignant gliomas are subdivided into anaplastic astrocytomas, mixed gliomas, and oligodendrogliomas (WHO grade III) and glioblastoma (WHO grade IV).

PRESENTATION AND CLINICAL FEATURES OF PEDIATRIC GLIOMAS

As with most other central nervous system tumors, the presentation of pediatric glioma depends upon the age of the child, as well as the histology and location of the lesion. Brain tumors in infants often produce nonspecific symptoms, such as irritability, lethargy, failure to thrive, and macrocephaly. In older children, localizing symptoms and signs are more common. Such presentations along with the rapidity of symptom onset can be helpful in predicting the location as well as the histology of the tumor [1]. Whereas low-grade lesions often present with an insidious onset of symptoms over a period of months or with a long history of seizures, high-grade lesions generally present with a more rapid symptom progression. Seizures are the presenting symptom in approximately 30% of malignant cerebral gliomas, less than with low-grade lesions. Signs of increased intracranial pressure and focal neurological deficits are seen in most patients. In 5% to 10% of patients, the presentation may be associated with sudden neurological deterioration, which, in most cases, reflects intratumoral hemorrhage. Clinical presentations for specific glioma types are discussed in the following text.

Gliomas of Cerebral Hemispheres

Hemispheric gliomas typically present with seizures and/or focal neurological deficits, such as hemiparesis, hemisensory deficits, or aphasia, depending on the site of the lesion [13–16]. The high incidence of seizures is due to the irritation of the cortical gray matter by these tumors, and was the only presenting symptom in 30% of the patients in the reported literature. Tumors that involve the cortical surface have a markedly higher incidence of seizures compared with those without cortical involvement. In addition, indolent glioma types such as dysembryoplastic neuroepithelial tumors, oligodendrogliomas, and gangliogliomas, which commonly involve the cortex of the temporal lobe, often have a history of seizures refractory to treatment with antiepileptic medications. In these patients, the first seizure usually occurs before 20 years of age. The history of presentation with seizures is also often the case with pleomorphic xanthoastrocytomas, and less commonly so in more malignant lesions. Neurological examination is often normal during the interictal period, although 90% of the patients who present with seizures eventually have cognitive changes. Nonlocalizing complaints can also be seen at initial presentation. These include headache, nausea, emesis, visual changes, or gait disturbances. Depending on the tumor location, focal neurological deficits such as hemiparesis, hemianesthesia, or aphasia can also occur. Raised intracranial pressure with papilledema can be present with more rapidly growing tumors, and may manifest as bulging of fontanelles or macrocephaly in infants and young children. In a previous report of 71 patients at our institution with hemispheric low-grade astrocytomas, oligodendrogliomas, and oligoastrocytomas, the most common presenting symptoms were seizures ($n = 41$), headache ($n = 29$), vomiting ($n = 22$), and hemiparesis ($n = 16$) [17]. Less common symptoms included visual loss ($n = 11$), lethargy ($n = 10$), personality changes ($n = 8$), aphasia ($n = 6$), and hemisensory complaints ($n = 4$). The most common finding on examination was papilledema, which was detected in 19 children. Various focal findings were detected in 32 children. Symptoms and signs of increased intracranial pressure and focal neurological deficits appear to be less commonly seen among children diagnosed in the magnetic resonance imaging (MRI) era, reflecting the earlier detection of these tumors at a less symptomatic stage.

As mentioned previously, the characteristic mode of presentation for benign neuroepithelial tumors, such as gangliogliomas and dysembryoplastic neuroepithelial tumors, is with partial complex seizures. However, desmoplastic infantile ganglioglioma, which characteristically presents during the first year of life, often manifests with signs of increased intracranial pressure, such as a bulging fontanelle, reflecting the large size of these lesions at diagnosis [1]. Subependymal giant cell astrocytomas also characteristically present with symptoms of increased intracranial pressure secondary to ventricular dilatation from obstruction of the foramen of Monro or with seizures and hemiparesis from involvement of the overlying frontal cortex. In addition, with the widespread availability of MRI for screening evaluations of children with tuberous sclerosis, such tumors are now often detected at a presymptomatic stage.

Diencephalic (Visual Pathway) Gliomas

The presentation of visual pathway gliomas is influenced by the direction of tumor growth and the resulting compression of adjacent structures. Several classification schemes have been described for these tumors including one that primarily takes into account the preoperative MRI appearance, and divides these tumors into prechiasmatic optic nerve gliomas, diffuse chiasmatic glioma, and exophytic chiasmatic-hypothalamic glioma. Thus, tumors of the optic pathway can present with symptoms of neurologic, ophthalmic, neuropsychologic, and endocrine deficits resulting either from mass effect or from infiltration by the tumor, depending on the predominant mode of growth. Thorough neuro-ophthalmologic, neuro-endocrine, and neuro-psychological evaluation should therefore be undertaken as a part of initial assessment of these patients. Although some of these symptoms may be easily assessed, others such as visual loss may be difficult to detect in very young children. Nystagmus and strabismus are often the first signs of visual compromise in infants (see Figure 31.1). Fundoscopy may reveal papilledema with

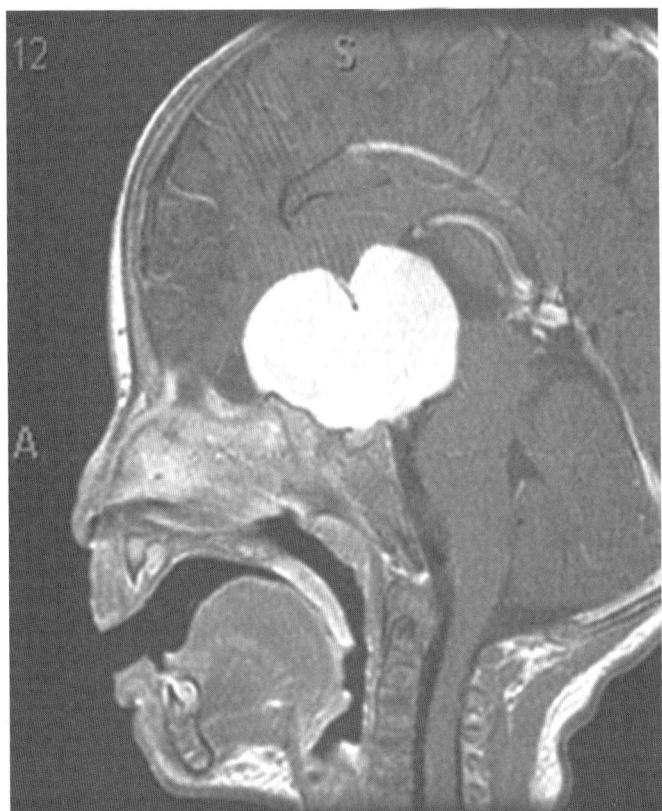

Figure 31.1 Contrast-enhanced T1-weighted MRI of the brain showing bright enhancement in an optic pathway glioma. The patient was a 4-month-old girl who presented with failure to thrive and nystagmus.

venous congestion, although in long standing cases, optic atrophy may be seen.

In children with neurofibromatosis type 1, asymptomatic tumors may be diagnosed on routine MRI screening. In such patients, diffuse chiasmatic gliomas may produce a decrease in visual acuity and bilateral visual field deficits that occur so gradually as to be undetectable by the patients themselves. Endocrinological disturbances and hydrocephalus may rarely be present as well. Exophytic chiasmatic-hypothalamic gliomas can have three different patterns of presentation depending on age. In children younger than 2 years of age, macrocephaly, failure to thrive, diencephalic syndrome, and visual failure are the common forms of presentation. The tumors are typically massive on radiological imaging, and emergent cerebrospinal fluid diversion may be warranted in cases of severe hydrocephalus. In patients between 2 and 5 years of age, endocrinological disturbances (short stature or precocious puberty commonly) are the most frequent presentations, although visual deficits may also be apparent. In tumors with extension into the third ventricle, hydrocephalus may be present with resulting symptoms of increased intracranial pressure. Less common presentations prompting evaluation include hemiparesis, seizures, loss of developmental milestones, or a deteriorating academic performance. Finally, in older children and young adults, visual complaints are the most common presentations. A thorough endocrinological work-up is also essential as hypopituitarism is common.

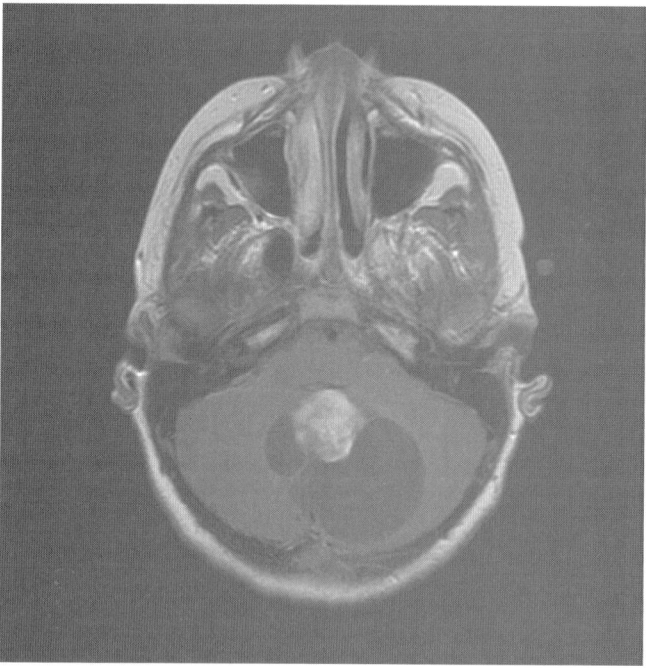

Figure 31.2 Contrasted T1-weighted MRI demonstrates a strongly enhancing, para-median cerebellar mass, which is typical in appearance for a pilocytic astrocytoma in a child. The patient was a 14-year-old boy who presented with a history of frontal headaches for several months.

Brainstem Gliomas

Brainstem gliomas mostly occur during childhood and adolescence, with 77% of patients less than 20 years of age [18]. Depending on their location and appearance on MRI, these tumors can be divided into diffuse (which are biologically and often histologically malignant, and characteristically involve the pons), cervicomedullary (72% low-grade astocytomas), focal (limited to the medulla, midbrain, or pons, 66% low-grade astrocytomas), and dorsally exophytic (mostly pilocytic astrocytomas or, less commonly, gangliogliomas). Whereas low-grade brainstem gliomas often present with focal deficits or symptoms from obstructive hydrocephalus, malignant lesions usually manifest with multiple, rapidly progressive lower cranial nerve deficits and long tract findings, such as hemiparesis or quadriparesis. Diffuse lesions can usually be diagnosed on MRI without the need for biopsy for tissue diagnosis.

Cerebellar Astrocytomas

Most children with cerebellar astrocytomas have hydrocephalus at the time of presentation secondary to compression of the fourth ventricle. Accordingly, the usual presenting symptoms include headache and vomiting (along with papilledema on clinical examination), because of increased intracranial pressure (see Figure 31.2). Gait disturbances (ataxia) and diplopia are also commonly seen either from raised intracranial pressure or from compression of cerebellum or brainstem. Other cranial neuropathies or motor system abnormalities are less common. In some children, there can be a more insidious presentation that may consist of neck pain (due to herniation of the cerebellar tonsils through the foramen magnum) or changes in behavior as a result of hydrocephalus. In advanced cases, coma or respiratory and/or circulatory arrest can result from brainstem compression. Generally, the duration of symptoms does not significantly affect the prognosis in these children, although patients with direct brainstem invasion (those more likely to present with cranial neuropathies or hemiparesis) appear to do worse because such lesions are more difficult to resect completely.

TREATMENT

Although a detailed discussion of the treatment of pediatric gliomas is beyond the scope of this chapter, a brief description follows so that late sequelae can be put in appropriate context. For most cerebral hemisphere gliomas, gross total resection is the mainstay of treatment [19]. Biopsy (usually stereotactic) is reserved for tumors that cannot be resected because of their location (deep-seated, basal ganglia, or thalamic tumors) or those with extensive involvement of the cerebrum. In addition to surgery, radiation and/or chemotherapy are used for high-grade tumors [19–21]. Radiation therapy is generally used only in children older than 3 years of age because of a significant risk of developmental delay and psychomotor retardation in younger patients. Chemotherapy, on the other hand, can be used in both younger and older children, and has been demonstrated to delay disease progression, compared to the use of surgery and irradiation alone [22]. Chemotherapy is also commonly administered for patients with recurrent disease.

The management of gliomas of the visual pathways is still controversial. Although surgical resection has been recommended for selected lesions (e.g., small prechiasmatic lesions or large exophytic tumors with significant local mass effort), the role of surgery may be limited for many optic pathway lesions. This is the case for most chiasmatic and hypothalamic tumors because of risk of damage to these structures. Chemotherapy has been increasingly used in recent years for the treatment of these tumors as a first-line modality and also to delay the use of radiation in patients younger than 5 years of age [23–25]. In older children, radiation is used if the disease progresses in spite of treatment or for tumor spread within the neuraxis [26].

For brainstem gliomas, the role of surgery is limited. For diffuse gliomas, radiotherapy without a biopsy is the currently accepted treatment, with no role for chemotherapy outside of clinical trials at the present time [19,27,28]. For focal (i.e., benign) brainstem tumors, the approach and extent of surgical resection depends on the location of the tumor and degree of involvement of the surrounding brainstem. Irradiation and/or chemotherapy are reserved mainly for recurrent low-grade tumors.

For cerebellar astrocytomas, surgical excision is the primary treatment with gross total resection as the goal [29–31]. Radiation treatment has no role after gross total resection of benign astrocytomas, but can be considered when there is unresectable recurrent disease [32,33].

LATE SEQUELAE

Some of the most difficult problems that arise as a result of treatment for childhood brain tumors manifest several years after diagnosis, which mandates long-term multidisciplinary follow-up. Serial measurements of IQ in young children who received whole brain irradiation have shown a gradual decline in intelligence during the first 2 years after treatment [34,35]. This appears to be less of a problem with focal irradiation, particularly if the medial temporal lobes and hypothalamus are outside the treatment volume. Cranial radiation has also been associated with carotid occlusive disease, particularly in patients irradiated for parasellar lesions, such as chiasmatic-hypothalamic gliomas. Endocrinopathies are also very common in children with such lesions [36]. Secondary neoplasms can also occur in children with a brain tumor, with an incidence range of 1% to 5% [37,38]. Most of these tumors are malignant gliomas, meningiomas, and sarcomas that occur within radiotherapy treatment fields 10 to 20 years after irradiation. An increased incidence of hematological malignancies has been noted after chemotherapy. Finally, surgery-related complications such as "cerebellar" mutism or posterior fossa syndrome can be encountered in some patients after resection of posterior fossa astrocytomas involving the cerebellar vermis [39–45].

REFERENCES

1. Pollack IF. Brain tumors in children. *N Engl J Med*. 1994;331:1500–1507.
2. Young JL Jr, Ries LG, Silverberg E, Horm JW, Miller RW. Cancer incidence, survival, and mortality for children younger than age 15 years. *Cancer*. 1986;58:598–602.
3. VandenBerg SR, May EE, Rubinstein LJ, et al. Desmoplastic supratentorial neuroepithelial tumors of infancy with divergent differentiation potential ("desmoplastic infantile gangliogliomas"). Report on 11 cases of a distinctive embryonal tumor with favorable prognosis. *J Neurosurg*. 1987;66:58–71.
4. Kleihues P, Burger, PC, Scheithauer BW, et al. *World Health Organization Histological Typing of Tumours of the Central Nervous System*. New York: Springer-Verlag; 1993.
5. Giannini C, Scheithauer BW, Burger PC, et al. Pleomorphic xanthoastrocytoma: what do we really know about it? *Cancer*. 1999;85:2033–2045.
6. Duffner PK, Burger PC, Cohen ME, et al. Desmoplastic infantile gangliogliomas: an approach to therapy. *Neurosurgery*. 1994;34:583–589; discussion 589.
7. Daumas-Duport C, Scheithauer BW, Chodkiewicz JP, Laws ER Jr, Vedrenne C. Dysembryoplastic neuroepithelial tumor: a surgically curable tumor of young patients with intractable partial seizures. Report of thirty-nine cases. *Neurosurgery*. 1988;23:545–556.
8. Berger MS, Keles GE, Geyer JR. Cerebral hemispheric tumors of childhood. *Neurosurg Clin N Am*. 1992;3:839–852.
9. Xu GF, O'Connell P, Viskochil D, et al. The neurofibromatosis type 1 gene encodes a protein related to GAP. *Cell*. 1990;62:599–608.
10. Basu TN, Gutmann DH, Fletcher JA, Glover TW, Collins FS, Downward J. Aberrant regulation of ras proteins in malignant tumour cells from type 1 neurofibromatosis patients. *Nature*. 1992;356:713–715.
11. Pollack IF, Mulvihill JJ. Special issues in the management of gliomas in children with neurofibromatosis 1. *J Neurooncol*. 1996;28:257–268.
12. Identification and characterization of the tuberous sclerosis gene on chromosome 16. *Cell*. 1993;75:1305–1315.
13. Jenkin RD, Boesel C, Ertel I, et al. Brain-stem tumors in childhood: a prospective randomized trial of irradiation with and without adjuvant CCNU, VCR, and prednisone. A report of the Childrens Cancer Study Group. *J Neurosurg*. 1987;66:227–233.
14. Kretschmar CS, Tarbell NJ, Barnes PD, Krischer JP, Burger PC, Kun L. Pre-irradiation chemotherapy and hyperfractionated radiation therapy 66 Gy for children with brain stem tumors. A phase II study of the Pediatric Oncology Group, Protocol 8833. *Cancer*. 1993;72:1404–1413.
15. Dunkel IJ, Garvin JH Jr, Goldman S, et al. High dose chemotherapy with autologous bone marrow rescue for children with diffuse pontine brain stem tumors. Children's Cancer Group. *J Neurooncol*. 1998;37:67–73.
16. Jennings MT, Sposto R, Boyett JM, et al. Preradiation chemotherapy in primary high-risk brainstem tumors: phase II study CCG-9941 of the Children's Cancer Group. *J Clin Oncol*. 2002;20:3431–3437.
17. Pollack IF, Claassen D, al-Shboul Q, Janosky JE, Deutsch M. Low-grade gliomas of the cerebral hemispheres in children: an analysis of 71 cases. *J Neurosurg*. 1995;82:536–547.
18. Packer RJ, Nicholson HS, Vezina LG, Johnson DL. Brainstem gliomas. *Neurosurg Clin N Am*. 1992;3:863–879.
19. Broniscer A, Gajjar A. Supratentorial high-grade astrocytoma and diffuse brainstem glioma: two challenges for the pediatric oncologist. *Oncologist*. 2004;9:197–206.
20. Lu Z, Cao Y, Chang L. [Post-operative radiotherapy of glioma in the cerebral hemisphere in adult--a retrospective study of 326 cases]. *Zhonghua Zhong Liu Za Zhi*. 1995;17:67–70.
21. Miyagami M, Tsubokawa T. [Chemotherapy with ACNU and radiation therapy in malignant glioma in cerebral hemisphere of adult]. *Gan To Kagaku Ryoho*. 1990;17:1447–1453.
22. Sposto R, Ertel IJ, Jenkin RD, et al. The effectiveness of chemotherapy for treatment of high grade astrocytoma in children: results of a randomized trial. A report from the Childrens Cancer Study Group. *J Neurooncol*. 1989;7:165–177.
23. Rosenstock JG, Packer RJ, Bilaniuk L, Bruce DA, Radcliffe JL, Savino P. Chiasmatic optic glioma treated with chemotherapy. A preliminary report. *J Neurosurg*. 1985;63:862–866.
24. Mantadakis E, Raissaki M, Danilatou V, Kambourakis A, Stiakaki E, Kalmanti M. Remission of a chiasmatic glioma in a non-NF1 patient

after brief chemotherapy with vincristine and carboplatin: case report and literature review. *J Neurooncol.* 2004;67:95–100.
25. Gnekow AK, Kortmann RD, Pietsch T, Emser A. Low grade chiasmatic-hypothalamic glioma-carboplatin and vincristin chemotherapy effectively defers radiotherapy within a comprehensive treatment strategy—report from the multicenter treatment study for children and adolescents with a low grade glioma—HIT-LGG 1996—of the Society of Pediatric Oncology and Hematology (GPOH). *Klin Padiatr.* 2004;216:331–342.
26. Alshail E, Rutka JT, Becker LE, Hoffman HJ. Optic chiasmatic-hypothalamic glioma. *Brain Pathol.* 1997;7:799–806.
27. Broniscer A, Leite CC, Lanchote VL, Machado TM, Cristofani LM. Radiation therapy and high-dose tamoxifen in the treatment of patients with diffuse brainstem gliomas: results of a Brazilian cooperative study. Brainstem Glioma Cooperative Group. *J Clin Oncol.* 2000;18:1246–1253.
28. Broniscer A, Iacono L, Chintagumpala M, et al. Role of temozolomide after radiotherapy for newly diagnosed diffuse brainstem glioma in children: results of a multiinstitutional study (SJHG-98). *Cancer.* 2005;103:133–139.
29. Abdollahzadeh M, Hoffman HJ, Blazer SI, et al. Benign cerebellar astrocytoma in childhood: experience at the Hospital for Sick Children 1980–1992. *Childs Nerv Syst.* 1994;10:380–383.
30. Schneider JH Jr, Raffel C, McComb JG. Benign cerebellar astrocytomas of childhood. *Neurosurgery.* 1992;30:58–62; discussion 62–63.
31. Morreale VM, Ebersold MJ, Quast LM, Parisi JE. Cerebellar astrocytoma: experience with 54 cases surgically treated at the Mayo Clinic, Rochester, Minnesota, from 1978 to 1990. *J Neurosurg.* 1997;87:257–261.
32. Sgouros S, Fineron PW, Hockley AD. Cerebellar astrocytoma of childhood: long-term follow-up. *Childs Nerv Syst.* 1995;11:89–96.
33. Saunders DE, Phipps KP, Wade AM, Hayward RD. Surveillance imaging strategies following surgery and/or radiotherapy for childhood cerebellar low-grade astrocytoma. *J Neurosurg.* 2005;102:172–178.
34. Radcliffe J, Packer RJ, Atkins TE, et al. Three- and four-year cognitive outcome in children with noncortical brain tumors treated with whole-brain radiotherapy. *Ann Neurol.* 1992;32:551–554.
35. Ellenberg L, McComb JG, Siegel SE, Stowe S. Factors affecting intellectual outcome in pediatric brain tumor patients. *Neurosurgery.* 1987;21:638–644.
36. Livesey EA, Hindmarsh PC, Brook CG, et al. Endocrine disorders following treatment of childhood brain tumours. *Br J Cancer.* 1990;61:622–625.
37. Dirks PB, Jay V, Becker LE, et al. Development of anaplastic changes in low-grade astrocytomas of childhood. *Neurosurgery.* 1994;34:68–78.
38. Hawkins MM. Second primary tumors following radiotherapy for childhood cancer. *Int J Radiat Oncol Biol Phys.* 1990;19:1297–1301.
39. Steinbok P, Cochrane DD, Perrin R, Price A. Mutism after posterior fossa tumour resection in children: incomplete recovery on long-term follow-up. *Pediatr Neurosurg.* 2003;39:179–183.
40. Pollack IF, Polinko P, Albright AL, Towbin R, Fitz C. Mutism and pseudobulbar symptoms after resection of posterior fossa tumors in children: incidence and pathophysiology. *Neurosurgery.* 1995;37:885–893.
41. Orlov Iu A, Zentani S. [Postoperative mutism in children with the posterior fossa tumors]. *Zh Vopr Neirokhir Im N N Burdenko.* 2001:6–9; discussion 10.
42. Ildan F, Tuna M, Erman T, Gocer AI, Zeren M, Cetinalp E. The evaluation and comparison of cerebellar mutism in children and adults after posterior fossa surgery: report of two adult cases and review of the literature. *Acta Neurochir (Wien).* 2002;144:463–473.
43. Gelabert-Gonzalez M, Fernandez-Villa J. Mutism after posterior fossa surgery. Review of the literature. *Clin Neurol Neurosurg.* 2001;103:111–114.
44. Ferrante L, Mastronardi L, Acqui M, Fortuna A. Mutism after posterior fossa surgery in children. Report of three cases. *J Neurosurg.* 1990;72:959–63.
45. Pollack IF. Posterior fossa syndrome. *Int Rev Neurobiol.* 1997;41:411–432.

32 Presentation and Clinical Features of Brainstem Tumors

Paul Graham Fisher

While more common in children, with a median age of presentation around 7 years, gliomas of the brainstem have been reported in adults up to 70 years of age. There is an increased frequency of brainstem gliomas in patients with neurofibromatosis 1, though such tumors can be remarkably asymptomatic with an indolent course [1,2]. Indeed, the term "brainstem glioma" is an imprecise descriptor that incorrectly suggests that all these tumors behave the same. Key to the diagnosis of any brainstem tumor is an appreciation of the pathology, clinical presentation, and radiographic appearance, so that an appropriate evaluation can be performed and therapy initiated accordingly.

PATHOLOGY

While biopsy for histological diagnosis is seldom sought today in brainstem tumors, an understanding of what is known from past studies about pathological subtypes of brainstem tumors is still critical to diagnosis and treatment. At least three-quarters or more of brainstem tumors are diffuse astrocytomas, typically the high-grade glioblastoma and anaplastic astrocytoma (WHO grade 3), or sometimes the well-differentiated, fibrillary astrocytoma (WHO grade 2) [3]. These tumors have a particular predisposition for the ventral pons. Whether this proclivity stems from precursor stem cells at that location or the cellular microenvironment is an area of current investigation. Regardless, these diffuse pontine gliomas can metastasize within the neuraxis. The frequency of such spread is poorly defined.

Less commonly, focal gliomas occur at the dorsal pons, midbrain, or cervicomedullary junction [3]. These tumors are usually circumscribed pilocytic astrocytomas (WHO grade 1) or less often gangliogliomas (WHO grades 1 or 2). Tectal gliomas are focal tumors of the dorsal midbrain, sometimes extending to the thalamus. Pathology for these lesions is often indeterminate between a pilocytic astrocytoma and a well-differentiated diffuse astrocytoma.

Rarely, other tumors occur in the brainstem. Infants and very young children may harbor an atypical teratoid/rhabdoid tumor or embryonal tumor (i.e., primitive neuroectodermal tumor). Older children and young adults may develop a hemangioblastoma, especially in the setting of von Hippel-Lindau disease. Other, non-neoplastic considerations include cavernous or arteriovernous malformation, demyelinating diseases (e.g., multiple sclerosis, acute disseminated encephalomyelitis, and central pontine myelinolysis), focal brain stem encephalitis (Bickerstaff encephalitis) and, rarely, tuberculoma, parasitic cyst, or other infectious masses.

CLINICAL PRESENTATION

The presentation of the patient with a brainstem tumor correlates closely with the underlying pathology and anatomical location.

Since diffuse astrocytomas arise most commonly in the ventral pons and grow posteriorly, affected patients present almost explosively with multiple cranial neuropathies, particularly of the abducens or facial nerve, resulting in esotropia or facial weakness, respectively. Indeed, the finding of abducens palsy at presentation is a rather sensitive but nonspecific indicator of a diffuse glioma [3]. The triad of cranial neuropathy, long tract signs (weakness, hyperreflexia, or Babinski sign), and cerebellar findings (ataxia or dysmetria) present for less than a month is highly specific to diffuse pontine gliomas [4]. Hydrocephalus is rare at diagnosis.

Patients with focal gliomas have a more insidious presentation and can be misdiagnosed initially as having gastrointestinal reflux, sleep-disordered breathing, wry neck, orthopedic problems, or ocular disorders. They may also present with emesis, or younger children may demonstrate failure to thrive. These patients usually have a long history, often greater than 6 months, of localizing signs, such as isolated cranial neuropathy and contralateral hemiparesis, isolated ptosis, or longstanding ataxia. Again, hydrocephalus is uncommon at presentation except with tectal gliomas. Tumors arising in the tectal region obstruct the aqueduct of Sylvius, leading to increased intracranial pressure and hydrocephalus, but rarely all the ocular findings of Parinaud's Syndrome (limited upgaze, light-near dissociation of pupillary reflexes, and convergence retraction nystagmus) are seen with nearby pineal neoplasms, such as germ cell tumor, pineoblastoma, or pineocytoma.

RADIOGRAPHIC APPEARANCE

High-quality magnetic resonance imaging (MRI) of brainstem tumors is essential to diagnosis, and has supplanted computed tomography (CT). The CT appearance of brainstem tumors is variable. Most tumors are isodense or hypodense, enhance poorly to moderately after contrast, and lack calcification [5]. Further, definition by CT is obscured by artifact from absorption of x-rays by the adjacent petrous bone. MRI is not subject to such bony artifact, and has greater sensitivity. The specific ability of MRI to localize a tumor precisely and demonstrate its extent of spread, as well as to differentiate among the various tumor types, clearly makes MRI the imaging modality of choice in brainstem tumors.

For the diffusely infiltrative pontine glioma, a convex or protuberant ventral border of the brainstem on the sagittal image may be the most obvious clue to the presence of a brainstem tumor, and, when present, strongly suggests the diagnosis of a brainstem glioma (see Figure 32.1). On transverse and other planar images, this diffuse tumor is poorly marginated, rarely enhances or enhances poorly to heterogeneously with gadolinium, and occupies more than 50% of the axial diameter of the pons (see Figure 32.2) [3,6,7]. The diffuse tumor, which infiltrates and expands the brain stem, is shown as increased signal on T2-weighted and fluid-attenuated inversion recovery MRI sequences. Abnormal signal may be noted extending to the midbrain and/or pons. How much of this signal abnormality represents tumor versus edema is debatable, but infiltration of tumor cells is present throughout all these abnormal signal areas. When gross enlargement of the pons is present, other indirect signs of diffuse glioma are also seen on MRI, including tumor engulfment of the basilar artery and effacement of the prepontine cistern [3].

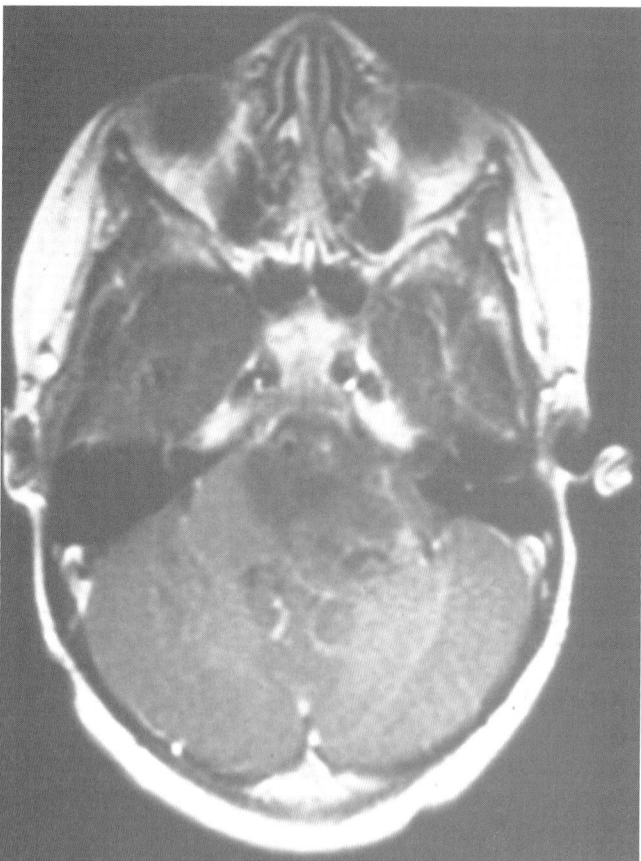

Figure 32.2 T1-weighted transverse MRI with gadolinium contrast revealing obliteration of the pons with a diffuse nonenhancing glioma, notable for engulfment of the basilar artery anteriorly.

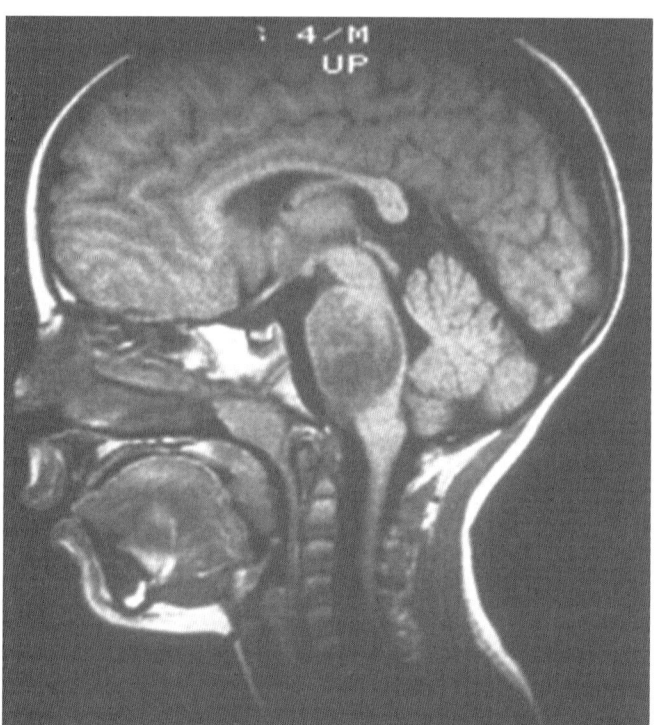

Figure 32.1 T1-weighted sagittal MRI with hypointense signal and expansion of the ventral edge in a diffuse pontine glioma.

As noted earlier, focal brain stem tumors are more discrete on MRI, with little or no surrounding infiltration or edema. These tumors may be cystic or solid. A focal tumor is typically well marginated, often enhances homogeneously with contrast, and occupies less than 50% of the axial diameter of the midbrain or medulla (see Figure 32.3), or arises from the dorsum of the pons.

Other histological types are rather uncommon and are not always stereotypical in appearance. Primitive neuroectodermal tumors of the pons are often isointense and tend not to enhance with gadolinium [8]. Occurring typically at the cervicomedullary junction, hemangioblastomas are often cystic, along with a solid portion that displays marked contrast enhancement [9]. Within the solid component, the large blood vessels of hemangioblastoma create a characteristic signal void on T1-weighted or spin echo imaging. Gradient echo imaging or magnetic resonance angiography may display this finding better.

Proton magnetic resonance spectroscopy can provide insight to the biology of brain stem tumors based on the small set of metabolites detected in the human brain [10]. The most prominent brain spectrum peaks are N-acetyl aspartate, creatine, and choline. N-acetyl aspartate is a neuronal marker and is generally decreased in tumors. The creatine peak includes creatine and phosphocreatine and is often normal or decreased in neoplastic tissue. Choline

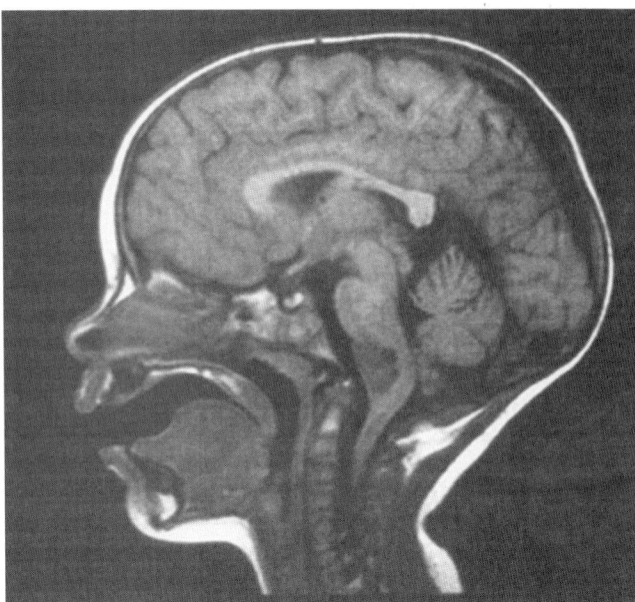

Figure 32.3 T1-weighted sagittal MRI without gadolinium demonstrating a focal medullary tumor, found at surgery to be a pilocytic astrocytoma.

reflects the metabolism of membrane turnover, and often is increased in tumors. In addition, peaks from lactate and mobile lipids are often elevated in malignant tumors, especially with necrosis. Thus, magnetic resonance spectroscopy is being used to differentiate brain stem glioma from brain stem enlargement associated with neurofibromatosis type 1 or necrosis with tumor response to therapy [11].

Fluorodeoxyglucose positron emission tomography (FDG PET) scanning has not been widely applied to the diagnosis of brain stem tumors, because the tumor size is smaller than cerebral gliomas and the PET findings are often indeterminate. As with other gliomas, the principle indication for FDG PET is to distinguish viable tumor from post-treatment changes. High FDG accumulation compared to adjacent brain indicates residual or recurrent tumor, whereas low or absent FDG uptake is observed in areas of necrosis. Nevertheless, FDG PET findings are not entirely consistent in differentiating tumor from treatment effects.

Prospective studies examining these modalities and other newer techniques, such as perfusion and diffusion MR sequences and diffusion tensor imaging, are accumulating data helpful to differentiate treatment change from disease progression [12]. These imaging methods provide quantitative physiological and functional information to complement the anatomical visualization provided by conventional imaging.

Magnetic resonance perfusion measures regional blood volume and flow reflecting the vascular nature of neoplasms [13]. Algorithms to develop relative vessel size maps and also determine a voxel-by-voxel estimate of the relative radius of tumor microvasculature are also evolving [14,15]. Serial changes in tumor vascularity may be a valuable method to monitor effectiveness of therapy, especially as new biological agents with anti-angiogenic properties

are introduced. Diffusion tensor imaging provides visualization and quantitative characterization of the major white matter pathways in the brain. It has been used to study supratentorial tumors and early data demonstrate its value in brain stem lesions to guide operative intervention in focal gliomas and to characterize white matter tracts in diffuse gliomas [16–19].

DIAGNOSTIC EVALUATION

Clinical presentation, combined with brain MRI with gadolinium, usually allows for clear differentiation between diffuse astrocytomas, focal gliomas, and other entities. Over the past two decades, for patients with diffuse pontine gliomas, biopsy has not been performed and radiotherapy, plus or minus chemotherapy, has been administered in the absence of a histological verification [20].

Recently there has been renewed consideration and enthusiasm for biopsy of the pontine tumors, not only to confirm histology—typically diffuse astrocytoma grades 2 through 4—but also to provide biological data on molecular receptors and pathways as targeted therapies evolve and are tested. In a series of stereotactic biopsy of 24 diffuse pontine tumors, there was no long-term procedural morbidity. Grade 3 or 4 astrocytoma was diagnosed in 22 patients, grade 2 astrocytoma in 1, and pilocytic astrocytoma in 1 [21]. Two patients exhibited mild and transient postoperative complications.

Regardless of biopsy, a thorough but limited evaluation should be considered for every patient with a brainstem tumor. A general physical examination should be performed to search for retinal angiomata, seen with von Hippel-Lindau disease, and café-au-lait spots or Lisch nodules, noted in neurofibromatosis type 1. If there is a consideration of infection or demyelination, a lumbar puncture for evaluation of the cerebrospinal fluid for inflammatory findings, such as pleocytosis, increased protein, IgG index, and oligoclonal bands, along with cytology, should be performed to help distinguish among the foregoing possibilities. Nonetheless, lumbar puncture is not routinely indicated as a staging test for brainstem gliomas, as metastasis is rather uncommon. There is no consensus regarding the need for a spine MRI for staging. There is typically no need for additional evaluation, such as staging by bone scan or bone marrow biopsy.

As this evaluation is conducted during the postoperative period, if the patient had already been placed on steroids, such as dexamethasone, to mitigate vasogenic edema, an effort should be made to taper or remove steroids, if possible. Patients started preoperatively on prophylactic antiepileptic drugs can have these compounds tapered and stopped if seizures occurred [22].

REFERENCES

1. Molloy PT, Bilaniuk LT, Vaughan SN, et al. Brainstem tumors in patients with neurofibromatosis type 1: a distinct clinical entity. *Neurology.* 1995;45:1897–1902.
2. Ullrich N, Raja AI, Irons MB, Kieran MW, Goumnerova L. Brainstem lesions in neurofibromatosis type 1. *Neurosurgery.* 2007;61:762–766.

3. Fisher PG, Breiter SN, Carson BS, et al. A clinicopathologic reappraisal of brain stem tumor classification: identification of pilocytic astrocytoma and fibrillary astrocytoma as distinct entities. *Cancer.* 2000;89:1569–1576.
4. Sanford RA, Freeman CR, Burger P, Cohen ME. Prognostic criteria for experimental protocols in pediatric brainstem gliomas. *Surg Neurol.* 1988;30:276–280.
5. Bilaniuk L, Zimmerman R, Littman P, et al. Computed tomography of brain stem gliomas in children. *Radiology.* 1980;134:89–95.
6. Fischbein NJ, Prados MD, Wara W, et al. Radiologic classification of brain stem tumors: correlation of magnetic resonance imaging with clinical outcome. *Pediatr Neurosurg.* 1996;24:9–23.
7. Moghrabi A, Kerby T, Tien RD, Friedman HS. Prognostic value of contrast-enhanced magnetic resonance imaging in brainstem gliomas. *Pediatr Neurosurg.* 1995;23:293–298.
8. Zagzag D, Miller DC, Knopp E, et al. Primitive neuroectodermal tumors of the brainstem: investigation of seven cases. *Pediatrics.* 2000;106:1045–1053.
9. Anson JA, Glick RP, Crowell RM. Use of gadolinium-enhanced magnetic resonance imaging in the diagnosis and management of posterior fossa hemangioblastomas. *Surg Neurol.* 1991;35:300–304.
10. Taylor JS, Ogg RJ, Langston JW. Proton MR spectroscopy of pediatric brain tumors. *Neuroimaging Clin N Am.* 1998;8:753–779.
11. Broniscer A, Gajjar A, Bhargava R, et al. Brain stem involvement in children with neurofibromatosis type 1: role of magnetic resonance imaging and spectroscopy in the distinction from diffuse pontine glioma. *Neurosurgery.* 1997;40:331–337.
12. Packer RJ, Zimmerman RA, Kaplan A, et al. Early cystic/necrotic changes after hyperfractionated radiation therapy in children with brain stem gliomas. Data from the Childrens Cancer Group *Cancer.* 1993;71:2666–2674.
13. Tzika AA, Astrakas LG, Zarifi MK, et al. Spectroscopic and perfusion magnetic resonance imaging predictors of progression in pediatric brain tumors. *Cancer.* 2004;100:1246–1256.
14. Schmainda KM, Rand SD, Joseph AM, et al. Characterization of a first-pass gradient-echo spin-echo method to predict brain tumor grade and angiogenesis. *AJNR Am J Neuroradiol.* 2002;25:1524–1532.
15. Sorensen AG, Patel S, Harmath C, et al. Comparison of diameter and perimeter methods for tumor volume calculation. *J Clin Oncol.* 2001;19:551–557.
16. Sinha S, Bastin ME, Whittle IR, et al. Diffusion tensor MR imaging of high-grade cerebral gliomas. *AJNR Am J Neuroradiol.* 2002;23:520–527.
17. Field AS, Alexander AL, Wu YC, et al. Diffusion tensor eigenvector directional color imaging patterns in the evaluation of cerebral white matter tracts altered by tumor. *J Magn Reson Imaging.* 2004;20:555–562.
18. Phillips NS, Sanford RA, Helton KJ, et al. Diffusion tensor imaging of intraaxial tumors at the cervicomedullary and pontomedullary junctions: report of two cases. *J Neurosurg.* 2005;103(6 suppl):557–562.
19. Helton KJ, Phillips, NS, Sanford RA, et al. Diffusion tensor imaging of tract involvement in children with pontine tumors. *AJNR Am J Neuroradiol.* 2006;27:786–793.
20. Albright AL, Packer RJ, Zimmerman R, et al. Magnetic resonance scans should replace biopsies for the diagnosis of diffuse brain stem gliomas: a report from the Children's Cancer Group. *Neurosurg.* 1993;33:1026–1029.
21. Roujeau T, Machado G, Garnett MR, et al. Stereotactic biopsies of diffuse pontine lesions in children. *J Neurosurg.* 2007;107(1 suppl):1–4.
22. Glantz MJ, Cole BF, Forsyth PA, et al. Practice parameter: anticonvulsant prophylaxis in patients with newly diagnosed brain tumors. Report of the Quality Standards Subcommittee of the American Academy of Neurology. *Neurology.* 2000;54:1886–1893.

33 Presentation and Clinical Features of Tumors of the Skull Base and Cranial Nerves

Mario Ammirati and Hekmat Khodr Zarzour

INTRODUCTION

Skull base tumors are tumors located at the base of the skull, irrespective of their site of origin. Skull base tumors may be divided into tumors primarily originating from the skull base or tumors invading the skull base secondarily. Meningiomas, pituitary tumors, and vestibular schwannomas are the most common primary benign neoplasms of the skull base whereas chordomas and chondrosarcomas are the most common primary malignant neoplasms of the skull base. Pituitary tumors are addressed in a subsequent chapter. Distant metastases from solid and nonsolid tumors or tumors that invade the skull base from surrounding areas such as the orbit, sinonasal area (ie, nose and sinusal cavities), and head and neck comprise tumors that involve the skull base secondarily. Prostate and breast cancer are the most common cancers that metastasize to the skull base, followed by lung cancer and lymphoma [1]. Among malignant orbital tumors, rhabdomyosarcoma, a common malignant intraorbital tumor of children, may invade the skull base, whereas orbital meningiomas and osteomas, mainly found in adults, represent the most common benign orbital tumors extending to the skull base. Cancer of the sinonasal tract (including esthesioneuroblastoma), nasopharynx (squamous and non squamous carcinoma), oropharynx, and ear may also invade the skull base.

In this chapter we present an overview of these tumors and their clinical presentation, and briefly discuss approaches to treatment.

EPIDEMIOLOGY

It is difficult to calculate the exact incidence of skull base tumors. Clearly, meningiomas, pituitary tumors, and vestibular schwannomas are the most common benign skull base tumors [2]. Considering that about 40% to 50% of meningiomas involve the skull base, and that the clinical incidence of meningiomas is 4.5/100,000 per year, then the incidence of skull base meningiomas would be about 2/100,000 per year [2,3]. Combining that with the known incidence of pituitary tumor of about 1/100,000 per year, and with that of acoustic schwannomas of about 1/100,000 per year, one may estimate a combined incidence for benign skull base tumor of about 4/100,000 per year [2,4].

This incidence is not that dissimilar from the incidence of primary malignant brain tumors, which has been estimated to be about 6.5/100,000 per year [2].

Data for skull base metastases are scant. One study quotes a 4% occurrence of skull base metastases in cancer patients [1]. Considering the fact that according to the American Cancer Society, 1,372,910 new patients were diagnosed with cancer in United States in 2005 and that the US population was about 300,000,000, that would give an incidence of skull base metastases of about 18/100,000 per year [1]. Certainly the incidence of skull base metastases is not negligible!

CLINICAL PRESENTATION: GENERAL CONSIDERATIONS

Three factors affect the clinical presentation of skull base tumors: location, growth rate/type, and the route of invasion or the path through which the tumor reaches the skull base [5–7]. For example, perineurial invasion of the skull base typical of squamous cell carcinoma and nonsquamous cell carcinoma (adenoid cystic carcinoma) of the head and neck gives rise to a specific neuropathy, even with absent or minimal tumor bulk. Olfactory groove meningiomas, on the other hand, may attain a gigantic size and yet the patient may be minimally or only mildly symptomatic because of the slow growth of these tumors and of the ability of the brain to adapt to this growth. The opposite is true for esthesioneuroblastomas—due to their high growth rate, patients become symptomatic at a much lower volume, even though the location is similar to olfactory groove meningiomas. Meningiomas of the upper clivus may give rise to symptoms, such as VI nerve palsy, even when they are very small (less than 1 cm) because of their location; the same occurs with meningiomas or schwannomas originating at the skull foramina, such as the foramen ovale, or with small vestibular schwannomas located at the fundus of the internal acoustic meatus. En plaque meningiomas, by virtue of their carpet-like infiltrative growth, become symptomatic at a very small volume as well.

Tumor bulk, infiltration, edema, or any combination of these three can cause generalized and/or focal symptoms. The cranium has a fixed volume that is divided into compartments by relatively inelastic dura, and changes in intracranial pressure caused by the tumor produce both generalized and focal symptoms, which commonly overlap. Brain herniation (cingulate, transtentorial, uncal, upward trans-tentorial, and tonsillar) occurs as tissue moves from areas of higher to areas of lower pressure to accommodate the elevated intracranial volume. Brain herniation can be chronic or acute, associated with minor or major symptoms and signs, depending on how quickly the tumor and tumor-related edema impair arterial, venous, and cerebrospinal fluid pathways.

In most cases, increased intracranial pressure causes generalized symptoms that may include headache, decreased level of consciousness, and also confusion, memory loss, nausea, and vomiting [5–7].

Focal symptoms, on the other hand, are caused by direct compression and infiltration of surrounding tissue and vary relative to the location of the lesion in the central nervous system and the degree of mass effect, infiltration, and/or edema. Common focal symptoms are focal seizures, which include temporal lobe seizures, weakness, numbness, speech and visual disturbances, problems with gait and stance, and double vision.

Headache is the most frequent nonspecific symptom associated with brain tumors. It occurs in approximately 41% of patients with all types of brain tumors, and is present in 23% to 56% of patients at the time of diagnosis [6,7]. Headache associated with nausea and vomiting usually indicates increased intracranial pressure and is generally worse in the morning because hypoventilation and horizontal position during sleep aggravate brain edema. Rapidly enlarging lesions may produce sudden severe headache not observed in cases of slow-growing lesions [5]. In most cases, headaches resemble tension headaches, whereas in some cases, migraine. Headache may also be present in the absence of increased intracranial pressure and is then due to direct tumor invasion or compression of the cranial nerves, vessels, dura, or periosteum. Seizures are the second most frequent symptom, occurring in 9% to 50% of patients with brain tumors [5,6]. Primary generalized tonic-clonic seizures are nonlocalizing, whereas focal seizures and temporal lobe seizures may point to a specific location within the cerebrum.

Nonspecific mental changes include confusion and memory loss, emotional lability, inertia, reduced initiative and spontaneity, and blunted affect [6,7].

It is uncommon for tumors of the skull base to present with symptoms related to elevated intracranial pressure, unless the tumor produces acute hydrocephalus or is a malignant, rapidly growing tumor, such as esthesioneuroblastoma.

CLINICAL PRESENTATIONS: SPECIAL CONSIDERATIONS

Meningiomas

General Considerations

Meningiomas are the most common primary skull base tumors. Meningiomas are thought to originate from the arachnoidal cap cells, cells that form the outer lining of the arachnoid membrane. The female/male ratio is 2.2 [2]. The World Health Organization has classified meningiomas in three grades: benign, atypical, and anaplastic (grade I, II, and III, respectively), based on their histological features [8]. The risk of 5-year recurrence after total excision is 5%, 40%, and 50% to 80% for World Health Organization grades I, II, and III, respectively. The median survival of grade III meningiomas is only 2 years [8]. World Health Organization grade II and III meningiomas are rare among skull base meningiomas [9]. Invasion of the dura related to the origin of the meningiomas or invasion of other mesodermal structures, such as bone and temporal muscle, may make the total removal of meningiomas more difficult or even impossible, but in and out of itself does not confer to the meningiomas a more aggressive behavior [10]. Symptoms and signs vary depending on the location of the main bulk of the meningioma.

Optic Nerve Meningiomas

Optic nerve meningiomas represent about 2% of all orbital tumors, 1% to 2% of all meningiomas, and 4% of all skull base meningiomas [10]. The most common presenting symptom is painless, progressive loss of visual acuity or visual field deficits that can usually be traced back to 1 to 5 years before presentation [11]. Optic atrophy, various degree of disk edema, and the presence of opticociliary shunt vessels are the most common signs [11].

Olfactory Groove Meningiomas

Olfactory groove meningiomas have classically been associated with primary optic atrophy on the side of the lesion and contralateral papilledema (ie, Foster-Kennedy syndrome). However, this syndrome is rare and was observed only in seven Cushing patients [12]. This is not surprising because olfactory groove meningiomas are rarely located on one side. These tumors tend to present, even when they have attained a considerable size. Compression of the orbitofrontal cortex bilaterally gives rise to behavioral and cognitive dysfunction. Consequently, patients present with personality changes, including impaired judgment, abnormal behavior, and a generalized lack of interest, consistent with an abulic/apathetic state. This constellation of symptoms/signs appears to be much more common than decreased sense of smell or decreased vision [10]. In a series of 157 patients with olfactory groove meningiomas reported by Dolenc in 2003, 99 patients had frontal symptoms, 80 demonstrated left or right anosmia independent of tumor size, and 41 with tumors larger than 5 cm had diminished vision [13].

Suprasellar Meningiomas

Suprasellar meningiomas arise most frequently from the planum sphenoidale or from the tuberculum sellae, even though occasionally they may originate from the diaphragma sellae. Compression of the optic nerves and/or chiasm is the rule; hence decreased vision and visual field abnormalities are the most common presenting symptoms and signs. The visual disturbance is asymmetric in most cases and begins with a unilateral decrease in central visual acuity or bilateral visual field defects. Usually the interval between onset of symptoms and diagnosis is shorter for suprasellar than for olfactory groove meningiomas, because of their closer relationship with the optic apparatus.

Sphenoid Wing Meningiomas

Sphenoid wing meningiomas need to be divided into medial, middle, and lateral sphenoid wing subgroups. Each type has a different pattern of growth and hence a different set of presenting symptoms. Medial sphenoid wing meningiomas, also referred to as clinoidal meningiomas, grow mainly toward the parasellar area, exhibiting a close relationship with the supraclinoid internal carotid artery and its branches, and with the optic apparatus (optic nerve, chiasm, and tract). The most common presenting symptom is decreased vision and/or visual field abnormalities. Some tumors have an en-plaque type of growth, with diffuse invasion of the orbit and cavernous sinus, as well as of the dura and bone of the middle cranial fossa and/or the orbit. They may reach the pterygopalatine fossa and the infratemporal fossa either by direct invasion of the dura/bone or by foraminal spread. In addition to visual problems, this type of tumor growth may be associated with proptosis, facial pain, and extra-ocular movement abnormalities. Middle and lateral sphenoid wing meningiomas may present with a globular type of growth and, in this case, headache and/or seizures are the most common presenting symptoms; or they may diffusely infiltrate the greater wing of the sphenoid. In this latter case they exhibit an en-plaque type of growth with diffuse invasion of the orbit, pterygopalatine fossa, and infratemporal fossa. Decreased vision, facial pain, and proptosis are the most common signs [10].

Incisural Meningiomas

When describing skull base meningiomas, we prefer the term incisural meningiomas to that of tentorial meningiomas. Indeed, we group with incisural meningiomas those meningiomas whose main bulk is located in the lateral (middle) incisural space [14]. Those meningiomas sitting on the tentorium or at the junction of the tentorium and the falx (falcotentorial meningiomas) are not, in our opinion, to be classified as skull base meningiomas. By and large, these latter tumors do not have relationships with the basal subarachnoid cisterns and hence their clinical presentation is different from that of incisural meningiomas. Incisural meningiomas may extend anteromedially toward the anterior incisural space, anterolaterally in the region of the cavernous sinus and medial middle fossa, laterally over the posterior aspect of the petrous pyramid, inferomedially over the clivus and inferolaterally in the cerebellopontine cistern. The most common presenting symptom is facial pain due to compression of the Vth cranial nerve.

Trigeminal Meningiomas

In most cases these present with pain involving the trigeminal nerve distribution, either as typical or atypical trigeminal neuralgia. The most common presenting sign is decreased facial sensation, mediated by Vth nerve dysfunction. Anterior growth of the tumor may involve the cavernous sinus, with double vision and/or exophthalmos whereas posteroinferior extension into the cerebellopontine angle causes hypoacusis, gait disturbance, and facial paresis. Delfini et al [15] in 1992 reported a series of 16 patients with meningiomas of Meckel cave. Trigeminal neuralgia, typical or atypical, was the first symptom in 10 patients (62.5%). At admission, trigeminal symptoms were present in 15 patients (93.7%); in 7 patients (43.7%), trigeminal dysfunction was shared with malfunction of other cranial nerves. Primary Meckel cave meningiomas are uncommon tumors, accounting for less then 1% of all intracranial meningiomas [16]. In 1997, Samii et al [16] reported 21 cases of meningiomas originating in Meckel cave. In most patients trigeminal nerve neuralgia was the most common symptom (75% of the cases) and the average time from the beginning of symptoms to diagnosis was 3.3 years.

Clival Meningiomas

Meningiomas involving the lower third of the clivus are more properly classified as craniospinal meningiomas; their presentation will be described in the craniospinal meningioma section. Meningiomas involving the upper and middle third of the clivus are rare. They present with double vision due to compromise of the abducens nerve, mild contralateral weakness, and hyperreflexia due to brain stem compression [10]. With growth, these tumors may involve the petroclival area and/or the posterolateral incisural space, giving rise to symptoms typical of meningiomas in those locations.

Petroclival Meningiomas

Meningiomas whose main bulk is located over the petrous apex and the upper clivus are considered petroclival meningiomas. Frequently they spill over the incisura superiorly, as well as over the middle clivus inferiorly, or over the pyramid posteriorly. By the time they become symptomatic, these tumors have often attained a relatively large size (more than 2.5 cm). We reported on a series of 24 patients with petroclival meningioma [17]. The average interval between the onset of symptoms and diagnosis was 2.5 years, with an average tumor size of 2.5 cm. The most common presenting symptoms were gait disturbances, decreased hearing, and mild weakness as a result of brain stem compression. Van Havenbergh et al [18] reported a retrospective study of 21 conservatively treated patients with petroclival meningiomas. All patients were observed for more then 4 years. The most common symptoms were headache, gait disturbance, visual disturbance, hearing loss, vertigo, trigeminal neuropathy, mental changes, and facial palsy. Another clinical series spanning a 10-year period reports headache, vertigo lack of coordination, and loss of hearing as the most common presenting symptoms [19]. Paresis of various degrees was present in 34% of patients on admission.

Posterior Pyramid Meningiomas (Cerebellopontine Angle Meningiomas)

Meningiomas involving the posterior aspect of the petrous pyramid grow in the cerebellopontine cistern. The cerebellopontine cistern is limited medially by the pons, laterally by the posterior aspect of the petrous pyramid, superior by the ambient cistern, inferiorly by the lateral cerebellomedullary cistern, anterior by the clivus, and posteriorly by the anterior surface of the cerebellum. The trigeminal nerve is contained in the rostral aspect of the cistern enveloped by its own arachnoidal sheath. Cranial nerves VII, VIII, and V and the anterior-inferior cerebellar artery with its labyrinthine branch are contained in the cistern. Meningiomas in this area present with different symptoms and signs according to their location with respect to the internal acoustic meatus. Those tumors located anterior to it present with abnormal hearing, whereas those located posterior to the internal acoustic meatus present with gait disturbance. Decreased cranial nerve VIII function and cerebellar signs are the corresponding neurological findings [10]. Occasionally hydrocephalus may be present with its accompanying signs and symptoms. The median interval between the onset of symptoms and the diagnosis is about 1 year [10].

Jugular Foramen Meningiomas

Jugular foramen meningiomas are very rare. One series reported their frequency at 1.3% of skull base meningiomas [10]. Indeed, most jugular foramen tumors are represented by paragangliomas (58.8%) followed by schwannomas (16.6%) and by meningiomas (9.8%) [20]. The most common presenting signs and symptoms are those due to malfunction of the lower cranial nerves; hence, hoarseness, difficulty in swallowing, and different degrees of IXth and Xth cranial nerve malfunction [10].

Craniospinal Meningiomas

Patients with craniospinal meningiomas usually have a long standing history of suboccipital pain, often ascribed to degenerative disease of the cervical spine. By the time the tumor is diagnosed, 41% of patients may have a negative neurological examination [21]. One series reported leg weakness as the most common symptom, and paraparesis as the most common sign [10]. Bassiouni et al [22] reported a series of 25 patients with meningiomas of the foramen magnum. The most frequent symptoms were cervico-occipital pain (72%) and gait disturbance (32%). Ataxic gait was demonstrable in 48% of the patients.

Cavernous Sinus Meningiomas

Meningiomas primarily originating in the cavernous sinus are rare; on the other hand, secondary invasion of the cavernous sinus by medial sphenoid wing meningiomas, incisural meningiomas, and petroclival meningiomas is not uncommon. When the cavernous sinus is involved by a meningioma, double vision or facial pain are the most common symptoms, whereas malfunction of cranial nerves III, IV, V and VI are the most common signs.

Schwannomas

General Considerations

Schwannomas arise from the Schwann cells of the nerve sheath. Vestibular schwannomas are the most common type of intracranial schwannoma (90% of cases), followed by trigeminal schwannomas (0.8–8% of cases) and facial schwannomas (2.5%) [23,24]. Occasionally schwannomas may involve other cranial nerves. Symptoms depend on the affected nerve. Schwannomas represent 8% of all intracranial neoplasm [23]. The male-to-female ratio is around 1 [2].

Vestibular Schwannomas

The annual incidence of vestibular schwannomas is about 0.8 to 1.1/100,000, representing 6% of all intracranial neoplasms and 60% to 78% of cerebellopontine angle tumors seen clinically [3,4]. The other cerebellopontine angle tumors include meningiomas (14.4%), epidermoids (4.4%), facial schwannomas, lipomas, and metastatic lesions [25].

Four percent are bilateral and associated with neurofibromatosis 2 (NF-2) [26]. The exact point on the eighth nerves where central myelin becomes peripheral myelin is variable. Brigeral and Farkashidy [27] in 1980, reporting on the examination of 23 nerves, stated that this transition zone (from neuroglial to Schwann cell) was medial to the porus in 56% of cases, at the porus in 18%, and within the internal auditory canal in 26% of cases. Hearing loss, especially manifested as reduced speech discrimination when talking on the phone, is one of the earliest symptoms. It can be complete or incomplete, gradual or sudden [28]. The audiometric findings in about 60% of cases are nonspecific [26]. Other symptoms such as tinnitus, dizziness, gait disturbance, and nystagmus may occur. In a study of 122 patients with vestibular schwannomas reported by Kentala et al [26], hearing loss was the most common symptom (94% of patients), followed by tinnitus in 83%, vertigo in 49%, imbalance in 10%, facial numbness in 4%, and visual changes and otalgia both occurring in 1% of patients. Vertigo can be felt consistently or intermittently, lasting from minutes to hours. In most cases vertigo attacks are mild to moderate.

Vertigo in vestibular schwannomas patients differ from that in patients with other diseases that attack the vestibular system because of the absence of nausea in 63% [26]. Tumor size correlates well with the occurrence of headache and neurologic symptoms such as gait disturbance and facial paresis, but not with hearing loss and tinnitus [26]. Indeed, small tumors growing mainly toward the fundus of the internal acoustic meatus may severely compress and damage the nerve at a very early stage; another mechanism responsible for hearing loss in a small tumor may be compromise of the labyrinthine artery. On the other hand tumors growing mainly outside the internal acoustic meatus can cause serious neurological symptoms with normal or mild hearing change.

Trigeminal Schwannomas

Trigeminal schwannomas are the second most common intracranial schwannoma. Trigeminal schwannomas are very rare, representing only 0.07% to 0.36% of all intracranial tumors, and 0.8% to 8% of intracranial schwannomas [23,29]. In one study 50% arose within the middle cranial fossa, 30% within the posterior cranial fossa, and 20% in between [29]. The most common symptoms are facial pain, typical or atypical trigeminal neuralgia, disturbance of sensation in the trigeminal nerve distribution, and headache [29]. Other symptoms such as facial spasm, hearing disturbance, seizures, diplopia, tinnitus, gait disturbance, and/or facial paresis are rare [29].

Schwannomas in Other Skull Base Locations

Schwannomas involving other cranial nerves are rare. Facial schwannoma represent only 2.5% of all intracranial schwannomas, and mostly present with facial palsy [23]. Schwannomas involving the lower cranial nerves (IX-X-XI) are even rarer and present with dysphagia, dysphonia, and glossopharyngeal pain [23]. Hypoglossal schwannomas are very unusual, presenting with unilateral lingual atrophy and palsy [30].

Craniopharyngiomas

Craniopharyngiomas are extra-axial, usually intra-arachnoidal, slow-growing, histologically benign tumors. In the sixth week of a normal pregnancy, the connection between Rathke pouch and the oral cavity (craniopharyngeal duct) disappears; however, rest of this involuted duct may give rise to craniopharyngiomas. Squamous metaplasia of the developing pituitary can also be the origin of craniopharyngioma. There are two histological subtypes of craniopharyngioma, namely classic adamantinomatous tumors, which make up 95% of pediatric cases, and the papillary squamous epithelium subtype that is mainly found in adults [31–33]. Craniopharyngiomas typically have a combination of cystic, solid, and calcified components. The clinical incidence of craniopharyngioma is 0.1/100,000 per year [2]. They account for approximately 0.7% of all primary brain tumors, with a male-to-female ratio of about 1 [2]. There are two age peaks, one at 5 to 14 and the other at 50 to 74 years [33]. They are the most common tumors to involve the pituitary-hypothalamic area in children, representing 90% of sellar-suprasellar pathology [31]; however, 50% of craniopharyngiomas are diagnosed in adults [33]. Craniopharyngiomas are also classified by location. Sellar lesions (11%) are usually small and expand the sella turcica, prechiasmatic lesions (51%) push the optic nerves and chiasm posteriorly, and retrochiasmatic lesions (36%) push the chiasm forward against the tuberculum sellae and fill the third ventricle [32].

The most common symptoms associated with craniopharyngiomas reflect alteration of the hypothalamic-pituitary axis, compromise of the hypothalamus, infringement on the visual pathways, and hydrocephalus. Hence, hypotalamopituitary compromise results in precocious puberty in children and growth failure and hypogonadism, respectively, in children and adults. Hypothalamic compromise gives rise to inappropriate secretion of antidiuretic hormone, diabetes insipidus, anorexia or hyperphagia, emotional lability, intermittent confusion, hypersomnia, decreased arousal, and apathy. Visual compromise may become evident as a visual field cut and/or as decreased visual acuity. Hydrocephalus declares itself with headache, nausea, vomiting, and a decreased level of consciousness. Headache, nausea, and vomiting are more common in children than in adults, likely due to the higher frequency of hydrocephalus in this population. All other symptoms are equally present in adults and children [33]. The interval between the onset of symptoms and diagnosis is highly variable ranging from weeks to years and does not seem to be age dependent [33].

At diagnosis, endocrine dysfunction is found in up to 80% of pediatric patients; reduced GH secretion is present in up to 75% of pediatric patients followed by FSH/LH deficiency (40% of patients), and ACTH and TSH deficiency (25% of pediatric patients) [34]. According to some studies, the rate of demonstrable endocrinological abnormalities is the same in children and adults [33].

Epidermoid/Dermoid

Dermoids and epidermoids are benign congenital cystic lesions thought to arise from entrapment of ectodermal cells at the time of neural groove closure, between the third and fifth weeks of embryonic life. That would account for the midline location of most dermoid cysts. Inclusion of ectoderm at a later developmental stage during the formation of the secondary cerebral vesicles could explain the lateral location of most epidermoid cysts [35–44]. Occasionally, epidermoids and dermoids have been thought to arise from iatrogenic, traumatic, and nontraumatic, implantation of skin fragments [35]. Occasional reports of malignant epidermoid and dermoid are present in the literature [35]. While the lining of epidermoid cysts is composed of simple squamous epithelium supported by collagen, the lining of dermoid cysts contains sebaceous material, sweat glands, and hair follicles. The inside of the cyst contains the remnants of exfoliated cells (keratinous material and cholesterol) in both types of cysts in addition to the secretion of sebaceous glands entangled in hairs in dermoid cysts.

Epidermoids account for 0.2% to 1.8% of brain tumors and usually occur in the cerebellopontine angle and in the parasellar region [36]. The clinical symptoms in most cases start in the late 30s and early 40s. Occasionally, epidermoids of the parasellar region may be extradurally located. Symptoms include hearing loss, dizziness, gait disturbance, trigeminal neuralgia, tinnitus, diplopia, visual impairment, apathy, headache, diplopia, trigeminal neuralgia, hypoacusia, and/or gait ataxia. In the case of paraseller growth, headache, visual disturbance, facial pain, and seizures are common symptoms, with hypothalamic-pituitary dysfunction being very rare. It is rare for epidermoids to rupture or cause hydrocephalus [40].

Dermoids are generally present in younger patients: the average age at presentation is 15 years for dermoids cysts versus 35 years for epidermoids [36]. Intracranial dermoid cysts represent 0.04% to 0.6% of primary brain tumors [37]. They are four to ten times less common than intracranial epidermoid cysts, with a female predominance [36,38].

In contrast to epidermoid cysts, dermoid cysts are located more often in the midline than in the lateral position. Most intracranial dermoids are located in the vermis and IV ventricle; and occasionally in the suprasellar cistern and subfrontal areas. Occasionally, dermoids may be completely extradural [39]. Suprasellar tumors can cause visual and endocrinological symptoms, whereas parasellar tumors may be associated with cranial nerve dysfunction and seizures. If dermoids become infected or ruptured, the dermal contents may be released into the ventricular or subarachnoid spaces and cause chemical or bacterial meningitis. This is a very serious complication that needs emergent treatment. Dermoids seem to rupture more frequently than epidermoids. The most common signs of rupture are headache (31.8%), seizures (29.5%), transient hemiparesis (15.9%), chemical meningitis (6.9%) psychosyndrome (4.5%), visual disturbance (4.5%), and death (2.3%) [38]. Hydrocephalus is unusual [40].

Chordomas and Chondrosarcomas

Chordomas are neoplasms that develop from remnants of the notochord. Their annual incidence is 0.03/100,000, which represents 0.2% of all intracranial neoplasm and 3% of malignant bone tumors [2,3].

Chordomas are generally located in the midline, as would be expected given their notochordal embryological origin. About 50% of chordomas are located in the sacrococcygeal region, 35% in the cranium, and 15% located elsewhere in the spine [45–51]. Cranial chordomas are usually extradural, at least in the beginning, thought to originate from the spheno-occipital synchondrosis and from there they may spread to the surrounding areas including the sellar-parasellar region, the middle fossa, the posterior fossa, and the nasopharynx. Occasionally chordomas may be located in the nasopharynx or solely intradurally.

Chondrosarcomas represent 0.02% to 0.03% of all intracranial neoplasms [2,43]. They are thought to originate from mesenchymal cells or from the embryonic cartilaginous matrix of the skull. They are usually located in a paramedian location and tend to favor the sphenopetroclival area. Their relationships with the dura and growth pattern are similar to that of chordomas Overall, they have a better prognosis than chordomas.

Both chordomas and chondrosarcomas are more frequent in men than women, the male-to-female ratio being about 1.5 [2]. Clinical presentation of chordomas and chondrosarcomas are similar and depend on location and size. Visual impairment (decreased visual acuity and/or blurred vision), double vision, and headache are the most common presenting symptoms whereas compromise of cranial nerve VI is the most common presenting sign. Tinnitus, vertigo, hearing loss, dysarthria, facial numbness, dysphagia (occasionally from retropharyngeal tumor extension), hemiparesis, and neck pain have all been reported.

Chemodectomas (Paragangliomas or Glomus Tumors)

General Considerations

Paragangliomas are benign neoplasms originating from neural crest derivatives, the paraganglia. In the head and neck, paraganglioma are located at the carotid bifurcation (carotid body tumors), at the superior vagal ganglion (glomus jugulare tumors), at the auricular branch of the vagus (glomus tympanicum tumors), and at the inferior vagal ganglion (glomus vagalis tumors). Even though glomus tympanicum tumors may extend into the skull base, it is the glomus jugulare tumors that are commonly grouped with skull base tumors.

Glomus Jugulare Tumors

They represent 0.03% of all neoplasms and 0.6% of head and neck tumors and arise within the jugular foramen (pars venosa), predominantly in the fifth and sixth decades of life [44]. Women are affected three to six times more commonly than men. They are very rare, encapsulated, slow-growing, usually benign, hypervascular tumors that tend to invade the temporal bone as they grow.

Jackson in 1990 reported on 67 patients with glomus jugulare tumors; the most common symptom were pulsatile tinnitus (73%), vertigo (23%), unsteadiness (5%), palsy of the facial nerve (21%), and lower cranial nerve palsy IX-XII (10%) [45]. In 4% of patients the tumors were functional and produced clinically significant levels of catecholamines, mimicking pheochromocytoma symptoms (hypertension, blood pressure fluctuations; tachycardia, sweating, chest pain, tremors, feeling of anxiety) [45]. Ramina in 2004 reported on 58 patients with glomus jugulare tumors; the most common presenting symptoms were pulsatile tinnitus and hearing loss [20].

Skull Base Invasion from Surrounding Areas and Skull Base Hematogenous Metastases

General Considerations

There are numerous tumors that invade the skull base from surrounding structures, either by direct extension or by insidious spread through the many fissures spanning the skull base and surrounding areas. Among sinonasal malignancies, squamous cell carcinomas and adenoid cystic carcinomas may involve the skull base (and from there the dura and the brain) by direct invasion or perineurial/foraminal spread. Esthesioneuroblastoma (olfactory neuroblastoma) often involves the cribriform plate and the skull base in general. In addition, cancers of the oropharynx, the nasopharynx, and the ear may all invade the skull base [3,46]. Rhabdomyosarcoma is the most common malignant tumor of childhood to invade the skull base from the orbit, whereas meningiomas and osteomas are most common in adults, and are the most frequent benign tumors to spread to the skull base from the orbit.

Data are scant on the frequency of hematogenous skull base metastases. According to Laigle-Donadey and colleagues, skull base metastases occur in 4% of patients with cancer [1]. Metastatic tumors accounted for less than 0.55% in 734 patients with all types of cranial base tumors operated at the George Washington University Medical Center between 1993 and 1997 [47]. Autopsy data seem to indicate a higher incidence of skull base metastases; Jung et al [48] studying 249 temporal bones taken from patients with a known history of cancer found evidence of metastases in 24% of them with breast, lung, and prostate being the most common cancers. Roessmann et al [49] examined 60 sella turcica specimens taken from patients with a known history of cancer and found evidence of metastases in 26.6% of them with breast and lung being the most common primary cancers. Gloria-Cruz et al [50] found temporal bone metastases in 22% (47 of 212) of patients with solid systemic cancer (thus excluding lymphoma, leukemia, and multiple myeloma); in 29 patients the temporal bone was involved bilaterally. Again breast (21%), lung (12%), and prostate (5%) were the major causes and only 36% of their patients had no metastases-related symptom while 40% had hearing loss [50].

The large difference between clinical incidence and autopsy results seems to be due to the fact that most skull base metastases are asymptomatic or their symptoms are not recognized. In this context, the 4% incidence reported by Laigle-Donadey et al [1] seems to be reasonable. They accrued 279 patients with skull base metastases from 1963 to 2003: 38.5% of them had prostate cancer, 20.5% breast cancer, 8% lymphoma, and 6% lung cancer. While skull base invasion from border areas may occur early in the course of the disease, is topographically related to the original neoplasm, and is seldom missed on radiological investigation, hematogenous metastases occur in the late stage of the primary disease, can occur in any location of the skull base, and frequently can be missed if the metastases do not compress or invade cranial-vascular structures of the skull base or if one does not actively looks for them.

Greenberg et al [1] described five clinical syndromes due to secondary skull base involvement: middle fossa (35%), occipital condyle (21%), jugular foramen (16%), parasellar (16%), and orbital (17%). However 33% of skull base metastases were in other locations than the ones associated with the five described syndromes. Clinical observations support the description of seven clinical syndromes related to secondary skull base involvement either by direct (contiguous) spread or by hematogenous metastases.

Orbital Syndrome

Frontal pain is the first manifestation of this syndrome; it is due to supraorbital nerve involvement. Further involvement of the orbit and its content causes diplopia, proptosis, and in later stages, exophthalmos, edema, and vision compromise. The initial symptoms are a result of selective involvement of the roof and the lateral wall of the orbit.

Anterior Fossa Syndrome

In most cases it begins with a frontal headache associated with seizures, mental changes, and apathy. Ophthalmoplegia, proptosis, and preorbital swelling can also be seen.

Sellar-Parasellar Syndrome

Frontal pain, unilateral or bilateral headache, ophthalmoplegia, diplopia, visual problems, and endocrinologic disturbance can all be seen. Anatomically this syndrome is due to cavernous sinus and pituitary involvement, with the cavernous sinus component being most common.

Middle Fossa Syndrome

This presents with pain involving the second and third division of the trigeminal nerve; this pain may be preceded by numbness in the same distribution. Occasionally, masseter and pterygoid muscles weakness may be seen as well as different degree of facial nerve function compromise. Anatomically, this syndrome is due to involvement of the foramen rotundum and ovale and of the geniculate ganglion area.

Jugular Foramen Syndrome

Hoarseness, dysphagia, and paralysis of the sternocleidomastoid and upper part of the trapezius muscles are the hallmark of this syndrome. Occasionally, Horner syndrome and pain behind the ear and in the cervical area may be present. Compromise of the jugular foramen nerves and the carotid canal is the anatomical substrate of this syndrome.

Occipital Condyle Syndrome

This syndrome is due to functional failure of the occipito-atlas joint and it manifests clinically with severe local suboccipital and upper cervical pain exacerbated by any type of cervical movement. Ipsilateral tongue atrophy and paresis when present indicates involvement of the hypoglossal nerve in its canal.

Posterior Fossa Syndrome

This syndrome is due to bulky disease present in the basal posterior cranial fossa. It manifests itself with numbness and tingling in the fingers, spastic weakness of the extremities, hyperreflexia, and gaits difficulties. It is due to brain stem compression. It may be associated with involvement of all the cranial nerves present in the posterior fossa (sixth through twelfth) with the corresponding clinical symptoms (double vision, facial weakness, decreased hearing, and hoarseness, dysphagia, and tongue compromise).

GENERAL TREATMENT PHILOSOPHY

Management of skull base tumors has significantly changed in the past decade due to the unequivocal understanding that radiosurgery, and/or fractionated stereotactic radiotherapy, is able to control most meningiomas and vestibular schwannomas. Even in patients presenting with mass effect and when surgery is the most appropriate treatment modality, the quest for a total tumor removal must be tempered by the knowledge that residual tumor could be monitored for growth using magnetic resonance imaging (MRI) and, may be very well controlled with radiotherapy. Furthermore, a better understanding of the natural history of vestibular schwannomas vis-à-vis our exquisite imaging resolution is putting in question the need for treating patients with small intracanalicular tumors (only 17% of which will grow to extracanalicular tumor) or patients with extrameatal tumors smaller than 20 mm (only 29% of which will ever grow more than 2 mm). The same considerations apply even more so to the treatment of malignant skull base tumors, where cure is elusive.

REFERENCES

1. Laigle-Donadey F, Taillibert S, Martin-Duverneuil N, Hilbrand J, Delattre JY. Skull base metastases. *J Neurooncol*. 2005;75:63–69.
2. Central brain tumor registry of the United States (CBTRUS) 2006.
3. Morita A, Piergras DG. *Tumors of the skull base*. In Pierre JV, George WB, eds. Neuro-oncology part II: Gliomas and Other primary Tumors of the Brain and Spinal Cord. Newyork: Elsevier; 1997.
4. Propp JM, McCarthy BJ, Davis FG, Preston-Martin S. Descriptive epidemiology of vestibular schwannomas. *Neurol Clin*. 2007;25(4):867–890.
5. Lang FL, Chang EL, Abi-Said D, Wildrick DM, Sawaya R. Metastatic brain tumors. In: Winn HR, ed. *Youmans Neurological Surgery*. 5th ed. Philadelphia, PA: WB Saunders; 2004:1077–1095.
6. Wilne SH, Ferris RC, Nathwani A, Kennedy CR. The presenting features of brain tumours: a review of 200 cases. *Arch Dis Child*. 2006;91:502–506.
7. Hamilton W, Kernick D. Clinical features of primary brain tumours: a case-control study using electronic primary care records. *Br J Gen Pract*. 2007;57(542):695–699.
8. Riemenschneider MJ, Perry A, Reifenberger G. Histological classification and molecular genetics of meningiomas. *Lancet Neurol*. 2006;5(12):1045–1054.
9. Sade B, Chahlavi A, Krishnaney A, Nagel S, Choi E, Lee JH. World health organization grades II and III meningiomas are rare in the cranial base and spine. *Neurosurgery*. 2007;61(6):1194–1198.
10. Samii M, Ammirati M. *Surgery of skull base meningiomas*. Berlin, Germany: Springer-Verlag; 1992.
11. Eddleman CS, Liu JK. Optic nerve sheath meningioma: current diagnosis and treatment. *Neurosurg Focus*. 2007;23(5):E4.
12. Cushing H, Eisenhardt C. *Meningiomas. Their classification, regional behavior, life history and surgical end results*. Hafner, New York; 1962.
13. Dolenc VV. Skull and skull base tumors. In: Winn HR, ed. *Youmans Neurological Surgery*. 5th ed. Philadelphia, PA: WB Saunders; 2004:1265–1281.
14. Ono M, Ono M, Rhoton AL Jr, Barry M. Microsurgical anatomy of the region Tentorial incisura. *J Neurosurg*. 1984;60(2):365–399.
15. Delfini R, Innocenzi G, Ciappetta P, Domenicuccu M, Cantore G. Meningioma of Meckel's cave. *Neurosurgery*. 1992;31(6):1000–1006; discussion 1006–1007.
16. Samii M, Carvalho GA, Tatagiba M, Matthies C. Surgical management of meningiomas originating in Meckel's cave. *Neurosurgery*. 1997;41(4):767–775.
17. Samii M, Ammirati M, Mahran A, Bini W, Sepehrnia A. Surgery of petroclival meningiomas: report of 24 cases. *Neurosurgery*. 1989;24:12–17.
18. Van Havenbergh T, Carvalho G, Tatagiba M, Plets C, Samii M. Natural history of petroclival meningiomas. *Neurosurgery*. 2003;52(1):55–64.
19. Bambakidis NC, Kakarla UK, Kim LJ, et al. Evolution of surgical approaches in the treatment of petroclival meningiomas: a retrospective review. *Neurosurgery*. 2007;61(5 suppl 2):202–211.
20. Ramina R, Maniglia JJ, Fernandes YB, et al. Jugular foramen tumors: diagnosis and treatment. *Neurosurg Focus*. 2004;17(2):E5.
21. Meyer FB, Ebersold MJ, Reese DF. Benign tumors of the foramen magnum. *J Neurosurg*. 1984;61:136–142.
22. Bassiouni H, Ntoukas V, Asgari S, Sandalcioglu EI, Stolke D, Seifert V. Foramen magnum meningiomas: clinical outcome after microsurgical resection via a posterolateral suboccipital retrocondylar approach. *Neurosurgery*. 2006;59(6):1177–1187.
23. Matthies C, Samii M. Acoustic neuromas (vestibular schwannoma). In: Berger MS, Prados MD, eds. *Textbook of neuro-oncology*. Philadelphia, PA: WB Saunders; 2005:321–329.
24. Ayoubi S, Al-Mefty O. Nonacoustic schwannomas of the cranial nerves. In: Berger MS, Prados MD, eds. *Textbook of neuro-oncology*. Philadelphia, PA: Saunders; 2005:330–350.
25. Thapa BK, Hossain BK, Khair A, et al. A clinical review of large cerebello pontile angle tumors. *Bangladesh Med Res Counc Bull*. 2003;29(1):23–28.
26. Kentala E, Pyykko I. Clinical picture of vestibular schwannoma. *Auris Nasus Larynx*. 2001;28:15–22.
27. Bridger MW, Farkashidy J. The distribution of neuroglia and Schwann cells in the 8th nerve of man. *J Laryngol otol*. 1980;94(12):1353–1362.
28. Sampath P, Long DM. Acoustic neuroma. In: Winn HR, ed. *Youmans Neurological Surgery*. 5th ed. Philadelphia, PA: WB Saunders; 2004:1147–1168.
29. Shrivastava RK, Sen C, Post KD. Trigeminal schwannomas. In: Winn HR, ed. *Youmans Neurological Surgery*. 5th ed. Philadelphia, PA: WB Saunders; 2004:1343–1350.
30. Beldarrain GM, Canton FG, Garcia-Monco JC. Hypoglossal schwannoma: an uncommon cause of twelfth-nerve palsy. *Neurologia*. 2000;15(4):182–183.
31. Jagannathan J, Kanter AS, Sheehan JP, Jane JA Jr, Laws ER Jr. Benign brain tumors: sellar/parasellar tumors. *Neurol Clin*. 2007;25:1231–1249.
32. Mehta V, Black PM. Craniopharyngioma in the adult. In: Winn HR, ed. *Youmans Neurological Surgery*. 5th ed. Philadelphia, PA: WB Saunders; 2004:1207–1222.
33. Karavitaki N, Cudlip S, Adams CBT, Wass JAH. Craniopharyngiomas. *Endocr Rev*. 2006;27(4):371–397.
34. Jagannathan J, Dumont AA, Jane JA, Laws ER. Pediatric sellar tumors: diagnostic procedures and management. *Neurosurg Focus*. 2005;18(6a):E6.
35. Russell DS, Rubinstein LJ. Tumors and tumor-like lesions of maldevelopmental origin. In Russell DS, Rubinstein LJ, eds. *Pathology of Tumours of the Nervous System*. 5th ed. Baltimore: Williams & Wilkings; 1988:690–695.
36. Gumerlock MK. Epidermoid, dermoid, and neuroenteric cysts. In: Winn HR, ed. *Youmans Neurological Surgery*. 5th ed. Philadelphia, PA: WB Saunders; 2004:1223–1230.
37. Johnson DG, Stemper SJ, Withers TK. Case report: ruptured "giant" supratentorial dermoid cyst. *J Clin Neurosci*. 2005;12(2):198–201.
38. Stendel R, Pietilä TA, Lehmann K, Kurth R, Suess O, Brock M. Ruptured intracranial dermoid cysts. *Surg Neurol*. 2002;57(6):391–398.
39. Ammirati M, Delgado M, Slone HW, Ray-Chaudhury A. Extradural dermoid tumor of the petrous apex. *J Neurosurg*. 2007;107(2):426–429.
40. Abramson RC, Morawetz RB, Schlitt M. Case report: multiple complications from an intracranial epidermoid cyst: case report and literature review. *Neurosurgery*. 1989;24(4):574–578.
41. Sekhar LN, Chanda A, Chandrasekar K, Wright DC. Chordoma and chondrosarcoma. In: Winn HR, ed. *Youmans Neurological Surgery*. 5th ed. Philadelphia, PA: WB Saunders; 2004:1283–1294.
42. Forsyth PJ, Cascino TL, Shaw EG, Brend W. Intracranial chordomas: a clinicopathological and prognostic study of 51 cases. *J Neurosurg*. 1993;78:741–747.
43. Hyun Cho Y, Hoon Kim J, Kwang Khang S, Lee JK, Jin Kim C. Chordomas and chondrosarcomas of the skull base: comparative analysis of clinical results in 30 patients. *Neurosurg Rev*. 2008;31:35–43.
44. Teixeira A, Al-Mefty O, Husain MM. Paragangliomas of the skull base. In: Berger MS, Prados MD, eds. *Textbook of neuro-oncology*. Philadelphia, PA: WB Saunders; 2005,:366–370.

45. Jackson CG, Harris PF, Glasscock ME, et al. Diagnosis and management of paragangliomas of the skull base. *Am J Surg*. 1990;159:389–393.
46. Sheehan JM, Jane JA. Esthesioneuroblastoma. In: Winn HR, ed. *Youmans Neurological Surgery*. 5th ed. Philadelphia: WB Saunders; 2004:1333–1342.
47. Morita IP, Sekhar LN, Wright DC. Current concept in the management of tumors of the skull base. *Cancer Control*. 1998;5:138.
48. Jung TT, Jun BH, Shea D, et al. Primary and secondary tumors of the facial nerve. A temporal bone study. *Arch Otolaryngol Head and Neck Surg*. 1986;112:1269–1273.
49. Roessmann U, Kaufman B, Friede RL. Metastatic lesions in the sella turcica and pituitary gland. *Cancer*. 1970;25:478–480.
50. Gloria-Cruz TI, Schachern PA, Paparella MM, Adams GL, Fulton SE. Metastases to the temporal bones from primary nonsystemic malignant neoplasms. *Arch Otolaryngol Head Neck Surg*. 2000;126:209–214.
51. Stangerup SE, Caye-Thomasen P, Tos M, Thomsen J. The natural history of vestibular schwannoma. *Otol Neurotol*. 2006:27:547–552.

34 Presentation and Clinical Features of Tumors of the Pituitary and Sellar Region

Edward R. Laws, John A. Jane, Jr., Jay Jagannathan, and Laurence Katznelson

INTRODUCTION

Sellar and parasellar lesions include a diverse group of tumors. The majority of tumors in this region are pituitary adenomas, although dysembryogenic lesions of the midline, such as Rathke's cleft cysts, also occur. The differential diagnosis of suprasellar lesions includes craniopharyngiomas, germinomas, dermoid/epidermoid cysts, meningiomas, lipomas, teratomas, metastases, and hamartomas (see Table 34.1). Recent advances in microsurgery, surgical endoscopy, neuroimaging, and molecular biology have changed the diagnosis and management of pituitary tumors [1,2]. In this chapter, we focus on the clinical presentation of these diverse pathological entities.

EPIDEMIOLOGY

Pituitary adenomas are the most common cause of pituitary malfunction in adults. They represent 15% to 20% of surgically treated primary brain tumors, with a low incidence in childhood that increases during adolescence [3]. Although the incidence varies according to age, sex, and ethnic group, between 0.5 and 10.7 per 100,000 in the population are diagnosed annually with a pituitary adenoma [4]. Autopsy series indicate that pituitary tumors are quite common and that nearly 25% of the population may harbor undiagnosed adenomas. Most of these tumors are less than 3 to 5 mm in diameter and would not require medical or surgical intervention. Women are reported to harbor pituitary tumors more frequently than men, and this may reflect the relative contribution of prolactinomas and adrenocorticotropic hormone (ACTH)-secreting tumors, which both have a female predominance.

Among the varying classes of adenomas, prolactinomas and clinically nonfunctioning adenomas are the most frequent. They account for nearly two-thirds of all pituitary tumors. With a peak incidence in women between the ages of 20 and 50. Prolactin (PRL)-secreting adenomas also account for 40% to 60% of functioning adenomas and are the most common subtype of pituitary tumor diagnosed in adolescents.

Growth hormone (GH)-secreting adenomas represent nearly 30% of all functioning tumors. Nearly three quarters of GH-secreting adenomas are macroadenomas. Approximately 40 to 60 individuals per million have acromegaly. Between 3 and 4 new cases per million are diagnosed annually. Most present in their third to fifth decades after they have been developing symptoms and signs for many years. Acromegaly is associated with an increased incidence of cardiovascular, respiratory, cerebrovascular, and malignant disease. Accordingly, studies report an increased risk of mortality compared to the unaffected population. Although some studies report a higher incidence of several cancers, others have only suggested an increase risk of colon cancer. Clearly, there is an increased risk of colon polyps in acromegaly. There is some evidence that mortality risk may be different between the sexes, but other reports find similar degrees of increased mortality in both sexes. Still others report increased risk of death in men from cardiovascular, respiratory, cerebrovascular, and malignant disease, but primarily from cerebrovascular disease in women.

ACTH-secreting adenomas account for 15% to 25% of all functioning adenomas and are the most common pituitary tumors diagnosed in prepubertal children. The majority are microadenomas. Approximately 39 individuals per million have Cushing's disease (CD) and the annual incidence is estimated at 2.4 per million. CD is more common in women, who tend to present in their third and fourth decades. There is a high incidence of hypertension and diabetes mellitus as well as higher vascular disease–related mortality.

Craniopharyngiomas account for the majority (~90%) of neoplasms other than pituitary adenomas arising in the pituitary region [5,6]. Most of these tumors arise from Rathke's pouch—a cystic diverticulum that originates from between the anterior and posterior pituitary gland. Patients with craniopharyngiomas have a bimodal age distribution during the first and second decade of life and then again in the fifth; and there is no apparent gender predilection. Most originate in the intrasellar and suprasellar region (70%) with solely intrasellar lesions (10%) occurring less frequently.

CLINICAL PRESENTATION AND DIAGNOSTIC EVALUATION—NONFUNCTIONING PITUITARY ADENOMAS AND CRANIOPHARYNGIOMAS (SEE TABLE 34.2)

Symptoms and clinical signs of tumors in the region of the sella turcia depend upon the type and size of the tumor and age of the patient. The patient may be asymptomatic

Table 34.1 Differential Diagnosis of Sellar and Suprasellar Mass Lesions

Pituitary adenoma
Craniopharyngioma
Meningioma
Rathke cleft cyst
Arachnoid cyst
Lymphocytic hypophysitis
Germinoma
Epidermoid, dermoid tumor
Langhans cell granulomatosis (histiocytosis X)
Chordoma, chondrosarcoma
Glioma (optic chiasm, hypothalamic)
Hamartoma
Granular cell tumor
Pituicytoma
Metastatic carcinoma
Lymphoma, leukemia, plasmacytoma
Sarcoid
Tuberculoma
Pituitary abscess

Table 34.2 Clinical Manifestations of Nonfunctioning Pituitary Adenomas, Craniopharyngiomas, Sellar and Parasellar Meningiomas, and other Hormonally Silent Masses

Headache
Visual loss, visual field deficit
Hypopituitarism (fatigue, sexual dysfunction)
Anemia
Mental changes

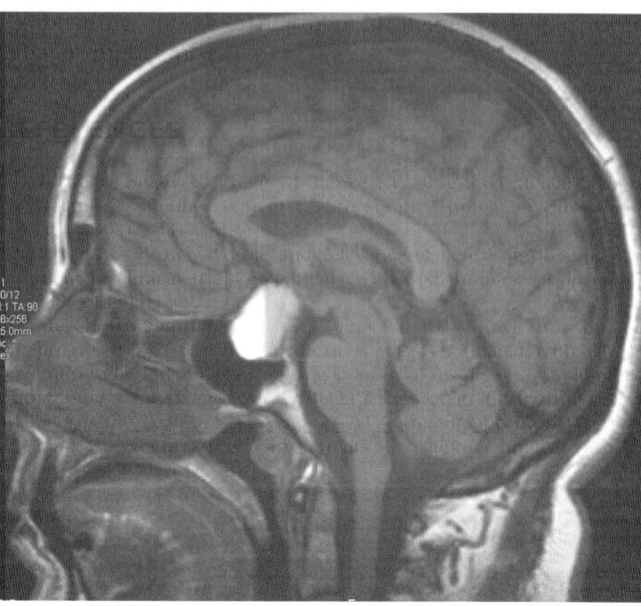

Figure 34.1 Saggital MRI of pituitary tumor apoplexy. Note the fluid level in the hemorrhagic cystic adenoma. Imaging was done with the patient in the supine position. The posterior pituitary "bright spot" is not visualized in this adult patient with an intrasellar lesion.

and the lesion discovered during imaging for an unrelated condition.

Mass effect from a sellar tumor may produce variable endocrinological and neurological manifestations. Diminished growth velocity or short stature is a common feature in many children harboring pituitary adenomas; this may be accompanied by delayed puberty or hypogonadism [7]. Mass effect can also result in galactorrhea from hyperprolactinemia resulting from disturbance of the pituitary stalk and loss of inhibition of PRL (i.e., stalk effect) by dopamine produced in the hypothalamus. Visual changes, including diminished acuity or visual field deficits, may result from compression of the optic apparatus, or hemorrhage. Mass effect producing increased intracranial pressure (ICP) may evoke headache, nausea, vomiting, and papilledema, especially in the setting of macroadenomas, with or without pituitary apoplexy (see Figure 34.1). Memory problems and behavioral changes may also be seen. Suprasellar lesions may block cerebrospinal fluid (CSF) pathways at the foramina of Monroe and lead to symptomatic hydrocephalus.

Neurological disturbances, such as headache and visual field defects, along with manifestations of endocrine deficiency are the common presenting symptoms of sellar region tumors. These tumors can often stretch the diaphragma sellae and cause headaches. Obstruction of the cerebral aqueduct and the foramen of Monroe may also occur, making a CSF-shunting procedure necessary. Large tumors with lateral growth may compress the mesial aspect of the temporal lobes and cause seizures. At diagnosis, endocrine dysfunction is found in many patients. Reduced GH secretion is the most frequent endocrinopathy, and can be present in more than 75% of patients. This is followed by FSH/LH deficiency with hypogonadism, which can occur in 40% of patients, and ACTH and thyroid-stimulating hormone (TSH) deficiency, which is present in about 25%. Diminished libido, anemia, and loss of vitality are common symptoms, most commonly noted in men.

Both premature sexual development in the first decade of life and pubertal delay in adolescent patients can occur as endocrine manifestations of sellar region tumors [8,9].

HORMONALLY ACTIVE PITUITARY ADENOMAS: CD (SEE TABLE 34.3)

The clinical manifestations of CD are a consequence of hypercortisolemia. The clinical presentation remains highly variable, with signs and symptoms ranging from subtle to obvious [10]. Physical manifestations of CD include facial plethora, atrophic striae in the abdomen, legs and arms, muscle weakness, hypertension, and osteoporosis. The most striking finding is central adiposity [11]. Bone mineral density (BMD) and metabolism in children and adults with CD reveal marked osteopenia. Recent reports indicate that a long period of time (>2 years) is necessary to restore bone mass after a cure from CD, so other therapeutic approaches are often implemented to limit bone loss and accelerate bone recovery in these patients.

Children with CD may have impaired carbohydrate tolerance (although diabetes mellitus is uncommon). Unfortunately, diagnosis is often delayed as growth

Table 34.3 Clinical Manifestations of Cushing Disease

Weight gain—centripetal obesity
Hirsutism
Hypertension
Diabetes mellitus, glucose intolerance
Osteoporosis, osteopenia
Proximal myopathy
Dorsal fat pad, supraclavicular fat pad enlargement
Moon facies
Thin skin, easy bruising
Acne, dermatitis
Pigmentation of knuckles, elbows, neck
Amenorrhea
Mental changes, cognitive, psychopathy, irritability
Growth arrest (children)
Fatigue
Sleep apnea
Headache

Table 34.4 Clinical Manifestations of Acromegaly

Enlargement of hands, feet, facial features, jaw
Hyperhidrosis
Hypertension
Glucose intolerance
Gigantism (children and adolescents)
Fatigue
Arthropathies
Cardiomyopathy
Dental malocclusion
Skin tags
Colon polyps
Tongue enlargement, snoring, sleep apnea
Headache

retardation may be the only perceptible symptom for several years. Excessive adrenal androgens may cause acne and excessive hair growth. Hypercortisolism may cause pubertal delay in adolescent patients. Interestingly, young patients with CD may present with neuropsychiatric symptoms that differ from those of adult patients. Frequently, they tend to be obsessive and are high performers in school.

The differential diagnosis of CD includes adrenal tumors, ectopic ACTH production (rare in the pediatric population), and ectopic corticotrophin-releasing hormone (CRH)-producing tumors. In a child/adolescent with suspected CD the diagnosis may be problematic not only because these tumors are often not evident on magnetic resonance (MR) imaging, but because pseudo-Cushing's states can be difficult to distinguish definitively from true CD. Pseudo-Cushing's syndrome results in a hypercortisolemic state and may also include biochemical and physical features indistinguishable from those of CD, and is found mostly in patients with depression, obesity, and excessive alcohol intake. Although the precise mechanism underlying pseudo-CD remains unclear, this syndrome appears to be centrally mediated and may involve excessive hypothalamic secretion of CRH. Of note, this condition resolves with treatment of the underlying disease. Hence, the initial examination of a patient suspected of having CD should include screening for disorders that result in pseudo-Cushing's syndrome.

HORMONALLY ACTIVE PITUITARY ADENOMAS: GH-SECRETING ADENOMAS (SEE TABLE 34.4)

In adults, chronic GH hypersecretion causes acromegaly. Hallmarks of acromegaly include hyperostosis and hypertrophy of soft tissues. In children and adolescents with open epiphyseal plates, GH hypersecretion leads to gigantism [12–14]. The two disorders may be considered along a spectrum of GH excess with manifestations determined by the age of disease onset. The clinical overlap between gigantism and acromegaly with approximately 10% of acromegalics exhibiting tall stature and the majority of giants eventually demonstrating features of acromegaly supports this hypothesis [15].

HORMONALLY ACTIVE PITUITARY ADENOMAS: PRL-SECRETING ADENOMAS (SEE TABLE 34.5)

The clinical manifestations of PRL-secreting adenomas vary depending on the age and gender of the patient. Prepubertal children generally present with a combination of headache, visual disturbance, growth failure, and primary amenorrhea. Adolescent and adult women more commonly present with amenorrhea and galactorrhea. Although men may experience galactorrhea, they more often present secondary to tumor mass effect and report headache, visual disturbance, diminished libido, sexual dysfunction and loss of vitality [16].

DIAGNOSTIC EVALUATION OF SELLAR LESIONS

All patients suspected of harboring a tumor in the region of the sella turcica should undergo a complete neurological, ophthalmological, endocrinological, and imaging evaluation. A careful neurological examination is performed, especially noting any focal neurological deficits, including cranial neuropathies. All patients old enough to cooperate should undergo formal visual field testing, visual acuity testing, and dilated fundoscopic examination. Each facet of the hypothalamic-pituitary-end organ axis should be assessed with appropriate laboratory evaluation, including tests for diabetes insipidus, when indicated [16].

Determination of the possible presence of a functioning pituitary adenoma should be made, and serum PRL levels should be evaluated in all patients with pituitary and parasellar tumors. Mild elevation (levels up to 150–200 ng/ml) may be due to a stalk effect (loss of inhibition), but levels greater than 200 ng/mL suggest the presence of a PRL-secreting adenoma. Further assessment for a hyperfunctioning pituitary lesion includes an evaluation for Cushing's syndrome. In a subject with suspected Cushing's syndrome, screening tests including 24-hour urine free cortisol excretion and cortisol response to a 1 mg overnight

Table 34.5 Clinical Manifestations of Prolactinomas

Amenorrhea
Galactorrhea
Infertility
Sexual dysfunction, loss of libido
Headache
Fatigue

dexamethasone suppression test are routinely performed. If these tests are abnormal, further dexamethasone testing using graded doses of dexamethasone and measurement of serum ACTH are performed to confirm the diagnosis. In a subject with suspected acromegaly, an oral glucose tolerance test (OGTT) and/or measurement of serum insulin-like growth factor-1 (IGF-1) should be performed. Inability to suppress GH to < 1 ng/ml following an OGTT and/or an elevated serum IGF-1 (normalized for gender and age) are suggestive of the diagnosis of acromegaly [14].

In the setting of a sellar mass, it is highly important to assess pituitary function to exclude hypopituitarism that would necessitate hormone replacement [6,12]. Assessment of the pituitary-adrenal axis is most critical, as adrenal insufficiency can be life threatening. Adrenal function is assessed by a morning serum cortisol measurement, or, preferably, dynamic testing using a cortrosyn stimulation test or insulin tolerance test. Thyroid function is evaluated by measuring free thyroxine, total thyroxine, and TSH. The presence of a low or low normal free-thyroxine level in the setting of a low or low normal TSH is consistent with central hypothyroidism. The pituitary-gonadal axis is assessed by determination of the presence of menstrual cycles in a woman of childbearing age, or hypogonadotropic testosterone deficiency in a male. It is notable that diabetes insipidus is rarely present in a subject with a pituitary adenoma, and the presence of diabetes insipidus suggests a diagnosis other than pituitary adenoma. The presence of GH deficiency can be highly suggested by a low serum IGF-1, but provocative testing using an insulin tolerance test, glucagon, or an arginine/GH-releasing hormone stimulation test may be necessary to assess GH reserve.

Imaging is carried out with dedicated MR imaging of the sellar region. At times, a computed tomographic (CT) scan may be useful to assess the degree of aeration of the sella, particularly in younger patients where the sella has not yet become fully pneumatized. The CT also demonstrates calcifications that help differentiate a Rathke's cleft cyst from craniopharyngioma in patients who present with cystic sellar/parasellar lesions. It facilitates identification of bony abnormalities (such as sphenoid septations, bone dehiscence) before surgery.

SURGICAL ANATOMY OF THE SELLAR REGION AND DIAGNOSTIC IMAGING

An understanding of sellar and parasellar anatomy and development is critical to the diagnosis of pathology in this region. The pituitary gland is composed of anterior and posterior lobes that develop separately before fusing during embryogenesis. The anterior lobe (adenohypophysis) arises from Rathke's pouch in the primordial stomodium and then migrates along the craniopharyngial duct to the sella. The posterior lobe (neurohypophysis) arises from an evagination of the developing inferior third ventricle which then migrates downward into the sella. The sella turcica is a goblet-like depression in the sphenoid bone bounded anteriorly and inferiorly by the sphenoid sinus, laterally by the cavernous sinuses, posteriorly by the dorsum sellae, and superiorly by the diaphragma sellae and suprasellar cistern.

In normal adults the adenohypophysis appears isointense to cerebral white matter on standard T1-weighted MR images. The neurohypophysis may appear hyperintense to the adenohypophysis on T1-weighted images, because of the effect of stored neurosecretory granules on relaxation time. This hyperintense region, the so-called posterior pituitary "bright spot", is evident in up to 90% of children but is less consistently observed in adults (see Figure 34.1), and is rarely seen in patients with macroadenomas of the pituitary.

Parasellar anatomy is visualized best on contrast-enhanced MR images [17]. The cavernous sinus, which lies directly lateral to the pituitary gland, enhances after the administration of gadolinium (Gd). Its enhancement is normally greater than that of the adjacent pituitary gland so that the border between the gland and the cavernous sinus can often be discerned. The internal carotid artery within the cavernous sinus appears as a signal void on magentic resonance imaging (MRI) images because the protons within flowing blood do not produce detectable signal on T1- or T2-weighted pulse sequences. On sagittal images the carotid siphon may be seen in profile, and in coronal images it is seen in cross-section as several round flow voids. Within the enhanced cavernous sinus, portions of cranial nerves III, IV, V, and VI may rarely be identified on the coronal or axial images. In coronal images, cranial nerve III lies lateral and slightly superior to the carotid artery. The course of cranial nerve VI parallels the internal carotid artery in axial images.

Since the anatomy of the sphenoid sinus is critical in the majority of surgical approaches to the sella, this warrants special mention. In spite of the complex anatomy and important surgical relationships of the sphenoid sinus, very few reports have focused on it. The sphenoid sinus is extremely variable with respect to size, shape, and relation to the sella. Oftentimes it contains septations, which can complicate its surgical anatomy, and can contain varying degrees of pneumatization, particularly in pediatric patients.

The sphenoid sinus has been described as being postsellar, presellar, or conchal. The postsellar type of sphenoid sinus is well pneumatized with bulging of the sellar floor into the sinus. The presellar type of sinus is situated in the anterior sphenoid bone and does not penetrate beyond the perpendicular plate of the tuberculum sellae. The conchal type of sphenoid sinus does not reach into the body of the sphenoid bone, and its anterior wall is separated from the sella turcica by approximately 10 mm of cancellous bone. In cases of extensive pneumatization, the maxillary nerve may bulge into the lateral wall of the sphenoid sinus. In extreme cases, the nerve may be entirely surrounded by pneumatization.

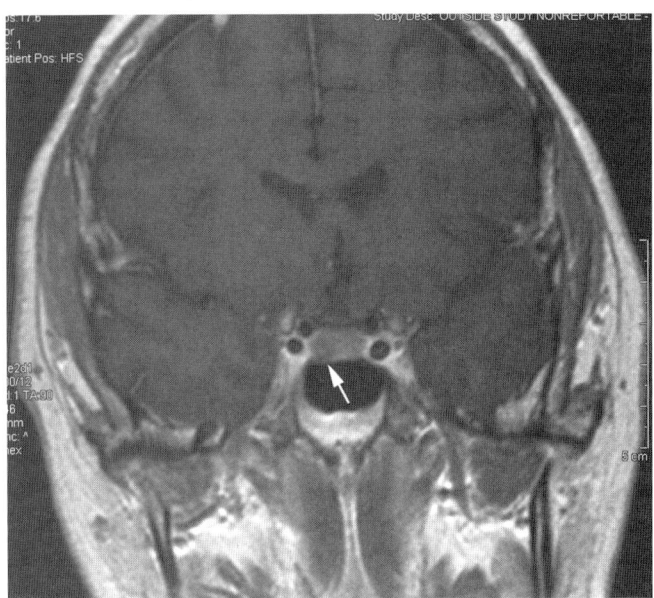

Figure 34.2 Coronal MRI demonstrating a pituitary microadenoma in a patient with Cushing's disease.

Identifying the ostia of the sphenoid sinus is critical for both endoscopic and microscopic approaches to the pituitary (see section on transsphenoidal surgery). The ostia are usually located in the sphenoethmoidal recess, medial to the superior or supreme turbinate where they can usually be seen well with the endoscope. The floor of sphenoid sinus is occasionally composed of ridges that cover the vidian nerve. The medial and superior walls are usually smooth, and the superior wall may balloon outward from pressure of the sella turcica.

Two bulges on the lateral wall of the sinus are of considerable clinical significance. They are produced by the optic nerve and the internal carotid artery. Depending on the degree of pneumatization, these two bulges may be barely noticeable or very obvious.

MR imaging is the most sensitive method of radiographic assessment of the pituitary, although the sensitivity of this technique in detecting small pituitary lesions is variable, and can be as low as 0.22 cm in patients with CD (see Figure 34.2).

In cases where T1-weighted MR imaging is negative or equivocal, a variety of more sensitive imaging techniques have shown promise in detecting adenomas in secretory tumors. An angiogram, CTA, or MRA may be used in cases where an aneurysm or pseudoaneurysm is suspected, and diffusion weighted imaging may be used in cases where an epidermoid tumor is suspected. Special MR sequences are helpful in diagnosing specific tumor subtypes, particularly secretory adenomas. This is particularly relevant in CD, where tumors are often undetectable on MR imaging. Spoiled gradient-recalled acquisition in the steady state (SPGR) MR imaging involves acquiring thin sections of 1 mm thickness (compared with 2.5–3 mm on standard SE sequences), using a spoiler gradient to shorten repetition time. The SPGR technique allows for substantial improvement in the spatial resolution of images that are acquired.

In a study of 30 children with CD, Batista et al. reported the overall probability that postcontrast SE-MR imaging would be positive in a child with surgically proven CD was 25%, while the probability of postcontrasted SPGR–MR imaging on the same patient was 71% [18]. Similar data have been reported in adults as well.

Dynamic MR imaging takes advantage of a tumor's characteristic slow constant enhancement when compared to the normal pituitary. Studies have demonstrated that the timing of postcontrast imaging is critical in diagnosing an adenoma, since the adenoma–normal pituitary maximal contrast following Gd injection may occur in some cases within seconds and last for only a few minutes. Modern MR technology now allows further dynamic studies, such as acquisition of images within seconds after the injection of Gd, allowing dynamic MR imaging to capture the early maximal contrast differences between tumors and normal pituitary tissue.

CONCLUSION

Prognosis for patients with sellar tumors depends upon patient status, comorbid conditions, tumor size, extension and functional histotype. Serial clinical, ophthalmological, endocrinological, and radiological evaluations are required for patients with nonfunctioning tumors. Children and adolescents should have careful monitoring of height, weight, and pubertal status. A qualified neuroendocrine team should screen patients for hypothyroidism, adrenal insufficiency, diabetes insipidus, and other endocrinopathies at regular intervals, and hormone replacement should be administered if needed. A postoperative MRI should be performed within 3 months of treatment, and yearly thereafter to evaluate for tumor recurrence or for residual tumor that is present.

For hormonally active tumors, surveillance measures should include the steps outlined above, as well as specific attention to ensure that the hormonal hypersecretion remains normalized.

REFERENCES

1. Barker FG II, Klibanski A, Swearingen B. Transsphenoidal surgery for pituitary tumors in the United States, 1996–2000: mortality, morbidity, and the effects of hospital and surgeon volume. *J Clin Endocrinol Metab*. 2003;88:4709–4719.
2. Laws ER, Sheehan JP. *Pituitary Surgery: A Modern Approach*. Basel, NY: Karger; 2006.
3. Ezzat S, Asa SL, Couldwell WT, et al. The prevalence of pituitary adenomas: a systematic review. *Cancer*. 2004;101:613–619.
4. Haupt R, Magnani C, Pavanello M, Caruso S, Dama E, Garre ML. Epidemiological aspects of craniopharyngioma. *J Pediatr Endocrinol Metab*. 2006;19(suppl 1):289–293.
5. Bunin GR, Surawicz TS, Witman PA, Preston-Martin S, Davis F, Bruner JM. The descriptive epidemiology of craniopharyngioma. *J Neurosurg*. 1998;89:547–551.
6. Sklar CA. Craniopharyngioma: endocrine abnormalities at presentation. *Pediatr Neurosurg*. 1994;21(suppl 1):18–20.
7. Richmond IL, Wilson CB. Parasellar tumors in children. I. Clinical presentation, preoperative assessment, and differential diagnosis. *Childs Brain*. 1980;7:73–84.
8. Cannavo S, Venturino M, Curto L, et al. Clinical presentation and outcome of pituitary adenomas in teenagers. *Clin Endocrinol (Oxf)*. 2003;58:519–527.

9. Jagannathan J, Dumont AS, Jane JA Jr. Diagnosis and management of pediatric sellar lesions. *Front Horm Res.* 2006;34:83–104.
10. Arnaldi G, Angeli A, Atkinson AB, et al. Diagnosis and complications of Cushing's syndrome: a consensus statement. *J Clin Endocrinol Metab.* 2003;88:5593–5602.
11. Reitmeyer M, Vance ML, Laws ER Jr. The neurosurgical management of Cushing's disease. *Mol Cell Endocrinol.* 2002;197:73–79.
12. Katznelson L, Kleinberg D, Vance ML, et al. Hypogonadism in patients with acromegaly: data from the multi-centre acromegaly registry pilot study. *Clin Endocrinol (Oxf).* 2001;54:183–188.
13. Molitch ME. Clinical manifestations of acromegaly. *Endocrinol Metab Clin North Am.* 1992;21:597–614.
14. Vance ML. Endocrinological evaluation of acromegaly. *J Neurosurg.* 1998;89:499–500.
15. Laws ER Jr. Acromegaly and gigantism. In: Wilkins RH, Rengechary SS, eds. *Neurosurgery.* New York, NY: McGraw Hill; 1985: 864–867.
16. Abboud CF, Laws ER Jr. Clinical endocrinological approach to hypothalamic-pituitary disease. *J Neurosurg.* 1979;51:271–291.
17. Davis WL, Lee JN, King BD, Harnsberger HR. Dynamic contrast-enhanced MR imaging of the pituitary gland with fast spin-echo technique. *J Magn Reson Imaging.* 1994;4:509–511.
18. Batista D, Courkoutsakis NA, Oldfield EH, Griffin KJ, Keil M, Patronas NJ, Stratakis CA. Detection of adrenocorticotropin-secreting pituitary adenomas by magnetic resonance imaging in children and adolescents with Cushing disease. *J Clin Endocrinol Metab.* 2005;90:5134–5140.

35 Presentation and Clinical Features of Spinal Cord Tumors

Herbert H. Engelhard, III, Edward Andrew Michals, and John Lee Villano

INTRODUCTION

Primary spinal cord (SC) tumors are relatively rare, representing 4% to 6% of all central nervous system (CNS) tumors [1–4], which corresponds roughly to their proportion of weight of neural tissue. The most common presenting symptoms are pain (back and/or radicular) and motor or sensory loss [4]. Primary SC tumors are organized based on their anatomy in relation to the dura, and whether or not they arise from the substance of the SC itself. SC tumors occur more commonly in older adults, with nerve sheath tumors (e.g., schwannomas and neurofibromas), meningiomas, astrocytomas, and hemangioblastomas forming the majority of cases (see Figure 35.1) [1]. SC tumors are less common in children, with neuroepithelial tumors (e.g., gliomas and ependymomas) representing the majority of the pediatric cases [1]. Most primary SC tumors are low grade, with older adults having a higher percentage of the higher grade tumors [1,4]. This results in the 65 and older age group having the poorest outcome [1]. Combining all histologies, survival for primary SC tumors at 5 years is 71% [1]. Matched for grade, astrocytomas are the most aggressive of the SC tumors. Unlike the situation within the brain, glioblastoma of the SC is exceedingly rare [4].

Magnetic resonance imaging (MRI) is the imaging modality of choice when there is the clinical suspicion of a SC tumor. Nearly all patients with tumor receive surgery for tissue diagnosis, or for definitive treatment, with the goal of complete resection, when it can be safely accomplished [4]. Some patients with intrinsic lesions of the SC (not proven to be tumor) are watched very closely with serial neurological examination and MRI, given the significant risks of surgery in this group of patients, where it is not definitively known that the lesion is a neoplasm. Although surgery is the primary treatment for SC tumors, radiation therapy also plays an important role in treating patients with malignant SC tumors either in the definitive or adjuvant setting following subtotal resection. Currently, chemotherapy is largely limited to treating refractory SC tumors [5,6].

Other lesions of the SC can mimic the presentation of SC tumor. Non-neoplastic, nontraumatic causes of SC symptoms and signs (i.e., myelopathy) include inflammatory, infectious, vascular, metabolic, spondylitic, and other causes. Additional serum and spinal fluid tests may complement MRI of the SC to help determine the underlying cause of myelopathy. In children, an extended period of back pain can often be caused by a serious problem and should be investigated [7].

INCIDENCE AND TUMOR HISTOLOGY

Primary tumors of the SC, spinal meninges, or cauda equina are relatively uncommon. Only about 5% of all primary CNS tumors are primary SC tumors or arise from the spinal meninges [1–4]. The overall incidence of SC tumors is 0.74 per 100 000 person-years, and therefore a little more than 2200 cases per year in the United States would be expected [1]. The incidence rate is lowest in children (0.26) and peaks in the 75- to 84-year age group (1.80). Rates are slightly higher in females (0.58–0.77) than in males (0.42–0.33), and higher in non-Hispanic whites than in Hispanics or non-Hispanic blacks [1]. In a recent multi-institutional study of 430 patients with primary intraspinal tumors, the mean age was 49.3 years, with a range of 1 to 93 years [4]. Only 6.3% of the patients were younger than 15 years; 57% were female and 43% male; and 78.6% were classified as being white, 8.6% black, 8.6% Hispanic, 1.4% Asian, and 2.8% other or unknown. Patients with SC tumor were found to be (on average) younger than patients having primary brain tumors [4].

Meningioma is the most common SC tumor, accounting for approximately 30% of cases. SC meningioma is primarily a disease of the elderly and has a striking female gender preference, with a male:female ratio of 0.29 [1,4,8,9]. Occurring slightly less than meningioma, schwannomas and ependymomas have similar incidence, representing approximately one quarter of patients [1,4,8,10,11]. Although both have median age at diagnosis in the forties, ependymomas have a wider age distribution and constitute nearly a quarter of SC tumors in children. Ependymomas have consistently demonstrated a male gender preference, with a male:female ratio of approximately 1.57 [1,9,11]. In children, astrocytomas are the most common SC tumor [1,3,4,9,12]. In all age groups, a wide variety of other histologies may rarely be encountered (see Figure 35.2). Overall, major SC histologies include the following: meningioma, ependymoma, schwannoma, astrocytoma, lymphoma and plasmacytoma, other glioma, lipoma and other benign unclassified tumors, hemangioblastoma, chordoma, teratoid and dermoid, neurofibroma, glioblastoma,

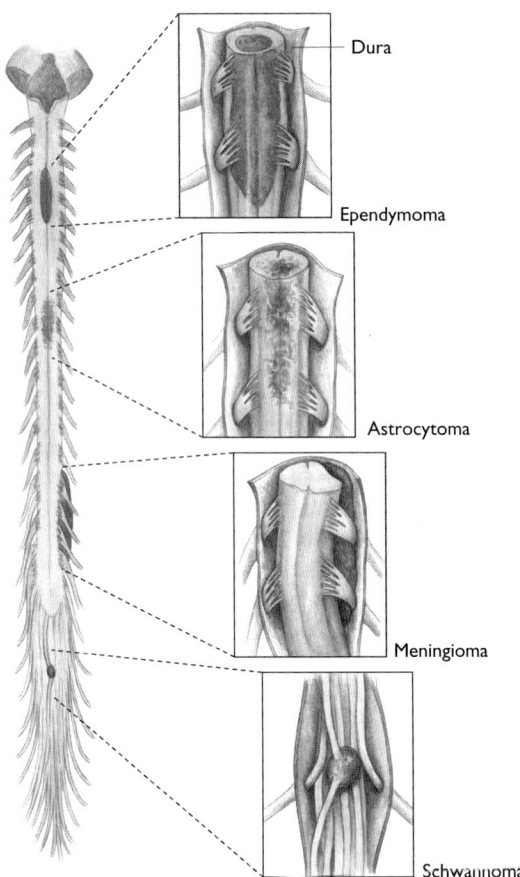

Figure 35.1 Examples of tumors in the intramedullary, extramedullary intradural, and extradural compartments.

oligodendroglioma, primitive neuroectodermal tumor, and other tumors [4].

COMPARTMENTS AND ANATOMY

Classically, primary SC tumors have been divided into three groups: (a) intramedullary (occurring within the SC itself), (b) extramedullary intradural, and (c) extradural. Common intramedullary tumors include astrocytomas and ependymomas. Meningiomas are usually extramedullary, but within the dura. Meningiomas may also occur in the epidural space [13]. Other intradural extramedullary tumors are the schwannoma and filum terminale ependymoma. About half of spinal ependymomas arise from the intradural portion of the filum terminale [8], most of which are of the myxopapillary histologic subtype. Nerve sheath tumors are also intradural and include the schwannoma and neurofibroma. Generally, a schwannoma occurs alongside the nerve root (and may splay it out into a thin sheet), whereas with a neurofibroma, the tumor cells and nerve fibers are intertwined in a fusiform fashion [8]. Cauda equina tumors, in addition to myxopapillary ependymoma, include schwannoma, lymphoma/plasmacytoma, meningioma, dermoid/lipoma, and other tumors including gliomas such as paraganglioma [4,14].

Anatomically, tumors in and around the SC may involve the bone, epidural space, nerve roots and intervertebral foramen, subdural or *intradural* (leptomeningeal) space, and/or the SC itself. Tumors of the bone may be anterior (arising from the vertebral body) and/or posterior (involving the lamina and/or spinous processes). Tumors that are posterior and/or posterolateral are surgically easier to remove (by laminectomy) than those directly in front

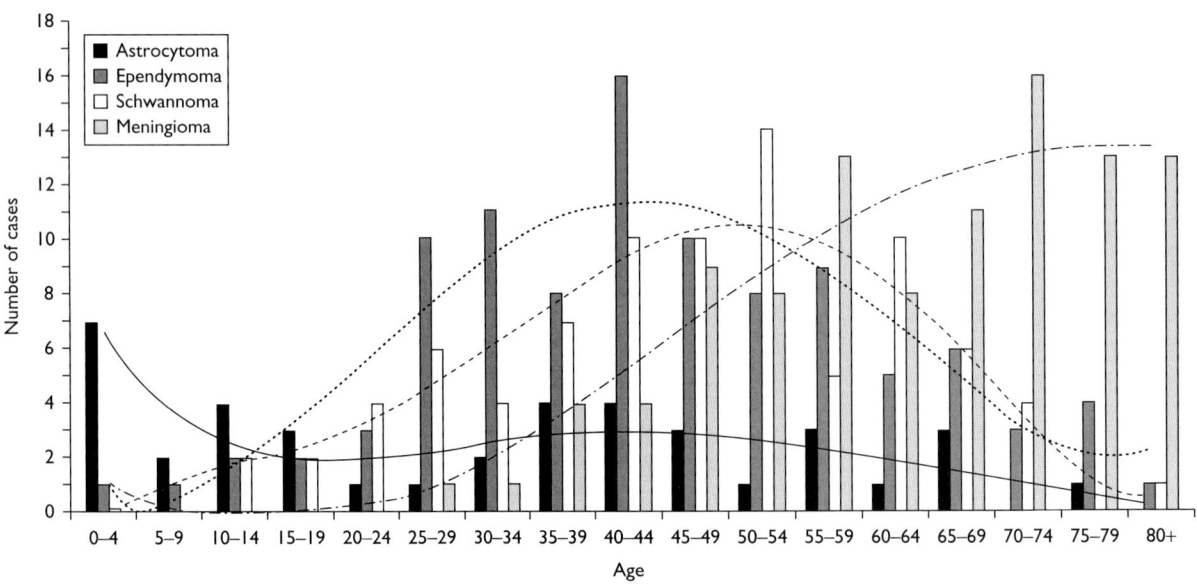

Figure 35.2 Age distribution of patients with spinal cord (SC) tumor. Astrocytomas are represented by the solid black bars, connected by a solid line; ependymomas are represented by hatched bars, connected by a dotted line; schwannomas are represented by dark dotted bars, connected by a dashed line; and meningiomas are represented by light dotted bars, connected by a dot and dash line. The trendlines are polynomial.

of the SC. Surgery for intradural tumors inherently runs a higher risk of postoperative spinal fluid leak. Surgery of tumors within the substance of the SC (i.e., intramedullary) poses the highest risk of permanent neurologic deficit, especially if there is not a distinct plane between tumor and non-neoplastic tissue. This being said, most patients do recover well from surgery [4]. Tumors may occur in a combination of compartments, for example, the bone and epidural space or schwannomas (most arise from nerve roots before leaving dura) that arise as the nerve root leaves the dural sac and has both an intradural and extradural component—dumbbell tumor [10].

ETIOLOGY

The etiology for primary SC tumor is largely unknown. An established risk factor for developing acoustic neuromas and intracranial gliomas and meningiomas is high-dose ionizing radiation, which increases the risk by a factor of 3 to 10, with a latency period of 10 years or more. Much of these data have been derived from the Israel tinea capitis cohort (new and prospective immigrants who were treated for scalp fungal infection) [15], a Swedish study of children treated with ionizing radiation for hemangiomas of the skin (40% of which were on the head or neck [16]), and the Childhood Cancer Survivor Study (this study lacked localization of radiation) [17]. Although not well established, it is likely that high-dose ionizing radiation to the spine may also increase the risk of developing SC tumors. Lumbosacral lipomas are considered to be more a spinal dysraphism than a true neoplasm and are not considered here [18].

Genetic factors undoubtedly influence the susceptibility to the development of a primary SC tumor. Persons with neurofibromatosis type 2 (NF2; locus 22q12) nearly all have bilateral vestibular schwannomas, but often the most debilitating manifestation is that of a SC tumor, which occurs in two thirds of patients or more [19]. The most common SC tumor in NF2 patients is schwannoma, which usually originates within the intravertebral (i.e., spinal) canal [20]. Less commonly, spinal meningiomas and intramedullary astrocytoma and ependymomas are thought to occur in at least 10% of patients with NF2 [21].

Loss of the *von Hippel-Lindau* gene (VHL; locus 3p25), which occurs in 1:36 000 (similar frequency as NF2), can lead to CNS hemangioblastomas involving the cerebellum or spine [22]. Nearly one fourth of intramedullary hemangioblastomas have the VHL syndrome [23]. These are highly vascular tumors where feeding arteries can often be visualized. They are pathologically similar to clear cell renal cell cancers. Presentation is usually from symptoms of local growth, but occasionally significant hemorrhage can be the inciting event [24].

CLINICAL PRESENTATION AND GENERAL OVERVIEW

The symptoms and signs of patients with primary SC tumors vary according to (a) anatomic compartment (as described earlier), (b) histology, and (c) level of involvement of the SC, that is, whether the tumor involves the high cervical, cervical, thoracic, and/or lumbar level, or the cauda equina. Of these three factors, the *level* of involvement best predicts the patient's presentation, yet the initial diagnosis of a SC tumor may still be challenging even for experienced clinicians.

Overall, the most common symptoms (in order of frequency) have been pain, extremity weakness, numbness and/or tingling, difficulty with coordination and/or balance, and urinary incontinence [4,14,25–29]. Symptoms reported in patients with primary SC tumors are listed in the left-top column of Table 35.1 [4]. The most frequently detected neurological signs include motor findings (weakness, fasciculations, and/or atrophy), decreased sensation, and difficulty with gait. The neurologic signs found to be associated with intraspinal tumors are listed in the left-lower column of Table 35.1 [4].

Table 35.1 Symptoms and Signs of Primary Intraspinal Tumors, According to Major Histologic Subgroup[a]

	Astrocytoma	Ependymoma	Schwannoma	Meningioma	Overall
Symptoms					
Pain	45.0	60.6	63.7	42.3	52.2
Weakness and/or paralysis	65.0	49.5	33.0	63.5	52.0
Numbness and/or tingling	52.5	52.5	34.1	50.0	45.9
Coordination and/or balance	30.0	14.1	16.5	47.1	26.5
Urinary incontinence	17.5	13.1	5.5	16.3	13.0
Fatigue	15.0	6.1	2.2	4.8	5.9
Fecal incontinence	10.0	7.1	1.1	5.8	5.0
Weight change	10.0	2.0	2.2	1.9	3.3
Signs					
Weakness, fascics, atrophy	35.0	30.3	20.0	35.6	30.9
Decreased sensation	30.0	34.3	16.7	38.5	29.8
Difficulty with gait	20.0	16.2	13.3	35.6	21.8
Increased reflexes (lower)	30.0	16.2	13.3	36.9	22.9
Increased reflexes (upper)	17.5	3.0	4.4	12.6	8.8
Babinski sign	7.5	4.0	2.2	17.5	8.1
Altered alertness	12.5	5.1	2.2	10.6	6.4
Change in facial sensation	7.5	2.0	3.3	4.9	3.3

All figures are in %.

[a] From Engelhard et al [4].

Symptoms and signs may relate to spinal root (i.e., dermatomal) involvement, dysfunction of the SC itself (myelopathy), or a combination of the two. Although pain is often a cardinal feature, particularly with sensory root compression, intramedullary lesions of the SC may be painless. *Axial* pain may be a symptom, localized primarily to the cervical, thoracic, or lumbar region. Nondermatomal symptoms and signs of SC dysfunction (i.e., nonradicular) may relate to tumor involvement directly or indirectly with the motor and/or sensory SC tracts (see Figure 35.3). Such tracts are *laminated* with centrally located cervical fibers within the SC and peripheral sacral fibers [30]. Lesions affecting the SC at a particular level may generally cause motor, sensory, and or reflex disturbances at any level below such involvement.

Motor symptoms may include weakness, heaviness, changes in gait, and cramping or muscle spasms, and clinical signs of weakness, spasticity and increased tone, atrophy, and fasciculations. Control of respiration may be affected because the diaphragm is innervated by the C3–5 nerve roots. The main sensory symptoms are numbness and paresthesia. Sensory signs relate to the different sensory modalities, such as pain (pinprick), light touch, position sense, vibratory sensation, and discrimination of hot and cold. Determination of a relative sensory *level* provides a key finding for localizing the level of the tumor and/or associated cyst or syrinx. The term *relative* is used because the patient may be able to sense the testing below that dermatomal level (for instance to pinprick), but the sensation is not as acute as would be expected normally. The Romberg sign is a sensory finding indicating relative loss of position sense in the lower extremities. Imaging of the SC may reveal that the lesion is higher in the SC, than what would be expected by the level of the relative loss of sensation. Loss of facial sensation may occur with higher cervical SC tumors (characterized by "onion skin" pattern on the face) because of the spinal location of the nucleus of the fifth (trigeminal) cranial nerve, and descending sensory fibers.

Alterations in reflexes may commonly be seen as signs of a SC tumor, or other SC diseases. Reflexes are divided into two categories: superficial reflexes and deep tendon (muscle stretch) reflexes. Abnormal superficial reflexes include the classic Hoffman and Babinski signs (and their numerous named counterparts) and also the abdominal, cremasteric, and anal reflexes. Deep tendon reflexes are commonly checked at the wrist, biceps, triceps, knee, and ankle. Autonomic nervous system dysfunction may occur with SC tumors and involve bowel, bladder, sexual, and other sympathetic and/or parasympathetic functions.

CLINICAL PRESENTATION: COMPARTMENT

Many classic SC syndromes have been described. The most well-known of these include the central cord syndrome and the Brown-Séquard syndrome. Combinations of symptoms and signs may be confusing, adding to the difficulty in diagnosis. The clinical presentation of lesions of the foramen magnum (such as a meningioma) or cervical tumors extending into the brainstem can be especially challenging.

Each spinal root has a dorsal (sensory) and ventral (motor) component, which combine before exiting at the neural foramina. Tumor compression of the dorsal root would be expected to correspond to pain and/or sensory loss to the affected dermatome. Most SC schwannomas arise from the sensory root [8]. Sacrificing such a root (at surgery) may not necessarily cause an increased sensory deficit. Individual patients may vary in the precise distribution of their dermatomal patterns, and overlap may occur. The "radicular" pain from sensory root (or ganglion) compression is often described as being sharp or shooting; it may be aggravated by particular activities. The sensory loss usually involves pain and or light touch and may be accompanied by paresthesia or dysesthesia.

Ventral root (motor) dermatomal involvement can present with weakness and decreases in tone and bulk (i.e., atrophy). However, such changes may not be as pronounced as with spinal motor tract involvement, because the major muscle groups are innervated by multiple roots, for example, the quadriceps femoris. Autonomic

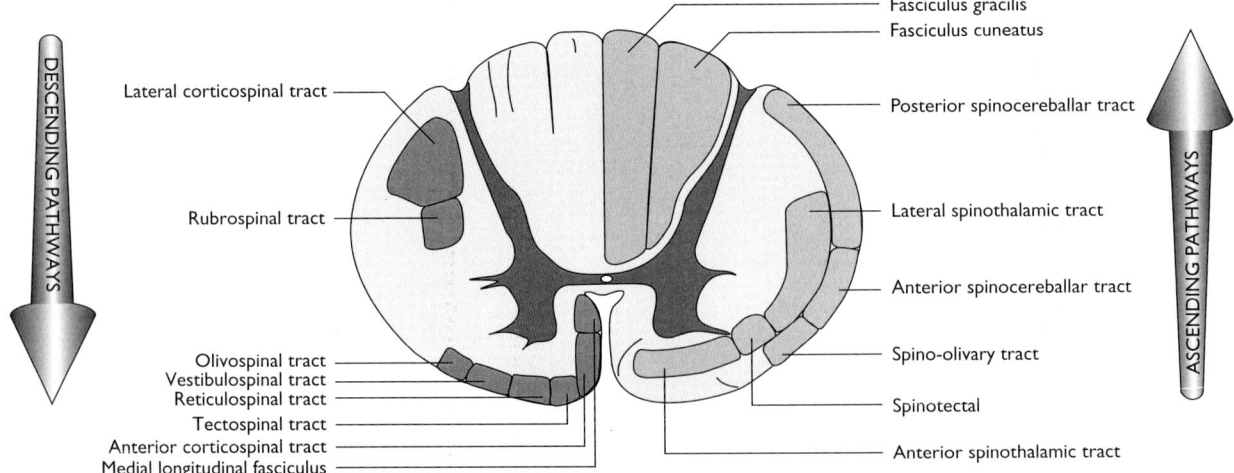

Figure 35.3 Major motor and sensory tracts of the spinal cord (cross section).

dysfunction, such as a Horner syndrome, may also occur with SC root involvement. Unlike the situation described earlier, deep tendon reflexes are *decreased* when the specific nerve *root* is involved, usually unilaterally. The biceps reflex corresponds to C5–6, triceps to C7–8, patellar reflex to L2–4, and ankle jerk (Achilles) to the S1 level.

A patient with a SC tumor may show a *combination* of effects, on careful neurologic examination, that is, a decreased deep tendon reflex and unilateral loss of sensation at the level of the tumor, and increased tone and generalized weakness below the level of the tumor due to generalized myelopathy. SC tumors (particularly intramedullary tumors) may cause an associated syringomyelia (cyst within the SC) or have an associated tumor cyst. The occurrence of either of these may cause more widespread findings both in terms of symptomatology and on neurologic exam.

The SC typically terminates at L1–2 at the conus medullaris, and at that level and distally, the exiting nerve roots form the cauda equina. A majority of patients with tumors of the cauda equina report significant radicular pain (with or without back pain), followed by numbness and/or tingling, weakness and/or paralysis, urinary incontinence, and/or fecal incontinence [4,14,27,31,32]. On examination, sensory deficits, leg weakness, and/or abolition of reflexes may be found [4,14]. The main differential diagnosis is with a herniated disc, lumbar stenosis, or a synovial cyst. The occurrence of tumors at the conus or cauda equina may interfere with sexual function. However, the full-blown cauda equina syndrome is very rarely seen in patients with cauda equina tumors [4].

NEURORADIOGRAPHIC FINDINGS

Intramedullary Tumors

Because of their rare incidence, SC tumors are not usually suspected until after an imaging study demonstrates their presence. MRI is the preferred imaging study and localizes the exact levels the tumor spans and the spinal compartment [33,34]. MRI identifies the constituents of the tumor and demonstrates the presence or absence of cystic, solid, and/or hemorrhagic components. This provides information required for surgical biopsy/resection, serial imaging, radiation and chemotherapy, or additional testing. Usually, MRI with and without contrast provides sufficient information; infrequently, however, postmyelogram computed tomography (CT) scanning may be necessary particularly to evaluate the bony elements and stability of the spine.

The common imaging features of all intramedullary tumors are cord expansion with narrowing of the surrounding cerebrospinal fluid (CSF) spaces and contrast enhancement of the solid component of tumors. Differences in radiographic appearance among astrocytomas, ependymomas, and hemangioblastoma include the site of the epicenter of the tumor, the clarity of the cord tumor interface, the presence or absence of blood products, and the presence and relative size of cystic spaces within the tumor.

Ependymomas originate centrally from the ependymal remnants of the central canal. The appearance of ependymomas reflects the location of this origin, the tendency to displace normal SC rather than infiltrate it, and the characteristic presence of cysts and hemorrhage (see Figure 35.4). On MRI, an ependymoma is seen as a well-demarcated mass with a clear interface between it and the normal spinal tissue. The presence of cord cysts of varying sizes within an ependymoma must be distinguished from cord edema that can extend beyond the capsule inferiorly and superiorly within the SC. The cystic components of the tumor are lower than normal cord on T1-weighted image (T1WI), markedly higher in signal than normal cord on T2-weighted image (T2WI) and does not enhance. The rim of the ependymoma is often hemorrhagic, and components are black on all sequences owing to hemosiderin deposition. Also, imaging of the entire spine axis is needed for concerns of dropped metastases.

The imaging of astrocytomas reflects their pattern of growth and pathologic appearance. Although astrocytomas are easily visualized with MRI, distinguishing normal cord from tumor is difficult because the tumor has numerous fibrils radiating in all directions and infiltrating normal tissues. The tumors have predominately low to isointense signal on T1WIs, high signal on T2WI, and greater than 90% enhance after the administration of

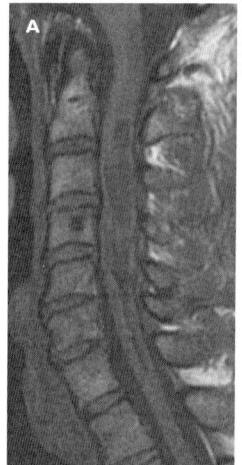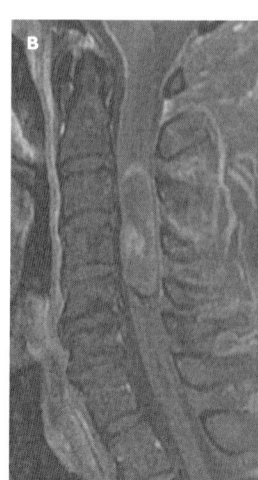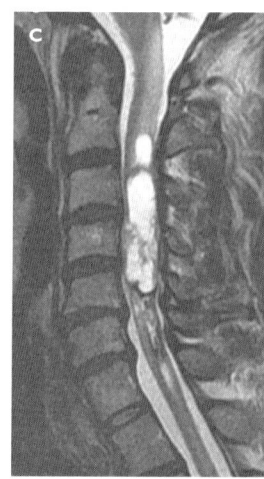

Figure 35.4 A 51-year-old male has a typical ependymoma. The tumor is relatively difficult to visualize on the noncontrast sagittal T1-weighted image (T1WI) **(A)**. After the administration of contrast, the tumor wall and the solid portions of the tumor enhance **(B)**. On the T2-weighted image (T2WI), the cystic areas are bright, the cord edema above and below the tumor is slightly less bright, and the hemorrhage in the tumor wall is dark **(C)**.

contrast. When cysts are present, the cystic portions are lower in signal on T1WI and higher in signal on T2WI and do not enhance with contrast.

In a typical hemangioblastoma, the large cystic portion is isodense to low signal on the T1WI and bright on the T2WI. The small nodule is usually eccentrically positioned in the dorsal aspect of the cord, and nodule is isointense on the T1WI and enhances intensely on the postcontrast images. The enhancing nodules have a predilection for the posterior third of the SC and may be quite superficial and can appear to be extramedullary. Although the most common appearance is a small enhancing nodule associated with a large intramedullary cyst, the nodule may be present without a cyst, an appearance that is often seen in the multiple tumors of VHL.

Extramedullary Tumors

The intradural extramedullary tumors of the spinal canal share many imaging similarities and can be difficult to distinguish preoperatively from one another [34,35]. All intradural extramedullary tumors displace the SC and widen the adjacent CSF space. The signal characteristics are fairly similar, with all generally isointense on T1WI and intensely enhance after the administration of contrast. The relationship of the tumor to the dura, nerves, and neural foramina may be helpful in distinguishing nerve sheath tumors from meningioma.

The three types of nerve sheath tumors are schwannoma, neurofibroma, and malignant nerve sheath tumor. Their common imaging features are an intimate association with the nerves and neural foramina and intense enhancement. The imaging differences between the types of nerve sheath tumors are the shape of the tumor, the presence of cystic degeneration in the larger schwannomas, and the relationship to the nerve root. When a nerve sheath extends into the neural foramina, the tumor exerts pressure and smoothly widens the neural foramina, which can be seen on CT or MRI. The portions of the tumor extends on both sides of the neural foramina grow larger in size compared with the tumor in the foramina because the bone constrains the growth. This forms a dumbbell-shaped neurofibroma or schwannoma.

Schwannomas tumors displace the cord and expand the adjacent CSF spaces. Like all nerve sheath tumors, schwannomas are intimately associated with the nerves in the lateral recess and/or neural foramina and can have a dumbbell configuration (see Figure 35.5). The tumor mass arises eccentrically from the nerve sheath. Schwannomas have a variable appearance on MRI. Schwannomas are typically isointense to slightly hyperintense on T1WI and bright on T2WI. After the administration of contrast, schwannomas enhance. The tumors can either be homogenous or heterogeneous and are related to the extracellular matrix. In addition, larger tumors can outgrow their blood supply and have central necrosis.

Neurofibromas are usually multiple, rarely solitary, tumors and are associated with neurofibromatosis type 1 (NF1). The nerve is affected longitudinally along its course, and it is typically diffusely widened rather than supporting

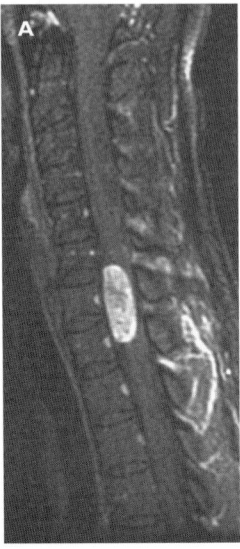
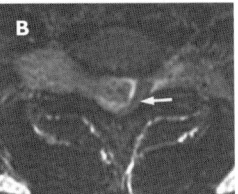

Figure 35.5 A 25-year-old female has a typical "dumbbell" schwannoma that enhances on the sagittal T1-weighted image (T1WI) **(A)**. The schwannoma displaces the spinal cord to the right (arrow) and expands the C7-T1 neuroforamina **(B)**.

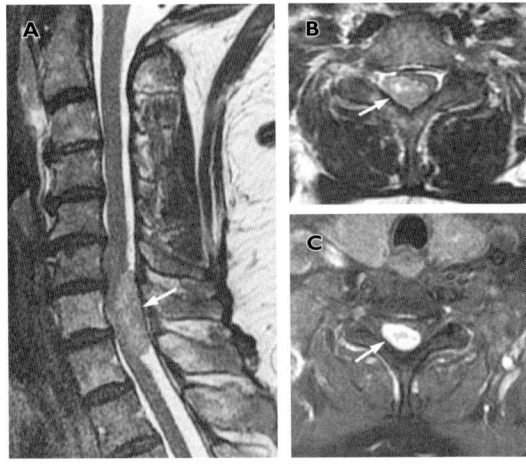

Figure 35.6 A 57-year-old female has a typical meningioma between C7 and T1. The mass (arrows) is intradural extramedullary and displaces the spinal cord, widens the cerebrospinal fluid (CSF) space next to the cord, and attaches broadly to the dura, which is best seen on the sagittal T2-weighted image (T2WI) **(A)**. The deformity and displacement of the cervical spinal cord is best seen on the axial T2WI **(B)** and axial postcontrast T1-weighted image (T1WI) **(C)**.

an eccentric bulbous tumor mass. Neurofibromas usually originate on the peripheral side of the dorsal root ganglia, but they can span and widen the neural foramina as well and have a dumbbell shape.

The typical meningioma is an intensely enhancing well-circumscribed intradural extramedullary mass with a broad dural attachment in a middle aged female that displaces, but does not invade, the cord. These masses are most commonly seen in the thoracic spine but can be anywhere in the neural axis. Meningiomas are isointense to slightly hypointense on T1WI and have a regular, but heterogeneous, appearance. On T2WI, meningiomas are isointense to slightly hyperintense relative to the SC and are well-demarcated by the surrounding bright CSF. After contrast administration, meningiomas enhance intensely and uniformly and may have a dural tail (see Figure 35.6).

SUMMARY

Patients with SC tumors may present with fascinating symptoms and signs, which may become more apparent on detailed neurologic examination. Diagnostic testing can be helpful in discriminating SC tumors from other lesions or conditions of the SC, such as multiple sclerosis or transverse myelitis. The most common SC tumor types are the meningioma, ependymoma, and schwannoma.

REFERENCES

1. Schellinger KA, Propp JM, Villano JL, McCarthy BJ. Descriptive epidemiology of primary spinal cord tumors. *J Neurooncol.* 2008;87:173–179.
2. Helseth A, Mork SJ. Primary intraspinal neoplasms in Norway, 1955 to 1986. A population-based survey of 467 patients. *J Neurosurg.* 1989;71:842–845.
3. Kaye AH, Giles GG, Gonzales M. Primary central nervous system tumours in Australia: a profile of clinical practice from the Australian Brain Tumour Register. *Aust N Z J Surg.* 1993;63:33–38.
4. Engelhard HH, Villano JL, Porter KR, et al. Clinical presentation, histology and treatment of 430 patients with primary tumors of the spinal cord, spinal meninges or cauda equina. *J Neurosurg-Spine.* 2010;13(1):67–77.
5. Fouladi M, Hunt DL, Pollack IF, et al. Outcome of children with centrally reviewed low-grade gliomas treated with chemotherapy with or without radiotherapy on Children's Cancer Group high-grade glioma study CCG-945. *Cancer.* 2003;98:1243–1252.
6. Chamberlain MC. Salvage chemotherapy for recurrent spinal cord ependymona. *Cancer.* 2002;95:997–1002.
7. Afshani E, Kuhn JP. Common causes of low back pain in children. *Radiographics.* 1991;11:269–291.
8. McCormick PC, Post KD, Stein BM. Intradural extramedullary tumors in adults. *Neurosurg Clin N Am.* 1990;1:591–608.
9. Preston-Martin S. Descriptive epidemiology of primary tumors of the spinal cord and spinal meninges in Los Angeles County, 1972–1985. *Neuroepidemiology.* 1990;9:106–111.
10. Conti P, Pansini G, Mouchaty H, et al. Spinal neurinomas: retrospective analysis and long-term outcome of 179 consecutively operated cases and review of the literature. *Surg Neurol.* 2004;61:34–43; discussion 44.
11. McCormick PC, Torres R, Post KD, Stein BM. Intramedullary ependymoma of the spinal cord. *J Neurosurg.* 1990;72:523–532.
12. Lowe GM. Magnetic resonance imaging of intramedullary spinal cord tumors. *J Neurooncol.* 2000;47:195–210.
13. Frank BL, Harrop JS, Hanna A, Ratliff J. Cervical extradural meningioma: case report and literature review. *J Spinal Cord Med.* 2008;31:302–305.
14. Waldron JN, Laperriere NJ, Jaakkimainen L, et al. Spinal cord ependymomas: a retrospective analysis of 59 cases. *Int J Radiat Oncol Biol Phys.* 1993;27:223–229.
15. Sadetzki S, Chetrit A, Freedman L, et al. Long-term follow-up for brain tumor development after childhood exposure to ionizing radiation for tinea capitis. *Radiat Res.* 2005;163:424–432.
16. Karlsson P, Holmberg E, Lundberg LM, et al. Intracranial tumors after radium treatment for skin hemangioma during infancy—a cohort and case-control study. *Radiat Res.* 1997;148:161–167.
17. Neglia JP, Robison LL, Stovall M, et al. New primary neoplasms of the central nervous system in survivors of childhood cancer: a report from the Childhood Cancer Survivor Study. *J Natl Cancer Inst.* 2006;98:1528–1537.
18. La Marca F, Grant JA, Tomita T, McLone DG. Spinal lipomas in children: outcome of 270 procedures. *Pediatr Neurosurg.* 1997;26:8–16.
19. Eldridge R, Parry D. Vestibular schwannoma (acoustic neuroma). Consensus development conference. *Neurosurgery.* 1992;30:962–964.
20. Parry DM, Eldridge R, Kaiser-Kupfer MI, et al. Neurofibromatosis 2 (NF2): clinical characteristics of 63 affected individuals and clinical evidence for heterogeneity. *Am J Med Genet.* 1994;52:450–461.
21. Mautner VF, Tatagiba M, Lindenau M, et al. Spinal tumors in patients with neurofibromatosis type 2: MR imaging study of frequency, multiplicity, and variety. *Am J Roentgenol.* 1995;165:951–955.
22. Tory K, Brauch H, Linehan M, et al. Specific genetic change in tumors associated with von Hippel-Lindau disease. *J Natl Cancer Inst.* 1989;81:1097–1101.
23. Wizigmann-Voos S, Plate KH. Pathology, genetics and cell biology of hemangioblastomas. *Histol Histopathol.* 1996;11:1049–1061.
24. Richard S, Campello C, Taillandier L, et al. Haemangioblastoma of the central nervous system in von Hippel-Lindau disease. French VHL Study Group. *J Intern Med.* 1998;243:547–553.
25. Baleriaux DL. Spinal cord tumors. *Eur Radiol.* 1999;9:1252–1258.
26. Constantini S, Houten J, Miller DC, et al. Intramedullary spinal cord tumors in children under the age of 3 years. *J Neurosurg.* 1996;85:1036–1043.
27. McCormick PC, Stein BM. Intramedullary tumors in adults. *Neurosurg Clin N Am.* 1990;1:609–630.
28. Stein BM. Intramedullary spinal cord tumors. *Clin Neurosurg.* 1983;30:717–741.
29. Vinken PJ, Bruyn GW. *Tumours of the Spine and Spinal Cord. Pt. I-II.* Amsterdam: North-Holland; 1975.
30. Snell RS. *Clinical Neuroanatomy.* Philadelphia: Lippincott Williams & Wilkins; 2006.
31. Bagley CA, Gokaslan ZL. Cauda equina syndrome caused by primary and metastatic neoplasms. *Neurosurg Focus.* 2004;16:e3.
32. Wippold FJ II, Smirniotopoulos JG, Pilgram TK. Lesions of the cauda equina: a clinical and pathology review from the Armed Forces Institute of Pathology. *Clin Neurol Neurosurg.* 1997;99:229–234.
33. Van Goethem JW, van den Hauwe L, Ozsarlak O, et al. Spinal tumors. *Eur J Radiol.* 2004;50:159–176.
34. Koeller KK, Rosenblum RS, Morrison AL. Neoplasms of the spinal cord and filum terminale: radiologic-pathologic correlation. *Radiographics.* 2000;20:1721–1749.
35. Beall DP, Googe DJ, Emery RL, et al. Extramedullary intradural spinal tumors: a pictorial review. *Curr Probl Diagn Radiol.* 2007;36:185–198.

36 Supportive Care in Neuro-Oncology

Herbert B. Newton

INTRODUCTION

The modern treatment of patients with brain tumor usually involves a team approach from a dedicated group of physicians, nurses, and support staff who specialize in various aspects of neuro-oncology [1]. Although the focus of the treatment team will be on therapeutic strategies to control tumor growth (e.g., surgical resection, radiotherapy, chemotherapy), many other facets of care are necessary and will involve patient support and symptom management, in an effort to maintain quality of life. The challenge for the treatment team begins at the moment of diagnosis, when appropriate information must be communicated to the patient and family. Recent research suggests that there are several important factors that should be considered when imparting a new cancer diagnosis [2]. It is critical that the physician use simple, nontechnical language in a nonpatronizing manner, with a warm and caring tone. Every effort should be made to empathize with the emotions the patient is experiencing. The physician should sit close to the patient and maintain good eye contact. It is also permissible to initiate physical contact, in an effort to provide comfort. A quiet, private, and comfortable room should be used for the meeting, where interruptions and distractions can be minimized. Many patients also find it helpful when the physician gives some kind of warning that bad news is forthcoming and does not rush through the ensuing discussion.

The role of support is crucial for patients with brain tumor and their families, and it continues until the patient is cured or, more often, succumbs to his or her disease [3]. The most important initial form of support is information and education about the diagnosis. At the moment the patient and family hear the words "brain tumor," they enter into a crisis mode and often feel a loss of control, fear of the unknown, and sense of helplessness. To regain some aspect of control of their lives, they need to learn as much as possible about the disease and form a partnership with their physician, taking an aggressive and active role in the plan for treatment and recovery. Informational brochures and other written materials are helpful, as are the websites of organizations that provide services and resources for patients with brain tumor and families, such as the North American Brain Tumor Coalition [3]. The Coalition is a network of charitable organizations dedicated to the cure of brain tumors, and it includes the American Brain Tumor Association, the Brain Tumor Foundation for Children, the Brain Tumor Foundation of Canada, the Brain Tumor Society, the Children's Brain Tumor Foundation, the National Brain Tumor Foundation, the Pediatric Brain Tumor Foundation of the United States, and the Preuss Foundation. During the course of a devastating illness such as a brain tumor, the patient's family will usually be the greatest source of support and comfort as well as active caregivers in the home setting [3,4]. In this context, family members often take on the role of information seekers and patient advocates. It is important to note that family caregivers are also at risk for depression and other signs of stress and require a strong support network to function effectively in this role [5]. Other sources of support for the patient and caregivers include the nurses of the treatment team, oncological social workers, Chaplains affiliated with the hospital or from the private sector, and hospital-based support groups (brain tumor specific or general).

The remaining sections of this chapter will review the various aspects of supportive care that may be necessary in the management of patients with brain tumor.

SEIZURES AND ANTICONVULSANT THERAPY

Seizure activity is a frequent complication in neuro-oncology patients and often compromises quality of life by the restriction of driving privileges, through seizure-related injuries, loss of time at work, and anxiety related to subsequent ictal events [1,6–8]. In addition, quality of life can be further affected by the side effects, drug interactions, and expenses incurred by the use of antiepileptic drugs (AEDs). Seizures occur at presentation in 20% to 50% of patients with primary brain tumor (PBT) and metastatic brain tumor (MBT) [1,6,9]. It is important to note that more than 25% of adults between 25 and 64 years of age with newly diagnosed seizures will have an underlying brain tumor [6]. At the time of tumor progression, seizure activity often becomes more frequent and severe, affecting another 10% to 20% of patients. The overall incidence of seizures is highest in patients with PBT of low histological grade and slow growth potential and becomes less frequent in those with high-grade PBT and MBT. For example, approximately 80% to 90% of patients with oligodendrogliomas and ganglioglioma will have seizures, whereas patients with more malignant PBT like anaplastic astrocytoma and glioblastoma multiforme (GBM) carry a risk for seizure activity of 68% and 33%, respectively [8]. Younger patients (e.g., children and young adults) tend to have a higher incidence of seizure activity when the tumors are supratentorial in location. In general, supratentorial tumors are most likely to cause seizures, especially when located within or near the cortex. Multifocal or bihemispheric tumors are also known to cause frequent ictal events. Seizures are much less common with tumors that are deep-seated or confined to the white matter.

Patients with low-grade tumors typically manifest seizures that are equally divided between partial motor, partial complex, and secondarily generalized varieties [6–8]. For patients with high-grade gliomas or brain metastases, focal motor seizures are the predominant variety, with less common secondarily generalized and complex partial seizures. The neurological examination tends to be relatively normal and nonfocal in patients with seizures from low-grade tumors. In contrast, patients with high-grade PBT and MBT are more likely to have seizure activity associated with focal neurological deficits on examination [6,7].

The pathophysiological mechanisms underlying tumor-associated seizures (TASs) remain unclear [8,10,11]. Recent evidence using direct brain recordings of electrical activity suggests that TAS originate from intact, non-infiltrated, neural tissue adjacent to tumors and not from within the tumor mass itself [10]. Histologically, epileptogenic regions of brain demonstrate gliosis and mild reactive astrocytosis, without evidence for tumor cells. It is now theorized that these peritumoral epileptogenic foci develop an imbalance between excitatory and inhibitory inputs, owing to multifactorial alterations in the local milieu from the tumor. The intracellular and extracellular pH is slightly alkaline in peritumoral tissues, which enhances excitatory neuronal pathways and induces a 30% reduction of activity in gamma amino butyric acid (GABA)-ergic inhibitory pathways [10]. In biopsy samples from peritumoral epileptic foci, the number of GABA- and somatostatin-containing neurons is decreased [12]. Similar biopsy studies have noted an elevated concentration of glutamine, the direct precursor of glutamate, in peritumoral epileptogenic foci [13]. Glutamine is taken up and secreted by normal glia and glioma cells, thus providing a large reservoir of precursor for peritumoral neurons to convert to glutamate. In addition, recent evidence suggests that glioma cells directly secrete glutamate, causing significantly increased, excitotoxic concentrations in peritumoral tissues [14,15]. In vitro experiments have demonstrated extensive N-methyl D-aspartate (NMDA) and α-amino-3-hydroxy-5-methyl-4-isoxazolepropionic acid (AMPA) receptor stimulation and delayed Ca^{2+}-dependent cell death in exposed neurons. These reports suggest that exposure of peritumoral neurons to chronically elevated concentrations of glutamate could contribute to neuronal injury, abnormalities of neuronal circuitry, and the development of epileptiform activity. Other peritumoral alterations that may contribute to epileptogenic potential include increased extracellular Fe^{3+}, dysfunction of astrocytic syncytial gap junctions due to the infiltration of tumor cells, and the presence of proinflammatory cytokines (e.g., tumor necrosis factor-α), which can increase membrane excitability [8].

The diagnosis of a seizure in a patient with a brain tumor is usually a clinical diagnosis, based on the history and description of the symptom complex from the patient and family members [1,6–8]. Testing with routine electroencephalography (EEG) is not helpful in most patients, because only 25% to 33% will demonstrate any focal interictal epileptiform activity. Prolonged EEG monitoring (with or without a video component) may be more helpful in diagnosing seizures in confusing or subtle cases. Once a patient with a malignant PBT has had a seizure, 50% to 75% will continue to have seizures [7]. In one half of the active seizure group, ictal events will occur more than once per month, whereas another 25% will have events more than once per week, despite the use of AED. The presence of seizure activity does not impact on the overall survival of patients with brain tumor [6]. However, patients who present with a seizure or have long-standing seizures do have a more favorable prognosis. There are several explanations for this phenomenon, including the increased likelihood that the tumor will be an oligodendroglioma, which typically have longer survival times, and that seizures will often lead to a more prompt work-up and earlier diagnosis, when the tumor is smaller and more amenable to surgical resection. Patients with chronic seizures that develop a new pattern, with frequent "breakthrough" activity, may relate to a change in the tumor such as bleeding or dedifferentiation into a more rapidly growing and more malignant lesion. It is also possible to have a "flare-up" of seizure activity, in otherwise well-controlled patients, at the onset of certain therapies that may cause irritation to surrounding brain, such as at the initiation of external beam radiotherapy and with certain forms of chemotherapy (e.g., gliadel wafers, intra-arterial cisplatin).

There is general consensus that any patient with a brain tumor with a well-documented, unequivocal seizure (generalized or focal) should be placed on an AED (see Table 36.1) [1,6–10]. For adult patients with generalized seizures, phenytoin, carbamazepine, and valproate have relatively equivalent efficacy for reducing seizure activity [16,17]. Similarly, all three drugs are effective for partial motor, partial sensory, and partial complex seizures. However, a comparative trial of carbamazepine and valproate has demonstrated better control of complex partial seizure activity with carbamazepine [18]. Monotherapy with phenytoin, carbamazepine, or valproate should be the initial management approach in most patients [1,16,17]. In some patients, a second drug must be added if high therapeutic concentrations of several of the first-line drugs are unable to control seizure activity. Phenytoin or carbamazepine in combination with valproate is a common strategy. Alternatively, one of the new anticonvulsants (e.g., levetiracetam, gabapentin, topiramate, zonisamide) could be added to one of the first-line agents [19–21]. Levetiracetam may be an excellent choice, because initial experience suggests it is effective and well tolerated in patients with brain tumor and has minimal potential to interact with other drugs such as corticosteroids or chemotherapy agents [21,22]. Ongoing studies will determine if levetiracetam and other new agents might be appropriate for first-line use or as secondary, stand-alone

Table 36.1 Antiepileptic Drugs Commonly Used for Treatment of Seizures in Patients with Brain Tumor

Drug	Dose (mg/day)	Metabolism	Enzyme Inducing	Bound Mechanism	Fraction (%)
Traditional AEDS					
Phenytoin	300–400	Hepatic +++	+++	Sodium channel	90–95
Carbamazepine	800–1600	Hepatic +++	+++	Sodium channel	75
Valproic acid	1000–3000	Hepatic +++	No; inhibitory	Sodium channel; enhanced GABA	80–90
Phenobarbital	90–180	Hepatic +++	+++	EAA antagonist; enhanced GABA	45
Newer AEDS					
Felbamate	2400–3600	Hepatic ++	+	EAA antagonist; enhanced GABA	25
Lamotrigine	100–500	Hepatic +++	None	Sodium channel	55
Gabapentin	1800–3600	Renal +++	None	Enhanced GABA	<5
Topiramate	200–400	Hepatic +	None	Sodium channel; EAA antagonist; enhanced GABA	9–17
Tiagabine	32–56	Hepatic +++	None	Enhanced GABA	95
Oxcarbazine	600–1800	Hepatic +++	+	Sodium channel	40
Levetiracetam	1000–3000	Renal ++	None	N-type calcium channels	<10
Zonisamide	100–400	Hepatic ++	None	Sodium and calcium channels; enhanced GABA	40

Adapted from refs. 6, 10, 16, and 17.

Abbreviations: +, mild; ++, moderate; +++, severe; AED, antiepileptic drug; EAA, excitatory amino acid; GABA, gamma amino butyric acid.

agents. Serum drug concentrations must be monitored and optimized in all patients whenever possible (e.g., phenytoin, carbamazepine, valproate).

In the brain tumor population, seizures remain difficult to control despite the use of AED. Patients who present with seizures tend to be more refractory to therapy than those who develop seizures later in the course of their disease [6,7]. In general, recurrent seizure activity is common, despite aggressive anticonvulsant therapy. Patient compliance can contribute to this problem and is frequently suboptimal. In many patients with a recent seizure, anticonvulsant levels are subtherapeutic. Further complicating the situation is that patients with brain tumor are more susceptible to AED toxicity and side effects, including cognitive impairment, hepatotoxicity, myelosuppression, skin rashes (including Stevens-Johnson syndrome), and interactions with concomitant medications [6]. Several AEDs (e.g., phenytoin carbamazepine, phenobarbital) enhance hepatic microsomal P-450-mediated metabolism of concomitant medications. This is especially problematic for patients receiving chemotherapy (e.g., nitrosoureas, temozolomide, irinotecan, paclitaxol, methotrexate), leading to lower tissue concentrations and reduced efficacy [6,23]. Some of the newer AEDs (e.g., levetiracetam, gabapentin) do not enhance the hepatic P-450 system and may be better choices in selected patients.

Anticonvulsant drugs are frequently administered to patients with brain tumor at the time of diagnosis or after craniotomy, as prophylaxis for potential seizure activity [6]. This practice was given early support in the literature, despite the fact that the data in these reports were modest at best [24,25]. All subsequent reports on the use of AED prophylaxis do not support this practice, including a randomized, blinded, placebo-controlled trial of valproate in patients with newly diagnosed PBT and MBT [26–30]. In this study, the odds ratio for a seizure in the valproate arm relative to the placebo arm was 1.7 ($p = 0.3$) [30]. Most authors would now recommend withholding implementation of AED in newly diagnosed patients until a seizure has been documented. This approach is supported by a recent meta-analysis by Glantz and associates for the American Academy of Neurology [31]. In addition, for patients who have not had a seizure and have received AED for craniotomy, tapering and discontinuing the AED after the first postoperative week is recommended [31].

CORTICOSTEROIDS

The use of corticosteroids is often necessary in patients with PBT and MBT to control symptoms caused by increased intracranial pressure (e.g., headache, nausea and emesis, confusion, weakness) [1,9,32]. Peritumoral edema is the principal cause of elevated intracranial pressure and is mediated through numerous mechanisms, including the leaky neovasculature associated with tumor angiogenesis, as well as increased permeability induced by factors secreted by the tumor and surrounding tissues, such as oxygen free radicals, arachidonic acid, glutumate, histamine, bradykinin, atrial natriuretic peptide, and vascular endothelial growth factor (VEGF) [33–35]. Dexamethasone is the high-potency steroid used most often to treat the edema associated with brain tumors [1,32]. It has several advantages over other synthetic glucocorticoids, including a longer half-life, reduced mineralocorticoid effect, lower incidence of cognitive and behavioral complications, and diminished inhibition of leukocyte migration [36]. The mechanisms by which dexamethasone and other glucocorticoids reduce peritumoral edema remain unclear. It is known that both PBT and MBT have high concentrations of glucocorticoid receptors. The effects of these drugs on tumor-induced edema are most likely mediated through binding to these receptors, with subsequent transfer to the nucleus and the expression of novel genes [35]. In a recent magnetic resonance imaging study, dexamethasone was able to induce a dramatic reduction in blood-tumor barrier permeability and regional cerebral blood volume, without significant alteration of cerebral blood flow or the degree of edema [37]. The inhibition of production and/or release of vasoactive factors secreted by tumor cells and endothelial cells, such as VEGF and prostacyclin, appears to be involved in this process [34,35]. In addition, glucocorticoids appear to inhibit the reactivity of endothelial cells to several substances that induce capillary permeability.

The exact dose of steroids necessary for each patient will vary depending on the histology (i.e., benign or malignant), size and location of the tumor, and amount of peritumoral edema. In general, most patients with malignant tumors will require between 8 and 16 mg of dexamethasone per day to remain clinically stable. The lowest dose of steroid that can control the patient's pressure-related symptoms should be used [1,32]. This approach will minimize some of the toxicity and complications that can arise from long-term corticosteroid usage, which includes oral candidiasis, hyperglycemia, peripheral edema, proximal myopathy, gastritis, infection, osteopenia, weight gain, bowel perforation, and psychiatric or behavioral changes (e.g., euphoria, hypomania, depression, psychosis, sleep disturbance) [1,38–43]. Patients with dexamethasone-induced proximal myopathy will often improve when the dosage is reduced [42,43]. In addition, the proximal leg muscles can usually be strengthened if the patient is placed on a lower extremity exercise regimen. Some authors have also reported an improvement in the myopathy when dexamethasone is replaced by an equivalent dosage of prednisone or hydrocortisone. The neuropsychiatric complications of steroids can often be improved by dosage reduction or discontinuation of the drug [41]. For those patients in whom continued steroid usage is necessary, symptomatic pharmacological intervention is appropriate. For example, patients experiencing steroid-induced delerium or psychosis will often improve with low-dose haloperidol (0.5–1.0 mg po, im, or iv), titrated to control symptoms. Steroid-induced sleep disturbances often respond to dosage reduction or by eliminating any doses after dinner. In refractory cases, the use of a hypnotic medication at bedtime (e.g., triazolam, 0.25 mg) will often be of benefit. Corticosteroid-induced osteoporosis is a common problem, affecting 30% to 50% of patients receiving treatment for a year or more [38,44,45]. Patients on long-term dexamethosone require a preventive program to minimize osteoporosis, including calcium and vitamin D supplements and weight-bearing exercises. These measures should be started early, because bone loss is greatest in the first 2 to 4 months of chronic steroid treatment. For patients on long-term steroid therapy (i.e., ≥3 months), or in those with established osteoporosis or evidence of an osteoporotic fracture, bisphosphonate therapy (e.g., risedronate, 2.5–5.0 mg/day; alendronate, 5–10 mg/day) should be added to the regimen of calcium and vitamin D supplements [45].

Patients with brain tumor can be immunosuppressed for a variety of reasons, including long-term steroid use, immunomodulatory factors secreted by the tumor, and the effects of chemotherapy [36,38]. Chronic steroid usage can lead to lymphopenia, mainly through a reduction in the concentration of CD4+ T cells, and an associated increased risk of systemic infection. Recent studies suggest that patients with brain tumor on chronic steroids are at substantial risk for *Pneumocystis carinii* pneumonia (PCP), a serious infection with a 50% to 55% case fatality rate. In a recent pair of reports reviewing the Johns Hopkins experience over the past 20 years, Grossman and colleagues noted that the rate of PCP in patients with PBT was less than 1.0% [46,47]. However, of all HIV-negative patients with PCP over the past 5 years, the percentage with PBTs had increased from 22% to 40% (half of which were primary central nervous system lymphoma [PCNSL]). In fact, it appears that patients with PCNSL are at particular risk for developing PCP, possibly because of the recent widespread use of methotrexate-based chemotherapy regimens, which can significantly reduce CD4+ T cell counts [47]. The authors did not recommend PCP prophylaxis for every patient with brain tumor on long-term steroids or chemotherapy. Rather, they suggested careful monitoring of all patients for the onset of lymphopenia, including an assessment in high-risk cases of the concentration of CD4+ T cells. For those high-risk patients with lymphopenia and CD4 counts below 200 cells/mL, a prophylactic anti-PCP regimen should be instituted [47]. The most commonly used prophylactic antibiotic is trimethoprim–sulphamethoxazole (TMP-SMX, 160 + 800 mg), at a dose of one double strength tablet per day. For patients with a sulpha allergy or deleterious interactions between TMP-SMX and other drugs (e.g., methotrexate), alternative prophylactic medications include pentamidine (300 mg/month by nebulizer) and dapsone (100 mg/day by mouth).

High-dose steroid usage frequently produces oral candidiasis, and prophylactic measures to avoid this are highly recommended. One possible measure is the use of clotrimazole troches.

GASTRIC ACID INHIBITORS

Patients with brain tumor on long-term dexamethasone are at increased risk for gastrointestinal complications (i.e., gastritis, ulceration, bowel perforation), although there remains some debate in the literature regarding ulcer formation [32,38,40]. A comprehensive review of the topic would suggest that ulcer prophylaxis is appropriate, because the incidence of ulcer formation is increased in patients with advanced malignant disease [48]. Patients at risk should be treated prophylactically with a gastric acid inhibitor such as ranitidine hydrochloride (150 mg po bid), famotidine (20 mg po bid), or omeprazole (20–40 mg po qd) [49,50]. These medications can be discontinued after the patient has been completely tapered off dexamethasone.

THROMBOEMBOLIC COMPLICATIONS AND ANTICOAGULATION

The risk of thromboembolism (i.e., deep venous thrombosis [DVT], pulmonary embolism [PE]) is high in patients with cancer, with an antemortem incidence of symptomatic events approaching 15% [51,52]. However, at autopsy, the incidence rates are much higher, between 45% and 50% in some series. For patients with brain tumors, the risk for DVT and PE appears to be even higher than in the general cancer population [52–54]. In the perioperative period, the overall incidence of thrombosis after brain tumor resection was 45%, as detected by 125I-labeled fibrinogen scans [53]. The incidence varied depending on the tumor type and was 72%, 60%, and 20% for patients with meningioma, GBM, and MBT, respectively. The high incidence of thromboembolism in patients with meningioma was unexpected, considering their generally benign natural history, and suggested that tumor biology may play a predominant role in risk for perioperative DVT and PE. Thromboembolic risk continues to remain high in patients with brain tumor after the perioperative period (i.e., beyond 6 weeks). A meta-analysis of patients with malignant glioma by Marras and colleagues noted a DVT incidence rate that ranged from 0.013 to 0.023 per patient-month of follow-up, corresponding to overall rates of 7% to 24% [55]. The only prospective study included in the analysis followed 75 patients until death and had a DVT incidence rate of 24% (0.015 DVT/patient-month) [56]. In addition to biological factors related to individual tumor histology, several clinical factors are also associated with increased risk of DVT and PE, including arm paresis, leg paresis, history of prior DVT or PE before tumor diagnosis, longer operative time, and presence of GBM [54,55,57]. Other less important factors that may also be relevant are older age, larger tumor size, and the use of chemotherapy.

If patients with a PBT or MBT develop a thromboembolic event, should they be treated with conventional anticoagulation approaches, or is that too dangerous and should they, instead, receive an inferior vena cava filter (VCF) without anticoagulation? The important question at the core of this dilemma is the risk of intratumoral hemorrhage while receiving anticoagulant therapy. This is a common problem for the neuro-oncology treatment team and continues to be studied in the literature. In general, the risk for symptomatic hemorrhage into a primary or MBT is quite low during conservative anticoagulation with heparin and coumadin [54,56–61]. Most authors report a hemorrhage rate of 2% to 3% for PBT and 5% to 7% for MBT. To minimize the potential for intratumoral hemorrhage, the parameters for heparin and coumadin therapy need to be very conservative, with PTT and PT values in the 1.5 to 2.0 times control range [57]. Once the patient has shifted completely over to coumadin, the INR should be maintained between 1.5 and 2.5 [54,59].

A more recent approach to treating a thromboembolic event would be to use a low-molecular-weight heparin (LMWH) [51,62]. The LMWHs (e.g., enoxaparin, dalteparin) are composed of fragments of unfractionated heparin produced by controlled enzymatic or chemical depolymerization, yielding chains with an average molecular weight of 5000 Da. In comparison with unfractionated heparin, LMWHs have a more predictable anticoagulant response because of better bioavailability, a longer half-life, and more dose-dependent clearance [62]. In addition, the LMWHs can be administered subcutaneously in the outpatient setting and do not require monitoring of coagulation status. When used in clinical trials of patients with DVT, LMWHs (e.g., enoxaparin, 100 U/kg bid) have proved as effective or more effective than unfractionated heparin, with a lower hemorrhage rate [62]. Meta-analyses of the clinical trial data conclude, in general, that LMWHs are more effective and safer than unfractionated heparin. However, the aforementioned studies have not included patients with brain tumor. Clinical trials to more specifically evaluate the safety and efficacy of LMWH in patients with brain tumor have not been completed.

The utility of VCF in brain tumor and other patients with cancer remains controversial [63]. Several studies have demonstrated a significant complication rate for VCF in patients with PBT and MBT (range 40–62%) and suggest that biological factors related to the tumor may be involved [60,61]. Complications after VCF placement include filter thrombosis, recurrent DVT, recurrent PE, and thrombosis of the inferior vena cava. Patients receiving anticoagulation had a lower recurrence rate of PE and DVT. Although most authors now suggest that acute and long-term anticoagulation is superior to VCF placement for patients with brain tumor with DVT and/or PE, selected patients should still be considered for this approach. Patients with large regions of intratumoral hemorrhage, impaired neurological function and excessive risk for falling episodes, and gastrointestinal bleeding should be evaluated for VCF placement instead of anticoagulation.

DYSPHAGIA AND SWALLOWING DISORDERS

Dysphagia and disorders of swallowing are common in patients with neurological disease and can be associated with stroke, multiple sclerosis, motor neuron disease, neurodegenerative disorders, and structural lesions such as a brain tumor [64–70]. Swallowing dysfunction can lead to serious morbidity from malnutrition, dehydration, and aspiration pneumonia. There remains a paucity of literature regarding the incidence and presentation of dysphagia in the brain tumor population. It must be remembered that oral and/or oropharyngeal candidiasis often produces dysphagia, and this must be adequately treated. The most well-described presentation involves dysfunction of the brainstem, either from compression to or growth within this region [64,71,72]. Tumors that can induce dysphagia in this manner include brainstem glioma, brainstem metastases, ependymoma, choroid plexus papilloma, large pineal region tumors (i.e., pinealoma, astrocytoma), and neoplasms of the cerebellopontine angle such as acoustic schwannoma and meningioma. Direct tumor compression causes impairment of the brainstem circuitry that underlies swallowing, including the nucleus tractus solitarius, ventromedial reticular formation, and cranial nerve motor efferents (V3, VII, IX, X, XII, and ansa cervicalis) [73–75]. Other reports contend that unilateral, supratentorial tumors can also cause dysphagia [76,77]. In a prospective analysis of dysphagia in patients with PBT and a set of non–brain tumor neurological controls, Newton and colleagues noted that 17 of 117 (14.5%) patients with tumor complained of swallowing problems [77]. Formal swallowing assessment of the symptomatic cohort revealed that most patients significantly underestimated their degree of dysfunction. It was also noted that symptomatic patients with decreased level of alertness (LOA) were more likely to have abnormalities during bedside and videofluoroscopic testing. Twelve of the 17 symptomatic patients (70.5%; GBM, 7) had large and diffuse, unilateral, supratentorial lesions with surrounding edema and mass effect, often associated with decreased LOA. The neuroanatomical basis for dysphagia from a unilateral lesion remains unclear. However, it is probably due to a combination of several factors, including reduced awareness of oral sensory feedback cues during mastication in patients with reduced LOA, contralateral weakness of the face and tongue, and oral apraxia with impaired motor programming ability for oral-lingual feeding behavior.

Based on the available literature, it would seem prudent to routinely screen all patients with brain tumor for dysphagic symptoms, especially in the latter stages of their disease, with or without reduced LOA. All symptomatic patients should undergo a formal swallowing evaluation, even when the complaint seems trivial [77]. The initial bedside screening examination can assess oral and laryngeal function and identify patients at risk for aspiration [78]. In addition, bedside testing can allow modification of eating behavior to diminish the risk of aspiration. Further examination is often needed after the initial bedside evaluation to allow more detailed assessment of the swallowing mechanism, such as delays during the pharyngeal swallow, the degree of laryngeal elevation, pharyngeal symmetry, pooling or coating of pharyngeal recesses, and silent aspiration. The modified barium swallow is used for this assessment and can accurately reveal the abnormalities of the swallowing mechanism, the degree of aspiration, and how best to modify the diet [77–80].

Management of patients with dysphagic brain tumor can often be a complex issue. Patients must be able to demonstrate the necessary cognitive and communication skills to actively participate in a swallowing management program [78,80]. Patients with tumor with diminished LOA or significant cognitive alterations may be unable to pursue complex rehabilitation strategies similar to those used for patients with other neurologic disorders (e.g., stroke). In those patients with adequate LOA, swallowing rehabilitation should be pursued. If compensatory techniques do not improve oral efficiency, an alternate route of nutrition may be required, such as a gastric feeding tube.

CONCLUSIONS

Although the focus of the treatment team will be on curative or stabilizing therapy for most patients, it will still be very important for the treating physician to be aware of the many aspects of supportive care outlined earlier. Common problems related to seizure control, toxicity of anticonvulsants and corticosteroids, prophylaxis and treatment of thromboembolic complications, and swallowing must be assiduously monitored in every patient.

REFERENCES

1. Newton HB. Primary brain tumors: review of etiology, diagnosis, and treatment. *Am Fam Phys.* 1994;49:787–797.
2. Ptacek JT, Ptacek JJ. Patients' perceptions of receiving bad news about cancer. *J Clin Oncol.* 2001;19:4160–4164.
3. Feldman GB. The role of support in treating the brain tumor patient. In: Black PM, Loeffler JS, eds. *Cancer of the Nervous System.* Cambridge: Blackwell Science;1997:335–345.
4. Given BA, Given CW, Kozachik S. Family support in advanced cancer. *CA Cancer J Clin.* 2001;51:213–231.
5. Nijboer C, Tempelaar R, Triemstra M, van den Bos GAM, Sanderman R. The role of social and psychologic resources in caregiving of cancer patients. *Cancer.* 2001;91:1029–1039.
6. Glantz M, Recht LD. Epilepsy in the cancer patient. In: Vecht CJ, ed. *Handbook of Clinical Neurology, Vol. 25 (69): Neuro-Oncology, Part III.* Amsterdam: Elsevier Science;1997:9–18.
7. Moots PL, Maciunas RJ, Eisert DR, Parker RA, Laporte K, Abou-Khalil B. The course of seizure disorders in patients with malignant gliomas. *Arch Neurol.* 1995;52:717–724.
8. Elisevich K. Epilepsy and low-grade gliomas. In: Rock JP, Rosenblum ML, Shaw EG, Cairncross JG, eds. *The Practical Management of Low-Grade Primary Brain Tumors.* Philadelphia: Lippincott Williams & Wilkins;1999:149–169.
9. Newton HB. Neurological complications of systemic cancer. *Am Fam Physician.* 1999;59:878–886.
10. Schaller B, Rüegg SJ. Brain tumor and seizures: pathophysiology and its implications for treatment revisited. *Epilepsia.* 2003;44:1223–1232.
11. Ettinger AB. Structural causes of epilepsy. Tumors, cysts, stroke, and vascular malformation. *Neurol Clin.* 1994;12:41–56.
12. Highland MM, Berger MS, Kunkel DD, Franck JE, Ghatan S, Ojemannn GA. Changes in gamma-aminobutyric acid and somatostatin in epileptic cortex associated with low-grade gliomas. *J Neurosurg.* 1992;77:209–216.
13. Bateman DE, Hardy JA, McDermott JR, Parker DS, Edwardson JA. Amino acid neurotransmitter levels in gliomas and their relationship to the incidence of epilepsy. *Neurol Res.* 1988;10:112–114.
14. Ye ZC, Sontheimer H. Glioma cells release excitotoxic concentrations of glutamate. *Cancer Res.* 1999;59:4383–4391.
15. Behrens PF, Langemann H, Strohschein R, Draeger J, Hennig J. Extracellular glutamate and other metabolites in and around RG2 rat glioma: an intracerebral microdialysis study. *J Neuro-Oncol.* 2000;47:11–22.
16. Brodie MJ, Dichter MA. Antiepileptic drugs. *New Engl J Med.* 1996;334:168–175.
17. Britton JW, So EL. Selection of antiepileptic drugs: a practical approach. *Mayo Clin Proc.* 1996;71:778–786.
18. Mattson RH, Cramer BS, Collins JF; Department of Veterans Affairs Epilepsy Cooperative Study Group. A comparison of valproate with carbamazepine for the treatment of complex partial seizures and secondarily generalized tonic-clonic seizures in adults. *New Engl J Med.* 1992;327:765–771.
19. Dichter MA, Brodie MJ. New antiepileptic drugs. *New Eng J Med.* 1996;334:1583–1590.
20. Rosenfeld WE. Topiramate: a review of preclinical, pharmacokinetic, and clinical data. *Clin Therap.* 1997;19:1294–1308.
21. Newton HB, Goldlust S, Pearl D. Retrospective analysis of the efficacy and tolerability of levetiracetam in brain tumor patients. *J Neuro-Oncol.* 2006;78:99–102.
22. Newton HB, Dalton J, Goldlust S, Pearl D. Retrospective analysis of the efficacy and tolerability of levetiracetam in metastatic brain tumor patients. *J Neuro-Oncol.* 2007;8:293–296.
23. Vecht CJ, Wagner GL, Wilms EB. Interactions between antiepileptic and chemotherapeutic drugs. *Lancet Neurol.* 2003;2:404–409.
24. North JB, Penhall RK, Hanieh A, Frewin DB, Taylor WB. Phenytoin and postoperative epilepsy. A double-blind study. *J Neurosurg.* 1983;58:672–677
25. Boarini DJ, Beck DW, VanGilder JC. Postoperative prophylactic anticonvulsant therapy in cerebral gliomas. *Neurosurg.* 1985;16:290–292.
26. Cohen N, Strauss G, Lew R, Silver D, Recht L. Should prophylactic anticonvulsants be administered to patients with newly-diagnosed cerebral metastases? A retrospective analysis. *J Clin Oncol.* 1988;6:1621–1624.
27. Franceschetti S, Binelli S, Casazza M, et al. Influence of surgery and antiepileptic drugs on seizures symptomatic of cerebral tumours. *Acta Neurochir.* 1990;103:47–51.
28. Shaw MDM. Post-operative epilepsy and the efficacy of anticonvulsant therapy. *Acta Neurochir Suppl.* 1990;50:55–57.
29. Foy PM, Chadwick DW, Rajgopalan N, Johnson AL, Shaw MDM. Do prophylactic anticonvulsant drugs alter the pattern of seizures after craniotomy? *J Neurol Neurosurg Psych.* 1992;55:753–757.
30. Glantz MJ, Cole BF, Friedberg MH, et al. A randomized, blinded, placebo-controlled trial of divalproex sodium prophylaxis in adults with newly diagnosed brain tumors. *Neurology.* 1996;46:985–991.
31. Glantz MJ, Cole BF, Forsyth PA, et al. Practice parameter: anticonvulsant prophylaxis in patients with newly diagnosed brain tumors.

Report of the Quality Standards Subcommittee of the American Academy of Neurology. *Neurology.* 2000;54:1886–1893.
32. Newton HB, Turowski RC, Stroup TJ, McCoy LK. Clinical presentation, diagnosis, and pharmacotherapy of patients with primary brain tumors. *Ann Pharmacother.* 1999;33:816–832.
33. Ohnishi T, Sher PB, Posner JB, Shapiro WB. Capillary permeability factor secreted by malignant brain tumor. Role in peritumoral edema and possible mechanism for anti-edema effect of glucocorticoids. *J Neurosurg.* 1990;72:245–251.
34. Del Maestro RF, Megyesi JF, Farrell CL. Mechanisms of tumor-associated edema: a review. *Can J Neurol Sci.* 1990;17:177–183.
35. Samdani AF, Tamargo RJ, Long DM. Brain tumor edema and the role of the blood-brain barrier. In: Vecht CJ, ed. *Handbook of Clinical Neurology, Vol. 23 (67): Neuro-Oncology, Part I.* Amsterdam: Elsevier Science;1997:71–102.
36. Mukwaya G. Immunosuppressive effects and infections associated with corticosteroid therapy. *Pediatr Infect Dis J.* 1988;7:499–504.
37. Østergaard L, Hochberg FH, Rabinov JD, et al. Early changes measured by magnetic resonance imaging in cerebral blood flow, blood volume, and blood-brain barrier permeability following dexamethasone treatment in patients with brain tumors. *J Neurosurg.* 1999;90:300–305.
38. Lester RS, Knowles SR, Shear NH. The risks of systemic corticosteroid use. *Dermatol Clin.* 1998;16:277–286.
39. Weissman DE, Dufer D, Vogel V, Abeloff MD. Corticosteroid toxicity in neuro-oncology patients. *J Neuro-Oncol.* 1987;5:125–128.
40. Fadul CE, Lemann W, Thaler HT, Posner JB. Perforation of the gastrointestinal tract in patients receiving steroids for neurologic disease. *Neurology.* 1988;38:348–352.
41. Stiefel FC, Breitbart WS, Holland JC. Corticosteroids in cancer: neuropsychiatric complications. *Cancer Investig.* 1989;7:479–491.
42. Dropcho EJ, Soong SJ. Steroid-induced weakness in patients with primary brain tumors. *Neurology.* 1991;41:1235–1239.
43. Batchelor TT, Taylor LT, Thaler HT, Posner JB, DeAngelis LM. Steroid myopathy in cancer patients. *Neurology.* 1997;48:1234–1238.
44. Joseph JC. Corticosteroid-induced osteoporosis. *Am J Hosp Pharm.* 1994;51:188–197.
45. McIlwain HH. Glucocorticoid-induced osteoporosis: pathogenesis, diagnosis, and management. *Preventive Med.* 2003;36:243–249.
46. Mahindra AK, Grossman SA. *Pneumocystis carinii* pneumonia in HIV negative patients with primary brain tumors. *J Neuro-Oncol.* 2003;63:263–270.
47. Mathew BS, Grossman SA. *Pneumocystis carinii* pneumonia prophylaxis in HIV negative patients with primary CNS lymphoma. *Cancer Treat Rev.* 2003;29:105–119.
48. Ellershaw JE, Kelly MJ. Corticosteroids and peptic ulceration. *Palliative Med.* 1994;8:313–319.
49. Garnett WR, Garabedian-Ruffalo SM. Identification, diagnosis, and treatment of acid-related diseases in the elderly: implications for long-term care. *Pharmacotherapy.* 1997;17:938–958.
50. Sachs G. Proton pump inhibitors and acid-related diseases. *Pharmacotherapy.* 1997;17:22–37.
51. Lee AYY, Levine MN. Management of venous thromboembolism in cancer patients. *Oncol.* 2000;17:409–421.
52. Gomes MPV, Deitcher SR. Diagnosis of venous thromboembolic disease in cancer patients. *Oncol.* 2003;17:126–139.
53. Sawaya R, Zuccarello M, Elkalliny M, Nighiyama H. Postoperative venous thromboembolism and brain tumors: part I. Clinical profile. *J Neuro-Oncol.* 1992;14:119–125.
54. Hamilton MG, Hull RD, Pineo GF. Venous thromboembolism in neurosurgery and neurology patients: a review. *Neurosurg.* 1994;34:280–296.
55. Marras LC, Geerts WH, Perry JR. The risk of venous thromboembolism is increased throughout the course of malignant glioma. An evidence-based review. *Cancer.* 2000;89:640–646.
56. Brandes AA, Scelzi E, Salmistraro E, et al. Incidence and risk of thromboembolism during treatment of high-grade gliomas: a prospective study. *Eur J Cancer.* 1997;33:1592–1596.
57. Quevedo JF, Buckner JC, Schmidt JL, Dinapoli RP, O'Fallon JR. Thromboembolism in patients with high-grade glioma. *Mayo Clin Proc.* 1994;69:329–332.
58. Ruff RL, Posner JB. The incidence and treatment of peripheral venous thrombosis in patients with glioma. *Ann Neurol.* 1983;13:334–336.
59. Altshuler E, Moosa H, Selker RG, Vertosick FT. The risk and efficacy of anticoagulant therapy in the treatment of thromboembolic complications in patients with primary brain tumors. *Neurosurg.* 1990;27:74–77.
60. Levin JM, Schiff D, Loeffler JS, Fine HA, Black PML, Wen PY. Complications of therapy for venous thromboembolic disease in patients with brain tumors. *Neurology.* 1993;43:1111–1114.
61. Schiff D, DeAngelis LM. Therapy of venous thromboembolism in patients with brain metastases. *Cancer.* 1994;73:493–498.
62. Weitz JI. Low-molecular-weight heparins. *New Engl J Med.* 1997;337:688–698.
63. Dorfman GS. Evaluating the roles and functions of vena caval filters: will data be available before or after these devices are removed from the market? *Radiology.* 1992;185:15–17.
64. Buchholz D. Neurologic causes of dysphagia. *Dysphagia.* 1987;1:152–156.
65. Kirshner HS. Causes of Neurogenic dysphagia. *Dysphagia.* 1989;3:184–188.
66. Barer DH. The natural history and functional consequences of dysphagia after hemispheric stroke. *J Neurol Neurosurg Psychiatry.* 1989;52:236–241.
67. Lieberman AN, Horowitz L, Redmond P, Pachter L, Lieberman I, Leibowitz M. Dysphagia in Parkinson's disease. *Am J Gastroenterol.* 1980;74:157–160.
68. Daly DD, Code CF, Anderson HA. Disturbances of swallowing and esophageal motility in patients with multiple sclerosis. *Neurology.* 1962;59:250–256.
69. Robbins J. Swallowing in ALS and motor neuron disease. *Neurol Clin.* 1987;5:213–229.
70. Buchholz D. Neurologic evaluation of dysphagia. *Dysphagia.* 1987;1:187–192.
71. Frank Y, Schwartz SB, Epstein NE, Beresford HR. Chronic dysphagia, vomiting and gastroesophageal reflux as manifestations of a brain stem glioma: a case report. *Pediatr Neurosci.* 1989;15:265–268.
72. Straube A, Witt TN. Oculo-bulbar myasthenic symptoms as the sole sign of tumour involving or compressing the brain stem. *J Neurol.* 1990;237:369–371.
73. Cunningham ET, Donner MW, Jones B, Point SM. Anatomical and physiological overview. In: Jones B, Donner MW, eds. *Normal and Abnormal Swallowing. Imaging in Diagnosis and Therapy.* New York: Springer-Verlag;1991:7–32.
74. Dodds WJ, Stewart ET, Logemann JA. Physiology and radiology of the normal oral and pharyngeal phases of swallowing. *Am J Roentgenol.* 1989;154:953–963.
75. Sessle BJ, Henry JL. Neural mechanisms of swallowing: neurophysiological and neurochemical studies on brain stem neurons in the solitary tract region. *Dysphagia.* 1989;4:61–75.
76. Meadows JC. Dysphagia in unilateral cerebral lesions. *J Neurol Neurosurg Psych.* 1973;36:853–860.
77. Newton HB, Newton C, Pearl D, Davidson T. Swallowing assessment in primary brain tumor patients with dysphagia. *Neurology.* 1994;44:1927–1932.
78. Emick-Herring B, Wood P. A team approach to neurologically based swallowing disorders. *Rehabil Nurs.* 1990;15:126–132.
79. Dodds WJ, Logemann JA, Stewart ET. Radiologic assessment of abnormal oral and pharyngeal phases of swallowing. *Am J Roentgenol.* 1990;154:965–974.
80. Bloch AS. Nutritional management of patients with dysphagia. *Oncol.* 1993;7:127–137.

37
Ethical Issues in Neuro-Oncology

Herbert B. Newton

INTRODUCTION

The discipline of neuro-oncology is quite broad and encompasses a diverse group of diseases that can involve any region of the central or peripheral nervous system. For the purposes of the current discussion, the focus will be on patients with primary brain tumors and metastatic brain tumors. In adults, the survival of patients with high-grade primary brain tumors (e.g., glioblastoma multiforme, anaplastic astrocytoma) is poor, ranging from 12 to 30 months [1]. Similarly, the majority of patients with brain metastases have multiple lesions, with an associated length of survival of 6 months or less [2]. In addition to poor survival, most patients with brain tumor are further compromised by their disease because of neurologic deficits (e.g., dysphasia, hemiparesis, hemianopsia), impaired cognition and memory, and seizure activity [1,2].

There are several basic ethical principles that will be referred to frequently during this discussion which require definition [3–5]. The most important ethical principles are respect for autonomy, justice, beneficence, and nonmaleficence. *Respect for autonomy* refers to recognition by the physician of the patient's right and ability to make his or her own decisions. These decisions are unique, are influenced by the patient's value system, and may differ from what is advised by the physician. *Justice* relates to fairness and what people are legitimately entitled to once they enter the medical system. In this context, justice demands that patients with brain tumors have access to care (e.g., treatment, pain control, nutritional support) equal to patients with other diseases that may have a less grave prognosis. *Beneficence* refers to actions by the physician toward the patient that will maximize positive outcomes and avoid unnecessary pain, injury, and suffering. These activities can include treatment of the cancer and extension of quality survival, control of pain and other disease-related symptoms, and interpersonal support. *Nonmaleficence* means that the physician should "do no harm" while providing care to the patient. This principle has a broad scope and can refer to many issues, including withholding relevant diagnostic or prognostic information, improper treatment of pain, inappropriate undertreatment, and persistent overtreatment.

Physicians usually have an ethical position or frame of reference that incorporates these basic ethical principles. The most common ethical stance is that in which the physician makes a decision based on an assessment of the good or bad consequences of each course of action. This ethical position, called *consequentialism* or *utilitarianism*, justifies a given decision by comparing probable good or benefit with potential harm or pain [6].The second most common ethical position, *respect for persons*, relies heavily on the ethical principles of autonomy and respect [7,8]. This approach emphasizes the importance of allowing patients to be involved in all decisions about their care and treatment. An alternative to *respect for persons* is *paternalism*, in which the physician assumes that all decisions should be made for the good of the patient, without regard to his or her specific wishes or needs [3,4,6].

DISCUSSING DIAGNOSIS AND PROGNOSIS

It is often difficult to be honest with a patient when discussing a new diagnosis as devastating as cancer, especially when it is a brain tumor [3,7,8]. In fact, a survey of ethical issues in the oncology literature determined that *truth-telling* was the most commonly debated subject [8]. Between 1961 and 1979, most physicians took the paternalistic approach and withheld information regarding diagnosis and prognosis to maintain hope and minimize psychological damage to their patients. Since 1979, attitudes have changed so that many physicians now prefer to reveal accurate information about their patient's diagnosis and prognosis [8]. This trend away from paternalism, toward a more "patient-oriented" or "respect for persons" approach when discussing diagnosis and prognosis, is important because the vast majority of patients want to know as much as possible about their disease, treatment options, and chances of survival.

The diagnosis of a brain tumor usually has a devastating effect on patients and family members [5].They are generally shocked and frightened when they hear the diagnosis and begin to contemplate the potential for severe neurological impairment, loss of employment, loss or separation from loved ones, pain, and premature death. It is important that the physician conduct the diagnostic interview properly, because recent research suggests that patient perception of physician behavior during this interview can be a significant predictor of subsequent psychological adjustment to cancer [8,9]. Most patients want their spouse or significant other present during the diagnostic interview; less often, the patient prefers to be alone. The physician should discuss the diagnosis using plain language, in a compassionate manner that is commensurate with the patient's level of education and medical sophistication. It is inappropriate to use excessive medical jargon and euphemistic terminology or to avoid words like "tumor," "malignancy," or "cancer." An honest, caring, down-to-earth approach by the physician is more likely to foster mutual trust, respect, and confidence. The type of tumor should be discussed thoroughly, including a brief description of where the tumor is located in the brain, the size of the mass, type of cells the tumor is derived from, and what functions might be affected by further growth. Whether the tumor is malignant or not (i.e., is it cancer?) and the chances for cure or extended survival should be explained. Other information related to prognosis, neurological status, and quality of life (QOL) should be discussed, including seizure activity (e.g., how well they can be controlled, types of seizures, medications), driving, need for follow-up examinations and computed tomography/magnetic resonance imaging scans, pain (e.g., should it be expected, can it be controlled), and, most importantly, the likelihood of dying from the brain tumor. For many patients, a detailed discussion of the prognosis and what to expect during treatment are even more important than information about the diagnosis. Finally, after the interview has been completed, it is helpful to provide patient education brochures that review in more detail the patient's specific type of brain tumor, radiation therapy (RT), chemotherapy, coping strategies, and how to maintain hope. Improving patient education has also been found to significantly improve the psychological adjustment to cancer.

It is often difficult for the physician caring for a patient with brain tumor to balance the ethically appropriate duty to convey accurate information about diagnosis and prognosis with the equally important responsibility to nurture and maintain hope. This dilemma was the crux of the problem that led many physicians in the past to adopt a paternalistic approach to truth-telling [8,9]. However, it is now clear that a more honest and accurate diagnostic interview does not remove hope and is more likely to strengthen the physician-patient relationship. The physician should explore what hope means to each patient, because it can represent many different things, some of which will be separate from the hope for cure or lengthy survival.

TO TREAT OR NOT TO TREAT?

For most patients with a brain tumor, the decision whether or not to pursue treatment will not involve an ethical debate. The majority of patients elect some type of treatment to "control" or "beat" their cancer. Nearly all patients with a brain tumor receive some form of surgical intervention [1]. The majority of patients with malignant tumors will also undergo RT and, in some cases, chemotherapy. However, other important issues may arise, such as which hospital or clinic is most appropriate to administer their therapy (e.g., local hospital vs specialized cancer center); how aggressive the treatment should be; whether to pursue standard therapy or an experimental clinical trial; how sick they might be during various treatments; and the complications that could occur during those treatments. Ethical questions regarding therapy usually arise in several specific circumstances: in elderly patients, in patients of any age who are severely compromised by central nervous system or systemic disease, and in patients who refuse therapy that could be potentially curative or life-sustaining [5,10]. Age alone should not be a consideration in treatment decisions for a patient with brain tumor. If an elderly patient wants to pursue some form of therapy, the physician should honor these wishes in accordance with the ethical principles of autonomy and justice. However, depending on the patient's medical and neurological condition, not all treatment modalities may be appropriate (e.g., surgical resection, full-course RT, intense chemotherapy). Some authors advocate a less aggressive approach to treatment in older patients with poor prognostic signs such as significant neurologic disability, concomitant debilitating medical conditions, and low performance status [10]. In this subgroup of patients, a biopsy or subtotal resection, followed by an accelerated course of external beam RT, may be appropriate for palliation. Within this same subgroup of elderly patients with primary or metastatic brain tumors and poor prognostic indicators, are individuals in whom nontreatment is more acceptable than treatment, even though this could lead to an earlier death. Although life is still precious, they may not have the desire "to fight" their disease and undergo potentially exhausting and toxic therapy. In a rational adult, the decision to forego treatment can be justified on the basis of the principles of autonomy, beneficence, and nonmaleficence [11]. Allowing a dignified, peaceful death without the ravages of active treatment may be acting to "promote the good," according to the patient's unique ethical position, even though these views may be contrary to those of the physician. The physician should respect the wishes of the patient and attempt to maximize other health goals, such as pain control. There is a legal precedent in support of the rights of rational adults to refuse treatment: the principle of self-determination [11]. If the patient is not competent to make a treatment decision, then the issues should be discussed with the appropriate surrogate (i.e., spouse, parents, or whoever has the Durable Power of Attorney for Health Care). The Durable Power of Attorney for Health Care designates a person to make medical decisions for the patient, according to the patient's value system, should he or she become incompetent. This process is referred to as the doctrine of substituted judgment. An alternative approach is to use the doctrine of best interest, in which the physician takes a course of action that he or she feels is in the patient's best overall interest, while considering issues such as social and religious values.

Although uncommon at the time of presentation, there are some cases in which the patient is so neurologically devastated by the brain tumor (e.g., intratumoral hemorrhage, tumor-related stroke, multifocal disease, leptomeningeal spread) that it may be ethically appropriate to recommend nontreatment as the most reasonable option. The final decision regarding therapy should be made in accordance with the wishes of the patient and family, using the principles of autonomy, beneficence, and nonmaleficence for guidance.

Occasionally, there are patients who refuse treatment even though they may be neurologically intact and have good prognostic indicators. The reasons for this course of action vary and include religious beliefs (e.g., Christian scientists), misconceptions regarding the efficacy or toxicity of therapy, and personal control issues. The personal control issues can sometimes manifest themselves as the patients "taking charge" of their illness and not being "forced" into undergoing potentially toxic therapy, even though this may hasten death. This position is often very frustrating and disheartening for the treating physician, especially if the patient is young and could expect extended survival with aggressive therapy. In some cases, the spouse or family may be helpful in convincing the patient to allow therapy. However, as with the elderly patient with brain tumor, the physician must ultimately respect the wishes of the patient according to the ethical principles of autonomy and beneficence. Legally, the rational patient is within his or her right to refuse therapy based on the principle of self-determination, even when the action results in a more rapid death [11].

QOL DURING AND AFTER THERAPY

In recent years, there has been an increased awareness of, and interest in, QOL of oncology patients, including those with brain tumors [12,13]. QOL refers to the physical, psychological, and social domains of health as perceived by the patient and influenced by the patient's own unique beliefs and expectations. Significant aspects of QOL include physical concerns and symptoms (e.g., pain), functional ability, family well-being, treatment satisfaction, sexuality and intimacy, and social functioning. Because of its subjective nature, perceived QOL may vary widely among patients who have similar levels of health. Numerous instruments have been devised to quantify the various aspects of QOL, so that different treatment modalities can be compared for their impact on the patient. Performance status measurements (e.g., Karnofsky scale [KPS]) can also be used as a more global determination of a patient's QOL. QOL issues are important to the oncologic physician from an ethical point of view in terms of beneficence and nonmaleficence: the treatment should provide potential benefit to the patient (e.g., extend survival, reduce pain, improve function) while keeping complications and deleterious side effects to an acceptable minimum [3].

The potential impact of each treatment modality on QOL should be explained to the patient and family using nontechnical and easily understood terms. Surgical intervention of some sort (i.e., biopsy, subtotal resection, gross total resection) is attempted in roughly 98% of all patients with brain tumor [1]. Of the many complications that can arise during surgery, the creation or exacerbation of a neurological deficit (e.g., hemiparesis, dysphasia, dysphagia) is most likely to compromise QOL. For patients with malignant astrocytomas, this can occur in a significant percentage of cases (i.e., 5–10%), because of the highly infiltrative nature of these neoplasms and their propensity to develop postoperative edema. Other complications of surgery that could affect QOL and should be discussed include hemorrhage, meningitis, and wound infection. RT is used in most patients with malignant primary, metastatic, and progressive inoperable benign brain tumors [1,2]. In many studies, RT has had a relatively benign impact on QOL; no differences were found between QOL of patients who had received surgery alone versus those who had undergone surgery and RT. However, others have noted significant impairment of short-term memory and cognition in many patients with brain tumor after RT [12,13]. These long-term neurological sequelae of RT, when they occur, have a negative impact on QOL. Other complications of RT that could affect QOL to a lesser extent and should be discussed include cytopenia, scalp dermatitis, transient exacerbation of neurological deficits, nausea and emesis, and loss of appetite.

It is now standard treatment in many cancer centers to use chemotherapy for malignant gliomas, because it has recently been shown to extend survival in a meta-analysis [1,14]. Many chemotherapy regimens have toxicities and potential complications that could adversely affect QOL, including pancytopenia, infection, hemorrhage, and organ-related damage (e.g., pulmonary fibrosis, peripheral neuropathy, nephropathy, hearing loss) [15]. Although some studies have been unable to detect a negative impact of chemotherapy on QOL, other reports suggest it may impair general cognitive function. Chemotherapy can also reduce QOL by requiring frequent blood draws and numerous visits to the hospital, causing generalized fatigue, and adding to psychosocial isolation.

In general, KPS correlates with psychosocial measurements of QOL in patients with brain tumor [13]. For patients with low-grade tumors, KPS and QOL typically improve after therapy and remain stable unless there is recurrence of disease or late treatment-related toxicity. Patients with high-grade tumors usually experience an improvement in KPS and QOL after they recuperate from initial therapy (i.e., surgery and RT), which then remains stable for 6 to 10 months. At this juncture, tumor recurrence or physical deterioration due to treatment usually causes a reduction of QOL and KPS in many patients. If depression occurs at any time after diagnosis, QOL will be adversely affected. Psychosocial measures of QOL are more sensitive to the presence of depression than the KPS score. It is imperative that the physician monitor closely for depression, because it can be effectively treated in most patients.

WHEN IS IT APPROPRIATE TO STOP THERAPY?

The decision to stop therapy is often very difficult for patients, their family members, and the treating physician [4,5]. It signals the "beginning of the end," when all reasonable hope for cure or prolonged stabilization is gone and the patient's death is imminent. These decisions usually arise when the patient has just progressed through the latest protocol and has often suffered further neurological deterioration. In many cases, the neurological status is quite poor, to a degree that functional ambulation, cognition, and verbal interaction are severely compromised.

Although there are often other treatment options that could be offered, the physician must state clearly and honestly that further therapy will not significantly affect outcome. In this situation, it is critical to weigh the adverse effects of further therapy on QOL against the potential benefits for improvement of QOL and prolongation of survival, which would be extremely limited. The physician must reassure the patient and family that the termination of active treatment does not mean the physician will abandon them. Even though the focus of subsequent care will shift to comfort, pain relief, and symptom control, the physician will remain actively involved in the patient's care. In addition to questions about the potential for extension of survival, many patients and family members want to know if further treatment might improve neurological function. In other words, could the patients' current neurological status be reversed somewhat to enhance QOL for the time they have left? Neurological function is rarely restored or improved at these late stages of disease; it would be optimistic even to expect further therapy to stabilize the patient's condition.

Because QOL is so subjective and the behavior of brain tumors can be so variable, the proper time to stop treatment will differ from patient to patient. Some patients accustomed to a high level of function cannot tolerate living their life in a severely compromised fashion while suffering the rigors of treatment. For others, the alterations of function and lifestyle are more easily accepted, so that simple survival is adequate, with less regard for the quality of existence.

Is it ethically appropriate to terminate therapy? If the physician has explained the situation properly and is acting in accordance with the wishes of the patient or family (or whoever has the DPHAC), the decision would be consistent with the principles of respect for autonomy, beneficence, and nonmaleficence [3,4,16]. The physician would be acting to allow a more dignified, peaceful death without the rigors of active therapy. Active treatment is terminated to "promote the good," which is to let the patient die on his or her own terms. It would be ethically improper and contrary to the principle of nonmaleficence for the physician to coerce or force the patient into undergoing further therapy.

SHOULD HOSPICE CARE BE IMPLEMENTED?

The hospice movement originated in England in the 1960s when Dr. Cicely Saunders founded the first multidisciplinary hospice to care for terminally ill patients [17–19]. The movement expanded and eventually spread to the United States in the 1970s. In England, most of the hospice care was administered within inpatient facilities, whereas in the United States, the care was shifted, whenever possible, to the home setting. Because of the success of the early hospice programs, the Congress passed legislation resulting in the establishment of the Medicare Hospice Benefit in 1982. The Medicare Hospice Benefit subsidizes care for terminally ill patients with a life expectancy of 6 months or less, as certified by their attending physician and the hospice medical director. In addition to the life expectancy criteria, other qualifications for Medicare Hospice Benefit include eligibility for Medicare (i.e., at least 65 years of age or certified as disabled), foregoing further aggressive or "curative" therapy, being able to receive most care in the home, and having a primary caregiver present at home. The Medicare Benefit will continue to pay for patients who live longer than 6 months, as long as the attending physician continues to certify the patient is terminally ill. Most patients admitted to hospice do not live longer than the typical 6 months allowed by the Medicare Benefit. In fact, the majority of patients die within 4 to 6 weeks, suggesting that physicians are not referring their patients to hospice care early enough [19]. Recent statistics show that more than one half of all terminally ill patients with cancer in the United States are not being offered hospice services at all or are entering hospice care too late to achieve maximal benefit [18]. Patients with brain tumor should be referred to hospice as soon as aggressive, curative therapy has been discontinued and the primary goal becomes comfort. Hospice care works best when there is time for members of the hospice team to develop meaningful relationships with the patient and family (i.e., over weeks to months).

The purpose of hospice care is to provide medical, psychosocial, and spiritual support for terminally ill patients and their families. This is an especially critical time when hope for cure is lost and anxiety about the future is overwhelming. Hospice care attempts to alleviate the physical and emotional suffering of the patient with brain tumor. Hope for cure is shifted to hope for maximizing dignity, comfort, QOL, and the process of enjoying each remaining day to its fullest. In addition, support is provided for the family members, who are also suffering and attempting to cope with the imminent loss of their loved one. One of the most common fears about advanced incurable cancer is isolation from family and loved ones. The presence of the hospice care team, especially in the home setting, alleviates this fear and ensures that isolation and loneliness are minimized.

The author feels strongly that the use of hospice is an important aspect of the complete care of virtually all patients with malignant brain tumors and many with progressive, benign brain tumors. It should be offered to all patients in the terminal stages of their disease once efforts to halt the progression of the malignancy have ceased. In addition to expertise at treating many aspects of cancer-related pain, hospice nurses can also effectively manage some of the problems specific to patients with brain tumor, such as swallowing difficulties and seizures. During the terminal phases of disease, many patients cannot take oral anticonvulsants properly, either because of neurological compromise of the swallowing mechanism or a reduced level of consciousness. It is often helpful for the hospice nurse to administer these medications rectally as a suspension. Sublingual valium drops can also be used, if needed, to augment seizure control.

CONCLUSIONS

This review has attempted to highlight a few of the many ethical issues that may arise during the care of neuro-oncological patients, in particular, those with brain tumors. As a group, these patients are very fragile and require a physician who has great compassion and empathy as well as excellent medical skills. Furthermore, it is important that the physicians have an understanding of basic ethical theory and the ability to apply medical ethics to the clinical setting. Frequent consideration of important principles such as respect for autonomy, beneficence, and nonmaleficence will guide the physician during the ethical decision-making process and improve his or her ability to make appropriate choices.

REFERENCES

1. Newton HB. Primary brain tumors: review of etiology, diagnosis, and treatment. *Am Fam Phys.* 1984;49:787–797.
2. Patchell RA. Metastatic brain tumors. *Neurol Clin.* 1995;13:915–925.
3. Latimer E. Ethical challenges in cancer care. *J Palliative Care.* 1992;8:65–70.
4. Smith TJ, Bodurtha JN. Ethical considerations in oncology: balancing the interests of patients, oncologists, and society. *J Clin Oncol.* 1995;13:2464–2470.
5. Vick NA, Wilson CB. Total care of the patient with a brain tumor. With considerations of some ethical issues. *Neurol Clin.* 1985;3:705–710.
6. Vanderpool HY, Weiss GB. Ethics and cancer: a survey of the literature. *South Med J.* 1987;80:500–506.
7. Gert B, Culver CM. Moral theory in neurologic practice. *Sem Neurol.* 1984;4:9–14.
8. Butow PN, Kazemi JN, Beeney LJ, Griffin AM, Dunn SM, Tattersall MHN. When the diagnosis is cancer. Patient communication experiences and preferences. *Cancer.* 1996;77:2630–2637.
9. Sardell AN, Trierweiler SJ. Disclosing the cancer diagnosis. *Cancer.* 1993;72:3355–3365.
10. Halperin EC. Malignant gliomas in older adults with poor prognostic signs. *Oncol.* 1995;9:229–238.
11. Nelson WA, Bernat JL. Decisions to withhold or terminate treatment. *Neurol Clin.* 1989;7:759–774.
12. Sachsenheimer W, Piotrowski W, Bimmler T. Quality of life in patients with intracranial tumors on the basis of Karnofsky's performance status. *J Neuro-oncol.* 1992;13:177–181.
13. Mackworth N, Fobair P, Prados MD. Quality of life self-reports from 200 brain tumor patients: comparisons with Karnofsky performance scores. *J Neuro-oncol.* 1992;14:243–253.
14. Fine HA, Dear KBG, Loeffler JS, Black PM, Canellos GP. Meta-analysis of radiation therapy with and without adjuvant chemotherapy for malignant gliomas in adults. *Cancer.* 1993;71:2585–2597.
15. Patterson W, Perry MC. Chemotherapeutic toxicities: a comprehensive overview. *Contemp Oncol* 1993;3(7):56–64.
16. Bernat JL, Goldstein ML, Viste KM. The neurologist and the dying patient. *Neurol.* 1996;46:598–599.
17. Rhymes J. Hospice care in America. *JAMA.* 1990;264:369–372.
18. Kinzbrunner BM. Ethical dilemmas in hospice and palliative care. *Support Care Cancer.* 1995;3:28–36.
19. Von Gunten CF, Neely KJ, Martinez J. Hospice and palliative care: program needs and academic issues. *Oncology.* 1996;10:1070–1074.

38 Role of Support Groups and Caregivers in Neuro-Oncology

Sarah R. G. Gupta

ROLE OF SUPPORT GROUPS AND CAREGIVERS IN NEURO-ONCOLOGY

The Unique Impact of Brain Tumors

The center of cognitive, emotional, and physical functioning, the brain is one of our most important organs. It is also one of the least understood. Based on these factors, the potential effects of brain tumors and their treatments are unique to other tumors in the body.

Like all ailments, brain tumors are a trauma to the mind and body. But, unlike other ailments, brain tumors affect the very center that processes this trauma. Patients and caregivers are faced with the overwhelming tasks of understanding the diagnosis and treatment, identifying and learning to cope with changes in the patient, while at the same time educating others on this process. Although there are parallels, their challenges are distinct from those of patients and caregivers diagnosed with other types of tumors. They benefit most from resources aware of, and sensitive to, these distinct challenges.

Support Groups and Caregivers: A Constellation of Care

A person sits in front of you, sharing his or her symptoms, questions, and fears. You listen, assess, and propose treatment options, drawing from your professional experience and knowledge. In this exchange, as a provider, you have a choice. You can treat the person in front of you as a single, disconnected individual, or you can treat him or her as a member of a constellation consisting of family, friends, colleagues, neighbors, communities, and beyond.

The reverse is true, as well. A patient can see his or her provider as a single, disconnected individual, or as a member of a constellation consisting of professional colleagues, support staff, and mentors, not to mention family, friends, and communities. Just as you as a provider draw information, strength, and support from your constellation, patients draw information, strength, and support from theirs. A comprehensive treatment plan incorporates a patient's constellation or facilitates connection to other resources if they do not already exist.

Illness of any type carries a physical, emotional, and psychological impact. Looking at an illness through only one lens limits perspective and scope of treatment. A comprehensive plan integrates professionals and resources capable of addressing all aspects of the illness.

Most neuro-oncology providers have so many patients that they are unable to spend extensive time with each. Creating a fusion of medical, psychological, and social resources widens the continuum of care, spreading the responsibility among many as opposed to one. Caregivers and support groups are two resources posing great potential benefits to people coping with a brain tumor diagnosis.

ROLE OF SUPPORT GROUPS

Support groups provide a forum for discussing the emotional, physical, and social aspects of brain tumors and their treatments. In their day-to-day lives, people coping with a brain tumor diagnosis may not have access to others who are comfortable or even familiar with the issues they face. Being among people who personally identify with the realities of brain tumors and their treatments often allows for a deeper and more honest exchange of emotion and information. There is less need to hold back with others who are living under similar circumstances.

A support group may also reinforce good communication between patients, caregivers, and their doctors. If patients and caregivers feel inhibited around their doctors, a support group can bolster their confidence and resolve by helping them figure out what issues to raise and how to approach their doctors with such concerns. In addition, for patients and caregivers who are hesitant to ask questions because they are afraid they will not like the answers, learning how others have dealt with this may help.

Location

Brain tumor support groups are often held within hospitals or treatment centers, but they can also occur in community-based settings such as nonprofit organizations, mental health clinics, churches, and homes. Support groups also exist online. Some online support groups are formally organized and facilitated by a center or organization, whereas others come together organically as people seek connections through the Internet. People with mobility or transportation issues, as well as those who feel uncomfortable talking about personal issues in public, may gravitate toward online support groups.

At times, support groups crop up naturally. Consider, for instance, the waiting room in a radiation oncology clinic. People who see each other five days a week, for five to six weeks at a time, tend to connect. The physical act of recognizing people undergoing similar experiences creates an environment of mutual support.

Format

With most formally run, face-to-face, brain tumor support groups, meetings are held once or twice a month, for 1 to 3 hours. Some are loosely structured, allowing group members to arrive and decide on topics to be discussed, based on their experiences. In others, topics are preselected by the facilitator to spark discussion around particular issues. Presenters with expertise in certain areas of brain tumor diagnosis and treatment may also be invited to speak to the group. Most brain tumor support groups are open-ended, meaning they are ongoing and people can come and go as it fits for them, as opposed to close-ended, where the group runs within certain dates and members must join at a certain time to participate.

Most formally organized support groups emphasize the importance of confidentiality. Group members are asked to respect each other's privacy. This builds a sense of safety, affording people the ability to speak without fear that what they share will go outside the group. Members who violate confidentiality agreements may be asked to leave the group. Groups offered through treatment centers or organizations often have their own specific rules governing confidentiality.

Support groups are not for everyone. Some people find listening to the stories of others stressful. Others do not like to share intimate details of their lives. What is most important is to get people connected to the type of support that fits best for their personality and style. Options for people who are not open to attending a support group include individual counseling, literature, and books on tape, as well as one-on-one peer networks.

Facilitation

Professionally facilitated groups are often led by a member of the medical or mental health professions: a doctor, nurse, or social worker. Other groups are facilitated by a patient, caregiver, or individual who has experienced a brain tumor diagnosis but who may not have formal training relevant to leading a support group; these are referred to as peer-facilitated groups. Groups facilitated by someone with group leadership experience, as well as a background in neuro-oncology, are preferable. Despite their many positive aspects, support groups can sometimes be a source of misinformation and stress. An experienced facilitator, with neuro-oncology experience, will be more equipped to effectively counter misinformation and manage stress. In addition, when caregivers and patients have a good working relationship with their treatment team, the treatment team can also provide a credible frame of reference for issues raised in support group discussions.

Conclusions

A brain tumor diagnosis can be an incredibly isolating and scary experience. Support groups connect people with others and encourage open dialogue about concerns and questions. They pose great potential benefits for the treatment team by giving patients, and the people around them, tools they need to cope with the realities of brain tumor diagnosis. The following resources provide information on brain tumor-specific support groups, as well as other groups relevant to brain tumors:

1. American Brain Tumor Association, www.abta.org, 800.886.2282
2. American Cancer Society, www.cancer.org, 800.227.2345
3. Cancer Care, www.cancercare.org, 800.813.4673
4. National Brain Tumor Society, www.braintumor.org, 800.770.8287
5. T.H.E. Brain Trust, www.braintrust.org, 877.252.8480
6. The Wellness Community, www.thewellnesscommunity.org, 888.793.WELL (9355)

ROLE OF CAREGIVERS

Take a moment to think about the amount of time patients spend with their caregivers versus any one member of their treatment team. No one knows the whole patient better than the people he or she spends time with in his or her natural environments and states. A neuro-oncologist is the expert when it comes to neurology, brain tumors, and the application of treatments, but the caregiver is the expert when it comes to the interface between all of these elements and this specific patient.

Patients and professionals must typically maintain a certain level of decorum when interacting. Although this decorum serves a purpose and is, in most cases, necessary, it can limit uninhibited and honest exchange of information. Caregivers and patients often do not need to maintain this decorum with each other. They see each other at their worst and best. They have made some form of commitment to resolve conflict and support and communicate effectively with each other.

With any relationship, clear boundaries and limits are necessary. The treatment team is grounded in one paradigm and the caregiver in another. The caregiver cannot take the place of the neuro-oncologist, and vice versa. This is how the system works. But, ideally, the caregiver and neuro-oncologist reach a place where they respect the ways in which they are each uniquely qualified to care for the patient.

Doctors cannot often afford the time to become intimately familiar with the lives of their patients. This is one of the areas where caregivers can help to fill in gaps. Competent and invested caregivers have great potential to shoulder some of the burden of care.

Caregivers

When you envision a typical caregiver, you may see a partner, adult child, or parent. Factors like population migration, changing family roles, and socioeconomic trends have changed the face of the typical caregiver. Friends, siblings, neighbors, religious community members, and extended family members are all examples of the type of people serving as caregivers for people diagnosed with brain tumors. Caregivers may also be individuals employed through an agency or private arrangement, with no previous personal relationship to the patient.

Roles and Responsibilities

A caregiver is someone who attends to the emotional and nonmedical needs of an ill or dependent person. Often, patients have a team of people providing care, with one particular person identified as the primary caregiver. This is the ideal scenario, with one person acting as the point of contact with the treatment team, providing an orderly and centralized conduit for exchanging information. Caregivers are also the patient's historian. Patient history is an important component of the treatment plan, and caregivers were often direct witnesses to that history.

Caregivers often help patients with their activities of daily living and are frequently in the best position to assist with nonmedical aspects of medication regimens, symptom tracking, therapy, and rehabilitation. The span of responsibility depends on the patient's cognitive, emotional, and physical condition. Under optimal circumstances, patients actively participate in these processes and work together with their caregivers to report their experiences and observations to their treatment team. When patients are unable to participate fully in this feedback, doctors must rely on the people who see them the most and know them the best. Even when patients are able to cognitively and physically participate in their treatment, caregivers should be relied upon as more objective observers. Patients may not notice or be willing to acknowledge all the various ways they change as a result of diagnosis and treatment.

Addressing the emotional and social needs of patients involves an entirely different, but equally important, array of activities. Listening, keeping company, and reassuring through touch and word are examples. A chronic and debilitating illness can have a devastating impact on emotional health. Patients need people in their lives who can compassionately frame any negative behaviors or emotions they manifest. Most people are capable of unconditional positive regard and empathy, but it is usually a patient's caregiver who commits to providing this day in and day out, no matter what.

Communication

Good communication and trust are cornerstones in any relationship. As with any new long-term relationship, people connected through a treatment plan need to get to know each other. Effective communication and trust-building should be a focus at the onset of the treatment plan. Patients, caregivers, and providers need to feel like they can talk to and be heard by one another. Patients and caregivers must also trust in the competence and expertise of their providers, while providers must trust in the ability of their patients and caregivers to provide them with accurate information and to follow through on treatment.

The patient's needs are rightfully central in the treatment plan. But it behooves both patients and providers to allow for a percentage of focus on the caregivers. Caregivers' concerns may differ from those of patients. As a provider, it is essential for you to allow them the opportunity to express their questions. Emphasize that this is a learning process, and educate them on what to look for as possible signs of improvement or deterioration. Provide or direct them to literature and materials geared toward nonmedical professionals. Let them know that the information they provide is critical to the success of the treatment plan, and offer specific examples of the type of information needed. Allow time for caregivers to become familiar with the diagnosis, treatment, and their role. It is a new role and not one they likely chose. People need time to adjust to the emotional, physical, and social changes inherent to the role of caregiver.

Professionals in all fields must be very clear on the rules and regulations governing a patient's right to confidentiality. To facilitate communication with a patient's primary caregiver(s), it is very important to have all necessary releases of information in place. Providers may need to prompt patients and caregivers on releases of information, as they are often preoccupied with the multitude of stressors associated with diagnosis.

Support

Like patients, caregivers require emotional support and information. To prevent burnout, connect caregivers with resources that focus on specifically on their issues and needs. For anyone thrust into a new role, not knowing what to expect and prepare for can be a setup for problems as time passes. There are a number of organizations, groups, books, articles, and professionals focused on informing and supporting caregivers. Figure out resources that may fit for caregivers, in terms of their style and personality, and get them connected as early as possible. Stress the importance of effective and healthful coping right from the start.

Conclusions

Although engaging caregivers can be an intense and complicated process, the benefits of successful engagement far outweigh the costs. A well-rounded treatment plan cultivates and maximizes the strengths and wisdom of caregivers and their relationship with the patient. There are a number of caregiver advocacy, information, and support resources, some specifically focused on brain tumors. These include the following:

1. American Brain Tumor Association, www.abta.org, 800.886.2282

2. Family Caregiver Alliance, www.caregiver.org, 800.445.8106
3. National Brain Tumor Society, www.braintumor.org, 800.770.8287
4. National Family Caregivers Association, www.nfcacares.org, 800.896.3650
5. T.H.E. Brain Trust, Brain Tumor Caregivers Online Support Group, www.braintrust.org

CONCLUSIONS

Caregivers and support groups can be of great benefit to neuro-oncologists and other members of the brain tumor treatment team. Integrating these resources into the treatment plan supports the whole patient by making a place for the emotional and social aspects of the diagnosis, as well as the physical. Patients are parents, partners, siblings, children, friends, colleagues, and neighbors. They are also members of the brain tumor community. They enter the consultation room with a number of existing and potential connections to people and resources which can be of great support to both them and their treatment. A treatment plan incorporating these resources is well-rounded and more potent, with improved outcomes for both patients and providers.

ADDITIONAL READINGS

Institute of Medicine (IOM). *Cancer Care for the Whole Patient: Meeting Psychosocial Health Needs*. Washington, DC: The National Academies Press; 2007.

Meier A, Lyons EJ, Frydman G, Forlenza M, Rimer B. How cancer survivors provide support on cancer-related internet mailing lists. *J Med Internet Res.* 2007;9(2):e12 (Accessed January 8, 2008, at http://www.pubmedcentral.nih.gov/articlerender.fcgi?artid=1874721).

Penson RT, Talsania SHG, Chabner BA, Lynch TJ Jr. Help me help you: support groups in cancer therapy. *The Oncologist.* 2004;9(2):217–225 (Accessed January 8, 2008, at http://theoncologist.alphamedpress.org/cgi/content/full/9/2/217).

Scherbring MJ. Effect of caregiver perception of preparedness on burden in an oncology population. *Oncol Nurs Forum.* 2002;29(6):E70-E76 (Accessed January 8, 2008, at http://ons.metapress.com/content/p485413560758634/fulltext.pdf).

39 Neurocognitive Function and Quality of Life

Christina A. Meyers

Children, adolescents, and adults with brain tumors experience a variety of adverse symptoms that negatively affect their ability to function. In addition to cognitive impairment, they may experience neurological signs and symptoms, fatigue, mood disturbance, sleep disturbance, and sexual dysfunction. Maintaining patient's quality of life (QOL) through preservation of function and symptom reduction is of paramount importance in the care of persons diagnosed with brain tumors. Unfortunately, management of this disease remains difficult and long-term survival, if achieved, is often accompanied by significant disability. In addition, survival and QOL are key criteria to meet when assessing the therapeutic effectiveness of brain tumor treatments, and freedom from symptomatic progression in itself represents benefit. Longer life and better life should be integrated; QOL should no longer be a secondary consideration, although it will likely require a change in culture for this integration to occur.

Neurocognitive impairment in patients with primary brain tumor is extremely common, with 91% of patients having at least one area of deficit compared to the normal population and 71% demonstrating at least three deficits [1]. Neurocognitive symptoms compromise perceived QOL, lead to affective distress, diminish the ability to function in academic, vocational, and household roles, and result in reduced overall functioning and increased caregiver burden. Improved understanding of the nature, course, and persistence of neurocognitive symptoms is an issue of critical importance, particularly given the expected growth in the number of survivors who will understandably want to return to the roles and activities they engaged prior to their diagnosis.

Neurocognitive assessment is useful for (a) understanding what cognitive problems exist prior to initiation of treatment, both to intervene more proactively and to establish a baseline by which the effects of disease and treatment can be established; (b) appreciating the extent to which different antineoplastic treatment regimens improve neurocognitive function (due to better tumor control) or have short- or long-term neurotoxicity; (c) improving patient care by clarifying differential diagnostic possibilities (e.g., depression vs impaired executive or frontal lobe functions); and (d) guiding therapeutic interventions, including pharmacological and behavioral strategies aimed at reducing the functional disability associated with tumor and treatment-related cognitive dysfunction.

The feasibility and tolerability of neurocognitive assessment in patients with brain tumor have been well demonstrated and neurocognitive outcomes are increasingly being incorporated into clinical trials of new antineoplastic agents [2]. Furthermore, cognitive dysfunction predicts survival better than clinical prognostic factors alone in patients with primary brain tumors, leptomeningeal disease, and parenchymal brain metastases [3–5].

CONTRIBUTIONS TO NEUROCOGNITIVE DYSFUNCTION

There are numerous sources that contribute to the etiology of cognitive impairment in patients with brain tumor, including tumor effects, treatment effects, host factors, and even factors unrelated to the diagnosis of brain tumor (e.g., history of head injury) [6]. The specific neurocognitive and neurological deficits are naturally related to the location of the tumor (e.g., verbal memory and language impairments associated with left hemisphere tumors, and visual-perceptual impairments associated with right hemisphere tumors). Although these focal deficits are typically less dramatic than those observed in patients with lesions of more acute onset, such as a stroke, certain additional symptoms such as impaired frontal lobe executive functions (the capacity for intentional behavior, planning and organization skills, mental flexibility, abstraction, accurate self-awareness, and personality), neurobehavioral slowing, and fatigue are ubiquitous in patients with brain tumors regardless of location [7].

Lesion momentum is also a significant factor in the presentation of neurocognitive deficits in patients with brain tumor. For instance, a patient with a glioblastoma that developed from a low-grade astrocytoma over an extended period of time may have fewer cognitive problems than a person with a primary glioblastoma that became rapidly symptomatic. Figure 39.1 displays the profile of neurocognitive function in patients with low-grade and high-grade gliomas [8].

EFFECT OF NEUROCOGNITIVE DEFICITS ON FUNCTION

For many patients with brain tumor, changes in cognition and personality are the most problematic and concerning

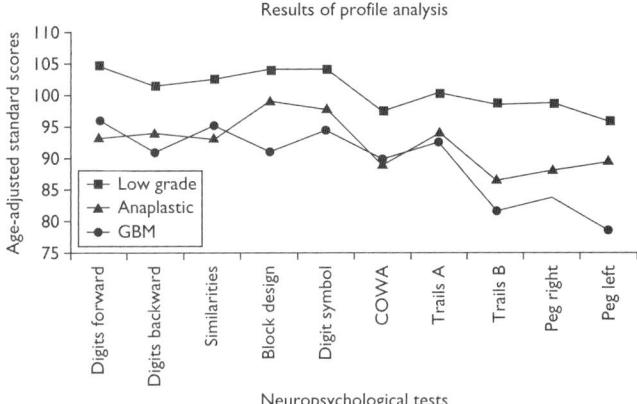

Figure 39.1 Relationship between cognitive impairment and tumor grade in presurgical brain tumor patients. From Gleason and Meyers [8].

symptoms to manage. For example, in a recent editorial highlighting patient perspectives on brain metastases from breast cancer, one woman commented, "My first thought was not my brain! To me, that meant I would lose me. The threat of dying was not uppermost in my fears but losing my identity and becoming totally dependent on someone else for personal needs" [9].

Unfortunately, the majority of individuals with primary brain tumors do suffer from neurocognitive, emotional, and behavioral difficulties that compromise their independence and interfere with their academic, vocational, and/or social pursuits. For instance, maintaining employment after diagnosis and treatment for a brain tumor is an exception, not a rule. Only 18% of patients return to work full-time and 10% return to work part-time after a brain tumor diagnosis and treatment [10]. This finding was echoed in a recent survey conducted by the National Brain Tumor Foundation. Of 277 patients with brain tumor who responded to the online survey, 91% were employed prior to diagnosis, but only 33% were working postdiagnosis. Moreover, 62% of caregivers surveyed ($n = 224$) reported making work adjustments (e.g., leave of absence, increased use of vacation time, and decreased hours) and 16% quit their jobs. Nearly half of all respondents (48%) reported downward shifts in household income [11]. Prior research has demonstrated that, more often than not, neurocognitive difficulties and not physical disabilities prevent patients with brain tumor from returning to work [12].

INTERVENTIONS

To appropriately target interventions, patients should undergo a neuropsychological assessment to objectively characterize the pattern and severity of cognitive impairment and to identify areas of preserved cognitive ability. Targets for intervention are developed that take into account the patient's cognitive strengths and weaknesses, emotional and functional status, medical circumstances and prognosis, and level of insight and motivation. Assessment of additional factors that may be contributing to the patient's cognitive difficulties (i.e., emotional distress and fatigue) should also be performed with referrals to appropriate services for management as needed.

Cognitive Rehabilitation

Despite the often bleak prognosis and outlook associated with the diagnosis, many patients with brain tumor can enjoy improved levels of independence and functioning if provided appropriate assistance to manage the impact of cognitive symptoms on their daily life. In fact, interventions designed to minimize the adverse cognitive consequences of this disease and its treatment represent a significant opportunity to improve patient's QOL, regardless of the stage of their illness. In 2000, the Brain Tumor Progress Review Group, cosponsored by the National Cancer Institute and the National Institute of Neurologic Disorders and Stroke, issued a specific call to review cognitive interventions used in other rehabilitation-related disciplines (e.g., acquired brain injury and stroke) to determine whether evidenced-based interventions could be used successfully with patients with brain tumor [13]. So far, answers to this call have remained limited.

Unfortunately, primary cancer centers rarely offer cognitive rehabilitation services to brain tumor survivors and traditional rehabilitation hospitals rarely target such individuals due to concerns about poor prognosis [12]. A multidisciplinary approach, incorporating pharmacological, cognitive, behavioral, and rehabilitative therapies, has the potential to maximize everyday functioning, coping, and adjustment with the ultimate goal of maintaining the highest level of functioning for the longest possible time. For some patients, cognitive and vocational rehabilitation can be very effective, with shorter stays, lower treatment costs, and better overall outcome in terms of independence and productivity compared with patients with traumatic brain injuries [14].

The goals of cognitive rehabilitation for adults and children treated for brain tumors depend upon a number of factors that relate not only to the identified areas of cognitive deficit but also to medical treatment and prognosis. At one end of the continuum are patients with aggressive tumors where the expected survival is limited. For these patients, significant morbidity is not unusual and maximizing QOL is the goal. In this setting, rehabilitation efforts are most efficiently directed at acute compensatory interventions. Compensatory interventions may include making accommodations in the patient's home and hospital environment to increase structure and decrease demands for planning and decision making. In addition, some patients may be able to learn new skills, such as using a personal digital assistant or memory notebook, to compensate for cognitive deficits. Even patients in terminal care can benefit from methods to enhance their orientation and social interactions. This approach is similar to that outlined in patients with progressive dementias in which the underlying neuropathology is not the target of the intervention and cognitive deficits are managed and compensated for, rather than "cured" or "rehabilitated" in the traditional sense [15]. Treatment goals, duration, and intensity must be extremely flexible in these cases to accommodate the changing needs of the patient and his/her family.

At the other end of the continuum in terms of medical prognosis are patients with tumors that are quite responsive to therapy. For example, among children with standard risk medulloblastoma, the 5-year survival rate approaches 80%. The goals of cognitive rehabilitation are more appropriately directed at long-term endpoints such as successful graduation from high school or college and the future ability to function independently as an adult. Within the past decade, many academic medical centers have developed specialized clinics for long-term survivors of childhood cancers, including brain tumors, that are focused on neurological, endocrinological, neuropsychological, and QOL issues. The timing of rehabilitation efforts depends upon the developmental stage of the child at diagnosis, as their deficits may emerge over time. The child might fail to demonstrate normal cognitive development when different brain regions initially affected by treatment are supposed to mature [16]. Some treatments, such as cranial radiation, may have a delayed impact on general intellectual development. Therefore, periodical neuropsychological assessment is often recommended. Only recently have multicenter randomized clinical trials to validate the efficacy of cognitive/behavioral rehabilitation approaches have been instituted [17]. The continued development of such specialized research endeavors is necessary to disseminate standardized, effective approaches to cognitive rehabilitation and to facilitate innovations in this area.

Pharmacologic Strategies

Neurobehavioral slowing is the hallmark of frontal lobe dysfunction and treatment-related adverse effects in patients with brain tumor. The syndrome of neurobehavioral slowing is generally due to involvement of the monoamine pathways of the frontal brain stem reticular system. In addition, catecholamines have an important role in the modulation of attention and working memory. Stimulant treatment (i.e., methylphenidate) has been reported to be useful in the treatment of concentration difficulties, psychomotor retardation, and fatigue frequently seen in patients with brain tumor and has helped to elevate mood as well [18]. A conservative dose of 10 mg twice a day significantly improved cognitive function as assessed by objective tests, and doses in excess of 60 mg twice a day were well-tolerated. Subjective improvements included improved gait, increased stamina and motivation to perform activities, and improved bladder control. There were no significant side effects, and many patients taking steroids were able to decrease their dose.

Methylphenidate can also be beneficial in childhood survivors of brain tumors. Thompson et al [19] were the first to report the beneficial effects of methylphenidate on attention in a randomized, double-blind trial of survivors of childhood cancer. Mulhern et al [20] conducted a randomized, double-blind, 3-week home crossover trial of 1 week each of placebo, low-dose methylphenidate (0.3 mg/kg to maximum of 10 mg), and moderate-dose methylphenidate (0.6 mg/kg to maximum of 20 mg). At the end of each week, parents and teachers rated the child's behavior and side effects. Compared to placebo, significant improvements in both cognitive and social ratings by teachers, and to a lesser extent parents, were observed with methylphenidate [20]. Whether this ultimately facilitates academic achievement among survivors of childhood cancer who have attentional problems is not yet known.

Although methylphenidate has relatively transient and minimal side effects, the drug may be contraindicated for some, and in such cases, clinicians may defer to alternative pharmacologic treatments. Modafinil, a novel vigilance promoting agent, is commonly used to treat excessive daytime somnolence associated with narcolepsy and idiopathic hypersomnia. The effectiveness of modafinil for alleviating fatigue in patients with brain tumor has been examined in a pilot study involving 15 patients with primary brain tumors [21]. Roughly, two thirds of patients studied reported moderate to significant improvements in cancer-related fatigue following 10 weeks of treatment with modafinil (200 mg daily, increased to 300 mg after 4 weeks in nonresponders). Twenty-six percent reported no or minimal effect despite dose escalation. Adverse effects (anxiety and dizziness) were mild, with the exception of one patient who required discontinuation of medication secondary to encephalopathy. Further study is clearly warranted.

There has also been an interest in assessing the potential benefits of pharmacologic agents used in other neurological disorders, such as Alzheimer disease, for patients with brain tumor. Shaw et al [22] reported on an open-label, Phase II clinical trial of donepezil a acetylcholinesterase inhibitor commonly used in the treatment of Alzheimer-related dementia, in 35 patients who had undergone partial or whole-brain cranial irradiation for primary or metastatic brain tumors at least 6 months prior to enrolment. A 24-week course of donepezil (5 mg daily for 6 weeks and then increased to 10 mg daily for 18 weeks) was associated with improvements in neurocognitive functioning (attention and memory) and brain-specific symptoms reflecting QOL (as measured by the Functional Assessment of Cancer Therapy—Brain Module). A Phase III randomized, double-blind, placebo-controlled, multicenter trial of donepezil was being conducted at the time of this writing, and investigation of other agents used in the treatment of dementia (e.g., memantine) are in clinical trials.

There is great interest in developing treatments focused on radiation injury to the brain. One recent study examined the effect of megadose α-tocopherol (vitamin E; 1000 IU twice per day) in a group of patients with nasopharyngeal carcinoma who had undergone standard treatment with radiation and later developed temporal lobe radiation necrosis [23]. These patients had significant memory impairment hypothesized to be related to free radical generation and tissue peroxidation in the brain. Vitamin E has been demonstrated in nonhuman studies to inhibit lipid peroxidation, reduce cell death in hypoxic neurons, and decrease degeneration of hippocampal cells after ischemia [24]. Using an open-label, nonrandomized, treatment versus control design, Chan et al [25] demonstrated an improvement in memory and executive functions in these patients after 1 year of dietary supplementation with vitamin E.

There are several other strategies that have been suggested to treat radiation-induced cognitive dysfunction. Low molecular weight heparin has been investigated to prevent venous thromboembolism in patients with brain tumor, and it may also have a beneficial effect on cognitive function by reducing ischemia associated with brain radiation [25]. In addition, there is growing evidence that cognitive impairment and other adverse cancer-related symptoms may be due in part to a cancer or treatment-induced inflammatory response (i.e., the induction of inflammatory cytokines) [26,27]. Radiation therapy is thought to induce the release of inflammatory cytokines that may cause more widespread brain injury [28]. It is possible that modulating cytokines and their receptors may ameliorate or protect against the development of radiation injury. Cytokine antagonists and antiinflammatory agents are being investigated for their antineoplastic properties; close monitoring of cognitive function and symptoms during these trials may also shed light on their ability to attenuate symptoms [29].

The cognitive decline seen in patients treated with brain radiation may also be caused by hippocampal dysfunction resulting from decreased hippocampal neurogenesis, proliferation, and increased apoptosis [30]. Neural stem cell advances hold promise for a host of neurological disorders and may at some point serve as vehicles for brain tumor treatments [31,32]. Newer approaches using neural stem cells or new agents that stimulate neurogenesis of stem cells normally residing in the brain are on the horizon [30,33]. A recent study of resected tissue from patients undergoing tumor surgery provided evidence of stem cells in the subventricular zone [34]. This work has implications for neuroregenerative approaches, although it is not known how the functionality of neural stem cells is affected by cancer treatment to the brain. Another approach evaluated the introduction of transplanted oligodendrocytes to stimulate remyelination of damaged neural cells [35]. Groves et al [35] described a process by which they were able to expand purified populations of oligodendrocyte type-2 astrocytes in vitro. When these cells were injected into demyelinated lesions of rat spinal cords, remyelination occurred. However, little data currently exist with transplantation in humans.

Prophylactic Treatment Approaches

Since patients with brain tumor often experience patterns of impairment that follow a somewhat predictable course based on tumor characteristics (e.g., lesion location and histology) and treatment plan (e.g., surgery followed by chemotherapy and/or radiation), the possibility of intervening with patients and caregivers *prior* to the emergence of neurocognitive disabilities offers exciting possibilities for prophylactic behavioral rehabilitation and pharmacological and psychoeducational strategies. Providing the patients with strategies to deal with cognitive impairments prior to their emergence may be efficient and cost-effective. Because of their focus on primary and secondary prevention of neurocognitive and emotional symptoms, such strategies may be considered *"prehabilitation"* as opposed to "rehabilitation." The goal of prehabilitative interventions in patients with brain tumor would be (a) to protect the brain from further neurocognitive compromise associated with progression of disease and cancer treatment; (b) to implement compensatory behavioral strategies designed to circumvent probable problems before they progress to life-limiting disabilities; and (c) to decrease patient and caregiver distress by introducing supportive counseling and psychoeducational programs. This "prehabilitation" model may be applied to individuals with extracerebral disease and fits particularly well with current plans for delivering quality cancer care in light of enhanced focus on issues of cancer survivorship [36].

Emotional Distress and Fatigue

Depression and adjustment disorders are extremely common in patients with brain tumor and can be related to preexisting or recurrent mood disorders, the direct effects of the disease in the brain, adjustment medications such as steroids, or psychological reactions to the devastating situation. Comprehensive studies of QOL in patients with brain tumor reveal increased emotional reactivity, lowered frustration tolerance, depression, anxiety, and reduced family functioning [37]. Patients with brain tumor experience significant emotional distress at rates higher than those associated with nearly all other cancer disease sites [38]. The prevalence of depression and emotional distress is underdiagnosed in patients with brain tumor, and it occurs throughout the course of disease [39]. In this study, 93% of patients report depressive symptoms, while only 15% of patients were identified as depressed by their treating physicians. Patients and their caregivers also need psychosocial support throughout the illness.

Assessment and effective intervention for emotional distress in patients with brain tumor is complicated by the subjective nature of symptoms, multifactorial etiologies, and disease-associated compliance problems. Despite these problems, many studies have shown that psychosocial interventions can have a positive impact on the psychological distress experienced by patients with brain tumor. A meta-analysis of controlled outcome studies demonstrated that psychosocial interventions have a positive impact on QOL in adult patients with cancer and that many different forms of intervention are beneficial [40]. The study found that the duration of the intervention emerged as a more relevant variable than the specific type of psychosocial intervention. Some of the more common approaches are individual psychotherapy or counseling, support groups, and psychoeducational activities. Pharmacologic therapies (e.g., antidepressants, psychostimulants, and anticonvulsants) are also employed. The type of psychosocial intervention selected must be made based on available resources, patient preference, and the nature of the psychosocial stressors being targeted by treatment.

An easy and cost-effective way to screen patients and caregivers for emotional concerns is the National Comprehensive Cancer Network's Distress Thermometer and Problem List. This tool uses a 0 to 10 scale that can be completed quickly and includes a list of problems that indicate possible reasons for the distress. Used in conjunction with clinical assessment by the primary oncology team, such tools can be a valuable means for evaluating depression, anxiety, and other QOL symptoms in the clinical setting and represent a time and cost-effective method to inform decisions about what support services will be most appropriate [41].

Fatigue is the one of most common adverse symptoms experienced by patients with brain tumor. Cancer-related fatigue has been defined by the National Comprehensive Cancer Network as "a distressing persistent, subjective sense of tiredness or exhaustion related to cancer or cancer treatment that is not proportional to recent activity and interferes with usual functioning" [42]. In addition to physical tiredness, a cognitive aspect of fatigue involving decreased concentration and reduced alertness is being increasingly recognized as a component of cancer-related fatigue. Fatigue can have adverse effects on cognitive function and mood and impaired cognitive functioning and mood disorders may also cause fatigue. Comprehensive management of fatigue requires a multidimensional approach that recognizes the myriad of factors that may contribute to the fatigue experienced by patients with cancer, including anemia, coexisting medical problems (e.g., infection, renal insufficiency, and dehydration), hormonal disturbances, deconditioning, inadequate pain management, medication side effects, sleep disorders, underlying mood disorders, and cognitive symptoms [43].

Education

To provide a healthcare environment in which patients with brain tumor and their caregivers have access to best support practices requires a professional network that promotes evidence-based support practices throughout the continuum of care. Patient and family education is also extremely important. Potential neurobehavioral symptoms may not be explained to the patient, sometimes because the primary physician is not aware of the impact of even subtle symptoms on social and vocational functioning. Patients who experience these symptoms may wonder if they are mentally ill or inaccurately attribute their symptoms to other causes. The more knowledgeable the patients and their families are about the disease, treatment, and expected problems, the more effective the intervention process will be. Even simple coping strategies, such as taking intermittent naps, writing notes, and taking special care to plan and organize activities, may be of benefit.

CONCLUSIONS

Many patients with brain tumor have the ability to improve their function at home and in vocational and leisure pursuits and enjoy an improved level of independence and QOL given the right support. We must be ready to meet the needs of these survivors and their caregiving milieu. Effective and proactive intervention strategies are a critical component throughout and following brain tumor treatment. As primary therapy becomes more effective and more patients experience long-term remissions, assessment of neurocognitive function and QOL and establishing effective treatment strategies will gain even greater importance.

REFERENCES

1. Tucha O, Smely C, Preier M, Lange KW. Cognitive deficits before treatment among patients with brain tumors. *Neurosurgery.* 2000;47:324–333.
2. Meyers C, Brown P. Role and relevance of neurocognitive assessment in clinical trials of patients with CNS tumors. *J Clin Oncol.* 2006;24:1305–1309.
3. Meyers CA, Smith JA, Bezjak A, et al. Neurocognitive function and progression in patient with brain metastases treated with whole-brain radiation and motexafin gadolinium: results of a randomized phase III trial. *J Clin Oncol.* 2004;22:157–165.
4. Sherman AM, Jaeckle K, Meyers CA. Pretreatment cognitive performance predicts survival in patients with leptomeningeal disease. *Cancer.* 2002;15:1311–1316.
5. Meyers CA, Hess KR, Yung WKA, Levin VA. Cognitive function as a predictor of survival in patients with recurrent malignant glioma. *J Clin Oncol.* 2000;18:646–650.
6. Scheibel RS, Meyers CA, Levin VA. Cognitive dysfunction following surgery for intracerebral glioma: influence of histopathology, lesion location, and treatment. *J Neurooncol.* 1996;30:61–69.
7. Anderson SW, Damasio H, Tranel D. Neuropsychological impairments associated with lesions caused by tumor or stroke. *Arch Neurol.* 1990;47:397–405.
8. Gleason AC, Meyers CA. Relationship between cognitive impairment and tumor grade in pre-surgical patients with primary brain tumors [abstract]. *J Int Neuropsychol Soc.* 2002;8:274.
9. Mayer M. A patient perspective on brain metastases in breast cancer. *Clin Cancer Res.* 2007;13:1623–1624.
10. Fobair P, Mackworth N, Varghese A, Prados M. Quality of life issues among 200 brain tumor patients treated at the University of California in San Francisco, interviewed 1988. Brain Tumor Conference: A Living Resource Guide; 1990.
11. Patterson H. *Nobody can Afford a Brain Tumor: The Financial Impact of Brain Tumors on Patients and Families: A Summary of Findings.* Watertown, MA: National Brain Tumor Foundation; 2007.
12. Meyers CA, Boake C. Neurobehavioral disorders experienced by brain tumor patients: Rehabilitation strategies. *Cancer Bull.* 1993;45:362–364.
13. National Cancer Institute, National Institute of Neurological Disorders and Stroke (November, 2000). Report of the Brain Tumor Progress Review Group. http://planning.cancer.gov/pdfprgreports/2000braintumor.pdf.
14. Sherer M, Meyers CA, Bergloff P. Efficacy of postacute brain injury rehabilitation for patients with primary malignant brain tumors. *Cancer.* 1997;80:250–257.
15. Attix D. An integrated model for geriatric neuropsychological intervention. In: Attix D, Welsh-Bomer K, eds. *Geriatric Neuropsychology Assessment and Intervention.* New York: Guilford Press; 2006:241–60.
16. Mulhern RK, Butler RW. Neurocognitive sequelae of childhood cancers and their treatment. *Pediatr Rehabil.* 2004;7:1–14.
17. Butler RW, Copeland DR. Attentional processes and their remediation in children treated for cancer: a literature review and the development of a therapeutic approach. *J Intl Neuropsychol Soc.* 2002;8:115–124.
18. Meyers CA, Weitzner MA, Valentine AD, Levin VA. Methylphenidate improves cognition, mood, and function of brain tumor patients. *J Clin Oncol.* 1998;16:2522–2527.
19. Thompson SJ, Leigh L, Christensen R, et al. Immediate neurocognitive effects of methylphenidate on learning-impaired survivors of childhood cancer. *J Clin Oncol.* 2001;19:1802–1808.
20. Mulhern RK, Khan RB, Kaplan S, et al. Short-term efficacy of methylphenidate: a randomized, double-blind, placebo-controlled trial among survivors of childhood cancer. *J Clin Oncol.* 2004;22:4795–4803.
21. Nasir S. Modafinil improves fatigue in primary brain tumor patients [abstract]. *Neuro Oncol.* 2003;5:335
22. Shaw EG, Rosdhal R, D'Agostino RB, et al. Phase II study of donepezil in irradiated brain tumor patients: effect on cognitive function, mood, and quality of life. *J Clin Oncol.* 2006;24:1415–1420.
23. Chan AS, Cheung M-C, Law SC, Chan JH. Phase II study of alpha-tocopherol in improving the cognitive function of patients with temporal lobe radionecrosis. *Cancer.* 2003;100(2):398–404.

24. Yoshida S, Busto R, Watson BD, Santiso M, Ginsberg MD. Postischemic cerebral lipid peroxidation in vitro: modification by dietary Vitamin E. *J Neurochem.* 1985;44:593–601.
25. Glantz MJ, Burger PC, Friedman AH, Radtke RA, Massey EW, Schold SC Jr. Treatment of radiation-induced nervous system injury with heparin and warfarin. *Neurology.* 1994;44:2020–2027.
26. Meyers CA, Albitar M, Estey E. Cognitive impairment, fatigue, and cytokine levels in patients with acute myelogenous leukemia or myelodysplastic syndrome. *Cancer.* 2005;104:788–793.
27. Lee B, Dantzer R, Langley K, et al. A cytokine-based neuroimmunological mechanism of cancer-related symptoms. *Neuroimmunomodulation.* 2004;11:279–292.
28. Shaw EG. Central nervous system overview. In: Gunderson LL, Tepper JE, eds. *Clinical Radiation Oncology.* Philadelphia, PA: Churchill-Livingstone; 2000.
29. Raz A. Is inhibition of cyclooxygenase required for the anti-tumorigenic effects of nonsteroidal, anti-inflammatory drugs (NSAIDs)? In vitro versus in vivo results and the relevance for the prevention and treatment of cancer. *Biochem Pharmacol.* 2002;63:343–347.
30. Monje ML, Mizumatsu S, Fike JR, Palmer TD. Irradiation induces neural precursor-cell dysfunction. *Nat Med.* 2002;8:955–962.
31. Kim SU. Genetically engineered human neuronal stem cells for brain repair in neurological diseases. *Brain Dev.* 2007;29:193–201.
32. Mapara KY, Stevenson CB, Thompson RC, Ehtesham M. Stem cells as vehicles for the treatment of brain cancer. *Neurosurg Clin N Am.* 2007;18:71–80.
33. Rezvani M, Birds DA, Hodges H, Hopewell JW, Milledew K, Wilkinson JH. Modification of radiation myelopathy by the transplantation of neural stem cells in the rat. *Radiat Res.* 2002;156:408–412.
34. Sanai N, Tramontin AD, Quinones-Hinojosa A, et al. Unique astrocyte ribbon in adult human brain contains neural stem cells but lacks chain migration. *Nature.* 2004;427:740–744.
35. Groves AK, Barnett SC, Franklin RJ, et al. Repair of demyelinated lesions by transplantation of purified O-2A progenitor cells. *Nature.* 1993;362:453–455.
36. Rowland J, Hewitt M, Ganz P. Cancer survivorship: A new challenge in delivering quality cancer care. *J Clin Oncol.* 2006;24:5101–5104.
37. Weitzner MA, Meyers CA. Cognitive functioning and quality of life in malignant glioma patients: a review of the literature. *Psychooncology.* 1997;6:169–177.
38. Zabora J, BrintzenhofeSzoc K, Curbow B, Hooker C, Piantadosi S. The prevalence of psychological distress by cancer site. *Psychooncology.* 2001;10:19–28.
39. Litofsky NS, Farace E, Anderson F Jr, Meyers CA, Huang W, Laws ER Jr; the Glioma Outcomes Project. Depression in patients with high-grade glioma: results of the Glioma Outcomes Project. *Neurosurgery.* 2004;54:358–366.
40. Rehse B, Pukrop R. Effects of psychosocial interventions on quality of life in adult cancer patients: meta analysis of 37 published controlled outcome studies. *Patient Educ Counsel.* 2003;50:179–186.
41. National Comprehensive Cancer Network. Standards of care for distress management, DIS-3. Version 1.205. http://www.nccn.org. Accessed September 3, 2005.
42. National Comprehensive Cancer Network. *Cancer-Related Fatigue.* NCCN Clinical Practice Guidelines in Oncology Version 2. Fort Washington, PA: National Comprehensive Cancer Network; 2007.
43. Valentine AD, Meyers CA. Cognitive and mood disturbance as causes and symptoms of fatigue in cancer patients. *Cancer.* 2001;92:1694–1698.

40 Neuropsychological Sequelae of Adult Brain Tumors

Martin Klein

INTRODUCTION

Standard therapeutic options for brain tumors include surgery, radiotherapy, and chemotherapy. Unfortunately, these same therapies pose risks of neurotoxicity, the most common long-term complications being radiation necrosis, chemotherapy-associated leukoencephalopathy, and cognitive deficits. These side effects remain difficult to predict, but are associated with risk factors that include patient age, therapeutic modality and dosage, genetic background, and idiosyncratic predispositions. Indices of cognitive function and health-related quality of life (QOL) have become increasingly important in clinical trials in patients with brain tumor for three reasons. First, although information on progression-free survival and objective response on computed tomography (CT) or magnetic resonance imaging (MRI) may be highly relevant in trials with patients with glioma, they do not directly inform us on the clinical situation of the patient. Second, the patient's physical function and ability to do activities of daily living do not reflect the patient's cognitive status and QOL. Finally, the main rationale for selecting a given treatment may be related to neurotoxic (e.g., cognitive) side effects and effect on QOL.

Deficits in cognitive function in patients with brain tumor may be caused by cerebral cortical lesions but, because of the widespread cortical-subcortical connections, may also result from subcortical white-matter disease or even from damage to cerebellar structures as is the case in patients with posterior fossa tumors [1,2]. Cognitive decline that might ultimately lead to dementia negatively affects the patient's QOL and well-being [3,4].

Epilepsy is the main effect of low-grade glioma, and patients have a long survival [5]. In these long-surviving patients, there is a growing concern that cognitive decline is caused by tumor and treatment effects. Consequently, cognitive function and QOL are increasingly incorporated as secondary outcome measures in clinical trials in patients with low-grade glioma. This is also true for patients with high-grade glioma, such as chemotherapy-responsive oligodendroglial tumors, and for patients with glioblastoma, whose prognosis has moderately improved in recent years by radiotherapy plus concomitant and adjuvant temozolomide [6,7].

As is the case in patients with non–central nervous system (CNS) cancer, cognitive function has independent prognostic significance in patients with high-grade and low-grade glioma. [8–11]. Assessment of cognitive function may help clinicians to decide which treatment should be selected. Moreover, cognitive deterioration indicates tumor progression before signs of disease recurrence are evident on CT or MRI [4,12,13].

CAUSES OF COGNITIVE DEFICITS

Cognitive deficits in patients with brain tumor can be caused by the tumor, by tumor-related epilepsy and its treatment (surgery, radiotherapy, antiepileptics, chemotherapy, or corticosteroids), and by psychological distress. More likely, a combination of these factors will contribute to cognitive dysfunction. Also, tumor regrowth (either locally or diffusely), leptomeningeal metastasis, or metabolic disturbances might negatively affect cognitive function.

Brain Tumor as the Cause of Cognitive Deficits

In addition to seizures, motor or sensory deficits, and increased intracranial pressure, patients with brain tumor can present with cognitive complaints and deficits. In patients with primary CNS lymphoma or gliomatosis cerebri, which are rare brain tumors, cognitive deficits are a prominent clinical feature. This is also true for patients with slowly growing tumors—such as low-grade glioma and World Health Organization (WHO) grade I meningiomas—most of whom present with seizures. Rapidly growing, high-grade tumors, on the other hand, lead to signs of increased intracranial pressure and neurological deficits, which might overshadow more subtle cognitive deficits [14]. In most studies on cognitive function in patients with brain tumor, conclusions on the role of the tumor cannot easily be made, because data are only gathered after treatment. Nevertheless, Tucha et al have found cognitive disturbances before treatment, including surgery, in 91% of 139 patients with diverse brain tumors [15]. These findings were corroborated by the same group in a study consisting of patients with meningioma only [16]. Results from other studies in patients with low-grade and high-grade glioma and meningioma also indicate that the tumor itself is an important contributor to cognitive deficits [17–19]. Patients with tumors in the dominant hemisphere furthermore have more cognitive deficits than those with nondominant hemisphere lesions [18,20–22].

However, patients with glioma tend to have more global cognitive deficits, unlike patients with stroke who tend to have site-specific deficits. This may be explained by a diffuse growth of tumor cells infiltrating normal brain tissue [23]. Additionally, acute neurotransmitter changes and chronic degeneration of fiber tracts caused by damage to certain brain areas may impair neuronal responses in remote undamaged cortical regions (i.e., diaschisis) [24]. Diaschisis in patients with brain tumor might be attributed to both tumor and treatment effects. However, given the brain plasticity and functional compensation seen after stroke, congenital malformations, or brain injury, infiltration by gliomas might lead to reshaping or local reorganization of functional networks [25].

Evidently, cognitive deficits may also be caused by recurrent tumor growth. Deterioration in cognitive function may be the first manifestation of tumor recurrence, even before structural changes are seen on CT or MRI [4,12].

Surgery as the Cause of Cognitive Deficits

Surgery for brain tumors is used to establish the histological diagnosis and to alleviate neurological symptoms through the reduction of tumor mass. Thus, surgery is beneficial to cognitive function or does not further deteriorate already compromised cognitive functioning. In a mixed histology group of patients with tumors in the frontal or temporal lobes, for example, Tucha et al demonstrated cognitive impairment already to be present at the time of diagnosis in the majority of patients and not to increase after surgery [15]. A later study in patients with frontal meningiomas also indicates that the surgical removal of frontal meningiomas does not additionally impair patients' cognitive functioning [16]. However, patients with meningioma with tumors in the dominant hemisphere and those using antiepileptic drugs (AEDs) might be more at risk to develop cognitive deficits [19,22].

Surgery and perioperative injuries may cause (mainly transient) neurological deficits owing to damage of normal surrounding tissue. Many neurosurgeons are therefore hesitant to operate on patients with tumors in eloquent brain areas. According to Scheibel et al, surgery in patients with glioma leads to focal cognitive deficits, in contrast to more diffuse cognitive disturbances caused by radiotherapy and chemotherapy [26]. Studies that use intraoperative image guiding and functional mapping in patients with low-grade glioma in eloquent brain locations showed a high percentage of postoperative cognitive deficits [25,27]. However, most of these deficits resolved within 3 months, presumably owing to the plasticity of the normal brain [25]. Patients with brain tumors have widespread disturbances in resting state functional connectivity between remote brain areas. Global slowing of resting state brain activity in patients with low-grade glioma has been associated with neurocognitive deficits [28,29]. To study how tumor treatment affects functional connectivity, magnetoencephalography recordings before and after tumor resection were analyzed in 15 newly diagnosed patients with primary brain tumor [30]. Functional connectivity changed in a complex manner after tumor resection, depending on frequency band and functional connectivity type. Post hoc analyses established a significant decrease of interhemispheric connectivity in the theta band after tumor resection. This result proved to be robust and was not influenced by radiotherapy or a variety of tumor- and patient-related factors.

In line with these data, a study on a large group of patients with low-grade glioma, who had surgery or biopsy at least 1 year before, indicated that surgery did not contribute to long-lasting cognitive disability [17]. In patients with high-grade glioma, the cognitive deficits after surgery were probably not caused by surgery or perioperative causes (e.g., general anesthesia) [18]. By contrast, surgery in patients with histologically proven versus suspected low-grade glioma had a negative effect on cognitive function and QOL in a case-matched control study [31].

Radiotherapy as the Cause of Cognitive Deficits

The risk of permanent CNS toxicity, which typically becomes detectable after an asymptomatic latency period, continues to influence clinical treatment decisions. Interindividual differences in sensitivity result in a certain variability of the threshold dose and preclude administration of a guaranteed safe dose, even in the current era of high-precision image-guided radiotherapy. Cognitive deficits attributed to radiotherapy were first reported in children treated for acute leukemia or brain tumors. This bias was partly caused by a larger vulnerability of the developing brain for neurotoxic side effects of radiotherapy [32]. In adults with gliomas, brain metastases, primary CNS lymphoma, and nasopharyngeal malignancies and in patients with small-cell lung carcinoma who had prophylactic irradiation of the brain, reports on radiation toxicity emerged later [33]. In contrast to these reports, radiotherapy may, like any other treatment for brain tumors, also improve cognitive function. However, the therapeutic index in the nervous system is low, because the radiation dose required for tumor control is very close to, if not higher than, the toxic dose for neighboring tissues. To describe neurotoxicity caused by radiotherapy, a distinction is made between acute encephalopathy, early-delayed encephalopathy, and late-delayed encephalopathy.

Acute radiation encephalopathy develops within 2 weeks of the start of radiotherapy, caused by vasogenic edema after disruption of the blood-brain barrier. This may result in headache, somnolence, and worsening of preexisting neurological deficits. Corticosteroids rapidly ameliorate this reversible disorder.

One to six months after completion of radiotherapy, early-delayed radiation encephalopathy may occur. This encephalopathy may be difficult to distinguish from early tumor progression. Apart from drowsiness and worsening of the neurological disorder, a transient cognitive impairment may occur [34]. A return to normal baseline results normally occurs within 12 months. A reversible demyelination associated with blood-brain barrier disruption is supposed to explain this disorder. There is no indication that this encephalopathy is a harbinger of the more severe late-delayed encephalopathy. Studies in patients with glioma by Armstrong et al and Vigliani et al have showed an initial decline in cognitive functioning after radiotherapy with a complete resolution at 12 months [35–37]. These findings are in line with an animal study that showed acute and reversible effect of radiation on cell proliferation, neurogenesis, and cell death [38].

In contrast to the early complications, late-delayed encephalopathy is an irreversible and serious disorder. This complication follows radiotherapy by several months to many years and may take the form of local radionecrosis or diffuse leukoencephalopathy and cerebral atrophy. Cognitive disturbances are the hallmark of the diffuse encephalopathy [39]. The severity of cognitive deficits ranges from mild or moderate cognitive deficits all the way to cognitive deterioration leading to dementia. Patients with mild to moderate cognitive deficits have attention or short-term memory disturbances as main features. Both the clinical picture and the incidence of this complication are hard to define exactly as studies on this subject vary greatly in the neuropsychological test procedures, the populations studied, and the duration of follow-up [33,39,40]. There is a relation, to some extent, between cognitive status and imaging abnormalities such as cerebral atrophy and leukoencephalopathy [41,42]. Brain atrophy and white-matter lesions are most likely to occur in patients treated with whole-brain radiotherapy and in older patients [43]. According to a large review of clinical studies, fairly severe cognitive deterioration, leading to dementia with mainly subcortical features, occurred in at least 92 of 748 patients treated with radiotherapy [44]. The results are progressive mental slowing and deficits in attention and memory, with less common features such as gait abnormalities, urinary incontinence, and apathy. In these cases, MRI shows diffuse atrophy with ventricular enlargement as well as severe confluent white-matter abnormalities [45]. Clinically, dysfunction of other systems may also occur, including pyramidal or extrapyramidal signs [39].

The pathophysiology of the white-matter abnormalities is not completely understood [46]. Both vascular structures and glial cells are thought to be the target of late radiation damage, as histological examination reveals both demyelination and vascular damage. In the glial hypothesis, oligodendrocytes are the primary target of radiation damage resulting in demyelination, whereas the vascular hypothesis is based on histological proof of blood-vessel dilatation and wall thickening with hyalinization, endothelial cell loss, and a decrease in vessel density leading to white-matter necrosis. The pathogenesis is probably far more complex and may also involve injury to the neurogenic cell population that exists in the dentate subgranular zone of the hippocampus associated with memory formation [39,45]. With regard to prevention or even repair of radiation damage, a number of promising studies have been performed recently [38,47,48].

Several radiation and host factors determine the risk of this diffuse leukoencephalopathy. Nearly all patients with glioma are treated with focal brain radiotherapy as opposed to whole-brain radiotherapy, which used to be the norm. Although a fraction dose of at most 2 Gy is considered "safe," total safety is not possible [17,49].

A commonly overlooked late complication of cranial radiotherapy in adults is endocrine dysfunction caused by damage to the hypothalamic-pituitary axis. Only a few studies have been done in adults, and these indicate that most patients have clinical or subclinical endocrine dysfunction. The link between abnormal test results and clinical features is unclear, but adrenal insufficiency and thyroid as well as growth hormone dysfunction in adults can result in cognitive deficits [50].

Late Encephalopathy in Patients With Low-Grade Glioma

The first study of long-term survivors of low-grade glioma in which a standardized series of cognitive tests was used showed that all 14 patients tested, who were without clinical and radiological signs of tumor progression, had cognitive and affective disturbances [51]. As all 14 patients had been treated with focal radiotherapy, radiotherapy was thought to be a major contributor to the deficits observed. However, a follow-up study by the same authors showed that the cognitive deficits in patients with low-grade glioma who had been treated with early radiotherapy were not different from those of a control group of patients with low-grade glioma who had not been treated with radiotherapy [52]. It was therefore concluded that the observed cognitive impairment in glioma survivors could not be attributed to focal radiotherapy and was caused by either the tumor itself or other treatment factors. Also in a more recent study of 195 survivors of low-grade glioma, the use of radiotherapy was associated with poor cognitive function on only a few tests and not restricted to one specific cognitive domain [17]. Clear cognitive disability in the memory domain, however, was found in a subgroup of 18 patients who received fraction doses above 2 Gy. Compared with healthy people and patients with hematological malignancies, cognitive deficits were common in survivors of low-grade glioma (radiated and nonradiated), but were more frequently related to other disease and treatment factors than to radiotherapy.

A number of other studies point to the same conclusion. Armstrong et al reported on a prospective study regarding cognitive function and MRI in 26 patients with low-grade glioma [53]. On follow-up, only a specific decline in visual memory could be demonstrated in 50% of patients. White-matter abnormalities on T2-weighted MRI emerged from 6 months onwards, but did not progress after 3 years from baseline. Torres et al showed subtle cognitive deficits in patients with low-grade tumors that were already present at the start of radiotherapy without further decline during a 2-year follow-up [54]. Brown et al reported on repeated Mini Mental State Examination scores in 101 patients with a median follow-up of 7.4 years after radiotherapy [55]. Although only a few patients had a cognitive deterioration after radiotherapy, the authors stated that a more discriminating cognitive assessment might reveal a degree of cognitive decline that is not apparent with the use of the Mini Mental State Examination. In a later study in which this group did perform extensive neurocognitive testing before radiotherapy and at ~18-month intervals for as long as 5 years after completing radiotherapy, test scores prior to radiotherapy were below average compared with age-specific norms [56]. At the second evaluation, however, the groups' mean test scores were higher than their initial performances on all psychometric measures, although the improvement was not statistically significant.

In contrast to the studies mentioned above, Surma-aho et al reported on 28 long-term survivors of low-grade glioma (mean follow-up of 7 years) who had more cognitive deficits after early radiotherapy than a control group of 23 patients (mean follow-up of 10 years) who had no radiotherapy [57]. Moreover, leukoencephalopathy on MRI was more severe in the group with postoperative irradiation. They concluded that radiotherapy in patients with low-grade glioma poses a significant risk of long-term leukoencephalopathy and cognitive impairment. Although the follow-up period in this study is longer than that in many other studies, 19 of 28 patients had whole-brain radiotherapy. A more recent follow-up of the study by Klein et al demonstrated that all tumor progression-free irradiated low-grade glioma patients had cognitive deterioration 13 years after radiotherapy, while all non-irradiated patients remained stable [17,42]. Moreover, an increase in radiological abnormalities was found only in the irradiated group.

Given the complexity of radiation-induced changes, single target interventions might not suffice. Future interventions might vary with patient age, elapsed time from radiotherapy, and toxicity type. Potential components include several drugs that interact with neurodegeneration, cell transplantation (into the CNS itself, the blood stream, or both) and creation of reparative signals, and a permissive microenvironment, for example, for cell homing.

Late Encephalopathy in Patients With High-Grade Glioma

As many patients with high-grade glioma are treated with both radiotherapy and chemotherapy after surgery, the cause of cognitive deficits in long-term survivors is even more difficult to determine than in patients with low-grade glioma. Early reports of long-term survivors of high-grade glioma without signs of tumor regrowth all pointed to radiotherapy as the main cause of cognitive deficits [58,59]. However, Kleinberg et al observed a good performance status and (subjective) memory function in 30 patients with glioma (most of whom had high-grade tumors) who had all been treated with radiotherapy [60]. Most patients were able to return to work after radiotherapy. In a prospective trial, Trojanowski et al assessed the effectiveness of combined treatment with lomustine (CCNU) and radiotherapy, and the use of radiotherapy alone [61]. The quality of survival was measured by a series of cognitive tests. Patients' cognitive functions improved after treatment followed by a rapid decline caused by tumor progression, but no treatment-related cognitive deterioration was reported. Also, Taylor et al prospectively studied cognitive function in patients with high-grade glioma, but they only used the Mini Mental State Examination as an outcome measure in 550 of a total number of 701 patients [62]. These patients had all been treated with radiotherapy and chemotherapy. In patients without tumor progression on follow-up there was no clear trend in cognitive decline. These findings are corroborated by more recent studies that furthermore suggest that the use of AEDs might additionally affect the already compromised cognitive functions [63,64].

Results of other studies, however, indicated moderate to severe cognitive deficits in survivors of high-grade glioma [65,66]. Archibald et al did sequential and extensive neuropsychological testing in two groups of long-term survivors treated with radiotherapy and chemotherapy [65]. Moderate to severe cognitive disturbances were generally evident by the first assessment. In some patients, a further decline developed during follow-up and only few patients were capable of fully independent living. These results, like the results from more recent studies, indicate that the tumor itself also has a prominent role in the cause of cognitive decline [18,20]. As far as reirradiation at the time of tumor progression of high-grade gliomas is concerned, modern conformal treatment options yield an acceptable probability of radionecrosis given the limited volume of normal brain tissue exposure [67].

Late Encephalopathy in Other Brain Tumors or Extracranial Malignancies

Radiotherapy is the mainstay in the treatment of patients with brain metastases of extracranial tumors. The risk of developing a devastating late-delayed encephalopathy caused by whole-brain radiotherapy has been estimated to range between 1.9% and 5.1% [49]. In particular, the use of high daily fractions (over 2 Gy) is thought to be detrimental. Prophylactic cranial irradiation for small-cell lung carcinoma has also been the subject of much debate over the past decades [39]. As an example of the multifactorial nature of the causes of neurological dysfunction, one study revealed that 97% of patients with limited stage small-cell lung cancer were found to experience neurocognitive decline before the delivery of prophylactic cranial irradiation [68,69]. Several reports of patients who received whole-brain radiotherapy for metastasis suggest that tumor progression correlates more closely with diminished neurocognitive functioning than does the delivery of whole-brain radiotherapy [70,71]. A landmark study of patients randomized to undergo surgical resection with or without whole-brain radiotherapy revealed that foregoing the radiotherapy increased death due to neurological causes, exposing patients to tumor induced loss of mental and physical abilities [72]. Regine et al confirmed the concern that these intracranial recurrences produce symptomatic neurological deficits [73].

Relatively little information is available on the outcome of patients with meningioma. A recent study showed the majority of patients with WHO grade I meningiomas to be affected by cognitive deficits that could partly be explained by the use of AEDs [19]. A study in which patients with WHO grade I meningiomas at least 1 year following surgery were compared to patients who had surgery followed by radiotherapy suggests that additional radiotherapy does not have additional deleterious effects on neurocognitive outcome [74].

The incidence of late-delayed radiation encephalopathy in immunocompetent patients with primary CNS lymphoma is high and may give rise to devastating cognitive decline [75,76]. Omuro et al found a 5-year cumulative incidence of neurotoxicity of 24% which increased over time [76]. Neurotoxicity presented as a rapidly progressive subcortical dementia characterized by psychomotor slowing, executive and memory dysfunction, behavioral changes, gait ataxia, and incontinence. Reasons for this high incidence are the median age of over 60 years of patients with primary CNS lymphoma, the necessity to give whole-brain treatment in contrast to local treatment for glioma, and the increasing use of chemotherapeutic agents. Whether an additional characteristic of primary CNS lymphoma (e.g., its angiocentric nature) makes patients with these tumors more susceptible to leukoencephalopathy and cognitive side effects than patients with other brain tumors is unknown. Mainly owing to the high risk of developing delayed neurotoxicity due to the combined treatment in elderly patients, chemotherapy alone is nowadays recommended as initial treatment [77]. In this respect, it is important to note that the introduction of temozolomide in combination treatment yielded a comparable efficacy as other standard regimens, with the advantage of a favorable toxicity profile and absence of intrathecal chemotherapy [78].

Even patients with nasopharyngeal carcinomas treated with radiotherapy may run the risk of developing temporal lobe radionecrosis associated with cognitive dysfunction [79]. The use of a megadose of α-tocopherol (vitamin E) may partially reduce the commonly found cognitive side effects [80].

Medical Therapy as the Cause of Cognitive Deficits

Antiepileptic Drugs

Epileptic seizures are the first symptom of an intracranial tumor in 30% to 90% of patients and can substantially affect daily life, even if the tumor is under control. Apart from tumor type, tumor location and peritumoral and genetic changes affect the mechanism of seizures in patients with brain tumor [81]. In a large study, one or more AEDs were taken by 71% of patients with low-grade glioma to prevent seizures [82].

Risks of cognitive side effects of AEDs can add to previous damage by surgery or radiotherapy, and therefore appropriate choice and dose of AED are crucial. The older AEDs (phenytoin, carbamazepine, and valproic acid) are known to decrease cognitive functioning [83,84]. These drugs may result in impairments of attention and cognitive slowing, which can subsequently have effects on memory by reducing the efficiency of encoding and retrieval [84]. Several newer AEDs (e.g., gabapentin, lamotrigine, and levetiracetam) appear to have fewer adverse cognitive effects than the older agents, though additional comparisons between new AEDs are required to fully assess the cognitive side effect profile of these newer anticonvulsant agents. Of the newer agents, topiramate is associated with the greatest risk of cognitive impairment, although this risk is decreased with slow titration and low target doses [85,86].

Apart from AEDs, cognitive function may also be negatively affected by the seizures themselves [87]. The importance of (the older) AEDs as a risk factor for cognitive deficits has been reported in a study on low-grade glioma; in a group of 156 long-term survivors without signs of tumor recurrence, deficits in information processing speed, psychomotor functioning, executive function, and working memory capacity were significantly related to the use of AEDs [82]. As patients in this study who took AEDs had cognitive disturbances even in the absence of seizures, the use of drugs primarily affects cognitive function.

Chemotherapy

The effect of chemotherapy on neurocognitive function is not well understood. Apart from the ability of chemotherapy to enter the brain across the blood-brain barrier, DNA damage and shortened telomere length resulting from chemotherapy, problems with neural repair such as the presence of apolipoprotein E4 alleles, and decreased neurotransmitter activity as potential mechanisms underlying neurocognitive deficits in patients with cancer, problems with cytokine regulation might provide an important explanation for compromised neurocognitive functioning [88].

Classical adjuvant chemotherapy, administered sequentially with radiotherapy and usually with nitrosourea (carmustine and lomustine) in patients with brain tumor has been thought ineffective for a long time. A meta-analysis comprising over 3000 patients showed that this kind of adjuvant chemotherapy may result in a very modest 5% increase in 2-year survival [89]. In recent years, the role of chemotherapy in glioma has been met with renewed interest mainly due to the improved outcome of patients with glioblastoma treated with concurrent radiotherapy and temozolomide followed by adjuvant temozolomide and due to the recognition of the sensitivity to chemotherapy of 1p/19q loss oligodendrogliomas [90].

Potential late CNS neurotoxic side effects of chemotherapy may be difficult to discern from radiotherapy, because most patients treated with chemotherapy have already been treated with radiotherapy or are even treated with radiotherapy concomitantly [91,92]. In contrast to the late radiation encephalopathy, side effects of chemotherapy on the CNS tend to arise during, or shortly after, the chemotherapy [92].

Neurotoxicity to the CNS may be increased by giving drugs intraarterially, especially in combination with osmotic blood-brain barrier disruption, meant to increase the local concentration of chemotherapy in the brain [93,94]. Modern delivery techniques might prevent some of the neurotoxicity, however [95]. Neurotoxicity may also be increased by chemotherapy given after, or even during, radiotherapy [96,97]. In these cases, the chemotherapeutic drugs also reach higher concentrations in normal brain tissue due to leakage of the blood-brain barrier caused by radiotherapy. In this way, radiation may potentiate the toxic effects of chemotherapy [92]. Finally, intrathecal chemotherapy, compared with systemically applied chemotherapy, has a higher likelihood of causing CNS toxicity [98]. The increased risk of cognitive deficits after chemotherapy in combination with the apolipoprotein E4 alleles also suggests a genetic role in chemotherapy-induced cognitive decline [99].

Only few data are available on the cognitive side effects of temozolomide. Preliminary data suggest cognitive status to remain stable in the course of the disease in patients with glioblastoma without tumor recurrence [100]. Furthermore, comparisons with patients treated only with radiotherapy suggests that multimodality radiotherapy plus temozolomide treatment yields equivalent neurocognitive outcome 6 to 8 months after the start of the treatment.

In the chemotherapeutic treatment of primary CNS lymphoma, methotrexate can cause cognitive side effects [101]. Methotrexate can reach significant CNS concentrations when given in high intravenous doses or when given intrathecally. An acute encephalopathy with seizures, confusion, and cognitive deficits may develop, which resolves spontaneously. In its chronic form, the encephalopathy resembles late-delayed radiation toxicity, clinically, on imaging, and on histological examination. There is evidence that cognitive impairment in adult patients with tumor after chemotherapy is comparable to the effects after cranial irradiation [102]. Radiotherapy, either before or during the chemotherapy, will increase the risk of the chronic encephalopathy [97]. The incidence of encephalopathy in primary CNS lymphoma only treated with systemic chemotherapy is unknown, but leukoencephalopathy on MRI may be present in 50% of patients, although no significant cognitive side effects in patients were found [103].

Patients with leptomeningeal metastases from solid extracranial tumors or from hematological malignancies may be treated with focal radiotherapy on the symptomatic site of disease in combination with intrathecal chemotherapy with methotrexate and cytarabine. Cognitive side effects of treatment are most likely to occur when radiotherapy precedes or is given concomitantly with chemotherapy [98].

Steroids

Corticosteroids—of which dexamethasone is most commonly used to treat brain tumors—may cause mood disturbances and (infrequently) psychosis. Steroid dementia is a reversible cause of cognitive deficits even in the absence of psychosis. Recent data suggest that the cognitive deficits are due to neurotoxic effects on both the hippocampal and the prefrontal areas [104] Both short-term and long-term use of steroids have been associated with cognitive deficits [105]. More than likely, cognitive deficits in patients with brain tumor will be alleviated by steroids owing to the resolution of brain edema.

Mood Disorder as a Cause of Cognitive Deficits

It comes as no surprise that patients with brain tumor have feelings of anxiety, depression, and future uncertainty as psychological reactions to the disease [51,106,107]. Patients with high-grade glioma report higher levels of panic, depression, anxiety, and fear of death than patients with low-grade glioma [108]. Mood changes are more common in patients with brain tumor than in patients with other neurological diseases and might be related to tumor location [109–111]. These mood disturbances may lead to deficits in attention, vigilance, and motivation that subsequently affect several cognitive domains [112]. As patients with extracranial tumors do not have structural brain lesions that cause cognitive deficits, neuropsychological disturbances in these patients are more likely related to mood disorders than to CNS lesions.

CONCLUSION

Cognitive function is increasingly regarded as an important endpoint in patients with brain tumor. An important rationale for the selection of a given brain tumor treatment may be related to cognitive side effects and effect on QOL. Although assessment of cognitive function in long-term surviving patients with brain tumor has become crucial, a clearer understanding is needed of the brain mechanisms that might be associated with cognitive deficits resulting from tumor and/or treatment. Certain areas of the brain (e.g., hippocampal formation) may be more vulnerable to damage with these treatments. Although once thought that tumor and treatment only had local effects, more recent studies furthermore suggest that the entire brain is affected and changes in brain structure or functioning can be observed outside of the area primarily involved.

The role of radiotherapy—for a long time thought to be the main cause of cognitive deficits in patients with brain tumors—has been extensively studied. Rather than lowering dosages, which may be ineffective in treating the tumor, prophylactic interventions may begin prior to adjuvant therapies and before impairments occur. An important finding from several studies in low-grade glioma is that, although radiotherapy has to some extent an adverse effect on cognitive function, other tumor and treatment factors deserve more attention.

REFERENCES

1. Cantelmi D, Schweizer TA, Cusimano MD. Role of the cerebellum in the neurocognitive sequelae of treatment of tumours of the posterior fossa: an update. *Lancet Oncol.* 2008;9(6):569–576.
2. Timmann D, Daum I. Cerebellar contributions to cognitive functions: a progress report after two decades of research. *Cerebellum.* 2007;6(3):159–162.
3. Heimans JJ, Taphoorn MJB. Impact of brain tumour treatment on quality of life. *J Neurol.* 2002;249:955–960.
4. Meyers CA, Hess KR. Multifaceted end points in brain tumor clinical trials: cognitive deterioration precedes MRI progression. *Neuro Oncol.* 2003;5(2):89–95.
5. Wessels PH, Weber WE, Raven G, Ramaekers FC, Hopman AH, Twijnstra A. Supratentorial grade II astrocytoma: biological features and clinical course. *Lancet Neurol.* 2003;2(7):395–403.
6. van den Bent MJ, Taphoorn MJ, Brandes AA, et al. Phase II study of first-line chemotherapy with temozolomide in recurrent oligodendroglial tumors: the European Organization for Research and Treatment of Cancer Brain Tumor Group Study 26971. *J Clin Oncol.* 2003;21(13):2525–2528.
7. Stupp R, Mason WP, van den Bent MJ, et al. Radiotherapy plus concomitant and adjuvant temozolomide for glioblastoma. *N Engl J Med.* 2005;352(10):987–996.
8. Anstey KJ, Mack HA, von Sanden C. The relationship between cognition and mortality in patients with stroke, coronary heart disease, or cancer. *Eur Psychol.* 2006;11(3):182–195.
9. Klein M, Postma TJ, Taphoorn MJB, et al. The prognostic value of cognitive functioning in the survival of patients with high-grade glioma. *Neurology.* 2003;61(12):1796–1799.
10. McCarter H, Furlong W, Whitton AC, et al. Health status measurements at diagnosis as predictors of survival among adults with brain tumors. *J Clin Oncol.* 2006;24(22):3636–3643.
11. Brown PD, Buckner JC, O'Fallon JR, et al. Importance of baseline mini-mental state examination as a prognostic factor for patients with low-grade glioma. *Int J Radiat Oncol Biol Phys.* 2004;59(1):117–125.

12. Armstrong CL, Goldstein B, Shera D, Ledakis GE, Tallent EM. The predictive value of longitudinal neuropsychologic assessment in the early detection of brain tumor recurrence. *Cancer.* 2003;97(3):649–656.
13. Meyers CA, Hess KR, Yung WK, Levin VA. Cognitive function as a predictor of survival in patients with recurrent malignant glioma. *J Clin Oncol.* 2000;18(3):646–650.
14. Deangelis LM. Brain tumors. *N Engl J Med.* 2001;344(2):114–123.
15. Tucha O, Smely C, Preier M, Lange KW. Cognitive deficits before treatment among patients with brain tumors. *Neurosurgery.* 2000;47(2):324–333.
16. Tucha O, Smely C, Preier M, Becker G, Paul GM, Lange KW. Preoperative and postoperative cognitive functioning in patients with frontal meningiomas. *J Neurosurg.* 2003;98(1):21–31.
17. Klein M, Heimans JJ, Aaronson NK, et al. Effect of radiotherapy and other treatment-related factors on mid-term to long-term cognitive sequelae in low-grade gliomas: a comparative study. *Lancet.* 2002;360(9343):1361–1368.
18. Klein M, Taphoorn MJ, Heimans JJ, et al. Neurobehavioral status and health-related quality of life in newly diagnosed high-grade glioma patients. *J Clin Oncol.* 2001;19(20):4037–4047.
19. Dijkstra M, van Nieuwenhuizen D, Stalpers LJ, et al. Late neurocognitive sequelae in patients with WHO grade I meningioma. *J Neurol Neurosurg Psychiatry.* 2009;80(8):910–915.
20. Hahn CA, Dunn RH, Logue PE, King JH, Edwards CL, Halperin EC. Prospective study of neuropsychologic testing and quality-of-life assessment of adults with primary malignant brain tumors. *Int J Radiat Oncol Biol Phys.* 2003;55(4):992–999.
21. Inskip PD, Tarone RE, Hatch EE, et al. Laterality of brain tumors. *Neuroepidemiology.* 2003;22(2):130–138.
22. Yoshii Y, Tominaga D, Sugimoto K, et al. Cognitive function of patients with brain tumor in pre- and postoperative stage. *Surg Neurol.* 2008;69(1):51–61.
23. Anderson SW, Damasio H, Tranel D. Neuropsychological impairments associated with lesions caused by tumor or stroke. *Arch Neurol.* 1990;47(4):397–405.
24. Witte OW. Lesion-induced plasticity as a potential mechanism for recovery and rehabilitative training. *Curr Opin Neurol.* 1998;11(6):655–662.
25. Duffau H, Capelle L, Denvil D, et al. Functional recovery after surgical resection of low grade gliomas in eloquent brain: hypothesis of brain compensation. *J Neurol Neurosurg Psychiatry.* 2003;74(7):901–907.
26. Scheibel RS, Meyers CA, Levin VA. Cognitive dysfunction following surgery for intracerebral glioma: influence of histopathology, lesion location, and treatment. *J Neurooncol.* 1996;30(1):61–69.
27. Duffau H, Capelle L, Denvil D, et al. Usefulness of intraoperative electrical subcortical mapping during surgery for low-grade gliomas located within eloquent brain regions: functional results in a consecutive series of 103 patients. *J Neurosurg.* 2003;98(4):764–778.
28. Bosma I, Douw L, Bartolomei F, et al. Synchronized brain activity and neurocognitive function in patients with low-grade glioma: A magnetoencephalography study. *Neuro Oncol.* 2008;10(5):734–744.
29. Bosma I, Stam CJ, Douw L, et al. The influence of low-grade glioma on resting state oscillatory brain activity: a magnetoencephalography study. *J Neurooncol.* 2008;88(1):77–85.
30. Douw L, Baayen H, Bosma I, et al. Treatment-related changes in functional connectivity in brain tumor patients: a magnetoencephalography study. *Exp Neurol.* 2008;212(2):285–290.
31. Reijneveld JC, Sitskoorn MM, Klein M, Nuyen J, Taphoorn MJ. Cognitive status and quality of life in patients with suspected versus proven low-grade gliomas. *Neurology.* 2001;56(5):618–623.
32. Crosley CJ, Rorke LB, Evans A, Nigro M. Central nervous system lesions in childhood leukemia. *Neurology.* 1978;28(7):678–685.
33. Vigliani MC, Duyckaerts C, Delattre JY. Radiation-induced cognitive dysfunction in adults. In: Vecht CJ, ed. *Handbook of Clinical Neurology.* Amsterdam, The Netherlands: Elsevier Science, BV; 1997:371–388.
34. Costello A, Shallice T, Gullan R, Beaney R. The early effects of radiotherapy on intellectual and cognitive functioning in patients with frontal brain tumours: the use of a new neuropsychological methodology. *J Neurooncol.* 2004;67(3):351–359.
35. Armstrong CL, Mollman J, Corn BW, Alavi J, Grossman M. Effects of radiation therapy on adult brain behavior: evidence for a rebound phenomenon in a phase I trial. *Neurology.* 1993;43:1961–1965.
36. Armstrong CL, Ruffer J, Corn BW, DeVries K, Mollman J. Biphasic patterns of memory deficits following moderate-dose partial-brain irradiation: neuropsychologic outcome and proposed mechanisms. *J Clin Oncol.* 1995;13:2263–2271.
37. Vigliani MC, Sichez N, Poisson M, Delattre JY. A prospective study of cognitive functions following conventional radiotherapy for supratentorial gliomas in young adults: 4-year results. *Int J Radiat Oncol Biol Phys.* 1996;35(3):527–533.
38. Ben Abdallah NM, Slomianka L, Lipp HP. Reversible effect of X-irradiation on proliferation, neurogenesis, and cell death in the dentate gyrus of adult mice. *Hippocampus.* 2007;17(12):1230–1240.
39. Béhin A, Delattre JY. Neurologic sequelae of radiotherapy of the nervous system. In: Schiff D, Wen PY, eds. *Cancer Neurology in Clinical Practice.* Totowa, NJ: Humana Press; 2003:173–192.
40. Roman DD, Sperduto PW. Neuropsychological effects of cranial radiation: current knowledge and future directions. *Int J Radiat Oncol Biol Phys.* 1995;31(4):983–998.
41. Postma TJ, Klein M, Verstappen CC, et al. Radiotherapy-induced cerebral abnormalities in patients with low-grade glioma. *Neurology.* 2002;59(1):121–123.
42. Klein M. Long term follow-up of cognition in irradiated low grade glioma patients. In: *Perspectives in Central Nervous System Malignancies III* Warsaw, Poland; 2007.
43. Swennen MH, Bromberg JE, Witkamp TD, Terhaard CH, Postma TJ, Taphoorn MJ. Delayed radiation toxicity after focal or whole brain radiotherapy for low-grade glioma. *J Neurooncol.* 2004;66(3): 333–339.
44. Crossen JR, Garwood D, Glatstein E, Neuwelt EA. Neurobehavioral sequelae of cranial irradiation in adults: a review of radiation-induced encephalopathy. *J Clin Oncol.* 1994;12:627–642.
45. Monje ML, Palmer T. Radiation injury and neurogenesis. *Curr Opin Neurol.* 2003;16(2):129–134.
46. Sheline GE, Wara WM, Smith V. Therapeutic irradiation and brain injury. *Int J Radiat Oncol Biol Phys.* 1980;6:1215–1228.
47. Thotala DK, Hallahan DE, Yazlovitskaya EM. Inhibition of glycogen synthase kinase 3 beta attenuates neurocognitive dysfunction resulting from cranial irradiation. *Cancer Res.* 2008;68(14):5859–5868.
48. Fan Y, Liu Z, Weinstein PR, Fike JR, Liu J. Environmental enrichment enhances neurogenesis and improves functional outcome after cranial irradiation. *Eur J Neurosci.* 2007;25(1):38–46.
49. DeAngelis LM, Delattre JY, Posner JB. Radiation-induced dementia in patients cured of brain metastases. *Neurology.* 1989;39:789–796.
50. Falleti MG, Maruff P, Burman P, Harris A. The effects of growth hormone (GH) deficiency and GH replacement on cognitive performance in adults: a meta-analysis of the current literature. *Psychoneuroendocrinology.* 2006;31(6):681–691.
51. Taphoorn MJB, Heimans JJ, Snoek FJ, et al. Assessment of quality of life in patients treated for low-grade glioma: a preliminary report. *J Neurol Neurosurg Psychiatry.* 1992;55(5):372–376.
52. Taphoorn MJB, Schiphorst AK, Snoek FJ, et al. Cognitive functions and quality of life in patients with low-grade gliomas: the impact of radiotherapy. *Ann Neurol.* 1994;36(1):48–54.
53. Armstrong CL, Hunter JV, Ledakis GE, et al. Late cognitive and radiographic changes related to radiotherapy: initial prospective findings. *Neurology.* 2002;59(1):40–48.
54. Torres IJ, Mundt AJ, Sweeney PJ, et al. A longitudinal neuropsychological study of partial brain radiation in adults with brain tumors. *Neurology.* 2003;60(7):1113–1118.
55. Brown PD, Buckner JC, O'Fallon JR, et al. Effects of radiotherapy on cognitive function in patients with low-grade glioma measured by the folstein mini-mental state examination. *J Clin Oncol.* 2003;21(13):2519–2524.
56. Laack NN, Brown PD, Ivnik RJ, et al. Cognitive function after radiotherapy for supratentorial low-grade glioma: a North Central Cancer Treatment Group prospective study. *Int J Radiat Oncol Biol Phys.* 2005;63(4):1175–1183.
57. Surma-aho O, Niemela M, Vilkki J, et al. Adverse long-term effects of brain radiotherapy in adult low-grade glioma patients. *Neurology.* 2001;56(10):1285–1290.
58. Hochberg FH, Slotnick B. Neuropsychologic impairment in astrocytoma survivors. *Neurology.* 1980;30:172–177.
59. Lieberman AN, Foo SH, Ransohoff J, et al. Long term survival among patients with malignant brain tumors. *Neurosurgery.* 1982;10:450–453.
60. Kleinberg L, Wallner K, Malkin MG. Good performance status of long-term disease-free survivors of intracranial gliomas. *Int J Radiat Oncol Biol Phys.* 1993;26:129–133.
61. Trojanowski T, Peszynski J, Turowski K, et al. Quality of survival of patients with brain gliomas treated with postoperative CCNU and radiation therapy. *J Neurosurg.* 1989;70(1):18–23.

62. Taylor BV, Buckner JC, Cascino TL, et al. Effects of radiation and chemotherapy on cognitive function in patients with high-grade glioma. *J Clin Oncol.* 1998;16(6):2195–2201.
63. Bosma I, Vos MJ, Heimans JJ, et al. The course of neurocognitive functioning in high-grade glioma patients. *Neuro Oncol.* 2007;9(1):53–62.
64. Brown PD, Jensen AW, Felten SJ, et al. Detrimental effects of tumor progression on cognitive function of patients with high-grade glioma. *J Clin Oncol.* 2006;24(34):5427–5433.
65. Archibald YM, Lunn D, Ruttan LA, et al. Cognitive functioning in long-term survivors of high-grade glioma. *J Neurosurg.* 1994;80(2):247–253.
66. Schmidinger M, Linzmayer L, Becherer A, et al. Psychometric- and quality-of-life assessment in long-term glioblastoma survivors. *J Neurooncol.* 2003;63(1):55–61.
67. Mayer R, Sminia P. Reirradiation tolerance of the human brain. *Int J Radiat Oncol Biol Phys.* 2008;70(5):1350–1360.
68. Komaki R, Meyers CA, Shin DM, et al. Evaluation of cognitive function in patients with limited small cell lung cancer prior to and shortly following prophylactic cranial irradiation. *Int J Radiat Oncol Biol Phys.* 1995;33(1):179–182.
69. Van Oosterhout AGM, Boon PJ, Houx PJ, ten Velde GPM, Twijnstra A. Follow-up of cognitive functioning in patients with small cell lung cancer. *Int J Radiat Oncol Biol Phys.* 1995;31:911–914.
70. Li J, Bentzen SM, Renschler M, Mehta MP. Regression after whole-brain radiation therapy for brain metastases correlates with survival and improved neurocognitive function. *J Clin Oncol.* 2007;25(10):1260–1266.
71. Laack NN, Brown PD. Cognitive sequelae of brain radiation in adults. *Semin Oncol.* 2004;31(5):702–713.
72. Patchell RA, Tibbs PA, Regine WF, et al. Postoperative radiotherapy in the treatment of single metastases to the brain: a randomized trial. *JAMA.* 1998;280(17):1485–1489.
73. Regine WF, Huhn JL, Patchell RA, et al. Risk of symptomatic brain tumor recurrence and neurologic deficit after radiosurgery alone in patients with newly diagnosed brain metastases: results and implications. *Int J Radiat Oncol Biol Phys.* 2002;52(2):333–338.
74. van Nieuwenhuizen D, Klein M, Stalpers LJ, Leenstra S, Heimans JJ, Reijneveld JC. Differential effect of surgery and radiotherapy on neurocognitive functioning and health-related quality of life in WHO grade I meningioma patients. *J Neurooncol.* 2007;84(3):271–278.
75. Correa DD, Maron L, Harder H, et al. Cognitive functions in primary central nervous system lymphoma: literature review and assessment guidelines. *Ann Oncol.* 2007;18(7):1145–1151.
76. Omuro AM, Ben-Porat LS, Panageas KS, et al. Delayed neurotoxicity in primary central nervous system lymphoma. *Arch Neurol.* 2005;62(10):1595–1600.
77. Mohile NA, Abrey LE. Primary central nervous system lymphoma. *Neurol Clin.* 2007;25(4):1193–1207.
78. Omuro AM, Taillandier L, Chinot O, Carnin C, Barrie M, Hoang-Xuan K. Temozolomide and methotrexate for primary central nervous system lymphoma in the elderly. *J Neurooncol.* 2007;85(2):207–211.
79. Cheung MC, Chan AS, Law SC, Chan JH, Tse VK. Impact of radionecrosis on cognitive dysfunction in patients after radiotherapy for nasopharyngeal carcinoma. *Cancer.* 2003;97(8):2019–2026.
80. Chan AS, Cheung MC, Law SC, Chan JH. Phase II study of alpha-tocopherol in improving the cognitive function of patients with temporal lobe radionecrosis. *Cancer.* 2004;100(2):398–404.
81. van Breemen MS, Wilms EB, Vecht CJ. Epilepsy in patients with brain tumours: epidemiology, mechanisms, and management. *Lancet Neurol.* 2007;6(5):421–430.
82. Klein M, Engelberts NHJ, Van der Ploeg HM, et al. Epilepsy in low-grade gliomas: the impact on cognitive functioning and quality of life. *Ann Neurol.* 2003;54(4):514–520.
83. Drane LD, Meador KJ. Cognitive and behavioral effects of antiepileptic drugs. *Epilepsy Behav.* 2002;3(5S):49–53.
84. Meador KJ. Cognitive outcomes and predictive factors in epilepsy. *Neurology.* 2002;58(8S5):21–26.
85. Meador KJ. Cognitive and memory effects of the new antiepileptic drugs. *Epilepsy Res.* 2006;68(1):63–67.
86. Meador KJ, Gevins A, Loring DW, et al. Neuropsychological and neurophysiologic effects of carbamazepine and levetiracetam. *Neurology.* 2007;69(22):2076–2084.
87. Dodrill CB. Progressive cognitive decline in adolescents and adults with epilepsy. *Prog Brain Res.* 2002;135:399–407.
88. Ahles TA, Saykin AJ. Candidate mechanisms for chemotherapy-induced cognitive changes. *Nat Rev Cancer.* 2007;7(3):192–201.
89. Glioma Meta-Analysis Group. Chemotherapy in adult high-grade glioma: a systematic review and meta-analysis of individual patient data from 12 randomised trials. *Lancet.* 2002;359:1011–1018.
90. van den Bent MJ. Adjuvant treatment of high grade gliomas. *Ann Oncol.* 2006;17(suppl 10):186–190.
91. Keime-Guibert F, Napolitano M, Delattre JY. Neurological complications of radiotherapy and chemotherapy. *J Neurol.* 1998;245:695–708.
92. Wen PY. Central nervous system complications of cancer therapy. In: Schiff D, Wen PY, eds. *Cancer Neurology in Clinical Practice.* Totowa, NJ: Humana Press; 2003:215–231.
93. Shapiro WR, Green SB. Reevaluating the efficacy of intra-arterial BCNU. *J Neurosurg.* 1987;66(2):313–315.
94. Shapiro WR, Green SB, Burger PC, et al. A randomized comparison of intra-arterial versus intravenous BCNU, with or without intravenous 5-fluorouracil, for newly diagnosed patients with malignant glioma. *J Neurosurg.* 1992;76(5):772–781.
95. Bellavance MA, Blanchette M, Fortin D. Recent advances in blood-brain barrier disruption as a CNS delivery strategy. *AAPS J.* 2008;10(1):166–177.
96. DeAngelis LM, Yahalom J, Thaler HT, Kher U. Combined modality therapy for primary CNS lymphoma. *J Clin Oncol.* 1992;10(4):635–643.
97. Philips PC. Methotrexate toxicity. In: Rottenberg DA, ed. *Neurological Complications of Cancer Treatment.* Boston: Butterworth-Heinemann; 1991:115–134.
98. Boogerd W. Leptomeningeal metastasis in solid tumours: Is there a role for intrathecal therapy? *Eur J Cancer Suppl* 2007;5(5):41–51.
99. Ahles TA, Saykin AJ, Noll WW, et al. The relationship of APOE genotype to neuropsychological performance in long-term cancer survivors treated with standard dose chemotherapy. *Psychooncology.* 2003;12(6):612–619.
100. Hilverda K, Heimans JJ, Bosma I, et al. Neurocognitive functioning in GBM patients during treatment with radiotherapy and temozolomide: Initial findings. In: 8th Congress of the European Association for Neurooncology; September 12–14, 2008; Barcelona, Spain.
101. Harder H, Holtel H, Bromberg JE, et al. Cognitive status and quality of life after treatment for primary CNS lymphoma. *Neurology.* 2004;62(4):544–547.
102. Welzel G, Steinvorth S, Wenz F. Cognitive effects of chemotherapy and/or cranial irradiation in adults. *Strahlenther Onkol.* 2005;181(3):141–156.
103. Fliessbach K, Urbach H, Helmstaedter C, et al. Cognitive performance and magnetic resonance imaging findings after high-dose systemic and intraventricular chemotherapy for primary central nervous system lymphoma. *Arch Neurol.* 2003;60(4):563–568.
104. Wolkowitz OM, Lupien SJ, Bigler E, Levin RB, Canick J. The "steroid dementia syndrome": an unrecognized complication of glucocorticoid treatment. *Ann N Y Acad Sci.* 2004;1032:191–194.
105. Keenan PA, Jacobson MW, Soleymani RM, Mayes MD, Stress ME, Yaldoo DT. The effect on memory of chronic prednisone treatment in patients with systemic disease. *Neurology.* 1996;47(6):1396–1402.
106. Cull A, Hay C, Love SB, Mackie M, Smets E, Stewart M. What do cancer patients mean when they complain of concentration and memory problems? *Br J Cancer.* 1996;74:1674–1679.
107. Stewart AL, Ware JE, eds. *Measuring Functioning and Well-Being: The Medical Outcomes Study Approach.* Durham, NC: Duke University Press; 1992.
108. Lilja A, Hagstadius S, Risberg J, Salford LG, Smith GJW, Ohman R. Frontal lobe dynamics in brain tumor patients: a study of regional blood flow and affective changes before and after surgery. *Neuropsychiatry Neuropsychol Behav Neurol.* 1992;5:294–300.
109. Andrewes DG, Kaye A, Murphy M, et al. Emotional and social dysfunction in patients following surgical treatment for brain tumour. *J Clin Neurosci.* 2003;10(4):428–433.
110. Meyers CA, Berman SA, Scheibel RS, Hayman A. Case report: acquired antisocial personality disorder associated with unilateral left orbital frontal lobe damage. *J Psychiatry Neurosci.* 1992;17(3):121–125.
111. Pringle AM, Taylor R, Whittle IR. Anxiety and depression in patients with an intracranial neoplasm before and after tumour surgery. *Br J Neurosurg.* 1999;13(1):46–51.
112. Anderson SI, Taylor R, Whittle IR. Mood disorders in patients after treatment for primary intracranial tumours. *Br J Neurosurg.* 1999;13(5):480–485.

41 Neuropsychological Sequelae Associated with Pediatric Brain Tumors: What We've Learned Over the Past 40 Years

Sarah C. Carpentieri

This chapter provides a summary of the progress of the field over the past four decades, with specific focus on the identification of patient-, tumor-, and treatment-related risk factors associated with declines in various domains of neuropsychological functioning. Young age at diagnosis and treatment, more aggressive treatment (e.g., greater doses and volumes of irradiation), and significant preirradiation factors can adversely impact neuropsychological development. It is difficult to predict, however, which children will be the most vulnerable to erosion of neuropsychological functioning, but since the majority of survivors require some educational intervention, deficits in neuropsychological functioning can have a significant impact on academic progress, educational attainment, and quality of life. During the last decade, there has been a greater emphasis on identifying the fundamental biological mechanisms that are associated with changes in neuropsychological functioning. Most recently, there has also been a focus on designing pharmacological and cognitive remediation interventions to specifically address areas of neuropsychological vulnerability and/or deficit.

Pediatric brain tumors, malignant and nonmalignant, account for ~20% of all childhood malignancies. They are second only to the leukemias in terms of incidence and are the most common of the solid tumors. In 2005, the Central Brain Tumor Registry of the United States estimated that there would be 3410 new cases diagnosed that year in children younger than 20 years of age, 76% of which would be in children less than 15 years of age [1]. With an overall incidence of 4.3 cases per 100,000 person-years, these tumors are slightly more common in males than in females (1.2:1) and occur more frequently in white children. Peak incidence of diagnosis declines through childhood and adolescence, with the highest incidence in children who are 4 years of age and younger and the lowest incidence in adolescents who are 15 to 19 years old. Different histologies have different age distributions; pilocytic astrocytomas and medulloblastomas are the most common in children between 0 and 14 years of age, accounting for 21% and 17%, respectively, of all brain tumors in that age group. In adolescents who are 15 to 19 years old, pilocytic astrocytomas and pituitary tumors are the most common, accounting for

Table 41.1 Incidence and Survival Rate for Pediatric Brain Tumors (Ages 0–19 years)[a]

Tumor Type	Incidence Rates	Relative Survival Rates	
		5-year	10-year
Pilocytic astrocytoma	0.83	94	93
Medulloblastoma	0.62	56	48
Glioma, malignant NOS	0.41	31	27
Astrocytoma NOS	0.25	77	73
Ependymoma	0.24	55	47
Glioblastoma	0.13	19	16
Anaplastic astrocytoma	0.09	51	45

[a] From ref. [1].

14% and 10%, respectively, of all brain tumors in that age group. While overall 5-year survival rates ranges from 63% (for ages 0–14) to 65% (for ages 15–19), rates vary widely across histology and location (see Table 41.1).

In 2000, it was estimated that there were more than 26,000 children diagnosed with brain tumor living in the United States [1]. With advances in treatment and increases in survival and cure rates, assessment of neuropsychological sequelae and long-term functional outcome has become more important. Assessment of these sequelae is an integral component when evaluating risks and benefits associated with treatment, providing accurate information for families of children newly diagnosed with a brain tumor, developing long-range education and behavioral management plans, and assisting the family in planning for an independent and fulfilling future for their child within the context of specific physical, cognitive, behavioral, and/or emotional vulnerabilities or limitations.

PEDIATRIC NEUROPSYCHOLOGY: THE PAST 40 YEARS

From a neurodevelopmental perspective, there are 10 broad domains of neuropsychological functioning (see Table 41.2). The most common method used to document neurocognitive effects in children treated for brain tumors

Table 41.2 Domains of Neuropsychological Functioning

Domain	Description
Intellectual functioning	Tests[a] of intellectual development (IQ)
Language processing	Tests of expressive language, receptive language, comprehension, fluency, phonological processing
Visual processing	Tests of visual functioning, perceptual organization, and visuomotor integration
Learning and memory	Tests of learning, short-term and long-term recall, retrieval and recognition in both verbal and visual domains
Motor functioning	Tests of dominant and nondominant fine motor speed, dexterity, coordination, quality of motor output
Processing speed	Tests of speed of information processing, reaction time
Attention	Tests of attention (sustained, selective, divided)
Executive functioning	Tests of organization, planning, inhibition, and flexibility
Achievement	Tests of academic skill acquisition in various areas of reading, math, spelling, listening skills
Neurobehavioral	Mental status exam, completion of inventories of behavioral, emotional, or psychosocial functioning by parent, child and/or teacher

[a] Tests are standardized and provide age-referenced norms for comparison

has been an Intelligence Quotient (IQ) test. IQ tests are standardized on large numbers of the general population and have a normative mean score of 100 with SDs of 15 or 16. Scaled scores are derived, which reflect the child's current level of functioning relative to same-age peers.

The study of the neuropsychological functioning of children with brain tumors has been an ongoing effort for the past four decades and is characterized by an increasing sophistication of study design (with the incorporation of various treatment and/or technological advances) as well as an effort to identify the fundamental biological mechanisms that are associated with changes in neuropsychological functioning in this population. The first studies describing the neuropsychological functioning of children after diagnosis and treatment of brain tumors were conducted in the late 1960s and 1970s with reports on general neurocognitive and neurobehavioral functioning of survivors. Over the next 2 decades, the identification of patient-, tumor-, and treatment-related risk factors associated with declines in cognitive functioning and academic achievement began in earnest. Numerous studies explored the impact of age at diagnosis and treatment, radiation therapy (RT), and tumor location on neuropsychological functioning at various intervals post diagnosis and treatment. Some investigators have focused on "late effects" (the emergence of neuropsychological deficits 2–4 years after diagnosis), and others moved beyond IQ and academic achievement measures to focus on other domains of neuropsychological functions, specifically memory, attention, and processing speed. During the last decade, neuropsychological research has continued to document the impact of patient-, tumor-, and treatment-related risk factors on IQ and achievement, with a greater emphasis on understanding the neurobiological and genetic markers that are associated with greater neuropsychological dysfunction, and on designing effective cognitive rehabilitation programs.

RISKS FOR NEUROPSYCHOLOGICAL DEFICITS

The analysis of risk factors for neurocognitive impairments among patients treated for brain tumors can be complex because of the number and variety of sources of brain damage. In general, young age at diagnosis, young age at treatment, more aggressive central nervous system (CNS) therapy, and tumor-associated factors are the most commonly cited risk factors.

Age at Diagnosis

The association between younger age at diagnosis and lower neurodevelopmental and cognitive functioning began to emerge in studies conducted in the 1980s and 1990s [2–5]. Infants diagnosed with brain tumors can be particularly vulnerable, as 75% or more have exhibited significant developmental delays at diagnosis, prior to either radiation or chemotherapy [6,7]. While the definition of "younger" and "older" varied across studies, significantly lower IQ scores at diagnosis, compared to older children, have been documented in patients younger than 5, 6, or 7 years at diagnosis [8–11]. In addition to IQ, younger age at diagnosis appears to be associated with deficits in memory and selective attention [9]. These findings suggest that infants and younger children may be more neurodevelopmentally vulnerable to the effects of the tumor, surgery, or perioperative factors than older children and adolescents.

Age at RT Treatment

The significant relationship between younger age at treatment and poorer intellectual outcome has been well documented across individual studies and reviews of the literature [12–17]. While a greater incidence of mental retardation has been reported for children treated with RT in the first year of life and for those who were under 3 years at treatment, the "safe" age to irradiate the brain has not been determined [18,19]. In an analysis of IQ data from 22 studies, children younger than 4 years of age at treatment were the most vulnerable to intellectual loss, showing a 14-point deficit in IQ (73.4 vs 87.0) compared to older children [16]. In a unique analysis of a cohort of 62 children treated with radiotherapy for primary intracranial tumors, investigators found that the age of the child at the time of treatment was the most powerful determinant of ultimate IQ [20]. Children who were younger than 5 years of age at treatment were at greatest risk (mean IQ = 72), those between 6 and 10 years were at intermediate risk (mean IQ = 93), and those between 11 and 15 years were functioning solidly in the average range (mean IQ = 107). The prevailing opinion is that children under 4 to 5 years are at greater risk for treatment-related neurocognitive impairments, as they are exposed to potentially neurotoxic agents during a time when, both anatomically and functionally, the CNS is rapidly developing.

Impact of RT

The progressive adverse effects of cranial irradiation therapy (CRT) on IQ are well-known and have been documented at various time intervals since treatment, in comparison to those who received local RT and in comparison to those who did not receive RT. Several independent studies have documented IQ decline in children with medulloblastoma at 5-years posttreatment with CRT. Investigators have reported that 20% of these children had IQs above 90, 40% to 50% had IQs below 80, and 31% had IQs below 70 [21–24]. By 10-years posttreatment, only 10% had IQs above 90 and 85% had IQs below 80 [21,23]. Children treated with CRT for medulloblastoma consistently showed declines in IQ over time, with the potential level of IQ deterioration as great as 25 to 30 points [17,22,25]. In an integrative analysis across 22 studies, patients receiving RT had IQ levels at least 12 to 14 points lower than those not receiving RT, and children who did not receive RT did not show significant decline in IQ over time [16,26]. More recently, in a long-term (median 8 years) follow-up study of 126 children younger than 4 years old at diagnosis, Fouladi et al found significant declines in IQ for children treated with CSI (−1.34 points/year) and for local RT (−0.51 points/year) in comparison to those not treated with RT (0.91 points/year) [27]. In addition, at a minimum of 5-years posttreatment, 71% of patients treated with CSI and 23% of those treated with local RT had IQs below 70.

In addition to IQ declines, children with medulloblastomas treated with CSI are vulnerable to other neuropsychological deficits. In a cohort of medulloblastoma survivors (mean follow-up time 12.2 years), Ribi et al found that 79% of the children exhibited significant deficits in attention and processing speed, 88% exhibited significant deficits in learning and memory, 56% in language, 50% in visual perception, and 64% in executive functioning [28]. Similarly, two more recent studies of children treated for medulloblastoma have found attention deficits (especially in selective attention), slower processing speed, and difficulties in working memory as well as verbal memory impairments (consisting of both retrieval and recognition deficits) [29,30].

The emergence of "late effects" and their relationship to age at diagnosis has been observed in children receiving CRT. IQ declines appear to be inversely correlated with age, with younger children showing the greatest loss of intelligence [26,31,32]. While significant declines can be documented as early as the first year, investigators have found that at 2 years posttreatment, children younger than 7 years at diagnosis and treated with CRT exhibited a mean decline in Full-Scale IQ (FSIQ) of 25 or 27 points [26,31,32]. In addition, after treatment with CRT, memory difficulties as well as deficits in fine motor, visual-motor, and visual-spatial skills were noted [26]. Age at diagnosis and time since treatment have been shown to make separable contributions to intellectual functioning. Dennis et al found that Performance IQ varied with chronological age of the child at diagnosis, but subsequently was relatively constant in magnitude; Verbal IQ, however, was less sensitive to age at diagnosis, but more sensitive to time since treatment [33].

Researchers have also focused on the relationship between age at diagnosis, radiotherapy dose, and IQ decline, with most finding that while both standard and reduced dose CRT are associated with IQ decline, higher exposure is associated with greater decline, especially in younger children [11,34–36]. More specifically, Mulhern et al found younger patients receiving standard dose (36 Gy) CRT had IQ scores 13 to 15 points lower than either older children receiving standard CRT or younger children receiving reduced dose (23.4 Gy) CRT [34]. Moreover, their IQ scores were 22 points lower than older children receiving reduced dose. An analogous pattern of differences between groups was also found with regard to measures of attention and academic achievement [34]. Similarly, IQ declines of 17 points over a 4-year period have been documented in a cohort of children treated with reduced dose CRT, with children younger than 7 years at CRT losing a mean of 21 IQ points over the 4-year period [36]. While IQ declines associated with RT appear to be consistent over time, the magnitude of the decline does seem to vary with dose and age at treatment. Silber et al analyzed their data and suggested that a statistical model using initial IQ, age at treatment, and the dose of CRT could forecast final IQ [37]. They demonstrated that a 10-year-old child would score 12 points higher than a 3-year-old child at equivalent doses of irradiation. The most recent studies on the progressive impact of RT indicate that FSIQ decreases 1 to 4 points per year (depending on age at RT and RT dose) and continues for a number of years with total decreases in the 15 to 20 point range [36,38–40]. However, younger children treated with higher doses of CRT can be vulnerable to greater declines.

Tumor Location

Since tumors of the cerebellum and brain stem account for about half of all pediatric brain tumors, posterior fossa and medulloblastoma have been the subject of a large number of investigations [1]. In a 1994 literature review, however, supratentorial tumors were found to have a greater impact on neuropsychological development and functioning than infratentorial tumors [17]. Similarly, various independent studies have reported greater IQ declines in patients with hemispheric tumor location in comparison to patients with midline tumors, third ventricle tumors, and posterior fossa tumors [8,12,41].

In addition to IQ declines, other site-specific deficits have been reported. Temporal lobe tumor location has been associated with lobe-specific verbal memory and visual memory deficits and, subsequent to memory difficulties, with lower reading and spelling achievement and generally poorer neuropsychological functioning [3,42,43]. In children treated for craniopharyngioma, many investigators report IQs in the average range [44,45]. However, Carpentieri et al identified specific memory deficits, in both verbal and visual domains, despite average

IQ [44]. Moreover, their findings suggest that the memory difficulties do not lie in the initial processing, encoding, or storage of the information, but in the retrieval of the information.

Severe deficits in working memory have been associated with thalamic tumors, and tumor extension to the hypothalamus has been associated with greater cognitive deficits [19,46]. More recently, investigators have found that children with third ventricle tumors were more impaired on verbal recall tasks and those with cerebellar tumors were more impaired on attention tasks [47]. In a follow-up study on a similar group of patients, Micklewright et al reported that children with cerebellar tumors exhibited significant auditory attentional impairments and those with third ventricle tumors exhibited encoding and retrieval deficits [48].

In children with posterior fossa tumors, numerous studies have found impairments in IQ, memory, language, attention, and academic skills, as well as signs and symptoms associated with damage to the cerebellum, including poor visual-motor and visuospatial functioning as well as problems with fine and gross motor steadiness, speed and coordination, and poor problem-solving skills [3,22,26,28,29,33,49,50]. However, these impairments have been observed in groups that have also undergone CRT, which makes it difficult to parse out the specific impact of tumor location. In children with cerebellar tumors treated with surgery-only, impaired fine motor speed and functioning, impaired visual-spatial functioning, attention deficits, poor problem-solving skills, and impaired executive function (including planning and sequencing) have been reported [51–53]. While poor expressive language and verbal memory have been observed, speech difficulties, including disfluency and slow speech, have been documented in children with posterior fossa tumors, regardless of radiation treatment [52,54]. Cerebellar lesion location can also impact functioning; children with right cerebellar tumors have exhibited auditory sequential memory and language-processing deficits and those with left cerebellar tumors had exhibited spatial and visual sequential memory deficits [55]. In addition, lesions of the vermis have been associated with dysregulation of affect and with speech/language disorders [52,55]. In sum, cerebellar lesions can result in neuropsychological dysfunction, and some have suggested these deficits are indicative of cerebellar cognitive affective syndrome in children.

Impact of Pre-RT Factors

There is increasing recognition that pre-RT factors, including tumor infiltration and the trauma, associated with surgical resection can play some role in the neuropsychological functioning of patients with brain tumor. While some researchers examining the relationship between surgery-only and IQ have reported lower IQs and school problems and cognitive decline, others have found improvements in IQ scores for children with posterior fossa tumors [9,56,57]. Most recently, in the context of average FSIQ, Carpentieri et al documented slower processing speed and motor output, poor visuospatial processing, and decreased verbal memory as well as significantly lower Performance IQs postsurgical resection in almost half of the children who had been treated with surgery only [58]. Moreover, the finding that 79% of the group exhibited a deficiency in some area of cognitive functioning while only a few were severely impaired suggests that a mild-to-moderate level of neuropsychological morbidity is not uncommon post-surgery. Similarly, Steinlin et al reported problems in attention, memory, and processing speed in the context of intact global intellectual ability [59]. While FSIQ has generally been reported to be in the average range, Beebe et al described a four-point loss in FSIQ 3 months postoperatively [60].

Secondary preoperative and postoperative deficits have been shown to adversely affect neuropsychological performance [17,61]. In one study, investigators found that 70% to 80% of children had IQs above 90 one to two years after surgery when no postoperative complications occurred, but only 20% to 40% had IQs above 90 if postoperative complications did occur [21]. At variance with earlier studies that did not find a significant relationship between hydrocephalus and later IQ, recent investigations do report an association [9,12,19,41,62,63]. In one study, hydrocephalus was one of four significant predictors of lower IQ, and in another, changes in IQ score, both before and after RT, were significantly correlated with the extent and treatment of hydrocephalus at the time of diagnosis [62,63]. While seizures can be a presenting complaint for children with brain tumors, the impact of seizure activity has not been a focus of research, but those investigators who have addressed it have observed that the presence of seizures or their inadequate control can negatively impact neuropsychological functioning [3,43,64,65].

NEUROCOGNITIVE CORRELATES

As treatment methods improve and survival increases for children with brain tumors, concerns have been raised about declines in cognitive functioning. Possible causes of IQ decline include a dementing process, loss of skills, the failure to acquire new cognitive skills at a developmentally appropriate rate, or a slowing in the acquisition and assimilation of new knowledge compared to same-age peers. It is difficult, however, to predict which children will be more vulnerable to erosion of cognitive functioning. Since children with IQ within the normal range can still be at risk for learning difficulties, there may be other mediating neurocognitive factors that increase a child's vulnerability to concurrent and future learning issues without significantly impacting performance on IQ measures. Neuropsychological tests of higher level function, such as IQ and achievement, may be useful to document current functioning, but may be less effective in forecasting risk for later functional declines because they are not sensitive enough to capture or quantify changes that will impact later neurocognitive functioning. Since up to 45% of the age-related improvements that occur in intelligence are directly accounted for by normal age-related improvements in processing speed and working memory, in theory, adequate performance on IQ and achievement measures requires adequate performance on prerequisite processes, such as memory, attention, and processing speed. Slower processing speed, memory difficulties, and/or poor attention therefore should impact the rate of acquisition of new skills and knowledge, resulting in IQ decline secondary to slower acquisition of skills and knowledge, rather than actual loss of skills and knowledge. Verbal memory difficulties have predicted low reading and spelling achievement, slower processing speed has been associated with lower IQ, and IQ decline has been associated with developmentally slower than normal rate of learning, rather than loss of previously acquired knowledge [25,43,58]. In children treated for posterior fossa tumors, deficits in attention and memory are seen simultaneously with IQ deficits, and their pattern of severity (more severe deficits associated with younger age at CRT) is similar to that seen with IQ [25]. However, it is unclear whether these deficits actually predate or cause declines in IQ and achievement or, like declines in IQ and achievement, are simply another reflection of the general compromise of the CNS after treatment. More work is needed to find measures that can provide predictive validity for determining the nature and extent of future declines in higher order neuropsychological functioning.

BIOLOGIC FOUNDATIONS OF NEUROPSYCHOLOGICAL DECLINE

With recent advances in quantification methods, researchers exploring the biological basis of neurocognitive decline are investigating the relationship between white matter abnormalities and IQ and other measures of neuropsychological functioning. The pathophysiology of CNS damage induced by radiation is not fully understood, especially with regard to the vulnerability of white matter to injury. Recent research indicates that white matter loss may be attributable to the adverse effects of ionizing irradiation on the microvasculature of endothelial cells or to axonal demyelination after oligodendrocytic death. In a series of studies by researchers at St Jude Children's Research Hospital of survivors of medulloblastoma, significant decreases in the volume of cerebral white matter and volume of corpus callosum have been documented and the extent of these decreases has been correlated with irradiation dose [66–72]. In addition, relationships have been found between decreases in volume of white matter and lower IQ and attention difficulties, as well as between hippocampal volumes and memory dysfunction [70–72]. Volume of white matter has been found to explain 70% of the association between IQ score and age at time of RT, and microscopic damage in normal-appearing white matter has been associated with poor intellectual functioning [69,73]. In addition, white matter appears to be deferentially sensitive to RT by location, which can also impact neuropsychological functioning [74]. With these findings, the specific neurobiological substrate for neuropsychological deficits associated with CRT is unknown, but may be related to a loss of normal white matter, the failure to develop normal white matter at an age-appropriate rate, microscopic damage within normal-appearing white matter, a greater radiosensitivity of white matter in specific areas, or some combination of two or more of these factors.

A more recent finding is the polymorphisms in the glutathione S-transferase (GST) genes, more specifically, the significant relationship between glutathione S-transferase Mu 1 (GSTM1) polymorphisms and development of intellectual decline in children treated with medulloblastoma treated with CRT. GSTs belong to a family of isoenzymes, highly heterogeneous proteins expressed in virtually all tissues, including the brain [75]. They catalyze the glutathione conjugation of a variety of electrophilic compounds, including carcinogens, mutagens, cytotoxic drugs, and their metabolites [76]. Accordingly, they catalyze the detoxification of alkylating agents and platinum compounds that are used in medulloblastoma chemotherapy, detoxify free oxygen radicals formed spontaneously or by chemotherapy drugs and radiation, and can sequester alkylating agents and steroids by direct binding [75,76]. In a recent study, Barahmani et al found that patients with the *GSTM1* null genotype exhibited declining IQ scores but those with *GSTM1* nonnull genotype did not [77]. A follow-up study also shows that patient with the GSTM1 null genotype have significant declines in memory and speed of information processing.

IMPACT OF NEUROPSYCHOLOGICAL FUNCTIONING ON QUALITY OF LIFE

Given the neuropsychological sequelae in survivors of pediatric brain tumors, particularly the incidence of IQ below 70 (consistent with functioning in the "impaired" range) and the emergence of learning disabilities or neuropsychological deficits, the need for special education services is not unexpected. Earlier studies documented that about one-third of the survivors had IQs below 70 and 87% to 94% were categorized as either "slow" or had been given a diagnosis of learning disability and estimated that 11% to 75% of survivors, depending on age at diagnosis and treatment, required some form of special education services in the schools [9,24,49,50,64,78–80]. The most recent estimates of children in the United States indicates that while 50% of brain tumor survivors required special education services, 70% of those diagnosed before age 5 years will require services. In addition, boys are 13 times more likely than their brothers to be in special education and girls are 30.5 times more likely to be in special education than their female siblings [81]. In the classroom setting, difficulties in attention, concentration, and memory and/or processing speed can impede the acquisition of new knowledge and impact academic progress. While some difficulties appear to be related to tumor location (e.g., slower psychomotor speed among children treated for posterior fossa tumors or memory difficulties associated with temporal lobe location), others can be associated with treatment (e.g., lower IQ, or attention problems associated with CRT) and learning problems can also occur despite normal IQ [22,43,49].

Difficulties in neuropsychological functioning can impact psychosocial functioning and can manifest in behavioral and/or emotional problems that may be evident primarily in the home environment, but may also impact functioning in the classroom setting. While the continuum of psychosocial problems observed in association with brain tumors can range from very general behavioral and adjustment problems to more severe emotional dysfunction, two of the more common concerns expressed by parents are academic adjustment difficulties and socialization difficulties (lack of social competency and greater social isolation) [2,9,41,49,80–85]. Difficulties with socialization can be secondary to the neuropsychological deficits in attention, memory, and speed of information processing, which negatively impact the ability to interact with peers in an effective and age-appropriate manner. In the school setting, teachers have also endorsed academic concerns, and socialization concerns but do not generally endorse significant behavioral or emotional concerns [80,84,85].

As they transition into young adulthood, most brain tumor survivors do graduate from high school, but at lower rates than sibling controls or general population and are much less likely to attend college [64,81]. In a recent study, Mitby et al found that 18% of the 1637 brain tumor survivors in their cohort did not graduate high school and 77% did not earn a college degree [81]. Vocationally, adult survivors of childhood brain tumors typically exhibit significantly lower rates of employment in comparison to other cancer survivors and the general population [64,81]. In addition, some survivors may not be able to live independently and, as a group, are much less likely to get married (men more so than women) and are more likely to get divorced than the general population [81].

INTERVENTIONS

The development of empirically validated interventions for neuropsychological deficits has proceeded slowly, with focus on either reducing the neuropsychological toxicity of therapy or by rehabilitating unavoidable deficits via cognitive rehabilitation or pharmacotherapy. Recent studies have assessed the feasibility of using cognitive remediation principles with impaired survivors, and recent pilot data indicate significant improvements in some areas [86,87]. Pharmacological interventions have primarily focused on the effectiveness of methylphenidate (Ritalin) in improving attention difficulties, which impact overall cognitive functioning. Results of several studies have shown some improvements with Ritalin in some areas of attention and learning, but not in other areas [25,86]. Lastly, when available and accessible, school intervention programs can be helpful in transitioning a child back into school and providing support for school-related concerns. Many school intervention programs emphasize regular communication between parents, medical providers, and school personnel, as well as social facilitation between the child and his peers to promote positive peer relations and limit psychosocial difficulties. Some school intervention programs will also help facilitate getting the child into resource or special education placements if needed. Depending on the level of the child's learning needs, placements are typically categorized under Other Health Impaired or a 504 plan and are provided through the school district in the child's local public school [88].

CONCLUSION

In summary, over the past four decades, research on children with brain tumors has shown that poor neuropsychological functioning is associated with a variety of patient-, tumor-, and treatment-related factors. Young age at diagnosis and treatment, more aggressive treatment (e.g., greater doses and volumes of RT), and significant pre-RT factors can adversely impact neuropsychological development. At this time, however, it continues to be difficult to predict which children will be the most vulnerable to erosion of cognitive functioning and which mediating neurocognitive factors may increase a child's vulnerability to concurrent and future learning issues. Current investigations are focused on identifying the relationship between neurobiological and polymorphic factors and neuropsychological functioning. With improvements in treatments and increasing survival rates, larger numbers of survivors are reentering the school environment after their treatment. Many of these children require special education services, which are delivered by the child's local school district, and should be individualized to meet the child's specific needs. At the present time, there are no nationally standardized cognitive rehabilitation programs designed to address their specific learning deficits in a more comprehensive manner. However, as more information is earned about neurocognitive correlates and biological foundations of neurpsychological functioning, effective cognitive rehabilitation programs can be designed, with emphasis on remediating global deficits that may impact all brain tumor survivors, as well as more specific location or treatment-related deficits.

ACKNOWLEDGMENTS

The author dedicates this chapter to the memory of Raymond K. Mulhern, PhD, a wonderful mentor, trusted colleague, and valued friend.

REFERENCES

1. Central Brain Tumor Registry of the United States. Statistical Report: *Primary Brain Tumors in the United States.* Hinsdale, IL: Central Brain Tumor Registry of the United States; 2006.
2. Copeland DR, Fletcher JM, Pfefferbaum-Levine B, Jaffe N, Reid H, Maor M. Neuropsychological sequelae of childhood cancer in long-term survivors. *Pediatrics.* 1985;75:745–753.
3. Mulhern RK, Kovnar EH, Kun LE, Crisco JJ, Williams JM. Psychologic and neurologic function following treatment for childhood temporal lobe astrocytoma. *J Child Neurol.* 1988;3(1):47–52.
4. Walter AW, Mulhern RK, Gajjar A, et al. Survival and neurodevelopmental outcome of young children with medulloblastoma at St Jude Children's Research Hospital. *J Clin Oncol.* 1999;17(12):3720–3728.
5. Moore BD, Copeland DR, Reid H, Levy B. Neuropsychological basis of cognitive deficits in long-term survivors of childhood cancer. *Arch Neurol.* 1992;49(8):809–817.
6. Mulhern RK, Horowitz ME, Kovnar EH, Langston J, Sanford RA, Kun LE. Neurodevelopmental status of infants and young children treated for brain tumors with pre-irradiation chemotherapy. *J Clin Oncol.* 1989;7(11):1660–1666.
7. Stargatt R, Rosenfeld JV, Anderson V, Hassall T, Maixner W, Ashley D. Intelligence and adaptive function in children diagnosed with brain tumour during infancy. *J Neurooncol.* 2006;80(3):295–303.

8. Fouladi M, Wallace D, Langston JW, et al. Survival and functional outcome of children with hypothalamic/chiasmatic tumors. *Cancer.* 2003;97(4):1084–1092.
9. Mulhern RK, Kun LE. Neuropsychologic function in children with brain tumors. III. Interval changes in size months following treatment. *Med Pediatr Oncol.* 1985;13(6):318–324.
10. George AP, Kuehn SM, Vassilyadi M, et al. Cognitive sequelae in children with posterior fossa tumors. *Pediatr Neurol.* 2003;28(1):42–47.
11. Mulhern RK, Palmer SL, Merchant TE, et al. Neurocognitive consequences of risk-adapted therapy for childhood medulloblastoma. *J Clin Oncol.* 2005;23(24):5511–5519.
12. Ellenberg L, McComb JG, Siegel SE, Stowe S. Factors affecting intellectual outcome in pediatric brain tumor patients. *Neurosurg.* 1987;21:638–644.
13. Dennis M, Spiegler BJ, Hoffman HJ, Hendrick EB, Humphreys RP, Becker LE. Brain tumors in children and adolescents-I. Effects on working, associative and serial-order memory of IQ at tumor onset and age of tumor. *Neuropsychologia.* 1991;29(9):813–827.
14. Moore BD, Ater JL, Needle MN, Slopis JM. Neuropsychological profile of children with neurofibromatosis, brain tumor, or both. *J Child Neuro.* 1994;9(4):368–377.
15. Copeland DR, deMoor C, Moore BD 3rd, Ater JL. Neurocognitive development of children after a cerebellar tumor in infancy: A longitudinal study. *J Clin Oncol.* 1999;17(11):3476–3486.
16. Mulhern RK, Hancock J, Fairclough D, Kun L. Neuropsychological status of children treated for brain tumors: A critical review and integration. *Med Pediatr Oncol.* 1992;20(3):181–191.
17. Ris MD, Noll RB. Long-term neurobehavioral outcome in pediatric brain-tumor patients: review and methodological critique. *J Clin Exp Neuropsychol.* 1994;16(1):21–42.
18. Raimondi AJ, Tomita T. Brain tumors during the first year of life. *Childs Brain.* 1983;10(3):193–207.
19. Danoff BF, Cowchock FS, Marquette C. Assessment of the long term effects of primary radiation therapy for brain tumors in children. *Cancer.* 1982;49:1580–1586.
20. Jannoun L, Bloom HJ. Long-term psychological effects in children treated for intracranial tumors. *Int J Radiat Oncol Biol Phys.* 1990;18(4):747–753.
21. Hoppe-Hirsch E, Brunet L, Laroussinie F, et al. Intellectual outcome in children with malignant tumors of the posterior fossa: influence of the field of irradiation and quality of surgery. *Childs Nerv Syst.* 1995;11(6):340–345; discussion 345–346.
22. Duffner PK, Cohen ME, Thomas P. Late effects of treatment on the intelligence of children with posterior fossa tumors. *Cancer.* 1983;51:233–237.
23. Hoppe-Hirsch E, Renier D, Lellouch-Tubiana A, Sainte-Rose C, Pierre-Kahn A, Hirsch JF. Medulloblastoma in childhood: progressive intellectual deterioration. *Childs Nerv Syst.* 1990;6(2):60–65.
24. Hirsch JF, Renier D, Czernichow P, BenVeniste L, Pierre-Kahn A. Medulloblastoma in childhood: survival and functional results. *Acta Neurologica.* 1979;48:1–15.
25. Mulhern RK, Merchant TE, Gajjar A, Reddick WE, Kun LE. Late neurocognitive sequelae in survivors of brain tumours in childhood. *Lancet Oncol.* 2004;5(7):399–408.
26. Packer RJ, Sutton LN, Atkins TE, et al. A prospective study of cognitive function in children receiving whole-brain radiotherapy and chemotherapy: 2-year results. *J Neurosurg.* 1989;70(5):707–713.
27. Fouladi M, Gilger E, Kocak M, et al. Intellectual and functional outcome of children 3 years old or younger who have CNS malignancies. *J Clin Oncol.* 2005;23(28):7152–7160.
28. Ribi K, Relly C, Landolt MA, Alber FD, Boltshauser E, Grotzer MA. Outcome of medulloblastoma in children: long-term complications and quality of life. *Neuropediatrics.* 2005;36(6):357–365.
29. Reeves CB, Palmer SL, Reddick WE, et al. Attention and memory functioning among pediatric patients with medulloblastoma. *J Pediatr Psychol.* 2006;31(3):272–280.
30. Nagel BJ, Delis DC, Palmer SL, Reeves C, Gajjar A, Mulhern RK. Early patterns of verbal memory impairment in children treated for medulloblastoma. *Neuropsychology.* 2006;20(1):105–112.
31. Radcliffe J, Packer R, Atkins TE, Bunin G. Three and four year cognitive outcome in children with noncortical brain tumors treated with whole brain radiotherapy. *Ann Neurol.* 1992;32(4):551–554.
32. Radcliffe J, Bunin GR, Sutton LN, Goldwein JW, Phillips PC. Cognitive deficits in long-term survivors of childhood medulloblastoma and other noncortical tumors: age-dependent effects of whole brain radiation. *Int J Dev Neurosci.* 1994;12(4):327–334.
33. Dennis M, Spiegler BJ, Hetherington CR, Greenberg ML. Neuropsychological sequelae of the treatment of children with medulloblastoma. *J Neuro-Oncol.* 1996;29:91–101.
34. Mulhern RK, Kepner JL, Thomas PR, Armstrong FD, Friedman HS, Kun LE. Neuropsychologic functioning of survivors of childhood medulloblastoma randomized to receive conventional or reduced-dose craniospinal irradiation: a Pediatric Oncology Group study. *J Clin Oncol.* 1998;16(5):1723–1728.
35. Grill J, Renaux VK, Bulteau C, et al. Long-term intellectual outcome in children with posterior fossa tumors according to radiation doses and volumes. *Int J Radiat Oncol Biol Phys.* 1999;45(1):137–145.
36. Ris MD, Packer R, Goldwein J, Jones-Wallace D, Boyett JM. Intellectual outcome after reduced-dose radiation therapy plus adjuvant chemotherapy for medulloblastoma: a Children's Cancer Group study. *J Clin Oncol.* 2001;19(15):3470–3476.
37. Silber JH, Radcliffe J, Peckman V, et al. Whole brain irradiation and decline in intelligence: The influence of dose and age on IQ score. *J Clin Oncol.* 1992;10(9):1390–1396.
38. Palmer SL, Goloubeva O, Reddick WE, et al. Patterns of intellectual development among survivors of pediatric medulloblastoma: a longitudinal analysis. *J Clin Oncol.* 2001;19(8):2302–2308.
39. Palmer SL, Gajjar A, Reddick WE, et al. Predicting intellectual outcome among children treated with 35–40 Gy craniospinal irradiation for medulloblastoma. *Neuropsychology.* 2003;17(4):548–555.
40. Spiegler BJ, Bouffet E, Greenberg ML, Rutka JT, Mabbott DJ. Change in neurocognitive functioning after treatment with cranial radiation in childhood. *J Clin Oncol.* 2004;22(4):706–713.
41. Kun LE, Mulhern RK. Neuropsychologic function in children with brain tumors II. Serial studies of intellect and time after treatment. *Am J Clin Oncol.* 1983;6(6):651–656.
42. Cavazzutti V, Winston K, Baker R, Welch K. Psychological changes following surgery for tumors in the temporal lobe. *J Neurosurg.* 1980;53:618–626.
43. Carpentieri SC, Mulhern RK. Patterns of memory dysfunction among children surviving temporal lobe tumors. *Arch Clin Neuropsych.* 1994;8:345–357.
44. Carpentieri SC, Waber DP, Scott RM, et al. Memory deficits among children with craniopharyngiomas. *Neurosurgery.* 2001;49(5):1053–1057.
45. Riva D, Pantaleoni C, Devoti M, Saletti V, Nichelli F, Giorgi C. Late neuropsychological and behavioural outcome of children surgically treated for craniopharyngioma. *Childs Nerv Syst.* 1998;14(4–5):179–184.
46. Dennis M, Spiegler BJ, Obonsawin MC, Maira BL, Cowell C. Brain tumors in children and adolescents-III. Effects of radiation and hormone status on intelligence and on working, associative ad serial-order memory. *Neuropsychologia.* 1992;30(3):257–275.
47. King TZ, Fennell EB, Williams L, et al. Verbal memory abilities of children with brain tumors. *Child Neuropsychol.* 2004;10(2):76–88.
48. Micklewright JL, King TZ, Morris RD, Morris MK. Attention and memory in children with brain tumors. *Child Neuropsychol.* 2007;13(6):522–527.
49. LeBaron S, Zeltzer PM, Seltzer LK, Scott S, Marlin AE. Assessment of quality of survival in children with medulloblastoma and cerebellar astrocytoma. *Cancer.* 1988;62(6):1215–1222.
50. Spunberg JJ, Chang CH, Goldman M. Quality of long-term survival following irradiation for intracranial tumors in children under the age of two. *Int J Radiat Oncol Biol Phys.* 1981;7(6):727–736.
51. Rønning C, Sundet K, Due-Tønnessen B, Lundar T, Helseth E. Persistent cognitive dysfunction secondary to cerebellar injury in patients treated for posterior fossa tumors in childhood. *Pediatr Neurosurg.* 2005;41(1):15–21.
52. Levisohn L, Cronin-Golomb A, Schmahmann JD. Neuropsychological consequences of cerebellar tumor resection in children: cerebellar cognitive affective syndrome in a pediatric population. *Brain.* 2000;123(5):1041–1050.
53. Riva D, Pantaleoni C, Milani N, Fossati Belani F. Impairment of neuropsychological functions in children with medulloblastomas and astrocytomas in the posterior fossa. *Childs Nerv Syst.* 1989;5(2):107–110.
54. Huber JF, Bradley K, Spiegler B, Dennis M. Long-term neuromotor speech deficits in survivors of childhood posterior fossa tumors:

54. effects of tumor type, radiation, age at diagnosis, and survival years. *J Child Neurol.* 2007;22(7):848–854.
55. Riva D, Giorgi C. The cerebellum contributes to higher functions during development: evidence from a series of children surgically treated for posterior fossa tumours. *Brain.* 2000;123:1051–1061.
56. Hirsch JF, Sainte Rose C, Pierre-Kahn A, Pfister A, Hoppe-Hirsch E. Benign astrocytic and ooligodendrocytic tumors of the cerebral hemispheres in children. *J Neurosurg.* 1989;70(4):568–572.
57. Mulhern RK, Heideman RL, Khatib ZA, Kovnar EH, Sanford RA, Kun LE. Quality of survival among children treated for brain stem glioma. *Pediatr Neurosurg.* 1994;20(4):226–232.
58. Carpentieri SC, Waber DP, Pomeroy SL, et al. Neuropsychological functioning after surgery in children treated for brain tumor. *Neurosurgery.* 2003;52(6):1348–1356.
59. Steinlin M, Imfeld S, Zulauf P, et al. Neuropsychological long-term sequelae after posterior fossa tumour resection in childhood. *Brain.* 2003;126(9):1998–2008.
60. Beebe DW, Ris MD, Armstrong, et al. Cognitive and adaptive outcome in low-grade pediatric cerebellar astrocytomas: evidence of diminished cognitive and adaptive functioning in National Collaborative Research Studies (CCG 9891/POG 9130). *J Clin Oncol.* 2005;23(22):5198–5204.
61. Kao GD, Goldwein JW, Schultz DJ, Radcliffe J, Sutton L, Lange B. The impact of perioperative factors on subsequent intelligence quotient deficits in children treated for medulloblastoma/posterior fossa primitive neuroectodermal tumors. *Cancer.* 1994;74(3):965–971.
62. Reimers TS, Ehrenfels S, Mortensen EL, et al. Cognitive deficits in long-term survivors of childhood brain tumors: Identification of predictive factors. *Med Pediatr Oncol.* 2003;40(1):26–34.
63. Merchant TE, Lee H, Zhu J, et al. The effects of hydrocephalus on intelligence quotient in children with localized infratentorial ependymoma before and after focal radiation therapy. *J Neurosurg.* 2004;101(suppl 2):159–168.
64. Syndikus I, Tait D, Ashley S, Jannoun L. Long-term follow-up of young children with brain tumors after irradiation. *Int J Radiat Oncol Biol Phys.* 1994;30(4):781–787.
65. Macedoni-Luksic M, Jereb B, Todorovski L. Long-term sequelae in children treated for brain tumors: impairments, disability, and handicap. *Pediatr Hematol Oncol.* 2003;20(2):89–101.
66. Reddick WE, Russell JM, Glass JO, et al. Subtle white matter volume differences in children treated for medulloblastoma with conventional or reduced dose craniospinal irradiation. *Magn Reson Imaging.* 2000;18(7):787–793.
67. Palmer SL, Reddick WE, Glass JO, Gajjar A, Goloubeva O, Mulhern RK. Decline in corpus callosum volume among pediatric patients with medulloblastoma: longitudinal MR imaging study. *AJNR Am J Neuroradiol.* 2002;23(7):1088–1094.
68. Mulhern RK, Reddick WE, Palmer SL, et al. Neurocognitive deficits in medulloblastoma survivors and white matter loss. *Ann Neurol.* 1999;46(6):834–841.
69. Mulhern RK, Palmer SL, Reddick WE, et al. Risks of young age for selected neurocognitive deficits in medulloblastoma are associated with white matter loss. *J Clin Oncol.* 2001;19(2).472–479.
70. Reddick WE, White HA, Glass JO, et al. Developmental model relating white matter volume to neurocognitive deficits in pediatric brain tumor survivors. *Cancer.* 2003;97(10):2512–2519.
71. Mulhern RK, White HA, Glass JO, et al. Attentional functioning and white matter integrity among survivors of malignant brain tumors of childhood. *J Int Neuropsychol Soc.* 2004;10(2):180–189.
72. Nagel BJ, Palmer SL, Reddick WE, et al. Abnormal hippocampal development in children with medulloblastoma treated with risk-adapted irradiation. *AJNR Am J Neuroradiol.* 2004;25(9):1575–1582.
73. Mabbott DJ, Noseworthy MD, Bouffet E, Rockel C, Laughlin S. Diffusion tensor imaging of white matter after cranial radiation in children for medulloblastoma: correlation with IQ. *Neuro Oncol.* 2006;8(3):244–252.
74. Qiu D, Kwong DL, Chan GC, Leung LH, Khong PL. Diffusion tensor magnetic resonance imaging finding of discrepant fractional anisotropy between the frontal and parietal lobes after whole-brain irradiation in childhood medulloblastoma survivors: reflection of regional white matter radiosensitivity? *Int J Radiat Oncol Biol Phys.* 2007;69(3):846–851.
75. Terrier P, Townsend AJ, Coindre JM, Triche TJ, Cowan KH. An immunohistochemical study of pi class glutathione S-transferase expression in normal human tissue. *Am J Pathol.* 1990:137(4): 845–853.
76. Hayes JD, Pulford DJ. The glutathione S-transferase supergene family: regulation of GST and the contribution of the isoenzymes to cancer chemoprotection and drug resistance. *Crit Rev Biochem Mol Biol.* 1995;30(6):445–600.
77. Barahmani N, Carpentieri S, Li XN, et al. Glutathione S-Transferase M1 and T1 polymorphisms may predict adverse effects after therapy in children with medulloblastoma. *NeuroOncol.* 2009;11(3):292–300.
78. Duffner PK, Krischer JP, Sanford RA, et al. Prognostic factors in infants and very young children with intracranial ependymomas. *Pediatr Neurosurg.* 1998;28(4):215–222
79. KunLE, MulhernRK, Crisco JJ. Quality of life in children treated for brain tumors. Intellectual, emotional and academic function. *J Neurosurg.* 1983;58(1):1–6.
80. Carpentieri SC, Meyer EA, Delaney BL, et al. Psychosocial and behavioral functioning among pediatric brain tumor survivors. *J Neurooncol.* 2003;63(3):279–287.
81. Mitby PA, Robison LL, Whitton JA, et al. Childhood Cancer Survivor Study Steering Committee. Utilization of special education services and educational attainment among long-term survivors of childhood cancer: a report from the Childhood Cancer Survivor Study. *Cancer.* 2003;97(4):1115–1126.
82. Mulhern RK, Carpentieri SC, Shema S, Stone P, Fairclough D. Factors associated with social and behavioral problems among children recently diagnosed with brain tumor. *J Pediatr Psychol.* 1993;18(3):339–350.
83. Carpentieri SC, Mulhern RK, Douglas S, Hanna S, Fairclough D. Behavioral resiliency among children surviving brain tumors: A longitudinal study. *J Clin Child Psychol.* 1993;22(2):236–246.
84. Radcliffe J, Bennett D, Kazak AE, Phillips PC. Adjustment in childhood brain tumor survival: child, mother, and teacher report. *J Pediatr Psychol.* 1996;21(4):529–539.
85. Vannatta K, Gartstein MA, Short A, Noll RB. A controlled study of peer relationships of children surviving brain tumors: teacher, peer, and self ratings. *J Pediatr Psychol.* 1998;23(5):279–287.
86. Butler RW, Copeland DR. Attentional processes and their remediation in children treated for cancer: a literature review and the development of a therapeutic approach. *J Int Soc Neuropsychol.* 2002;8:115–124.
87. Butler RW, Haser JK. Neurocognitive effects of treatment for childhood cancer. *Ment Retard Dev Disabil Res Rev.* 2006;12(3):184–191.
88. Thompson SJ, Leigh L, Christensen R, et al Immediate neurocognitive effects of methylphenidate on learning-impaired survivors of childhood cancer. *J Clin Oncol.* 2001;19:1802–1808.

42 Rehabilitation of Central Nervous System Tumors

Subhadra L. Nori

Cancer is a disease process characterized by uncontrolled growth and spread of malignant cells. Although the exact etiology remains unclear, proposed modes include both internal and external factors such as chemicals, viruses, radiation exposure, hormones, and inherited mutations. The basic treatment of cancer consists of chemotherapy, radiation therapy, hormonal therapy, and immunotherapy. The American Cancer Society estimated that 18,500 malignant tumors of the brain and spinal cord have been reported during 2005. There were 10,620 men and 7880 women, of which 12,760 people died of their disease. Brain tumors account for 1.3% of cancer-related deaths.

OVERVIEW OF REHABILITATION

Physical Medicine and Rehabilitation (PMR) is a specialty that deals with disabilities, impairments, and handicaps that are a result of either acute or chronic diseases. According to 1980 World Health Organization classification, impairment is a physiological dysfunction or anatomic loss; disability is a functional consequence. Handicap is a physical condition that interferes with the patient's ability to lead a normal life in social, cultural, educational, or vocational pursuits. Handicap may prevent a person's full participation in personal relationships, family, and social roles.

In 1971, the National Cancer Act was introduced. Rehabilitation approaches were introduced as an objective in this legislation, which led to research and development. In 1972, the National Cancer Institute introduced four objectives at the National Cancer Rehabilitation Planning Conference, which consisted of the following:

1. Psychological support
2. Optimization of physical function
3. Vocational counseling
4. Optimization of social functioning

Cancer rehabilitation is a process that assists the patient in obtaining the above four goals, within the limits of the scope of the disease and/or its treatment consequences. In 1981, Dietz introduced the following goals to be included in the rehabilitation process: preventative, restorative, supportive, and palliative [1].

1. Preventative rehabilitation: Achievement of maximal function in patients with a good prognosis for cure or remission (e.g., respiratory therapy preoperatively and crutch walking instruction to an amputee).
2. Restorative rehabilitation: Restoration of previous functional status by means of therapeutic exercises, modalities, and devices.
3. Supportive rehabilitation: When no residual major disability is expected. Supportive rehabilitation can be offered to offset a steady decline in function, for example, provision of activities of daily living (ADL) devices, adaptive self-care equipment, range of motion (ROM) exercises, and so on.
4. Palliative rehabilitation: To maintain comfort and function during terminal stages of the disease. Periodic assessment of patients' progress and responses should be made. Appropriate goals should be selected at different stages of the disease. Especially with pediatric patients, family, parents, and close friends must be included in the instruction and treatment. Only by gaining the confidence of the patient, especially the young, can therapy be successful.

In 1978, Lehman et al [2] investigated a variety of cancers and found that more than 50% of patients had problems associated with PMR.

APPROACH TO REHABILITATION

As in any other disease process, cancer rehabilitation should be approached as a comprehensive multidisciplinary team process. The availability of professionals from various disciplines is crucial. Patients and family members must participate actively in this process. Together the team must approach the needs of the patients and family members in a realistic manner within the realm of cancer and its effects. An example of a typical team is as follows:

Physicians

Clinicians from several specialties, such as primary care medicine, neuro-oncology, oncology, neurology, neurosurgery, and surgical oncology make significant contributions to the care of the patient.

Physiatrist

A physiatrist is a PMR specialist, with specific training in the rehabilitation of various musculoskeletal diseases.

He or she serves as a liaison between the team members, such as physical therapy, occupational therapy, and speech therapy, thereby providing the leadership of patient management. In addition, a physiatrist also performs electrodiagnostic testing (e.g., electromyogram) to diagnose neuromuscular causes for weakness and numbness.

Nurse

Rehabilitation nurses are pivotal in cancer care. They provide interventions such as carryover of exercises, ADLs, mobility, self-care devices, speech, and swallowing techniques. They also provide emotional support for the family and patients. They are responsible for skin care, bladder and bowel management, and finally home care.

Social Worker/Case Manager

Social workers provide counseling, access to community resources, and financial assistance, and actively assist in discharge planning.

Psychologist

The psychologist assists patients in dealing with psychological stress. The psychologist's interventions help the patients overcome depression associated with the disease, thereby assisting their capability in making proper decisions.

Physical Therapist

Physical therapists assist in evaluating the patient's muscle strength, mobility, and joint ROM. They provide interventions that include therapeutic exercises and assistive devices for mobility training, such as crutches, walkers, and canes. They are also licensed to use various therapeutic modalities to control pain, for example, heat, cold, and therapeutic ultrasound.

Occupational Therapist

Occupational therapists evaluate the patient's ability to carry on self-care activities (i.e., ADLs), such as homemaking, dressing, bathing, and eating. They provide assistive and adaptive devices, such as weighted utensils, long-handled shoehorns; and driving with adaptive devices to make up for deficiencies with gross and fine motor hand coordination. They provide mobility devices such as wheelchairs when a patient loses hand function due to neurological or surgical consequences, and provide splinting to maintain hand function.

Dietician

A dietician addresses the nutritional requirements of the patient, such as nutritional supplements and alternative foods.

Speech Therapist

A speech therapist provides evaluation and treatment of disorders of speech and language for patients with brain tumors, head and neck cancers, and similar malignancies. They provide treatment for dysphasia, dysarthria, and aphasia. Speech communication defects due to laryngectomy can also be facilitated (e.g., by use of electrolarynx). Other methods such as esophageal and laryngeal speech are also taught to appropriate patients. In addition, speech therapists are important for the evaluation and treatment of swallowing disorders and dysphagia in selected patients.

Vocational Counselors

In some centers, vocational counselors assist patients in returning to their jobs or finding an alternative form of employment, if necessary.

COMMON FUNCTIONAL DEFICITS

Frontal Lobe Tumors

Patients with frontal lobe tumors present with variable slowing of fine motor coordination of the contralateral hand. Drawing a person, writing one's name, buttoning and unbuttoning one's shirt, and similar ADLs may be used to uncover and asses fine motor deficits. Primitive grasp and sucking reflexes may be noted with this syndrome. Dysphagia to liquids can be assessed during drinking of water. Patients with left-sided frontal lobe tumors can experience nonfluent dysphasia and apraxia of lip, tongue, or hand movements.

Temporal Lobe

Impairment in recent memory, homonymous quadrantanopsia, perceptual problems, and spatial disorientation can be seen. Fluent Wernicke-type aphasia is commonly seen when the dominant temporal lobe is involved.

Parietal Lobe

Sensory and perceptual functions are affected to a greater extent than motor functions. Hemianesthesia and hemisensory abnormalities occur with deep-seated tumors. Agnosia and dressing apraxia are also common.

Brainstem

Multiple cranial nerve abnormalities (typically contralateral to the motor deficits) associated with ataxia and hemiparesis comprise the presenting picture. Cranial nerve palsies may present as dysphagia, visual deficits, hearing loss, and facial numbness. When the brain is affected, headache, cognitive changes, gait abnormalities, seizures, nausea, and vomiting can be seen. Bilateral cortical dysfunction presents as cognitive changes. All of these symptoms are a result of increased intracranial pressure (ICP) and/or invasion of the brain and spinal cord.

DEFICITS RELATED TO TREATMENT

Steroids

High-dose steroids used to reduce brain edema of the brain may lead to many side effects, of which the one most pertaining to our field is proximal myopathy. Steroid-induced proximal myopathy may interfere with activities such as rising from a low chair, sofa, toilet seat, and so on. Therapeutic exercises and living modification such as a high toilet chair and high chair are beneficial. These symptoms are usually reversible.

Radiation Therapy

The typical dose is between 5000 and 6000 cGY. Symptoms such as loss of hair, transient worsening of neurological symptoms, nausea, vomiting, headache, and loss of taste are reported. Ten percent of long-term survivors may develop dementia and urinary incontinence. Long-term survivors may suffer from cognitive impairments.

Myelopathy

A transient myelopathy is known to occur in patients receiving radiotherapy to the spinal cord, typically developing after a latent period of 1 to 30 months, with a peak at 4 to 6 months after treatment. These symptoms subside quickly over the next 2 to 9 months [3]. The patient complains of an electric shock–like feeling radiating from the cervical spine downwards to the extremities (i.e., Lhermitte sign). These paresthesias are symmetrical and are caused by tension on demyelinated and hypersensitive fibers of the upper spinal cord.

Delayed radiation myelopathy is a permanent and irreversible condition that is reported in 1% to 12% of patients [4–6]. The onset is between 9 and 18 months after completion of treatment. The dose and schedule of radiotherapy seem not to have any bearing on this condition. With higher doses, the latent period can be shortened. Signs and symptoms may be acute or insidious and may include paresthesias in the lower extremities, sphincter dysfunction, partial Brown-Sequard syndrome, paraplegia, and quadriplegia. The posterior columns and superficial lateral tracts are involved. Vascular changes, including arteriolar necrosis and vascular occlusion, occur.

Endocrine Deficiencies

Endocrine deficiencies occur after radiation therapy for tumors of the central nervous system (CNS), especially when the treatment field involves the hypothalamic-pituitary axis. Growth hormone disorders are common if the ventro-medical nucleus of the hypothalamus, the site of growth hormone–releasing factor, is included in the treatment port. Irradiation may cause spinal column injury if administered during periods of rapid growth or during puberty; spinal deformities may be severe. Vertebral body deformities, such as kyphosis and scoliosis, may be noted.

Chemotherapy

A variety of different drugs and drug combinations have been shown to have activity in the treatment of brain tumors [7–11]. Active drugs include temozolomide, cisplatin, cyclophosphamide, vincristine, and methotrexate. Methotrexate may cause significant leukoencephalopathy, especially when used after radiation therapy. Chemotherapy-induced neuropathies are generally distal and symmetrical. Autonomic neuropathies are caused by vincristine and cisplatin and may be severe enough to mimic spinal cord involvement. Cytarabine (Ara-C) is also known to cause brachial plexopathy. Because of distal axonal degeneration, vincristine neuropathy tends to be prolonged. Sensory complaints of paresthesias, numbness, neuropathic pain, and foot drop have been associated with vincristine toxicity. Peripheral neuropathies and plexopathies are also a result of vincristine and cisplatin toxicity. Encephalopathies, cerebellar syndromes, myopathies, and stroke-like syndromes may also occur after the administration of various chemotherapeutic drugs.

Postsurgical Sequelae

Irritability, confusion, lethargy, and sometimes seizures are known to occur in the immediate postoperative phase. Postoperative neurologic morbidity may be correlated with the segment of spinal cord that is involved with the neoplasm. Dissection within the cervical spinal cord may be associated with significant morbidity. For example, anterior–horn cell dysfunction as evidenced by atrophy of the muscle groups of the upper extremity is not uncommon.

Tumors that are located in the lower spinal segments from T9 to T12 have the greatest incidence of postoperative neurologic morbidity. This is due to compression of regional gray matter. If the tumor extends into the conus medullas, significant postoperative sphincteric dysfunction follows. In patients who have undergone extensive laminectomy, postoperative muscle retraction, paraspinal muscle denervation, and spinal deformities may occur.

Remediation is provided via handling that incorporates stimulation of the cortical tracts involving the use of different tasks to improve visual perceptions. Early programmed activities designed to minimize inactivity and disuse, and to maintain proprioceptive and sensory stimuli should be started.

GENERAL EFFECTS OF CANCER ON FUNCTION

Cancer in itself causes weakness, pain, and lethargy, thereby making the patient prone to bed rest. The functional recovery is affected by metabolic and physiologic changes associated with prolonged bed rest. Bone loss leads to hypercalcemia. Muscle atrophy follows rapidly after bed rest, leading to an inability to walk. Changes in muscle physiology and fiber type have been documented. Pressure ulcers follow as a result of depletion of soft tissue. Bed rest alone depletes the patient's strength day by day in the immobilized parts; contractures may soon follow. Other medical complications, such as deep venous thrombosis and pulmonary embolus, are common. Another important impairment is pressure palsy. Peroneal mononeuropathy and ulnar mononeuropathy are commonly seen in cachectic patients on prolonged bed rest.

Joint Contractures

A majority of patients with cancer suffer from pain. To avoid the pain these patients tend to position their joints in a fixed way, which leads to the formation of joint contractures. Collagen fibers, ligaments, and tendons undergo a shortening contracture. Heel cords, hips, knees, elbows, and shoulders are the most common areas affected. Therapeutic exercises and joint ROM exercises should be prescribed for these patients. Other modalities, such as heat and cold, may be used to release these contractures. Motor point blocks with phenol have been helpful in some chronically contracted patients. Splinting of the upper extremity by an occupational therapist will help maintain the hand or foot in its proper anatomical position. Other orthotic devices are also used.

Bleeding Problems

Thrombocytopenia can be a side effect of both chemotherapy and radiotherapy. A platelet count below 10,000 mm^3 is hazardous because of potential intratumoral and intra-articular bleeding below this level. Exercise should be performed only under careful vigilance in patients with thrombocytopenia. Some centers do not allow any activity for platelet counts below 10,000 mm^3.

REHABILITATION INTERVENTIONS

Hemiparesis and Hemiplegia

Activities that enhance or maintain the musculoskeletal status of the affected side, including passive ROM, and positive and sensory education should be implemented by the therapist.

Facilitation techniques are used to promote motor recovery. Inhibition techniques discourage abnormal posturing and other unwanted reflex patterns commonly seen in upper motor neuron deficits. Ambulation training can be achieved by the use of pediatric walkers, crutches, canes, and wheelchairs.

Cognitive-Perceptual Interventions

Remediation is provided via handling that incorporates stimulation of the cortical tracts involving the use of different tasks to improve visual perceptions. Early programmed activities designed to minimize inactivity and disuse, and to maintain proprioceptive and sensory stimuli should be started.

Adaptive Equipment

The therapist should teach adaptive techniques and prescribe adaptive devices to support patient function. For example, a body jacket can be worn after surgical treatment of metastatic disease of the spine (see Figure 42.1). These adaptive aids include braces, dressers, reachers, dressing aids, and bathroom equipment. Positioning of upper extremities by means of slings, splints, and orthotic devices is important because these aids prevent contractures. Upper extremity orthotics may aid in substituting for lost function.

Therapeutic Exercises

These patients have increased metabolic demands and impaired protein-sparing mechanisms. Inactivity and the effect of chemotherapy and other treatment modalities further decrease lean body mass and muscle endurance. Therefore, any method that spares protein breakdown and enhances incorporation of protein into lean muscle is beneficial.

Lemon and colleagues found that 40% to 50% of submaximal exercise maintains nitrogen equilibrium [12]. High-intensity endurance programs with high Vo_2 max increase protein needs and therefore are unsuitable for cancer patients.

Carefully selected aerobic, ROM stretching, isokinetic, and isometric exercises can be used in patients with cancer. These exercises are generally safe. Some guidelines for precautions are given in Table 42.1.

Walkers are also available in lightweight models, with or without gliding devices, to allow a debilitated person to walk with a broad base of support. Adding weights to these walkers aids in the ambulation for patients with ataxia, by providing a fixed point of stability and proprioceptive feedback.

Spinal Cord Involvement

The degree of functional impairment usually corresponds to the level of spinal segment involvement as shown in Table 42.2. A patient with C5 quadriplegia will be able to bring food to the mouth, but needs assistance for most ADLs. A patient with C8-T1 quadriplegia will have intact hand function. For safe ambulation, the hip and knee extension

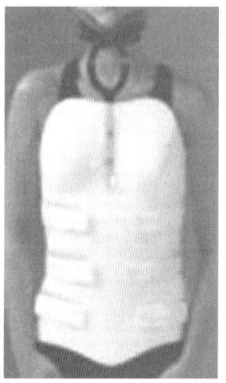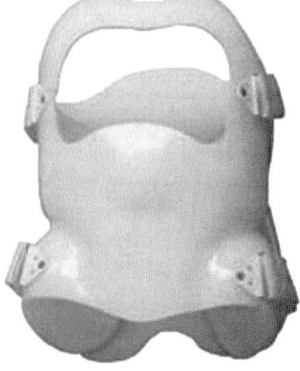

Figure 42.1 Body jacket. Provides external stability to the thoracic spine and chest.

Table 42.1 Exercise Guidelines and Precautions for Cancer Patients

Medical Problems	Laboratory Values	Recommendation
Thrombocytopenia		
Normal values	30,000–50,000 ml	Active exercise/ROM
Platelets 150,000–450,000/ml		Light weights (1–2 lb) (no heavy resistance/isokinetics)
		Ambulation
		Self-care activity
	20,000–30,000 ml	Gentle exercise (passive or active)
		Ambulation and self-care with assistance as needed for endurance/balance safety
	Less than 20,000 ml	Minimal or cautious exercise/activity
		Essential ADLs only
Anemia		
Normal values (6 m–6 y)	Hematocrit < 25%	Light ROM exercise, isometrics
Hematocrit 37–47%	Heomglobin < 8 g/dL	Avoid aerobic or progressive programs
Hemoglobin 12–16 g/dL	Hematocrit 25–35%	Essential ADLs: assistance as needed for safety
	Hemoglobin 8/10 g/dL	Light aerobics, light weights (1–2 lb)
	Hematocrit > 35%	Ambulation and self-care as tolerated
	Hemoglobin > 10 g/dL	Resistance exercise ambulation self-care as tolerated
Bony metastasis		
Plain X-ray findings	>50% cortex involved	No exercise
High risk indicated by the following:	25–50% cortex involved	Touch down: not weight-bearing, use crutches, walker
Cortical lesions > 2.5–3 cm		Active ROM exercise (no twisting)
>50% cortical involvement		No stretching
Painful lesions, unresponsive to radiation	0–25% cortex involved	Partial weight bearing
		Light aerobic exercise
		Avoid lifting/straining activity
		Full weight bearing
Pulmonary dysfunction		
Pulmonary function tests	<50% of predicted FEV_1 or diffusion capacity	No aerobic exercise
Chest radiograph	50–75% of predicted FEV_1 or diffusion capacity	Light aerobic exercise
	75% + of predicted FEV_1 or diffusion capacity	Most programs fine
	Large plural effusions or multiple	ROM
	Pericardial effusions or multiple	Few submaximal isometrics
	Metastases to lungs	Consult cardiologist and oncologist
Cardiac dysfunction		
Ejection fraction	Low	Low aerobics
Electrocardiogram	Recent premature ventricular contractions	No aerobics
	Fast atrial arrhythmia	Consult cardiologist
	Ventricular arrhythmia	
	Ischemic pattern	
Electrolyte abnormalities		
Na+ (133–148 mEq/L)	<130	No exercise requires treatment
K+ (3–6 mEq/L)	<3.0 (hypokalemic)	No exercise requires treatment
Ca^2 (8/8–10.4 mg/100 mL)	>6.0 (hyperkalemia)[a]	
Endocrine dysfunction		
Diabetes on insulin	Monitor carefully as exercise	
	May potentiate response to insulin	

[a] Often associated with arrhythmias and muscle weakness.

Abbreviations: ADL, activities of daily living; FEV_1, forced expiratory volume in 1 second; ROM, range of motion.

Adapted, with permission from Gerber LH. Rehabilitation of cancer patient. In: Devita VT, Hellman S, Rosenberg SA, eds. Cancer: Principles and Practice of Oncology. 5th ed. Philadelphia: Lippincott-Raven Publishers; 1997:table 56–15.

Table 42.2 Spinal Cord Levels: Functional Relationships

Level of Involvement	Intact Key Muscle	Function
C4	Neck muscles	Unassisted breathing
C5	Biceps	Able to bring hand to mouth
C6	Wrist extensors	Light grasp through tenodesis effect
C7	Elbow extensors	Lift self-weight
		Shift during transfers
C8T1	Hand intrinsics	Hand function
Lower thoracic	Hip-knee extensor	Ambulation possible with long leg brace
Lower lumbar	Ankle dorsiflexion	Ambulation with ankle-foot orthosis

strength should be at least 3/5. Extensive bracing crossing the knee should be avoided in the cancer patient, because the brace consumes a great deal of energy for ambulation, which will be taxing to the already debilitated person. Ankle-foot orthotics (see Figure 42.2) made of lightweight polypropylene or laminated plastic can be used in patients with lower extremity weakness. These devices provide stability to the ankle joint and may prevent falls.

Bladder Management

Spinal cord damage results in either upper motor neuron bladder or lower motor neuron bladder dysfunction,

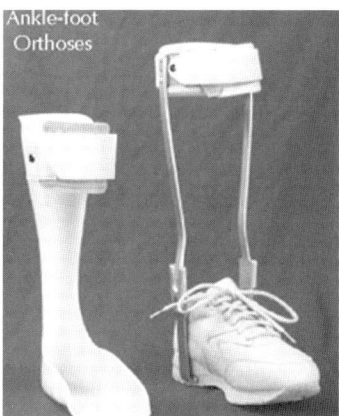

Figure 42.2 Ankle-foot orthotics. Provides stability to ankle joint, aids in propulsion, and prevents falls in patients with a foot drop.

depending on the level of involvement. In a flaccid or lower motor neuron bladder, the goal should be to keep the bladder as empty as possible to avoid infection caused by retention of urine, as well as hydronephrosis and pyelonephrosis.

As early as possible the patient and family members should be taught intermittent catherization, as frequently as every 3 to 4 hours. Other methods, such as manipulation, can also be taught. Outlet obstruction can be managed by an adrenergic blocking agent, such as phenoxybenzamine. A parasympathomimetic agent may be of use in cases of flaccid bladder. A patient with both flaccid bladder and outlet obstruction may need both medications. Consultation with a urologist may be necessary in a patient who requires urodynamic evaluation. If all else fails, a suprapubic cystostomy or intraurethral resection or external sphincterotomy may become necessary. By keeping the urine pH acidic, stone promotion and infection can be avoided.

Bowel Management

Bowel management can be instituted by the use of laxative stool softeners, and bulking agents. A selected time either in the morning or in the evening after food intake makes use of the gastrocolic reflex and establishes a bowel regimen.

Spasticity

Spasticity is a disabling component of many nervous system diseases including brain tumors, cerebral palsy, traumatic encephalopathy with spinal cord involvement, congenital abnormalities, and degenerative disorders of the CNS. Spasticity is defined as a velocity-dependent increase in resistance to passive stretch seen in concert with the other components of the upper motor neuron syndrome [13,14].

Spasticity has been of interest for more than 100 years. Because it can cause disabling impairments in function, patients experience muscle tone abnormalities coupled with shortening contractures of the joints. This may lead

Table 42.3 Ashworth Scale

Grade	
1	No increased tone
2	Slightly increased tone, manifested by a catch and release or minimal resistance when the affected part is moved in flexion or extension
3	Marked increase in tone through most of ROM, but affected parts are easily moved
4	Considerable increase in tone; passive movement is difficult
5	Affected parts rigid in flexion and extension

Abbreviation: ROM, range of motion.

Table 42.4 Assistance Scale

Grade	
5	Maintains independently without assistance
4	Maintains with unilateral upper extremity support or requires intermittent contact by therapist for balance only
3	Maintains with bilateral upper extremity support or requires constant contact by therapist for balance only
2	Full external support of one person
1	Cannot be placed

to progressive joint subluxation and dislocations. Whether or not spasticity needs to be treated depends on its effect on functional impairment. In many cases, although clinically present spasticity may contribute very little to the patient's disability, elimination of spasticity may not provide a functional advantage. Evaluation of spasticity may be performed using the Ashworth Scale (see Table 42.3) or the Assistance Scale (see Table 42.4).

Treatment

A wide variety of options are available for the treatment of generalized spasticity; physical therapists utilize manual stretching, serial casting, and tone reduction techniques. Occupational therapists provide assistive devices and splinting.

Drug therapy using Baclofen orally and even intrathecally via an infusion pump is now a common clinical practice. Baclofen inhibits both monosynaptic and polysynaptic reflexes at the spinal level, and decreases excitatory neurotransmitter release from the primary afferent terminal. Dantrolene reduces muscle action potential–induced release of calcium into the sacroplasmic reticulum, decreasing the force produced by excitation-contraction coupling. Liver toxicity is a potential side effect. Other medication such as benzodiazepines and trizanadines are also useful.

For more focal areas with spasticity, botox injections, musculocutaneous blocks, and phenol blocks with 2% to 6% aqueous phenol solutions may be considered. Surgical procedures, such as selective dorsal rhizotomy, may offer permanent alleviation of spasticity. The SPlit Anterior Tibial Transfer (SPLATT) procedure consists of splitting the anterior tibialis tendon, distally, which is then tunneled and attached to the third cuneiform and cuboid bones. This provides eversion, thus giving a solid platform. Achilles tendon lengthening is conjointly performed, thus reducing toe pointing equinus posture. This can dramatically improve the gait of a hemiplegic patient.

Functional Outcomes

Several studies have been published on functional outcomes of patients with brain and spinal cord tumors [15,16]. The three most common brain tumors have been found to be glioblastoma, meningioma, and astrocytoma. Patients with low-grade gliomas survived 5 to 8 years. Those with high-grade gliomas had a short survival time of 9 to 18 months. Huang and coworkers compared brain tumors to strokes. No statistically significant differences were seen in functional independence measures (FIM). Another study by O'Dell et al compared patients with tumors and traumatic brain injury, with similar results.

Outcomes for Patients with Malignant Epidural Cord Compression

Catz et al [17] discovered that the most important criterion was the level of ambulation at the time of admission, which correlates closely with final outcome. Those who were ambulatory at admission remained so at discharge. In a study by Hirabayashi et al [18], factors that affected survival after surgery included pretreatment neurologic status, the most important factor being the primary tumors site. Increased susceptibility to infection, bed sores, and immobility related comorbidities contribute to shorter survival. The survival time was longer in patients who could walk after surgery than those who could not. Symptoms of even minor signs of cord compression should be followed immediately by imaging studies. If cord compression is diagnosed early, treated outcomes are better. McKinley and colleagues found that nontraumatic spinal cord injury patients present with less severe neurologic impairment compared with traumatic spinal cord injury patients [19]. These patients are usually older than 50 years. Despite the age, these patients were able to be discharged to their home. He also reported that neoplastic cord injury had a significantly lower length of stay than traumatic injury; however, their FIM scores were lower. The median survival of these patients was 11 months after onset of neurological symptoms. The outcome depended on FIM scores at admission, tumor type, and level of the lesion. Eriks et al [20] found that patients with epidural spinal cord compressions were admitted for less time than those with spinal cord compression due to other causes. Patients with epidural metastasis survived longer. One year after discharge, 52% of these patients were still alive, with an average survival duration of 1472 days.

SUMMARY

Patients suffering from CNS malignancy not only suffer from the effects of the tumor and its location, but also from the consequences of its treatment. Other factors including cognitive impairment, fatigue, and psychological consequences, such as depression and the fear of death, may lead to poor participation in therapy. Therefore, the rehabilitation process should be a team approach working with not only the patient, but also all of the family members.

Timely diagnosis of deficits and consequences of treatment should be identified. Proper orthotic devices should be designed and encouragement should be provided to use them since the usage of these devices may prevent further progression and prevent potential complications, such as fractures in a patient with spinal metastasis. The approach should be practical and realistic. As more cancers are diagnosed at earlier stages, more survivors are seen today than ever before; therefore, rehabilitation interventions may improve functional outcomes.

REFERENCES

1. Dietz JH. *Rehabilitation Oncology.* New York, NY: John Wiley & Sons; 1981.
2. Lehmann JF, Delisa JA, Warren CG, et al. Cancer rehabilitation: assessment of need, development and evaluation of a model of care. *Arch Phys Med Rehabil.* 1978;59(9):410–419.
3. Leibel SA, Guten PH, Davis RL. Tolerance of the brain and spinal cord. In: Guten PH, ed. *Radiation Injury to the Nervous System.* New York, NY: Raven Press; 1991:239–256.
4. Albers JW. Adverse effects of antineoplastic therapy on peripheral nervous system. *Am Assoc Electromyography Electrodiag.* 1983;C:37–47.
5. Schulthesis TE, El-Mahdi AM. Statistical analysis of two hundred radiation myelopathy cases. *Proc 7th Int Cong Radiat Res.* 1983;D:3–41.
6. Garden FH. Radiation injury to the spinal cord and peripheral nerves. *Phys Med Rehabil State Art Rev.* 1994;8:405–411.
7. Wheeler JS Jr, Siroky MB, Bell R, et al. Vincristine-induced bladder neuropathy. *J Urol.* 1982;130(2):342.
8. Rosenfeld CS, Broden LE. Cisplatin-induced autonomic neuropathy. *Cancer Treat Rep.* 1984;68(4):659.
9. Raphaelson MI, Steven JC, Newman RP. Vincristine neuropathy with bowel and bladder atony, mimicking spinal cord compression. *Cancer Treat Rep.* 1983;67(6):604.
10. Salner AL, Botnick LE, Herzog AG, et al. Revisable brachial plexopathy following radiation therapy for breast cancer. *Cancer Treat Rep.* 1981;65(9–10):797.
11. Forman A. Peripheral neuropathy in cancer patients: clinical types, etiology, and presentation. *Oncology.* 1990;4:85–89.
12. Lemon PWR, Dolly DG, Yaraseske KE. Effect of intensity on protein utilization during prolonged exercise (abstract). *Med Sci Sports Exerc.* 1984;16:157.
13. Young RR. The physiology of spasticity and its response to therapy. *Ann NY Acad Sci.* 1988;531:146.
14. Katz RT. Management of spasticity. *Am J Phys Med Rehabil.* 1988;67(3):108.
15. Huang ME, Cifu DX, Keyser-Marcus L. Functional outcome after brain tumor and acute stroke: a comparative analysis. *Arch Phys Med Rehabil.* 1998;79(11):1386–1390.
16. O'Dell MW, Barr K, Spanier D, Warnick RE. Functional outcome of inpatient rehabilitation in persons with brain tumors. *Arch Phys Med Rehabil.* 1998;79(12):1530–1534.
17. Catz A, Goldin D, Fishel B, et al. Recovery of neurologic function following nontraumatic spinal cord lesions in Israel. *Spine.* 2004;29(20):2278–2282; discussion 2283.
18. Hirabayashi H, Ebara S, Kinoshita T, et al. Clinical outcome and survival after palliative surgery for spinal metastases: palliative surgery in spinal metastases. *Cancer.* 2003;97(2):476–484.
19. McKinley WO, Huang ME, Tewksbury MA. Neoplastic vs. traumatic spinal cord injury:an inpatient rehabilitation comparison. *Am J Phys Med Rehabil.* 2000;79(2):138–144.
20. Eriks IE, Angenot EL, Lankhorst GJ. Epidural metastatic spinal cord compression: functional outcome and survival after inpatient rehabilitation. *Spinal Cord.* 2004;42(4):235–239.

43 Palliative Care in Neuro-Oncology

Nina D. Wagner-Johnston and Stuart A. Grossman

INTRODUCTION

Palliative care is comprehensive care, which encompasses the patient's physical, psychological, and social domains and is ultimately aimed at maximizing quality of life for patients and their families. Palliative care generally refers to any form of medical care or treatment that concentrates on reducing the severity of disease symptoms rather than providing a cure. This was recently described in a WHO statement as "an approach that improves the quality of life of patients and their families facing the problems associated with life-threatening illness." In some cases, palliative treatments may be used to alleviate the side effects of curative treatments, such as relieving the nausea associated with chemotherapy. Although the concept of palliative care is not new, physicians have traditionally concentrated on aggressively trying to cure patients. However, over the past 20 years the focus on a patient's quality of life has gained substantial ground. In this chapter, special attention will be given to the unique features of palliative care as they relate directly to patients with neuro-oncologic disorders.

TUMOR-RELATED SIDE EFFECTS

The most common symptoms observed in patients with primary or metastatic brain tumors are related to increased intracranial pressure (ICP) or site-specific symptoms related to the location of the tumor. Increased ICP usually occurs as a result of the expanding tumor mass and the associated peritumoral edema. Occasionally symptoms will rapidly progress if there is an acute hemorrhage into the tumor or if the tumor or edema compresses cerebrospinal fluid (CSF) flow pathways leading to the development of acute hydrocephalus. Increased ICP may result in headache, drowsiness, visual deficits, nausea, vomiting, nuchal rigidity, and occasional sixth nerve palsy. Site-specific symptoms vary by tumor location and can include motor, sensory, visual, language, speech, hearing, balance, gait, and memory disturbances.

Headache is the most common nonspecific symptom in patients with high-grade gliomas occurring as the initial symptom in more than 40% of patients. These are often intermittent, deep, pressure-like and are typically worse in the morning and improve during the day. Drowsiness and psychomotor retardation are also frequent manifestations of increased ICP. These are frequently characterized by an inability to complete routine tasks, faulty insight, emotional lability, forgetfulness, and may degenerate into frank confusion and dementia. Generalized and focal seizures are common and may result from increased ICP, local irritation of neural tissue by the tumor or resultant brain edema, or a combination of both.

Site-specific symptoms result from compression or destruction of functional brain or nerves exiting from the central nervous system. Frontoparietal lesions are often associated with motor and sensory losses, inferior frontal or posterior parietotemporal lesions may result in expressive or receptive language dysfunction, posterior fossa lesions produce ataxia and gait disturbances, frontal and temporal lesions are often associated with apathy, personality changes, and memory loss, while bifrontal lesions can cause urinary incontinence.

Spinal lesions may result in pain and neurologic deficits related to the location of the tumor in the spinal cord. Paralysis below the level of involvement and bladder and bowel incontinence are frequent complications of progressing spinal malignancies. Leptomeningeal involvement by cancer frequently presents with headaches and nuchal rigidity that can occur with obstruction of CSF flow pathways and the resultant increased ICP or from direct invasion of the pial surfaces. In addition, seizures and focal neurologic deficits, including cranial neuropathies, are common in patients with neoplastic meningitis.

Palliation of the above symptoms can be challenging. Surgery is often very effective at debulking tumor or evacuating an intratumoral hematoma with the resultant rapid resolution of increased ICP. Similarly acute hydrocephalus can be rapidly alleviated if tumor debulking opens a compressed CSF flow pathway (ie, the 4th ventricle in a patient with a cerebellar tumor) or if the CSF is drained externally (eg, ventriculo-peritoneal shunt). Dexamethasone is also effective at reducing increased ICP by restoring the integrity of the blood-brain barrier and thereby reducing the flow of serum proteins and the associated influx of water into brain parenchyma. Patients with significant T2 or fluid-attenuated inversion recovery abnormalities on magnetic resonance imaging scans are most likely to respond to dexamethasone. The maximum effect of glucocorticoids occurs in 5 to 7 days. As a result, symptomatic patients are often given high doses of dexamethasone initially to determine if this approach will be useful and to reverse symptoms as soon as possible. The dose is thereafter tapered as tolerated. Severe headaches due to increased ICP are often best treated with surgery or dexamethasone for the reasons stated above. Although not preferred, conventional analgesics may be necessary for palliation while awaiting a response from the steroids, or in situations where surgery and/or dexamethasone are not options or are ineffective. Anticonvulsants are indicated in patients who have had focal or generalized seizures but are not recommended prophylactically. Anticonvulsants that induce hepatic P450 enzymes have been shown to dramatically affect the metabolism of many chemotherapeutic agents. Therefore these are not recommended as first-line therapy in patients who are likely to be treated with chemotherapy.

TREATMENT-RELATED SIDE EFFECTS

Antineoplastic therapies administered to patients with neoplasms of the central nervous system can result in complications that can severely affect a patient's quality of life. Surgical complications can result in strokes, bleeds, infections, or neurologic deficits from operating in eloquent brain. These may require reoperation, intensive rehabilitation, or antibiotics. Radiation will cause alopecia within the treatment field and often results in significant fatigue that can be severe enough to generate excessive somnolence that may last for weeks. Patients frequently complain of a loss of appetite and food tasting "different" during and after radiation. In addition, radiation therapy frequently injures the blood-brain barrier resulting in more edema, mass effect, and symptoms relating to this. This is frequently reflected in magnetic resonance imaging scans done after radiation therapy, which generally show increased contrast enhancement, T2/fluid attenuated inversion recovery signal, and mass effect. Symptoms related to this occur most commonly toward the completion of radiation to the brain, often last for 3 months or more, and frequently require increased glucocorticoid doses to control the associated symptoms.

The most commonly prescribed chemotherapeutic agent to patients with brain tumors is temozolomide. This agent is associated with modest nausea and vomiting that is generally well controlled with modern antiemetics. Its dose-limiting toxicity is myelosuppression, which occurs in about 20% of patients receiving daily temozolomide (75 mg/m^2/day) during the 6 weeks of radiation therapy. The associated thrombocytopenia can be severe requiring platelet transfusions for months in approximately 5% of patients. Temozolomide has also been associated with significant immunosuppression and as a result prophylaxis against *Pneumocystis jiroveci* pneumonia is recommended with its use.

Many patients remain dependent on glucocorticoids for long periods of time. The side effects associated with steroids are often more troublesome than the toxicities of the chemotherapy. The immunosuppressive and antipyretic effects of these agents can lead to serious infectious complications. Acneiform rash, weight gain, fluid retention, and changes in body habitus can affect a patient's self-image. One of the most disabling complications is a proximal myopathy that can lead to falls and inactivity. Early enrollment in a physical therapy program may prevent or delay the onset. Suggestions that uncontrolled hyperglycemia may be associated with worse cancer outcomes underscores the need to emphasize improved glycemic control [1].

DYSPNEA

Unlike many other malignancies where the onset of dyspnea is frequently associated with disease progression, dyspnea in the neuro-oncology patient is most frequently caused by pulmonary embolism. Advanced age, large tumor size, leg paresis, and ABO blood group have been identified as risk factors for venous thromboembolism in patients with malignant gliomas [2–4]. Although concerns for the risk of intracranial bleeding with anticoagulation are real, treatment with heparin and warfarin are usually well tolerated by these patients and venal caval filters are rarely required. The platelet count should be maintained at 50,000/μL during anticoagulation therapy. *P jiroveci* pneumonia should also be on the differential when a patient presents with dyspnea. Patients treated with temozolomide, radiation, and steroids have dramatically reduced CD4 counts explaining their susceptibility to *P jiroveci* pneumonia [5,6]. Since the mortality rate even with appropriate therapy approaches 50%, prophylaxis is strongly encouraged.

Education about the expected breathing patterns in the patient's final hours will help prepare the family so that the experience may not be quite so distressful. The "death rattle," often present in the final hours of life, is caused by pooling of secretions in the trachea and larynx. Treating with anticholinergics and withholding parenteral fluids will prevent the production of new secretions.

DELIRIUM

Terminal delirium, often associated with hallucinations, is common in cancer patients and particularly problematic in the neuro-oncology patient. Subclinical seizures and adverse reactions to medications, including steroids, antiepileptics, and opioids should be considered. Delirium frequently worsens at night. Reinforcing the sleep-wake cycle, providing a familiar environment, and eliminating unnecessary sedating medications will decrease the intensity of delirium. Neuroleptics are also effective for the treatment of delirium and terminal restlessness [7,8].

CARE OF THE DYING PATIENT

The end of life can be difficult for this patient population. Patients may be unable to communicate their needs or feelings. Progressive confusion, disorientation, and somnolence are common and many patients are distraught by their extraordinary dependence. The vast majority of patients experience mild depressive symptoms [9]. Demoralized patients do not typically require treatment with antidepressants though appropriate referrals for counseling may be beneficial [10].

Many patients become increasingly lethargic and die peacefully. However, headaches, nausea, and vomiting from increased ICP, seizures, and bedsores are not infrequent. Controlling the symptoms of increased ICP and prevention of seizures are paramount during this phase of the illness. Increasing doses of glucocorticoids may transiently reduce ICP but could also prolong the illness.

With increasing sedation, patients may have difficulty swallowing. Gastrostomy tube placements and parenteral nutrition can assist in sustaining nutrition but are associated with significant discomfort and risks of complications. The routine use of enteral or parenteral nutrition for quality of life or survival in these scenarios is not supported by evidence [11]. These alternatives might be considered, however, as a means for administering glucocorticoids and antiepileptics if alternate routes are not feasible.

END-OF-LIFE PLANNING

Hospice

Hospice is a program designed to provide comprehensive, multidisciplinary care for patients at the end of their lives. Eligibility under the Medicare Hospice Benefit includes a physician-certified expected prognosis of less than 6 months and treatment that is oriented toward quality of life [12]. Most hospice care is provided at home although it can also be delivered in the nursing home setting when long-term care is needed. Hospice does not provide 24-hour care. Inpatient hospices are available for patients who have active symptom management needs or are actively dying. When considering hospice, it is helpful to review the ongoing treatments in efforts to both minimize family caregiving burden and maximize the benefit-risk ratio of the current interventions. In the neuro-oncology patient, physicians are confronted with the difficult decision of when to discontinue corticosteroids. In the setting of irreversible altered consciousness, steroids may simply prolong a burdensome situation.

Caregiver Issues

The natural history of most primary brain tumors heralds devastating changes for patients and their families. Many patients present with seizures or visual impairment and are unable to drive a car from the time they are diagnosed with the illness. Others cannot dress, walk, eat, or bathe independently. Cognitive deficits, expressive and receptive aphasias, short-term memory deficits, motor deficits, and a propensity to fall can make it impossible for some patients to remain unsupervised for even short periods of time. The sudden and extreme dependence on family and friends, along with the potential loss of mental function and communicative capacity place great stresses on patients and their families. Caregivers often need to adjust their work schedules to provide care. These circumstances often lead to significant financial hardships. As a result, patients and families must have a broad range of medical and social support services. Caregivers report feeling alone in their decisions and ill prepared for the tasks assumed [13]. Symptoms including stress, lack of sleep, feeling overwhelmed, and contemplating suicide require specific management [14]. Following death, the caregiver is faced with readjusting to life without their loved one. His or her previously developed sense of purpose may be in question and the transition to a redefined role is difficult. Family-focused grief therapy may assist in preventing maladaptive grieving [15,16].

CONCLUSION

Caring for patients with neuro-oncologic disorders is complex often requiring multidisciplinary input. The progressive loss of neurologic function and the management of seizures are often of major concern to patients and family members. Optimal palliation requires that the etiology for each tumor or treatment-related symptom be assessed to prescribe appropriate interventions. The role of caregivers in this patient population is critical given the many challenges confronting a patient dying of a brain tumor. Mindfulness of the extreme burden on the caregiver and provision of psychosocial support is key. Embracing these challenges and providing excellent palliative care can be one of the most rewarding aspects of treating patients with neuro-oncologic disorders.

REFERENCES

1. Richardson LC, Pollack LA. Therapy insight: Influence of type 2 diabetes on the development, treatment and outcomes of cancer. *Nat Clin Pract Oncol.* 2005;2(1):48–53.
2. Ruff RL, Posner JB. Incidence and treatment of peripheral venous thrombosis in patients with glioma. *Ann Neurol.* 1983;13(3):334–336.
3. Sawaya R, Zuccarello M, Elkalliny M, Nishiyama H. Postoperative venous thromboembolism and brain tumors: part I. Clinical profile. *J Neurooncol.* 1992;14(2):119–125.
4. Streiff MB, Segal J, Grossman SA, Kickler TS, Weir EG. ABO blood group is a potent risk factor for venous thromboembolism in patients with malignant gliomas. *Cancer.* 2004;100(8):1717–1723.
5. Stupp R, Dietrich PY, Ostermann Kraljevic S, et al. Promising survival for patients with newly diagnosed glioblastoma multiforme treated with concomitant radiation plus temozolomide followed by adjuvant temozolomide. *J Clin Oncol.* 2002;20(5):1375–1382.
6. Hughes MA, Parisi M, Grossman S, Kleinberg L. Primary brain tumors treated with steroids and radiotherapy: low CD4 counts and risk of infection. *Int J Radiat Oncol Biol Phys.* 2005;62(5):1423–1426.
7. Lacasse H, Perreault MM, Williamson DR. Systematic review of antipsychotics for the treatment of hospital-associated delirium in medically or surgically ill patients. *Ann Pharmacother.* 2006;40(11):1966–1973.
8. Kehl KA. Treatment of terminal restlessness: a review of the evidence. *J Pain Palliat Care Pharmacother.* 2004;18(1):5–30.
9. Litofsky NS, Farace E, Anderson F Jr, Meyers CA, Huang W, Laws ER Jr. Depression in patients with high-grade glioma: results of the Glioma Outcomes Project. *Neurosurgery.* 2004;54(2):358–366; discussion 66–67.
10. Coyne JC, Palmer SC, Shapiro PJ. Prescribing antidepressants to advanced cancer patients with mild depressive symptoms is not justified. *J Clin Oncol.* 2004;22(1):205–206; author reply 6–8.
11. Dy SM. Enteral and parenteral nutrition in terminally ill cancer patients: a review of the literature. *Am J Hosp Palliat Care.* 2006;23(5):369–377.
12. Gazelle G. Understanding hospice—an underutilized option for life's final chapter. *N Engl J Med.* 2007;357(4):321–324.

13. Teschendorf B, Schwartz C, Ferrans CE, O'Mara A, Novotny P, Sloan J. Caregiver role stress: when families become providers. *Cancer Control.* 2007;14(2):183–189.
14. Deeken JF, Taylor KL, Mangan P, Yabroff KR, Ingham JM. Care for the caregivers: a review of self-report instruments developed to measure the burden, needs, and quality of life of informal caregivers. *J Pain Symptom Manage.* 2003;26(4):922–953.
15. Cherlin EJ, Barry CL, Prigerson HG, et al. Bereavement services for family caregivers: how often used, why, and why not. *J Palliat Med.* 2007;10(1):148–158.
16. Kissane DW, McKenzie M, Bloch S, Moskowitz C, McKenzie DP, O'Neill I. Family focused grief therapy: a randomized, controlled trial in palliative care and bereavement. *Am J Psychiatry.* 2006;163(7):1208–1218.

44 Imaging of Brain Tumors

Yair Safriel and Volker Wilhelm Walter Stieber

INTRODUCTION

The uses of imaging in brain tumor evaluation include diagnostic assessment, differentiation of tumor and adjacent functional brain, localization for surgery and radiation therapy treatment planning, differentiation of radiation necrosis and tumor necrosis, and assessment of treatment response. Future roles may include grading and predicting outcomes.

COMPUTED TOMOGRAPHY

In a modern spiral (helical) computed tomography (CT) scan, the patient is moved through a rotating, continuous fan-beam exposure, and a block of data in the form of a corkscrew or helix is obtained. High heat–capacity X-ray tubes, subsecond tube rotation times, sophisticated detector technologies, and real-time image reconstruction computer hardware and software allow rapid, large-volume, multi-image acquisition. CT does not have the same degree of soft-tissue resolution of brain parenchyma as magnetic resonance imaging (MRI) but its ability to depict blood and calcium, as well as the ventricular system, is useful for rapid assessment in the unstable patient. Once the patient's condition has stabilized, the brain imaging modality of choice is MRI of the brain with and without gadolinium enhancement. Patients with contraindications to MRI, such as severe claustrophobia, a pacemaker, or severe obesity, may have to undergo a contrast-enhanced CT scan instead of MRI.

MAGNETIC RESONANCE IMAGING

One or more orthogonal magnetic field gradients are imposed upon the patient while exciting nuclear spins with radiofrequency (RF) pulses. The image is formed primarily on the basis of the nuclear magnetic resonance (NMR) signal from the protons of water. Signal intensity is a function of the water concentration and relaxation times (T1 and T2). Paramagnetic metal ions, as a result of their unpaired electrons, act as MRI contrast agents by decreasing the T1 and T2 relaxation times of nearby water protons. If the time between successive scans is short, regions associated with a Gd+++ ion appear bright when water appears as a dark background.

For both benign and malignant central nervous system (CNS) tumors, MRI is the gold standard for imaging [1]. T1-weighted images with intravenous contrast provide excellent visualization of contrast-enhancing tumors such as meningiomas, glioblastomas, and brain metastases. T2-weighted images generally demonstrate areas of edema, and T1-weighted fluid attenuation inversion recovery (FLAIR) images better delineate infiltration by low- or high-grade gliomas. Table 44.1 summarizes some distinctive findings useful in the diagnosis of a variety of CNS tumors. In radiation therapy, treatment planning MRI registration with the treatment planning CT scan is essential for target definition [2–4].

MRI of the entire neural axis is required for the staging of tumors with a high propensity for spread within the CNS by involvement of the cerebrospinal fluid (CSF), leptomeninges (i.e., coverings of the brain), or spinal cord. In the initial evaluation of a patient with suspected metastatic spinal cord compression it is critical to image the entire spine, as 25% of these patients have spinal cord compression verified at multiple levels by MRI, and approximately two-thirds of these have involvement of different regions of the spine [5]. In addition, a sensory level present on patient evaluation may be two or more segments different from the actual lesion on MRI in 28% of patients, and four or more levels distant from the lesion in 21% of patients [5].

Additional imaging studies that can reflect the biologic characteristics of tumors, such as metabolism, proliferation, oxygenation, and blood flow, as well as the function of surrounding the normal brain include diffusion weighted imaging (DWI), diffusion tensor imaging (DTI), perfusion imaging, magnetic resonance spectroscopy (MRS), and functional MRI (fMRI). After radiation therapy, positron emission tomography (PET) scans and MRI spectroscopy may assist in differentiating active tumor from radionecrosis.

Diffusion Weighted Imaging

DWI is dependent on the movement of protons in water. It attempts to quantify cellularity based on the premise that water diffusivity within the extracellular compartment is inversely related to the content and attenuation of the constituents of the intracellular space. DWI in brain tumors putatively assesses cellularity and therefore indirectly

Table 44.1 Distinctive Image Findings by Tumor Type

Tumor	Location (Most Frequent)	CT	Edema	Well vs. Poorly Circumscribed	Homo- vs. Heterogeneous Signal Intensity	MRI T1	T2	Contrast Enhancement	Other
Pilocytic astrocytoma (WHO grade I) (Figure 44.1)	Cerebellum Thalamus Third ventricle		Minimal	Well		Hypointense cysts	Hyperintense cysts	Intense nodules	
Subependymal giant cell astrocytoma (WHO grade I) (Figure 44.2)	Lateral ventricle near foramen of Monro				Heterogeneous		Hypointense	Yes	
Pleomorphic xanthoastrocytoma (WHO grade I) (Figure 44.3)	Temporal Parieto-occipital					Hypo- to isointense	Hyperintense	Yes	
Astrocytoma (WHO grade II) (Figures 44.4 and 44.5)		50% have calcification		Well	Homogeneous	Hypointense	Hyperintense	No	
Anaplastic astrocytoma (WHO grade III) (Figures 44.6 and 44.7)			Moderate	Intermediate	Heterogeneous	Heterogeneous	Heterogeneous		
Brainstem glioma (Figure 44.8)	pons > midbrain > medulla			Either		Hypointense	Hyperintense	Usually not	
Glioblastoma multiforme (WHO grade IV) (Figure 44.9)			Significant	Poorly		Heterogeneous	Heterogeneous (better defined with T2 FLAIR)	Yes	Hemorrhage
Oligodendroglioma (Figures 44.10 and 44.11)	Frontal Temporal	Calcification Calvarial erosion	Significant in high-grade	Low-grade: well High-grade: poorly	Heterogeneous	Isointense	Hyperintense	50% demonstrate faint enhancement	Often extend to cortical surface
Medulloblastoma (Figure 44.12)	Midline in young lateral in adults			Well	Homogeneous	Hyperintense	Isointense to gray matter		Cysts & necrosis more common in adults
Ependymoma (Figure 44.13)	Posterior fossa in children Spinal cord in adults	50% have calcifications	Mild		Both	Hypo- to isointense	Hyperintense	Yes	Cysts more common in supratentorial
Ganglioglioma & gangliocytoma (Figure 44.14)	Temporal Parieto-occipital also thalamic, cerebellar, optic nerve	Calcifications		Well		Hyperintense	Hyperintense	Yes, solid component	Cystic component common
Meningioma (Figure 44.15)	Extra-axial, dural-based	Hyperostosis	Variable	WHO Gr I-II: well WHO Gr III: poorly	Homogeneous	Hypo- to isointense	Isointense	Yes	Dural tail
Craniopharyngioma (Figure 44.16)	(supra-)sellar	Calcifications Enlarged sella		Well		Hypointense to isointense	Hyperintense	Yes, solid component	
Hemangioblastoma (Figure 44.17)	Posterior fossa		Little	Well		Isointense	Hyperintense	Yes, solid component	Small solid nodule Large cyst
Primary CNS lymphoma (Figures 44.18 and 44.20)	Immunocompetent: single peripheral lesion Immunosuppressed: multiple deep lesions		Yes	Either	Homogeneous	Hypo- to isointense	Hyperintense	Intense	

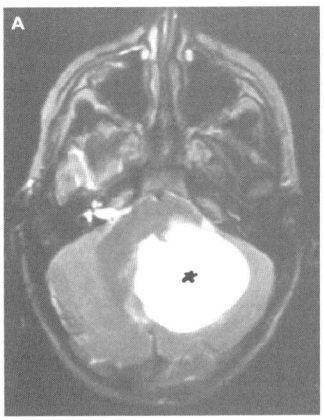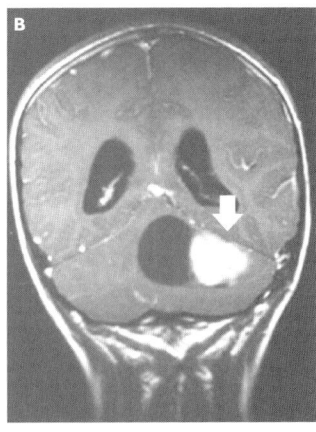

Figure 44.1 Pilocytic astrocytoma: Axial FLAIR **(A)** and postcontrast T1 coronal **(B)** images show a pilocytic astrocytoma with a typical T2 hyperintense/T1 hypointense cyst (asterisk) and an enhancing nodule (arrow). Hemangioblastoma is the primary imaging differential diagnosis.

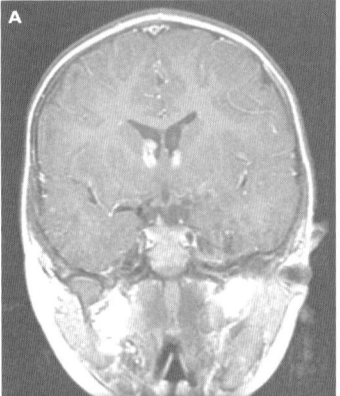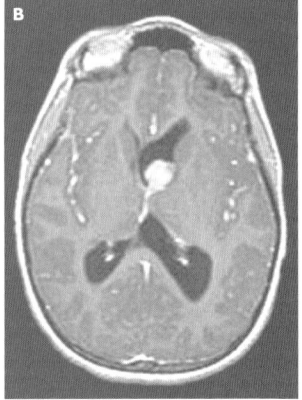

Figure 44.2 Subependymal giant cell astrocytoma. **(A)** Post contrast T1 coronal image show bilateral tumors in a patient with tuberous sclerosis. **(B)** Axial post-contrast T1 image shows left sided tumor.

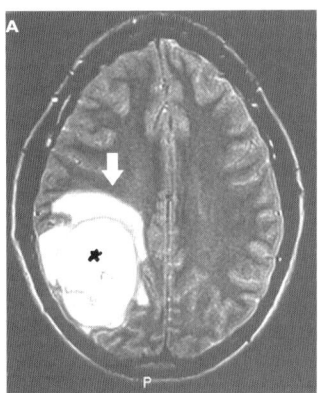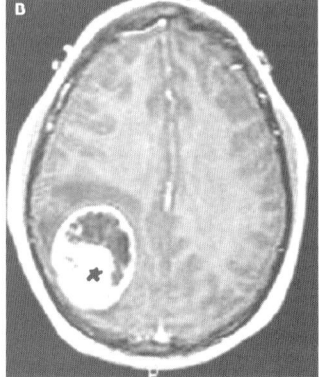

Figure 44.3 Pleomorphic xanthoastrocytoma: **(A)** T2 axial and **(B)** T1 postcontrast axial image shows a T2 hyperintense, enhancing tumor (asterisk) in the right supramarginal and angular gyrus region with surrounding edema (arrow).

may roughly correlate with grade, postoperative injury, peritumoral edema, and integrity of white matter tracts (Figure 22).

The apparent diffusion coefficient (ADC) measures water diffusion and, therefore, often mirrors changes in DWI signal. The main determinant of the ADC is the extracellular volume fraction [6]. In tumors there are two processes that can affect the extracellular volume fraction: vasogenic edema and the increased cellularity of tumors. The higher the tumor cellularity (and therefore the greater the volume of intracellular space), the lower is the ADC because of decreased water diffusivity, caused by a relative reduction in extracellular space for protons to move about.

Grading Tumors

Generally tumors have higher ADC values compared with the normal brain [7–16]. ADC in high-grade gliomas is significantly lower than in the less cellular low-grade gliomas [10,11,17,18]. Grading in this manner remains investigational because of substantial overlap in ADC values among different grades of glioma, likely because of tissue heterogeneity associated with gliomas across different grades, within the same grade, and even within a single tumor. ADC values have also been correlated with cellularity of nonglial brain tumors.

Postoperative Injury

Any process that results in acute intracellular swelling and subsequent decrease in the surrounding extracellular space can lead to reduced proton diffusion in the brain. Thus, areas of immediate postoperative diffusion abnormality can be easily misinterpreted as tumor recurrence. A new area of contrast enhancement observed on postcontrast T1-weighted images after glioma surgery should therefore be interpreted in comparison to an immediate postoperative DWI.

Assessing Edema

In general, the nonenhancing area of abnormality surrounding the enhancing tumor core is referred to as peritumoral edema. In gliomas this represents both vasogenic edema (implying reversible reactive changes rather than permanent cellular damage) and infiltrating tumor cells that are behind the blood-brain barrier (BBB) and usually invade the white matter tracts. ADC alone currently cannot discriminate pure white matter water (vasogenic edema) from brain water with scattered foci of microscopic and isolated tumor cells (infiltrative edema) because of the inherent limitation of spatial resolution of DWI [19].

Assessing the Integrity of White Matter Tracts

Another Application of DWI in brain tumors is the use of fractional anisotropy (FA) maps derived from DTI to determine the integrity of white matter tracts in the vicinity of a brain tumor. For DWI it is assumed that water diffuses

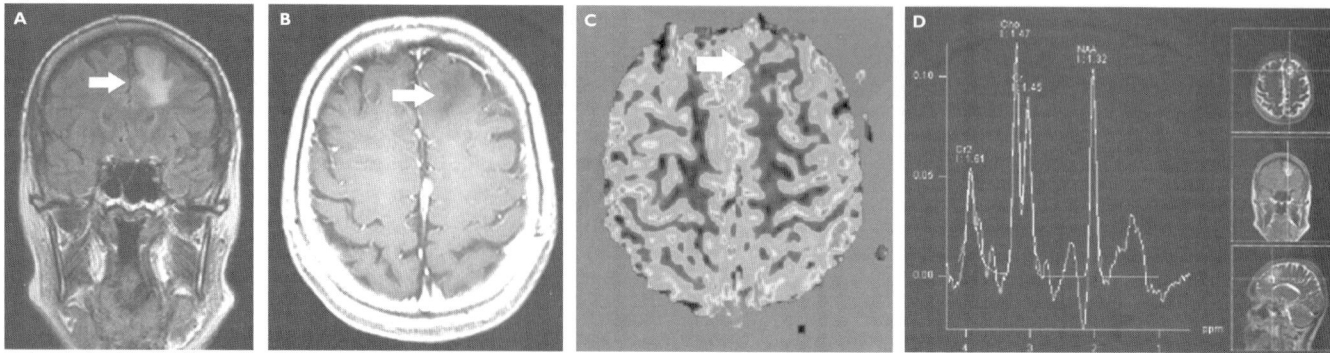

Figure 44.4 Grade II astrocytoma: **(A)** FLAIR axial image and **(B)** T1 postcontrast axial image showing small lesion in left frontal region (arrows). Axial DSC rCBV perfusion map **(C)** shows lesion to have mild increased rCBV (arrow). Long TE (TE = 135) CSI MRS **(D)** shows slight elevation of Cho/Cr ratio. *See color insert.*

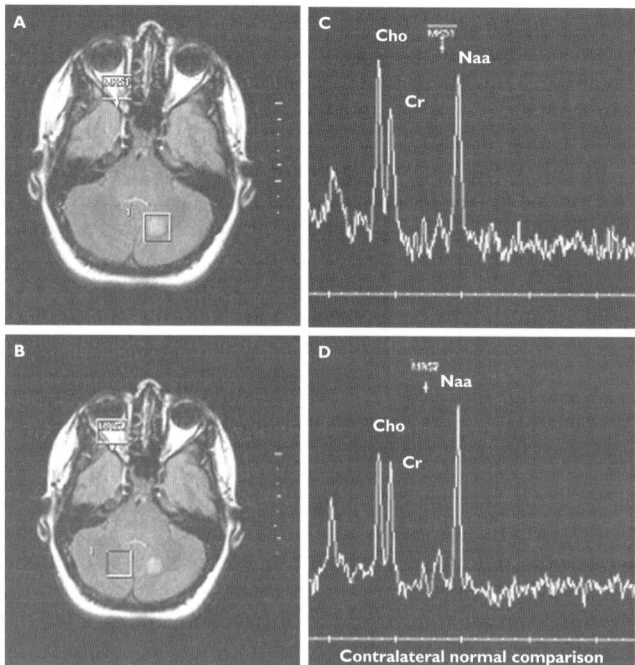

Figure 44.5 Grade II astrocytoma: **(A)** Axial FLAIR image shows a small left dentate nucleus hyperintensity that did not enhance (not shown). **(B)** Single voxel long (TE = 135) MRS (the voxel is the area inside the white box on A) shows mild elevation of the Cho:Cr ratio and mild decrease of Naa:Cr ratio. There is inversion of the Naa:Cho ratio. **(C)** and **(D)** MRS with same parameters from the contralateral normal dentate nucleus for comparison shows normal spectra.

in all directions, that is, diffusion is isotropic. In the brain, there is anisotropic diffusion, largely attributed to myelin and axons. The differential degree of water diffusivity that is maximal parallel to and minimal perpendicular to the long axes of axonal bundles and the myelin sheath allows the assessment of fiber track orientation. Anisotropic diffusion can be described by a tensor made up of a matrix of numbers derived from diffusion measurements in at least six independent diffusion-encoding directions to calculate orientation-dependent diffusion in all spatial directions for each image voxel. This is characterized by three eigenvectors (direction) and three eigenvalues (magnitude). The direction of the largest eigenvalue, referred to as the principal axis of diffusion, can be color-coded to provide directionally encoded color maps.

The reduction in fractional anisotropy correlates with cell density [20,21] and the proliferation index of the glioma [20].

- Where a tumor has displaced a white matter tract, it has a different color hue on the directionally encoded color maps with normal FA values compared with the contralateral side.
- Where tumor has infiltrated, the FA is reduced compared with the contralateral side and the color hues are abnormal. DTI can correctly identify tumor infiltration with an overall sensitivity of 98% and specificity of 81% [22].
- Where tumor has completely disrupted a tract, the latter is not identifiable on either FA or directionally encoded color maps [23].

There is marked regional heterogeneity in response to treatment [24,25].

Perfusion MRI

Perfusion MRI attempts to study and quantify brain tumor vasculature. It is putatively used to assess the degree of tumor angiogenesis and capillary permeability, both of which are presumed biologic correlates of malignancy, grading, and prognosis; quantitative estimates of microvascular permeability have been shown to correlate with brain tumor grade [26–29]. There are three main methods to study brain perfusion: dynamic susceptibility contrast imaging (DSCI); dynamic contrast enhancement (DCE); and arterial spin labeling (ASL), an experimental methodology which provides actual quantitative values of cerebral blood flow.

Dynamic Susceptibility Contrast Imaging

DSCI relies on the T2 signal drop caused by the passage of a gadolinium-containing contrast agent through the

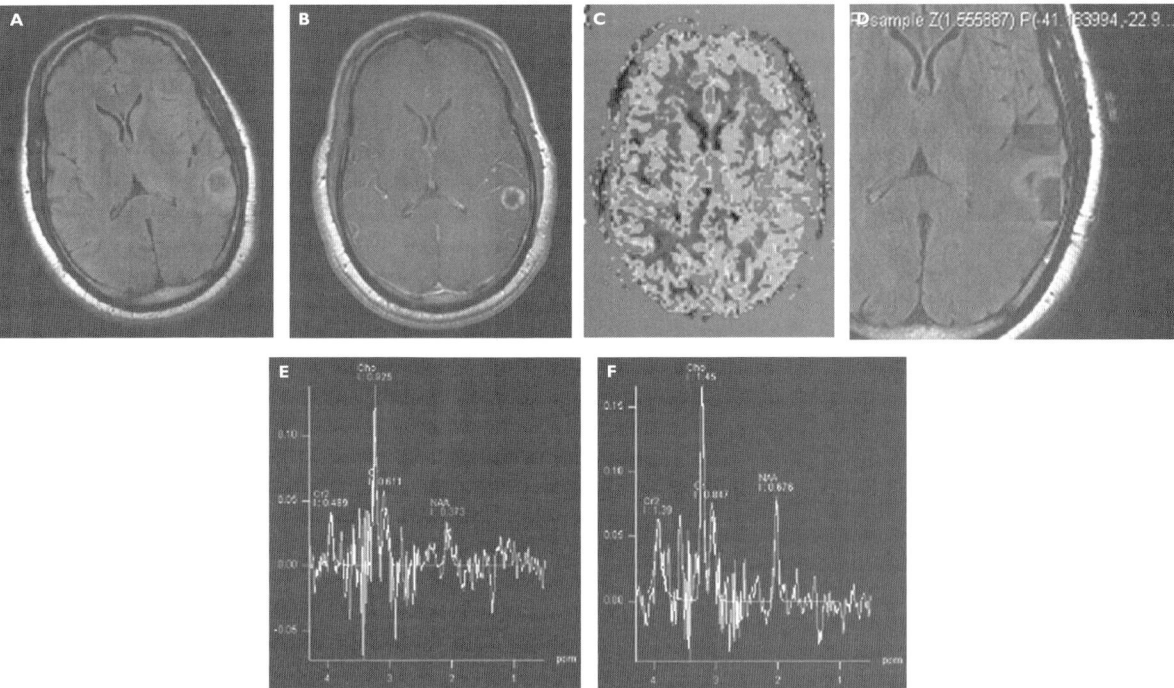

Figure 44.6 Grade III astrocytoma: **(A)** FLAIR axial image and **(B)** T1 postcontrast axial image showing small lesion in left medial occipital gyrus. **(C)** Axial DSC rCBV perfusion map (red denotes higher rCBV) shows lesion to have mild increased rCBV (arrow) as compared with the contralateral side. 3D Spectroscopy **(D)** choline map superimposed upon the FLAIR axial image shows heterogeneity in the tumor with the outer regions showing greater cell turn over (red) as compared to the medial portions of the tumor. Individual spectra from within the tumor confirm much lower Naa values and slightly higher Cho/Cr ratio at the outer **(E)** than inner **(F)** portions of the tumor. *See color insert.*

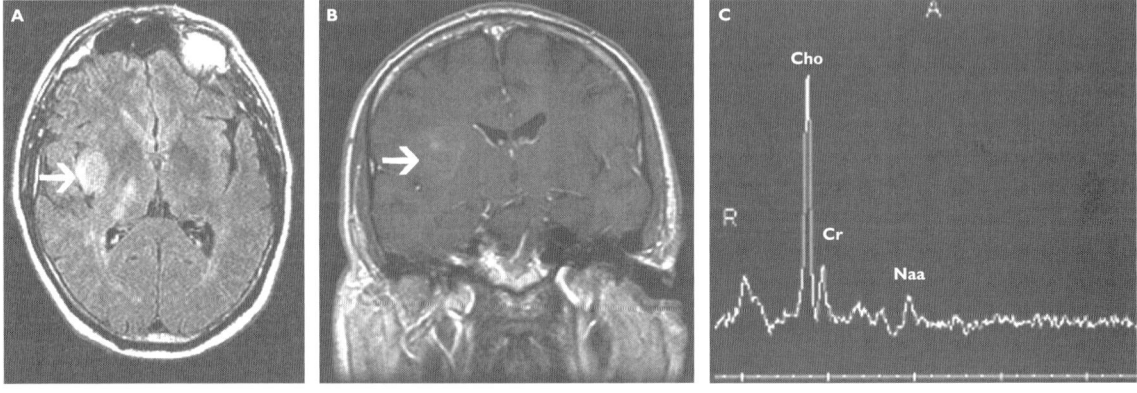

Figure 44.7 Grade III astrocytoma. **(A)** T2 axial image and **(B)** T1 postcontrast axial image showing left insular mass with mild enhancement and mild mass effect (arrow). Single voxel (TE = 135) spectroscopy **(C)** from within the tumor shows significant decrease in Naa and elevation of Cho denoting neuronal destruction and increased cell turn over.

tissues. The drop in signal is proportional to the concentration of the contrast agent and the tissue vascularity.

More quantitative measures involve the calculation of the relative cerebral blood volume (rCBV = volume of blood in the voxel/mass of tissue within the voxel). In the absence of recirculation and contrast material leakage, CBV is proportional to the area under the contrast agent concentration-time curve and thus does not provide an absolute measurement. Because of the nonlinear relationship between the signal change and gadolinium contrast, it is necessary to express the measurement relative to a standard reference, usually the contralateral white matter.

It is not certain what an elevated rCBV represents histologically, though in tumors it correlates with tumor vascularity as assessed by nonquantitative scales of histological vascularity [30–35]. Some studies suggest a possible

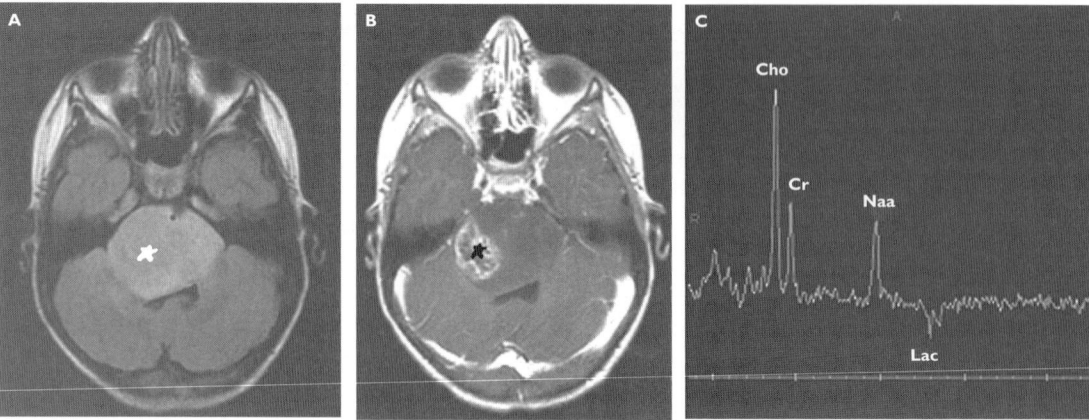

Figure 44.8 Brain stem grade III glioma: **(A)** FLAIR axial image and **(B)** T1 postcontrast axial image showing lesion expanding pons with irregular enhancement. Single voxel (TE = 135) spectroscopy **(C)** from within the tumor shows decrease in Naa and elevation of Cho denoting neuronal destruction and increased cell turn over. Lactate inverted double peak (lac) denotes rapid cell turnover and anaerobic metabolism.

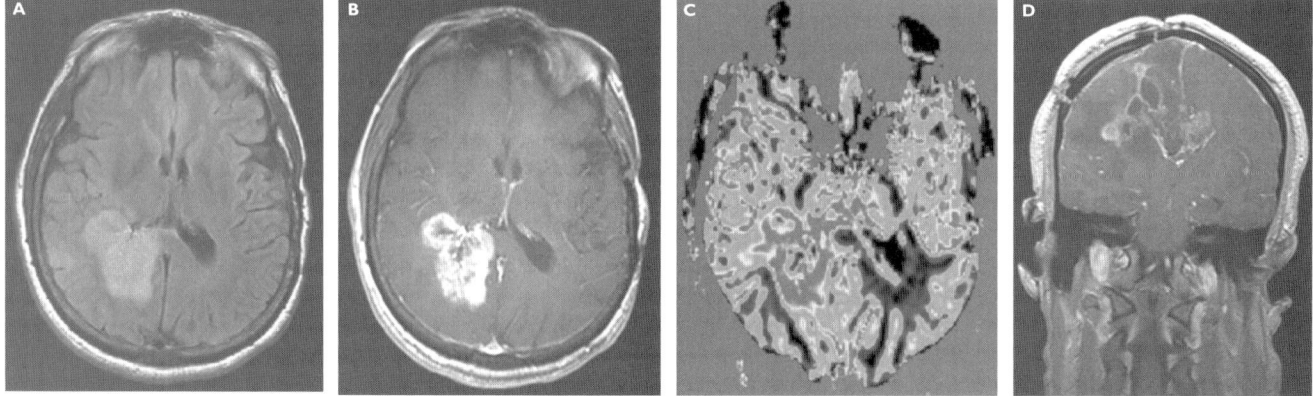

Figure 44.9 Grade IV astrocytoma: **(A)** FLAIR axial image and **(B)** T1 postcontrast axial image showing irregularly enhancing lesion in the right forceps major invading the splenium of the corpus callosum. **(C)** Axial DSC rCBV perfusion map (areas in red are higher rCBV) shows lesion to have markedly increased rCBV (arrow) as compared with the contralateral side. Coronal T1 postcontrast image **(D)** from another patient shows a grade IV astrocytoma crossing the midline via the corpus callosum—the so called butterfly glioma. *See color insert.*

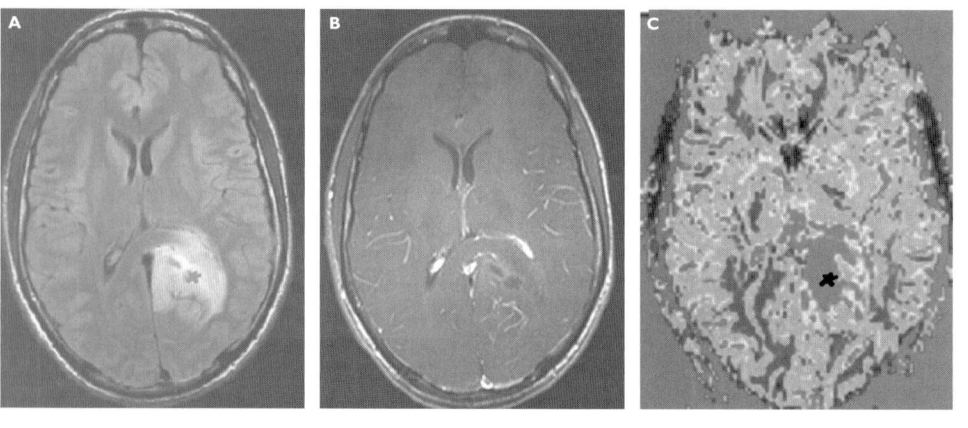

Figure 44.10 Oligodendroglioma with 1q/p19 loss exhibit greater rCBV and may appear radiologically more aggressive than those tumors without this mutation. **(A)** FLAIR axial image and **(B)** T1 postcontrast axial image showing left lingual gyrus mass (asterisk) with relatively mild enhancement deforming and invading the splenium of the corpus callosum. Axial DSC rCBV perfusion map **(C)** shows lesion (asterisk) to have markedly increased rCBV (areas in red are higher rCBV) as compared with the contralateral side. *See color insert.*

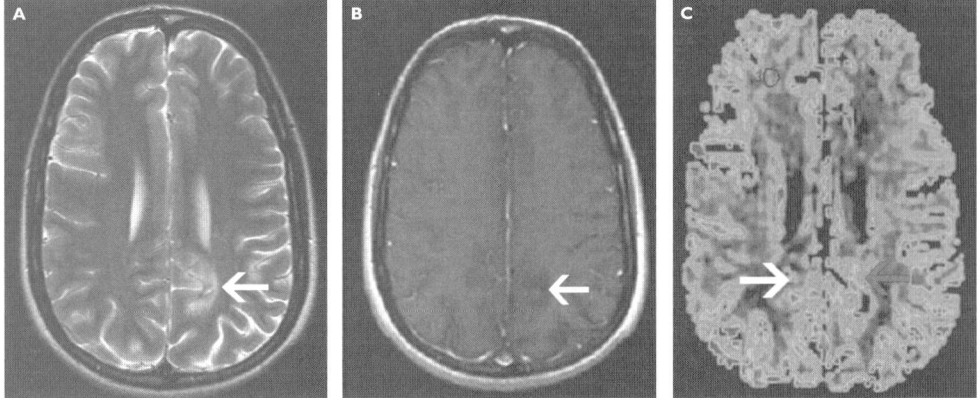

Figure 44.11 Oligodendroglioma without 1q/p19 loss exhibit only mild rCBV elevation and may appear radiologically less aggressive than those tumors without this mutation. **(A)** T2 axial image and **(B)** T1 postcontrast axial image showing left cingulate gyrus mass without enhancement (red arrow). **(C)** Axial DSC rCBV perfusion map (areas in red are higher rCBV) shows lesion to have only minimally increased rCBV (red arrow) as compared with the contralateral side (white arrow). *See color insert.*

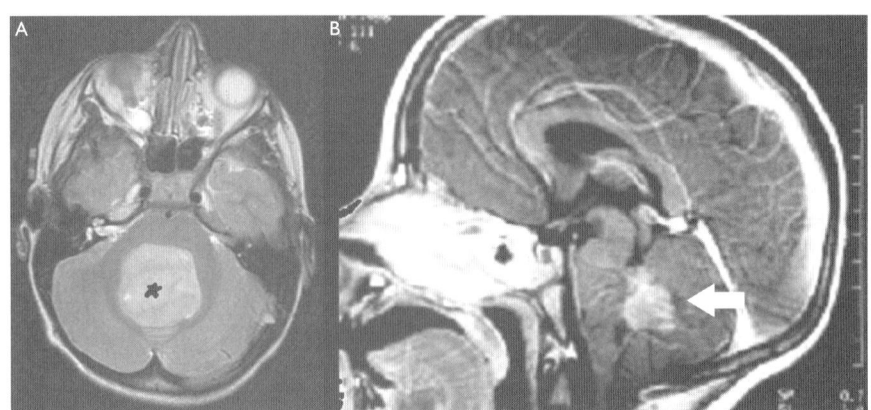

Figure 44.12 Medulloblastoma: **(A)** Axial T2 image showing hyperintense mass in fourth ventricle (asterisk). **(B)** Postcontrast T1 sagittal image of another patient shows enhancement within a fourth ventricle medulloblastoma (arrow).

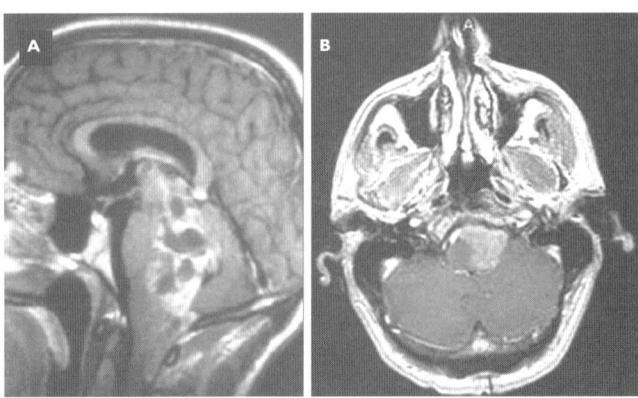

Figure 44.13 Ependymoma: Postcontrast T1 sagittal **(A)** and axial **(B)** images show two posterior fossa ependymomas.

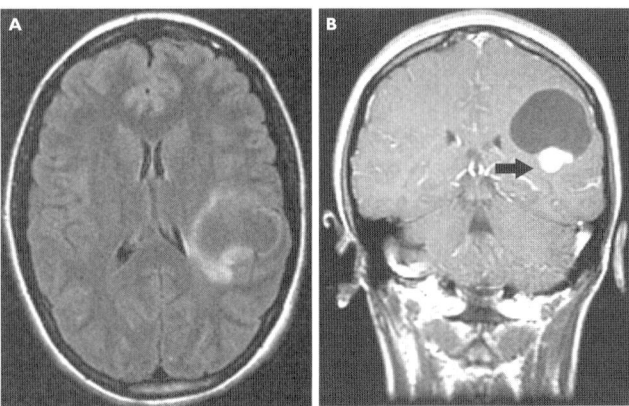

Figure 44.14 Ganglioglioma: Axial FLAIR **(A)** and post-contrast T1 coronal **(B)** images show a ganglioglioma with an enhancing nodule (asterisk). Pilocytic astrocytoma or hemangioblastoma are the primary imaging differential diagnosis.

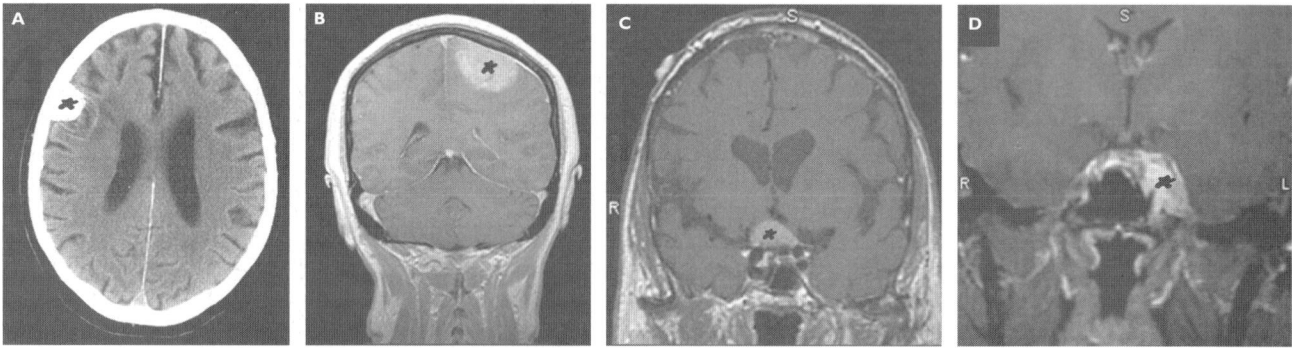

Figure 44.15 Meningioma: **(A)** Noncontrast CT showing a calcified right frontal extra axial meningioma (asterisk). **(B)** T1 contrast enhanced coronal image with an enhancing left parietal extra axial meningioma (asterisk). **(C)** T1 contrast enhanced coronal image with an enhancing planum sphenoidale extra axial meningioma (asterisk). **(D)** T1 contrast enhanced coronal image with an enhancing left cavernous sinus meningioma (asterisk).

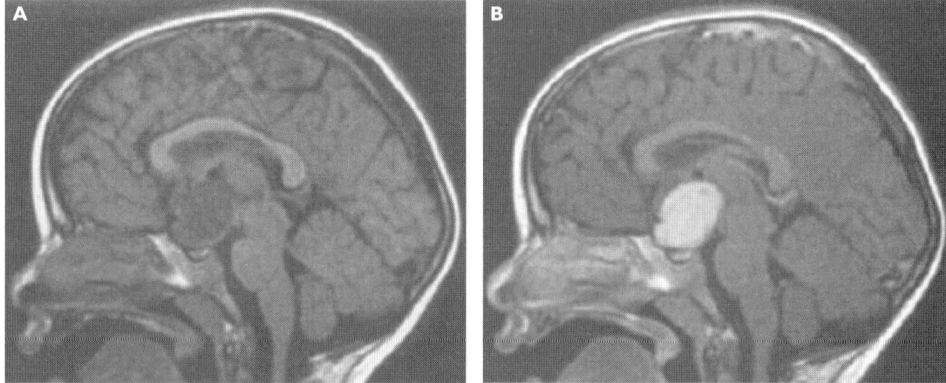

Figure 44.16 Craniopharyngioma. **(A)** Pre and **(B)** postcontrast T1 sagittal images show a sellar and suprasellar Craniopharyngioma.

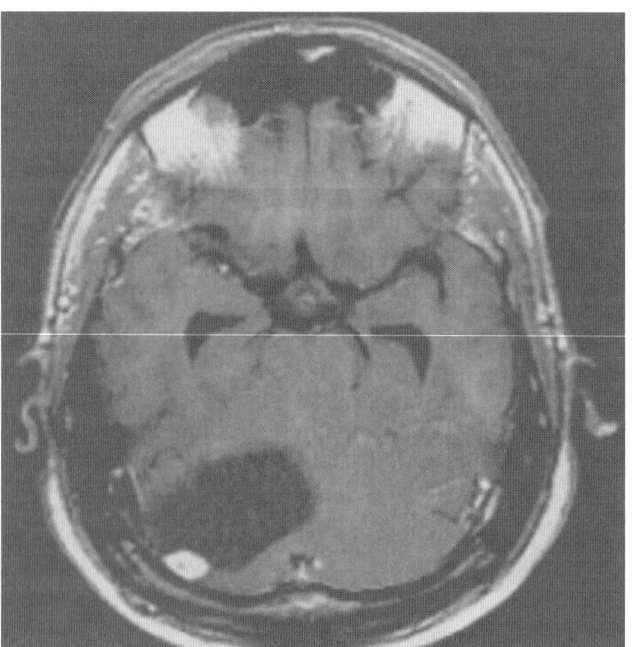

Figure 44.17 Hemangioblastoma: Axial postcontrast T1 image shows a hemangioblastoma with an enhancing nodule. Pilocytic astorcytoma or ganglioglioma are the primary imaging differential diagnosis.

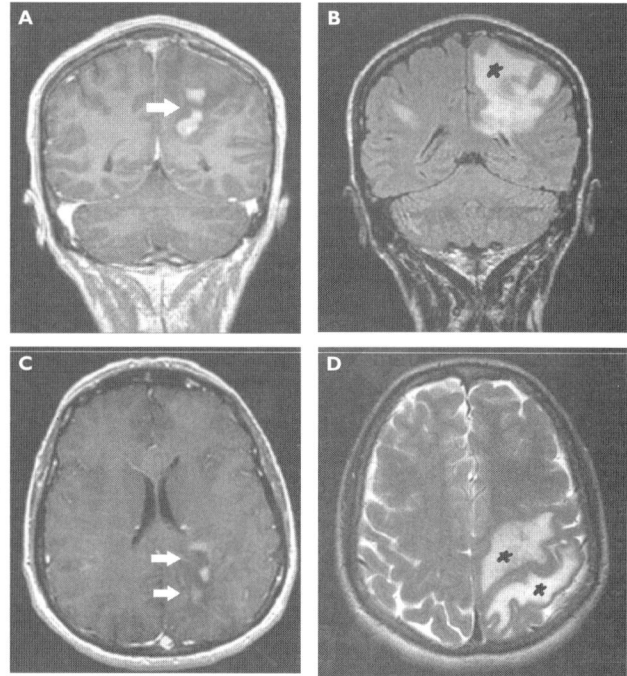

Figure 44.18 Lymphoma: **(A)** coronal postcontrast T1, **(B)** coronal FLAIR, **(C)** axial postcontrast T1, and **(D)** axial T2 images show a left parietal enhancing tumor (arrow) with adjacent edema (asterisk).

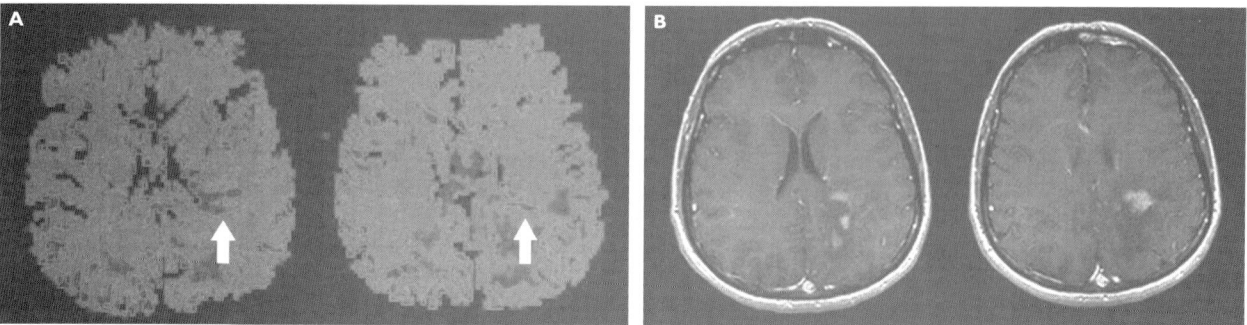

Figure 44.19 Lymphoma: **(A)** Axial DSC rCBV perfusion map (areas in red are higher rCBV) shows lesion to have increased rCBV (arrow) as compared with the contralateral side (white arrow). Note that the areas of maximal increased rCBV do not always correspond to the areas of enhancement on the axial T1 postcontrast **(B)** images. In biopsy planning or treatment assessment, it is the areas of increased rCBV that denotes viable tumor as enhancement is a function of blood brain barrier breakdown that may be caused by factors other than the tumor. See *color insert*.

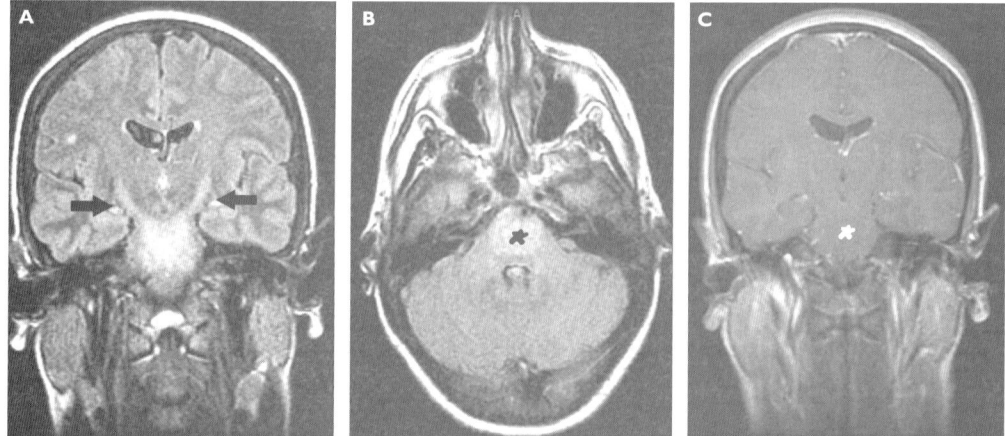

Figure 44.20 Brain stem lymphoma: **(A)** Coronal and **(B)** axial FLAIR show signal hyperintensity that expands the brain stem and pons (asterisk) with extension up the long tracts (arrows). There is only faint enhancement on the **(C)** postcontrast T1 coronal image (asterisk).

role in distinguishing high-grade tumors from lower-grade gliomas [30,36]. A reduction of rCBV during radiotherapy is a predictor for a better prognosis [37]. These changes can even be detected after only 1 week of radiotherapy (Figure 44.23). Dose-related reduction in perfusion can also be detected in the irradiated normal brain surrounding gliomas. Potentially this may be a marker for normal brain radiation injury.

Glioma grading using rCBV should be limited to fibrillary astrocytomas because other gliomas, most notably oligodendrogliomas, may have high rCBV regardless of grade and could be falsely graded as a higher-grade tumor [36,38] (Figures 44.10 and 44.11). In addition, studies show marked overlap of rCBV with different tumor grades, making grading in an individual patient inaccurate [32,34,35,39]. Choroid plexus tumors are nonastrocytic gliomas that arise from the choroid plexus within the ventricular system of the brain. These highly vascular tumors are composed of highly leaky capillaries without a BBB, which causes avid enhancement on T1-weighted images after contrast administration. Because there is no BBB, intravascular compartmentalization of contrast is not possible due to almost simultaneous transition of the contrast agent from intravascular to interstitial space, making rCBV measurements of choroid plexus tumors unreliable.

Nonglial tumors include meningiomas, which are highly vascular tumors. Selection of patients for preoperative embolization, which is limited to dural vessels, and surgical planning for pial-supplied meninigiomas, which tend to bleed more during surgery, may be helped by the use of DSCI. Primary cerebral lymphoma (PCL) can mimic malignant primary gliomas, brain metastases, and infections on conventional MRI (Figure 44.19). On DWI, PCL shows reduced diffusion, presumably due to high cellularity of the tumor. On DSCI, PCL tends to show elevated rCBV, but less than glioblastoma. Metastatic brain tumors contain highly leaky capillaries.

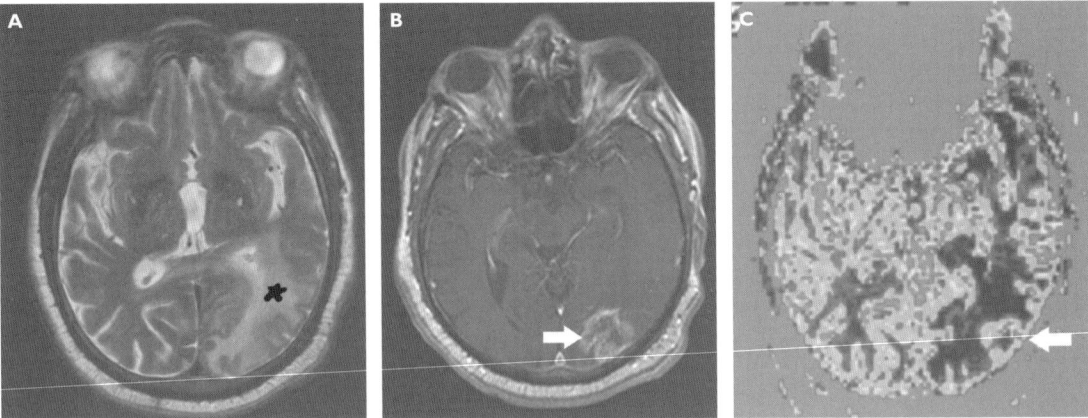

Figure 44.21 Metastatic disease: **(A)** T2 axial image and **(B)** T1 postcontrast axial image showing an enhancing lesion in left occipital region (arrow) with adjacent edema (asterisk). Axial DSC rCBV perfusion map **(C)** shows lesion to have increased rCBV (arrow) surrounded by decreased rCBV. Metastases typically have low rCBV in the peritumoral edema whereas primary brain neoplasms have normal or even increased rCBV in the peritumoral region. *See color insert.*

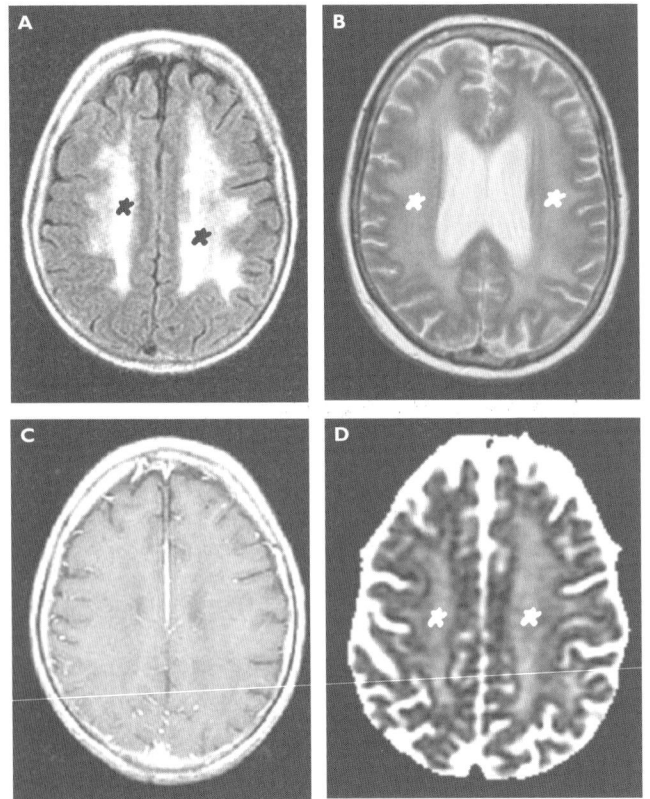

Figure 44.22 Posttreatment changes: **(A)** Axial FLAIR, **(B)** axial T2, **(C)** axial postcontrast T1, and **(D)** and axial ADC map derived from DWI shows diffuse non enhancing white matter signal changes without mass effect and that show higher ADC values compatible with postradiation demyelination (asterisk).

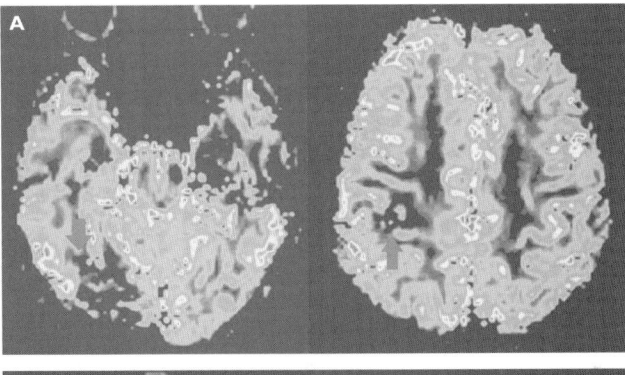

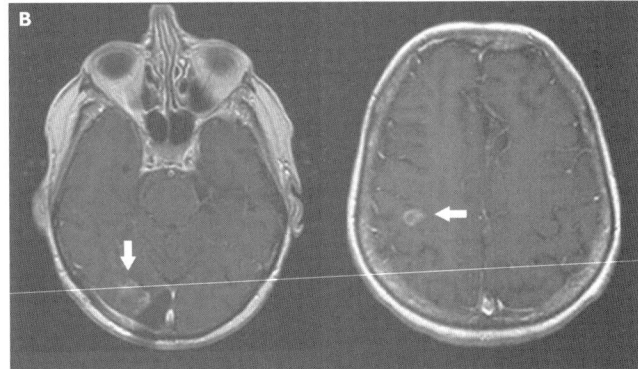

Figure 44.23 Postradiation changes: **(A)** Axial DSC rCBV perfusion map (dark areas are lower rCBV) shows areas that enhance on the axial T1 postcontrast **(B)** images to have low rCBV (arrow) as compared with the contralateral side (white arrow). Residual or recurrent tumor would be expected to show increased rCBV. *See color insert.*

Hence, DSC perfusion MRI is useful in differentiating these from primary gliomas, as rCBV measurements within the vasogenic edema of metastasis are significantly lower than those within the infiltrative edema of gliomas [33] (Figure 44.21).

Dynamic Contrast Enhancement

DCE perfusion MRI consists of repeated imaging with a rapid T1-weighted sequence to measure changes in signal intensity as a bolus of gadolinium diffuses across the damaged BBB, measuring the shape of the contrast agent concentration curve in blood plasma, referred to as the arterial input function, and a time course of accumulation of contrast agent in tissue from individual voxels. Compared to DSC MRI, DCE MRI offers better spatial resolution, and is resistant to susceptibility artifacts. This technique may be a useful method of studying the microcirculation of tumors. Consensus recommendations and guidelines propose that DCE MRI be used as a primary imaging method to assess antiangiogenic and antivascular therapeutic agents [40].

The most widely used DCE MRI quantitative parameter is the transfer constant K_{trans}, a quantitative measure of the degree of increase in T1 due to accumulation of contrast in tissue. K_{trans} describes the relationship between the time course of blood plasma contrast concentration (arterial input function) and contrast concentration changes occurring in the voxel. It is limited by either vascular blood flow or permeability. In brain tumors, the blood flow to the tumor is often hampered by an abnormal tumor vasculature, so the uptake of contrast by tumor is mainly limited by blood flow, not by permeability. With increasing glioma grade, there is higher likelihood of T1-weighted contrast enhancement of the tumor and increasing K_{trans} correlates strongly with glioma grade [28,41–43].

Magnetic Resonance Spectroscopy

MRS is based on the principle of chemical shift as protons will spin slower in water than in fat. The frequency differences are used and expressed as a ppm scale where the resonant frequency is related to a reference frequency. Proton spectroscopy acquisition sequences require water suppression as the concentration of water protons is >10,000 times greater than that of other substances. At 1.5 Tesla (T), the most commonly seen peaks differ greatly between the normal brain and gliomas, and these are listed below in order of parts-per-million (ppm):

Mobile Lipids

A double peak at 0.9 ppm (methyl lipid) and 1.3 ppm (methylene lipid). These substances are only found using short TEs unless they are grossly elevated. Mobile lipids are not seen in the normal brain but are increased with necrosis when cellular death results in membranes break down and lipid droplets are formed in necrotic/perinecrotic areas [44]. Lipid is therefore commonly seen in malignant tumors and is associated with the degree of malignancy and presence of necrosis [45,46]. In standard 1H-MR spectroscopy acquisition, the peaks of lactate and mobile lipids overlap and are often treated as a single metabolite, though each represents very different tumor biology and measure of tissue viability:

- The regions of lactate most likely represent areas of hypoxic but viable tumor.
- The regions of mobile lipid represent necrotic nonviable tissue.

Spectral editing is necessary to detect the intensity of lactate and mobile lipid metabolites separately and reliably by using long TE MRS or lactate editing [47]. In malignant gliomas, the lipid peak appears to provide the best marker of proliferation, and with increasing grade there is an increase in the lactate/lipid peak [45,46,48,49].

1. Lactate—1.33 ppm. This signal peak is usually below the level of detection in the normal brain. Lactate is the end product of the nonoxidative glycolysis and rises in disorders of energy metabolism from an increase in nonoxidative glycolysis. Within tumors there is disruption of normal glucose metabolism and a significant degree of hypoxia, resulting in elevated lactate levels [45,50,51] (Figure 44.8).

2. *N*-acetyl aspartate (NAA)—2.02 ppm. This is the largest spectral peak. Immunocytochemistry has shown that NAA is predominantly localized to neurons [52]. This peak provides a measure of "neuronal density" and is a surrogate marker of neuronal integrity, which is reduced in disorders that result in axonal loss. Due to the lack of viable neurons within a tumor, gliomas demonstrate a marked reduction in the NAA peak and in the NAA/Cr ratio [45,46,51]. With increasing grade there is a reduction in NAA [22,45,46,49,53,54] (Figures 44.5 to 44.8). After treatment, the lactate/NAA ratio is a strong predictor of response to radiotherapy and overall survival [55].

3. Glutamate and glutamine (Glx)—2.1 to 2.4 ppm and 3.6 to 3.8 ppm (composite peak). These signals are difficult to separate at 1.5 T. Elevated glutamate levels lead to excitotoxic cell damage. Increased glutamine synthesis occurs as a result of increased blood ammonia levels.

4. Creatine (Cr and PCr)—3.02 ppm. This signal is made up of both creatine and phosphocreatine. Both of these compounds are involved in ATP generation and energy metabolism. The amount of creatine and phosphocreatine appears to be relatively constant in the normal brain, so it is used as a *reference signal*. The concentrations of other metabolites are often expressed as the ratio of the peak areas compared with the creatine peak. Total creatine levels are lower in tumors than in the normal brain [56,57]. In malignant gliomas, grade increases with the Cho/Cr ratio [45,46,48,49,53,58] (Figures 44.4 to 44.7).

5. Choline (Cho)—3.24 ppm. It is made up from glycerophosphocholine (GPC), phosphocholine (PC), and a small amount of free choline. These choline compounds are involved in membrane synthesis and degradation. The choline peak correlates with cell density [49,59]. Increased choline occurs with disorders causing increased membrane turnover, expressed as an increase in the Cho/Cr and Cho/NAA ratios [45,46,51,53,54]. In malignant gliomas, grade increases with the Cho/Cr ratio [45,46,48,49,55,58] (Figures 44.4 to 44.8). In one image-guided biopsy study, the normalized choline ratios and the Cho/NAA correlated with the degree of tumor infiltration [51].

MR spectroscopy in glioma grading has not been proven to be accurate enough to replace tissue diagnosis and grading. While it is very accurate in the differentiation of high- and low-grade gliomas [60–63], it has diminished diagnostic accuracy in the differentiation between grade III and grade IV gliomas [64]. The sensitivity and specificity of MRS for accurately detecting high-grade gliomas prior to biopsy is 87.7% and 93.3%, respectively (Setzer 2007) (Figure 44.24).

Three-dimensional magnetic resonance spectroscopy (3DMRS) may be used to assess the choline-to-*N*-acetyl-

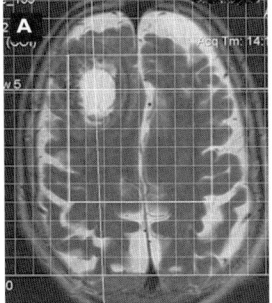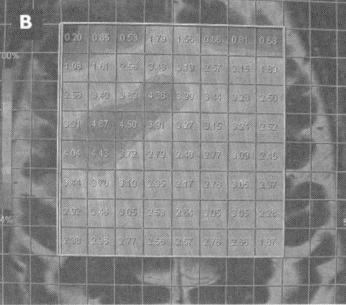

Figure 44.24 3D MRS—Biopsy guidance. Axial T2 image **(A)** demonstrates a necrotic right frontal lesion. In larger lesions such as this one in the right frontal region it may be difficult for the surgeon to obtain a viable biopsy, especially post treatment. Using a 3D MR spectroscopy choline map **(B)** can guide surgical biopsy to the areas of greatest cell turnover denoted in red. *See color insert.*

aspartate index (CNI). It has been shown that this volume appears to more accurately represent infiltrative tumor (compared to conventional MRI) for the purposes of radiation therapy treatment planning [65]. Using 1 cm² voxel resolution MRS at 1.5 T field strength to measure tumor metabolite concentration and metabolite ratios (Cho/NAA, Cr/NAA, Cho/Cr), a relative choline/NAA ratio (*aka* CNI) of 2 is significantly correlated with the presence of tumor [66–71]. Comparison of volumes of microscopic tumor infiltration as defined by T2 changes on conventional MRI versus the CNI showed a median increase of 14% in volume size compared to anatomic MRI [65].

After completion of treatment, accurate evaluation of MRI changes may be difficult, as necrosis and tumor progression often have similar appearances, that is, enhancement on T1-weighted MR images with an increase in surrounding edema (Figure 44.25). This is especially problematic in the setting of dose escalation [72]. Differentiating treatment-related new contrast enhancement from that due to tumor progression, while difficult [73], is important, since early post-treatment MRI-based tumor progression appears to predict median survival [74]. An abnormal increase in the choline peak >50% of the contralateral brain or a choline/creatine ratio >2 have moderate to high sensitivity (64–95%) and high specificity (82–100%) for differentiating active tumor from therapy-related necrosis [75–77]. 3DMRS may also be useful in differentiating between necrosis and viable tumor [78–83]. The CNI volume also correlates inversely with the time to onset of new contrast enhancement after radiation therapy [65]. In fact, the presence of a tumor spectrum and CNI on 3DMRS appears to predict both the presence of tumor and clinical progression thereof [54,65]. The pattern of change of CNI-based volumes after therapy and its correlation to treatment effects and disease progression is not known at this time.

Functional Magnetic Resonance Imaging

When an area of the brain is active, there is a corresponding increase in blood flow not matched by an increase in oxygen extraction, so the concentration of deoxyhemoglobin

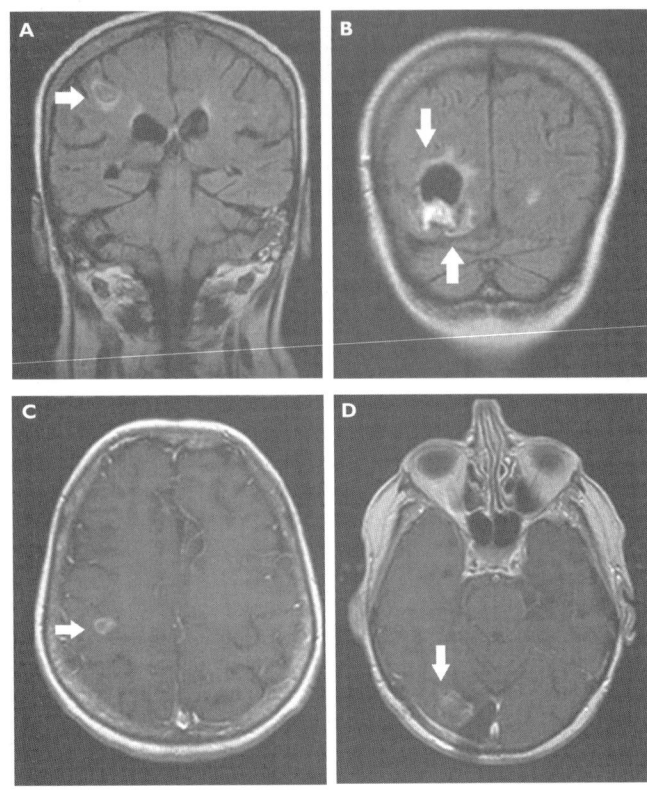

Figure 44.25 Posttreatment changes: **(A)** and **(B)** coronal FLAIR, **(C)** and **(D)** axial T1 postcontrast images in a patient post radiation treatment for metastatic disease show multiple signal abnormalities on the FLAIR images that enhance (arrows). With anatomic MRI alone, it is not possible to distinguish post treatment changes from recurrent or residual disease.

is reduced. As deoxyhemoglobin is paramagnetic there is a change in the T2 signal. This change, referred to as blood oxygen level–dependent contrast (BOLD), is detected by the MR sequence.

fMRI has only limited functionality in surgical planning for the resection of infiltrative gliomas, as some areas that are activated are not necessarily essential to avoid in order to prevent a neurological deficit. In addition, the BOLD signal is lost adjacent to gliomas [84,85]. fMRI also provides no information regarding the relationship of white matter tracts to the tumor. The accuracy of fMRI in mapping language tasks is poorer than motor studies and usually will require the assessment of multiple language tasks [86]. For language paradigms the intrasubject repeatability is, at best, 40% [87]; for bilingual patients there is evidence that there are different areas responsible for each language function [88]. Motor activation has better repeatability but the size of the regions activated by a finger-tapping task varies by about 50% [89].

Novel Contrast Agents

Most MR contrast agents are limited to reporting only anatomical detail. Newer, experimental agents potentially capable of reporting on physiological status and metabolic activity [90] are summarized in Table 44.2.

Table 44.2 Novel Contrast Agents

Type of Agent	Mechanism of Action	Proposed Use
Enzyme-activated agents	An enzyme substrate (sugar) occupies all coordination sites on the agent, inhibiting water access to the paramagnetic ion. The contrast agent is irreversibly turned "on" when β-galactosidase cleaves the sugar. As a result, water becomes accessible to the ion	Used in vivo to monitor gene expression
Calcium-activated agents	A reversible contrast agent incorporates a calcium-binding domain. The stronger binding affinity of Ca++ to the domain allows water access to the Gd+++	Mapping brain function and signal transduction
pH-activated agents	These contrast agents have a sulfonamide nitrogen. At high pH, the deprotonated amine chelates Gd+++. This prevents water access to the ion, resulting in a low MR signal. At low pH, the agent is protonated and unable to chelate the paramagnetic ion. Water access to the ion is restored, resulting in a detectable signal	Markers for abnormal tissue
pO2-activated agent	The oxidation state of a europium ion (Eu+++) is varied to trigger the signal on and off by the environmental pO2. Eu+++ is reduced to Eu++ (isoelectronic with Gd+++), which enhances the observed MR signal upon reduction. The oxidation state of the metal is directly related to the pO2, allowing for quantitative determination	The blood oxygen level–dependent (BOLD) signal could be used for noninvasive mapping of human brain function
Protein binding of an agent	The contrast agent consists of a human serum albumin (HSA) binding inhibitor group, an HSA binding group, and a chelated Gd+++ ion. Relaxivity is enhanced by covalent and noncovalent interaction with a protein (large molecule), which occurs after enzymatic cleavage of a peptide The ability to detect enzymatic cleavage is dictated by the agent binding to HSA	Not yet certain in CNS
T2-activated agent	The agent enhances T2 relaxation by the simultaneous detection of a specific oligonucleotide sequence. To target a specific oligonucleotide sequence, a crosslinked iron oxide (CLIO) agent is synthesized with an oligonucleotide sequence complementary to that of a target sequence	Detection of specific oligonucleotide sequences in tumor DNA
Chemical exchange saturation transfer (CEST)	These agents can be switched on and off externally with an applied RF pulse, directed at the frequency of one of the proton pool resonances. This causes saturation transfer to the water resonances which decreases the bulk water intensity. This method allows for external manipulation of the signal intensity	Not yet certain in CNS

PET IMAGING

When a positron-emitting radionuclide decays, the positron interacts with an electron, yielding two photons that travel in almost opposite directions, the detection of which yields a tomographic reconstruction of the region of their origin. The most commonly used tracer is 18F-fluorodeoxyglucose (FDG), which is transported into cells by a glucose transporter and remains trapped there in relative proportion to their energy metabolism.

Indications

Theoretical uses for PET imaging in brain tumor evaluation include tumor grading, localization for surgery and radiation therapy treatment planning, differentiating radiation necrosis from tumor, assessing treatment response, and predicting outcomes. In practical use, however, FDG PET use is not a part of the standard clinical management of brain tumor patients. Highly malignant brain tumors usually show increased FDG uptake in comparison to the surrounding brain parenchyma, but inherent limitations, such as low-resolution and high-background glucose metabolism of normal gray matter structures, result in little useful information compared to other imaging modalities. The ability of 18F-FDG PET to differentiate recurrent tumor from radiation necrosis is limited due to inadequate sensitivity and specificity [91,92]. FDG PET can have some prognostic importance [93,94] but its role in assessing response to chemotherapy or radiotherapy remains limited [95].

Tracers which provide a measurement of amino acid (AA) transport and incorporation (methyl-[11C]-L-methionine (MET) or evaluation of DNA synthesis (18F-labeled O-(2) fluoroethyl-L-tyrosine (FET)) are still only in limited clinical use. Amino acid positron emission tomography (AA-PET) has higher sensitivity and specificity for the diagnosis of gliomas than CT and MRI. The similar characteristics of different AA tracers imply that the clinical results with one tracer can be extrapolated to others; limited data support this contention.

MET-PET

MET-PET has been utilized for a quarter century [96]. Tissue correlation studies in patients with suspected brain tumors show a sensitivity of 87% and a specificity of 75% to 89%. This results in correct tumor classification in approximately 80% of cases [97–99]. Surgical studies have also shown that, when compared to MRI, MET-PET can detect infiltrating glioma cells outside the T2 hyperintense areas, potentially impacting the planning of surgical resection or stereotactic biopsy in 80% of patients [100,101]. After tumor resection, MET volume extends beyond the MRI contrast-enhancing regions in 74% of patients, indicating residual tumor, and in 69% of cases MRI contrast enhancement extends beyond the volume of MET uptake, suggesting postoperative BBB disturbance [102,103]. Overall, MET uptake corresponds to MRI-Gd enhancement in only 13% of cases. In a small prospective study in patients with recurrent gliomas treated with stereotactic fractionated radiotherapy, this methodology translated into a significant improvement in survival when MET-PET was integrated into target volume delineation, in comparison to patients treated using CT/MRI alone [104].

FET-PET

Unfortunately, the short half time of 11C limits the use of MET-PET to centers with on-site cyclotrons. The AA analogue 18F-labeled O-(2) FET is an attractive alternative. Tyrosine can be radiolabelled with fluorine-18, an isotope with a physical half-life of 110 minutes. It can be synthesized with high radiochemical yields allowing large-scale production, and thus can be distributed to PET imaging centers without an on-site cyclotron [105,106]. Preliminary clinical studies using 18F-FET-PET for human brain tumors have shown results analogous to those for 11C-MET-PET [107,108]. Tissue correlation studies in patients with suspected brain tumors have shown that the sensitivity and specificity of FET-PET are, respectively, 88% to 92% and 81% to 88% in the diagnosis of gliomas, 100% and 81% for MR spectroscopy in the same patients, and 93% and 94% when combining the two [109,110]. However, as FET-PET cannot reliably distinguish between neoplastic and non-neoplastic ring-enhancing intracerebral lesions, histological confirmation is mandatory [111].

SPECT

The use of single-photon emission tomography (SPECT) in brain tumors is limited. Thallium (Tl) is the most studied tracer and there appears to be a relationship between 201Tl uptake and tumor grade, though not definitive enough for accurate diagnosis [112,113]. 99mTc-Sestamibi also cannot accurately differentiate tumors according to grade [114]. Comparison of FET-PET and 3–123I-iodo-alpha-methyl-L-tyrosine SPECT (IMT-SPECT) shows a high correlation between the two methods in imaging for the tumor extent [115,116]. However, the resolution of FET-PET is significantly higher. In comparison to 1H-MRS, IMT-SPECT appears to have slightly higher sensitivity, specificity, and accuracy in diagnosing malignant gliomas [76], as well as in target volume delineation in nonresected [117] and resected [118] patients. One small prospective study in patients with recurrent gliomas treated with stereotactic fractionated radiotherapy demonstrated a significant improvement in survival when IMT-SPECT was integrated into target volume delineation [104]. Focal IMT-SPECT uptake after tumor resection is highly correlated with poor survival, confirming that these tracers are reliable markers for residual tumor [119].

MULTICHANNEL MAGNETOENCEPHALOGRAPHY IMAGING

Multichannel magnetoencephalography (MEG) reflects intracellular electric current flow in the brain, providing direct information of neural activity [120]. It has mainly been used for functional brain mapping of the primary cortex by measuring evoked magnetic fields. Potential applications of this technology in the management of brain tumors may include [104,121]:

- Localizing areas of normally functioning brain for purposes of surgical and/or radiation therapy treatment planning [122,123].
- Localizing areas of involved brain not apparent on conventional imaging [124]
- Integration of these data with other imaging modalities to determine if changes in MEG function are due to tumor invasion or mass effect (i.e., reversible or irreversible). For example, a study of MEG in brain tumor patients treated with tumor resection with or without radiation therapy showed that the pathology underlying a particular wave pattern was not the result of the presence of the tumor bulk but due to the structural damage caused by the tumor to the surrounding brain parenchyma [125]. A study of MEG + MR spectroscopy suggested that preserved metabolically active cortical tissue with remaining NAA signal and increased pathological magnetic activities under lactic acidosis could be interpreted as a border zone between normal and seriously damaged brain tissue [124]. Post-treatment studies can also help differentiate between deficits caused by tumor mass effect and by tumor invasion [125].

SERIAL ASSESSMENT OF BRAIN TUMORS

Initial Assessment

Serial imaging studies should be used to evaluate changes in size of contrast-enhancing tumors [126]. These can be either two- or three-dimensional, using diameter-based measurements on a single axial section containing the largest diameter of tumor, or computer-assisted volumetric analysis. Postoperatively, baseline gadolinium-enhanced MRI should be performed within the first 72 hours following surgery to minimize postoperative enhancement along the margin of the surgical cavity [127].

Two-Dimensional Methods

Response Evaluation Criteria in Solid Tumors (RECIST) measure the longest single linear enhancing diameter across a lesion in the axial plane [128]. The minimal measurable lesion diameter is 10 mm or at least twice the imaging section thickness, which requires the use of 3 mm, skip 0 mm gadolinium-enhanced T1-weighted images (standard 5 mm, skip 1 mm, result in a minimal diameter of 12 mm). Cystic or necrotic regions and leptomeningeal involvement are considered nonmeasurable.

Macdonald Criteria measure two orthogonal diameters on a single axial section [129]. The first is the maximal enhancing tumor diameter on a single axial gadolinium-enhanced T1-weighted section; the second is the largest perpendicular diameter measured on the same image. The product of the two diameters is calculated, and the measurements are repeated with each scan.

Table 44.3 Comparison of Response Criteria for Different Measurement Approaches

	RECIST (Single Diameter)	RECIST-Based Volume	Macdonald (Orthogonal Diameters)	Macdonald-Based Volume
Methodology	Single longest diameter		Product of orthogonal diameters on section with largest tumor area	
CR	Resolution of all-enhancing tumor	Resolution of all-enhancing tumor	Resolution of all-enhancing tumor	Resolution of all-enhancing tumor
PR (percentage change from baseline)	≥30% decrease in sum of maximal diameters	≥66% decrease in volume	≥50% decrease in product of two orthogonal diameters	≥65% decrease in volume
SD	All others	All others	All others	All others
PD (percentage change from nadir)	≥20% increase in sum of maximal diameters	≥73% increase in volume	≥25% increase in product of orthogonal diameters	≥40% increase in volume

The volumes assume a spherical tumor calculated from a single diameter or two orthogonal diameters using the formula $V = (4/3) \pi r^3$. For multiple lesions, this response assesses the sum of longest diameters/volumes of multiple measurable lesions

Volumetric Methods

Quantitative correlations between 2D and volumetric measurements are difficult as linear measurement on a single axial image cannot account for highly irregular shapes, nodular growth patterns, cystic areas, and central necrosis [130–133]. As changes in volume may only have a slight effect on tumor diameter, volume changes up to 59% can go undetected [134]. Thus, for the same tumor, depending on whether RECIST or MacDonald criteria are used, corresponding changes in their volumes (estimated using the formula for a sphere, $V = (4/3) \pi r^3$) can vary significantly (Table 44.3). For MRI, standardized volumetric assessments may be feasible using validated computerized automated pattern recognition algorithms [135].

Post-Treatment Response Assessment

Clinically significant changes should be confirmed by serial imaging at 4 weeks. In clinical trials they are defined as complete response (CR); partial response (PR); stable disease (SD); and progressive disease (PD). Inhibitors of vascular endothelial growth factor (VEGF) produce a rapid decrease in the degree of contrast enhancement within malignant gliomas and in the extent of surrounding hyperintense T2-weighted signal intensity [136]. These effects, which are consistent with decrease in the permeability of tumor capillaries, make it exceedingly difficult to use conventional measures of tumor size.

SUMMARY

Significant advances have been made in brain images since the introduction of the CT scan in 1970. Simple anatomic images showing only blood, brain, and bone have been enhanced by a variety of modalities showing anatomic detail and biologic function at ever-increasing levels of detail.

REFERENCES

1. Ricci PE, Dungan DH. Imaging of low- and intermediate-grade gliomas. *Semin Radiat Oncol.* 2001;11(2):103–112.
2. Munley MT, Kearns WT, Hinson WH, et al. Bioanatomic IMRT treatment planning with dose function histograms. *Int J Radiat Oncol Biol Phys.* 2002;54:126.
3. Nuutinen J, Sonninen P, Lehikoinen P, et al. Radiotherapy treatment planning and long-term follow-up with [(11)C]methionine PET in patients with low-grade astrocytoma. *Int J Radiat Oncol Biol Phys.* 2000;48(1):43–52.
4. Pirzkall A, Larson DA, McKnight TR, et al. MR-Spectroscopy results in improved target delineation for high-grade gliomas. *Int J Radiat Oncol Biol Phys.* 2000;48:115.
5. Husband DJ, Grant KA, Romaniuk CS. MRI in the diagnosis and treatment of suspected malignant spinal cord compression. *Br J Radiol.* 2001;74(877):15–23.
6. Latour LL, Svoboda K, Mitra PP, Sotak CH. Time-dependent diffusion of water in a biological model system. *Proc Natl Acad Sci USA.* 1994;91(4):1229–1233.
7. Brunberg JA, Chenevert TL, McKeever PE, et al. In vivo MR determination of water diffusion coefficients and diffusion anisotropy: correlation with structural alteration in gliomas of the cerebral hemispheres. *AJNR Am J Neuroradiol.* 1995;16(2):361–371.
8. Bulakbasi N, Kocaoglu M, Ors F, Tayfun C, Uçöz T. Combination of single-voxel proton MR spectroscopy and apparent diffusion coefficient calculation in the evaluation of common brain tumors. *AJNR Am J Neuroradiol.* 2003;24(2):225–233.
9. Castillo M, Smith JK, Kwock L, et al. Apparent diffusion coefficients in the evaluation of high-grade cerebral gliomas. *AJNR Am J Neuroradiol.* 2001;22:60–64.
10. Guo AC, Cummings TJ, Dash RC, Provenzale JM. Lymphomas and high-grade astrocytomas: comparison of water diffusibility and histologic characteristics. *Radiology.* 2002;224(1):177–183.
11. Kono K, Inoue Y, Nakayama K, et al. The role of diffusion weighted imaging in patients with brain tumors. *AJNR Am J Neuroradiol.* 2001;22(6):1081–1088.
12. Krabbe K, Gideon P, Wagn P, et al. MR diffusion imaging of human intracranial tumours. *Neuroradiology.* 1997;39:483–489.
13. Lam WW, Poon WS, Metreweli C. Diffusion MR imaging in glioma: does it have any role in the pre-operation determination of grading of glioma? *Clin Radiol.* 2002;57(3):219–225.
14. Maier SE, Bogner P, Bajzik G, et al. Normal brain and brain tumor: multicomponent apparent diffusion coefficient line scan imaging. *Radiology.* 2001;219(3):842–849.
15. Stadnik TW, Chaskis C, Michotte A, et al. Diffusion-weighted MR imaging of intracerebral masses: comparison with conventional MR imaging and histologic findings. *AJNR Am J Neuroradiol.* 2001;22(5):969–976.
16. Tien RD, Felsberg GJ, Friedman H, Brown M, MacFall J. MR imaging of high-grade cerebral gliomas: value of diffusion-weighted echoplanar pulse sequences. *AJR Am J Roentgenol.* 1994;162(3):671–677.
17. Filippi CG, Edgar MA, Ulug AM, Prowda JC, Heier LA, Zimmerman RD. Appearance of meningiomas on diffusion-weighted images: correlating diffusion constants with histopathologic findings. *AJNR Am J Neuroradiol.* 2001;22(1):65–72.

18. Sugahara T, Korogi Y, Kochi M, et al. Usefulness of diffusion-weighted MRI with echo-planar technique in the evaluation of cellularity in gliomas. *J Magn Reson Imaging*. 1999;9(1):53–60.
19. Eis M, Els T, Hoehn-Berlage M, et al. Quantitative diffusion MR imaging of cerebral tumor and edema. *Acta Neurochir Suppl (Wien)*. 1994;60:344–346.
20. Beppu T, Inoue T, Shibata Y, et al. Fractional anisotropy value by diffusion tensor magnetic resonance imaging as a predictor of cell density and proliferation activity of glioblastomas. *Surg Neurol*. 2005;63:56–61.
21. Stadlbauer A, Ganslandt O, Buslei R, et al. Gliomas: histopathologic evaluation of changes in directionality and magnitude of water diffusion at diffusion-tensor MR imaging. *Radiology*. 2006;240(3):803–810.
22. Price SJ, Jena R, Burnet NG, et al. Improved delineation of glioma margins and regions of infiltration with the use of diffusion tensor imaging: an image-guided biopsy study. *AJNR Am J Neuroradiol*. 2006;27:1969–1974.
23. Witwer BP, Moftakhar R, Hasan KM, et al. Diffusion-tensor imaging of white matter tracts in patients with cerebral neoplasm. *J Neurosurg*. 2002;97(3):568–575.
24. Hall DE, Moffat BA, Stojanovska J, et al. Therapeutic efficacy of DTI-015 using diffusion magnetic resonance imaging as an early surrogate marker. *Clin Cancer Res*. 2004;10(23):7852–7859.
25. Moffat BA, Chenevert TL, Lawrence TS, et al. Functional diffusion map: a noninvasive MRI biomarker for early stratification of clinical brain tumor response. *Proc Natl Acad Sci USA*. 2005;102(15):5524–5529.
26. Law M, Yang S, Babb JS, et al. Comparison of cerebral blood volume and vascular permeability from dynamic susceptibility contrast-enhanced perfusion MR imaging with glioma grade. *AJNR Am J Neuroradiol*. 2004;25:746–755.
27. Provenzale JM, Wang GR, Brenner T, Petrella JR, Sorensen AG. Comparison of permeability in high-grade and low-grade brain tumors using dynamic susceptibility contrast MR imaging. *AJR Am J Roentgenol*. 2002;178(3):711–716.
28. Roberts HC, Roberts TP, Brasch RC, et al. Quantitative measurement of microvascular permeability in human brain tumors achieved using dynamic contrast-enhanced MR imaging: correlation with histologic grade. *AJNR Am J Neuroradiol*. 2000;21:891–899.
29. Roberts HC, Roberts TP, Ley S, et al. Quantitative estimation of microvascular permeability in human brain tumors: correlation of dynamic Gd-DTPA-enhanced MR imaging with histopathologic grading. *Acad Radiol*. 2002;9 (suppl 1):S151-S155.
30. Aronen HJ, Gazit IE, Louis DN, et al. Cerebral blood volume maps of gliomas: comparison with tumor grade and histologic findings. *Radiology*. 1994;191(1):41–51.
31. Aronen HJ, Pardo FS, Kennedy DN, et al. High microvascular blood volume is associated with high glucose uptake and tumor angiogenesis in human gliomas. *Clin Cancer Res*. 2000;6(6):2189–2200.
32. Knopp EA, Cha S, Johnson G, et al. Glial neoplasms: dynamic contrast-enhanced T2*-weighted MR imaging. *Radiology*. 1999;211(3):791–798.
33. Law M, Cha S, Knopp EA, Johnson G, Arnett J, Litt AW. High-grade gliomas and solitary metastases: differentiation by using perfusion and proton spectroscopic MR imaging. *Radiology*. 2002;222(3):715–721.
34. Shin JH, Lee HK, Kwun BD, et al. Using relative cerebral blood flow and volume to evaluate the histopathologic grade of cerebral gliomas: preliminary results. *AJR Am J Roentgenol*. 2002;179(3):783–789.
35. Sugahara T, Korogi Y, Kochi M, et al. Correlation of MR imaging-determined cerebral blood volume maps with histologic and angiographic determination of vascularity of gliomas. *AJR Am J Roentgenol*. 1998;171(6):1479–1486.
36. Lev MH, Ozsunar Y, Henson JW, et al. Glial tumor grading and outcome prediction using dynamic spin-echo MR susceptibility mapping compared with conventional contrast-enhanced MR: confounding effect of elevated rCBV of oligodendrogliomas [corrected]. *AJNR Am J Neuroradiol*. 2004;25(2):214–221.
37. Cao Y, Tsien CI, Nagesh V, et al. Survival prediction in high-grade gliomas by MRI perfusion before and during early stage of RT [corrected]. *Int J Radiat Oncol Biol Phys*. 2006;64(3):876–885.
38. Cha S, Tihan T, Crawford F, et al. Differentiation of low-grade oligodendrogliomas from low-grade astrocytomas by using quantitative blood-volume measurements derived from dynamic susceptibility contrast-enhanced MR imaging. *AJNR Am J Neuroradiol*. 2005;26(2):266–273.
39. Sugahara T, Korogi Y, Kochi M, Ushio Y, Takahashi M. Perfusion-sensitive MR imaging of gliomas: comparison between gradient-echo and spin-echo echo-planar imaging techniques. *AJNR Am J Neuroradiol*. 2001;22(7):1306–1315.
40. Leach MO, Brindle KM, Evelhoch JL, et al. Assessment of antiangiogenic and antivascular therapeutics using MRI: recommendations for appropriate methodology for clinical trials. *Br J Radiol*. 2003;76 Spec No 1:S87-S91.
41. Lüdemann L, Grieger W, Wurm R, Budzisch M, Hamm B, Zimmer C. Comparison of dynamic contrast-enhanced MRI with WHO tumor grading for gliomas. *Eur Radiol*. 2001;11(7):1231–1241.
42. Patankar TF, Haroon HA, Mills SJ, et al. Is volume transfer coefficient (K(trans)) related to histologic grade in human gliomas? *AJNR Am J Neuroradiol*. 2005;26(10):2455–2465.
43. Roberts HC, Roberts TP, Bollen AW, Ley S, Brasch RC, Dillon WP. Correlation of microvascular permeability derived from dynamic contrast-enhanced MR imaging with histologic grade and tumor labeling index: a study in human brain tumors. *Acad Radiol*. 2001;8(5):384–391.
44. Rémy C, Fouilhé N, Barba I, et al. Evidence that mobile lipids detected in rat brain glioma by 1H nuclear magnetic resonance correspond to lipid droplets. *Cancer Res*. 1997;57(3):407–414.
45. Murphy M, Loosemore A, Clifton AG, et al. The contribution of proton magnetic resonance spectroscopy (1HMRS) to clinical brain tumour diagnosis. *Br J Neurosurg*. 2002;16:329–334.1
46. Negendank WG, Sauter R, Brown TR, et al. Proton magnetic resonance spectroscopy in patients with glial tumors: a multicenter study. *J Neurosurg*. 1996;84(3):449–458.
47. Star-Lack J, Spielman D, Adalsteinsson E, Kurhanewicz J, Terris DJ, Vigneron DB. In vivo lactate editing with simultaneous detection of choline, creatine, NAA, and lipid singlets at 1.5 T using PRESS excitation with applications to the study of brain and head and neck tumors. *J Magn Reson*. 1998;133(2):243–254.
48. McBride DQ, Miller BL, Nikas DL, et al. Analysis of brain tumors using 1H magnetic resonance spectroscopy. *Surg Neurol*. 1995;44(2):137–144.
49. Nafe R, Herminghaus S, Raab P, et al. Preoperative proton-MR spectroscopy of gliomas–correlation with quantitative nuclear morphology in surgical specimen. *J Neurooncol*. 2003;63(3):233–245.
50. Allen N. Oxidative metabolism of brain tumors. *Prog Exp Tumor Res*. 1972;17:192–209.
51. Croteau D, Scarpace L, Hearshen D, et al. Correlation between magnetic resonance spectroscopy imaging and image-guided biopsies: semiquantitative and qualitative histopathological analyses of patients with untreated glioma. *Neurosurgery*. 2001;49(4):823–829.
52. Simmons ML, Frondoza CG, Coyle JT. Immunocytochemical localization of N-acetyl-aspartate with monoclonal antibodies. *Neuroscience*. 1991;45(1):37–45.
55. Tarnawski R, Sokol M, Pieniazek P, et al. 1H-MRS in vivo predicts the early treatment outcome of postoperative radiotherapy for malignant gliomas. *Int J Radiat Oncol Biol Phys*. 2002;52(5):1271–1276.
53. Law M, Yang S, Wang H, et al. Glioma grading: sensitivity, specificity, and predictive values of perfusion MR imaging and proton MR spectroscopic imaging compared with conventional MR imaging. *AJNR Am J Neuroradiol*. 2003;24:1989–1998.
54. McKnight TR, von dem Bussche MH, Vigneron DB, et al. Histopathological validation of a three-dimensional magnetic resonance spectroscopy index as a predictor of tumor presence. *J Neurosurg*. 2002;97(4):794–802.
56. Howe FA, Barton SJ, Cudlip SA, et al. Metabolic profiles of human brain tumors using quantitative in vivo 1H magnetic resonance spectroscopy. *Magn Reson Med*. 2003;49(2):223–232.
58. Sijens PE, Oudkerk M. 1H chemical shift imaging characterization of human brain tumor and edema. *Eur Radiol*. 2002;12:2056–2061.
59. Gupta RK, Cloughesy TF, Sinha U, et al. Relationships between choline magnetic resonance spectroscopy, apparent diffusion coefficient and quantitative histopathology in human glioma. *J Neurooncol*. 2000;50(3):215–226.
57. Meyerand ME, Pipas JM, Mamourian A, Tosteson TD, Dunn JF. Classification of biopsy-confirmed brain tumors using single-voxel MR spectroscopy. *AJNR Am J Neuroradiol*. 1999;20(1):117–123.
60. Astrakas LG, Zurakowski D, Tzika AA, et al. Noninvasive magnetic resonance spectroscopic imaging biomarkers to predict the clinical grade of pediatric brain tumors. *Clin Cancer Res*. 2004;10(24):8220–8228.

61. Fountas KN, Kapsalaki EZ, Vogel RL, et al. Noninvasive histologic grading of solid astrocytomas using proton magnetic resonance spectroscopy. *Stereotact Funct Neurosurg.* 2004;82:90–97.
62. Huang Y, Lisboa PJ, El-Deredy W. Tumour grading from magnetic resonance spectroscopy: a comparison of feature extraction with variable selection. *Stat Med.* 2003;22(1):147–164.
63. Lukas L, Devos A, Suykens JA, et al. Brain tumor classification based on long echo proton MRS signals. *Artif Intell Med.* 2004;31(1):73–89.
64. Herminghaus S, Dierks T, Pilatus U, et al. Determination of histo-pathological tumor grade in neuroepithelial brain tumors by using spectral pattern analysis of *in vivo* spectroscopic data. *J Neurosurg.* 2003;98(1):74–81.
65. Pirzkall A, Li X, Oh J, et al. 3D MRSI for resected high-grade gliomas before RT: tumor extent according to metabolic activity in relation to MRI. *Int J Radiat Oncol Biol Phys.* 2004;59(1):126–137.
66. Graves EE, Nelson SJ, Vigneron DB, et al. A preliminary study of the prognostic value of proton magnetic resonance spectroscopic imaging in gamma knife radiosurgery of recurrent malignant gliomas. *Neurosurgery.* 2000;46(2):319–26; discussion 326.
67. Graves EE, Pirzkall A, Nelson SJ, Larson D, Verhey L. Registration of magnetic resonance spectroscopic imaging to computed tomography for radiotherapy treatment planning. *Med Phys.* 2001;28(12):2489–2496.
68. McKnight TR, Noworolski SM, Vigneron DB, Nelson SJ. An automated technique for the quantitative assessment of 3D-MRSI data from patients with glioma. *J Magn Reson Imaging.* 2001;13(2):167–177.
69. Nelson SJ, Graves E, Pirzkall A, et al. In vivo molecular imaging for planning radiation therapy of gliomas: an application of 1H MRSI. *J Magn Reson Imaging.* 2002;16(4):464–476.
70. Pirzkall A, McKnight TR, Graves EE, et al. MR-spectroscopy guided target delineation for high-grade gliomas. *Int J Radiat Oncol Biol Phys.* 2001;50(4):915–928.
71. Pirzkall A, Nelson SJ, McKnight TR, et al. Metabolic imaging of low-grade gliomas with three-dimensional magnetic resonance spectroscopy. *Int J Radiat Oncol Biol Phys.* 2002;53(5):1254–1264.
72. Stieber V, Tatter S, Lovato J, et al. A phase I dose escalating study of intensity modulated radiation therapy (IMRT) for the treatment of glioblastoma multiforme (GBM). *Int J Radiat Oncol Biol Phys.* 2004;(suppl 1):261.
73. Stieber V, Tatter S, Mikkelsen T, et al. A Phase I dose-escalation trial of GliaSite brachytherapy with conventional radiation therapy for newly diagnosed glioblastoma multiforme. J Clin Oncol. 2005;23:1570.
74. Barker FG 2nd, Davis RL, Chang SM, Prados MD. Necrosis as a prognostic factor in glioblastoma multiforme. *Cancer.* 1996;77(6):1161–1166.
75. Ando K, Ishikura R, Nagami Y, et al. [Usefulness of Cho/Cr ratio in proton MR spectroscopy for differentiating residual/recurrent glioma from non-neoplastic lesions]. *Nippon Igaku Hoshasen Gakkai Zasshi.* 2004;64(3):121–126.
76. Plotkin M, Eisenacher J, Bruhn H, et al. 123I-IMT SPECT and 1H MR-spectroscopy at 3.0 T in the differential diagnosis of recurrent or residual gliomas: a comparative study. *J Neurooncol.* 2004;70(1):49–58.
77. Träber F, Block W, Flacke S, et al [1H-MR Spectroscopy of brain tumors in the course of radiation therapy: Use of fast spectroscopic imaging and single-voxel spectroscopy for diagnosing recurrence]. *Rofo.* 2002;174(1):33–42.
78. Dowling C, Bollen AW, Noworolski SM, et al. Preoperative proton MR spectroscopic imaging of brain tumors: correlation with histo-pathologic analysis of resection specimens. *AJNR Am J Neuroradiol.* 2001;22(4):604–612.
79. Kamada K, Houkin K, Abe H, Sawamura Y, Kashiwaba T. Differentiation of cerebral radiation necrosis from tumor recurrence by proton magnetic resonance spectroscopy. *Neurol Med Chir (Tokyo).* 1997;37(3):250–256.
80. Nelson SJ, Huhn S, Vigneron DB, et al. Volume MRI and MRSI techniques for the quantitation of treatment response in brain tumors: presentation of a detailed case study. *J Magn Reson Imaging.* 1997;7(6):1146–1152.
81. Nelson SJ, Vigneron DB, Dillon WP. Serial evaluation of patients with brain tumors using volume MRI and 3D 1H MRSI. *NMR Biomed.* 1999;12(3):123–138.
82. Schlemmer HP, Bachert P, Henze M, et al. Differentiation of radiation necrosis from tumor progression using proton magnetic resonance spectroscopy. *Neuroradiology.* 2002;44(3):216–222.
83. Taylor JS, Langston JW, Reddick WE, et al. Clinical value of proton magnetic resonance spectroscopy for differentiating recurrent or residual brain tumor from delayed cerebral necrosis. *Int J Radiat Oncol Biol Phys.* 1996;36(5):1251–1261.
84. Holodny AI, Schulder M, Liu WC, Maldjian JA, Kalnin AJ. Decreased BOLD functional MR activation of the motor and sensory cortices adjacent to a glioblastoma multiforme: implications for image-guided neurosurgery. *AJNR Am J Neuroradiol.* 1999;20(4):609–612.
85. Ulmer JL, Krouwer HG, Mueller WM, Ugurel MS, Kocak M, Mark LP. Pseudo-reorganization of language cortical function at fMR imaging: a consequence of tumor-induced neurovascular uncoupling. *AJNR Am J Neuroradiol.* 2003;24(2):213–217.
86. Roux FE, Boulanouar K, Lotterie JA, Mejdoubi M, LeSage JP, Berry I. Language functional magnetic resonance imaging in preoperative assessment of language areas: correlation with direct cortical stimulation. *Neurosurgery.* 2003;52(6):1335–1345; discussion 1345.
87. Rutten GJ, Ramsey NF, van Rijen PC, van Veelen CW. Reproducibility of fMRI-determined language lateralization in individual subjects. *Brain Lang.* 2002;80(3):421–437.
88. Roux FE, Trémoulet M. Organization of language areas in bilingual patients: a cortical stimulation study. *J Neurosurg.* 2002;97(4):857–864.
89. Ramsey NF, Tallent K, van Gelderen P, Frank JA, Moonen CT, Weinberger DR. Reproducibility of human 3D fMRI brain maps acquired during a motor task. *Hum Brain Mapp.* 1996;4(2):113–121.
90. Meade TJ, Taylor AK, Bull SR. New magnetic resonance contrast agents as biochemical reporters. *Curr Opin Neurobiol.* 2003;13(5):597–602.
91. Chao ST, Suh JH, Raja S, Lee SY, Barnett G. The sensitivity and specificity of FDG PET in distinguishing recurrent brain tumor from radionecrosis in patients treated with stereotactic radiosurgery. *Int J Cancer.* 2001;96(3):191–197.
92. Ricci PE, Karis JP, Heiserman JE, Fram EK, Bice AN, Drayer BP. Differentiating recurrent tumor from radiation necrosis: time for re-evaluation of positron emission tomography? *AJNR Am J Neuroradiol.* 1998;19(3):407–413.
93. Barker FG 2nd, Chang SM, Valk PE, Pounds TR, Prados MD. 18-Fluorodeoxyglucose uptake and survival of patients with suspected recurrent malignant glioma. *Cancer.* 1997;79(1):115–126.
94. De Witte O, Levivier M, Violon P, et al. Prognostic value positron emission tomography with [18F]fluoro-2-deoxy-D-glucose in the low-grade glioma. *Neurosurgery.* 1996;39(3):470–476; discussion 476.
95. Spence AM, Mankoff DA, Muzi M. Positron emission tomography imaging of brain tumors. *Neuroimaging Clin N Am.* 2003;13(4):717–739.
96. Bergström M, Collins VP, Ehrin E, et al. Discrepancies in brain tumor extent as shown by computed tomography and positron emission tomography using [68Ga]EDTA, [11C]glucose, and [11C]methionine. *J Comput Assist Tomogr.* 1983;7(6):1062–1066.
97. Braun V, Dempf S, Weller R, Reske SN, Schachenmayr W, Richter HP. Cranial neuronavigation with direct integration of (11)C methionine positron emission tomography (PET) data – results of a pilot study in 32 surgical cases. *Acta Neurochir (Wien).* 2002;144(8):777–782; discussion 782.
98. Herholz K, Hölzer T, Bauer B, et al. 11C-methionine PET for differential diagnosis of low-grade gliomas. *Neurology.* 1998;50(5):1316–1322.
99. Kracht LW, Miletic H, Busch S, et al. Delineation of brain tumor extent with [11C]L-methionine positron emission tomography: local comparison with stereotactic histopathology. *Clin Cancer Res.* 2004;10(21):7163–7170.
100. Miwa K, Shinoda J, Yano H, et al. Discrepancy between lesion distributions on methionine PET and MR images in patients with glioblastoma multiforme: insight from a PET and MR fusion image study. *J Neurol Neurosurg Psychiatr.* 2004;75(10):1457–1462.
101. Pirotte B, Goldman S, Dewitte O, et al. Integrated positron emission tomography and magnetic resonance imaging-guided resection of brain tumors: a report of 103 consecutive procedures. *J Neurosurg.* 2006;104(2):238–253.
102. Grosu AL, Lachner R, Wiedenmann N, et al. Validation of a method for automatic image fusion (BrainLAB System) of CT data and 11C-methionine-PET data for stereotactic radiotherapy using a LINAC: first clinical experience. *Int J Radiat Oncol Biol Phys.* 2003;56(5):1450–1463.
103. Grosu AL, Weber WA, Riedel E, et al. L-(methyl-11C) methionine positron emission tomography for target delineation in resected

high-grade gliomas before radiotherapy. *Int J Radiat Oncol Biol Phys.* 2005;63:64–74.
104. Grosu AL, Weber WA, Franz M, et al. Reirradiation of recurrent high-grade gliomas using amino acid PET (SPECT)/CT/MRI image fusion to determine gross tumor volume for stereotactic fractionated radiotherapy. *Int J Radiat Oncol Biol Phys.* 2005;63:511–519.
105. Hamacher K, Coenen HH. Efficient routine production of the 18F-labelled amino acid O-2–18F fluoroethyl-L-tyrosine. *Appl Radiat Isot.* 2002;57(6):853–856.
106. Wester HJ, Herz M, Weber W, et al. Synthesis and radiopharmacology of O-(2-[18F]fluoroethyl)-L-tyrosine for tumor imaging. *J Nucl Med.* 1999;40(1):205–212.
107. Langen KJ, Jarosch M, Mühlensiepen H, et al. Comparison of fluorotyrosines and methionine uptake in F98 rat gliomas. *Nucl Med Biol.* 2003;30(5):501–508.
108. Weber WA, Wester HJ, Grosu AL, et al. O-(2-[18F]fluoroethyl)-L-tyrosine and L-[methyl-11C]methionine uptake in brain tumours: initial results of a comparative study. *Eur J Nucl Med.* 2000;27(5):542–549.
109. Floeth FW, Pauleit D, Wittsack HJ, et al. Multimodal metabolic imaging of cerebral gliomas: positron emission tomography with [18F]fluoroethyl-L-tyrosine and magnetic resonance spectroscopy. *J Neurosurg.* 2005;102(2):318–327.
110. Pauleit D, Floeth F, Hamacher K, et al. O-(2-[18F]fluoroethyl)-L-tyrosine PET combined with MRI improves the diagnostic assessment of cerebral gliomas. *Brain.* 2005;128(Pt 3):678–687.
111. Floeth FW, Pauleit D, Sabel M, et al. 18F-FET PET differentiation of ring-enhancing brain lesions. *J Nucl Med.* 2006;47(5):776–782.
112. Oriuchi N, Tamura M, Shibazaki T, et al. Clinical evaluation of thallium-201 SPECT in supratentorial gliomas: relationship to histologic grade, prognosis and proliferative activities. J Nucl Med. 1993;34:2085–2089.
113. Sun D, Liu Q, Liu W, Hu W. Clinical application of 201Tl SPECT imaging of brain tumors. *J Nucl Med.* 2000;41(1):5–10.
114. Bénard F, Romsa J, Hustinx R. Imaging gliomas with positron emission tomography and single-photon emission computed tomography. *Semin Nucl Med.* 2003;33(2):148–162.
115. Langen KJ, Ziemons K, Kiwit JC, et al. 3-[123I]iodo-alpha-methyl-tyrosine and [methyl-11C]-L-methionine uptake in cerebral gliomas: a comparative study using SPECT and PET. *J Nucl Med.* 1997;38(4):517–522.
116. Pauleit D, Floeth F, Tellmann L, et al. Comparison of O-(2–18F-fluoroethyl)-L-tyrosine PET and 3–123I-iodo-alpha-methyl-L-tyrosine SPECT in brain tumors. *J Nucl Med.* 2004;45(3):374–381.
117. Grosu AL, Weber W, Feldmann HJ, et al. First experience with I-123-alpha-methyl-tyrosine spect in the 3-D radiation treatment planning of brain gliomas. *Int J Radiat Oncol Biol Phys.* 2000;47(3):517–526.
118. Grosu AL, Feldmann H, Dick S, et al. Implications of IMT-SPECT for postoperative radiotherapy planning in patients with gliomas. *Int J Radiat Oncol Biol Phys.* 2002;54(3):842–854.
119. Weber WA, Dick S, Reidl G, et al. Correlation between postoperative 3-[(123)I]iodo-L-alpha-methyltyrosine uptake and survival in patients with gliomas. *J Nucl Med.* 2001;42(8):1144–1150.
120. Papanicolaou AC. An introduction to magnetoencephalography with some applications. *Brain Cogn.* 1995;27(3):331–352.
121. Babiloni F, Mattia D, Babiloni C, et al. Multimodal integration of EEG, MEG and fMRI data for the solution of the neuroimage puzzle. *Magn Reson Imaging.* 2004;22(10):1471–1476.
122. Aoyama H, Kamada K, Shirato H, et al. Integration of functional brain information into stereotactic irradiation treatment planning using magnetoencephalography and magnetic resonance axonography. *Int J Radiat Oncol Biol Phys.* 2004;58(4):1177–1183.
123. Kamada K, Houkin K, Takeuchi F, et al. Visualization of the eloquent motor system by integration of MEG, functional, and anisotropic diffusion-weighted MRI in functional neuronavigation. *Surg Neurol.* 2003;59(5):352–361; discussion 361.
124. Kamada K, Möller M, Saguer M, et al. A combined study of tumor-related brain lesions using MEG and proton MR spectroscopic imaging. *J Neurol Sci.* 2001;186(1–2):13–21.
125. de Jongh A, Baayen JC, de Munck JC, Heethaar RM, Vandertop WP, Stam CJ. The influence of brain tumor treatment on pathological delta activity in MEG. *Neuroimage.* 2003;20(4):2291–2301.
126. Miller AB, Hoogstraten B, Staquet M, et al. Reporting results of cancer treatment. *Cancer.* 1981;47:207–214.
127. Forsyth PA, Petrov E, Mahallati H, et al. Prospective study of postoperative magnetic resonance imaging in patients with malignant gliomas. *J Clin Oncol.* 1997;15:2076–2081.
128. Therasse P, Arbuck SG, Eisenhauer EA, et al. New guidelines to evaluate the response to treatment in solid tumors. European Organization for Research and Treatment of Cancer, National Cancer Institute of the United States, National Cancer Institute of Canada. *J Natl Cancer Inst.* 2000;92(3):205–216.
129. Macdonald DR, Cascino TL, Schold SC Jr, Cairncross JG. Response criteria for phase II studies of supratentorial malignant glioma. *J Clin Oncol.* 1990;8(7):1277–1280.
130. Galanis E, Buckner JC, Maurer MJ, et al. Validation of neuroradiologic response assessment in gliomas: measurement by RECIST, two-dimensional, computer-assisted tumor area, and computer-assisted tumor volume methods. *Neuro-oncology.* 2006;8(2):156–165.
131. Shah GD, Kesari S, Xu R, et al. Comparison of linear and volumetric criteria in assessing tumor response in adult high-grade gliomas. *Neuro-oncology.* 2006;8(1):38–46.
132. Sorensen AG, Patel S, Harmath C, et al. Comparison of diameter and perimeter methods for tumor volume calculation. *J Clin Oncol.* 2001;19(2):551–557.
133. Warren KE, Patronas N, Aikin AA, Albert PS, Balis FM. Comparison of one-, two-, and three-dimensional measurements of childhood brain tumors. *J Natl Cancer Inst.* 2001;93(18):1401–1405.
134. Filipek PA, Kennedy DN, Caviness VS Jr. Volumetric analyses of central nervous system neoplasm based on MRI. *Pediatr Neurol.* 1991;7(5):347–351.
135. Tate AR, Majós C, Moreno A, Howe FA, Griffiths JR, Arús C. Automated classification of short echo time in *in vivo* 1H brain tumor spectra: a multicenter study. *Magn Reson Med.* 2003;49(1):29–36.
136. Pope WB, Lai A, Nghiemphu P, Mischel P, Cloughesy TF. MRI in patients with high-grade gliomas treated with bevacizumab and chemotherapy. *Neurology.* 2006;66(8):1258–1260.

PART IV: NEUROANATOMY AND NEUROSURGERY

45 Functional Neuroanatomy

Sameer A. Sheth, Bradley R. Buchbinder, and Fred G. Barker, II

INTRODUCTION

Compartmentalization of the brain along contours that delineate functional boundaries presupposes a unique correspondence between brain structure and function. The notion that the brain is parceled into distinct areas that each subserve a particular function had dubious origins. This concept was first proffered in the late 18th century by the Viennese physician Franz Joseph Gall, who demonstrated to his own (and others') satisfaction that the brain's various constituent "mental organs" were dedicated to distinct cognitive faculties and that the development of these mental organs could be traced on the patient's skull [1]. Despite the tremendous failure of his theory of phrenology, Gall's idea of functional topography laid the groundwork for future localization endeavors by others after an initial period of reaction against cerebral localization [2–6].

The aim of this chapter is to portray the functional anatomy of the brain and spinal cord by giving a survey of the functional neuroanatomy most relevant for neuro-oncology and neurosurgery. The first section provides a brief overview of functional neuroimaging techniques, including magnetoencephalography and transcranial magnetic stimulation, functional magnetic resonance imaging, and diffusion tensor imaging, with an emphasis on preoperative planning.

The following sections cover the functional neuroanatomy of the cerebral lobes, including the frontal, parietal, temporal, and occipital lobes. Whereas some authors distinguish the hippocampal formation (HF) as part of a separate limbic lobe, it is included here in the discussion of the temporal lobe because of its clinical relevance to temporal lobe lesions and surgery. Within each section, we delineate the anatomical boundaries of the region. Particular attention is paid to not only the eloquent cortical areas but also the subcortical white matter tracts that project to and from them, as disruption of these deep tracts can cause significant functional impairment. The function of the region is then described, along with clinical manifestations or syndromes that can arise from damage to the region. We also mention the surgical approaches to lesions situated within the area, contributions from preoperative functional imaging, and techniques for minimizing postoperative deficit while maximizing resection.

PREOPERATIVE FUNCTIONAL MAPPING

Magnetoencephalography and Transcranial Magnetic Stimulation

The field of noninvasive functional brain imaging arguably began with the development of electroencephalography (EEG), pioneered in the late 1920s [7]. The cortical mantle can be macroscopically modeled as an electrical dipole based on net current flow into sink layers and out of source layers. The EEG is thought to represent summated postsynaptic potentials of the soma and dendrites of pyramidal cells in cortical layers III through V [8]. Although it is still used extensively for monitoring epileptiform activity, its relatively low spatial resolution precludes EEG from common use for functional localization for operative planning.

Cortical electrical currents generate extremely weak but detectable magnetic fields, which can be imaged using magnetoencephalography (MEG) [9]. The patient performs an assigned task while cortical magnetic fields are acquired and averaged. The availability of exquisitely sensitive magnetic field detectors called SQUIDs (superconducting quantum interference devices) [10] has made MEG a practical reality. Due to the way in which the magnetic fields are detected, MEG is preferentially sensitive to tangentially oriented neurons, which are often in sulci [11]. An important advantage of MEG over EEG is the head's relatively uniform permeability to magnetic fields [12]. Whereas the brain, skull, and scalp conduct electrical potentials differentially and thereby degrade EEG spatial resolution, magnetic fields are less distorted. This property offers improved spatial resolution for MEG although it is still limited to several millimeters at best.

Volumetric magnetic resonance imaging (MRI) data can be coregistered with MEG data, giving a superimposed functional map on an anatomical map [13]. This combined modality, called magnetic source imaging, has been successfully used to map motor cortex in patients whose anatomy is distorted by mass effect from nearby tumors [14]. Preoperative localization compares favorably with intraoperative electrocortical stimulation mapping (ESM) [15].

Transcranial magnetic stimulation (TMS) is a disruption-based technique that uses rapidly alternating magnetic fields to induce electrical currents within a targeted volume of cerebral cortex [16]. With proper timing, this process can produce either a positive stimulus or a temporary lesion in the underlying cortex. TMS has been used to identify motor and language cortices for preoperative planning [17].

Functional Magnetic Resonance Imaging

Increased neuronal activity in a region of the brain triggers local changes in oxygen metabolism and blood flow [18]. Although this hemodynamic response has been recognized since the late 19th century [19,20], it was not until 100 years later that it was harnessed for practical clinical use. In the early 1990s, the changes in blood oxygenation that accompany the hemodynamic response to neuronal activity were used as the basis for endogenous contrast in MRI studies, giving rise to the field of functional MRI (fMRI) [21–24]. The increase in local cerebral blood flow that follows neuronal activation increases tissue oxygen content, decreasing the relative amount of deoxyhemoglobin in the local environment. Because deoxyhemoglobin is paramagnetic, its reduction results in an increased signal strength in T2*-weighted images. This technique, termed blood oxygenation level dependent (BOLD) fMRI, is presently the most commonly used form of fMRI.

Whereas early fMRI studies demonstrated its utility for identifying sensorimotor cortex, the field has developed rapidly, and more recent work evidences its ability to delineate the fine architecture of complex functions such as language and memory [25] as well as a range of more complex mental functions such as religious experience, emotion, and belief [26]. fMRI can provide extremely useful information for preoperative planning in patients with lesions in or near eloquent regions, as their functional anatomy can be quite distorted. Loading the data into an intraoperative navigation system can also aid the surgeon when operating on such lesions [27].

Although fMRI is used to measure neuronal activity, it is important to keep in mind that the signal is actually an indicator of the hemodynamic response to neuronal activation and therefore subject to the limitations of neurovascular coupling. First, there are significant differences in vascular architecture between different regions of neocortex and between neocortex and archicortex (i.e., hippocampus), making cross-regional comparisons difficult [28]. Second, fMRI signals tend to be spatially biased towards vasculature, especially medium to large draining veins, rather than the parenchyma [29]. Third, fMRI is an activation-based technique and identifies not only regions that are essential for the chosen task but also regions that are coactivated, potentially yielding false positives.

Diffusion Tensor Imaging

Contemporaneously with the emergence of BOLD fMRI, MRI was also being used to measure the diffusion properties of water [30]. In contrast to diffusion in a homogenous solution, which occurs isotropically in all directions, diffusion may be restricted in certain directions in an inhomogeneous environment. In media containing paths along which water molecules can migrate, such as white matter tracts, diffusion is not isotropic, with a preferential orientation to the movement along the tracts. This diffusion anisotropy can be measured and used to reconstruct the course of these putative tracts through space in a process called diffusion tensor imaging (DTI) [31]. Although DTI is strictly speaking a purely anatomical technique, a combination with classical anatomical knowledge can ascribe functional significance to the identified tracts, which can be extremely useful when interpreted properly.

It is important to appreciate the limitations of DTI and the three-dimensional fiber maps it produces. Because of its inherent limited spatial resolution (on the order of a few mm), individual axons cannot be identified. Where there are no local axonal bundles of sufficient size and uniform orientation, each DTI voxel represents a meaningless average of axons traveling in different directions (i.e., just noise with no "signal").

As more sophisticated analyses are developed, the role of DTI for clinically relevant subcortical tractography is increasing. When combined with intraoperative navigation, recent studies have demonstrated its utility for identifying and sparing important tracts in motor and language areas [32,33]. The integration of motor tracts identified by DTI into the intraoperative navigation system increased extent of resection of high-grade gliomas and decreased postoperative deficit, compared with routine navigation alone, in another recent series [34]. DTI may also have utility in mapping tracts important for functions that are difficult to monitor intraoperatively, such as visual pathways.

FRONTAL LOBE

Primary Motor

Primary motor cortex is located on the precentral gyrus (Figures 45.1 and 45.2) and is somatotopically arranged in the well-known homunculus distribution, with the lower extremity on the medial aspect of the hemisphere, the upper extremity on the superior aspect of the convexity, and the face on the inferior aspect of the convexity of the frontal lobe. Efferent fibers from primary motor cortex collect in the corona radiata and further narrow into the posterior limb of the internal capsule. Somatotopic organization is maintained in the internal capsule, with fibers to the face near the genu in the corticobulbar tract and fibers to the upper and lower extremities progressively more posterior. In the midbrain these tracts are the ventral-most layer of the cerebral peduncles and are arranged similarly, with face fibers medially and leg fibers laterally. Approximately one third to one half of the corticospinal

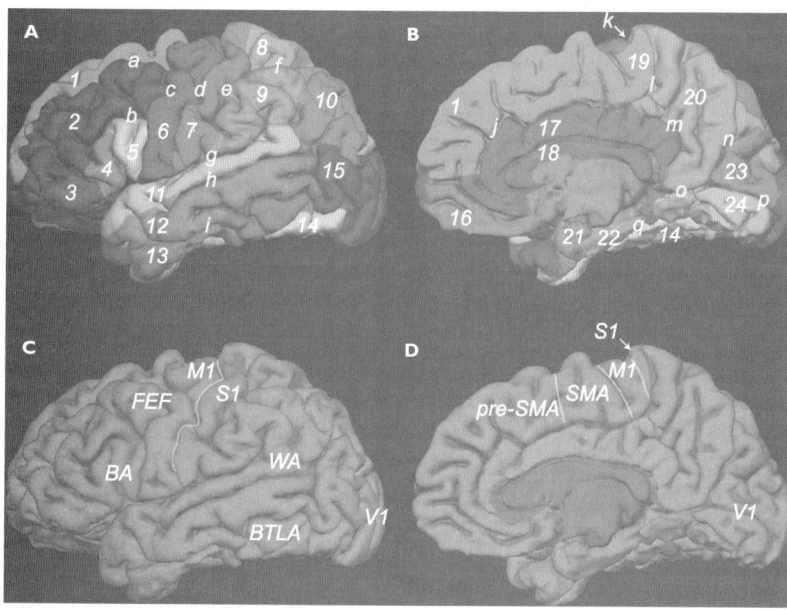

Figure 45.1 Brain surface gyral, sulcal, and functional anatomy. The lateral (**A**) and mesial (**B**) brain surface is shown, with gyri identified by white numbers and sulci by yellow letters. 1. Superior frontal gyrus; 2. middle frontal gyrus; 3. inferior frontal gyrus (IFG) pars orbitalis; 4. IFG pars triangularis; 5. IFG pars opercularis; 6. precentral gyrus; 7. postcentral gyrus; 8. superior parietal lobule; 9. supramarginal gyrus of inferior parietal lobule; 10. angular gyrus of inferior parietal lobule; 11. superior temporal gyrus; 12. middle temporal gyrus; 13. inferior temporal gyrus; 14. fusiform gyrus; 15. lateral occipital gyrus; 16. medial orbitofronal cortex; 17. cingulate gyrus; 18. corpus callosum; 19. paracentral lobule; 20. precuneus; 21. entorhinal cortex; 22. parahippocampal gyrus; 23. cuneus; 24. lingual gyrus. a. superior frontal sulcus; b. inferior frontal sulcus; c. precentral sulcus; d. central sulcus; e. postcentral sulcus; f. intraparietal sulcus; g. Sylvian fissure; h. superior temporal sulcus; i. inferior temporal sulcus; j. cingulate sulcus; k. central sulcus; l. marginal branch of cingulate sulcus; m. subparietal sulcus; n. parieto-occipital sulcus; o. anterior calcarine sulcus; p. calcarine sulcus; q. collateral sulcus. Panels (**C**) and (**D**) respectively show lateral and medial surfaces with classical functional regions highlighted. BA, Broca's area; FEF, frontal eye fields; M1, primary motor cortex; S1, primary sensory cortex; WA, Wernicke's area; BTLA, basal temporal language area; V1, primary visual cortex; SMA, supplementary motor area; pre-SMA, pre-supplementary motor area. *See color insert.*

tract fibers originate from primary motor cortex, with other contributions from supplementary and premotor cortex, primary sensory cortex, and parietal association cortex [35].

The central sulcus can be identified using a variety of anatomical landmarks [36–39]. It is the sulcus immediately posterior to the precentral sulcus, which in turn can be identified as the termination of the horizontally oriented superior and inferior frontal sulci (Figure 45.2F). Whereas the precentral sulcus is often interrupted by the middle frontal gyrus, the central sulcus is usually continuous along the convexity. It is capped superiorly by the paracentral lobule and inferiorly by the subcentral gyrus, which connect the pre- and postcentral gyri (Figure 45.1B). The latter gyrus also usually separates the central sulcus from the Sylvian fissure [36]. The central sulcus can also be identified as the posterior boundary of the precentral "omega-shaped knob" that demarcates the motor hand region [37] (Figure 45.2F). On sagittal or axial images, the marginal branch of the cingulate sulcus continues posteriorly and superiorly toward the vertex (Figures 45.1B). Immediately anterior to its intersection with the vertex is a notch formed by the central sulcus [38] (Figures 45.1B and 45.9B).

The location of the central sulcus may be obscured by the presence of a mass lesion and surrounding vasogenic edema. On T2-weighted MRI images, however, the cortical thickness of the anterior bank of the central sulcus is approximately twice that of the posterior bank [39]. This feature allows reliable identification of the central sulcus despite distorting edema.

The phase reversal of somatosensory evoked potentials (SSEPs) across the central sulcus is a reliable intraoperative indicator of its position. During contralateral medial nerve stimulation, the 20 ms latency somatosensory evoked potential recorded by subdural electrodes reverses phases from a positive precentral peak to a negative postcentral peak across the central sulcus (N20-P20 phase reversal) [40].

Damage to primary motor cortex or the descending tracts results in contralateral paresis or paralysis. For this reason, aggressive resection of lesions in this region, and in eloquent cortex in general, was to a large degree avoided in the past. The meticulous application of ESM, which has

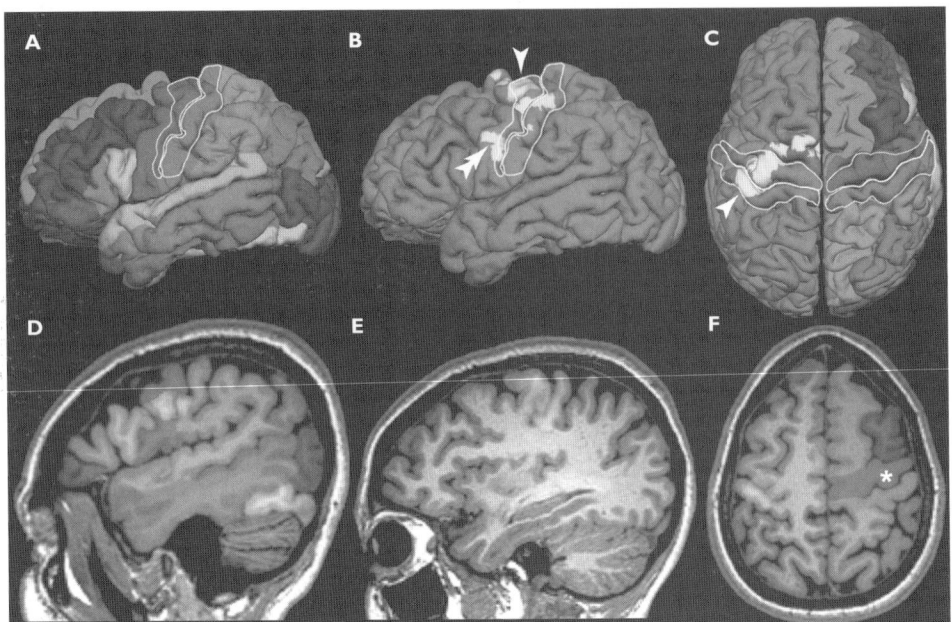

Figure 45.2 Sensorimotor functional anatomy. Panel **(A)** shows the lateral cortical surface with primary sensorimotor cortex demarcated as in Figure 45.1. Functional MRI activations during hand clenching (arrowhead) and tongue movement (double arrowhead) tasks are shown superimposed over the lateral **(B)** and superior **(C)** surfaces. Note that motor tasks such as hand clenching typically activate both primary motor and primary somatosensory cortex. Panel **(D)** shows a sagittal T1-weighted slice through the tongue activation, showing its proximity to Broca's area. Panels **(E)** and **(F)** show sagittal and axial slices through the hand activation, respectively. Task-induced SMA activation can be seen anterior to primary motor cortex in **(C)** and **(F)**. The omega-shaped knob demarcating the hand region of sensorimotor cortex is denoted by an asterisk in **(F)**. Of note, the orientation of panel **(F)** is opposite that of radiological convention (the fMRI activation is on the left side), in order to visually correspond with **(C)**, which is a top-down view. See color insert.

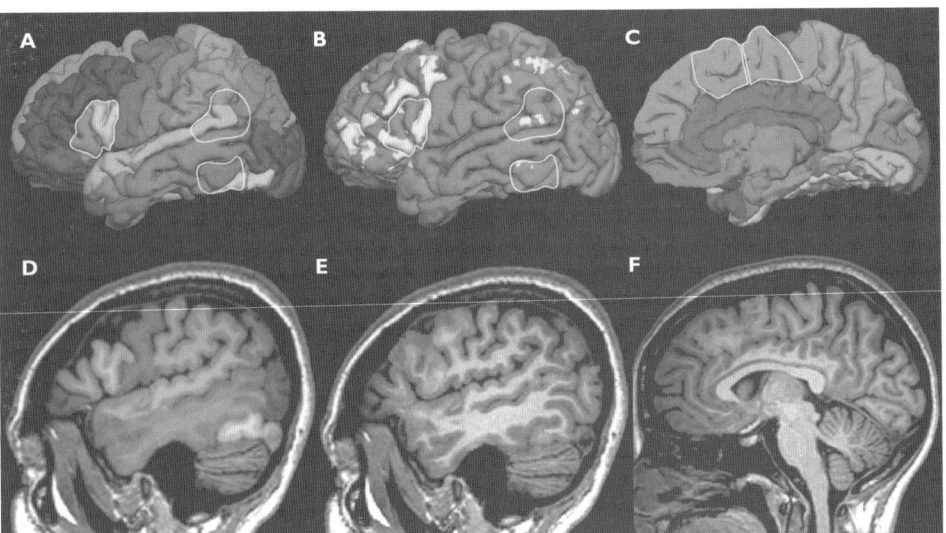

Figure 45.3 Language surface functional anatomy. Panel **(A)** shows the lateral cortical surface with classical language regions demarcated as in Figure 45.1, including Broca's area anteriorly, Wernicke's area posteriorly, and the basal temporal language area (BTLA) inferiorly. Functional MRI activations during a visually presented covert verb generation task are shown over the lateral surface in **(B)**. The SMA and pre-SMA are demarcated on the mesial surface in **(C)**. Panel **(D)** shows gyral anatomy in a lateral T1-weighted sagittal slice. Activation of Broca's area, Wernicke's area, and the BTLA, as well as other prefrontal regions is seen on a lateral sagittal slice **(E)**, and activation of pre-SMA and SMA on a mesial slice **(F)**. See color insert.

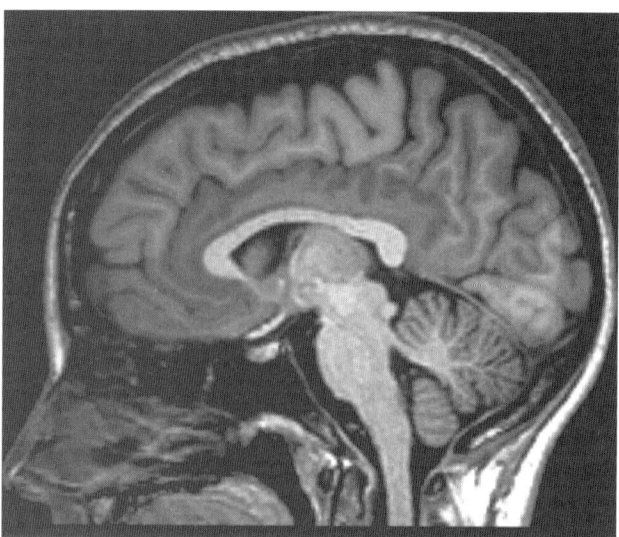

Figure 45.4 Visual surface functional anatomy. A sagittal paramedian T1-weighted slice is shown with a superimposed functional MRI activation during a visual task (flashing checkerboard). The activation is centered over primary visual cortex (banks of the calcarine sulcus) and extends into higher order visual cortices in the occipital lobe. The color scheme corresponds to that in Figure 45.1. *See color insert.*

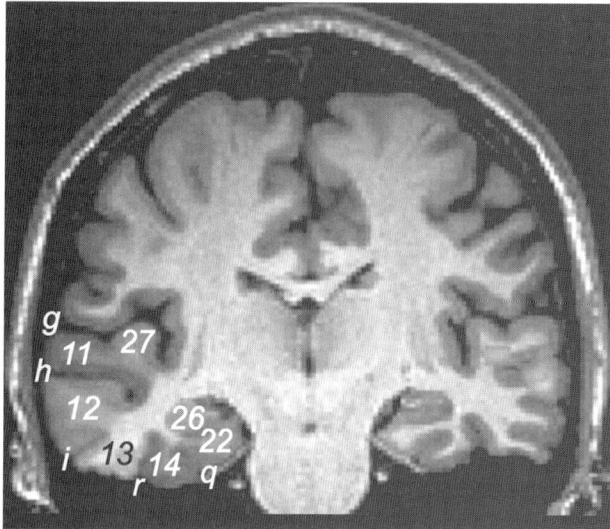

Figure 45.5 Temporal lobe and auditory surface functional anatomy. A coronal T1-weighted slice is shown, with temporal lobe gyri indicated with white numbers and sulci with yellow letters, continuing the same identification scheme as in Figure 45.1. 11. Superior temporal gyrus; 12. middle temporal gyrus; 13. inferior temporal gyrus; 14. fusiform gyrus; 22. parahippocampal gyrus; 26. hippocampal formation; 27. Heschl's gyrus (primary auditory cortex). g. Sylvian fissure; h. superior temporal sulcus; i. inferior temporal sulcus; q. collateral sulcus; r. lateral occipitotemporal sulcus. Functional MRI activation during an auditory task (passive listening to short tones) is shown on the left side, activating primary auditory cortex in the base of Heschl's gyrus as well as auditory association cortices in the superior temporal gyrus. Although the activation was bilateral, only the left side is shown for clarity. *See color insert.*

been used to identify eloquent cortex since the late 19th century [41], increases the safety of neurosurgical procedures in this region [42–44]. More recently, larger series showed greater extent of resection of primary motor lesions with decreased long-term postoperative motor deficits [45,46]. Functional anatomy is often distorted due to a lesion's mass effect. Preoperative fMRI of motor cortex is well characterized and can help identify shift or even reorganization of brain function [47,48] (Figure 45.9). When merged into an intraoperative navigation environment, it can help identify distorted surface anatomy during surgical resection [49].

ESM of the subcortical fibers of the corticospinal tract is also instrumental to preserving function, as disruption of these fibers will produce the same deficits as disruption of the cortex (Figure 45.6). Several recent studies have emphasized the importance of subcortical mapping in preserving function [27,50]. DTI tractography is a noninvasive method of delineating white matter tracts. Interfacing DTI maps with intraoperative navigation systems may help the surgeon predict the location of important tracts around which careful stimulation mapping is warranted [32,34,51].

Optical intrinsic signal imaging is a perfusion-based technique similar to fMRI in that it detects hemodynamic changes resulting from neuronal activation [52,53]. It affords high spatial and temporal resolution and can be used intraoperatively to map functional cortex in real time [54–56]. Although still an investigational tool, it may prove useful for delineating borders of eloquent regions [57,58].

Supplementary Motor and Presupplementary Motor

The supplementary motor area (SMA) is located on the medial wall of the frontal lobe, just anterior to the lower extremity representation in primary motor cortex [35] (Figures 45.1D and 45.3). Its posterior boundary is the precentral sulcus and inferior boundary is cingulate sulcus. The lateral boundary is not sharply demarcated but is in the vicinity of the superior frontal sulcus. The anterior boundary is similarly indistinct, approximately 5 cm anterior to precentral sulcus [59]. As is primary motor cortex, SMA is organized somatotopically, with regions corresponding to leg, arm, and face proceeding anteriorly [35,60].

Neurons in SMA project reciprocally to primary motor cortex and are also the source of a significant fraction of corticospinal tract axons. Stimulation studies suggest that SMA coordinates complex, multijoint, or bilateral movements, rather than innervating single specific muscle groups [61]. Damage to the SMA produces a characteristic constellation of deficits known as SMA syndrome, characterized by expressive speech disturbance and contralateral hemiparesis. The language deficit ranges from diminished spontaneous speech to mutism and is most common in dominant hemisphere SMA lesions [62]. Both motor and language deficits tend to improve weeks to months after injury [59,62–64].

Preservation of function during approach to lesions in SMA is challenging. Electrocortical stimulation mapping of SMA is possible, but higher currents are required

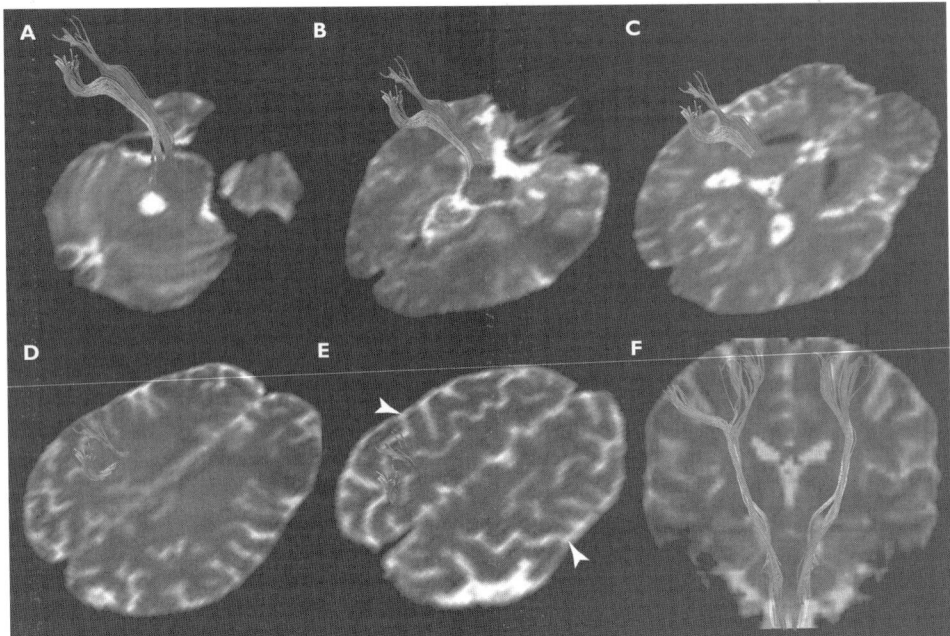

Figure 45.6 Sensorimotor white matter tractography. Diffusion tensor imaging tractography maps of the descending motor corticospinal tract (orange) and ascending somatosensory tracts (yellow; the posterior column-medial lemniscus and spinothalamic systems are not distinguishable) are shown with cross sectional axial T2-weighted slices at various levels through their course. Motor fibers travel in the basis pontis **(A)** and the cerebral peduncles of the midbrain **(B)** ventral to the sensory fibers. Both systems travel through the posterior limb of the internal capsule **(C)** and corona radiata **(D)**. The motor fibers originate largely from the precentral gyrus and sensory fibers terminate in the postcentral gyrus **(E)**. The central sulcus is indicated by arrowheads. The entire course of these motor and sensory systems through the brain and brainstem can be appreciated on the coronal slice **(F)**. *See color insert.*

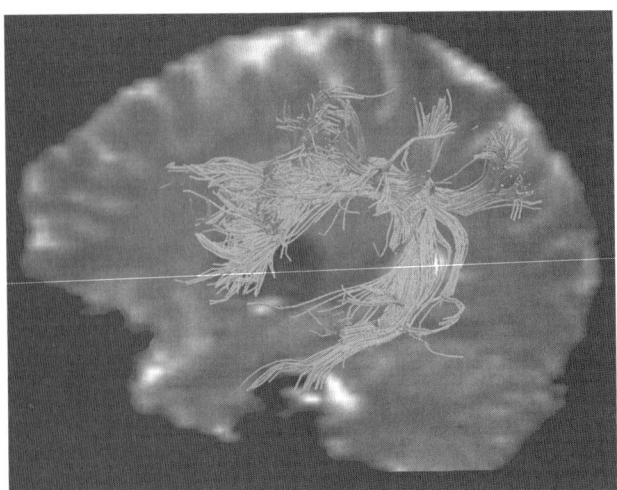

Figure 45.7 Superior longitudinal fasciculus white matter tractography. The superior longitudinal fasciculus (SLF) was constructed using DTI and shown overlaid on a sagittal T2-weighted image. The central tract follows an arcuate course around the Sylvian fissure, with fiber bundles penetrating the temporal, parietal, and frontal lobes. Connections mediated by the SLF allow regulation of motor behavior, visuo-spatial attention, and language articulation. *See color insert.*

compared to primary motor cortex [65]. Furthermore, lack of intraoperative ESM-induced movements does not guarantee lack of postoperative deficit [64]. Even though SMA syndrome deficits are usually self-limited, quality of life in patients with high-grade gliomas, whose survival is measured in months, may be unacceptably diminished by an injury to this region during surgery. Limiting the resection to the solid, enhancing region of a high-grade glioma, without disruption of presumably functional neighboring parenchyma, has been shown to reduce the incidence of SMA syndrome [59].

In monkeys, there is strong evidence for a distinct motor region rostral to the SMA, termed the pre-SMA (Figures 45.1D and 45.3). This region is involved in preparatory movements and, in contrast to SMA, has no projections to primary motor cortex or spinal cord. Functional imaging data supports the existence of a similar region in humans, located rostral to SMA, in a plane rostral to the anterior commissure [65]. Pre-SMA in humans appears to be involved in movements requiring a high level of cognitive control, selection from among a variety of choices, and early stages of skill acquisition.

The SMA, as well as surrounding areas on the medial wall of both hemispheres, is also involved in micturition. Functional imaging studies identify this region during the urge to void [66] and in voluntary

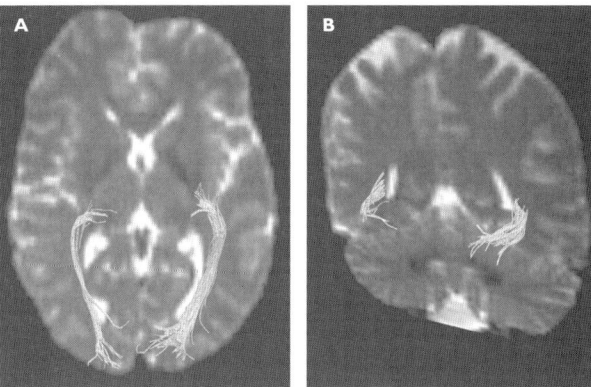

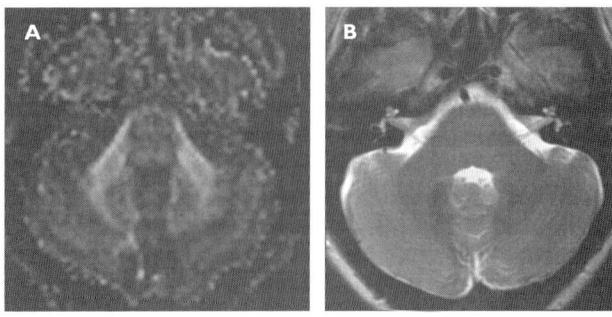

Figure 45.8 Optic radiations white matter tractography. Fibers of the optic radiations, as estimated using DTI, are shown overlaid on an axial (**A**) and coronal (**B**, as viewed from anterior) T2-weighted slice. The fibers course posteriorly from the posterolateral thalamus (lateral geniculate nucleus), along the lateral edge of the temporal and occipital horns of the lateral ventricles, toward the occipital lobe (A). Their relation to the lateral wall of the temporal horns can be appreciated in (B). *See color insert.*

Figure 45.10 Brain stem white matter tractography. An axial DTI map through the level of the pons is shown with colors indicating principal fiber directions (red, left-right; green, anterior-posterior; blue, superior-inferior) (**A**). An axial T2-weighted slice through the same region is provided for anatomical reference (**B**). The corticospinal tract (blue) runs rostro-caudally in the basis pontis, amongst the pontine nuclei. The pontocerebellar fibers (red) cross horizontally ventral and dorsal to the corticospinal tract. Fibers traveling in the middle cerebellar peduncle (green) to the cerebellum course postero-laterally. The pontine tegmentum contains numerous tracts running rostro-caudally (blue), including the medial lemniscus, spinothalamic tract, medial longitudinal fasciculus, and others. *See color insert.*

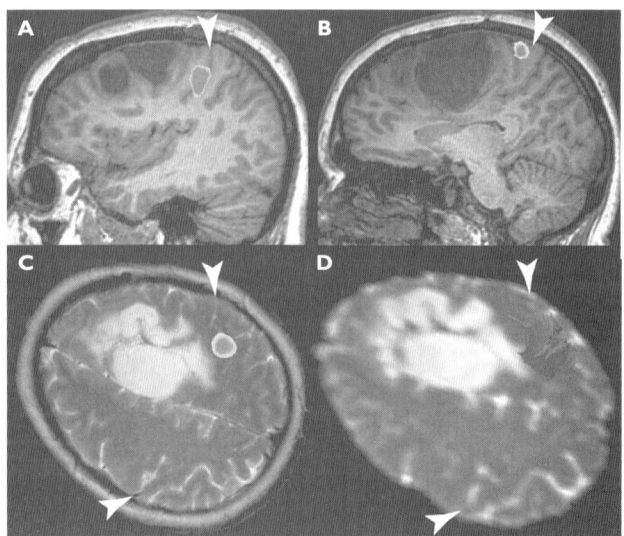

Figure 45.9 Identification of functional anatomy distorted by a mass lesion using fMRI and DTI. Despite the presence of this left frontal tumor (anaplastic oligodendroglioma, WHO grade III/IV), fMRI activations of the hand (**A,C**) and foot (**B,D**) sensorimotor regions were reliably identifiable. DTI maps were also able to determine the trajectory of primary motor and somatosensory white matter tracts, which course through the posterior T2 signal abnormality. The central sulcus is denoted with arrowheads. The availability of this functional information can help identify distorted anatomy intraoperatively and assist in preservation of function during resection. *See color insert.*

Frontal Eye Fields

The frontal eye fields reside in the middle frontal gyrus, near the intersection of the superior frontal sulcus and precentral sulcus, as confirmed by functional imaging [69,70] and electrical stimulation studies [69,71] (Figure 45.1C). The frontal eye fields generate eye saccades in the contralateral direction, via connections with the paramedian pontine reticular formation. Lesions to the frontal eye fields produce gaze preference toward the side of the lesion as contralateral saccadic eye movement is impaired. This deficit is usually self-limited and resolves within weeks to months [72].

Broca's Area

The French physician Paul Broca was one of the early pioneers of the field of functional anatomy. His demonstration of the correspondence between a dense expressive aphasia in his patient "Tan" (thus named because that was the only word he could utter) and the postmortem finding of a lesion in the patient's posterior left inferior frontal gyrus provided the first solid evidence of functional localization within the brain [3]. Broca's area is now classically described as the pars opercularis and pars triangularis of the dominant hemisphere inferior frontal gyrus (Figures 45.1C and 45.3). Detailed electrocortical stimulation and functional imaging studies have shown, however, that there is considerable variability in the location of this region between individuals [26,73].

Broca's area is considered to subserve the generation site of motor programs that control the particular sequences of orofacial movements required to produce speech. These programs are executed by the neighboring face region of primary motor cortex, which is immediately posterior to

control of voiding [67]. Damage to this region, even unilaterally, produces voiding disturbances such as detrussor hyperreflexia, dyssynergy, and uninhibited sphincter relaxation [68].

Broca's area. Lesions produce an expressive aphasia known as Broca's aphasia, characterized by decreased fluency and phrase length, impaired prosody and syntax, and difficulty with naming and repetition [74]. In the extreme case, there may be complete mutism. Comprehension of speech is generally preserved. Broca's area is connected to other language, motor, and association areas by important white matter tracts within the insula, described in more detail in the next section.

Given the high stakes involved, improvements in the techniques to approach lesions in this area have been the goal of substantial work in the past two decades, beginning with the seminal work of Ojemann, Berger, and colleagues [73]. Comparing their own results with and without awake ESM of language function, Duffau et al. [75] have suggested that intraoperative mapping significantly improves resection and reduces postoperative deficit. The importance of mapping has been reaffirmed by several groups [76–78]. Consistent with the growing emphasis on subcortical mapping, recent work has also focused on preservation of language-related white matter tracts [46,50,79,80].

The utility of preoperative functional imaging data for guiding surgery near Broca's area is mixed. fMRI has not been shown to correlate accurately enough with ESM in this region to be the exclusive guide for resection [81–83], possibly due to the vascular bias and false positive errors mentioned earlier (see Functional Magnetic Resonance Imaging). Thus, although it may not supplant the gold standard ESM, fMRI may have some utility in limiting the extent of ESM required. DTI-assisted neuronavigation, on the other hand, may be useful for identifying essential white matter tracts deep to Broca's area when combined with ESM [33].

Insula

Buried deep to the Sylvian fissure and covered by the frontal, parietal, and temporal opercula, the insula overlies the site of fusion of the diencephalon and telencephalon. Its location and proximity to middle cerebral artery branches in the Sylvian fissure make direct study via ESM difficult, but the insula appears to be involved in gustatory sensation and autonomic control. The insula is also intimately related to the basal ganglia and the internal, external, and extreme capsules, which lie just deep to it. Therefore damage to the insula is often accompanied by some disruption of these nuclei and tracts as well as to middle cerebral artery branches. The resulting contralateral weakness and language disturbance is likely at least partially attributable to this collateral damage.

The extreme capsule is a white matter tract that lies just medial to the insula and lateral to the claustrum. The original anatomical studies described its function rather vaguely, containing projection fibers connecting association regions in the frontal, temporal, and parietal lobes [84]. A recent fiber-tracing study in monkeys provides a new view of this fiber bundle [85]. According to this study, the extreme capsule links areas in the monkeys that are homologous to Wernicke's and Broca's areas in humans. Functional imaging and cytoarchitectonic postmortem analyses have provided some support for this paradigm shift [86,87]. Previous work has considered the arcuate fasciculus to be the principal connection between these language areas and its disruption the classic cause of conduction aphasia. This disconnection syndrome, originally described by Geschwind [88], is characterized by repetition errors with preserved comprehension and fluency. Further work will determine whether the extreme capsule indeed subserves this important function, which would imply that preserving its fibers may be important for avoiding disconnection deficits.

TEMPORAL LOBE

Wernicke's Area

Wernicke's area comprises the posterior two thirds of the superior temporal gyrus in the dominant hemisphere (Figures 45.1C and 45.3). Immediately adjacent to primary auditory cortex, the language association cortex in Wernicke's area parses the auditory stream into the comprehensible quanta known as words. Lesions here produce a receptive aphasia, known as Wernicke's aphasia, characterized by difficulty with language comprehension, production of fluent but nonsensical speech with neologisms and paraphasic errors, and occasionally associated with anosognosia. Prosody and grammar are usually unimpaired.

Wernicke's area is connected to Broca's area by white matter tracts thought to be within the extreme capsule or arcuate fasciculus, as described earlier. In addition, there are important connections with associative language regions in the inferior parietal lobule of the ipsilateral parietal lobe. This region in the posterior temporal lobe is also in close proximity to the optic radiations projecting from the lateral geniculate nucleus to primary visual cortex. Disruption of subcortical tracts in this region is therefore often associated with both receptive aphasia and contralateral visual field cut.

Basal Temporal Language Area

The basal temporal language area (BTLA) consists of the inferior and basal region of the dominant hemisphere temporal lobe (Figures 45.1C and 45.3). Stimulating via subdural electrodes in an epileptic patient, Luders first localized the BTLA to the left fusiform gyrus [89]. Later studies demonstrated that the BTLA can also encompass a broader area, including the inferior temporal gyrus and parahippocampal gyrus [90,91]. Anteroposteriorly, it may extend from 1 to 6 cm posterior to the temporal tip and mediolaterally from 1.5 to 6 cm from the lateral edge of the temporal lobe [91]. Damage to this region produces speech arrest or anomia. Intraoperative ESM of the BTLA using naming paradigms may be used to identify and spare this region [92].

Primary Auditory

Heschl's transverse gyri, the site of primary auditory cortex, are straight finger-like gyri on the superior surface of the temporal lobe medial to the superior temporal gyrus

(Figure 45.5). Auditory information sensed in the cochlea is transmitted within the cochlear division of cranial nerve VIII to the dorsal and ventral cochlear nuclei and ascends bilaterally in the lateral lemnisci to reach the inferior colliculi, where the pathways again partially decussate and ascend via the medial geniculate nuclei to auditory cortex.

Fiber tracts connecting the caudal superior temporal gyrus to the dorsal frontal lobes appear to be responsible for conveying auditory spatial information and assist in controlling the orientation of the body and head to auditory stimuli [85]. The same monkey tract-tracing study mentioned earlier suggests that this fiber bundle is the arcuate fasciculus and that its primary function is actually auditory spatial awareness rather than nonarticulatory language.

Because of the decussations in the auditory system, lesions beyond the cochlear nuclei do not produce unilateral hearing loss. Damage to the arcuate fasciculus might be predicted to cause difficulty with auditory localization, but this phenomenon has not been well described in the neuro-oncology literature.

Optic Radiations

Axons leaving the lateral geniculate nucleus travel posteriorly to primary visual cortex within the optic radiations (Figure 45.8). The more superior fibers of the optic radiation pass directly posteriorly, in the inferior parietal lobe, to primary visual cortex. The more inferior bundle of fibers first course anteriorly, laterally, and inferiorly within the temporal lobe before sweeping posteriorly to the occipital lobe, in a structure known as Meyer's loop [93]. These fibers curve over the temporal and occipital horns of the lateral ventricle, about 3 to 4 mm lateral to the ventricle [94].

Damage to the entire optic radiation produces a contralateral homonymous hemianopia, as may be the case for deep-seated parietal lesions. Temporal lobe lesions or surgeries that result in disruption of Meyer's loop produce a contralateral superior quadrantanopia. The anterior extent of Meyer's loop has been a source of controversy. Since Penfield's estimation of 60 mm from the temporal tip [95], this estimated distance has been decreasing. A recent study of temporal lobectomy patients places the anterior extent at just 24 mm from the frontal pole of the temporal lobe [96]. The fibers therefore cap the anterior tip of the temporal horn of the lateral ventricle. This study estimates the posterior extent of Meyer's loop to end 79 mm from the frontal pole and representation of the macula at 54 mm. They also found a linear correlation between extent of resection and degree of field defect. Given the significant intersubject variability, preoperative identification of the anatomy of an individual's optic radiations would be useful. Although not yet clinically used for this role, DTI has been shown to delineate these tracts in a research setting [97].

Hippocampal Formation

The HF contains the subiculum, hippocampus (with cornu ammonis fields), and dentate gyrus. Some sources refer to the entire formation as the hippocampus. This formation is located in the medial temporal lobe and forms the medial wall of the temporal horn of the lateral ventricle (Figure 45.5). It is continuous with the parahippocampal gyrus, which continues posteriorly and is separated from the rest of the temporal lobe laterally by the collateral suclus. There are reciprocal connections between the HF and association cortices from much of the brain. The major outputs from the HF pass through the fornix, which sweeps along the curve of the lateral ventricle to end in the mammillary bodies of the thalamus.

Damage to the HF bilaterally or sometimes unilaterally on the dominant side typically produce anterograde amnesia, as evidenced by the well-known case of H.M., who suffered profound anterograde and mild retrograde amnesia following bilateral mesial temporal lobectomy for intractable seizures [98]. Temporal lobectomy studies suggest that resection of the nondominant HF does not typically impair verbal memory [99,100]. Dominant HF resection (anterior temporal lobectomy and amygdalohippocampectomy), however, produces progressive verbal memory deterioration for 2 years after surgery, followed by a plateau [100].

PARIETAL LOBE

Primary Somatosensory

Primary somatosensory cortex is located on the postcentral gyrus and arranged in the somatotopy of the homunculus, similar to the motor strip [101] (Figure 45.1). In the spinal cord and brain stem, somatosensory information from the body below the face is carried rostrally in the posterior column-medial lemniscus (proprioception and light touch) and spinothalamic (pain, temperature) tracts (more details below). These fibers synapse in the ventral posterior lateral nucleus of the thalamus (Figure 45.6).

Facial sensation is mediated by fibers of the trigeminal nerve (CN V), whose cell bodies are within the trigeminal (gasserian) ganglion. Proprioception and light touch sensation is carried by fibers that synapse in the main sensory nucleus of CN V and then ascend in the trigeminal lemniscus, analogous to the dorsal column-medial lemniscus pathway. Pain and temperature sensation is carried by fibers that synapse in the spinal nucleus of CN V and then ascend in the trigeminothalamic tract, analogous to the spinothalamic pathway. These fibers synapse in the ventral posterior medial nucleus of the thalamus. Efferents from the thalamus ascend in the posterior limb of the internal capsule toward primary somatosensory cortex.

The primary function of this system is somatic sensation, but up to a third of corticospinal tract fibers also originate here, so damage can result in contralateral motor as well as sensory deficits. The approach to lesions is similar to that for lesions in primary motor cortex, as the pre- and postcentral gyri are often grouped together as sensorimotor cortex.

INFERIOR PARIETAL LOBULE

The inferior parietal lobule consists of the supramarginal gyrus, which caps the posterior limit of the Sylvian fissure, and the angular gyrus, which caps the posterior limit of the superior temporal sulcus (Figure 45.1). In the dominant hemisphere, this region is intimately related to Wernicke's area and is involved in language comprehension. It functions as a lexicon, mapping auditory information streams into meaningful language. In addition, this region is required for visual information to be mapped to meaning during reading [74].

Damage to the dominant inferior parietal lobule does not usually cause a purely receptive aphasia such as damage to Wernicke's area does, but rather difficulty with reading and writing (alexia and agraphia) or anosognosia [85]. It may also produce Gerstmann syndrome, characterized by agraphia, acalculia, finger agnosia, and left–right confusion.

The inferior parietal lobule has important subcortical connections with the dorsolateral prefrontal cortex, via parts of the superior longitudinal fasciculus (Figure 45.7). Via this and other connections, the angular gyrus appears to negotiate spatial awareness and attention, and the supramarginal gyrus helps control and monitor articulatory aspects of speech [85].

Given the higher order functions of these areas, they are not routinely amenable to intraoperative ESM and must usually be identified anatomically.

OCCIPITAL LOBE

Primary Visual

Primary visual cortex is located on the banks of the calcarine fissure on the medial wall of the occipital lobe (Figures 45.1 and 45.4). The cortex is organized retinotopically, with the fovea represented at the occipital pole and more peripheral regions of the retina represented successively anteriorly along the calcarine sulcus. The superior bundle of optic radiations projects to the superior bank and the inferior bundle (including Meyer's loop) to the inferior bank. Damage to the superior bank therefore causes contralateral inferior quadrantanopia, and damage to the inferior bank causes contralateral superior quadrantanopia. Loss of an entire unilateral calcarine cortex causes contralateral homonymous hemianopia. Bilateral lesions of primary visual cortex can cause cortical blindness or Anton syndrome. This syndrome of visual anosognosia is characterized by objective loss of visual perception on confrontational testing but subjective unawareness of the deficit.

Association regions of visual cortex are arranged concentrically outward from primary visual cortex and process higher order aspects of visual perception. One such canonical process is the distinction between identification of an object's location and form. These separate processes are classically ascribed to the dorsal occipito-parietal stream ("Where" pathway) and the ventral occipito-temporal stream ("What" pathway). The former identifies aspects of spatial localization and movement, whereas the latter identifies specifics of form such as color or shape as well as facial recognition.

fMRI has been used extensively in the research setting to study visual field architecture in primary and higher order visual cortices [102], but its use for clinical mapping has been limited (Figure 45.4). Basic limitations such as vascular contamination and decreased specificity, true for fMRI in motor and language cortices (see Functional Magnetic Resonance Imaging earlier), are still pertinent. In addition, corroboration of fMRI activations with intraoperative electrocorticography is particularly challenging in visual cortex. Stimulation using light emitting diode goggles [49] is cumbersome, and measurement of visual evoked potentials using electrode grids is difficult along the deep surface of the calcarine sulcus [103,104].

BRAINSTEM

The brainstem consists of the medulla, pons, and midbrain, and evolutionarily represents the most ancient region of the brain. Its contents can be generally categorized into four groups: cranial nerve circuitry, cerebellar circuitry, long white matter tracts, and reticular circuitry [74]. This chapter covers cranial nerve nuclei briefly, including a description of safe entry zones into the brain stem and floor of the 4th ventricle.

Cranial Nerve Circuitry

During embryological development, the sulcus limitans separates the medioventral motor nuclei from the dorsolateral sensory nuclei, an organizational pattern maintained in the adult brainstem. The somatic motor nuclei are midline nuclei that innervate the extraocular and intrinsic tongue muscles and include oculomotor (CN III), trochlear (IV), abducens (VI), and hypoglossal (XII). The extraocular nuclei are interconnected with the vestibular nuclei via the medial longitudinal fasciculus, which runs just ventral to the periaqueductal gray matter in the midbrain and along the ventral medial border of the 4th ventricle in the pons.

The branchial motor nuclei innervate muscles derived from the branchial arches and include the trigeminal motor (V), facial (VII), nucleus ambiguus (IX, X), and spinal accessory (XI). They are ventrolateral to the somatic motor nuclei in the tegmentum, except for XI, which is in the rostral spinal cord.

The parasympathetic nuclei send preganglionic fibers to nonstriated muscle and include the Edinger-Westphal nucleus (III), superior (VII) and inferior (IX) salivatory nuclei, and the dorsal motor nucleus of the vagus (X). Postganglionic fibers innervate the pupil constrictor and ciliary muscles (III), salivary and lacrimal glands (VII, IX), and cardiac and digestive smooth muscle (X).

The visceral sensory system includes only the nucleus solitarius and is the most medial of the sensory nuclei. Special visceral afferents (VII, IX, X) provide taste sensation and project to the rostral nucleus solitarius (gustatory nucleus), whereas general visceral afferents (IX, X) provide cardiorespiratory and gastrointestinal sensation and project to the caudal nucleus soliarius (cardiorespiratory nucleus).

General somatic facial sensation is subserved by CN V and, to a much lesser extent, VII, IX, and X, which project to the trigeminal nucleus complex. These fibers transmit sensations of proprioception, touch, pain, and temperature from the face, sinuses, pharynx, and meninges.

Special somatic facial sensation refers to audition and vestibular sense, which are transmitted by CN VIII to the cochlear and vestibular nuclei, respectively. Other special senses are olfaction and vision, whose nuclei are in the cerebrum and taste, which was discussed in the section concerning the insula.

Surgical approaches to the brainstem must respect the cranial nerve nuclei and interconnecting tracts. In general, if the lesion reaches the brainstem surface, it is approached at that point. Deep lesions in the rostral and lateral pons may be approached via a retromastoid suboccipital craniotomy. An incision is made in the ventrolateral brainstem, between the root entry zones of CN V and CN VII/VIII, lateral to the corticospinal tract [105]. This approach minimizes risk of injury to CN nuclei V through VII, the descending motor fibers, and the medial longitudinal fasciculus.

Deep lesions in the dorsal pons or medulla may be approached through the floor of the 4th ventricle. Anatomical and morphometrical studies by Bogucki et al. [106,107] have delineated safe entry zones in this region. The surface landmarks that must be identified include the obex (inferior point of 4th ventricle and entry point into spinal cord central canal), median sulcus (midline), hypoglossal triangle (caudal medial elevation corresponding to XII nucleus), vagal triangle (elevation just lateral to hypoglosal triangle corresponding to X dorsal motor nucleus), and vestibular area (elevation lateral and rostral to vagal triangle corresponding to VIII nuclei). The facial colliculus must also be identified, but if it is not easily visible, its rostral margin is 19.5 mm (± 1.5) rostral to obex. Using these landmarks, there are two safe entry regions, one caudal and one rostral to the facial colliculus [106,107]. The infrafacial safe entry zone boundaries are caudally, the rostral margin of the hypoglossal triangle; laterally, the vestibular area; and rostrally, the facial colliculus. The suprafacial safe entry zone boundaries are caudally, the facial colliculus; laterally, the cerebellar peduncles and lateral wall of the 4th ventricle; and rostrally, the frenulum and rostral extent of the 4th ventricle. The medial boundary for both is 2 mm lateral to the median sulcus, to avoid the medial longitudinal fasciculus.

Long White Matter Tracts

The most important descending white matter tracts are the corticospinal and corticobulbar tracts, which run in the middle third of the cerebral peduncles in the midbrain (Figure 45.6 and 45.10). The former continues though the basis pontis and culminates in the pyramids of the medulla, where it decussates and forms the lateral corticospinal tract of the spinal cord (see below).

The prominent ascending tracts are the dorsal column-medial lemniscus and spinothalamic tract. The former remains ipsilateral in the spinal cord and synapses on the gracile (lower extremity) or cuneate (upper extremity) nuclei in the caudal medulla. Postsynaptic fibers cross in the internal arcuate fibers just ventral to the central canal and ascend in the medial lemniscus. The medial lemniscus moves laterally as it enters the pons and lies lateral to the red nucleus in the midbrain. The spinothalamic tract is part of the anterolateral system (which also includes the spinoreticular and spinomesencephalic tracts), which is already crossed and postsynaptic within the brainstem. This system remains lateral throughout its course. Both ascending systems synapse in the ventral posterior lateral nucleus of the thalamus (Figure 45.6).

Lesions in or damage to the ventral pons can disrupt descending motor pathways, producing the locked-in syndrome in which sensation and cognition are preserved but motor control to the head and body are absent.

Reticular Circuitry

The reticular formation is a system of nuclei and tracts that runs within the brainstem tegmentum. Rostrally it is continuous with the subthalamus and lateral hypothalamus and caudally with the intermediate zone of the spinal cord. The rostral reticular formation, within the upper pons and midbrain, modulates consciousness and awareness. Lesions here can therefore produce coma. The caudal reticular formation, within the lower pons and medulla, coordinates reflex and autonomic functions. Damage here can cause autonomic instability, cardiac dysrhythmia, and abnormal respiration.

SPINAL CORD

Descending Tracts

Descending spinal cord tracts can be generally divided into lateral and medial tracts. Lateral tracts include the lateral corticospinal and rubrospinal tracts, and medial tracts include the anterior corticospinal, vestibulospinal, reticulospinal, and tectospinal tracts. Lateral tracts synapse on motor neurons in the lateral aspect of the anterior horn and control distal muscles in the extremities, whereas medial tracts synapse on medial anterior horn cells and control proximal trunk muscles.

The most clinically important descending tract is the lateral corticospinal tract, which carries fibers that decussate in the medullary pyramids. The fibers maintain their somatotopic organization, with upper extremity fibers medial to lower extremity fibers. This tract lies in the lateral white matter column of the spinal cord and synapses on anterior horn motor neurons at the level of the target muscle group.

Ascending Tracts

The main ascending tracts are the dorsal column-medial lemniscus path, which mediates light touch, proprioception, and vibration and the spinothalamic tract, which mediates pain and temperature sensation. The cell bodies for both lie in the dorsal root ganglia and send axons through the dorsal root entry zone into the dorsal horn of the spinal cord.

Fibers in the dorsal column-medial lemniscus path ascend in the ipsilateral posterior column, with lower extremity fibers in the more medial gracile fasciculus and upper extremity fibers in the more lateral cuneate fasciculus. They synapse upon the respective nuclei in the caudal medulla before crossing.

Fibers in the spinothalamic tract synapse immediately upon entering the dorsal horn, in the lamina of the dorsal horn. Some ascend or descend in Lissauer's tract for a few segments before crossing the gray matter to enter the contralateral tract, which is ventrolateral to the anterior horn. The lower extremity is represented most laterally within this tract and the upper extremity most medially. The postsynaptic fibers ascend through the midbrain to the ventral posterior lateral nucleus of the thalamus.

Surgical resection of intramedullary spinal lesions is usually accomplished via a posterior approach. If the lesion reaches the surface pia, the myelotomy may be performed there in a manner similar to brainstem lesions. Otherwise, a midline myelotomy through the dorsal median sulcus is generally preferred [108]. The sulcus is midway between the two dorsal root entry zones and may have veins emerging from the raphe. Myelotomy at the dorsal root entry zone is less commonly used [109].

REFERENCES

1. Gall FJ, Spurzheim JG. Anatomie et physiologie du système nerveux en général, et du cerveau en particulier, avec des observations sur la possibilité de reconnoître plusieurs dispositions intellectuelles et morales de l'homme et des animaux, par la configuration de leurs têtes. Paris: Schoell, F., 1810–1819.
2. Flourens MJP. Recherches expérimentales sur les propriétés et les fonctions du système nerveux, dans les animaux vertébrés. Paris: Crevot; 1824.
3. Broca P. Remarques sur le siége de la faculté du langage articulé, suivies d'une observation d'aphemie. *Bulletins de la société anatomique de Paris*. 1861;36:330–357.
4. Fritsch G, Hitzig E. Über die elektrische Erregbarkeit des Grosshirns. *Arch Anat Physiol Wiss Med*. 1870;37:300–332.
5. Wernicke C. *Der aphasische Symptomenconplex: Eine psychologische Studies auf anatomischer Basis*. Breslau: Kohn and Weigert; 1874.
6. Ferrier D. *The Functions of the Brain*. London: Smith, Elder; 1876.
7. Berger H. Uber das elektrekephalogramm des menschen. *Arch Psychiatr Nervenkr*. 1929;87:527–570.
8. Lewine JD, Orrison WW. Clinical electroencephalography and event-related potentials. In: Orrison WW, Lewine JD, Sanders JA, Hartshorne MF, eds. *Functional Brain Imaging*. St. Louis: Mosby; 1995.
9. Cohen LB, Keynes RD, Hille B. Light scattering and birefringence changes during nerve activity. *Nature*. 1968;218:438–441.
10. Zimmerman JE, Thiene P, Harding JT. Design and operation of stable rf-based superconducting quantum interference devices and a note on the properties of perfectly clean metal contacts. *J Appl Physiol*. 1970;41:1572–1580.
11. Lounasmaa OV, Hamalainen M, Hari R, Salmelin R. Information processing in the human brain: magnetoencephalographic approach. *Proc Natl Acad Sci U S A*. 1996;93:8809–8815.
12. Lewine JD, Orrison WW. Magnetoencephalography and magnetic source imaging. In: Orrison WW, Lewine JD, Sanders JA, Hartshorne MF, eds. *Functional Brain Imaging*. St Louis: Mosby; 1995.
13. Wheless JW, Castillo E, Maggio V, et al. Magnetoencephalography (MEG) and magnetic source imaging (MSI). *Neurologist*. 2004;10:138–153.
14. Kirsch HE, Zhu Z, Honma S, Findlay A, Berger MS, Nagarajan SS. Predicting the location of mouth motor cortex in patients with brain tumors by using somatosensory evoked field measurements. *J Neurosurg*. 2007;107:481–487.
15. Schiffbauer H, Berger MS, Ferrari P, Freudenstein D, Rowley HA, Roberts TP. Preoperative magnetic source imaging for brain tumor surgery: a quantitative comparison with intraoperative sensory and motor mapping. *Neurosurg Focus*. 2003;15:E7.
16. Pascual-Leone A, Walsh V, Rothwell J. Transcranial magnetic stimulation in cognitive neuroscience—virtual lesion, chronometry, and functional connectivity. *Curr Opin Neurobiol*. 2000;10:232–237.
17. Devlin JT, Watkins KE. Stimulating language: insights from TMS. *Brain*. 2007;130:610–622.
18. Sheth S, Nemoto M, Guiou M, Walker M, Pouratian N, Toga AW. Linear and nonlinear relationships between neuronal activity, oxygen metabolism, and hemodynamic responses. *Neuron*. 2004;42:347–355.
19. James W. *Principles of Psychology*. New York: Henry Holt; 1890.
20. Roy C, Sherrington C. On the regulation of the blood supply of the brain. *J Physiol Lond*. 1890;11:85:108.
21. Ogawa S, Lee TM, Kay AR, Tank DW. Brain magnetic resonance imaging with contrast dependent on blood oxygenation. *Proc Natl Acad Sci U S A*. 1990;87:9868–9872.
22. Ogawa S, Tank DW, Menon R, et al. Intrinsic signal changes accompanying sensory stimulation: functional brain mapping with magnetic resonance imaging. *Proc Natl Acad Sci U S A*. 1992;89:5951–5955.
23. Bandettini PA, Wong EC, Hinks RS, Tikofsky RS, Hyde JS. Time course EPI of human brain function during task activation. *Magn Reson Med*. 1992;25:390–397.
24. Kwong KK, Belliveau JW, Chesler DA, et al. Dynamic magnetic resonance imaging of human brain activity during primary sensory stimulation. *Proc Natl Acad Sci U S A*. 1992;89:5675–5679.
25. Bookheimer S. Pre-surgical language mapping with functional magnetic resonance imaging. *Neuropsychol Rev*. 2007;17:145–55.
26. Harris S, Sheth SA, Cohen MS. Functional neuroimaging of belief, disbelief, and uncertainty. *Ann Neurol*. 2008;63(2):141–147.
27. Keles GE, Lundin DA, Lamborn KR, Chang EF, Ojemann G, Berger MS. Intraoperative subcortical stimulation mapping for hemispherical perirolandic gliomas located within or adjacent to the descending motor pathways: evaluation of morbidity and assessment of functional outcome in 294 patients. *J Neurosurg*. 2004;100:369–375.
28. Zeineh MM, Engel SA, Bookheimer SY. Application of cortical unfolding techniques to functional MRI of the human hippocampal region. *Neuroimage*. 2000;11:668–683.
29. Frahm J, Merboldt KD, Hanicke W, Kleinschmidt A, Boecker H. Brain or vein—oxygenation or flow? On signal physiology in functional MRI of human brain activation. *NMR Biomed*. 1994;7:45–53.
30. Le Bihan D, Breton E, Lallemand D, Grenier P, Cabanis E, Laval-Jeantet M. MR imaging of intravoxel incoherent motions: application to diffusion and perfusion in neurologic disorders. *Radiology*. 1986;161:401–407.
31. Mori S. Principles, methods, and applications of diffusion tensor imaging. In: Toga AW, Mazziota JC, eds. *Brain Mapping: The Methods*. San Diego, CA: Academic Press; 2002:379–398.
32. Berman JI, Berger MS, Chung SW, Nagarajan SS, Henry RG. Accuracy of diffusion tensor magnetic resonance imaging tractography assessed using intraoperative subcortical stimulation mapping and magnetic source imaging. *J Neurosurg*. 2007;107:488–494.
33. Bello L, Gambini A, Castellano A, et al. Motor and language DTI fiber tracking combined with intraoperative subcortical mapping for surgical removal of gliomas. *Neuroimage*. 2008;39:369–382.
34. Wu JS, Zhou LF, Tang WJ, et al. Clinical evaluation and follow-up outcome of diffusion tensor imaging-based functional neuronavigation: a prospective, controlled study in patients with gliomas involving pyramidal tracts. *Neurosurgery*. 2007;61:935–948; discussion 948–949.
35. Nolte J. *The Human Brain: An Introduction to its Functional Anatomy*. St. Louis, MO: Mosby; 2002.
36. Naidich TP, Valavanis AG, Kubik S. Anatomic relationships along the low-middle convexity: Part I—Normal specimens and magnetic resonance imaging. *Neurosurgery*. 1995;36:517–532.
37. Yousry TA, Schmid UD, Alkadhi H, Schmidt D, Peraud A, Buettner A, Winkler P. Localization of the motor hand area to a knob on the precentral gyrus. A new landmark. *Brain*. 1997;120:141–157.
38. Gonzales-Portillo G. Localization of the central sulcus. *Surg Neurol*. 1996;46:97–99.
39. Biega TJ, Lonser RR, Butman JA. Differential cortical thickness across the central sulcus: a method for identifying the central sulcus in the presence of mass effect and vasogenic edema. *AJNR Am J Neuroradiol*. 2006;27:1450–1453.
40. Romstock J, Fahlbusch R, Ganslandt O, Nimsky C, Strauss C. Localisation of the sensorimotor cortex during surgery for brain tumours: feasibility and waveform patterns of somatosensory evoked potentials. *J Neurol Neurosurg Psychiatry*. 2002;72:221–229.

41. Boling W, Oliver A, Fabinyi G. Historical contributions to the modern understanding of function in the central area. *Neurosurgery.* 2002;50:1296–1309; discussion 1309–1310.
42. Berger MS, Ojemann GA. Intraoperative brain mapping techniques in neuro-oncology. *Stereotact Funct Neurosurg.* 1992;58:153–161.
43. Berger MS, Ojemann GA, Lettich E. Neurophysiological monitoring during astrocytoma surgery. *Neurosurg Clin N Am.* 1990;1:65–80.
44. LeRoux PD, Berger MS, Haglund MM, Pilcher WH, Ojemann GA. Resection of intrinsic tumors from nondominant face motor cortex using stimulation mapping: report of two cases. *Surg Neurol.* 1991;36:44–48.
45. Ebeling U, Schmid UD, Ying H, Reulen HJ. Safe surgery of lesions near the motor cortex using intra-operative mapping techniques: a report on 50 patients. *Acta Neurochir (Wien).* 1992;119:23–28.
46. Carrabba G, Fava E, Giussani C, et al. Cortical and subcortical motor mapping in rolandic and perirolandic glioma surgery: impact on postoperative morbidity and extent of resection. *J Neurosurg Sci.* 2007;51:45–51.
47. Fandino J, Kollias SS, Wieser HG, Valavanis A, Yonekawa Y. Intraoperative validation of functional magnetic resonance imaging and cortical reorganization patterns in patients with brain tumors involving the primary motor cortex. *J Neurosurg.* 1999;91:238–250.
48. Lehericy S, Duffau H, Cornu P, et al. Correspondence between functional magnetic resonance imaging somatotopy and individual brain anatomy of the central region: comparison with intraoperative stimulation in patients with brain tumors. *J Neurosurg.* 2000;92:589–598.
49. Schulder M, Maldjian JA, Liu WC, et al. Functional image-guided surgery of intracranial tumors located in or near the sensorimotor cortex. *J Neurosurg.* 1998;89:412–418.
50. Duffau H, Capelle L, Sichez N, et al. Intraoperative mapping of the subcortical language pathways using direct stimulations. An anatomo-functional study. *Brain.* 2002;125:199–214.
51. Berman JI, Berger MS, Mukherjee P, Henry RG. Diffusion-tensor imaging-guided tracking of fibers of the pyramidal tract combined with intraoperative cortical stimulation mapping in patients with gliomas. *J Neurosurg.* 2004;101:66–72.
52. Sheth SA, Nemoto M, Guiou M, et al. Columnar specificity of microvascular oxygenation and volume responses: implications for functional brain mapping. *J Neurosci.* 2004;24:634–641.
53. Grinvald A, Lieke E, Frostig RD, Gilbert CD, Wiesel TN. Functional architecture of cortex revealed by optical imaging of intrinsic signals. *Nature.*1986;324:361–364.
54. Haglund MM, Ojemann GA, Hochman DW. Optical imaging of epileptiform and functional activity in human cerebral cortex. *Nature.* 1992;358:668–671.
55. Pouratian N, Sicotte N, Rex D, et al. Spatial/temporal correlation of BOLD and optical intrinsic signals in humans. *Magnetic Res Med.* 2002;47:766–776.
56. Pouratian N, Sheth SA, Martin NA, Toga AW. Shedding light on brain mapping: advances in human optical imaging. *Trends Neurosci.* 2003;26:277–282.
57. Haglund MM, Hochman DW. Imaging of intrinsic optical signals in primate cortex during epileptiform activity. *Epilepsia.* 2007;48:65–74.
58. Pouratian N, Sheth S, Bookheimer SY, Martin NA, Toga AW. Applications and limitations of perfusion-dependent functional brain mapping for neurosurgical guidance. *Neurosurgical Focus.* 2003;15:1–8.
59. Russell SM, Kelly PJ. Incidence and clinical evolution of postoperative deficits after volumetric stereotactic resection of glial neoplasms involving the supplementary motor area. *Neurosurgery.* 2003;52:506–516; discussion 515–516.
60. Mitz AR, Wise SP. The somatotopic organization of the supplementary motor area: intracortical microstimulation mapping. *J Neurosci.* 1987;7:1010–1021.
61. Fried I, Katz A, McCarthy G, et al. Functional organization of human supplementary motor cortex studied by electrical stimulation. *J Neurosci.* 1991;11:3656–3666.
62. Krainik A, Lehericy S, Duffau H, et al. Postoperative speech disorder after medial frontal surgery: role of the supplementary motor area. *Neurology.* 2003;60:587–594.
63. Laplane D, Talairach J, Meininger V, Bancaud J, Orgogozo JM. Clinical consequences of corticectomies involving the supplementary motor area in man. *J Neurol Sci.* 1977;34:301–314.
64. Rostomily RC, Berger MS, Ojemann GA, Lettich E. Postoperative deficits and functional recovery following removal of tumors involving the dominant hemisphere supplementary motor area. *J Neurosurg.* 1991;75:62–68.
65. Picard N, Strick PL. Motor areas of the medial wall: a review of their location and functional activation. *Cereb Cortex.* 1996;6:342–353.
66. Kuhtz-Buschbeck JP, van der Horst C, Pott C, et al. Cortical representation of the urge to void: a functional magnetic resonance imaging study. *J Urol.* 2005;174:1477–1481.
67. Zhang H, Reitz A, Kollias S, Summers P, Curt A, Schurch B. An fMRI study of the role of suprapontine brain structures in the voluntary voiding control induced by pelvic floor contraction. *Neuroimage.* 2005;24:174–180.
68. Sakakibara R, Hattori T, Yasuda K, Yamanishi T. Micturitional disturbance after acute hemispheric stroke: analysis of the lesion site by CT and MRI. *J Neurol Sci.* 1996;137:47–56.
69. Lobel E, Kahane P, Leonards U, et al. Localization of human frontal eye fields: anatomical and functional findings of functional magnetic resonance imaging and intracerebral electrical stimulation. *J Neurosurg.* 2001;95:804–815.
70. Grosbras MH, Laird AR, Paus T. Cortical regions involved in eye movements, shifts of attention, and gaze perception. *Hum Brain Mapp.* 2005;25:140–154.
71. Blanke O, Spinelli L, Thut G, et al. Location of the human frontal eye field as defined by electrical cortical stimulation: anatomical, functional and electrophysiological characteristics. *Neuroreport.* 2000;11:1907–1913.
72. Ringman JM, Saver JL, Woolson RF, Adams HP. Hemispheric asymmetry of gaze deviation and relationship to neglect in acute stroke. *Neurology.* 2005;65:1661–1662.
73. Ojemann G, Ojemann J, Lettich E, Berger M. Cortical language localization in left, dominant hemisphere. An electrical stimulation mapping investigation in 117 patients. *J Neurosurg.* 1989;71:316–326.
74. Blumenfeld H. *Neuroanatomy Through Clinical Cases.* Sunderland, MA: Sinauer Associates; 2002.
75. Duffau H, Lopes M, Arthuis F, et al. Contribution of intraoperative electrical stimulations in surgery of low grade gliomas: a comparative study between two series without (1985–96) and with (1996–2003) functional mapping in the same institution. *J Neurol Neurosurg Psychiatry.* 2005;76:845–851.
76. Meyer FB, Bates LM, Goerss SJ, et al. Awake craniotomy for aggressive resection of primary gliomas located in eloquent brain. *Mayo Clin Proc.* 2001;76:677–687.
77. Low D, Ng I, Ng WH. Awake craniotomy under local anaesthesia and monitored conscious sedation for resection of brain tumours in eloquent cortex—outcomes in 20 patients. *Ann Acad Med Singapore.* 2007;36:326–331.
78. Benzagmout M, Gatignol P, Duffau H. Resection of World Health Organization Grade II gliomas involving Broca's area: methodological and functional considerations. *Neurosurgery.* 2007;61:741–752; discussion 752–753.
79. Duffau H, Capelle L, Denvil D, et al. Usefulness of intraoperative electrical subcortical mapping during surgery for low-grade gliomas located within eloquent brain regions: functional results in a consecutive series of 103 patients. *J Neurosurg.* 2003;98:764–778.
80. Bello L, Gallucci M, Fava M, et al. Intraoperative subcortical language tract mapping guides surgical removal of gliomas involving speech areas. *Neurosurgery.* 2007;60:67–80; discussion 80–82.
81. Reinges MH, Krings T, Meyer PT, et al. Preoperative mapping of cortical motor function: prospective comparison of functional magnetic resonance imaging and [15O]-H2O-positron emission tomography in the same co-ordinate system. *Nucl Med Commun.* 2004;25:987–997.
82. Picht T, Wachter D, Mularski S, et al. Functional magnetic resonance imaging and cortical mapping in motor cortex tumor surgery: complementary methods. *Zentralbl Neurochir.* 2008;69:1–6.
83. Roux FE, Boulanouar K, Lotterie JA, Mejdoubi M, LeSage JP, Berry I. Language functional magnetic resonance imaging in preoperative assessment of language areas: correlation with direct cortical stimulation. *Neurosurgery.* 2003;52:1335–1345; discussion 1345–1347.
84. Berke JJ. The claustrum, the external capsule and the extreme capsule of Macaca mulatta. *J Comp Neurol.* 1960;115:297–321.
85. Schmahmann JD, Pandya DN. *Fiber Pathways of the Brain.* New York, NY: Oxford University Press; 2006.

86. Duffau H, Gatignol P, Mandonnet E, Peruzzi P, Tzourio-Mazoyer N, Capelle L. New insights into the anatomo-functional connectivity of the semantic system: a study using cortico-subcortical electrostimulations. *Brain.* 2005;128:797–810.
87. Amunts K, Weiss PH, Mohlberg H, et al. Analysis of neural mechanisms underlying verbal fluency in cytoarchitectonically defined stereotaxic space—the roles of Brodmann areas 44 and 45. *Neuroimage.* 2004;22:42–56.
88. Geschwind N. Selected papers on language and the brain. In: Cohen RS, MW Wartofsky, eds. *Boston Studies in the Philosophy of Science.* Vol. 16. Boston, MA: Reidel; 1974.
89. Luders H, Lesser RP, Hahn J, et al. Basal temporal language area demonstrated by electrical stimulation. *Neurology.* 1986;36:505–510.
90. Burnstine TH, Lesser RP, Hart J, et al. Characterization of the basal temporal language area in patients with left temporal lobe epilepsy. *Neurology.* 1990;40:966–970.
91. Schaffler L, Luders HO, Morris HH, Wyllie E. Anatomic distribution of cortical language sites in the basal temporal language area in patients with left temporal lobe epilepsy. *Epilepsia.* 1994;35:525–528.
92. Pouratian N, Bookheimer S, Rubino G, Martin NA, Toga A. Category-specific naming deficit identified by intraoperative stimulation mapping and postoperative neuropsychological testing. *J Neurosurg.* 2003;99:170–176.
93. Meyer A. The connections of the occipital lobes and the present status of the cerebral visual affections. *Trans Assoc Am Physicians.* 1907;22:7–15.
94. Kretschmann HJ, Weinrich W. *Neurofunctional Systems: 3D Reconstructions with Correlated Neuroimaging.* New York, NY: Thieme Medical Publishers, 1998.
95. Penfield W. Temporal lobe epilepsy. *Br J Surg.* 1954;41:337–343.
96. Barton JJ, Hefter R, Chang B, Schomer D, Drislane F. The field defects of anterior temporal lobectomy: a quantitative reassessment of Meyer's loop. *Brain.* 2005;128:2123–2133.
97. Taoka T, Sakamoto M, Iwasaki S, et al. Diffusion tensor imaging in cases with visual field defect after anterior temporal lobectomy. *AJNR Am J Neuroradiol.* 2005;26:797–803.
98. Scoville WB, Milner B. Loss of recent memory after bilateral hippocampal lesions. *J Neurol Neurosurg Psychiatry.* 1957;20:11–21.
99. Rausch R, Kraemer S, Pietras CJ, Le M, Vickrey BG, Passaro EA. Early and late cognitive changes following temporal lobe surgery for epilepsy. *Neurology.* 2003;60:951–959.
100. Alpherts WC, Vermeulen J, van Rijen PC, da Silva FH, van Veelen CW. Verbal memory decline after temporal epilepsy surgery: A 6-year multiple assessments follow-up study. *Neurology.* 2006;67: 626–631.
101. Penfield W, Rasmussen T. *The Cerebral Cortex of Man: A Clinical Study of Localization of Function.* New York, NY: Macmillan; 1950.
102. Wandell BA, Dumoulin SO, Brewer AA. Visual field maps in human cortex. *Neuron.* 2007;56:366–383.
103. Roux FE, Ibarrola D, Lotterie JA, Chollet F, Berry I. Perimetric visual field and functional MRI correlation: implications for image-guided surgery in occipital brain tumours. *J Neurol Neurosurg Psychiatry.* 2001;71:505–514.
104. Kamada K, Todo T, Morita A, et al. Functional monitoring for visual pathway using real-time visual evoked potentials and optic-radiation tractography. *Neurosurgery.* 2005;57(1 suppl):121–127.
105. Zausinger S, Yousry I, Brueckmann H, Schmid-Elsaesser R, Tonn JC. Cavernous malformations of the brainstem: three-dimensional-constructive interference in steady-state magnetic resonance imaging for improvement of surgical approach and clinical results. *Neurosurgery.* 2006;58:322–330.
106. Bogucki J, Czernicki Z, Gielecki J. Cytoarchitectonic basis for safe entry into the brainstem. *Acta Neurochir (Wien).* 2000;142:383–387.
107. Bogucki J, Gielecki J, Czernicki Z. The anatomical aspects of a surgical approach through the floor of the fourth ventricle. *Acta Neurochir (Wien).* 1997;139:1014–1019.
108. Fischer G, Brotchi J, Mahla K. Surgical management of intramedullary spinal cord tumors in adults. In: Schmidek H, Roberts D, eds. *Schmidek and Sweet's Operative Neurosurgical Techniques: Indications, Methods, and Results.* Vol. 1. Philadelphia, PA: Elsevier; 2006.
109. Jallo GI, Kothbauer KF, Epstein FJ. Intrinsic spinal cord tumor resection. *Neurosurgery.* 2001; 49:1124–1128.

46 Skull Base Anatomy, Pathology, and Approaches: An Overview

Burak Sade and Joung H. Lee

INTRODUCTION

Tumors arising from or involving the cranial base pose significant challenges to surgeons due to specific anatomical considerations related to their locations. Traditionally, many of these lesions have been considered inoperable or difficult to access, and their postoperative outcomes have been reported to be suboptimal. This has been in part due to the proximity of these lesions to critical neurovascular structures such as the cranial nerves, major arteries and venous sinuses of the brain, as well as critical structures such as the optic apparatus, cavernous sinus or the brainstem. In addition, in order to reach these relatively deeply located lesions, the amount of brain retraction has been a concern utilizing the traditional neurosurgical techniques. With the advent of special "skull base techniques," such lesions became surgically more manageable over the last few decades.

This chapter aims to overview the very basics of the most common tumors of the skull base, its pertinent anatomical features, and brief descriptions of skull base techniques that can be utilized in the surgical management of these lesions. Certain tumors of the skull base, which are mainly managed by head and neck surgeons, will be excluded. The biological characteristics of the tumors mentioned here will not be the main focus of the chapter. To enhance the understanding of the reader, the "skull base" will be reviewed in four sections: the anterior, middle, and posterior cranial fossae, as well as the central skull base.

ANTERIOR FOSSA

Anatomy

The anterior cranial fossa is formed by the ethmoid, sphenoid, and frontal bones [1]. Medially, it covers the nasal cavity, as well as the frontal, sphenoid, and ethmoid sinuses (Figure 46.1). Laterally, it covers the orbits. The olfactory nerve filaments pass through the cribriform plate of the ethmoid bone. The gyri recti and gyri orbitalis of the frontal lobes sit over the anterior cranial fossa.

Pathology

Meningiomas

By far, the most common intracranial tumor encountered in the anterior cranial base is meningioma. Approximately,

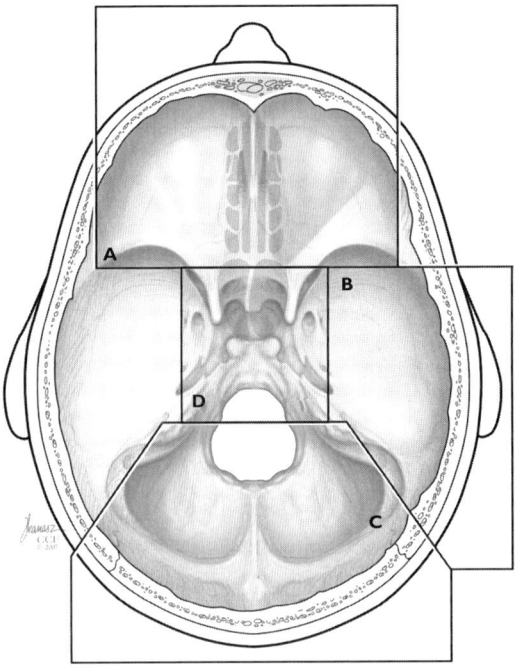

Figure 46.1 Overview of the skull base. **(A)** Anterior fossa, **(B)** middle fossa, **(C)** posterior fossa, and **(D)** central skull base.

7% to 8% of all intracranial meningiomas arise from the anterior cranial base [2]. These include meningiomas of the olfactory groove (Figure 46.2), planum sphenoidale, and orbital roofs. Meningiomas arising from the tuberculum sellae or anterior clinoid process will be discussed in the section of the central skull base. Because of their location, anterior fossa meningiomas may reach a relatively large size before they get detected. Most common symptoms of these tumors at the time of presentation include headache, seizure, personality/mood changes, fatigue, anosmia, and in advanced cases, visual loss.

Sinonasal Tumors

Owing to the neighboring paranasal sinuses and nasal cavity, tumors originating from these structures can at times warrant involvement of skull base neurosurgeons. The most common tumors of this type are adenocarcinomas, squamous cell carcinomas, esthesioneuroblastomas, and malignant melanomas originating from the sinonasal mucosa. Other tumors such as adenoid cystic or undifferentiated carcinoma can also be seen, but with much less frequency. Neurosurgical involvement is usually indicated in patients with tumoral involvement of the dura, olfactory nerve, or the brain. Sole involvement of the anterior fossa floor itself may or may not require neurosurgical intervention depending on the extent of the tumor invasion. In cases that require neurosurgical intervention, the surgery results in direct communication of the sinonasal cavity with intracranial space, implications of which will be discussed under surgical approaches to the anterior cranial base. Figure 46.3 shows intracranial extension of adenocarcinoma of the ethmoid sinus. Management of this type of pathology frequently requires adjuvant chemotherapy and radiotherapy either preoperatively or postoperatively.

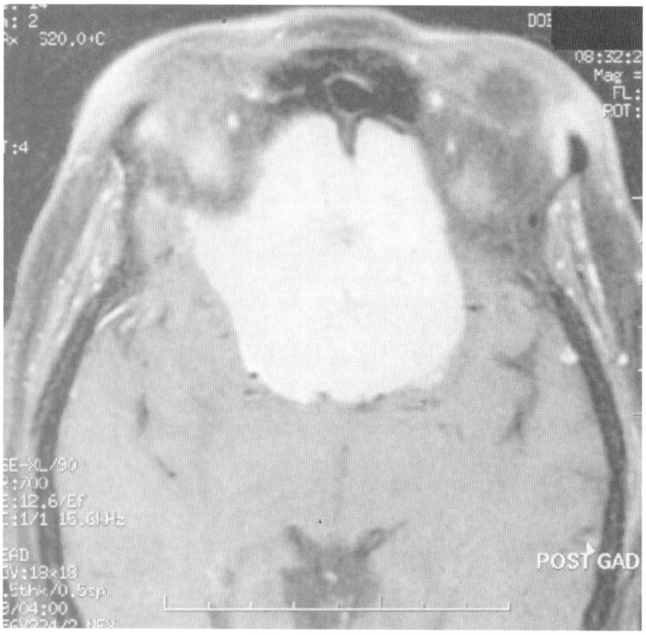

Osseous Tumors

Tumors of osseous origin may be encountered along the anterior cranial base such as fibrous dysplasia, ossifying fibroma, osteoma, and aneurismal bone cyst. These lesions usually involve a significant part of the anterior cranial fossa and therefore, similar to sinonasal tumors, their resection may result in direct communication of the sinonasal cavity with intracranial space. Figure 46.4 shows a case with extensive involvement of the anterior cranial fossa by an osteoid osteoma. Primary malignant bone tumors such as chordomas or chondrosarcomas will be mentioned in the central skull base section.

Orbital Tumors

Certain tumors of the orbit have traditionally been accepted in the domain of skull base surgery. Although these orbital tumors are not strictly classified as anterior cranial fossa tumors, the surgical approach in the management of these tumors often requires a route through the anterior fossa/orbital roof. Cavernous angiomas (aka hemangiomas) are the most common type of these lesions. Other common lesions of interest to neurosurgeons include meningiomas.

Surgical Approaches to the Anterior Cranial Base

Surgical approach is selected based on the type of the suspected pathology, size of the tumor, anatomical features of that particular patient, as well as the goals of the procedure in mind.

For lesions that are completely intradural, such as the majority of meningiomas, a bifrontal, unifrontal, or frontotemporal approach may be utilized. Surgical management of lesions with extensive extradural component often results in direct communication of the sinonasal structures with the intracranial space. In the case of sinonasal

Figure 46.2 A large olfactory groove meningioma with significant compression of the brain.

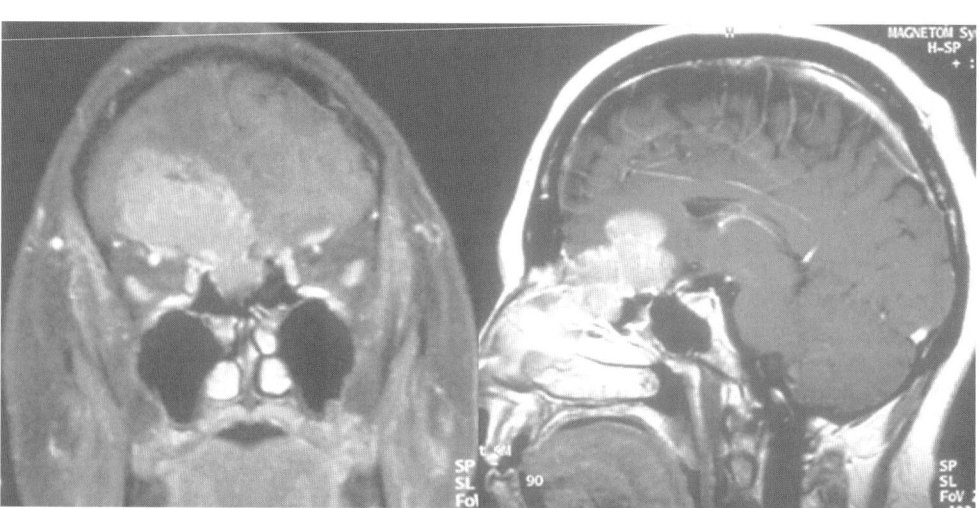

Figure 46.3 Adenocarcinoma of the ethmoid sinus with extensive involvement of the anterior cranial fossa and right frontal lobe.

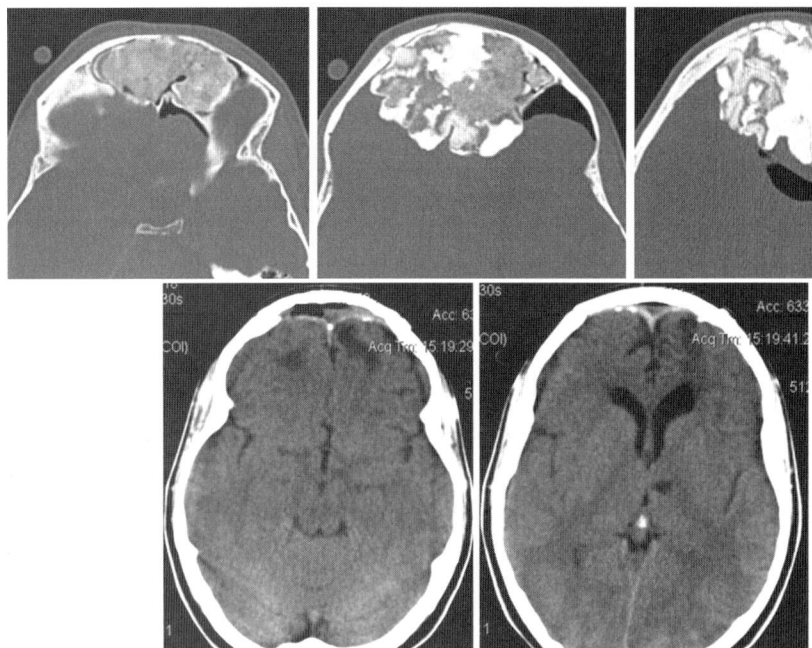

Figure 46.4 Osteoid osteoma of the anterior cranial fossa, originating from the frontal sinuses. Note the hypodense appearance of spontaneous pneumocephalus as a result of the defect on the sinus wall caused by the tumor. The calvarium is also affected. The last 2 images show after resection of the tumor and reconstruction of the skull base and frontal calvarium.

tumors, the bifrontal approach is usually combined with a lateral rhinotomy exposure, transnasal endoscopic approach, or removal of the orbital rim in the case of transbasal approach [3,4]. Regardless of the chosen approach, reconstruction of the dura and skull base would be of paramount importance in these cases to avoid potential complications such as cerebrospinal fluid rhinorrhea and pneumocephalus. For this purpose, tissues such as fat, vascularized pericranial flap or commercially available synthetic/semisynthetic materials can be utilized [5].

MIDDLE FOSSA

Anatomy

The middle cranial fossa is formed by the greater wing of the sphenoid bone as well as the squamous and petrous part of the temporal bone [1] (Figure 46.1). There are multiple foramina through which important neurovascular structures enter/exit the skull. Of significance, the middle meningeal artery enters the skull through the foramen spinosum. The maxillary and mandibular divisions of the trigeminal nerve exit the skull via foramina rotundum and ovale, respectively. Through these structures, the middle cranial fossa is in communication with the infratemporal fossa. The greater superficial petrosal nerve, a branch of the facial nerve, exits the temporal bone through the facial hiatus along the superior surface of the petrous bone. Medial and lateral to this structure are the internal carotid artery and the eustachian tube in a deeper plane, respectively. Other structures embedded in the temporal fossa floor include the cochlea, the superior semicircular canal of the labyrinth with the arcuate eminence being its superior projection, and tegmen, under which the middle ear cavity resides. The anterior two thirds of the temporal lobe sits over the middle cranial fossa.

Pathology

Meningiomas

As in the case for anterior cranial fossa, the most common intracranial tumor encountered in the middle cranial base is meningioma. Meningiomas arising from the middle or lateral sphenoid wing (Figure 46.5), floor of the middle fossa, as well as the temporal bone constitute about 8% of all intracranial meningiomas [2]. These lesions may present with headache, seizure, memory problems, or if they invade the sphenoid bone and enter into the orbit, may present with exophthalmos or diplopia.

Other Tumors

In rare occasions, invasive head and neck malignancies may show intracranial extension through the bony foramina into the middle fossa. Facial nerve schwannomas or glomus tympanicum are most often encountered as otologic problems; however, these may extend intracranially by eroding the superior surface of the petrous bone. Schwannoma of the greater superficial petrosal nerve has been reported to present as a middle fossa mass [6]. Despite being an intraaxial tumor, gliosarcoma of the temporal lobe may invade the skull base floor and may extend into the infratemporal fossa, presenting as a middle cranial fossa tumor [7]. In addition, although rarely, dermoid/epidermoid cysts may occur in the middle fossa as well.

Surgical Approaches to the Middle Cranial Base

Surgical approaches for tumoral lesions involving the middle cranial fossa depends on the type and size of the lesion, extent of the involvement, as well as the goal of the procedure.

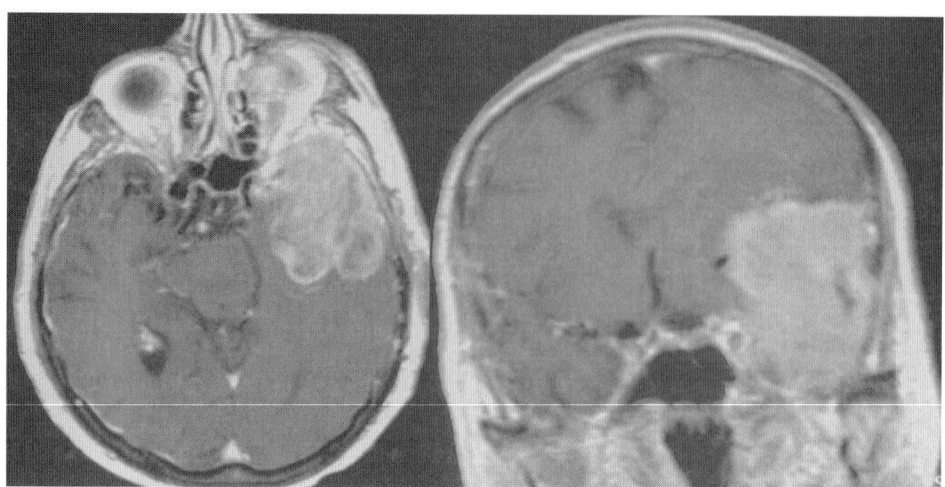

Figure 46.5 Sphenoid wing meningioma on the left with significant mass effect.

For primary intracranial tumors, a frontemporal or temporal craniotomy is usually adequate. At times, drilling of the middle fossa floor may be indicated in lesions extending into the infratemporal fossa. In our experience, zygomatic osteotomy is rarely indicated for lesions involving solely the middle cranial fossa. Exposure of the intracanalicular and labyrinthine segments of the facial nerve, as well as the geniculate ganglion, can be achieved with an extradural middle cranial fossa approach. Glomus tympanicum tumors or facial nerve schwannomas that involve more distal segments of the nerve require a transmastoid approach and involvement of an otologist.

POSTERIOR FOSSA

Anatomy

The posterior cranial fossa is formed anteriorly by the clivus, superiorly by the tentorium, laterally by the posterior surfaces of the petrous bones, and posteriorly by the occipital bone. Inferiorly, through the foramen magnum the brainstem exits the cranium and continues as the spinal cord within the spinal canal. The posterior fossa harbors the cerebellum, brainstem, and numerous cranial nerves. Of note is the cerebellopontine angle, which is the lateral aspect of the posterior fossa in which all critical neurovascular structures such as the cranial nerves from trigeminal to accessory nerve, as well as the superior cerebellar, anterior inferior cerebellar, posterior inferior cerebellar, and vertebral arteries are located. Cranial nerves from 7 to 12 leave the skull through foramina in the posterior cranial fossa, namely, the facial and vestibulocochlear nerves via the internal auditory canal; glossopahryngeal, vagal, and accessory nerves through the jugular foramen; and hypoglossal nerve through the hypoglossal canal. It is important to remember that the torcula, straight sinus, and both transverse sinuses reside within the tentorial dural folds. The transverse sinus becomes sigmoid sinus on both sides, which also exit the skull via the jugular foramen and become the internal jugular vein in the neck. The part of the posterior fossa anterior to the internal auditory canal will be discussed under the section of central skull base.

Pathology

Vestibular Schwannomas

Schwannomas arising from the vestibular component of the vestibulocochlear nerve are by far the most common type of intracranial schwannomas (Figure 46.6). They mainly occupy the cerebellopontine angle and may extend into the internal auditory canal and expand it in various degrees. The primary symptom of this type of tumor is hearing loss. Dizziness, gait imbalance, and tinnitus are also frequent, either due to the involvement of the vestibular nerve and/or to the compression of the brainstem. As the tumor grows, facial numbness and retroauricular pain may also develop. Facial weakness and diplopia are seen rarely and only in large tumors. Lower cranial nerve palsy is exceedingly rare.

Meningiomas

Meningiomas can occur in various parts of the posterior fossa. Among these are posterior petrous bone, inferior surface of the tentorium (Figure 46.7), as well as posterior foramen magnum. Their presentation depends on the size and their involvement of the cranial nerves and can range from headache to various cranial nerve deficits.

Other Tumors

The posterior cranial fossa, cerebellopontine angle in particular, is a fairly common location for epidermoid and dermoid cysts. In fact, a significant number of these lesions occupy more than one cranial compartment, extending superiorly to the parasellar cisterns and the middle cranial fossa. In rare occasions, invasive head and neck malignancies may show intracranial extension through the petrous bone into the posterior fossa. Schwannomas of the jugular foramen arise from one of the three cranial nerves that exit the skull through this foramen, most commonly arising from the glossopharyngeal nerve. They are far less frequent than vestibular schwannomas. Another distinct tumoral entity of the posterior fossa is glomus jugulare tumors. These tumors, which originate from the jugular

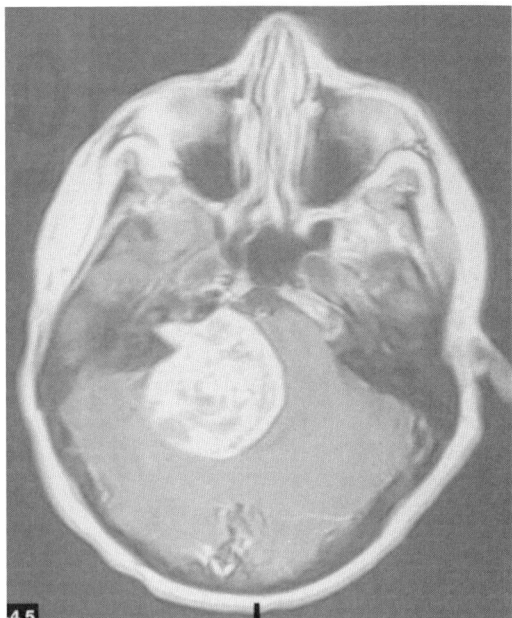

Figure 46.6 Vestibular schwannoma on the right with full extension into the internal auditory canal and significant compression of the brainstem.

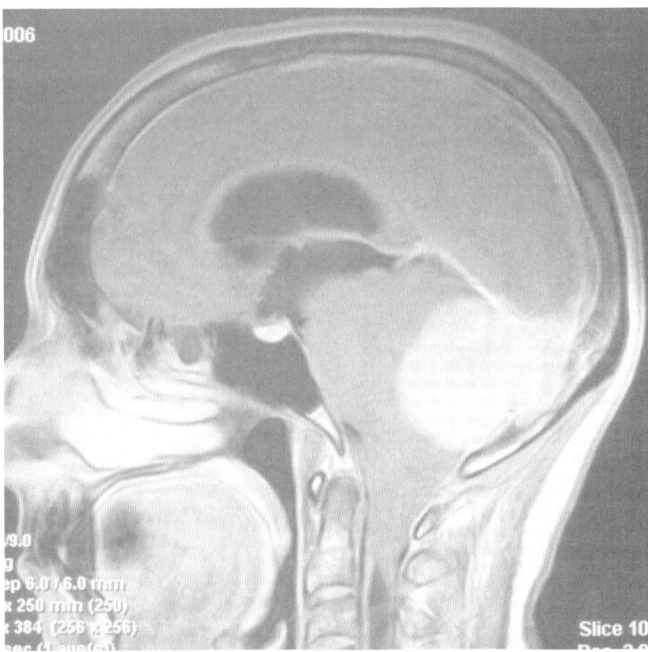

Figure 46.7 Posterior fossa meningioma arising from the inferior surface of the tentorium. Note the hydrocephalus, descent of cerebellar tonsils below the level of the foramen magnum, and syrinx formation at the cervical spinal cord, secondary to the tumor.

foramen, usually have components extending into the posterior fossa and inferiorly into the superior neck.

Surgical Approaches to the Posterior Cranial Base

The most commonly used approaches to gain access to the posterior fossa include midline suboccipital craniectomy/ craniotomy or, if the cerebellopontine angle or the lateral posterior fossa is involved, suboccipital retrosigmoid approach. Using these two approaches, the majority of the lesions at the level of the foramen magnum, cerebellontine angle, posterior petrous surface, and inferior surface of the tentorium can be accessed. For lesions involving the internal auditory canal, the posterior wall of the canal may have to be removed. For schwannomas or meningiomas involving the jugular foramen, or for glomus jugulare tumors, a more extensive approach requiring mastoidectomy and neck exposure may be required [8].

CENTRAL SKULL BASE

Anatomy

The central skull base is depicted in the area D of Figure 46.1. This area defines the deepest and, therefore, surgically most challenging part of the skull base. It includes the regions of tuberculum sellae, anterior clinoid process, posterior clinoid process, cavernous sinus, tentorial incisura, ventral petrous bone, clivus, and anterior foramen magnum.

This area harbors some of the most critical neurovascular structures of the skull base such as the optic nerves, internal carotid arteries, cavernous sinus, pituitary gland, basilar artery and its branches, as well as the brainstem. The proximity or involvement of these neurovascular structures to the tumors arising in this location critically influence the clinical presentation, surgical decision making, and operative outcome.

Pathology

Meningiomas

Similar to other skull base locations, meningiomas constitute the majority of intracranial tumors located at the central skull base. As with other locations, their presentations vary with their size and with their location. For example, tuberculum sellae meningiomas (Figure 46.8) often present with uni- or bilateral visual acuity loss and/or field defects, whereas foramen magnum meningiomas (Figure 46.9) may present with gait imbalance.

Schwannoma

The second most common cranial nerve to be involved with schwannomas is the trigeminal nerve (Figure 46.10). It can arise from any segment of the nerve and therefore may be intradural or extradural (within the cavernous sinus) or both. Schwannomas of this location usually present with some degree of retroorbital pain and facial numbness. In some instances, facial pain in the form of trigeminal neuralgia, or atypical facial pain, can also be encountered.

Chordoma/Chondrosarcoma/Fibrous Dysplasia

Chordoma and chondrosarcomas are rare tumors; however, they are the most common primary malignant bone tumors of the skull base. Chordomas arise from the embryologic remnants of notochord, whereas chondrosarcomas

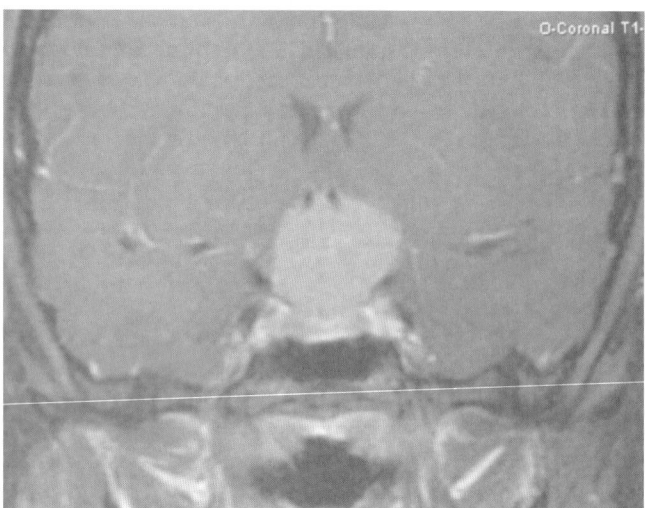

Figure 46.8 Coronal view of a tuberculum sellae meningioma. Note the internal carotid arteries on both sides of the tumor and the pituitary gland underneath.

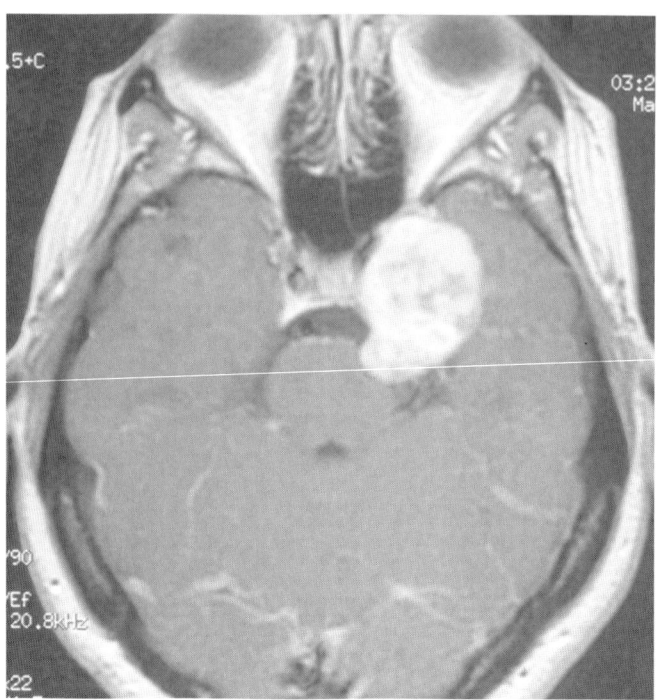

Figure 46.10 A trigeminal schwannoma on the left. The bulk of the tumor is within the cavernous sinus, with extension into the posterior fossa.

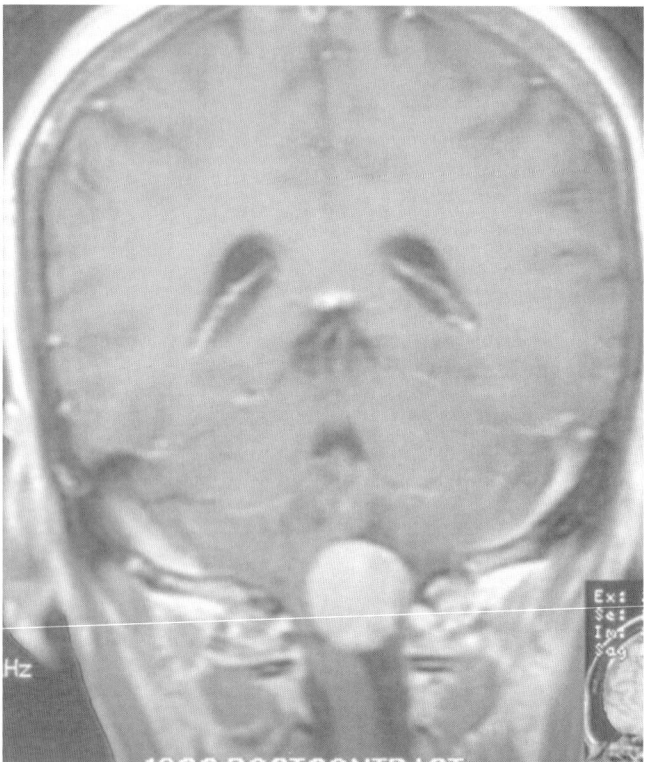

Figure 46.9 Foramen magnum meningioma with severe compression of the craniocervical junction.

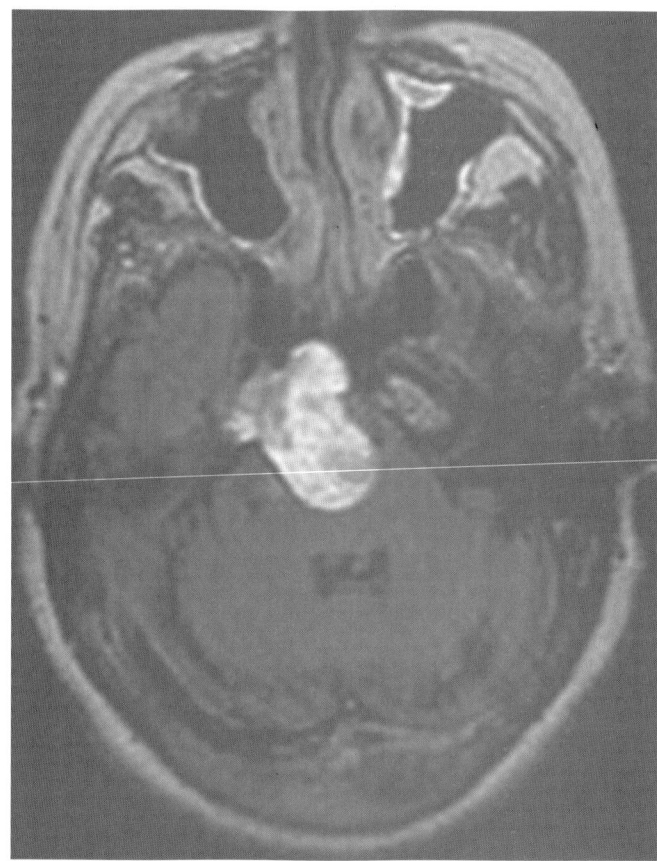

Figure 46.11 Chondrosarcoma of the right petrous-clival region in a patient who presented with a right-sided abducens nerve palsy due to the compression of the nerve at the Dorello's canal.

(Figure 46.11) originate from the synchondral cartilage tissues of the skull base. Fibrous dysplasia, which is often included in the differential diagnosis of the bony lesions of the skull base, is a result of the arrest of the bone maturation in the lamellar/woven stage, rather than being a real neoplastic process.

Other Tumors

Craniopharyngiomas arise from the embryologic remnants of the Rathke's cleft at the level of the pituitary stalk. Their appearance and consistency can be very heterogeneous, that is, cystic versus solid, soft versus densely calcified, sellar versus suprasellar versus intraventricular, and therefore pose great challenges in the surgical decision-making process. Pituitary adenomas arise from the adenohypophysis of the pituitary gland. Depending on their hormone-status, size, and growth extent, they may present with hormonal disturbances, visual complaints or signs, and symptoms of cavernous sinus invasion. As discussed previously, epidermoid/dermoid cysts may commonly involve the parasellar/central skull base region.

Surgical Approaches to the Central Skull Base

There are several skull base approaches to access the central skull base depending on the type and size of the tumor, the goal of the procedure, and the part of the central skull base that needs to be exposed.

For example, extradural anterior clinoidectomy, initially described by Dolenc [9] for the vascular lesions of the cavernous sinus, can provide various operative advantages in tumors around the optic nerves, peri- or subchiasmatic lesions, or tumors located in the interpedincular cistern such as tuberculum sellae, anterior clinoid meningiomas, as well as craniopharyngiomas [10–13]. At the same time, it is an invaluable technique in the surgical management of cavernous sinus tumors such as trigeminal schwannomas or meningiomas. It may or may not be combined with orbito-zygomatic approach in which the superior and lateral rims of the orbit is removed along with the zygoma [14].

For lesions involving the sella, sphenoid sinus, or suprasellar area, such as the pituitary adenomas, transnasal transspehnoidal approach either microscopically or endoscopically is most frequently favored [15–17]. In addition to the parasellar area, endoscopic endonasal approach has been utilized for other parts of the central skull base such as the clivus [18,19].

Lesions involving the tentorial incisura, petroclival region, or ventral petrous region are among the most difficult to reach. In addition to the middle and posterior fossa approaches described above, transpetrous approaches, each of which involves drilling and removing different parts of the petrous bone, may also be utilized [20–22]. These approaches may be tailored according to the need of the patient and can be used in combination with other techniques such as the suboccipital retrosigmoid approach.

To reach the caudal aspect of the central skull base, which includes the clivus and anterior foramen magnum, a far lateral approach can be utilized by additional removal of a part of the occipital condyle [23]. This gives additional room to the surgeon with much less need for retraction to the craniocervical junction.

SUMMARY

Tumors of the skull base constitute a heterogeneous group. Therefore surgical management of each patient should be regarded as a unique challenge. Various techniques of skull base surgery should serve as important tools in the neurosurgeon's armamentora and these should be tailored for each patient to achieve the operative goals and to optimize the surgical outcome.

REFERENCES

1. Rhoton AL Jr. The anterior and middle cranial base. *Neurosurgery.* 2002;51(suppl 4):S273–302.
2. Lee JH, Sade B, Choi E, Golubic M, Prayson R. Meningothelioma as the predominant histological subtype of midline skull base and spinal meningioma. *J Neurosurg.* 2006;105:60–64.
3. Batra PS, Citardi MJ, Worley S, Lee JH, Lanza DC. Resection of anterior skull base tumors: comparison of combined traditional and endoscopic techniques. *Am J Rhinol.* 2005;19:521–528.
4. Fliss DM, Abergel A, Cavel O, Margalit N, Gil Z. Combined subcranial approaches for excision of complex anterior skull base tumors. *Arch Otolaryngol Head and Neck Surg.* 2007;133:888–896.
5. Liu JK, Niazi Z, Couldwell WT. Reconstruction of the skull base after tumor resection: an overview of methods. *Neurosurg Focus.* 2002;12(5):e9.
6. Sade B, Lee JH. Recovery of low-frequency sensorineural hearing loss following resection of a greater superficial petrosal nerve schwannoma. *J Neurosurg.* 2007;107:181–184.
7. Sade B, Prayson RA, Lee JH. Gliosarcoma with infratemporal fossa extension. *J Neurosurg.* 2006;105:904–907.
8. Jackson CG, Kaylie DM, Coppit G, Gardner EK. Glomus jugulare tumors with intracranial extension. *Neurosurg Focus.* 2004;17(2):E7.
9. Dolenc VV. Direct microsurgical repair of intracavernous vascular lesions. *J Neurosurg.* 1983;58:824–831.
10. Evans JJ, Hwang YS, Lee JH. Pre- versus post-anterior clinoidectomy measurements of the optic nerve, internal carotid artery and opticocarotid triangle: a cadaveric morphometric study. *Neurosurgery.* 2000;46:1018–1023.
11. Lee JH, Sade B, Park BJ. A surgical technique for the removal of clinoidal meningiomas. *Neurosurgery.* 2006;59(1 suppl 1):ONS108–114.
12. Sade B, Kweon CY, Evans JJ, Lee JH. Enhanced exposure of the oculomotor triangle following extradural anterior clinoidectomy: a comparative anatomical study. *Skull Base.* 2005;15:57–62.
13. Yonekawa Y, Ogata N, Imhof HG, et al. Selective extradural anterior clinoidectomy for supra and parasellar processes. *J Neurosurg.* 1997;87:636–642.
14. Zabramski JM, Kiris T, Snkhla SK, Cabiol J, Spetzler RF. Orbitozygomatic craniotomoy. *J Neurosurg.* 1998;89:336–341.
15. De Divitiis E, Cavallo LM, Cappabianca P, Esposito F. Extended endoscopic endonasal transsphenoidal approach for the removal of suprasellar tumors: part 2. *Neurosurgery.* 2007;60:46–58; discussion 58–59.
16. Hardy J. Transspehnoidal microsurgery of the normal and pathological pituitary. *Clin Neurosurg.* 1969;16:185–217.
17. Jho HD, Alfieri A. Endoscopic endonasal pituitary surgery: evolution of surgical technique and equipment in 150 operations. *Minim Invasive Neurosurg.* 2001;44:1–12.
18. Jho HD, Ha HG. Endoscopic endonasal skull base surgery, part 3—the clivus and posterior fossa. *Minim Invasive Neurosurg.* 2004;47(1):16–23.
19. Solares CA, Fakhri S, Batra PS, Lee J, Lanza DC. Transnasal endoscopic resection of lesions of the clivus: a preliminary report. *Laryngoscope.* 2005;115:1917–1922.
20. Abdel Aziz KM, Sanan A, van Loveren HR, Tew JM Jr, Keller JT, Pensak ML. Petroclival meningiomas: predictive parameters for transpetrosal approaches. *Neurosurgery.* 2000;47:139–152.
21. Al-Mefty O, Ayoubi S, Smith RR. The petrosal approach: indications, technique, and results. *Acta Neurochir (Wien).* 1991;53:166–170.
22. Sekhar LN, Schessel DA, Bucur SD, Raso JL, Wright DC. Partial labyrinthectomy petrous apicectomy approach to neoplastic and vascular lesions of the petroclival area. *Neurosurgery.* 1999;44:537–552.
23. Baldwin HZ, Miller GM, van Loveren HR, Keller JT, Daspit CP, Spetzler RF. The far lateral/combined supra- and infratentorial approach. *J Neurosurg.* 1994;81:60–68.

47 Surgical Navigation

Gene H. Barnett

INTRODUCTION

Surgical navigation (SN; "frameless stereotaxy") has become a mainstay in the surgical diagnosis and management of most cranial tumors (Figure 47.1). This procedure is capable of providing almost instantaneous information on location, orientation, and guidance based on pre- and intraoperatively acquired images. Although most commonly used to provide guidance to a lesion, for the purpose of either biopsy or resection, when used properly SN can be an important, effective aid in safely maximizing the extent of resection of intra-axial tumors, particularly gliomas. Coregistration of different types of image data can provide a wealth of information for surgery deeper than surface and lesion features, including vascular anatomy, cortical function, and demonstration of white matter tracts.

This chapter reviews the basics of cranial navigation, and then discusses the uses of navigation for craniotomy and optimization of tumor resection, as well as strategies and outcomes from navigation-directed brain biopsy and related procedures. Advanced applications, particularly as they pertain to imaging, are also presented. It is hoped that the reader will gain a better understanding of the benefits that SN can provide in cranial surgery for brain tumor, as well as some of its limitations.

BASICS OF CRANIAL SN

Frame Stereotaxy

The roots of SN date back a century to the invention of the first stereotactic frame for cranial neurosurgery [1]. Nearly 40 years were required for this technology to be adapted to human neurosurgery by Spiegal and Wycis [2]. Shortly thereafter, there was a proliferation of frames, typically using ventriculography and brain atlases to target structures deep in the brain, particularly for the treatment of movement disorders and chronic pain. The advent of better medical therapies, particularly l-dopa for Parkinson disease, led to a steep decline in the number of such stereotactic procedures.

Nonetheless, it was at this time that the model for the future advances in frame and "frameless" cranial stereotaxy was set as follows: (a) exploiting the skull as an exoskeleton that remained in a fixed position in relation to intracranial brain structures; (b) using an externally applied coordinate system that had a rigid relationship to the skull (here a frame); (c) imaging to derive a coordinate for a target point(s); and (d) an apparatus to direct an instrument (or anything else) to that target based on the coordinate system.

A renaissance of stereotaxy occurred when some of these frames were adapted to exploit the spatial information inherent in computed tomography (CT) and, later, magnetic resonance imaging (MRI) scans [3,4]. Image-guided frame stereotaxy allowed for targeting of lesions in the brain for the purposes of biopsy, catheter placement, radiosurgery and, later, surgical resection [5–20]. During the 1980s and early 1990s a wealth of information was obtained on how to safely perform procedures using this technology, the outcomes, and a comparison of these results with those from conventional procedures [21–26]. Craniotomy using frame stereotaxy, however, was never embraced by mainstream neurosurgery, likely due to it being logistically cumbersome, mathematically intensive, and because of its inability to identify locations or structures deep in the brain.

Types of Navigation Systems

The convergence of three technological advances in the late 1980s allowed for the development of the first practical surgical navigation systems (SNS), at the time best known as "frameless stereotaxy": (a) CT and MRI scanners were now capable of generating spatially accurate 3D image data; (b) computers that could manipulate these large image data sets were now available at reasonable prices; and (c) accurate 3D digitizers that could serve as spatial input devices to these computers in the operating room were now manufactured.

The general concept of this navigation system was to translate ("transform") the image coordinate set (typically a Cartesian x,y,z system) to a coordinate system that represented the patient's head and brain in the operating room, and vice versa. This registration process was usually done by identifying several landmarks on the image set and touching those same landmarks with the digitizing device. Anatomic landmarks typically resulted in localization accuracy of several millimeters, applied scalp markers ("fiducials") resulted in accuracy of a few millimeters, and markers secured to the skull could result in accuracy

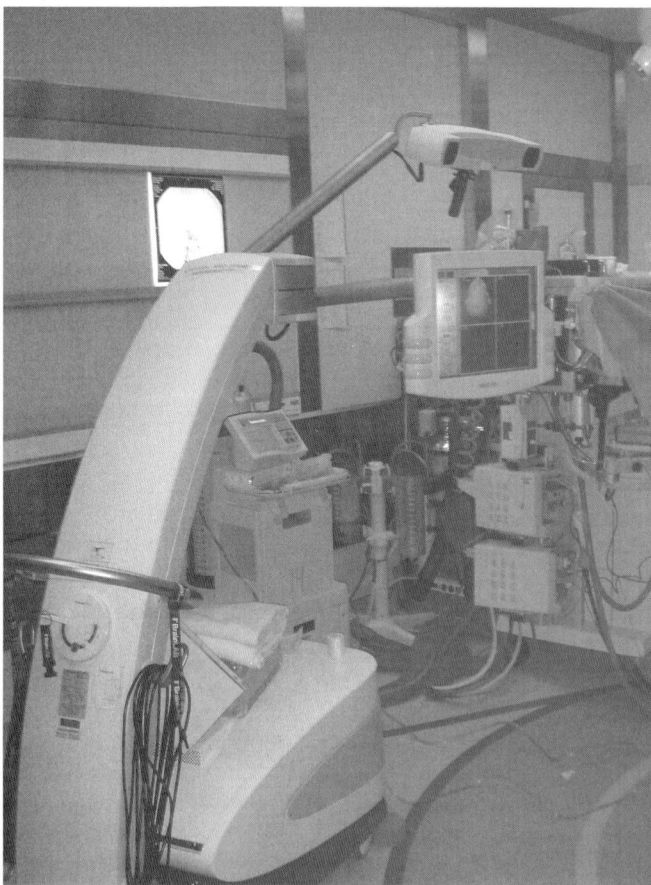

Figure 47.1 Contemporary surgical navigation system in use for brain tumor surgery. These systems display image data for the purposes of localization, orientation, and guidance.

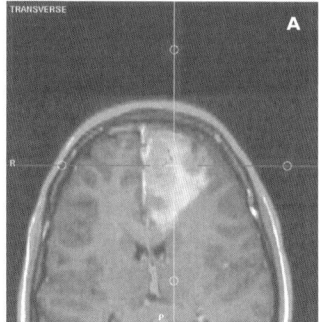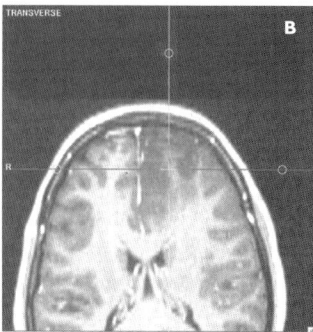

Figure 47.2 **(A)** Coregistration of low-resolution fluid attenuation inversion recovery MRI (color) with high-resolution T1-weighted volume image (gray) renders the low-grade glioma (orange-white) far more visible than with the **(B)** grayscale volume image alone.

that was submillimetric and potentially superior to that obtained using image-guided frame procedures [27–30]. Laser scanning of facial features could even be registered to imaging, resulting in reasonably accurate navigation nearby, although most accurate near the face [31].

Initially, the first digitizers used ultrasonic pulses or multiarticulated arms [32–38]. Infrared technology eventually became the standard, using infrared emitting diodes, passive infrared reflectors, or a combination of these technologies, usually detected by a stereoscopic camera array [39–43]. Sound or light requires clear "line-of-sight" between the detector and the pointing device (wand, adapted tool, endoscope [44], operating microscope, etc). Magnetic and electromagnetic systems [45,46] have also been developed that are not affected by line-of-sight; however, uncertainties due to potential interference of metal in or near the surgical field seemed to limit their appeal in cranial neurosurgery. Initially, in order to be able to move the head during the surgical procedure, either the detector had to be mechanically linked to the head or a reference that was also "seen" by the detector needed to track the patient's head [32,33]. Today, most of these dynamic reference frames are secured to the fixation device (FD) that secures the patient's head during the surgical procedure.

Image displays include localization (usually presented on coronal, transverse, and sagittal images), orientation (usually using planes containing the axis of the pointing device and a plane(s) perpendicular to this axis and selectable/identifiable depth), and guidance. Guidance came relatively late to these systems [47], but most now allow for the selection of target points and the option to define a trajectory to that point, with some visual means of directing an instrument to that target point along that trajectory. Images are typically presented on flat panel displays either attached to the navigation system or mounted from ceiling-mounted arms, but image data may also be presented through the surgical microscope or using head-mounted displays [48].

Coregistration

Navigation systems generally use high-resolution MRI (typically T1-weighted with or without contrast) or CT images for their primary display. Contemporary SNSs allow for multiple image sets to be "coregistered" to these primary image sets by automated, manual, or combination techniques [5,49,50]. CT or MR angiography or venography can provide useful information on brain vascular anatomy. Fluid attenuation inversion recovery (FLAIR) or T2-weighted images allow for clearer identification of low-grade tumors and regions of edema than T1-weighted studies (Figure 47.2). Functional MRI may provide localization information on critical speech, motor, sensory, and visual cortex [51]. Positron emission tomography [52] or magnetic resonance spectroscopy [53] can generate spatial data on the metabolic and chemical behavior of a brain lesion.

Perhaps the most exciting, recent development in navigation is the ability to navigate using information on white matter fiber tract anatomy generated by diffusion tensor imaging (DTI) MRI [54]. Subcortical navigation employs representations of relevant fiber tracks that may be critical for normal brain functions such as optic radiations, corticobulbar/spinal, and arcuate fasciculus (Figure 47.3).

In reality, surgical planning and intraoperative navigation often use a combination of several of the aforementioned imaging techniques to determine surgical risk prior to surgery, and to minimize risk during surgery.

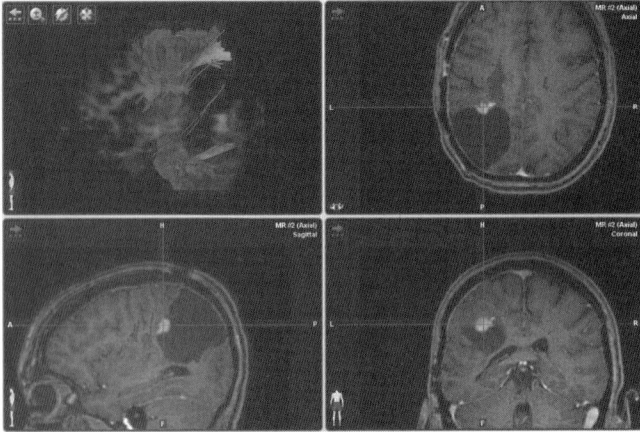

Figure 47.3 Diffusion tensor image (DTI)–generated fiber tracking showing relationship of critical white matter tracks to tumor.

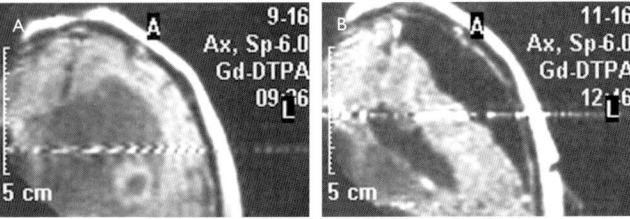

Figure 47.4 Images of glioma **(A)** before and **(B)** during resection monitored by intraoperative MRI—note the extent of brain shift and small amount of residual enhancing tumor.

Brain Shift and Tissue Deformation

A significant limitation of SNSs employing preoperative imaging is that the brain/skull relationship becomes dynamic once the dura is breached, thereby allowing cerebrospinal fluid to escape [16–18,55–57]. As the brain behaves like a fluid, it will begin to slowly flow—generally downward along the vector of gravity (Figure 47.4). This effect is most pronounced over the convexities (cerebral and cerebellar) and is less of a factor along the interhemispheric fissure or other areas where the brain surface is tightly tethered to rigid structures such as the falx. Tumor resection itself causes local deformations that may render preoperatively acquired imaging inaccurate or misleading to the unwary, as the tumor cavity will collapse with tumors undergoing piecemeal resection. The SNS will, however, display the preoperative size and location of the tumor, often suggesting there is more tumor to be resected than exists, thereby risking surgical trespass into areas beyond the intended limits of the lesion. Complicating matters further, deep structures that have been displaced inward due to tumor mass may actually move outwards, against the force of gravity, once the mass has been decompressed. Practical strategies to manage brain shift and tissue deformation are outlined in Table 47.1.

These strategies are often effective to help achieve the intended extent of resection in many cases—but not all. Another strategy to improve upon the limitations of preoperative image data focuses on acquisition of intraoperative image data. Intraoperative ultrasound, CT, and MRI

Table 47.1 Strategies to Manage Brain Shift and Deformation

1. Use vertical surgical trajectory. This does not prevent brain shift, but makes it easier for the surgeon to compensate for shift as it directs the major effect of movement (due to CSF loss) in one direction—downward.
2. Avoid early cyst or ventricular puncture.
3. Remove tumor in an en bloc fashion (or as few large pieces) rather than piecemeal.
4. Minimize use of diuretics.
5. Operate near critical areas first (when preoperative imaging is most representative of intraoperative status).
6. Place markers in brain (catheters, cottonoids, etc.) at periphery of intended resection using SNS at beginning of case [58,59].
7. Fill cavity with cotton balls in an effort to reestablish original tumor volume, to help identify regions that may harbor residual tumor.

have all been used to this end, either alone or to update SNS image data [49,58–72]. An exhaustive analysis of the pros and cons of each of these intraoperative imaging methods is beyond the scope of this chapter; however, a few points merit discussion. Intraoperative ultrasound is relatively inexpensive, does not expose operating room personnel to potentially hazardous energy, and does not require room modifications or special surgical equipment. Many, however, find these images difficult to interpret and even neurosurgeons experienced in the technique may find that they have substantially underestimated the amount of residual tumor. Coregistration of intraoperative ultrasound to preoperative imaging using SNSs may help mitigate these problems. Intraoperative MRI is expensive (device cost, room modifications, MRI-compatible/safe surgical/anesthesia equipment). It can, however, produce detailed images that may aid surgical resection or identify the true location of an instrument, such as a biopsy probe, with respect to the intended target. Many intraoperative MRIs incorporate SNSs, and the output of virtually all can be imported into an SNS and coregistered to intraoperative images. Intraoperative CT is used infrequently in this setting, but may become more important as a means of confirming critical catheter placement for convection-enhanced delivery (CED) [73,74].

CRANIOTOMY FOR TUMOR

Minimal Access Craniotomy

Prior to the advent of stereotaxy-guided craniotomy, the conventional surgical belief was that the "only good craniotomy is a large craniotomy." Largely, this was related to these procedures being exploratory in nature, even in the early era of diagnostic CT or MRI. Localizing tumors that are not apparent on the surface was often difficult and was inferred by identification of altered surface appearance (discoloration, widened gyri, arterialized veins), atypical firmness on palpation, or sounding with probes such as brain needles. Stereotaxy allowed for accurate guidance to lesions and minimizing the size of cranial access. Tumors that reach the cerebral convexity surface usually require a craniotomy that provides exposure to the entire involved surface, except for certain locations such as the frontal poles (where accessing the posterior/superior border of the tumor may be sufficient). These minimal access craniotomies appear to be associated with lower wound morbidity and shorter hospital stays than conventional craniotomies for tumors [75].

Resection Control

The impact of the extent of resection on outcome in glioma surgery has been controversial. The preponderance of evidence and a single randomized trial (resection vs. biopsy in elderly patients with glioblastoma) support that near-total resection of most gliomas improves tumor control and longevity, although this is still not universally accepted [61,76–78]. It is the author's opinion that an SNS can be an important tool to optimize safe resection when using the methods outlined earlier to manage brain shift and tissue deformation. A randomized trial of enhancing intracerebral tumors failed to demonstrate such a benefit [79]; however, the number of patients in the study was probably insufficient to exclude a type-II statistical error. The tumors were of mixed types and it is not clear whether the surgeons using SNSs employed these key strategies. Resection control is usually less of an issue for metastatic disease as the tumors are typically distinguishable from the adjacent brain, although exceptions exist, while even superficially well-demarcated gliomas typically blend imperceptibly into the brain at depth.

General SNS-Assisted Craniotomy Technique [32,80,81]

Preoperative imaging is obtained and coregistration of different image types (as determined by the judgment of the surgeon) performed. At least one scan is usually performed with scalp-applied markers (fiducials) that serve as reference marks during surgery. Critical structures (cortical, tracts, vessels, etc.) are identified and a surgical trajectory defined. After induction of anesthesia, the patient is positioned so as to minimize brain shift and the navigation system registered to the scalp fiducials. It is also critical to avoid compression or stretch of neck veins so as not to artificially elevate intracranial pressure and extra brain swelling. If high intracranial pressure is anticipated, diuretics may be considered (the author prefers furosemide as opposed to osmotic diuretics), the head elevated, and the craniotomy positioned/dural opening located such that if the brain herniates, it does not result in critical brain.

Ideally, for gliomas, the surgical trajectory should be near vertical if significant brain shift is expected. The author generally prefers a linear or "lazy-S" incision over the craniotomy as opposed to small or large flaps. Exceptions include the use of bicoronal incisions for anterior frontal approaches to avoid forehead incisions, and lateral frontal lesions that may require curved incisions, largely for cosmetic reasons. The navigation wand is used to map the surgical trajectory and define the location of this incision, and a narrow hair clip performed along the incision [82]. The area is widely prepped with antiseptic, and adjacent hair draped off with drapes secured with surgical staples. The scalp is incised, underlying muscle (if any) managed as appropriate, and retractors placed. The SNS is used to define the location and boundaries of the craniotomy flap. At this point, some surgeons place reference marks on the skull in the event that navigation registration may be lost during the procedure. The bone flap is elevated and the dura opened. In most cases, a cruciate incision is made, with the base of each leaflet retracted with a suture to maximize exposure of the underlying cortex. Dural openings near major dural sinuses should account for draining veins—often well visualized during surgical planning.

The SNS is used to confirm the expected surface anatomy. If the tumor extends to the surface, microsurgical resection is commenced, using the principles outlined in Table 47.1. If deep, a surgical corridor is created to the tumor. In most cases, fixed brain retraction is not necessary and the corridor can be maintained with cottonoids, and by retraction with the suction and bipolar instrument. When retraction is necessary, it should be used judiciously, aiming to minimize trauma to the adjacent brain. Cylindrical retractors have been devised to assist with access to deep intra-axial or ventricular tumors. At times, a nasal speculum can be employed to maintain the corridor. Access to some subcortical tumors (particularly metastasis) may be best provided by opening the nearby sulcus rather than entering the apex of the gyrus. When practical, the tumor should be removed in one or a few large pieces to minimize the impact of tissue deformation. Navigation may be used to help determine or confirm the extent of resection using the cotton ball technique outlined in Table 47.1. When resection has been completed and hemostasis insured, the dura is approximated, the epidural space sealed with a fibrin glue and cellulose sponge, and the bone secured with titanium plates and screws with the aim of producing a positive extradural pressure to prevent cerebrospinal fluid leakage. A subgaleal drain may be used, particularly for bicoronal or other flaps. The overlying tissues are closed conventionally, the hair washed, and a dressing stapled in place. Full head wraps are rarely needed.

SNSs and Awake Technique

Certain cases require the patient to be awake for portions of the resection due to the critical location of the tumor. Awake craniotomy dictates a few modifications to the methods outlined earlier, and use of navigation necessitates some alterations to the general technique of awake craniotomy. Typically, the patient is positioned in a lateral, fetal position to optimize comfort and prevent the patient from trying to sit upright during the procedure. (Note that this position may accentuate brain shift problems for certain tumors.) The FD is secured to the patient's head (to provide a point of attachment for the dynamic reference frame); however, it is not secured to the operating room table. Rather, the head and FD can rest on a pillow to allow for limited movement of the patient's head and minimize the risk of tearing away from the fixation pins that rigid fixation might potentiate.

Instead of attempting an en bloc fixation, after the patient is awakened and the function mapped, piecemeal resection is generally performed, starting at the least critical portion of the tumor and working toward the most critical. Subcortical stimulation may be used during resection to try to identify critical white matter tracts nearby (ideally identified by DTI fiber tracking preoperatively). Resection is generally completed when the resection goal is achieved, a new deficit is encountered, or subcortical stimulation identifies critical tracts. Exceptions to this paradigm include resection of or through the supplementary motor area where a profound temporary deficit may develop. Again, intraoperative mapping and preoperative imaging may help the surgeon decide when to continue or abort the procedure.

Other Tumors

SN may be useful when performing craniotomy for extra-axial tumors such as meningiomas, large schwannomas, and pituitary tumors. For meningiomas, an SNS can be used to tailor an optimal craniotomy for convexity or falcine lesion, avoid venous or air sinuses, and locate critical structures deeper than the tumor intraoperatively such as large cranial nerves or arteries [83,84]. Guidance to the sella and avoidance of lateral structures such as the carotid arteries and cavernous sinuses may be facilitated by SNSs for pituitary surgery.

BIOPSY AND RELATED PROCEDURES

Biopsy

Frame stereotactic and freehand biopsy has been supplanted by SNS-directed biopsy by many neurosurgical oncologists [12,25,27,68,85,86]. In the author's opinion, virtually any lesion accessible by frame biopsy can be accessed equally well (if not better) using frameless methodologies when proper technique is used. While scalp-applied fiducials may be used for surgical registration in most cases, certain cases may warrant use of skull-applied fiducials (Table 47.2).

A detailed review of technique has been published elsewhere [27,87]. Briefly, a high-resolution planning and navigation scan(s) is obtained and the target and trajectory are defined. Typically, the center of the most abnormal area of the lesion (even if necrotic) is selected. Exceptions include non-enhancing tumors where blood volume or magnetic resonance spectroscopy indicates a region that is more likely to be of higher grade so as to minimize the risk of underestimating tumor grade due to sampling error. Trajectories are determined to minimize risk of violating a vascular structure (visible vessels, traversing multiple pial/ependymal planes), avoiding critical cortex/tracts, and minimizing the length of the trajectory (in descending order of importance) (Figure 47.5).

Table 47.2 Lesions Where Skull Fiducials Should Be Considered

1. Posterior fossa tumors
2. Small (<1 cm) targets
3. Targets near critical vascular structures

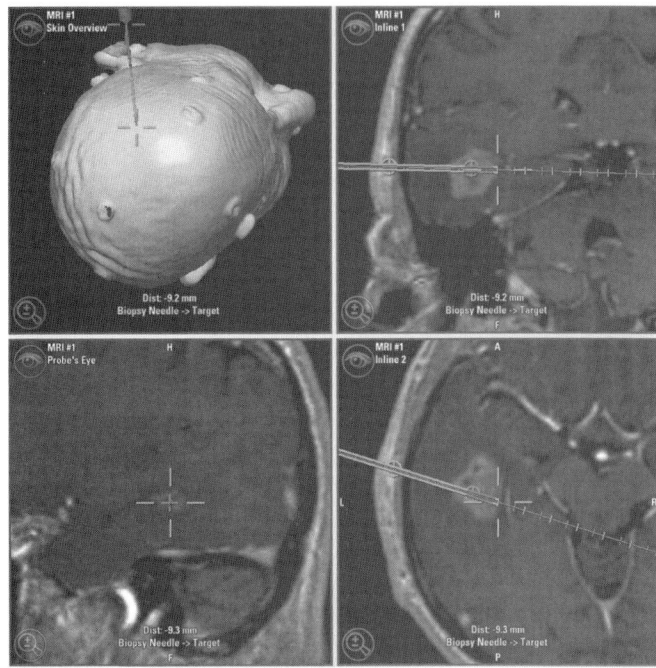

Figure 47.5 Biopsy of intracerebral tumor as directed and monitored by surgical navigation system.

The author prefers that the patient be under a general anesthetic. After surgical registration, the surgical trajectory is mapped onto the patient's scalp. A small zone of hair is clipped, the area cleansed, a small incision made, and a twist drill or bur hole fashioned. The side-cutting biopsy instrument is advanced to the target, guided by a device set using the SNS [88]. One or two specimens are obtained and sent for frozen section or smear analysis, along with a portion retained for permanent section. If not diagnostic, the depth of the instrument is adjusted (usually deeper) at 5 to 10 mm increments until diagnostic tissue is obtained, undue bleeding occurs, or unexpected findings are encountered [89]. By targeting the center of the lesion, the lesion is "impaled" on the outer sheath of the biopsy instrument and shift is unlikely to be of consequence. Also, the diagnostic rim is likely to be encountered eventually. If the outer rim of an enhancing lesion is targeted, the small but real inaccuracy of localization may lead to the instrument actually being outside the tumor, particularly if the tumor is small. Intraoperative pathology consultation is considered essential as the first specimen is often not diagnostic using this methodology. Bleeding observed at biopsy may be managed by head elevation, instrument irrigation and mechanical clearing (to prevent blockage by clot), blood pressure control, and, at times, instillation of thrombin [90]. After withdrawal of the biopsy instrument, the wound is closed, the head cleansed, a dressing applied, and the patient awakened; the patient is then transferred to recovery where a CT scan without contrast is obtained about 2 hours thereafter. If excessive bleeding is not encountered at surgery, the patient has no new deficit, and the CT shows little if any blood, the patient may be transferred to a regular room (or even discharged home under certain circumstances) [91].

Related Procedures

A number of procedures related to SNS brain biopsy are used in the practice of neurosurgical oncology. These include tumor cyst aspiration, placement of an intratumoral cyst catheter with subgaleal Ommaya reservoir, brachytherapy, biventricular catheter placement for obstructive hydrocephalus, and endoscopic procedures such as biopsy. Laser interstitial thermal therapy (LITT) or third ventriculostomy. All of these may be successfully performed using SNS planning and guidance.

An emerging role for SNS is the placement of catheters for intracerebral drug delivery via CED [73,74]. Many unanswered questions remain regarding optimal catheter location for CED, but it appears that extratumoral location is preferred over intratumoral placement; catheters need to be situated away from sulci, ventricles, tumor cavities as well as entry points; and flow patterns related to preferential flow along white matter tracts need to be considered. Computerized paradigms are being developed to help assist the surgeon with planning catheter targeting. Brain shift occurring between sequential placement of catheters also appears to be an important consideration. Formal, widely accepted methodologies for placement of CED catheters have yet to be defined.

FUTURE USES OF SNSS IN NEURO-ONCOLOGY

Although already possible in the laboratory and with normal brains, the ability to coregister brain image data in a plastic (i.e., non-rigid) manner could allow for automated anatomical identification of normal structures and, with appropriate modeling, "morphing" of preoperative images accounting for brain shift and local tissue deformations with sparse intraoperative information, obviating the need for high-resolution CT or MRI intraoperative imaging [92]. The robust image processing and general computing capacity of SNSs is often idle unless it is actively used for surgical planning or episodically for navigation during surgery. As such, networked SNSs could be used as neuro-oncology management systems, coregistering brain images across time with volumetric assessments of tumor burden to quantify the impact of medical and radiotherapies. The addition of robotic effectors, models of physical tissue characteristics and appropriate algorithms could make SNSs serve as the core of surgical simulators, robotics assistants, and telesurgery systems for brain tumor surgery [93–95]. To a certain extent, the future capabilities of these systems are limited only by our imagination.

SUMMARY

Proper use of SNSs for preoperative planning and intraoperative navigation may extend the operability of primary or secondary brain tumors by allowing for minimal or optimal craniotomy size, optimizing safe access, and maximizing the extent of surgical resection. Navigation has become a mainstay in performing stereotactic brain biopsy and a number of related procedures in the management of the neuro-oncology patient as well as emerging procedures such as CED of antitumoral agents. A thorough understanding of the principles, capabilities, and limitations of these systems optimizes their use by surgeons in the diagnosis and treatment of patients with brain tumors.

REFERENCES

1. Horsley VA, Clarke RH. The structure and functions of the cerebellum examined by a new method. *Brain* 1908;31:45–85.
2. Spiegel EA, Wycis HT, Marks M, Lee AJ. Stereotaxic apparatus for operations on the human brain. *Science*. 1947;106(2754):349–350.
3. Brown RA. A computerized tomography-computer graphics approach to stereotaxic localization. *J Neurosurg*. 1979;50(6):715–720.
4. Laitinen LV, Liliequist B, Fagerlund M, Eriksson AT. An adapter for computed tomography-guided stereotaxis. *Surg Neurol*. 1985;23(6):559–566.
5. Alexander E, Kooy HM, van Herk M, et al. Magnetic resonance image-directed stereotactic neurosurgery: use of image fusion with computerized tomography to enhance spatial accuracy. *J Neurosurg*. 1995;83(2):271–276.
6. Apuzzo ML, Chandrasoma PT, Cohen D, Zee CS, Zelman V. Computed imaging stereotaxy: experience and perspective related to 500 procedures applied to brain masses. *Neurosurgery*. 1987;20(6):930–937.
7. Barnett GH, McKenzie RL, Ramos L, Palmer J. Nonvolumetric stereotaxy-assisted craniotomy. Results in 50 consecutive cases. *Stereotact Funct Neurosurg*. 1993;61(2):80–95.
8. Bernstein M, Gutin PH. Interstitial irradiation of brain tumors: a review. *Neurosurgery*. 1981;9(6):741–750.
9. Bernstein M, Parrent AG. Complications of CT-guided stereotactic biopsy of intra-axial brain lesions. *J Neurosurg*. 1994;81(2):165–168.
10. Bosch DA, Rähn T, Backlund EO. Treatment of colloid cysts of the third ventricle by stereotactic aspiration. *Surg Neurol*. 1978;9(1):15–18.
11. Chandrasoma PT, Smith MM, Apuzzo MLJ. Stereotactic biopsy in the diagnosis of brain masses: comparison of results of biopsy and resected surgical specimen. *Neurosurgery*. 1989;24:160–165.
12. Kelly PJ, Earnest F, Kall BA, Goerss SJ, Scheithauer B. Surgical options for patients with deep-seated brain tumors: computer-assisted stereotactic biopsy. *Mayo Clin Proc*. 1985;60(4):223–229.
13. Kelly PJ, Daumas-Duport C, Kispert DB, Kall BA, Scheithauer BW, Illig JJ. Imaging-based stereotaxic serial biopsies in untreated intracranial glial neoplasms. *J Neurosurg*. 1987;66(6):865–874.
14. Kelly PJ, Kall BA, Goerss SJ. Results of computed tomography-based computer-assisted stereotactic resection of metastatic intracranial tumors. *Neurosurgery*. 1988;22:7–17.
15. Kelly PJ. Computer-assisted stereotaxis: new approaches for the management of intracranial intra-axial tumors. *Neurology*. 1986;36(4):535–541.
16. Kelly PJ. Stereotactic resection: general principles. In: *Tumor Stereotaxis*. Philadelphia: W.B. Saunders, 1991:268–295.
17. Kelly PJ. Volumetric stereotactic surgical resection of intra-axial brain mass lesions. *Mayo Clin Proc*. 1988;63(12):1186–1198.
18. Mundinger F, Ostertag CB, Birg W, Weigel K. Stereotactic treatment of brain lesions. Biopsy, interstitial radiotherapy (iridium-192 and iodine-125) and drainage procedures. *Appl Neurophysiol*. 1980;43(3–5):198–204.
19. Rogers LR, Barnett G. Percutaneous aspiration of brain tumor cysts via the Ommaya reservoir system. *Neurology*. 1991;41(2):279–282.
20. Whittle IR, Denholm SW, Elshunnar K. CT-guided stereotactic neurosurgery using the Brown-Roberts-Wells system: experience with 125 procedures. *Aust N Z J Surg*. 1991;61(12):919–928.
21. Grunert P, Ungersböck K, Bohl J, Kitz K, Hopf N. Results of 200 intracranial stereotactic biopsies. *Neurosurg Rev*. 1994;17(1):59–66.
22. Gutin PH, Phillips TL, Wara WM, et al. Brachytherapy of recurrent malignant brain tumors with removable high-activity iodine-125 sources. *J Neurosurg*. 1984;60(1):61–68.
23. Hahn JF, Levy WJ, Weinstein MJ. Needle biopsy of intracranial lesions guided by computerized tomography. *Neurosurgery*. 1979;5(1):11–15.
24. Kulkarni AV, Guha A, Lozano A, Bernstein M. Incidence of silent hemorrhage and delayed deterioration after stereotactic brain biopsy. *J Neurosurg*. 1998;89(1):31–35.

25. Lee T, Kenny BG, Hitchock ER, et al. Supratentorial masses: stereotactic or freehand biopsy? *Br J Neurosurg.* 1991;5(4):331–338.
26. Soo TM, Bernstein M, Provias J, Tasker R, Lozano A, Guha A. Failed stereotactic biopsy in a series of 518 cases. *Stereotact Funct Neurosurg.* 1995;64(4):183–196.
27. Barnett GH, Miller DW, Weisenberger J. Frameless stereotaxy with scalp-applied fiducial markers for brain biopsy procedures: experience in 218 cases. *J Neurosurg.* 1999;91(4):569–576.
28. Maciunas RJ, Galloway RL, Latimer J, et al. An independent application accuracy evaluation of stereotactic frame systems. *Stereotact Funct Neurosurg.* 1992;58(1–4):103–107.
29. Vrionis FD, Foley KT, Robertson JH, Shea JJ. Use of cranial surface anatomic fiducials for interactive image-guided navigation in the temporal bone: a cadaveric study. *Neurosurgery.* 1997;40(4):755–63; discussion 763.
30. Wang MY, Maurer CR, Fitzpatrick JM, Maciunas RJ. An automatic technique for finding and localizing externally attached markers in CT and MR volume images of the head. *IEEE Trans Biomed Eng.* 1996;43(6):627–637.
31. Marmulla R, Hassfeld S, Lüth T, Mühling J. Laser-scan-based navigation in cranio-maxillofacial surgery. *J Craniomaxillofac Surg.* 2003;31(5):267–277.
32. Barnett GH, Kormos DW, Steiner CP, Weisenberger J. Use of a frameless, armless stereotactic wand for brain tumor localization with two-dimensional and three-dimensional neuroimaging. *Neurosurgery.* 1993;33(4):674–678.
33. Barnett GH, Kormos DW, Steiner CP, Weisenberger J. Intraoperative localization using an armless, frameless stereotactic wand. Technical note. *J Neurosurg.* 1993;78(3):510–514.
34. Friets EM, Strohbehn JW, Hatch JF, Roberts DW. A frameless stereotaxic operating microscope for neurosurgery. *IEEE Trans Biomed Eng.* 1989;36(6):608–617.
35. Golfinos JG, Fitzpatrick BC, Smith LR, Spetzler RF. Clinical use of a frameless stereotactic arm: results of 325 cases. *J Neurosurg.* 1995;83(2):197–205.
36. Roberts DW, Strohbehn JW, Hatch JF, Murray W, Kettenberger H. A frameless stereotaxic integration of computerized tomographic imaging and the operating microscope. *J Neurosurg.* 1986;65(4):545–549.
37. Sipos EP, Tebo SA, Zinreich SJ, Long DM, Brem H. In vivo accuracy testing and clinical experience with the ISG Viewing Wand. *Neurosurgery.* 1996;39(1):194–202.
38. Watanabe E, Watanabe T, Manaka S, Mayanagi Y, Takakura K. Three-dimensional digitizer (neuronavigator): new equipment for computed tomography-guided stereotaxic surgery. *Surg Neurol.* 1987;27(6):543–547.
39. Germano IM, Villalobos H, Silvers A, Post KD. Clinical use of the optical digitizer for intracranial neuronavigation. *Neurosurgery.* 1999;45(2):261–9.
40. Heilbrun MP, McDonald P, Wiker C, Koehler S, Peters W. Stereotactic localization and guidance using a machine vision technique. *Stereotact Funct Neurosurg.* 1992;58(1–4):94–98.
41. Kato A, Yoshimine T, Hayakawa T, et al. A frameless, armless navigational system for computer-assisted neurosurgery. Technical note. *J Neurosurg.* 1991;74(5):845–849.
42. Maciunas RJ, Galloway RL, Fitzpatrick JM, Mandava VR, Edwards CA, Allen GS. A universal system for interactive image-directed neurosurgery. *Stereotact Funct Neurosurg.* 1992;58(1–4):108–113.
43. Smith KR, Frank KJ, Bucholz RD. The NeuroStation–a highly accurate, minimally invasive solution to frameless stereotactic neurosurgery. *Comput Med Imaging Graph.* 1994;18(4):247–256.
44. Rhoten RL, Luciano MG, Barnett GH. Computer-assisted endoscopy for neurosurgical procedures: technical note. *Neurosurgery.* 1997;40(3):632–7.
45. Rubino GJ, Farahani K, McGill D, Van De Wiele B, Villablanca JP, Wang-Mathieson A. Magnetic resonance imaging-guided neurosurgery in the magnetic fringe fields: the next step in neuronavigation. *Neurosurgery.* 2000;46(3):643–53.
46. Suess O, Kombos T, Kurth R, et al. Intracranial image-guided neurosurgery: experience with a new electromagnetic navigation system. *Acta Neurochir (Wien).* 2001;143(9):927–934.
47. Barnett GH, Steiner CP, Weisenberger J. Target and trajectory guidance for interactive surgical navigation systems. *Stereotact Funct Neurosurg.* 1996;66(1–3):91–95.
48. Barnett GH, Steiner CP, Weisenberger J. Adaptation of personal projection television to a head-mounted display for intra-operative viewing of neuroimaging. *J Image Guid Surg.* 1995;1(2):109–112.
49. Pallatroni H, Hartov A, McInerney J, et al. Coregistered ultrasound as a neurosurgical guide. *Stereotact Funct Neurosurg* 1999;73(1–4):143–147.
50. Pelizzari CA, Chen GT, Spelbring DR, Weichselbaum RR, Chen CT. Accurate three-dimensional registration of CT, PET, and/or MR images of the brain. *J Comput Assist Tomogr.* 1989;13(1):20–26.
51. Cosgrove GR, Buchbinder BR, Jiang H. Functional magnetic resonance imaging for intracranial navigation. *Neurosurg Clin N Am.* 1996;7(2):313–322.
52. Kraus GE, Bernstein TW, Satter M, Ezzeddine B, Hwang DR, Mantil J. A technique utilizing positron emission tomography and magnetic resonance/computed tomography image fusion to aid in surgical navigation and tumor volume determination. *J Image Guid Surg.* 1995;1(6):300–307.
53. Chernov MF, Muragaki Y, Ochiai T, et al. Spectroscopy and navigation. *J Neurosurg.* 2005;102(2):402–403.
54. Nimsky C, Ganslandt O, Fahlbusch R. Implementation of fiber tract navigation. *Neurosurgery* 2006;58(4 Suppl 2):ONS-292–303.
55. Hill DL, Maurer CR, Maciunas RJ, Barwise JA, Fitzpatrick JM, Wang MY. Measurement of intraoperative brain surface deformation under a craniotomy. *Neurosurgery.* 1998;43(3):514–526.
56. Nabavi A, Black PM, Gering DT, et al. Serial intraoperative magnetic resonance imaging of brain shift. *Neurosurgery.* 2001;48(4):787–797.
57. Nimsky C, Ganslandt O, Cerny S, Hastreiter P, Greiner G, Fahlbusch R. Quantification of, visualization of, and compensation for brain shift using intraoperative magnetic resonance imaging. *Neurosurgery.* 2000;47(5):1070–1079.
58. Hassenbusch SJ, Anderson JS, Pillay PK. Brain tumor resection aided with markers placed using stereotaxis guided by magnetic resonance imaging and computed tomography. *Neurosurgery.* 1991;28(6):801–805.
59. Yoshikawa K, Kajiwara K, Morioka J, et al. Improvement of functional outcome after radical surgery in glioblastoma patients: the efficacy of a navigation-guided fence-post procedure and neurophysiological monitoring. *J Neurooncol.* 2006;78(1):91–97.
60. Barnett GH: Compact MRI for intraoperative neurosurgical imaging and navigation. *Acta Neurochir (Wien).* 2000;142:1169–1210.
61. Berger MS. Intraoperative MR imaging: making an impact on outcomes for patients with brain tumors. *AJNR Am J Neuroradiol.* 2001;22(1):2.
62. Bernstein M, Al-Anazi AR, Kucharczyk W, Manninen P, Bronskill M, Henkelman M. Brain tumor surgery with the Toronto open magnetic resonance imaging system: preliminary results for 36 patients and analysis of advantages, disadvantages, and future prospects. *Neurosurgery.* 2000;46(4):900–907.
63. Black PM, Moriarty T, Alexander E, et al. Development and implementation of intraoperative magnetic resonance imaging and its neurosurgical applications. *Neurosurgery.* 1997;41(4):831–842.
64. Bohinski RJ, Kokkino AK, Warnick RE, et al. Glioma resection in a shared-resource magnetic resonance operating room after optimal image-guided frameless stereotactic resection. *Neurosurgery.* 2001;48(4):731–742.
65. Fahlbusch R, Ganslandt O, Nimsky C. Intraoperative imaging with open magnetic resonance imaging and neuronavigation. *Childs Nerv Syst.* 2000;16(10–11):829–831.
66. Hadani M, Spiegelman R, Feldman Z, Berkenstadt H, Ram Z. Novel, compact, intraoperative magnetic resonance imaging-guided system for conventional neurosurgical operating rooms. *Neurosurgery.* 2001;48(4):799–807; discussion 807.
67. Knauth M, Wirtz CR, Tronnier VM, Aras N, Kunze S, Sartor K. Intraoperative MR imaging increases the extent of tumor resection in patients with high-grade gliomas. *AJNR Am J Neuroradiol.* 1999;20(9):1642–1646.
68. Koivukangas J, Louhisalmi Y, Alakuijala J, Oikarinen J. Ultrasound-controlled neuronavigator-guided brain surgery. *J Neurosurg.* 1993;79(1):36–42.
69. Lunsford LD, Kondziolka D, Bissonette DJ. Intraoperative imaging of the brain. *Stereotact Funct Neurosurg.* 1996;66(1–3):58–64.
70. Schulder M, Liang D, Carmel PW. Cranial surgery navigation aided by a compact intraoperative magnetic resonance imager. *J Neurosurg.* 2001;94(6):936–945.

71. Steinmeier R, Fahlbusch R, Ganslandt O, et al. Intraoperative magnetic resonance imaging with the magnetom open scanner: concepts, neurosurgical indications, and procedures: a preliminary report. *Neurosurgery.* 1998;43(4):739–747.
72. Wirtz CR, Bonsanto MM, Knauth M, et al. Intraoperative magnetic resonance imaging to update interactive navigation in neurosurgery: method and preliminary experience. *Comput Aided Surg.* 1997;2(3–4):172–179.
73. Bobo RH, Laske DW, Akbasak A, Morrison PF, Dedrick RL, Oldfield EH. Convection-enhanced delivery of macromolecules in the brain. *Proc Natl Acad Sci USA.* 1994;91(6):2076–2080.
74. Sampson JH, Brady ML, Petry NA, et al. Intracerebral infusate distribution by convection-enhanced delivery in humans with malignant gliomas: descriptive effects of target anatomy and catheter positioning. *Neurosurgery.* 2007;60(2 suppl 1):ONS89–98; discussion ONS98.
75. Bingaman WE, Barnett GH. Social and economic impact of surgical navigation systems. In: Barnett GH, Roberts DW, Maciunas RJ, eds. *Image Guided Neurosurgery. Clinical Applications of Surgical Navigation.* St. Louis, MO: Quality Medical Publishing; 1998.
76. Berger MS, Deliganis AV, Dobbins J, Keles GE. The effect of extent of resection on recurrence in patients with low grade cerebral hemisphere gliomas. *Cancer.* 1994;74(6):1784–1791.
77. Curran WJ, Scott CB, Horton J, et al. Does extent of surgery influence outcome for astrocytoma with atypical or anaplastic foci (AAF)? A report from three Radiation Therapy Oncology Group (RTOG) trials. *J Neurooncol.* 1992;12(3):219–227.
78. Vuorinen V, Hinkka S, Färkkilä M, Jääskeläinen J. Debulking or biopsy of malignant glioma in elderly people—a randomised study. *Acta Neurochir (Wien).* 2003;145(1):5–10.
79. Willems PW, Taphoorn MJ, Burger H, Berkelbach van der Sprenkel JW, Tulleken CA. Effectiveness of neuronavigation in resecting solitary intracerebral contrast-enhancing tumors: a randomized controlled trial. *J Neurosurg.* 2006;104(3):360–368.
80. Barnett GH. The role of image-guided technology in the surgical planning and resection of gliomas. *J Neurooncol.* 1999;42(3):247–258.
81. Murphy MA, Barnett GH, Kormos DW, Weisenberger J. Astrocytoma resection using an interactive frameless stereotactic wand: an early experience. *J Clin Neurosci.* 1994;1(1):33–37.
82. Winston KR. Hair and neurosurgery. *Neurosurgery.* 1992;31(2):320–329.
83. Barnett GH, Steiner CP, Weisenberger J. Intracranial meningioma resection using frameless stereotaxy. *J Image Guid Surg.* 1995;1(1):46–52.
84. Barnett GH. Use of surgical navigation systems for resection of intracranial meningiomas. In: Barnett GH, Robert DW, Maciunas RJ, eds. *Image-Guided Surgery: Clinical Applications of Surgical Navigation System.* St. Louis, MO: Quality Medical Publishers, 1998.
85. Di Lorenzo N, Esposito V, Lunardi P, Delfini R, Fortuna A, Cantore G. A comparison of computerized tomography-guided stereotactic and ultrasound-guided techniques for brain biopsy. *J Neurosurg.* 1991;75(5):763–765.
86. Goldstein S, Gumerlock MK, Neuwelt EA. Comparison of CT-guided and stereotaxic cranial diagnostic needle biopsies. *J Neurosurg.* 1987;67(3):341–348.
87. Barnett GH. Brain biopsy and related procedures using surgical navigation systems. In: Barnett GH, Robert DW, Maciunas RJ eds. *Image-Guided Surgery: Clinical Applications of Surgical Navigation System.* St.Louis, MO: Quality Medical Publishers, 1998.
88. Hall WA, Liu H, Truwit CL. Navigus trajectory guide. *Neurosurgery.* 2000;46(2):502–504.
89. Brainard JA, Prayson RA, Barnett GH. Frozen section evaluation of stereotactic brain biopsies: diagnostic yield at the stereotactic target position in 188 cases. *Arch Pathol Lab Med.* 1997;121(5):481–484.
90. Chimowitz MI, Barnett GH, Palmer J. Treatment of intractable arterial hemorrhage during stereotactic brain biopsy with thrombin. Report of three patients. *J Neurosurg.* 1991;74(2):301–303.
91. Kaakaji W, Barnett GH, Bernhard D, Warbel A, Valaitis K, Stamp S. Clinical and economic consequences of early discharge of patients following supratentorial stereotactic brain biopsy. *J Neurosurg.* 2001;94(6):892–898.
92. Miga MI, Roberts DW, Kennedy FE, et al. Modeling of retraction and resection for intraoperative updating of images. *Neurosurgery.* 2001;49(1):75–84; discussion 84.
93. Glauser D, Fankhauser H, Epitaux M, Hefti JL, Jaccottet A. Neurosurgical robot Minerva: first results and current developments. *J Image Guid Surg.* 1995;1(5):266–272.
94. Koyama H, Uchida T, Funakubo H, Takakura K, Fankhauser H. Development of a new microsurgical robot for stereotactic neurosurgery. *Stereotact Funct Neurosurg.* 1990;54–55:462–467.
95. Nathoo N, Cavusoglu MC, Vogelbaum MA, Barnett GH. In touch with robotics: neurosurgery for the future. *Neurosurgery.* 2005;56(3):421–433.

48 Stereotactic Brain Biopsy

S. Bulent Omay and Michael A. Vogelbaum

INTRODUCTION

Despite scientific and technological progress in the diagnosis and treatment of cancer, malignant gliomas remain deadly with few, modestly effective treatment options available. Treatment options, which include microsurgery with navigation and/or real time imaging, radiosurgery, radiotherapy and chemotherapy, are becoming increasingly complex and tumor subtype specific. Furthermore, an increased use of advanced imaging modalities at the screening stage means that lesions are now often discovered at a significantly earlier phase of their growth. Defining an optimal, multifaceted therapeutic strategy is now a key strategy in neurooncology and this strategy places a premium on acquiring as much radiographic and tissue marker data as possible. The advancing imaging technologies currently available, alone, are still not able to establish a diagnosis with the necessary reliability to support therapeutic decision-making. Preoperative diagnosis based only on clinical and radiological findings may be incorrect in more than one-third of patients with intra-axial brain lesions [1]. Therefore, strategies for treating these malignant lesions are most effective when based upon histopathologic diagnoses, and evaluate tissue-based molecular and genetic markers, rather than upon clinical and radiographic findings alone. This continued requirement for diagnostic tissue is the reason why the acquisition of tissue is still a necessity to plan and execute a patient- and tumor-specific treatment protocol [2].

Lesions that cause mass effect and/or those that are easily accessible in relatively functionally silent areas of the brain may be resected as a first step in the treatment plan and thereby produce diagnostic tissue. However, those lesions that cannot be approached by standard craniotomy without an inordinate risk of neurological morbidity, or a lesion in a patient whose general medical status precludes craniotomy, or a situation where medical therapy would likely be superior to operative resection (e.g., primary central nervous system [CNS] lymphoma) may be best diagnosed with a more limited procedure than a craniotomy [3]. In these situations, and others, diagnostic tissue can be obtained using stereotactic brain biopsy (SBB). As much as an SBB can be useful in the situations described earlier, it has a major limitation in that gliomas are histologically heterogeneous; hence it is impossible to reveal the full histopathological profile of a tumor by a single stereotactic biopsy. As will be described more fully, there is a need to perform "subtargeting" within a bulk of tumor to obtain the most metabolically active tissue or that with the most malignant histological features. The ability to localize these subparts within a tumor with the aid of advanced imaging as a guide will help to produce more informative biopsy results. This increase in diagnostic information, in turn, will lead to improvements in developing patient-specific treatment plans [4].

STEREOTACTIC BRAIN BIOPSY, THE LEXICON

Biopsy is defined as "the removal and examination of tissue, cells, or fluids from the living body" [5]. For the clarity of this discussion, the word biopsy will be used only to refer to the removal and not the examination of the live tissue in this chapter. Biopsy is a diagnostic procedure. It is invasive and involves risks, but it still serves as the gold standard diagnostic test for most malignant diseases.

Stereotaxis in Greek means movement [6]; in biology it designates a specific movement pattern defined as "An orientation movement in response to stimulation by contact with a solid body" [7]. *Stereotactic* is defined as "involving, being, utilizing, or used in a surgical technique for precisely directing the tip of a delicate instrument (as a needle) or beam of radiation in three planes using coordinates provided by medical imaging (as computed tomography [CT]) in order to reach a specific locus in the body (as a tumor in the brain or breast)" [5]. SBB uses the earlier mentioned 3D coordinate system to locate, get access, and execute a biopsy for brain lesions.

A BRIEF HISTORY OF SURGICAL STEREOTAXIS

Horsley and Clarke pioneered the field of stereotaxy in 1908, with their invention of an apparatus to create lesions in the cerebellum of the rat [8]. The next major development was the Spiegel-Wycis apparatus in the late 1940s, designed to create lesions for psychiatric and movement disorders [9,10]. It used pneumoencephalography to localize intracranial reference points. Ernest Spiegel, a neurologist, and Henry Wycis, a neurosurgeon, also developed a frame which used rigid skull fixation and a probe with an angular degree of freedom to approach the target from a varied trajectory. This early use of neuroradiological localization allowed human application of this technology. Its first clinical use was to produce therapeutic lesions in medial globus pallidus to treat Huntington's chorea [9,10].

Modern stereotactic surgery was introduced with the coupling of newly developed computer techniques and CT technology in the late 1970s and early 1980s. CT images permitted the accurate localization of targets in the brain, while the reflection of these coordinates to stereotactic space was made possible by the developing software technologies. Later, magnetic resonance imaging (MRI) also became available for use in SBB. Arc-based frames, such as the Leksell device, the Riechert-Mundinger system, the Brown-Roberts-Wells system, and the newer Cosman-Roberts-Wells system increased the popularity of SBB by making it possible to reach a target from an infinite number of trajectories based on the same arc [2].

The past 10 to 15 years has brought the development of frameless surgical navigation systems that are commonly replacing the frame-based stereotaxy systems [11]. The development of powerful computers and image processing software programs with sufficient complexity to interact with the neurosurgeon represented another major technological advance leading to more widespread use of stereotaxis for the diagnosis and treatment of brain lesions [12].

TARGETS AND TECHNIQUES

Brain biopsy is the surgical act involving the patient, the neurosurgeon, the technology and its related equipment to locate or "to define where to aim," and the technology and its related equipment to navigate correctly or to "define how to aim." Progress in these two areas ("where" and "how") has revolutionized SBB, leading to improved diagnostic success and decreased morbidity.

Locating the Target: Where to Aim

Because SBB relies on the definition of a target as defined on a radiological study, understanding the types of information one can obtain from current imaging techniques, as well as the limitations that come with each technique, is essential to maximize the chance for obtaining the most relevant pathological tissue and to minimize the chance for avoidable morbidity. These various imaging modalities provide information that ranges from pure anatomical detail to assessments of metabolic or biochemical properties of the involved tissues.

Computerized Tomography

CT was a pioneering tool in neuroradiology in the sense that it made possible the direct visualization of the brain. CT results in source images perpendicular to the long axis of the brain. X-ray photons are initially collimated into a thin fan-shaped beam that is attenuated by the patient being imaged. The attenuation profile of this fan beam is recorded by detectors. These attenuation values, which reflect the density and atomic number of various tissues, are usually expressed as relative attenuation coefficients, or Hounsfield units (HUs). By definition, the HU of water is zero, and that for air is –1000. Typically, the HU of soft tissues ranges from 10 to 50 [13]. These values are represented in the image produced by the CT software. It has been reported that CT scans will detect 90% of all brain tumors [14] but small tumors less than 0.5 cm in size, tumors adjacent to bone such as pituitary tumors, clival tumors, and vestibular schwannomas may be missed by CT scans [14]. CT scanners provide images at standard matrix sizes of 512 × 512 pixels, and in some instances, 1024 × 1024 pixels, to yield an effective pixel size of less than 0.2 to 0.4 mm at a 22 cm field-of-view for the head [15]. This submillimeter precision provides a high degree of accuracy for stereotactic targeting. Recent advances in scanning technology now permit simultaneous acquisition of multiple images during a single rotation of the x-ray tube, therefore CT has become faster to acquire images and expose the patients to less radiation [16]. Because CT images are computer generated, data making up the axial images can be reformatted in the coronal, sagittal, or oblique planes or as a 3-D image, although some resolution may be lost. Although CT is surpassed by MRI for the detection of small or nonenhancing lesions, it still remains a useful tool for several reasons including increased speed of image acquisition, lower cost, and for being nonmagnetic. The latter feature makes CT the most useful in the evaluation of patients who have conditions that are incompatible with MRI, such as those with pacemakers or other indwelling metallic devices [16].

CT scanners do have a number of disadvantages. Patients are exposed to ionizing radiation and iodine-based contrast agents (although lower doses of contrast are needed with the newer multidetector scanners). Imaging artifacts can interfere with accurate interpretation. In particular, images of the brain stem and posterior fossa are often degraded by "streak artifacts" from the surrounding dense bone of the skull base. Images can be severely degraded by patient motion. Fortunately, unlike MRI scans, individual CT images degraded by motion can be rapidly reacquired [16]. On the other hand, CT imaging is not prone to have the imaging distortions, which is an intrinsic weakness of MRI [17]. CT is more spatially accurate than MRI and often can be used to confirm the spatial accuracy of MRI images used for stereotactic planning.

Magnetic Resonance Imaging

The introduction of MRI has deeply affected the practice of surgical neurooncology. MRI is now the gold standard imaging tool for the diagnosis, treatment, and follow up of brain tumors. The physics of MRI is based on the fact that under a magnetic field of sufficient power, the protons in water molecules, regardless of their initial localization, lay either parallel or antiparallel to the vector of the magnetic field. A radiofrequency pulse excites these protons and dislodges them out of the orderly alignment. They fall to their resting state with the cessation of the pulse, only by emitting the radiofrequency energy gained during the pulse excitation, which is detected by the sensors of the MRI scanner, and transformed into a 3D image [14].

MRI is better able to detect smaller lesions, define cystic and hemorrhagic components within a tumor, create images in three axes, and provide visualization of the posterior fossa particularly with respect to the anatomic relationships of a lesion with critical neurovascular structures than is CT [14]. On the other hand, because the technique relies on the application of a homogenous magnetic field, any paramagnetic materials within the field (e.g., dental implants, shrapnel, and surgical devices) can produce alterations that lead to phantom lesions or distortions of the spatial fidelity of the image. The latter limitation is of particular importance with regard to stereotactic targeting as it can lead to biopsy probe trajectory errors and unexpected morbidity.

Despite its well-defined soft tissue contrast, capability of multiplanar image acquisition, and noninvasive nature, MRI is largely limited to depicting morphologic abnormalities. Conventional MRI is limited in its ability to reliably grade gliomas before surgery. Contrast enhancement on postcontrast T1-weighted images is one of the most common methods for assessing glioma grade. Contrast enhancement is not synonymous with malignancy, and less aggressive tumors such as pilocytic astrocytomas and meningiomas often are avidly enhancing tumors. Hence, grading based solely on conventional MRI is unreliable [18]. In addition, nonspecificity is an intrinsic problem in MRI. Different disease processes can appear similar, and a single disease entity may have varied imaging findings. The metabolic or functional brain cannot be adequately evaluated based on "anatomic" MRI alone. As a consequence of this deficiency of conventional MRI, several physiology-based MRI methods have been developed and have become a part of an imaging armamentarium to improve tumor characterization [18].

Magnetic Resonance Spectroscopy

As discussed earlier, MRI best provides structural information about the brain and any malignant tissues but it does not do much more than that in terms of delineating the heterogeneous nature of gliomas. The currently used methods of T2-weighted MRI and contrast-enhanced T1-weighted MRI are not specific for tumors and can result in ambiguous or misleading results [19–21]. The ability to recognize the border zone between tumor and normal brain tissue is one of the major obstacles in planning surgery for high-grade tumors, and conventional MRI is not capable of overcoming this limitation [19].

Magnetic resonance spectroscopy (MRS) provides qualitative and quantitative information about brain metabolism and tissue composition. This functional analysis is based on detecting variations in the precession frequencies of spinning protons in a magnetic field. One factor influencing the resonance frequency is the chemical environment of the individual proton. Protons in different cerebral metabolites can be accurately separated on this basis, and the position of these metabolites can be displayed as a spectrum. On the spectroscopy plot, the y-axis corresponds to relative quantity, whereas the x-axis position of a given metabolite reflects the degree of "chemical shift" of the metabolite with respect to a designated reference metabolite, and it is expressed in units of parts per million (ppm). The area under the peak is determined by the number of protons that contributed to the MR signal [13].

The major metabolites detected in the CNS are N-acetyl aspartate (NAA), a neuronal marker; choline, a marker for cellularity and cell membrane turnover; creatine, a marker for energy metabolism; and lactate, a marker for anaerobic metabolism [13]. In MRS studies, the most notable peak is that of NAA, which is a marker of mature neuronal density and viability and is therefore decreased in tumor tissue because malignant cells in a tumor replace healthy neurons. Choline is one of the most important peaks for analyzing brain tumors, reflecting the metabolism of cellular membrane turnover. The choline peak is increased in all malignant primary and secondary brain tumors. Low-grade gliomas show slightly decreased NAA and slightly increased choline peaks. The level of choline activity is usually compared to levels of creatine activity; an elevated ratio of choline to creatine suggests the presence of a tumor [19,22]. Another metabolite that is useful in evaluating intracranial malignancy is lactate. The presence of lactate indicates that the normal metabolic respiration of tissue has been altered. This situation occurs in highly active and cellular lesions that outgrow their blood supply, entering an anaerobic metabolic state. Pilocytic astrocytomas display unique features: despite their benign nature and histology, MRS maps of these tumors show lactate peaks without necrosis [19,23,24]. Tumors that are necrotic or areas of treatment-induced necrosis exhibit lipid metabolites, which can also be identified with MRS. In an untreated tumor, lipid is usually an indicator of high-grade malignancy [19,25]. The typical pattern of a high-grade malignancy demonstrates a spectrum with an elevated choline-to-creatine ratio and a depressed NAA peak [19].

MRS imaging, which is usually focused on the region of interest, provides biochemical information as opposed to structural. Metabolite maps can be fused with routine anatomical MRI images facilitating correlation of functional and structural information. Since the MRS metabolite pattern of the normal brain at a given age is known and predictable, deviation from the expected normal metabolite pattern can give additional information about tumor composition, the grade of a malignancy, and any change over time. Tumor recurrence and change in biological degree of malignancy may also be seen with MRS [13,19]. Thus, MRS can reduce the need for biopsy of multiple different areas of brain tumors, which can increase the risk of procedural-related complications. By coupling MRS with conventional MRI, neuronavigation systems provide biochemical imaging data in the context of the structural imaging thereby giving the surgeon the ability to specifically target biochemically abnormal portions of the tumor tissue for biopsy.

The acquisition of MRS involves first defining the 3D volume of interest (VOI) to be studied. Localization of VOI can be done by either single voxel or chemical shift technique. In single voxel spectroscopy, a small region (usual minimum of 1 cm^3) of brain is used to obtain metabolic information. It is a fast and easy technique, but limited by tissue coverage. Chemical shift imaging, on the other hand, offers larger coverage and improved signal detection. For brain tumors, chemical shift imaging is preferable because of its ability to provide metabolic information on a larger target area. This method does, however, require longer imaging time and complex data processing. It is important to recognize, however, that the minimum voxel size for MRS is 1 cm³, whereas a biopsy tissue specimen may be smaller than 1 mm³. This discrepancy in size must be kept in mind when choosing a biopsy site based on MRS and interpretation of biopsy result.

There are several important limitations associated with clinical application of proton MRS for brain tumor imaging. First, due to limitations in MRS voxel size, entire tumor volume may not be covered by this modality. Consequently, important areas of tumor may be left out of the MRS analysis. Second, there is no one specific MRS characteristic that designates a tumor as malignant, and nonspecific spectral findings are common. MRS data processing remains a time-consuming procedure, especially in case of multidimensional datasets, and requires offline workstation and sophisticated software programs. Further studies are needed to improve MRS acquisition and data interpretation before it can be incorporated into the routine of clinical brain tumor–imaging protocols [18].

MR Perfusion

MR perfusion involves the rapid venous injection of gadolinium contrast material with imaging through a focused volume of tissue, starting before arrival of contrast material and continuing during the passage of contrast through the region of interest. MR perfusion makes it possible to make the calculation of physiologic parameters such as cerebral blood volume (CBV), mean transit time, cerebral blood flow, and tissue permeability. These parameters can then be analyzed and interpreted at the same time as conventional anatomical imaging and spectroscopic data. This technique is useful in the evaluation of benign and malignant intracranial and skull base tumors, but it is probably most widely used as a method to distinguish radionecrosis from recurrent tumor when evaluating new enhancement on a standard anatomic MRI. MR perfusion parameters, particularly permeability, are sensitive to tumoral angiogenesis and may be useful in grading of primary brain neoplasia, as well as monitoring the effects of therapy on neovascular proliferation. Another use is to assist the surgeon in identifying the most aggressive portions of a tumor so that optimal biopsy locations can be chosen [26].

The progressive increase in relative CBV from low-grade to high-grade tumors is consistent with studies showing that microvascular density in low-grade astrocytomas is significantly lower than in anaplastic astrocytomas or glioblastomas [18]. On the other hand, relative CBV measurements can and do vary considerably because of the histopathologic heterogeneity inherent in the gliomas. Therefore, maps of relative CBV of gliomas should not be interpreted without a parallel evaluation of conventional MR images, which can provide other valuable information, such as the integrity of the blood-brain barrier or the degree and characteristics of T2 abnormality [18]. Perfusion MRI is also highly sensitive to susceptibility artifacts because of

echoplanar and T2 effect of the technique. Therefore any paramagnetic or ferromagnetic material can cause severe artifact, particularly near the brain-bone-air interface near the middle cranial fossa or posterior fossa. Perfusion MRI of tumors in these locations is, therefore, intrinsically limited and challenging [18].

Positron Emission Tomography

Positron emission tomography (PET) scans consist of computer-generated cross-sectional images of the distribution and local concentration of a radiopharmaceutical. Energy metabolism is a central function of all tissues, including tumors, and can be measured with PET. The glucose analogue radiotracer ^{18}F-deoxyglucose (FDG) is most commonly used to measure the rate of local glucose metabolism, and most malignant tumors show high FDG uptake. PET scanning with this agent gives a spatially localized measurement of brain glucose metabolism [27]. Areas of high metabolic activity (i.e., cerebral cortex, deep gray nuclei) demonstrate greater radiopharmaceutical uptake than areas of low metabolic activity, such as white matter or cerebrospinal fluid. Anatomic resolution is not as good as with CT or MRI, however. The major advantage of PET imaging is that it is extremely versatile, providing information about brain perfusion, glucose metabolism, receptor density, and, ultimately, brain function [13].

FDG uptake has been associated with histological tumor grade and survival in primary and recurrent gliomas, but this association has been weak with relatively high false-positive and false-negative rates [27–32]. FDG uptake in low-grade gliomas is usually similar to that of normal white matter, whereas many grade III anaplastic gliomas have a FDG uptake similar to or exceeding that of normal gray matter. Untreated glioblastomas also tend to have high uptake of FDG, which might be heterogeneous throughout the tumor. Glucose consumption in normal brain tissue is reduced in most patients with malignant brain tumors, contributing to an increased tumor-to-reference uptake ratio [33]. A problem with the use of FDG for the diagnosis of tumors in the brain is the high glucose metabolism of normal gray matter, which exceeds that of most other organs apart from the heart. Thus, the localization of brain tumors with FDG-PET alone is difficult, or impossible, and co-registration and fusion of FDG-uptake images with structural scans is required for the reliable separation of the tumor from normal brain tissue [27,34].

The thymidine analog 39-deoxy-39–18F-fluorothymidine (FLT) PET is another tracer for PET which was developed as a noninvasive method to evaluate tumor cell proliferation [35]. Uptake of 18F-FLT is related to thymidine kinase-1 activity, an enzyme expressed during the DNA synthesis phase of the cell cycle [36]. Thymidine kinase-1 activity is high in proliferating cells and low in quiescent cells. Although 18F-FLT appears to have limited sensitivity, uptake of 18F-FLT by tumors correlates with Ki-67, in brain tumors [35]. Thus, 18F-FLT has the potential to monitor treatment response and to serve as a prognostic marker. It has also been shown that combined use of MRI and 18F-FET PET significantly improves the identification of tumor tissue [33].

Accessing the Target: How to Aim

As discussed earlier, SBB is indicated in a number of clinical conditions including: (a) when surgical decision-making will be heavily influenced by the histologic nature of the lesion; (b) for lesions that are located deep within the brain or in eloquent cortex, surgically unresectable and diffusely infiltrating, or cystic and causing significant mass effect on surrounding neural structures in which case aspiration may result in decompression of CNS tissue and restoration of function; (c) to determine the pathology of multiple intracranial lesions; and (d) when cytoreductive surgery would not be beneficial to the patient [36–38].

As with any neurosurgical procedure, the preoperative workup should anticipate potential causes of avoidable morbidity. All patients should have a recent preoperative imaging not only for targeting the lesion, but also for reducing the likelihood of inadvertent biopsy of a vascular lesion or an adjacent blood vessel. Detailed imaging can also alert the surgeon to the possibility of a vascularized tumor, which might be more safely approached via an open surgical procedure. A systemic cancer evaluation should be considered if the radiographic appearance is suggestive of a metastatic lesion. The patient should have a general medical workup including the coagulation profile to prevent an unforeseen adverse event. Aspirin should be stopped at least 5 days before the procedure; longer times may be required to clear long-circulating, irreversible antiplatelet agents such as clopidogrel.

Attention to detail, with the procedure performed in a stereotypical fashion by an experienced and well-rehearsed team, is an absolute necessity for all stereotactic biopsies [2]. Unlike open surgical procedures, SBBs are performed without the surgeon directly visualizing the brain and/or target area. Instead, he/she must rely on the use of technology for guidance. The lack of a direct line of sight to the target during SBB prevents the surgeon from being able to recognize targeting errors at the site of the biopsy during the procedure. In particular, small angular errors become progressively amplified as a function of the depth of the lesion from the surface of the cranium. What seems to be a simple and straightforward procedure can be associated with significant morbidity if not performed rigorously.

Frameless versus Frame-Based SBB

Stereotactic procedures can be categorized into frame-based and frameless procedures.

Frame-based SBB involves application of a rigid frame directly to the patient's skull under local anesthesia using screws. Stereotactic imaging is performed after the fixation of the frame to the patient. At this point, the specific techniques for translating the imaging data into a 3D map of the framespace depends upon the type of frame and image guidance system used. However, in general, the procedure involves the use of an imaging adapter that is attached to the frame to produce reference points in each image slice that encode the images with the quantitative information necessary to translate the position of the target into mathematical coding.

In frameless SBB, images are obtained after either surface-applied scalp fiducials or, in some cases, skull implanted fiducials are placed. The application of fiducials is often done the day of or the day before the procedure. The stereotactic images are transferred to planning station in the operation room. At the time of the procedure, the patient's head is placed in a head-holder to which a reference array, which is visible to the navigation system, is attached. A stereotactic probe is used to register the scalp fiducials to the navigation system at which point stereotactic targeting can be performed.

Surgical Navigation Technology

Most surgical navigation technologies have image fusion capabilities. This means that the earlier mentioned specialized MRI, metabolic and molecular imaging modalities can be fused to a standard stereotactic CT or MRI, thereby, creating an anatomically coregistered image set that presents the surgeon with anatomic, metabolic, and molecular data simultaneously. These data sets can be manipulated for planning the optimal trajectory and target. Target and trajectory planning is conducted based on the fused images to optimize diagnostic yield and to minimize risk and morbidity [11]. The target and entry site selection are the critical events during the stereotactic biopsy.

Target selection in the case of malignant lesions requires the balancing of a number of factors that may affect diagnostic yield. A central site may be selected in homogeneous lesions to avoid the confusion caused by reactive astrocytes in the periphery. However, because most malignant lesions are inhomogeneous, central biopsies may be prone to return nondiagnostic necrotic tissue. In these cases, a more peripheral biopsy of the enhancing region is more likely to provide a diagnostic specimen. Use of fused anatomic and metabolic imaging technology may help to improve targeting within subparts of the lesion, but this remains more of a research interest than a widely used clinical tool at this point in time [2,39–41].

Entry point selection is also influenced by a number of factors and must be individualized to each patient and lesion. In general, one selects an entry point that provides the most direct path to the lesion via an overlying gyrus. Using modern surgical navigation systems, one can examine the trajectory provided by an individual entry point-target combination. Care must be taken to examine the various images along the probe path to avoid any intervening critical neural or vascular structures. Trajectories that traverse pial or ependymal interfaces, especially in the depths of sulci, are to be particularly avoided, because of the high vascularity of these areas [2]. One should also plan for a trajectory that will allow for sampling multiple points within a lesion so that the biopsy probe can simply be advanced as necessary if initial biopsies are nondiagnostic. Alternatively, some surgeons will create a larger opening that will allow the use of multiple separate trajectories.

Brain biopsy can also be executed with the use of intraoperative MRI (iMRI). The main benefits of this approach are that preoperative imaging is not necessary (although it can be made available for co-registration with the intraoperative images) and biopsy probe can be visualized within the target in real time. Brain shift is usually minimal in biopsy procedures but in the rare occasion where a cyst is drained simultaneously or a large volume of cerebrospinal fluid is lost, reliability of surgical navigation system, which is based only on pre-operative imaging, may become questionable. However, the high cost of acquisition and siting of iMRI equipment and the cost of MRI-compatible surgical instruments limit the availability of this approach [11]. In addition, some iMRI systems also do not provide the high-quality and detailed imaging that is available with conventional diagnostic MRI devices.

The Biopsy Procedure

The biopsy procedure may be performed under light sedation with local anesthesia or under general anesthesia. After an optimal entry point-target combination is chosen a small skin incision is made. The length of the skin incision depends upon the type of cranial opening that will be performed. Some surgeons place burr holes and open the dura under direct vision, whereas others may perform an image-guided twist drill craniostomy and open the dura sharply with a spinal needle or bluntly with an electrocautery probe. Depending upon the type of surgical navigation system used, either measurements from the dura to the target are made and the depth the biopsy instrument should be advanced is calculated, the biopsy instrument is itself equipped with markers that allow it to be tracked in real time by the image guidance system, or the tip of the instrument is visualized using an iMRI system. A number of instruments can be used for tissue acquisition such as needle core device, side-cutting aspirator, spiral needle, side-cutting needle, and cup forceps. Occasional bleeding may be seen from the cannula; in most cases this bleeding will stop with continued irrigation or head elevation. After initial specimen(s) are obtained, and the cannula is left in place while a neuropathologist performs a frozen section diagnosis. When the specimen is considered adequate for final diagnosis after tissue processing for permanent sections, the cannula is withdrawn and the wound is irrigated and closed. If a frame was used, it is removed at this time. A CT scan is recommended in the first few postoperative hours to confirm accurate targeting of the lesion (usually an air bubble can be seen at the biopsy site), and also to provide early diagnosis of a postoperative hemorrhage [2].

COMPLICATIONS

Stereotactic biopsy is a safe procedure in experienced hands, but it can still be a cause of morbidity and even mortality. Reported morbidity includes seizures, hemorrhage, stroke, new neurologic deficits, cerebrospinal leakage, brain infection, pin-site infection, tumor seeding, and lack of diagnosis [37,42]. Biopsy of vascular lesions can be catastrophic. Similarly, extremely vascular tumors, such as metastatic renal cell carcinoma, hemangioblastoma, choriocarcinoma, and metastatic melanoma, are best approached through other means if suspected. In fact, if a metastatic lesion is suspected, a search for and biopsy of an extracranial source is probably the most appropriate means of management. Identification of a major blood vessel close to the lesion can be a cause for concern, as would location close to the vessel-rich Sylvian fissure, cavernous sinus, or brain-pial interface. An analysis of more than 3800 cases reported in the literature reveals an overall morbidity rate of 3.2% and a mortality rate of 0.6% [2].

The most common complication is hemorrhage at the biopsy site, which is symptomatic in 1 to 2% of all cases [2,11]. This complication is associated with the inability of the surgeon to directly visualize the target, which is inherent to this type of minimal access procedure. In many cases, damage to small blood vessels in the trajectory of the biopsy is unavoidable, but both frame-based and frameless stereotaxy systems coupled with surgical navigation systems can help reduce the incidence of this complication [11]. It is important to note that the presence of a bleeding diathesis will not necessarily result in a hemorrhage, but it can turn a minor event into a catastrophe [2].

A second area of morbidity is a new neurological deficit that is unrelated to whether an area of hemorrhage is present on the postoperative imaging study. In these cases, damage is related to trauma to the surrounding brain or edema caused directly by the biopsy. The chances for this complication may be reduced by limiting the number of needle insertions during the biopsy, and by utilizing the least traumatic means of sample acquisition.

Edema can also be caused by interruption of an intervening draining vein; in rare cases, these veins can be seen on a preoperative MRI and thereby avoided. Other, less common types of morbidity include seizures and postoperative infections [2].

As a rule of thumb, for any biopsy procedure it is important to consider the risk of hemorrhage and stroke with each individual biopsy sample obtained. The chance of a definitive diagnosis and grading must be weighed against the risk of an ensuing complication to the patient. Judicious selection of the number and location of biopsy samples necessary to make an accurate diagnosis is critically important [43].

CONCLUSION

Brain biopsy will continue to be the gold standard for diagnosing brain tumors until noninvasive technologies evolve to the point where they can provide the same degree of diagnostic accuracy. Until then the technology and procedures underlining SBB will continue to evolve to improve target planning, by incorporating an increasingly diverse set of imaging data into the target selection process, and decrease procedural morbidity.

REFERENCES

1. Friedman WA, Sceats DJ, Nestok BR, Ballinger WE. The incidence of unexpected pathological findings in an image-guided biopsy series: a review of 100 consecutive cases. *Neurosurgery.* 1989;25(2):180–184.
2. Krieger MD, Chandrasoma PT, Zee CS, Apuzzo ML. Role of stereotactic biopsy in the diagnosis and management of brain tumors. *Semin Surg Oncol.* 1998;14(1):13–25.

3. Sawin PD, Hitchon PW, Follett KA, Torner JC. Computed imaging-assisted stereotactic brain biopsy: a risk analysis of 225 consecutive cases. *Surg Neurol.* 1998;49(6):640–649.
4. Preul MC, Leviver MC, Caramanos Z, Arnold DL, Wikler D, Goldman S. Metabolic and functional imaging of brain tumors. In: Kaye H, Laws ER, eds. *Brain tumors.* New York: Churchill Livingstone; 2001.
5. Merriam-Webster Medical Dictionary [Internet]. Springfield, MA: Merriam-Webster, Incorporated; ©2003. Biopsy; ©2003 [cited 2008 Jan 20]; http://www2.merriam-webster.com/cgi-bin/mwmednlm&book=Medical&va=Biopsy
6. Willems PW, van der Sprenkel JW, Tulleken CA, Viergever MA, Taphoorn MJ. Neuronavigation and surgery of intracerebral tumours. *J Neurol.* 2006;253(9):1123–1136.
7. Access Science Encyclopedia of Science & Technology Online. [Internet]: McGraw-Hill; ©2007 Stereotaxis; [cited 2008 Jan 20]; http://www.accessscience.com/search.aspx?searchStr=stereotaxis
8. Horsley V, Clarke RH: The structure and functions of the cerebellum examined by a new method. *Brain.* 1908;31:45–124.
9. Nashold BS. The history of stereotactic neurosurgery. *Stereotact Funct Neurosurg.* 1994;62(1–4):29–40.
10. Spiegel EA, Wycis HT, Marks M, Lee AJ. Stereotaxic Apparatus for Operations on the Human Brain. *Science.* 1947;106:349–350.
11. Siomin V, Barnett GH. Brain biopsy and related procedures. In: Barnett GH, Maciunas RJ, Roberts DW, eds. *Computer Assisted Neurosurgery.* New York: Taylor and Francis Group, LLC: 2006.
12. Linskey ME. The changing role of stereotaxis in surgical neuro-oncology. *J Neurooncol.* 2004;69:35–54.
13. Bradbury MS, Williams DW III. Brain and its coverings. In: Chen MYM, Pope TL Jr, Ott DJ, eds. *Basic Radiology.* [Internet]: McGraw-Hill Companies; ©2004 [cited 2008 Jan 10]; http://www.accessmedicine.com/content.aspx?aID=2270780
14. Wen P, Teoh SK, Black PM. Clinical Imaging and laboratoy diagnosis of brain tumors. In: Kaye H, Laws ER, eds. *Brain Tumors.* New York: Churchill Livingstone; 2001.
15. Kim PE, Zee CS. Imaging of the cerebrum. *Neurosurgery.* 2007;61[SHC (suppl 1)]:SHC-123–SHC-146.
16. Debnam JM, Ketonen L, Hamberg LM, Hunter GJ. Current techniques used for the radiologic assessment of intracranial neoplasms. *Arch Pathol Lab Med.* 2007;131(2):252–260.
17. Landil A. Accuracy of stereotactic localisation with magnetic resonance compared to CT Scan: experimental findings. *Acta Neurochir (Wien).* 2001;143: 593–601.
18. Cha S. Update on brain tumor imaging. *Current Neurology and Neuroscience Reports.* 2005, 5:169–177.
19. Stadlbauer A, Moser E, Gruber S, et al. Improved delineation of brain tumors: an automated method for segmentation based on pathologic changes of 1H-MRSI metabolites in gliomas. *Neuroimage.* 2004;23(2):454–461.
20. Dowling C, Bollen AW, Noworolski SM, et al. Preoperative proton MR spectroscopic imaging of brain tumors: correlation with histopathologic analysis of resection specimens. *AJNR Am J Neuroradiol.* 2001;22(4):604–612.
21. Kondziolka D, Lunsford LD, Martinez AJ. Unreliability of contemporary neurodiagnostic imaging in evaluating suspected adult supratentorial (low-grade) astrocytoma. *J Neurosurg.* 1993;79(4):533–536.
22. Stadlbauer A, Nimsky C, Buslei R, et al. Proton magnetic resonance spectroscopic imaging in the border zone of gliomas: correlation of metabolic and histological changes at low tumor infiltration–initial results. *Invest Radiol.* 2007;42(4):218–223.
23. Ganslandt O, Stadlbauer A, Fahlbusch R, et al. Proton magnetic resonance spectroscopic imaging integrated into image-guided surgery: correlation to standard magnetic resonance imaging and tumor cell density. *Neurosurgery.* 2005;56(2 Suppl):291–298.
24. Rock JP, Hearshen D, Scarpace L, et al. Correlations between magnetic resonance spectroscopy and image-guided histopathology, with special attention to radiation necrosis. *Neurosurgery.* 2002;51(4):912–919.
25. Li X, Lu Y, Pirzkall A, McKnight T, Nelson SJ. Analysis of the spatial characteristics of metabolic abnormalities in newly diagnosed glioma patients. *J Magn Reson Imaging.* 2002;16(3):229–237.
26. Provenzale JM, Mukundan S, Barboriak DP. Diffusion-weighted and perfusion MR imaging for brain tumor characterization and assessment of treatment response. *Radiology.* 2006;239(3):632–649.
27. Herholz K, Coope D, Jackson A. Metabolic and molecular imaging in neuro-oncology. *Lancet Neurol.* 2007;6(8):711–724.
28. Padma MV, Said S, Jacobs M, et al. Prediction of pathology and survival by FDG PET in gliomas. *J Neurooncol.* 2003;64(3):227–237.
29. De Witte O, Levivier M, Violon P, et al. Prognostic value positron emission tomography with [18F]fluoro-2-deoxy-D-glucose in the low-grade glioma. *Neurosurgery.* 1996;39(3):470–476.
30. Barker FG, Chang SM, Valk PE, Pounds TR, Prados MD. 18-Fluorodeoxyglucose uptake and survival of patients with suspected recurrent malignant glioma. *Cancer.* 1997;79(1):115–126.
31. Patronas NJ, Di Chiro G, Kufta C, et al. Prediction of survival in glioma patients by means of positron emission tomography. *J Neurosurg.* 1985;62(6):816–822.
32. Alavi JB, Alavi A, Chawluk J, et al. Positron emission tomography in patients with glioma. A predictor of prognosis. *Cancer.* 1988;62(6):1074–1078.
33. Pauleit D, Floeth F, Hamacher K, et al. O-(2-[18F]fluoroethyl)-L-tyrosine PET combined with MRI improves the diagnostic assessment of cerebral gliomas. *Brain.* 2005;128:678–687.
34. Pirotte B, Goldman S, Dewitte O, et al. Integrated positron emission tomography and magnetic resonance imaging-guided resection of brain tumors: a report of 103 consecutive procedures. *J Neurosurg.* 2006;104(2):238–253.
35. Chen W, Cloughesy T, Kamdar N, et al. Imaging proliferation in brain tumors with 18F-FLT PET: comparison with 18F-FDG. *J Nucl Med.* 2005;46(6):945–952.
36. Chen W. Clinical applications of PET in brain tumors. *J Nucl Med.* 2007;48(9):1468–1481.
37. Bernstein M, Parrent AG. Complications of CT-guided stereotactic biopsy of intra-axial brain lesions. *J Neurosurg.* 1994;81(2):165–168.
38. Hall WA. The safety and efficacy of stereotactic biopsy for intracranial lesions. *Cancer.* 1998;82(9):1749–1755.
39. Burtscher IM, Skagerberg G, Geijer B, Englund E, Ståhlberg F, Holtås S. Proton MR spectroscopy and preoperative diagnostic accuracy: an evaluation of intracranial mass lesions characterized by stereotactic biopsy findings. *AJNR Am J Neuroradiol.* 2000;21(1):84–93.
40. Son BC, Kim MC, Choi BG, et al. Proton magnetic resonance chemical shift imaging (1H CSI)-directed stereotactic biopsy. *Acta Neurochir (Wien).* 2001;143(1):45–49.
41. Hall WA, Liu H: Magnetic resonance spectroscopy-guided biopsy of intracranial tumors. *Tech Neurosurg.* 2002;7:291–298.
42. Kondziolka D, Lunsford LD. The role of stereotactic biopsy in the management of gliomas. *J Neurooncol.* 1999;42(3):205–213.
43. Shastri-Hurst N, Tsegaye M, Robson DK, Lowe JS, Macarthur DC. Stereotactic brain biopsy: an audit of sampling reliability in a clinical case series. *Br J Neurosurg.* 2006;20(4):222–226.

49 Intraoperative Anatomical Imaging

Salvatore M. Zavarella and Michael Schulder

INTRODUCTION

The ability to bring digital imaging technology into the operating room (OR) has transformed the practice of brain tumor surgery. Although other forms of intraoperative imaging had been tried, the seminal development probably was the introduction of intraoperative MRI (iMRI) at the Brigham and Women's Hospital in 1995 (Figure 49.1) [1,2]. In the first decade of the 21st century, intraoperative imaging techniques have become regular features in the neurosurgical OR. Integrated imaging and navigation systems have provided the surgeon with objective data by which to guide surgery in real time or close to it [3–7].

Anatomical imaging as we know it began in 1895 with Wilhelm Roentgen's discovery that x-rays could image boney anatomy [8]. X-rays alone rarely provided information regarding intracranial tumors, except for the occasional calcified lesion. In 1919, Walter Dandy described ventriculography in which cerebrospinal fluid (CSF) was drained and replaced with air, oxygen, or helium, allowing for better resolution of intracranial structures via x-ray [9]. In 1927, Egas Moniz performed the first cerebral angiogram [10]. This method was a huge leap in its ability to visualize vascular anatomy including the vascular blush often associated with intracranial tumors.

The modern era of neurosurgical imaging arrived in the early 1980s with the use of computed tomography (CT) and several years later, magnetic resonance imaging (MRI), in frame-based stereotaxy [11–13]. Because of ergonomic limitations of the stereotactic frame, surgical navigation systems (also known as "frameless stereotaxy") have gained popularity and become a fixture in the OR [14,15].

The limitations of preoperative imaging in neuronavigational frame-based and frameless stereotaxy became quickly evident as these rigid nonupdatable images are prone to inaccuracies in localizing lesions after dural opening, CSF leakage, and tumor removal [16]. The push for real-time updatable intraoperative imaging of cranial anatomy became vital to improving the morbidity and mortality in patients with complex intracranial lesions. In an attempt to answer these important issues, Lunsford, in 1982, described the first use of a dedicated real-time intraoperative CT (iCT) for use in a stereotactic OR environment [17]. The correlation between intraoperative ultrasound (iUS) and image-guided surgery was then described in 1986 [18].

With the era of MRI-guided stereotactic neurosurgery underway, and with the limited soft tissue resolution of iCT and iUS, many investigators and clinicians began looking toward the implementation of iMRI to aid in intracranial surgery [19]. By 1997, Black et al [16] in conjunction with General Electric Medical Systems (Waukesha, Wisconsin) pioneered the use of a 0.5T iMRI at Brigham and Women's Hospital in Boston (Figure 49.1).

Since this time there have been great advances in the imaging of intraoperative anatomical structures for use in many kinds of neurosurgical therapy. Recently, intraoperative imaging has been utilized for therapies ranging from tumor biopsy and removal (especially glioma and hormonally inactive pituitary tumors), aneurysm clipping and AVM debulking, monitoring during surgery for the treatment of refractory epilepsy, functional cortical mapping, and a vast array of spine treatments. This chapter will discuss recent advances, technical issues, cost, clinical results, and future directions in the use of iCT, US, angiography, and MRI.

INTRAOPERATIVE IMAGING: THE RATIONALE

Tumor Invasion

Microneurosurgical techniques have advanced since the advent of the operating microscope in the early 1960s [20]. This technology has enabled neurosurgeons the ability to visually navigate deep anatomical structures allowing for tumor debulking with significant decreases in morbidity and mortality. However, the rate-limiting step in complete microsurgical tumor extirpation has been the inability of the aided eye to discern microscopic tumor cell invasion. Many tumors lack distinctive capsules and as a result the surgeon has difficulties discriminating between intact and neoplastic brain. This leads to either (a) inadequate resection as the surgeon is not able to visualize microscopic tumor burden, or (b) the lack of definitive margins and the desire for complete removal, leading the surgeon to unnecessarily aggressive surgery and leaving the patient with a deficit [21]. This is particularly true for patients with

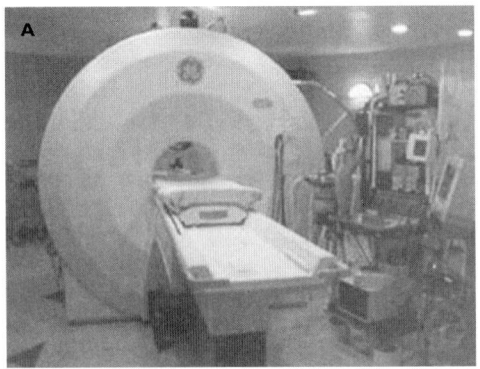 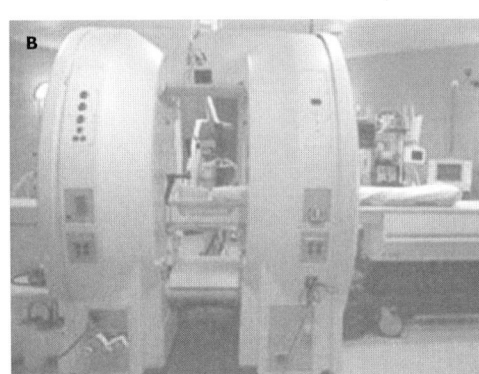

Figure 49.1 The Signa 0.5 T "double doughnut" iMRI. Courtesy of Elsevier Science [145].

gliomas, and especially so for low-grade tumors, due to their propensity to blend into and appear identical to surrounding normal brain [22–25]. At the same time, recent evidence from multiple groups suggest that a more rigorous resection translates into longer survival for patients with both low- and high-grade gliomas [26–29]. Another application of intraoperative imaging for tumor resection control is in the trans-sphenoidal resection of pituitary tumors, where the approach through the pathology limits the ability to assess extent of resection, even with endoscopic guidance [30].

Thus, intraoperative imaging has a critical role to play in facilitating maximal removal of intracranial tumors, while minimizing the iatrogenic creation of new neurological deficits.

Brain Shift

Another critical issue addressed by intraoperative imaging is that of brain shift during intracranial surgery. During neurosurgical procedures brain parenchyma and its associated vasculature are prone to 1 cm or more of shift due to the egress of CSF, gravity, and edema associated with either the pathology or the procedure [31,32]. This displacement renders preoperative imaging utilized for stereotactic navigation less than optimal for navigation in the brain itself. Intracranial shift becomes more pronounced and more difficult to predict as tumor resection proceeds [21].

As shift occurs and the initial resection cavity is altered by tumor removal, difficulties arise for the surgeon in locating small areas of residual tumor enclosed by a collapsing cavity. Continually updatable real-time images allow for precise location of these concealed tumor burden areas and minimize the effects of excess brain retraction [33,34].

INTRAOPERATIVE IMAGING TECHNOLOGIES

Intraoperative Ultrasound

Recent years have brought considerable technological advances in the image quality and ease of iUS. However, as Unsgaard et al [35] point out in their 2006 review, many neurosurgeons have a reluctance to implement iUS into their practice because of past experiences. They go on to point out a few myths such as inferior image quality, the necessity for larger craniotomies to accommodate the iUS probe, limited use at the finish of most cases due to further loss of image quality, and finally the difficulties in interpreting and understanding the imaging results. However, they and others demonstrate in multiple reports that nearly all tumors can be depicted by iUS in the initial phases of surgery [36–42] and that image quality is either equal to or sometimes superior to preoperative MRI [43,44]. They state that in their experience craniotomies do not need to be extended to optimize image acquisition, that with simple adjustments good image quality can be maintained, and that the learning curve for iUS, including 3D iUS, is fast because images can be displayed in the same planes as preoperative MRI, thereby making navigational integration much easier [43].

Image Quality

US probes utilize a particular frequency to obtain spatial resolution and thus resolve target images. The radial and lateral resolutions equal the pulse length and width, respectively. For example, in using a 5 MHz phase probe, the radial resolution is around 0.5 mm and the lateral resolution is around 1.0 mm. In addition to the radial and lateral resolutions, there is an elevation resolution that accounts for the depth of an image in a certain plane. For a 5 MHz probe this resolution is around 2 mm. As frequencies are escalated, resolution increases but with a loss in tissue penetration [35]. US image quality has improved due to technological advances allowing for probes to be tuned to a range of frequencies facilitating good optical resolution at multiple depths. For example, a 5 MHz probe with a range from 4 to 8 MHz gives an optimal depth range from 2.5 to 6 cm and thus would be suitable for most neurosurgical applications. However for more superficial supratentorial lesions, posterior fossa lesions, and spinal medullary pathologies, a 10 MHz probe, yielding an optimal depth range from 0.5 to 4 cm, would yield the greatest image resolution.

Studies have shown that most parenchymal brain tumors are hyperechoic on iUS; also, there is a correlation between positive residual tumor found on iUS (when neurosurgeons had felt there was complete resection) and positive tumor histopathology of samples taken at these tumor margins [44,45]. Except in patients who had undergone prior irradiation, Hammoud et al and others demonstrated that clear tumor margins are easily discernable on iUS from surrounding normal brain parenchyma [41,46–49]. The difficulty in differentiating edema from solid tumor on iCT and MRI has been reported to be easily resolvable by iUS [50].

There have been reports stating difficulties with iUS in certain scenarios. Blood clots within a tumor cavity, especially at the end of a surgery, may yield hyperechoic bands and be interpreted as residual tumor. Resection procedures can lead to irregular surfaces in tumor beds contributing to an echotexture that resembles that of residual disease. It needs to be understood that echoic rims are seen at distal cyst walls and these rims are identical to those seen in a tumor cavity filled with saline. Disruptions in the blood-brain barrier lead to extravasations of contrast agents and can be a confusing factor in interpretation of iUS images. Finally, low specificity can be attributed to the acoustic phenomenon in which air is found between the probe and the dura [41,42,45,51].

Applications of iUS

Strowitzki et al [52] comment on the use of iUS during intracranial burr hole procedures. They note indications ranging from tapping of the ventricular system, tapping of intracranial cysts, biopsy of intracranial tumors, evacuation of intracranial abscesses, and evacuation of intracerebral hematomas. Their study essentially established the basis for minimally invasive iUS neuronavigation utilizing a single burr hole technique as being efficient, easy-to-use, and safe.

Auer described the use of iUS in stereotactic neuronavigation to guide the tip of a neurosurgical endoscope to a set depth within the brain parenchyma [53,54]. Other groups took the concept one step further in describing an integrated iUS probe with their neuroendoscope creating an instrument for US-guided endoscopic neurosurgery [55,56].

Much time has been spent in understanding the use of iUS for cranial neurosurgery; however, there is also a significant role for this imaging modality in the treatment of spinal cord pathologies and deformities. Some groups have commented on their use of iUS for visualization of an anterior compressive mass from a posterior approach. It has been used to asses the reduction of bony deformities and canal compromise in posterolateral decompression [57–59]. The utility of iUS in identifying intradural spinal tumor before and after resection is similarly well known.

Another important use of iUS is in visualizing the intracranial vasculature. Various neurosurgeons have reported that intraoperative microvascular Doppler sonography is a safe, effective, reliable, and cost-effective method for documenting the patency of vessels, arterial branches, and major perforators as well as the complete occlusion of cerebral aneurysms. This information can be of critical importance in the planning and performance of intradural tumor surgery [60–64].

iUS and Neuronavigation Systems

There have been many 2D iUS systems that have been integrated into a neuronavigational platform [43,65–72]. With these systems preoperative MRI images were obtained and iUS was utilized during the duration of the case. These iUS images were correlated to the preoperative MRI in a neuronavigational manner to aid the surgeon in correctly orienting and elucidating the data received from the iUS. These systems, such as *CAS Navigator* (SUN Microsystems, Mountain View, CA) [67], or the *SMN* (Carl Zeiss Inc, Oberkochen, Germany) [69], utilize two monitors and do not overlay the iUS images on the preoperative MRI.

A newer approach presents a novel iUS neuronavigational system, featuring a high-resolution US probe, directly incorporated into a commercially available neuronavigation platform (BrainLAB, Heimstetten, Germany) [73]. This device incorporates the IGSonic probe, which has a frequency of 5.0 to 7.5 MHz and a penetration depth of 120 mm. This "one-platform system" is the first of its kind that overlays iUS images on the preoperative navigational-based CT or MRI. The touch screen can be draped in a sterile fashion so that the surgeon can manipulate registration settings and recalibration of the probe if needed. Initial iUS images are obtained (acquisitions take between 30 seconds and 2 minutes) and are fused using a gray-scale for the preoperative imaging modality and a green-scale for the iUS images. Miller et al [74] compared this technology to conventional nonnavigated US and concluded that the integration of this technology into a navigation system facilitates a superior anatomical understanding than conventional US. A key limitation of this approach is that brain shift, even though easily visualized, cannot be compensated for with the current image fusion technology.

3-Dimensional iUS, Applications, and Future Developments

A new alternative to 2D iUS is the use of real-time updateable 3D reconstructed images to aid in navigation as seen in Figure 49.2. These volumes can be acquired in seconds with the benefit of the probe not being in the field of operation [35]. The creation of the 3D US volumes can be done either by video grabbing of 2D US images [75,76] or by reconstructing the volume from 100 to 200 2D images made by moving the US probe over the area of interest [77]. The display of 3D volumes is the same as for any conventional neuronavigation system and can also be shown as an anaglyphic stereoscopic projection [41,78].

Technological advances indicate a great potential for iUS. Development of neurosurgically dedicated probes with thinner image planes and greater depth capability as well as contrast agents such as thin-shelled micro bubbles will improve image quality [35]. One limitation and need for refinement of 3D iUS is that the integration of real time 3D imaging into a neuronavigational system has not yet been made commercially available.

There is great promise for the use of iUS in everyday neurosurgical intervention due to the flexibility, cost, ease and safety of use, and wide scope of application. Particularly with anticipated future developments, this

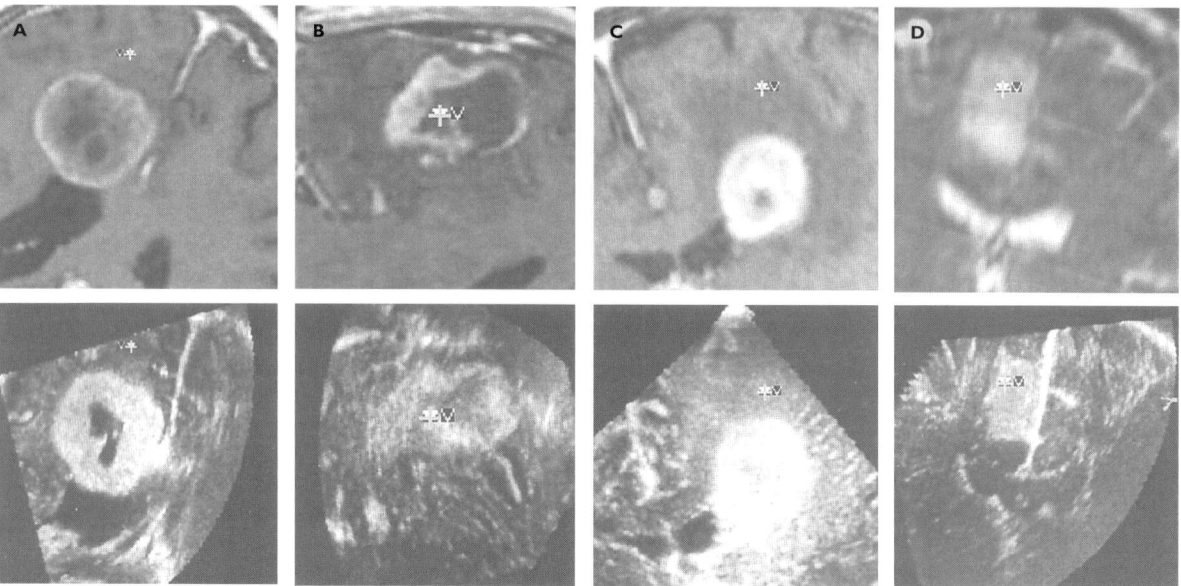

Figure 49.2 3D iUS with neuronavigational capacity. Slices from all 3D volume scans shown on the screen simultaneously during resection of a glioblastoma, preoperative MRI **(A)**, initial 3D iUS volume at the start of the case, 3D iUS volume at the middle of the case **(C)**, 3D iUS volume toward the end of the resection. Arrows indicate residual tumor tissue. The single-slice display feature allows for 3D volumes to be correlated to the preoperative MRI slice orientation without needing to take into consideration patient orientation on the table. Courtesy of Lippincott, Williams, and Wilkins [44].

technology can add tremendously to the neurosurgeons' imaging armamentarium.

Intraoperative CT

Computed axial tomography is a widely used imaging modality in the initial, diagnostic, and follow-up management and treatment of neurological patients with both cranial and spinal pathologies. In 1979, the first intraoperative use of CT was described in a single case in which the entire operation for a recurrent glioma was performed on a CT scanner table. At the end of the case, this method enabled the neurosurgeons to conclude that there was no residual tumor detected on CT scan [79]. Its use within an intraoperative environment has been described by many groups since then [79–86]. These groups utilized this modality when asking certain specific questions such as estimation of residual tumor during radical resection. The ability of iCT to delineate boney structures also is very useful for imaging the spinal column for the localization of surgical levels and in the placement of instrumentation [5].

Intraoperative CT in Cranial Neurosurgery

There have been many CT-based systems that have been utilized for the intraoperative imaging of anatomy. Kabuto et al [84] designed a motorized rail-track system for mobilization of the CT gantry, and the longitudinal motion of the OR table can be controlled by a foot pedal enabling this group to image without altering the surgical workspace. Some groups utilized a mobile CT scanner adapted to neurosurgical requirements and made use of this just as any other intraoperative tool, enabling the surgeon to move the iCT gantry rather than the OR table during data acquisition (Figure 49.3) [80,82,83]. Other groups utilized the CT scanner table as an OR table and in performing their neurosurgical procedures [86,87]. Some groups even had exclusively developed OR CT scanners [81,85,88].

No matter the system that was used, all reports of iCT have advocated its use in the everyday practice of neurosurgery. One group utilized a mobile iCT system and found that 10 of 36 cases, or 28%, showed residual tumor on iCT that would have otherwise have been overlooked [82]. The Broggi group went on to state that in 23 of 27 cases iCT verified residual tumor [89]. This group also utilized iCT in the verification of the correct stereotactic positioning of deep brain electrodes in relation to the planned target. They went on to state that 21 of 23 such cases were verified as correct by iCT. Gumprecht and Lementa also found iCT as highly helpful in detecting residual tumor. They found that in 27 of 43 patients with glioma there was residual tumor found on iCT and that in 13 of these cases they were able to resume surgery until complete resection was achieved. However, they found that in comparing iCT to postoperative MRI there was residual tumor demonstrated in six cases by MRI; of these six cases, three cases, or 6.8%, could have gone on to a more complete tumor removal [83].

With an understanding of the benefits iCT offers the neurosurgeon in visualizing anatomic structures, residual tumor, displacement of catheters, clot formation during the course of the neurosurgical procedure, and so on, it is important to next weigh the alteration on work flow

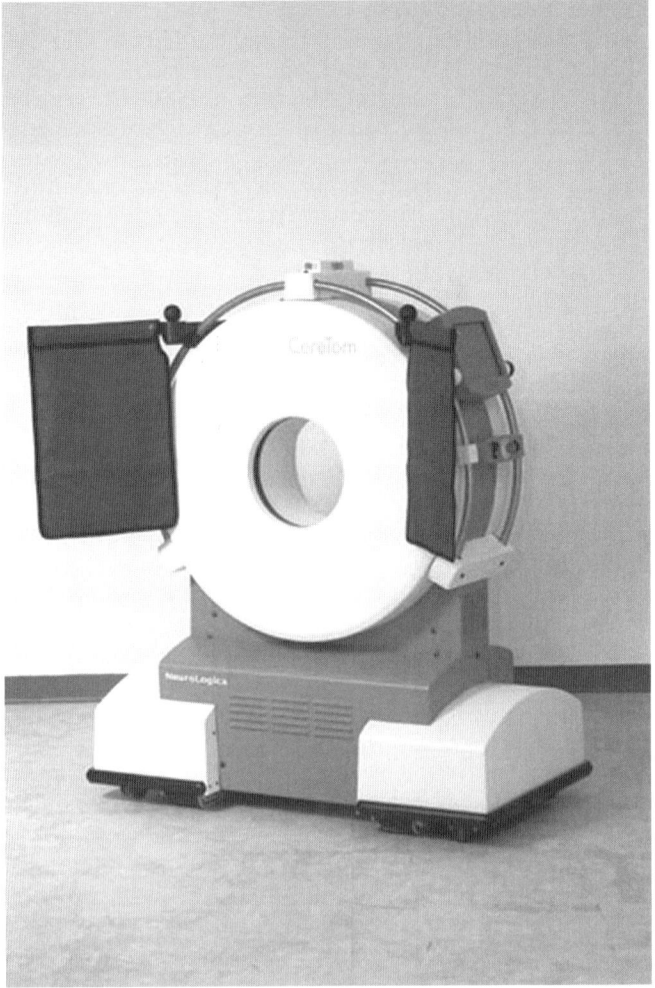

Figure 49.3 The CereTom intraoperative/intensive care unit CT scanner. Courtesy of NeuroLogica.

and ergonomics of the procedures being performed while using iCT. Implementing iCT into everyday neurosurgical routine can be a daunting task because of the cost of an integrated iCT neuronavigational system, ergonomic limitations due to size, the ability to complete all neurosurgical tasks and interventions in one room, and how the use of this tool affects other individuals involved, including anesthesiologists, other OR staff, and neuroradiologists. Matula et al [90] presented an interesting view on the topic. They divided workflow into four main stages: the preparation process, the treatment process, the quality process, and the release process. On comparing a group treated with iCT and neuronavigation with another group with very similar pathology treated without neuronavigation, they found that for the arm of patients treated with iCT and neuronavigation the total elapsed time from the preparation process to the release process was actually 20% shorter or, in other words, a single OR saves an average of 55 hours per 6 months. The total operating time is longer, on the average of about 30 minutes, but the total time of treatment is the factor that is decreased [90].

ICT offers the neurosurgeon many advantages, including resection control of brain tumors, compensation for brain shift, and the ability to rule out intraoperative complications; it can also be used in applications including biopsies, catheter placements, cyst aspirations, tumor removal, and anatomic imaging of the spine. Most importantly, this imaging tool offers the neurosurgeon a safe imaging modality that increases procedural precision and accuracy [82]. These benefits must be weighed against the ergonomics of operating in the iCT environment, in particular the use of ionizing radiation. The surgeons and other OR staff need to wear lead shielding during imaging, or to otherwise protect themselves from radiation. In addition, the patient is exposed to possibly multiple scan sessions and the concomitant irradiation [91].

Intraoperative MRI

It has been more than a decade since iMRI was introduced [1]. As mentioned previously intraoperative imaging presents great benefits for the surgeon in many venues of neurosurgical interventions. The neurosurgeon is able to monitor changes that occur superficially, subcortically, or deep in the vicinity of a lesion and thus alter technique or approach [14,92]. iMRI gives the neurosurgeon the ability to make objective decisions as to the progress of surgery and the physical global status of the brain in terms of hydocephalus, hemorrhage, edema, and so on in a very detailed and precise manner [16]. However, this modality, depending on the imager type and magnetic field strength, alters OR environment and dynamics considerably. Special MRI-compatible anesthesia equipment needs to be implemented to reduce noise. Depending on the magnet strength, some surgical equipment may need to be MRI compatible. Draping of the patient and aseptic technique need to be altered [93–95]. Here we will discuss the use, effect, and benefit of iMRI, the various types of imagers that are currently available, and the future prospects for this technology.

Low-Field iMRI Approaches

It is well established that there is a direct relationship between the strength of the magnet within the MRI and image resolution of anatomic structures. iMRI systems possessing a magnetic field less than 0.5 Tesla (T) are considered low-field imagers. There have been many imagers that have fallen into this category, starting from the 0.2 T University of Heidelberg and Erlangen systems (Magnetom Open by Siemens) whereby a twin OR concept was employed with one room for imaging and another room as the conventional OR. The University of California concept employed the same 0.2 T magnet into a conventional one-room OR suite [96–98].

In 2001, a group at the University of Cincinnati Medical Center presented the concept of a 0.3 T two-room operating suite whereby the room that housed the 0.3 T magnet (AIRIS II by Hitachi) could be used for both intraoperative imaging and routine diagnostic imaging [99]. In that same month, the Hadani group presented a novel concept of a 0.12 T freely movable iMRI system (PoleStar N-10) with the ability to be positioned under the OR table [100]. This adoption allowed the free use of standard neurosurgical instruments and significantly increased the ergonomic ease of the operating field. Other groups subsequently added this technology to their centers [101,102]. More recently, in 2006, one of these groups reported the introduction of the expanded 0.15 T PoleStar N-20 (Medtronic Navigation, Louisville, CO) iMR imager with a wider gap between poles and a more ergonomic gantry (Figures 49.4, 49.5, and 49.6) [103].

Another group from the Oulu University Hospital in Finland presented their use of a horizontal 0.23 T iMR imager stating that the main advantage of their system is the ability to operate next to the scanner without having to move the patient into the magnetic fringe fields [104].

Mid-Field iMRI Approaches

This group of iMR imagers refers primarily to the 0.5 T system, the first iMRI to be developed. These 0.5 T imagers, termed the "double doughnut" (Signa SP from GE, Milwaukee, WI), were the first iMR imagers introduced into the market at the Brigham and Women's Hospital in Boston (Figure 49.1) [16]. This system had the important advantage of image, stereotactic, and surgical space being one and the same. However, the 56 cm gap between the two vertical poles, difficulties in positioning, the need to place the magnet out of the main OR area, and the requirement that all instruments had to be MRI compatible made acceptance of this device limited. The image quality elicited from this imager was adequate as seen in Figure 49.7. It is no longer marketed commercially by the vendor.

High-Field iMRI Approaches

There have been essentially three 1.5 T iMR imaging concepts introduced. The first was the University of Calgary system (now marketed by IMRIS, Winnipeg, Manitoba) in which the unit is moved on a ceiling-mounted track into the surgical suite when intraoperative imaging is needed [105]. The second iMR imager, the Magnetom Sonata by Siemens, was pioneered at the University of Erlangen–Nurnberg. This system incorporates a general-purpose 1.5 T magnet into an OR setting. The OR table has rotational capabilities enabling both operating position and imaging positions [106]. The last 1.5 T system was described by Tummala et al [107] whereby a general-purpose MR imager is present in the OR suite. The patient is transported to a designated distance away from the imager for tumor resection; when imaging is needed he/she is then transported on a floating tabletop to the imager (Figure 49.8).

One concept that has integrated iMRI at 1.5 T, iCT, and x-ray is the MRI/x-ray/OR suite (MRXO) from the Tokai University School of Medicine in Japan (Figure 49.9). This suite consists of three stations located in three separate but connected rooms. The OR-angiography suite is located in the middle, and on either side are the iMRI and iCT bays. During the interventional procedure if intraoperative imaging is necessary the patient is transported from the center OR room to the adjacent imaging rooms on a specifically designed movable tabletop. The 1.5 T iMRI can be used for various indications (Figure 49.10) [108].

Several centers have begun the implementation of iMRI using 3 T magnets (T. Kaibara, C. Raftopoulos, N. Pamir, personal communication). These systems require patients to be transported from the OR itself to an adjacent imaging suite, which is used for diagnostic imaging at other times.

Effect on Resection

There is a literature advocating for the use of iMRI in improving the surgical outcome in patients with intracranial neoplasms, especially glioma and pituitary adenomas [21,107,109–118]. iMRI has been coupled with endoscopy in transphenoidal surgery to safely visualize the optic chiasm and internal carotid artery surrounding the pituitary during extirpation of adenomas [119–121]. This use of iMRI has further aided the neurosurgeon for the removal of epileptogenic foci [122–125]. In cervical spine surgery, iMRI can yield quality images leading to safer and more accurate procedures [126]. iMRI has aided the neurosurgeon in evacuation of hypertensive hematomas in the basal ganglia and thalamus [127,128] as well as puncture and aspiration of cystic lesions [129–131].

The most important aspect in determining the effect of iMRI on the extent of resection is to correlate its use with clinical outcomes. As stated previously, evidence exists that for patients with gliomas of any grade, a smaller volume of postoperative residual tumor carries a significant survival advantage. In this light, Nimsky et al [114] found that in 20% of cases surgeons felt they achieved gross total resection when in fact iMRI evidenced the contrary. Another study found that the mean survival time for patients with glioblastoma was 15.7 months after total resection and no residual tumor versus 8.6 months for those with residual [29]. The Claus group did a similar

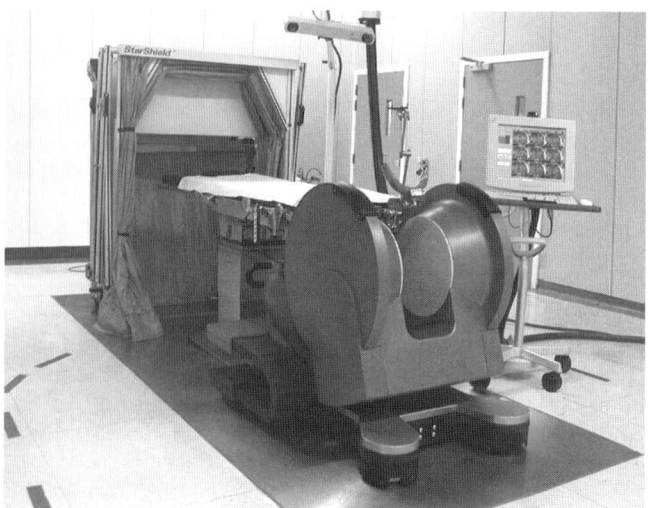

Figure 49.4 Polestar N-20 0.15 T iMRI by Medtronic. Electromagnetic shielding is seen in the background. This feature encloses the iMRI unit and patient, obviating the need to shut off unfiltered electrical sources during image acquisition.

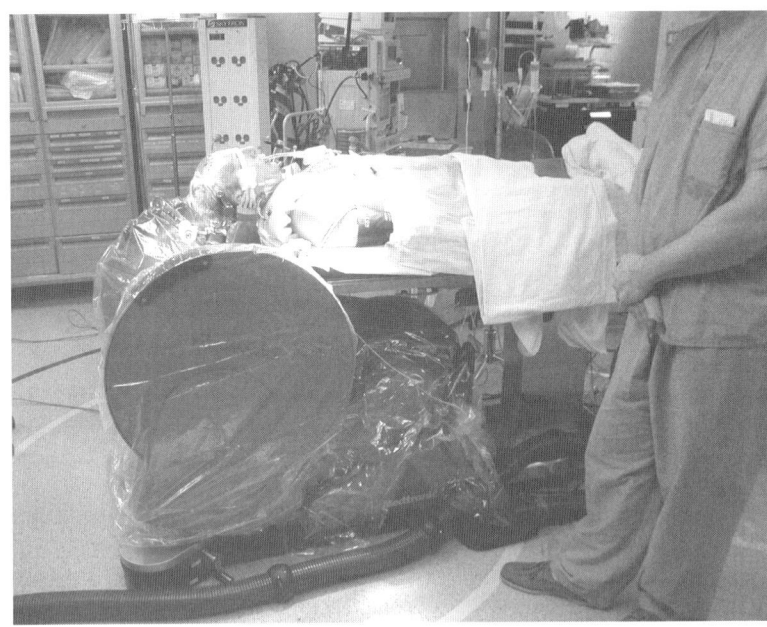

Figure 49.5 Patient positioning utilizing the Polestar N-20 0.15 T iMRI by Medtronic. The mobile compact gantry is easily placed under the OR table when not in use, and when imaging is needed the poles are elevated into position.

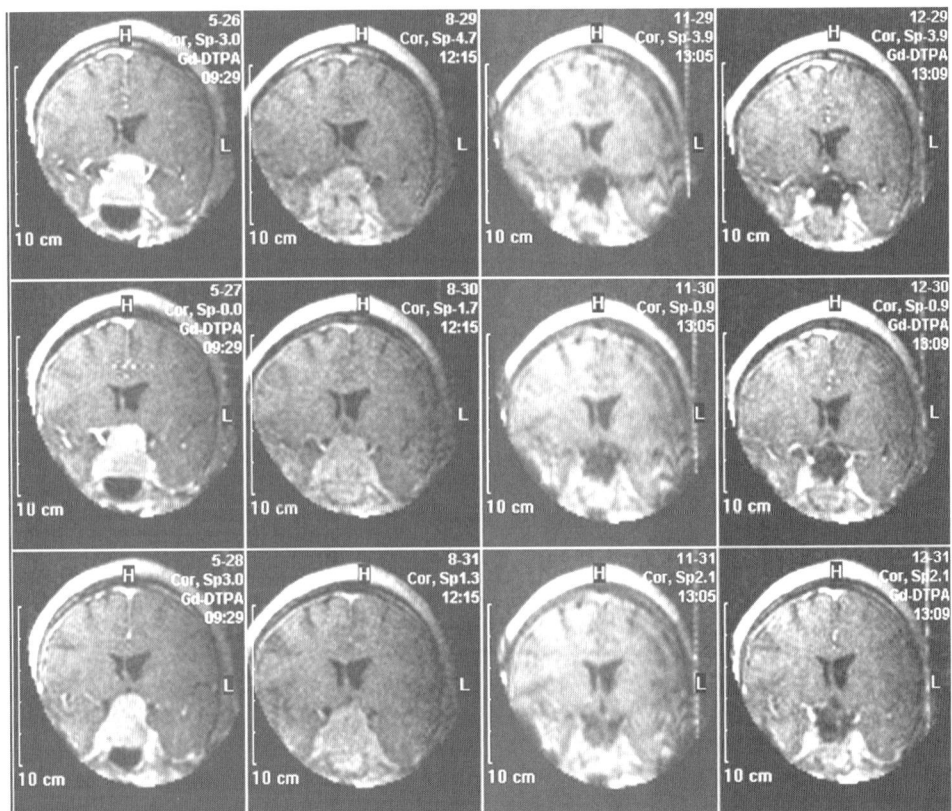

Figure 49.6 Polestar N-20 0.15 T by Medtronic iMRI scans of a patient pituitary adenoma. Comparative scans show progression through operation.

study on patients with low-grade glioma. They found that during a median follow-up of 3 years the risk of recurrence was found to be 1.4 times higher and the risk of death was 4.9 fold higher in the subtotal resection arm of patients, as compared with patients who underwent complete resection. They go on to state that the 1-year, 2-year, and 5-year age-adjusted and histologic-adjusted death rates are significantly lower than national databases in patients who underwent iMRI-guided resection of their glioma, suggesting a possible association between the use of iMRI in directing surgical resection and an increase in patient survival [132].

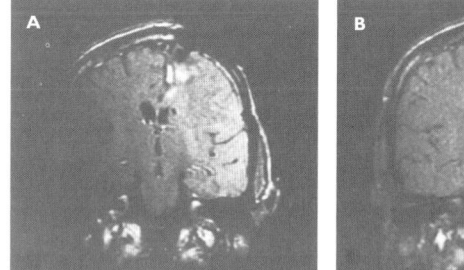
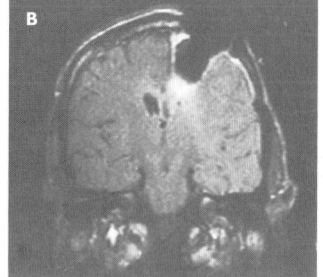
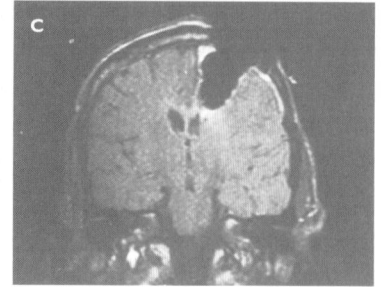

Figure 49.7 Low-grade astrocytoma resection utilizing the Signa 0.5 T "double doughnut." Preoperative **(A)**, intraoperative **(B)**, and postoperative **(C)** images. Courtesy of Elsevier Science [145].

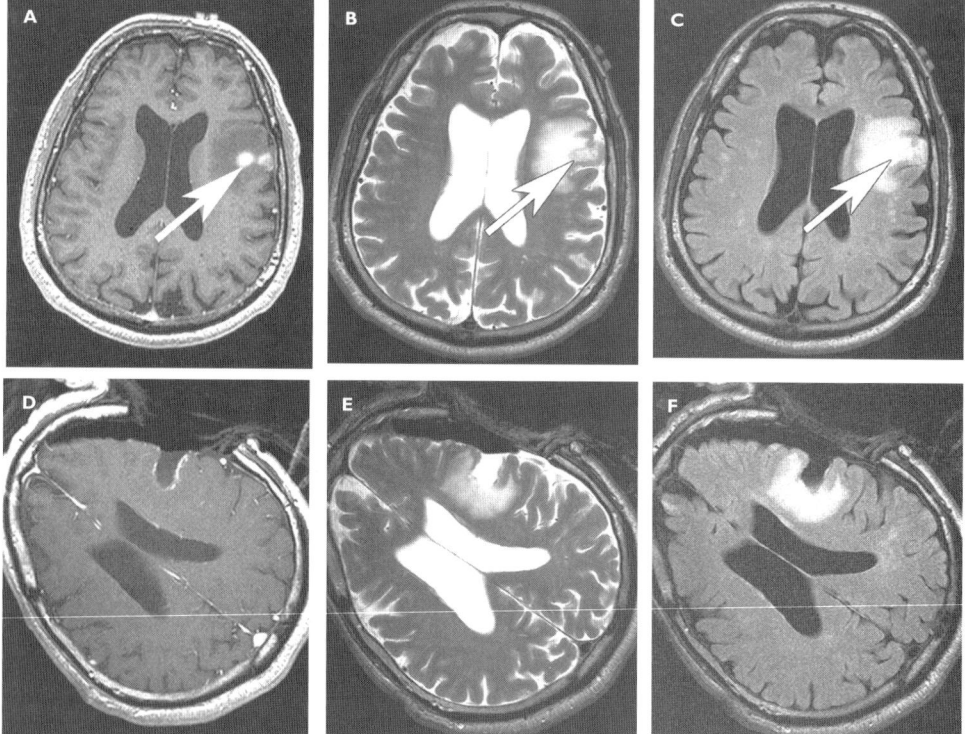

Figure 49.8 1.5 T iMRI images of a patient with a left-sided glioblastoma. Preoperative T1 **(A)**, T2 **(B)**, and fluid-attenuated inversion-recovery (FLAIR) **(C)** sequences show contrast-enhanced areas as indicated by the arrows. **D to F** demonstrate iMRI images with the same respective pulse sequences obtained in A to C confirming complete removal of all contrast-enhancing tumor. Courtesy of RSNA [146].

Effect on Length of Surgery

Any intraoperative imaging modality chosen will affect the OR work flow and thus operative time. Use of the mobile PoleStar iMRI added an average of about 1.6 extra hours per surgery [109]. On utilizing the PoleStar N-20, the same group noted that the added time was on average 1.1 hours with an average of 2.3 imaging sessions per surgery [103]. Another group noted that operative time using a high-field iMRI system was about 6 hours 47 minutes whereas conventional procedures for the same type of pathology averaged about 4 hours 45 minutes [93]. This group found that in the patients who underwent surgery with the high-field iMR imager, of the extra 122 minutes, 100 minutes or 83% of the added time was devoted strictly to imaging. They also go on to state that there is no significant difference in time spent in the postoperative recovery unit between the study arms.

Effect on Surgical Instruments

Interference that degrades iMRI quality can result from the proximity of ferromagnetic instrumentation to the surgical and imaging field, and by the presence of unfiltered electrical sources during scanning. Interference leads to poor image quality and can render the iMRI image data useless. Anesthesia machines (respirator/patient monitor) must be MRI compatible to limit interference, but also so they can continue to operate during imaging, off of alternating current if need be. Also, as life-support equipment, there should be no chance of a malfunction induced by the use of iMRI at any point during the procedure. Another major source of interference comes from surgical devices such as electrocautery, ultrasonic aspirators, drills, microscopes, and various light sources. These devices need to be turned off and their power sources unplugged during imaging, unless a separate method for electrical isolation

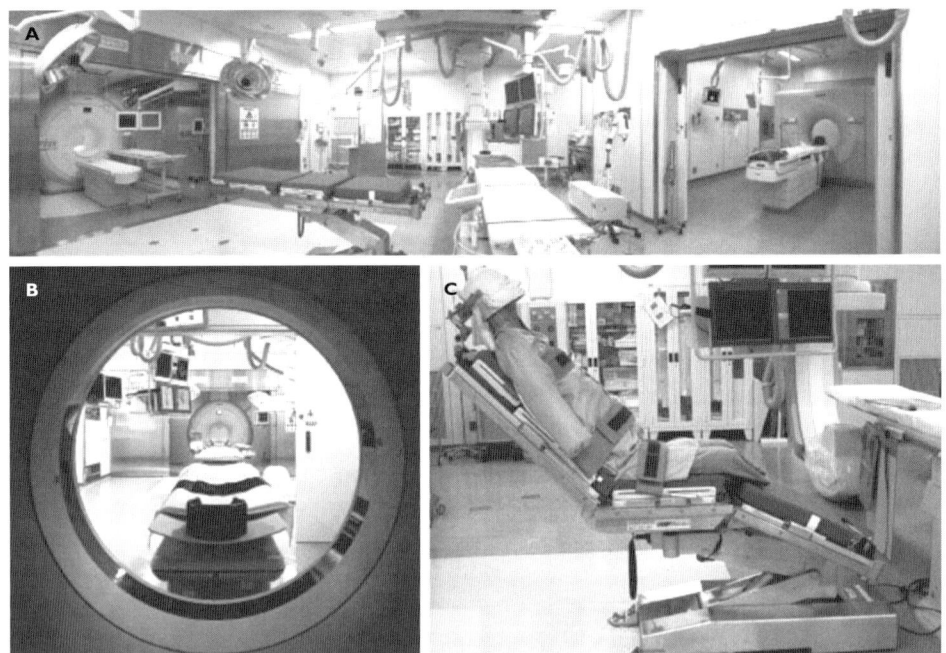

Figure 49.9 (A) Panoramic view of the entire MRXO suite. The center room is the fully compatible OR-angiography bay. iMRI is located on the left and iCT is located on the right. Patients are transported on a movable tabletop between rooms for intraoperative imaging. (B) An in-line view from the CT scanner through the OR-angiography room and into the MRI room. (C) MRI-compatible tabletop is mounted on a mobile operating table. This table facilitates a multitude of patient positions. Courtesy of New Medicine in Japan [108].

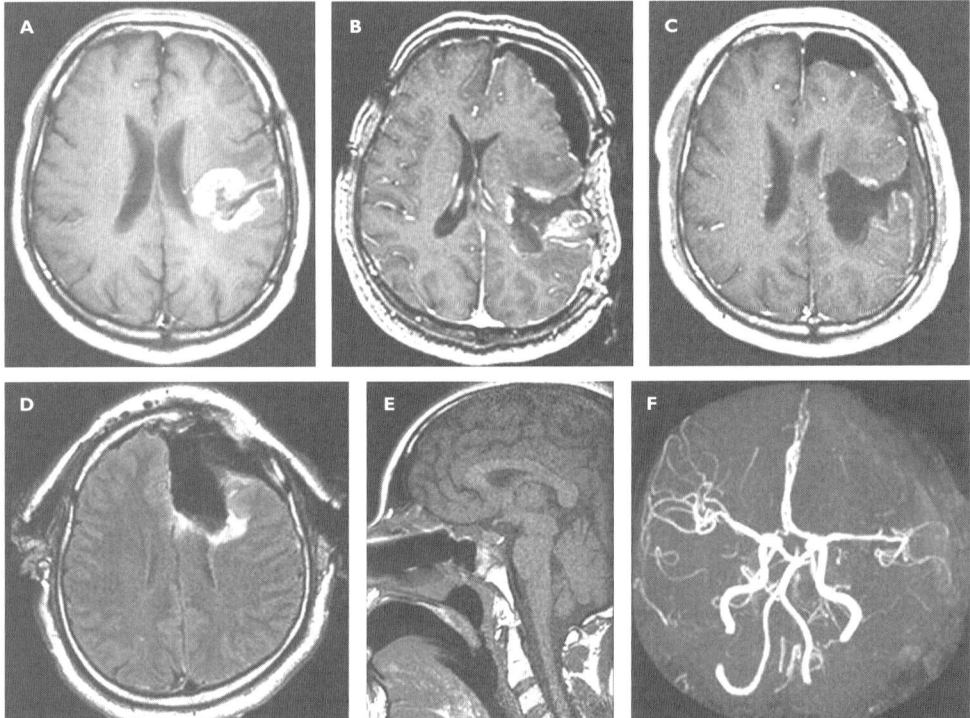

Figure 49.10 MRXO (A) Preoperative contrast-enhanced T1-weighted MRI of a recurrent World Health Organization (WHO) Grade III astrocytoma. (B) iMRI showing residual tumor. (C) Postoperative MRI showing nearly complete resection. (D) FLAIR iMRI of an astrocytoma (WHO III) evidencing remaining tumor in the resection cavity. (E) T1-weighted iMRI showing an MRI-compatible instrument nearing a pituitary adenoma. (F) Magnetic resonance imaging (MRI) of intracranial vascular anatomy. Courtesy of AANS [108].

of the magnet has been established [133]. As noted earlier, many current high-field iMRI systems require that the patient move into another room entirely.

Patient safety is a critical consideration in the implementation of iMRI. Iron-based alloys, when brought into the magnetic field, quickly become projectiles. The higher the strength of the magnetic field, the more attention must be paid to avoid the introduction of potentially dangerous ferrous objects near the magnet. With some low-field strength systems, such as the PoleStar N-20, the magnetic attraction is directed away from the surgical field [134].

Contrast Agents

Although a benefit of iMRI is that the surgeon has the capability to use paramagnetic contrast agents during the operative procedure to detect residual tumor enhancement, these images must be interpreted with great care.

Table 49.1 Comparison of Intraoperative Imaging Modalities

	Image Quality	Ease of Use	Effect on Instruments	Ergonomics	Cost
iUS	- Excellent solid vs. cystic differentiation	- No problem with fringe magnetic fields or ionizing radiation	- Conventional instruments can be used	- Units can easily be moved around OR	$250,000–$400,000
	- Truly real-time	- Easily draped and can quickly be moved in and out of operating field	- Can be coupled and attached to widely used surgical tools, that is, CUSA	- Probes are small enough to be placed within the sterile field	
	- Ability to assess flow information/ patency in blood vessels				
	- 3D capabilities				
	- Limited penetration beyond 5 cm and no bone penetration				
	- Orientation and spatial resolution are limited and difficult to interpret				
	- Resection and tumor margins can be indistinguishable from normal surrounding brain				
iCT	- Excellent bone-tissue contrast	- Operated by existing OR staff or technician	- Conventional instruments can be used	- Easily portable and can be stored in a closet	$500,000–$1,000,000
	- Sensitive and specific for hemorrhage, edema and postoperative hematoma	- Lead garments for shielding need to be worn by staff			
	- Limited soft tissue contrast	- Can be used in both ICU and OR settings			
Low-field iMRI	- Adequate to good as compared to high-field systems	- Operated by existing OR staff or technician	- Most conventional surgical instruments can be used	- Can be installed into an existing OR suite and less obtrusive than high field systems	$1,000,000
Low field (0.15 T)	- Low SNR	- Weighs 750 lbs so it is recommended that 2+ individuals from OR staff aid in moving	- Electronically powered surgical equipment needs to be powered off and unplugged during imaging	- Can be stored under OR table when not in use	
	- Limited field of view (0.15 T)	- Adds on average 1.1 hrs to OR time	- Special iMRI compatible anesthesia machines need to be utilized		
	- Limited functional imaging capabilities	- Patient requires ear protection			
High-field iMRI	- Superior image quality	- Needs special radiology technician to run	- All surgical tools and equipment need to be iMRI compatible unless patient is being transported a safe distance away from iMR imager	- Needs to be built into OR suite or patient needs to be transported out of OR to area where iMR imager is located	$4,000,000–$6,000,000
High field (1.5 T to 3 T)	- Capable of functional imaging		- Special iMRI-compatible anesthesia machines need to be utilized		

CUSF, cavitron ultrasonic surgical aspirator.

As the blood-brain barrier is further disrupted during surgery, these contrast agents have the propensity to leak into the resection cavity, giving the illusion of residual tumor. This "pseudo-enhancement" is more pronounced as time elapses from injection to iMR imaging. This phenomenon can be alleviated, to a certain extent, by imaging soon after injection and limiting the number of injections during the course of an operation [29,97]. The surgeon must recognize this feature so as to avoid unnecessary and potentially harmful resection of functionally important brain.

iMRI-Based Neuronavigation

The technique of surgical navigation, or "frameless stereotaxy" based on a patient's preoperative MRI, is ubiquitous in neurosurgical centers around the world. As noted, application of this method is limited due to the elements of brain shift and degree of resection during the surgical procedure (this of course holds true for CT-based navigation as well). The advantage of iMRI-based neuronavigation is that the images can be continually updated during the surgical procedure and new navigational data sets can be based off the most recent scans (Figure 49.6). In centers that use technology in which the patient can be operated on within the imaging space (such as the PoleStar system), optical navigation over repetitive imaging is the method of choice [100,101,135–140]. In some centers, preoperatively acquired magnetoencephalography and functional MRI data have been incorporated into neuronavigation [135].

Future Developments

As more sophisticated and ergonomically favorable imagers with higher field strength are developed, the capabilities to do functional, perfusion, diffusion, and MRI spectroscopy will become standard practice. Diffusion-tensor imaging will then enable the neurosurgeon to generate images of important white matter tracts in near-real time, as has been reported by Nimsky et al [141–144] (Figure 49.11). The goal will be for the routine acquisition of multiple datasets that will provide a comprehensive anatomical, functional, and biological map of the brain during intracranial surgery [145,146] (Table 49.1).

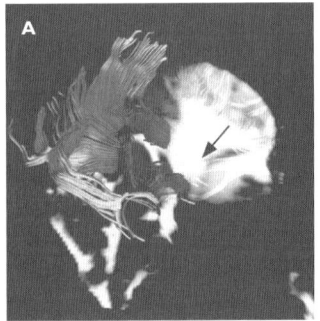 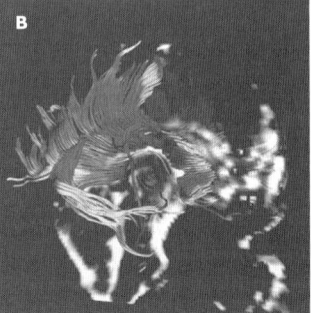

Figure 49.11 Tractography of a patient with a right frontal WHO Grade III oligoastrocytoma. **(A)** preoperative tractography image showing marked depression and discontinuity (black arrow) of anterior corpus callosal fibers. **(B)** Intraoperative tractography image after tumor removal showing shifting of the anterior corpus callosal fibers to a normal anatomic position with a loss of discontinuity. Courtesy of Lippincott, Williams, and Wilkins [141].

CONCLUSION

Progress in neurosurgery has been marked by a decreasing amount of guesswork. Most of this improvement has been fueled by advances in imaging, beginning with x-rays and ventriculography, followed by angiography and moving into the digital imaging era of CT and MRI. The logic of intraoperative imaging is obvious. Modern neurosurgical practice mandates imaging before and after surgery. Who, then, would not want to have that information readily at hand during the surgery itself? Only issues of cost and ergonomics, and questions regarding the effect on outcomes, have limited the growth of intraoperative imaging technology.

We believe that the advantages of iUS, iCT, and iMRI are obvious and that as these are demonstrated in rigorous studies, and as the technology becomes increasingly versatile and accessible, intraoperative imaging will be a ubiquitous feature of the neurosurgical OR.

REFERENCES

1. Jolesz FA, Blumenfeld SM. Interventional use of magnetic resonance imaging. *Magn Reson Q.* 1994;10(2):85–96.
2. Jolesz FA, Kikinis R. Intraoperative imaging revolutionizes therapy. *Diagn Imaging (San Franc).* 1995;17(9):62–68.
3. Ebmeier K, Giest K, Kalff R. Intraoperative computerized tomography for improved accuracy of spinal navigation in pedicle screw placement of the thoracic spine. *Acta Neurochir Suppl.* 2003;85:105–113.
4. Foley KT, Smith MM. Image-guided spine surgery. *Neurosurg Clin N Am.* 1996;7(2):171–186.
5. Foley KT, Simon DA, Rampersaud YR. Virtual fluoroscopy: computer-assisted fluoroscopic navigation. *Spine.* 2001;26(4):347–351.
6. Kahn T, Schmidt F, Mödder U. [MR imaging-guided interventions]. *Radiologe.* 1999;39(9):741–749.
7. Bradley WG. Achieving gross total resection of brain tumors: intraoperative MR imaging can make a big difference. *AJNR Am J Neuroradiol.* 2002;23(3):348–349.
8. Robinson D, On E, Hadas N, Halperin N, Hofman S, Boldur I. Microbiologic flora contaminating open fractures: its significance in the choice of primary antibiotic agents and the likelihood of deep wound infection. *J Orthop Trauma.* 1989;3(4):283–286.
9. Dandy WE. Rontgenography of the brain after the injection of air into the spinal canal. *Ann Surg.* 1919;70(4):397–403.
10. Moniz E. L'encephalographie arterielle, son importance dans la localisation des tumeurs cerebrales [in French]. *Review Neural.* 1927;2:72–90.
11. Ganslandt O, Behari S, Gralla J, Fahlbusch R, Nimsky C. Neuronavigation: concept, techniques and applications. *Neurol India.* 2002;50(3):244–255.
12. Lee JY, Lunsford LD, Subach BR, Jho HD, Bissonette DJ, Kondziolka D. Brain surgery with image guidance: current recommendations based on a 20-year assessment. *Stereotact Funct Neurosurg.* 2000;75(1):35–48.
13. Wirtz CR, Tronnier VM, Bonsanto MM, Hassfeld S, Knauth M, Kunze S. Neuronavigation. Methods and prospects. *Nervenarzt.* 1998;69(12):1029–1036.
14. Ganslandt O, Steinmeier R, Kober H, et al. Magnetic source imaging combined with image-guided frameless stereotaxy: a new method in surgery around the motor strip. *Neurosurgery.* 1997;41(3):621–627; discussion 627.
15. Wirtz CR, Tronnier VM, Bonsanto MM, et al. Image-guided neurosurgery with intraoperative MRI: update of frameless stereotaxy and radicality control. *Stereotact Funct Neurosurg.* 1997;68:39–43.
16. Black PM, Moriarty T, Alexander E, et al. Development and implementation of intraoperative magnetic resonance imaging and its neurosurgical applications. *Neurosurgery.* 1997;41(4):831–842; discussion 842.
17. Lunsford LD. A dedicated CT system for the stereotactic operating room. *Appl Neurophysiol.* 1982;45(4–5):374–378.

18. Koivukangas J, Kelly PJ. Application of ultrasound imaging to stereotactic brain tumor surgery. *Ann Clin Res*. 1986;47(suppl 18):25–32.
19. Nimsky C, Ganslandt O, Fahlbusch R. 1.5 T: intraoperative imaging beyond standard anatomic imaging. *Neurosurg Clin N Am*. 2005;16(1):185–200, vii.
20. Sutherland GR, Kaibara T. Neurosurgical suite of the future. III. *Neuroimaging Clin N Am*. 2001;11(4):593–609.
21. Oh DS, Black PM. A low-field intraoperative MRI system for glioma surgery: is it worthwhile? *Neurosurg Clin N Am*. 2005;16(1):135–141.
22. Black PM. The present and future of cerebral tumor surgery in children. *Childs Nerv Syst*. 2000;16(10–11):821–828.
23. Hall WA, Martin AJ, Liu H, et al. High-field strength interventional magnetic resonance imaging for pediatric neurosurgery. *Pediatr Neurosurg*. 1998;29(5):253–259.
24. Lam CH, Hall WA, Truwit CL, Liu H. Intra-operative MRI-guided approaches to the pediatric posterior fossa tumors. *Pediatr Neurosurg*. 2001;34(6):295–300.
25. Vitaz TW, Hushek S, Shields CB, Moriarty T. Intraoperative MRI for pediatric tumor management. *Acta Neurochir Suppl*. 2003;85:73–78.
26. Berger MS, Rostomily RC. Low grade gliomas: functional mapping resection strategies, extent of resection, and outcome. *J Neurooncol*. 1997;34(1):85–101.
27. Johannesen TB, Langmark F, Lote K. Progress in long-term survival in adult patients with supratentorial low-grade gliomas: a population-based study of 993 patients in whom tumors were diagnosed between 1970 and 1993. *J Neurosurg*. 2003;99(5):854–862.
28. Sakata K, Hareyama M, Komae T, et al. Supratentorial astrocytomas and oligodendrogliomas treated in the MRI era. *Jpn J Clin Oncol*. 2001;31(6):240–245.
29. Wirtz CR, Knauth M, Staubert A, et al. Clinical evaluation and follow-up results for intraoperative magnetic resonance imaging in neurosurgery. *Neurosurgery*. 2000;46(5):1112–20; discussion 1120.
30. Rajaraman V, Schulder M. Postoperative MRI appearance after transsphenoidal pituitary tumor resection. *Surg Neurol*. 1999;52(6):592–598; discussion 598.
31. Hata N, Nabavi A, Wells WM, et al. Three-dimensional optical flow method for measurement of volumetric brain deformation from intraoperative MR images. *J Comput Assist Tomogr*. 2000;24(4):531–538.
32. Nabavi A, Black PM, Gering DT, et al. Serial intraoperative magnetic resonance imaging of brain shift. *Neurosurgery*. 2001;48(4):787–797; discussion 797.
33. Nimsky C, Ganslandt O, Hastreiter P, Fahlbusch R. Intraoperative compensation for brain shift. *Surg Neurol*. 2001;56(6):357–364; discussion 364.
34. Nimsky C, Ganslandt O, Cerny S, Hastreiter P, Greiner G, Fahlbusch R. Quantification of, visualization of, and compensation for brain shift using intraoperative magnetic resonance imaging. *Neurosurgery*. 2000;47(5):1070–1079; discussion 1079.
35. Unsgaard G, Rygh OM, Selbekk T, et al. Intra-operative 3D ultrasound in neurosurgery. *Acta Neurochir (Wien)*. 2006;148(3):235–253; discussion 253.
36. Auer LM, van Velthoven V. Intraoperative ultrasound (US) imaging. Comparison of pathomorphological findings in US and CT. *Acta Neurochir (Wien)*. 1990;104(3–4):84–95.
37. Chandler WF, Knake JE, McGillicuddy JE, Lillehei KO, Silver TM. Intraoperative use of real-time ultrasonography in neurosurgery. *J Neurosurg*. 1982;57(2):157–163.
38. Le Roux PD, Berger MS, Wang K, Mack LA, Ojemann GA. Low grade gliomas: comparison of intraoperative ultrasound characteristics with preoperative imaging studies. *J Neurooncol*. 1992;13(2):189–198.
39. Regelsberger J, Lohmann F, Helmke K, Westphal M. Ultrasound-guided surgery of deep seated brain lesions. *Eur J Ultrasound*. 2000;12(2):115–121.
40. Rubin JM, Dohrmann GJ. Intraoperative neurosurgical ultrasound in the localization and characterization of intracranial masses. *Radiology*. 1983;148(2):519–524.
41. Unsgaard G, Ommedal S, Rygh OM, Lindseth F. Operation of arteriovenous malformations assisted by stereoscopic navigation-controlled display of preoperative magnetic resonance angiography and intraoperative ultrasound angiography. *Neurosurgery*. 2005;56(suppl 2):281–290; discussion 281.
42. van Velthoven V, Auer LM. Practical application of intraoperative ultrasound imaging. *Acta Neurochir (Wien)*. 1990;105(1–2):5–13.
43. Unsgaard G, Gronningsaeter A, Ommedal S, Nagelhus Hernes TA. Brain operations guided by real-time two-dimensional ultrasound: new possibilities as a result of improved image quality. *Neurosurgery*. 2002;51(2):402–411; discussion 411.
44. Unsgaard G, Ommedal S, Muller T, Gronningsaeter A, Nagelhus Hernes TA. Neuronavigation by intraoperative three-dimensional ultrasound: initial experience during brain tumor resection. *Neurosurgery*. 2002;50(4):804–812; discussion 812.
45. Chacko AG, Kumar NK, Chacko G, Athyal R, Rajshekhar V. Intraoperative ultrasound in determining the extent of resection of parenchymal brain tumours–a comparative study with computed tomography and histopathology. *Acta Neurochir (Wien)*. 2003;145(9):743–748; discussion 748.
46. Hammoud MA, Ligon BL, elSouki R, Shi WM, Schomer DF, Sawaya R. Use of intraoperative ultrasound for localizing tumors and determining the extent of resection: a comparative study with magnetic resonance imaging. *J Neurosurg*. 1996;84(5):737–741.
47. Enzmann DR, Wheat R, Marshall WH, et al. Tumors of the central nervous system studied by computed tomography and ultrasound. *Radiology* 1985;154(2):393–399.
48. LeRoux PD, Berger MS, Ojemann GA, Wang K, Mack LA. Correlation of intraoperative ultrasound tumor volumes and margins with preoperative computerized tomography scans. An intraoperative method to enhance tumor resection. *J Neurosurg*. 1989;71(5, pt 1):691–698.
49. Quencer RM, Montalvo BM. Intraoperative cranial sonography. *Neuroradiology*. 1986;28(5–6):528–550.
50. Brant-Zawadzki M, Badami JP, Mills CM, Norman D, Newton TH. Primary intracranial tumor imaging: a comparison of magnetic resonance and CT. *Radiology*. 1984;150(2):435–440.
51. Suramo I, Päivänsalo M, Vuoria P. Shadowing and reverberation artifacts in abdominal ultrasonography. *Eur J Radiol*. 1985;5(2):147–151.
52. Strowitzki M, Moringlane JR, Steudel W. Ultrasound-based navigation during intracranial burr hole procedures: experience in a series of 100 cases. *Surg Neurol*. 2000;54(2):134–144.
53. Auer LM. Ultrasound stereotaxic endoscopy in neurosurgery. *Acta Neurochir Suppl (Wien)*. 1992;54:34–41.
54. Auer LM. Intraoperative ultrasound as guide for neurosurgical endoscopic procedures. *Acta Radiol Suppl*. 1986;369:164–166.
55. Yamakawa K, Kondo T, Yoshioka M, Takakura K. Ultrasound guided endoscopic neurosurgery–new surgical instrument and technique. *Acta Neurochir Suppl*. 1994;61:46–48.
56. Strowitzki M, Kiefer M, Steudel WI. A new method of ultrasonic guidance of neuroendoscopic procedures. Technical note. *J Neurosurg*. 2002;96(3):628–632.
57. Eismont FJ, Green BA, Berkowitz BM, Montalvo BM, Quencer RM, Brown MJ. The role of intraoperative ultrasonography in the treatment of thoracic and lumbar spine fractures. *Spine*. 1984;9(8):782–787.
58. Garfin SR, Mowery CA, Guerra J, Marshall LF. Confirmation of the posterolateral technique to decompress and fuse thoracolumbar spine burst fractures. *Spine*. 1985;10(3):218–223.
59. Vincent KA, Benson DR, McGahan JP. Intraoperative ultrasonography for reduction of thoracolumbar burst fractures. *Spine*. 1989;14(4):387–390.
60. Akdemir H, Oktem IS, Tucer B, Menkü A, Basaslan K, Günaldi O. Intraoperative microvascular Doppler sonography in aneurysm surgery. *Minim Invasive Neurosurg*. 2006;49(5):312–316.
61. Akdemir H, Oktem S, Menkü A, Tucer B, Tugcu B, Günaldi O. Image-guided microneurosurgical management of small arteriovenous malformation: role of neuronavigation and intraoperative Doppler sonography. *Minim Invasive Neurosurg*. 2007;50(3):163–169.
62. Bailes JE, Tantuwaya LS, Fukushima T, Schurman GW, Davis D. Intraoperative microvascular Doppler sonography in aneurysm surgery. *Neurosurgery*. 1997;40(5):965–970; discussion 970.
63. Kapsalaki EZ, Lee GP, Robinson JS, Grigorian AA, Fountas KN. The role of intraoperative micro-Doppler ultrasound in verifying proper clip placement in intracranial aneurysm surgery. *J Clin Neurosci*. 2008;15(2):153–157.
64. Marchese E, Albanese A, Denaro L, Vignati A, Fernandez E, Maira G. Intraoperative microvascular Doppler in intracranial aneurysm surgery. *Surg Neurol*. 2005;63(4):336–342; discussion 342.
65. Comeau RM, Fenster A, Peters TM. Intraoperative US in interactive image-guided neurosurgery. *Radiographics*. 1998;18(4):1019–1027.

66. Giorgi C, Casolino DS. Preliminary clinical experience with intraoperative stereotactic ultrasound imaging. *Stereotact Funct Neurosurg.* 1997;68(1–4, Pt 1):54–58.
67. Hata N, Dohi T, Iseki H, Takakura K. Development of a frameless and armless stereotactic neuronavigation system with ultrasonographic registration. *Neurosurgery.* 1997;41(3):608–613; discussion 613.
68. Hirschberg H, Unsgaard G. Incorporation of ultrasonic imaging in an optically coupled frameless stereotactic system. *Acta Neurochir Suppl.* 1997;68:75–80.
69. Jödicke A, Springer T, Böker DK. Real-time integration of ultrasound into neuronavigation: technical accuracy using a light-emitting-diode-based navigation system. *Acta Neurochir (Wien).* 2004;146(11):1211–1220.
70. Koivukangas J, Louhisalmi Y, Alakuijala J, Oikarinen J. Ultrasound-controlled neuronavigator-guided brain surgery. *J Neurosurg.* 1993;79(1):36–42.
71. Nikas DC, Hartov A, Lunn K, Rick K, Paulsen K, Roberts DW. Coregistered intraoperative ultrasonography in resection of malignant glioma. *Neurosurg Focus.* 2003;14(2):e6.
72. Trobaugh JW, Richard WD, Smith KR, Bucholz RD. Frameless stereotactic ultrasonography: method and applications. *Comput Med Imaging Graph.* 1994;18(4):235–246.
73. Tirakotai W, Miller D, Heinze S, Benes L, Bertalanffy H, Sure U. A novel platform for image-guided ultrasound. *Neurosurgery.* 2006;58(4):710–718; discussion 710.
74. Miller D, Heinze S, Tirakotai W, et al. Is the image guidance of ultrasonography beneficial for neurosurgical routine? *Surg Neurol.* 2007;67(6):579–587; discussion 587.
75. Letteboer MM, Willems PW, Viergever MA, Niessen WJ. Brain shift estimation in image-guided neurosurgery using 3-D ultrasound. *IEEE Trans Biomed Eng.* 2005;52(2):268–276.
76. Trantakis C, Meixensberger J, Lindner D, et al. Iterative neuronavigation using 3D ultrasound. A feasibility study. *Neurol Res.* 2002;24(7):666–670.
77. Gronningsaeter A, Kleven A, Ommedal S, et al. SonoWand, an ultrasound-based neuronavigation system. *Neurosurgery* 2000;47(6):1373–1379; discussion 1379.
78. Hernes TA, Ommedal S, Lie T, Lindseth F, Langø T, Unsgaard G. Stereoscopic navigation-controlled display of preoperative MRI and intraoperative 3D ultrasound in planning and guidance of neurosurgery: new technology for minimally invasive image-guided surgery approaches. *Minim Invasive Neurosurg.* 2003;46(3):129–137.
79. Shalit MN, Israeli Y, Matz S, Cohen ML. Intra-operative computerized axial tomography. *Surg Neurol.* 1979;11(5):382–384.
80. Butler WE, Piaggio CM, Constantinou C, et al. A mobile computed tomographic scanner with intraoperative and intensive care unit applications. *Neurosurgery.* 1998;42(6):1304–1310; discussion 1310.
81. Engle DJ, Lunsford LD. Brain tumor resection guided by intraoperative computed tomography. *J Neurooncol.* 1987;4(4):361–370.
82. Grunert P, Müller-Forell W, Darabi K, et al. Basic principles and clinical applications of neuronavigation and intraoperative computed tomography. *Comput Aided Surg.* 1998;3(4):166–173.
83. Gumprecht H, Lumenta CB. Intraoperative imaging using a mobile computed tomography scanner. *Minim Invasive Neurosurg.* 2003;46(6):317–322.
84. Kabuto M, Kubota T, Kobayashi H, et al. Intraoperative CT imaging system using a mobile CT scanner gantry mounted on floor-embedded rails for neurosurgery. *No To Shinkei.* 1998;50(11):1003–1008.
85. Lunsford LD, Parrish R, Albright L. Intraoperative imaging with a therapeutic computed tomographic scanner. *Neurosurgery.* 1984;15(4):559–561.
86. Patil A, Kumar P, Leibrock L, Gelber B, Aarabi B. The value of intraoperative scans during CT-guided stereotactic procedures. *Neuroradiology.* 1992;34(5):453–456.
87. Shalit MN, Israeli Y, Matz S, Cohen ML. Experience with intraoperative CT scanning in brain tumors. *Surg Neurol.* 1982;17(5):376–382.
88. Okudera H, Kobayashi S, Kyoshima K, Gibo H, Takemae T, Sugita K. Development of the operating computerized tomographic scanner system for neurosurgery. *Acta Neurochir (Wien).* 1991;111(1–2):61–63.
89. Broggi G, Ferroli P, Franzini A, et al. CT-guided neurosurgery: preliminary experience. *Acta Neurochir Suppl.* 2003;85:101–104.
90. Matula C, Rössler K, Reddy M, Schindler E, Koos WT. Intraoperative computed tomography guided neuronavigation: concepts, efficiency, and work flow. *Comput Aided Surg.* 1998;3(4):174–182.
91. Slomczykowski M, Roberto M, Schneeberger P, Ozdoba C, Vock P. Radiation dose for pedicle screw insertion. Fluoroscopic method versus computer-assisted surgery. *Spine.* 1999;24(10):975–982; discussion 983.
92. Jolesz FA, Kikinis R, Talos IF. Neuronavigation in interventional MR imaging. Frameless stereotaxy. *Neuroimaging Clin N Am.* 2001;11(4):685–693, ix.
93. Archer DP, McTaggart Cowan RA, Falkenstein RJ, Sutherland GR. Intraoperative mobile magnetic resonance imaging for craniotomy lengthens the procedure but does not increase morbidity. *Can J Anaesth.* 2002;49(4):420–426.
94. Silverman SG, Jolesz FA, Newman RW, et al. Design and implementation of an interventional MR imaging suite. *AJR Am J Roentgenol.* 1997;168(6):1465–1471.
95. Tronnier VM, Wirtz CR, Knauth M, et al. Intraoperative computer-assisted neuronavigation in functional neurosurgery. *Stereotact Funct Neurosurg.* 1996;66(1–3):65–68.
96. Rubino GJ, Farahani K, McGill D, Van De Wiele B, Villablanca JP, Wang-Mathieson A. Magnetic resonance imaging-guided neurosurgery in the magnetic fringe fields: the next step in neuronavigation. *Neurosurgery.* 2000;46(3):643–653; discussion 653.
97. Steinmeier R, Fahlbusch R, Ganslandt O, et al. Intraoperative magnetic resonance imaging with the magnetom open scanner: concepts, neurosurgical indications, and procedures: a preliminary report. *Neurosurgery.* 1998;43(4):739–747; discussion 747.
98. Wirtz CR, Bonsanto MM, Knauth M, et al. Intraoperative magnetic resonance imaging to update interactive navigation in neurosurgery: method and preliminary experience. *Comput Aided Surg.* 1997;2(3–4):172–179.
99. Bohinski RJ, Kokkino AK, Warnick RE, et al. Glioma resection in a shared-resource magnetic resonance operating room after optimal image-guided frameless stereotactic resection. *Neurosurgery.* 2001;48(4):731–742; discussion 742.
100. Hadani M, Spiegelman R, Feldman Z, Berkenstadt H, Ram Z. Novel, compact, intraoperative magnetic resonance imaging-guided system for conventional neurosurgical operating rooms. *Neurosurgery.* 2001;48(4):799–807; discussion 807.
101. Schulder M, Sernas TJ, Carmel PW. Cranial surgery and navigation with a compact intraoperative MRI system. *Acta Neurochir Suppl.* 2003;85:79–86.
102. Kanner AA, Vogelbaum MA, Mayberg MR, Weisenberger JP, Barnett GH. Intracranial navigation by using low-field intraoperative magnetic resonance imaging: preliminary experience. *J Neurosurg.* 2002;97(5):1115–1124.
103. Schulder M, Salas S, Brimacombe M, et al. Cranial surgery with an expanded compact intraoperative magnetic resonance imager. Technical note. *J Neurosurg.* 2006;104(4):611–617.
104. Yrjänä SK, Tuominen J, Koivukangas J. Intraoperative magnetic resonance imaging in neurosurgery. *Acta Radiol.* 2007;48(5):540–549.
105. Sutherland GR, Kaibara T, Louw D, Hoult DI, Tomanek B, Saunders J. A mobile high-field magnetic resonance system for neurosurgery. *J Neurosurg.* 1999;91(5):804–813.
106. Nimsky C, Ganslandt O, von Keller B, Fahlbusch R. Preliminary experience in glioma surgery with intraoperative high-field MRI. *Acta Neurochir Suppl.* 2003;88:21–29.
107. Tummala RP, Chu RM, Liu H, Truwit CL, Hall WA. Optimizing brain tumor resection. High-field interventional MR imaging. *Neuroimaging Clin N Am.* 2001;11(4):673–683.
108. Matsumae M, Koizumi J, Fukuyama H, et al. World's first magnetic resonance imaging/x-ray/operating room suite: a significant milestone in the improvement of neurosurgical diagnosis and treatment. *J Neurosurg.* 2007;107(2):266–273.
109. Schulder M, Carmel PW. Intraoperative magnetic resonance imaging: impact on brain tumor surgery. *Cancer Control.* 2003;10(2):115–124.
110. Schulder M, Catrambone J, Carmel PW. Intraoperative magnetic resonance imaging at 0.12 T: is it enough? *Neurosurg Clin N Am.* 2005;16(1):143–154.
111. Schulder M, Liang D, Carmel PW. Cranial surgery navigation aided by a compact intraoperative magnetic resonance imager. *J Neurosurg.* 2001;94(6):936–945.
112. Black PM, Alexander E, Martin C, et al. Craniotomy for tumor treatment in an intraoperative magnetic resonance imaging unit. *Neurosurgery.* 1999;45(3):423–431; discussion 431.

113. Knauth M, Wirtz CR, Tronnier VM, Aras N, Kunze S, Sartor K. Intraoperative MR imaging increases the extent of tumor resection in patients with high-grade gliomas. *Am J Neuroradiol.* 1999;20(9):1642–1646.
114. Nimsky C, Ganslandt O, Buchfelder M, Fahlbusch R. Glioma surgery evaluated by intraoperative low-field magnetic resonance imaging. *Acta Neurochir Suppl.* 2003;85:55–63.
115. Schulder M, Jacobs A, Carmel PW. Intraoperative MRI and adjuvant radiosurgery. *Stereotact Funct Neurosurg.* 2001;76(3–4):151–158.
116. Martin AJ, Hall WA, Liu H, et al. Brain tumor resection: intraoperative monitoring with high-field-strength MR imaging-initial results. *Radiology.* 2000;215(1):221–228.
117. Schneider JP, Schulz T, Schmidt F, et al. Gross-total surgery of supratentorial low-grade gliomas under intraoperative MR guidance. *Am J Neuroradiol.* 2001;22(1):89–98.
118. Darakchiev BJ, Tew JM, Bohinski RJ, Warnick RE. Adaptation of a standard low-field (0.3-T) system to the operating room: focus on pituitary adenomas. *Neurosurg Clin N Am.* 2005;16(1):155–164.
119. Fahlbusch R, Ganslandt O, Buchfelder M, Schott W, Nimsky C. Intraoperative magnetic resonance imaging during transsphenoidal surgery. *J Neurosurg.* 2001;95(3):381–390.
120. Pergolizzi RS, Nabavi A, Schwartz RB, et al. Intra-operative MR guidance during trans-sphenoidal pituitary resection: preliminary results. *J Magn Reson Imaging.* 2001;13(1):136–141.
121. Nimsky C, von Keller B, Ganslandt O, Fahlbusch R. Intraoperative high-field magnetic resonance imaging in transsphenoidal surgery of hormonally inactive pituitary macroadenomas. *Neurosurgery.* 2006;59(1):105–114; discussion 105.
122. Schwartz TH, Marks D, Pak J, et al. Standardization of amygdalohippocampectomy with intraoperative magnetic resonance imaging: preliminary experience. *Epilepsia.* 2002;43(4):430–436.
123. Kelly JJ, Hader WJ, Myles ST, Sutherland GR. Epilepsy surgery with intraoperative MRI at 1.5 T. *Neurosurg Clin N Am.* 2005;16(1):173–183.
124. Buchfelder M, Nimsky C. Intraoperative low-field MR imaging in epilepsy surgery. *Arq Neuropsiquiatr.* 2003;61(suppl 1):115–122.
125. Buchfelder M, Fahlbusch R, Ganslandt O, Stefan H, Nimsky C. Use of intraoperative magnetic resonance imaging in tailored temporal lobe surgeries for epilepsy. *Epilepsia.* 2002;43(8):864–873.
126. Kaibara T, Hurlbert RJ, Sutherland GR. Transoral resection of axial lesions augmented by intraoperative magnetic resonance imaging. Report of three cases. *J Neurosurg.* 2001;95(suppl 2):239–242.
127. Bernays RL, Seifert B, Kollias SS, Valavanis A, Yonekawa Y. Near-real-time guidance using intraoperative magnetic resonance imaging for radical evacuation of hypertensive hematomas in the basal ganglia. *Neurosurgery.* 2001;49(2):478.
128. Bernays RL, Kollias SS, Romanowski B, Valavanis A, Yonekawa Y. Near-real-time guidance using intraoperative magnetic resonance imaging for radical evacuation of hypertensive hematomas in the basal ganglia. *Neurosurgery.* 2000;47(5):1081–1089; discussion 1089.
129. Kollias SS, Bernays RL. Interactive magnetic resonance imaging-guided management of intracranial cystic lesions by using an open magnetic resonance imaging system. *J Neurosurg.* 2001;95(1):15–23.
130. Vitaz TW, Hushek S, Shields CB, Moriarty T. Changes in cyst volume following intraoperative MRI-guided Ommaya reservoir placement for cystic craniopharyngioma. *Pediatr Neurosurg.* 2001;35(5):230–234.
131. Nimsky C, Ganslandt O, Hofmann B, Fahlbusch R. Limited benefit of intraoperative low-field magnetic resonance imaging in craniopharyngioma surgery. *Neurosurgery.* 2003;53(1):72–80; discussion 80.
132. Claus EB, Horlacher A, Hsu L, et al. Survival rates in patients with low-grade glioma after intraoperative magnetic resonance image guidance. *Cancer.* 2005;103(6):1227–1233.
133. Levivier M, Wikler D, De Witte O, Van de Steene A, Balériaux D, Brotchi J. PoleStar N-10 low-field compact intraoperative magnetic resonance imaging system with mobile radiofrequency shielding. *Neurosurgery.* 2003;53(4):1001–1006; discussion 1007.
134. Jolesz FA, Morrison PR, Koran SJ, et al. Compatible instrumentation for intraoperative MRI: expanding resources. *J Magn Reson Imaging.* 1998;8(1):8–11.
135. Gralla J, Ganslandt O, Kober H, Buchfelder M, Fahlbusch R, Nimsky C. Image-guided removal of supratentorial cavernomas in critical brain areas: application of neuronavigation and intraoperative magnetic resonance imaging. *Minim Invasive Neurosurg.* 2003;46(2):72–77.
136. Kaibara T, Saunders JK, Sutherland GR. Advances in mobile intraoperative magnetic resonance imaging. *Neurosurgery.* 2000;47(1):131–137; discussion 137.
137. Moriarty TM, Quinones-Hinojosa A, Larson PS, et al. Frameless stereotactic neurosurgery using intraoperative magnetic resonance imaging: stereotactic brain biopsy. *Neurosurgery.* 2000;47(5):1138–1145; discussion 1145.
138. Nimsky C, Ganslandt O, Kober H, Buchfelder M, Fahlbusch R. Intraoperative magnetic resonance imaging combined with neuronavigation: a new concept. *Neurosurgery.* 2001;48(5):1082–1089; discussion 1089.
139. Tuominen J, Yrjänä SK, Katisko JP, Heikkilä J, Koivukangas J. Intraoperative imaging in a comprehensive neuronavigation environment for minimally invasive brain tumour surgery. *Acta Neurochir Suppl.* 2003;85:115–120.
140. Vahala E, Ylihautala M, Tuominen J, et al. Registration in interventional procedures with optical navigator. *J Magn Reson Imaging.* 2001;13(1):93–98.
141. Nimsky C, Ganslandt O, Hastreiter P, et al. Preoperative and intraoperative diffusion tensor imaging-based fiber tracking in glioma surgery. *Neurosurgery.* 2005;56(1):130–137; discussion 138.
142. Nimsky C, Ganslandt O, Merhof D, Sorensen AG, Fahlbusch R. Intraoperative visualization of the pyramidal tract by diffusion-tensor-imaging-based fiber tracking. *Neuroimage.* 2006;30(4):1219–1229.
143. Nimsky C, Grummich P, Sorensen AG, Fahlbusch R, Ganslandt O. Visualization of the pyramidal tract in glioma surgery by integrating diffusion tensor imaging in functional neuronavigation. *Zentralbl Neurochir.* 2005;66(3):133–141.
144. Nimsky C, Ganslandt O, Fahlbusch R. Implementation of fiber tract navigation. *Neurosurgery.* 2006;58(4, suppl 2):ONS-292.
145. Alexander E. Optimizing brain tumor resection. Midfield interventional MR imaging. *Neuroimaging Clin N Am.* 2001;11(4):659–672.
146. Nimsky C, Ganslandt O, Von Keller B, Romstöck J, Fahlbusch R. Intraoperative high-field-strength MR imaging: implementation and experience in 200 patients. *Radiology.* 2004;233(1):67–78.

50 Intraoperative Molecular Imaging

Walter Stummer and Jörg-Christian Tonn

RATIONALE FOR INTRAOPERATIVE IMAGING

Accumulating data support that completeness of resection improves outcome in patients bearing a malignant glioma [1]. Not only does resection itself appear to influence survival, novel medical therapies will probably also rely on resections being as complete as possible for these therapies to be as beneficious as possible. In this context it was observed that concomitant radiochemotherapy followed by adjuvant chemotherapy was most efficacious in patients treated by complete resections as compared with incomplete resections or biopsy [2].

Nevertheless, the goal of removing all of contrast-enhancing tumor on magnetic resonance imaging (MRI) in published surgical series with early postoperative imaging has been reached only in less than 30% of cases [3–5], one important reason being that viable tumor tissue at the margin of a resection cavity is often difficult to distinguish intraoperatively and may be missed. A number of technical adjuncts to surgery have been explored to solve this problem, such as intraoperative MRI [6], neuronavigation [7], and ultrasound [8]. However, only neuronavigation has been subjected to a prospectively randomized trial [9] in which efficacy for improving resections could not be demonstrated. Another promising tool, intraoperative MRI, is expensive, somewhat demanding in its use and not widely available, whereas ultrasound is prone to artifacts, and image interpretation is highly dependent on the investigator's experience. Therefore, none of these methods have evolved into a standard for surgery on malignant gliomas with the aim of optimizing resection.

Ideally, a tool useful for enhancing intraoperative discrimination and resections of malignant gliomas by improving visualization would have to be specific, economical, simple, and fast to use with real-time visualization. Intraoperative imaging with modern fluorescent markers for highlighting tumor appears to have the potential for achieving these aims. Provided that the fluorochrome specifically highlights tumor tissue, fluorescence imaging can be incorporated into standard operating microscopes, giving the opportunity for real-time tumor resection under direct control of the surgeon.

FLUORESCENT AGENTS PREVIOUSLY USED FOR INTRAOPERATIVE IMAGING

Attempts to enhance contrast of malignant glioma tissue by intravenous administration of fluorescent markers have been described as early as 1948 [10] using fluorescein as the first compound explored for fluorescence-guided resections. In fact, fluorescein has been explored in a number of studies [11,12] to date and has been observed at high concentrations within malignant brain tissue. However, tumor demarcation using fluorescein is not entirely specific, because fluorescein within the plasma enters the brain via the defective blood-brain barrier in the tumor [12] and fluorescence outside the tumor has been observed [11,12]. Also, fluorescein has been observed to highlight tissue unspecifically in brain tissue exposed to blood during surgery. Intraoperative fluorescence-guided resection of malignant gliomas using fluorescein has not been tested in large controlled trials. It has not been determined whether the method is specific enough for enhancing resection, and, more importantly, whether it causes additional neurological deficits. The pitfall of unspecific intraoperative fluorescence accumulation theoretically affects all other fluorochromes that are given intravenously and are present in blood, such as porphyrins [13,14] or their derivatives, such as m-tetrahydroxyphenylchlorin [15]. More recently, fluorescein conjugated with albumin has been explored with fluorescence-guided resections delayed to more than 24 hours after application [16,17]. These conjugates appear to be selectively accumulated by malignant glioma cells, thus increasing specificity as opposed to intravenous fluorescein. However, only clinical pilot series regarding this method have been presented to date.

Finally, a number of groups have investigated the value of endogenous fluorochromes for delineation of tumor by their specific pattern of autofluorescence emission, with focus on spectral shape, signal amplitude, or fluorescence lifetimes of autofluorescence [18–20]. Several biomolecules involved in both functional and metabolic processes (coenzymes, flavins, lipopigments, porphyrins) and in histological organization (constitutive proteins, cellular density) [20] act as endogenous fluorochromes and may be expressed differently within glioma tissue. Utilizing these fluorochromes for fluorescence delineation of gliomas would have the distinct advantage that exogenous compounds would not have to be administered. However, the necessary technology is complex, requiring multiphoton microscopy and fluorescence lifetime imaging (4D microscopy). At present, these methods are on the verge of leaving the lab bench to being explored more conclusively in patients.

FLUORESCENCE-GUIDED SURGERY USING 5-AMINOLEVULINIC ACID

5-aminolevulinic acid (5-ALA) differs from both exogenously administered fluorochromes, such as fluorescein, and endogenous fluorochromes, the detection of which is technically demanding. ALA is the body's own metabolite in the heme biosynthesis pathway. Experimental and clinical studies have shown colorless and nonfluorescent ALA to be taken up by malignant glioma cells, where it is converted into strongly fluorescing porphyrins. [21]. Using specifically modified surgical microscopes, the resulting fluorescence can be utilized for resecting residual malignant glioma tissue (Figure 50.1) [22,23].

In contrast to exogenous fluorochromes or autofluorescence detection, 5-ALA has so far undergone structured development, resulting in marketing approval within Europe. Thus, 5-ALA is the most widely and most intensely investigated drug used for fluorescence-guided surgery of malignant gliomas at present. Its development has not only given insight into the efficacy and safety of 5-ALA for fluorescence-guided resections, but has also strengthened the current concept of cytoreductive therapy as the initial step in the treatment of patients with malignant gliomas.

Efficacy of Fluorescence-Guided Resections Using 5-ALA

The pivotal study for approval of ALA was a randomized phase III trial comparing standard microsurgery followed by radiotherapy with fluorescence-guided resection followed by radiotherapy (study sponsor: Medac GmbH, Wedel, Germany). The study not only focused on the efficacy of ALA-induced fluorescence for enhancing resections, but also closely scrutinized neurological function to assess any undesired deterioration. Eligible patients had to suffer from malignant gliomas considered to be "completely" resectable by the participating surgeons. "Complete" resection was assumed if contrast-enhancing tumor was no longer visible on early postoperative MRI, obtained within 72 hours after surgery. Details of the study are given elsewhere [24].

The study was able to demonstrate early postoperative MRI to be devoid of residual contrast-enhancing tumor in 65% of patients with glioblastoma multiforme in the ALA group compared to only 36% in the control (white light) arm. This important primary result demonstrated that resections using conventional microsurgery were much less effective in terms of "complete" resection of contrast-enhancing glioma tissue compared to fluorescence-guided resections. In the longer term, Kaplan-Meier analyses revealed significantly prolonged progression-free survival in ALA patients compared to white light alone with cumulative 6-month progression-free survival rates of 41% and 21% ($p < 0.01$). Survival on the other hand, which was a secondary study aim, was only marginally prolonged (13.5 vs. 15.2 months, $p = 0.1$). In retrospect it became evident that the study was underpowered to demonstrate differences in survival and, since control patients also had complete resections in 35%, the increase to 65% complete resections in the study arm might not have been large enough to elicit statistical differences in survival, if the effect of resection on survival was not overwhelming. Importantly, survival results suffered from a bias in augmental therapies which favored the control arm. This was particularly evident for repeat surgery, which was more frequent and occurred earlier in white light compared to ALA-patients (12-month rate 33 vs. 22%, $p = 0.0331$). A similar observation, albeit not quite significant, was made

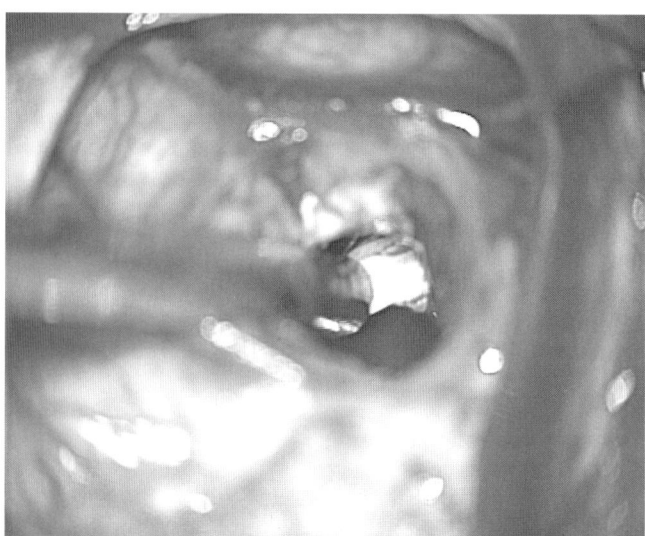 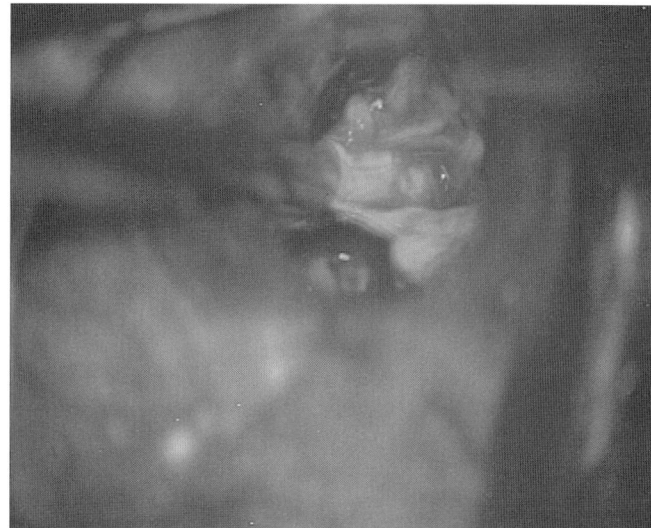

Figure 50.1 Visualization of residual tumor through intraoperative fluorescence imaging with 5-ALA. *See color insert.*

for the initiation of chemotherapy with temozolamide which was given less frequently in ALA patients (52 vs. 42%, $p = 0.06$; data submitted). Thus, the ALA study not only demonstrated efficacy regarding resection with ALA, but also demonstrated long-term benefits from improving resections. Finally, restratification of patients according to resection status strikingly confirmed the prognostic influence of complete vs. incomplete resections (17.9 vs. 12.9 months, $p = 0.0001$). In multivariate analysis, the overall survival advantage noted for patients without contrast-enhancing tumor remained significant ($p = 0.0006$), in addition to age ($p = 0.01$), Karnowsky Performance Score (KPS) ($p = 0.006$) [25].

Safety Profile of Fluorescence-Guided Resections Using 5-ALA

From a strictly toxicological perspective, few side-effects were identified for the use of ALA. Twenty-four hours after surgery gamma glutamyl transpeptidase, alanine transaminase, and aspartate aminotransferase were significantly elevated in patients from the ALA group compared to white light patients, but no longer than 7 days after surgery. We interpret this observation to indicate a greater metabolic burden for the liver rather than being a transient liver disease.

From a neurological perspective, there was a tendency for patients in the ALA arm to be worse 48 hours after surgery ($p = 0.05$) according to the National Institutes of Health-stroke scale, which was used as measure for acute changes in neurological function in the ALA study. No significant differences were noted at later points of time. Also there was a tendency toward a misbalance in the most frequently reported severe adverse events (ALA group vs. WL group): hemiparesis (2.9% vs. 1.5%,) and aphasia (3.0% vs. 0%, $p = 0.25$). Importantly, all patients with a report of postoperative aphasia had already suffered aphasia before surgery, which had not responded completely to steroids. This observation was important, since it helped to identify those patients with a greater risk for a permanent neurological deficit as being those patients in whom tumor infiltration and destruction of eloquent brain rather than functional impairment by tumor-related edema was the reason for a preoperative impairment in function.

On the other hand, median KPS 6 weeks after surgery was 90% for both treatment groups. At 6 months, the rate of patients with KPS deterioration to values less or equal to 60 was 27.7% in the ALA group compared to 31.3% in the WL group, ruling out an overall impairment of global function through enhanced resections using 5-ALA.

In summary, the trade-off between possible dangers of enhanced resection regarding neurological functions and clinical benefit (prolonged progression-free survival) appeared favorable.

Practical Implementation of 5-ALA Fluorescence-Guided Surgery

Dosage and Time of ALA Application

Fluorescence-guided resection using ALA has only been tested in a controlled setting using an oral dose of 20 mg 5-ALA/kg bodyweight in combination with dexamethasone (3×4 mg per day for 2 days). Dexamethasone pretreatment is believed to be crucial for the efficacy and safety profile observed in the phase III study, because dexamethasone probably influences ALA uptake and fluorescence yields by tightening the blood-brain barrier. Lower doses of 5-ALA (0.2 and 2 mg/kg) have been tested in a double-blinded, prospectively randomized trial (medac trial MC-ALS.8-I/GLI, unpublished data) but found to generate much less fluorescence and were thus abandoned. Higher doses have not been tested for fluorescence-guided resections of malignant gliomas of the brain. However, systemic side effects with higher doses of 5-ALA, as used for other indications, have been reported. Higher doses of 40 mg/kg bodyweight or more have been observed to induce hypotension, nausea, vomiting and increases in plasma liver enzymes [25–28]. On the other hand, since porphyrin-IX fluorescence using 20 mg 5-ALA/kg bodyweight has proved adequate for efficient detection and/or resection of malignant gliomas, there does not appear to be any necessity for increasing fluorescence intensity by augmenting the 5-ALA dosage.

In practice, 5-ALA is given to patients orally 2.5 to 3.5 hours before induction of anesthesia. The time point of administration was derived from initial in vivo experiments using the C6-glioma model in the rat with peak fluorescence being observed approximately 6 hours after administration [21]. For surgery on patients it was calculated that induction of anesthesia, positioning of the patient, draping, and craniotomy would take approximately 1.5 to 2 hours. Allowing another hour for removal of the clearly discernable tumor core, the surgeons would be involved 3 to 3.5 hours in the operation before fluorescence-guidance becomes necessary. Pharmacokinetic assessments performed in the medac phase I/II study (MC-ALS.8-I/GLI, unpublished data) have demonstrated complete absorption of the total 5-ALA dose within 1 hour of oral administration, so that the solution can be expected to have passed the intestine at the time point of anesthesia induction.

On the other hand, fluorescence in human malignant gliomas appears to be very stable. In our experience in a number of cases that were unexpectedly delayed, an unperturbed fluorescence impression was obtained even 12 to 16 hours after administration of 5-ALA.

Light Protection

Sensitization of the skin has been reported after systemic application of 5-ALA [26–28]. In contrast to traditional sensitizers, fortunately skin sensitization due to 5-ALA is short, with a duration of approximately 24 hours. In our practice and as previously recommended for patients in the phase III ALA trial, direct exposure of patients to sunlight or strong room light has to be avoided for 24 hours. Between the time point of 5-ALA administration and induction of anesthesia, low levels of ambient light are permitted. In our opinion the most vulnerable period is during the induction of anesthesia and the positioning of the patient for surgery, before draping. During this phase of bustling activity in the neurosurgical operating room, direct illumination by overhead lighting is often unavoidable. We try at least to prevent direct illumination of the patients' skin by the operating lights and keep the patient covered as early and consequently as possible. Low levels of ambient light are permitted during the postoperative period. Restrictions regarding light exposure are withdrawn 24 hours after 5-ALA administration. Observing these precautions, no severe skin reactions in terms of significant sunburn have been observed, although several patients have had slight rubor of the skin lasting 2 to 3 days.

Equipment

Adequate equipment for the visualization of porphyrin fluorescence is of utmost importance for successfully implementing fluorescence-guided resections. In modern neurosurgical practice, the surgical microscope is indispensable. Therefore, fluorescence imaging hardware has to be adapted to the microscope.

In the medac study MC-ALS.3/GLI, only the Zeiss NC4 system with its particular combination of excitation light source, excitation filter, microscope optics, and emissions filters was tested for safety and efficacy. All participating centers were equipped with identical microscopes. Whether the results from this study can be extended to equipment supplied by alternate microscope manufacturers is unknown. If alternate equipment were more sensitive, it might pick up tissue autofluorescence or diffuse porphyrin fluorescence not seen with the Zeiss system, leading to greater resection volumes, which might jeopardize safety. If alternate equipment were less sensitive, this might result in less radical resections. Thus, caution is warranted in this regard.

At present, other major microscope producers are offering surgical microscopes for fluorescence-guided resections, such as Möller-Wedel and Leica. Zeiss company has equipped the Pentero™ system with an optional module for fluorescence-guided resection with 5-ALA.

Implementation During Surgery

Apart from necessary precautions regarding light exposure, the course of the normal operation does not differ greatly from conventional microneurosurgical operations. Anesthesia induction, patient positioning, draping, and craniotomy are performed in the usual fashion. As in other operations, neuronavigation can be a useful adjunct for planning craniotomy or locating tumors, which do not reach the cortical surface. Alternatively, for initial localization of tumor, sonography may be used. At times, even when the cortical surface appears inconspicuous, switching to blue excitation light may allow discrimination of subcortical tumor extensions, providing a valuable guide for initial corticotomy. For surgery in eloquent brain regions, we have repeatedly used awake craniotomy for language mapping or for surgery in the vicinity of the motor cortex; this has never interacted negatively with fluorescence-guided resections (Figure 50.2). Apart from initial localization, neuronavigation or sonography has never been of additional help for defining tumor borders. However, sonography has been helpful in defining gross anatomy, for instance when operating on temporal tumors extending toward the basal ganglia. In this situation, sonography is useful for delineating the Sylvian fissure and insula to define the plane for termination of resection before entering the basal ganglia. It must be borne in mind that tissue fluorescence gives only two-dimensional information on tumor extensions and does not prevent the surgeon from following the tumor into eloquent brain. While intact neurological function does not seem likely to be located within strong fluorescent tissue, surgical manipulations may lead to remote damage, away from the immediate resection site, for instance by damaging blood vessels traversing the tumor. Therefore, 5-ALA is a tool that helps discriminate tumor, but it is at the surgeon's discretion as to whether all the fluorescing tissue encountered should be removed.

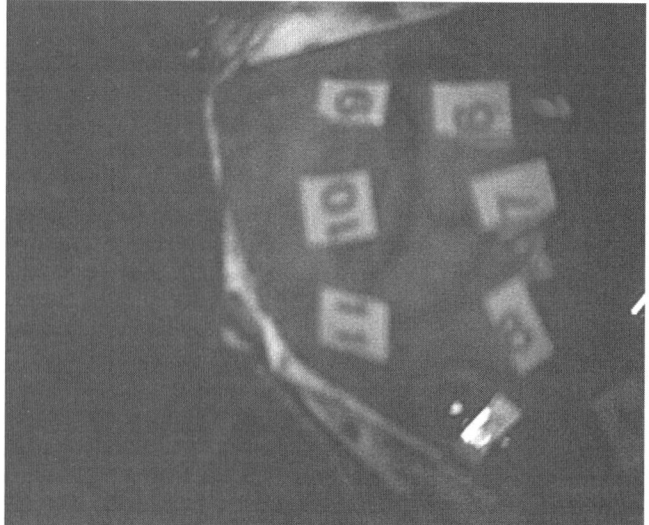
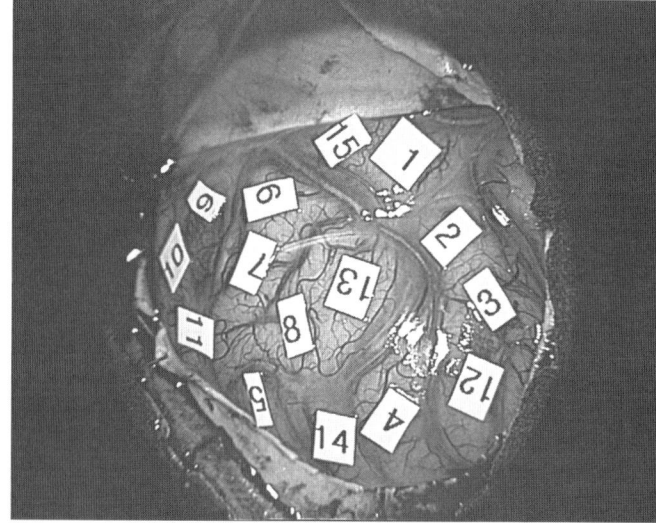

Figure 50.2 Combining fluorescence for visualizing the cortical extension of the tumor with language mapping for determining function. See *color insert*.

There are of course different methods for operating on a malignant glioma. The surgeon might prefer to remove necrotic and easily distinguishable solid tumor regions first, predominantly under white light, and then to remove marginal residual tumor using fluorescence-guided resection. Alternately, the surgeon might choose to remain in fluorescing tumor margins at the resection plane. We use simple suction or the ultrasound aspirator for removing tumor. Blood in the resection cavity quenches the fluorescence signal but can easily be removed by suction to give an impression of the fluorescence quality of the tissue. In this respect, fluorescence-guided resection is a dynamic process. Conditions do not have to be optimized for demonstrating fluorescence. Rather, switching from normal to blue excitation light in the microscope is manually repeatedly performed during the course of the operation. Toward the end, longer periods of the operation can be performed using blue excitation light alone. If unspecific oozing gets too strong and impairs fluorescence detection, white light illumination with its greater detail is used for coagulating vessels. However, the technique of fluorescence-guided resection requires some experience with this tool. This should be gained by hands-on training and observation at sites or with surgeons being acquainted with it already.

Photobleaching

There has been some concern about photobleaching of porphyrins by microscope illumination, which might destroy tissue fluorescence and impair sensitivity. We have examined this issue in detail in earlier work [29] and found photobleaching to be much slower than anticipated. Under operating light conditions, fluorescence decayed to 36% in 25 minutes for violet blue and 87 minutes for white light. Moreover, during surgery, microscope light is usually directed at a small part of the resection cavity, whereas other parts are often covered by coagulated blood or cotton patties. Still, mild fluorescence may be bleached in exposed regions of the tumor which are not removed immediately and may be missed. In this situation fluorescence may be refreshed by suction and removal of superficial cell layers.

How Far to Resect?

Past investigations (medac Study MC-ALS.28/GLI, unpublished data) have demonstrated the extent of 5-ALA-derived fluorescence accumulation to exceed the area of contrast enhancement observed on MRI. Thus, ALA-derived fluorescence appears to be more sensitive in delineating residual tumor. MC-ALS.28/GLI has further led to assume in general that infiltrated brain tissue in these regions might be functionally deficient. Furthermore, slight disruption of the blood-brain barrier for small molecules such as 5-ALA will have to be expected in fluorescing tissue regions. Disruption of the blood-brain barrier regarding small molecules is a prerequisite for ALA uptake into the brain. Disruption will also preclude a normal milieu interieur with intact function. On the other hand, going beyond this region might lead to neurological deficits. It is also evident that tissue manipulation, such as coagulation or shearing, might result in damage to neighboring brain regions, with subsequent neurological deficits. Furthermore, blood vessels supplying adjacent, eloquent brain regions might be damaged, leading to distant ischemia, resulting in neurological deficits. Again, it is in the responsibility of the surgeon to decide how far he/she is prepared to remove fluorescing tissue. ALA should not replace a critical awareness of cerebral anatomy, vascular supply, and function of the brain region, in which resections are performed.

In the phase III ALA trial there was a slight preponderance of neurological deterioration in the ALA arm 48 hours after the procedure [24]. Further analysis demonstrated deterioration to have occurred almost exclusively in patients having preoperative neurological deficits that were not completely responsive to steroid pretreatment. Steroid pretreatment was obligatory within that trial. This observation strongly cautions against attempts at "radical" resection in such patients, whose tumors had already caused structural damage in eloquent brain regions, rather than impaired function through edema alone.

Pitfalls

In some of the studies on fluorescence-guided resections using ALA, incompletely resected tumors were observed, in which anatomical location did not preclude complete resection. An analysis of the images pertaining to these patients revealed "overhanging resection margins" to be a common problem herein. During the course of resecting tumors surgeons tend to undercut the cortex, leaving residual tumor under the margins, that is, outside the surgeon's direct field of vision. It is important to be aware of this phenomenon, to prevent missing substantial portions of the tumor. A second problem can frequently be encountered in tumors with cystic portions and slender margins of enhancement. Opening the cysts leads to the collapse of parts of the tumor, which in some cases might be missed. Finally, wrongly placed craniotomies have been identified as the main factor precluding complete resection of contrast-enhancing tumor.

Other pitfalls were observed when patient's histology did not conform to the expectancy of a malignant glioma, for example, abscess, metastasis, vasculitis and lymphoma. In the experience of the authors, both abscesses and metastases are sometimes surrounded by a region with weak, unspecific fluorescence accumulation. While the source of this fluorescence is unclear, it is crucial to be aware of this phenomenon to avoid fluorescence-guided resections in perifocal tissue in these entities. Patients with lymphoma and necrotizing vasculitis were also observed to demonstrate strong fluorescence accumulation within their lesions, possibly related to inflammatory or neoplastic cells. Because of this experience, we recommend obtaining frozen sections at an early stage of the procedure in any unclear cases to prevent unnecessary damage. Similarly, stereotactic biopsy might be performed ahead of definite surgery to clarify diagnosis in ambiguous MR images. Finally, some cases of gliosarcoma have been observed to show modest fluorescence accumulation within those areas of the tumor with predominantly solid texture, although

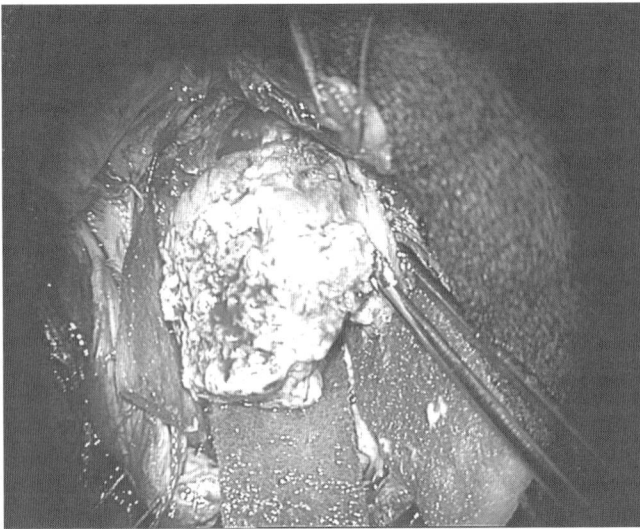 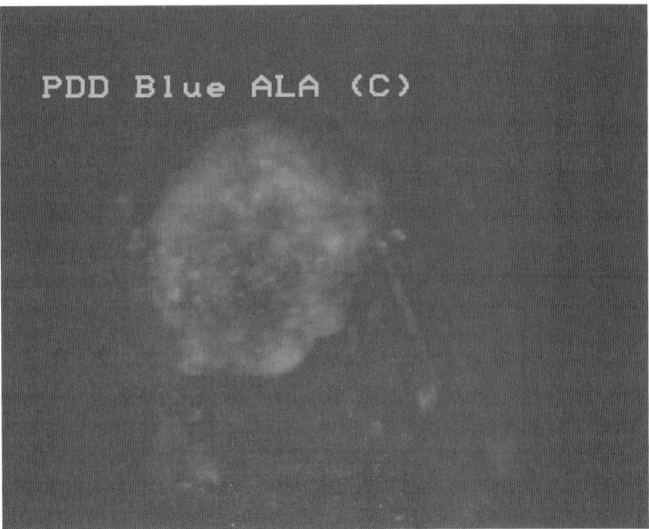

Figure 50.3 Atypical meningioma. Left: white light, Right: blue-violet illumination. *See color insert.*

infiltrating tumor beyond that had revealed the expected fluorescence.

Ambient light within the operating room will interfere with the fluorescence signal. Neon lighting contains substantial amounts of light within the red and infrared spectrum. This will be selected by the filters in the microscope in the observation light path and will make the entire cavity and brain appear red. Standard operating room lights are less of a problem in this regard, because their red and infrared wavelengths are blocked more effectively. In our practice, we turn off all light sources except the surgical lights, which are diverted away from the surgical cavity toward the instrument trays. Of course the operating rooms have to be darkened with respect to daylight.

We have found it helpful to reduce the microscope's light intensity under white light to aid fast adaptation to violet-blue excitation light. Modern neurosurgical microscopes have excessive white light in any case and reducing this by 50% to 70% does little to reduce image quality under white light. This is especially important for the Zeiss Pentero system, which features an excess of normal white light, the intensity of which can easily be reduced to 25%. Even in standard neurosurgical procedures it is wise to reduce illumination intensity (which in addition reduces thermal stress on the tissue as well) and to reserve the full capabilities of this system for deep-seated procedures and/or procedures with high magnification. For fluorescence-guided resections, however, the system should automatically switch to full intensity in the "blue light mode" to have the highest possible intensity of violet-blue excitation light.

Future Applications

Recently, a number of investigators have indicated usefulness of 5-ALA-induced fluorescent porphyrins in other neurosurgical entities apart from malignant glioma, such as spinal medullary ependymoma [30] or recurrent, atypical meningioma [31]. The latter has been our experience, too (Figure 50.3).

Apart from its usefulness for fluorescence-guided resections, the fluorescent metabolite of ALA, protoporphyrin IX, appears to have a strong potential as photosensitizer useful for photodynamic therapy of malignant gliomas. The photosensitizing properties of this compound has been investigated in vitro [32,33] and in vivo [34,35], and selective destruction of sensitized malignant glioma tissue has been noted. Thus, ALA-induced protoporphyrin IX accumulation in malignant glioma cells appears to render these selectively susceptible to phototherapy, provided they are exposed to sufficient light. An overview of the technical approach to the problem of treating deep-seated tumors is given elsewhere [36]. This technique utilizes a software platform for 3D planning and stereotactic implantation of light diffusers into sensitized malignant glioma tissue. The first patient subjected to this method harbored the distant recurrence of a previously resected glioblastoma multiforme treated by adjuvant radio- and chemotherapy, which was unresponsive to second-line interventions. She responded dramatically to 5-ALA phototherapy and remained without recurrence more than 56 months after treatment [37]. A randomized study is presently being planned to further elucidate this promising therapy.

REFERENCES

1. Stummer W, Reulen HJ, Meinel T, et al. Extent of resection and survival in glioblastoma multiforme: identification of and adjustment for bias. *Neurosurgery.* 2008;62(3):564–576; discussion 564.
2. Van den Bent MJ, Stupp R, Mason W, Mirimanoff RO, Lacombe D, Gorlia T. Impact of the extent of resection on overall survival in newly-diagnosed glioblastoma after chemo-irradiation with temozolamide: further analysis of EORTC study 26981. *Eur J Cancer.* 2005;(suppl 3):134 (abstract).
3. Albert FK, Forsting M, Sartor K, Adams HP, Kunze S. Early postoperative magnetic resonance imaging after resection of malignant glioma: objective evaluation of residual tumor and its influence

on regrowth and prognosis. *Neurosurgery*. 1994;34(1):45–60; discussion 60.

4. Kowalczuk A, Macdonald RL, Amidei C, et al. Quantitative imaging study of extent of surgical resection and prognosis of malignant astrocytomas. *Neurosurgery*. 1997;41(5):1028–1036; discussion 1036.

5. Shrieve DC, Alexander E 3rd, Black PM, et al. Treatment of patients with primary glioblastoma multiforme with standard postoperative radiotherapy and radiosurgical boost: prognostic factors and long-term outcome. *J Neurosurg*. 1999;90(1):72–77.

6. Nimsky C, Ganslandt O, Buchfelder M, Fahlbusch R. Intraoperative visualization for resection of gliomas: the role of functional neuronavigation and intraoperative 1.5 T MRI. *Neurol Res*. 2006;28(5):482–487.

7. Wirtz CR, Albert FK, Schwaderer M, et al. The benefit of neuronavigation for neurosurgery analyzed by its impact on glioblastoma surgery. *Neurol Res*. 2000;22(4):354–360.

8. Lindner D, Trantakis C, Renner C, et al. Application of intraoperative 3D ultrasound during navigated tumor resection. *Minim Invasive Neurosurg*. 2006;49(4):197–202.

9. Willems PW, Taphoorn MJ, Burger H, Berkelbach van der Sprenkel JW, Tulleken CA. Effectiveness of neuronavigation in resecting solitary intracerebral contrast-enhancing tumors: a randomized controlled trial. *J Neurosurg*. 2006;104(3):360–368.

10. Moore GE, Peyton WT. The clinical use of fluorescein in neurosurgery; the localization of brain tumors. *J Neurosurg*. 1948;5(4):392–398.

11. Kuroiwa T, Kajimoto Y, Ohta T. Comparison between operative findings on malignant glioma by a fluorescein surgical microscopy and histological findings. *Neurol Res*. 1999;21(1):130–134.

12. Shinoda J, Yano H, Yoshimura S, et al. Fluorescence-guided resection of glioblastoma multiforme by using high-dose fluorescein sodium. Technical note. *J Neurosurg*. 2003;99(3):597–603.

13. Yang VX, Muller PJ, Herman P, Wilson BC. A multispectral fluorescence imaging system: design and initial clinical tests in intra-operative Photofrin-photodynamic therapy of brain tumors. *Lasers Surg Med*. 2003;32(3):224–232.

14. Stummer W, Götz C, Hassan A, Heimann A, Kempski O. Kinetics of Photofrin II in perifocal brain edema. *Neurosurgery*. 1993;33(6):1075–1081; discussion 1081.

15. Zimmermann A, Ritsch-Marte M, Kostron H. mTHPC-mediated photodynamic diagnosis of malignant brain tumors. *Photochem Photobiol*. 2001;74(4):611–616.

16. Kremer P, Wunder A, Sinn H, et al. Laser-induced fluorescence detection of malignant gliomas using fluorescein-labeled serum albumin: experimental and preliminary clinical results. *Neurol Res*. 2000;22(5):481–489.

17. Ichioka T, Miyatake S, Asai N, et al. Enhanced detection of malignant glioma xenograft by fluorescein-human serum albumin conjugate. *J Neurooncol*. 2004;67(1–2):47–52.

18. Leppert J, Krajewski J, Kantelhardt SR, et al. Multiphoton excitation of autofluorescence for microscopy of glioma tissue. *Neurosurgery*. 2006;58(4):759–767; discussion 759.

19. Toms SA, Lin WC, Weil RJ, Johnson MD, Jansen ED, Mahadevan-Jansen A. Intraoperative optical spectroscopy identifies infiltrating glioma margins with high sensitivity. *Neurosurgery*. 2005;57(4 suppl):382–391; discussion 382.

20. Croce AC, Fiorani S, Locatelli D, et al. Diagnostic potential of autofluorescence for an assisted intraoperative delineation of glioblastoma resection margins. *Photochem Photobiol*. 2003;77(3):309–318.

21. Stummer W, Stocker S, Novotny A, et al. *In vitro* and *in vivo* porphyrin accumulation by C6 glioma cells after exposure to 5-aminolevulinic acid. *J Photochem Photobiol B*. 1998;45(2–3):160–169.

22. Stummer W, Stepp H, Möller G, Ehrhardt A, Leonhard M, Reulen HJ. Technical principles for protoporphyrin-IX-fluorescence guided microsurgical resection of malignant glioma tissue. *Acta Neurochir (Wien)*. 1998;140(10):995–1000.

23. Stummer W, Novotny A, Stepp H, Goetz C, Bise K, Reulen HJ. Fluorescence-guided resection of glioblastoma multiforme by using 5-aminolevulinic acid-induced porphyrins: a prospective study in 52 consecutive patients. *J Neurosurg*. 2000;93(6):1003–1013.

24. Stummer W, Pichlmeier U, Meinel T, et al. Fluorescence-guided surgery with 5-aminolevulinic acid for resection of malignant glioma: a randomised controlled multicentre phase III trial. *Lancet Oncol*. 2006;7(5):392–401.

25. Herman MA, Webber J, Fromm D, Kessel D. Hemodynamic effects of 5-aminolevulinic acid in humans. *J Photochem Photobiol B, Biol*. 1998;43(1):61–65.

26. Mlkvy P, Messmann H, Regula J, et al. Sensitization and photodynamic therapy (PDT) of gastrointestinal tumors with 5-aminolaevulinic acid (ALA) induced protoporphyrin IX (PPIX). A pilot study. *Neoplasma*. 1995;42(3):109–113.

27. Regula J, MacRobert AJ, Gorchein A, et al. Photosensitisation and photodynamic therapy of oesophageal, duodenal, and colorectal tumours using 5 aminolaevulinic acid induced protoporphyrin IX-a pilot study. *Gut*. 1995;36(1):67–75.

28. Fan KF, Hopper C, Speight PM, Buonaccorsi G, MacRobert AJ, Bown SG. Photodynamic therapy using 5-aminolevulinic acid for premalignant and malignant lesions of the oral cavity. *Cancer*. 1996;78(7):1374–1383.

29. Stummer W, Stocker S, Wagner S, et al. Intraoperative detection of malignant gliomas by 5-aminolevulinic acid-induced porphyrin fluorescence. *Neurosurgery*. 1998;42(3):518–525; discussion 525.

30. Shimizu S, Utsuki S, Sato K, Oka H, Fujii K, Mii K. Photodynamic diagnosis in surgery for spinal ependymoma. Case illustration. *J Neurosurg Spine*. 2006;5(4):380.

31. Kajimoto Y, Kuroiwa T, Miyatake S, et al. Use of 5-aminolevulinic acid in fluorescence-guided resection of meningioma with high risk of recurrence. Case report. *J Neurosurg*. 2007;106(6):1070–1074.

32. Zelenkov P, Baumgartner R, Bise K, et al. Acute morphological sequelae of photodynamic therapy with 5-aminolevulinic acid in the C6 spheroid model. *J Neurooncol*. 2007;82(1):49–60.

33. Karmakar S, Banik NL, Patel SJ, Ray SK. 5-Aminolevulinic acid-based photodynamic therapy suppressed survival factors and activated proteases for apoptosis in human glioblastoma U87MG cells. *Neurosci Lett*. 2007;415(3):242–247.

34. Inoue H, Kajimoto Y, Shibata MA, et al. Massive apoptotic cell death of human glioma cells via a mitochondrial pathway following 5-aminolevulinic acid-mediated photodynamic therapy. *J Neurooncol*. 2007;83(3):223–231.

35. Hirschberg H, Sun CH, Krasieva T, Madsen SJ. Effects of ALA-mediated photodynamic therapy on the invasiveness of human glioma cells. *Lasers Surg Med*. 2006;38(10):939–945.

36. Beck TJ, Kreth FW, Beyer W, et al. Interstitial photodynamic therapy of nonresectable malignant glioma recurrences using 5-aminolevulinic acid induced protoporphyrin IX. *Lasers Surg Med*. 2007;39(5):386–393.

37. Stummer W, Beck T, Beyer W, et al. Long-sustaining response in a patient with non-resectable, distant recurrence of glioblastoma multiforme treated by interstitial photodynamic therapy using 5-ALA: case report. *J Neurooncol*. 2008;87(1):103–109.

51 Intraoperative Functional Mapping

R. Mark Richardson and Mitchel S. Berger

INTRODUCTION

The resection of tumors located within or adjacent to eloquent cortical regions is often necessary to alleviate focal neurological deficits that are secondary to mass effect and increased intracranial pressure. In addition, there is growing evidence that greater extent of tumor resection correlates with increased time to tumor progression and overall survival for glioma patients, for both low- and high-grade gliomas [1–5]. The surgical aim is to achieve maximal tumor removal without producing permanent morbidity. To accomplish this goal, neurophysiological mapping of functional areas is critical for minimizing the morbidity associated with removing abnormal tissue from eloquent cortex.

Here we present techniques for intraoperative cortical and subcortical stimulation mapping to maximize safe removal of tumors located in motor and language cortex. Cortical stimulation techniques have been adapted from the pioneering methods of Penfield and Boldrey [6], whereas localization of subcortical motor and sensory tracts was first described by Berger and Ojemann [7].

MOTOR-FUNCTION MAPPING DURING ASLEEP CRANIOTOMY

Indications

Hemispheric tumors located within or adjacent to rolandic cortex, supplementary motor area, corona radiata, internal capsule, and uncinate fasciculus constitute the major indications for intraoperative motor-function mapping. Regardless of the degree of tumor infiltration, swelling, apparent necrosis, and gross distortion by the tumor mass, functional cortex and subcortical white matter may be located within the tumor itself or the adjacent infiltrated brain [8]. Due to the risk of damaging descending motor pathways, subcortical stimulation mapping is required in addition to cortical mapping. When using stimulation mapping methods to identify subcortical pathways, the surgeon is able to achieve an acceptable risk of permanent motor deficits in patients with gliomas that are within or adjacent to motor tracts.

Preoperative Neurological Evaluation

Although motor mapping will often not be useful in patients with severe hemiparesis, if antigravity movement is present preoperatively it is usually possible to stimulate both cortical and subcortical motor pathways intraoperatively. In children younger than 6 years of age, who may have cortical electrical inexcitability, somatosensory-evoked potentials must be available and used to identify the central sulcus via phase reversal.

Preoperative Functional Imaging

A volumetric magnetic resonance imaging (MRI) scan is obtained preoperatively for use with an intraoperative navigational system. The relationship of the tumor to primary motor cortex is assessed by identifying the central or rolandic sulcus on the rostral cuts of the axial T2-weighted MRI scan. This landmark is always present, regardless of mass effect, and is a reliable marker for the motor strip located within the gyrus directly anterior to the sulcus. The motor cortex can be found on midsagittal cuts by following the cingulate sulcus posteriorly and superiorly to its termination, at which point the motor cortex is directly anterior to this sulcus. On far lateral images, the inferior to mid portion of the motor cortex is localized to a region bisected by a perpendicular line drawn from the posterior corner of the insular triangle. Each of these MRI landmarks is useful for determining the proximity of the lesion to the motor cortex preoperatively.

Preoperative functional imaging of primary motor cortex is best achieved currently by magnetic source imaging (MSI), in which the source localization of functional cortical areas by magnetoencephalography (MEG) is coregistered with an anatomic MRI scan [9,10]. MEG is used to detect the magnetic field associated with neuronal activity itself, rather than relying on an indirect correlate such as the hemodynamic response upon which functional magnetic resonance imaging (fMRI) is based. MEG is generated by dipole currents associated with dendritic excitatory and inhibitory postsynaptic potentials, which produce frequency specific oscillations whose rhythms change upon brain activation. In this way, the somatosensory cortex and motor cortex are reliably localized preoperatively (Figure 51.1).

As mentioned, resecting brain tumors involves the risk of damaging the descending subcortical motor pathways. Diffusion tensor image (DTI) fiber tracking is a noninvasive MRI technique that can delineate the subcortical course of

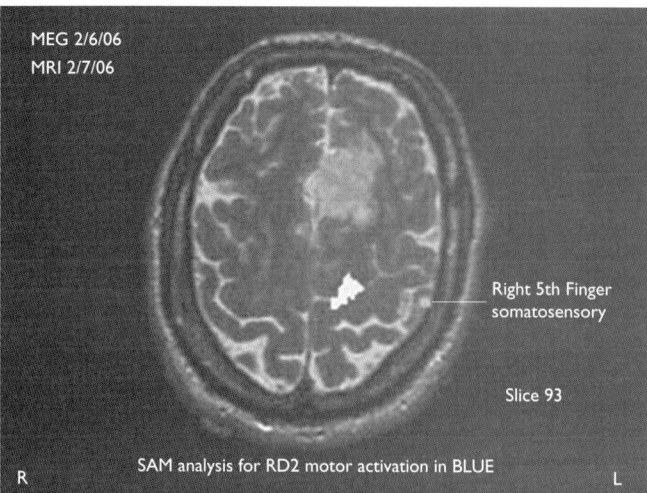

Figure 51.1 Magnetic source imaging demonstrating localization of the somatosensory cortex involving the right fifth finger. The white matter tract to the inside of the MSI point depicts a subcortical pathway subserving the motor cortex.

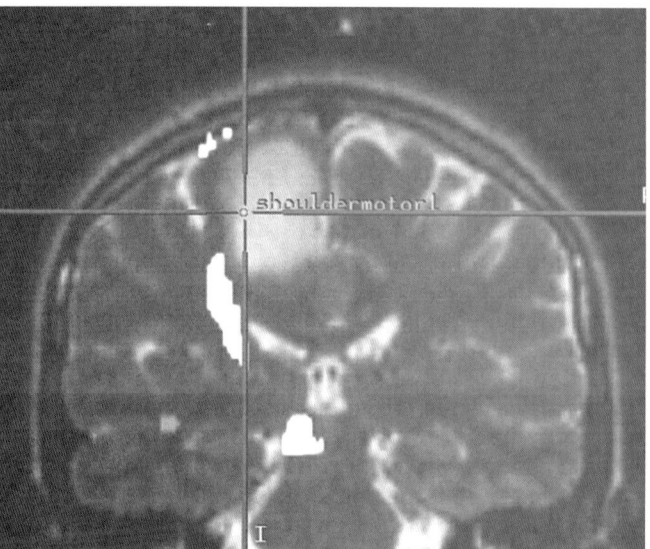

Figure 51.2 This is a diffusion tensor image showing the subcortical motor pathway within the corona radiata adjacent to the tumor. This particular component of the subcortical pathway subserves motor function involving the shoulder. The point within the crosshairs represents stimulation mapping of subcortical shoulder motor responses as depicted by the intraoperative navigation system.

the motor pathway by modeling three-dimensional local water diffusion along axonal membranes. DTI is used to visualize descending motor pathways starting from a functional cortical site and extending through the corona radiata, posterior limb of the internal capsule, and cerebral peduncle [11] (Figure 51.2). Fiber tracts delineated using DTI can be used to identify the motor tract in deep white matter and define a safety margin around the tract during tumor resection, a method that has been validated using intraoperative subcortical stimulation mapping of the motor tract and MSI [12]. DTI tractography, however, may be limited by tract termination or deviation in regions of peritumoral vasogenic edema and, therefore, should always be used in combination with intraoperative stimulation mapping.

Surgical Technique

After the dura is opened, and the patient's contralateral arm, leg, and face are uncovered to observe for movement, stimulation mapping begins with identification of the motor cortex. A bipolar electrode (5-mm spacing, 60 Hz, 1-ms phase duration) is placed on the surface of the brain for 2 to 3 seconds with a current amplitude between 2 and 16 mA. The motor strip is stimulated in the asleep patient with a starting current of 4 mA and increased in 2 mA increments until a motor response is visually identified. A current above 16 mA has never been necessary to evoke sensory or motor responses and should be avoided. The current is reduced to 2 mA when stimulating the awake patient and is raised in 1-mA increments for eliciting responses from both the motor and sensory cortex. At this point, cold Ringer's lactate solution should be available for immediate irrigation of the stimulated cortex should a focal motor seizure develop. This usually will abruptly stop the seizure activity originating from the irritated cortex, without the need for short-acting barbiturates (205). Multichannel electromyography recording may be used for greater sensitivity in detecting muscle movements (249), allowing the use of a lower stimulation current and decreasing the risk of stimulation-induced seizure activity. Stimulated brain sites are marked with sterile numbered tickets, or in some cases, a strip electrode (Figure 51.3A and 51.3B). First, eliciting responses in the face and hand identifies the inferior aspect of the rolandic cortex. For leg-motor cortex, a strip electrode may be inserted along the falx and stimulated using the same current applied to the lateral cortical surface to evoke leg-motor movements. This maneuver is safe due to lack of bridging veins between the falx and the leg motor cortex. Similarly, a subdural strip electrode may be used to locate the motor strip when the craniotomy is near but not overlying this cortex.

Once the motor cortex is defined, the resection proceeds with identification of the descending tracts using similar stimulation parameters. Functional white matter axons are depolarized using the same current parameters applied to the cortex (Figure 51.4A and 51.4B). When movements or paresthesias are evoked, the resection should cease because of the close proximity of intact functional pathways (current spread with bipolar stimulation is 2–3 mm from the electrode contacts). Following completion of tumor resection, a final stimulation of previously identified cortical motor sites confirms that underlying functional tracts have been preserved, which is equally valuable information in cases where subcortical responses are not obtained. The presence of intact cortical and subcortical motor pathways implies that any surgery-related deficit would likely be transient, with resolution in days to weeks. In the senior author's experience with surgery for hemispheric gliomas within or adjacent to the rolandic cortex, patients whose subcortical pathways were identified with stimulation mapping were more prone to develop an additional (temporary or permanent) motor deficit (27%) than were those

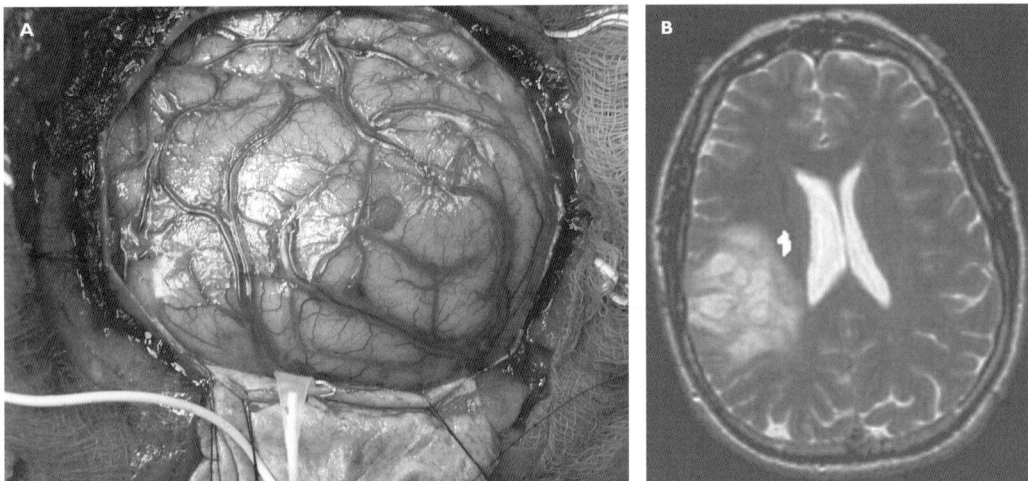

Figure 51.3 Exposed cortical surface demonstrating the region of the face motor cortex in the nondominant hemisphere. When the face motor cortex is stimulated, no responses are seen. Thus, a strip electrode (under the reflected dura) is inserted to identify the non-exposed hand and forearm motor cortex (A). A T2-axial MRI scan depicts the tumor seen in (A) with the underlying subcortical tract inserted using diffusion tensor image (B).

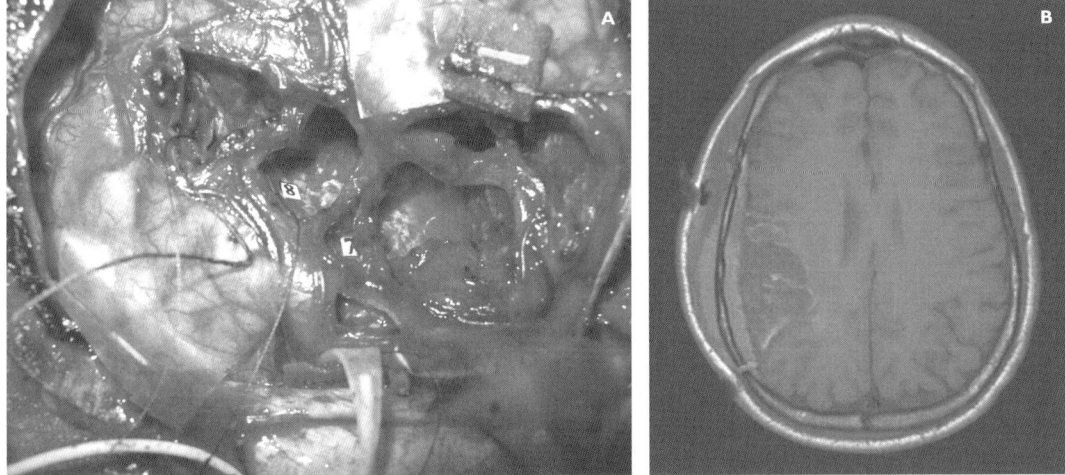

Figure 51.4 Subcortical sites depicted using stimulation mapping of the tumor that is resected in (A). Ticker numbers 8 and 7 represent subcortical stimulation-induced movement of the hand and forearm, respectively. Postoperative scan (B) demonstrates resection cavity with blood outlining the perimeter of the resection margins.

in whom subcortical pathways could not be identified (13.1%) [13]. Similarly, motor deficits that lasted more than 3 months occurred in 7.4% of the patients whose subcortical pathways were identified, compared to 2.1% of those without subcortical responses, although very few patients have been left with a dense paresis using this method.

LANGUAGE FUNCTION MAPPING DURING AWAKE CRANIOTOMY

Indications

Due to the discrete localization of essential language areas in the individual patient and great variation in their location across the population, an awake craniotomy with cortical stimulation mapping is indicated for any lesion involving the dominant temporal, mid- to posterior-frontal, and mid- to anterior-parietal lobes. Stimulation mapping has shown that multiple discrete areas in perisylvian cortex of the dominant hemisphere as essential for language functions, with separation of areas for different aspects of language, including naming in two languages, different semantic classes, naming compared to reading, and language from verbal memory [14]. Sites where stimulation repeatedly interferes with naming have been localized to focal areas of approximately 1 cm^2 in the dominant hemisphere cortex, frequently with one such site in perisylvian inferior frontal cortex and several others in temporoparietal cortex [15]. The exact location of these sites in the language-dominant hemisphere varies substantially across the patient population, particularly in temporoparietal cortex, with random distribution within the temporal lobe and in the inferior posterior frontal and anterior inferior parietal lobes. In addition, no specific region of the temporal-lobe cortex may be found to be essential for language function in nearly half of all patients (42–55%) [15,16].

With regard to bilingual patients, cortical stimulation studies have demonstrated the existence of both shared and distinct language-specific cortical centers. In one study of 25 bilingual patients, primary and secondary language representations were similar in total cortical extent, but differed in anatomical distribution [17]. Secondary sites were located exclusively in the posterior temporal and parietal regions, whereas sites for the primary language were found throughout the mapped region. Other studies in bilingual patients have demonstrated both common and separate cortical anomia areas for both languages in temporoparietal and frontal areas [18], anomia sites for the second acquired language that were always colocalized with anomia sites in the first acquired language [19], and anomia sites for each language that were always distinct and separate [20]. For these reasons, it is advisable to individually speech map each language in which the patient is fluent.

Preoperative Neurological Evaluation

Patients with dominant-hemisphere tumors in close proximity to language sites are ideal candidates for an awake craniotomy. Note that patients with significant vasogenic edema and mass effect from their tumor may not be candidates for an awake craniotomy due to the potential for cerebral herniation out of the dural opening. Despite the use of osmotic diuretics, awake patients are at risk for developing alterations in arterial CO_2 that may compromise the safety of the planned craniotomy and tumor resection. Swelling, herniation, and contusion may occur and lead to termination of the procedure.

The left hemisphere is dominant for language in 85% of the population, with right-sided dominance present in 6% and bilateral representation present in 9%. About 98% to 99% of right-handed individuals have left-sided language dominance. Thus, a Wada (intracarotid amytal) test is used almost entirely for verifying cerebral dominance in left-handed patients.

Those patients who undergo intraoperative mapping for language sites should be preoperatively tested for language errors by presenting the individual with a series of visual slides with common objects and words to be named and read, respectively. After confirming that the face motor cortex and Broca's area are functional by asking the patient to protrude the tongue and count to 10, the slides of common objects and words are shown. Patients must be able to name common objects with a baseline error rate lower than 25%, with each slide presented at least three times. In patients who have moderate-to-severe dysphasia in either comprehension or expression, successful language mapping will not be possible. Therefore, these patients may either be asleep during surgery, without any attempt to do more than an internal decompression, or be challenged with steroids and diuretics for 7 to 10 days and reevaluated regarding their baseline naming error rate. An alternative approach is to biopsy the tumor, confirm histopathology, and radiate the lesion to reduce its size or stabilize its growth, in hopes of producing functional recovery sufficient to allow for intraoperative mapping.

Preoperative Functional Imaging

Literature describing the correlation between cortical sites identified with language fMRI and those found by direct cortical stimulation at the time of surgery show variable agreement in localization [21], and, therefore, fMRI is not routinely used for preoperative planning. DTI studies of the superior longitudinal, inferior fronto-occipital and uncinatus fasciculi, reconstructed from anatomical landmarks, have depicted tracts occurring mostly at the periphery in high-grade gliomas, but frequently located inside the tumor mass in low-grade gliomas [22]. A high correlation (97%) between DTI fiber tracking and intraoperative subcortical stimulation was noted, suggesting that the combined use of these modalities may decrease the duration of surgery, resulting in less patient fatigue and intraoperative seizures. As we move into an era of functional imaging to preoperatively map descending language pathways, it becomes important to keep in mind that the pathways identified are purely anatomical and may not reflect the true functionality of the axonal bundles identified.

Neuroanesthetic Regimen

Before surgery, most patients receive midazolam (2 mg) and fentanyl (50–100 μg). During craniotomy surgery, propofol (50–100 μg per kilogram of body weight per minute) and remifentanil (0.05–0.2 μg per kilogram per minute) are given for sedation. No anesthesia is administered during mapping. When mapping is complete, sedatives are given again, typically dexmedetomidine (0.7–2.0 μg per kilogram per hour) administered with remifentanil (0.05–0.1 μg per kilogram per minute).

Surgical Technique

The initial primary goal during an awake craniotomy is to have a cooperative patient for speech-mapping purposes. It is imperative that the patient be kept comfortably sedated when mapping is not being performed. The propofol and remifentanil infusion is titrated for patient sedation during the incision and craniotomy. Once the bone flap is removed, the dura is infiltrated with local anesthetic along the middle meningeal artery. The dura should remain closed until the patient is awake and alert; otherwise, coughing and straining during emergence from propofol may cause the brain to herniate outward, especially if tumor edema and mass effect are present. All sedatives are then discontinued to restore the patient to an awake, cooperative state. During cortical mapping of language function, no sedatives are administered. If seizures occur during cortical mapping and are not controlled with cold Ringer's lactate solution, propofol can be given for seizure suppression.

After the motor pathways have been identified, the electrocorticography (ECoG) equipment is placed on the field and attached to the cranium. ECoG is used to monitor for after discharges induced by bipolar electrode stimulation of the cortex (Figure 51.5). The presence of after-discharge potentials indicates that the stimulation current is too high and must be decreased by 1 to 2 mA until no after-discharge potential is present following stimulation. Using the ideal stimulation current, object-naming slides are presented and changed every 4 seconds, and the patient is expected to correctly name the object during stimulation mapping. The answers are carefully recorded, and each cortical site is checked 3 times to ensure that there is no anomic or dysnomic stimulation-induced error. All cortical sites essential for naming are marked on the surface of the brain with sterile numbered tickets. Sites for reading may similarly be identified, following the presentation of slides showing single words. In addition, the patient is asked to count from 1 to 50 while the stimulation probe is placed near the inferior aspect of the motor strip to identify Broca's area. Interruption of counting (complete speech arrest), without oropharyngeal movement, localizes Broca's area. Speech arrest is usually localized to the area directly anterior to the face motor cortex within a few centimeters. On occasion, however, stimulation-induced speech arrest can be found anteriorly in the pars opercularis or above the face motor cortex in the inferior frontal gyrus. Throughout language mapping, ECoG is continuously monitored for after-discharge spikes to alleviate the possibility that naming errors are caused by the propagated effects of current spread or ongoing cortical depolarization (Figure 51.6A–51.6E).

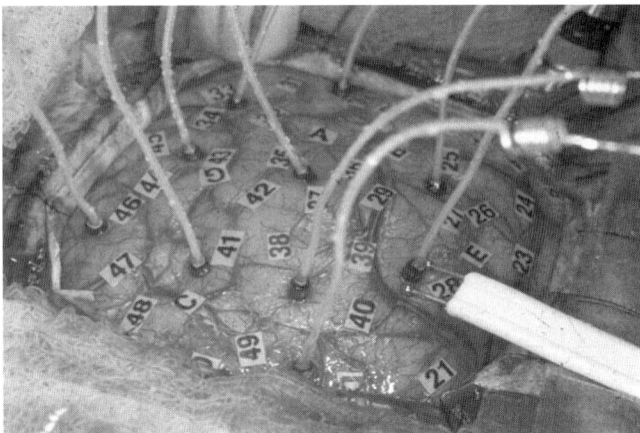

Figure 51.5 Electrocorticography equipment is shown in place, with the electrodes touching the cortical surface and the bipolar electrode stimulating around the electrode to identify after-discharge potentials.

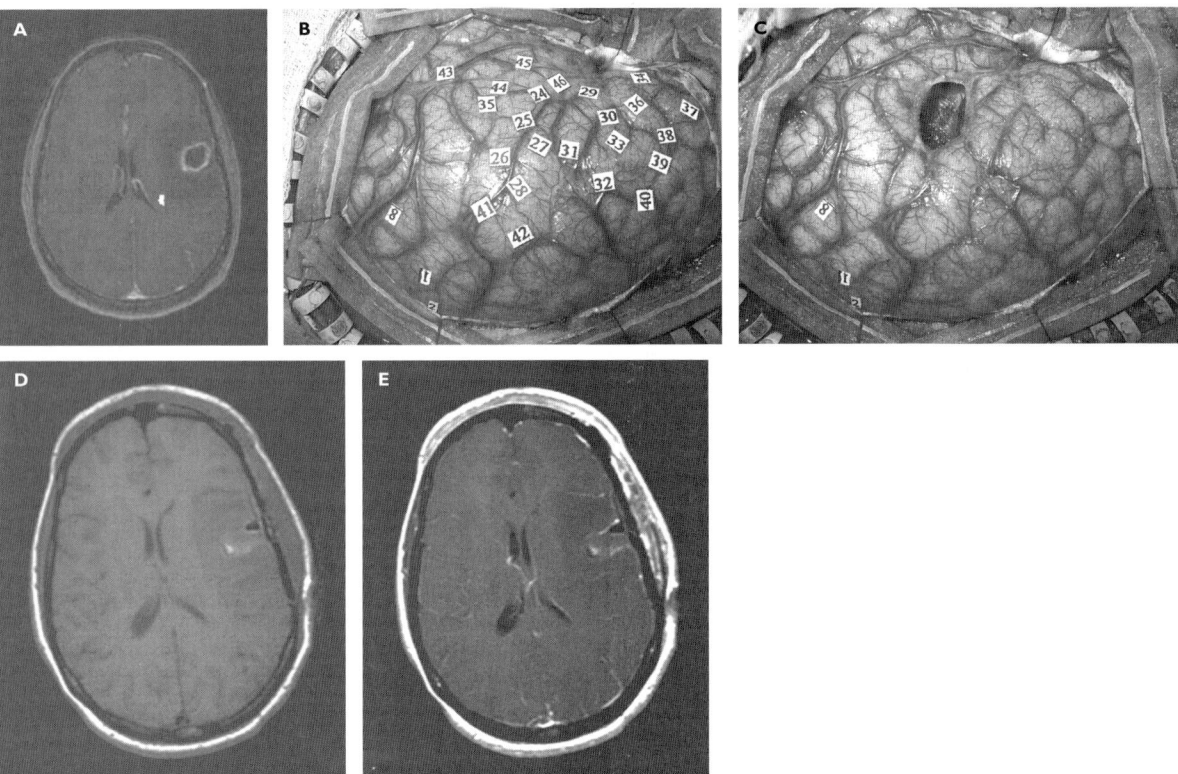

Figure 51.6 Preoperative MRI scan showing a moderate-sized contrast-enhancing necrotic tumor involving the posterior aspect of the inferior frontal lobe in the dominant hemisphere **(A)**. Intraoperative map **(B)** demonstrating the sensory cortex involving the mouth (#8) as well as the face motor cortex (#1 and 2). No sites for speech arrest, stimulation-induced anomia, or alexia were seen in the rest of the frontal lobe in any of the numbers depicted. Postresection intraoperative photograph showing resection of the tumor within the negatively mapped cortex **(C)**. Postoperative MRI scans **(D and E)** demonstrating the resection cavity with blood products following gross total resection of the high-grade glioma.

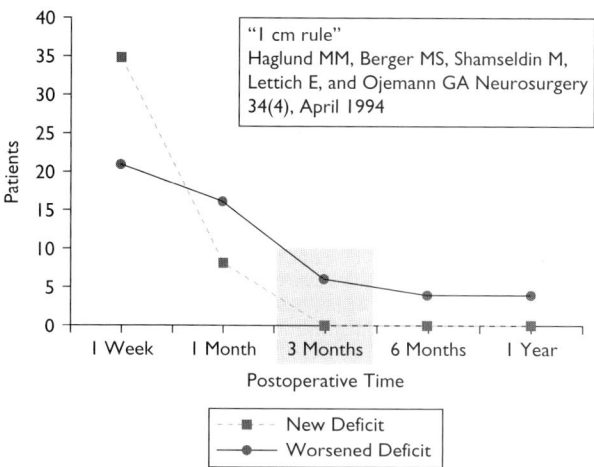

Figure 51.7 Postresection deficits based on the "1-centimeter rule." Language is preserved when the resection does not encroach within 1 cm of an essential language site. Although deficits may occur temporarily, no new deficits are seen following 3 months from surgery.

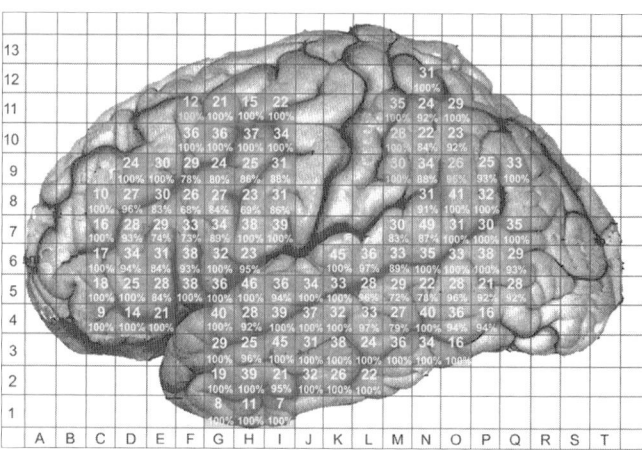

Figure 51.8 Cumulative negative mapping sites showing the number of times each cortical region was stimulated and the likelihood (percentage) that a site is negative for language with stimulation mapping [16].

Subcortical stimulation may also be used for detection of eloquent white matter bundles that are essential for language function [23]. Routine use of subcortical language-site identification has been reported to result in the identification of language-related cortical sites in 59% of patients [22]. In the group of patients in whom a subcortical language site was identified during resection, the likelihood of developing a permanent deficit was 3.8% (7% in patients with a preexisting language deficit), independent of histology and location. When no subcortical sites were found at the time of surgery, no permanent deficits were noted, indicating that when a subcortical response is reliably detected, resection must stop. Cortical stimulation studies have shown that the distance of the resection margin from the nearest language site is likely the most important variable in predicting improvement in preoperative language deficits, duration of postoperative language deficits, and permanence of postoperative language deficits [24]. If the distance of the resection margin from the nearest language site is >1 cm, significantly fewer permanent language deficits occur (Figure 51.7).

In line with these principles, the resection strategy does not require that stimulation-induced language sites be found within the field of exposure. The senior author recently reported language-function outcomes after glioma resection in 250 consecutive patients who underwent craniotomies tailored to limit cortical exposure, where tumor resection was directed by localization of the cortical regions that were not associated with stimulation-induced language or motor function [16]. This study again revealed tremendous variability in the localization of language sites, which went well beyond the classic anatomical boundaries of Broca's area, most typically involving areas contiguous with the face motor cortex, although many were located several centimeters from the sylvian fissure. In this group of patients, 42% had no positive language sites in their field of exposure. Historically, it was thought essential to identify areas where language was located before any nonfunctional area could be safely resected; however, only 1.6% of all patients had a persistent language deficit 6 months after surgery (92.9% of patients with an initial decrease in language function had complete recovery). This "negative mapping" strategy eliminates the surgeon's dependence on positive control sites, which allows minimal cortical exposure, less extensive intraoperative mapping, and a more efficient neurosurgical procedure (Figure 51.8).

SUMMARY

Identification of functional cortical areas in patients with brain tumors provides the neurosurgeon with the ability to achieve aggressive resections while preserving neurological function. The localization of intracerebral tumors via mapping of functional cortical and subcortical tracts has become an important tool in the preoperative assessment of patients with intrinsic cerebral tumors. The advantages of combining functional imaging information with a surgical navigation system are optimized when combined with intraoperative cortical and subcortical mapping. An analysis of the recent ECoG data showing task-specific changes in the spatial pattern of neuronal oscillations [25]. shows that it may be possible to localize function by correlating alterations in these rhythms with various behavioral tasks administered at the time of surgery rather than by directly stimulating cortical tissue.

REFERENCES

1. Berger MS, Deliganis AV, Dobbins J, Keles GE. The effect of extent of resection on recurrence in patients with low grade cerebral hemisphere gliomas. *Cancer.* 1994;74(6):1784–1791.
2. Keles GE, Anderson B, Berger MS. The effect of extent of resection on time to tumor progression and survival in patients with glioblastoma multiforme of the cerebral hemisphere. *Surg Neurol.* 1999;52(4):371–379.
3. Keles GE, Lamborn KR, Berger MS. Low-grade hemispheric gliomas in adults: a critical review of extent of resection as a factor influencing outcome. *J Neurosurg.* 2001;95(5):735–745.

4. Lacroix M, Abi-Said D, Fourney DR, et al. A multivariate analysis of 416 patients with glioblastoma multiforme: prognosis, extent of resection, and survival. *J Neurosurg.* 2001;95(2):190–198.
5. Smith JS, Chang EF, Lamborn KR, et al. Role of extent of resection in the long-term outcome of low-grade hemispheric gliomas. *J Clin Oncol.* 2008;26(8):1338–1345.
6. Penfield W, Boldrey, E. Somatic motor and sensory representation in the cerebral cortex of man as studied by electrical stimulation. *Brain.* 1937;60:389–443.
7. Berger MS, Kincaid J, Ojemann GA, Lettich E. Brain mapping techniques to maximize resection, safety, and seizure control in children with brain tumors. *Neurosurgery.* 1989;25(5):786–792.
8. Skirboll SS, Ojemann GA, Berger MS, Lettich E, Winn HR. Functional cortex and subcortical white matter located within gliomas. *Neurosurgery.* 1996;38(4):678–684; discussion 684.
9. Gallen CC, Sobel DF, Waltz T, et al. Noninvasive presurgical neuromagnetic mapping of somatosensory cortex. *Neurosurgery.* 1993;33(2):260–268; discussion 268.
10. Benzel EC, Lewine JD, Bucholz RD, Orrison WW. Magnetic source imaging: a review of the Magnes system of biomagnetic technologies incorporated. *Neurosurgery.* 1993;33(2):252–259.
11. Berman JI, Berger MS, Mukherjee P, Henry RG. Diffusion-tensor imaging-guided tracking of fibers of the pyramidal tract combined with intraoperative cortical stimulation mapping in patients with gliomas. *J Neurosurg.* 2004;101(1):66–72.
12. Berman JI, Berger MS, Chung SW, Nagarajan SS, Henry RG. Accuracy of diffusion tensor magnetic resonance imaging tractography assessed using intraoperative subcortical stimulation mapping and magnetic source imaging. *J Neurosurg.* 2007;107(3):488–494.
13. Keles GE, Lundin DA, Lamborn KR, Chang EF, Ojemann G, Berger MS. Intraoperative subcortical stimulation mapping for hemispherical perirolandic gliomas located within or adjacent to the descending motor pathways: evaluation of morbidity and assessment of functional outcome in 294 patients. *J Neurosurg.* 2004;100(3):369–375.
14. Ojemann GA. The neurobiology of language and verbal memory: observations from awake neurosurgery. *Int J Psychophysiol.* 2003;48(2):141–146.
15. Ojemann G, Ojemann J, Lettich E, Berger M. Cortical language localization in left, dominant hemisphere. An electrical stimulation mapping investigation in 117 patients. *J Neurosurg.* 1989;71(3):316–326.
16. Sanai N, Mirzadeh Z, Berger MS. Functional outcome after language mapping for glioma resection. *N Engl J Med.* 2008;358(1):18–27.
17. Lucas TH, McKhann GM, Ojemann GA. Functional separation of languages in the bilingual brain: a comparison of electrical stimulation language mapping in 25 bilingual patients and 117 monolingual control patients. *J Neurosurg.* 2004;101(3):449–457.
18. Roux FE, Trémoulet M. Organization of language areas in bilingual patients: a cortical stimulation study. *J Neurosurg.* 2002;97(4):857–864.
19. Walker JA, Quiñones-Hinojosa A, Berger MS. Intraoperative speech mapping in 17 bilingual patients undergoing resection of a mass lesion. *Neurosurgery.* 2004;54(1):113–117; discussion 118.
20. Bello L, Acerbi F, Giussani C, et al. Intraoperative language localization in multilingual patients with gliomas. *Neurosurgery.* 2006;59(1):115–125; discussion 115.
21. Roux FE, Boulanouar K, Lotterie JA, Mejdoubi M, LeSage JP, Berry I. Language functional magnetic resonance imaging in preoperative assessment of language areas: correlation with direct cortical stimulation. *Neurosurgery.* 2003;52(6):1335–1345; discussion 1345.
22. Bello L, Gallucci M, Fava M, et al. Intraoperative subcortical language tract mapping guides surgical removal of gliomas involving speech areas. *Neurosurgery.* 2007;60(1):67–80; discussion 80.
23. Duffau H, Capelle L, Sichez N, et al. Intraoperative mapping of the subcortical language pathways using direct stimulations. An anatomo-functional study. *Brain.* 2002;125(pt 1):199–214.
24. Haglund MM, Berger MS, Shamseldin M, Lettich E, Ojemann GA. Cortical localization of temporal lobe language sites in patients with gliomas. *Neurosurgery.* 1994;34(4):567–576; discussion 576.
25. Canolty RT, Edwards E, Dalal SS, et al. High gamma power is phase-locked to theta oscillations in human neocortex. *Science.* 2006;313:1626–1628.

52 Endoscopy

Johnathan A. Engh, Amin B. Kassam, Daniel M. Prevedello, and Paul A. Gardner

INTRODUCTION

The introduction of the microscope to neurosurgery represented a fundamental paradigm shift by providing superior light and magnification than the prior visualization tools. This dawned an era for the neurosurgeon to pursue the resection of complex intracranial tumors and, more important, facilitated the dissection of the circle of Willis. Over the ensuing decades, further refinements led to an improved understanding of the detailed microenvironment and, in particular, the vasculature and microcirculation of the brain. Pioneers such as Walter Dandy, Peter Jannetta, Ted Kurze, Al Rhoton, Bill Hitselberger, and Gazi Yaşargil led the way in improving this understanding, facilitating the path for a generation of neurosurgeons to follow. The fundamental properties that the microscope offered were light and magnification delivered across a corridor in a coned view creating the focal distance.

The endoscope was originally developed in 1806 by Bozzini. The first endoscopes were illuminated by candlelight for use in natural body cavities such as the rectum and the bladder [1]. It wasn't until the 1920s that Lespinasse and Dandy introduced the endoscope into the ventricular space for the treatment of hydrocephalus via fulguration of the choroid plexus [2]. There are two fundamental methods of using the endoscope for visualization. The first uses a fiber-optic pathway to transmit light and magnification to a camera. The fiber-optic visualization that is provided is primarily used during through-channel endoscopy. It is important to note that because this procedure involves working within the endoscope itself, it can prove to be constraining and limiting, possibly precluding true bimanual dissection.

By contrast, a rod-lens endoscope provides light and magnification through a rod lens to a camera. In this case, the endoscope is used only for visualization, and dissection is accomplished by a bimanual technique parallel to the endoscope. As a result, the fundamental principles of microsurgery can then be applied to the endoscope. This is in contrast to through-channel endoscopy.

With the evolution of the endoscope, surgeons began to take advantage of its ability to provide light and magnification directly at the source. This property is analogous to that of a flashlight as opposed to the cone of light associated with a microscope. To optimize the advantages of this technology, neurosurgeons began to incorporate the endoscope into microsurgical procedures, performing endoscopic-assisted microsurgery [3]. Over time, this then led to using the endoscope exclusively and solely for visualization and in turn the emergence of endoneurosurgery as a distinct field.

The endoscope has emerged as a versatile and independent instrument for many applications within the cranial space. Broadly, these applications can be divided into endonasal approaches (expanded endonasal approach) to the skull base and transcranial endoscopic surgery. These transcranial applications can be divided into conventional intraventricular approaches and, as more recent developments evidence, intra-axial approaches. Therefore, it is important that we discuss the various techniques of endoneurosurgery, which we will do so as detailed under the subheadings of endoscopic endonasal approaches (EEAs) and transcranial approaches, subdivided into sections on intraventricular and intra-axial approaches.

Before we embark on such a discussion, however, it is imperative that we first discuss the techniques of dissection that are used in endoneurosurgery. The tried and true techniques of microsurgery must be adhered to when using an endoscope for visualization. Specifically, microsurgical principles of bimanual dissection with internal debulking, followed by extracapsular dissection and early isolation of neurovascular structures, form the tenets of all resection principles, regardless of which equipment being used, an endoscope or a microscope. Therefore, it becomes, in our opinion, vital that any endoscopic tumor resection be able to allow for bimanual dissection.

ENDOSCOPIC SKULL-BASE SURGERY

Since the feasibility of purely endoscopic, endonasal, pituitary tumor resection was demonstrated over a decade ago, [4] applications of the EEA have been developed in a series of modular approaches to extend from the crista galli to the odontoid process in the sagittal (between the carotids) plane (Figure 52.1) and from the sella through the infratemporal fossa and jugular foramen in the coronal and paramedian (lateral to the carotids) plane (Figure 52.2) [5–9]. Each

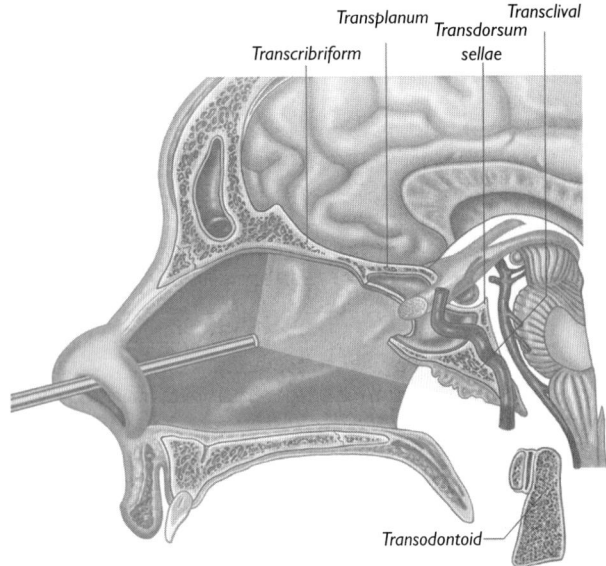

Figure 52.1 The endoscopic endonasal approach in the sagittal plane, featuring operative corridors from the subfrontal region (transcribriform) to the foramen magnum and below (transodontoid). Reprinted with permission from Kassam et al [1].

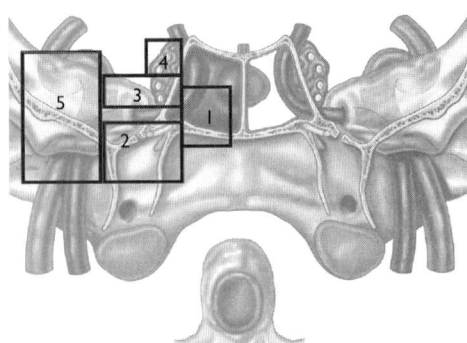

Figure 52.2 The endoscopic endonasal approach in the coronal plane, illustrating the five anatomic zones of paramedian structures lateral to the sella. The critical anatomic landmark in these approaches is the carotid artery, which compartmentalizes the five zones. Zone 1 is the medial pterygoid approach, zone 2, petrous apex approach; zone 3, quadrangular approach; zone 4, cavernous sinus approach; and zone 5, lateral pterygoid approach. Refer to the text for details Reprinted with permission from Kassam et al [5].

anatomic module is designed around the adjacent neurovascular structures. Collaboration between the otolaryngologist and the neurosurgeon is critical to the successful completion of expanded endonasal approaches. These operations truly represent "team surgery," a dynamic process of both visualization and tumor resection. We do not advocate the use of an endoscopic holder; rather, we prefer dynamic team surgery, akin to that of a pilot and a copilot working together to fly a plane. Cases are ideally performed in a dedicated neuroendoscopy suite, with video monitors available for both surgeons to have adequate visualization, and with a dedicated neuroanesthesia team possessing experience with these procedures. All patients are given a preoperative dose of a third- or fourth-generation cephalosporin (alternative broad-spectrum antibiotic if allergic), and this antibiotic is continued until any nasal packing is discontinued postoperatively. Postoperative infections are quite rare using this protocol; the authors have encountered a less than 2% incidence of postoperative bacterial meningitis in more than 800 cases to date.

Venous hemostasis for endonasal approaches is most often achieved through the use of warm saline irrigation (~40°C). Focal application of Avitene (Davol, Inc., Cranston, RI) on a cottonoid sponge or bone wax on a cottonoid sponge is effective for cavernous sinus and bony bleeding, respectively. Arterial bleeding is stopped using endoscopic bipolar cautery. In the event of a major vessel tear, the combined efforts of both surgeons are required to isolate the location of bleeding with maintenance of visualization and subsequently coagulate or ligate the vessel with a clip.

Access for EEA is binarial, with room for up to four instruments at a time (including the endoscope). Intraoperative image guidance is used to provide radiographic feedback coincident with visualized anatomic landmarks; these images are especially useful as teaching tools for novice endoscopists and surgeons in training. In addition, intraoperative image guidance is an indispensable tool for ensuring adequate exposure of the lesion of interest prior to dural opening. Taking the extra time to remove bone from the skull base is critical for safe intradural tumor surgery. In addition, it should be noted that the fundamental microsurgical principles of internal debulking, meticulous sharp dissection, and isolation of critical structures are as important (if not more so) to endoscopic skull-base surgery as they are to traditional skull-base surgery [10].

General Considerations of Exposure

We recommend a bilateral exposure for all EEA modules. This involves resection of the right middle turbinate followed by a wide sphenoidotomy. The left middle turbinate is lateralized and the sphenoidotomy is converted to a bilateral approach. The posterior one-third of the nasal septum is subsequently resected, a key step for appropriate exposure. This dissection technique allows for bimanual dissection without pushing the septum, which behaves as a curtain into the endoscope.

Sagittal Midline Approaches

Transsellar

The most common application of EEA is the transsellar approach for pituitary surgery. Following enlargement of the natural ostium of the sphenoid sinus, a wide bilateral sphenoidotomy that extends to the medial pterygoid plates laterally, superiorly to the planum sphenoidale, and inferiorly to the clival recess (Figure 52.3) provides the working corridor. This wide opening provides room for the endoscope to be freely maneuvered without being encumbered by bone or dissecting instruments. This creates a single rectangular cavity always consisting of a "sinus and a half." In the case of transsellar approaches, the opening consists of a complete sphenoid sinus (including the lateral

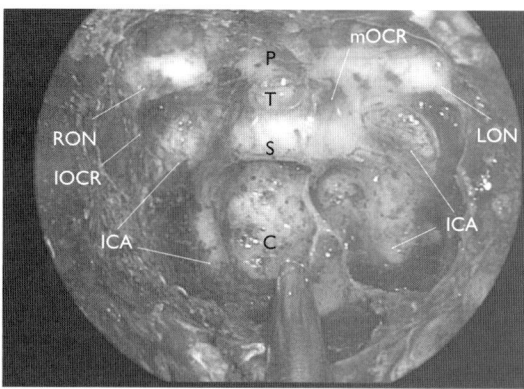

Figure 52.3 Demonstrating of the floor of the sella (S), clival recess (C), tuberculum sellae (T), planum sphenoidale (P), right optic nerve (RON), left optic nerve (LON), internal carotid artery (ICA), lateral opticocarotid recess (lOCR), and medial opticocarotid recess (mOCR), following bilateral wide sphenoidotomies, partial ethmoidectomies, and upper clivectomy for exposure of the midline skull base. The wide view is essential to avoid injury to neurovascular structures, during tumor resection.

recess) and half of a posterior ethmoid sinus. This allows for visualization of critical landmarks such as the medial optic-carotid recess, carotid prominence, and optic-nerve prominence [8].

Bone is drilled from the sellar floor, and the dura is opened in cruciate fashion, with attention to the inferior margin of the sella first. After an adequate specimen has been sent to pathology, a combination of two teardrop-suction devices can be used to deliver the tumor using "two-suction" technique (usually a 4 and 6 French suction or a 6 and 8 French suction). Fibrous bands are sharply divided. Care is taken to preserve the diaphragma sellae and to avoid damaging the normal pituitary gland, which is best differentiated from tumor by small microvessels on the surface of the gland. Though most commonly used on adenomas, these resection techniques are also useful for meningiomas and other sellar lesions. Figure 52.4 demonstrates the appearance of pre- and postoperative MRI following the complete resection of a pituitary macroadenoma by using the expanded endonasal approach.

Transplanum/Transcribriform

If the bony dissection from the sella is extended rostrally across the tuberculum sellae, then a transplanum approach can be performed. The superior intercavernous sinus lies immediately underneath the tubercular strut. Posterior ethmoidectomies provide access to the planum. It is imperative not to transgress the anterior limits of the posterior ethmoidal arteries, in order to avoid anosmia. Bony removal of the medial clinoid and lateral tubercular strut provides immediate control of the internal carotid arteries; the dura can then be opened safely for the removal of anterior skull base lesions such as planum meningiomas, suprasellar macroadenomas, and craniopharyngiomas. During resection, the critical neurovascular structures of the anterior skull base are viewed within the endoscope millimeters from the target (Figure 52.5). For lesions extending even

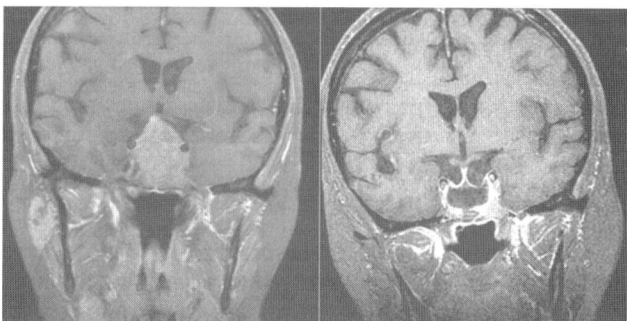

Figure 52.4 Pre- and postoperative coronal MRI scans with contrast enhancement, demonstrating complete resection of a pituitary macroadenoma by using the expanded endonasal approach. Reprinted with permission from Kassam et al [6].

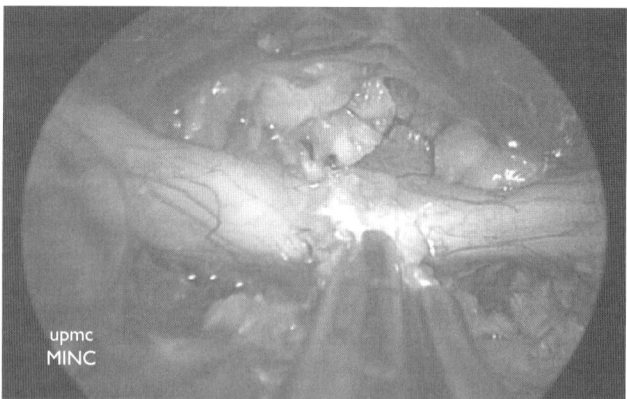

Figure 52.5 During the resection of a planum meningioma, the tumor is carefully removed from the optic chiasm while visualizing the anterior cerebral arteries and the anterior communicating artery directly above the chiasm. This visualization helps prevent injury to perforating vessels during tumor resection.

more anteriorly, a transcribriform approach can provide access to the crista galli or, if necessary, the frontal sinus. The anatomic boundaries of this module involve the entire ethmoid sinus (anterior and posterior) and the posterior half of the frontal sinus. The lateral margins of this rectangular box extend through the lamina papyracea to the periorbita creating a single cavity. Cauterization of the ethmoidal arteries provides rapid and immediate devascularization of the overlying pathology. This module is most commonly used for the resection of olfactory groove meningiomas and esthesioneuroblastomas [6].

Transclival

Caudal extension of the transsphenoidal approach provides access into the entire clivus. Transclival approaches are best divided into three modules: the superior third of the clivus (sella, dorsum, and posterior clinoid), the middle third of the clivus (Dorello's canal to the jugular foramen), and the inferior third of the clivus (below the jugular foramen). The superior clivus extends from the posterior clinoids to Dorello's canal. Removal of the superior clivus can

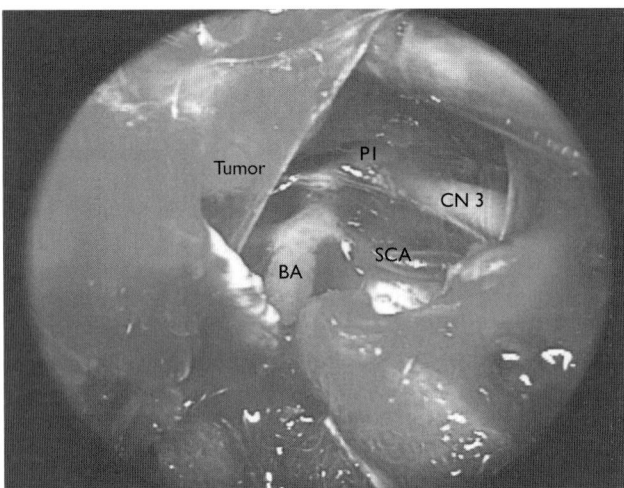

Figure 52.6 During resection of a craniopharyngioma, the interpeduncular recess is visualized endoscopically, including the basilar artery (BA), a duplicated superior cerebellar artery (SCA), the oculomotor nerve (CN 3), and the first segment of the posterior cerebral artery (PI). Tumor is superior and anterior to the vessel complex. The arachnoid over the PI and the SCA represents Liliequist's membrane.

Table 52.1 Segments of the Carotid and Critical Anatomical Landmarks

Segment	Anatomic Landmark
Paraclinoid	Medial clinoid
Anterior genu	Medial pterygoid
Horizontal segment	Vidian nerve
Ascending carotid	Eustachian tube

be used to gain access to lesions directly behind the pituitary gland (e.g., retroinfundibular craniopharyngiomas and germ-cell tumors) via pituitary transposition [11]. Although performing a pituitary transposition risks the development of hypopituitarism, it provides a more direct midline view of these lesions obviating manipulation of the critical neurovascular structures such as the oculomotor nerve and basilar artery that guard the interpeduncular fossa. For example, Figure 52.6 demonstrates the appearance of the interpeduncular recess during resection of a craniopharyngioma. The key anatomic landmarks here are the posterior clinoids, and the most common tumors treated are petroclival meningiomas and retrochiasmatic craniopharyngiomas.

The middle third of the clivus is bound laterally by the paraclival internal carotid artery (ICA), and it extends from the cavernous sinus to the foramen lacerum. The key anatomic landmark for this module is the medial pterygoid plate and the vidian nerve that mark the location of the lacerum segment of the ICA. It is imperative to stay between the medial pterygoids to avoid injury. Removal of this portion of the clivus is generally part of a panclival exposure for the resection of clival chordomas, chondrosarcomas, petroclival meningiomas, and some sinonasal tumors [8]. Further extension of the clivectomy inferiorly exposes the foramen magnum. Foramen magnum meningiomas and some chordomas require such an inferior extension of the endonasal approach for adequate resection.

Coronal/Paramedian-Plane Approach

The coronal/paramedian plane is defined as that portion of the ventral skull base that is located lateral to the carotid artery as it courses to the ventral skull base. The carotid artery as it rises along the skull base is best thought of in four segments. From the most proximal segment, this represents the parapharyngeal carotid that extends from a caudal to rostral direction and then enters the carotid canal at the posterior genu. The next segment is the horizontal segment that traverses horizontally across the petrous bone until it reaches the anterior genu. The anterior genu represents the third segment, which is located at the level of foramen lacerum, and the carotid artery then turns vertically to form the paraclival segment. This enters the cavernous sinus and then extends into the fourth component represented by the paraclinoid segment. Each of these segments has a critical anatomic landmark (Table 52.1). Therefore, the coronal plane is not a straight vertical plane but rather is a plane that is widest at the base, as the parapharyngeal carotids have the most distance between them, and narrowest at the top, as the paraclinoid segments have the least amount of space in between them. Furthermore, the coronal plane can be divided into an anterior coronal plane at the level of the anterior cranial fossa, a middle coronal plane at the level of the infratemporal and middle cranial fossa, and a posterior coronal plane at the level of the parapharyngeal carotid and posterior fossa.

Anterior

The anterior coronal plane really represents a variety of anterior transorbital modules that extend and open the lamina papyracea, which is line with the principles of the previous transcribriform approach. In this case, the lamina papyracea and the periorbita are opened and the intraorbital intraconal space can then be accessed. Often, these require transconjunctival incisions to mobilize the muscles to allow for endoscopic resection of intraconal pathology.

Middle

The middle coronal plane is occupied as that portion that extends lateral to the paraclival carotid artery. Traveling from a medial to a lateral direction, this involves traversing through the pterygopalatine fossa, the infratemporal fossa, and then into the temporal fossa. In this middle coronal plane, regions are divided into five zones on the basis of their anatomic location along the ICA (Figure 52.2). Zone 1 is the medial petrous apex approach, which essentially represents the lateral extension of a transclival approach. The vidian artery, nerve, and the medial pterygoid plate are used to gain access to the lacerum segment of the ICA, and then the vessel is mobilized laterally to provide access to the petrous apex.

The zone 2 approaches target the petrous bone beneath the ICA, that is, subpetrous/infrapetrous approach. Following identification of the lacerum segment of the ICA, bony dissection is extended laterally underneath the horizontal segment of the petrous carotid artery. Zone 3, also known as the quadrangular space approach, provides direct access to the anterior portion of Meckel's cave. This involves extension of the zone 2 approach into the space above the petrous carotid artery (suprapetrous approach), keeping the paraclival ICA medially and V2 laterally. The abducent nerve lies within the superior margin of this space. Further superior lateral extension allows access into zone 4, the cavernous sinus approach. Unlike the zone 3 approach, this approach has a relatively high risk of cranial neuropathy, and is not often performed, unless the patient already has a cavernous sinus syndrome. Further lateral extension along the midcoronal plane allows access to the infratemporal fossa, that is, zone 5. Working lateral to the petrous carotid, the surgeon can dissect into the infratemporal fossa [5]. It should be noted that this approach should only be undertaken by a team with significant endoscopic and vascular surgical experience.

Posterior

Further caudal extension along these paramedian planes occur lateral to the parapharyngeal carotid. These exposures generally involve identification of the parapharyngeal carotid by utilizing the Eustachian tube, which allows for bilateral extension. These posterolateral paramedian extensions provide access to the medial occipital condyle, hypoglossal canal, and jugular foramen sequentially from a medial to lateral direction. A variety of anatomic nuances and landmarks for this are represented by the location of the parapharyngeal carotid, posterolateral to the torus of the Eustachian tube. The most common lesions treated in this region are sinonasal carcinomas, jugulare foramen schwannomas, and a small subset of glomus jugulare lesions. Occasionally, cerebrovascular lesions, such as vertebral basilar aneurysms, can also be treated using this approach.

Reconstruction

The principles of reconstruction following endonasal surgery have undergone significant evolution. The original approaches utilized a series of autologous grafts, such as fat grafts, and synthetic grafts, such as a variety of dural substitutes. These required a varying degree of revascularization to occur over a protracted period of time to create a watertight seal. As a result, the initial experiences were very disappointing with a relatively high rate of cerebrospinal fluid (CSF) leak. Much like the case in open skull-base surgery, it's the evolution of vascularized pedicle reconstruction that really allowed for open cranial-base surgery to become a stand-alone specialty. It was only after vascularized tissue was developed, such as the pericranial flap, that open skull-base surgery became a viable option for treating disease in this location. Similarly, in the case of endonasal surgery, the development of the nasoseptal flap, in our opinion, has represented a sentinel event, as this allows for immediate vascularized reconstruction in a robust and consistent manner [12]. The current preferred technique involves a series of inlay grafts to reconstruct the arachnoid barriers consisting of a collagen matrix such as DuraGen (Integra LifeSciences, Plainsboro, NJ). Of note, these should not be used in isolation to reconstruct the dura. We instead use a nasoseptal flap that is harvested during the initial exposure. This uses a submucoperichondrial periosteal dissection with a vascularized flap that is pedicled on the posterior nasoseptal artery. The flap is then stored either in the maxillary antrum or the clivus during the resection. The flap is then mobilized and used as an onlay reconstruction, following the inlay reconstruction described previously. The flap is then held in position with a buttress by using a nasoseptal balloon to hold it in place. This provides for immediate, rapid vascularization in the majority of cases (Figure 52.7). Our experience with this technique has shown a CSF leak rate of 5.4% following endonasal surgery, which is comparable to data from reconstruction following conventional open skull-base surgery [13].

TRANSCRANIAL ENDOSOPIC APPROACHES

Endoscopic Intraventricular Surgery

Intraventricular tumors are a small subset of brain tumors on the whole, but they represent some of the first intracranial tumors to be removed using an endoscopic approach. Common pathologies include colloid cysts, subependymomas, central neurocytomas, choroid plexus tumors, meningiomas, and subependymal giant-cell astrocytomas. As

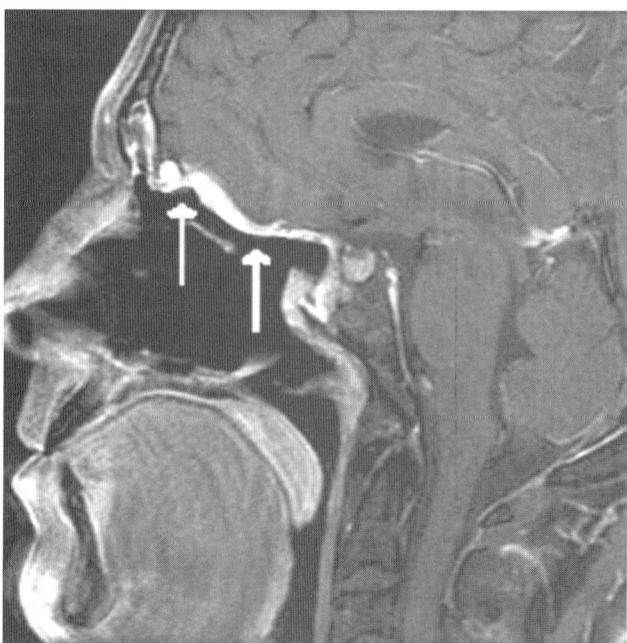

Figure 52.7 Postoperative, sagittal, contrast-enhanced MRI scan demonstrating brisk enhancement of the pedicled nasoseptal flap (NSF), following endoscopic endonasal tumor resection of an esthesioneuroblastoma of the ventral skull base.

is the case with skull-base tumors, the principles of intraventricular tumor resection remain constant: All tumors should be resected with the best visualization possible, damage to surrounding neural structures should be minimized using microsurgical techniques, and the anatomy of the patient should determine the safest corridor into the tumor.

The first endoscopic intraventricular tumor resections were performed using through-channel fiber-optic endoscopes. Resection is carried out within a fluid medium, and instruments are introduced through the working channel of the endoscope. Large lesions and calcified lesions are difficult to resect using this technique. Therefore, some authors have suggested that the limitations of through-channel endoscopy are intraventricular tumors that are less than 2 cm in length, friable, noncalcified, and nonvascular [14–16].

To overcome the limitations of through-channel endoscopy, the use of a rod-lens endoscope was developed. In this case, the endoscope is used only as a visualization tool that allows the surgeon to work parallel to the scope. The key advantage of this technology is the surgeon's ability to operate with both hands, using the microsurgical principles explained earlier. Specifically, we use stereotactic guidance to place an 11.5-mm transparent, cylindrical conduit transcortically into the ventricle [17]. This device is called the neuroendoport (Figure 52.8) The ventricle is cannulated using a bullet-shaped dilator, which is passed over a brain needle. Following removal of the dilator, the transparent conduit is left behind, and CSF is aspirated to create an air medium for endoscopy. The fundamental difference in this technique is the ability to work in an air medium rather than a fluid medium, coupled with the ability to use standard bimanual microsurgical techniques. Microsurgical instruments modified for endosurgery are passed parallel to the endoscope within the port, thereby specifically allowing for the piecemeal resection of large and complex lesions while still maintaining the principles of microsurgical technique (Figure 52.9).

The patient is positioned supine on an intraoperative computed tomography (CT) scanner bed, intubated, and administered perioperative antibiotics, 10 mg of dexamethasone, and an appropriate dose of anticonvulsants. The patient is placed into a Leksell G (Elekta Instruments, Stockholm, Sweden) stereotactic frame, and a preoperative CT is performed. Frameless stereotaxis may also be used. Performing the operation on a CT scanner bed provides not only the convenience of the targeting scan but also the ability to perform an immediate postoperative scan before leaving the operating room. The planning CT scan is used to delineate a trajectory into the ventricle. A small craniotomy is performed (~2.5 cm), either by using a trephine or a high-speed air drill. Following the craniotomy, the dura is opened in cruciate fashion. Hemostasis is obtained, and a 5- to 6-mm cortisectomy is performed. The brain needle is then passed through the cortisectomy, and the dilating device with the neuroendoport attached is passed over the needle. Essentially this represents the Seldinger technique. The entire device is anchored to the stereotactic frame to ensure pinpoint accuracy. Care is taken to avoid excessive evacuation of CSF prior to final positioning of the conduit.

A 4-mm rod-lens endoscope is brought into the field and secured rigidly on a custom-designed holder with a dynamic arm (Armand Holder, KLS Martin, Jacksonville, FL). This holder allows the endoscope to be docked against the edge of the port and out of the way of microsurgical instruments. However, the port and the endoscope are repositioned multiple times to facilitate the resection of tumors considerably larger in size than the 11.5-mm port itself. To remove larger lesions, the scope must maintain its ability to move with at least 4 degrees of freedom, thus essentially becoming steerable.

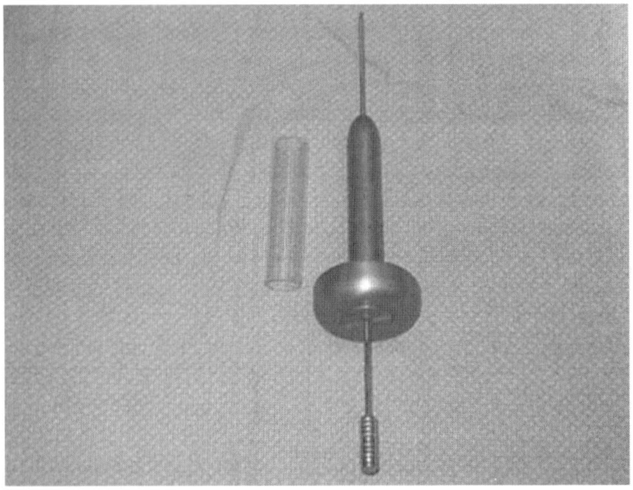

Figure 52.8 Transparent conduit (left) and bullet-shaped dilator with brain needle for the performance of "neuroendoport" surgery. The conduit is 11.5 mm wide and varies in length between 5.5 and 6.5 cm, depending on the depth of the target selected. The conduit is placed on the dilator during the initial tumor cannulation; upon removal of the dilator, the conduit is left behind.

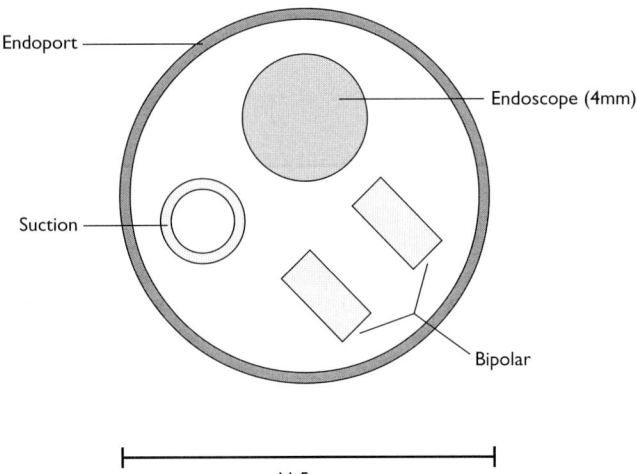

Figure 52.9 Schematic cross-sectional view of the 11.5-mm diameter endoscopic port featuring the endoscope, the bipolar cautery, and a suction device all working within the same space. Bimanual dissection and microsurgical technique are performed through this port, although the learning curve is steep.

Colloid cysts are the most common intraventricular masses seen in our practice. For patients with symptomatic lesions or lesions >7 mm in size, resection is generally recommended. Rather than a microsurgical transcortical or transcallosal approach, the completely endoscopic approach can be performed through a small cortisectomy to achieve resection. The dilator allows the port to be placed parallel to white matter fascides, creating radial retraction and minimizing focal trauma. Following removal of the port, these fascides tend to recover their native position. Stereotactic guidance is critical to avoid positioning the head of the caudate nucleus between the port and the lesion due to a poor trajectory. Following visualization of the lateral ventricle, a septostomy is performed to maximize relaxation of the ventricles. A 0.5-cm cottonoid sponge is placed at the foramen of Monro to prevent bleeding into the ventricular system, and the tumor is resected using the standard microsurgical techniques of sharp dissection and bipolar coagulation. Special care is taken to avoid thermal injury to the internal cerebral vein or the thalamostriate vein and to avoid manipulation of the fornix immediately anterior and superior to the foramen of Monro. Complete resection of the cyst is performed, including the cyst wall, following evacuation of cyst contents (Figure 52.10). We believe that by being able to use bimanual microsurgical techniques, more complete resections are feasible than with through-channel endoscopy.

Other intraventricular tumors can vary in difficulty of resection, depending on location and friability. Subependymomas tend to have relatively low vascularity and low viscosity; therefore, they are quite amenable to endoscopic removal. The most difficult intraventricular tumors to remove endoscopically are calcified intraventricular meningiomas. However, with meticulous microsurgical technique and sharp dissection, these tumors can be devascularized and safely removed piecemeal, despite minimal manipulation of surrounding white matter. Ultrasonic aspirators have also been developed for endoneurosurgery application. For very large tumors, staged resection is performed (Figure 52.11).

At the conclusion of the resection, the intraventricular region is irrigated with warm saline, and any bleeding is controlled with bipolar cautery or Avitene on a cottonoid sponge. A ventriculostomy catheter may be left in the ventricle if there is thought to be a high risk of postoperative hydrocephalus, though this is rarely needed. Intraoperative CT scanning can be performed either after dural closure or after skin closure, according to the surgeon's preference, to rule out any postoperative hemorrhage.

Completely Endoscopic Intra-axial Tumor Resection

One of the essentials of successful endoscopy is the presence of a medium through which light may pass in order for the target to be visualized. In the case of intraparenchymal tumors, such a natural cavity is lacking; as a result, endoscopic techniques for these lesions are far less developed than they are for skull-base tumors and intraventricular tumors. Though surgeons have reported on using the endoscope as an adjunct to the microscope following intra-axial tumor resection, [18] very few have attempted completely endoscopic tumor resection while operating on intraparenchymal tumors. However, the endoscope offers an ideal, minimally invasive approach to deep-seated pathology; for this reason, the authors have pursued its use for intra-axial tumors in recent years. The ability to dilate white matter along fiber tracts creates corridors into deep-seated lesions, preserving not only critical cortical structures but also underlying white matter connections.

In 1980, the endoscope was used to target intraparenchymal lesions while mounted onto a stereotactic frame [19,20]. A visualization medium was created for the endoscope by a tulip-shaped retractor, which dissected away white matter to allow light into the cavity. In 1990, Otsuki and colleagues reported on the use of a bullet-shaped dilator to create a medium for endoscopic resection of intra-axial tumors [21]. Their dilator was also attached to a stereotactic frame. Multiple tumors were removed using this approach. Despite the precision of the stereotactic-assisted endoscopic method, this technique is lacking in the ability to dissect around large tumors at multiple angles. The more versatile solution for such tumors is to use an endoscopic port with frameless image guidance. In our experience, this tube is allowed to be a modular instrument; at multiple times during the resection of the tumor,

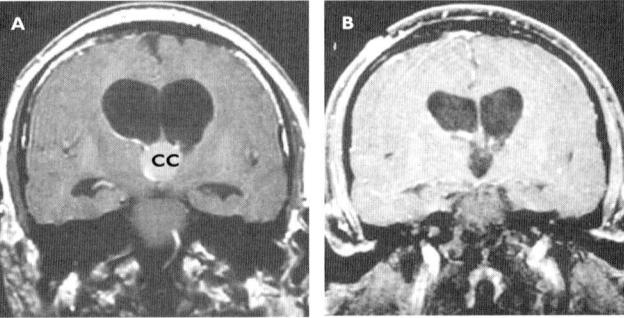

Figure 52.10 (A) Pre- and (B) postoperative coronal contrast-enhanced MR images depicting a colloid cyst before and after complete endoscopic resection.

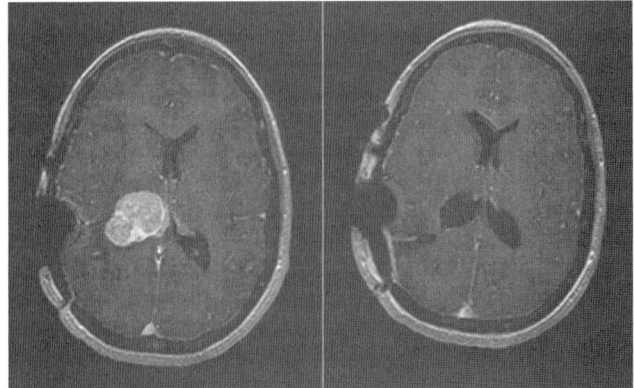

Figure 52.11 Pre- and postoperative contrast-enhanced axial MR images depicting a recurrent 3.5-cm intraventricular meningioma that was completely endoscopically resected in two stages.

the angle of the tube and the endoscope is changed to improve the view of the lesion, all through a minimal cortisectomy and a single cannulation, that is, a steerable conduit facilitating optimum visualization of the target while permitting bimanual microsurgery.

The completely endoscopic tumor resection begins with a 2.5-cm craniotomy, targeted according to preoperative image guidance. Patients are preloaded with dexamethasone, antibiotics, and anticonvulsants. The patient is fixated in a rigid, radiolucent head holder on the intraoperative CT scanner bed. Following the craniotomy, the cruciate dural opening and cortisectomy are identical to the intraventricular technique. Rather than cannulate the ventricle, the dilator device with overlying port is passed over a brain needle into the base of the tumor of interest (Figure 52.12). Upon withdrawal of the dilator, the port is held in place, and any cystic component of the tumor typically delivers itself into the port. It is important to note that the deepest portion of the tumor is cannulated first. This creates a central core within the tumor of negative pressure/low pressure. The outside of the port has much higher pressure, and this pressure gradient delivers the tumor into the port. The tumor is then removed from the deepest parts first, with progressive decannulation. When combined with steerability, this allows for large tumors to be delivered through small corridors.

The endoscope is introduced into the field, and teardrop suctions (usually 6 French and 8 French) are used to aspirate tumor with the previously described two-suction technique. Generally, the surgeon searches for an interface between the tumor and surrounding white matter (Figure 52.13). Then, using one suction to aspirate tumor and the other to provide countertraction, the tumor is removed piecemeal. Bleeding is controlled either with warm saline irrigation, Avitene sponges, or bipolar cautery. At the risk of being redundant, it is important to reiterate the fundamental tenant of intra-axial neuroendoport surgery: The regional increase in intracranial pressure surrounding the tumor is exploited to allow the tumor to deliver itself into the port. As the tumor collapses, the conduit is slowly decannulated from the brain to allow residual superficial tumor to fall into view for removal. Resection generally proceeds from deep to superficial, opposite to microscopic techniques. The port is dynamically manipulated throughout the procedure to ensure maximal resection. However, white matter injury is minimized by the use of the cylindrical conduit. Figure 52.14 presents a schematic of some common cannulation sites for deep tumors.

During resection, image guidance is a useful tool to confirm the location of the port and to guide subsequent trajectory adjustments. For example, Figure 52.15 demonstrates the port adjacent to the falx during the resection of a parietal metastasis. This image confirmed the surgeon's suspicion to move anteriorly along the falx in order to continue tumor resection. In addition, the image guidance allowed for planning of a trajectory that did not endanger the ipsilateral motor strip, inferior parietal lobule, or visual cortex.

At the conclusion of the endoscopic resection, the operative field is dried with warm saline irrigation by using bipolar cautery only when necessary. Following decannulation, the cortical defect is covered with a small piece of DuraGen (Integra LifeSciences, Plainsboro, NJ). The dura is approximated over the collagen matrix, and a head CT is performed prior to the completion of wound closure. In certain cases, intravenous contrast is given to visualize any residual enhancing tumor prior to leaving the operating room.

Using the endoscopic port, the disturbance to surrounding white matter appears to be minimal relative to

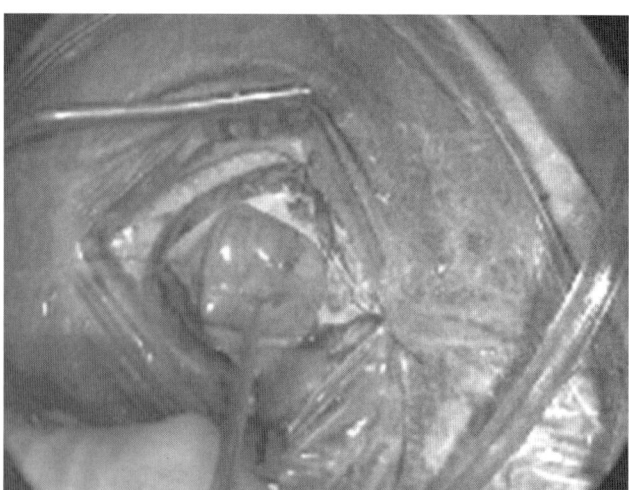

Figure 52.12 Cannulation of a right frontal tumor using the endoscopic port. Following a cruciate dural opening, a 5- to 6-mm cortisectomy is performed. The image-guidance probe (Stryker, Inc., Kalamazoo, MI) is used to determine the trajectory (pictured above). Next, the brain needle is passed through the cortisectomy site, and then the dilating device is placed over the needle, creating a 11.5-mm conduit. Following withdrawal of the dilator, the port is left within the parenchyma.

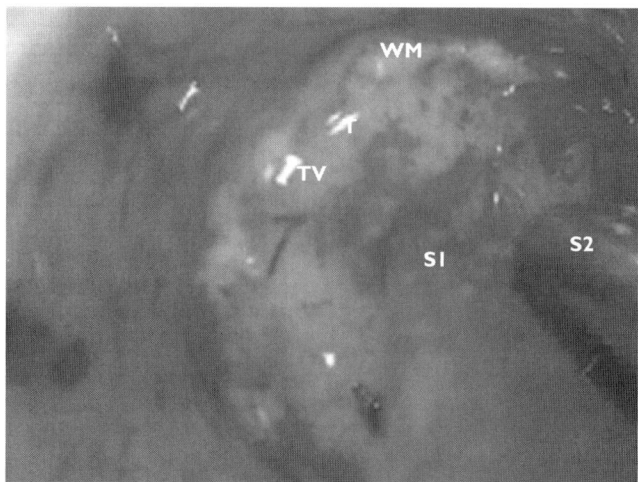

Figure 52.13 Intraoperative endoscopic view of resection of a glioblastoma via a completely endoscopic technique. Note the interface between white matter (WM) and tumor (T) and the thrombosed vein (TV) within the tumor. The two suctions (S1 and S2) are used to dissect and aspirate tumor, with excellent endoscopic visualization. The view of the white matter through the transparent conduit is noted to the left edge of the photograph.

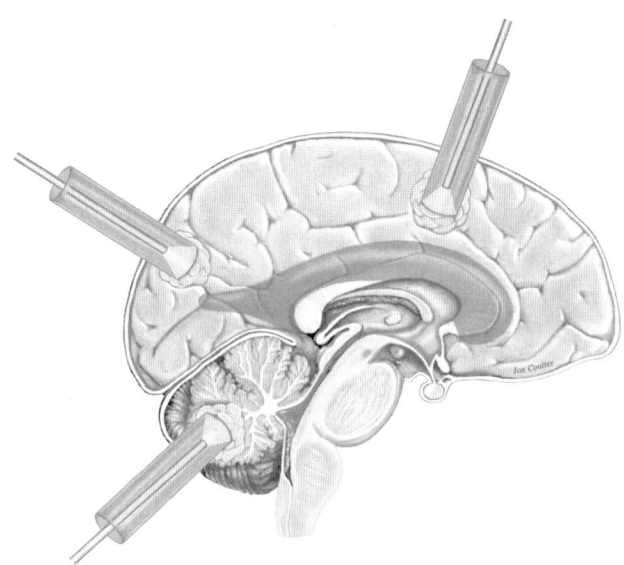

Figure 52.14 Schematic diagram of common cannulation trajectories for intraparenchymal brain tumors. A transcoronal approach is shown for a frontal tumor, a transparietooccipital approach is shown for an occipital tumor, and a transcerebellar approach is shown for a cerebellar tumor. The tube represents the endoscopic resection port, and the endoscope with the expanding cone of light is shown illuminating the tumor bed. In addition, a variety of transtemporal and other approaches are feasible for completely endoscopic tumor resection.

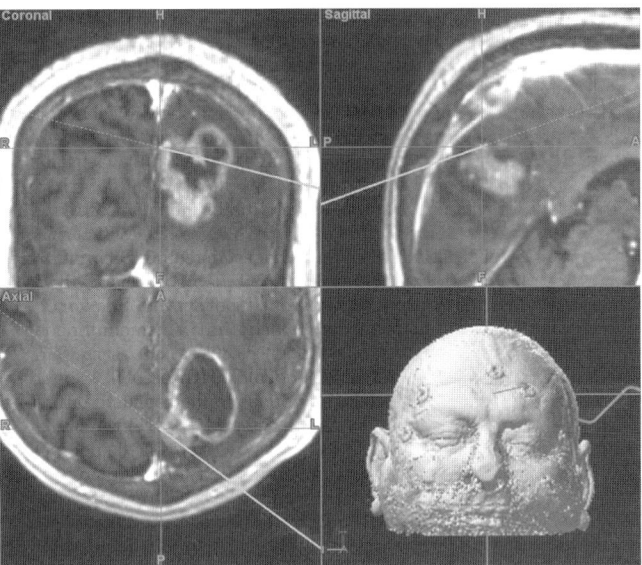

Figure 52.15 Intraoperative image guidance scan demonstrating resection of a left parietal metastasis (Stryker, Inc., Kalamazoo, MI). This image was used to guide dissection in an anterior and inferior direction, facilitating near-total metastasis resection.

standard microsurgical techniques. As opposed to the spatulas and retractors used for the microscope, the port is designed to dilate white matter tracts rather than transect them. The ultimate goal is to create a paradigm of parafascicular surgery, instead of transfascicular surgery. For large or deep lesions beneath the cortical mantle, both primary and metastatic, the neuroendoport appears to be an effective and safe alternative to the microscope in our early experience.

CONCLUSION

The rod-lens endoscope has become an effective and independent visualization instrument for the resection of both extra- and intra-axial brain tumors. In many cases, the endoscope has distinct advantages over the microscope for the treatment of specific tumors, including improved visualization and a telescopic light source. At all times, the operative corridor into the lesion of interest is dictated by the surrounding neurovascular structures. Prevention of iatrogenic damage to surrounding structures during tumor removal is critical to procedural success. As smaller corridors into larger lesions are realized the surgeon maintains the ability to maximize effective resection and minimize surgical trauma. The endoscope is now accepted as an effective tool in mainstream procedures for skull-base and intraventricular neurosurgery and is beginning to grow as an independent instrument for intra-axial tumor surgery. Continued experience and outcomes data, combined with consideration of the needs of individual patients, will allow future surgeons to decide which brain tumors are the most suitable for endoscopic resection. There will always be a role for microscope visualization, and the endoscope is complementary. However, it is more important that the basic principles of microsurgery are not compromised, notwithstanding which visualization tool is selected for use, for example, an endoscope or a microscope.

REFERENCES

1. Reuter HJ. *Philipp Bozzini and Endoscopy in the 19th Century*. Stuttgart: Max Nitze Museum; 1988.
2. Abbott R. History of neuroendoscopy. *Neurosurg Clin N Am*. 2004;15:1–7.
3. Perneczky A, Fries G. Endoscope-assisted brain surgery: part I-evolution, basic concept, and current technique. *Neurosurgery*. 1998;42:219–225.
4. Carrau RL, Jho HD, Ko Y. Transnasal-transsphenoidal endoscopic surgery of the pituitary gland. Laryngoscope. 1996;106:914–918.
5. Kassam AB, Gardner P, Snyderman C, Mintz A, Carrau R. Expanded endonasal approach: fully endoscopic, completely transnasal approach to the middle third of the clivus, petrous bone, middle cranial fossa, and infratemporal fossa. Neurosurg Focus. 2005;19(1):E6.
6. Kassam A, Snyderman CH, Mintz A, Gardner P, Carrau RL. Expanded endonasal approach: the rostrocaudal axis. Part I. Crista galli to the sella turcica. *Neurosurg Focus*. 2005;19(1):E3.
7. Kassam A, Snyderman CH, Mintz A, Gardner P, Carrau RL. Expanded endonasal approach: the rostrocaudal axis. Part II. Posterior clinoids to the foramen magnum. *Neurosurg Focus*. 2005;19(1):E4.
8. Kassam AB, Snyderman CH, Carrau RL, et al. *The Expanded Endonasal Approach to the Ventral Skull Base: Sagittal Plane*. Tuttlingen, Germany: Endo-Press; 2007.
9. Kassam AB, Snyderman C, Gardner P, Carrau R, Spiro R. The expanded endonasal approach: a fully endoscopic transnasal approach and resection of the odontoid process: technical case report. *Neurosurgery*. 2005;57(1 suppl):E213.
10. Prevedello DP, Kassam AB, Snyderman C, et al. Endoscopic cranial base surgery: ready for prime time? *Clin Neurosurg*. 2007;54:48–57.
11. Kassam A, Prevedello D, Thomas AJ, et al. Endoscopic endonasal pituitary transposition for transdorsum sellae approach to the interpeduncular cistern. *Neurosurgery*. 2008;62(3 suppl 1):57–72.

12. Hadad G, Bassagasteguy L, Carrau RL, et al. A novel reconstructive technique after endoscopic expanded endonasal approaches: vascular pedicle nasoseptal flap. *Laryngoscope.* 2006;116:1882–1886.
13. Kassam A, Thomas A, Carrau RL, et al. Endoscopic reconstruction of the cranial base using a pedicled nasoseptal flap. *Neurosurg.* 2008 Jul;63(ONS Suppl 1):44–52; discussion 52–53.
14. Gaab MR, Schroeder HW. Neuroendoscopic approach to intraventricular lesions. *J Neurosurg.* 1998;88:496–505.
15. Hellwig D, Bauer BL, Schulte M, Gatscher S, Riegel T, Bertalanffy H. Neuroendoscopic treatment of colloid cysts of the third ventricle: the experience of a decade. *Neurosurgery.* 2003;52:525–531.
16. Souweidane M. Endoscopic management of pediatric brain tumors. *Neurosurg Focus.* 2005;18(6):E1.
17. Harris AE, Hadjipanayis CG, Lunsford LD, Lunsford AK, Kassam AB. Microsurgical removal of intraventricular lesions using endoscopic visualization and stereotactic guidance. *Neurosurgery.* 2005;56(1 suppl):125–132.
18. Teo C, Nakaji P. Application of endoscopy to the resection of intra-axial tumors. *Op Tech Nsgy.* 2005;8:179–185.
19. Jacques S, Shelden CH, McCann GD, Freshwater DB, Rand R Computerized three-dimensional stereotaxic removal of small central nervous system lesions in patients. *J Neurosurg.* 1980;53:816–820.
20. Shelden CH, McCann G, Jacques S, et al. Development of a computerized microstereotaxic method for localization and removal of minute CNS lesions under direct 3-D vision: technical report. *J Neurosurg.* 1980;52:21–27.
21. Otsuki T, Jokura H, Yoshimoto T. Stereotactic guiding tube for open-system endoscopy: a new approach for the stereotactic endoscopic resection of intra-axial brain tumors. *Neurosurgery.* 1990;27:326–330.

53 Transsphenoidal

Ashok R. Asthagiri, Adam S. Kanter, Edward H. Oldfield, and John A. Jane, Jr.

Neoplastic transformation within the adenohypophysis is a frequent event that generally results in the formation of histologically benign adenomas. A meta-analysis of radiographic and postmortem studies provides the true prevalence rate of a pituitary adenoma, that nearly one in five persons among the general population harbors this ailment [1]. The majority of these lesions are small, incidental tumors and are clinically silent, but the remainder constitutes 10% to 15% of all symptomatic intracranial tumors treated by neurosurgeons [2]. The chapter aims to provide a systematic review of the current diagnostic methods and treatment alternatives utilized in the management of the more common subtypes of symptomatic pituitary adenomas.

CLINICAL PRESENTATION

The clinical presentation of symptomatic pituitary adenomas varies significantly, depending on the underlying pathological subtype. Broadly, pituitary adenomas may be characterized on the basis of causes for presentation and their functional hormone-secreting status (Table 53.1). Tumors that produce prolactin (PRL), growth hormone (GH), thyroid-stimulating hormone (TSH), and adrenocorticotropic hormone (ACTH) typically present with the remote effects of hormone hypersecretion. In addition, these functioning tumors may enlarge to the extent they cause local mass effect due to the insidious progression of systemic hormonal sequelae. Iatrogenic disruption of the end-organ target of pituitary hormone hypersecretion may lead the "functional" adenoma to cause symptoms through local mass effect alone. Nonfunctioning adenomas present clinically with signs of mass effect on adjacent structures, including the optic chiasm (bitemporal hemianopsia), neurovascular elements coursing through the cavernous sinus (ophthalmoplegia, facial numbness), native pituitary gland (hypopituitarism), and dura mater investing the sella (headaches).

FUNCTIONAL ADENOMAS

PRL-Secreting Adenomas

PRL-secreting tumors account for 40% of all pituitary adenomas and are the most common subtype of functional adenoma. Circulating PRL excess results in gonadal and sexual dysfunction, the effects of which vary according to the patient's age and sex. In adult women, disruption of the hypothalamic-pituitary-gonadal axis is caused by minor elevations in PRL and results in secondary amenorrhea and galactorrhea (Forbes-Henneman-Griswold-Albright syndrome). In adult men, the cardinal symptoms are reduced libido, dysfunctional semen production, and sexual impotence. Larger tumors with higher pretreatment serum PRL levels are more common in men [3,4]. This may be secondary to the different sequelae of excess PRL production between the sexes or a greater awareness of the symptoms by women. However, the possibility of a more

Table 53.1 Pituitary Adenomas are Characterized on the Basis of Their Clinical Presentation and Functional Hormone-Secreting Status

	Mass Effect	**Endocrinopathy**
Functional adenoma	• ACTH adenoma (after bilateral adrenalectomy—Nelson syndrome) • TSH adenoma • Plurihormonal adenomas[a]	• Prolactinoma (Forbes–Albright syndrome in women, impotence and infertility in men) • TSH adenoma • ACTH adenoma (Cushing disease) • GH adenoma (acromegaly/gigantism)
Nonfunctional adenoma	• Null-cell adenoma • Gonadotropin-secreting adenomas • Silent subtype III adenomas* • Oncocytomas[a]	• Nonfunctional adenomas may cause endocrinopathies due to mass effect on the normal pituitary gland (hypopituitarism) and stalk compression effect (increased circulating prolactin)

[a] A review of clinical presentation, diagnosis, and treatment of these lesions is beyond the scope of this chapter.

aggressive disease course in men has not been excluded. Consequently, it follows that men more frequently present with visual-field disturbances and hypopituitarism. Pubertal-age patients, like their adult counterparts, not only display a similar gamut of symptoms but can also present with pubertal delay. Children typically present with visual disturbance, headache, and hypopituitarism (growth failure) rather than due to the effects of hormone hypersecretion.

Diagnosis of a PRL-secreting adenoma in the setting of hyperprolactinemia relies on the exclusion of secondary causes of circulating-hormone elevation and subsequent radiographic confirmation of the presence of a tumor. Normal circulating levels of PRL in men is <20 µg/L and <25 µg/L in women. Physiologic increases in PRL levels occur during pregnancy (up to a 10-fold increase), after exercise, eating, and rarely after breast examination (Table 53.2). Serum PRL levels may also elevate as a result of impaired clearance from renal failure or hepatic insufficiency. Pharmacologic causes of secondary hyperprolactinemia (metoclopramide, phenothiazines, butyrophenones, risperidone, monoamine oxidase inhibitors, tricyclic antidepressants, serotonin-reuptake inhibitors, verapamil, reserpine, methyldopa, estrogen) typically result in levels between 25 µg/L and 100 µg/L that readily return to normal levels within days of drug cessation [5]. Exclusion of these secondary causes should prompt further evaluation with pituitary-region-specific gadolinium-enhanced magnetic resonance imaging (MRI).

Identification of a sellar-based lesion in the setting of hyperprolactinemia does not guarantee the diagnosis of a prolactinoma. Large, nonfunctioning adenomas and other lesions in the area (Rathke cleft cyst, craniopharyngioma) may cause elevations in serum PRL levels (25–200 µg/L) from stalk compression and disruption of dopamine (PRL inhibitory factor) transport. Once PRL levels reach 200 µg/L, a diagnosis of prolactinoma is more certain. A subset of PRL-secreting macroadenomas that produce very high levels of serum PRL may masquerade as nonfunctioning tumors exhibiting stalk compression effect, with serum PRL levels returning at <100 µg/L. This laboratory artifact, termed the "hook effect," is readily apparent when serial dilutions of the serum samples are performed [6].

The therapeutic goals in the treatment of prolactinomas are (a) to return PRL levels to gender-specific norms, with resolution of gonadal and sexual dysfunction, and (b) to resolve symptoms due to mass effect. The primary management of most prolactinomas is medical therapy with dopamine-receptor agonists. Unlike other adenohypophysial hormones, the physiologic control of PRL production is mediated via tonic inhibition through dopamine activation of the D2 receptor. Cabergoline, an ergot-alkaloid derivative, is the drug of choice for initial pharmacotherapy because it has been shown to be more effective in lowering PRL levels to normal and reducing tumor size and having fewer side effects when compared to bromocriptine [7,8]. One exception may be in pregnancy, where the safety of bromocriptine therapy has been more widely studied and thus is preferred by some practitioners and patients. Pergolide, a synthetic ergot-alkaloid derivative that required only once-daily dosing, was recently withdrawn from the US market due to side effects of cardiac-valve fibrosis associated with its use at high doses in the treatment of Parkinson disease [9]. Similar findings have been reported with high-dose Cabergoline therapy, suggesting care in its administration. Nevertheless, it is not clear whether the low doses used in the treatment of prolactinomas will carry the same risks.

Surgery for treatment of prolactinomas is rarely curative and, therefore, should be reserved for cases of resistance or intolerance to medical therapy and for those in whom long-term drug treatment is not acceptable. Specific circumstances, as in the case of unstable pituitary apoplexy, or lesions causing rapidly progressive visual loss, may also necessitate surgical decompression. Radiation therapy also assumes a secondary role in the management of prolactinomas. Historically, fractionated radiotherapy was utilized in the treatment of recurrent or residual pituitary tumors. Due to the prolonged latency for effect and risk to adjacent structures, there has been a strong movement toward the utilization of stereotactic radiosurgical (SRS) techniques (LINAC, Gamma Knife). SRS is generally reserved for the subset of patients with tumors that are refractory to both medical and surgical therapy.

GH-Producing Adenomas

GH-producing adenomas represent approximately 30% of all hormonally active tumors and, depending on the age of onset of hypersecretion, cause acromegaly and/or gigantism. Due to the gradual onset of symptoms, diagnosis of acromegaly is often delayed for a period of 8 to 10 years. This provides an explanation for the high proportion (60%) of these tumors that are identified as macroadenomas (>10 mm) at initial diagnosis [10–12]. Acromegaly presents with soft-tissue hypertrophy and skeletal hyperostosis that manifest with characteristic facial (frontal bossing, prognathism, teeth separation) and skin changes (increased thickness and oily and sweaty skin), large joint arthropathy (axial and appendicular), and peripheral nerve-entrapment syndromes (carpal-tunnel syndrome). Systemic findings in acromegaly include development of biventricular cardiac hypertrophy, insulin resistance and diabetes mellitus, hypertension, and a possible increased risk of malignancy. The clinical presentation of gigantism is more overt due to gross changes in stature that are evident due to GH excess before epiphyseal closure. Hyperprolactinemia and its endocrinologic sequelae occur in 30% of patients, due to stalk compression effect or cosecretion of both hormones

Table 53.2 Common Causes of Hyperprolactinemia and Associated Typical Serum Prolactin Levels

Cause of Hyperprolactinemia	Typical Serum Prolactin Level (µg/L)
Pregnancy	25–250
Pharmacotherapy	25–100
Tumors resulting in stalk effect	25–200
Macroprolactinoma	>200

(mammosomatotroph adenomas). In addition to their direct endocrinologic effect, many GH-producing pituitary adenomas display signs of local mass effect resulting from growth allowed by subtle systemic disease progression.

The biologic effects of excess GH secretion are mediated through the increased hepatic production of insulin-like growth factor I (IGF-1). Because IGF-1 has a prolonged serum half-life, serum levels remain the same throughout the day despite pulsatile variations in serum GH levels. Normal serum levels of IGF-1 vary with gender and age. When normalized for sex and age, the measurement of serum IGF-1 level serves as an ideal screening test. The current international consensus for the diagnosis of acromegaly recommends a nadir GH level of more than 1 µg/L during standard, Oral Glucose Tolerance Test in conjunction with clinical suspicion and high adjusted IGF-1 levels [13]. Subsequent to laboratory evaluation, diagnosis of a pituitary source of GH hypersecretion is confirmed with gadolinium-enhanced MRI.

The primary goals in the management of acromegaly are (a) to restore GH and IGF-I values to the normal range for age and sex, with reduction in morbidity and mortality associated with this elevation, (b) to resolve symptoms due to mass effect, and (c) to completely and permanently eradicate the tumor. Surgical resection, typically via the transsphenoidal route, is the preferred initial treatment because it provides an opportunity for rapid and complete normalization of GH secretion. Surgical management of macroadenomas and those exhibiting invasion are associated with approximately 50% success in achieving normalization of GH secretion, whereas surgeries performed on microadenomas have higher success rates (70%) [14–20]. Reported recurrence rates after successful surgery have ranged from 0% to 19%, emphasizing the need for long-term endocrinologic and radiologic surveillance despite apparently curative surgery [19,21–23]. Treatment of persistent or recurrent GH elevation warrants consideration for reoperation, employing medical therapy, and/or radiotherapy.

Medical treatment can play an integral role in the management of acromegaly through reduction of IGF-1 production. Somatostatin analogues (octreotide, lanreotide), and their long-acting depot forms, inhibit GH secretion via the somatostatin-receptor subtypes 2 and 5 [24]. A meta-analysis reviewing their utilization in the treatment of acromegaly revealed reduction of GH levels and normalization of IGF-1 levels in 48% and 42% of acromegalic patients, respectively [25]. In addition, a measurable tumor-volume reduction was observed in approximately 36% of patients and tumor enlargement during treatment occurred rarely (<2%) [26]. Dopamine agonists (bromocriptine, cabergoline) are also used to inhibit pituitary GH secretion, though the mechanism that mediates the reduction remains less clear. Studies evaluating the efficacy of dopamine agonist therapy reported relatively lower rates of GH response and normalization of IGF-1 levels, though responses are better in GH/PRL cosecreting tumors and in patients with lower pretreatment IGF-1 levels [27]. Whereas somatostatin analogues and dopamine agonists indirectly reduce IGF-1 levels through reduction of GH levels, pegvisomant works at the peripheral target as a GH-receptor antagonist. This directly inhibits hepatic IGF-1 production but has no effect on the pituitary adenoma itself. The lack of IGF-1 feedback inhibition results in an increase in GH production but does not appear to cause a trophic response in the pituitary tumor, at least in the comparatively short duration of available studies. Recent studies show that pegvisomant is effective in achieving normalization of IGF-1 levels in 89% to 97% of patients [28,29]. Although none of these medical treatments are curative, they may serve as a primary treatment option for patients in whom surgery is not feasible, as a short-term bridge to relieve the effects of persistent GH and IGF-1 elevation while awaiting surgery, or, as an adjunct to radiotherapy, following unsuccessful surgery or recurrence.

Radiotherapy remains an important therapeutic alternative in patients with surgically and medically refractory acromegaly. Stereotactic radiosurgery offers single-fraction delivery, faster hormonal response, and excellent control of tumor growth (>95%) [30]. Conformity and steep dose falloff minimize radiation effect to adjacent neurovascular structures. Conventional fractionated radiotherapy offers similar efficacy in control of tumor growth (>95%) but theoretically may take longer to product the desired effect. It is available regardless of the size of the field of therapy and can be used for tumors that are close to the optic nerves and chiasm. Thus, it is an option in certain circumstances in which radiosurgery is not a good choice due to tumor size or contiguity of the tumor to the optic system. Because both methods of radiotherapy show variable efficacy in controlling GH and IGF-1 levels, concomitant medical therapy is often used [20,31].

Adrenocorticotropin-Secreting Adenomas

Adrenocorticotropin (ACTH)-secreting adenomas account for approximately 15% to 25% of all functional pituitary adenomas and are responsible for two-thirds of all cases of Cushing syndrome. In response to hypersecretion of ACTH, the adrenal cortex increases production of glucocorticoids that results in profound metabolic changes and systemic sequelae. The characteristic habitus of Cushing disease (central obesity, thin extremities, buffalo hump, supraclavicular fat pad) develops from the central mobilization of adipose tissue. Thinning of skin, proximal muscle wasting, easy bruisability, and large violaceous striae are result of the catabolic effects of excess glucocorticoids. Hypercortisolemia also results in hypertension, psychiatric disorders, osteoporosis, insulin resistance, and diabetes mellitus. Although well characterized, the gradual onset of this cluster of signs and symptoms is easily overlooked.

Biochemical screening in search for support of a diagnosis of Cushing syndrome is initially performed with measurement of 24-hour urinary-free cortisol, a low-dose dexamethasone suppression test, measurement of late night salivary-cortisol levels and/or measurement of midnight serum cortisol. If Cushing syndrome is confirmed, the next step in the evaluation is measurement of serum ACTH levels. Cushing disease and occult ectopic sources of ACTH production are associated with normal to moderately elevated serum ACTH levels, whereas suppressed ACTH levels are indicative of an intrinsic adrenal lesion.

Next, the integrity of the hypothalamic-pituitary-adrenal axis is evaluated with high-dose dexamethasone testing. Semblance of feedback inhibition is maintained in most cases of Cushing disease (80–90%) and serum cortisol levels decrease, whereas ectopic tumors are not usually sensitive to feedback inhibition by high-dose dexamethasone. Additional testing that may support the diagnosis of Cushing disease include responses to corticotrophin-releasing hormone (CRH) and desmopressin. Although neither the dexamethasone suppression tests nor the CRH stimulation test are independently highly specific, they each have a positive predictive value high enough to be useful if the results are positive [32,33]. A pituitary-region-specific and gadolinium-enhanced MRI should be performed in all patients with ACTH-dependent Cushing syndrome. Even with the current advances in MRI technology, up to 38% of microadenomas may remain unvisualized [34–36]. The sensitivity and accuracy of MRI is appreciably enhanced by using certain MRI imaging techniques. Discordant cases in which MRI does not reveal a discrete lesion and biochemical evaluation of the source of ACTH-dependant Cushing syndrome is equivocal or suggests the presence of a pituitary source should be further evaluated with bilateral inferior petrosal sinus sampling (IPSS) with CRH stimulation. As the petrosal sinus drains venous blood from the tumor in the region of the pituitary and sellar region, a gradient of petrosal–peripheral ACTH levels, representing secretion of ACTH by the tumor in the presence of suppression of the normal corticotrophs, is generated in Cushing disease. Utilizing a threshold ratio greater than 2 at baseline, and greater than 3 with CRH stimulation, the sensitivity and specificity of bilateral IPSS with CRH stimulation in identifying a pituitary source for ACTH hypersecretion approaches 95% (Figure 53.1) [37,38].

Patients who are subject to false-negative extrapituitary localization of disease origin often undergo bilateral adrenalectomy and may present later with effects of a rapidly growing sellar neoplasm. The lack of end-organ feedback inhibition creates a trophic environment for the growth of a previously occult ACTH-secreting pituitary adenoma. These patients with Nelson syndrome, the combination of very high levels of serum ACTH and progressive tumor growth, lack features of cortisol excess but typically harbor an aggressive pituitary adenoma that causes local mass effect in conjunction with hyperpigmentation due to increased melanocyte-stimulating hormone production, a byproduct of increased ACTH production from the division of the common precursor molecule—proopiomelanocortin (POMC).

Transsphenoidal adenomectomy is the treatment of choice in the management of Cushing disease because it provides an opportunity for rapid and complete normalization of ACTH secretion and complete tumor elimination. Although various institutions utilize different standards in determining success rates, a recent review of reports published since 1995, with a minimum of 40 patients and 6-month follow-up, found overall success rates to be 68% to 98%, with recurrence rates varying from 5% to 11.5% [39]. As expected, immediate surgical remission rates are higher among patients with microadenomas as opposed to those with macroadenomas or those displaying invasion.

Medical management of Cushing disease is generally not considered a first-line option but is frequently used to temporize the effects of hypercortisolemia preoperatively and in conjunction with radiotherapy while waiting for effect. Attempts to modulate ACTH secretion with dopamine agonists, GABA agonists, somatostatin analogues, and serotonin antagonists have rarely demonstrated clinical efficacy. Pharmacotherapy in Cushing disease has been most successful in the reduction of cortisol production through the use of adrenal-enzyme inhibitors. Ketaconazole, a potent inhibitor of 17,20-lyase and 17α-hydroxylase, usually produces a biochemical remission via inhibiting cortisol production. The most common adverse effect from therapy is hepatotoxicity that necessitates monitoring of liver function while receiving treatment. In cases where stand-alone ketaconazole therapy is ineffective, not tolerated, or is overcome, additional adrenal-enzyme inhibitors (metyrapone, aminoglutethimide) or adrenolytic agents (mitatone) may be utilized for further medical control of cortisol levels. However, these medical therapies that simulate bilateral adrenalectomy also have the potential to induce enhanced ACTH secretion and tumor growth, as in Nelson syndrome following surgical adrenalectomy. Thus, they are most commonly used while awaiting the effects of irradiation therapy, or in certain instances in preparation for surgery.

Residual and recurrent disease after pituitary surgery is usually treated with fractionated radiation therapy. Long-term results indicate biochemical remission in 53% to 100% of patients and excellent control of tumor growth in patients with Cushing disease [40–42]. Because of the impetus for more conformal dosing and the convenience of single dosing, stereotactic radiosurgery has been increasingly used in the adjunctive treatment of Cushing disease over the past decade. Infrequently, biochemical remission may not be attained despite surgery, radiotherapy, and pharmacotherapy. To curtail the significant deleterious effects of hypercortisolemia, the need for bilateral adrenalectomy may arise. When this is performed, many centers also use pituitary irradiation to reduce the incidence of

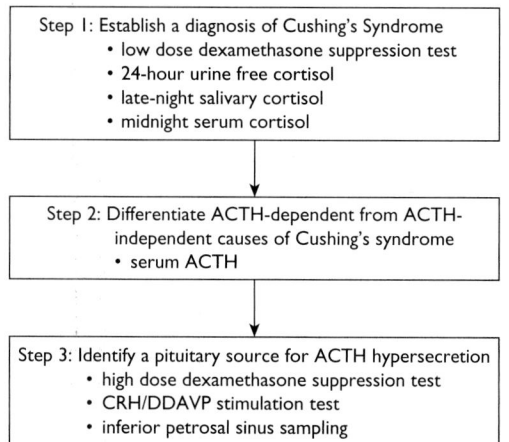

Figure 53.1 Approach to the diagnosis of Cushing syndrome.

Nelson syndrome and those that do not use close monitoring with serial ACTH measurement and sellar imaging with MRI to detect the possible development of Nelson's syndrome.

Thyrotropin (TSH)–Secreting Adenomas

Thyrotropin-secreting adenomas are rare and account for less than 2% of all pituitary adenomas [43,44]. Most patients present with a protracted development of secondary hyperthyroidism (weight loss, palpitations, tremulousness, difficulty in sleeping, excessive sweating, and fatigue) and imaging reveals a macroadenoma in greater than 90% of patients. At the time of diagnosis, 40% of lesions display extensive invasion into parasellar and suprasellar locations [45,46]. Less frequently, overt symptoms of hyperthyroidism may lead to the discovery of a microadenoma. Occasional cosecretion of mammosomatroph-derived hormones (GH, PRL) may result in clinical features associated with these respective hormone excesses.

The biochemical diagnosis of a TSH adenoma begins with the initial demonstration of an unsuppressed serum TSH in the setting of high-circulating levels of free thyroxine (FT4) and tri-iodothyronine (T3) levels. The lack of feedback inhibition is confirmed with a short T3 suppression test that reveals a lack in suppression of circulating TSH levels. Normal controls generally suppress TSH levels to <10% baseline [47]. These tumors cause loss of normal circadian rhythmicity in serum TSH levels (levels increase at night) and is further supportive of autonomous TSH secretion. Key to the biochemical diagnosis of a TSH-secreting adenoma is distinguishing this entity from the syndrome of pituitary resistance to thyroid-hormone feedback, a rare autosomal dominant disorder characterized by a similar circulating TSH, FT4, and T3 profile [48]. Octreotide administration suppresses TSH secretion in patients with adenomas because of the high concentration of somatostatin receptors found in these tumors. A thyrotropin-releasing hormone (TRH) stimulation test usually does not increase TSH secretion in adenomas but causes an exaggerated response in patients with pituitary resistance to thyroid hormone. The TSH molecule is composed of a unique β-subunit and an α-subunit common to TSH, luteinizing hormone (LH), follicle-stimulating hormone (FSH), and human chorionic gonadotropin (HCG). As tumors secrete excess α-subunit compared to TSH, evaluation of the baseline serum α-subunit levels and α-subunit/TSH ratio (α-subunit/TSH molar ratio) typically reveals higher levels in patients harboring pituitary TSH-secreting adenomas [49].

The therapeutic goals in the treatment of TSH adenomas are to (a) obviate the effects of TSH hypersecretion, (b) resolve symptoms due to mass effect, and (c) eliminate the tumor. Regardless of the initial treatment chosen for addressing the adenoma, medical therapy (β-blocker and antithyroid agent) is instituted initially to reduce the effect of excessive thyroid hormones. The initial form of definitive therapy in the treatment of most TSH-secreting adenomas is surgery. The advantages of surgery include immediate elimination of mass effect and the potential for a complete and curative resection. Because of high variability in patient selection, duration of follow-up and criteria for biochemical remission and reported surgical remission rates vary from 0% to 80% [45–47,50,51]. Tumors operated upon with extensive extrasellar invasion are associated with higher morbidity, mortality, and incomplete removal.

Currently, medical therapy is typically used in patients who fail surgical management or whose systemic conditions preclude operative intervention. The majority of tumors display somatostatin receptors and are amenable to treatment with somatostatin analogs. Indeed, somatostatin analog therapy normalizes thyroid function in 75% to 96% of patients and induces tumor shrinkage in up to 50% of patients [43,47,52,53]. In patients who have persistent elevation of TSH despite surgery and medical therapy or who cannot tolerate medical therapy for one reason or another, radiation therapy or radiosurgery remain an option.

NONFUNCTIONING ADENOMAS

Nonfunctioning adenomas (gonadotropin-secreting, null-cell adenoma, silent subtype III, oncocytomas) comprise approximately one-third of most large, unselected pituitary-adenoma surgical series and almost universally present due to symptoms of local mass effect. Their effect on the normal pituitary gland often leads to subclinical hypopituitarism. A thorough evaluation of the entire hypothalamic-pituitary axis reveals reduced GH levels in more than 85% of patients, reduced gonadotropin levels in 70%, reduced ACTH levels in 30%, and reduced thyrotropin levels in 25%. A balance in PRL secretion may occur by offsetting stalk compressive effect with native lactotroph dysfunction yielding less frequent hyperprolactinemia than expected with these macroadenomas (40% of patients) [54–62]. Treatment paradigms centered on relieving mass effect are shared between most subtypes of nonfunctioning adenomas and will be discussed in aggregate.

Gonadotropin-Secreting Adenomas

Gonadotropin-producing adenomas constitute the vast majority of nonfunctioning pituitary adenomas. Due to the rather insidious onset of symptoms and limited hormonal effects from gonadotropin secretion in the most patients, these tumors are brought to clinical attention typically due to symptoms of mass effect, such as visual loss, anterior pituitary-derived hormone deficiencies, and headaches. Few patients harbor tumors that cause dramatic increases in circulating levels of FSH, LH, and/or α-subunit proteins. When present in young women, replacement of cyclical variations in gonadotropic hormones with persistent hypersecretion and downregulation of the gonadotropin-releasing hormone (GnRH) receptor of the normal gonadotrophs leads to ovarian failure rather than stimulation, and thus secondary amenorrhea with normal pubertal development and secondary sexual characteristics may develop. Gonadotropin-producing adenomas are most common among elderly males who generally present with progressive visual loss and headaches. These tumors are exceptionally rare in children.

Biochemical diagnosis is of secondary importance due to the imperative need to treat symptomatic mass effect. Pretreatment laboratory diagnosis rests on the findings of elevated FSH, LH, or α-subunit proteins, though these may be masked by physiologic increases in women living in postmenopausal phase. In these circumstances, paradoxical stimulation of gonadotropin release with TRH administration may help delineate the secretory function of the tumor. Regardless of the biochemical diagnosis, all gonadotropin (and nonfunctioning) adenomas share a common treatment paradigm that involves surgical decompression, at which time immunohistochemical and ultrastructural classification is performed.

Null-Cell Adenoma

Null-cell adenomas have no endocrinologic, immunohistochemical, or ultrastructural features of specific adenohypophyseal cell differentiation and thus present with symptoms and signs from direct invasion of adjacent structures or due to mass effect on the normal pituitary gland and stalk and/or the adjacent optic nerves or chiasm. In general, these tumors occur primarily in adults, with a slight male preponderance. Biochemical evaluation is performed to evaluate pituitary function and to detect hypopituitarism. As with other nonfunctioning adenomas, radiologic evaluation reveals that extrasellar extension is common.

Treatment of Nonfunctioning Adenomas

The primary goals in the treatment of symptomatic nonfunctioning adenomas are (a) decompression of neurovascular structures, (b) restoration/preservation of the hypothalamic-pituitary endocrine axis, and (c) tumor elimination and prevention of recurrence. Because these lesions almost universally come to clinical attention due to signs of mass effect, prompt surgical decompression is the treatment of choice. A subset of tumors may display significant lateral suprasellar extension, necessitating transcranial approaches to allow adequate removal of tumor. A more routine option is to perform transsphenoidal surgery, as it yields low morbidity and mortality rates and improves visual symptoms in most (60–91%) of the patients who present with visual deterioration [63–66]. Preoperative hypopituitarism often improves after surgical decompression, but detection of it and diagnosis of persistent or new hypopituitarism requires close endocrinologic follow-up for adequate replacement therapy. Long-term recurrence rates (10–15%) after complete transsphenoidal resection of tumors depend on the duration of follow-up, particularly in the absence of radiation therapy approaches. In contrast, recurrence rates exceed 55% in patients with subtotal resection and who did not undergo radiation therapy, emphasizing the need for long-term radiologic surveillance in these patients [67]. Postsurgical residual tumor, inaccessible regions of tumor extension (cavernous sinus), and local recurrences without symptoms of mass effect are typically treated with radiotherapy. Active debate regarding the merits of conventional fractionated radiotherapy and radiosurgery still exist, but both appear to offer excellent tumor growth-control rates (>90%).

ATYPICAL PITUITARY ADENOMA AND PITUITARY CARCINOMA

Pituitary carcinoma, a pituitary tumor with distant metastasis, is a rare clinical entity that constitutes 0.2% of all pituitary adenomas reported in surgical series [68]. Approximately, 150 cases have been reported in the previous literature. These tumors typically present as invasive macroadenomas with signs and symptoms of hormone excess and local mass effect. ACTH (46%) and PRL (33%) hypersecretion are the most commonly identified functional variants, and endocrinologically nonfunctioning tumors comprise 15% to 20% of cases [69]. The hallmark of pituitary carcinoma is distant metastasis, whether manifested systemically via hematogenous spread or within the craniospinal compartment along cerebrospinal pathways. The symptoms related to metastases are site specific.

The diagnosis of pituitary carcinoma is a clinical and radiologic diagnosis, as opposed to one delineated by pathological evaluation; thus, a diagnosis of "carcinoma in situ" is not possible. The pathogenesis of pituitary carcinomas remains unclear, and immunohistochemical markers that histologically distinguish pituitary "carcinoma in situ" from their more benign counterparts remain elusive. In 2000, the World Health Organization Classification addressed the difficulty in identifying tumors with increased potential for anaplastic conversion and developed the intermediate classification of atypical pituitary adenomas. These tumors are characterized by increased proliferative activity (Ki-67 >3%) and p53 overexpression. It is presumed that accrual of genetic alterations and transformation from benign tumors accounts for many cases of pituitary carcinoma, but the possibility of de novo formation of these tumors is also likely.

Because disseminated disease is required for diagnosis of pituitary carcinoma, survival is generally poor, with 66% of patients surviving less than 1 year [70]. Limited success has been achieved with surgery and adjunctive therapies, although occasional long-term survivors are reported. The primary role for surgery in sellar lesions and central nervous system-related metastasis is decompression of symptomatic lesions. Treatment of functional tumors and their hypersecretion syndromes with hormone-modulating agents (bromocriptine, cabergoline, somatostatin analogs, pegvisomant) has generally met with failure because most of these tumors have already escaped hormonal suppression [71]. Attempts to treat pituitary carcinoma with cytotoxic chemotherapy (carmustine, temazolamide, cisplatin and etoposide, cyclophosphamide, and adriamycin +/- adriamycin) have been limited to anecdotal reports that have shown variable efficacy and duration of effect, though in a few patients a surprising response has been observed [72–74]. Conventional radiotherapy has had moderate success in the local control of CNS metastasis, but there is no data to support that it may improve prognosis. Until more effective pharmacotherapy is available in the treatment of pituitary carcinoma, independently tailored multimodal therapy targeted at symptomatic or progressive lesions remains the primary guideline in management.

CONCLUSION

Given their high prevalence, the pituitary adenomas represent the most common cause behind pituitary dysfunction and disease and particularly in adult population. The clinical presentation of pituitary tumors and their management varies significantly, depending on the underlying clinical and pathological subtype of adenoma involved. The proper evaluation, diagnosis, treatment, and surveillance of pituitary disease require the expertise and coordination of a multidisciplinary clinical team, including a primary care physician, endocrinologist, ophthalmologist, oncologist, neurosurgeon, radiologist, and pathologist. Concurrently, advances in medical therapeutics, surgical techniques, and radiotherapy have improved safety and efficacy in the management of pituitary adenomas. As the armamentarium of diagnostic and therapeutic modalities continues to expand, it has become ever-more critical that there be consistency in the criteria for diagnosis and remission in the management of these complex lesions.

REFERENCES

1. Ezzat S, Asa SL, Couldwell WT, et al. The prevalence of pituitary adenomas: a systematic review. *Cancer*. 2004;101(3):613–619.
2. Kovacs K, Horvath E. *Tumors of the Pituitary Gland. Atlas of Tumor Pathology, Second Series, Fascicle 21*. Washington, DC: Armed Forces Institute of Pathology; 1986.
3. Ho KY, Evans WS, Thorner MO. Disorders of prolactin and growth hormone secretion. *Clin Endocrinol Metab*. 1985;14(1):1–32.
4. Ma W, Ikeda H, Yoshimoto T. Clinicopathologic study of 123 cases of prolactin-secreting pituitary adenomas with special reference to multihormone production and clonality of the adenomas. *Cancer*. 2002;95(2):258–266.
5. De Rivera JL, Lal S, Ettigi P. Effect of acute and chronic neuroleptic therapy on serum prolactin levels in men and women of different age groups. *Clin Endocrinol*. 1976;5(3):273–282.
6. St-Jean E, Blain F, Comtois R. High prolactin levels may be missed by immunoradiometric assay in patients with macroprolactinomas. *Clin Endocrinol*. 1996;44(3):305–309.
7. Webster J, Piscitelli G, Polli A, et al. The efficacy and tolerability of long-term cabergoline therapy in hyperprolactinaemic disorders: an open, uncontrolled, multicentre study. *Clin Endocrinol (Oxf)*. 1993;39(3):323–329.
8. Sarno AD, Landi ML, Cappabianca P, et al. Resistance to cabergoline as compared with bromocriptine in hyperprolactinemia: prevalence, clinical definition, and therapeutic strategy. *J Clin Endocrinol Metab*. 2001;86(11):5256–5261.
9. Horvath J, Fross RD, Kleiner-Fisman G, et al. Severe multivalvular heart disease: a new complication of the ergot derivative dopamine agonists. *Mov Disord*. 2004;19(6):656–662.
10. Thapar K, Kovacs K, Muller PJ. Clinical-pathological correlations of pituitary tumours. *Baillieres Clin Endocrinol Metab*. 1995;9(2):243–270.
11. Molitch ME. Clinical manifestations of acromegaly. *Endocrinol Metab Clin North Am*. 1992;21(3):597–614.
12. Jadresic A, Banks LM, Child DF. The acromegaly syndrome: relation between clinical features, growth hormone values and radiological characteristics of the pituitary tumours. *Q J Med*. 1982;51(202):189–204.
13. Giustina A, Barkan A, Casanueva FF, et al. Criteria for cure of acromegaly: a consensus statement. *J Clin Endocrinol Metab*. 2000;85(2):526–529.
14. Van 't Verlaat JW, Nortier JW, Hendriks MJ, et al. Transsphenoidal microsurgery as primary treatment in 25 acromegalic patients: results and follow-up. *Acta Endocrinol (Copenh)*. 1988;117(2):154–158.
15. Freda PU, Wardlaw SL, Post KD. Long-term endocrinological follow-up evaluation in 115 patients who underwent transsphenoidal surgery for acromegaly. *J Neurosurg*. 1998;89(3):353–358.
16. Grisoli F, Leclercq T, Jaquet P. Transsphenoidal surgery for acromegaly—long-term results in 100 patients. *Surg Neurol*. 1985;23(5):513–519.
17. Leavens ME, Samaan NA, Jesse RH Jr, Byers RM. Clinical and endocrinological evaluation of 16 acromegalic patients treated by transsphenoidal surgery. *J Neurosurg*. 1977;47(6):853–860.
18. Swearingen B, Barker FG II, Katznelson L, et al. Long-term mortality after transsphenoidal surgery and adjunctive therapy for acromegaly. *J Clin Endocrinol Metab*. 1998;83(10):3419–3426.
19. Kreutzer J, Vance ML, Lopes MB, Laws ER Jr. Surgical management of GH-secreting pituitary adenomas: an outcome study using modern remission criteria. *J Clin Endocrinol Metab*. 2001;86(9):4072–4077.
20. Goffman TE, Dewan R, Arakaki R, Gorden P, Oldfield EH, Glatstein E. Persistent or recurrent acromegaly: long-term endocrinologic efficacy and neurologic safety of postsurgical radiation therapy. *Cancer*. 1992;69(1):271–275.
21. Beauregard C, Truong U, Hardy J, Serri O. Long-term outcome and mortality after transsphenoidal adenomectomy for acromegaly. *Clin Endocrinol (Oxf)*. 2003;58(1):86–91.
22. Biermasz NR, Van Dulken H, Roelfsema F. Ten-year follow-up results of transsphenoidal microsurgery in acromegaly. *J Clin Endocrinol Metab*. 2000;85(12):4596–4602.
23. De P, Rees DA, Davies N, et al. Transsphenoidal surgery for acromegaly in Wales: results based on stringent criteria of remission. *J Clin Endocrinol Metab*. 2003;88(8):3567–3572.
24. Lamberts SWJ, van der Lely AJ, de Herder WW, Hofland LJ. Octreotide. *N Engl J Med*. 1996;334(4):246–254.
25. Freda PU, Katznelson L, van der Lely AJ, Reyes CM, Zhao S, Rabinowitz D. Long-acting somatostatin analog therapy of acromegaly: a meta-analysis. *J Clin Endocrinol Metab*. 2005;90(8):4465–4473.
26. Melmed S, Sternberg R, Cook D, et al. A critical analysis of pituitary tumor shrinkage during primary medical therapy in acromegaly. *J Clin Endocrinol Metab*. 2005;90(7):4405–4410.
27. Abs R, Verhelst J, Maiter D, et al. Cabergoline in the treatment of acromegaly: a study in 64 patients. *J Clin Endocrinol Metab*. 1998;83(2):374–378.
28. Trainer PJ, Drake WM, Katznelson L, et al. Treatment of acromegaly with the growth hormone-receptor antagonist pegvisomant. *N Engl J Med*. 2000;342(16):1171–1177.
29. van der Lely AJ, Hutson RK, Trainer PJ, et al. Long-term treatment of acromegaly with pegvisomant, a growth hormone receptor antagonist. *Lancet*. 2001;358(9295):1754–1759.
30. Sheehan JP, Niranjan A, Sheehan JM, et al. Stereotactic radiosurgery for pituitary adenomas: an intermediate review of its safety, efficacy, and role in the neurosurgical treatment armamentarium. *J Neurosurg*. 2005;102(4):678–691.
31. Sheehan JP, Jagannathan J, Pouratian N, Steiner L. Stereotactic radiosurgery for pituitary adenomas: a review of the literature and our experience. *Front Horm Res*. 2006;34:185–205.
32. Patronas N, Bulakbasi N, Stratakis CA, et al. Spoiled gradient recalled acquisition in the steady state technique is superior to conventional postcontrast spin echo technique for magnetic resonance imaging detection of adrenocorticotropin-secreting pituitary tumors. *J Clin Endocrinol Metab*. 2003;88(4):1565–1569.
33. Batista D, Courkoutsakis NA, Oldfield EH, et al. Detection of adrenocorticotropin-secreting pituitary adenomas by magnetic resonance imaging in children and adolescents with cushing disease. *J Clin Endocrinol Metab*. 2005;90(9):5134–5140.
34. Colombo N, Loli P, Vignati F, Scialfa G. MR of corticotropin-secreting pituitary microadenomas. *AJNR Am J Neuroradiol*. 1994;15(8):1591–1595.
35. Doppman JL, Frank JA, Dwyer AJ, et al. Gadolinium DTPA enhanced MR imaging of ACTH-secreting microadenomas of the pituitary gland. *J Comput Assist Tomogr*. 1988;12(5):728–735.
36. Dwyer AJ, Frank JA, Doppman JL, et al. Pituitary adenomas in patients with Cushing disease: initial experience with Gd-DTPA-enhanced MR imaging. *Radiology*. 1987;163(2):421–426.
37. Oldfield EH, Doppman JL, Nieman LK, et al. Petrosal sinus sampling with and without corticotropin-releasing hormone for the differential diagnosis of Cushing's syndrome. *N Engl J Med*. 1991;325(13):897–905.

38. Newell-Price J, Trainer P, Besser M, Grossman A. The diagnosis and differential diagnosis of Cushing's syndrome and pseudo-Cushing's states. *Endocr Rev.* 1998;19(5):647–672.
39. Kelly DF. Transsphenoidal surgery for Cushing's disease: a review of success rates, remission predictors, management of failed surgery, and Nelson's Syndrome. *Neurosurg Focus.* 2007;23(3):E5.
40. Estrada J, Boronat M, Mielgo M, et al. The long-term outcome of pituitary irradiation after unsuccessful transsphenoidal surgery in Cushing's disease. *N Engl J Med.* 1997;336(3):172–177.
41. Mahmoud-Ahmed AS, Suh JH. Radiation therapy for Cushing's disease: a review. *Pituitary.* 2002;5(3):175–180.
42. Tsang RW, Brierley JD, Panzarella T, Gospodarowicz MK, Sutcliffe SB, Simpson WJ. Role of radiation therapy in clinical hormonally-active pituitary adenomas. *Radiother Oncol.* 1996;41(1):45–53.
43. Beck-Peccoz P, Brucker-Davis F, Persani L, Smallridge RC, Weintraub BD. Thyrotropin-secreting pituitary tumors. *Endocr Rev.* 1996;17(6):610–638.
44. Greenman Y, Melmed S. Thyrotropin-secreting pituitary tumors. In: Melmed S, ed. *The Pituitary.* Cambridge: Blackwell Publishing;1995: 546–558.
45. Sanno N, Teramoto A, Osamura RY. Thyrotropin-secreting pituitary adenomas. Clinical and biological heterogeneity and current treatment. *J Neurooncol.* 2001;54(2):179–186.
46. McCutcheon IE, Weintraub BD, Oldfield EH. Surgical treatment of thyrotropin-secreting pituitary adenomas. *J Neurosurg.* 1990;73(5):674–683.
47. Brucker-Davis F, Oldfield EH, Skarulis MC, Doppman JL, Weintraub BD. Thyrotropin-secreting pituitary tumors: diagnostic criteria, thyroid hormone sensitivity, and treatment outcome in 25 patients followed at the National Institutes of Health. *J Clin Endocrinol Metab.* 1999;84(2):476–486.
48. Refetoff S, Weiss RE, Usala SJ. The syndromes of resistance to thyroid hormone. *Endocr Rev.* 1993;14(3):348–399.
49. Kourides IA, Ridgway EC, Weintraub BD. Thyrotropin-induced hyperthyroidism: use of alpha and beta subunit levels to identify patients with pituitary tumors. *J Clin Endocrinol Metab.* 1977;45(3):534–543.
50. Laws ER, Vance ML, Jane JA Jr. TSH adenomas. *Pituitary.* 2006;9(4): 313–315.
51. Ness-Abramof R, Ishay A, Harel G, et al. TSH-secreting pituitary adenomas: follow-up of 11 cases and review of the literature. *Pituitary.* 2007;10(3):307–310.
52. Caron P, Arlot S, Bauters C, et al. Efficacy of the long-acting octreotide formulation (Octreotide-LAR) in patients with thyrotropin-secreting pituitary adenomas. *J Clin Endocrinol Metab.* 2001;86(6):2849–2853.
53. Kuhn JM, Arlot S, Lefebvre H, et al. Evaluation of the treatment of thyrotropin-secreting pituitary adenomas with a slow release formulation of the somatostatin analog lanreotide. *J Clin Endocrinol Metab.* 2000;85(4):1487–1491.
54. Arafah BM. Reversible hypopituitarism in patients with large nonfunctioning pituitary adenomas. *J Clin Endocrinol Metab.* 1986;62(6): 1173–1179.
55. Colao A, Cerbone G, Cappabianca P, et al. Effect of surgery and radiotherapy on visual and endocrine function in nonfunctioning pituitary adenomas. *J Endocrinol Invest.* 1998;21(5):284–290.
56. Comtois R, Beauregard H, Somma M, Serri O, Aris-Jilwan N, Hardy J. The clinical and endocrine outcome to trans-sphenoidal microsurgery of nonsecreting pituitary adenomas. *Cancer.* 1991;68(4):860–866.
57. Dekkers OM, Pereira AM, Roelfsema F, et al. Observation alone after transsphenoidal surgery for nonfunctioning pituitary macroadenoma. *J Clin Endocrinol Metab.* 2006;91(5):1796–1801.
58. Ebersold MJ, Quast LM, Laws ER Jr. Long-term results in transsphenoidal removal of nonfunctioning pituitary adenomas. *J Neurosurg.* 1986;64(5):713–719.
59. Greenman Y, Ouaknine G, Veshchev I, Reider-Groswasser II, Segev Y, Stern N. Postoperative surveillance of clinically nonfunctioning pituitary macroadenomas: markers of tumour quiescence and regrowth. *Clin Endocrinol (Oxf).* 2003;58(6):763–769.
60. Mortini P, Losa M, Barzaghi R, Boari N, Giovanelli M. Results of transsphenoidal surgery in a large series of patients with pituitary adenoma. *Neurosurgery.* 2005;56(6):1222–1233.
61. Nomikos P, Ladar C, Fahlbusch R, Buchfelder M. Impact of primary surgery on pituitary function in patients with non-functioning pituitary adenomas—a study on 721 patients. *Acta Neurochir (Wien).* 2004;146(1):27–35.
62. Tominaga A, Uozumi T, Arita K, Kurisu K, Yano T, Hirohata T. Anterior pituitary function in patients with nonfunctioning pituitary adenoma: results of longitudinal follow-up. *Endocr J.* 1995;42(3):421–427.
63. Black McL P, Zervas NT, Candia GL. Incidence and management of complications of transsphenoidal operation for pituitary adenomas. *Neurosurgery.* 1987;20(6):920–924.
64. Cohen AR, Cooper PR, Kupersmith MJ. Visual recovery after transsphenoidal removal of pituitary adenomas. *Neurosurgery.* 1985;17(3):446–452.
65. Powell M. Recovery of vision following transsphenoidal surgery for pituitary adenomas. *Br J Neurosurg.* 1995;9(3):367–373.
66. Trautmann JC, Laws ER Jr. Visual status after transsphenoidal surgery at the Mayo clinic. 1971–1982. *Am J Ophthalmol.* 1983;96(2):200–208.
67. Chang EF, Zada G, Kim S, et al. Long-term recurrence and mortality after surgery and adjuvant radiotherapy for nonfunctional pituitary adenomas. *J Neurosurg.* 2008;108(4):736–745.
68. Pernicone PJ, Scheithauer BW, Sebo TJ, et al. Pituitary carcinoma: a clinicopathologic study of 15 cases. *Cancer.* 1997;79(4):804–812.
69. Ragel BT, Couldwell WT. Pituitary carcinoma: a review of the literature. *Neurosurg Focus.* 2004;16(4):E7.
70. Lopes MBS, Scheithauer BW, Schiff D. Pituitary carcinoma: diagnosis and treatment. *Endocrine.* 2005;28(1):115–121.
71. Kaltsas GA, Nomikos P, Kontogeorgos G, Buchfelder M, Grossman AB. Clinical review: diagnosis and management of pituitary carcinomas. *J Clin Endocrinol Metab.* 2005;90(5):3089–3099.
72. Kaiser FE, Orth DN, Mukai K, Oppenheimer JH. A pituitary parasellar tumor with extracranial metastases and high, partially suppressible levels of adrenocorticotropin and related peptides. *J Clin Endocrinol Metab.* 1983;57(3):649–653.
73. Kaltsas GA, Mukherjee JJ, Plowman PN, Monson JP, Grossman AB, Besser GM. The role of cytotoxic chemotherapy in the management of aggressive and malignant pituitary tumors. *J Clin Endocrinol Metab.* 1998;83(12):4233–4238.
74. McCutcheon IE, Pieper DR, Fuller GN, Benjamin RS, Friend KE, Gagel RF. Pituitary carcinoma containing gonadotropins: treatment by radical excision and cytotoxic chemotherapy: case report. *Neurosurgery.* 2000;46(5):1233–1240.

54 Spinal Neoplasms

Patrick C. Hsieh, John H. Chi, Ali Bydon, and Ziya L. Gokaslan

INTRODUCTION

Neoplasms involving the vertebral column can be primary tumors arising from the elements of the spinal column or metastatic tumors reaching the spine from distant sites. Whereas primary vertebral column tumors are rare, metastatic spinal tumors are quite common. Both medical and surgical management of primary and metastatic spinal tumors can be quite different. Therefore, in the management of vertebral column tumors, it is paramount to identify the origin of the lesion and obtain an accurate hisotological diagnosis. Although one can occasionally diagnose a lesion based on the combination of clinical history, physical examination, and imaging findings, an absolute tissue diagnosis is important and can only be obtained through histopathological examination on a biopsied specimen. With tissue diagnosis, one can properly elucidate the aggressiveness and the natural history of the disease and its likelihood to respond to chemotherapy and/or radiation therapy. It also allows the surgeons to decide on the appropriate surgical strategy to treat the lesion.

PRIMARY SPINAL TUMORS

Primary spinal tumors can be benign or malignant. Primary tumors of the vertebral column are exceedingly rare. Only less than 10% of all primary bony tumors arise from the vertebral column [1]. Commonly occurring benign and malignant spinal tumors are listed in Table 54.1.

Clinical Presentation and Workup

In general, patients with primary spinal tumors typically present at a younger age than those with metastatic spinal tumors. Several of the primary spinal tumors are in fact counterparts of more common pediatric and adolescent primary bone tumors that are usually seen in other skeletal regions. They include Ewing's sarcoma, osteosarcoma, osteoblastoma, and giant-cell tumors. The overwhelming majority of patients with primary spinal tumor present with pain. In one series, almost 85% of patients with primary spinal tumor were found to have pain [2]. Pain related to neoplastic disease may be difficult to differentiate from other benign conditions. Nevertheless, accurate and timely diagnosis of primary spinal neoplasm is critical. Inaccurate diagnosis or delay in diagnosis can have significant impact on prognosis.

Pain related specifically to neoplastic disease is often worse at night and occurs even at rest [3]. However, pain associated with primary spine tumors can also be axial or mechanical in nature, or radicular if spinal roots are irritated. Progressive neurological deficits can be associated with both benign and malignant primary spinal neoplasms; however, substantial impingement of neural elements or pathological fractures can signify a more aggressive lesion. Spinal deformity can occur in patients with primary spinal tumor, but it is unusual for these patients to have gross spinal instability. Nevertheless, one classical presentation of patients with osteoid osteoma is painful scoliosis [4].

Young patients with protracted spinal pain, back pain that is worse at night, back pain at rest, or any neurological deficits should prompt a medical workup for spinal tumors. Plain radiographs are often used for the initial workup. Plain radiographs can localize the lesion and it can be diagnostic in certain cases. However, plain films require approximately 50% loss of mineralization to allow detection of osteolytic lesions [5]. Computed tomography (CT) and magnetic resonance imaging (MRI) are the tests of choice to help precisely define the location of the lesion and the extent of the disease. Findings from these tests are oftentimes complementary to each other. MRI allows for finer resolution and details of soft tissues imaging. Therefore it allows enhanced delineation of the relationship between the tumor and neural elements (Figure 54.1). On the other hand, CT scans allow for better assessment of bony destruction and the osseous architecture of the involved and surrounding spine (Figure 54.2). Moreover, several of the primary spinal neoplasms have characteristic imaging finding on plain films, CT scan, and MRI. A complement of the characteristic findings from all these modalities can potentially result in the diagnosis of a primary spinal tumor without further unnecessary testing or procedures. The primary example of this is an aneurismal bone cyst (ABC) with its characteristic findings of cystic structures with fluid-fluid levels from blood degradation products on MRI and CT (Figure 54.3). Identifying the characteristic CT and MRI imaging findings that is consistent with an ABC can eliminate the need for a tissue biopsy and avoid the potential complication of a hematoma. Yet it is also known that other malignant primary bone tumors

Table 54.1 Primary Neoplasms of the Vertebral Column

Benign Primary Spine Tumors	Malignant Primary Spine Tumors
Hemanigioma	Ewing sarcoma
Osteoid osteoma	Osteogenic sarcoma
Osteoblastoma	Chordoma
Osteochondroma	Chondrosarcoma
Chondroblastoma	Mesenchymal sarcoma
Aneurysmal bone cyst	Plasmacytoma
Eosinophilic granuloma	
Giant-cell tumor	

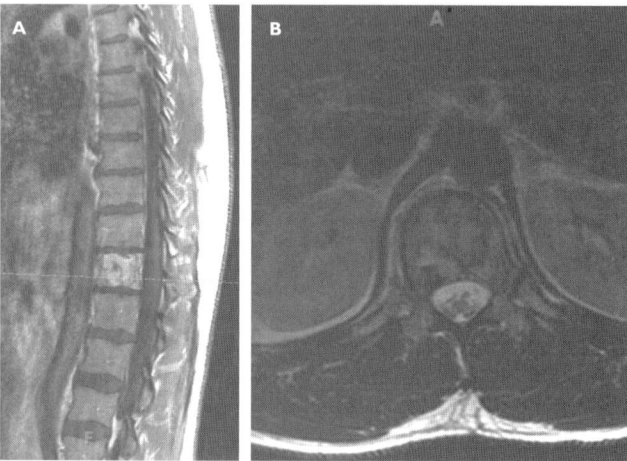

Figure 54.1 (A) Sagittal T1 MRI with contrast of thoracic giant-cell tumor. (B) Axial T2 MRI of thoracic giant-cell tumor.

such as osteogentic sarcoma may be ABC component as part of the lesion, occasionally leading to misinterpretation on biopsy specimens.

In addition to the radiographs, CT scan, and MRI, other imaging techniques that can be used include bone scan, positron emission tomography (PET) scan, and angiography. A bone scan is a nuclear medicine study that can help to identify new areas of bone growth or breakdown as a result of tumor growth. The lesion can be considered "cold" or "hot," depending on the amount of local cell activity and function in the osteocytes. In general, bone scans have high sensitivity but poor specificity. Nevertheless, lesions that are small and not well visualized with plain radiographs, CT scan, or MRI, can be detected with a bone scan such as osteoid osteomas [6,7]. PET scan is another nuclear medicine imaging technique that involves the use of a radioactive tracer that is metabolically active. The most commonly used tracer is 18-fluorodeoxyglucose (18F-FDG). Following injection, it accumulates and becomes concentrated in the neoplasm. PET scan is a common imaging technique used in oncology [6–14]. PET scan has high sensitivity and it provides both anatomic and functional information regarding a lesion. Angiography can be used for diagnostic and therapeutic purposes. For diagnosis, angiography can help to aid the diagnosis of a highly vascular lesion, such as an ABC. In addition, in can help to determine the anatomy and extent of blood flow to a lesion prior to any surgical intervention (Figure 54.4). Lesions including ABC, hemangiomas, giant-cell tumors, and large sarcomas are often associated with increased vascularity that can result in significant perioperative blood loss. Preoperative embolization for these cases can reduce intraoperative blood loss and perioperative morbidity [15–32].

Chemotherapy and Radiation Therapy

In general, chemotherapy has a limited role in the management of primary spinal neoplasms. Chemotherapy is typically administered as an adjunct to surgical resection of malignant spinal tumors or in patients with systemic disease. Neoadjuvant chemotherapy has been shown to have favorable results in the treatment of Ewing's sarcoma and osteogenic sarcoma [33–48]. Patients with certain primary spinal tumors can benefit from neoadjuvant or postoperative radiation [33–48]. Adjuvant radiation therapy has been shown to benefit patients with giant-cell tumor, residual hemiangioma, chordoma, Ewing's sarcoma, and osteogenic sarcoma [49–58]. However, many of the primary spinal tumors have poor response to radiotherapy and in general, the low-grade tumors have an inferior response rate compared to high-grade tumors.

The most common form of delivery of radiation therapy to the spine is external beam radiation. However, radiation toxicity to the spinal cord is of great concern because of the proximity of the cord and the high dose radiation required to attain local tumor control. In addition, although rare, radiation exposure to surrounding tissues leading to radiation-induced sarcoma is a concern for patients with benign tumors that are likely to be long-term survivors.[4] Recent advancements in radiation therapy have improved the ability to deliver higher dose radiation therapy to the tumors while limiting radiation exposure to the spinal cord and surrounding tissues. Theses advancements include proton beam therapy and conformal radiation therapy such as intensity-modulated radiation therapy (IMRT) and other stereotactic radiosurgery techniques. Currently, there is still limited data on the long-term efficacy of these advanced radiotherapy techniques in the management of primary spinal tumors, and future clinical studies incorporating these therapeutic modalities will be extremely valuable.

Surgical Management

Indications for surgical treatment of primary spinal neoplasms include severe pain, spinal cord compression, spinal instability, and tumor resection for cure or long-term disease control. The goal of surgery is to provide neural decompression, maintain spinal stability, and provide wide surgical resection when possible to achieve long-term tumor control and potential for cure.

Treatment for primary spinal tumors is often dictated by histology of the tumor, the location of the tumor, and the extent of tumor invasion [59,60]. For benign lesions, appropriate surgical resection can result in cure, but not every benign lesion warrants a surgical resection. For instance, hemangiomas are found in 10% to 12% of the general population and they are most often asymptomatic. Similarly, incidental osteoid osteoma can be managed

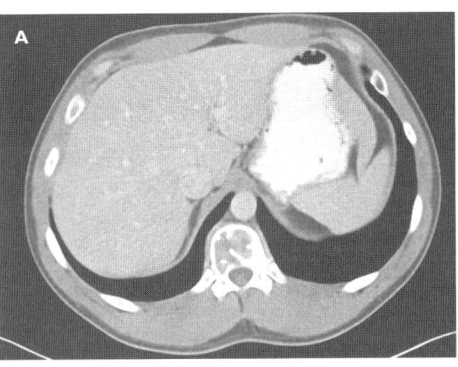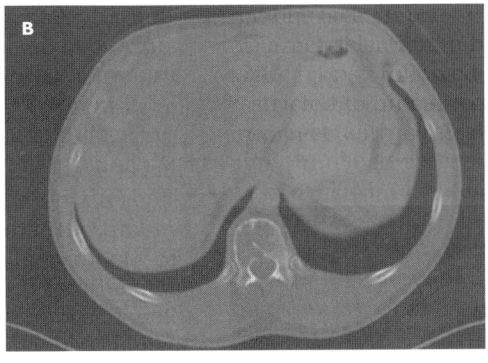

Figure 54.2 (**A**) Axial CT of thoracic giant-cell tumor in soft tissue window. (**B**) Axial CT of thoracic giant-cell tumor in bone window.

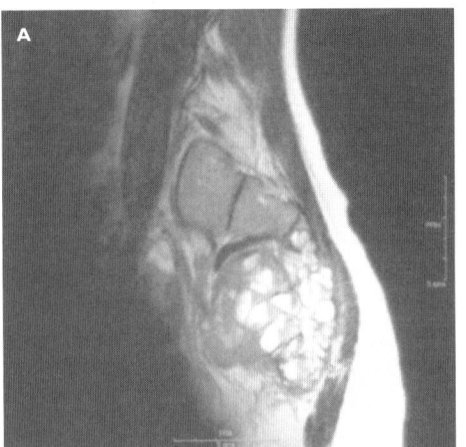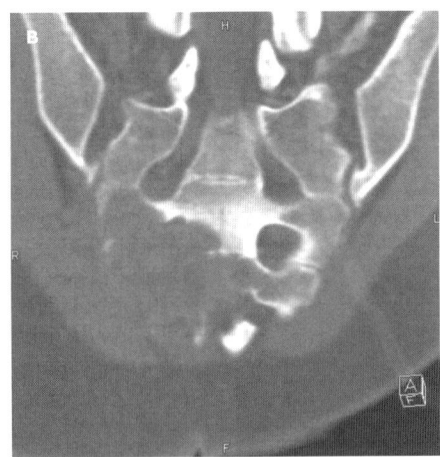

Figure 54.3 (**A**) MRI imaging of aneurysmal bone cyst (ABC) demonstrating fluid-fluid level with the vertebral body. (**B**) CT imaging of aneurysmal bone cyst (ABC) demonstrating the cystic and expansile lesion with vertebral body scalloping of vertebral body and posterior elements.

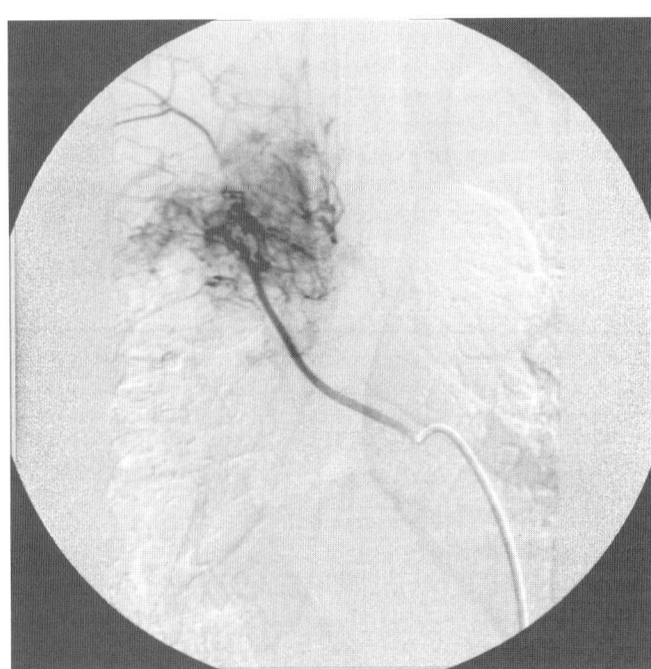

Figure 54.4 Angiogragm demonstrating extensive vascularity of a hepatocelluar metastatic tumor requiring preoperative embolization.

conservatively and surgery is reserved for patients who exhibit pain symptoms refractory to medical therapy, painful scoliosis, or signs of tumor progression [61]. Certainly, a malignant histology for primary tumors almost always warrants surgical treatment. However, treatment strategies using neoadjuvant or adjuvant radiation and chemotherapy with surgery can be significantly affected by the knowledge of tumor histology. For instance, with Ewing's sarcoma, neoadjuvant chemotherapy and radiation therapy should first be attempted [34,36,37,44,45,49]. Early surgery for Ewing's sarcoma is indicated when there are neurological deficits, high-grade spinal cord compression, and failure to respond to neoadjuvant chemotherapy and radiation, or residual tumor following chemotherapy and radiation therapy. Similarly, in osteogenic sarcoma, neoadjuvant chemotherapy and radiation should be attempted first [39–43,52,53,56,58]. Neoadjuvant can significantly reduce the bulk of the tumor to decrease the magnitude of surgery and to improve the likelihood of achieving wide en bloc resection to improve local tumor control rate and the prospect for cure.

In primary sarcomas from extraspinal sites, long-term tumor control, tumor progression-free survival, and the potential for cure have been shown to correlate with the ability to achieve a marginal, wide, or radical en bloc tumor resection [62–68]. Accordingly, the goal of modern surgical treatment for primary spinal neoplasms is to achieve wide or marginal en bloc vertebral body resection (i.e., total en bloc spondylectomy [TES]). Over the recent decades, there is accumulating evidence that en bloc spondylectomy for primary spinal tumors can impart longer local tumor control rate, longer disease-free survival, and possible cure for chordomas and chondrosarcomas specifically [69–73].

The term "en bloc" resection signifies an attempt to remove the lesion in a single piece. In en bloc spondylectomy, the vertebral body is typically removed in a single piece, while the posterior arch is removed separately as a single piece. Spondylectomy was first described by Stener in 1971 [71] and since then, various reports supported improved local tumor control rate and disease-free survival with spondylectomy [69–73]. In the 1990s, Tomita et al further modified and popularized the TES originally described by Roy-Camille. In this procedure, en bloc spondylectomy with anterior and posterior spinal reconstruction is performed through an all posterior approach [60,74,75]. En bloc spondylectomy can be performed in a single level or up to three consecutive levels using this approach. Based on cadaveric study, Kawahara et al found that the single stage posterior TES approach can be achieved for lesions located from T1 to L2 and possibly L3 and L4 if the inferior vena cava and iliac vessels have been safely mobilized anteriorly [76]. To achieve en bloc spondylectomy with wide margins of resection, the tumor should be contained within the vertebral body with minimal to no paraspinal extension [59,60]. In addition, there should be no epidural disease, and at least one pedicle must be free of tumor.

Although the assumption is that the en bloc resection of a spinal tumor removes the lesion in its entirety, it does not equate to the classic en bloc radical resection of extremity tumors due to the presence of the neural element and spinal cord within the lesion, which may often be spared. Therefore, the extent of spine tumor resection should instead be designated as "marginal," "wide," or "radical" en bloc resection [59]. Any resection would be considered "intralesional" resection when the tumor capsule has been violated during the resection. On the other hand, a marginal en bloc resection involves removal of the tumor with dissection along the pseudocapsule without entrance into the tumor. In wide en bloc resection, a continuous layer of surrounding healthy tissue is removed along with the tumor. A radical en bloc resection requires removal of the tumor along with entire anatomical compartment of the tumor origin. It is not possible in the spine, given that it would require removal of the entire spine compartment from the skull base to the coccyx with its surrounding soft tissues.

The ability to accomplish marginal or wide en bloc resection of primary spinal tumors is largely based on the tumor location and extension. Weinstein, Boriani, and Biagini devised a classification system (WBB staging system) for primary spinal tumors based on concepts and terms accepted by most oncologists for other musculoskeletal tumor [59]. In this classification, the vertebra is divided into 12 sectors, numbered from 1 to 12 in a clockwise order and with the spinal canal as the center. In addition, the vertebral is also divided into five layers, ranging from the paravertebral extraosseous region to intradural involvement. Finally, the longitudinal extend of the tumor is defined by the number of spinal segments involved. The authors recommend surgical planning for primary spinal tumors should be based on this WBB staging system. Accordingly, neoplasms that are confined within the vertebral body or the posterior arch can be resected with marginal or wide en bloc resection. Moreover, tumors located eccentrically with unilateral pedicle and/or transverse process involvement with small paraspinal extension can be excised with marginal or wide en bloc resection with the sagittal resection technique [59]. On the other hand, those tumors with extensive epidural involvement are not good candidates for en bloc resection as the risk of neurological injury is high.

Surgical Technique

TES can be achieved through a combined anterior-posterior approach or an all posterior approach. In the posterior-only approach for TES, the patient is positioned prone unto a Jackson spinal frame® (OSI, Union City, California). Following incision, the paraspinal muscles are elevated from the spinous process, lamina, and transverse process of the tumor-involved level as well as two spinal levels above and below the the neoplastic level(s). Instrumentation is typically placed at two levels above and below the lesional level and wide laminectomy is performed at the level immediately above and below the lesion. Osteotomy is performed at the level above and below the lesion to remove the inferior and superior articulating processes respectively to expose the entire posterior element of involved level. In the thoracic spine, at the level of the tumor and the levels immediately above and below, the exposure is further extended laterally to expose approximately 4 to 5 cm of the ribs lateral to the costotransverse joint. The rib of the diseased level is dissected away from the intercostal muscles and the parietal pleura. The proximal rib is transected up to 4 to 5 cm lateral to the costotransverse joint.

Following removal of soft tissue attached to the inferior articulating process and pars interarticularis, a curved malleable saw guide is passed in a caudal-cephalad fashion and through the neuroforamina above the pedicle. Care should be taken to avoid injury to the exiting nerve root. A fine-threaded wire saw is passed through the guide and wrapped around the pedicle. This process is repeated for the contralateral pedicle. The pedicles are subsequently cut with reciprocating sawing motion using the fine-threaded wire saw. With bilateral pediculotomy completed, the entire posterior element is removed in an en bloc fashion Figure 54.5). In cases where there is unilateral pedicle involvement of the tumor, a posterior osteotomy can be performed through the ipsilateral lamina along with a contralateral pediculotomy to achieve disconnection of the posterior arch.

To initiate blunt dissection of the paraspinal tissues of the vertebral body, the segmental vessels should first be identified. The spinal branch of the segmental artery is identified, ligated, and divided. In the thoracic spine, the nerve roots of the affected level are also ligated and cut to provide additional exposure for vertebral body resection and removal of the body around the spinal cord. Meticulous blunt dissection is carried out using suction tips and blunt dissectors along the lateral wall to the anterior wall of the

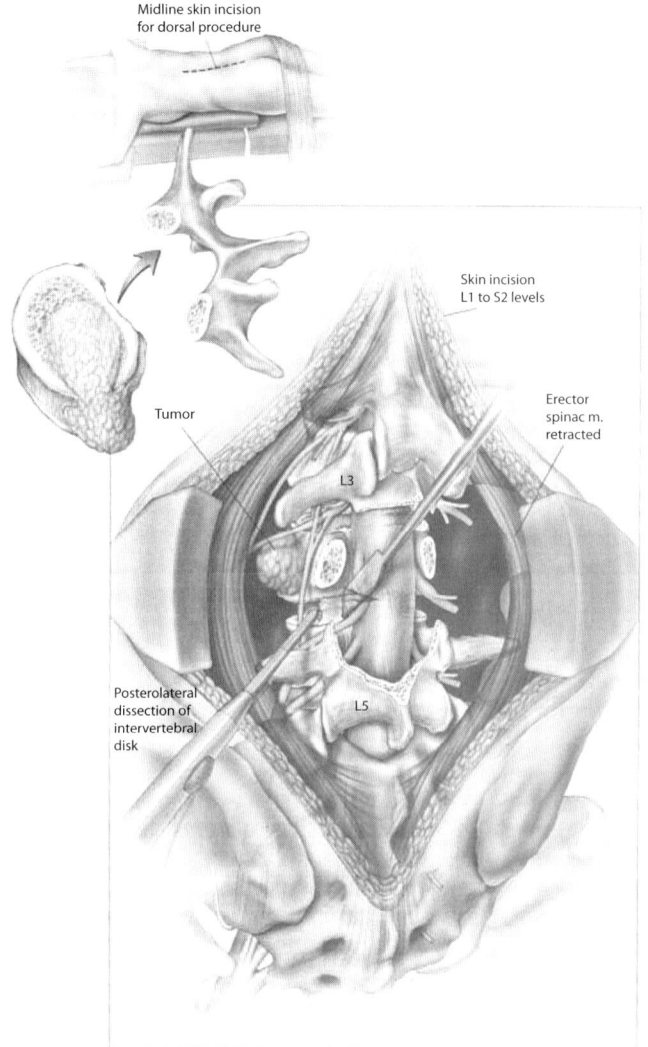

Figure 54.5 Artist illustration demonstrating en bloc spondylectomy through a posterior approach. Adapted from Marmor et al [81].

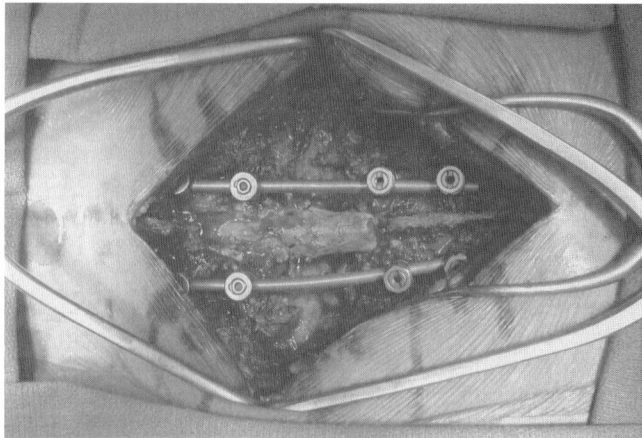

Figure 54.6 Intraoperative images from thoracic posterior total en bloc spondylectomy. A posterior view demonstrating the wide exposure of the thecal sac to allow safe en bloc resection of the vertebral body and placement of segmental instrumentation to maintain spinal stability.

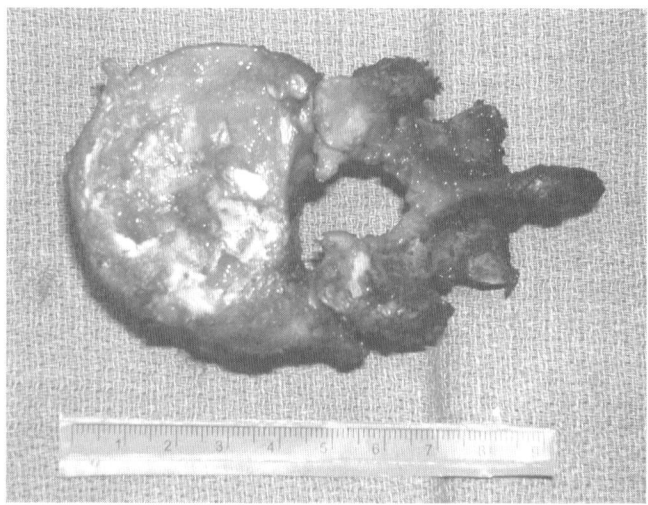

Figure 54.7 Surgical specimen demonstrating the total en bloc spondylectomy in 2 pieces.

vertebral body. Blunt dissection is performed along the tissue plane just dorsal to the segmental vessels at all times. This ensures that the dissection is performed dorsal to the great vessels during the anterior vertebral wall dissection to avoid inadvertent vascular injury. The aorta and vena cava is gently dissected away from the ventral vertebral body. Once the dissection is completed across the ventral vertebral body, a penrose drain is placed around the vertebral body to maintain the plane. A malleable blade is subsequently passed around the vertebral body over the penrose drain to maintain the exposure and to protect the paraspinal structures during the remainder of the TES.

The thecal sac is dissected from the venous plexus and posterior longitudinal ligament (PLL). Discectomy is performed above and below the affected level, using either fine-threaded wires or discectomy knives. The anterior longitudinal ligament (ALL) and PLL are excised at the level of the disectomies. Segmental instrumentation and temporary rods are placed with initiation of discectomy and detachment of the ligaments to ensure spinal stability (Figure 54.6). With completion of discectomy and excision of ALL and PLL, the vertebral body is detached and is removed en bloc by mobilizing it gently around the spinal cord (Figure 54.5).

With completion of TES (Figures 54.6 and 54.7), circumferential reconstruction of the involved level is required. Ventral reconstruction is typically performed with an interbody spacer. Several alternatives for interbody spacers can be considered and they include allograft, titanium mesh cylindrical cage, polyetheretherketones (PEEK) cages, and distractable titanium or PEEK cylindrical cage. With the advent of distractable cages, ventral reconstruction can be performed with greater ease. Distractable cages in undistracted state are more compact and can be manipulated in a restricted corridor and around the spinal cord with greater safety. Once in appropriate position, the cage is slowly distracted and fitted to bridge the intervertebral defect. Gentle distraction will allow for engagement and impaction of the cage to the vertebral end plates. However, overdistraction can occur and lead to vertebral fractures or overdistraction of posterior elements. One other additional concern for the use of the distractable cage is that long-term bony union is less likely and can be a concern for long-term survivors.

Despite reports of good clinical results with TES for spinal neoplasms, TES is a technically highly demanding procedure and is associated with significant perioperative risks [60,74,75,77–82]. The risks in TES include neurological injury and dural injury during pedicle resection and vascular injury to the aorta or vena cava during blunt dissection around the anterior vertebral body, which can be fatal. There is risk of spinal cord ischemia with manipulation and sacrifice of segmental vessels. Excessive bleeding from epidural plexus or vertebral body can occur. Finally, there is complete disconnection of the spine with spinal instability following completion of the spondylectomy that requires well-planned reconstruction. Moreover, despite the meticulous effort to remain extralesional, there is still inherent risk of tumor contamination of the field during pediculotomy [75]. However, the use of fine-threaded T-saw has been shown to decrease the risk of tumor contamination during pediculotomy in an animal model [83].

At times, en bloc resection is not achievable in the management of primary vertebral column tumors as a result of extension into surrounding anatomical structures. These structures include the dura, neural elements, major vessels, paraspinal musculature, and visceral organs. Tumor involvement in these structures will limit the ability to accomplish wide or marginal excision of the tumor without significant risk. In these cases, intralesional or piecemeal resection have been widely performed [84]. However, limitation of piecemeal resection includes difficulty to identify the margins of the tumor and it places surrounding tissues at risk for tumor contamination [75,84].

METASTATIC SPINAL TUMORS

Metastatic disease to the spine most commonly occurs in the vertebral body. Unlike primary spinal neoplasms, metastatic spinal tumor is a frequent disease encountered by the oncologist, radiation oncologist, and spine surgeons. Approximately 1.4 million new cases of cancer were diagnosed in the United States in 2007 [85] and about 18,000 new cases of metastatic spine tumors are encountered in North America annually [86]. The vertebral column is the most common site of skeletal metastasis. As oncological treatments continue to evolve and improve, life expectancy for cancer patients have increased and the prevalence of long-term cancer survivors continues to rise. With the incidence of spinal metastasis in cancer patients varying between 30% and 70%, [87] there will likely be increasing number of patients developing metastatic spine disease and epidural spinal cord compression [88].

Typical primary sites for spinal metastasis include lung, breast, prostate, kidney, melanoma, and hematopoietic cancers (Table 54.2). Since these various neoplasms have diverse response to radiation and chemotherapy, it is important to decipher the primary origin of metastatic

Table 54.2 Common Primary Origin of Metastatic Spinal Neoplasms

Lung cancer
Breast cancer
Prostate cancer
GI tract cancers
Renal cell carcinoma
Melanoma
Thyroid cancer
Lymphoma
Others: Unknown origin, multiple myeloma

origin. Tumors that are considered radiosensitive include small-cell lung cancer, multiple myeloma, germ-cell tumor, leukemia, and lymphoma. On the other hand, renal cell and melanoma metastasis are radioresistant. Patients with radiosensitive or chemosensitive metastatic tumor without neurological deficits or significant cord compression should be treated with radiation or chemotherapy as first line of treatment. However, patients with radioresistant neoplasms are unlikely to respond to radiotherapy and should be considered for upfront surgical resection.

Clinical Presentation and Workup

Similar to patients with primary spinal tumor, the overwhelming clinical presentation for metastatic spinal tumor is pain [86,88,89]. Pain related to metastatic spinal tumor can be local pain, neurogenic pain, or mechanical pain. Local pain or biologic pain is related to tumor involvement of spine with lytic destruction and periosteum expansion and mediated through prostaglandins. Local pain is often worse at night or in the early morning and with recumbence [3]. Neurogenic pain is typically related to direct nerve compression or invasion. Mechanical pain is related to spinal instability and is typically exacerbated with standing, ambulation, and performing activities.

Unlike patients with primary spinal tumor, patients with metastatic spinal tumors are far more likely to present with neurological symptoms. Presenting neurological deficits can range from radiculopathy to subtle myelopathy, or to complete spinal cord paralysis. Neurological deficits most often correlate with the severity of metastatic cord compression (Figure 54.8). Metastatic epidural spinal cord compression (MESCC) occurs in 5% to 10% of cancer patients [88,90,91] and approximately 25,000 new cases of symptomatic MESCC are diagnosed in the United States annually [92]. Severe metastatic epidural disease causes displacement and distortion of spinal cord, and it should be treated promptly to prevent progressive neurological deficits.

Patients with suspected metastatic spine disease should undergo prompt medical evaluation. Although plain radiographs can demonstrate shoulder bone erosions or osteoblastic changes, MRI is the gold standard imaging modality for diagnosis of metastatic spinal tumor. MRI has high sensitivity for detection of tumor and presents detailed resolution for soft tissue imaging. Typically, MRI with T1-weighted and T2-weighted sequences is obtained with a postcontrast T1-weighted sequence. The complement of these sequences allows for thorough interpretation

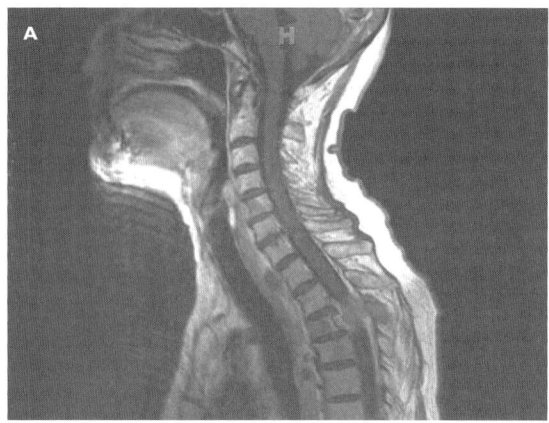 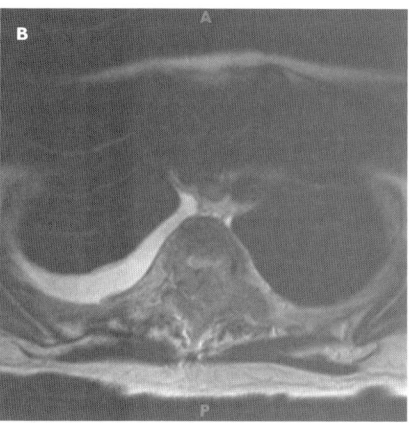

Figure 54.8 (A) Sagittal T1-weighted image with contrast of metastatic lung cancer to thoracic spine with epidural cord compression. (B) Axial T2-weighted image demonstrating high-grade spinal cord compression as a result of metastatic epidural tumor from same patient.

of the tumor anatomy and its relationship with surrounding structures, including the vertebral column, spinal cord, and nerve roots (Figure 54.8). On the other hand, CT scan provides the best information regarding the bony involvement, osseous architecture, and spinal stability. The combination of MRI and CT scan provides most effective method of evaluating patients with spinal metastases and MESCC [88].

Approximately 10% to 20% of patients can have metastatic spine disease as the initial presentation of cancer [93]. In those patients without prior history of neoplastic disease, a CT-guided biopsy should be obtained to acquire a histological diagnosis. Percutaneous CT-guided biopsy of spine has a diagnostic accuracy rate up to 93% [94–97]. An accurate diagnosis can have significant impact on treatment and overall prognosis.

Patients with metastatic spine disease should be evaluated for systemic disease burden and other areas of metastasis. Typical evaluation includes CT scan of chest, abdomen, and pelvis to rule out visceral metastatic lesions. The use of PET scan with 18F-fluorodeoxyglucose is gaining increasing popularity for metastatic survey and staging. Those with extensive metastatic disease and with life expectancy less than 3 months are typically not good surgical candidates for extensive spinal decompression and reconstruction. Tokuhashi et al presented a scoring system for the preoperative evaluation of metastatic spine tumor patient to help determine prognosis and life expectancy [98,99]. However, the process of estimating prognosis and life expectancy remains subjective. In addition, cancer patients should undergo preoperative medical clearance, and those with significant medical comorbidities may not be suitable surgical candidates.

Chemotherapy and Radiation Therapy

With the exception of selected chemosensitive tumors, chemotherapy has a limited role in the acute treatment of patients with symptomatic metastatic spine tumors. Chemosensitive tumors that can be considered for upfront chemotherapy include Ewing's sarcoma, osteogenic sarcoma, neuroblastoma, primitive neuroectodermal tumor (PNET), multiple myeloma, leukemia, and lymphoma. However, in the presence of neurological deficits or severe spinal cord compression, surgery or radiation therapies remain the treatment of choice.

Although corticosteroids are not chemotherapeutic agents, they can have several important activities against tumor effect and provide neuroprotection. The most commonly utilized corticosteroid in oncology is dexamethasone. Corticosteroids such as dexamethasone can have direct oncolytic effects on certain tumors such as lymphoma [100–103]. Second, administering dexamethasone in patients with metastatic tumors can rapidly improve their biological pain symptom [104]. Finally, the steroid can reduce vasogenic edema related to the tumor leading to prevention or reversal of neurological deficits prior to radiation or surgical treatment [100,105].

Radiation therapy has been considered by many to be the first line of therapy over half of the last century. Radiation therapy remains the first line of treatment for some radiosensitive metastatic tumors, and they include germ-cell tumors, leukemia, lymphoma, multiple myeloma, and small-cell lung cancer. Radiation has proven to be effective for pain improvement, maintenance of ambulatory status, and even improving neurological status in some nonambulatory patients [106–113]. Standard radiation treatment of metastatic spinal tumor consists of delivery of 30 Gy in 10 daily fractions of 3 Gy to the involved vertebral bodies with a surrounding margin. Although higher doses are more effective to achieve tumoricidal effects, the tolerance of spinal cord and caudal equina to radiation is the limiting factor for higher dose escalation. In addition, patients who have failed radiation treatment or have delayed local tumor recurrence following radiotherapy are not candidates for repeat radiotherapy due to risk of radiation-induced myelopathy.

In recent years, the advent of conformation radiotherapy modality such as IMRT and radiosurgery have improved the therapeutic ratio of radiotherapy. These advance modalities allows for delivery of higher conformal doses of radiation to the targeted tumor while minimizing radiation exposure to the surrounding tissues including the spinal cord and caudal equina. In 2007, Gerszten et al performed a prospective study on 393 patients with 500 lesions treated with Cyberknife (Accuray, Sunnyvale, California). In this study, with a mean maximum intratumoral dose of 20 Gy and a mean tumor volume of 46 ml, they found long-term pain improvement in 86% of the cohort, neurological improvement in 85% of the patients, and long-term radiographic tumor control in 90% of the cases when radiosurgery was used as the first line of therapy. Moreover, the long-term tumor control rate was 88% when radiosurgery was used as "salvage therapy" in those patients who failed prior conventional radiotherapy. The study provides Class II evidence of promising outcomes with radiosurgery in the treatment of metastatic tumor. Future randomized prospective studies to compare clinical outcomes following radiosurgery and surgery in metastatic spine disease will be extremely valuable.

Surgical Management

Indications for surgical intervention in metastatic spine disease include acute and progressive neurological deficits, severe cord compression, spinal instability, and failed radiation treatment. Other relative surgical indications include radioresistant tumor and severe pain refractory to medical therapy. Goals of surgery include circumferential neural decompression, excision of tumor, and maintaining or reestablishing spine stability. Unlike treatment goal for primary spinal neoplasm, cure is not achievable with spine surgery for metastatic disease. The primary treatment goal for metastatic spinal tumor is mainly palliation for neural protection, maintaining spinal stability, pain improvement, and local tumor control.

Early efforts in surgical treatment for metastatic spinal tumor were focused on decompressive laminectomies [114–123]. Because the majority of the metastatic spine disease involves the vertebral body, decompression by laminectomy results in poor ventral decompression and further destabilizes the spine. As a result, early clinical series comparing surgery to radiotherapy demonstrated poor results with surgical treatments. However, advancement in surgical techniques in modern spine surgery now allows aggressive circumferential decompression and spinal reconstruction. Various surgical approaches can be utilized to achieve circumferential decompression and spinal stabilization. The surgical route to use largely depends on the regional anatomy and the surgeon's expertise. Anterior approaches to the spine include anterolateral approach to the cervical spine, transthoracic approach to the thoracic spine, thoracolumbar approach to the lower thoracic spine and upper lumber spine, and transabdominal approach to the lumbosacral junction. Anterior approaches provide a more direct route to the vertebral body where most metastatic tumors reside, and it allows better visualization of the ventral epidural space. On the other hand, anterior approaches can be associated with significant approach-related morbidities, including injuries to visceral and vascular structures. Classic posterior approaches for treatment of metastatic spinal tumor include the transpedicular, costotransversectomy, or lateral extracavitary approaches for vertebral body resection. These approaches vary in their degree of bony resection in the lateral spine and ribs to allow for a more oblique trajectory to the vertebral body and the ventral epidural space for safer decompression around the spinal cord. The posterior approaches are familiar to most spine surgeons and allow circumferential decompression and stabilization in a single setting (Figure 54.9). In selected cases such as tumors involving the upper thoracic spine, anterior approaches are technically challenging and have significant approach-related morbidities. In these cases involving the upper thoracic spine, tumor resection is best performed through posterior approaches for circumferential decompression and spinal reconstruction (Figures 54.8 and 54.9). Nevertheless, the posterior-only approaches are typically limited to the thoracic spine and upper lumbar spine. Other potential complications with posterior approaches include spinal cord or nerve root injury, cerebrospinal fluid leak, segmental artery injury, spinal cord ischemia, and hemo- or pneumothorax.

In 2005, Patchell et al provided Class I data supporting surgical treatment of patients with symptomatic MESCC. In this landmark study, 101 patients with symptomatic MESCC, who were acceptable surgical candidates and had life expectancy greater than 3 months, were randomized to radiation therapy or surgery followed by radiation therapy. Patients with radiosensitive tumors such as lymphomas, leukemia, multiple myeloma, and germ-cell tumors were excluded from the study. In the surgical arm, the goal of surgery was to provide direct circumferential decompression of the spinal cord and stabilization of the spine in

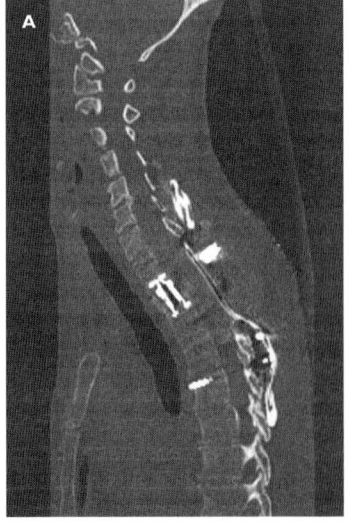
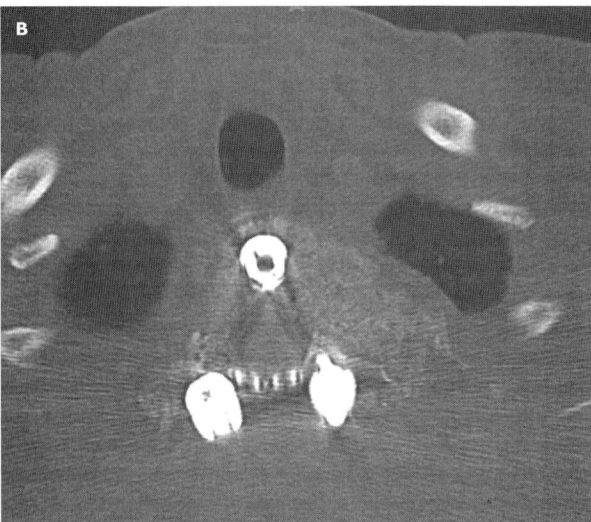

Figure 54.9 Postoperative sagittal **(A)** and axial **(B)** CT images demonstrating circumferential spinal reconstruction with anterior cage and posterior segmental instrumentations.

cases with spinal instability. The study demonstrated that the group of patients who underwent surgery and radiotherapy had significantly increased number of ambulatory patients than those who received radiation alone (84% vs. 57%, $P = 0.001$). In addition, the surgical group patients retained their ability to ambulate significantly longer than those patients treated with radiation (median 122 days vs. 13 days, $P = 0.003$). Furthermore, the study also demonstrated that surgery resulted in improved maintenance of continence, improved maintenance of neurological status using ASIA and Frankel scales, and longer survival time.

Although the goal of surgery for metastatic spine disease is palliation in majority of cases, in selected solitary metastatic tumor cases, the goal of surgery is to improve local tumor control and the potential for long-term survival. The role of TES in surgical management of metastatic spine tumors is controversial. However, Tomita et al have reported some success with TES in metastatic spine disease with lower local tumor recurrence rate and longer survival than those treated with intralesional piecemeal resection. Nevertheless, TES carries significant perioperative risks and are considered only in selected patients who have a solitary metastatic lesion from a slow growing neoplasm [74,79,80,124].

In recent years, vertebroplasty and kyphoplasty are two procedures that have gained increased popularity for the treatment of pain from pathological fractures [125]. Vertebroplasty and kyphoplasty are closely related procedures that involve injection of polymethylmethacrate (PMMA) cement in a semiviscous state into the vertebral body (Figure 54.10). Both procedures can be performed percutaneously and require the use of fluoroscopic imaging. Vertebroplasty and Kyphoplasty are have been routinely used for multiple myeloma, hemiangioma, and metastatic lesions with great success [125–127]. In one series of 56 patients with 65 vertebroplasty and 32 kyphoplasty, complete pain relief was reported in 84% of the patients following the procedures. At 1 month, analgesic requirement was significantly reduced and significant improvement in pain scores persisted after 1 year [128].

CONCLUSION

Appropriate management of vertebral column tumors is highly dependent on the histological diagnosis. It is important to differentiate primary spinal tumor from the metastatic tumor. In treatment of primary spinal neoplasms, the goal of treatment is to provide long-term tumor control and potential for cure. Aggressive surgical resection with wide or marginal en bloc spondylectomy is the treatment of choice when possible. On the other hand, in metastatic spine disease, disease cure is unlikely and the primary treatment goal is those cases is palliation. As a result, a multimodality approach with consideration for surgical treatment, radiation therapy, and chemotherapy is often required. Metastatic tumor patients with radiosensitive or chemosensitive tumors can be treated with radiation or chemotherapy as first line of therapy. Nevertheless, metastatic spine tumor patients with symptomatic epidural disease, neurological decline, spinal instability, or severe cord compression are best treated with circumferential decompression of spinal cord and stabilization of the spine.

REFERENCES

1. Unni KK. *Dahlin's Bone Tumors: General Aspects and Data on 11,087 Cases*. 5th ed. Philadelphia, PA: Lippincott Williams & Wilkins; 1996.
2. Weinstein JN. Surgical approach to spine tumors. *Orthopedics*. 1989;12(6):897–905.
3. Nicholas JJ, Christy WC. Spinal pain made worse by recumbency: a clue to spinal cord tumors. *Arch Phys Med Rehabil*. 1986;67(9):598–600.
4. Hitchon PW, Bilsky MH, Ebersold MJ. *Primary Bony Spinal Lesions*. 2nd ed. Philadelphia, PA: Elsevier; 2005.
5. O'Mara RE. Bone scanning in osseous metastatic disease. *JAMA*. 1974;229(14):1915–1917.
6. Schirrmeister H, Glatting G, Hetzel J, et al. Prospective evaluation of the clinical value of planar bone scans, SPECT, and (18) F-labeled NaF PET in newly diagnosed lung cancer. *J Nucl Med*. 2001;42(12):1800–1804.
7. Schirrmeister H, Guhlmann A, Elsner K, et al. Sensitivity in detecting osseous lesions depends on anatomic localization: planar bone scintigraphy versus 18F PET. *J Nucl Med*. 1999;40(10):1623–1629.
8. Schirrmeister H. Detection of bone metastases in breast cancer by positron emission tomography. *Radiol Clin North Am*. 2007;45(4):669–676, vi.
9. Buck AK, Schirrmeister H, Mattfeldt T, Reske SN. Biological characterisation of breast cancer by means of PET. *Eur J Nucl Med Mol Imaging*. 2004;31(suppl 1):S80-S87.
10. Hetzel M, Arslandemir C, Konig HH, et al. F-18 NaF PET for detection of bone metastases in lung cancer: accuracy, cost-effectiveness, and impact on patient management. *J Bone Miner Res*. 2003;18(12):2206–2214.
11. Schirrmeister H, Buck AK, Bergmann L, Reske SN, Bommer M. Positron emission tomography (PET) for staging of solitary plasmacytoma. *Cancer Biother Radiopharm*. 2003;18(5):841–845.
12. Schirrmeister H, Bommer M, Buck AK, et al. Initial results in the assessment of multiple myeloma using 18F-FDG PET. *Eur J Nucl Med Mol Imaging*. 2002;29(3):361–366.
13. Schirrmeister H, Buck A, Guhlmann A, Reske SN. Anatomical distribution and sclerotic activity of bone metastases from thyroid cancer assessed with F-18 sodium fluoride positron emission tomography. *Thyroid*. 2001;11(7):677–683.

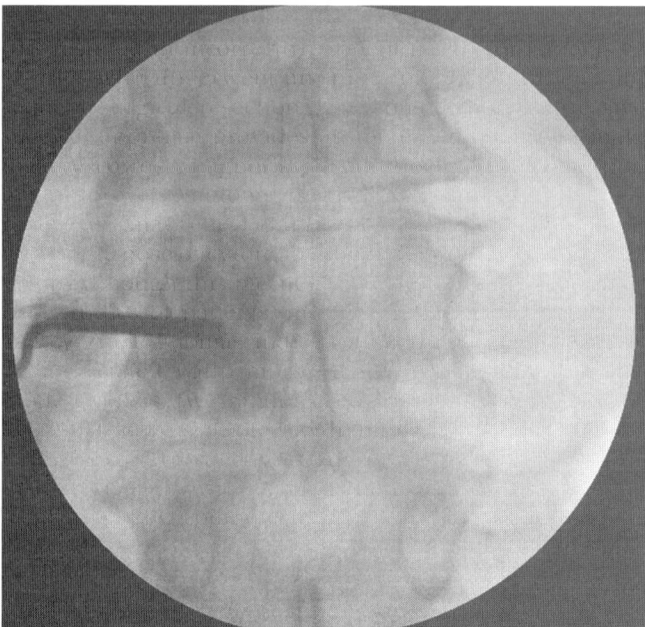

Figure 54.10 Fluoroscopic image demonstrating a vertebroplasty with transpedicular cannulation of the vertebral body with injection of PMMA cement.

14. Schirrmeister H, Guhlmann A, Kotzerke J, et al. Early detection and accurate description of extent of metastatic bone disease in breast cancer with fluoride ion and positron emission tomography. *J Clin Oncol.* 1999;17(8):2381–2389.
15. Trubenbach J, Nagele T, Bauer T, Ernemann U. Preoperative embolization of cervical spine osteoblastomas: report of three cases. *AJNR Am J Neuroradiol.* 2006;27(9):1910–1912.
16. Schirmer CM, Malek AM, Kwan ES, Hoit DA, Weller SJ. Preoperative embolization of hypervascular spinal metastases using percutaneous direct injection with n-butyl cyanoacrylate: technical case report. *Neurosurgery.* 2006;59(2):E431-E432.
17. Heary RF, Bono CM. Metastatic spinal tumors. *Neurosurg Focus.* 2001;11(6):e1.
18. Pogoda P, Linhart W, Priemel M, Rueger JM, Amling M. Aneurysmal bone cysts of the sacrum. Clinical report and review of the literature. *Arch Orthop Trauma Surg.* 2003;123(5):247–251.
19. Prabhu VC, Bilsky MH, Jambhekar K, et al. Results of preoperative embolization for metastatic spinal neoplasms. *J Neurosurg.* 2003;98(2)(suppl):156–164.
20. Papagelopoulos PJ, Currier BL, Shaughnessy WJ, et al. Aneurysmal bone cyst of the spine. Management and outcome. *Spine.* 1998;23(5):621–628.
21. Hess T, Kramann B, Schmidt E, Rupp S. Use of preoperative vascular embolisation in spinal metastasis resection. *Arch Orthop Trauma Surg.* 1997;116(5):279–282.
22. Gokaslan ZL. Spine surgery for cancer. *Curr Opin Oncol.* 1996;8(3):178–181.
23. Breslau J, Eskridge JM. Preoperative embolization of spinal tumors. *J Vasc Interv Radiol.* 1995;6(6):871–875.
24. Boriani S, Biagini R, De Iure F, et al. Primary bone tumors of the spine: a survey of the evaluation and treatment at the Istituto Ortopedico Rizzoli. *Orthopedics.* 1995;18(10):993–1000.
25. Olerud C, Jonsson H Jr., Lofberg AM, Lorelius LE, Sjostrom L. Embolization of spinal metastases reduces peroperative blood loss. 21 patients operated on for renal cell carcinoma. *Acta Orthop Scand.* 1993;64(1):9–12.
26. Konya A, Szendroi M. Aneurysmal bone cysts treated by superselective embolization. *Skeletal Radiol.* 1992;21(3):167–172.
27. King GJ, Kostuik JP, McBroom RJ, Richardson W. Surgical management of metastatic renal carcinoma of the spine. *Spine.* 1991;16(3):265–271.
28. Gellad FE, Sadato N, Numaguchi Y, Levine AM. Vascular metastatic lesions of the spine: preoperative embolization. *Radiology.* 1990;176(3):683–686.
29. Roscoe MW, McBroom RJ, St Louis E, Grossman H, Perrin R. Preoperative embolization in the treatment of osseous metastases from renal cell carcinoma. *Clin Orthop Relat Res.* 1989(238):302–307.
30. Disch SP, Grubb RL Jr., Gado MH, Strecker WB, Marbarger JP. Aneurysmal bone cyst of the cervicothoracic spine: computed tomographic evaluation of the value of preoperative embolization. Case report. *Neurosurgery.* 1986;19(2):290–293.
31. Graham JJ, Yang WC. Vertebral hemangioma with compression fracture and paraparesis treated with preoperative embolization and vertebral resection. *Spine.* 1984;9(1):97–101.
32. Esparza J, Castro S, Portillo JM, Roger R. Vetebral hemangiomas: spinal angiography and preoperative embolization. *Surg Neurol.* 1978;10(3):171–173.
33. Li WK, Lane JM, Rosen G, et al. Pelvic Ewing's sarcoma. Advances in treatment. *J Bone Joint Surg Am.* 1983;65(6):738–747.
34. Rosen G. Primary Ewing's sarcoma: the multidisciplinary lesion. *Int J Radiat Oncol Biol Phys.* 1978;4(5–6):527–532.
35. Rosen G. The current management of malignant bone tumours: where do we go from here? *Med J Aust.* 1988;148(8):373–377.
36. Rosen G, Caparros B, Nirenberg A, et al. Ewing's sarcoma: ten-year experience with adjuvant chemotherapy. *Cancer.* 1981;47(9):2204–2213.
37. Rosen G, Juergens H, Caparros B, Nirenberg A, Huvos AG, Marcove RC. Combination chemotherapy (T-6) in the multidisciplinary treatment of Ewing's sarcoma. *Natl Cancer Inst Monogr.* 1981(56):289–299.
38. Sundaresan N, Rosen G, Fortner JG, Lane JM, Hilaris BS. Preoperative chemotherapy and surgical resection in the management of posterior paraspinal tumors. Report of three cases. *J Neurosurg.* 1983;58(3):446–450.
39. Link MP. Adjuvant therapy in the treatment of osteosarcoma. *Important Adv Oncol.* 1986:193–207.
40. Link MP, Goorin AM, Miser AW, et al. The effect of adjuvant chemotherapy on relapse-free survival in patients with osteosarcoma of the extremity. *N Engl J Med.* 1986;314(25):1600–1606.
41. Link MP, Goorin AM, Horowitz M, et al. Adjuvant chemotherapy of high-grade osteosarcoma of the extremity. Updated results of the Multi-Institutional Osteosarcoma Study. *Clin Orthop Relat Res.* 1991(270):8–14.
42. Eilber F, Giuliano A, Eckardt J, Patterson K, Moseley S, Goodnight J. Adjuvant chemotherapy for osteosarcoma: a randomized prospective trial. *J Clin Oncol.* 1987;5(1):21–26.
43. Eilber FR. Adjuvant treatment of osteosarcoma. *Surg Clin North Am.* 1981;61(6):1371–1378.
44. Bacci G, Balladelli A, Forni C, et al. Adjuvant and neoadjuvant chemotherapy for Ewing sarcoma family tumors in patients aged between 40 and 60: report of 35 cases and comparison of results with 586 younger patients treated with the same protocols in the same years. *Cancer.* 2007;109(4):780–786.
45. Bacci G, Forni C, Longhi A, et al. Long-term outcome for patients with non-metastatic Ewing's sarcoma treated with adjuvant and neoadjuvant chemotherapies. 402 patients treated at Rizzoli between 1972 and 1992. *Eur J Cancer.* 2004;40(1):73–83.
46. Fayette J, Blay JY. Adjuvant chemotherapy in the treatment of sarcomas [in French]. *Bull Cancer.* 2006;93(3):257–261.
47. Goto T, Okuma T, Nakada I, Hozumi T, Kondo T. Preoperative adjuvant therapy for primary malignant bone tumors [in Japanese]. *Gan To Kagaku Ryoho.* 2007;34(11):1750–1754.
48. Hoffken K. Pre- and postoperative chemotherapy in bone and soft tissue tumors [in German]. *Langenbecks Arch Chir.* 1987;372:311–314.
49. Scully SP, Temple HT, O'Keefe RJ, Scarborough MT, Mankin HJ, Gebhardt MC. Role of surgical resection in pelvic Ewing's sarcoma. *J Clin Oncol.* 1995;13(9):2336–2341.
50. Brown AP, Fixsen JA, Plowman PN. Local control of Ewing's sarcoma: an analysis of 67 patients. *Br J Radiol.* 1987;60(711):261–268.
51. DeLaney TF, Park L, Goldberg SI, et al. Radiotherapy for local control of osteosarcoma. *Int J Radiat Oncol Biol Phys.* 2005;61(2):492–498.
52. Eilber FR, Grant T, Morton DL. Adjuvant therapy for osteosarcoma: preoperative and postoperative treatment. *Cancer Treat Rep.* 1978;62(2):213–216.
53. Ferguson WS, Goorin AM. Current treatment of osteosarcoma. *Cancer Invest.* 2001;19(3):292–315.
54. Hershey A, Bos GD, Stevens K. Successful treatment of spinal osteosarcoma with radiation and chemotherapy. *Orthopedics.* 1996;19(7):617–618.
55. Hristov B, Shokek O, Frassica DA. The role of radiation treatment in the contemporary management of bone tumors. *J Natl Compr Canc Netw.* 2007;5(4):456–466.
56. Papagelopoulos PJ, Galanis EC, Vlastou C, et al. Current concepts in the evaluation and treatment of osteosarcoma. *Orthopedics.* 2000;23(8):858–867; quiz 68–69.
57. Rao BN, Rodriguez-Galindo C. Local control in childhood extremity sarcomas: salvaging limbs and sparing function. *Med Pediatr Oncol.* 2003;41(6):584–587.
58. Suit HD. Radiotherapy in osteosarcoma. *Clin Orthop Relat Res.* 1975(111):71–75.
59. Boriani S, Weinstein JN, Biagini R. Primary bone tumors of the spine. Terminology and surgical staging. *Spine.* 1997;22(9):1036–1044.
60. Tomita K, Kawahara N, Baba H, Tsuchiya H, Fujita T, Toribatake Y. Total en bloc spondylectomy. A new surgical technique for primary malignant vertebral tumors. *Spine.* 1997;22(3):324–333.
61. Sansur CA, Pouratian N, Dumont AS, Schiff D, Shaffrey CI, Shaffrey ME. Part II: spinal-cord neoplasms—primary tumours of the bony spine and adjacent soft tissues. *Lancet Oncol.* 2007;8(2):137–147.
62. Brady MS, Gaynor JJ, Brennan MF. Radiation-associated sarcoma of bone and soft tissue. *Arch Surg.* 1992;127(12):1379–1385.
63. Dirix LY, Somville J, van Oosterom AT. Diagnosis and treatment of soft tissue sarcomas in adults. *Curr Opin Oncol.* 1996;8(4):289–298.
64. Dirix LY, Vermeulen P, De Wever I, Van Oosterom AT. Soft tissue sarcoma in adults. *Curr Opin Oncol.* 1997;9(4):348–359.
65. Enneking WF. A system of staging musculoskeletal neoplasms. *Clin Orthop Relat Res.* 1986(204):9–24.
66. Springfield DS, Schmidt R, Graham-Pole J, Marcus RB Jr., Spanier SS, Enneking WF. Surgical treatment for osteosarcoma. *J Bone Joint Surg Am.* 1988;70(8):1124–1130.
67. Heslin MJ, Lewis JJ, Nadler E, et al. Prognostic factors associated with long-term survival for retroperitoneal sarcoma: implications for management. *J Clin Oncol.* 1997;15(8):2832–2839.

68. Kraus DH, Dubner S, Harrison LB, et al. Prognostic factors for recurrence and survival in head and neck soft tissue sarcomas. *Cancer*. 1994;74(2):697–702.
69. Boriani S, Biagini R, De Iure F, Di Fiore M, Gamberini G, Zanoni A. Lumbar vertebrectomy for the treatment of bone tumors: surgical technique. *Chir Organi Mov*. 1994;79(2):163–173.
70. Roy-Camille R, Saillant G, Bisserie M, Judet T, Hautefort E, Mamoudy P. Total excision of thoracic vertebrae (author's transl) [in French]. *Rev Chir Orthop Reparatrice Appar Mot*. 1981;67(3):421–430.
71. Stener B. Total spondylectomy in chondrosarcoma arising from the seventh thoracic vertebra. *J Bone Joint Surg Br*. 1971;53(2):288–295.
72. Stener B. Complete removal of vertebrae for extirpation of tumors. A 20-year experience. *Clin Orthop Relat Res*. 1989;245:72–82.
73. Sundaresan N, Rosen G, Huvos AG, Krol G. Combined treatment of osteosarcoma of the spine. *Neurosurgery*. 1988;23(6):714–719.
74. Tomita K, Kawahara N, Baba H, Tsuchiya H, Nagata S, Toribatake Y. Total en bloc spondylectomy for solitary spinal metastases. *Int Orthop*. 1994;18(5):291–298.
75. Tomita K, Kawahara N, Murakami H, Demura S. Total en bloc spondylectomy for spinal tumors: improvement of the technique and its associated basic background. *J Orthop Sci*. 2006;11(1):3–12.
76. Kawahara N, Tomita K, Baba H, et al. Cadaveric vascular anatomy for total en bloc spondylectomy in malignant vertebral tumors. *Spine*. 1996;21(12):1401–1407.
77. Kawahara N, Tomita K, Matsumoto T, Fujita T. Total en bloc spondylectomy for primary malignant vertebral tumors. *Chir Organi Mov*. 1998;83(1–2):73–86.
78. Murakami H, Kawahara N, Abdel-Wanis ME, Tomita K. Total en bloc spondylectomy. *Semin Musculoskelet Radiol*. 2001;5(2):189–194.
79. Tomita K, Kawahara N, Kobayashi T, Yoshida A, Murakami H, Akamaru T. Surgical strategy for spinal metastases. *Spine*. 2001;26(3):298–306.
80. Tomita K, Toribatake Y, Kawahara N, Ohnari H, Kose H. Total en bloc spondylectomy and circumspinal decompression for solitary spinal metastasis. *Paraplegia*. 1994;32(1):36–46.
81. Marmor E, Rhines LD, Weinberg JS, Gokaslan ZL. Total en bloc lumbar spondylectomy. Case report. *J Neurosurg*. 2001;95(2 suppl):264–269.
82. Yao KC, Boriani S, Gokaslan ZL, Sundaresan N. En bloc spondylectomy for spinal metastases: a review of techniques. *Neurosurg Focus*. 2003;15(5):E6.
83. Abdel-Wanis Mel S, Tsuchiya H, Kawahara N, Tomita K. Tumor growth potential after tumoral and instrumental contamination: an in-vivo comparative study of T-saw, Gigli saw, and scalpel. *J Orthop Sci*. 2001;6(5):424–429.
84. Talac R, Yaszemski MJ, Currier BL, et al. Relationship between surgical margins and local recurrence in sarcomas of the spine. *Clin Orthop Relat Res*. 2002;397:127–132.
85. Society AC. *Cancer Facts & Figures 2007*. Atlanta, GA: American Cancer Society; 2007.
86. Gokaslan ZL, York JE, Walsh GL, et al. Transthoracic vertebrectomy for metastatic spinal tumors. *J Neurosurg*. 1998;89(4):599–609.
87. Weigel B, Maghsudi M, Neumann C, Kretschmer R, Muller FJ, Nerlich M. Surgical management of symptomatic spinal metastases. Postoperative outcome and quality of life. *Spine*. 1999;24(21):2240–2246.
88. Witham TF, Khavkin YA, Gallia GL, Wolinsky JP, Gokaslan ZL. Surgery insight: current management of epidural spinal cord compression from metastatic spine disease. *Nat Clin Pract Neurol*. 2006;2(2):87–94; quiz 116.
89. Helweg-Larsen S, Sorensen PS. Symptoms and signs in metastatic spinal cord compression: a study of progression from first symptom until diagnosis in 153 patients. *Eur J Cancer*. 1994;30A(3):396–398.
90. Gerszten PC, Welch WC. Current surgical management of metastatic spinal disease. *Oncology (Williston Park)*. 2000;14(7):1013–1024; discussion 24, 29–30.
91. Schaberg J, Gainor BJ. A profile of metastatic carcinoma of the spine. *Spine*. 1985;10(1):19–20.
92. Schiff D. Spinal cord compression. *Neurol Clin*. 2003;21(1):67–86, viii.
93. Schiff D, O'Neill BP, Suman VJ. Spinal epidural metastasis as the initial manifestation of malignancy: clinical features and diagnostic approach. *Neurology*. 1997;49(2):452–456.
94. Lis E, Bilsky MH, Pisinski L, et al. Percutaneous CT-guided biopsy of osseous lesion of the spine in patients with known or suspected malignancy. *AJNR Am J Neuroradiol*. 2004;25(9):1583–1588.
95. Babu NV, Titus VT, Chittaranjan S, Abraham G, Prem H, Korula RJ. Computed tomographically guided biopsy of the spine. *Spine*. 1994;19(21):2436–2442.
96. Ghelman B, Lospinuso MF, Levine DB, O'Leary PF, Burke SW. Percutaneous computed-tomography-guided biopsy of the thoracic and lumbar spine. *Spine*. 1991;16(7):736–739.
97. Stoker DJ, Kissin CM. Percutaneous vertebral biopsy: a review of 135 cases. *Clin Radiol*. 1985;36(6):569–577.
98. Tokuhashi Y, Matsuzaki H, Oda H, Oshima M, Ryu J. A revised scoring system for preoperative evaluation of metastatic spine tumor prognosis. *Spine*. 2005;30(19):2186–2191.
99. Tokuhashi Y, Matsuzaki H, Toriyama S, Kawano H, Ohsaka S. Scoring system for the preoperative evaluation of metastatic spine tumor prognosis. *Spine*. 1990;15(11):1110–1113.
100. Koehler PJ. Use of corticosteroids in neuro-oncology. *Anticancer Drugs*. 1995;6(1):19–33.
101. Pohl P, Oberhuber G, Dietze O, et al. Steroid-induced complete remission in a case of primary cerebral non-Hodgkin's lymphoma. *Clin Neurol Neurosurg*. 1989;91(3):247–250.
102. Posner JB, Howieson J, Cvitkovic E. "Disappearing" spinal cord compression: oncolytic effect of glucocorticoids (and other chemotherapeutic agents) on epidural metastases. *Ann Neurol*. 1977;2(5):409–413.
103. Pui CH, Costlow ME, Dahl GV, Rivera G, Murphy SB. Response of recurrent acute lymphoblastic leukemia to glucocorticoids: serial studies of receptor content, in vivo cytokinetic changes and clinical responses. *Leuk Res*. 1983;7(6):747–753.
104. Greenberg HS, Kim JH, Posner JB. Epidural spinal cord compression from metastatic tumor: results with a new treatment protocol. *Ann Neurol*. 1980;8(4):361–366.
105. Ikeda Y, Carson BS, Long DM. Therapeutic effects of topical dexamethasone on experimental brain tumours and peritumoural brain oedema. *Acta Neurochir Suppl (Wien)*. 1990;51:163–164.
106. Bilsky MH, Lis E, Raizer J, Lee H, Boland P. The diagnosis and treatment of metastatic spinal tumor. *Oncologist*. 1999;4(6):459–469.
107. Gilbert HA, Kagan AR, Nussbaum H, et al. Evaluation of radiation therapy for bone metastases: pain relief and quality of life. *AJR Am J Roentgenol*. 1977;129(5):1095–1096.
108. Poulsen HS, Nielsen OS, Klee M, Rorth M. Palliative irradiation of bone metastases. *Cancer Treat Rev*. 1989;16(1):41–48.
109. Tong D, Gillick L, Hendrickson FR. The palliation of symptomatic osseous metastases: final results of the Study by the Radiation Therapy Oncology Group. *Cancer*. 1982;50(5):893–899.
110. Kida A, Taniguchi S, Fukuda H, Sakai K. Radiation therapy for metastatic spinal tumors. *Radiat Med*. 2000;18(1):15–20.
111. Maranzano E, Latini P, Beneventi S, et al. Radiotherapy without steroids in selected metastatic spinal cord compression patients. A phase II trial. *Am J Clin Oncol*. 1996;19(2):179–183.
112. Maranzano E, Latini P, Perrucci E, Beneventi S, Lupattelli M, Corgna E. Short-course radiotherapy (8 Gy x 2) in metastatic spinal cord compression: an effective and feasible treatment. *Int J Radiat Oncol Biol Phys*. 1997;38(5):1037–1044.
113. Maranzano E, Trippa F, Chirico L, Basagni ML, Rossi R. Management of metastatic spinal cord compression. *Tumori*. 2003;89(5):469–475.
114. Apuzzo ML, Weiss MH, Minassian HV. Epidural spinal metastases: factors related to selection of cases for decompressive laminectomy. *Bull Los Angeles Neurol Soc*. 1977;42(2):63–70.
115. Bhalla SK. Metastatic disease of the spine. *Clin Orthop Relat Res*. 1970;73:52–60.
116. Crue BL, Felsoory A. Discussion of the indications for decompressive laminectomy in epidural spinal metastases. *Bull Los Angeles Neurol Soc*. 1977;42(2):71–76.
117. Hattori A. Laminectomy for spinal cord compression from metastatic tumor. *Nippon Geka Hokan*. 1976;45(2):175–180.
118. Iacovou JW, Marks JC, Abrams PH, Gingell JC, Ball AJ. Cord compression and carcinoma of the prostate: is laminectomy justified? *Br J Urol*. 1985;57(6):733–736.
119. Javid R, Belmusto L, Owens G. Results of surgical intervention for spinal cord compression due to metastatic tumors. *N Y State J Med*. 1965;65:409–411.
120. Nicholls PJ, Jarecky TW. The value of posterior decompression by laminectomy for malignant tumors of the spine. *Clin Orthop Relat Res*. 1985;201:210–213.
121. Slatkin NE, Posner JB. Management of spinal epidural metastases. *Clin Neurosurg*. 1983;30:698–716.

122. Solini A, Paschero B. Surgical management of spinal cord lesions due to metastases. *J Neurosurg Sci.* 1984;28(3–4):201–212.
123. Young RF, Post EM, King GA. Treatment of spinal epidural metastases. Randomized prospective comparison of laminectomy and radiotherapy. *J Neurosurg.* 1980;53(6):741–748.
124. Sakaura H, Hosono N, Mukai Y, Ishii T, Yonenobu K, Yoshikawa H. Outcome of total en bloc spondylectomy for solitary metastasis of the thoracolumbar spine. *J Spinal Disord Tech.* 2004;17(4):297–300.
125. Halpin RJ, Bendok BR, Liu JC. Minimally invasive treatments for spinal metastases: vertebroplasty, kyphoplasty, and radiofrequency ablation. *J Support Oncol.* 2004;2(4):339–351; discussion 52–55.
126. Cortet B, Cotten A, Boutry N, et al. Percutaneous vertebroplasty in patients with osteolytic metastases or multiple myeloma. *Rev Rhum Engl Ed.* 1997;64(3):177–183.
127. Cotten A, Dewatre F, Cortet B, et al. Percutaneous vertebroplasty for osteolytic metastases and myeloma: effects of the percentage of lesion filling and the leakage of methyl methacrylate at clinical follow-up. *Radiology.* 1996;200(2):525–530.
128. Fourney DR, Schomer DF, Nader R, et al. Percutaneous vertebroplasty and kyphoplasty for painful vertebral body fractures in cancer patients. *J Neurosurg.* 2003;98(1 suppl):21–30.

55 Spinal Cord Tumors

Sean J. Nagel, Kene T. Ugokwe, Paul Kim, and Edward C. Benzel

HISTORY

Patients diagnosed with intramedullary spinal cord tumors (IMSCT) have benefited remarkably from several breakthroughs adapted for neurosurgical practice over the past 50 years. From a surgical standpoint, the operating microscope and bipolar cautery have emboldened the neurosurgeon to aggressively resect IMSCT with an acceptably low risk of lasting morbidity. Similarly, the evolution of neuroimaging, specifically the advent of the magnetic resonance imaging (MRI), has been virtually invaluable as the cornerstone of perioperative management. Prior to these developments, the surgical goals advocated by most were palliative with few triumphs dotting the literature.

In a 1911 publication, Charles Elsberg championed a staged operative strategy; he initially performed a myelotomy and returned later once the tumor had delivered itself [1–3]. Another notable early report documenting the successful surgical treatment of intramedullary tumors came from the desk of Harvey Cushing. He presented his surgical series in 1927 of patients with intramedullary ependymomas [4,5]. Nearly a quarter of a century later, Greenwood detailed his experience resecting IMSCT with negligible neurologic injury. This feat predated the introduction of the operating microscope [2,6]. Today local control, if not cure, is a realistic goal in many cases through aggressive surgical resection.

EPIDEMIOLOGY

Although the exact incidence and prevalence of IMSCT is difficult to ascertain based on reported series, the relative frequency is between 2% and 8.5% of all central nervous system (CNS) tumors. Approximately 15% to 20% of adult spinal column tumors and 35% of spinal column tumors in children are IMSCT [5,7]. In general, IMSCT are found equally among men and women although appreciable gender differences do exist along some specific histologic lines [8].

EPENDYMOMA

In the adult population, ependymomas are the most common histologic type encountered, observed in approximately 60% of intramedullary spinal cord specimens. Perivascular pseudorosettes and true rosettes are reliable histologic findings [9]. Intramedullary ependymomas usually present in young adults or those nearing middle age. The cellular histologic subtype is the most frequently identified and is designated World Health Organization grade II neoplasm although more than one subtype is occasionally observed in the same lesion. The presence of vascular proliferation and an elevated mitotic index raises the grade to World Health Organization grade III or anaplastic ependymoma. Importantly, necrosis and intratumoral hemorrhage are not necessarily a harbinger of aggressive behavior [10]. Myxopapillary ependymomas are a histologically distinct subtype found almost exclusively in the filum terminale and generally are regarded as an intradural, extramedullary benign, but persistent, tumor.

ASTROCYTOMA

In the pediatric population, astrocytomas predominate, accounting for approximately 60% of IMSCT [5,11,12]. In addition, before the age of 10, nearly 90% of IMSCT will be astrocytomas [8]. In adults diagnosed with IMSCT, 20% of collected surgical specimens are astrocytomas, the vast majority of which are diagnosed before the age of 60 [5,13]. In either case, the proportion of high-grade lesions is fortunately quite low, representing 10% to 30% of spinal astrocytomas in the adult and 7% to 25% in the pediatric age group [12]. The Kernohan grading scheme is usually applied to astrocytomas arising in the spine [13]. In children, low-grade tumors are frequently pilocytic astrocytomas similar to their intracranial counterpart; conversely, the low-grade histologic subtype in adults is most often fibrillary [12,13]. Malignant astrocytomas (World Health Organization grades III, IV) are infrequent, infiltrate rapidly, and are uniformly fatal.

HEMANGIOBLASTOMA

Spinal cord hemangioblastomas account for 2% to 8% of IMSCT, are diagnosed 1.5 to 2 times more often in males, and frequently present between the ages of 33 and 35 [8,10,14]. Histologically, hemangioblastomas are characterized by a network of abundant capillaries interlaced with lipid laden stromal cells, the presumptive tumor precursor cell [15,16].

METASTASIS

Intramedullary spinal cord metastasis represents 1% to 3% of all IMSCT and only 8.5% of all CNS metastasis [17,18]. However, 57% of patients with known ISCM disease also have intracranial metastasis [17]. The bulk of ISCM, occurring in over 50% of cases, are attributed to lung cancer and more specifically small cell lung cancer [17,18]. A number of other pathologies contribute to the balance of cases with breast cancer and melanoma, isolated in 9% and 8% of patients respectively [19]. Metastatic disease secondary to a preexisting intracranial tumor, especially medulloblastoma, ependymoma, or glioma should be entertained where appropriate.

OTHER TUMORS

Approximately 1% of IMSCT are classified as ganglio-gliomas. The average age at presentation is 12. These tumors are characterized by mature neuronal and astrocytic cells populations. A review of the literature published in 2003 identified 40 reported cases of sub-ependymoma. This tumor type appears to be twice as common in men, usually presenting after the age of 40 [20]. Lipomas, not recognized as true neoplasms, are the most common dysembryogenic spinal cord lesion, diagnosed in 1% of patients. They occupy the subpial space and are therefore categorized as juxtamedullary. Other rare intramedullary tumors reported in the literature include schwannoma, germinoma, lymphoma, melanoma, primitive neuroectodermal tumor, and meningioma. Nonneoplastic considerations are cavernous angiomas, arteriovenous malformations, abscess, and dermoid or epidermoid cysts [19].

IMSCT GENETICS

Ependymoma

Ependymomas are believed to arise from the ependymal cells lining the brain and spinal cord. Genetic analysis of spinal cord ependymomas suggests that these tumors, though histologically similar, may be distinct entities based on genetic differences from intracranial ependymomas. Lending further support to a unique molecular biology is the more favorable clinical behavior observed in spinal ependymomas of similar grade [21,22]. Perhaps the most compelling evidence thus far, however, is based on the well-established association of patients with neurofibromatosis type II who are subsequently diagnosed with a CNS ependymoma. This association led to the discovery of sporadic mutations of the NF2 gene transcript, located on chromosome 22, that are often identified in patients with spinal cord ependymomas but not in intracranial ependymomas [21,22]. Similarly, LOH at 22q is also location specific [22]. Interestingly, there is evidence to suggest surgery should be used very sparingly in the management of asymptomatic IMSCT in patients with NF2 based on the indolent behavior observed when followed over several years [23].

Astrocytoma

Evidence supporting a unique cascade of detectable genetic events in the spontaneous development of spinal astrocytomas has not been as fruitful. The current consensus is that this tumor arises and upgrades to a more aggressive, incurable infiltrative tumor through a series of mutations, losses, and amplifications shown in intracranial gliomas [24]. Of note, patients with NF1 who are subsequently diagnosed with an IMSCT seem to be predisposed to the growth of an astrocytoma in contrast to patients with NF2 [13,17,24,25].

Hemangioblastoma

Patients with von Hipple-Lindau disease account for up to 20% to 30% of those eventually diagnosed with CNS hemangioblastomas; however, the genetic pathway is not necessarily shared with sporadic tumors. A "two-hit" hypothesis at the VHL gene leading to biallelic inactivation has been proposed to explain the occurrence of CNS hemangioblastomas in VHL-families [17]. In such patients, a germ line mutation at the VHL gene exists. In sporadic cases, loss of heterozygosity in the setting of a preexisting germ line mutation is much less common. All patients diagnosed with hemangioblastoma should be screened for VHL and the presence of a pheochromocytoma should be ruled out when surgery is anticipated [15].

PRESENTATION

Although no single complaint or examination finding reliably predicts the occurrence of an IMSCT, there are many frequently encountered signs and symptoms common to this population of patients. In certain instances, subtle abnormalities in the neurologic exam may yield useful clues regarding tumor type and location.

Ependymoma

In patients with ependymomas, for example, the indolent growth rate translates into months to years of unremitting symptoms [26]. Complaints are invariably disturbances in sensory function at or below the level of the lesion, specifically dysesthesias and paresthesias [26]. Radicular pain is not uncommon. Bowel and bladder dysfunction may predominate in some cases. Motor function is usually preserved until late in the course or if there is a delay in diagnosis or treatment. Preoperative ambulatory status, specifically the ability to walk unassisted is predictive of postoperative ambulatory status [27]. A sudden deterioration in neurologic function may indicate intratumoral hemorrhage. In a patient with subarachnoid hemorrhage of unknown etiology, intramedullary ependymoma should be ruled out [28].

Astrocytoma

Astrocytomas often present with pain along the neuroaxis, most commonly in a paravertebral distribution possibly related to venous congestion [13,19]. Radicular pain can mimic other causes and delay diagnosis especially when overlapping with common ailments in the abdomen and thorax. Other sensory deficits including dysesthesias and misfiring of the spinothalamic tract are routinely observed. Dorsal column dysfunction may indirectly impair the motor system; on the other hand, patients may present with an unequivocal gross motor deficit. IMSCT will characteristically impinge on the more medially located motor tracts of the upper extremities before threatening the lower extremities [13]. Although the sequence of symptoms may vary between ependymoma and astrocytoma, the temporal pattern is similar. A precipitous decline over the course of several months is suggestive of a high-grade astrocytoma [13,19].

Pediatric Spinal Cord Astrocytoma

Most pediatric patients with spinal cord astrocytomas are initially brought to attention complaining of pain. However, gait impairment, spinal deformity, torticollis, and regression of motor skills are oftentimes present [2,13]. Spinal deformity is evident in up to one third of patients [2]. In contrast to idiopathic scoliosis, the apex of the curve is often aligned to the left and when asymptomatic, may not be recognized until the patient is in young adulthood [13]. Signs and symptoms of hydrocephalous may also be observed in approximately 15% of patients; malignant tumors tend to aggravate this finding.

Other Tumors

The signs and symptoms of less common IMSCT do not vary significantly from more frequent tumors. Hemangioblastomas, usually positioned dorsally, are often associated with sensory complaints and symptomatic tumors are almost always associated with a syrinx. Patients with intramedullary spinal cord metastasis characteristically exhibit a shorter duration (<6 months) and rapid progression of debilitating symptoms [18]. This is likely secondary to the limited tolerance of the spinal cord in the setting of a rapidly expanding mass. A new sensory deficit usually alerts the patient initially; however, weakness, pain, and bowel and/or bladder deficits are often present on examination. In patients with known malignancy and a Brown-Sequard syndrome or complete cord transection, intramedullary spinal cord metastasis is a likely culprit [18]. Severe neurologic deficits are predictive of poor functional recovery mandating objective pretreatment grading [18].

IMAGING CHARACTERISITICS

Magnetic Resonance Imaging

MRI remains the modality of choice in detecting and differentiating intramedullary spinal cord lesions. Whereas other imaging techniques may have an expanded role under some circumstances, such as in preoperative planning using multiplanar reformatted CT, the diagnostic value is negligible in comparison. In a patient with an absolute contraindication to MRI, CT-myelography should be ordered and may demonstrate partial or complete block. Standard MRI sequences should include T1, T1 with gadolinium, and fast spin echo T2 formatted in axial and sagittal planes. In addition, gradient echo sequences may be beneficial in distinguishing areas marked with hemosiderin [28]. The utility of fluid attenuation inversion recovery in IMSCT imaging is of unknown benefit. Short time inversion recovery sequences are undervalued in revealing intramedullary pathology. Although it may be possible to identify an anatomic region of interest with the physical exam alone, the MRI should include several vertebral levels above and below the suspected area to ensure that a syrinx is not overlooked; routine complete neuroaxis imaging is rarely warranted, however, on initial assessment unless metastatic disease is a consideration [18].

Evaluating Operative Versus Nonoperative Lesions

The evaluation of an intramedullary lesion on MRI rests on determining if it is operative in nature. Nonsurgical lesions, such as spinal cord infarct, multiple sclerosis, sarcoidosis, amyloid, and transverse myelitis are often mistaken for tumors initially both on neuroimaging and clinical grounds including cerebrospinal fluid (CSF) studies [29,30,31] (Figure 55.1). On the T1-weighted images, tumors are usually hypo- or isointense to the spinal cord and are characterized by subtle or prominent cord expansion although acute nonoperative lesions may produce a similar effect. The complete absence of cord expansion should strongly dissuade the operative pursuit of

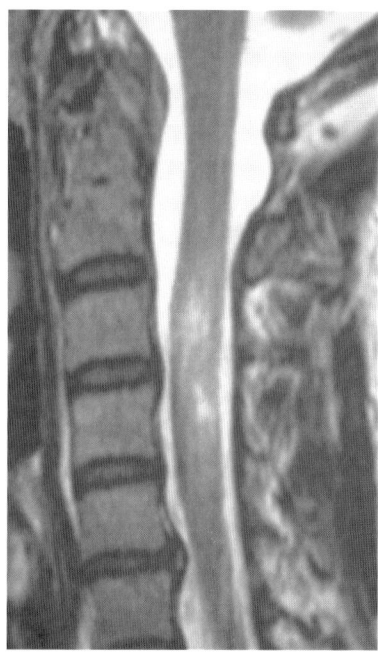

Figure 55.1 Sagittal T2-weighted MRI of the cervical spine showing subtle cord enlargement and variable, hyperintense signal in the spinal cord. The patient presented with rapid-onset quadriparesis and was later diagnosed with Devic's disease.

a neoplastic lesion [28,31]. Of note, the buildup of mucin in myxopapillary ependymomas likely contributes to the hyperintense signal seen on T1 and T2 MRI [32]. Many tumors will enhance uniformly with gadolinium, but this is not the rule and enhancement appears unrelated to histologic grade [28]. Tumor associated cysts are commonplace and may limit the differential. Areas of peritumoral edema are best observed on fast spin echo T2-weighted images but may impair the appreciation of the tumor-edema interface in light of the fact that most tumors are also often hyperintense on this sequence. A tumor-derived syrinx is often present in patients harboring IMSCT and is more frequently observed at higher vertebral levels [29].

Surgical Planning

In patients in whom surgery is imminent, whether for open biopsy or partial or complete resection of an IMSCT, it is necessary to identify and address several key radiographic features. The boundaries of the tumor along its long axis should be studied and correlated with the enclosing vertebral levels. Furthermore, on the axial sections, the relationship of the tumor to the cord substance should be used to plan the least destructive approach to the tumor with the myelotomy. Last, if the tumor is potentially a hemangioblastoma, preoperative embolization should be considered.

Distinguishing Ependymoma Versus Astrocytoma

At this time, only a surgical biopsy can reliably confirm the difference between an ependymoma and an astrocytoma, and distinguishing the two on MRI alone remains largely an academic exercise. Nevertheless, large series of patients with IMSCT have been collected and have identified several recognizable, consistent findings that may be useful during preoperative patient counseling and operative planning. Ependymomas are rarely eccentric and usually have well-defined borders. They have a tendency to occupy the cervicothoracic spinal cord and virtually always enhance with either a heterogeneous or a homogeneous pattern [26,33] (Figure 55.2). Nonenhancing cysts, both rostral and/or caudal, are the norm and usually resolve after resection; enhancing intratumoral cysts on the other hand may also be evident and should be included with resection [32]. Syringomyelia is observed in approximately 65% of ependymomas [29]. Hemorrhage, while not pathognomonic, is rarely seen with other IMSCT [32]. Pseudocapsule formation, identified on T1 or T2 as a hypointensity at the tumor margins is indicative of ependymoma [32,33]. By contrast, astrocytomas are usually infiltrative, eccentrically located tumors that take root predominantly in the cervical spine; rarely holocord tumors are observed, usually in children [32] (Figure 55.3). Associated cysts are less common [33].

Imaging Features of Hemangioblastoma

Hemangioblastomas appear isointense on T1-weighted images; an enhancing tumor nodule is evident after

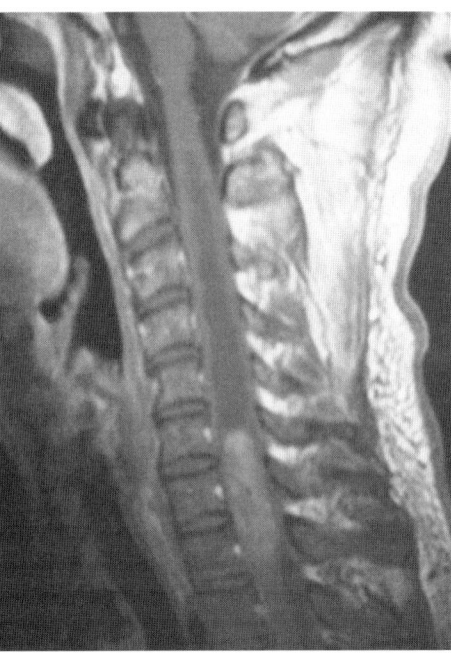

Figure 55.2 Preoperative, sagittal, gadolinium-enhanced T1 MRI of a patient with a histologically confirmed intramedullary ependymoma at the cervicothoracic junction. The tumor characteristically exhibits heterogeneous enhancement, central location, and an associated syrinx.

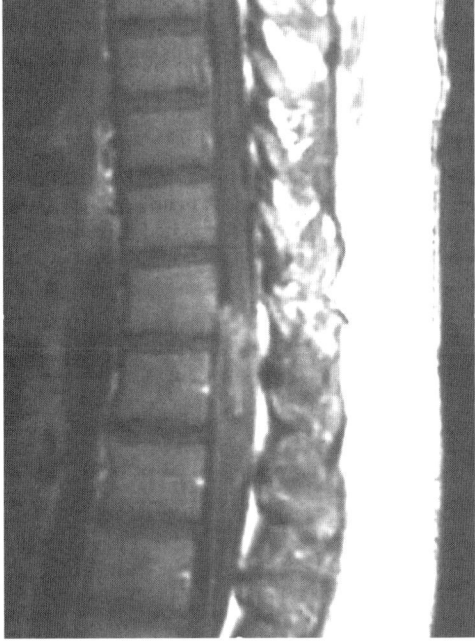

Figure 55.3 Sagittal, gadolinium-enhanced T1 MRI with infiltrating intramedullary spinal cord tumor. Histologic features were consistent with glioblastoma multiforme.

gadolinium is given. There is a preponderance of peritumoral edema often out of proportion to the size of the nodule and an associated syrinx is usually evident [28,33] (Figure 55.4A). The presence of flow voids favors, but is

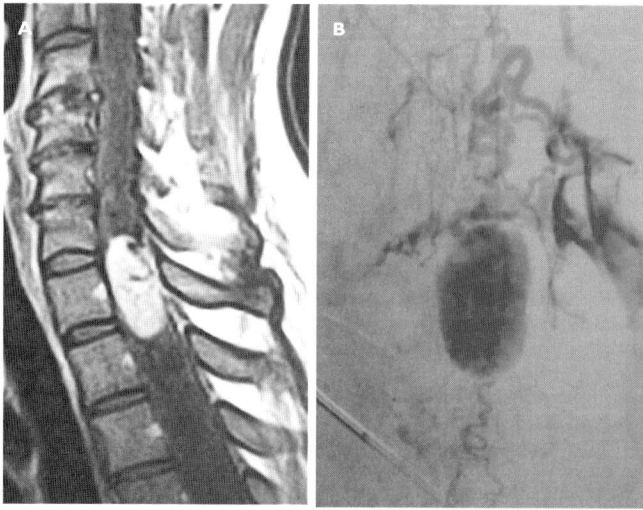

Figure 55.4 Sagittal, gadolinium enhanced cervical spine MRI demonstrating homogeneously enhancing mass with flow void (A). A preoperative angiogram was identified in the arterial supply and venous drainage (B). These findings are consistent with hemangioblastoma. This was confirmed surgically.

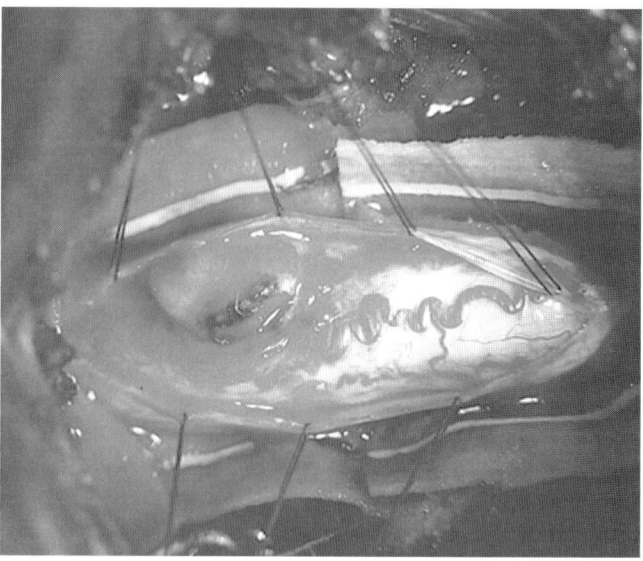

Figure 55.5 Intraoperative photograph of a hemangioblastoma with well-defined spinal cord–tumor boundary after pial splitting.

not diagnostic of hemangioblastomas. When hemangioblastoma is a diagnostic consideration, spinal angiography and more specifically embolization may augment the surgical resection of large, hypervascular tumors though this is debatable [15,34] (Figure 55.4B). Dedicated spinal magnetic resonance angiography may also be of value. Most tumors are fed by the posterior and lateral spinal arteries. Stable, asymptomatic hemangioblastomas can potentially be followed in patients with VHL [15].

Imaging Features of Gangliogliomas

Gangliogliomas are virtually always eccentrically located, have mixed signal characteristics on T1-weighted images, and often lack surrounding edema [33]. Bone remodeling and scoliosis are frequently associated with gangliogliomas. They frequently extend over multiple segments with holocord involvement in 15% [29].

Imaging Features of Nonglial Tumors

In considering the nonglial tumors, with the exception of hemangioblastoma, which to some extent is radiographically unique, the relative infrequency with which other IMSCT types are encountered do not appreciably lend themselves to tidy classification patterns in most instances. Metastasis may be found in multiple locations of the spinal cord in up to a third of patients; therefore, holocord imaging is suggested [29]. Metastases are less likely to have an associated cyst but are more likely to incite peritumoral edema [28] (Figure 55.4B).

PREOPERATIVE EVALUATION

Surgery is usually scheduled and promptly carried out after an IMSCT is diagnosed. As most of these patients are young adults or early middle age, a standard history and physical examination should capture the relevant medical information. Steroids are not routinely administered in the preoperative period unless the patient presents in a precipitous functional decline or if surgery is expected to be difficult with a high risk of neurological injury. Several retrospective series that address the surgical treatment of IMSCT point to preoperative neurological status as a significant predictor of postoperative functional outcome [35–37]. Preservation, rather than restoration, of neurological function is the expected outcome of uncomplicated surgery [35,36]. In a recent series of 78 patients who underwent surgical resection of IMSCT, nearly 35% had deteriorated from baseline following surgery [36]. Significant improvement of a severe or long-standing preoperative neurological deficit rarely occurs even after technically successful surgery. Surgical morbidity is amplified in patients with significant preoperative deficits and thus the surgical risk may actually be reduced in many patients with minimal neurological deficits. Taken together, early clinical diagnosis and definitive initial surgical treatment are critical to the management of most intramedullary tumors [38].

SURGICAL STRATEGY

Surgical Objectives

The nature of the tumor-spinal cord juncture determines the operative plan. Benign tumors, such as ependymomas and hemangioblastomas, are generally noninfiltrative lesions that exhibit a distinct tumor-spinal cord interface (Figure 55.5). As such, gross total resection (GTR) is the treatment of choice in these cases. Unlike the generally benign histology, circumscribed nature, and natural history of ependymomas and hemangioblastomas, astrocytomas display variable histology, spinal cord deformation, and behavior. Although some low-grade astrocytomas are well-circumscribed and are amenable to GTR, most exhibit spinal cord infiltration. Intraoperatively, there is rarely a definitive, identifiable dissection plane sequestering tumor from spinal cord. Whereas GTR may be achieved and recognized intraoperatively in some cases, the extent of resection in astrocytomas is often uncertain and ill-defined in most cases. Furthermore, aggressive resection beyond what is clearly tumor risks loss of neurological function from resection of infiltrated, yet functionally viable, spinal cord parenchyma.

Correlation between the extent of resection and tumor control in astrocytomas has not been definitively established [39,40]. Because preservation of neurological function, rather than GTR, is a more prudent treatment strategy in these cases, tumor removal should be limited to pathologic tissue that is clearly distinguishable from the surrounding spinal cord. In accordance, the extent of tumor resection varies; diffusely infiltrative lesions are often biopsied alone or debulked, whereas GTR may be possible in well-circumscribed cases.

The management of less common IMSCT is also dictated by the nature of the tumor-spinal cord interface. Metastatic spinal cord tumors usually appear as a well-circumscribed, focal mass amenable to GTR. Postresection radiation therapy, as used following resection of intracranial metastasis, may reduce the risk of local tumor recurrence. Intramedullary lipomas are inclusion tumors that are sharply demarcated from the spinal cord, yet are tightly adherent to functional spinal cord tissue at its margins. Conservative internal debulking of the tumor usually begets long-term clinical stability and satisfactory functional outcomes without significant progression of the tumor.

Intraoperative Monitoring

Although spinal cord monitoring is often used during surgery for IMSCT, its value remains debated. Recent literature suggests that long-term motor outcome may be improved by monitoring motor evoked potentials [41]. However, as aforementioned, preoperative neurological status is considered to be the most important variable affecting postoperative functional outcome. Patients who have no or minimal preoperative motor deficits are at small risk for neurological deterioration. Those with significant preexisting motor deficits are more likely to deteriorate postoperatively.

Operative Technique

Exposure

Surgery for IMSCT is performed in the prone position in nearly all cases. A dexamethasone bolus is administered at the start of the operation. A laminectomy is performed, spanning the rostral and caudal aspect of the solid portion of the tumor. The bony removal does not necessarily need to expose cysts rostral or caudal to the solid portion of the IMSCT unless the cyst wall enhances indicating an intratumoral cysts. The facet joints should be preserved if possible; delayed instability rarely occurs after laminectomy for IMSCT removal in adults. Laminoplasty, or instrumented

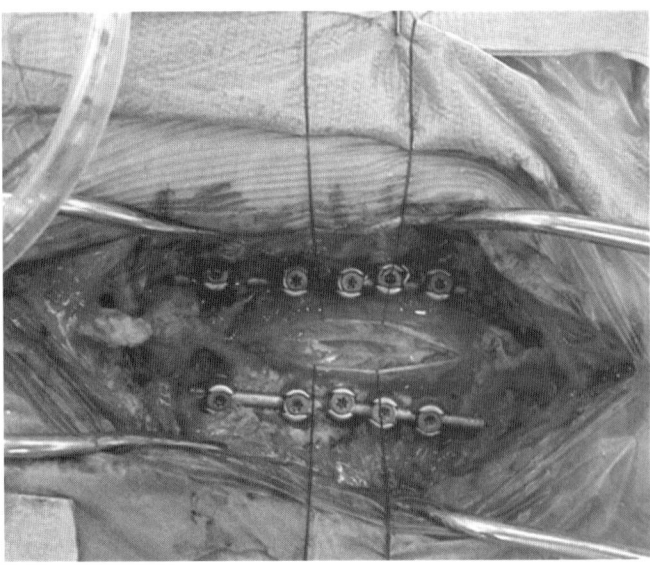

Figure 55.6 Intraoperative photograph taken immediately after midline myelotomy. The dura is retained with sutures to facilitate tumor removal.

fusion, is recommended when the laminectomy includes the apices of normal spine curvature (Figure 55.6). Intraoperative ultrasound, when available, can be used to accurately detect the tumor margins, confirming that the bony removal is sufficient.

Tumor Resection

The dura mater is usually opened in the midline; the spinal cord is often expanded, rotated, or distorted. Occasionally, the spinal cord overlying the tumor may be thinned or even transparent because of a large or eccentrically located tumor or cyst. Standard microsurgical techniques with suction and bipolar cautery are used together with a select set of specialized instruments that aid in minimizing surgical trauma to the normal spinal cord (Figure 55.7). The application of the Cavitron ultrasonic aspirator system has improved the resection of IMSCT [2]. This device uses high-frequency sound waves to fragment tumor tissue, which is then aspirated by a suction apparatus at the tip of the device. This facilitates intratumoral debulking. However, experience with intraoperative monitoring has shown that partial injury to the motor pathways is a risk with use of the Cavitron ultrasonic aspirator. It should be used to remove already partially detached tumor bulk rather than to resect tumor tissue that remains largely in situ within the spinal cord.

The microsurgical laser is an excellent tool for surgery of IMSCT. The Nd:YAG Contact LaserTM system (SLT, Montgomeryville, PA, USA) consists of a laser-suction combination that can be used like other microsurgical instruments. It is particularly useful for myelotomy and to demarcate the glial-tumor interface. Unlike bipolar cautery, it does not interfere with intraoperative monitoring. It is especially useful with firm IMSCT, which risk injury to adjacent normal spinal cord with excessive manipulation

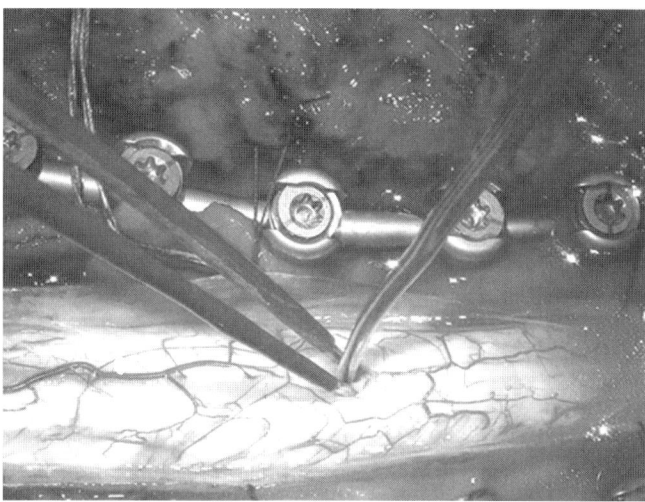

Figure 55.7 Intraoperative photograph demonstrating microdissection using bipolar cautery and suction. In this patient, the spinal instrumentation seen adjacent to the dura was implanted prior to dural opening.

[42]. The laser also simplifies internal debulking of spinal cord lipomas by vaporizing the fat.

Closure

Following tumor resection, lasting hemostasis should be achieved prior to closure of the dura. The dura mater and muscle fascia should be closed in watertight fashion to prevent CSF leakage. This is particularly important in patients who have been on high-dose systemic corticosteroids and/or those who have undergone previous surgery or radiation therapy, as they represent a high-risk group for wound dehiscence and other complications. Adjuvant therapy, when indicated, should begin no sooner than 6 weeks postoperatively to minimize the risk of wound breakdown.

POSTOPERATIVE CARE AND COMPLICATIONS

After a routine, uncomplicated stay in the postanesthesia care unit, most patients are transferred to the regular nursing floor unless autonomic instability or airway compromise is feared. MRI with gadolinium is completed within 24 hours. Patients with lumbar incisions are instructed to remain recumbent for 24 to 48 hours; conversely, those with cervical or thoracic incision are left upright. Patients should be mobilized early as tolerated. In those with marked deficits, early rehab referral is desirable. The same preventative measures used in those plagued with chronic spinal cord injuries are instituted immediately in patients who are bedridden secondary to tumor invasion.

Postoperative Disability

Nearly all patients experience dorsal column dysfunction postoperatively. This is likely an unavoidable consequence

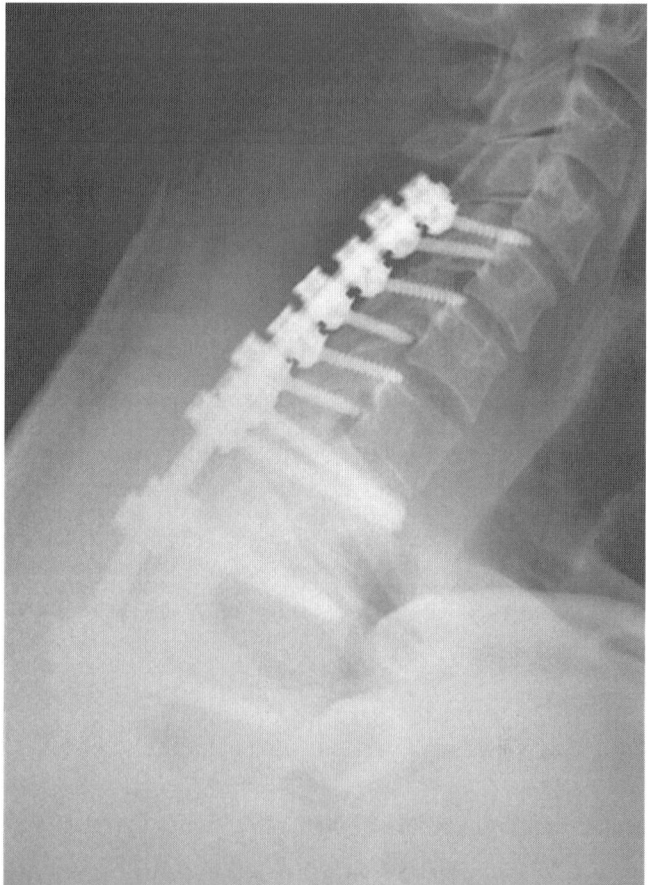

Figure 55.8 Postoperative lateral x-ray of the cervicothoracic junction. Spinal construct bridges the cervicothoracic junction to prevent delayed kyphotic deformity.

of dorsal midline myelotomy. Patients will often complain of numbness or paresthesias with relatively minimal objective discriminative or proprioceptive deficits. The subjective complaints usually improve with time, but may endure. Impaired joint position sense can lead to long-term disability. These patients may require aggressive physical therapy to maximize functional recovery and/or to compensate for acquired deficits. In addition, patients may experience unrelenting pain syndromes and autonomic perturbations. Such patients routinely complain of seasonal fluctuations, worse during cold weather months.

Prevention and Correction of Spinal Deformity

Although scoliosis and kyphosis are uncommon deformities after intradural surgery in adults, their relevance in children cannot be overstated. There is an increased incidence of developing a postoperative deformity requiring a second, stabilizing operation in children, ranging from 33% to 100% in selected series [2,43–45]. Although osteoplastic laminotomy is believed to reduce the incidence of spinal deformity in children, many surgeons still prefer instrumented fusion to prevent a postlaminectomy kyphotic deformity in the cervical spine (Figure 55.8). Conversely, there is considerably less risk in developing a kyphosis or instability necessitating a subsequent instrumented stabilization following laminectomy for resection of thoracic and lumbar IMSCT. It is thus imperative to follow-up children with serial plain x-rays. In addition, in patients who develop a late progressive deformity, a new MRI should be ordered to rule out tumor recurrence. Spinal deformity may also arise following radiation therapy used to treat IMSCT as well as extradural spine tumors. An increased rate of spinal deformity was associated with younger age at the time of radiation, doses greater than 20 Gy, and asymmetrical radiation fields [46,47]. Thus radiation treatment for IMSCT should not be considered a "noninvasive" alternative to surgery.

CSF Fistula

CSF leakage is infrequent after initial surgery for resection of IMSCT. However, after radiation, previous surgery, and/or high-dose systemic corticosteroid therapy, there is a significant risk for wound dehiscence and CSF fistula. When observed, plastic surgical techniques, including mobilization of paraspinal musculature for wound closure, have been successful. In addition, trapezius and latissimus flaps have been used for complex cervicothoracic wounds as other options for well-vascularized soft tissue to obliterate dead space and cover exposed, nonhealing wounds [48].

FUNCTIONAL OUTCOME

Functional outcomes following surgery for IMSCT are largely influenced by the preoperative neurological condition. Currently, the most commonly used clinical measure of neurologic function in patients with IMSCT was developed by McCormick et al [49] (Table 55.1).

Overall, the existing literature indicates that roughly 60% of patients undergoing resection for IMSCT remain at their preoperative functional grade [35,36,50]. Patients with only minimal deficit at presentation rarely fall more than one grade, whereas the risk for further decline in patients with moderate to severe preexisting deficits is magnified. Although there are conflicting reports in the literature, a number of studies have demonstrated previous treatment (surgery, radiotherapy, or chemotherapy), level and extent of tumor, or patient age did not independently affect functional outcome following surgery for IMSCT. However, other selected studies have demonstrated differences in functional outcome based on histopathology alone, with relatively more favorable functional outcomes in patients with vascular tumors versus those with tumors of neuroepithelial or glial origin [36].

OUTCOMES AND ADJUVANT THERAPY

Given the relatively rare incidence of IMSCT in the population, a comprehensive treatment strategy has yet to evolve due to insufficient evidence. The cumulative data suggests however, that surgical resection and specifically GTR is the first line and often the definitive treatment for the majority of low-grade, easily accessible IMSCT. The optimal postsurgical adjuvant therapy, if even necessary for IMSCT, has yet to be adequately evaluated in patients with GTR, subtotal resection (STR), or recurrence. This will likely be the case for some time. There is a growing body of literature addressing the utility of radiation in IMSCT although a consensus among the involved physicians on its true merits is lacking. Nevertheless, the role of radiation in IMSCT management is institutional if not directly physician driven at present. Chemotherapy is even less well studied and consequently has even fewer proponents.

Long-term Survival

The main determinant of long-term patient survival is the histopathologic diagnosis of the IMSCT. For low-grade tumors, length of survival is considerably longer than that reported for high-grade tumors. Several studies have demonstrated between 5- and 10-year survival rates at more than 90% and 80%, respectively, for low-grade tumors [35,36]. In contrast, one recent study revealed between 5- and 10-year survival rates of 24% and 18%, respectively, for high-grade tumors [35].

Another factor affecting long-term survival is the extent of tumor resection. Several retrospective studies have indicated that gross total or STR of low-grade gliomas yielded the longest intervals of progression-free survival in comparison to a minimal resection [35,36]. However, discrepancy exists regarding the definition of a gross total, subtotal, and minimal resection. In addition, the inherent difficulty in overcoming surgeon's bias and evaluating postoperative MRI render data from these retrospective studies suspect in many cases. While those patients developing spinal deformities following treatment for IMSCT tended to demonstrate worse survival characteristics, it is unclear as to whether this correlation was due to tumor recurrence or the effect of the deformity and the need for spinal stabilization in these patients.

Conventional Radiation

IMSCTs are typically controlled with ionizing radiation that is delivered to patients using a shaped photon beam generated by a linear accelerator. The length of the field to be radiated should encompass the tumor and one or two vertebral bodies above and below. The width of the field should cover the region between the transverse processes

Table 55.1 Modified McCormick Scale for Functional Evaluation of Patients with IMSCT

Grade	Explanation
I	Neurologically intact, ambulates normally, may have minimal dysesthesia
II	Mild motor or sensory deficit, maintains functional independence
III	Moderate deficit, limitation of function, independent with external aid
IV	Severe motor or sensory deficit, limitation of function, dependent
V	Paraplegic/quadriplegic, even if there is flickering movement

of the vertebral body of interest. To minimize the harmful effects of radiation on normal spinal cord, the radiation is fractionated in small, daily doses over several weeks. Further protection of normal spinal cord is afforded through the alignment of convergent radiation beams. When multidirectional radiation beams converge on a target, the energy is summated, yielding a stronger, concentrated exposure at the target. A radiation dose of 4500 to 5000 cGy administered in 180 to 200 cGy fractions (a standard dose for IMSCT) carries a 5% risk of permanent, potentially crippling spinal cord injury at 5 years [51–53]. Favorable prognostic factors following radiation include young age at diagnosis, low-grade primary tumors, and duration of symptoms prior to presentation.

Chemotherapy

There are a limited number of trials that have specifically compared postoperative chemotherapy regimens in patients with IMSCT. Most of the available information and recommendations are adapted from the literature focusing on intracranial tumors of similar histology.

Adjuvant Therapy in Ependymoma

The complete resection of ependymomas without adjuvant therapy, generally regarded as the initial treatment of choice, still results in a failure rate of approximately 10% or less according to several studies [54–58]. Surgery with postoperative radiation leads to survival rates of 50% to 100% at 5 and 10 years even in the presence of local failure [59–62]. At the Cleveland Clinic, we advocate routine neuroimaging following GTR. Failure to achieve GTR should prompt return to the operating room in most cases when the potential for neurologic injury is not the limiting factor. In patients with STR, where further surgery is deemed unsafe, radiation should be strongly considered. Benign ependymomas are treated with a total dose of up to 5040 cGy in 180 cGy fractions over 28 treatment days [63,64]. There is an expected correlation between the extent of resection and survival [49,65]. Hoshimaru et al [66] reported that in 36 patients with spinal cord ependymomas(34 had GTR and 2 had STR) at a mean follow-up of 56 months, 39% were neurologically improved, 47% were stable, and 14% were worse. Tumor recurrence warrants repeat surgical resection in most settings if possible followed by radiation.

Spinal cord ependymomas are relatively chemoresistant. Neoplastic cellular defenses includes the overproduction of the multidrug resistance gene (MDR1) and its product P-glycoprotein (Pgp) [67]. Most of the information available on the use of chemotherapy in managing spinal cord ependymomas is derived from the pediatric literature. In children less than 2 years of age with cranial and spinal ependymomas, chemotherapy plays a significant role because radiation therapy is fraught with problems including interference with normal growth and development. Certain studies have examined the treatment of intracranial ependymomas with "8-in-1 regimen" and carboplatin plus etoposide [68]. There have also been reports of treatment of intracranial ependymomas with cisplatin [69], carboplatin [70], or ifosfamide [71] in patients with recurrent tumors. It is unclear if and how this data can be applied to spinal cord tumors.

Adjuvant Therapy in Astrocytoma

In general, it may be difficult to obtain a GTR of astrocytomas of the spinal cord due to the infiltrative nature of the lesion. Whether a patient with evidence of residual tumor on postoperative neuroimaging should return to the operating room is debatable. In patients with intramedullary spinal cord pilocytic astrocytomas, GTR is more desirable than STR. Epstein et al [72] concluded that radiation therapy in the management of low-grade astrocytomas should be reserved for situations where only an STR was achieved. Survival outcomes in patients diagnosed with astrocytomas are not as promising as in ependymomas. In a series of 21 patients that were seen and treated, 15 patients received radiation therapy after biopsy or resection; the 5-year survival for patients with low-grade astrocytomas was only 57% [40]. When surgical resection is followed by postoperative radiation, the survival rate is reported to be 60% to 90% at 5 years [54,59,73,74]. The survival rate for high-grade astrocytomas is appalling. Surgery usually results in worsened or at best the same neurologic function as before intervention. The median survival after surgery is 6 months; this does not appear to be affected by the extent of surgical resection [72,75]. Patients with low-grade astrocytomas are treated similarly to those with benign ependymomas using a total dose of up to 5040 cGy in 180 cGy fractions over 28 treatment days [63,64]. High-grade astrocytomas are treated to a total dose of 5400 cGy with 180 cGy fractions [76]. Radiation doses that lead to functional and histologic cordotomy may improve survival up to 4 years after surgery [54,75].

The use of chemotherapy in spinal cord astrocytomas has not been as extensively studied as in intracranial astrocytomas. Allen reported on 8-in-1 chemotherapy for high-grade spinal astrocytomas [77]. The 8-in-1 chemotherapy refers to treatment with vincristine, carmustine, procarbazine, hydroxyurea, cisplatin, cytarabine, prednisone, and cyclophosphamide, all in a one-day regimen. The patients had two cycles of induction therapy that was followed by radiotherapy. After radiotherapy, the patients then received maintenance chemotherapy with eight cycles of the same regimen. The 5-year progression-free survival and overall survival were 48% ± 14% and 54% ± 14%, respectively. The authors were unable to observe a statistically significant benefit of the 8-in-1 regimen over CCNU and vincristine. Bouffet and Foreman have also reported the treatment of spinal cord astrocytomas with carboplatin and vincristine [78,79]. Bouffet presented a case report of a patient who had radiographic evidence of remission after treatment with carboplatin and vincristine.

Adjuvant Therapy in Hemangioblastomas

Surgical resection when feasible should be offered as first-line therapy in the management of hemangioblastoma arising in the spine. Following the surgical resection of spinal hemangioblastoma, more than 90% of patients improve or remain clinically stable. Five to 10% of patients worsen after surgical resection [55,80]. Radiation therapy is the treatment of choice for unresectable and incompletely resected hemangioblastomas. In patients with recurrent hemangioblastomas who are unable to tolerate further surgery, radiation therapy is also a potential treatment option. Most of the radiation data on hemangioblastomas is based on the available data on the treatment of cerebellar lesions. Smalley et al [81] reported their experience with 25 patients with intracranial hemangioblastomas. Nineteen patients had gross disease at the time of irradiation and six had evidence of residual microscopic disease. The 5-, 10-, and 15-year recurrence-free survival rates were 76%, 76%, and 42%, respectively. In their report, it was evident that better control was achieved with doses of at least 5000 cGy [81]. There is a limited role for chemotherapy in the management of spinal cord hemangioblastomas at present. Antiangiogenic treatment of hemangioblastomas with interferon α-2a and SU 5416 has been reported in patients with previously progressive hemangioblastomas [82]. However, this still falls within the realm of experimental therapy. Piribauer et al [83] also presented a case report of stabilization of a progressive cerebellar hemangioblastomas with thalidomide in a patient who underwent surgical resection three times with subsequent radiation therapy . In general, when patients present with spinal cord hemangioblastomas, surgical resection is often the treatment of choice even in the presence of recurrent disease.

Adjuvant Therapy in Intramedullary Spinal Cord Metastasis

Intramedullary spinal cord metastases are generally an indicator of advanced systemic disease and generally carry a very poor prognosis. Median survival following the diagnosis of an intramedullary spinal cord metastases is 19 weeks (range 3 weeks to 27 months) [84]. Patients receiving only steroids survived only 5 weeks on average whereas those receiving radiation only or radiation with chemotherapy had average survival of 15 weeks and 29 weeks, respectively [84]. Surgery may be an option in patients with limited systemic disease and no evidence of leptomeningeal spread. Traditionally however, radiation therapy and corticosteroids have been used in the treatment of intramedullary spinal cord metastases. Fractionated external radiation using 16.3 to 45.2 Gy in 5 to 25 fractions over 2 to 4 weeks has been postulated as an adequate protocol [85]. Chemotherapy regimens for intramedullary spinal cord metastases are the same as used for the primary tumor.

CONCLUSIONS

Surgery for IMSCT, once used solely for diagnosis, currently represents the most effective treatment method for the majority of intramedullary neoplasms [86]. Long-term tumor control or cure, with preservation of neurological function, is possible. Therefore, thorough preoperative planning, avoidance of errors intraoperatively, and establishing optimal postoperative conditions are the keys to successful management and outcomes. The benefits of adjuvant therapy are difficult to interpret but remain an important option in the multifaceted care necessary to treat these patients.

REFERENCES

1. Elsberg CA, Beer E. The operability of intramedullary tumors of the spinal cord. A report of two operations with remarks upon the extrusion of intraspinal tumors. *Am J Med Sci.* 1911;141:636–647.
2. Kothbauer KF. Neurosurgical management of intramedullary spinal cord tumors in children. *Pediatr Neurosurg.* 2007;43(3):222–235.
3. Jallo GI, Freed D, Epstein F. Intramedullary spinal cord tumors in children. *Childs Nerv Syst.* 2003;19(9):641–649.
4. Cushing H. The intracranial tumors of preadolescence. *Am J Dis Child.* 1927;33:551–584.
5. Cooper PR, Hida K. Intramedullary spinal cord tumors. In: Dickman CA, Fehlings MG, Gokaslan ZL (Eds.) *Spinal Cord and Spinal Column Tumors: Principles and Practices.* New York, NY: Thieme; 2006.
6. Greenwood J Jr. Total removal of intramedullary tumors. *J Neurosurg.* 1954;11(6):616–621.
7. Chi JH, Parsa AT. Intrinsic metastatic spinal cord tumors. In. Berger M, Prados M, eds. *Textbook of Neurooncology.* Philadelphia: Elsevier Saunders; 2005:531–534.
8. Parsa A, Tihan T, McCormick PC. Spinal axis tumors. In: Berger M, Prados M, eds. *Textbook of Neurooncology.* Philadelphia: Elsevier Saunders; 2005:476–484.
9. Schwartz T, Parsa AT, McCormick PC. Intramedullary ependymomas. In. Berger M, Prados M, eds. *Textbook of Neurooncology.* Philadelphia: Elsevier Saunders; 2005:497–500.
10. Tihan T, Chi JH, McCormick PC, Ames CP, Parsa AT. Pathologic and epidemiologic findings of intramedullary spinal cord tumors. *Neurosurg Clin N Am.* 2006;17(1):7–11.
11. Marmor E, Gokaslan ZL. Primary spinal cord tumors. In: Victor A. Levin (Ed.) *Cancer of the Nervous System.* New York: Oxford University Press; 2002.
12. Goldstein IM, Houten JK. Spinal cord astrocytoma: presentation, management and outcome. In: Berger M, Prados M, eds. *Textbook of Neurooncology.* Philadelphia: Elsevier Saunders; 2005:501–510.
13. Houten JK, Cooper PR. Spinal cord astrocytomas: presentation, management and outcome. *J Neurooncol.* 2000;47(3):219–224.
14. Lonser RR, Oldfield, EH. Spinal cord hemangioblastoma. In: Berger M, Prados M, eds. *Textbook of Neurooncology.* Philadelphia: Elsevier Saunders; 2005:501–510.
15. Lonser RR, Oldfield EH. Spinal cord hemangioblastomas. *Neurosurg Clin N Am.* 2006;17(1):37–44.
16. Vortmeyer AO, Gnarra JR, Emmert-Buck MR, et al. von Hippel-Lindau gene deletion detected in the stromal cell component of a cerebellar hemangioblastoma associated with von Hippel-Lindau disease. *Hum Pathol.* 1997;28(5):540–543.
17. Chi JH, Cachola K, Parsa AT. Genetics and molecular biology of intramedullary spinal cord tumors. *Neurosurg Clin N Am.* 2006;17(1):1–5.
18. Lee SS, Kim MK, Sym SJ, et al. Intramedullary spinal cord metastases: a single-institution experience. *J Neurooncol.* 2007;84(1):85–89.
19. Roonprapunt C, Houten JK. Spinal cord astrocytomas: presentation, management, and outcome. *Neurosurg Clin N Am.* 2006;17(1):29–36.
20. Sarkar C, Mukhopadhyay S, Ralte AM, et al. Intramedullary subependymoma of the spinal cord: a case report and review of literature. *Clin Neurol Neurosurg.* 2003;106(1):63–68.
21. Ebert C, von Haken M, Meyer-Puttlitz B, et al. Molecular genetic analysis of ependymal tumors. NF2 mutations and chromosome 22q loss occur preferentially in intramedullary spinal ependymomas. *Am J Pathol.* 1999;155(2):627–632.
22. Lamszus K, Lachenmayer L, Heinemann U, et al. Molecular genetic alterations on chromosomes 11 and 22 in ependymomas. *Int J Cancer.* 2001;91(6):803–808.
23. Patronas NJ, Courcoutsakis N, Bromley CM, Katzman GL, MacCollin M, Parry DM. Intramedullary and spinal canal tumors in patients with neurofibromatosis 2: MR imaging findings and correlation with genotype. *Radiology.* 2001;218(2):434–442.

24. Parsa AT, Fiore AJ, McCormick PC, Bruce JN. Genetic basis of intramedullary spinal cord tumors and therapeutic implications. *J Neurooncol.* 2000;47(3):239–251.
25. Lee M, Rezai AR, Freed D, Epstein FJ. Intramedullary spinal cord tumors in neurofibromatosis. *Neurosurgery.* 1996;38(1):32–37.
26. Chang UK, Choe WJ, Chung SK, Chung CK, Kim HJ. Surgical outcome and prognostic factors of spinal intramedullary ependymomas in adults. *J Neurooncol.* 2002;57(2):133–139.
27. Woodworth GF, Chaichana KL, McGirt MJ, et al. Predictors of ambulatory function after surgical resection of intramedullary spinal cord tumors. *Neurosurgery.* 2007;61(1):99–105; discussion 105.
28. Lowe GM. Magnetic resonance imaging of intramedullary spinal cord tumors. *J Neurooncol.* 2000;47(3):195–210.
29. Waldron JS, Cha S. Radiographic features of intramedullary spinal cord tumors. *Neurosurg Clin N Am.* 2006;17(1):13–19.
30. Brinar M, Rados M, Habek M, Poser CM. Enlargement of the spinal cord: inflammation or neoplasm? *Clin Neurol Neurosurg.* 2006;108(3):284–289.
31. Lee M, Epstein FJ, Rezai AR, Zagzag D. Nonneoplastic intramedullary spinal cord lesions mimicking tumors. *Neurosurgery.* 1998;43(4):788–94; discussion 794.
32. Kahan H, Sklar EM, Post MJ, Bruce JH. MR characteristics of histopathologic subtypes of spinal ependymoma. *AJNR Am J Neuroradiol.* 1996;17(1):143–150.
33. Bloomer CW, Ackerman A, Bhatia RG. Imaging for spine tumors and new applications. *Top Magn Reson Imaging.* 2006;17(2):69–87.
34. Shi HB, Suh DC, Lee HK, et al. Preoperative transarterial embolization of spinal tumor: embolization techniques and results. *AJNR Am J Neuroradiol.* 1999;20(10):2009–2015.
35. Constantini S, Miller DC, Allen JC, Rorke LB, Freed D, Epstein FJ. Radical excision of intramedullary spinal cord tumors: surgical morbidity and long-term follow-up evaluation in 164 children and young adults. *J Neurosurg.* 2000;93(2 suppl):183–193.
36. Sandalcioglu IE, Gasser T, Asgari S, et al. Functional outcome after surgical treatment of intramedullary spinal cord tumors: experience with 78 patients. *Spinal Cord.* 2005;43(1):34–41.
37. Cooper PR, Epstein F. Radical resection of intramedullary spinal cord tumors in adults. Recent experience in 29 patients. *J Neurosurg.* 1985;63(4):492–499.
38. McCormick PC, Anson JA. Intramedullary spinal cord tumors. In: Benzel EC, ed. *Spine Surgery: Techniques, Complications, Avoidance, and Management.* 2nd ed. Philadelphia: Elsevier Churchill Livingstone; 2005:939–947.
39. Rossitch E Jr, Zeidman SM, Burger PC, et al. Clinical and pathological analysis of spinal cord astrocytomas in children. *Neurosurgery.* 1990;27(2):193–196.
40. Sandler HM, Papadopoulos SM, Thornton AF Jr, Ross DA. Spinal cord astrocytomas: results of therapy. *Neurosurgery.* 1992;30(4):490–493.
41. Sala F, Palandri G, Basso E, et al. Motor evoked potential monitoring improves outcome after surgery for intramedullary spinal cord tumors: a historical control study. *Neurosurgery.* 2006;58(6):1129–1143; discussion 1129.
42. Jallo GI, Kothbauer KF, Epstein FJ. Contact laser microsurgery. *Childs Nerv Syst.* 2002;18(6–7):333–336.
43. Abbott R, Feldstein N, Wisoff JH, Epstein FJ. Osteoplastic laminotomy in children. *Pediatr Neurosurg.* 1992;18(3):153–156.
44. Tachdjian MO, Matson DD. Orthopedic aspects of intraspinal tumors in infants and children. *J Bone Joint Surg Am.* 1965;49:713–720.
45. Yasuoka S, Peterson HA, MacCarty CS. Incidence of spinal column deformity after multilevel laminectomy in children and adults. *J Neurosurg.* 1982;57(4):441–445.
46. Katzman H, Waugh T, Berdon W. Skeletal changes following irradiation of childhood tumors. *J Bone Joint Surg Am.* 1969;51(5):825–842.
47. Riseborough EJ, Grabias SL, Burton RI, Jaffe N. Skeletal alterations following irradiation for Wilms' tumor: with particular reference to scoliosis and kyphosis. *J Bone Joint Surg Am.* 1976;58(4):526–536.
48. Disa JJ, Smith AW, Bilsky MH. Management of radiated reoperative wounds of the cervicothoracic spine: the role of the trapezius turnover flap. *Ann Plast Surg.* 2001;47(4):394–397.
49. McCormick PC, Torres R, Post KD, Stein BM. Intramedullary ependymoma of the spinal cord. *J Neurosurg.* 1990;72(4):523–532.
50. Robinson CG, Prayson RA, Hahn JF, et al. Long-term survival and functional status of patients with low-grade astrocytoma of spinal cord. *Int J Radiat Oncol Biol Phys.* 2005;63(1):91–100.
51. Wara WM, Phillips TL, Sheline GE, Schwade JG. Radiation tolerance of the spinal cord. *Cancer.* 1975;35(6):1558–1562.
52. Phillips TL, Buschke F. Radiation tolerance of the thoracic spinal cord. *Am J Roentgenol Radium Ther Nucl Med.* 1969;105(3):659–664.
53. Fu KK, Phillips TL, Kane LJ, Smith V. Tumor and normal tissue response to irradiation in vivo: variation with decreasing dose rates. *Radiology.* 1975;114(3):709–716.
54. McLaughlin MP, Buatti JM, Marcus RB Jr, Maria BL, Mickle PJ, Kedar A. Outcome after radiotherapy of primary spinal cord glial tumors. *Radiat Oncol Investig.* 1998;6(6):276–280.
55. Rawlings CE 3rd, Giangaspero F, Burger PC, Bullard DE. Ependymomas: a clinicopathologic study. *Surg Neurol.* 1988;29(4):271–281.
56. Sonneland PR, Scheithauer BW, Onofrio BM. Myxopapillary ependymoma. A clinicopathologic and immunocytochemical study of 77 cases. *Cancer.* 1985;56(4):883–893.
57. Wen BC, Hussey DH, Hitchon PW, et al. The role of radiation therapy in the management of ependymomas of the spinal cord. *Int J Radiat Oncol Biol Phys.* 1991;20(4):781–786.
58. Guidetti B, Mercuri S, Vagnozzi R. Long-term results of the surgical treatment of 129 intramedullary spinal gliomas. *J Neurosurg.* 1981;54(3):323–330.
59. DeSousa AL, Kalsbeck JE, Mealey J Jr, Campbell RL, Hockey A. Intraspinal tumors in children. A review of 81 cases. *J Neurosurg.* 1979;51(4):437–445.
60. Waldron JN, Laperriere NJ, Jaakkimainen L, et al. Spinal cord ependymomas: a retrospective analysis of 59 cases. *Int J Radiat Oncol Biol Phys.* 1993;27(2):223–229.
61. Whitaker SJ, Bessell EM, Ashley SE, Bloom HJ, Bell BA, Brada M. Postoperative radiotherapy in the management of spinal cord ependymoma. *J Neurosurg.* 1991;74(5):720–728.
62. Shaw EG, Evans RG, Scheithauer BW, Ilstrup DM, Earle JD. Radiotherapeutic management of adult intraspinal ependymomas. *Int J Radiat Oncol Biol Phys.* 1986;12(3):323–327.
63. Wahab SH, Simpson JR, Michalski JM, Mansur DB. Long term outcome with post-operative radiation therapy for spinal canal ependymoma. *J Neurooncol.* 2007;83(1):85–89.
64. Rodrigues GB, Waldron JN, Wong CS, Laperriere NJ. A retrospective analysis of 52 cases of spinal cord glioma managed with radiation therapy. *Int J Radiat Oncol Biol Phys.* 2000;48(3):837–842.
65. Cooper PR. Outcome after operative treatment of intramedullary spinal cord tumors in adults: intermediate and long-term results in 51 patients. *Neurosurgery.* 1989;25(6):855–859.
66. Hoshimaru M, Koyama T, Hashimoto N, Kikuchi H. Results of microsurgical treatment for intramedullary spinal cord ependymomas: analysis of 36 cases. *Neurosurgery.* 1999;44(2):264–269.
67. Chou PM, Barquin N, Gonzalez-Crussi F, Ridaura Sanz C, Tomita T, Reyes-Mugica M. Ependymomas in children express the multidrug resistance gene: immunohistochemical and molecular biologic study. *Pediatr Pathol Lab Med.* 1996;16(4):551–561.
68. Fouladi M, Baruchel S, Chan H, et al. Use of adjuvant ICE chemotherapy in the treatment of anaplastic ependymomas. *Childs Nerv Syst.* 1998;14(10):590–595.
69. Sexauer CL, Khan A, Burger PC, et al. Cisplatin in recurrent pediatric brain tumors. A POG Phase II study. A Pediatric Oncology Group Study. *Cancer.* 1985;56(7):1497–1501.
70. Gaynon PS, Ettinger LJ, Baum ES, Siegel SE, Krailo MD, Hammond GD. Carboplatin in childhood brain tumors. A Children's Cancer Study Group Phase II trial. *Cancer.* 1990;66(12):2465–2469.
71. Chastagner P, Sommelet-Olive D, Kalifa C, et al. Phase II study of ifosfamide in childhood brain tumors: a report by the French Society of Pediatric Oncology (SFOP). *Med Pediatr Oncol.* 1993;21(1):49–53.
72. Epstein FJ, Farmer JP, Freed D. Adult intramedullary astrocytomas of the spinal cord. *J Neurosurg.* 1992;77(3):355–359.
73. Reimer R, Onofrio BM. Astrocytomas of the spinal cord in children and adolescents. *J Neurosurg.* 1985;63(5):669–675.
74. Kopelson G, Linggood RM. Intramedullary spinal cord astrocytoma versus glioblastoma: the prognostic importance of histologic grade. *Cancer.* 1982;50(4):732–735.
75. Cohen AR, Wisoff JH, Allen JC, Epstein F. Malignant astrocytomas of the spinal cord. *J Neurosurg.* 1989;70(1):50–54.
76. Isaacson SR. Radiation therapy and the management of intramedullary spinal cord tumors. *J Neurooncol.* 2000;47(3):231–238.
77. Allen JV, Avivner S, Yates AJ, et al. Treatment of high-grade spinal cord astrocytoma of childhood with '8-in-1' chemotherapy and radiotherapy: a pilot study of CCG-945. *J Neurosurg.* 1998;88:215–220.

78. Bouffet E, Amat D, Devaux Y, Desuzinges C. Chemotherapy for spinal cord astrocytoma. *Med Pediatr Oncol*. 1997;29(6):560–562.
79. Foreman NK, Hay TC, Handler M. Chemotherapy for spinal cord astrocytoma. *Med Pediatr Oncol*. 1998;30(5):311–312.
80. Lonser RR, Weil RJ, Wanebo JE, DeVroom HL, Oldfield EH. Surgical management of spinal cord hemangioblastomas in patients with von Hippel-Lindau disease. *J Neurosurg*. 2003;98(1):106–116.
81. Smalley SR, Schomberg PJ, Earle JD, Laws ER Jr, Scheithauer BW, O'Fallon JR. Radiotherapeutic considerations in the treatment of hemangioblastomas of the central nervous system. *Int J Radiat Oncol Biol Phys*. 1990;18(5):1165–1171.
82. Niemelä M, Mäenpää H, Salven P, et al. Interferon alpha-2a therapy in 18 hemangioblastomas. *Clin Cancer Res*. 2001;7(3):510–516.
83. Piribauer M, Czech T, Dieckmann K, et al. Stabilization of a progressive hemangioblastoma under treatment with thalidomide. *J Neurooncol*. 2004;66(3):295–299.
84. Connolly ES Jr, Winfree CJ, McCormick PC, Cruz M, Stein BM. Intramedullary spinal cord metastasis: report of three cases and review of the literature. *Surg Neurol*. 1996;46(4):329–37; discussion 337.
85. Schiff D, O'Neill BP. Intramedullary spinal cord metastases: clinical features and treatment outcome. *Neurology*. 1996;47(4):906–912.
86. McCormick PC, Stein BM. Intramedullary tumors in adults. *Neurosurg Clin N Am*. 1990;1(3):609–630.

56
Low-Grade Gliomas

Michael L. Di Luna, Joachim M. Baehring, and Joseph M. Piepmeier

INTRODUCTION

Approximately 2000 low-grade gliomas (LGGs) are diagnosed annually, accounting for 15% to 20% of primary central nervous system tumors [1]. Because these tumors are relatively uncommon, the literature provides mostly retrospective clinical reviews to guide management. Consequently, optimal treatment and the benefits of various interventions, including aggressive resection, remain subjective. Randomized clinical trials assessing the effect of radiation therapy (RT) for LGGs have shown that there is no dose-response to high-dose versus low-dose RT and adjuvant radiation will delay tumor recurrence, but will not prolong survival [2–4]. There is general consensus that the presumptive diagnosis of LGG based upon imaging is not sufficient to guide treatment, with few exceptions. Some subtypes of LGG may be cured by gross total resection (GTR) whereas others will require more extensive treatment regimens, and yet others have been treated conservatively for decades solely with symptomatic management. Currently, LGGs are treated with various regimens ranging from observation to biopsy and radiotherapy to radiosurgery to chemotherapy to gross resection or a combination of each. However, there is a growing consensus that surgical removal of the tumor can prolong survival. Toward this end, tumor surgeons have applied advancements in imaging, image-guided surgery and technology to improve surgical management of these lesions.

LGGs are the beginning of a fatal disease for most patients. Although the biological behavior of these lesions can be unpredictable, they commonly transform into high-grade tumors [5–7]. This is the most common cause of mortality. Most clinical reviews emphasize the importance of young age, high performance status, and preserved neurological function as predictors of a more favorable prognosis [8–11]. These reviews also note that aggressive surgery is associated with improved tumor control [12,13]. Some reports suggest that tumor size also influences survival with larger tumors having a worse prognosis. Over the past decade the routine use of 1p/19q deletion studies also divide most infiltrative low-grade tumors into clinically useful prognostic groups [14]. Tumors that contain deletions in these chromosomes have a more indolent course and longer survival. These clinical and genetic parameters currently are the primary source of information for anticipating outcome and directing treatment. Since the transition from a relatively slow-growing low-grade tumor to a rapidly fatal high-grade glioma is the major cause of mortality in this population, efforts to prevent or delay this biological change are the focus of treatment. In addition, because malignant transformation results from the accumulation of additional genetic mutations, laboratory studies are directed toward identifying those genetic events that cause tumor transformation.

Only a minority of LGGs are amenable to GTR [12]. Consequently, for most patients subtotal resection or biopsy plays a significant role in the management of these tumors. Long-term management of this disease highlights the importance of a comprehensive team approach to treatment including collaboration with neuroimaging for diagnosis, operative guidance, and sequential evaluations as well as comprehensive neuropathology. The focus of this chapter is the surgical management of adult LGGs with a discussion centered upon the various histological grades, advanced imaging, and modern surgical approaches.

PATHOLOGY

Traditionally, gliomas are classified based upon routine histology and immunohistochemistry. These standard diagnostic criteria correlate with biological activity, but also combine tumors with variable natural histories within the same classification. Classification scales (WHO, Ringertz, or St. Anne-Mayo) define the type of glioma based upon infiltration into normal brain, mitotic index, nuclear architecture (presence of atypia), endothelial proliferation, and necrosis [15]. The term *low-grade glioma* was reserved for a heterogeneous group of tumors that arise from neuroepithelial cells that resemble astrocytes, oligodendrocytes, or ependyma. These tumors have a low mitotic index (<5%). On the basis of the WHO classification (most commonly used), LGGs would include WHO class I and II tumors. Over the past decade there has been a gradual transition in the frequency of diagnosis of oligodendroglioma. Although in the past, most LGGs were considered to be from an astrocytic lineage, oligodendrogliomas have emerged as the more common subtype. The reasons for this change likely reflect the addition of routine glial fibrillary acidic protein staining, the recognition of

Table 56.1 Classification of Low-Grade Gliomas

Astrocytoma
Pilocytic astrocytoma
Pleomorphic xanthoastrocytoma
Subependymal giant cell astrocytoma
Oligodendroglioma
Oligoastrocytoma
Gliomatosis cerebri
Ependymoma (cellular, papillary, clear cell, tanycytic)
Choroid glioma of the third ventricle
Gangliocytoma
Dysembryoplastic neuroepithelial tumor
Ganglioglioma
Dysplastic gangliocytoma of cerebellum (Lhermitte-Duclos)
Dysplastic infantile astrocytoma/ganglioglioma

With permission from Yale Brain Tumor Center, New Haven, Connecticut.

"trapped" astrocytes that are not neoplastic, and the common application of 1p/19q deletion testing [7,15]. The diversity of tumors encompassed by the term LGGs is detailed in Table 56.1.

The most common tumors included in the WHO II classification are diffuse astrocytomas, oligodendrogliomas, or oligoastrocytomas [15]. However, there are a number of less common histological subtypes that also are considered to be low-grade glial neoplasms. These tumors include the pilocytic astrocytoma and its variant, the pilomyxoid astrocytoma, the subependymal giant cell astrocytoma, and the pleomorphic xanthoastrocytoma. Recent descriptions of a papillary glioneuronal tumor as well as variations in morphology with glial tumors expressing neuronal markers have been published [16]. These tumors tend to have an indolent course; however, further long-term assessment is needed before they can be appropriately classified by the WHO.

CLINICAL SIGNS AND SYMPTOMS

LGGs commonly reach clinical attention following the new onset of seizures [8–11,17]. These space-occupying lesions can exert mass-effect causing perturbations in neurological function (motor/sensory deficits, psychological changes, memory problems) or cerebrospinal fluid flow (obstructive hydrocephalus). Cerebral edema can result from both infiltration and mass-effect, leading to elevated intracranial pressure, neurological sequelae, and headache. Some studies suggest that the tumor cells themselves are neurotoxic (through cytokine and neurotransmitter release) and can elicit seizures by disruption of neuronal pathways or through local glutamate concentration/metabolism changes [18,19]. This may explain why seizure is among the most common presenting signs of a LGG [8–11,17]. Incidental discovery is not uncommon and with the increased use of and access to imaging, many physicians have encountered incidental, asymptomatic LGG in patients where a tumor was not suspected (e.g., trauma) [9,20].

LGGs are associated with Mendelian disorders and phakomatoses or neurocutaneous syndromes [15]. For example, low-grade astrocytomas are seen in Von Recklinghausen disease (neurofibromatosis type I) and

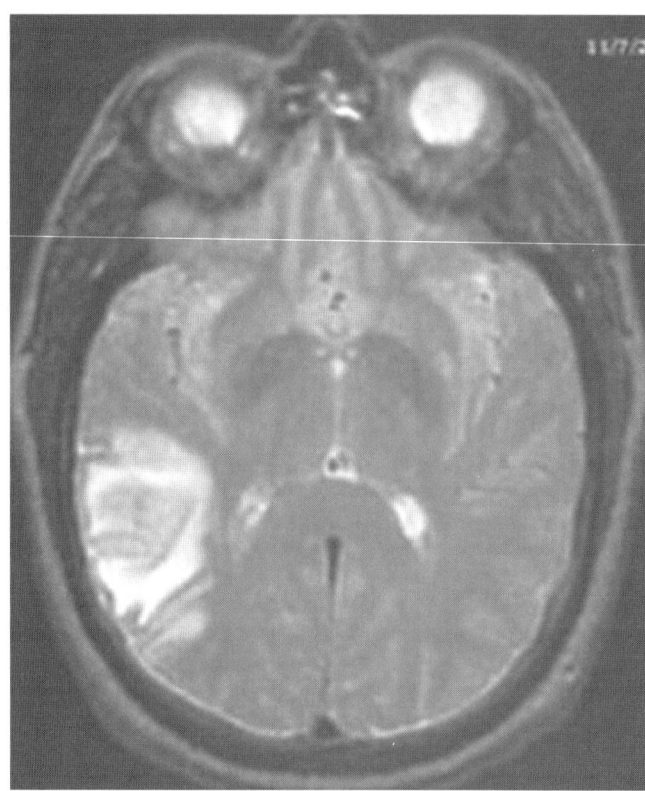

Figure 56.1 T2-weighted MRI demonstrating a diffuse mass lesion in a 56-year-old man with new onset of seizures. This lesion did not enhance with contrast and was considered to represent a low-grade glioma. Surgery revealed this to be granulomatous angitis.

subependymal giant cell astrocytomas are seen in tuberous sclerosis. Other than the set of genes which when mutated lead to these phenotypes, mutation of p53 or loss of 1p-19q are most commonly associated with LGGs.

IMAGING

Several studies question the reliability of imaging alone to diagnose a tumor and up to 30% to 50% will underestimate the grade of tumor or even result in misdiagnosis (Figure 56.1). LGGs commonly have characteristic magnetic resonance imaging (MRI) findings such as T1 shortening, T2 prolongation, calcification, and perifocal vasogenic edema [21–23]. Contrast enhancement on MRI can be found in 10% to 15% of infiltrative LGGs [7]. This is associated with a worse prognosis. Most of these lesions do not enhance with contrast on MRI and are best delineated on fluid attenuated inversion recovery or T2-weighted sequences. They commonly demonstrate an irregular border with surrounding white matter, exert mass effect, and extend to the cortical surface (Figure 56.2). Tumors with indistinct margins have been correlated with a 1p deletion [24] (Figure 56.3), whereas well-demarcated tumors have been characterized as identifying lesions with preserved 1p alleles. Although these topographical patterns are not specific, they can provide an estimate of the 1p status on preoperative images. Precise diagnosis of LGGs

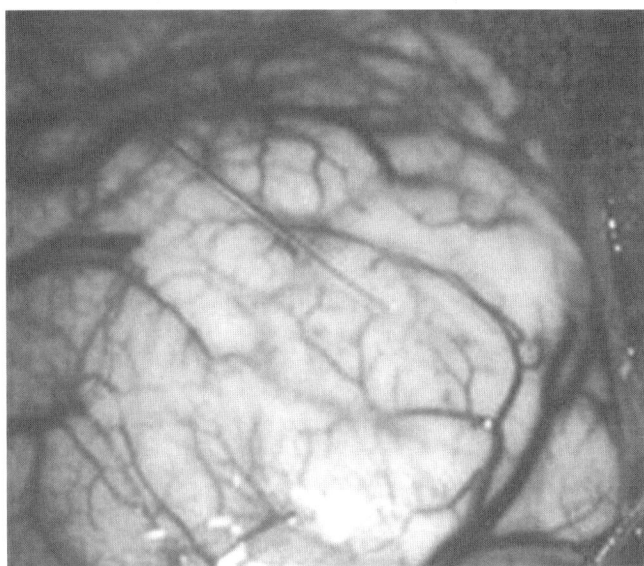

Figure 56.2 Intraoperative view of an oligodendroglioma extending to the cortical surface in the parietal lobe.

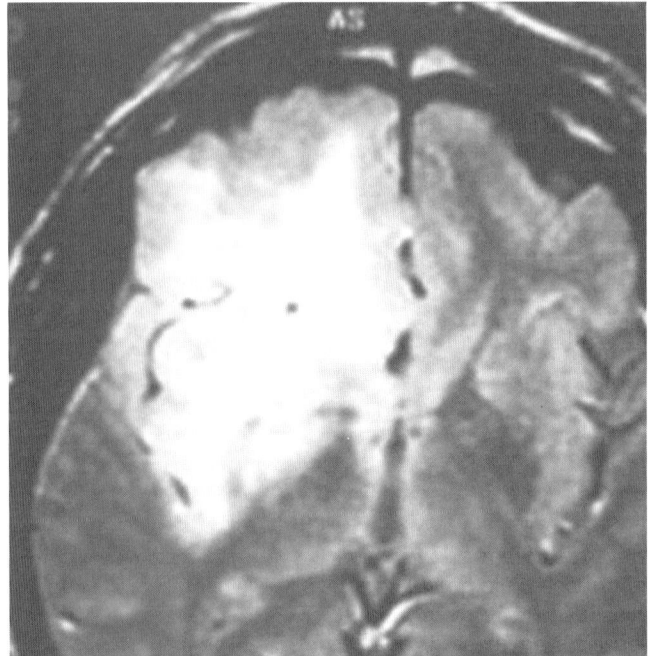

Figure 56.3 FLAIR MRI of an extensive low-grade glioma in the frontal lobe extending into the basal ganglia. This lesion could not be removed and was treated with a biopsy.

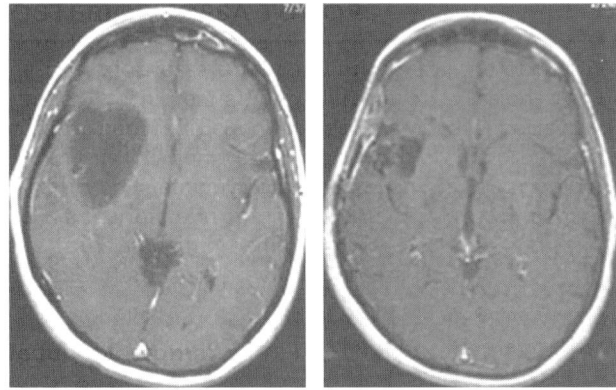

Figure 56.4 Pre- (left, FLAIR) and postoperative MRI (right, T1 with gadolinium) of an oligodendroglioma in the right Sylvian region.

requires immunohistochemical, cytogenetic, and molecular diagnosis for which procurement of adequate tissue is required.

Newer imaging techniques are proving to have some diagnostic power in the grading of gliomas. Perfusion weighted magnetic resonance (MR) imaging allows for noninvasive determination of relative tumor blood volume and is increasingly being used to grade gliomas [25–27].

Increased relative tumor blood volume compared with the contralateral normal brain identifies a LGG with higher proliferative capacity and more likely to transform into a high-grade lesion. While blood flow and volume heterogeneity exists within LGGs, MR perfusion can be correlated with cytogenetics and thus potentially predict outcome, further highlighting the importance of a comprehensive diagnosis which includes tissue [25].

STRATEGIES FOR SURGICAL MANAGEMENT

The principles that guide the surgical management of LGGs include obtaining sufficient tissue for accurate histological diagnosis, reducing tumor burden to improve quality of life (and perhaps treatment efficacy), and preservation of neurological function. However, GTR is only achieved in a minority of cases and is highly dependent upon the location and size of the tumor. Maximal resection can reduce the tumor burden if chemotherapy and/or radiotherapy are planned. Modern neurosurgical techniques have optimized the surgeon's ability to perform a range of procedures from accurate biopsy to maximal resection of the lesion while minimizing peri- and postoperative morbidity (Figure 56.4). LGGs often extend to the cortical surface and expand an involved gyrus. This local gyral expansion typically respects the sulci that demarcate the superficial extent of the tumor. In the subcortical area, gliomas are identified by alterations in color, consistency, and vascularity that are optimally viewed through intraoperative magnification. These tumors commonly blend with surrounding white matter making tumor margins difficult to identify (Figure 56.5).

BIOPSY

Stereotactic diagnostic biopsy is often the optimal procedure for inaccessible lesions (e.g., thalamus, basal ganglia) or lesions within eloquent cortex (language; primary motor cortex). The procedure is associated with minimal morbidity or complications compared to craniotomy and

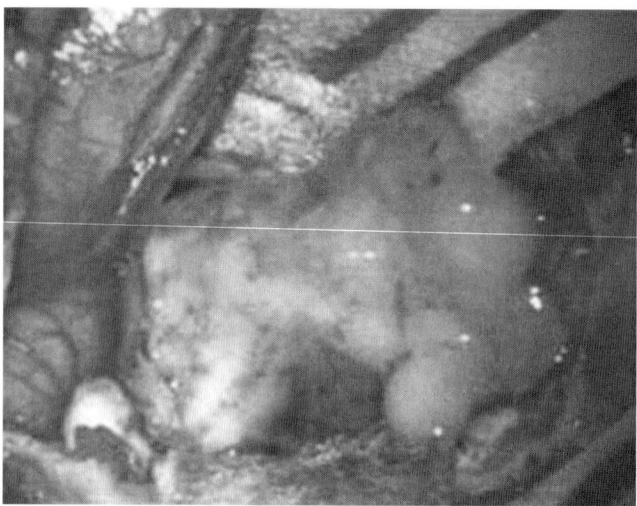

Figure 56.5 Intraoperative view of an oligodendroglioma during resection. The tumor is identified by its pearly gray color and firm consistency.

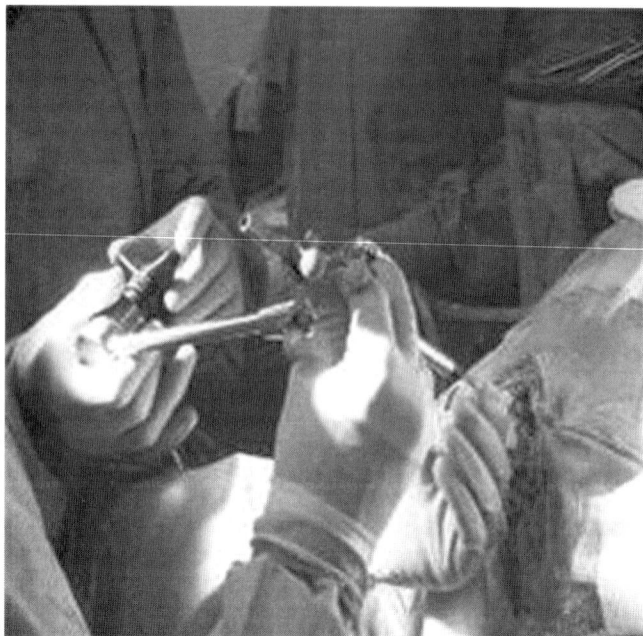

Figure 56.6 Intraoperative view of a stereotactic biopsy for a low-grade glioma.

can be performed under local anesthesia. In one study reviewing 7471 reported biopsies within the literature, the combined morbidity was 3.5%, the mortality rate was 0.7%, and the diagnostic yield was 91% [28]. Comorbidities (such as diabetes) and deeper lesions may be associated with increased operative morbidity, while prior seizure history does not increase risk of seizure after biopsy [29].

Typically, stereotactic biopsies are reserved for tissue diagnosis when the lesions are not amenable to removal. The reported accuracy of stereotactic biopsies (reliability and ability to accurately diagnose lesions and guide treatment) is generally high with some variability between large institutions (Figure 56.6). Diagnostic accuracy increases with the number of biopsy samples, though the increase in risk to the patient has not been determined [30,31]. In one study, 130 patients underwent stereotactic biopsy for brain lesions and 23 went further to have the lesions resected, the diagnostic yield of the initial biopsy (as compared to the subsequently resected lesions) was 94% [32]. Yet other institutions report less diagnostic reliability of stereotactic biopsy (compared to resection specimens in the same patient) with accuracies more in the 50% to 60% range [33,34]. It should be remembered that stereotactic biopsy specimens only represent a small portion of the lesion and, in the case of mixed lesions with high-grade regions, they may be limited by the probability of biopsy within the diagnostic high-grade region. The diagnostic yield of this procedure thus depends on target selection. Infiltrative brain tumor biopsies are best reviewed by an experienced neuropathologist to maximize the diagnostic potential from small samples of LGGs. The other diagnostic problem from stereotactic biopsies is found in diffuse regions of isolated tumor cells that may not produce sufficient evidence for some pathologists to render a diagnosis. Some oligodendrogliomas are composed of only isolated tumor cells without a discrete solid tumor mass early in the course of the disease [35] (Figure 56.7). These cases may be difficult to diagnose if the pathologist is not familiar with this

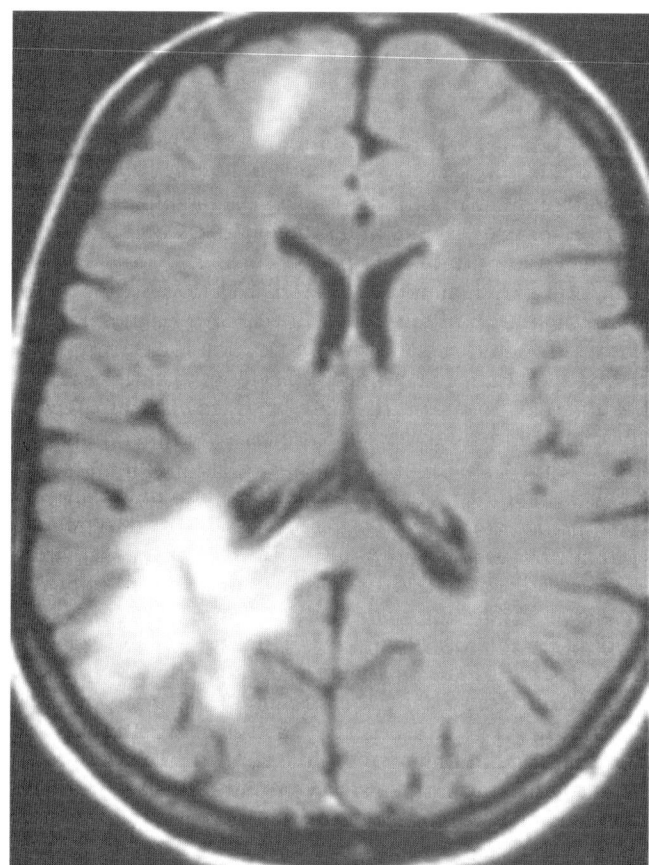

Figure 56.7 FLAIR MRI demonstrating a multifocal oligodendroglioma in the right parietal and frontal lobe. The biopsy demonstrated infiltrative tumor cells without a solid tumor mass.

growth pattern. An accurate diagnosis for these patients requires examination of both the pathological sample and the imaging. This collaborative interaction is typically performed with a Tumor Board where the clinical, imaging, and histopathology are reviewed.

SURGERY FOR LGGS

The consensus within the neurosurgical community is that a tissue diagnosis is required before treatment of LGGs. In addition, the majority consider GTR as the best option for longer progression-free survival (PFS) and longer overall survival compared to subtotal resection. The surgeon also should consider the psychological state of patients with central nervous system tumors and consultations should reflect the limited objective data that support the role of cytoreduction and GTR to reduce the risk of malignant transformation and increase the PFS [5–7,13,36]. Many patients will request a second opinion and this is encouraged.

Neurosurgery has developed a number of techniques to maximize patient safety and minimize morbidity, for removal of LGGs within difficult locations. Computer-assisted stereotaxy is now widely used in planning the approach to lesions while avoiding injury to adjacent eloquent structures. Resection and retraction of normal brain can often be minimized. Preoperative functional mapping of the cortex adjacent to tumors (through diffusion tensor imaging MRI (DTI) or functional MRI has better defined the topographical relationship between tumors and adjacent eloquent cortex. Neuronavigation systems can further assist the surgeon in the approach as well and during the resection in evaluating the extent of tissue removal (Figure 56.8). By referencing the surface anatomy of patients and/or co-registering image-defined data points to computed tomography or MRI, instruments (probes) can guide the angle and depth of resection. Although this technique does not replace knowledge of neuroanatomy, image guidance can provide further information about location (Figure 56.8).

Preoperative imaging using DTI or functional MRI is a sensitive (though not specific) technique for identifying critical structures adjacent to tumors. Images generated preoperatively with functional MRI through detection of increase in blood oxygen level delivery resulting from increased blood supply to activated cortical regions during tasks can be coregistered with neuronavigation equipment for more accurate intraoperative mapping. DTI can generate maps of white matter tracts by measuring directional diffusion. Fiber tracks delineated using DTI can be used to identify the motor tract in deep white matter and define a safety margin around the tract [37] (Figure 56.9). These images will show tracts that are either distorted or disrupted by lesions. These data can also be coregistered for intraoperative neuronavigation.

Cortical and subcortical mapping by direct intraoperative stimulation has been widely used in the resection of LGGs [38,39]. This technique requires not only a cooperative patient, but also an experienced team to obtain reliable information during testing. Although motor and language

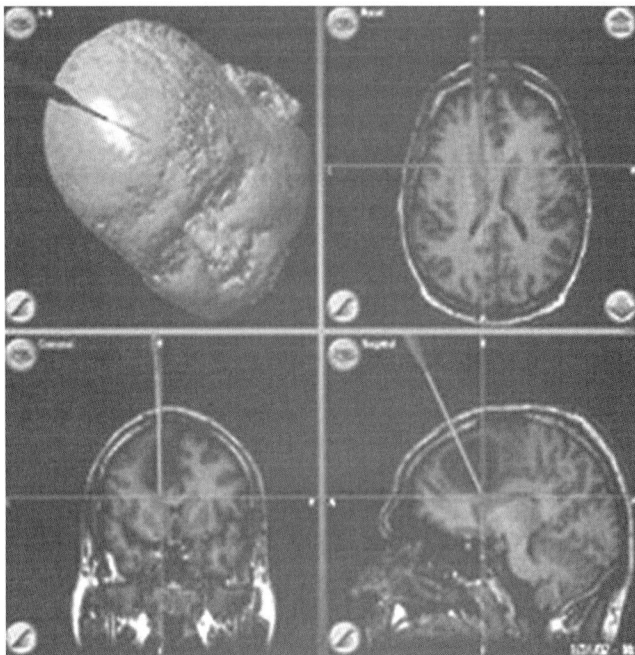

Figure 56.8 Stereotactic images during resection of a low-grade glioma in the frontal lobe. Note the probe demonstrates that surgery has reached the deepest part of the tumor.

testing can be relatively simple, variations in speech location, types of language processing in the brain, and more refined assessments of visuospatial orientation are gained from a broad experience in these techniques (Figure 56.10). Several reviews of clinical experience in the use of intraoperative brain mapping have demonstrated that LGGs often displace functional cortical and subcortical regions [40]. In addition, the slow growth of large tumors can result in significant variations in location of function that can only be determined by intraoperative assessment. Furthermore, there appears to be a capacity for functional plasticity that has emerged from LGG surgery. Most surgeons prefer bipolar stimulation between 4 and 10 mA. Once a stimulation threshold has been determined from the cortical surface, these same parameters are used for white matter track monitoring. Frequent testing is required to determine fiber track location. In experienced hands, intraoperative mapping has enhanced the ability to remove some tumors previously thought to be unresectable.

Intraoperative imaging (ioMRI) has been successfully utilized in a number of centers to evaluate the extent of resection before completion of the surgery. This technique is associated with improved survival and longer time to tumor recurrence [41]. The use of this technology can increase the chances of GTR in selected patients. A number of commercially available ioMRI systems are in use throughout North America and the world. This technology offers the opportunity to not only evaluate anatomic images, but also to measure the preservation of functional organization. Future intraopertive imaging will likely include co-registration of anatomic, functional, and metabolic imaging to better define the extent of the lesion

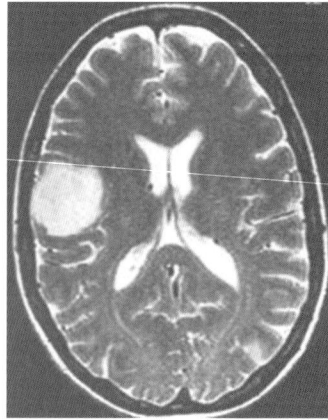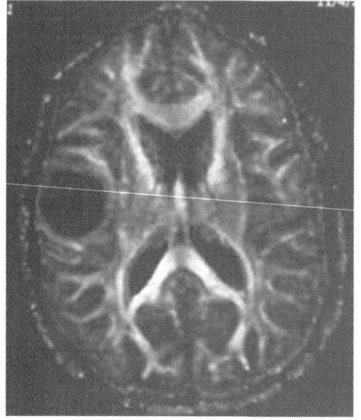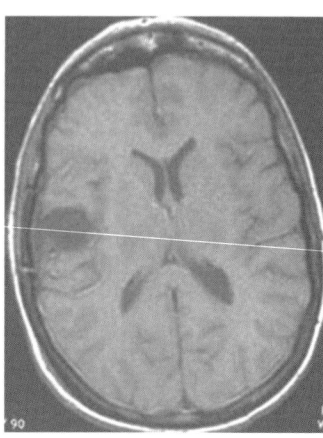

Figure 56.9 Preoperative T2-weighted MRI (left), fiber tractography based on DTI (middle) and T1-enhanced MRI (right) of an oligodendroglioma.

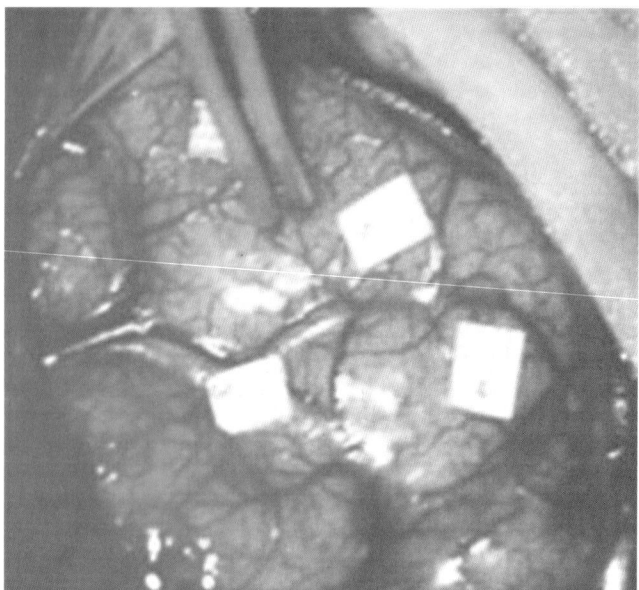

Figure 56.10 Intraoperative view of bipolar electrode stimulation and cortical mapping for removal of a low-grade glioma near primary language cortex.

and the more aggressive portion of a tumor with mixed histology.

EXTENT OF RESECTION AND OUTCOME

There are several potential benefits to aggressive resection of a LGG. Surgery may be associated with seizure reduction or elimination and improvement in quality of life as well as increased survival [42]. In a summary of the literature on surgery and variables associated with survival, Keles et al [12] estimated hazard ratios of 2.6 to 3.3 for less-than maximal resection. Patients with larger tumor volumes (categorized as >20 cc) preoperatively may have shortened PFS [36] and diminished overall survival [14]. A prospective trial examining the effect of RT demonstrated similar findings; however, the numbers and differences were far less striking. While the study was designed to compare low-dose and high-dose localized RT for supratentorial low-grade astrocytoma, multivariate analysis identified histologic subtype, tumor size, and age as the most significant prognostic factors and the subgroup that received a GTR had a marginal survival benefit over those who did not [2].

The difficulty in comparing outcomes after surgical resection of LGGs with the overall tumor population is the limited reporting of patient selection criteria, lack of inclusion of patients harboring small, nonenhancing LGGs that never undergo resection, and no uniformity in the assessment criteria of extent of resection. Most studies rely on the "surgeon's impression" of the resection based presumably on pre- and postoperative imaging. Other reports use volumetric calculations based upon computed tomography and MRI. Even with the current limitations in the literature, recent reports of outcomes in patients who received surgery with ioMRI demonstrated significantly improved long-term survival and decreased high-grade transition compared with historical controls [41]. It is appropriate to assume that the use of ioMRI increased the probability of more extensive resection and that had a beneficial influence on outcome.

ADJUVANT TREATMENT

The extent of resection for most patients with LGGs is less than a GTR. In addition, it must be remembered that an imaging-defined GTR does not preclude the likely infiltration of tumor cells beyond the region of tumor as delineated on MRI or computed tomography. For the vast majority of patients, surveillance imaging and clinical follow-up are necessary to monitor for tumor recurrence. In patients with persistent symptomatic tumor, adjuvant therapy may be required to control symptoms and to prevent progression or recurrence.

Neuro-oncologists remain divided as to the optimal use of adjuvant treatment modalities (chemotherapy, RT therapy) for *infiltrative* LGG (astrocytoma, oligodendroglioma). Early radiotherapy at the time of diagnosis extends PFS but does not increase overall survival [4]. As higher doses bear no benefit, standard radiotherapy is provided in 1.8 Gy fractions to a total dose of 50 to 54 Gy

[2,42,43]. There is accumulating evidence that chemotherapy with PCV or temozolomide is of benefit to patients with infiltrative LGG, especially oligodendroglioma with deletion of chromosome 1p [44–47]. Prospective randomized trials are ongoing (Radiation Therapy Oncology Group Study 98–02, European Organization for Research and Treatment of Cancer Study 22041). As the immediate and long-term effects of early therapy on quality of life have not been studied prospectively, no firm recommendations can be given. Prognostic factors of progression risk have been identified (age of 40 years or older, astrocytic subtype, largest diameter of the tumor equal to or greater than 6 cm, tumor crossing the midline, and presence of neurologic deficit before surgery) that may facilitate the decision-making process including multiple variables [48]. Chromosome 1p loss, or the combined loss of 1p and 19q, confers a survival benefit and predicts treatment response in oligodendrogliomas. We generally defer adjuvant therapy for LGG until there is a change in the radiographic growth pattern (acceleration of growth, imminent neurological complications from mass effect, nodular contrast enhancement in a previously nonenhancing neoplasm) or a neurological syndrome arises—typically, seizures—that fails to adequately respond to symptomatic therapy.

For *noninfiltrative* neoplasms, adjuvant radiation is reserved for patients with symptomatic residual disease after surgery or documented disease progression. Stereotactic radiation may be a reasonable alternative to conventional techniques in this setting.

LGG-Subtype-Based Approach

We follow asymptomatic patients with *astrocytomas* expectantly after surgery in quarterly and then half yearly intervals. At the time of radiographic progression or evolution of symptoms, radiotherapy is provided. Chemotherapy is reserved for disease progression after radiation. For *oligodendroglial and mixed glial tumors*, we likewise recommend a conservative approach after surgery. Selected patients with tumor infiltrating eloquent areas may benefit from "neoadjuvant" chemotherapy after stereotactic biopsy, especially if molecular analysis of biopsy material shows 1p loss. Life-long surveillance is warranted. External beam RT provided at initial diagnosis does not prolong overall survival irrespective of dose [2,43,49]. Predictors of unfavorable outcome have been identified and are used in clinical studies to select patients who may benefit from early therapy [48,50]. Undisputed is the need for adjuvant treatment for low-grade tumors giving rise to symptoms unresponsive to symptomatic measures or displaying radiographic progression. We prefer chemotherapy in patients with large tumors, especially if they are located in the dominant hemisphere. Radiation is provided at the time maximum tumor shrinkage has been achieved or at the time progression is noted after chemotherapy is completed. RT or chemotherapy for *pilocytic astrocytoma* is only provided in the rare event of progressive tumor growth or uncontrollable neurological symptoms in unresectable cases. For most patients with *pleomorphic xanthoastrocytoma*, complete resection is feasible. Adjuvant therapies are needed only for the few (less than 15–20%) whose tumors are anaplastic.

REFERENCES

1. 2005–2006 Primary brain tumors in the United States statistical report 1998–2002 years data collected. 2006. http://www.cbtrus.org/reports//2005–2006/2006report.pdf.
2. Shaw E, Arusell R, Scheithauer B, et al. Prospective randomized trial of low- versus high-dose radiation therapy in adults with supratentorial low-grade glioma: initial report of a North Central Cancer Treatment Group/Radiation Therapy Oncology Group/Eastern Cooperative Oncology Group study. *J Clin Oncol*. 2002;20(9):2267–2276.
3. Shaw EG, Tatter SB, Lesser GJ, Ellis TL, Stanton CA, Stieber VW. Current controversies in the radiotherapeutic management of adult low-grade glioma. *Semin Oncol*. 2004;31(5):653–658.
4. van den Bent MJ, Afra D, de Witte O, et al. Long-term efficacy of early versus delayed radiotherapy for low-grade astrocytoma and oligodendroglioma in adults: the EORTC 22845 randomised trial. *Lancet*. 2005;366(9490):985–990.
5. Leighton C, Fisher B, Bauman G, et al. Supratentorial low-grade glioma in adults: an analysis of prognostic factors and timing of radiation. *J Clin Oncol*. 1997;15(4):1294–1301.
6. Nakamura M, Konishi N, Tsunoda S, et al. Analysis of prognostic and survival factors related to treatment of low-grade astrocytomas in adults. *Oncology*. 2000;58(2):108–116.
7. Piepmeier J, Christopher S, Spencer D, et al. Variations in the natural history and survival of patients with supratentorial low-grade astrocytomas. *Neurosurgery*. 1996;38(5):872–878; discussion 8–9.
8. Engelhard HH. Current diagnosis and treatment of oligodendroglioma. *Neurosurg Focus*. 2002;12(2):E2.
9. Olson JD, Riedel E, DeAngelis LM. Long-term outcome of low-grade oligodendroglioma and mixed glioma. *Neurology*. 2000;54(7):1442–1448.
10. Schiff D, Brown PD, Giannini C. Outcome in adult low-grade glioma: the impact of prognostic factors and treatment. *Neurology*. 2007;69(13):1366–1373.
11. Stupp R, Janzer RC, Hegi ME, Villemure JG, Mirimanoff RO. Prognostic factors for low-grade gliomas. *Semin Oncol*. 2003;30 (6 suppl 19):23–28.
12. Keles GE, Lamborn KR, Berger MS. Low-grade hemispheric gliomas in adults: a critical review of extent of resection as a factor influencing outcome. *J Neurosurg*. 2001;95(5):735–745.
13. Lo SS, Cho KH, Hall WA, et al. Does the extent of surgery have an impact on the survival of patients who receive postoperative radiation therapy for supratentorial low-grade gliomas? *Int J Cancer*. 2001;96 suppl:71–78.
14. Kreth FW, Faist M, Rossner R, Volk B, Ostertag CB. Supratentorial World Health Organization Grade 2 astrocytomas and oligoastrocytomas. A new pattern of prognostic factors. *Cancer*. 1997;79(2):370–379.
15. Kleihues P, Cavenee WK. *International Agency for Research on Cancer. Pathology and Genetics of Tumours of the Nervous System*. Lyon: IARC Press; 2000.
16. Rosenblum MK. The 2007 WHO classification of nervous system tumors: newly recognized members of the mixed glioneuronal group. *Brain Pathol*. 2007;17(3):308–313.
17. Lebrun C, Fontaine D, Bourg V, et al. Treatment of newly diagnosed symptomatic pure low-grade oligodendrogliomas with PCV chemotherapy. *Eur J Neurol*. 2007;14(4):391–398.
18. Rothstein JD, Brem H. Excitotoxic destruction facilitates brain tumor growth. *Nat Med*. 2001;7(9):994–995.
19. Takano T, Lin JH, Arcuino G, Gao Q, Yang J, Nedergaard M. Glutamate release promotes growth of malignant gliomas. *Nat Med*. 2001;7(9):1010–1015.
20. Steiger HJ. Preventive neurosurgery: population-wide check-up examinations and correction of asymptomatic pathologies of the nervous system. *Acta Neurochir (Wein)*. 2006;148(10):1075–1083; discussion 1083.
21. Kondziolka D, Lunsford LD, Martinez AJ. Unreliability of contemporary neurodiagnostic imaging in evaluating suspected adult supratentorial (low-grade) astrocytoma. *J Neurosurg*. 1993;79(4):533–536.

22. Pace A, Vidiri A, Galie E, et al. Temozolomide chemotherapy for progressive low-grade glioma: clinical benefits and radiological response. *Ann Oncol.* 2003;14(12):1722–1726.
23. Scott JN, Brasher PM, Sevick RJ, Rewcastle NB, Forsyth PA. How often are nonenhancing supratentorial gliomas malignant? A population study. *Neurology.* 2002;59(6):947–949.
24. Megyesi JF, Kachur E, Lee DH, et al. Imaging correlates of molecular signatures in oligodendrogliomas. *Clin Cancer Res.* 2004;10(13):4303–4306.
25. Law M, Oh S, Johnson G, et al. Perfusion magnetic resonance imaging predicts patient outcome as an adjunct to histopathology: a second reference standard in the surgical and nonsurgical treatment of low-grade gliomas. *Neurosurgery.* 2006;58(6):1099–1107; discussion 1107.
26. Law M, Yang S, Wang H, et al. Glioma grading: sensitivity, specificity, and predictive values of perfusion MR imaging and proton MR spectroscopic imaging compared with conventional MR imaging. *AJNR Am J Neuroradiol.* 2003;24(10):1989–1998.
27. Preul C, Kuhn B, Lang EW, Mehdorn HM, Heller M, Link J. Differentiation of cerebral tumors using multi-section echo planar MR perfusion imaging. *Eur J Radiol.* 2003;48(3):244–251.
28. Hall WA. The safety and efficacy of stereotactic biopsy for intracranial lesions. *Cancer.* 1998;82(9):1749–1755.
29. McGirt MJ, Woodworth GF, Coon AL, et al. Independent predictors of morbidity after image-guided stereotactic brain biopsy: a risk assessment of 270 cases. *J Neurosurg* 2005;102(5):897–901.
30. Jain D, Sharma MC, Sarkar C, Deb P, Gupta D, Mahapatra AK. Correlation of diagnostic yield of stereotactic brain biopsy with number of biopsy bits and site of the lesion. *Brain Tumor Pathol* 2006;23(2):71–75.
31. Woodworth G, McGirt MJ, Samdani A, Garonzik I, Olivi A, Weingart JD. Accuracy of frameless and frame-based image-guided stereotactic brain biopsy in the diagnosis of glioma: comparison of biopsy and open resection specimen. *Neurol Res.* 2005;27(4):358–362.
32. Aker FV, Hakan T, Karadereler S, Erkan M. Accuracy and diagnostic yield of stereotactic biopsy in the diagnosis of brain masses: comparison of results of biopsy and resected surgical specimens. *Neuropathology.* 2005;25(3):207–213.
33. Jackson RJ, Fuller GN, Abi-Said D, et al. Limitations of stereotactic biopsy in the initial management of gliomas. *Neuro Oncol.* 2001;3(3):193–200.
34. McGirt MJ, Villavicencio AT, Bulsara KR, Friedman AH. MRI-guided stereotactic biopsy in the diagnosis of glioma: comparison of biopsy and surgical resection specimen. *Surg Neurol.* 2003;59(4):277–281; discussion 281–282.
35. Daumas-Duport C, Scheithauer BW, Kelly PJ. A histologic and cytologic method for the spatial definition of gliomas. *Mayo Clin Proc.* 1987;62(6):435–449.
36. Berger MS, Deliganis AV, Dobbins J, Keles GE. The effect of extent of resection on recurrence in patients with low grade cerebral hemisphere gliomas. *Cancer.* 1994;74(6):1784–1791.
37. Berman JI, Berger MS, Chung SW, Nagarajan SS, Henry RG. Accuracy of diffusion tensor magnetic resonance imaging tractography assessed using intraoperative subcortical stimulation mapping and magnetic source imaging. *J Neurosurg.* 2007;107(3):488–494.
38. Duffau H. Intraoperative cortico-subcortical stimulations in surgery of low-grade gliomas. *Expert Rev Neurother.* 2005;5(4):473–485.
39. Duffau H. New concepts in surgery of WHO grade II gliomas: functional brain mapping, connectionism and plasticity—a review. *J Neurooncol.* 2006;79(1):77–115.
40. Duffau H, Capelle L, Denvil D, et al. Usefulness of intraoperative electrical subcortical mapping during surgery for low-grade gliomas located within eloquent brain regions: functional results in a consecutive series of 103 patients. *J Neurosurg.* 2003;98(4):764–778.
41. Claus EB, Horlacher A, Hsu L, et al. Survival rates in patients with low-grade glioma after intraoperative magnetic resonance image guidance. *Cancer.* 2005;103(6):1227–1233.
42. Gunnarsson T, Olafsson E, Sighvatsson V, Hannesson B. Surgical treatment of patients with low-grade astrocytomas and medically intractable seizures. *Acta Neurol Scand.* 2002;105(4):289–292.
43. Karim AB, Maat B, Hatlevoll R, et al. A randomized trial on dose-response in radiation therapy of low-grade cerebral glioma: European Organization for Research and Treatment of Cancer (EORTC) Study 22844. *Int J Radiat Oncol Biol Phys.* 1996;36(3):549–556.
44. Brada M, Viviers L, Abson C, et al. Phase II study of primary temozolomide chemotherapy in patients with WHO grade II gliomas. *Ann Oncol.* 2003;14(12):1715–1721.
45. Buckner JC, Gesme D Jr, O'Fallon JR, et al. Phase II trial of procarbazine, lomustine, and vincristine as initial therapy for patients with low-grade oligodendroglioma or oligoastrocytoma: efficacy and associations with chromosomal abnormalities. *J Clin Oncol.* 2003;21(2):251–255.
46. Hoang-Xuan K, Capelle L, Kujas M, et al. Temozolomide as initial treatment for adults with low-grade oligodendrogliomas or oligoastrocytomas and correlation with chromosome 1p deletions. *J Clin Oncol.* 2004;22(15):3133–3138.
47. Quinn JA, Reardon DA, Friedman AH, et al. Phase II trial of temozolomide in patients with progressive low-grade glioma. *J Clin Oncol.* 2003;21(4):646–651.
48. Pignatti F, van den Bent M, Curran D, et al. Prognostic factors for survival in adult patients with cerebral low-grade glioma. *J Clin Oncol.* 2002;20(8):2076–2084.
49. Karim AB, Afra D, Cornu P, et al. Randomized trial on the efficacy of radiotherapy for cerebral low-grade glioma in the adult: European Organization for Research and Treatment of Cancer Study 22845 with the Medical Research Council study BRO4: an interim analysis. *Int J Radiat Oncol Biol Phys.* 2002;52(2):316–324.
50. Lebrun C, Fontaine D, Ramaioli A, et al. Long-term outcome of oligodendrogliomas. *Neurology.* 2004;62(10):1783–1787.

57 Pineal Gland Tumors

Gaetan Moise, Alfred T. Ogden, and Jeffrey N. Bruce

INTRODUCTION

The pineal region is an anatomically complex area consisting of multiple cell types capable of giving rise to neoplastic disease. The advent of modern microsurgical techniques has made tumors in this region surgically accessible with acceptable morbidity. The development of stereotactic-guidance for surgical and radiosurgical procedures as well as endoscopy have further expanded the tools available to treat pineal region tumors [1]. Creating a comprehensive treatment approach to these tumors is hindered by the diversity of pathologies, the relatively small number of patients affected, and the paucity of reliable outcomes data. Nonetheless, certain basic concepts for surgical management of any neoplastic process in the central nervous system can be applied:

1. Histopathological diagnosis is necessary and should be obtained by the safest, most accurate means possible.
2. Complete surgical excision for benign processes, while typically curative, should not produce undue morbidity.
3. Surgical debulking can play an important role in the facilitation of responses to adjuvant therapy.

ANATOMY OF THE PINEAL REGION

The pineal region, which contains the pineal body, is also known as the posterior incisural space or quadrigeminal cistern. The anterior wall is formed by the habenular trigone, habenular commissure and pineal body superiorly, the vermis inferomedially, and the superior cerebellar peduncles inferolaterally. The pineal body lies along the posterior wall of the third ventricle (i.e., the midbrain quadrigeminal plate formed by the superior and inferior colliculi). The splenium and tela choroidea form the roof of the quadrigeminal cistern. The thalami, crura of the fornices, and medial cerebral hemispheres bound the space laterally. At the apex of the tentorium, a thick sheet of arachnoid containing the precentral cerebellar vein separates the quadrigeminal cistern from the superior cerebellar cistern [2,3].

Venous structures carrying a majority of deep venous return of the brain are funneled through this region. The internal cerebral veins leave the velum interpositum (a potential space between the two membranous layers of the tela choroidea) and enter the pineal region superolateral to the pineal body, joining to form the great cerebral vein of Galen [4]. The basal veins of Rosenthal enter the region from the ambient cisterns and join the complex either at the internal cerebral veins or the vein of Galen. The internal occipital veins, pre-central cerebellar vein, and vermian vein all drain into the vein of Galen which courses to the straight sinus, formed within the dural leaves of the tentorium [2,5].

HISTORICAL REVIEW OF PINEAL REGION SURGERY

Given the anatomical complexity of the region, pineal tumors have always been among the most challenging of neurosurgical diseases. Without the advantages of high resolution imaging, operative microscopy, modern anesthesia, and neurocritical care, early surgical attempts at resection of pineal tumors were marred by poor outcomes. Walter Dandy, who spent years in a Johns Hopkins dog lab practicing the interhemispheric, transcallosal approach to the pineal region first described by Rorschach and Brunner [6], was the first to claim successful total resection of a pineal tumor in two of three patients, one of whom died 2 days after surgery [7]. At a time when neuroimaging was in its infancy, multiple surgeons made unsubstantiated claims regarding complete resection of pineal tumors as evidenced by lack of recurrence, resolution of symptoms, or intraoperative visual inspection.

During the following decades, new surgical approaches to the region were developed. Van Wagenen described a transcortical, transventricular approach to the pineal region in 1931 [8] while Horrax modified Dandy's approach by including occipital lobe resection for greater exposure [9]. The literature from this time is a testament to the almost uniformly poor outcomes of surgically treated patients. In Horrax's series of 22 pineal tumor patients, there were five perioperative mortalities and only two patients still alive by the time the report was published [10]. Suzuki's series of 19 patients included 3 perioperative deaths and 8 patients who were left vegetative [11].

Concurrently, reports of respectable clinical responses to radiation therapy for pineal tumors led most neurosurgeons and oncologists to advocate empiric radiation, with or without ventriculoperitoneal shunting. Surgical resection was reserved for patients who had failed to respond to radiation or those presenting *in extremis*. As most pineal region pathologies demonstrate relatively indolent growth and certain pathologies are highly radiosensitive (germinoma being the best example) this strategy produced 5-year survival rates as high as 70%. However, patients with radioresistant or benign pathologies were unnecessarily exposed to whole brain radiation.

The introduction of microsurgical instruments and usable operative microscopes brought significantly improved outcomes in pineal surgery. Two influential surgical series published in 1971 by Stein [12] and Jamieson [13] using an adaptation of the infratentorial supracerebellar approach and the occipital-transtentorial (OTT) approach, respectively, forced a radical rethinking of management of pineal region tumors. Modern surgical series on pineal region surgery have confirmed these improvements in safety and demonstrated that many tumors represent a mix of pathologies at time of presentation.

Several technologies have since been incorporated into the surgical management of pineal region tumors. Stereotaxy for biopsy of pineal region lesions has been validated in several retrospective series [14–18]. Neuroendoscopy, which offers a means to manage cerebrospinal fluid (CSF) obstruction and achieve tissue sampling/resection under direct visualization, has also been the focus of several series [19–23]. The refinement of stereotactic radiosurgery (SRS), and its potentially broad applications, makes it a potentially useful modality for pineal region tumors as well.

As a result of the improved safety of pineal-based surgical procedures and the known consequences of whole brain radiation, general practice in Western medicine has abandoned the prior convention of radiation before pathological confirmation. The small overall number of patients affected by pineal neoplasms, the diversity of tumors arising in this region, and the proliferation of new techniques and technologies have combined to create an imbalance between therapeutic options and comparative outcomes analysis.

PATHOLOGY

A wide range of pathologies involving the pineal region have been described [24]. Non-neoplastic entities such as vascular malformations, infectious lesions, or benign cysts can arise in this region. Neoplasia in this region falls into one of several broad categories (see Table 57.1): pineal parenchymal tumors (PPTs), germ cell tumors (GCTs), neuroectodermal tumors, meningeal tumors, metastases, and others [25]. PPTs are derived from the cells of the pineal gland itself. Neuroectodermal tumors are thought to arise from glia within the pineal gland or surrounding structures such as the brainstem or thalamus, ependymal cells along the posterior third ventricle, or choroid plexus. The presence of multiple arachnoidal planes including arachnoid cap cells in the tela choroidea allows for meningeal-based neoplastic transformation. Abnormal primitive cell rests retained in the pineal gland can give rise to GCTs.

Table 57.1 Pineal Region Tumor Classification

Pineal Parenchymal Tumors
  Pineocytoma
  Pineal parenchymal tumor of intermediate differentiation
  Pineoblastoma
Glial/Neuroectodermal
  Astrocytoma: Pilocytic, fibrillary, anaplastic, glioblastoma, oligodendroglioma
  Ependymoma
  Papillary tumor of the pineal region[a]
  Choroid plexus papilloma/carcinoma
  Neural: ganglioglioma
  Melanoma
Germ Cell Tumor
  Germinoma
  Embryonal carcinoma
  Endodermal sinus (Yolk Sac) tumor
  Teratoma
  Choriocarcinoma
Meningeal
  Meningioma
  Hemangiopericytoma
Other
  Metastasis
  Craniopharyngioma
  Dermoid/Epidermoid

[a] Cell of origin unclear.

Metastatic lesions can spread to any of multiple structures in the pineal region.

CLINICAL CONSIDERATIONS

Preoperative Workup

Patients presenting with unknown pineal region lesions require imaging and laboratory studies as part of the standard preoperative workup. Pre- and postcontrast, high-resolution magnetic resonance imaging is useful in formulating a differential diagnosis. The only tumor with pathognomonic imaging that would preclude the need for histological confirmation in the absence of demonstrated radiographic or clinical progression is a quadrigeminal plate/tectal glioma [26]. Nonetheless, magnetic resonance imaging provides the kind of detailed information on the relationship of the tumor to critical structures necessary for formulating a surgical strategy. In addition, neuroimaging allows for assessment of hydrocephalus to determine the need for CSF diversion.

Laboratory analysis of serum and CSF for the germ cell markers β-human chorionic gonadotropin and α-fetoprotein is also needed for appropriate workup of patients with pineal tumors. The presence of a pineal region mass and detectable CSF/serum levels of these markers is diagnostic of a malignant GCT [27]. When germ cell markers are elevated, a biopsy is not necessary before beginning chemotherapy and radiation. As germinomas are exquisitely radiosensitive and nongerminomatous malignant GCTs are typically chemo-sensitive, combinatorial radiation and chemotherapy can produce clinical and radiographic remission with 5-year survival rates close to

100% for germinomas and between 38% and 69% for non-germinomatous GCTs [28].

Hydrocephalus Management

Many patients with pineal region masses have some degree of obstructive (noncommunicating) hydrocephalus secondary to aqueductal compression at the time of initial neurosurgical evaluation. Therefore, control of CSF flow is a necessary step before direct surgical treatment of pineal region masses. As many patients in whom adequate tumor decompression is achieved do not need permanent CSF diversion, placement of an external ventricular drain immediately before pineal surgery with careful postoperative weaning is a reasonable strategy. For patients in whom only biopsy is performed, or patients who fail ventricular drain weaning, third ventriculostomy is the preferred method of treating hydrocephalus. Although first successfully performed in 1923 by Mixter [29], endoscopic third ventriculostomy (ETV) found widespread acceptance with the introduction of smaller, more reliable endoscopic equipment. Large case series demonstrate long-term success rates between 75% and 90% [19,30]. Ventriculoperitoneal shunts, which are prone to infection and failure requiring reoperation, should be reserved for patients who fail third ventriculostomy or whose tumor involves the floor of the third ventricle to such a degree as to make third ventriculostomy unsafe or unlikely to remain functional.

SURGICAL DECISION MAKING

Objectives of Surgery

Accurate histology is the goal of any surgical procedure involving an unknown pineal region mass. Histological diagnosis is the key to determining the need for further workup, radiotherapy or chemotherapy, and appropriate follow-up. Furthermore, it offers practitioners a means of estimating prognosis, which facilitates decision making. However, given the pathological heterogeneity of many pineal region lesions, acquisition of diagnostic tissue is not a simple matter.

Tumor debulking and/or complete resection may be a secondary surgical objective depending upon the diagnosis. For benign lesions, a complete resection can provide a surgical cure. However, for some pathologies, germinoma being the most studied, extent of resection has not been demonstrated to improve outcomes [27]. Thus, the decision to attempt maximal tumor resection at the time of surgery must balance the benefits of resection for a specific pathology with potential operative morbidity.

Stereotactic biopsy has several advantages including its relative lack of invasiveness and its low risk of complication [17,18]; additionally, when coupled with third ventriculostomy in patients with obstructive hydrocephalus, the total number of procedures is reduced [20,21]. The primary disadvantage of biopsy is a function of the limited amount of tissue obtained, which increases the potential for sampling error [31–33]. The heterogeneity on imaging of many lesions that arise from the pineal regions (see Figures 57.1 and 57.2) adds to the complexity of target selection in biopsy planning. A study of stereotactic biopsy followed by open surgery for resection (not restricted to pineal region tumors) found that biopsy was incorrect with clinical implications in ~7% of the cases,

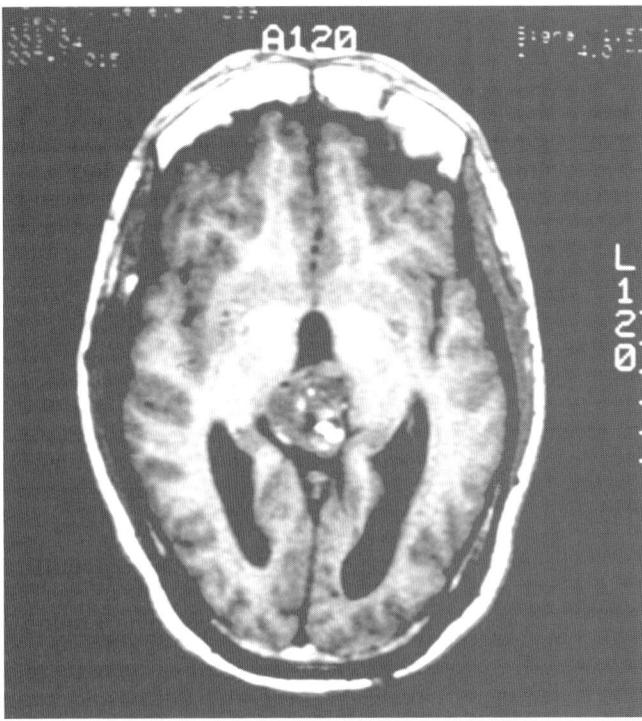

Figure 57.1 Axial noncontrast MRI demonstrating mixed signal intensity pineal region mass.

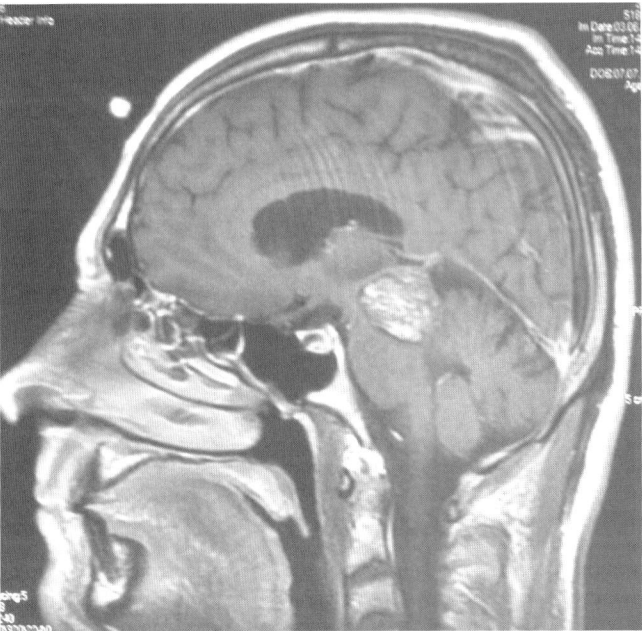

Figure 57.2 Sagittal T1-weighted contrast MRI demonstrating heterogeneously enhancing pineal region mass with evidence of intralesional hemorrhage.

and incorrect without clinical implications in 30% of cases [31].

Stereotactic biopsy is not a therapeutic procedure, so any morbidity derived from the procedure occurs in the absence of immediate therapeutic benefit. Although the mechanics of performing stereotactic biopsies are familiar to all neurosurgeons, and therefore widely available, the pineal region is a relatively dangerous region to biopsy because of its vascularity. Small choroidal arteries supply multiple structures, the majority of the deep drainage of the brain traverses the area, and malignant tumors in this region can parasitize this vascular supply. In addition, the biopsy trajectory requires passage through multiple pial surfaces. As a result, hemorrhage, the major potential complication of any stereotactic biopsy, may be more common after biopsies in this region.

Open microsurgery, while clearly more invasive than stereotactic biopsy, has the potential for greater complications. However, in experienced hands, open pineal region microsurgery can be performed with favorable outcomes, with most modern series reporting less than 10% mortality (see Table 57.2). The recent development of neurocritical care as a specialty has also improved postoperative management of these patients. Open surgery increases sample procurement, maximizes chances of accurate diagnosis, and provides the opportunity for maximal tumor removal, thereby potentially improving prognosis. For benign lesions, complete surgical resection offers the chance of cure [36,41,42,48–50]. In cases of obstructive hydrocephalus, maximal resection can re-establish anatomical CSF flow patterns, obviating the need for CSF diversion.

For malignant tumors, the relationship between degree of resection and outcome is not as easily determined. Theoretically, maximal tumor resection should improve the efficacy of adjuvant therapy, leading to improved long-term survival. Some studies have suggested a correlation for certain tumor types, but as most were small, retrospective, and have inadequate length of follow-up it is difficult to elucidate the relationship between surgery and survival in this population [51–56].

SURGICAL PROCEDURES

Stereotactic Biopsy

Stereotactic biopsy may be the appropriate first procedure in certain cases: patients with multiple lesions on imaging, patients whose medical condition preclude general anesthesia or lengthy procedures, and potentially patients carrying lesions with imaging highly suggestive of brainstem invasion thereby limiting the degree of achievable resection [25]. The procedure can typically be performed with sedation and local anesthesia, thereby avoiding the potential complications of intubation and general anesthesia.

Although frameless stereotaxy methods are becoming common neurosurgical adjuncts in many procedures, frame-based image-guided systems are the preferred method for stereotactic biopsy as they are simple and accurate. The planning software that accompanies the various stereotactic systems can be used to calculate a trajectory that avoids critical structures and minimizes crossing ventricular, cisternal, and gyral surfaces to reduce risk of hemorrhage and inaccuracy from shift or tissue deformation. The two most common stereotactic trajectories to the pineal region are an anterolateral-superior approach and a posterolateral-superior approach [57]. The anterolateral-superior trajectory starts anterior to the coronal suture and lateral to the mid-pupillary line and traverses the frontal lobe and internal capsule. The poster-lateral-superior trajectory starts in the region of the parieto-occipital junction and is most useful for tumors with significant lateral extension.

Theoretically, diagnostic accuracy should improve with larger sample volumes and increased numbers of

Table 57.2 Major Series of Open Microsurgery for Pineal Region Tumors

Authors	Year	Case No.	Approach	Patient Population	Pathology	GTR (%)	Mortality (%)	Major Morbidity (%)	Permanent Minor Morbidity (%)
Hoffman et al [34]	1983	61	TC/SCIT	Peds	All	NA	20	NA	NA
Neuwelt et al [35]	1985	13	OTT	Adult/peds	All	60%	0	0	20
Lapras et al [36]	1987	86	TC/OTT	Adult/peds	All	65	5.8[a]	5.8[a]	28
Edwards et al [37]	1988	36	TC/OTT/SCIT	Peds	All	NA	0	3.3	3.3
Pluchino et al [38]	1989	40	SCIT	Adult/peds	All	25	5	NA	NA
Luo et al [39]	1989	64	OTT	Adult/peds	All	21	10	NA	NA
Vaquero et al [40]	1992	29	TC/SCIT/OTT	Adult/peds	All	NA	11	NA	NA
Herrman et al	1992	49	TC/SCIT	Adult/peds	All	NA	8	NA	NA
Bruce and Stein [41]	1995	160	SCIT/TC/OTT	Adult/peds	All	45	4	3	19
Chandy et al [42]	1998	48	SCIT/OTT	Adult/peds	"benign lesions"	55	0	NA	NA
Kang et al [43]	1998	16	OTT/SCIT/TC	Adult/peds	All	37.5	0	0	19
Shin et al [44]	1998	21	OTT	Adult/peds	All	54.5	0	0	5
Konovalov et al [45]	2003	201	OTT/SCIT	Adult/peds	All	58	10[b]	NA	>20
Bruce et al [25]	2004	81	SCIT/TC/OTT	Adult/peds	All	47	1	2	NA
Desai et al [46]	2006	24	SCIT/TC	Adult/peds	Epidermoid cysts	25	0	NA	NA
Cuccia et al [47]	2006	11	OTT/?	Peds	Pinealoblastoma	18	0	18	NA

Abbreviations: GTR, gross total resection; OTT, occipital transtentorial; SCIT, supracerebellar-intfratentorial; TC, interhemispheric-transcallosal.

[a] Combined mortality/major morbidity 2.8% in last 40 patients.

[b] Mortality rate 1.8% for all cases after 1990 (168 surgical cases).

separate locations sampled. Determining the optimal number of core samples varies for individuals patients. Factors that should be considered include the pathologist's confidence on initial frozen section inspection, the patient's condition and ability to tolerate lengthening of the procedure, the incremental bleeding risk of successive biopsies, and degree of tumor heterogeneity.

Overall complication rates from stereotactic biopsy in the pineal region are similar to those in other regions of the brain [18,58]. Although hemorrhage rates in pineal biopsies are reportedly higher than in other brain regions, many are small and carry little clinical significance [14,15]. Analysis of published literature on pineal region stereotactic biopsies (see Table 57.3) reveals procedure-related mortality of less than 2% with a risk of major morbidity of 0% to 1.2%. The rate of "transient minor morbidity" is higher at 7% to 8.4%. The rate of diagnostically useful sample acquisition reported is 87% to 97%. This represents an overestimate of diagnostic accuracy as pathologic correlation of biopsy specimens with resection specimens demonstrates only an 89% correlation between diagnosis at biopsy versus diagnosis at time of resection [45].

Endoscopy

The use of endoscopy for management of pineal region masses was first described in 1973 [61] but reliable data on its use remain relatively sparse. ETV is generally the accepted procedure for management of obstructive hydrocephalus in this patient population. The greater controversy lies in the use of endoscopy for other applications such as biopsy or as an adjunct for surgical resection of pineal region masses. Studies exclusively examining endoscopic biopsy of pineal region masses in conjunction with ETV are few in number and have small patient numbers (see Table 57.4). As a result, it is difficult to make conclusions regarding its role in management of pineal region tumors. As the trajectories for pineal region biopsy and ETV vary significantly, use of a rigid endoscope almost always necessitates placement of two different burr holes and different trajectories performed at one sitting. Attempts at single-trajectory approaches for both ETV and pineal region biopsy appear to have a higher rate of nondiagnostic specimen acquisition [21].

Obtaining hemostasis is one of the more difficult aspects of endoscopic procedures as even minor amounts of bleeding can significantly impair visualization. As a result, bleeding at the time of initial procedure is most often the factor that leads to aborted biopsy attempts. Given the relatively small numbers reported in the literature, ETV remains the only proven role of endoscopic approaches for the management of pineal region tumors. Larger series of consecutively treated pineal tumors managed endoscopically will be needed to make useful comparisons to stereotactic biopsy or open microsurgery.

Stereotactic Radiosurgery

SRS is most often promulgated as part of a "minimally invasive approach" to pineal region tumors. Advocates of this strategy promote stereotactic biopsy (with CSF diversion procedures as needed) as the initial step to obtain histological diagnosis, followed by SRS and adjuvant chemotherapy for tumor control [60,63,68–70]. The major advantage of SRS with either gamma knife or LINAC technologies over whole brain radiation is the restriction of tissues exposed to damaging doses of radiation. This also is a potential negative in the treatment of malignant tumors in this region

Table 57.3 Major Series on Stereotactic Biopsy of Pineal Region Lesions

Authors	Year	Location	Number of Pineal Cases	Diagnostic Yield (%)	Mortality (%)	Major Morbidity (%)	Transient/Minor Morbidity (%)	Hemorrhage Rate (%)
Pecker et al [59]	1979	Pineal	25	NR	0	NR	NR	NR
Dempsey et al [60]	1992	Pineal	15	87	0	0	NR	13
Regis et al [17]	1996	Pineal	370	94	1.3	1.2	7	4.4
Kreth et al [16]	1996	Pineal	106	97	1.9	0	8.4	7.5
Konovalov et al [45]	2003	Pineal	61	82	1.6	NR	NR	NR
Apuzzo et al [58]	1987	Pineal/all	22/500 (all)	NR/95.6	0/0.2	0/1	NR	NR
Sawin et al [18]	1996	Pineal/all	7/225 (all)	NR	0/0.4	0/3.6	14/1.3	14
Field et al [15]	2001	Pineal/all	19/500 (all)	NA	0/0.2	0/1.2	0/NR	21

Table 57.4 Studies of Endoscopic Biopsy of Pineal Region Masses

Authors	Year	Cases	Diagnostic Yield (%)	Mortality (%)	Major Morbidity (%)	Transient Minor Morbidity (%)	Percentage Requiring VP Shunt
Ferrer et al [62]	1997	4	75	0	25	50	25
Oi et al [63]	2000	6	100	0	0	0	17
Gangemi et al [64]	2000	5	100	0	0	20	NR
Pople et al [65]	2001	34	94	0	2.9	2.9	74
Kim et al [20]	2004	5	100	0	NR	NR	0
Yamini et al [66]	2005	6	63	0	0	NR	63
Chernov et al [67]	2006	23	100	0	0	77	0

as diffuse metastatic spread is not addressed by this technique. Table 57.5 represents the available literature on SRS for the treatment of pineal region lesions. As the overall number of studies is small, the number of treated pathological entities large, and the time of follow-up relatively short, it is difficult to make treatment recommendations based on this literature.

Stereotactic brachytherapy using interstitial Iodine-125 or Iridium-192 has been described, but the data are too meager to draw useful conclusions about its role in pineal tumor management [16,75–77].

A few observations regarding the role of SRS can be made from the available literature. SRS targeted to the pineal region appears safe, that is, not associated with undue morbidity from the procedure itself. From the two studies on PPTs [68,74], treatment failures outside of the stereotactic target are common for malignant PPTs. This can be addressed with additional courses of SRS if focal metastatic lesions exist, or craniospinal radiotherapy if widespread. However, given the high failure rate, there is little evidence to support SRS over radical surgical resection and adjuvant therapy. Finally, SRS almost certainly has a role in the management of pineal region tumors, with potential utility for local control of benign lesions. Nonetheless, the demonstrated potential for malignant tumors in this region to metastasize limits the utility of this modality as a replacement for craniospinal radiation in the treatment of many types of pineal tumors.

Microsurgery

Open microsurgical procedures play an important role in the management of pineal region tumors. Open radical resection represents the best chance at cure for benign lesions as gross total resection may be achieved with non-infiltrative lesions (see Figures 57.3 and 57.4). Debulking before the institution of adjuvant therapies can improve response rates and reduce morbidity associated with tumor response to radiation or chemotherapy. For lesions that demonstrate incomplete or nonresponse to chemo or radiotherapy, some authors advocate 'second look' surgery to treat residual tumor. In addition, by increasing pathological yield, radical surgery offers the best chance at diagnostic accuracy which is used to guide therapeutic strategies, determine the need for further evaluation, and present prognostic information to patients.

A number of surgical approaches to the pineal region have been described, but two are primarily used: the supracerebellar-infratentorial or the OTT [12,41,78]. Although anatomical features of the patient and the lesion in question help determine which approach is best suited to an individual case, the best data suggest that the approaches are fairly equivalent, making surgeon preference a key consideration [79].

The supracerebellar-infratentorial approach makes use of a natural midline corridor between the cerebellum and the tentorium with relatively few interposed venous structures. The approach has the added benefit of aiding separation of tumor from deep venous structures and any attachments to the velum interpositum, often the most critical and difficult portions of surgery in this region.

The OTT is the most popular supratentorial approach; although a number of other supratentorial approaches have been described including the less commonly used posterior interhemispheric-transcallosal. The OTT approach offers excellent exposure to the pineal region, but does require occipital lobe retraction for adequate visualization which can result in postoperative visual problems that are typically reversible. The posterior interhemispheric approach, which requires transection of the posterior portion of the corpus callosum, is most frequently complicated by weakness or sensory deficits secondary to parietal lobe manipulation rather than a clinically relevant disconnection syndrome.

For any surgical approach to the pineal region, hemorrhage in the postoperative period is the most serious complication. Incomplete resection is a risk factor as remnants of malignant tumors with abnormal neovasculature have a greater propensity to bleed. Specific neurological complications with pineal region surgery include cerebellar signs such as ataxia, and brainstem or cranial nerve findings such as extraocular muscle dysfunction. Many postoperative neurological findings improve up to a year after surgery so long as no permanent anatomical disruption exists. Higher complication rates occur in patients who have previously been irradiated, patients with invasive or malignant tumors, and patients who present with focal neurological symptoms preoperatively [25,78,80]. Many modern series of open microsurgery do not include detailed descriptions of operative morbidity. The available data suggest that major morbidity from open microsurgery can be limited to less than 6%, but permanent minor morbidity rates of up to

Table 57.5 Major Series of Stereotactic Radiosurgery for Pineal Region Tumors

Authors	Year	Cases	Post-surgical	Modality	Tumor Types	Mean F/U (months)	CR (%)	PR (%)	NC (%)	PG (%)	Death (%)
Manera et al [71]	1996	11	NA	LINAC	All	12.4	NR	NR	NR	NR	0
Raco et al [70]	2000	22	NA	LINAC	All	NR	36	9	0	4.5	45
Kobayashi et al [69]	2001	33	11	GKRS	All	23.3	24	42	0	24	21
Amendola et al [72]	2005	20	NA	GKRS	All	NR	NR	NR	NR	NR	15
Lekovic et al [73]	2007	17	15	GKRS	All	31	11.8	47.1	35.3	5.9	18.8
Hasegawa et al [68]	2002	16	13	GKRS	PPT	61	29	50	6.2	0	5
Reyns et al [74]	2006	13	3	GKRS	PPT	34	25	50	16.7	8.3	16.7

Abbreviations: CR, complete response; NC, no change; PG, progression; PPT, pineal parenchymal tumors; PR, partial response.

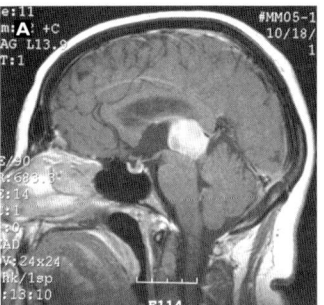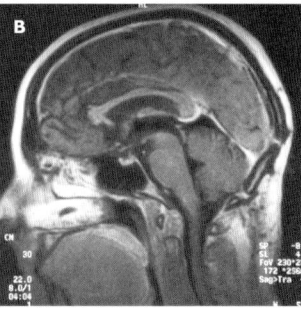

Figure 57.3 Pre- and postoperative sagittal T1-weighted contrast MRI demonstrating gross total resection of pineal region tumor using supracerebellar-infratentorial approach.

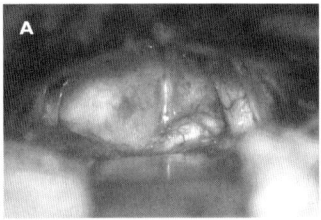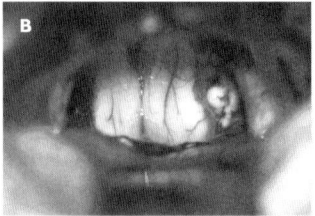

Figure 57.4 Pre- and postresection intraoperative photographs of pineal region tumor as seen via supracerebellar-infratentorial approach.

28% have been reported and represent an area of potential improvement (see Table 57.2).

Role of Surgery for Specific Pathologies

The role of surgical resection of pineal region tumors varies by histopathological diagnosis. Definitive statements for all tumor types are hampered by a relative lack of available evidence. Table 57.2 presents the results of the major surgical series in the literature. Difficulties in interpreting this literature include insufficient follow-up, inadequate assessment of degree of resection, lack of prospective studies, varied pathologies, and constantly changing adjuvant therapy strategies. Nonetheless, certain trends are discernable from the literature and are used to guide surgical and adjuvant therapies on a histology-specific basis.

For GCTs, the presence of serum and CSF markers (β-human chorionic gonadotropin and α-fetoprotein) allows diagnosis in many patients without need for biopsy. Most malignant GCTs, including germinomas, do not have elevated germ cell markers and therefore must have a tissue-derived diagnosis. Germinomas, the most common pineal region GCT, are highly radiosensitive with excellent 5-year survival, even with reduced-dose radiation as part of a combined chemoradiation strategy [28]. Hence, resective surgery is not typically useful for germinomas. Nongerminomatous GCTs are more radioresistant, but craniospinal radiation (upfront and at higher doses) as part of a combined chemoradiation strategy remains first-line therapy for these tumors after diagnosis (by tumor marker analysis or biopsy) [81,82]. If follow-up imaging demonstrates residual tumor and/or tumor markers do not decrease appropriately, many authors advocate a "second-look" open microsurgical strategy for the purposes of specimen acquisition to evaluate for evidence of residual malignancy on pathology (used to guide decision-making on further chemotherapy) and aggressive radical resection [83–87].

PPTs can demonstrate a wide spectrum of clinical behaviors ranging from benign (pineocytoma) to malignant (pineoblastoma) with a large intermediate category (PPT of intermediate differentiation [PPTID]) that reflects the struggle to improve grading so that it more accurately predicts prognosis [88,89]. A single patient's tumor can have a mix of histological patterns, open surgery for diagnosis and resection is extremely valuable. Although surgical cure is not possible, the best data available suggest maximal resection correlates with significant improvements in overall survival for malignant PPTs in conjunction with chemoradiation therapy [45,51].

Pineal region gliomas can arise from pineal gland itself or neighboring structures such as the thalamus or brainstem and range from low-grade to highly malignant. No clear management strategy for this group of tumors can be elucidated because of the paucity of data, the diversity of potential structural involvement, and the numerous tumor subtypes and grades possible. Obtaining tissue for diagnosis is necessary, but given the potentially infiltrative nature of these tumors, radical resection may not be feasible. Tectal gliomas represent an exceptional subset, with the sparse data available suggesting an indolent course, particularly for lesions below 1.5 cm in diameter [26,90–96]. Hence, current management strategies for tectal gliomas stress observation and symptomatic treatment of hydrocephalus with no absolute requirement to biopsy in the absence of clinical or radiographic progression.

For benign tumors in this area such as meningiomas and pineocytomas, resective surgery is the treatment of choice as it offers the best chance at long-term recurrence free survival without the need for adjuvant therapies [97]. Attempts at gross total resection should be tempered by efforts to avoid excess morbidity as slow growth rates coupled with the continued development of newer adjuvant therapies may produce equally good clinical outcomes in the future.

Adjuvant Therapy

A detailed analysis of available adjuvant therapy regimens for pineal region tumors is beyond the scope of this chapter. Nonetheless, in regards to several tumor classes found in the pineal region, several themes have started to emerge from the current literature (see Table 57.6). Intracranial GCTs are broadly categorized as germinomatous or nongerminomatous because of a potential difference in responsiveness to radiation therapy. For germinomatous tumors, radiation-only protocols have produced response rates greater than 90%, although the role of spinal radiation for prophylaxis remains controversial [98–101]. Concerns over the cognitive effects of radiation therapy and the lower response rates in nongerminomatous tumors have led to the development of platinum-based chemotherapy

Table 57.6 Basic Surgical Strategies for Pineal Region Tumors by Pathology

Pathology	Behavior	Surgical Strategy	Adjuvant Therapy
Benign tumors: meningioma, epidermoid	Slow-growing, symptoms derive from local compression.	Radical resection for attempted cure except pineal cysts, which may be observed unless symptomatic	None
Germinoma	Aggressive	Biopsy	Radiotherapy ± chemotherapy
Nongerminomatous GCT	Aggressive	Biopsy; 'Second-look' radical resection in cases of incomplete response to adjuvant therapy	Radiotherapy & chemotherapy
Pineocytoma	Indolent, although pediatric cases may behave more aggressively	Radical resection alone in adults with excellent long-term outcomes	Possibly radiation
Pineal parenchymal tumors of indeterminate differentiation; pineoblastoma	More aggressive in pediatric populations	Radical resection	Chemotherapy Craniospinal radiation in pt. >4 YO
Astrocytoma—Pineal gland	Varies by tumor grade	Complete surgical resection may provide long-term remission for lower-grade lesions.	Varies by tumor grade
Astrocytoma—Tectal/quadrigeminal plate	Indolent	Observation unless evidence of progressive behavior	Unclear

regimens which appear to be effective in both classes of GCTs, although a significantly high relapse rate after chemotherapy alone has led some to advocate for chemotherapy in combination with a reduced field and overall dose of radiation [27,84,102–105]. The continued presence of viable tumor on pathological analysis after second-look surgery in patients with pineal germ-cell tumors previously treated with combination radiation and platinum-based chemotherapy demonstrates the decreased responsiveness of nongerminomatous compared with germinomatous tumors and the need for improvement in adjuvant therapies for these tumors [87].

PPTs remain a classification in flux. The literature on adjuvant therapy specifically for PPTID is limited to three case reports [106–108]. As a result, most authors treat PPTID under a broader classification of malignant PPTs, a grouping that includes pinealoblastoma. In a study by Lutterback et al examining patterns of treatment in malignant PPTs, almost all patients underwent craniospinal irradiation and approximately a third had adjuvant chemotherapy in conjunction with radiation. Outcome was linked to presence of metastasis (by CSF sampling or on imaging), pathology (PPTID vs. pinealoblastoma), and presence of residual tumor after treatment [51]. Because of the relatively high rates of leptomeningeal and CSF metastasis (9%) and the significantly worse outcome associated with residual tumor, most authors agree that a diagnosis of PPTID or pinealoblastoma necessitates craniospinal irradiation and adjuvant chemotherapy regardless of extent of resection [97]. Most reports of chemotherapy for pinealoblastoma are platinum-based, but alkylating agents and topoisomerase inhibitors have been used alone or in combination. As pinealoblastoma of early childhood appear less responsive to current adjuvant therapy, this group is the focus of many investigational chemotherapy regimens [108,109].

Given their relative rarity, glial tumors of the pineal region are treated similarly to those located in other regions. Lower-grade astrocytomas are a controversial management issue as the extent of surgery and optimal timing of adjuvant therapy remain uncertain given the rare metastatic potential of these lesions and long latency before malignant degeneration [110]. Higher-grade astrocytomas of the region remain a reportable entity, with the most recent review suggesting that chemotherapy and radiation therapy may result in a slight improvement in prognosis [111]. Ependymomas demonstrate little response to known chemotherapy regimens, making postoperative radiation therapy standard for all higher-grade lesions as well as in cases of incomplete resection of lower-grade tumors [112]. In situations of complete resection of lower-grade lesions, radiation is occasionally deferred until evidence of recurrence.

Craniospinal Evaluation

The inability of neuroimaging to accurately determine pineal pathology is a linchpin of current surgical management strategies based on tissue acquisition for histological diagnosis [113]. However, neuroimaging is critical to oncological management of pineal region tumors. Histologically confirmed benign pathologies merit postoperative imaging to determine extent of resection as studies have demonstrated that surgeon's assessments are inaccurate [114,115]. Furthermore, given the potential for misdiagnosis secondary to sampling error, benign pathologies of the pineal region should be periodically imaged to ensure stability.

A histological diagnosis of pineal malignancy should prompt full craniospinal imaging for staging purposes. Contrast magnetic resonance imaging has replaced myelography as the diagnostic method of choice for identification of spinal lesions [116]. Evidence of leptomeningeal or focal spinal metastasis can prompt changes in adjuvant therapy and can be used to monitor treatment response in cases without metastatic spread [117]. For cases of pineal region malignancy with negative metastatic neuroimaging, obtaining CSF (if not done intraoperatively) is necessary as a subset of patients will have positive CSF dissemination in the absence of evidence on imaging [51]. Also, in the case of marker-positive GCTs, serum marker levels can be used to monitor therapeutic response [118].

CONCLUSION

Confirmation of histological diagnosis is critical in treating pineal region tumors as it guides all management decisions. Representative diagnostic tissue acquisition, either by stereotactic biopsy or open microsurgery, is the first and most important role of surgery in the pineal region. Stereotactic biopsy is simpler to perform and less invasive, but is also less accurate than open surgery, does not address potential CSF obstruction, and is not directly therapeutic. The development and refinement of endoscopy and SRS may adequately address these shortcomings, although the currently available data are inadequate to make universal treatment recommendations.

Open microsurgery remains the gold-standard for obtaining accurate diagnosis, albeit with greater potential complications than stereotactic biopsy. For low-grade and benign tumors, surgical resection almost certainly improves outcome while reestablishing anatomical CSF pathways for treatment of obstructive hydrocephalus. For malignant tumors, the role of open resective surgery is more complicated as it must be coordinated with evolving adjunctive therapeutic strategies. In the hands of experienced surgeons, with the support of neuroanesthesia and neurocritical care teams, radical resection of malignant pineal region tumors can be accomplished with low morbidity and mortality. Technological improvements in the tools available to neurosurgeons, coupled with neoadjuvant therapies should contribute to continued refinement of treatment options and improved outcomes for patients burdened with pineal region tumors.

REFERENCES

1. Bruce JN, Ogden AT. Surgical strategies for treating patients with pineal region tumors. *J Neurooncol.* 2004;69(1–3):221–236.
2. Ono M, Ono M, Rhoton AL Jr, Barry M. Microsurgical anatomy of the region of the tentorial incisura. *J Neurosurg.* 1984;60(2):365–399.
3. Rhoton AL Jr. Tentorial incisura. *Neurosurgery.* 2000;47(3 suppl):S131-S153.
4. Yamamoto I. Pineal region tumor: surgical anatomy and approach. *J Neurooncol.* 2001;54(3):263–275.
5. Ono M, Rhoton AL Jr, Peace D, Rodriguez RJ. Microsurgical anatomy of the deep venous system of the brain. *Neurosurgery.* 1984;15(5):621–657.
6. Rorschach H. Zur pathologie und operabilitat der zirbeldruse. *Beitr z klin Chir.* 1913;83:451.
7. Dandy W. An operation for the removal of pineal tumors. *Surg Gynec Obstet.* 1921;33:113–119.
8. Van Wagenen W. A surgical approach for the removal of certain pineal tumors. *Surg Gynec Obstet.* 1931;53:216–220.
9. Horrax G. Extirpation of a huge pinealoma from a patient with pubertas praecox: a new operative approach. *Arch Neurol Psychiatry.* 1950;37:385–397.
10. HORRAX G. Treatment of tumors of the pineal body; experience in a series of 22 cases. *Arch Neurol Psychiatry.* 1950;64(2):227–242.
11. Suzuki J IT. Surgical removal of pineals tumors pinealomas and teratomas. Experience in a series of 19 cases. *J Neurosurg.* 1965;17:815–823.
12. Stein BM. The infratentorial supracerebellar approach to pineal lesions. *J Neurosurg.* 1971;35(2):197–202.
13. Jamieson KG. Excision of pineal tumors. *J Neurosurg.* 1971;35(5):550–553.
14. Favre J, Taha JM, Burchiel KJ. An analysis of the respective risks of hematoma formation in 361 consecutive morphological and functional stereotactic procedures. *Neurosurgery.* 2002;50(1):48–56; discussion 56.
15. Field M, Witham TF, Flickinger JC, Kondziolka D, Lunsford LD. Comprehensive assessment of hemorrhage risks and outcomes after stereotactic brain biopsy. *J Neurosurg.* 2001;94(4):545–551.
16. Kreth FW, Schätz CR, Pagenstecher A, Faist M, Volk B, Ostertag CB. Stereotactic management of lesions of the pineal region. *Neurosurgery.* 1996;39(2):280–289; discussion 289.
17. Regis J, Bouillot P, Rouby-Volot F, Figarella-Branger D, Dufour H, Peragut JC. Pineal region tumors and the role of stereotactic biopsy: review of the mortality, morbidity, and diagnostic rates in 370 cases. *Neurosurgery.* 1996;39(5):907–912; discussion 912.
18. Sawin PD, Hitchon PW, Follett KA, Torner JC. Computed imaging-assisted stereotactic brain biopsy: a risk analysis of 225 consecutive cases. *Surg Neurol.* 1998;49(6):640–649.
19. Dusick JR, McArthur DL, Bergsneider M. Success and complication rates of endoscopic third ventriculostomy for adult hydrocephalus: a series of 108 patients. *Surg Neurol.* 2008;69(1):5–15.
20. Kim IY, Jung S, Moon KS, Jung TY, Kang SS. Neuronavigation-guided endoscopic surgery for pineal tumors with hydrocephalus. *Minim Invasive Neurosurg.* 2004;47(6):365–368.
21. O'Brien DF, Hayhurst C, Pizer B, Mallucci CL. Outcomes in patients undergoing single-trajectory endoscopic third ventriculostomy and endoscopic biopsy for midline tumors presenting with obstructive hydrocephalus. *J Neurosurg.* 2006;105(3 suppl):219–226.
22. Roopesh Kumar SV, Mohanty A, Santosh V, et al. Endoscopic options in management of posterior third ventricular tumors. *Childs Nerv Syst.* 2007;23(10):1135–1145.
23. Yurtseven T, Ersahin Y, Demirtas E, Mutluer S. Neuroendoscopic biopsy for intraventricular tumors. *Minim Invasive Neurosurg.* 2003;46(5):293–299.
24. Hirato J, Nakazato Y. Pathology of pineal region tumors. *J Neurooncol.* 2001;54(3):239–249.
25. Bruce JN. Pineal tumors. In: Winn H, ed. *Youman's Neurological Surgery.* Philadelphia: WB Saunders Company; 2004:1011–1029.
26. Daglioglu E, Cataltepe O, Akalan N. Tectal gliomas in children: the implications for natural history and management strategy. *Pediatr Neurosurg.* 2003;38:223–231.
27. Weiner HL, Finlay JL. Surgery in the management of primary intracranial germ cell tumors. *Childs Nerv Syst.* 1999;15(11–12):770–773.
28. Brandes AA, Pasetto LM, Monfardini S. The treatment of cranial germ cell tumours. *Cancer Treat Rev.* 2000;26(4):233–242.
29. Mixter W. Ventriculoscopy and puncture of the floor of the third ventricle. *Boston Med Surg J.* 1923;188:277–278.
30. Gangemi M, Mascari C, Maiuri F, Godano U, Donati P, Longatti PL. Long-term outcome of endoscopic third ventriculostomy in obstructive hydrocephalus. *Minim Invasive Neurosurg.* 2007;50(5):265–269.
31. Chandrasoma PT, Smith MM, Apuzzo ML. Stereotactic biopsy in the diagnosis of brain masses: comparison of results of biopsy and resected surgical specimen. *Neurosurgery.* 1989;24(2):160–165.
32. Kraichoke S, Cosgrove M, Chandrasoma PT. Granulomatous inflammation in pineal germinoma. A cause of diagnostic failure at stereotaxic brain biopsy. *Am J Surg Pathol.* 1988;12(9):655–660.
33. Mueller W, Schneider GH, Hoffmann KT, Zschenderlein R, von Deimling A. Granulomatous tissue response in germinoma, a diagnostic pitfall in endoscopic biopsy. *Neuropathology.* 2007;27(2):127–132.
34. Hoffman HJ, Yoshida M, Becker LE, Hendrick EB, Humphreys RP. Pineal region tumors in childhood. Experience at the Hospital for Sick Children. 1983. *Pediatr Neurosurg.* 1994;21:91–103; discussion 4.
35. Neuwelt EA. An update on the surgical treatment of malignant pineal region tumors. *Clin Neurosurg.* 1985;32:397–428.
36. Lapras C, Patet JD, Mottolese C, Lapras C Jr. Direct surgery for pineal tumors: occipital-transtentorial approach. *Prog Exp Tumor Res.* 1987;30:268–280.
37. Edwards MS, Hudgins RJ, Wilson CB, Levin VA, Wara WM. Pineal region tumors in children. *J Neurosurg.* 1988;68(5):689–697.
38. Pluchino F, Broggi G, Fornari M, Franzini A, Solero CL, Allegranza A. Surgical approach to pineal tumours. *Acta Neurochir (Wien).* 1989;96(1–2):26–31.
39. Luo SQ, Li DZ, Zhang MZ, Wang ZC, Zhong CW. Occipital transtentorial approach for removal of pineal region tumors: report of 64 consecutive cases. *Surg Neurol.* 1989;32(1):36–39.

40. Vaquero J, Ramiro J, Martínez R, Bravo G. Neurosurgical experience with tumours of the pineal region at Clinica Puerta de Hierro. *Acta Neurochir (Wien)*. 1992;116(1):23–32.
41. Bruce JN, Stein BM. Surgical management of pineal region tumors. *Acta Neurochir (Wien)*. 1995;134(3–4):130–135.
42. Chandy MJ, Damaraju SC. Benign tumours of the pineal region: a prospective study from 1983 to 1997. *Br J Neurosurg*. 1998;12(3):228–233.
43. Kang JK, Jeun SS, Hong YK, et al. Experience with pineal region tumors. *Childs Nerv Syst*. 1998;14(1–2):63–68.
44. Shin HJ, Cho BK, Jung HW, Wang KC. Pediatric pineal tumors: need for a direct surgical approach and complications of the occipital transtentorial approach. *Childs Nerv Syst*. 1998;14(4–5):174–178.
45. Konovalov AN, Pitskhelauri DI. Principles of treatment of the pineal region tumors. *Surg Neurol*. 2003;59(4):250–268.
46. Desai KI, Nadkarni TD, Fattepurkar SC, Goel AH. Pineal epidermoid cysts: a study of 24 cases. *Surg Neurol*. 2006;65(2):124–129.
47. Cuccia V, Rodríguez F, Palma F, Zuccaro G. Pinealoblastomas in children. *Childs Nerv Syst*. 2006;22(6):577–585.
48. Barnett DW, Olson JJ, Thomas WG, Hunter SB. Low-grade astrocytomas arising from the pineal gland. *Surg Neurol*. 1995;43(1):70–75; discussion 75.
49. MacKay CI, Baeesa SS, Ventureyra EC. Epidermoid cysts of the pineal region. *Childs Nerv Syst*. 1999;15(4):170–178.
50. Vaquero J, Ramiro J, Martínez R, Coca S, Bravo G. Clinicopathological experience with pineocytomas: report of five surgically treated cases. *Neurosurgery*. 1990;27(4):612–8; discussion 618.
51. Lutterbach J, Fauchon F, Schild SE, et al. Malignant pineal parenchymal tumors in adult patients: patterns of care and prognostic factors. *Neurosurgery*. 2002;51(1):44–55; discussion 55.
52. Matsutani M, Sano K, Takakura K, et al. Primary intracranial germ cell tumors: a clinical analysis of 153 histologically verified cases. *J Neurosurg*. 1997;86(3):446–455.
53. Mena H, Rushing EJ, Ribas JL, Delahunt B, McCarthy WF. Tumors of pineal parenchymal cells: a correlation of histological features, including nucleolar organizer regions, with survival in 35 cases. *Hum Pathol*. 1995;26(1):20–30.
54. Reddy AT, Janss AJ, Phillips PC, Weiss HL, Packer RJ. Outcome for children with supratentorial primitive neuroectodermal tumors treated with surgery, radiation, and chemotherapy. *Cancer*. 2000;88(9):2189–2193.
55. Schild SE, Scheithauer BW, Haddock MG, et al. Histologically confirmed pineal tumors and other germ cell tumors of the brain. *Cancer*. 1996;78(12):2564–2571.
56. Schild SE, Scheithauer BW, Schomberg PJ, et al. Pineal parenchymal tumors. Clinical, pathologic, and therapeutic aspects. *Cancer*. 1993;72(3):870–880.
57. Maciunas R. Stereotactic biopsy of pineal region lesions. In: Kaye A, Black P, eds. *Operative Neurosurgery*. London: Churchill Livingstone; 2000:841–845.
58. Apuzzo ML, Chandrasoma PT, Cohen D, Zee CS, Zelman V. Computed imaging stereotaxy: experience and perspective related to 500 procedures applied to brain masses. *Neurosurgery*. 1987;20(6):930–937.
59. Pecker J, Scarabin JM, Vallee B, Brucher JM. Treatment in tumours of the pineal region: value of sterotaxic biopsy. *Surg Neurol*. 1979;12(4):341–348.
60. Dempsey PK, Lunsford LD. Stereotactic radiosurgery for pineal region tumors. *Neurosurg Clin N Am*. 1992;3(1):245–253.
61. Fukushima T, Ishijima B, Hirakawa K, Nakamura N, Sano K. Ventriculofiberscope: a new technique for endoscopic diagnosis and operation. Technical note. *J Neurosurg*. 1973;38(2):251–256.
62. Ferrer E, Santamarta D, Garcia-Fructuoso G, Caral L, Rumià J. Neuroendoscopic management of pineal region tumours. *Acta Neurochir (Wien)*. 1997;139(1):12–20; discussion 20.
63. Oi S, Shibata M, Tominaga J, et al. Efficacy of neuroendoscopic procedures in minimally invasive preferential management of pineal region tumors: a prospective study. *J Neurosurg*. 2000;93(2):245–253.
64. Gangemi M, Maiuri F, Colella G, Buonamassa S. Endoscopic surgery for pineal region tumors. *Minim Invasive Neurosurg*. 2001;44(2):70–73.
65. Pople IK, Athanasiou TC, Sandeman DR, Coakham HB. The role of endoscopic biopsy and third ventriculostomy in the management of pineal region tumours. *Br J Neurosurg*. 2001;15(4):305–311.
66. Yamini B, Refai D, Rubin CM, Frim DM. Initial endoscopic management of pineal region tumors and associated hydrocephalus: clinical series and literature review. *J Neurosurg*. 2004;100(5 suppl Pediatrics):437–441.
67. Chernov MF, Kamikawa S, Yamane F, Ishihara S, Kubo O, Hori T. Neurofiberscopic biopsy of tumors of the pineal region and posterior third ventricle: indications, technique, complications, and results. *Neurosurgery*. 2006;59(2):267–77; discussion 267.
68. Hasegawa T, Kondziolka D, Hadjipanayis CG, Flickinger JC, Lunsford LD. The role of radiosurgery for the treatment of pineal parenchymal tumors. *Neurosurgery*. 2002;51(4):880–889.
69. Kobayashi T, Kida Y, Mori Y. Stereotactic gamma radiosurgery for pineal and related tumors. *J Neurooncol*. 2001;54(3):301–309.
70. Raco A, Raimondi AJ, D'Alonzo A, Esposito V, Valentino V. Radiosurgery in the management of pediatric brain tumors. *Childs Nerv Syst*. 2000;16(5):287–295.
71. Manera L, Régis J, Chinot O, et al. Pineal region tumors: the role of stereotactic radiosurgery. *Stereotact Funct Neurosurg*. 1996;66 suppl 1:164–173.
72. Amendola BE, Wolf A, Coy SR, Amendola MA, Eber D. Pineal tumors: analysis of treatment results in 20 patients. *J Neurosurg*. 2005;102 suppl:175–179.
73. Lekovic GP, Gonzalez LF, Shetter AG, et al. Role of Gamma Knife surgery in the management of pineal region tumors. *Neurosurg Focus*. 2007;23(6):E12.
74. Reyns N, Hayashi M, Chinot O, et al. The role of Gamma Knife radiosurgery in the treatment of pineal parenchymal tumours. *Acta Neurochir (Wien)*. 2006;148(1):5–11; discussion 11.
75. Julow J, Viola A, Major T. Review of radiosurgery of pineal parenchymal tumors. Long survival following 125-iodine brachytherapy of pineoblastomas in 2 cases. *Minim Invasive Neurosurg*. 2006;49(5):276–281.
76. Matsumoto K, Higashi H, Tomita S, Ohmoto T. Pineal region tumours treated with interstitial brachytherapy with low activity sources (192-iridium). *Acta Neurochir (Wien)*. 1995;136(1–2):21–28.
77. Peraud A, Goetz C, Siefert A, Tonn JC, Kreth FW. Interstitial iodine-125 radiosurgery alone or in combination with microsurgery for pediatric patients with eloquently located low-grade glioma: a pilot study. *Childs Nerv Syst*. 2007;23(1):39–46.
78. Stein BM, Bruce JN. Surgical management of pineal region tumors (honored guest lecture). *Clin Neurosurg*. 1992;39:509–532.
79. Campero A, Tróccoli G, Martins C, Fernandez-Miranda JC, Yasuda A, Rhoton AL Jr. Microsurgical approaches to the medial temporal region: an anatomical study. *Neurosurgery*. 2006;59(4 suppl 2):ONS279–307; discussion ONS307.
80. Bruce J, Stein B. Supracerebellar approaches in the pineal region. In: Apuzzo ML, ed. *Brain Surgery: Complication Avoidance and Management*. New York, NY: Churchill-Livingstone; 1993:511–536.
81. Choi JU, Kim DS, Chung SS, Kim TS. Treatment of germ cell tumors in the pineal region. *Childs Nerv Syst*. 1998;14(1–2):41–48.
82. Wolden SL, Wara WM, Larson DA, Prados MD, Edwards MS, Sneed PK. Radiation therapy for primary intracranial germ-cell tumors. *Int J Radiat Oncol Biol Phys*. 1995;32(4):943–949.
83. Calaminus G, Bamberg M, Harms D, et al. AFP/beta-HCG secreting CNS germ cell tumors: long-term outcome with respect to initial symptoms and primary tumor resection. Results of the cooperative trial MAKEI 89. *Neuropediatrics*. 2005;36(2):71–77.
84. Balmaceda C, Heller G, Rosenblum M, et al. Chemotherapy without irradiation–a novel approach for newly diagnosed CNS germ cell tumors: results of an international cooperative trial. The First International Central Nervous System Germ Cell Tumor Study. *J Clin Oncol*. 1996;14(11):2908–2915.
85. Buckner JC, Peethambaram PP, Smithson WA, et al. Phase II trial of primary chemotherapy followed by reduced-dose radiation for CNS germ cell tumors. *J Clin Oncol*. 1999;17(3):933–940.
86. Kochi M, Itoyama Y, Shiraishi S, Kitamura I, Marubayashi T, Ushio Y. Successful treatment of intracranial nongerminomatous malignant germ cell tumors by administering neoadjuvant chemotherapy and radiotherapy before excision of residual tumors. *J Neurosurg*. 2003;99(1):106–114.
87. Nakamura H, Takeshima H, Makino K, Kuratsu J. Evaluation of residual tissues after adjuvant therapy in germ cell tumors. *Pediatr Neurosurg*. 2007;43(2):82–91.
88. Jouvet A, Saint-Pierre G, Fauchon F, et al. Pineal parenchymal tumors: a correlation of histological features with prognosis in 66 cases. *Brain Pathol*. 2000;10(1):49–60.

89. Louis DN, Ohgaki H, Wiestler OD, et al. The 2007 WHO classification of tumours of the central nervous system. *Acta Neuropathol.* 2007;114(2):97–109.
90. Bowers DC, Georgiades C, Aronson LJ, et al. Tectal gliomas: natural history of an indolent lesion in pediatric patients. *Pediatr Neurosurg.* 2000;32(1):24–29.
91. Gómez-Gosálvez FA, Menor F, Morant A, et al. [Tectal tumours in paediatrics. A review of eight patients]. *Rev Neurol.* 2001;33(7):605–611.
92. Grant GA, Avellino AM, Loeser JD, Ellenbogen RG, Berger MS, Roberts TS. Management of intrinsic gliomas of the tectal plate in children. A ten-year review. *Pediatr Neurosurg.* 1999;31(4):170–176.
93. Guillamo JS, Monjour A, Taillandier L, et al. Brainstem gliomas in adults: prognostic factors and classification. *Brain.* 2001;124(pt 12):2528–2539.
94. Stark AM, Fritsch MJ, Claviez A, Dörner L, Mehdorn HM. Management of tectal glioma in childhood. *Pediatr Neurol.* 2005;33(1):33–38.
95. Ternier J, Wray A, Puget S, Bodaert N, Zerah M, Sainte-Rose C. Tectal plate lesions in children. *J Neurosurg.* 2006;104(6 suppl):369–376.
96. Yeh DD, Warnick RE, Ernst RJ. Management strategy for adult patients with dorsal midbrain gliomas. *Neurosurgery.* 2002;50(4):735–738; discussion 738.
97. Blakeley JO, Grossman SA. Management of pineal region tumors. *Curr Treat Options Oncol.* 2006;7(6):505–516.
98. Shikama N, Ogawa K, Tanaka S, et al. Lack of benefit of spinal irradiation in the primary treatment of intracranial germinoma: a multiinstitutional, retrospective review of 180 patients. *Cancer.* 2005;104(1):126–134.
99. Hardenbergh PH, Golden J, Billet A, et al. Intracranial germinoma: the case for lower dose radiation therapy. *Int J Radiat Oncol Biol Phys.* 1997;39(2):419–426.
100. Shibamoto Y, Sasai K, Oya N, Hiraoka M. Intracranial germinoma: radiation therapy with tumor volume-based dose selection. *Radiology.* 2001;218(2):452–456.
101. Smith AA, Weng E, Handler M, Foreman NK. Intracranial germ cell tumors: a single institution experience and review of the literature. *J Neurooncol.* 2004;68(2):153–159.
102. Allen JC, DaRosso RC, Donahue B, Nirenberg A. A phase II trial of preirradiation carboplatin in newly diagnosed germinoma of the central nervous system. *Cancer.* 1994;74(3):940–944.
103. Aoyama H, Shirato H, Ikeda J, Fujieda K, Miyasaka K, Sawamura Y. Induction chemotherapy followed by low-dose involved-field radiotherapy for intracranial germ cell tumors. *J Clin Oncol.* 2002;20(3):857–865.
104. Ushio Y, Kochi M, Kuratsu J, Itoyama Y, Marubayashi T. Preliminary observations for a new treatment in children with primary intracranial yolk sac tumor or embryonal carcinoma. Report of five cases. *J Neurosurg.* 1999;90(1):133–137.
105. Douglas JG, Rockhill JK, Olson JM, Ellenbogen RG, Geyer JR. Cisplatin-based chemotherapy followed by focal, reduced-dose irradiation for pediatric primary central nervous system germinomas. *J Pediatr Hematol Oncol.* 2006;28(1):36–39.
106. Anan M, Ishii K, Nakamura T, et al. Postoperative adjuvant treatment for pineal parenchymal tumour of intermediate differentiation. *J Clin Neurosci.* 2006;13(9):965–968.
107. Pusztaszeri M, Pica A, Janzer R. Pineal parenchymal tumors of intermediate differentiation in adults: case report and literature review. *Neuropathology.* 2006;26(2):153–157.
108. Senft C, Seifert V, Hermann E, Gasser T. Surgical treatment of cerebral abscess with the use of a mobile ultralow-field MRI. *Neurosurg Rev.* 2009;32(1):77–84; discussion 84.
109. Hinkes BG, von Hoff K, Deinlein F, et al. Childhood pineoblastoma: experiences from the prospective multicenter trials HIT-SKK87, HIT-SKK92 and HIT91. *J Neurooncol.* 2007;81(2):217–223.
110. Brown PD. Low-grade gliomas: the debate continues. *Curr Oncol Rep.* 2006;8(1):71–77.
111. Amini A, Schmidt RH, Salzman KL, Chin SS, Couldwell WT. Glioblastoma multiforme of the pineal region. *J Neurooncol.* 2006;79(3):307–314.
112. Reni M, Gatta G, Mazza E, Vecht C. Ependymoma. *Crit Rev Oncol Hematol.* 2007;63(1):81–89.
113. Reis F, Faria AV, Zanardi VA, Menezes JR, Cendes F, Queiroz LS. Neuroimaging in pineal tumors. *J Neuroimaging.* 2006;16(1):52–58.
114. Albert FK, Forsting M, Sartor K, Adams HP, Kunze S. Early postoperative magnetic resonance imaging after resection of malignant glioma: objective evaluation of residual tumor and its influence on regrowth and prognosis. *Neurosurgery.* 1994;34(1):45–60; discussion 60.
115. Kiwit JC, Floeth FW, Bock WJ. Survival in malignant glioma: analysis of prognostic factors with special regard to cytoreductive surgery. *Zentralbl Neurochir.* 1996;57(2):76–88.
116. Zee CS, Segall H, Apuzzo M, et al. MR imaging of pineal region neoplasms. *J Comput Assist Tomogr.* 1991;15(1):56–63.
117. Moon WK, Chang KH, Han MH, Kim IO. Intracranial germinomas: correlation of imaging findings with tumor response to radiation therapy. *AJR Am J Roentgenol.* 1999;172(3):713–716.
118. Fujimaki T, Mishima K, Asai A, et al. Levels of beta-human chorionic gonadotropin in cerebrospinal fluid of patients with malignant germ cell tumor can be used to detect early recurrence and monitor the response to treatment. *Jpn J Clin Oncol.* 2000;30(7):291–294.

58 Intraventricular Tumors

Shakeel A. Chowdhry, Jonathan P. Miller, and Alan R. Cohen

Intraventricular tumors are relatively rare, constituting less than 1% of all intracranial tumors. Certain notable exceptions withstanding, tumors of the ventricular system are often benign, slow-growing lesions. These features, coupled with the long-term compliance of the ventricles, provide opportunity for many intraventricular lesions to reach significant size before their initial presentation [1].

Patient presentation can vary considerably. Any patient with a new headache or significant change in the quality of chronic headache should be considered for possible structural intracranial abnormality including an intraventricular lesion. Additionally, focal neurological symptoms and cognitive or personality changes should prompt consideration for an intracranial neoplasm. Onset of symptoms may be acute, as with the classic drop attacks (sudden onset of severe headache, nausea and emesis, incontinence, imbalance, and loss of postural tone) described for intermittent obstructive hydrocephalus secondary to foramen of Monro obstruction classically by colloid cyst or, and far more likely, chronic as with cerebellar signs and nonspecific signs of elevated intracranial pressure associated with posterior fossa juvenile pilocytic astrocytoma in the pediatric population. Seizures are uncommon at the time of presentation, and may suggest extension of the tumor beyond the confines of the walls of the ventricle. Most intraventricular lesions will lead to the eventual development of hydrocephalus, which may result in headache and possibly (depending on acuity) nausea and emesis, somnolence and lethargy, and cognitive decline or personality change.

Physical exam findings vary considerably based upon the specific tumor type and location. Lesions affecting the lateral ventricles may result in an asymmetric hydrocephalus. Physical findings may include a subcortical hemiparesis with equal involvement of the arm and leg due to infiltration of the centrum semiovale.

Surgical approaches to intraventricular lesions are numerous. All approaches share the common goal of providing maximum access with the least disruption of normal anatomy, with careful attention paid to eloquent cortex and midline structures. The surrounding structures that encase the ventricles coupled with the often large size of the intraventricular lesion present a formidable challenge to even the most experienced surgeon.

The patient's presentation should be used to help select which approach should be undertaken. The patient's preoperative deficits, coupled with the size of the tumor, its location and its blood supply should all be factored into the decision process. For dominant hemisphere lesions, preoperative neuropsychological testing should be performed. Preoperative imaging generally includes magnetic resonance imaging. Stereotactic guidance, functional magnetic resonance imaging, and diffusion tensor imaging may assist in selection of a surgical route. Intraoperative mapping should be considered when appropriate.

SURGICAL APPROACHES TO THE LATERAL VENTRICLES

A thorough grasp of the complex anatomy surrounding the ventricular system is essential to understanding certain manifestations of a given intraventricular lesion as well as deciding upon the most favorable route for surgical resection. The shortest route to the lesion has been demonstrated to be an effective approach for surgical evacuation but is often fraught with critical neurologic structures, resulting in high morbidity. Often the most prudent route involves a slightly longer course aimed at avoiding key anatomical structures, as discussed in the later text.

Background

Less than 1% of all intracranial neoplasms originate within the lateral ventricles. Roughly one-half of all adult and one-quarter of all pediatric intraventricular neoplasms occur in the lateral ventricles. In adults, the atrium is the most common site for tumor formation, followed by the body, the frontal horn, and lastly, the temporal horn. In the pediatric population, the atrium is also the most common location, but it is followed by the frontal horn. The occipital horn and then the temporal horn are next in frequency, followed by panventricular lesions. By lesion type, the most common intraventricular tumor in the pediatric population is the subependymal giant cell astrocytoma, following in succession by choroid plexus papilloma, choroid plexus carcinoma, ependmoma, and astrocytoma.

ANTERIOR INTERHEMISPHERIC TRANSCALLOSAL APPROACH

This approach (Figure 58.1) provides access to lesions in the frontal horn, the anterior aspects of the third ventricle, and the body of the third ventricle.

Key Anatomy

This approach is commonly used to access lesions in the frontal horn, anterior body of the lateral ventricle, and the anterior third ventricle. The approach involves entering through the interhemispheric sulcus, located between the medial surfaces of the frontal, parietal, and occipital lobes. (see Figure 58.2) The interhemispheric sulcus contains the falx, a sickle-shaped dural fold that extends from its anterior attachment to the cribiform plate posteriorly where it fuses with the tentorium along the straight sinus. In the most superior aspect of the falx, the dural sheath separates to form the superior sagittal sinus. The anterior aspect of the falx is separated from the corpus callosum, but this distance disappears as one progresses posteriorly.

The relevant venous anatomy includes an understanding of frontal lobe venous drainage. The anteromedial, centromedial, and posteromedial frontal veins, along with the paracentral veins, drain superiorly into the superior sagittal sinus. These veins often join with the terminal end of veins from the lateral surface (the frontopolar; anterior, middle and posterior frontal; and precentral and central veins) before emptying in the superior sagittal sinus. The anterior pericallosal, paraterminal, and anterior cerebral veins drain into the inferior sagittal sinus or basal veins of Rosenthal [2–4].

Surgical Approach

The coronal suture serves as an important external landmark. Direct inferior extension of the coronal suture in the sagittal plane would often mark the midway point between the genu and splenium of the corpus callosum. A line drawn from the bregman to the external auditory meatus should pass through the foramen of Monro.

After intubation, some surgeons place a lumbar drain to assist in relaxation of the brain. The patient is positioned supine with the head fixed in the Mayfield pin headholder in an elevated and slightly flexed position, with care taken to ensure the internal jugular veins are not compressed. Often, a craniotomy overlying the nondominant hemisphere can provide access to either lateral ventricle.

We prefer a linear coronal scalp incision, although numerous other possibilities exist to obtain satisfactory exposure of the underlying bone. We use a quadrangular bone flap, the medial limb of which is on the midline. The bone flap extends 1 cm posterior to the bregma and 6 cm anterior to it. Multiple burrholes can be placed along the midline to facilitate dissection over the superior sagittal sinus. The bone flap extends 5 cm lateral to the midline.

The dura is tacked to the margins of the craniotomy, except medially, and then opened in a horseshoe fashion with the base toward the superior sagittal sinus. All draining cortical veins encountered should be preserved if possible. When necessary, veins anterior to the coronal suture can be divided without serious sequelae. Overly aggressive

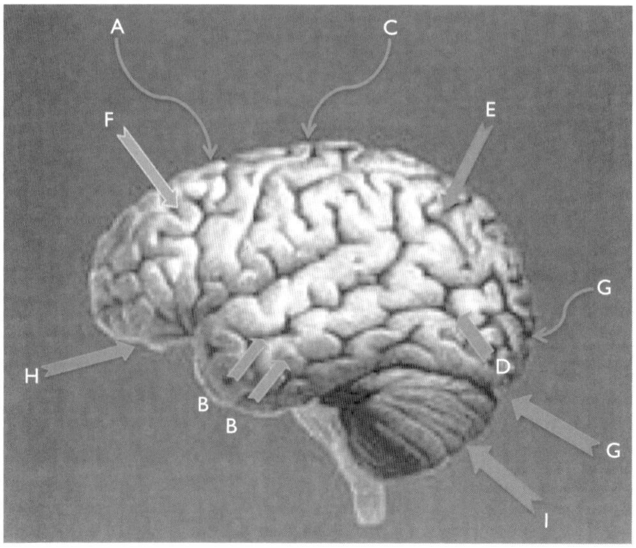

Figure 58.1 Common surgical approaches to the ventricles (A) Anterior interhemispheric transcallosal approach; (B) Middle temporal gyrus / Superior temporal gyrus approach; (C) Posterior interhemispheric transcingular approach; (D) Occipitotemporal sulcus approach; (E) Intraparietal sulcus / Superior parietal lobule approach; (F) Middle frontal gyrus / Superior frontal sulcus approach; (G) Supracerebellar infratentorial / Occipital transtentorial approach; (H) Subfrontal approach; (I) Approaches to the fourth ventricle

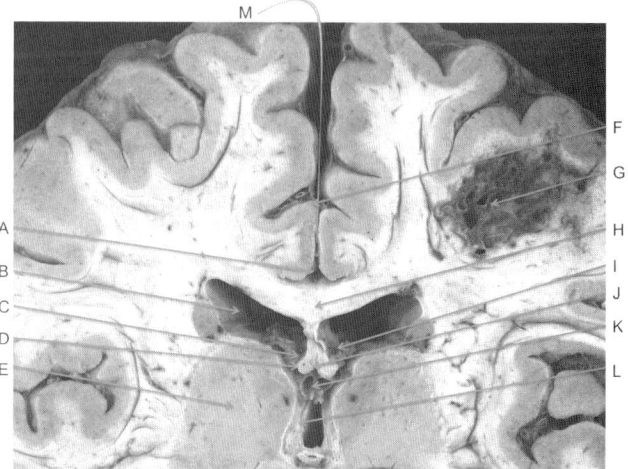

Figure 58.2 Interhemispheric transcallosal approach. Coronal slice of gross specimen from a patient with a left frontal Spetzler-Martin grade II arteriovenous malformation. A – Pericallosal artery. B – Right lateral ventricle. C – Taenia fornicis. This is transected in the traditional transchoroidal approach. D – Taenia thalami. This is divided in the subchoroidal approach. E – Thalamus. F – Callosomarginal artery. G – Arteriovenous malformation. H – Corpus callosum. I – Choroid plexus. J – Fornix. K – Internal cerebral vein. L – Ependyma of the third ventricle. M – Interhemispheric transcallosal route.

medial anchoring of the dura should be avoided to prevent the untoward occlusion of the superior sagittal sinus.

The arachnoid membrane is separated from the falx as the dissection is performed through the interhemispheric fissure. As the inferior aspect of the falx is encountered, the cingulate gyrus should be identified. The falx does not extend to the corpus callosum in this area, and the cingulate sulcus may be misinterpreted as the callosal sulcus.

The corpus callosum is identified by its striking white appearance. After the callosal sulcus is identified and callosal cistern is entered, the pericallosal arteries should be readily visible. They should be carefully separated. A 2 cm stretch of the anterior portion of the corpus callosum between the arteries is then coagulated with bipolar cautery before entry. Extension of the callosotomy posteriorly increases the risk for disconnection morbidity [5–12].

After the lateral ventricle has been entered, a septum pellucidotomy may be performed as necessary to allow cerebrospinal fluid drainage from the contralateral ventricle, thereby providing further brain relaxation. Orientation within the ventricle upon entry is most easily confirmed with identification of the choroid plexus and its relationship to the foramen of Monro, septal vein, and thalamostriate vein. This relationship is of particular importance when confronted with large intraventricular lesions or obstructive lesions that may distort the normal anatomy.

MIDDLE TEMPORAL GYRUS/SUPERIOR TEMPORAL SULCUS

This particular approach (Figure 58.1) provides access to lesions with the basal cisterns, the anterior temporal horn, the trigone, and the anterior third ventricle near the lamina terminalis.

Key Anatomy

The sylvian fissure is an infolding of eloquent cortex spanning between the basal frontal/parietal and superior temporal lobes. The superficial sylvian fissure consists of a stem and three rami. The stem extends medially from the semilunar gyrus of the uncus to the lateral end of the sphenoid ridge, then divides into the anterior horizontal, anterior ascending, and posterior rami on the lateral surface of the brain. The deep aspect of the sylvian fissure consists of an anterior, or sphenoidal, compartment and a posterior, or operculoinsular, compartment. The insula, or island of Reil, is the medial wall of the sylvian fissure. Radiographically, it is the covering of the mass of deep structures consisting the basal ganglia, thalamus, claustrum, and extreme, external and internal capsules. It is separated from the opercula by the circular sulcus of the insula. The insula, via the limen insulae, connects the temporal lobe to the posterior orbital gyrus. The limen insulae is the uncinate fasciculus with a thin covering of gray matter. As an anatomic landmark, it separates the sylvian fissure laterally from the carotid cistern medially [13].

As one extends inferiorly along the surface of the brain, the superior, middle, and inferior temporal gyri are encountered and are separated, respectively, by the superior and inferior temporal sulci.

An understanding of the course of the middle cerebral artery is essential for this approach. The middle cerebral artery extends from the bifurcation through the carotid cistern to pass through toward the temporal lobe, through the insular component of the sylvian fissure and then out over the lateral surface of the cerebrum [14]. The insular veins course along the surface of the insula and unite at the limen insulae to form the deep middle cerebral vein, which coalesces with the cerebral, olfactory, fronto-orbital, and inferior striate veins to constitute the first segment of the basal vein of Rosenthal, ultimately draining via the great vein of Galen and straight sinus into the torcular herophili [13].

Surgical Approach

Patient is placed in the supine position, and the head is fixed in the Mayfield head holder. The head is elevated, slightly extended, rotated, and tilted to bring the sylvian fissure parallel to the floor. Multiple skin incisions have been described. The temporalis fascia and muscle are reflected anteriorly. Muscle may be dissected with bipolar cautery; the authors prefer inferior to superior dissection with a periosteal elevator as separation of the muscle attachment in line with the muscle fibers to minimize bleeding. The temporalis muscle and fascia may be reflected with the galea or separately dissected and subsequently reflected. In the latter approach, care should be taken to protect the frontalis branch of the facial nerve.

A pterional craniotomy is performed in standard fashion. Adequate exposure of the temporal lobe is essential, often necessitating extension of the temporal portion of the craniotomy inferiorly under it is flush with the middle cranial fossa floor. Particularly large lesions or posteriorly located lesions may be better visualized with removal of the lateral orbital ridge. The dura is then opened with the base of the flap located superomedially.

The middle temporal gyrus approach requires a corticotomy to be made in the middle temporal gyrus. The white matter is then dissected posteriorly in parallel with the floor until the temporal horn of the lateral ventricle is reached. Others prefer dissection of the superior temporal sulcus. A corticotomy is made at the depth of the sulcus and then the white matter tracts are dissected until the ependyma of the lateral ventricle is reached. Finally, a **transsylvian approach** has also been described that involves dissection of the sylvian fissure in standard fashion with bipolar tips, blunt hooks, and an arachnoid knife. The basal cisterns are entered, and the inferior circular sulcus of the insula and the limen insulae are identified. The temporal horn can be reached by proceeding with dissection along the inferior circular sulcus, generally 1 cm posterior to the limen insulae.

POSTERIOR INTERHEMISPHERIC TRANSCINGULAR APPROACH

This approach (Figure 58.1) provides access to the atrium and occipital horn.

Key Anatomy

As one proceeds along the falx posteriorly, it comes in close contact with the corpus callosum. The posterior interhemispheric fissure is limited inferiorly by the tentorium cerebelli, medially by the falx cerebri, and laterally by the precuneus, cuneus, and lingual gyri. The medial portion of the parietal lobe comprises the precuneus along with the paracentral lobule posterior to the central sulcus. The cuneus is bounded by the parieto-occipital and calcarine sulci. The medial occipital lobe is formed by the cuneus and the medial lingual gyrus.

The calcarine sulcus is divided into posterior and anterior portions by the parieto-occipital sulcus. The anterior calcrine sulcus intercepts the isthmus of the cingulate gyrus. The anterior calcarine sulcus is crossed by the anterior cuneolinear gyrus, and it bulges into the medial wall of the atrium as the calcar avis. The carlacarin sulcus contains key branches of the posterior cerebral artery. The posterior calcarine sulcus is straddled by primary visual cortex on its upper and lower lips, while the anterior calcarine sulcus has primary visual cortex fibers running only on its inferior lip [15].

Of particular concern with this approach is injury to the optic radiations. The medial and superior walls of the atrium are free from optic radiation fibers. However, in the occipital horn, the medial wall alone is devoid of optic radiations.

Surgical Approach

The patient is positioned in a semiseated position with the head elevated, flexed, and secured in a Mayfield head holder. Others have described a three-quarters prone position. A horseshoe incision is followed by a craniotomy that exposes the superior sagittal sinus medially, allowing for gentle retraction of the falx and sinus as described earlier in the anterior interhemispheric approach. In general, exposure of the torcular herophili and transverse sinus is not necessary. The dura is opened in a horseshoe fashion and reflected medially toward the sinus. Sutures or retractors are placed as previously described.

During the interhemispheric approach, bridging veins are dissected and preserved if possible. If the vessels cannot be salvaged, they are coagulated with bipolar cautery and divided. The arachnoid membrane is separated from the falx, and the interhemispheric fissure is dissected following the falx and the parieto-occipital sulcus. The splenium and the calcarine sulcus are identified. Direct retraction over the calcarine sulcus is discouraged. Gentle retraction over the cuneus may be performed to create additional working space. Further room may be obtained by dissection of the parieto-occipital sulcus with separation of the precuneus from the cuneus. Visualization of the posterior cerebral artery (P3 segment) exiting the quadrigeminal cistern is often possible. The calcarine sulcus can be followed to the isthmus of the cingulate gyrus, where a corticotomy is performed, posterior and lateral to the splenium. Anterior and lateral dissection ultimately leads the surgeon into the atrium.

OCCIPITOTEMPORAL SULCUS APPROACH

This approach (Figure 58.1) provides access to lesions in the posterior temporal horn through the basal surface (thereby avoiding the theoretical risk of injury to optic radiations inherent in a superior or lateral approach).

Pertinent Anatomy

From lateral to medial, the basal surface of the temporal lobe consists of the inferior temporal gyrus, the occipitotemporal sulcus, the fusiform gyrus, the collateral (or fusiform sulcus), and the parahippocampal gyrus. The basal parietotemporal line delineates the basal surface of the temporal lobe from the occipital lobe. It extends from the preoccipital notch to the junction of the parieto-occipital and calcarine fissures. The occipitotemporal sulcus is located medial to the inferior temporal gyrus and points toward the collateral eminence; it is often fused anterior and posteriorly with the collateral sulcus [16].

Surgical Approach

Patient is positioned in a lateral decubitus position so that the zygoma is the most elevated portion of the head. Care is taken to ensure that venous outflow is not obstructed. A reverse question mark incision is made; some may prefer a horseshoe incision. A quadrilateral craniotomy extending to the floor of the middle cranial fossa is performed. The dura is opened in a horseshoe fashion and flapped laterally toward the skull base.

The inferior temporal gyrus is identified and followed. Gentle retraction may be necessary. The occipitotemporal sulcus (which points toward the collateral eminence) is identified and dissected, following its orientation until the temporal horn is entered.

INTRAPARIETAL SULCUS / SUPERIOR PARIETAL LOBULE APPROACH

This approach (Figure 58.1) provides access to lesions in the atrium.

Pertinent Anatomy

The intraparietal sulcus is located within the parietal lobe. It begins at the postcentral sulcus and travels posteriorly and inferiorly toward the occipital lobes, dividing the superior parietal lobule from the inferior parietal lobule (ie, the supramarginal and angular gyri). The sulcus approaches the roof of the atrium and the occipital horn. The intraparietal sulcus is continuous much less frequently on the right than on the left [16].

Surgical Approach

Patient is positioned supine in the slouched position with the head elevated, angled 30°, and secured in a Mayfield head holder. Alternatively, the patient may be placed in the prone position with the head facing the floor. A horseshoe incision is made, followed by a paramedian quadrangular craniotomy. Exposure of the superior sagittal sinus is not necessary, but it may be useful for orientation. The dura is opened and reflected medially. The intraparietal sulcus is oriented parallel to the midline and is easily identified. The sulcus is dissected beyond its base until the atrium is reached. Alternatively, the superior parietal lobule is identified and a corticotomy is made, utilizing routine dissection technique until the atrium is entered.

MIDDLE FRONAL GYRUS / SUPERIOR FRONTAL SULCUS APPROACH

This approach (Figure 58.1) provides access to the frontal horn of the lateral ventricle and the foramen of Monro.

Pertinent Anatomy

The frontal lobe consists of the superior frontal, middle frontal, and inferior frontal gyri as one travels laterally from the midline. These gyri are aligned in the anterior-posterior plane. The superior frontal sulcus is continuous in 36% of cases and separates the superior and middle frontal gyri [16]; the inferior frontal sulcus separates the middle frontal gyrus from the inferior frontal gyrus. As one travels posteriorly along the gyri, the supplemental motor area is transversed followed by the motor cortex. Injury to the supplemental motor area may result in the supplemental motor area syndrome, which is often self-limited.

Surgical Approach

Patient is positioned supine with the head slightly flexed. A horseshoe incision (or alternatively a coronal incision) is made, followed by a quadrangular craniotomy, with the flap extending no further than 2 cm behind the coronal suture. Exposure of the superior sagittal sinus is not necessary. The dura is opened in a horseshoe fashion or a stellate fashion depending upon preference. The middle frontal gyrus is identified and a vertical corticotomy is made. Alternately, the superior frontal sulcus can be dissected with the corticotomy made at the inferior base of the sulcus. The white matter tracts are dissected and coagulated until the ependymal lining of the frontal horn of the lateral ventricle is reached. The ventricle is entered and self-retaining retractors are placed.

SURGICAL APPROACHES TO THE THIRD VENTRICLE

Background

The vast majority of tumors affecting the third ventricle are astrocytomas that either form in the walls or floor of the third ventricle or originate in adjacent structures and affect the third ventricle by direct extension [5]. Most are low-grade lesions. Presenting symptoms are generally due to increased intracranial pressure secondary to hydrocephalus. Endocrinological disturbances and visual symptoms are typically uncommon with tumors arising within the third ventricle. When visual symptoms are present, they are generally due to extraventricular involvement or optic pathway compression resulting from ventricular distortion. Mass effect on the hypothalamus or hypothalamic involvement may result in the diencephalic syndrome (emaciation combined with hyperalertness, classically seen in infants) [17]. Posterior third ventricle lesions can cause mass effect on the tectum leading to Parinaud's syndrome or may obstruct cerebrospinal fluid flow.

Various tumors can occur in the third ventricle. In children, those with predilection for the anterior portion of the third ventricle include hypothalamic astrocytoma and suprasellar craniopharyngioma. Choroid plexus papilloma, germinoma, teratoma, and ependymoma are occasionally seen. The most common lesion seen in the anterior third ventricle in adults is the colloid cyst.

TRANSFORAMINAL, TRANSCHOROIDAL, AND INTERFORNICEAL APPROACHES

This approach provides access to the anterior two-thirds of the third ventricle.

Pertinent Anatomy

The foramen of Monro connects the lateral ventricles to the third ventricle. It is draped by the fornices and limited posteriorly by the thalamus. The genu of the internal capsule passes just lateral to the foramen. (see Figure 58.3)

The choroid plexus is a villous structure consisting of a stroma of leptomeningeal cells, blood vessels, and connective tissue that is lined by an ependyma-derived epithelium. It is located on the medial floor of the body of the lateral ventricle. It is attached medially to the body of the fornix and laterally to the thalamus by ependymal that covers the ventricular wall and the choroid plexus. The taenia fornix refers to the ependymal attachment between the choroid plexus and the fornix. The taenia choroidea refers to the attachment between the thalamus and choroid plexus.

The choroidal fissure extends between the body of the fornix and the thalamus, is lined by the two membranes of the tela choroidea, and is covered by the choroid plexus of the lateral ventricle.

Vasculature considerations involving the third ventricle include an appreciation for draining veins. The medial group drains primarily through the posterior septal veins. The lateral group drains mainly via the thalamostriate, the anterior and posterior caudate veins, and the superior thalamic veins. The anterior septal vein travels from the septum pellucidum posteriorly and medially to join the thalamostriate vein and superior choroidal veins in the velum interpositum, forming the internal cerebral veins. The thalamostriate vein runs in the striothalamic sulcus between the body of the caudate and the thalamus. It enters the choroidal

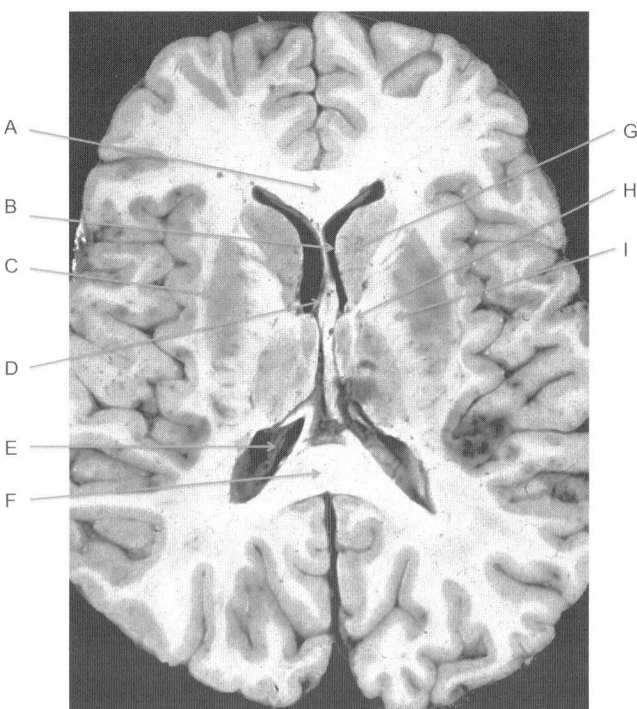

Figure 58.3 Axial slice of a gross specimen from a patient with thrombotic thrombocytopenic purpura. The close proximity of the genu of the internal capsule to the foramen of Monro can be easily appreciated. A – Anterior commissure. B – Left lateral ventricle. C – External capsule. D – Posterior septum pellucidum. E – Atrium of left lateral ventricle. F – Posterior commissure. G – Head of the left caudate nucleus. H – Genu of the left internal capsule as it nears the foramen of Monro. I – Left internal capsule.

fissure at or behind the foramen on Monro and pierces the inferior membrane of the tela choroidea to enter the velum interpositum and join the internal cerebral vein. The thalamostriate vein is covered by ependyma until it nears the choroid plexus; at this point, the tenia choroidea separates from the surface of the thalamus to cover the choroid plexus [4,18].

Surgical Approach

Transforaminal Approach

The initial aspects of this approach including entry into the lateral ventricle are covered in detail in the anterior transcallosal interhemispheric section. After entering the lateral ventricle, the foramen of Monro may be seen along with the choroid plexus and venous vasculature. Occasionally, the contralateral lateral ventricle may be entered inadvertently, and the choroid plexus, along with the thalamostriate and septal veins, are used to confirm orientation. The foramen of Monro is visualized rostral to the choroid plexus, and this channel may be used to resect tumors of the anterior third ventricle. The surgical corridor is limited by the size of the foramen of Monro, and care must be taken to limit retraction on the fornices and the thalamus. If further exposure is necessary, then the choroidal fissure may be opened as described in the following text. Additionally, in cases where the junction between the anterior septal and internal cerebral veins is posterior, the foramen of Monro may be safely enlarged in the posterior direction [19].

Additionally, the transforminal approach may be performed endoscopically. A right frontal burrhole craniotomy is performed with stereotactic navigation to ensure the proper entry angle to maximize tumor exposure. A small right frontal corticotomy is made and the endoscope is passed into the ipsilateral frontal ventricle [20–23].

Transchoroidal Approach

The thalamus, fornix, and the choroidal fissure are important anatomical structures to be identified in this approach. The taenia fornicis is opened, as described by Rhoton, to allow entry into the choroidal fissure. Others have utilized the taenia thalami to gain entry to the choroidal fissure (otherwise known as the **subchoroidal route**) [24], although this route carries a theoretical increased risk of injury to the thalamus. The superior membrane of the tela choroidea and the contents of the velum interpositum (ie, branches of the medial posterior choroidal artery and the internal cerebral vein) are readily visible. The superior membrane of the tela choroidea is then carefully opened, and dissection is performed between the two internal cerebral veins to prevent inadvertent injury to branches entering laterally (including the thalamostriate vein). The inferior membrane of the tela choroidea is identified and opened, allowing visualization of the massa intermedia and the space and floor of the third ventricle.

Dissection of the roof of the third ventricle may continue posteriorly in the choroidal fissure from the foramen of Monro until just above the pineal gland. If additional working space is needed, the foramen of Monro can be carefully expanded, but often requires sacrifice of the anterior septal vein and carries the earlier mentioned increased risk of morbidity from forniceal retraction [25–27].

Interforniceal Approach

This approach, popularized by Apuzzo, may also be utilized when the transforminal approach provides an insufficient operative corridor. This approach lends itself to large lesions that may cause bowing and partial separation of the fornices. It also may be used in patients with cavum septi pellucidi. As it involves potential manipulation of both fornices, it carries an increased risk of morbidity [12,18,28,29].

The anterior body of the lateral ventricle is entered as previously described in the transforminal approach. Orientation is confirmed with localization of the choroid plexus and the thalamostriate and septal veins. The septum pellucidum is identified, allowing for identification of midline between the two fornices (ie, the point of attachment of the septum to the fornices). The fornix is then carefully split. The superior membrane of the tela choroidea is opened allowing visualization of the vessels within the velum interpositum. Dissection is carried out between the internal cerebral veins posteriorly into the choroidal fissure as previously described. The inferior membrane of the tela choroidea is split to enter the cavity of the third ventricle [30–32].

SUPRACEREBELLAR INFRATENTORIAL APPROACH, OCCIPITAL TRANSTENTORIAL APPROACH

This approach (Figure 58.1), more often utilized to access the pineal region, can also provide access to the posterior portion of the third ventricle and is beyond the scope of this chapter.

SUBFRONTAL APPROACH

This approach (Figure 58.1), popularized by Suzuki, provides an alternate route to the anterior third ventricle [33,34].

SURGICAL APPROACHES TO THE FOURTH VENTRICLE

Background

Preoperative steroids may decrease vasogenic edema as well as alleviate headache and neck pain. Additionally, steroids may decrease the incidence and severity of aspectic meningitis and the posterior fossa syndrome, as well as decrease nausea and emesis allowing for improved hydration and nutrition before surgery [35–37].

Automatic retractor systems are useful. Intraoperative monitoring may be prudent when manipulation of the floor of the fourth ventricle, particularly in the region of the median eminence, is anticipated. The most sensitive measure of alteration of brainstem function is the pulse and blood pressure (cardiovascular reflexes are mediated by structures near the fourth ventricle, for example, the nucleus tractus solitarius and the dorsal motor nucleus of the vagus). Any alterations in vitals signs while working near the floor of the fourth ventricle should be considered a serious warning sign. Direct monitoring of brainstem function can be performed with brainstem auditory evoked responses. An auditory click is measured at earlobe and vertex electrodes. The click produces five waves that correspond, respectively, to the proximal cochlear nerve, the distal cochlear nerve, cochlear nucleus, superior olive, and lateral lemniscus/inferior colliculus. Demonstration of pontomesencephalic transmission of the impulse indirectly implies that brainstem function is intact. It is important to remember that this pathway is mostly lateral and may remain functional in spite of profound injury to the central core of the brainstem. Somatosensory evoked potentials follow sensory signals through the medial lemniscus, which is some distance from the fourth ventricle and as such considered to be less sensitive in detecting injury when operating in this area of the cranial vault. Lastly, electromyography with direct stimulation of the facial nerve or lateral rectus muscle may verify the integrity of the sixth and seventh cranial motor nerves in instances where tumor abuts or encases them.

Pertinent Anatomy

The superior cerebellar arteries exit the brainstem between cranial nerves IV and V (trochlear and trigeminal) to enter the cerebellomesencephalic fissure. After several sharp hairpin turns, the superior cerebellar arteries give rise to the precerebellar arteries which pass along the superior cerebellar peduncle to reach the superior fourth ventricle and dentate nucleus. Upon leaving the fissure, the arteries supply end branches to the surface of the tentorium cerebelli. Each anterior inferior cerebellar artery passes posteriorly around the pons before releasing branches to the nerves of the acoustic meatus and choroid plexus protruding from the foramen of Luschka. The anterior inferior cerebellar arteries supply the petrosal surface of the cerebellum. The posterior inferior cerebellar arteries (PICAs) are branches of the vertebral arteries. They course around the medulla to reach the cerebellar tonsils and lower half of the floor of the fourth ventricle. The PICAs then loop superiorly (caudal loop) at the caudal pole of the tonsil to ascend into the cerebellomedullary fissure. They course as far as the upper pole of the tonsil and then loop again inferiorly (cranial loop) over the inferior medullar velum. Branches of the PICA radiate from the borders of the tonsils to supply the suboccipital surface of the cerebellum.

Venous drainage from the superior fourth ventricle occurs primarily through the vein of Galen. The vein of the cerebellomesencephalic fissure (also known as the precentral cerebellar vein) is formed by the union of the paired veins of the superior cerebellar peduncle. The precentral cerebellar vein ascends through the quadrigeminal cistern to drain either directly into the vein of Galen or indirectly via the superior vermian vein. Venous drainage from the cerebellopontine fissure and lateral recess passes primarily into the superior petrosal sinus. The vein of the cerebellopontine fissure courses near the superior limb of the cerebellopontine fissure to drain ino the superior petrosal sinus rostral to the facial and glossopharnygeal nerves.

Inferior fourth ventricle drainage occurs mainly anteriorly through the superior petrosal sinus via the vein of the cerebellopontine fissure, although some drainage passes posteriorly into the tentorial sinuses en route to the torcular Herophili. The vein of the cerebellomedullary fissure originates on the lateral edge of the nodule and uvula and courses laterally near the telovelar junction to reach the cerebellopontine angle.

Surgical Approach

The safest and most direct approach to the fourth ventricle is via the midline suboccipital route. The operative corridor is somewhat superior directed and follows a trajectory parallel to the tentorium cerebelli. The patient may be positioned prone, sitting, or in the lateral oblique or "park bench" position. The patient should be properly padded and electrophysiological monitoring leads are placed. The head should be fixed in a Mayfield or Sugita head holder and registration performed in stereotactic navigation is being used. In situations where concern for postoperative obstructive hydrocephalus exists, a burrhole may be placed at the start of the procedure for ventriculostomy.

A midline incision extending from 1 cm above the external occipital protuberance to the midcervical region is made following routine shaving, sterile preparation, draping, and infiltration with local anesthetic. If the tumor extends laterally, a hockeystick incision allows for a wider craniotomy. We prefer to use sharp dissection in the midline plane following the avacular nuchal line. The fascia may be opened in a Y-shaped fashion with the lateral ends of the Y below the ligamentous insertion to allow for tight reapproximation. However, in cases of low set lesions where exposure up to the external occipital protuberance is not necessary, we prefer to remain in the avascular plane between the splenius capitus and the semispinalis capitis muscles. Exposure is generally performed down to C2. We prefer to place several burrholes and perform a suboccipital craniotomy extending to the foramen magnum inferiorly. When performing a craniotomy, care must be taken near the midline bone as it is often vascular and its keel may be fairly deep. C1 laminectomy is performed as needed.

At this point, retractors are placed and the microscope is engaged. Additional maneuvers are performed as necessary depending on the tension beneath the dura. The dura is generally opened in a Y-fashion, and care should be taken while crossing the inconstant occipital and annular sinuses, particularly in children. Bleeding from these sinuses, which may be profuse in children, is controlled with surgical clips. The arachnoid is then opened over the cisterna magna to allow for drainage of cerebrospinal fluid.

Techniques for intradural exposure and resection of the tumor vary depending upon the location and size of the tumor. Gentle separation of the cerebellar tonsils exposes the cerebellomedullary fissure through the vallecula providing a clear view of the inferior roof of the fourth ventricle. Extension superiorly is performed on the telovelar plane. Narrow malleable automatic retractors are useful to maintain the exposure. The caudal loops of the PICA may be appreciated inferiorly as they pass over the tonsils and the walls of the cerebellomedullary fissure. Exposure for lateral lesions may require removal of one tonsil, which may be performed by dividing the pedicle attaching the superolateral margin of the tonsil to the biventral lobule. Access to the lateral roof or recess can be aided by partial resection of the cerebellar hemisphere, although care should be taken not to violate the dentate nuclei. Cattonoid patties are carefully placed beneath the tumor to protect the floor of the fourth ventricle for tumors that are not adherent to the floor (Figure 58.1).

REFERENCES

1. Gokalp HZ, Yuceer N, Arasil E, et al. Tumours of the lateral ventricle. A retrospective review of 112 cases operated upon 1970–1997. *Neurosurg Rev.* 1988;21:126–137.
2. Nagata S, Rhoton AL Jr, Barry M. Microsurgical anatomy of the choroidal fissure. *Surg Neurol.* 1988;30:3–59.
3. Rhoton AL Jr. The lateral and third ventricle. *Neurosurgery.* 2002;51(suppl):207–271.
4. Villani RM, Tomei G. Transcallosal approach to tumors of the third ventricle. pp. 772–785.
5. Apuzzo MLJ, Zee CS, Breeze RE, Day JD. Anterior and mid-third ventricular lesions: a surgical overview. In Apuzzo MLJ, ed. *Surgery of the Third Ventricle*, 2nd ed. Baltimore: Williams and Wilkins; 1998:635–680.
6. Ehni G, Ehni B. Considerations in transforminal entry. In Apuzzo MLJ, ed. *Surgery of the Third Ventricle.* 2nd ed. Baltimore: Williams and Wilkins; 1998:391–419.
7. Garretson HD. Memory in man: a neurosurgeon's perspective. In Apuzzo MLJ, ed. *Surgery of the Third Ventricle.* 2nd ed. Baltimore: Williams and Wilkins; 1998:187–204.
8. Bogen JE. Physiological consequences of complete or partial commissural section. In Apuzzo MLJ, ed. *Surgery of the Third Ventricle.* 2nd ed. Baltimore: Williams and Wilkins; 1998:167–186.
9. Habib M. Syndromes de deconnexion calleuse et organization fonctionelle du corps calleux chez l'adulte. *Neurochirurgie.* 1998;44(suppl 1):102–109.
10. Nakasu Y, Isozumi T, Nioka H, Handa J. Mechanism of mutism following the transcallosal approach to the ventricles. *Acta Neurochir (Wien).* 1991;110:146–153.
11. Sauerwein HC, Lassonde M. Neuropsychological alterations after split-brain surgery. *J Neurosurg Sci.* 1997;41:59–66.
12. Villani R, Papagno C, Tomei G, Grimoldi N, Spagnoli D, Bello L. Transcallosal approach to tumors of the third ventricle. Surgical results and neuropsychological evaluation. *J Neurosurg Sci.* 1997;41:41–50.
13. Wolf BS, Huang YP. The insula and deep middle cerebral venous drainage system: normal anatomy and angiography. *Am J Roentgenol Radium Ther Nucl Med.* 1963;90:472–489.
14. Gibo H, Carver CC, Rhoton AL Jr, Lenkey C, Mitchell RJ. Microsurgical anatomy of the middle cerebral artery. *J Neurosurg.* 1981;54:151–169.
15. Margolis MT, Newton TP, Hoyt WF. The posterior cerebral artery, II: Gross and roentgenographic anatomy. In Newton TH, DG Potts, eds. *Radiology of the Skull and Brain.* Vol. 2. St. Louis: Mosby; 1974:1551–1576.
16. Ono M, Kubic S, Abernathey CD. *Atlas of the Cerebral Sulci.* Stuttgart: Georg Thieme Verlag; 1990.
17. Page RB. Functional anatomy of the human hypothalamus. In Apuzzo MLJ, ed. *Surgery of the Third Ventricle.* 2nd ed. Baltimore: Williams and Wilkins; 2002:233–251.
18. Apuzzo ML, Chikovani OK, Gott PS, et al. Transcallosal, interforncial approaches for lesions affecting the third ventricle: surgical considerations and consequences. *Neurosurgery.* 1982;10:547–554.
19. Ture U, Yasargil MG, Al-Mefty O. The transcallosal-transforaminal approach to the third ventricle with regard to the venous variations in this region. *J Neurosurg.* 1997;87:706–715.
20. Abdou MS, Cohen AR. Endoscopic treatment of colloid cysts of the third ventricle. Technical note and review of the literature. *J Neurosurg.* 1998;89:1062–1068.
21. Hellwig D, Bauer BL, Schulte M, Gatscher S, Riegel T, Bertalanffy H. Neuroendoscopic treatment for colloid cysts of the third ventricle: the experience of a decade. *Neurosurgery.* 2003;52:525–533; discussion 532–523.
22. Schroeder HW, Gaab MR. Endoscopic resection of colloid cysts. *Neurosurgery.* 2002;51:1441–1444; discussion 1444–1445.
23. Sgaramella E, Sotgiu S, Crotti FM. Neuroendoscopy: one year of experience—personal results, observations and limits. *Minim Invasive Neurosurg.* 2003;46:215–219.
24. Rhoton A. Microsurgical anatomy of the third ventricular region. In Apuzzo MLJ, ed. *Surgery of the Third Ventricle.* 2nd ed. Baltimore: Williams & Wilkins; 1998:89–158.
25. Lozier AP, Bruce JN. Surgical approaches to posterior third ventricular tumors. *Neurosurg Clin N Am.* 2003;14:527–545.
26. Rhoton AL Jr, Yamamoto I, Peace DA. Microsurgery of the third ventricle: part 2. Operative approaches. *Neurosurgery.* 1981;8:357–373.
27. Wen HT, Rhoton AL Jr, de Oliveira E. Transchoroidal approach to the third ventricle: an anatomic study of the choroidal fissure and its clinical application. *Neurosurgery.* 1998;42:1205–1217; discussion 1217–1209.
28. Gaffan D. Recognition impaired and association intact in the memory of monkeys after transection of the fornix. *J Comp Physiol Psychol.* 1974;86:1100–1109.
29. Gaffan D, Gaffan EA. Amnesia in man following transection of the fornix. A review. *Brain.* 1991;114(pt 6):2611–2618.

30. Apuzzo MLJ, Amar AP. Transcallosal interforniceal approach. In Apuzzo MLJ, ed. *Surgery of the Third Ventricle*. 2nd ed. Baltimore: Williams and Wilkins; 1998:421–452.
31. Winkler PA, Weis S, Buttner A, Raabe A, Amiridze N, Reulen HJ. The transcallosal interforniceal approach to the third ventricle: anatomic and microsurgical aspects. *Neurosurgery*. 1997;40:973–981; discussion 981–972.
32. Winkler PA, Weis S, Wenger E, Herzog C, Dahl A, Reulen HJ. Transcallosal approach to the third ventricle: normative morphometric data based on magnetic resonance imaging scans, with special reference to the fornix and forniceal insertion. *Neurosurgery*. 1999;45:309–317; discussion 317–309.
33. Suzuki J. The bifrontal anterior interhemispheric approach. In Apuzzo MLJ, ed. *Surgery of the Third Ventricle*. 2nd ed. Baltimore: Williams and Wilkins; 1998:489–515.
34. Suzuki J, Katakura R, Mori T. Interhemispheric approach through the lamina terminalis to tumors of the anterior part of the third ventricle. *Surg Neurol*. 1984;22:157–163.
35. Pollack IF, Polinko P, Albright AL, Towbin R, Fitz C. Mutism and pseudobulbar symptoms after resection of posterior fossa tumors in children: incidence and pathophysiology. *Neurosurgery*. 1995;37:885–893.
36. Van Calenbergh F, Van de Laar A, Plets C, Goffin J, Casaer P. Transient cerebellar mutism after posterior fossa surgery in children. *Neurosurgery*. 1995;37:894–898.
37. Wisoff JH, Epstein FJ. Pseudobulbar palsy after posterior fossa operation in children. *Neurosurgery*. 1984;15:707–709.

List of Color Plates

Figure 14.2	The microenvironment of infiltrating astrocytomas	i3
Figure 14.3	Pathologic features that define the microenvironment of glioblastoma	i3
Figure 14.4	Heterogeneity of pseudopalisades and adjacent brain tumor	i4
Figure 14.5	Intratumoral heterogeneity in a human glioblastoma	i4
Figure 16.2	Distinct stages of glioma neovascularization in a murine model	i5
Figure 16.4	Mobilization and recruitment of bone marrow-derived proangiogenic cells	i5
Figure 16.3	Tumor hypoxia selectively suppresses cellular energy metabolism	i6
Figure 16.6	Molecular signaling pathways targeted by antiangiogenic drugs	i7
Figure 17.6	Intracranial xenograft tumor	i8
Figure 18.1	An incidental middle fossa meningioma found at autopsy	i8
Figure 18.2	A histologically benign olfactory groove meningioma	i8
Figure 18.3	Arachnoid cap cells	i8
Figure 18.4	WHO grade I histological subtypes include meningothelial meningiomas	i9
Figure 18.5	Chordoid and clear cell meningiomas	i9
Figure 18.6	In the absence of chordoid or clear cell morphologies	i10
Figure 18.7	Tumors demonstrating varying characteristics	i10
Figure 18.8	The perivascular growth pattern of papillary meningiomas	i11
Figure 18.9	Epithelial membrane antigen immunohistochemistry	i11
Figure 18.10	Meningiomas that are WHO grade I by standard morphological criteria	i12
Figure 18.11	Fluorescent in situ hybridization	i12
Figure 19.1	Retroperitoneal schwannoma	i13
Figure 19.2	Cutaneous schwannoma	i13
Figure 19.3	Schwannoma, gross appearance	i13
Figure 19.4	Schwannoma, histology	i13
Figure 19.5	Schwannoma, histology	i14
Figure 19.6	Plexiform schwannoma, histology	i14
Figure 19.7	Cellular schwannoma, histology	i14
Figure 21.1	Neurofibromas	i15
Figure 21.2	Malignant peripheral nerve sheath tumor	i16
Figure 23.1	Pilocytic astrocytoma	i19
Figure 23.2	Pilomyxoid astrocytoma	i20
Figure 23.3	Angiocentric glioma	i20
Figure 23.4	Diffuse astrocytoma	i21
Figure 23.5	Gross glioblastoma	i21
Figure 23.6	PXA showing pleomorphic fibrillary astrocytes	i21
Figure 23.7	Macroscopic appearance of a cerebellar medulloblastoma	i22
Figure 23.8	Supratentorial primitive neuroectodermal tumor	i23
Figure 23.9	A large destructive, hemorrhagic and necrotic mass	i24
Figure 23.10	Ependymoma	i24
Figure 23.11	Gross appearance of an anaplastic ependymoma	i24
Figure 23.12	Choroid-plexus papilloma	i25
Figure 23.13	Choroid plexus carcinoma	i25
Figure 23.14	Ganglioglioma	i25
Figure 23.15	Desmoplastic infantile ganglioglioma/astroctyoma	i26
Figure 23.16	DNET showing the typical glioneuronal component	i26
Figure 23.17	Craniopharyngioma showing palisaded epithelial cells	i27

Figure 24.3	The activated RAS pathway in high-grade astrocytomas	i27
Figure 25.3	Histopathology of neuroblastoma tumors	i27
Figure 25.4	1p deletion in neuroblastoma detected by FISH	i28
Figure 25.5	N-myc amplification	i28
Figure 44.4C	Grade II astrocytoma	i28
Figure 44.6	Grade III astrocytoma	i28
Figure 44.9C	Grade IV astrocytoma	i29
Figure 44.10C	Oligodendroglioma with 1q/p19 loss	i29
Figure 44.11C	Oligodendroglioma without 1q/p19 loss	i29
Figure 44.19	Lymphoma	i29
Figure 44.21C	Metastatic disease	i30
Figure 44.23A	Postradiation changes	i30
Figure 44.24B	3D MRS—Biopsy guidance	i30
Figure 45.1	Brain surface gyral, sulcal, and functional anatomy	i31
Figure 45.2	Sensorimotor functional anatomy	i31
Figure 45.3	Language surface functional anatomy	i32
Figure 45.4	Visual surface functional anatomy	i32
Figure 45.5	Temporal lobe and auditory surface functional anatomy	i32
Figure 45.6	Sensorimotor white matter tractography	i33
Figure 45.7	Superior longitudinal fasciculus white matter tractography	i33
Figure 45.8	Optic radiations white matter tractography	i34
Figure 45.9	Identification of functional anatomy distorted by a mass lesion	i34
Figure 45.10	Brain stem white matter tractography	i35
Figure 50.1	Visualization of residual tumor	i35
Figure 50.2	Combining fluorescence for visualizing the cortical extension of the tumor	i35
Figure 50.3	Atypical meningioma	i36
Figure 60.3	Utility of MEG	i36
Figure 72.1	Perivascular growth pattern of a B-cell primary CNS lymphoma	i37
Figure 81.7	Mammalian cell survival curve	i37
Figure 81.8	Typical 3D conformal plan for a GBM	i38
Figure 81.10	Tomotherapy plan showing sparing of the hippocampus	i39
Figure 81.12	Fractional depth dose in water of a 170 MeV proton beam	i39
Figure 82.1	Comparison of dose plans for different volume definitions	i40
Figure 82.2	Example of MRI fusion	i41
Figure 87.1	Dosimetric comparison of proton therapy and IMRT	i42
Figure 88.1	Lateral skull film	i43
Figure 88.3	Comparisons of x-rays	i43
Figure 88.4	Isodose distribution for boost of the primary site in a child with medulloblastoma	i43
Figure 93.7	Stereotactic radiosurgery	i43
Figure 93.9	Fractionated stereotactic EBRT	i44
Figure 95.1	Example of proton therapy	i44
Figure 95.2	Color wash of the total dose delivered with proton therapy	i45
Figure 97.1	Comparison of whole ventricular treatment using opposed lateral fields	i45
Figure 98.2	Isodose plots superimposed on the treatment planning CT images for a parallel opposed shaped WBRT PCNSL field arrangement	i45
Figure 98.3	Isodose plots superimposed on treatment planning CT images for a parallel opposed shaped WBRT and whole orbit PCNSL field arrangement used when there is ocular involvement	i46
Figure 99.1	Central neurocytoma	i46
Figure 101.2B	Single-fraction stereotactic radiosurgery	i47
Figure 101.3	A situation with a rather large metastasis in the brain stem	i47
Figure 101.6	High-precision irradiation with fractionated stereotactic radiotherapy	i48

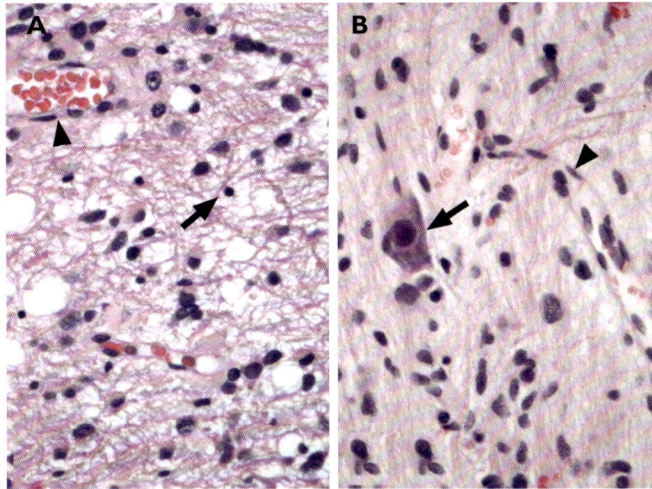

Figure 14.2 The microenvironment of infiltrating astrocytomas includes normal CNS structures that depend on tumor location. **(A)** The microenvironment of infiltrating tumors in the white matter includes axonal processes and myelin sheaths, oligodendrocytes (arrow), endothelial cells (arrowhead), astrocytes, and microglia. **(B)** Tumors that infiltrate the cortex or deep gray structures will also have a variety of neuronal cell bodies (arrow) and a prominent vasculature (arrowhead) within their immediate environment.

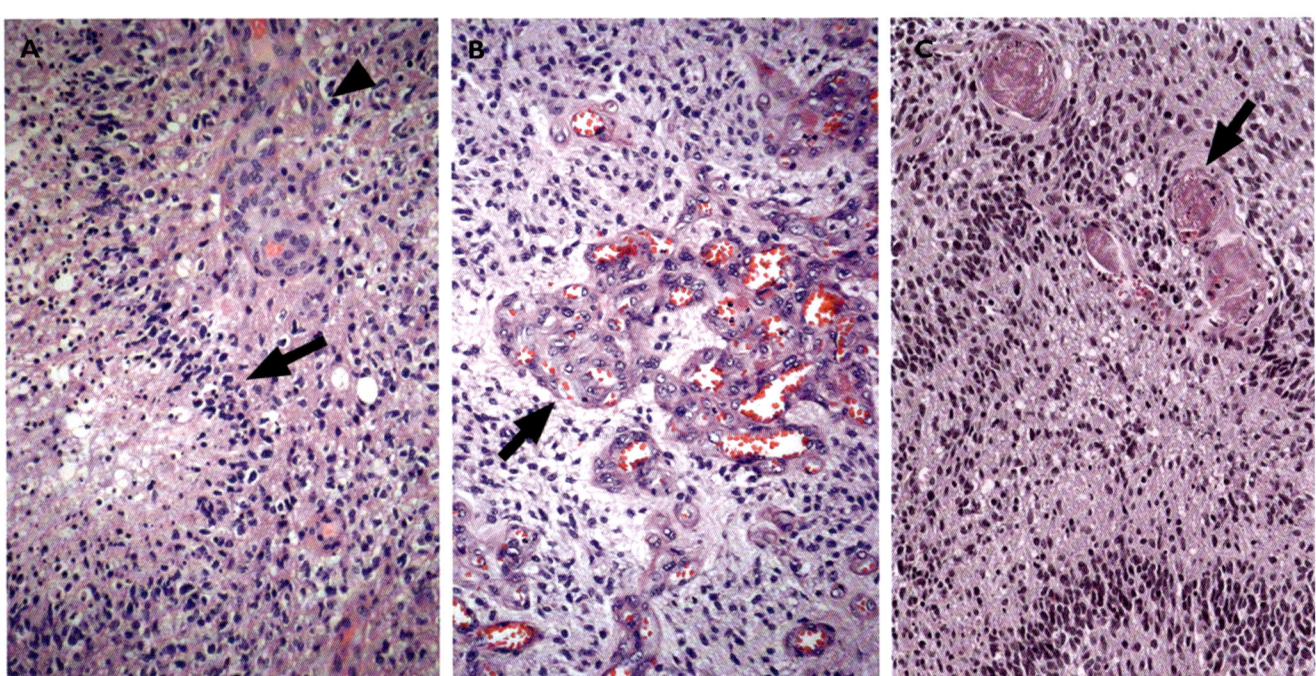

Figure 14.3 Pathologic features that define the microenvironment of glioblastoma. **(A)** Pseudopalisades (arrow) are characterized by a high cellular density of tumor cells that accumulate around a central zone of necrosis. (A,B) Microvascular hyperplasia (**B**, arrow) is a florid form of angiogenesis that can be noted in regions adjacent to necrosis but is also seen peripherally at the tumor's leading edge. **(C)** Intravascular thrombosis is present in nearly all GBMs and is usually identified adjacent to necrosis or within pseudopalisading cells associated with necrosis.

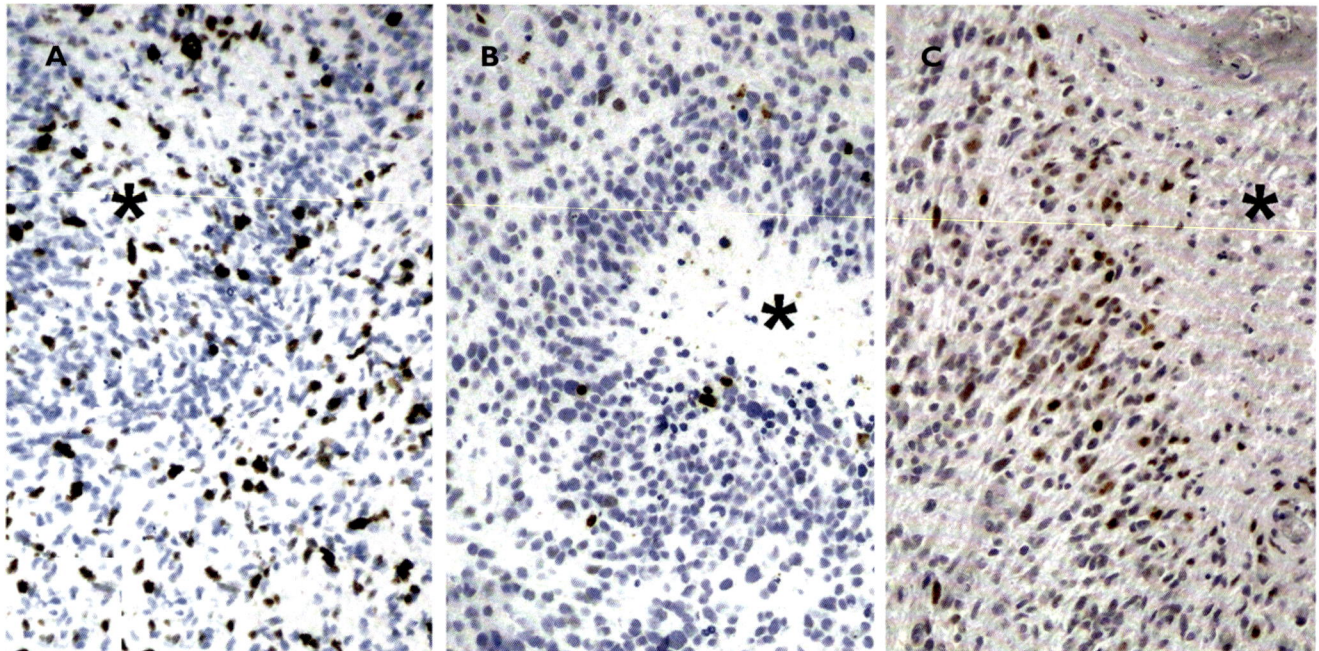

Figure 14.4 Heterogeneity of pseudopalisades and adjacent brain tumor. **(A)** Although the cells of the pseudopalisade around necrosis (*) have a higher cellular density than adjacent tumor cells, they have lower proliferation index as determined by immunohistochemistry for MIB-1 (nuclear stain). **(B)** Apoptotic cells are more frequent in pseudopalisading cells as determined by staining for cleaved caspase 3. **(C)** Cells adjacent to necrosis (*) express a high level of HIF-1α.

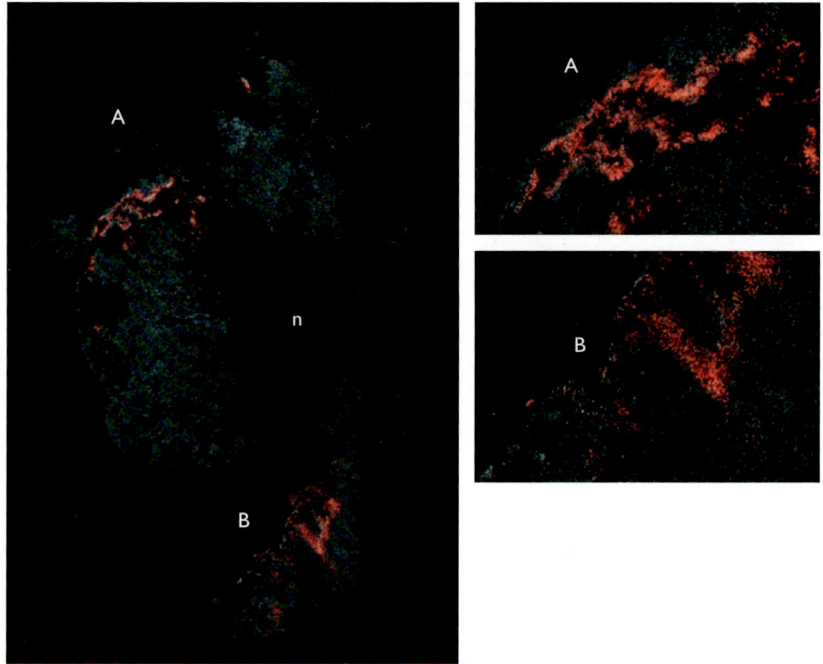

Figure 14.5 Intratumoral heterogeneity in a human glioblastoma. This image demonstrates the patterns, distributions, and levels of hypoxia (as measured by EF5 binding) in a human GBM. On the left is a tissue section (approximately 4 × 6 mm) from a GBM. A large portion of the central region is necrotic (n, macroscopic necrosis), but regions of viable oxic cells (green) are seen, even adjacent to this area. Two large areas of hypoxia (red regions A, B; also shown in detail (10×) on the right) are seen surrounding microscopic necrosis. Both regions are moderately hypoxic ($pO_2 \approx 0.5\%$ oxygen).

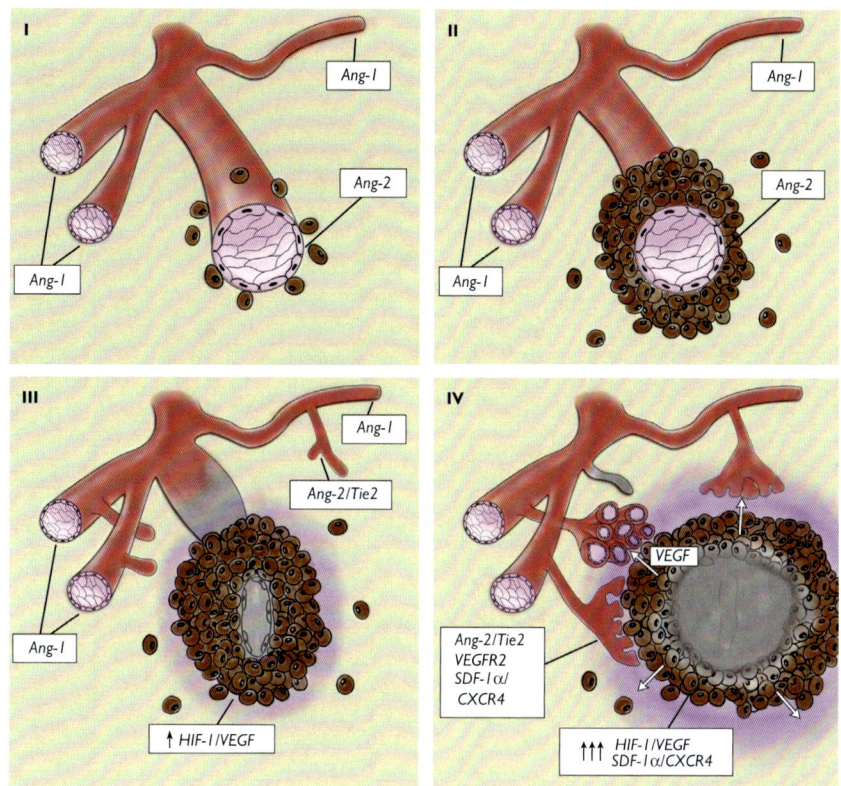

Figure 16.2 Distinct stages of glioma neovascularization in a murine model. Stage I (day 7 post-tumor implantation): Perivascular organization. Stage II (day 14): Tumor proliferation. Stage III (day 21): Vascular involution. Stage IV (day 28): Angiogenesis. Please refer to page 124 for the unabridged caption.

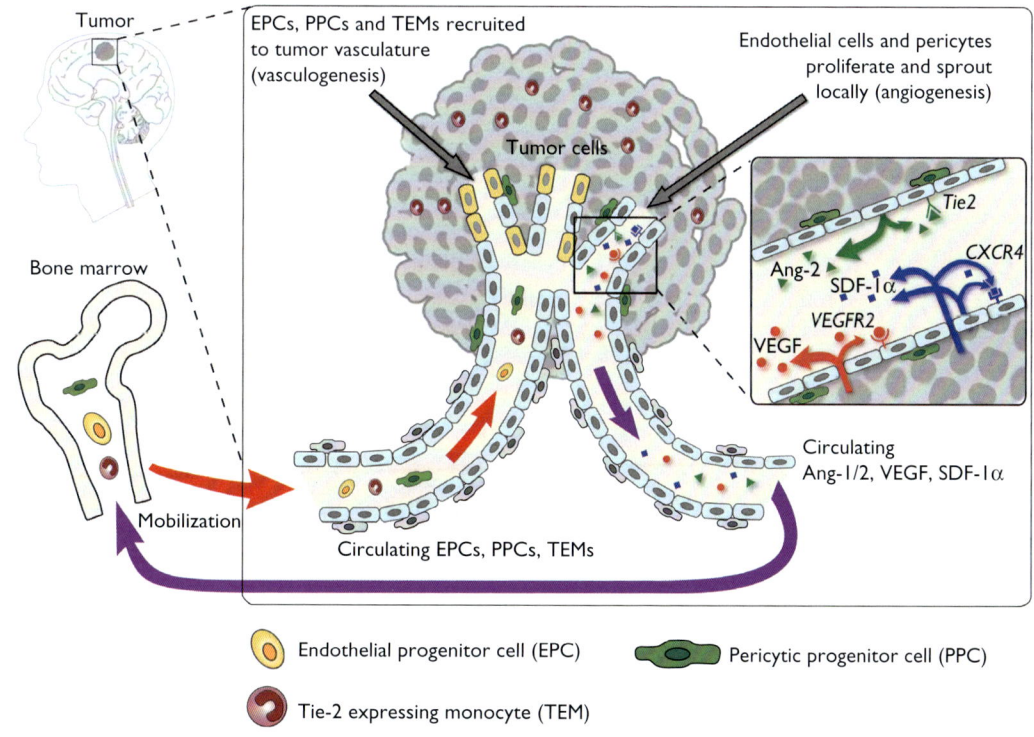

Figure 16.4 Mobilization and recruitment of bone marrow-derived proangiogenic cells to the site of tumor neovascularization. Solid tumors can produce and release cytokines into the systemic circulation that can mobilize various populations of proangiogenic cells from the bone marrow. Following entry in tumor tissues, these cell populations exert different roles in neovascularization, possibly by differentiating and maturing in the growing vasculature and/or stimulating angiogenesis locally in a paracrine manner. Please refer to page 131 for the unabridged caption.

Please note: Figure 16.3 follows on the next page.

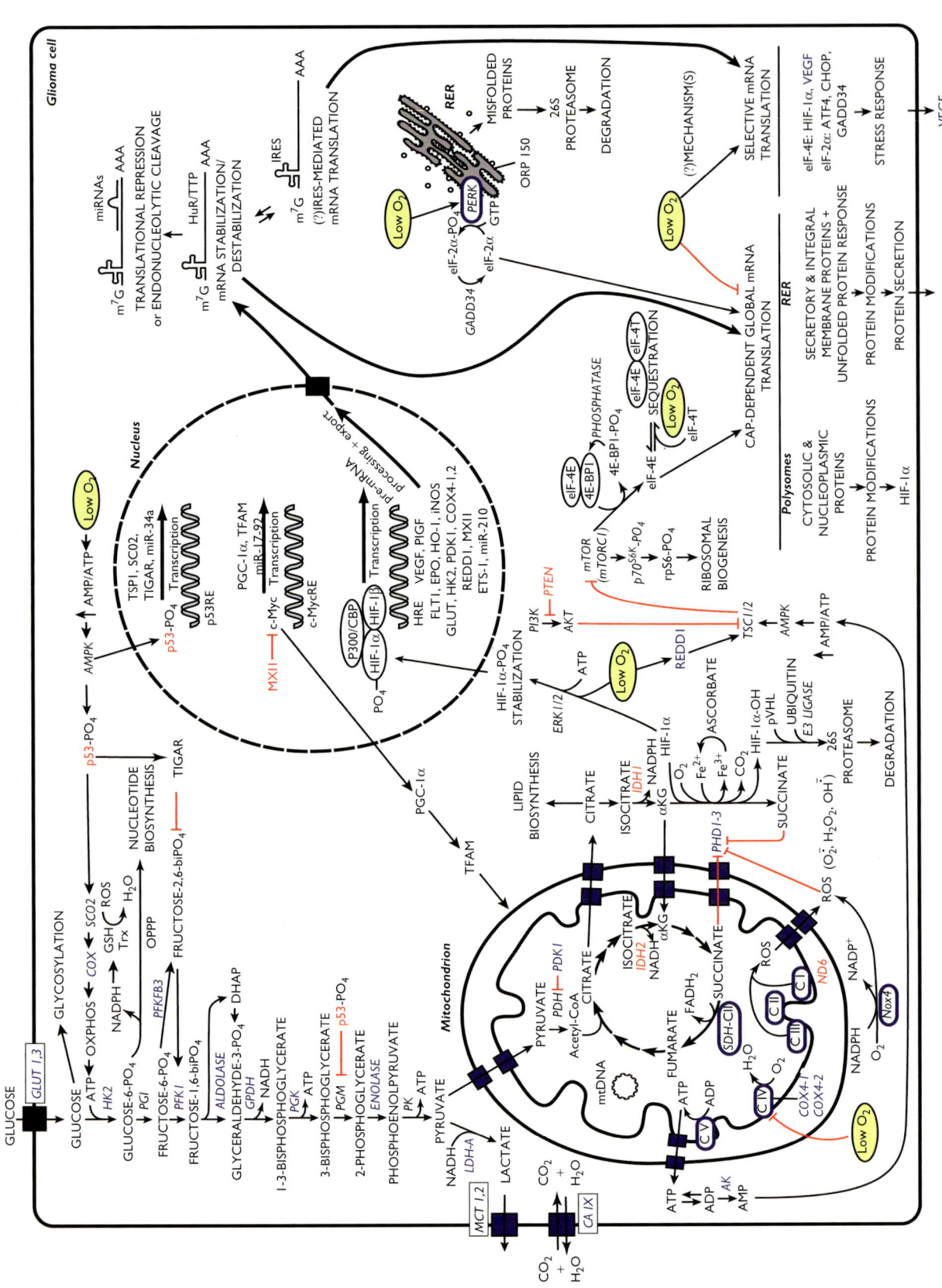

Figure 16.3 Tumor hypoxia selectively suppresses cellular energy metabolism and biosynthetic machinery through HIF-dependent and independent mechanisms. Tumor hypoxia and/or nonhypoxic oncogenic events have been implicated in regulating many of the genes responsible for the reprogramming of tumor energy metabolism and the selective translation of stress response proteins, including VEGF. In this diagram, gene products regulated by HIF-1 are indicated in BLUE, and genetic or chromosomal abnormalities in RED; the inhibitory effect of a product is indicated by a BLUNT ENDED RED LINE. Please refer to page 127 for the unabridged legend.

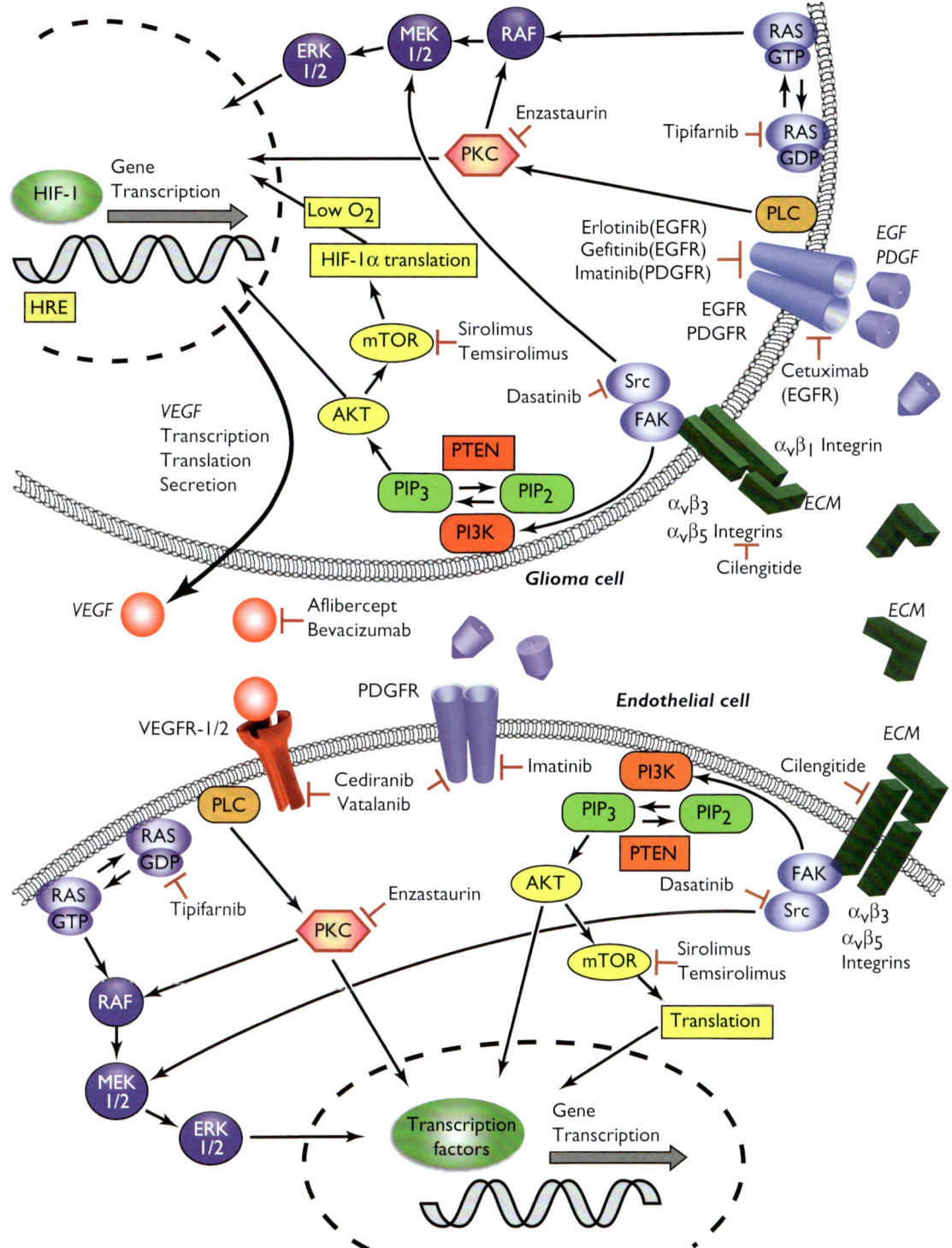

Figure 16.6 Molecular signaling pathways targeted by antiangiogenic drugs in clinical trials for malignant gliomas. During malignant transformation, common deregulation of growth factor signaling pathways lead to enhanced HIF-1-regulated expression of VEGF and other effector molecules in glioma cells (illustrated on top), that stimulate signaling pathways regulating angiogenesis in the tumor endothelium (at the bottom). These aberrations have become important potential targets of antiangiogenic therapy for malignant gliomas. Please refer to page 136 for the unabridged legend.

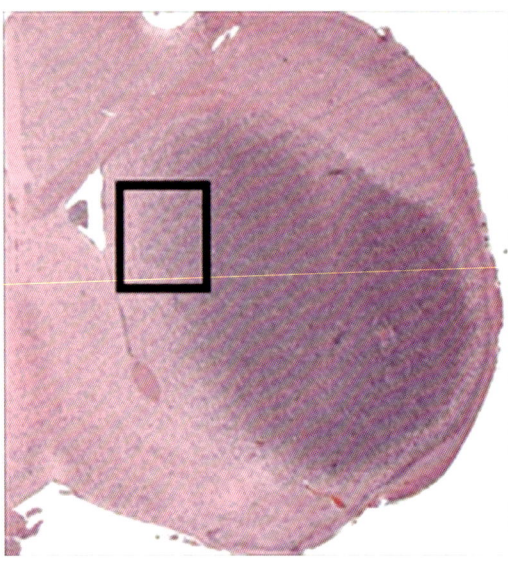

Figure 17.6 Intracranial xenograft tumor established from human GBM neurosphere culture. Growth is as a highly cellular mass with infiltrating cells at the tumor margin (black rectangle).

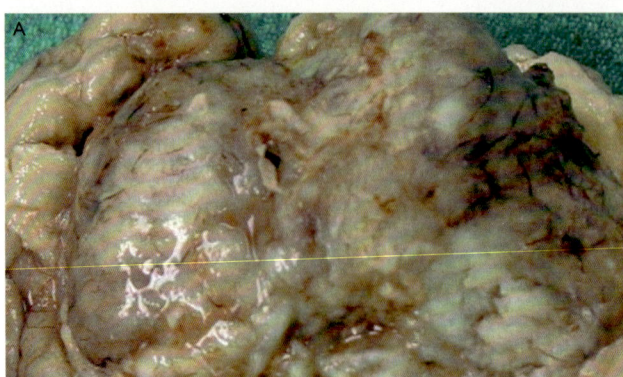

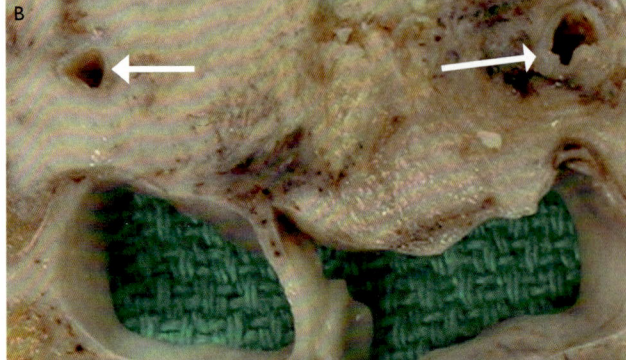

Figure 18.2 A histologically benign olfactory groove meningioma **(A)** encases the cavernous sinuses **(B, arrows)**, invades the skull, and grows into the sinuses.

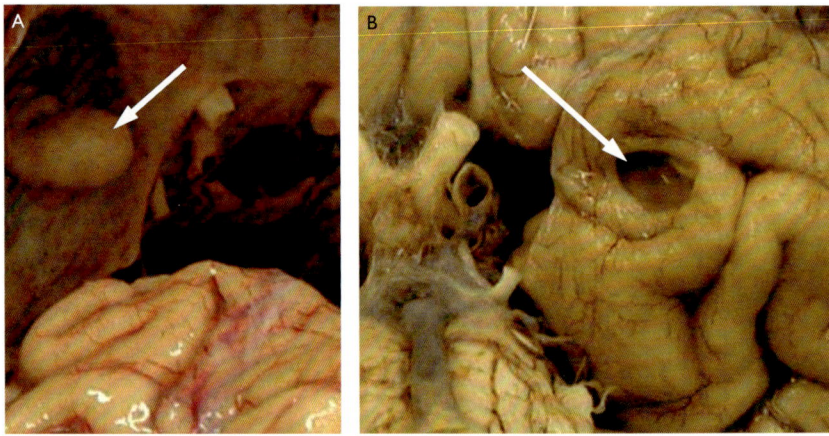

Figure 18.1 An incidental middle fossa meningioma found at autopsy **(A)** compresses but does not invade the inferior surface of the temporal lobe **(B)**.

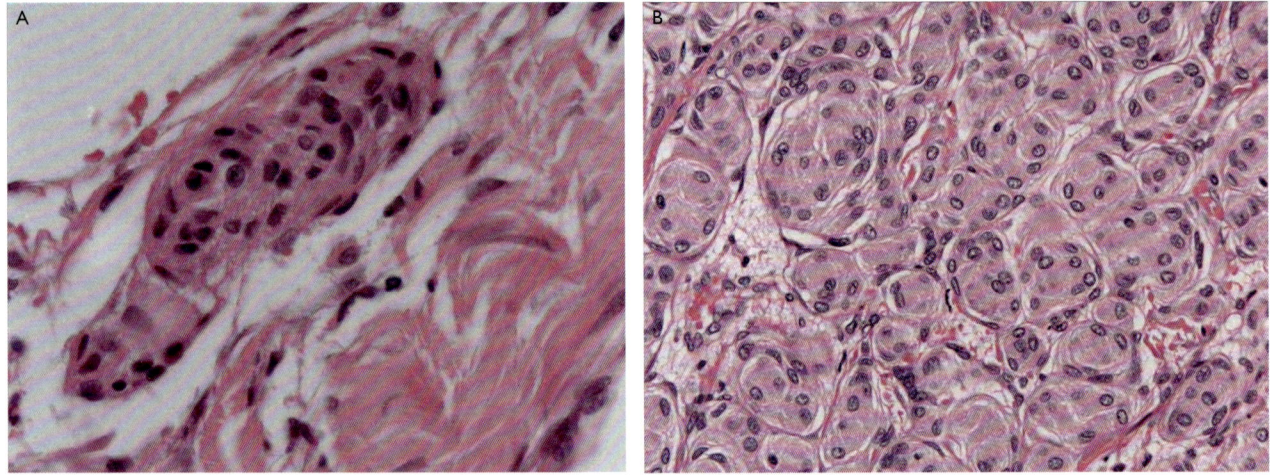

Figure 18.3 Arachnoid cap cells **(A)** and the whorls of a meningothelial meningioma **(B)** share both architecture and cytology.

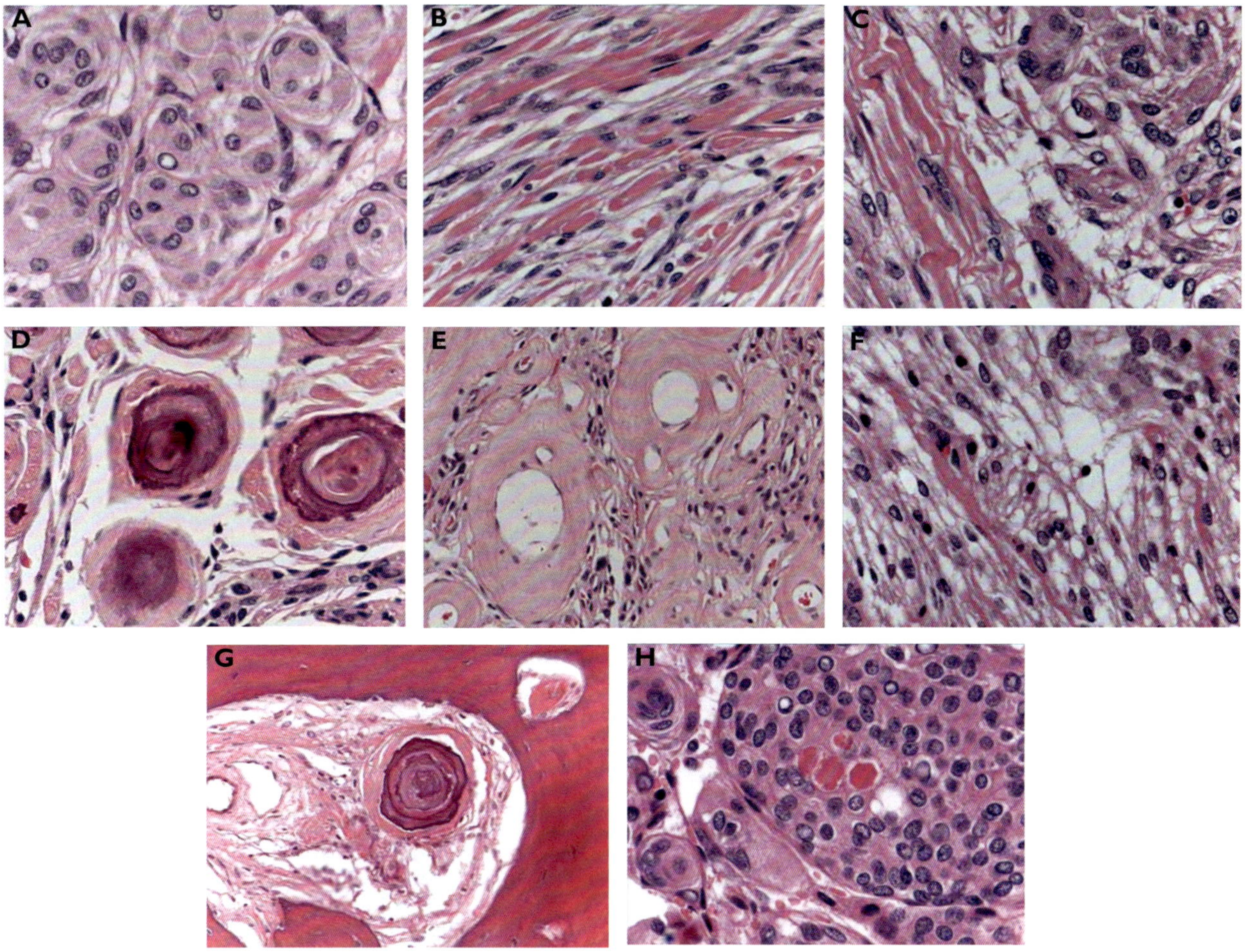

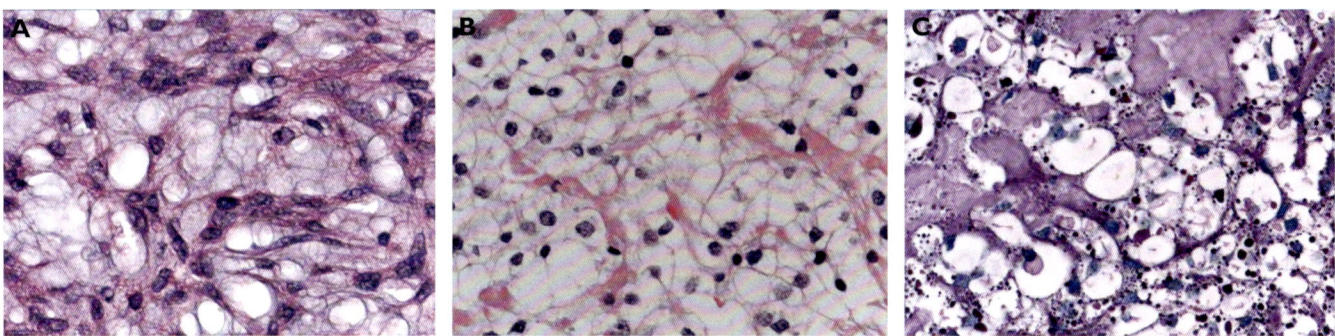

Figure 18.4 WHO grade I histological subtypes include meningothelial meningiomas **(A)**, fibroblastic meningiomas **(B)**, and transitional meningiomas with elements of both meningothelial and fibroblastic tumors **(C)**. Psammomatous meningiomas **(D)** have calcifications, angiomatous meningiomas have small vessels **(E)**, and microcystic meningiomas have a vacuolated background **(F)**. Metaplastic meningiomas demonstrate focal mesenchymal elements such as the bone seen here **(G)**. Secretory meningiomas demonstrate eosinophilic intracellular inclusions **(H)**.

Figure 18.5 Both chordoid **(A)** and clear cell meningiomas **(B, C)** are WHO grade II/atypical. The chordoid tumors feature a myxoid background with vacuolated cells, whereas in the clear cell variant, the cytoplasm of the tumor cells is glycogen rich, accounting for the stunning PAS positivity (C).

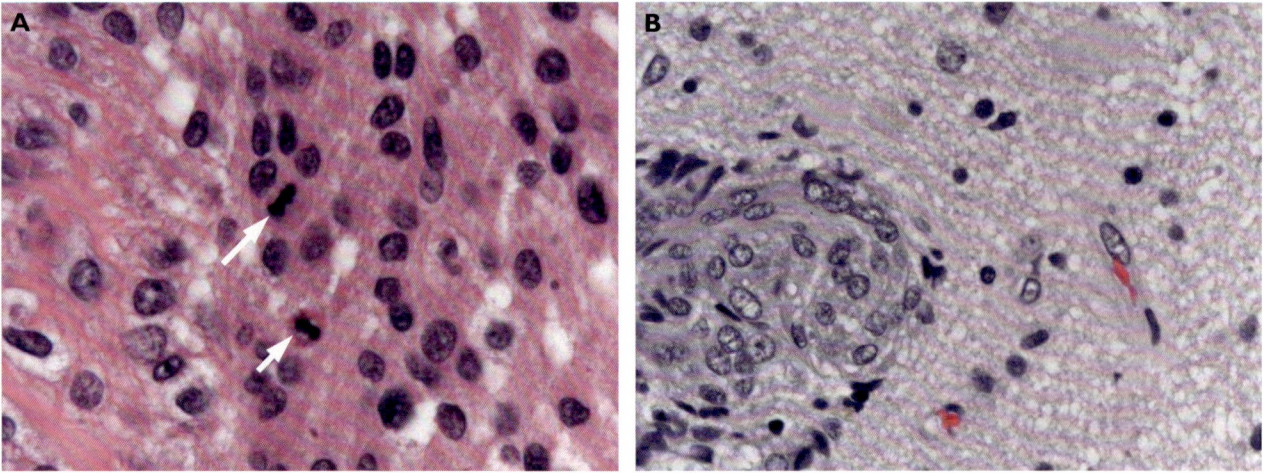

Figure 18.6 In the absence of chordoid or clear cell morphologies, either four mitoses/10 high-power fields **(arrows, A)** or brain invasion by tumor **(B)** is sufficient to make the diagnosis of atypical meningioma.

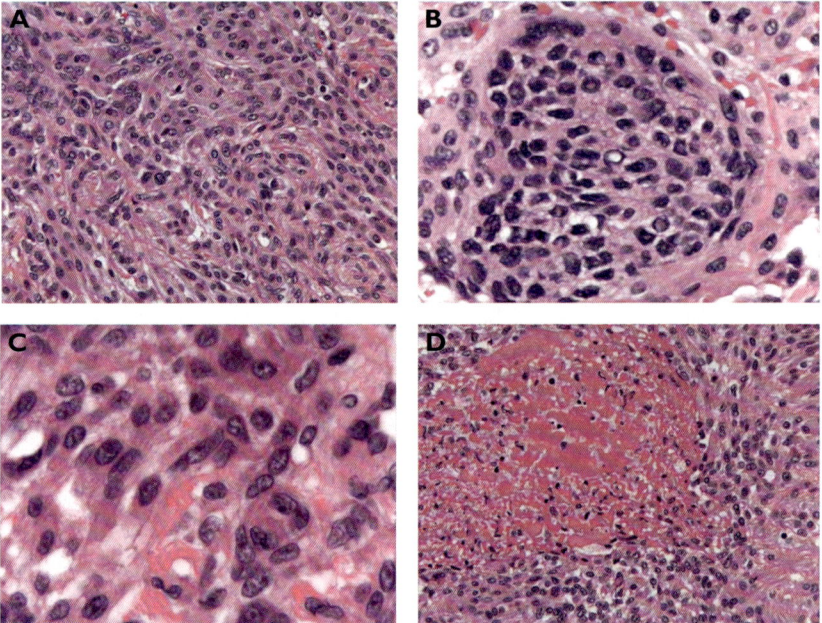

Figure 18.7 Tumors demonstrating three of the following: patternless growth **(A)**, hypercellularity, foci of small cells with high nuclear:cytoplasmic ratio **(B)**, prominent nucleoli **(C)**, or foci of necrosis **(D)** are also considered grade II/ atypical.

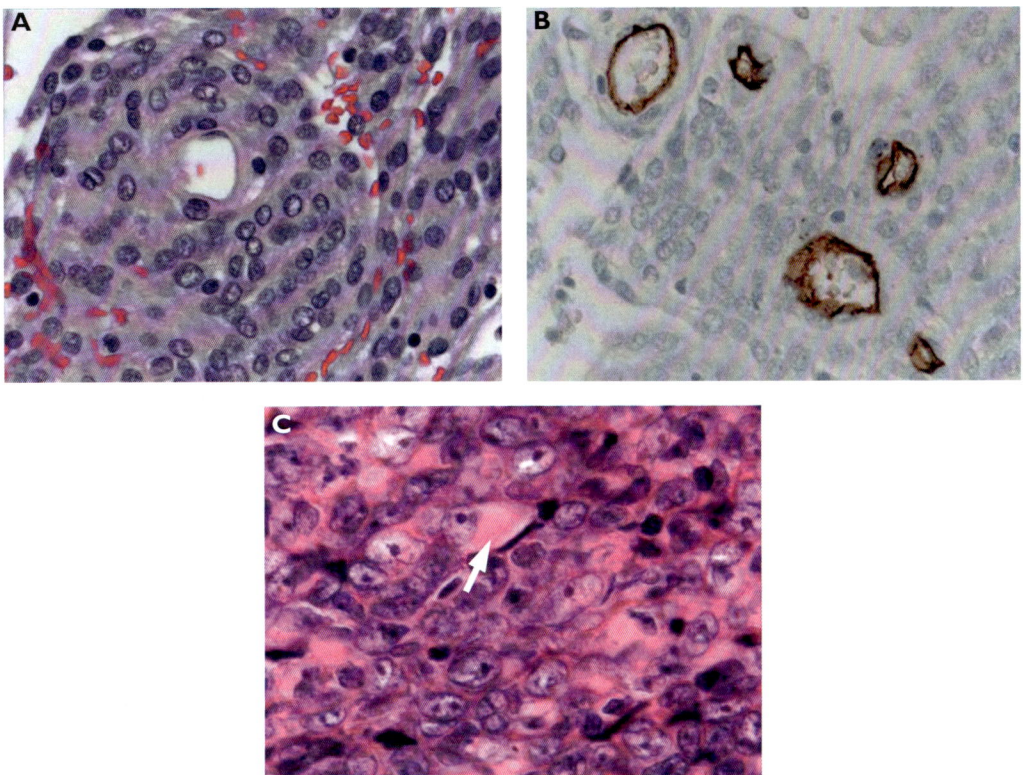

Figure 18.8 The perivascular growth pattern of papillary meningiomas can be seen with hematoxylin and eosin staining **(A)** but is even clearer with immunohistochemistry for CD34 **(B)** which clarifies the structure of the vascular cores. The intracytoplasmic inclusions of rhabdoid meningiomas **(C arrow)** are brightly eosinophilic.

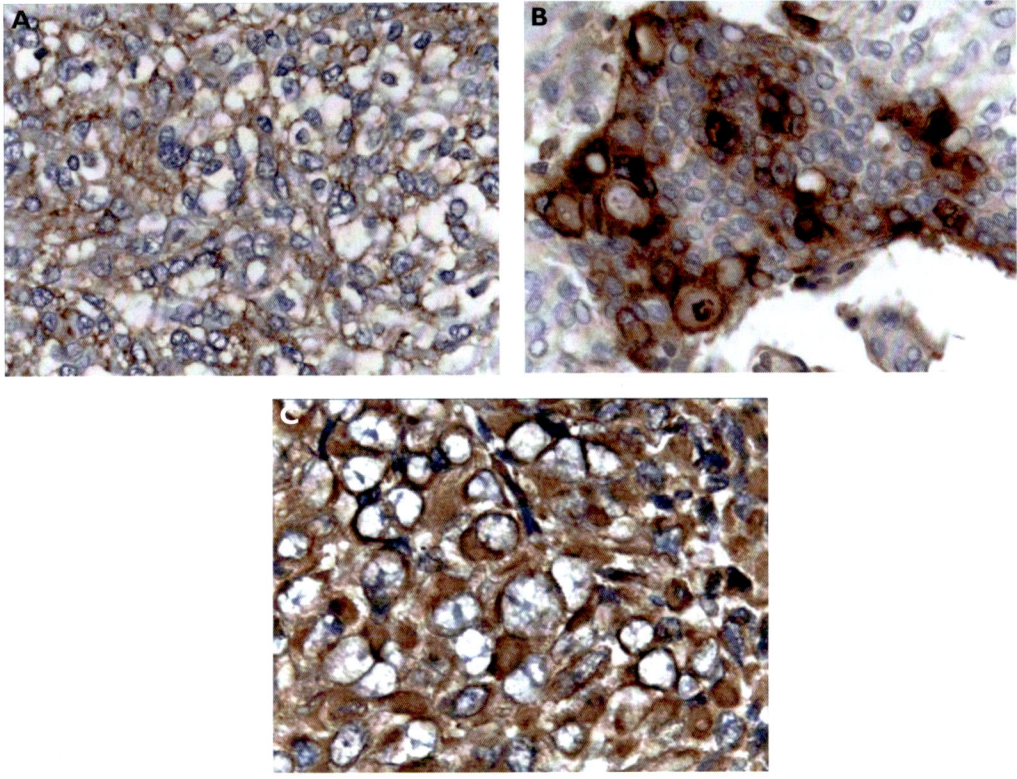

Figure 18.9 Epithelial membrane antigen immunohistochemistry stains most meningiomas **(A)**, whereas carcinoembryonic antigen is positive in secretory meningiomas **(B)** and vimentin marks the intracytoplasmic filamentous accumulations of rhabdoid meningiomas **(C)**.

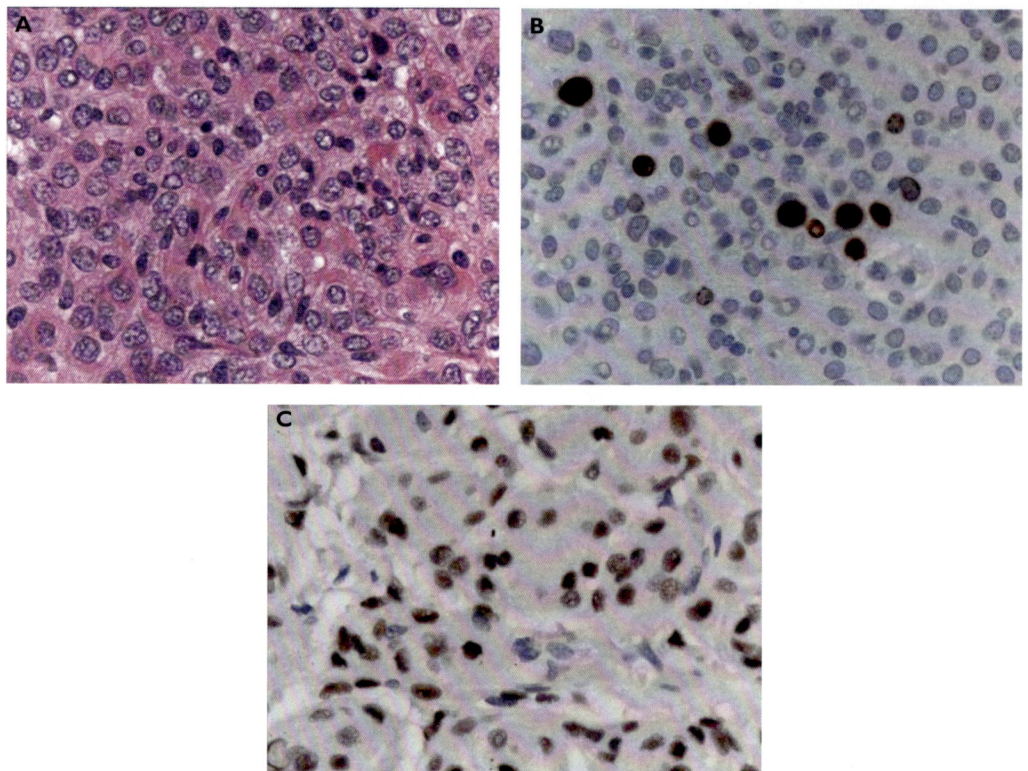

Figure 18.10 Meningiomas that are WHO grade I by standard morphological criteria **(A)** but have proliferation indices of 5% to 10% by MIB-1 staining **(B)** have an increased risk of early recurrence. Progesterone receptor expression can be demonstrated by immunohistochemistry in most meningiomas **(C)**.

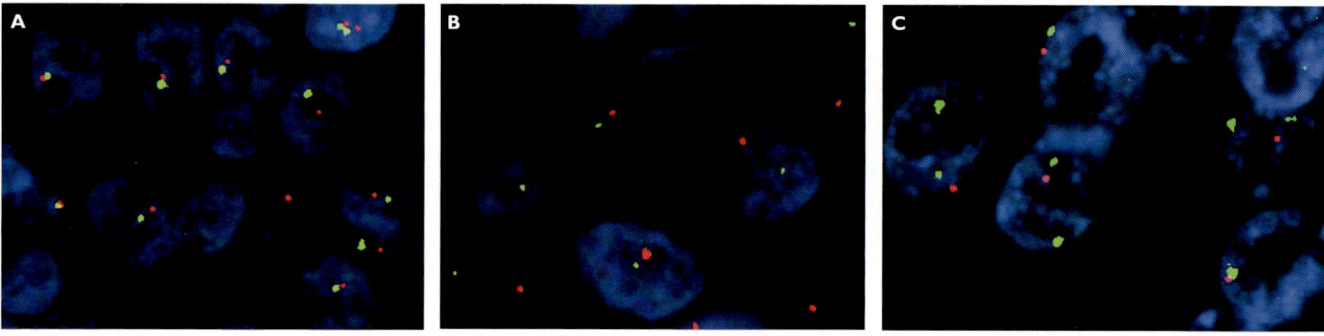

Figure 18.11 Fluorescent in situ hybridization (FISH) is used to detect chromosomal abnormalities in meningiomas. 22q deletion is demonstrated with a probe for NF2 (22q12) in red and another for BCR (22q11.2) in green. The presence of only one of each in most nuclei is consistent with either monosomy of chromosome 22 or a large 22q deletion **(A)**. Loss of both 1p and 14q is demonstrated with a probe for 1p32 labeled in green and another for 14q32 labeled in red. Again, most cells have one green and one red, consistent with deletions of both chromosomal regions **(B)**. Hemizygous deletion of 9p21 is shown with CEP9 (centromere enumerating probe for chromosome 9) in green (2 signals in most nuclei) and the p16 (CDKN2A) gene region (9p21) in red (1 signal in most cells) **(C)**. Courtesy of Arie Perry, MD, Department of Pathology, University of California at San Francisco.

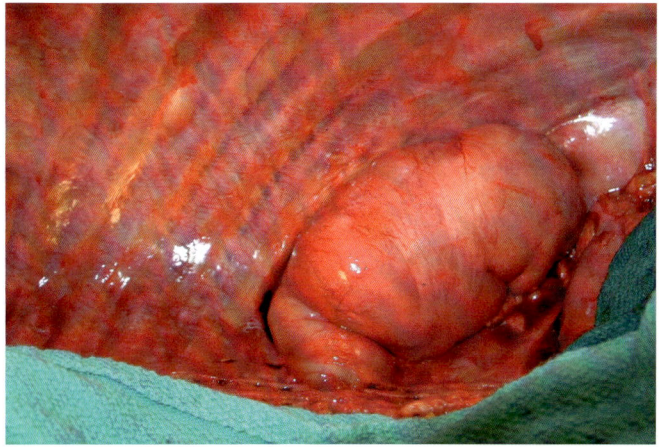

Figure 19.1 Retroperitoneal schwannoma. A large retroperitoneal schwannoma in an NF2 patient.

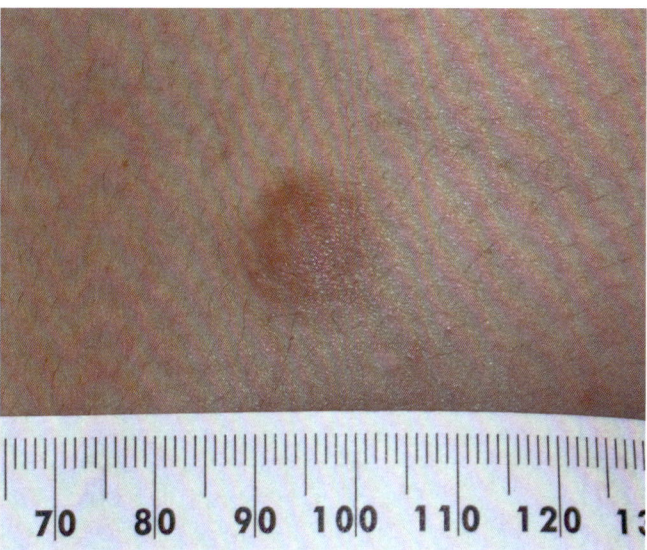

Figure 19.2 Cutaneous schwannoma. Cutaneous schwannomas often appear as discrete nodules under a mildly hyperpigmented skin. Cutaneous schwannomas are common in NF2.

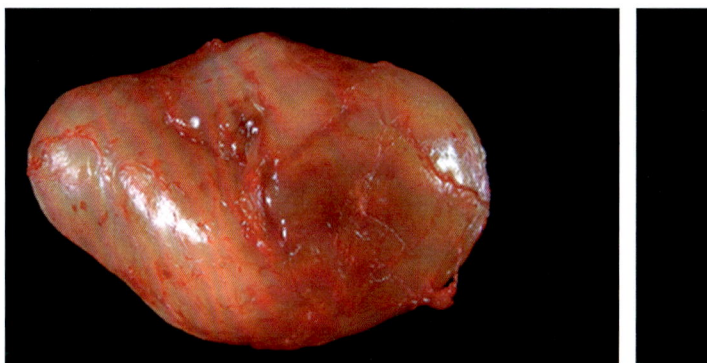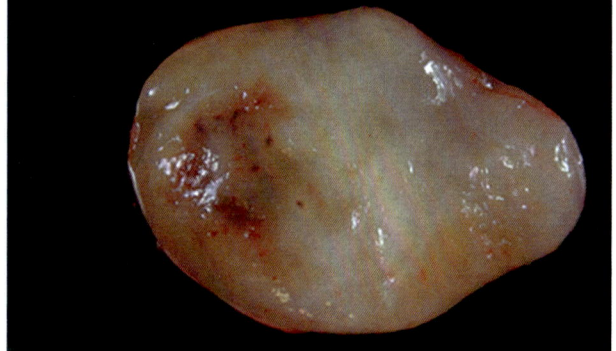

Figure 19.3 Schwannoma, gross appearance. Schwannomas are discrete, encapsulated tumors with smooth external surface (right). Cut surface may show areas of yellow (lipid rich) and red/brown (hemorrhages) discoloration (left).

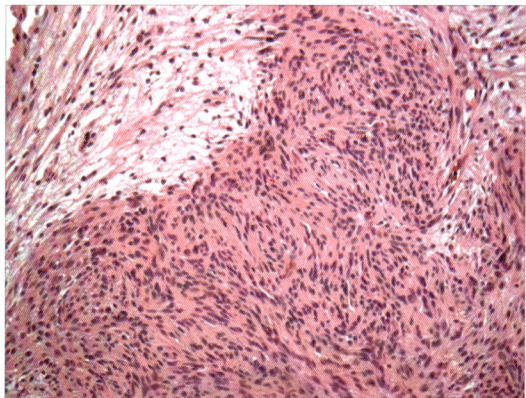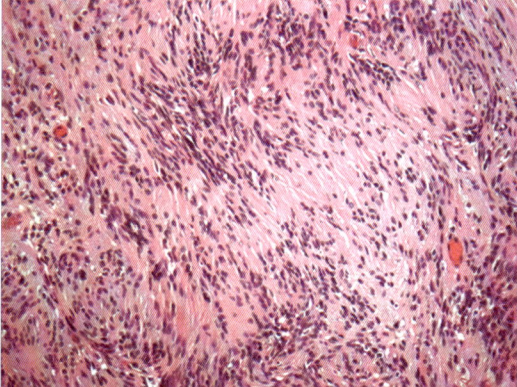

Figure 19.4 Schwannoma, histology. Typical features in schwannoma include a biphasic pattern of compact (Antoni A) and loose (Antoni B) areas (right) and nuclear palisades with formation of Verocay bodies (left).

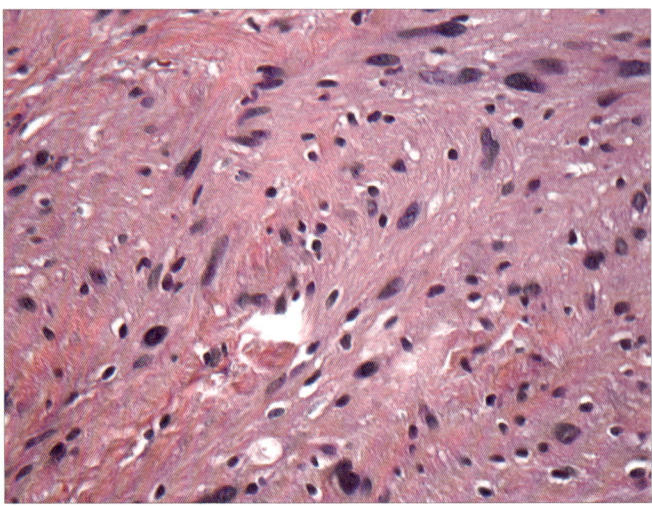

Figure 19.5 Schwannoma, histology. Large, hyperchromatic and atypical nuclei are often encountered in conventional schwannomas and are not indicative of malignant transformation.

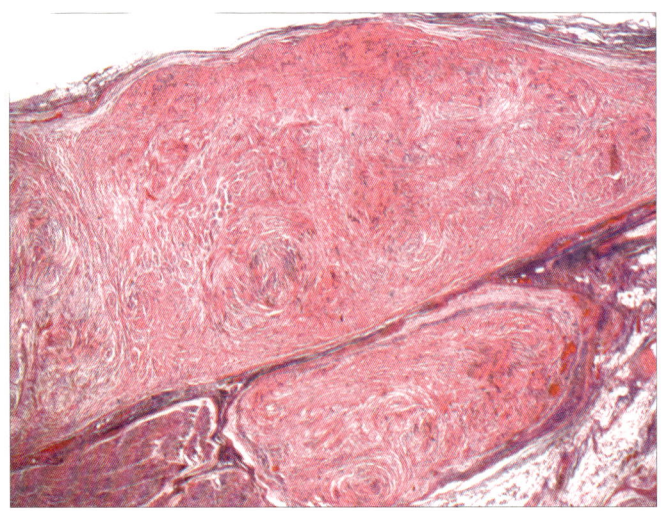

Figure 19.6 Plexiform schwannoma, histology. Expansion of multiple peripheral nerves by a plexiform schwannoma in an NF2 patient. Plexiform schwannomas may mimic the gross appearance of plexiform neurofibromas.

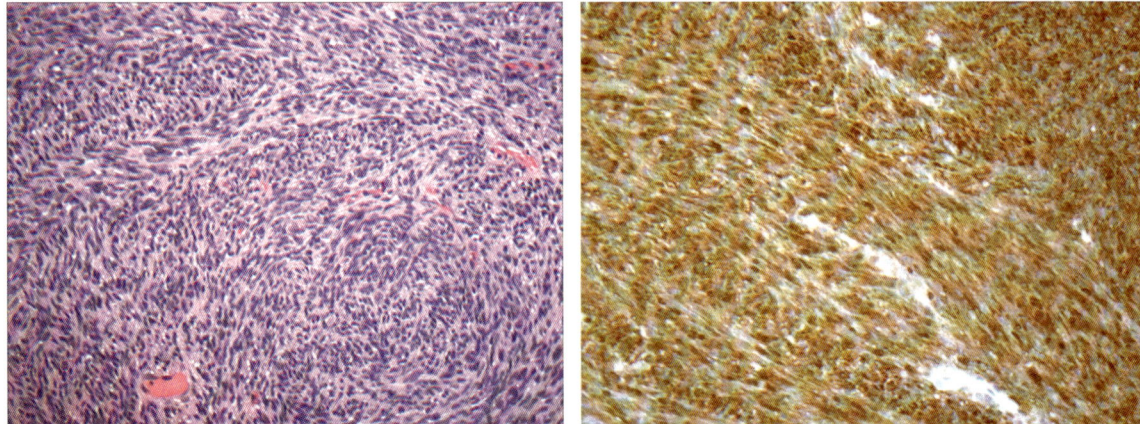

Figure 19.7 Cellular schwannoma, histology. Cellular schwannomas are cellular and mitotically active. Biphasic pattern and Verocay bodies are often absent (right). Diagnosis is confirmed by diffuse S100 immunostaining of the tumor (left).

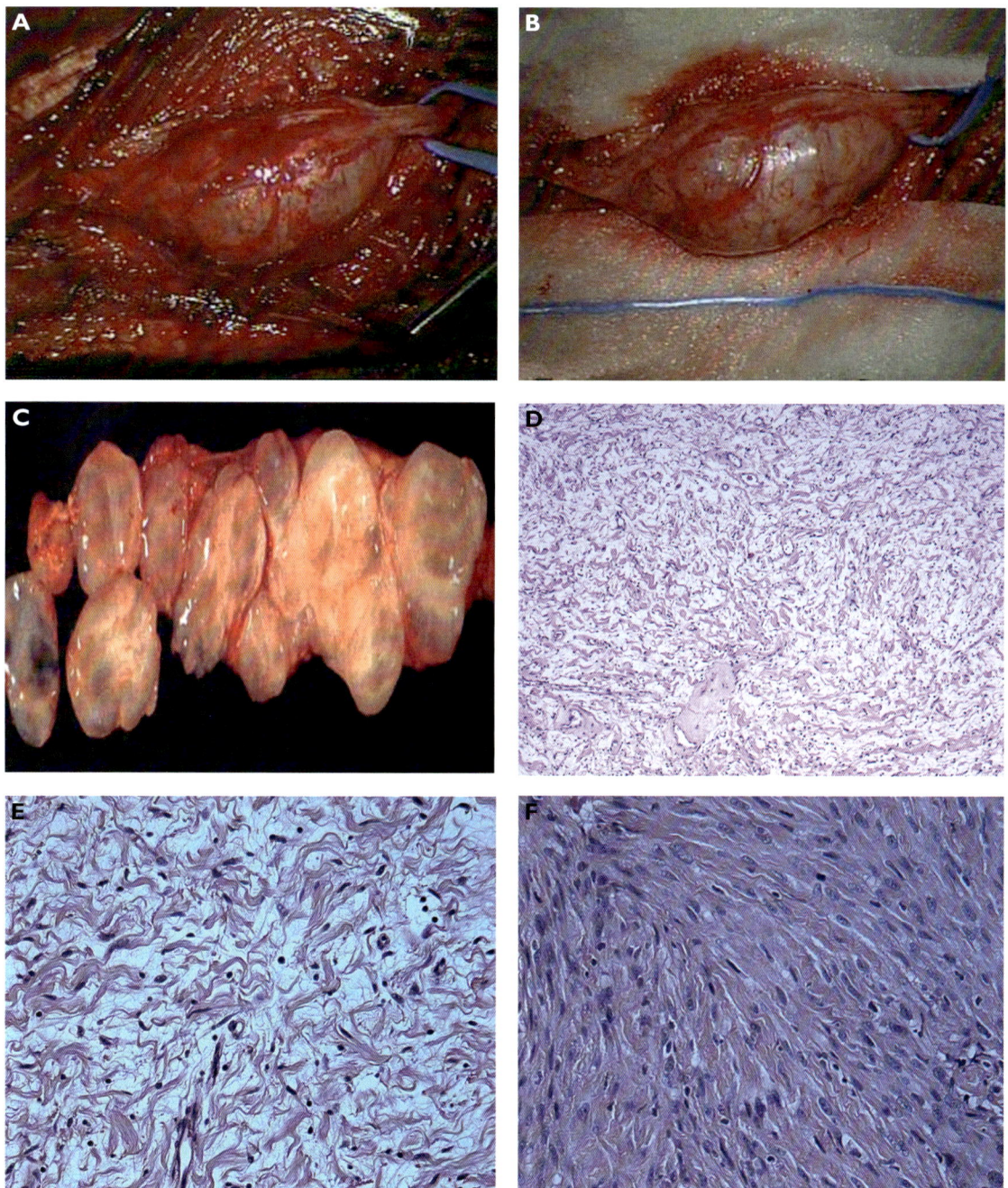

Figure 21.1 Neurofibromas often have a fusiform shape **(A, B)** because they tend to grow along a nerve. The cut surface often has a yellow-white or grey-tan, gelatinous appearance **(C)**. The consistency is often soft or only moderately firm. Microscopically, neurofibromas show wavy strands of collagen **(D)**, often without much architectural patterning. Higher magnification demonstrates that neurofibromas are proliferations of neoplastic Schwann cells as the predominant cellular element **(E)**, but also contain fibroblasts and perineurial cells. The collagenous fibers are sometimes described as resembling "shredded carrots." In an atypical neurofibroma **(F)**,

(*Continued*)

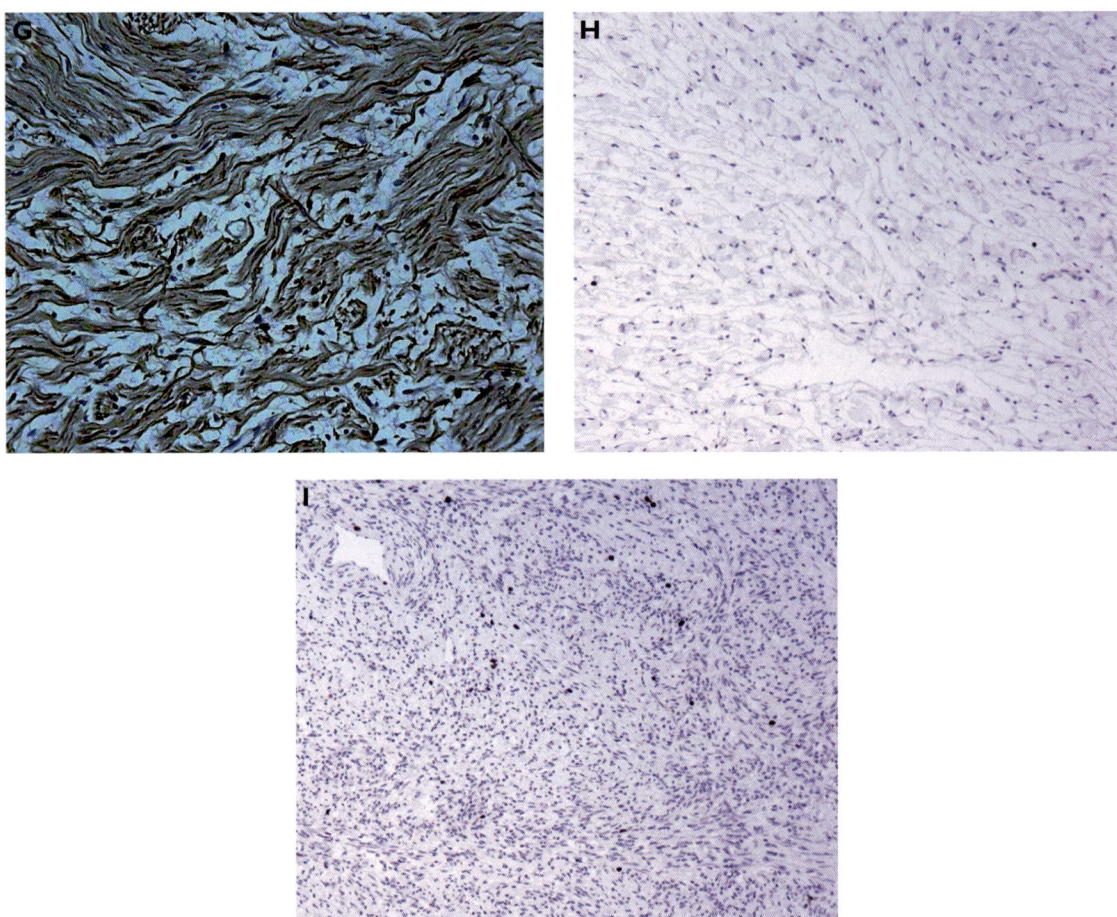

Figure 21.1 (*Continued*) there is increased cellularity and nuclear atypia. Neurofibromas are nearly always positive for S-100 **(G)**. The MIB-1 (KI-67) proliferation index is low in neurofibromas, labeling only 1% to 2% of nuclei **(H)**, but may reach 5% to 15 % in atypical neurofibromas **(I)**.

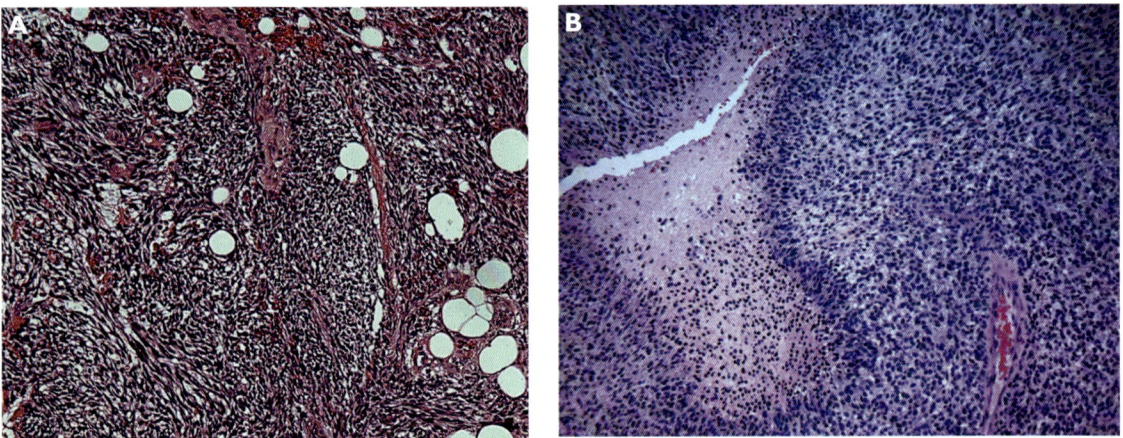

Figure 21.2 MPNST can often diffusely invade surrounding tissues so that adjacent structures such as adipose tissue become incorporated into the tumor **(A)**. Cellularity is high, and there are often well-delineated areas of "geographic" necrosis **(B)**.

(*Continued*)

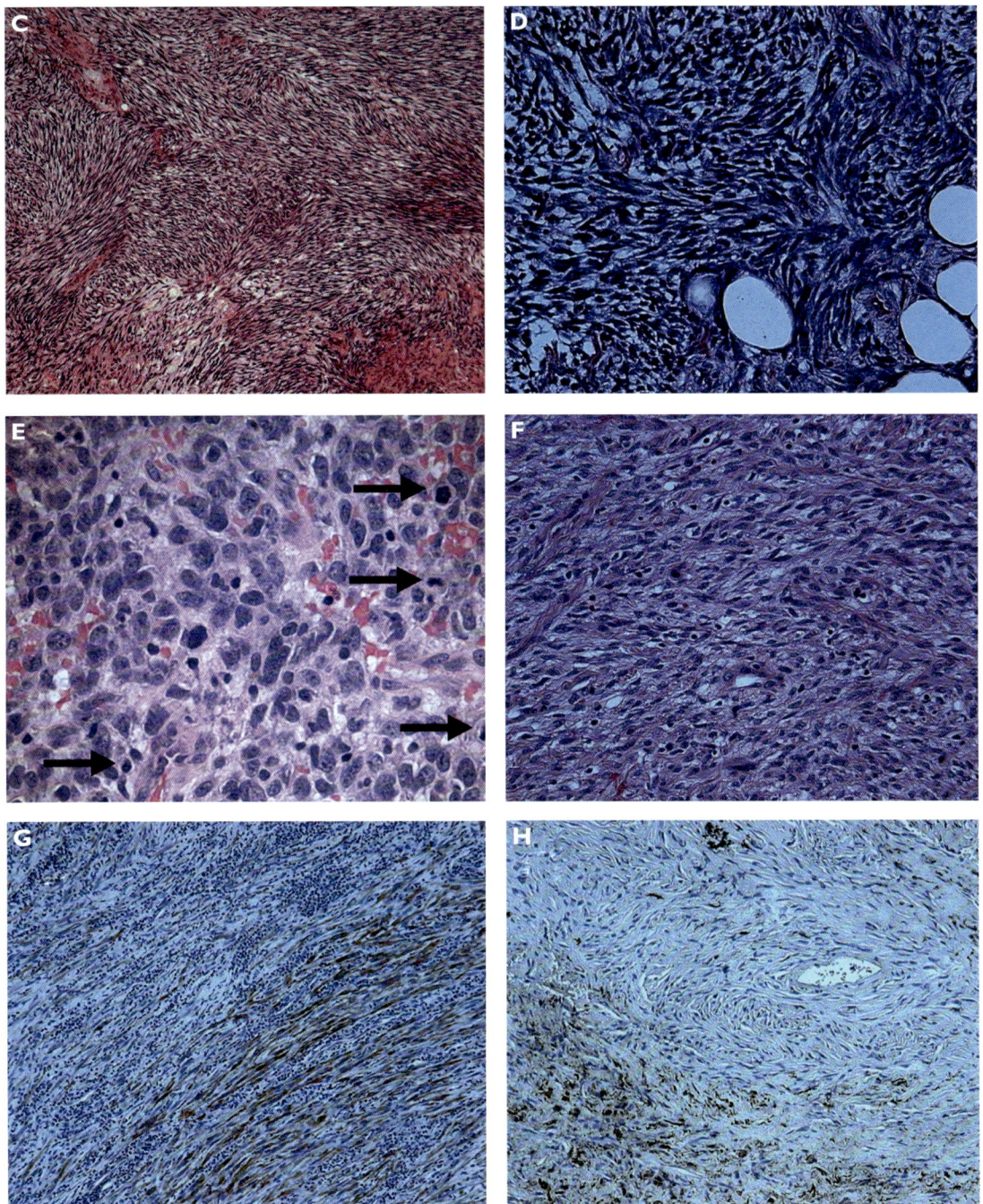

Figure 21.2 (*Continued*) A herringbone-type pattern of interlacing fascicles and sheets may be seen **(C)**, resembling fibrosarcoma. At higher magnification, cells are often spindle-shaped and have variable amounts of eosinophilic cytoplasm **(D)**. They have large, hyperchromatic nuclei and brisk mitotic activity **(E)**. In low-grade MPNST, there is no necrosis, cellularity tends to be lower, and nuclei are smaller **(F)**. One of several variant histological types is the so-called "MPNST with mesenchymal differentiation," here shown with immunoreactivity to smooth muscle actin (SMA; **G**). Reactivity for S-100 is inversely correlated with tumor grade and can be only focal in high-grade MPNSTs **(H)**.

(*Continued*)

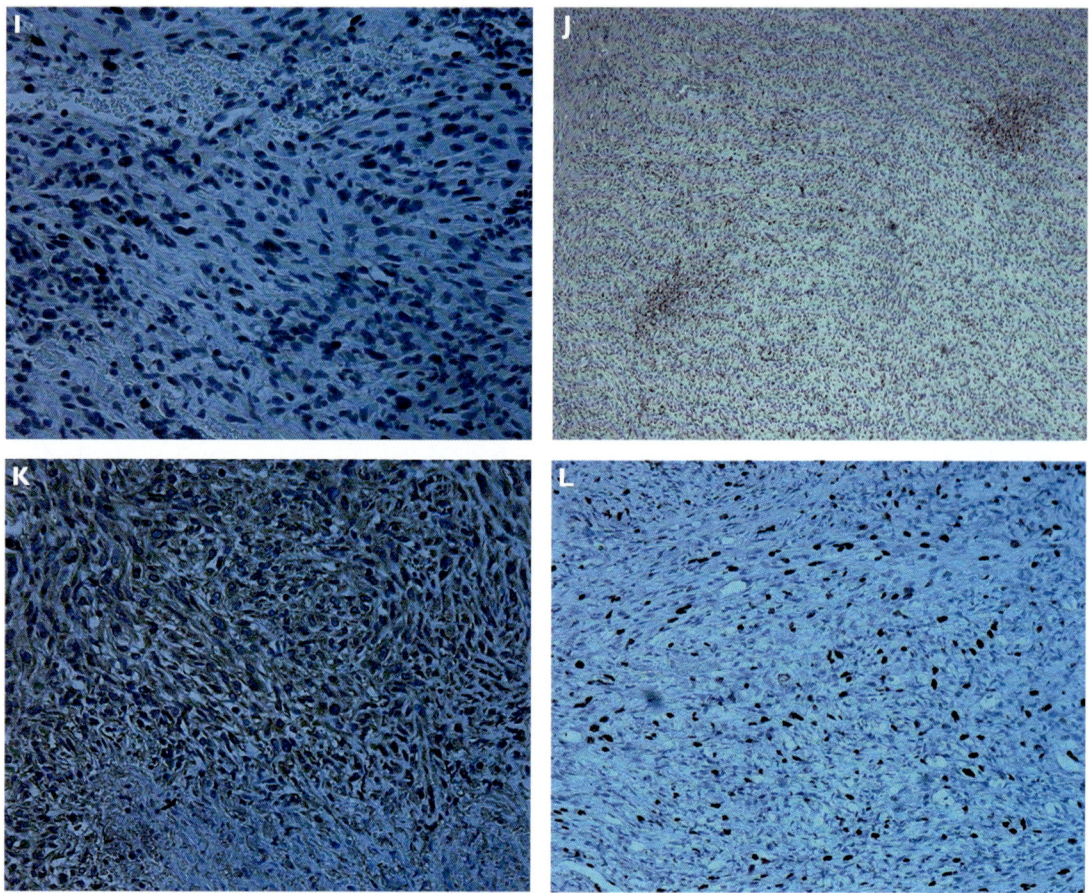

Figure 21.2 (*Continued*) Immunoreactivity for p53 is common in MPNST **(I)**. Intratumoral lymphocytes can give the appearance of increased cellularity and can be highlighted with a CD45 stain **(J)**. Vimentin is usually positive **(K)**. The KI-67 (MIB-1) proliferation index is markedly increased in high-grade MPNST, easily labeling 20% to 50% of nuclei **(L)**.

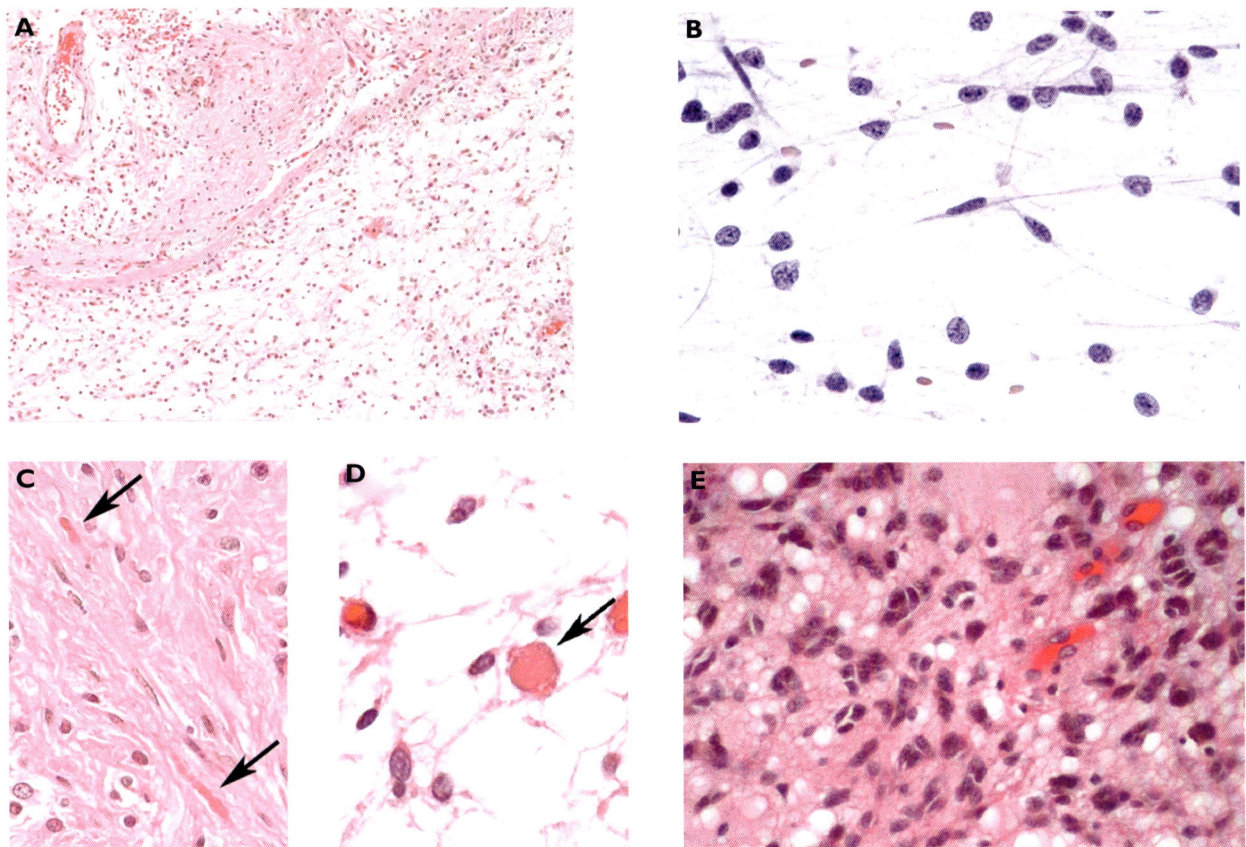

Figure 23.1 **(A)** Pilocytic astrocytoma showing a biphasic architecture, with both a loose, hypocellular pattern (lower right half) and a compact cellular pattern (upper left half). H&E, original magnification ×100. **(B)** A smear of a pilocytic astrocytoma showing bipolar hair-like processes that characterize the piloid cell. H&E, original magnification ×400. **(C)** Rosenthal fibers (arrows) scattered within the compact piloid component of a pilocytic astrocytoma. H&E, original magnification ×400. **(D)** Eosinophilic granular body (arrow) within a loose area in a pilocytic astrocytoma. H&E, original magnification ×600. **(E)** Pilocytic astrocytoma with scattered tumor cells showing degenerative changes, which include hyperchromatic and mild-to-moderate pleomorphic nuclei and multinucleation. H&E, original magnification ×400.

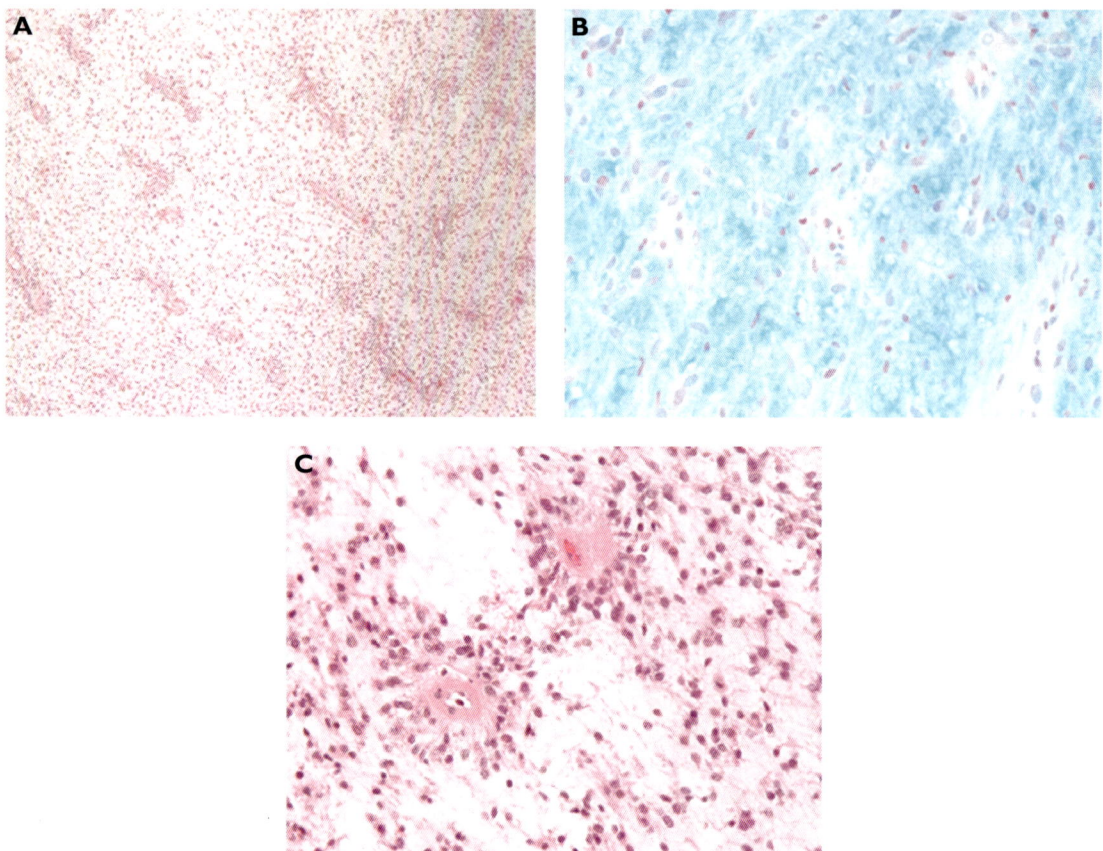

Figure 23.2 **(A)** Pilomyxoid astrocytoma showing a monophasic architecture. There is an impression of the angiocentric pattern at this low power, which is better seen at higher power (C). H&E, original magnification ×40. **(B)** Alcian blue highlights the prominent myxoid background of pilomyxoid astrocytoma. Original magnification ×200. **(C)** Angiocentric pattern of pilomyxoid astrocytoma. H&E, original magnification ×200.

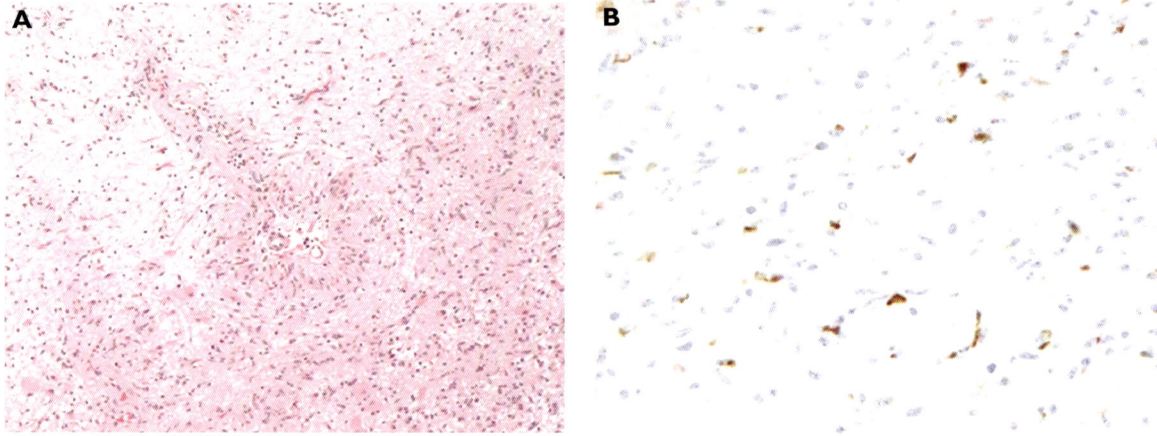

Figure 23.3 **(A)** Angiocentric glioma showing elongated astrocytic tumor cells. The angiocentric pattern is noted centrally. H&E, original magnification ×100. **(B)** A dot-like staining pattern with epithelial membrane antigen (EMA) immunohistochemistry is a characteristic feature of angiocentric glioma. Original magnification ×400.

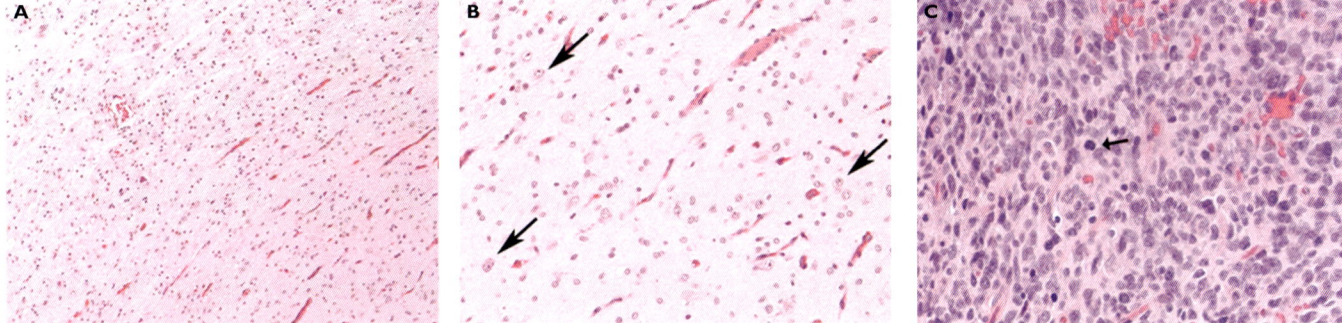

Figure 23.4 **(A)** At low power, diffuse astrocytoma can be recognized as areas of hypercellularity within the brain. H&E, original magnification ×100. **(B)** On higher power, entrapped neurons (arrows) can be seen demonstrating the infiltrative nature of the tumor. H&E, original magnification ×200. **(C)** Anaplastic astrocytoma showing markedly increased cellularity, nuclear pleomorphism, and mitosis (arrow). H&E, original magnification ×200.

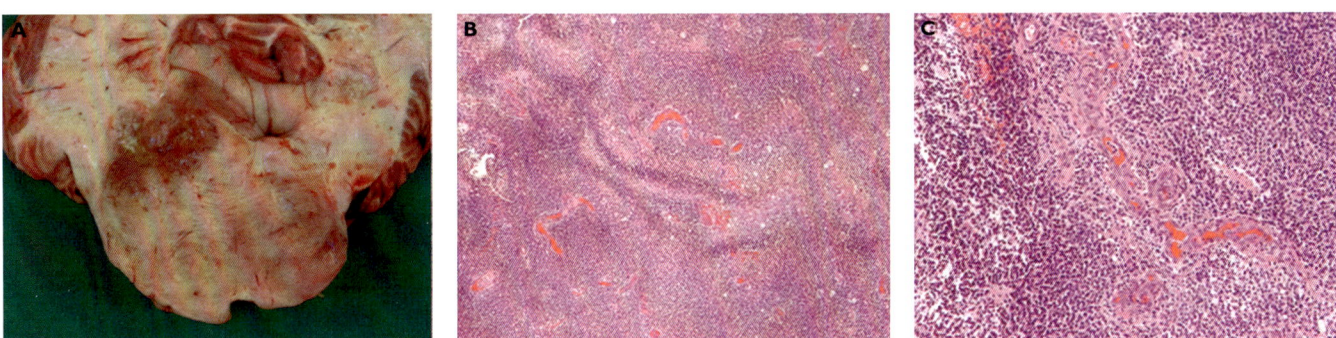

Figure 23.5 **(A)** Grossly, glioblastoma causes enlargement and distortion of the involved brain tissue. It is usually necrotic, hemorrhagic, and exhibits yellowish discoloration. Microscopically, the classical palisading of the neoplastic cells around areas of necrosis **(B)** and vascular endothelial proliferation **(C)** is seen. H&E, original magnification ×40 (B) and ×100 (C).

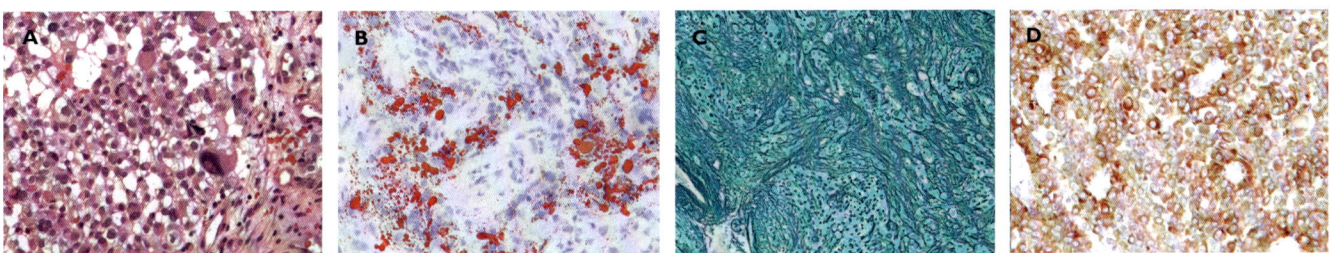

Figure 23.6 **(A)** PXA showing pleomorphic fibrillary astrocytes, including large, bizarre cells. H&E, original magnification ×200. **(B)** Oil red-O stain highlighting the intracellular lipid components in PXA. Original magnification ×200. **(C)** PXA typically exhibits an extensive reticulin network. Reticulin, original magnification ×40. **(D)** GFAP immunostain confirming the glial nature of the neoplastic cells in PXA. Original magnification ×200.

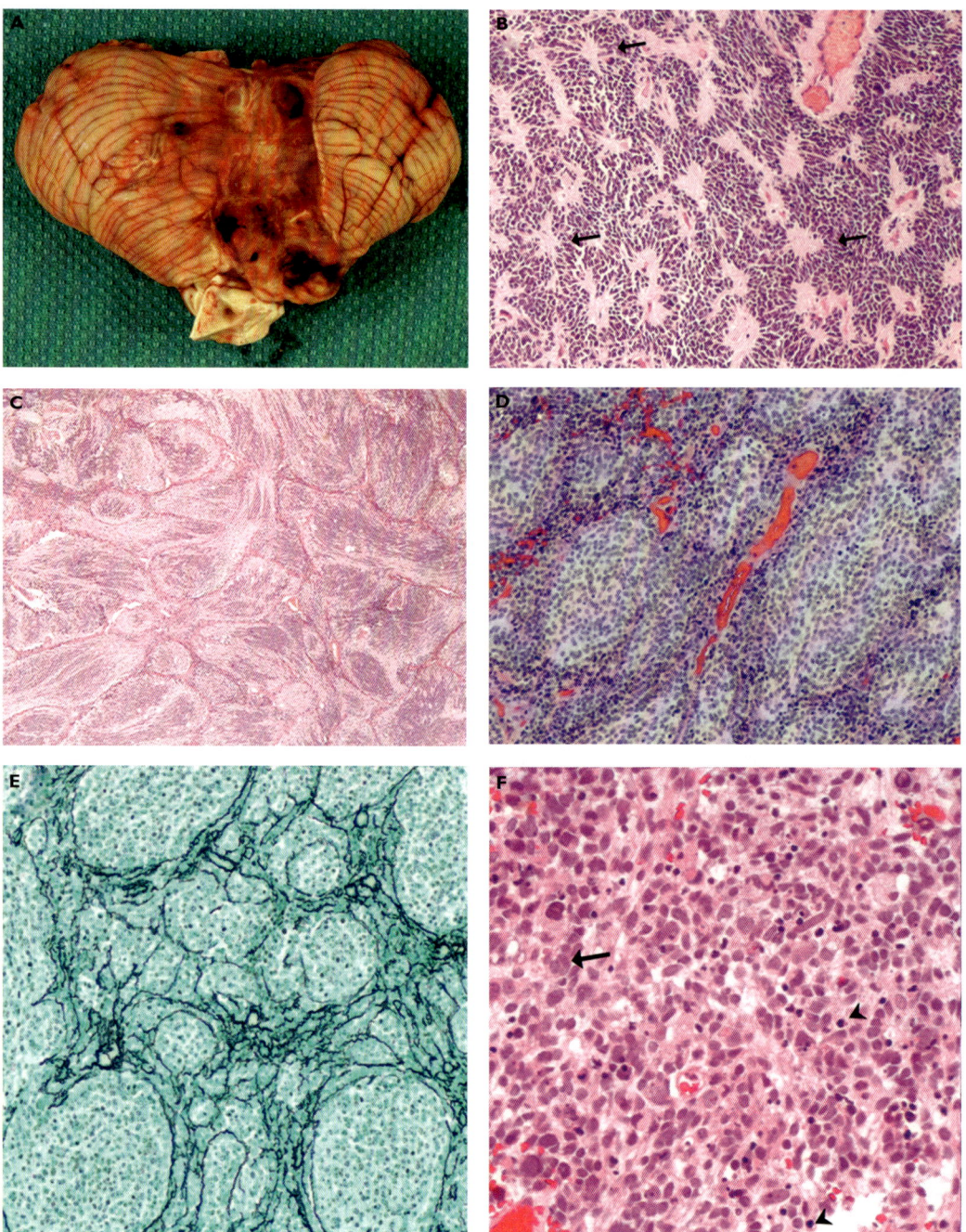

Figure 23.7 **(A)** Macroscopic appearance of a cerebellar medulloblastoma. **(B)** Small, round, blue cells arranged in rows and exhibiting Homer-Wright rosettes (arrows) in medulloblastoma. H&E, original magnification ×100. **(C)** Markedly prominent nodular pattern created by small, round, blue cells lying in a background of neuropil in medulloblastoma with extensive nodularity. H&E, original magnification ×40. **(D)** Desmoplastic medulloblastoma showing pale nodular areas in-between more cellular internodular regions. H&E, original magnification ×100. **(E)** Reticulin rich internodular regions in desmoplastic medulloblastoma. Reticulin, original magnification ×100. **(F)** Anaplastic medulloblastoma showing markedly pleomorphic cells, cell wrapping (arrow) and prominent apoptosis (arrowheads). H&E, original magnification ×200.

(Continued)

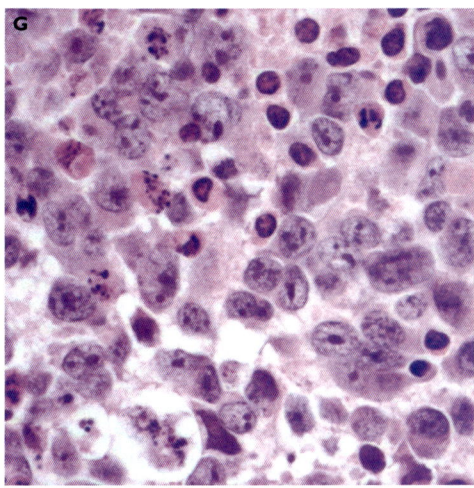

Figure 23.7 (*Continued*) **(G)** Large cell medulloblastoma showing large anaplastic cells with prominent nucleoli and vesicular chromatin. Note the prominent apoptosis. H&E, original magnification ×400.

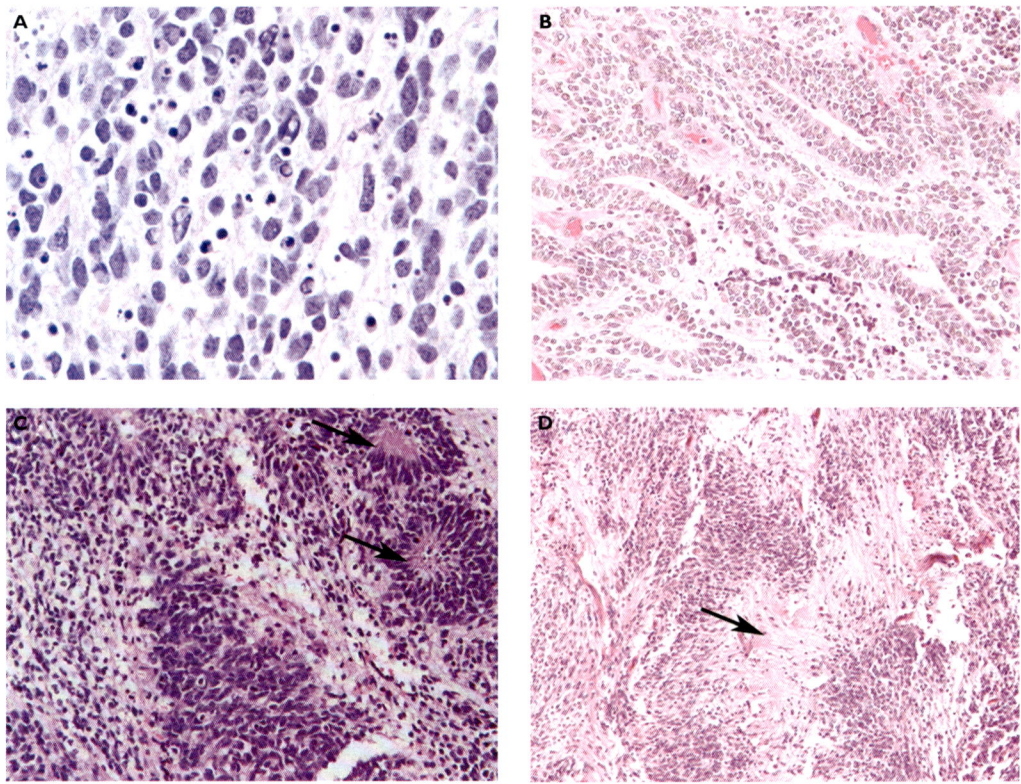

Figure 23.8 **(A)** sPNET showing a cellular neoplasm with hyperchromatic, anaplastic nuclei and numerous apoptotic bodies. H&E, original magnification ×200. **(B)** Medulloepithelioma showing the characteristic tubular structures mimicking the primitive neural tube. H&E, original magnification ×200. **(C)** Ependymoblastoma showing ependymoblastic, multilayered rosette formation (arrows) within sheets of round blue cells. H&E, original magnification ×200. **(D)** Embryonal tumor with abundant neuropil and true rosettes demonstrating the biphasic architecture with hypercellular regions abutting hypocellular fibrillar regions. H&E, original magnification ×100.

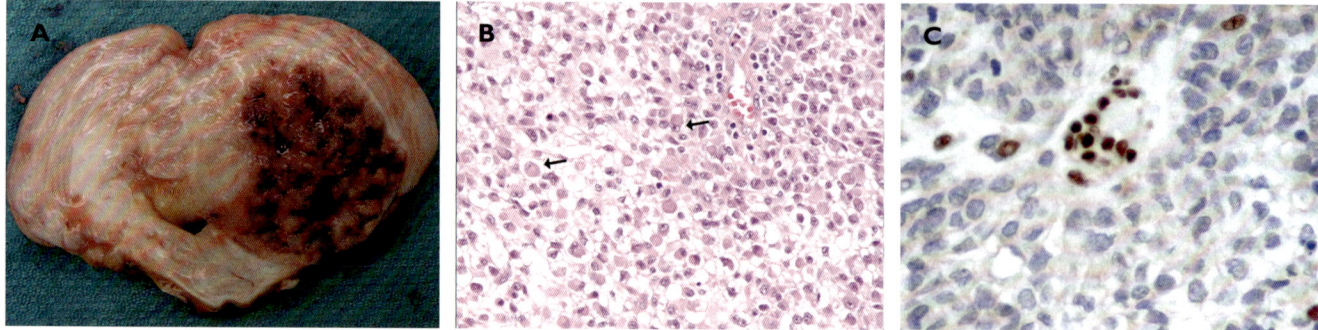

Figure 23.9 **(A)** A large destructive, hemorrhagic and necrotic mass occupying most of a cerebellar hemisphere that was found to be ATRT. **(B)** ATRT showing sheets of large pleomorphic cells, some of which exhibits globular cytoplasmic eosinophilic material that push the nucleus to the cell edges (arrows). Note the prominent nucleoli within vesicular nuclei. H&E, original magnification ×100. **(C)** In ATRT, the tumor cells are negative for INI-1. Also present are scattered lymphocytes and a vessel (center of the picture) that show normal, positive, nuclear staining for INI-1. Original magnification ×200.

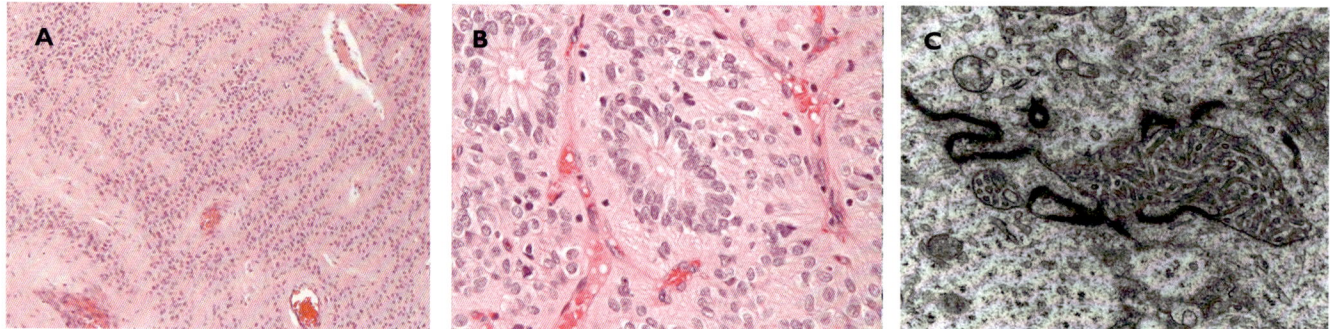

Figure 23.10 **(A)** Ependymoma showing small, bland cells within a fibrillary background. Note the perivascular nuclear-free zones that are a typical, low-power appearance of ependymoma. H&E, original magnification ×100. **(B)** True ependymal rosettes with the formation of lumens are sometimes found in ependymoma. H&E, original magnification ×200. **(C)** Ultrastructural features of an ependymoma showing microvilli in lumina and long intracellular junctions.

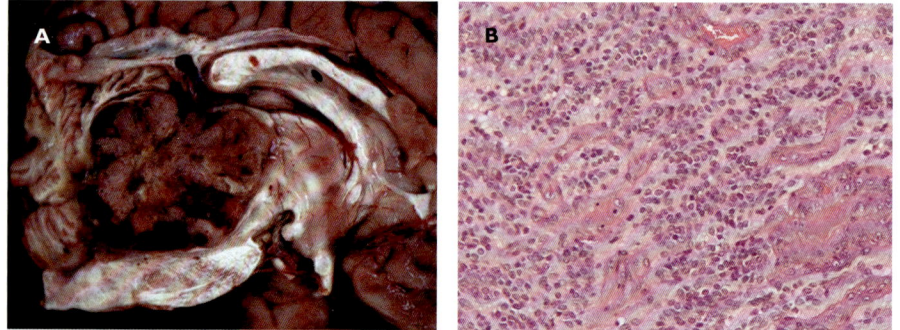

Figure 23.11 **(A)** Gross appearance of an anaplastic ependymoma showing a soft, fleshy, and well-demarcated mass protruding into the lumen of the fourth ventricle. **(B)** Anaplastic ependymoma showing increased cellularity and abundant vascular-endothelial proliferation.

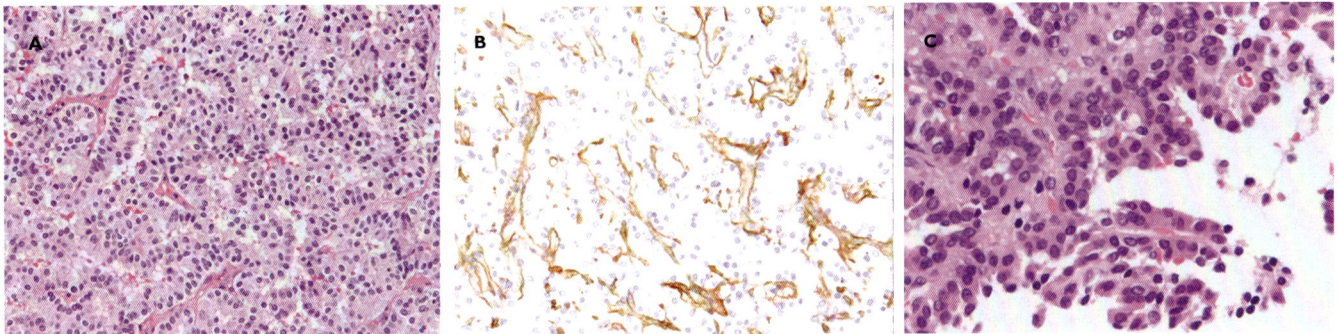

Figure 23.12 **(A)** Choroid-plexus papilloma showing the papillary architecture where the papillae are formed by fibrovascular stroma with overlying columnar epithelium. H&E, original magnification ×200. **(B)** Immunohistochemical staining for laminin highlighting the basement membrane in CPP. Original magnification ×200. **(C)** The epithelial cells lining the papillae are slightly crowded and exhibit minor atypical changes such as mild nuclear pleomorphism and hyperchromasia. H&E, original magnification ×400.

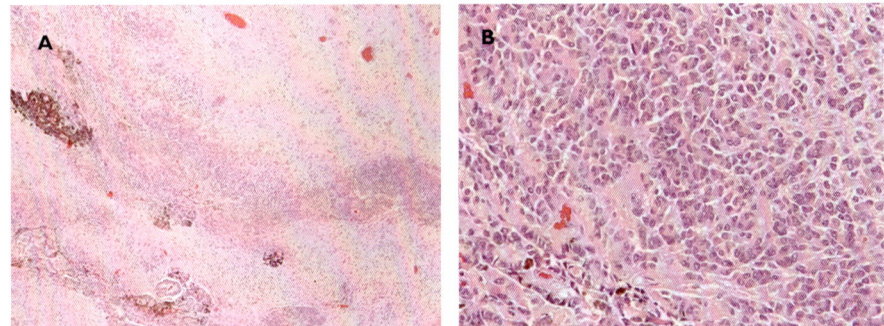

Figure 23.13 **(A)** Choroid plexus carcinoma showing sheets of anaplastic tumor cells that are invading adjacent brain tissue. Melanization of some of the tumor cells can be seen. H&E, original magnification ×40. **(B)** A higher-power view of the tumor showing nuclear atypia, blurring of the papillary pattern, and increased cell density compared with CPP. H&E, original magnification ×200.

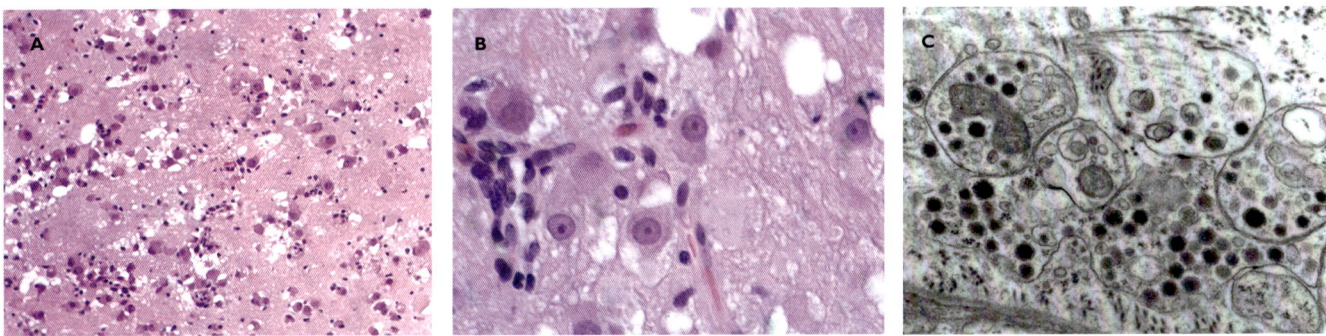

Figure 23.14 **(A)** Ganglioglioma showing scattered ganglion cells within a rich fibrillary background. H&E, original magnification ×40. **(B)** Ganglion cells are large cells with prominent nucleoli and abundant eosinophilic cytoplasm; some contain basophilic Nissl substance in the periphery of the cytoplasm. H&E, original magnification ×400. **(C)** Ultrastructurally, electron-dense neurosecretory vesicles can be seen in the cytoplasm of the tumor cells.

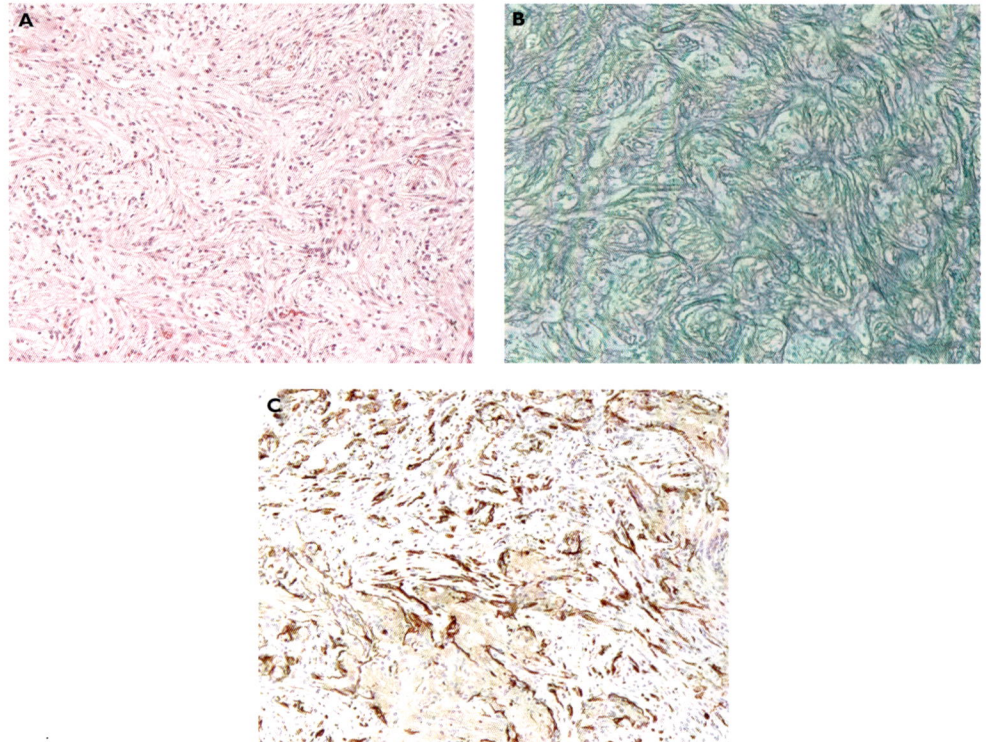

Figure 23.15 **(A)** Desmoplastic infantile ganglioglioma/astroctyoma showing fascicles of spindled astrocytes within a desmoplastic stroma that is highlighted with reticulin staining **(B)**. **(C)** Immunohistochemical staining is positive for GFAP. All pictures original magnification ×100.

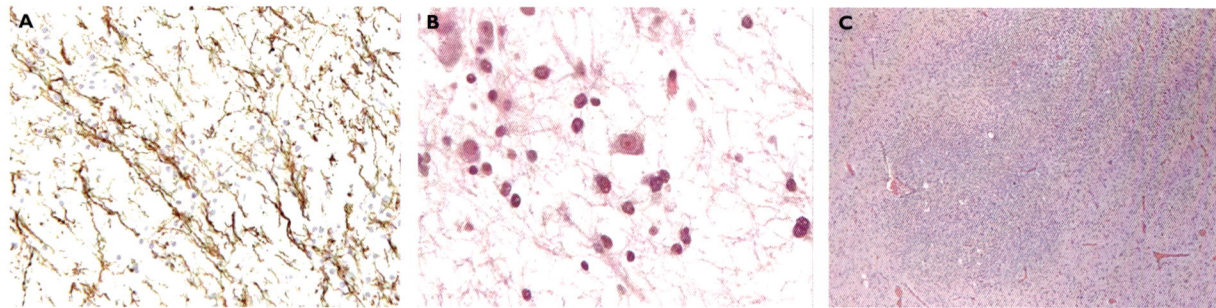

Figure 23.16 **(A)** DNET showing the typical glioneuronal component. The axons are highlighted with immunohistochemical staining for neurofilament. Original magnification ×200. **(B)** Within the hypocellular myxoid areas of DNET, scattered, floating neurons are present. H&E, original magnification ×400. **(C)** Tumor nodules within the cortex in a case of complex DNET. H&E, original magnification ×40.

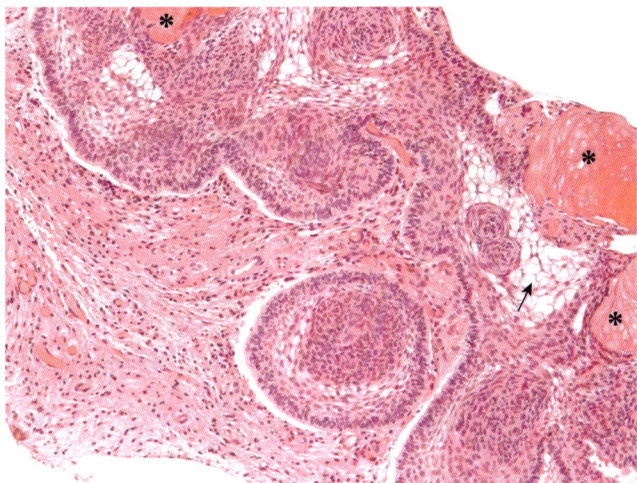

Figure 23.17 Craniopharyngioma showing palisaded epithelial cells, the loose stellate reticulum (arrow) and wet keratin (*). H&E, original magnification ×100.

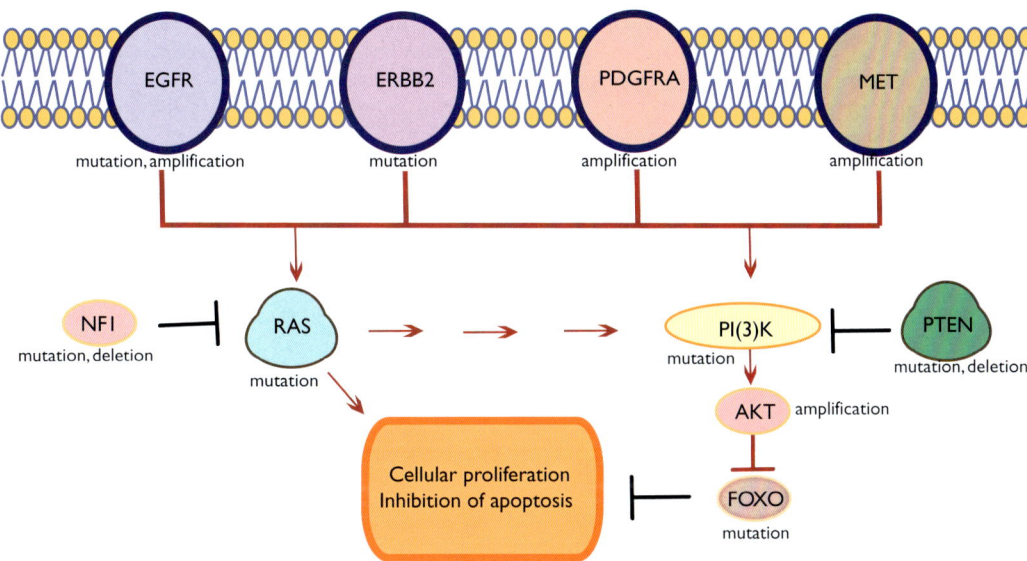

Figure 24.3 The activated RAS pathway in high-grade astrocytomas is illustrated. Arrows highlighted in *red* are activated, whereas those in *black* are suppressed. The net effect is cellular proliferation and inhibition of apoptosis.

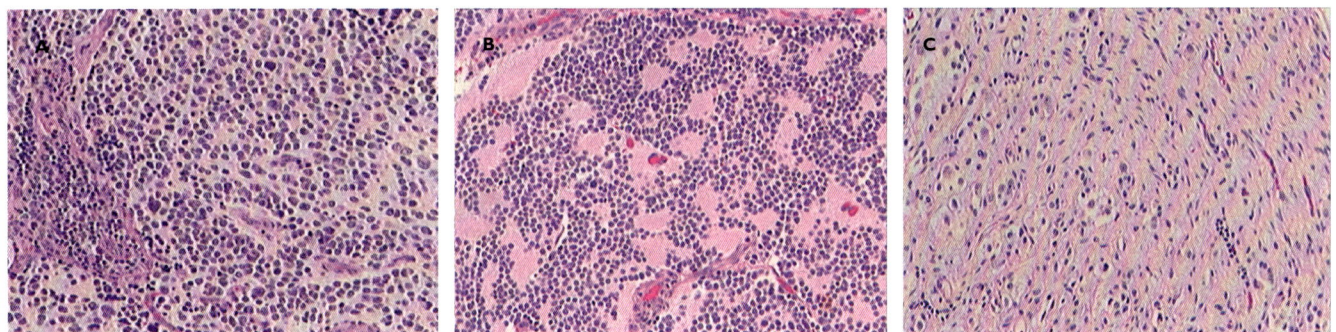

Figure 25.3 Histopathology of neuroblastoma tumors. **(A)** Neuroblastoma that is categorized as undifferentiated and stroma poor with a high MKI (mitosis–karryorhexis index), **(B)** Neuroblastoma that is poorly differentiated with a lower MKI and classic rosette formation of tumor cells. **(C)** Ganglioneuroblastoma with significant areas of well-differentiated larger cells, stroma rich, and dense neuropil. Images, courtesy of Dr. Paul Thorner, Department of Laboratory Medicine and Pathology, Hospital for Sick Children.

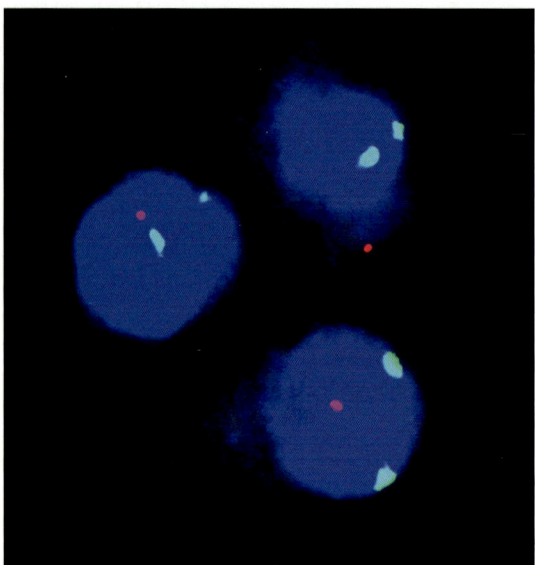

Figure 25.4 1p deletion in neuroblastoma detected by FISH (Fluourescence In situ hybridization). Tumor-cell nuclei are stained in blue (DAPI staining). Loss of 1p chromosome is demonstrated by staining of a single 1p allele in each cell (with a probe labeled with red fluorescence). By contrast, two 1q alleles are detected with the 1q probe labeled with light-blue fluorescence. Images provided by the Dr. Mary Shago, Cytogenetics Laboratory, Hospital for Sick Children, Toronto, Ontario.

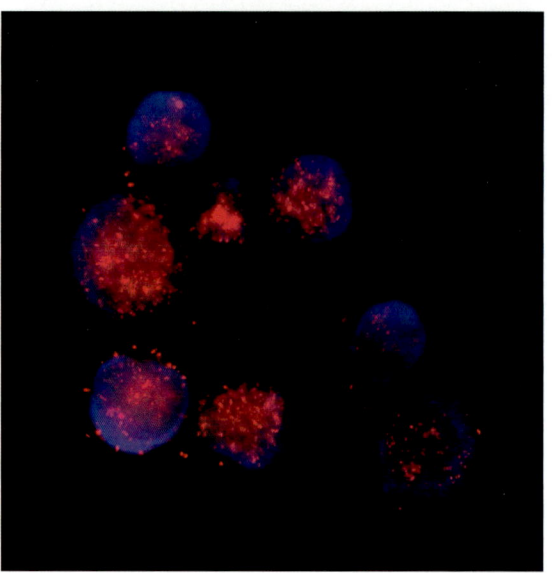

Figure 25.5 N-myc amplification. FISH using a probe to N-myc (labeled with red fluorescence) demonstrates high levels of N-myc in nuclei of tumor cells (nuclei are stained in blue). Amplification of N-myc is defined as greater than 10 copies of N-myc genes detected per cell as per the INRG (International Neuroblastoma Risk Group) guidelines. Images provided by the Dr. Mary Shago, Cytogenetics Laboratory, Hospital for Sick Children, Toronto, Ontario.

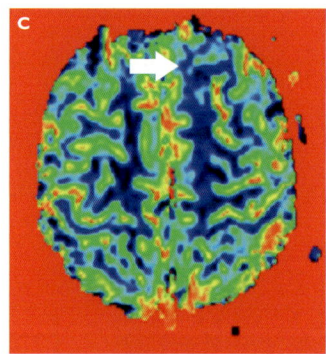

Figure 44.4C Grade II astrocytoma. Shows lesion to have mild increased rCBV (arrow). Long TE (TE=135) CSI MRS.

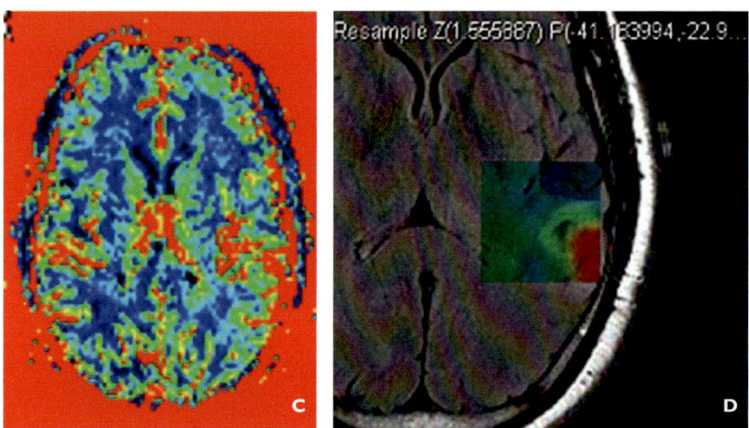

Figure 44.6 Grade III astrocytoma: **(C)** Axial DSC rCBV perfusion map (red denotes higher rCBV) shows lesion to have mild increased rCBV (arrow) as compared with the contralateral side. **(D)** 3D Spectroscopy choline map superimposed upon the FLAIR axial image shows heterogeneity in the tumor with the outer regions showing greater cell turn over (red) as compared to the medial portions of the tumor. Individual spectra from within the tumor confirm much lower Naa values and slightly higher Cho/Cr ratio at the outer.

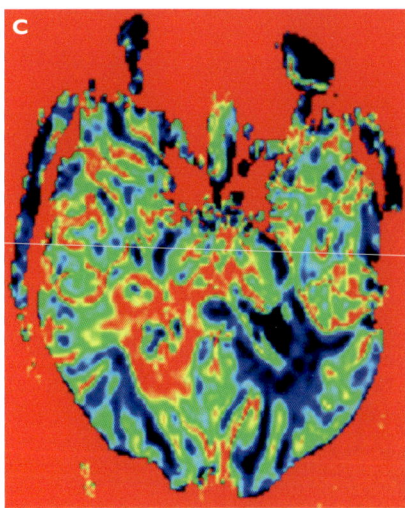

Figure 44.9C Grade IV astrocytoma: Axial DSC rCBV perfusion map (areas in red are higher rCBV) shows lesion to have markedly increased rCBV (arrow) as compared with the contralateral side.

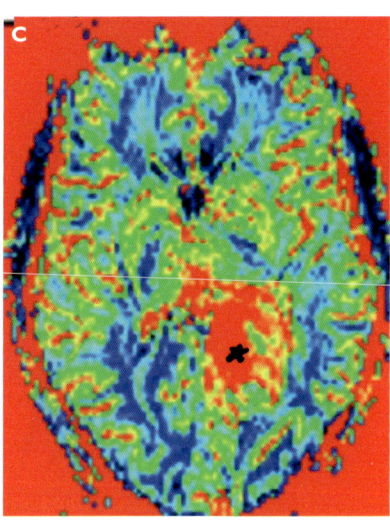

Figure 44.10C Oligodendroglioma with 1q/p19 loss exhibit greater rCBV and may appear radiologically more aggressive than those tumors without this mutation. Axial DSC rCBV perfusion map shows lesion (asterisk) to have markedly increased rCBV (areas in red are higher rCBV) as compared with the contralateral side.

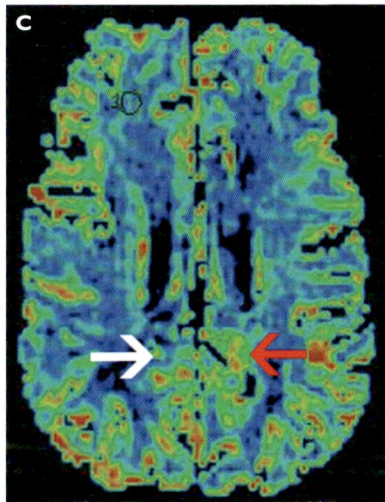

Figure 44.11C Oligodendroglioma without 1q/p19 loss exhibit only mild rCBV elevation and may appear radiologically less aggressive than those tumors without this mutation. Axial DSC rCBV perfusion map (areas in red are higher rCBV) shows lesion to have only minimally increased rCBV (red arrow) as compared with the contralateral side (white arrow).

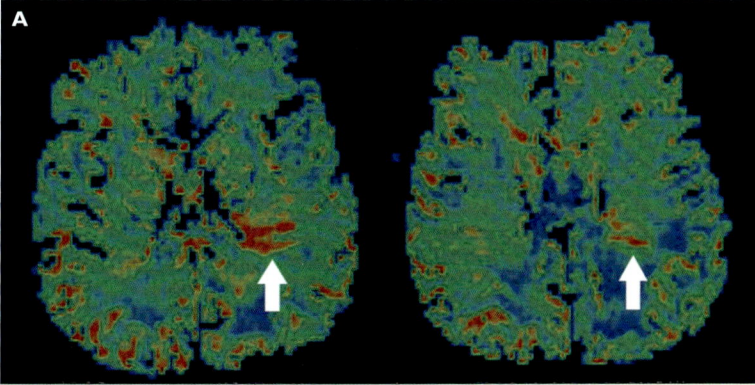

Figure 44.19 Lymphoma: **(A)** Axial DSC rCBV perfusion map (areas in red are higher rCBV) shows lesion to have increased rCBV (arrow) as compared with the contralateral side (white arrow).

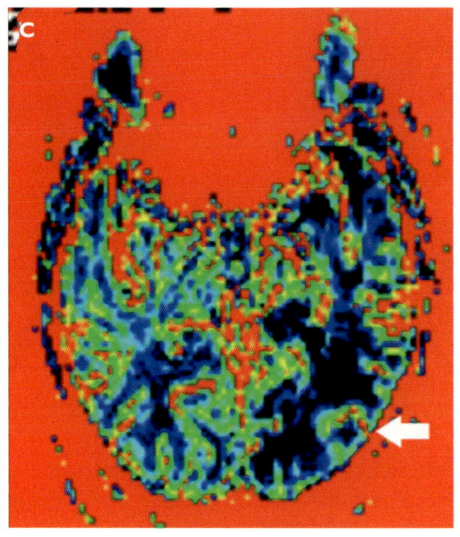

Figure 44.21C Metastatic disease: Shows lesion to have increased rCBV (arrow) surrounded by decreased rCBV. Metastases typically have low rCBV in the peritumoral edema whereas primary brain neoplasms have normal or even increased rCBV in the peritumoral region.

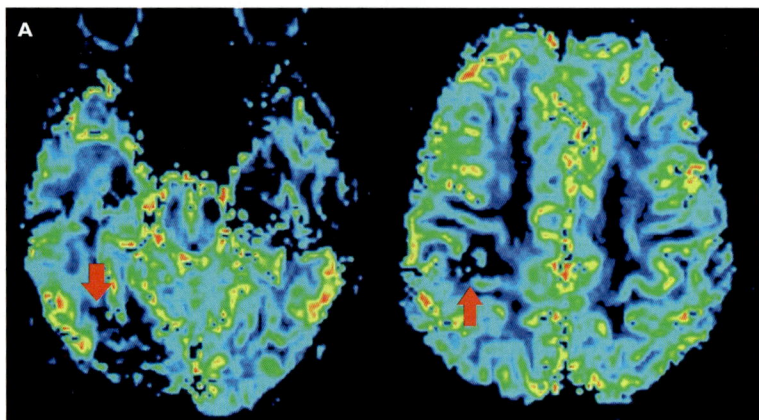

Figure 44.23A Postradiation changes: Axial DSC rCBV perfusion map (dark areas are lower rCBV) shows areas that enhance on the axial T1 postcontrast.

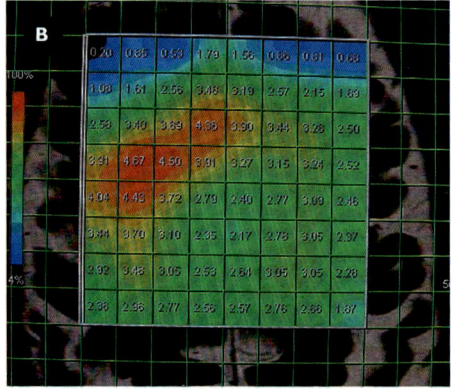

Figure 44.24B 3D MRS—Biopsy guidance. Using a 3D MR spectroscopy choline map can guide surgical biopsy to the areas of greatest cell turnover denoted in red.

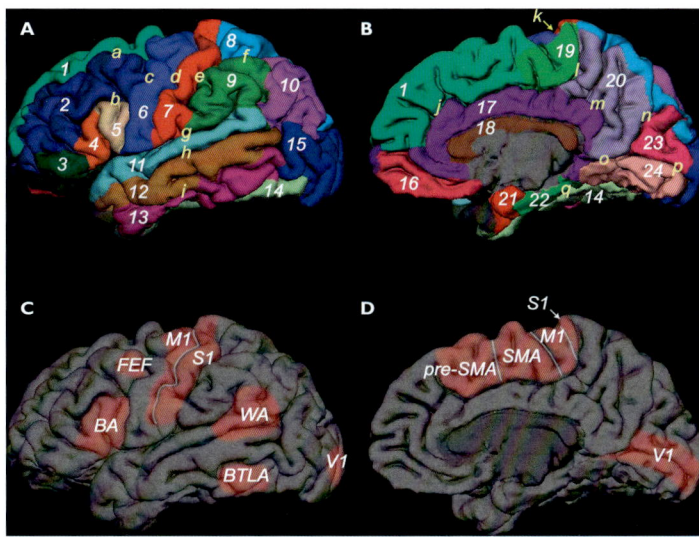

Figure 45.1 Brain surface gyral, sulcal, and functional anatomy. The lateral (**A**) and mesial (**B**) brain surface is shown, with gyri identified by white numbers and sulci by yellow letters. 1. Superior frontal gyrus; 2. middle frontal gyrus; 3. inferior frontal gyrus (IFG) pars orbitalis; 4. IFG pars triangularis; 5. IFG pars opercularis; 6. precentral gyrus; 7. postcentral gyrus; 8. superior parietal lobule; 9. supramarginal gyrus of inferior parietal lobule; 10. angular gyrus of inferior parietal lobule; 11. superior temporal gyrus; 12. middle temporal gyrus; 13. inferior temporal gyrus; 14. fusiform gyrus; 15. lateral occipital gyrus; 16. medial orbitofrontal cortex; 17. cingulate gyrus; 18. corpus callosum; 19. paracentral lobule; 20. precuneus; 21. entorhinal cortex; 22. parahippocampal gyrus; 23. cuneus; 24. lingual gyrus. a. superior frontal sulcus; b. inferior frontal sulcus; c. precentral sulcus; d. central sulcus; e. postcentral sulcus; f. intraparietal sulcus; g. Sylvian fissure; h. superior temporal sulcus; i. inferior temporal sulcus; j. cingulate sulcus; k. central sulcus; l. marginal branch of cingulate sulcus; m. subparietal sulcus; n. parieto-occipital sulcus; o. anterior calcarine sulcus; p. calcarine sulcus; q. collateral sulcus. Panels (**C**) and (**D**) respectively show lateral and medial surfaces with classical functional regions highlighted. BA, Broca's area; FEF, frontal eye fields; M1, primary motor cortex; S1, primary sensory cortex; WA, Wernicke's area; BTLA, basal temporal language area; V1, primary visual cortex; SMA, supplementary motor area; pre-SMA, pre-supplementary motor area.

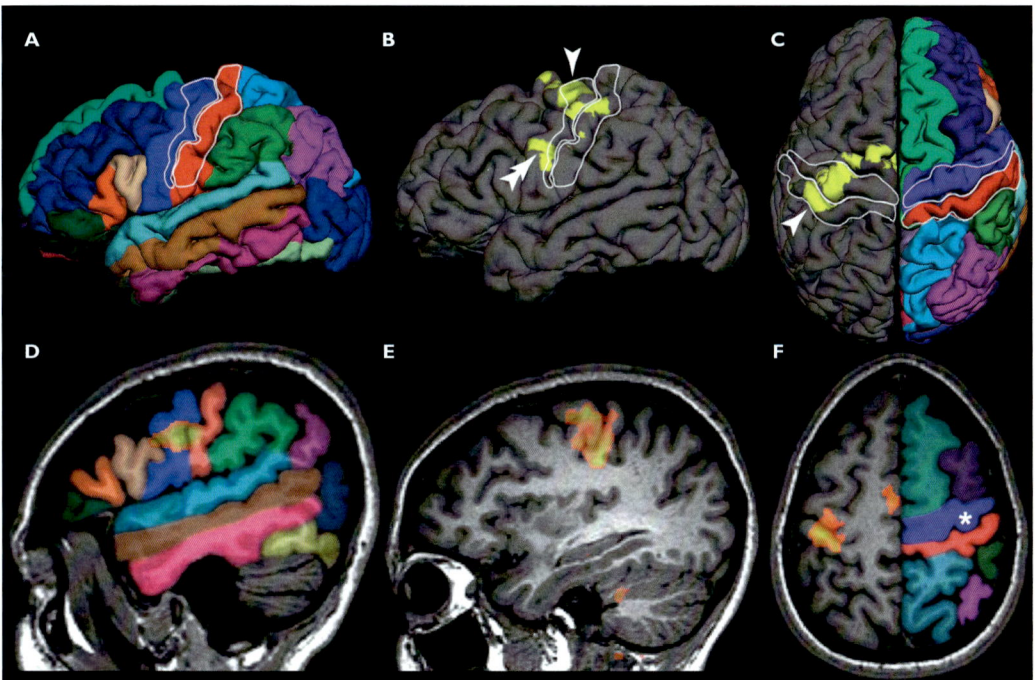

Figure 45.2 Sensorimotor functional anatomy. Panel (**A**) shows the lateral cortical surface with primary sensorimotor cortex demarcated as in Figure 45.1. Functional MRI activations during hand clenching (arrowhead) and tongue movement (double arrowhead) tasks are shown superimposed over the lateral (**B**) and superior (**C**) surfaces. Note that motor tasks such as hand clenching typically activate both primary motor and primary somatosensory cortex. Panel (**D**) shows a sagittal T1-weighted slice through the tongue activation, showing its proximity to Broca's area. Panels (**E**) and (**F**) show sagittal and axial slices through the hand activation, respectively. Task-induced SMA activation can be seen anterior to primary motor cortex in (**C**) and (**F**). The omega-shaped knob demarcating the hand region of sensorimotor cortex is denoted by an asterisk in (**F**). Of note, the orientation of panel (**F**) is opposite that of radiological convention (the fMRI activation is on the left side), in order to visually correspond with (**C**), which is a top-down view.

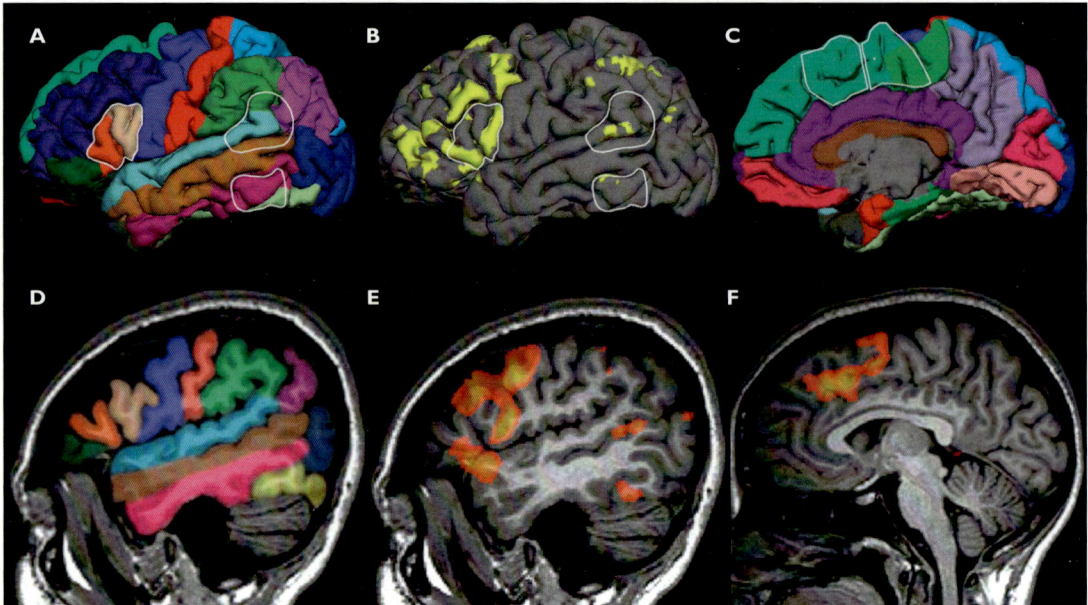

Figure 45.3 Language surface functional anatomy. Panel **(A)** shows the lateral cortical surface with classical language regions demarcated as in Figure 45.1, including Broca's area anteriorly, Wernicke's area posteriorly, and the basal temporal language area (BTLA) inferiorly. Functional MRI activations during a visually presented covert verb generation task are shown over the lateral surface in **(B)**. The SMA and pre-SMA are demarcated on the mesial surface in **(C)**. Panel **(D)** shows gyral anatomy in a lateral T1-weighted sagittal slice. Activation of Broca's area, Wernicke's area, and the BTLA, as well as other prefrontal regions is seen on a lateral sagittal slice **(E)**, and activation of pre-SMA and SMA on a mesial slice **(F)**.

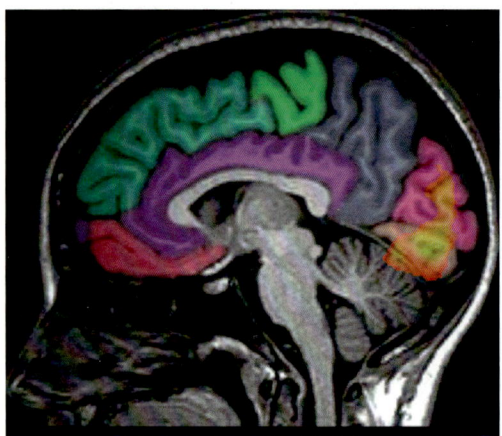

Figure 45.4 Visual surface functional anatomy. A sagittal paramedian T1-weighted slice is shown with a superimposed functional MRI activation during a visual task (flashing checkerboard). The activation is centered over primary visual cortex (banks of the calcarine sulcus) and extends into higher order visual cortices in the occipital lobe. The color scheme corresponds to that in Figure 45.1.

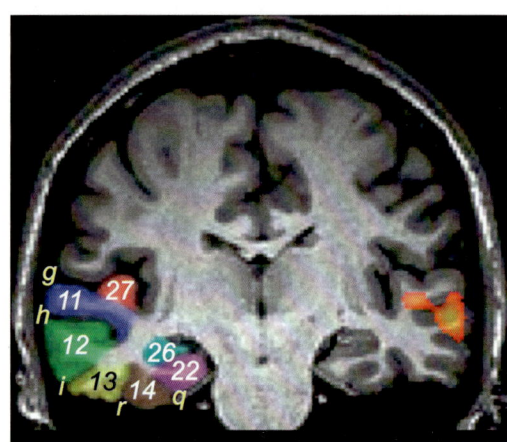

Figure 45.5 Temporal lobe and auditory surface functional anatomy. A coronal T1-weighted slice is shown, with temporal lobe gyri indicated with white numbers and sulci with yellow letters, continuing the same identification scheme as in Figure 45.1. 11. Superior temporal gyrus; 12. middle temporal gyrus; 13. inferior temporal gyrus; 14. fusiform gyrus; 22. parahippocampal gyrus; 26. hippocampal formation; 27. Heschl's gyrus (primary auditory cortex). g. Sylvian fissure; h. superior temporal sulcus; i. inferior temporal sulcus; q. collateral sulcus; r. lateral occipitotemporal sulcus. Functional MRI activation during an auditory task (passive listening to short tones) is shown on the left side, activating primary auditory cortex in the base of Heschl's gyrus as well as auditory association cortices in the superior temporal gyrus. Although the activation was bilateral, only the left side is shown for clarity.

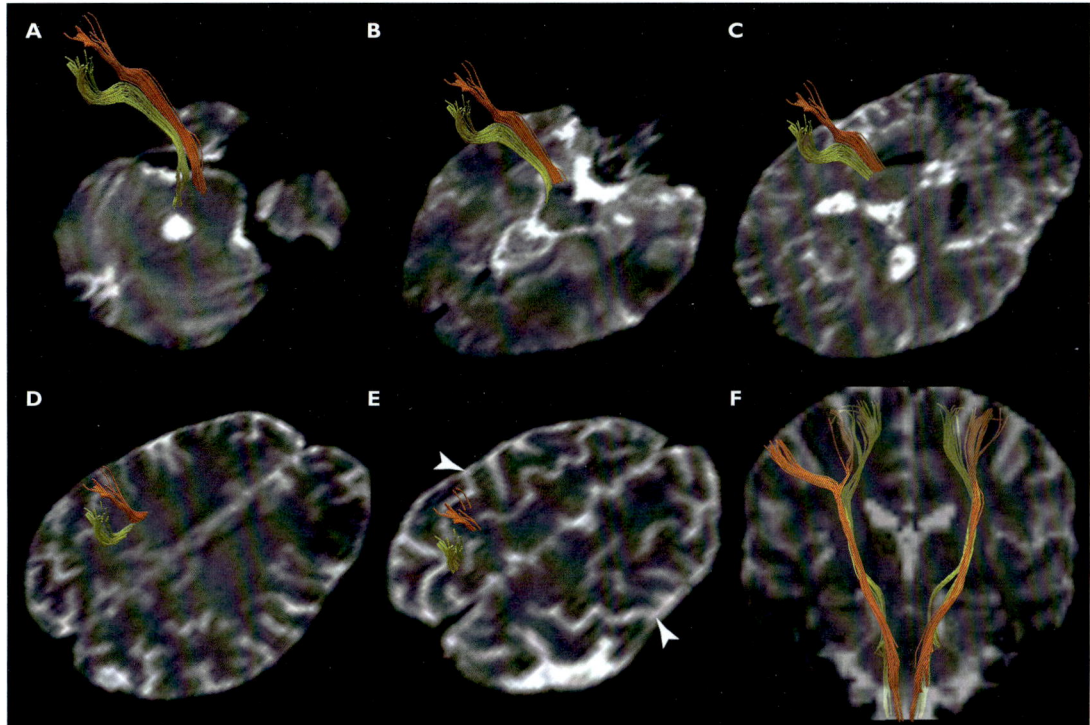

Figure 45.6 Sensorimotor white matter tractography. Diffusion tensor imaging tractography maps of the descending motor corticospinal tract (orange) and ascending somatosensory tracts (yellow; the posterior column-medial lemniscus and spinothalamic systems are not distinguishable) are shown with cross sectional axial T2-weighted slices at various levels through their course. Motor fibers travel in the basis pontis **(A)** and the cerebral peduncles of the midbrain **(B)** ventral to the sensory fibers. Both systems travel through the posterior limb of the internal capsule **(C)** and corona radiata **(D)**. The motor fibers originate largely from the precentral gyrus and sensory fibers terminate in the postcentral gyrus **(E)**. The central sulcus is indicated by arrowheads. The entire course of these motor and sensory systems through the brain and brainstem can be appreciated on the coronal slice **(F)**.

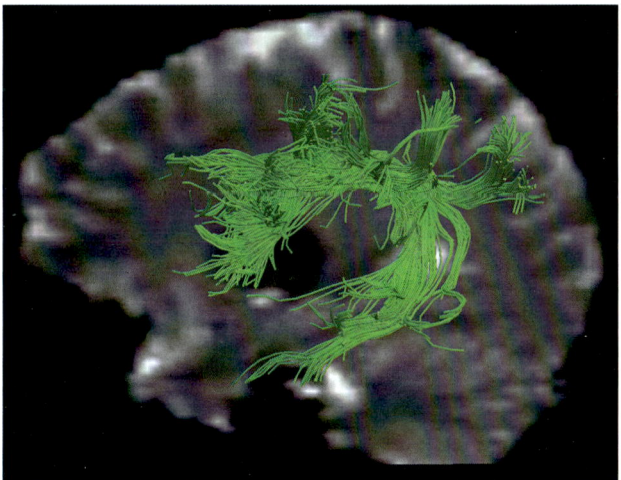

Figure 45.7 Superior longitudinal fasciculus white matter tractography. The superior longitudinal fasciculus (SLF) was constructed using DTI and shown overlaid on a sagittal T2-weighted image. The central tract follows an arcuate course around the Sylvian fissure, with fiber bundles penetrating the temporal, parietal, and frontal lobes. Connections mediated by the SLF allow regulation of motor behavior, visuospatial attention, and language articulation.

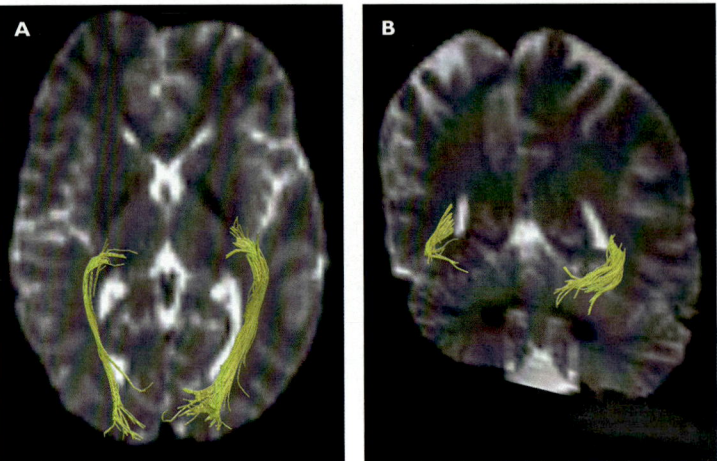

Figure 45.8 Optic radiations white matter tractography. Fibers of the optic radiations, as estimated using DTI, are shown overlaid on an axial (**A**) and coronal (**B**, as viewed from anterior) T2-weighted slice. The fibers course posteriorly from the posterolateral thalamus (lateral geniculate nucleus), along the lateral edge of the temporal and occipital horns of the lateral ventricles, toward the occipital lobe (A). Their relation to the lateral wall of the temporal horns can be appreciated in (B).

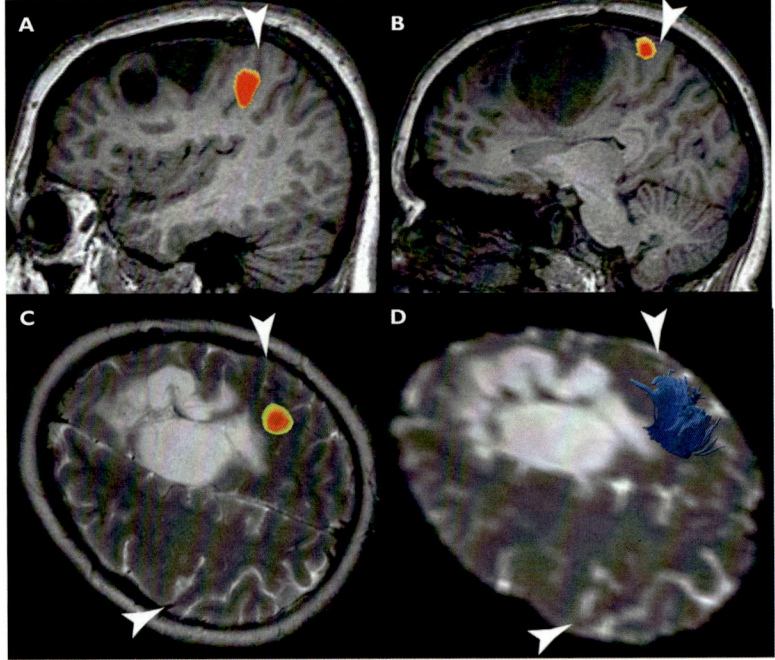

Figure 45.9 Identification of functional anatomy distorted by a mass lesion using fMRI and DTI. Despite the presence of this left frontal tumor (anaplastic oligodendroglioma, WHO grade III/IV), fMRI activations of the hand (**A,C**) and foot (**B,D**) sensorimotor regions were reliably identifiable. DTI maps were also able to determine the trajectory of primary motor and somatosensory white matter tracts, which course through the posterior T2 signal abnormality. The central sulcus is denoted with arrowheads. The availability of this functional information can help identify distorted anatomy intraoperatively and assist in preservation of function during resection.

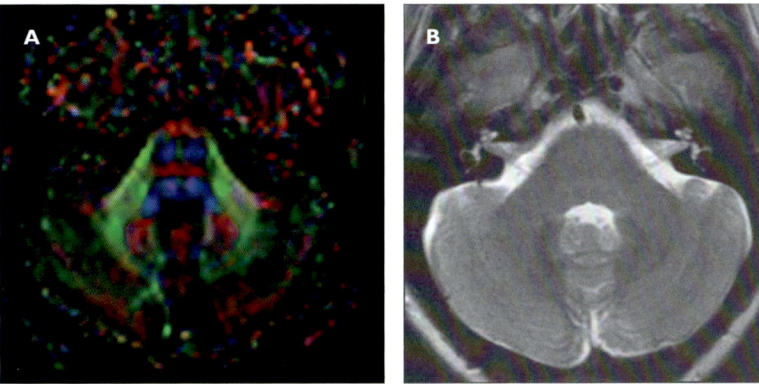

Figure 45.10 Brain stem white matter tractography. An axial DTI map through the level of the pons is shown with colors indicating principal fiber directions (red, left-right; green, anterior-posterior; blue, superior-inferior) **(A)**. An axial T2-weighted slice through the same region is provided for anatomical reference **(B)**. The corticospinal tract (blue) runs rostro-caudally in the basis pontis, amongst the pontine nuclei. The pontocerebellar fibers (red) cross horizontally ventral and dorsal to the corticospinal tract. Fibers traveling in the middle cerebellar peduncle (green) to the cerebellum course postero-laterally. The pontine tegmentum contains numerous tracts running rostro-caudally (blue), including the medial lemniscus, spinothalamic tract, medial longitudinal fasciculus, and others.

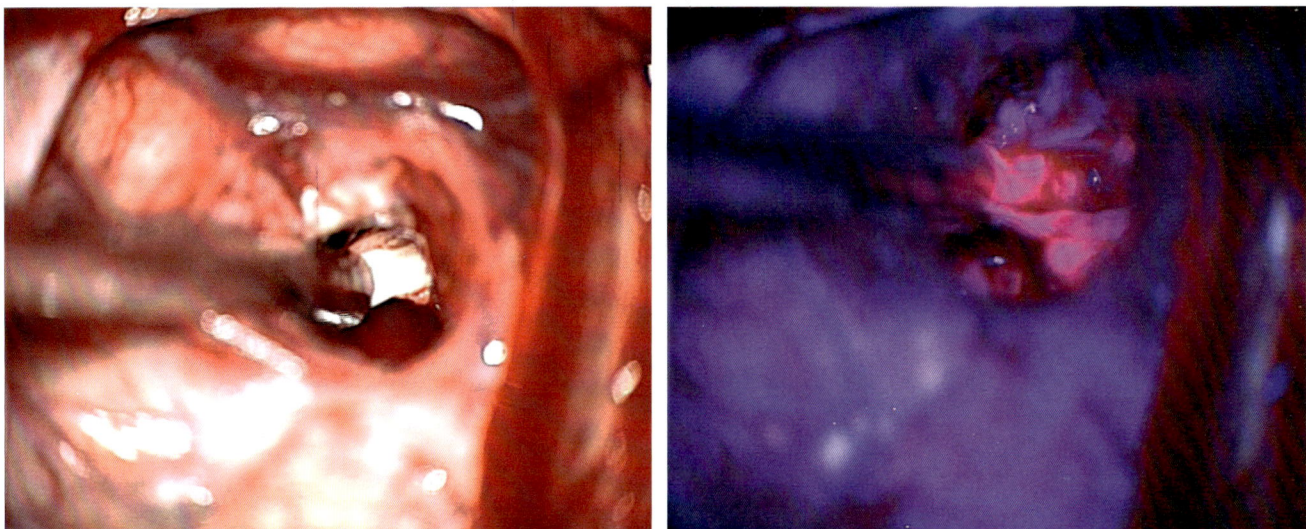

Figure 50.1 Visualization of residual tumor through intraoperative fluorescence imaging with 5-ALA.

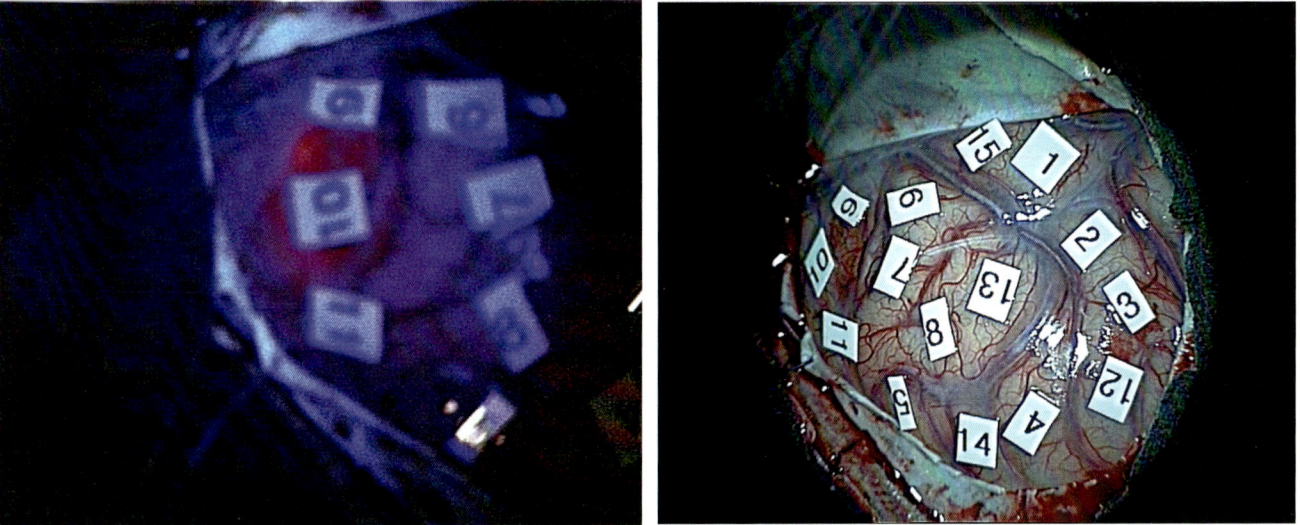

Figure 50.2 Combining fluorescence for visualizing the cortical extension of the tumor with language mapping for determining function.

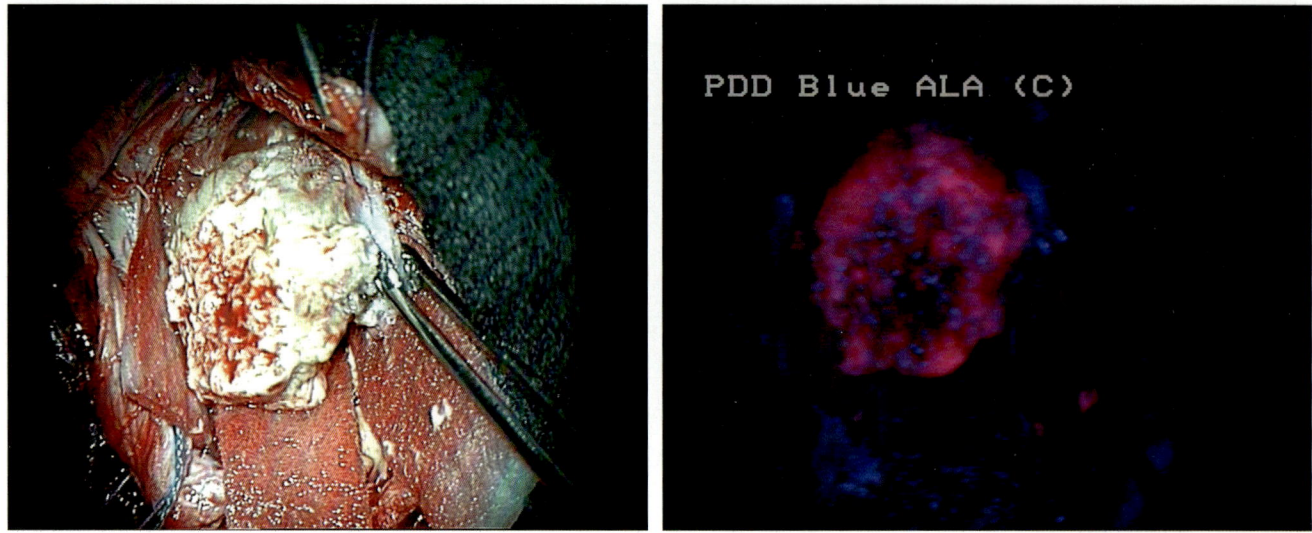

Figure 50.3 Atypical meningioma. Left: white light, Right: blue-violet illumination.

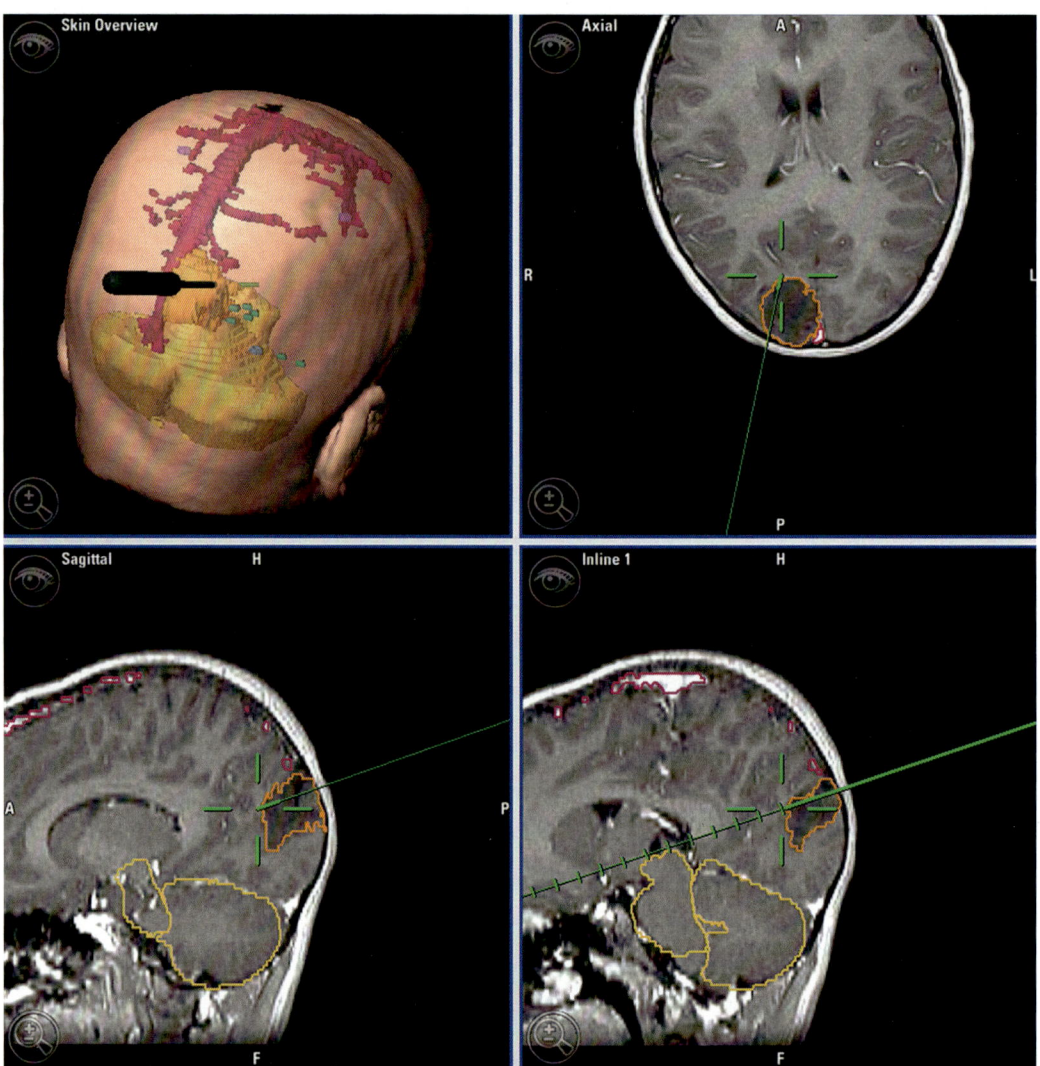

Figure 60.3 Utility of MEG demonstrated while linked to frameless stereotaxy in 8-year-old male with visual scintillations and right occipital tumor. The green squares to the right of the tumor mass (orange) represent the location of the interictal spike waves from the EEG. Using MEG, we can also map the visual evoked fields in the calcarine cortex, so as to attempt to preserve visual indices as best as possible.

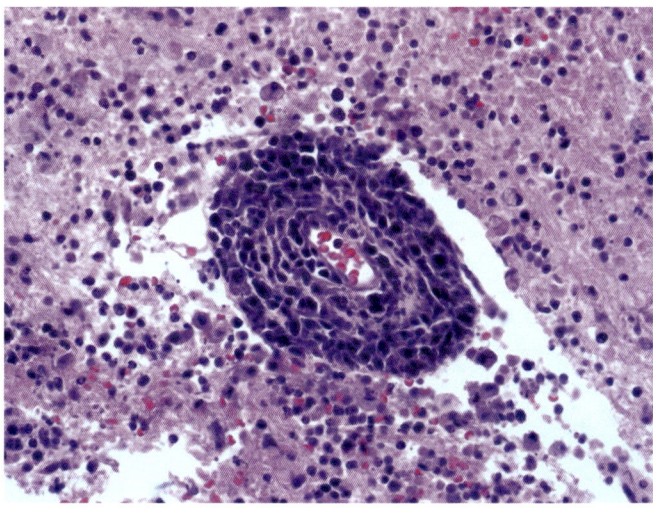

Figure 72.1 Perivascular growth pattern of a B-cell primary CNS lymphoma Hematoxylin Eosin at 400× magnification.

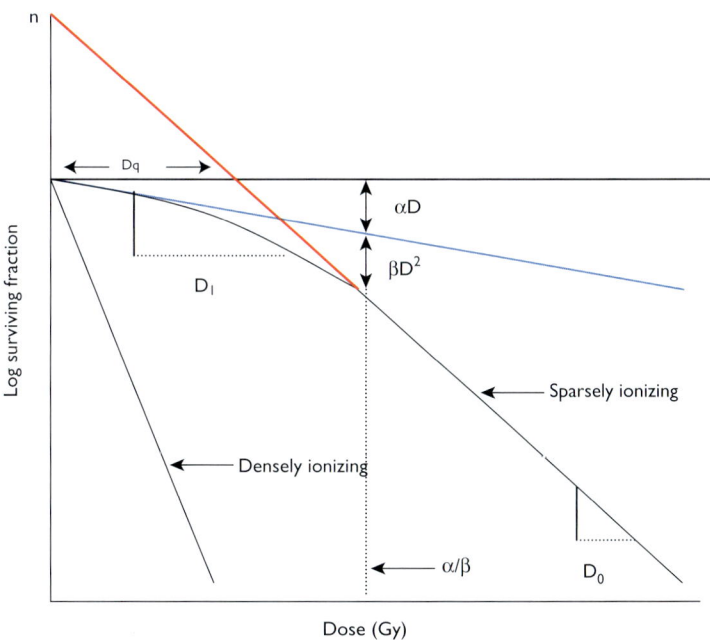

Figure 81.7 Mammalian cell survival curve for densely and sparsely ionizing radiation. D_q and n define the width of the shoulder region. D_1 is the initial slope where cell killing is proportional to dose (αD). D_0 represents the final slope where cell killing is proportional to the dose squared (βD^2). The α/β ratio for the cell population is defined when the linear (αD) component of cell killing is equal to the quadratic (βD^2).

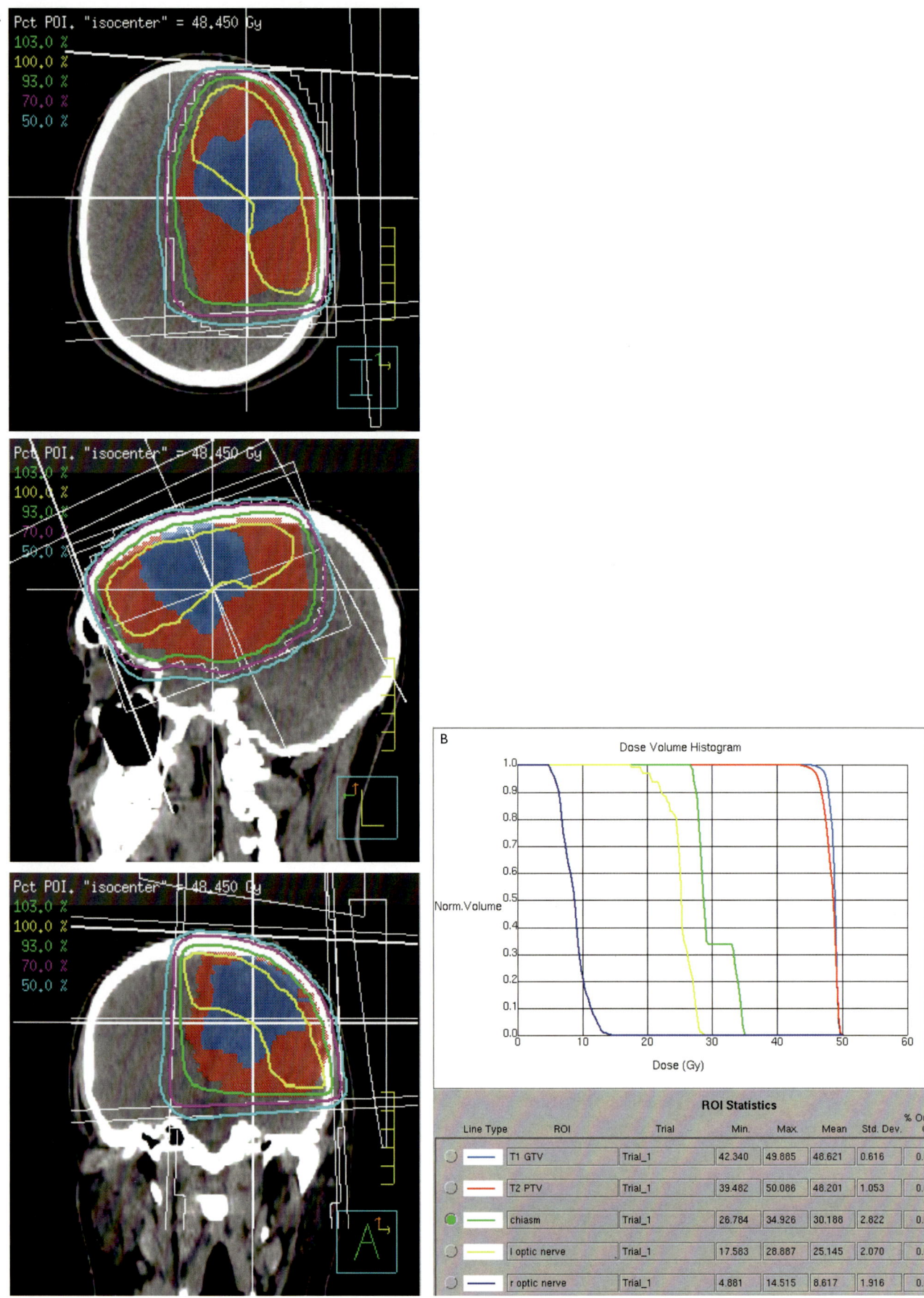

Figure 81.8 **(A)** Typical 3D conformal plan for a GBM. **(B)** Dose-volume histogram (DVH) showing the dose and volume related to the different structures within the treatment plan.

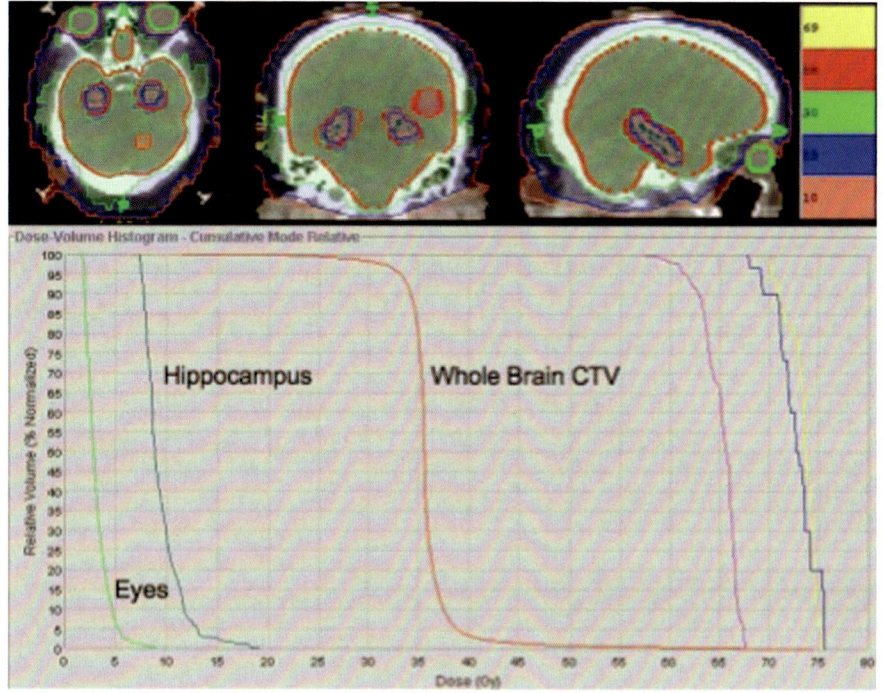

Figure 81.10 Tomotherapy plan showing sparing of the hippocampus while escalating doses to the metastatic tumors. This is done in an effort to simultaneously improving local control while sparing neurcognition.

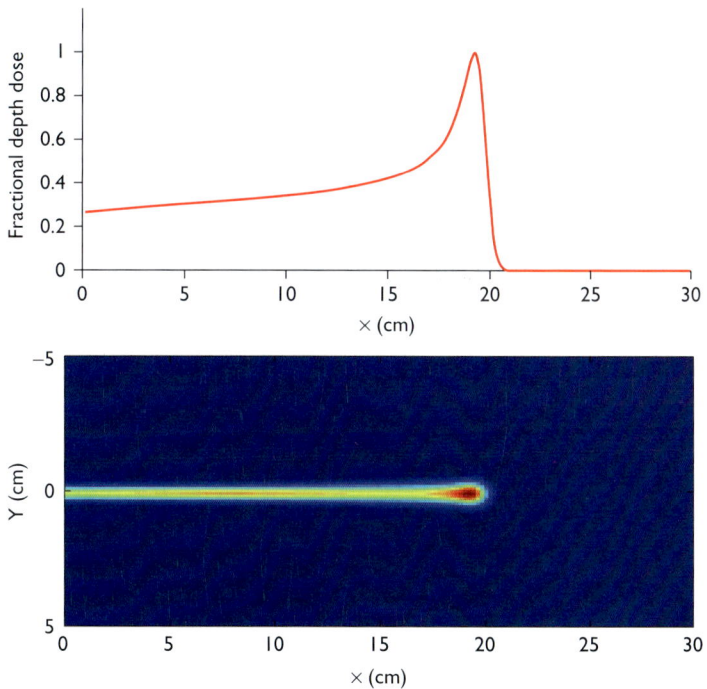

Figure 81.12 Fractional depth dose in water of a 170 MeV proton beam having a full width half maximum of 8mm. There is a rapid rise and then a fall off with little exit dose (Bragg Peak.) The associated proton pencil beam is shown below the fractional depth dose curve. (Courtesy of Wolfgang Tomè)

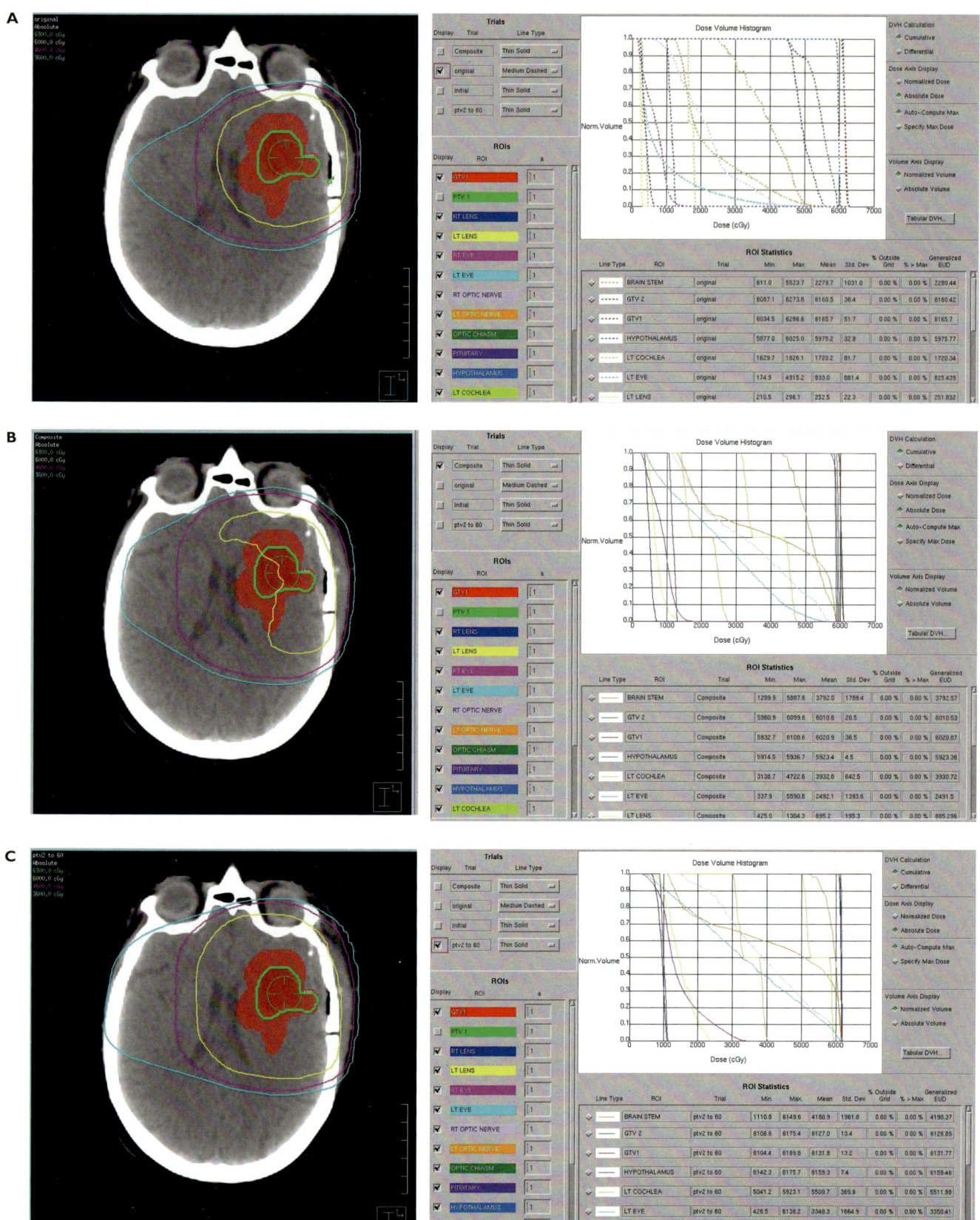

Figure 82.1 Comparison of dose plans for different volume definitions. **(A)** Dose plan using block margins per older RTOG studies. **(B)** Dose plan using dosimetric margins per RTOG 0525. **(C)** Dose plan using EORTC volume definition.

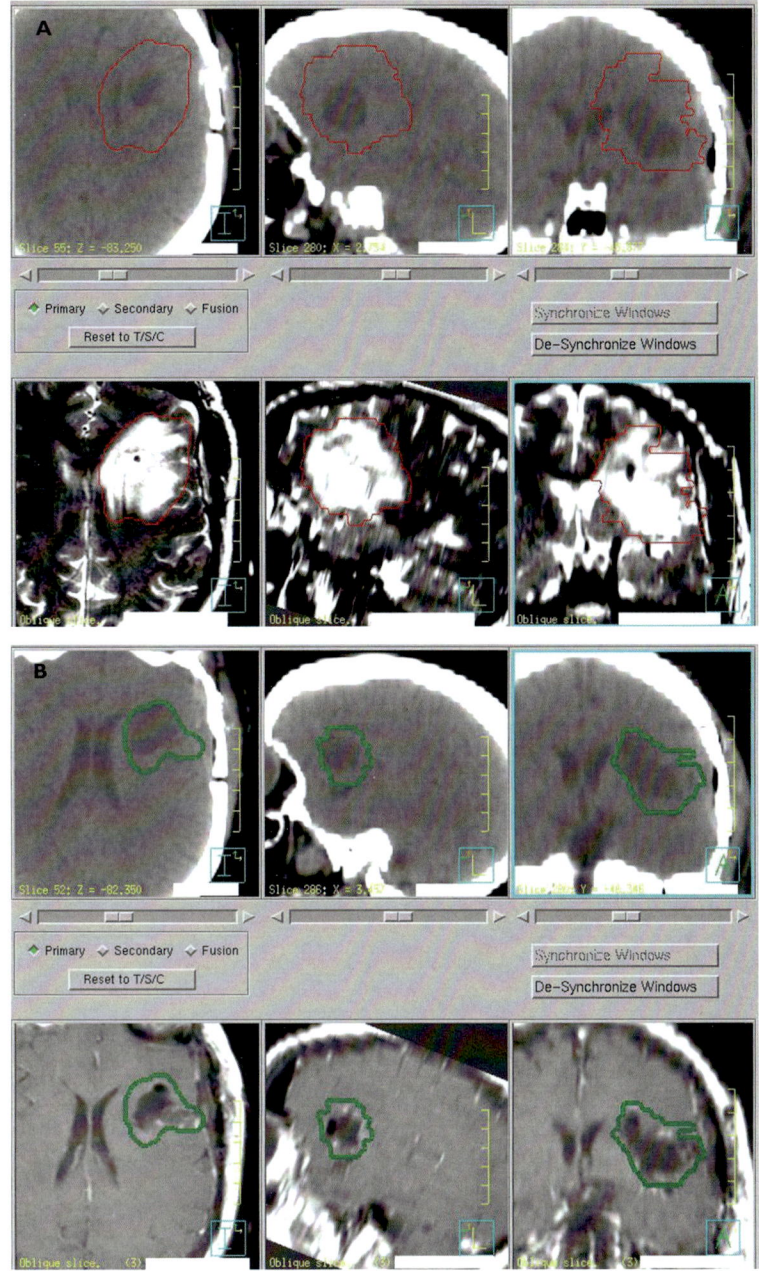

Figure 82.2 Example of MRI fusion. **(A)** MRI fusion for initial volume. **(B)** MRI fusion for boost volume.

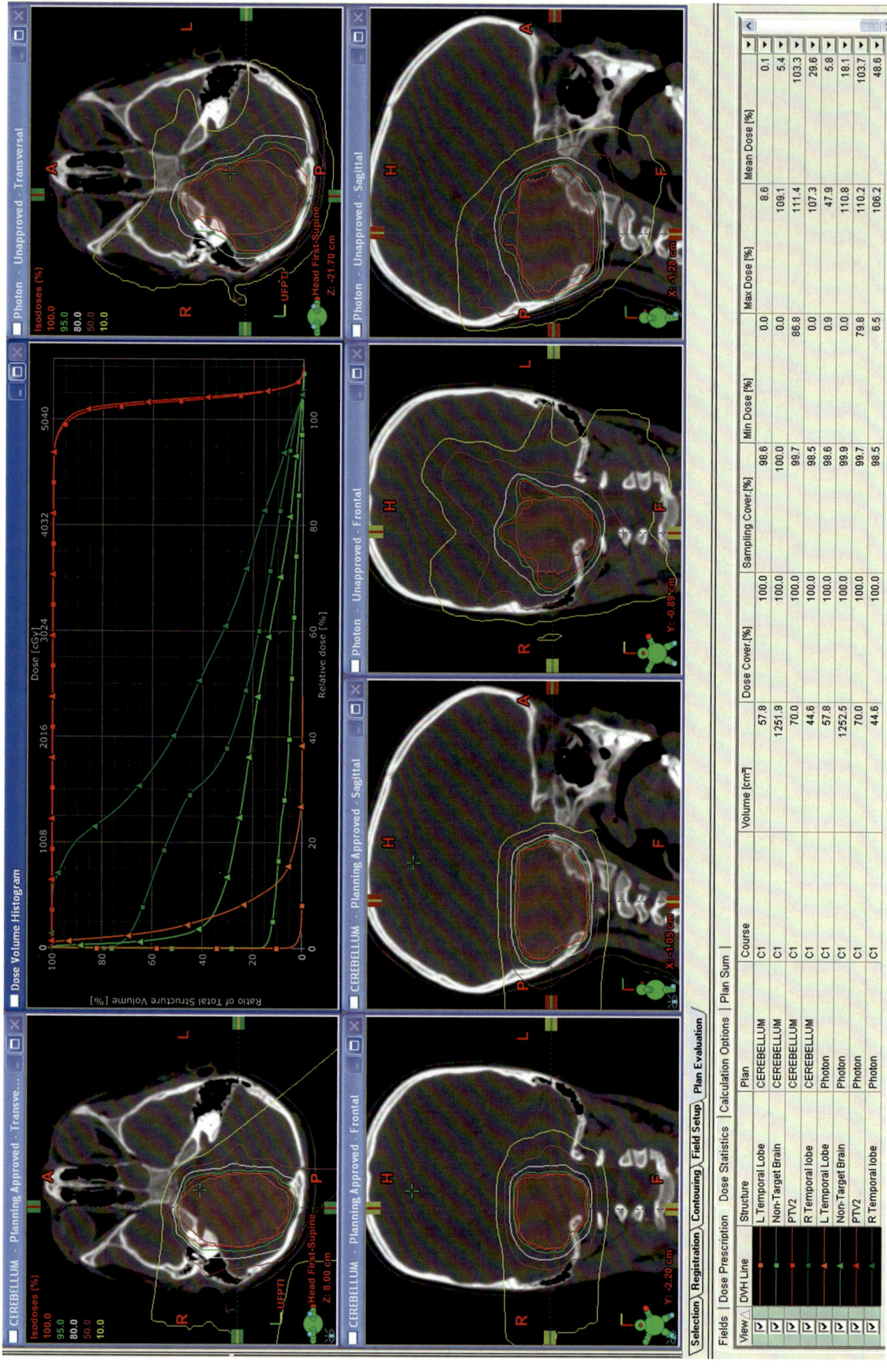

Figure 87.1 Dosimetric comparison of proton therapy and IMRT for a patient with LGG of the posterior fossa treated at the University of Florida Proton Therapy Institute.

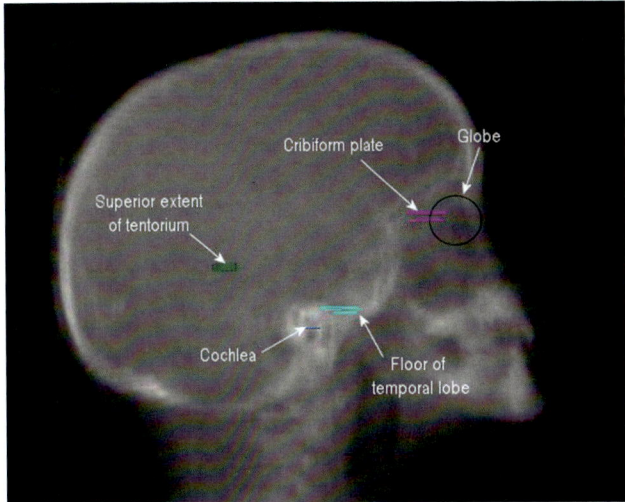

Figure 88.1 This lateral skull film is digitally reconstructed from a treatment planning CT scan. Note the positions of the cribiform plate and superior aspect of the posterior fossa, which can be easily identified on the CT planning study.

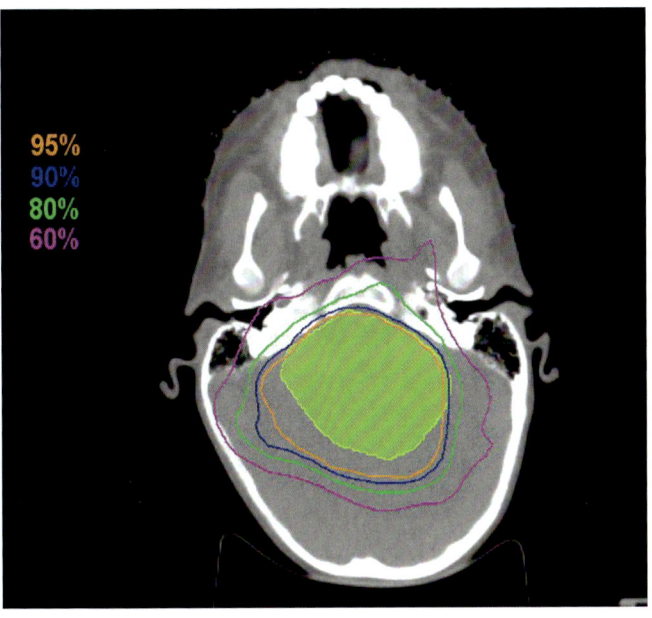

Figure 88.4 Isodose distribution for boost of the primary site in a child with medulloblastoma. Use of IMRT allows sparing of the cochlea and lateral temporal lobes.

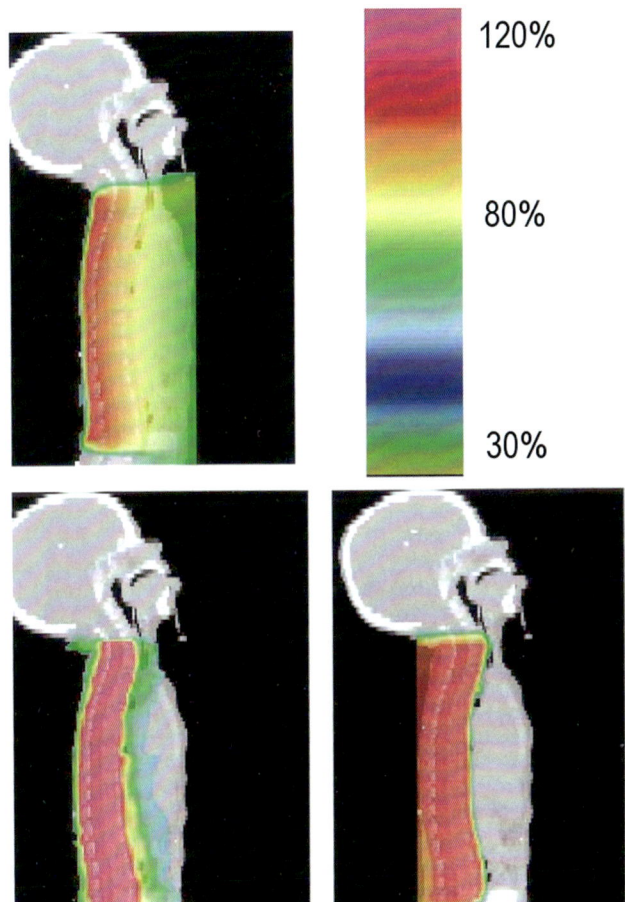

Figure 88.3 Comparisons of x-rays (upper left), IMRT (lower left), and proton (lower right) isodoses for CSI. Reprinted from Int J Rad Oncol Biol Phys, Vol 58:3, St. Clair WH, Adams JA, Bues M, et al., Advantage of protons compared to conventional x-ray or IMRT in the treatment of a pediatric patient with medulloblastoma, 731. © 2004 with permission from Elsevier.

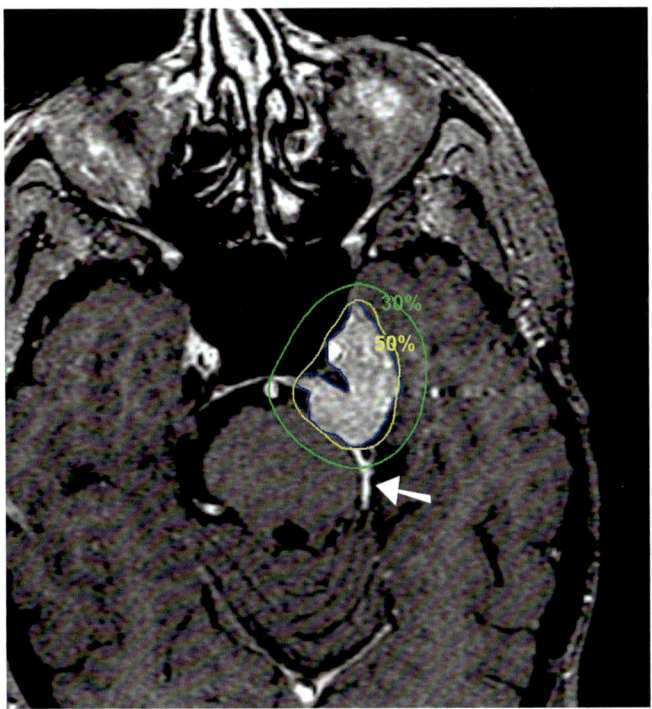

Figure 93.7 Stereotactic radiosurgery. Planning MRI for radiosurgery of a meningioma treated to 14 Gy at the 50% isodose. The prescription 50% and 30% isodose lines are included. The white arrow identifies a dural tail.

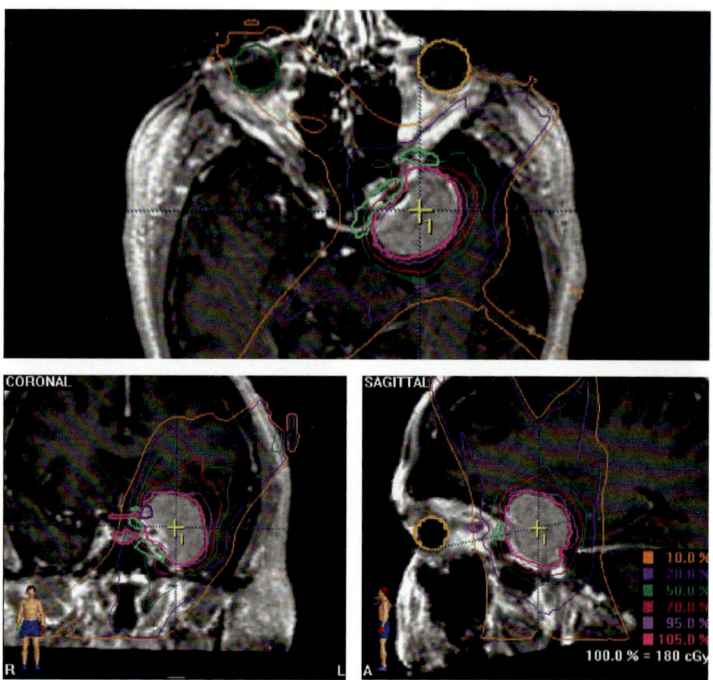

Figure 93.9 Fractionated stereotactic EBRT. Radiation therapy plan with isodoses. This paracavernous meningioma was treated to 54Gy in 30 fractions. The legend at the lower right hand corner illustrates percentage values for each of the pictured isodoses. Courtesy of Dennis Shrieve, MD, Chair of Radiation Oncology, Huntsman Cancer Institute, University of Utah.

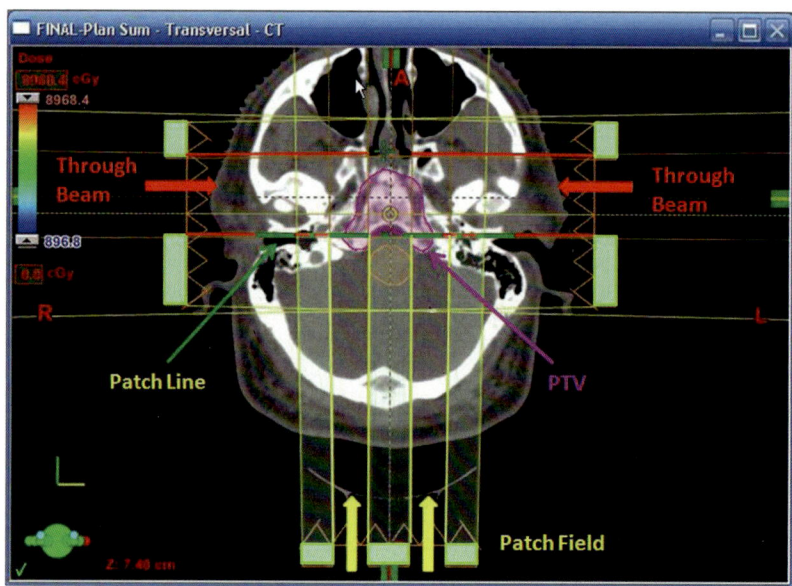

Figure 95.1 Example of proton therapy utilizing a combination of patch- and through-field techniques for treatment of clivus chordoma while sparing the brainstem.

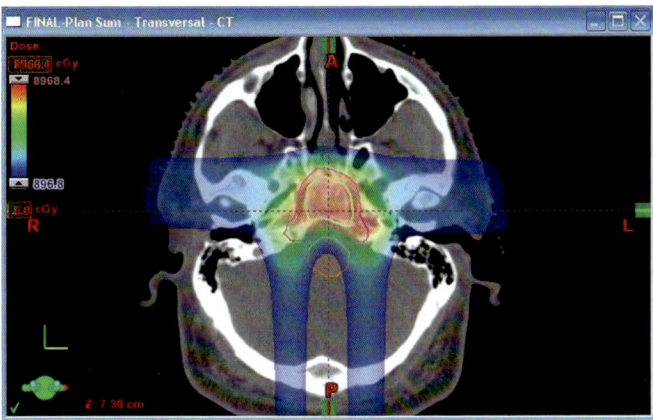

Figure 95.2 Color wash of the total dose delivered with proton therapy to treat a clivus chordoma.

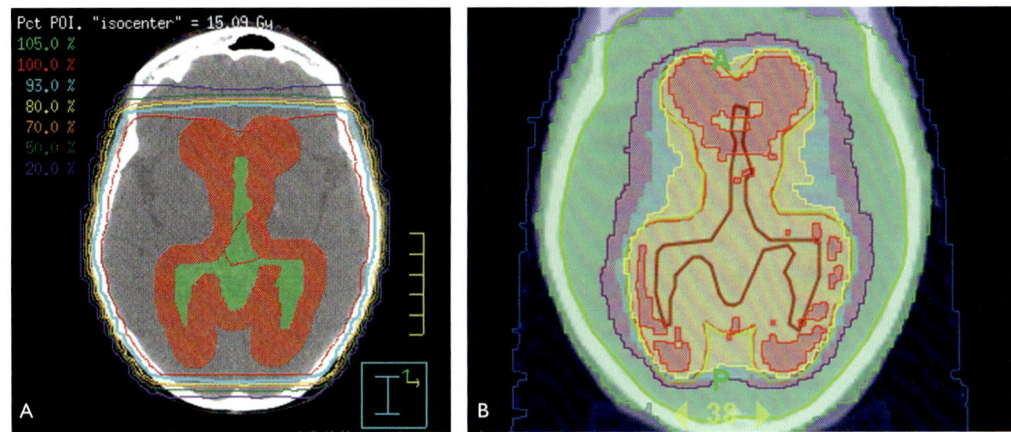

Figure 97.1 Comparison of whole ventricular treatment using opposed lateral fields **(A)** or with a tomotherapy IMRT plan **(B)**.

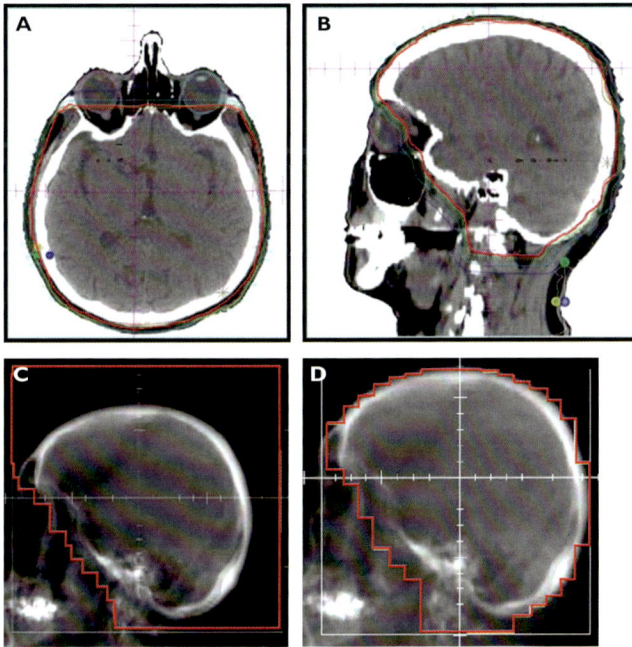

Figure 98.2 Isodose plots superimposed on the treatment planning CT images for a parallel opposed shaped WBRT PCNSL field arrangement (100% isodose line shown in red). The axial plot **(A)** demonstrates the desired coplanar anterior field edge in region of the posterior orbit, thereby avoiding divergence into contralateral orbit. Adequate coverage of the subarachnoid space is demonstrated on the sagital plot **(B)**. Typical WBRT multileaf collimation is demonstrated in image **(C)**. A "scalp block" multileaf collimation pattern is shown in image **(D)** that may be considered after 18 to 20 Gy has been delivered to the initial WBRT fields. Use of such a "scalp block" allows for adequate dose to subarachnoid space while lowering the probability of permanent convexity alopecia.

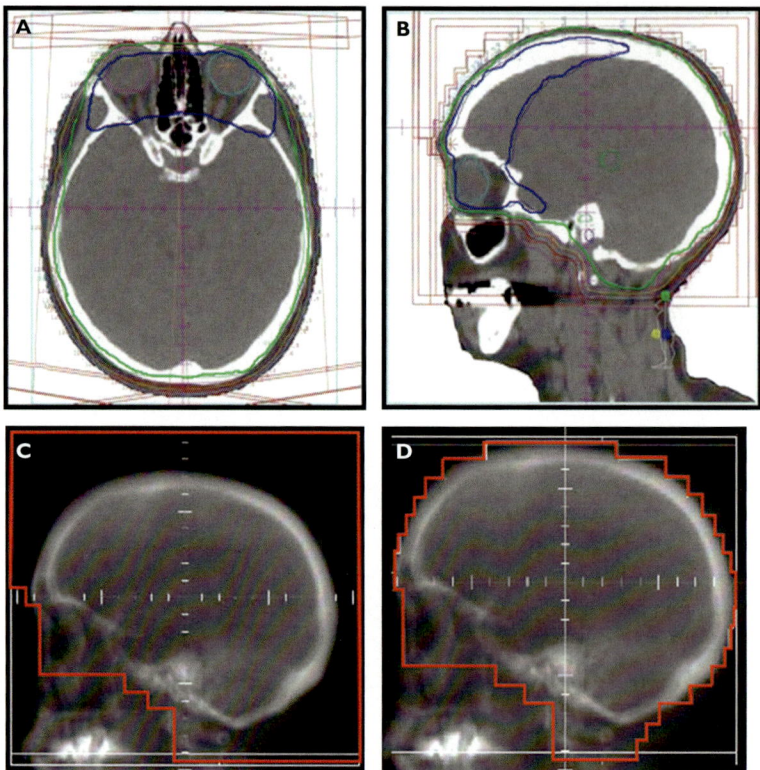

Figure 98.3 Isodose plots superimposed on treatment planning CT images for a parallel opposed shaped WBRT and whole orbit PCNSL field arrangement used when there is ocular involvement. The axial **(A)** and sagital **(B)** plots illustrate the dose inhomogeneity (volume encompassed by 110% isodose line shown in blue, 100% isodose line shown in green) that can occur when using typical WBRT arrangements. Compensating filters or "wedges" can be used to improve the homogeneity of dose in such cases. In addition, the total dose and fractionation scheme can be modified to lessen the risk of acute and late toxicity associated with such dosimetric inhomogeneity. Typical WBRT/orbit multileaf collimation pattern and WBRT/orbit "scalp block" multileaf collimation pattern are shown in images **(C)** and **(D)**, respectively.

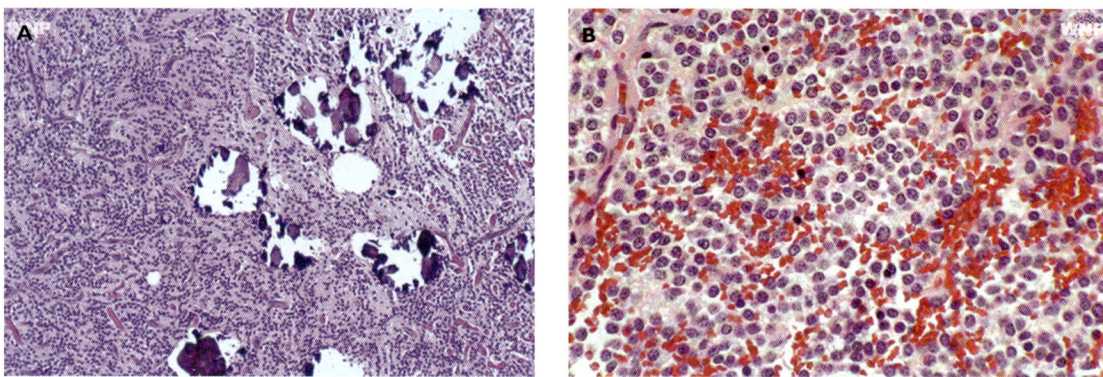

Figure 99.1 **(A)** Central neurocytoma. H&E stained slide demonstrating a cellular lesion composed of monomorphous small, round cells in a fibrillar background containing arborizing capillaries. Coarse calcifications are present. **(B)** Central neurocytoma. Higher power view demonstrating monomorphous, round nuclei with finely stippled chromatin, and inconspicuous nucleoli. Courtesy of Stephanie Koplin, MD, and Shahriar Salamat, MD, PhD, University of Wisconsin Department of Pathology.

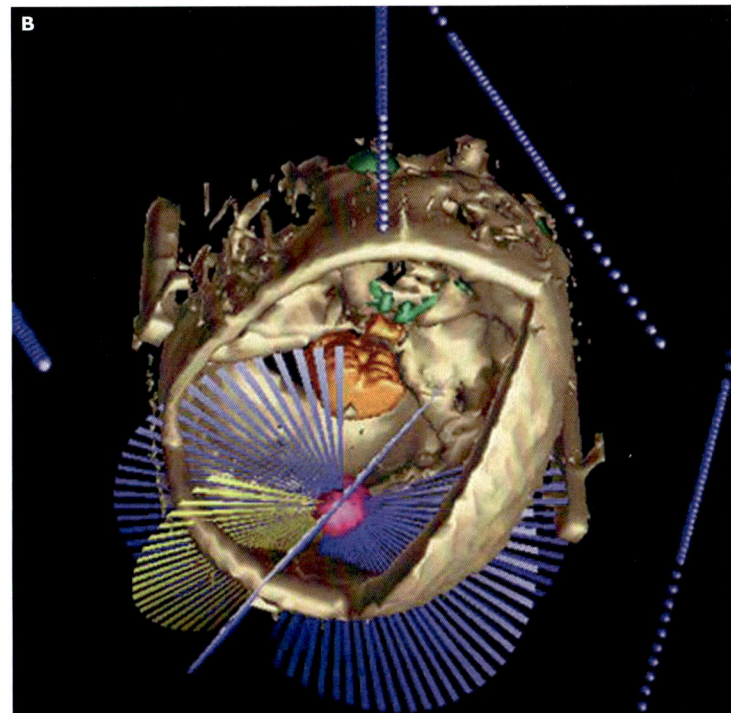

Figure 101.2B Single-fraction stereotactic radiosurgery for a single brain metastasis from kidney cancer. Immobilization is achieved with a stereotactic head ring fixed to the patient's skull. Treatment planning is based on CT/MRI image fusion. Small, well circumscribed lesions with very limited brain infiltration, such as brain metastasis, represent ideal targets for radiosurgery. In this case, a dose of 20 Gy was prescribed to the 45% isodose, which encloses the target volume. The lesion volume was 5 cc. Radiosurgery is characterized by a highly conformal dose distribution with very steep dose gradients toward the normal tissues. In this case, treatment was administered with a gamma knife. The follow-up MRI scans were taken 3 years after successful radiosurgery. Slight white matter changes are present in the irradiated region.

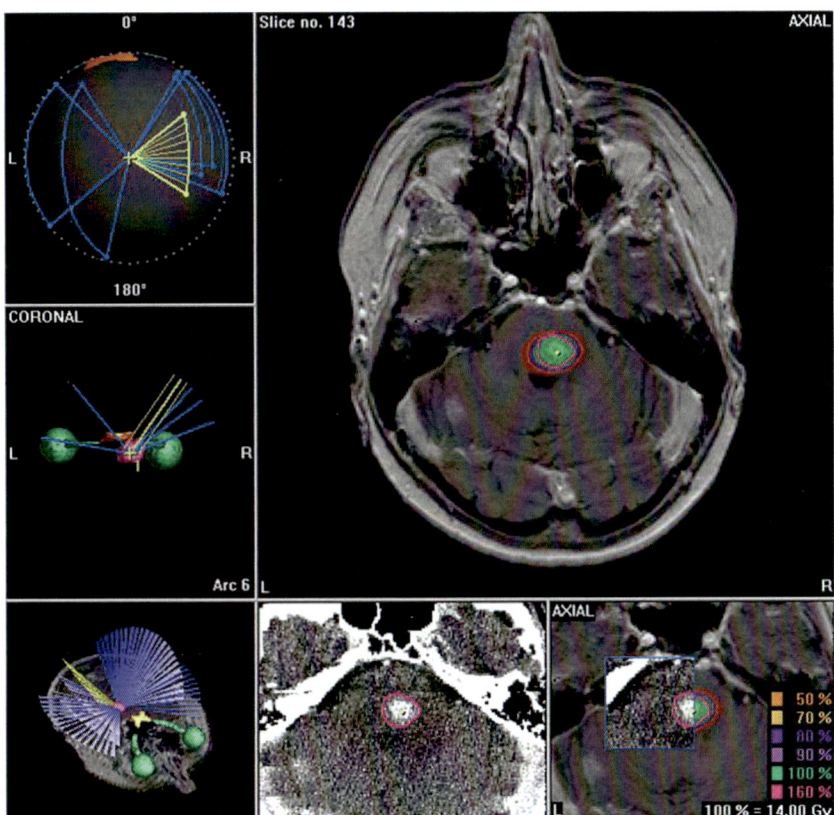

Figure 101.3 A situation with a rather large metastasis in the brain stem, where the therapeutic ratio of radiosurgery is small. The long-term tumor control probability with a margin dose of 14 Gy, as displayed here, is not satisfactory. Under such circumstances, fractionated stereotactic radiotherapy might be considered. The total dose will thus be administered in 5–7 fractions. Fractionated treatment requires the use of a removable non-invasive immobilization system attached to a stereotactic localization device rather than a classic stereotactic ring.

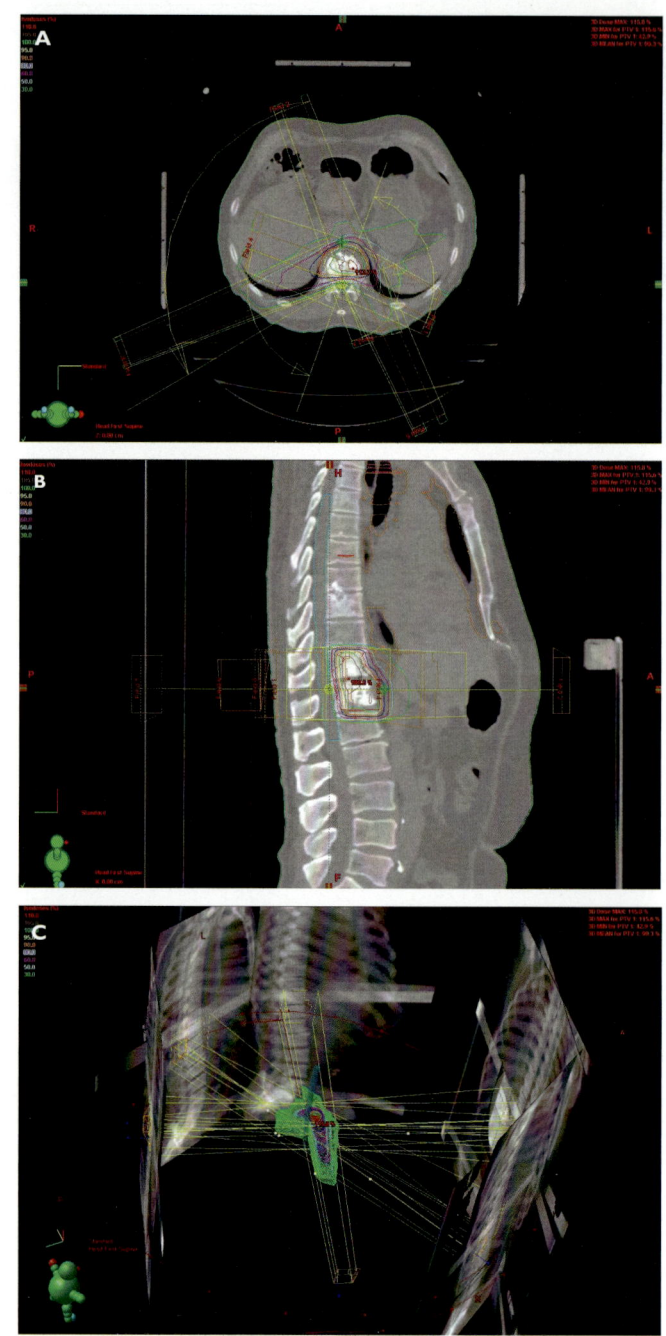

Figure 101.6 High-precision irradiation with fractionated stereotactic radiotherapy. The maximum dose delivered to the spinal cord was 27% of the prescribed dose.

59 Insular Tumors

Adam Wu and Frederick F. Lang

INTRODUCTION

Although insular tumors have historically been underreported due to the lack of familiarity with this region, it is now recognized that gliomas arising in the insular lobe are relatively common, comprising 25% of low-grade gliomas and 11% of glioblastomas multiforme [1]. Because the insula is surrounded by critical neural and vascular structures subserving sensory, motor, language, and cognitive functions, gliomas of the insula are often considered unresectable, and minimalist surgical interventions such as stereotactic biopsy are commonly recommended [2–4]. However, the pioneering work of Yasargil, demonstrating that radical resection of insular tumors is feasible, opened the door to more aggressive surgical approaches. Since his seminal publication, other series demonstrating good results have followed, and surgical resection of insular tumors is increasingly becoming part of the surgical repertoire of the neurosurgical oncologist [2,5–11]. Nevertheless, the surgical management of intrinsic tumors of the insula continues to pose special challenges as the two primary goals of brain tumor surgery, namely, maximal resection and preservation of neurologic function, frequently stand at odds with one another in insular tumors. The successful surgical treatment of insular tumors demands a solid knowledge of the surgical anatomy, pathology, classification, decision-making considerations, resection technique and strategies, complication avoidance, and outcomes. This chapter will review all of these areas of insular tumor surgery.

FUNCTIONS OF THE INSULA

The insula is part of the paralimbic mesocortex and is thought to function as a relay between limbic allocortex and neocortex [12]. As a result, it participates in multiple functions, including autonomic sensation, auditory-vestibular function, gestation, olfaction, and motor planning of speech in the dominant hemisphere [10], acting to integrate cognition with emotion. Studies using functional magnetic resonance imaging have shown that the anterior insula is activated in response to adverse occurrences in social interactions [13,14] and when assessing the intentions and emotional states of others [15,16]. Recent studies have implicated the anterior insula in the development of trust, and abnormal function in the region has been linked to borderline personality disorder [17]. Other reports have suggested a role in addictive behaviors, such as smoking [18].

Despite the potentially complex functions associated with the insula, work by Duffau et al [8] has demonstrated that most insular functions appear to be compensable through normal brain plasticity, and deficits directly associated with insular injury or removal generally are temporary. This is important for surgeons as it suggests that intrinsic tumors of the insula can be resected with minimal permanent deficit so long as the surrounding neural and vascular structures are preserved.

NORMAL ANATOMY OF THE INSULA

The insula lies deep relative to the sylvian fissure and is covered by the frontal, parietal, and temporal opercula, which include primary motor cortex, sensory cortex and, in the dominant hemisphere, language cortex (Broca's and Wernicke's areas) [9,12]. The topographic anatomy of the insula is shown in Figure 59.1. Three deep sulci separate the insula from the overlying opercular structures and form the anatomical boundaries of the insular cortex. The anterior, superior, and inferior peri-insular sulci separate the insula from the fronto-orbital, frontoparietal, and temporal opercula, respectively [12]. The peri-insular sulci are critical surgical landmarks as they define the insula as a three-sided pyramidal structure, the peak of which is called the insular apex. The insula is divided by the central insular sulcus into anterior and posterior portions. This central insular sulcus is often contiguous with the central sulcus of Roland. The anterior insula, which is the larger of the two portions, consists of the transverse, accessory, and three short insular gyri, while the posterior insula is composed of anterior and posterior long gyri. The limen insula lies in the anterobasal portion and joins the insular cortex with the anterior perforated substance [12].

Located deep relative to the insular cortex are the extreme capsule, the claustrum, and the external capsule that overlie the putamen and globus palidus. The internal capsule lies deep relative to these basal ganglia structures, except superiorly where it passes over the top of these structures below the superior insula within the corona radiata. The corona radiata, in which the corticospinal

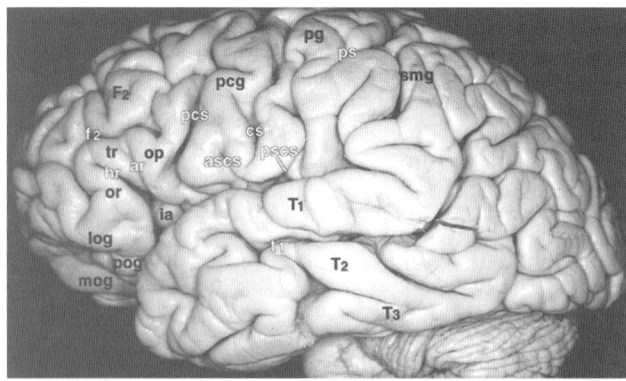

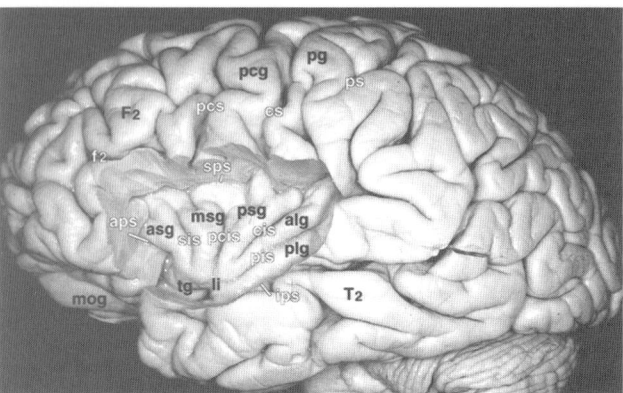

Figure 59.1 Photographs of brain specimens. Upper: The sylvian fissure is located in the lateral aspect of the left cerebral hemisphere. The frontoorbital, frontoparietal, and temporal opercula cover the insula. Lower: The insula is exposed, following excision of the opercula, to the level of the periinsular sulci. Abbreviations with white letters denote sulci and fissures. alg, anterior long insular gyrus; aps, anterior periinsular sulcus; ar, ascending ramus of sylvian fissure; ascs, anterior subcentral sulcus; asg, anterior short insular gyrus; cis, central insular sulcus; cs, central sulcus of Rolando; F2, middle frontal gyrus; f2, inferior frontal sulcus; hr, horizontal ramus of sylvian fissure; ia, insular apex; ips, inferior periinsular sulcus; li, limen insula; log, lateral orbital gyrus; mog, medial orbital gyrus; msg, middle short insular gyrus; op, pars opercularis of F3; or, pars orbitalis of F3; pcg, precentral gyrus; pcis, precentral insular sulcus; pcs, precentral sulcus; pg, postcentral gyrus; pis, postcentral insular sulcus; plg, posterior long insular gyrus; pog, posterior orbital gyrus; ps, postcentral sulcus; pscs, posterior subcentral sulcus; psg, posterior short insular gyrus; sis, short insular sulcus; smg, supramarginal gyrus; sps, superior periinsular sulcus; tg, transverse insular gyrus; tr, pars triangularis of F3; T1, superior temporal gyrus; T2, middle temporal gyrus; T3, inferior temporal gyrus; t1, superior temporal sulcus. Reprinted with permission from Ture et al [12].

tract runs, is located below the superior peri-insular sulcus, while below the inferior peri-insular sulcus lies the uncinate fasciculus, and an approach through the center of the insula leads into the putamen [9].

Figure 59.2 illustrates the intimate association the insula has with the middle cerebral artery (MCA) and its branches that essentially surround the insula. The M1 segment sits at the anteroinferior portion of the insula and gives rise to the lateral lenticulostriate arteries (LLA) that are small perforators that supply the basal ganglia and internal capsule. The M2 branches lie along the lateral surface of the insula, giving off short and medium perforating branches that supply the insular cortex, extreme capsule, claustrum, and external capsule but do not supply the basal ganglia or internal capsule. There are also long perforators arising from the M2 branches that can extend deep into the corona radiata and supply the corticospinal tract.

PATHOLOGICAL ANATOMY OF INSULAR TUMORS

Most insular tumors, except for the highest grade and most aggressive glioblastomas, have a tendency to respect the pial borders of the insula, expanding the insular cortex but not infiltrating across the peri-insular sulci into the surrounding opercula. When the gyri are expanded by tumor, they often cover the M2 branches that typically run in the sulci separating the gyri. Importantly, many insular gliomas respect the medial putamenal border and do not invade the basal ganglia [3]. When insular tumors extend beyond the limits of the insula itself, they tend to follow the subcortical U-fibers below the peri-insular sulci, once again respecting pial boundaries [9]. Insular gliomas extend into the temporal lobe through the uncinate fasciculus and into the frontobasal lobe via the inferior frontal tracts [9]. The respect for pial borders and the basal ganglia is what makes radical resection possible in many cases as the pial borders and surrounding sulci can be used to define the limits of the tumor (see below). However, it must be recognized that this growth pattern is most common in low-grade or anaplastic gliomas that are typically nonenhancing on MRI. In contradistinction, glioblastomas more commonly cross pial borders and more often violate the medial basal ganglia border, invading these deep structures.

Another critical aspect of insular tumor anatomy is that they receive most of their blood supply from the short and medium perforators arising from the M2 branches. In contrast, the LLA, which provide the main blood supply to the internal capsule, typically do not supply insular tumors but are pushed medially as the tumor expands. This pattern makes devascularization and resection of insular tumors possible without injury to the lenticulostriate vessels. However, this vascular pattern is most common in low-grade and some anaplastic gliomas, whereas glioblastomas tend to parasitize the lenticulostriate vessels. Thus ischemia of the corticospinal tract is more common in glioblastomas in which critical lenticulosriate vessels may be enveloped by tumor [2]. It must also be recognized that long perforators may arise from M2 branches supplying both the tumor and the corona radiata. These vessels, like the lenticulostriate perforators, must be preserved during tumor resection [19].

TYPES OF INSULAR GLIOMAS

As expected for intrinsic tumors, most insular tumors are gliomas although other pathologies have been reported. These results are summarized in Table 59.1. In terms of histology, most series report astrocytomas as the most

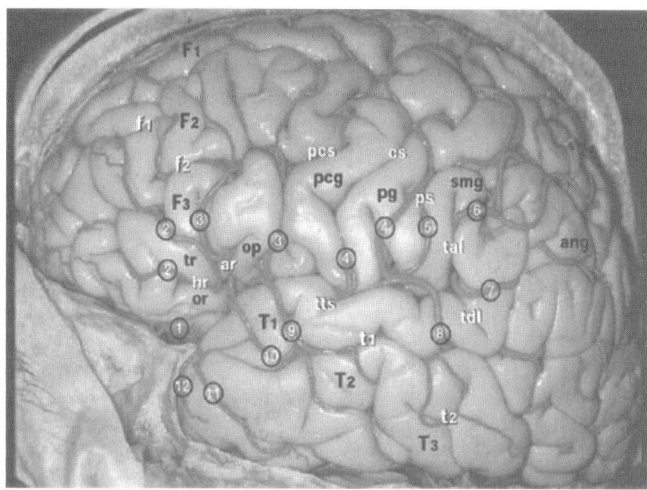
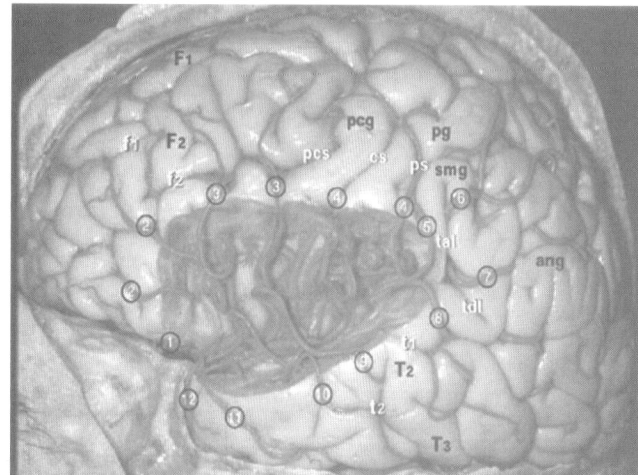
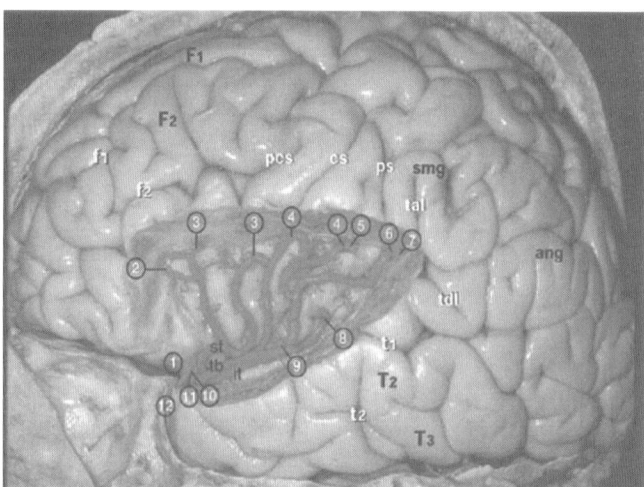

Figure 59.2 Photographs of brain specimens. Upper left: The lateral surface of the left hemisphere is supplied by the M4 and M5 segments of the MCA. Upper right: The same specimen is shown following removal of the entire opercula with preservation of all segments of the MCA. Lower: The same specimen. The M3, M4, and M5 segments of the MCA have been removed, and the M2 segment, which supplies the insula, has been preserved over the insular cortex. White letters denote sulci and fissures. 1, lateral orbitofrontal artery; 2, prefrontal artery; 3, precentral artery; 4, central artery; 5, anterior parietal artery; 6, posterior parietal artery; 7, angular artery; 8, temporooccipital artery; 9, posterior temporal artery; 10, middle temporal artery; 11, anterior temporal artery; 12, temporal polar artery; ang, angular gyrus; ar, ascending ramus of sylvian fissure; cs, central sulcus of Rolando; F1, superior frontal gyrus; F2, middle frontal gyrus; F3, inferior frontal gyrus; f1, superior frontal sulcus; f2, inferior frontal sulcus; hr, horizontal ramus of sylvian fissure; it, inferior trunk of M2 segment; op, pars opercularis of F3; or, pars orbitalis of F3; pcg, precentral gyrus; pcs, precentral sulcus; pg, postcentral gyrus; ps, postcentral sulcus; smg, supramarginal gyrus; st, superior trunk of M2 segment; T1, superior temporal gyrus; T2, middle temporal gyrus; T3, inferior temporal gyrus; t1, superior temporal sulcus; t2, inferior temporal sulcus; tal, terminal ascending limb of sylvian fissure; tb, temporal branch of the MCA; tdl, terminal descending limb of sylvian fissure; tr, pars triangularis of F3; tts, transverse temporal sulcus. Reprinted with permission from Ture et al [19].

frequent glial type, followed by oligodendrogliomas and mixed gliomas. In terms of tumor grade, in Yasargil's series of 150 insular tumors [3,20], there was a nearly equal distribution of glioblastomas (26%, WHO Grade IV), anaplastic gliomas (34%, WHO grade III), and low-grade gliomas (31%, WHO grade II). Later surgical series typically have a predominance of anaplastic and low-grade gliomas, with glioblastomas being significantly less represented.

In our own published series ($n = 47$), we observed a distribution of tumor grades similar to other series, with 15% glioblastomas, 31% anaplastic gliomas, and 49% low-grade gliomas [2,9]. Interestingly, there was a higher incidence of oligodendrogliomas (34%) and mixed gliomas (17%) in our series compared with earlier reports, reflecting an increased emphasis on identifying oligodendroglial differentiation for chromosome 1p/19q loss of heterozygosity determination. The decrease in the proportion of glioblastomas reported in our series and other contemporary series may be a result of refinement in selection criteria over time, with glioblastomas being treated more conservatively [2,10,14,21–23].

CLASSIFICATIONS OF INSULAR TUMORS

Yasargil proposed a general classification of all limbic and paralimbic tumors, summarized in Table 59.2 A, in which he considered insular tumors as a subset. In his classification, insular tumors were considered type 3 tumors. Yasargil further subdivided insular tumors into type 3a for tumors solely within the insula and type 3b for parainsular tumors and further subdivided these tumors into ones with frontal opercular involvement, temporal opercular involvement, and frontotemporal opercular involvement.

Table 59.1 Pathology of Intrinsic Tumors of the Insula, Summary of Literature

Tumor Type	Yasargil 1992 [3]	Zentner 1996 [6]	Vanacochla 1997 [11]	Lang 2001 [2] and Hentschel 2005 [9]	Duffau 2006 [8]	Neuloh 2007 [10]
	N = 150	N = 30	N = 28[a]	N = 47	N = 42	N = 84
Glioblastoma	39(26%)	8(27%)	3(11%)	7(15%)		15(18%)
Anaplastic						
Astrocytoma	40(27%)	5(17%)	4(15%)	9(19%)		36(43%)
Oligodendroglioma	6(4%)	1(3%)		5(11%)		
Mixed	5(3%)					
Total	51(34%)	6(20%)	4(15%)	14(30%)		36(43%)
Low grade						
Astrocytoma	33(22%)	9(30%)	19(68%)	4(9%)	NS	NS
Oligodendroglioma	9(6%)	1(3%)	2(7%)	11(23%)	NS	NS
Mixed	5(3%)	3(10%)		8(17%)	NS	NS
Total	47(31%)	13(43%)	21(75%)		42(100%)	33(39%)
Other	13(9%)	3(9%)			3(6%)	

[a] 28 surgeries, 23 patients.

Table 59.2A The Yasargil Classification of Limbic and Paralimbic Tumors

Type	Location	Subcategories
1	Temporal mediobasal	a. Medial temporal pole b. Amygdalar c. Hippocampal d. Parahippocampal
2	Cingulate gyrus	a. Anterior b. Middle c. Posterior

3	Insular and parainsular	a. Pure Insular
		  α. Anterior
		  β. Posterior
		  χ. Entire
		b. Insular-frontobasal
		c. Insular-temporal mediobasal
		d. Insular-frontobasal-septal and temporal mediobasal

4	Medial limbic association areas	a. Forniceal b. Septal c. Mammillary
5	Entire limbic system	

From Ref. 20.

Table 59.2B A Proposed Classification of Insular Tumors

Type	Location
I	Pure insular
II	With extension into frontal lobe
III	With extension into temporal lobe
IV	With extension into both frontal and temporal lobes

The largest tumors with extensive frontal and/or temporal lobe extension would be considered type 5 tumors in Yasargil's system [20].

We developed our own simplified classification system for tumors involving the insula (Table 59.2 B). Type I tumors are those that are purely within the boundaries of the insula. Type II tumors extend into the frontal lobe, type III tumors extend into the temporal lobe, and type IV tumors extend into both the frontal and temporal lobes. In our experience, a plurality (about 40%) of insular tumors are type I, involving only the insular lobe, with an approximately equal distribution of type II and type III tumors, and type IV tumors are rare [2,9]. This classification has the advantage that it defines whether resections of the temporal, frontal, or both lobes are needed for complete resection.

CLINICAL PRESENTATION OF PATIENTS WITH INSULAR GLIOMAS

Patients with insular glioma most commonly present with seizures and most are without any neurological signs on examination. In our series, 59% of patients presented with seizures and were neurologically intact [2]. Neurological findings, when present, include hemiparesis, speech disturbance, and neuropsychological deficits. The presence of such signs usually suggests a more aggressive pathology with infiltration of the tumor into critical structures [2,3,8].

Radiographically, many insular tumors are nonenhancing lesions on postgadolinium T1-weighted MRI and appear hyperintense on T2-weighted MR images. As with gliomas in other locations, the presence of enhancement suggests a higher grade lesion, typically glioblastoma multiforme. In our recently published series, 50% were nonenhancing on T1-weighted MRI [2].

SURGICAL DECISION MAKING

The goal of all brain tumor surgery is maximal removal of tumor with minimal neurological morbidity. The need to carefully balance these sometimes opposing goals is particularly marked for insular tumors because of the challenges of the complex anatomy and the fact that most patients have normal neurological function at presentation. In addition, most insular tumors are nonenhancing lesions on imaging studies. Thus decision making for resection of insular tumors often reflects approaches to nonenhancing tumors in general, which is an area of controversy in itself. Indeed, many neurosurgeons recommend a conservative strategy for nonenhancing tumors, particularly of the insula, deferring any surgical intervention until tumor progression occurs, citing the potential morbidity associated with surgical interventions in this region and the controversy surrounding the actual surgical benefit associated with surgical resection. When surgery is ultimately recommended, proponents of this conservative approach prefer stereotactic biopsy over radical resection.

However, we generally prefer early surgical intervention, rather than a "watch-and-wait approach" for nonenhancing tumors, including those in the insula, for several reasons. First, early surgical intervention allows determination of the histological tumor type, which is important because the prognosis of patients with astrocytomas is different from that of patients with oligodendrogliomas. Second, imaging studies do not reveal the grade of the tumor. Although most nonenhancing tumors are of low grade (WHO grade II), up to one third are anaplastic tumors (WHO grade III). Identifying these higher grade gliomas is important because the subsequent treatments are different from those of low-grade gliomas. Last, radiographic studies are uninformative about whether or not the tumor has loss of heterozygosity at 1p/19q. This information can only be obtained through tissue sampling. Because tumors with loss of heterozygosity at 1p/19q have a better prognosis and may be more responsive to chemotherapy, treatment options for these lesions are expanding; thus early identification of this molecular subtype is of increasing importance [21–23].

Likewise, we generally prefer maximal removal rather than stereotactic biopsy. Radical resection with sampling of large parts of the tumor increases the accuracy of diagnosis. Indeed, in a recent study from our institution, we found that an incorrect diagnosis was made on small stereotactic biopsies in 38% of patients and that this resulted in incorrect treatment in 26% of patients in a series who underwent an initial biopsy and then subsequent surgical resection [24]. Thus a more aggressive surgical approach provides an increased chance of making the correct diagnosis. In addition, radical resection may improve symptoms, particularly seizures, as well as relieve any mass effect of the lesion. Last, radical resection for the purpose of cytoreduction may prolong patient survival. Although this has never been proved in a randomized studies of patients, multiple retrospective analyses of low-grade gliomas indicate that the larger resections are associated with improved survival [25]. For higher grade gliomas, two randomized trials indicate that radical resection is associated with improved outcome [26,27]. Likewise, a retrospective study of 416 patients from our institution demonstrated that the extent of resection, as determined by computerized volumetric analyses, was significantly associated with improved outcome [28]. An algorithm used at our institution for the management of nonenhancing intraparenchymal brain tumors is shown in Figure 59.3.

Ultimately, the patient's age, clinical condition, presenting symptoms, and image-defined tumor anatomy must all be taken into account in making the decision for surgery. Although age is not itself a contraindication to surgery, elderly patients in poor medical condition with imaging suggestive of an insular glioblastoma generally do poorly, and may be candidates for more conservative measures [2]. In contrast, symptoms attributable to mass effect typically require surgical resection. Similarly, effective seizure control often requires near complete removal of the offending lesion [5].

Imaging studies provide critical information regarding the patient's specific anatomy and the relation of the tumor mass to surrounding vital structures, features which are critical to surgical decision making. The sharpness of the tumor borders as defined on T2-weighted MRI is a very important factor guiding surgical decisions. The presence of a sharp demarcation of T2 signal change at the medial border of the tumor correlates well with the presence of a readily identifiable dissection plane, which is vitally important for the successful complete removal of the tumor with preservation of function [2,4]. Tumors with diffuse margins on T2-weighted MRI engender less enthusiasm for radical resection, because the interface between the tumor and the brain is often more difficult to define. MRI also provides useful information with regard to the associated vascular anatomy around insular tumors. In particular, flow voids representing the lenticulostriate perforators can often be seen along the medial border of the tumor, providing the neurosurgeon with information about the intimacy of the relationship between these vital arteries and the medial extent of the intended resection [2].

SURGICAL CONSIDERATIONS FOR COMPLICATION AVOIDANCE

Prior to embarking on any surgical procedure, the surgeon must be cognizant of the potential anatomical, pathological, and physiological pitfalls that may contribute to complications. This truism is especially relevant to surgery for insular tumors. The major anatomic considerations for insular tumors are shown in Figure 59.4. Postoperative neurological deficits after insular tumor resection can be attributed to opercular retraction, manipulation of the MCA, interruption of perforating arteries, and direct injury to the internal capsule.

Opercular Retraction

In order to fully expose the insular lobe, significant retraction is sometimes necessary on the frontal and temporal opercula when the transsylvian approach is used. Edema, compressive ischemia to M3 branches, and resulting postoperative swelling may produce dysfunction of motor cortex, sensory cortex, Broca's area or Wernicke's area leading to motor, sensory, or speech impairments. To avoid these problems, Yasargil has gone so far as to recommend not using retractors at all, relying instead on dynamic retraction and cotton balls to keep the fissure open [3]. Other authors have used awake craniotomy and other forms of intraoperative monitoring, with repositioning of retractors until normal function is restored [2]. Unfortunately, the

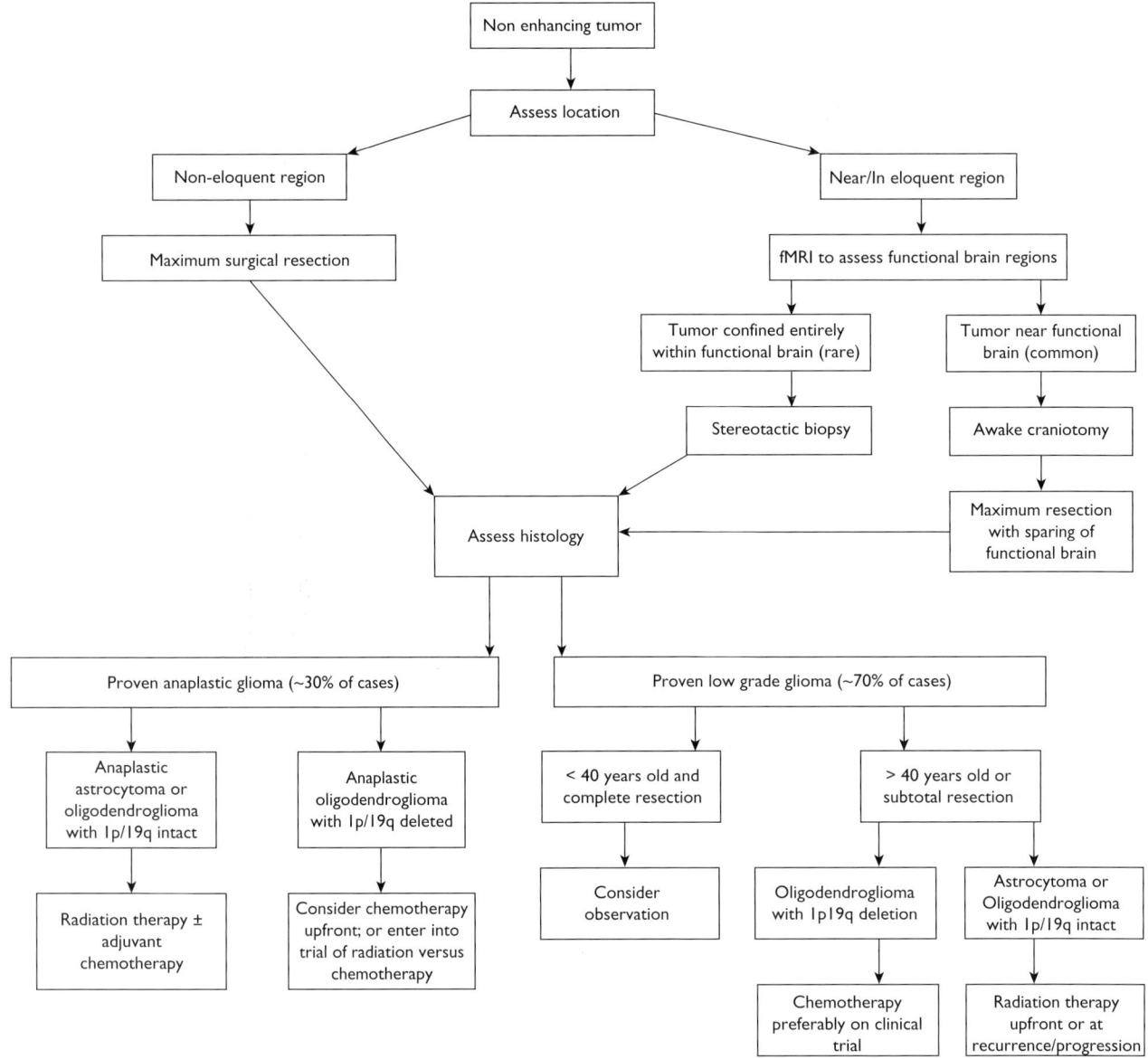

Figure 59.3 Diagram showing the M.D. Anderson Cancer Center algorithm for managing nonenhancing brain tumors. Reprinted with permission from Toms et al [4].

development of a deficit during awake craniotomy may result in the premature termination of the procedure and inadequate tumor resection, even if the deficit turns out to be transient [2]. An alternative option is to modify the transsylvian approach to include an opercular resection. Obviously this is ideal for tumors with frontal opercular extension in the nondominant hemisphere. Elective resection of the frontal operculum for tumors confined to the insula has also been suggested [7]. However, this option is less viable for tumors of the dominant hemisphere or if brain mapping determines that the frontal operculum is functional cortex. In our experience, most tumors confined to the insula can be removed without resection of the operculum.

MCA Manipulation

The MCA is draped over the surface of insular tumors and is particularly vulnerable to injury and excessive manipulation. For insular tumors of moderate and large size, the MCA is frequently enveloped entirely by tumor and therefore obscured from view, placing the artery at risk for injury during tumor dissection [2,3,11]. As stated above, the primary blood supply of most insular tumors arises from perforators originating along the undersurface of the M2 segment. If these perforators are torn from the parent vessel during dissection, the M2 segment is placed at risk. It is important therefore to individually coagulate and divide in a controlled manner each of these perforators.

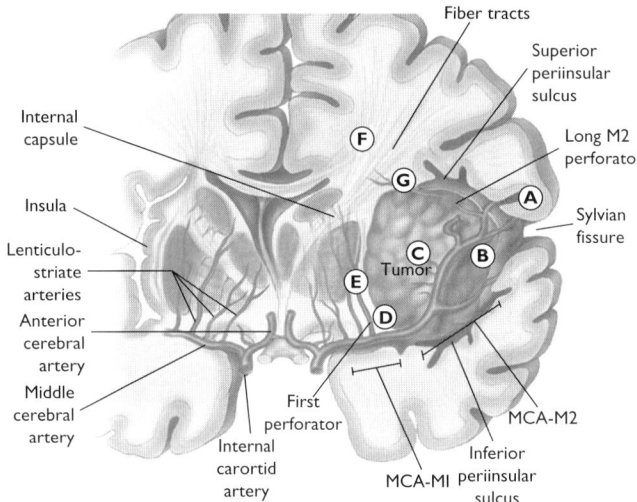

Figure 59.4 Surgical anatomy of insular tumors. The insular cortex and surrounding structure without (left side) and with (right side) an insular tumor (see text for details). (A) Frontal operculum can be injured during sylvian fissure splitting and secondary to retraction. (B) M2 branches may be buried within the tumor as the tumor expands the insular gyri. These vessels can be inadvertently coagulated if not correctly identified. (C) Multiple small vessels that arise from the undersurface of the M2 branches (short and medium M2 perforating arteries) are the main blood supply to insular tumors. These vessels can be torn from the M2, resulting in potential injury to the M2. These vessels are best approached subpially and must be individually coagulated and divided. (D) and (E) The lateral lenticulostriate arteries supply the internal capsule and often course along the medial side of the tumor. Injury to these vessels normally results in a dense hemiplegia. (F) The corona radiata with its motor and sensory fibers is vulnerable on the superior edge of the tumor. Inadvertent dissection deep to the superior periinsular sulcus can directly disrupt all or some of these fibers. (G) Long perforating arteries may arise from the M2 segment. Disruption of these vessels can result in hemiparesis because they supply the corona radiata. Reprinted with permission from Hentschel and Lang [9].

Manipulation of the MCA during tumor dissection can also predispose the vessel for the development of postoperative vasospasm, leading to ischemic injury to the brain areas in the MCA territory.

Perforating Vessels

The lateral lenticulostriate perforators supply the internal capsule and are vulnerable at the medial border of the tumor resection. They too can be enveloped by expanding tumor. To minimize the risk of injury to the LLAs and the subsequent development of hemiplegia, the most lateral LLA should be identified as early in the operation as possible (see below). The position of this vessel helps define the parasagittal plane that delimits the depths of the resection. In addition, the surgeon should be aware that the lenticulostriate perforators run in a plane parallel to the base of the tumor, whereas the perforators arising from the M2 run in a plane perpendicular to the tumor. This directionality can help in preserving these vessels.

Long perforators arising from the M2 branches are also at risk. These vessels supply the corona radiata, and their interruption may produce hemiparesis. It can be particularly challenging distinguishing these long M2 perforators from the short M2 perforators supplying the tumor that need to be divided. All large perforating branches arising from M2 branches overlying the posterior insula should be always be preserved [3,19].

Internal Capsule Injury

The internal capsule lies directly beneath the superior peri-insular sulcus and is vulnerable at the superior aspect of an insular tumor, where the motor fibers are not protected by the basal ganglia [2]. Dissection at the superior margin of the tumor extending beyond and deep relative to the superior peri-insular sulcus is therefore at risk of interrupting the corticospinal tract and producing hemiparesis. The most difficult cases are those wherein the tumor extends beyond the sulcal base. The use of intraoperative subcortical stimulation is probably the best adjunctive procedure for avoiding complications, but even this is not a fail-safe [7]. Careful anatomic dissection remains the best way of avoiding neurologic complications.

SURGICAL METHOD [9]

The transsylvian route is the preferred approach to the insula [3]. For tumors with frontal extension, a frontal opercular resection may be included, while tumors with temporal extension often require a temporal lobe resection, often a partial temporal lobectomy [7].

Position and Craniotomy

The patient may be positioned either in the lateral position or supine with the head turned 30° to 45°. In our experience, we have found that placing the patient's head at 45° is the best option because it allows the frontal and temporal opercula to "fall open," facilitating dissection. It also provides a better angle than do the other positions for viewing the most posterior aspect of these tumors.

A standard frontotemporal craniotomy is performed, with drilling of the sphenoid ridge, allowing for maximal access to the entire sylvian fissure (Figure 59.5). The dura is opened and flapped anteriorly. Computer-assisted neuronavigation and intraoperative ultrasound may be used to help define the tumor borders prior to opening the arachnoid. After exposure, the anatomic dissection of insular tumors is composed of five stages: (1) sylvian fissure dissection; (2) exposure of the MCA and all important branches; (3) dissection of the peri-insular sulci; (4) devascularisation of the tumor; and (5) resection of the tumor mass (Figure 59.6).

Sylvian Fissure Dissection

A long and wide splitting of the sylvian fissure along its entire length, typically 6 to 7 cm, is critical for adequate exposure. The tumor itself may facilitate opening of the

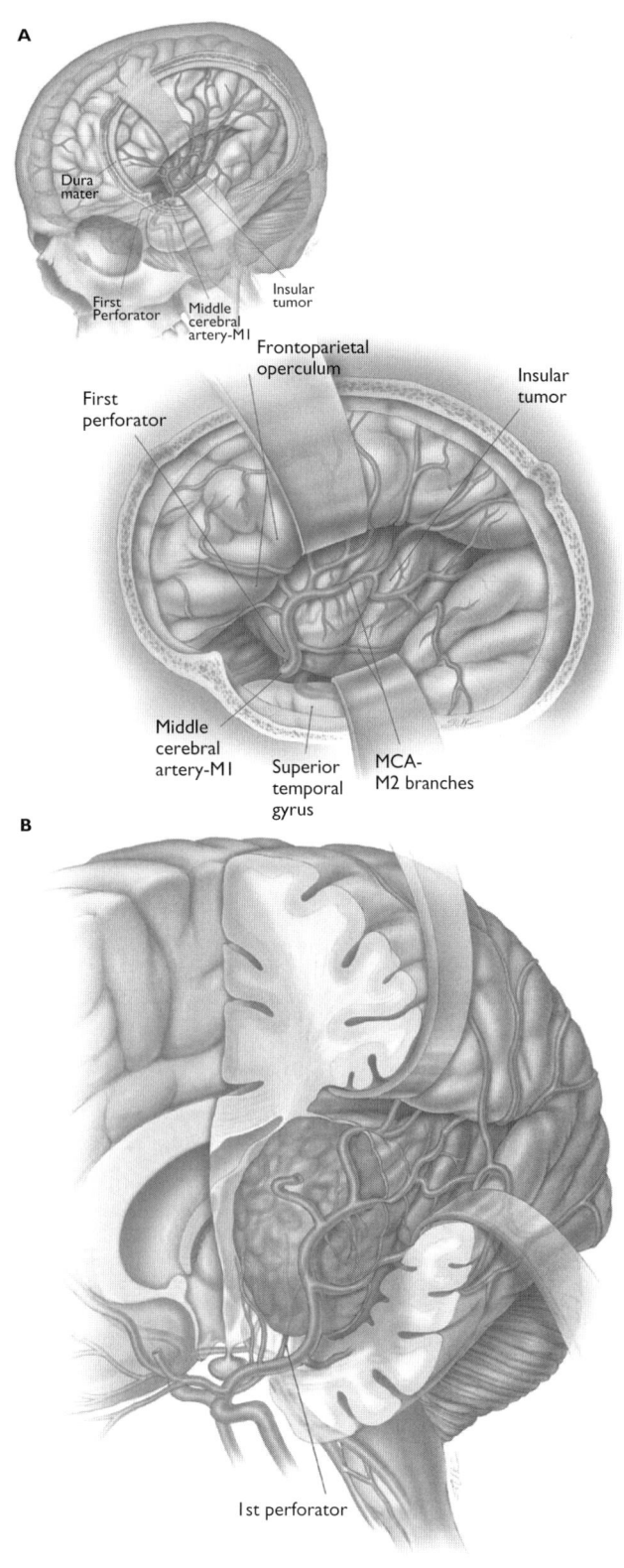

Figure 59.5 Surgical approach: Sylvian fissure dissection and MCA exposure. **(A)** Frontal temporal craniotomy is typically performed with adequate bone removal to visualize the frontal and temporal opercula as well as to allow for brain mapping. Note that in the typical operation, more exposure of the temporal tip than depicted is usually achieved, particularly if a temporal lobectomy is needed. The opening must allow for the exposure of the entire sylvian fissure. The MCAs typically lie with the insular sulci (especially the central insular sulcus) and may be buried because of tumor-induced expansion of the sulcus. **(B)** Critical feature of resecting insular tumors is to dissect to the base of the superior and inferior periinsular sulcus. This maneuver defines the extent of the tumor and helps to establish the depth of the tumor. In addition, identification of the first (most lateral) lenticulostriate artery is critical for defining the depth. The small tumor vessels arising from the M2 branches must be coagulated and cut. This devascularizes the tumor, aids in its resection, and prevents injury to the main M2 branches. Reprinted with permission from Hentschel and Lang [9].

fissure as an expanded insular apex often protrudes into the fissure. The initial split of the vertical portion of the fissure is followed by widening of the fissure, which is accomplished by following the dissection into the peri-insular sulci and separating the opercula from the surface of the insula. This will expose the surface of the tumor and the M2 branches. This is illustrated in figure 59.5.

MCA Exposure

As the sylvian fissure is split, the MCA branches are exposed. Early exposure of the MCA along its entire length, from the turn at the limen insula to the M3 segments at the surface of the peri-insular sulci, with identification of all important perforators, reduces the risk of MCA injury during subsequent tumor dissection. Branches engulfed by tumor are identified to prevent their inadvertent coagulation later in the procedure. The M2 branches are followed into the peri-insular sulci and isolated, allowing for the identification of the short perforators supplying the tumor, which can then be safely divided. Most critical of all is the identification of the origins of the LLAs. The most lateral (distal) LLA can be used as a mark for the medial margin of tumor resection and dissection deep relative to this vessel is discouraged (Figure 59.6) [2,3,20].

Peri-Insular Sulcus Dissection

The dissection of the peri-insular sulci begins concurrently with the end of the sylvian fissure dissection and the exposure of the distal MCA branches. We regard it as a separate stage in order to emphasize the importance of identifying the base of these sulci. As previously mentioned, the three peri-insular sulci delineate the boundaries of the insular lobe and separate the insula from the overlying opercula. Because most insular tumors expand the insula without infiltrating beyond, the peri-insular sulci define the boundaries of the tumor, as illustrated in Figure 59.6. Dissecting to the depth of each of these sulci is critical, as this depth frequently demarcates the deep margin of the tumor, and the plane between tumor and surrounding white matter is frequently best identified at the base of the sulcus.

Generally, dissection of the inferior peri-insular sulcus is straightforward, as large M2 vessels always run parallel

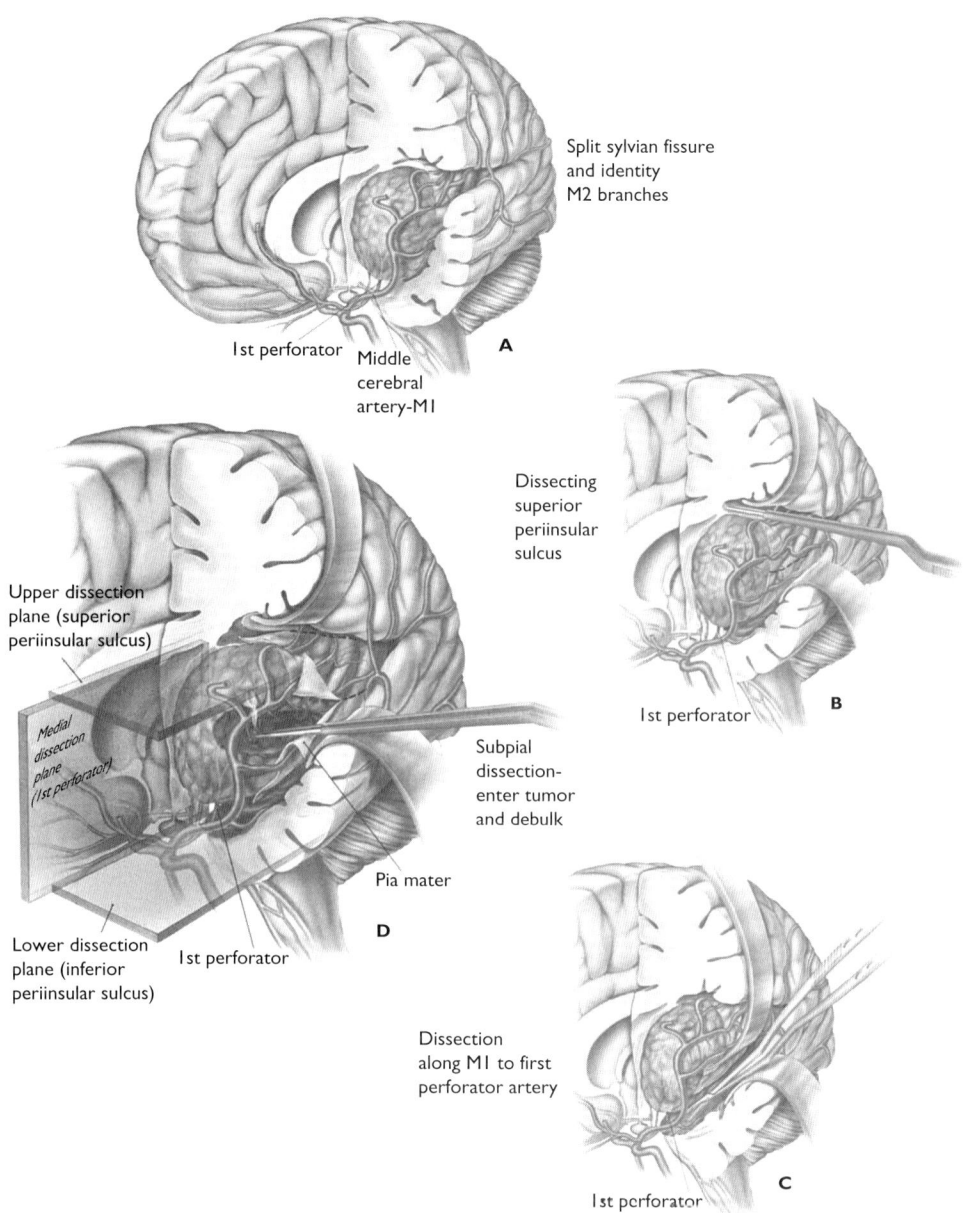

Figure 59.6 Surgical approach: peri-insular sulcus dissection and boundaries of resection. **(A)** Initial splitting of the sylvian fissure allows identification of the apex of the insula and the posterior extent of the tumor. The MCA vessels are often seen but may be encased by tumor. **(B)** The superior and inferior periinsular sulci are dissected to their bases to define the superior and inferior aspects of the tumor. **(C)** The MCA is dissected proximally until the first LLA is identified. This defines the deep plane of the tumor and protects the LLA from injury. The MCA is dissected in a proximal to distal direction. **(D)** Once the three planes of the tumor are defined, the tumor is resected in a subpial fashion with preservation of M2 vessels and coagulation of small M2 branches. Reprinted with permission from Lang et al [2].

to the sulcus and allow for easy separation of the temporal operculum from the insula. The insular vein lies at the base of this sulcus and can be coagulated. The anterior sulcus is similarly easy to define, as an M2 branch supplying the frontal lobe is usually present. This sulcus can seem quite deep, however, especially if the insular apex expands into the sylvian fissure. In contrast, the base of the superior peri-insular sulcus is the most difficult to reach. It is at this stage of the dissection that retraction of the frontal operculum is often required. The MCA vessels run perpendicular rather than parallel to this sulcus, increasing the difficulty of the dissection. In addition, the sulcus is usually quite deep and at a very superior angle. The mean distance from the insular apex to the superior peri-insular sulcus is normally 1.9 cm [19] but can be double this in some insular tumors [2]. Angulation of the operating microscope can help provide a better view of this region, allowing for the use of retraction to be minimized. Proper positioning of the patient also helps reduce the need for retraction. Some tumor debulking may be performed preceding deeper dissection in this region as well, to minimize retraction. The superior peri-insular sulcus also identifies the location where the internal capsule is at greatest risk, and the surgeon must be cognizant of the proximity of this important structure when working in this area.

Devascularization of the Tumor

After defining the margins of the dissection by exposing the bases of the peri-insular sulci and identifying the important vasculature within the operative field, it is critical to devascularize the tumor before beginning its actual resection. As previously mentioned, insular tumors draw their blood supply primarily from the short and medium M2 perforators that supply the normal insular cortex and white matter in which the tumor typically grows and expands. Each perforator must be identified, coagulated, and divided in turn, as avulsion of these vessels can lead to bleeding that is difficult to stop without injuring the critical parent vessel. The long M2 perforators, which make up about 5% of the perforating vessels, must be recognized and preserved at this point. Typically they are larger in diameter, do not taper, and arise from M2 branches overlying the posterior insula [2,19].

Removal of Tumor Mass

With the boundaries defined and the tumor devascularized, the removal of the tumor mass may now begin. Large sections of tumor within the tumor bulk between the overlying vessels may be removed nearly en bloc. Along the boundaries of the tumor, subpial dissection is recommended. This ensures that the resection stays within the anatomic confines of the expanded insular lobe. Also, the intact pia provides a barrier that helps to protect and limit manipulation of the overlying MCA branches [2].

Determining the medial extent of the resection is the greatest challenge. This is where the risk of injury to the LLAs is greatest. The bases of the peri-insular sulci and the most lateral LLA can be used as landmarks to define the deepest plane of the tumor and the medial tumor border (Figure 59.6). Intraoperative ultrasound may be used to help with this determination. Finally, the surgeon must be acutely aware of changes in the color, consistency, and texture of the tumor tissue, as this is often critical in determining when the medial resection should cease. It is important to maintain a level dissection and avoid dissecting too deeply in one area and too shallowly in another. We usually resect the anterior portion of the tumor first, followed by the central portion, and then the edges. Retraction should be minimized in the posterior-inferior aspect of the tumor, which lies near receptive speech areas on the dominant hemisphere, and the posterior-superior aspect of the tumor, which may lie close to primary motor areas of the frontal lobe. After tumor resection is complete, meticulous hemostasis is achieved. Closure of the craniotomy and skin incision may be performed in the standard manner.

INTRAOPERATIVE ADJUNCTS

A variety of intraoperative adjuncts have been used in an attempt to reduce the risk of complications in insular tumor surgery, including image-guided neuronavigation, intraoperative ultrasound, intraoperative MRI, awake craniotomy, direct stimulation of deep white matter tracts, and motor evoked potential (MEP) monitoring [2,10]. All have their advantages and disadvantages.

Neuronavigation can be used to maximize surgical resection. Frameless stereotactic methods are most helpful in localizing the tumor prior to opening the skull and in designing the craniotomy, but once the sylvian fissure has been split and part of the tumor removed, brain shift generally reduces their effectiveness in determining useful tumor margins. This is particularly true when approaching the most difficult aspect of the resection along the deep margin between the tumor and the basal ganglia. Intraoperative ultrasound is a useful tool because it allows for following the tumor in real time. However, it is susceptible to resection artifact, particularly at the deep margins of the tumor. Intraoperative MRI is another new technology that may overcome many of these difficulties but has not been fully evaluated to date.

To reduce neurological dysfunction, intraoperative cortical mapping of motor and speech functions using direct brain stimulation during awake craniotomy is particularly advantageous for reducing risk of motor or speech deficits. Nevertheless, awake craniotomy does not eliminate risk completely. Injuries may occur between tests, or damage to a structure may produce a deficit that is immediately irreversible. This is particularly true when the dissection encroaches on the internal capsule [2]. In the most recently published study, Neuloh reported the successful use of MEP monitoring under general anesthesia with a high degree of sensitivity for impending neurological injury. Specifically, no patients with normal MEP recordings throughout the procedure developed postoperative permanent neurologic deficits, and among patients with intraoperative MEP changes, no permanent deficits occurred in any of the cases where normal MEPs were restored by intraoperative interventions. However, the reported incidence of permanent postoperative deficits in this series was not substantially different from previously reported averages, despite the use of MEP monitoring [10].

SURGICAL OUTCOMES

Because the goals of surgery are maximal resection with minimal morbidity, outcomes are best defined in terms of these parameters. Table 59.3 summarizes the rates of neurological dysfunction and the extent of resection in the clinical series reported in the literature to date.

Neurologic Function

The most significant deficits associated with resection of insular tumors are hemiparesis and aphasia. These can be transient or permanent. The rate of transient neurologic deficit following insular tumor surgery is not insignificant, but the degree of the deficits is usually not severe. Zentner reported 63% neurological morbidity immediately postoperatively and 23% neurologic deficit at 3 months [6]. Vanacochla reported a rate for immediate postoperative deficits of 21% [11], Duffau reported 50% immediate postoperative hemiparesis, 24% aphasia, and 17% neuropsychological dysfunction [8]. Neuloh reported a rate of transient postoperative hemiparesis of 18% with the use of continuous intraoperative MEP monitoring [10]. In our series, we have found an immediate postoperative deficit rate of 34%, mostly mild speech dysfunction associated with resecting insular tumors from the dominant hemisphere [2,9].

However, most of these transient symptoms resolve, though the duration of recovery can be up to

Table 59.3 Extent of Resection and Clinical Outcome, Summary of Literature[a]

Published Series	n	Extent of Resection	Summary of Outcome
Yasargil 1992 [3]	57	Not reported	87% good outcome if benign 85% good outcome if malignant
Yasargil 1996 [20]	150	Not reported	93% good outcome if benign 89% good outcome if malignant
Zentner 1996 [6]	30	17% 100% resection 70% >80% resection 13% 50–80% resection	63% postoperative neurological morbidity 23% deficit 3 months postoperative 7% permanent deficit
Vanacochla 1997 [11]	28	71% complete resection 4% subtotal resection	21% postoperative deficit 9% requiring assistance long term
Duffau 2000 [7]	12	25% total resection 50% subtotal resection	58% postoperative deficit 8% deficit 3 months postoperative
Lang 2001 [2]	22	45% >90% resection 27% 75% to 90% resection	23% improved postoperative 41% unchanged postoperative 36% increased deficits postoperative 9% permanent deficit
Duffau 2002 [5]	11	27% total resection 64% subtotal resection	45% postoperative deficit No deficits 3 months postoperative 82% epilepsy class I
Hentschel 2005 [9]	36	Not reported	42% postoperative deficit 11% permanent deficit, all minor
Duffau 2006 [8]	42	74% total/subtotal resection	50% postoperative hemiparesis 24% postoperative aphasia 17% postoperative neuropsychological symptoms 7% deficits at 3 months postoperative

Neuloh 2007 [10]	84	100% critical resection with safe completion reported for all cases with stable MEPs
		56% cessation of critical resection with MEP deterioration or loss
			Overall
			  18% transient paresis
			  12% permanent paresis
			  6% severe permanent paresis
			Stable MEP
			  5% transient paresis
			Reversible MEP deterioration:
			  40% transient mild paresis
			  12% transient moderate paresis
			Irreversible MEP loss
			  100% permanent new paresis

Neuloh 2007 [29]	100	Not reported	8% permanent deficit, all with irreversible MEP loss, in monitored group 18% (n = 11) permanent deficit in group where reliable MEP monitoring could not be established

[a] some patients reported in more than one series by author(s).

Abbreviation: MEP, motor evoked potential.

4 to 12 weeks [8]. The rates of permanent deficits in the reported series ranged from 7% to 10% [2,6,8,9,11]. Yasargil reported that 93% of patients with low-grade tumors and 90% of patients with high-grade tumors ultimately had no or only minor deficits that did not interfere with independence, while the remainder of the patients in his series were able to return home, but required some assistance with daily activities [3,20]. Neuloh reported a rate of permanent deficit in operations utilizing MEP monitoring to be 8% compared with a rate of 23% for surgeries where MEP monitoring could not be instituted for technical reasons, but the number of cases without MEP monitoring was very small. The rate of severe disabling permanent deficit in monitored patients in this study was only 4% [10]. In our series of 47 patients, in which 66% of tumors were in the dominant hemisphere, the rate of permanent neurological motor deficits was only 9%, and no patient had permanent speech dysfunction [2,9].

Extent of Resection

Because most insular tumors do not show enhancement, complete resection is defined as removal of all the hyperintense signal evident on T2-wighted MR images. Comparisons of preoperative and postoperative images are critical to this analysis. A review of the literature demonstrates that 100% removal of all the hyperintense signal on T2-weighted images is difficult to achieve but that radical resection (>90%) is more common. Zentner reported achieving 100% tumor removal in 17% of patients, more than 80% removal in 70%, and 50% to 80% removal in 14% of cases [6]. Vanacochla reported 71% complete, 4% subtotal, and 25% partial resections, and after repeat operations in patients with incomplete initial resections, 87% of patients ultimately had complete resections [11]. Duffau reported a combined total and subtotal resection rate of 74% [8]. In all these series, the extent of resection was typically determined by comparing preoperative and postoperative MR images although the specific methods used in these determinations were often not defined. In our series, we measured the tumor volume on preoperative and postoperative MR images using a computer-based algorithm and found that we achieved a >90% resection in 45% of patients, 75% to 90% resection in 27%, and less than 75% in 27% of cases [2,9]. Thus a radical resection of >75% was achieved in 72% of cases.

An unsatisfactory extent of resection can usually be attributed to two main causes. The first is the development of new neurological dysfunction (during awake craniotomy) or changes in neuromonitoring during tumor dissection that prompt the surgeon to abort the resection prematurely for fear of producing permanent neurological deterioration [2]. In some instances, this is unavoidable due to the specific proximity of the tumor to important neural and vascular structures. In other cases, the intraoperative findings of concern are transient phenomena related to excessive retraction, vascular spasm, global or local hypoperfusion, or technical issues related to monitoring equipment. Although these changes are reversible and not necessarily related to impending risk of permanent injury, they may still compel the surgeon to abandon aggressive dissection prematurely. These circumstances can be minimized with careful and judicious technique. The second main cause of incomplete resection are local changes in the physical properties of the tumor, for instance, the appearance of a more fibrous texture [2] or the disappearance of a readily identifiable resection plane in areas near critical neuroanatomy, which make it difficult for the surgeon to confidently pursue further aggressive dissection in that area. In these instances, intraoperative localization with frameless stereotaxy and/or ultrasound can sometimes provide helpful information. Ultimately, the surgeon must apply appropriate clinical judgment in determining whether further resection is safe and/or necessary [29]. (Figure 59.7).

CONCLUSION

Insular tumors were once considered to be inoperable lesions. However, modern microsurgical techniques, based on a clear understanding of the normal and tumoral anatomy have made the successful extirpation of these tumors possible. Optimal tumor removal and the minimization of complications can be achieved by careful patient selection,

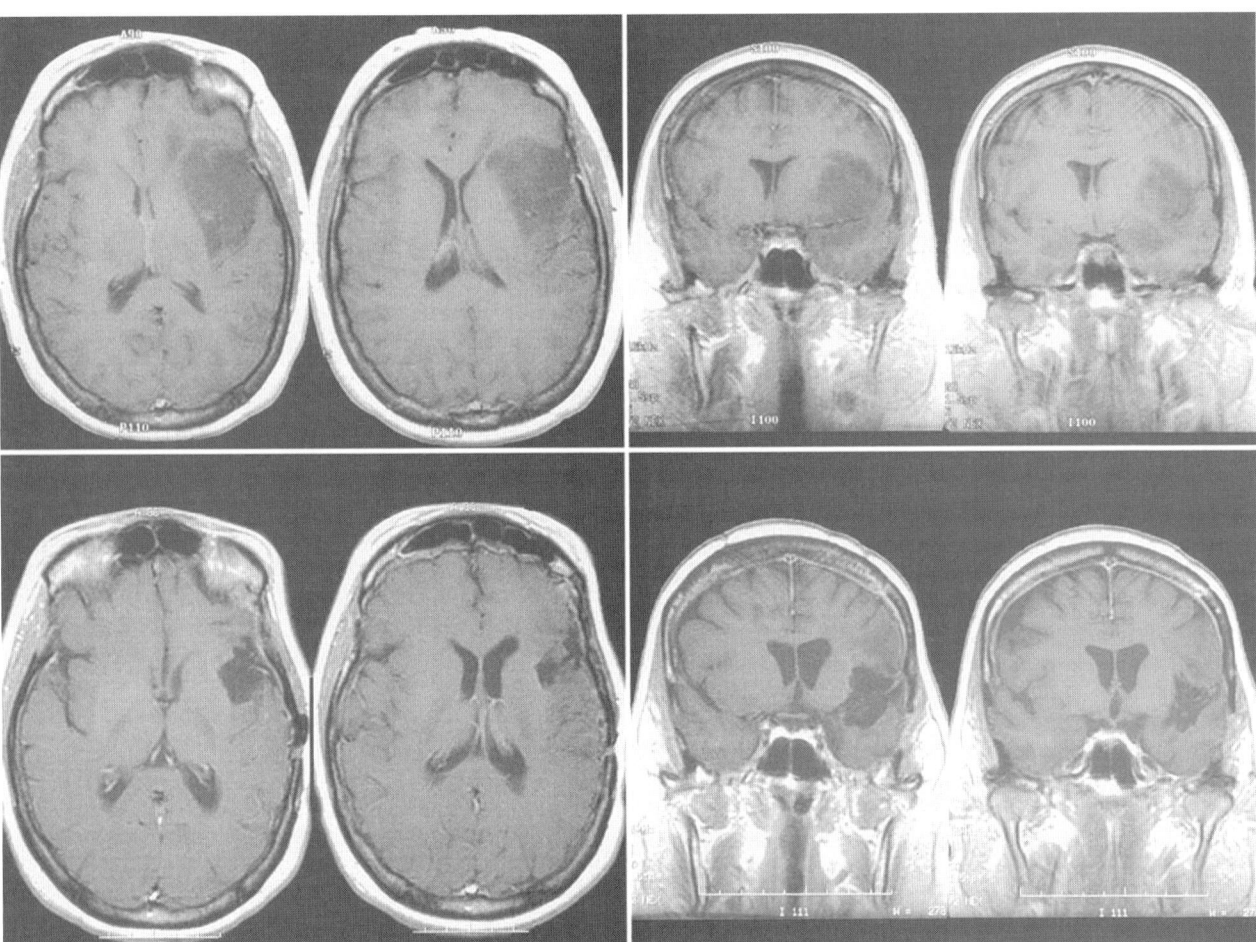

Figure 59.7 Axial (left) and coronal (right) T1-weighted MR images obtained before (upper) and after (lower) transsylvian resection of a purely insular tumor. A 99% resection was achieved. Reprinted with permission from Lang et al [2].

judicious use of appropriate intraoperative adjuncts, meticulous dissection, and a healthy respect for the pertinent anatomy. The successful treatment of insular tumors remains a test of the surgeon's clinical judgment and technical skill.

REFERENCES

1. Duffau H, Capelle L. Preferential brain locations of low-grade gliomas. *Cancer.* 2004;100:2622–2626.
2. Lang FF, Olansen NE, DeMonte F, et al. Surgical resection of intrinsic insular tumors: complication avoidance. *J Neurosurg.* 2001;95:638–650.
3. Yasargil MG, von Ammon K, Cavazos E, Doczi T, Reeves JD, Roth P. Tumours of the limbic and paralimbic systems. *Acta Neurochir (Wien).* 1992;118:40–52.
4. Toms SA, Weil RJ, Gupta A, Boulis NM, Prayson R, Lang FF. Clinical problem-solving: island intruder. *Neurosurgery.* 2008;62:920–929.
5. Duffau H, Capelle L, Lopes M, Bitar A, Sichez JP, van Effenterre R. Medically intractable epilepsy from insular low-grade gliomas: improvement after an extended lesionectomy. *Acta Neurochir (Wien).* 2002;144:563–573.
6. Zentner J, Meyer B, Stangl A, Schramm J. Intrinsic tumors of the insula: a prospective surgical study of 30 patients. *J Neurosurg.* 1996;85:263–271.
7. Duffau H, Capelle L, Lopes M, Faillot T, Sichez JP, Fohanno D. The insular lobe: physiopathological and surgical considerations. *Neurosurgery.* 2000;47:801–811.
8. Duffau H, Taillandier L, Gatignol P, Capelle L. The insular lobe and brain plasticity: lessons from tumor surgery. *Clin Neurol Neurosurg.* 2006;108:543–548.
9. Hentschel SJ, Lang FF. Surgical resection of intrinsic insular tumors. *Neurosurgery.* 2005;57:176–183.
10. Neuloh G, Pechstein U, Schramm J. Motor tract monitoring during insular glioma surgery. *J Neurosurg.* 2007;106:582–592.
11. Vanaclocha V, Saiz-Sapena N, Garcia-Casasola C. Surgical treatment of insular gliomas. *Acta Neurochir (Wien).* 1997;139:1126–1134.
12. Ture U, Yasargil DC, Al-Mefty O, Yasargil MG. Topographic anatomy of the insular region. *J Neurosurg.* 1999;90:720–733.
13. Sanfey AG, Rilling JK, Aronson JA, Nystrom LE, Cohen JD. The neural basis of economic decision-making in the Ultimatum Game. *Science.* 2003;300:1755–1758.
14. Zink CF, Tong Y, Chen Q, Bassett DS, Stein JL, Meyer-Lindenberg A. Know your place: neural processing of social hierarchy in humans. *Neuron.* 2008;58:273–283.
15. Adolphs R, Damasio H, Tranel D, Cooper G, Damasio AR. A role for somatosensory cortices in the visual recognition of emotion as revealed by three-dimensional lesion mapping. *J Neurosci.* 2000;20:2683–2690.
16. Carr L, Iacoboni M, Dubeau MC, Mazziotta JC, Lenzi GL. Neural mechanisms of empathy in humans: a relay from neural systems for imitation to limbic areas. *Proc Natl Acad Sci U S A.* 2003;100:5497–5502.
17. Meyer-Lindenberg A. Psychology. Trust me on this. *Science.* 2008;321:778–780.
18. Naqvi NH, Rudrauf D, Damasio H, Bechara A. Damage to the insula disrupts addiction to cigarette smoking. *Science.* 2007;315:531–534.
19. Ture U, Yasargil MG, Al-Mefty O, Yasargil DC. Arteries of the insula. *J Neurosurg.* 2000;92:676–687.
20. Yasargil MG. *Microneursurgery.* New York, NY: Thieme Medical Publishers; 1996.
21. Cairncross G, Berkey B, Shaw E, et al. Phase III trial of chemotherapy plus radiotherapy compared with radiotherapy alone for pure and mixed anaplastic oligodendroglioma: Intergroup radiation therapy oncology group trial 9402. *J Cin Oncol.* 2006;24:2707–2714.
22. Cairncross JG, Ueki K, Zlatescu MC, et al. Specific genetic predictors of chemotherapeutic response and survival in patients with anaplastic oligodendrogliomas. *J Natl Cancer Inst.* 1998;90:1473–1479.
23. Kanner AA, Staugaitis SM, Castilla EA, et al. The impact of genotype on outcome in oligodendroglioma: validation of the loss of chromosome arm 1p as an important factor in clinical decision making. *J Neurosurg.* 2006;104:542–550.
24. Jackson RJ, Fuller GN, Abi-Said D, et al. Limitations of stereotactic biopsy in the initial management of gliomas. *Neuro Oncol.* 2001;3:193–200.
25. Lang FF, Gilbert MR. Diffusely infiltrative low-grade glioma in adults. *J Clin Oncol.* 2006;24:1236–1245.
26. Stummer W, Pichlmeier U, Meinel T, et al. Fluorescence-guided surgery with 5-aminolevulinic acid for resection of malignant glioma: a randomised controlled multicentre phase III trial. *Lancet Oncol.* 2006;7:392–401.
27. Vuorinen V, Hinkka S, Farkkila M, Jaaskelainen J. Debulking or biopsy of malignant glioma in elderly people - a randomized study. *Acta Neurochir (Wien).* 2003;145:5–10.
28. Lacroix M, Abi-Said D, Fourney DR, et al. A multivariate analysis of 416 patients with glioblastoma multiforme: prognosis, extent of resection, and survival. *J Neurosurg.* 2001;95:190–198.
29. Neuloh G, Simon M, Schramm J. Stroke prevention during surgery for deep-seated gliomas. *Neurophysiol Clin.* 2007;37:383–389.

60 Pediatric Tumor Surgery

Shobhan Vachhrajani, Michael Ellis, and James T. Rutka

After hematological malignancies, central nervous system (CNS) neoplasms represent the most common cancers in children. Their heterogeneity, both in pathology and location, present an academic and technical challenge to the pediatric neurosurgeon. This chapter aims to address these concerns and provide a guide to surgical treatment for anatomically based groups of brain tumors: supratentorial, suprasellar, intraventricular, pineal region, and posterior fossa. It is hoped that the clinical nuances gleaned from this chapter will prove invaluable to the pediatric neurosurgeon embarking on such cases.

SUPRATENTORIAL TUMORS

Arguably the most significant challenge in managing supratentorial lesions in children is the large number of tumor types that face the pediatric neurosurgeon. Purely glial tumors, both high and low grade, as well as mixed glioneuronal tumors are common. We briefly discuss three types of supratentorial lesions here: gliomas, dysembryoplastic neuroepithelial tumors (DNET), and gangliogliomas. Surgical considerations of performing hemispheric tumor resections are also addressed.

Gliomas

Tumors of glial origin account for approximately 50% of all brain tumors in children, and their classification is based both on location within the brain and by grade [1]. Both of these characteristics impart prognostic significance. Low-grade hemispheric tumors represent 10% to 15% of all brain tumors in children, and high-grade gliomas in this region are much less common.

Clinical presentation of gliomas in children varies with grade and location. Children with low-grade lesions commonly present with nonspecific symptoms such as lethargy, irritability, macrocephaly, localizing and lateralizing findings, and failure to thrive in combination with symptoms related to increased intracranial pressure. Those with high-grade lesions present similarly although their time course is often shorter. Although uncommon, children in this group may also present with abrupt changes in neurological status secondary to intratumoral hemorrhage [2]. Radiographically, low-grade lesions are usually hypointense on T1-weighted magnetic resonance (MR) images and hyperintense on T2-weighted MR images with little to no contrast enhancement (Figure 60.1A). High grade lesions appear as irregular, infiltrative, ring-enhancing lesions that are hypointense on T1-weighted MR imaging and hyperintense on T2-weighted MR imaging. There is usually significant associated mass effect and surrounding edema (Figure 60.1B).

Gangliogliomas

Mixed glioneuronal tumors, including gangliogliomas, are a rare form of CNS neoplasm representing up to 2.5% of all brain tumors [1]. These lesions are comprised of dysplastic neurons and neoplastic glial cells with considerable heterogeneity in both of these cell lines. Occasionally due to clear cell morphology, differentiating these from DNET or oligodendroglioma can prove difficult [3,4].

Patients harboring these lesions present primarily with seizures, and these tumors may be found in up to 40% of those with chronic temporal lobe epilepsy [3,5–7]. Gangliogliomas typically behave in a biologically benign fashion; however, higher-grade lesions have been reported. Surgical therapy in this disease is directed at achieving long-term seizure control with complete lesionectomy providing Engel Class I seizure outcome in greater than 80% of patients (Figure 60.1C) [4]. Complete resection also minimizes the risk of tumor recurrence.

Dysembryoplastic Neuroepithelial Tumors

This group of lesions also falls within the group of mixed glioneuronal tumors and comprise approximately 0.5% of brain tumors in the pediatric age group [1]. As with gangliogliomas, childhood onset of medically intractable seizures are the major mode of presentation (Figure 60.1D). Resection of these lesions, either complete or incomplete, generally results in favorable seizure outcome; however, the outcome analysis is blurred by the heterogeneity of procedures performed. Previously published reports have, similar to gangliogliomas, displayed Engel Class I outcomes in up to 80% of patients although reports from our institution are not as favorable with only 62% of patients in this category at long-term follow-up [8,9]. Residual tumor is a significant predictor of poor long-term outcome, and total resection of the lesion is therefore recommended [9].

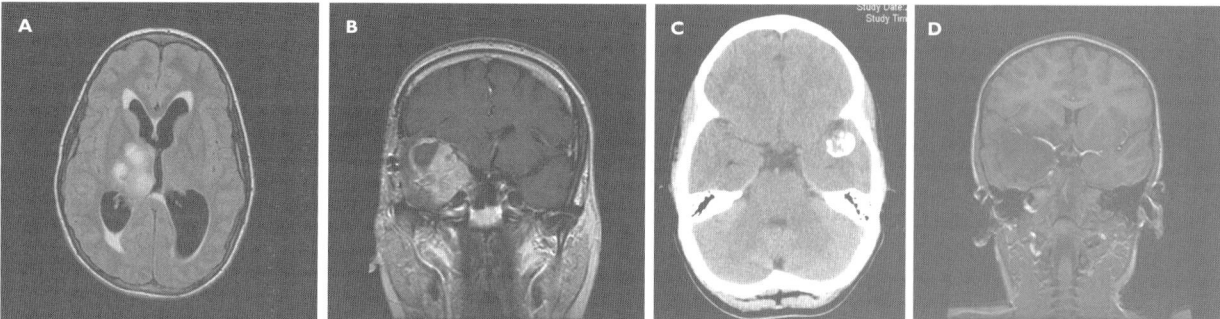

Figure 60.1 The varied appearance of pediatric supratentorial gliomas. **(A)** Axial FLAIR MRI in a 12-year-old male who presented with headaches and right hemiparesis. A diffuse, patchy lesion is seen in the right thalamus, which did not enhance with gadolinium. The lesion was biopsy-proven as low-grade astrocytoma. **(B)** Gadolinium-enhanced coronal MRI through the anterior temporal lobes showing densely enhancing right temporal tumor in an 11-year-old male who is a survivor of acute lymphocytic leukaemia in infancy. The lesion was removed and was an anaplastic astrocytoma. **(C)** Axial unenhanced CT scan in a 14-year-old female who presented with complex partial seizures with speech arrest. A calcified left temporal lesion is seen. Following preoperative brain mapping with functional MRI and MEG, the lesion was removed. It was a ganglioglioma. **(D)** Gadolinium-enhanced coronal MRI through the optic chiasm showing nonenhancing, diffuse lesion in the right temporal lobe, which crosses the Sylvian fissure in a 3-year-old male who presented with complex partial seizures. A right temporal lobectomy was performed, and the lesion proved to be a DNET.

Surgical Considerations

Complete surgical resection of the aforementioned lesions provides the best chance at survival, in the case of gliomas, and seizure-free outcome in the case of gangliogliomas and DNETs. The surgical challenge rests, however, in the safe resection of these intraparenchymal lesions given their intimacy with eloquent structures. The potential for long-term neuropsychological and developmental sequelae in children only compounds this concern. Advances in neuroimaging and functional evaluation have provided a means to safely achieve total surgical resection with minimal neurocognitive morbidity.

Neuronavigation

The use of neuronavigation is ubiquitous in neurosurgery, and its application to pediatric brain tumor surgery is especially important. The development of frameless stereotaxy has allowed for preoperative planning maximizing the accuracy of craniotomy and cortical incision placement along with the identification of vital neurovascular structures to be avoided during resection [10,11]. All of this information provides real time anatomical feedback to surgeons, consequently optimizing the degree of lesional resection while minimizing neurological injury (Figure 60.2).

This technology remains limited in its ability to predict intraoperative tissue shifts. Accordingly, intraoperative MRI has been employed in select cases; however, the expense associated with this technology has precluded its implementation in a widespread fashion [12]. Currently, intraoperative ultrasound provides the best available method for real-time tracking of the extent of resection. Future directions will likely consist of integrating intraoperative static imaging with functional techniques to optimally protect eloquent brain structures during tumor resection.

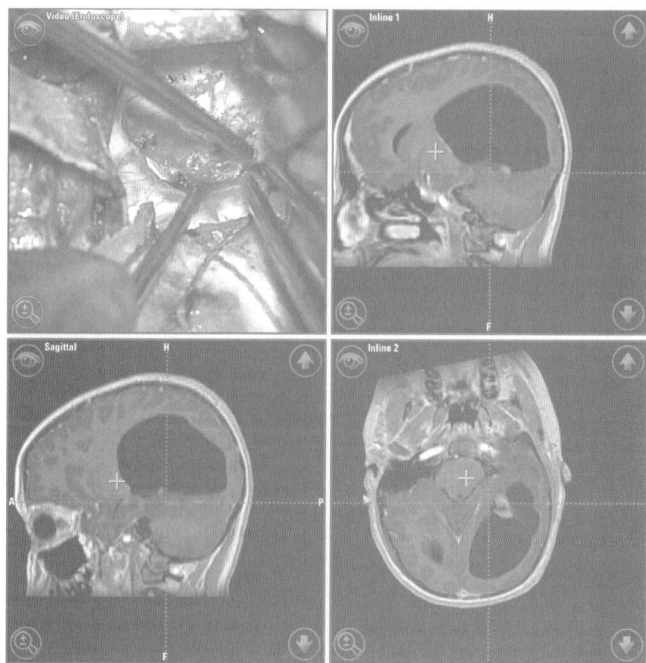

Figure 60.2 Intraoperative view of neurosurgical removal of left occipital pilocytic astrocytoma in 14-year-old male who presented with headaches, poor school performance, and right hemianopsia. The use of neuronavigation has facilitated the removal of deep-seated lesions such as this.

Functional Imaging

The creation of a functional brain map cannot be overstated in these patients, and several techniques are used as surgical adjuncts in this regard. Functional MRI has proven to be greatly beneficial in locating language, motor, and sensory regions of cortex using gradient echo sequences aimed at detecting changes in local blood flow correlated with cortical activation [13,14]. Patients are required to perform a variety of paradigms aimed at elucidating these areas. The ease with which such tasks are performed in adults is appreciable; however, it does raise some special concerns in children. Differences in the hemodynamic response to stimulation can lead to differential blood oxygenation level responses, and the hyperdynamic circulation of the child leads to increased noise in image acquisition. Similarly, differences in head circumference, skull thickness, and developmental changes in metabolism will all impact on the signals acquired. Finally, performance must be matched for age, and these inherent complexities influence the interpretation of functional MRI studies [15].

In lesions where seizure control represents the primary goal of surgery, magnetoencephalography (MEG) and magnetic source imaging (MSI) have become an integral part of surgical planning. MEG relies on changes in magnetic fields created by epileptogenic foci, and coupling of this data to structural imaging (MSI) creates an anatomical and functional map that can also be incorporated into stereotactic neuronavigational systems. Although the temporal resolution of MEG is similar to scalp electroencephalography, it has improved spatial resolution compared to electroencephalography and does not suffer from issues related to signal attenuation by the scalp or cranium [14]. Several groups have reported good correlation of functional MEG data with intraoperative electrocortical mapping, and its use in locating eloquent cortex near a variety of hemispheric lesions has also been widely reported [16–22]. Its application in facilitating maximal tumor resection with minimal violation of functional cortex is easily appreciated (Figure 60.3).

Finally, direct electrocortical stimulation remains the gold standard for brain mapping prior to surgical resection. The precentral and postcentral gyri as well as the premotor and supplementary motor areas can be mapped. Motor functions may be mapped with the patient under general anesthetic; however, language functions must be assessed with the patient awake [14]. This can prove difficult in the pediatric population.

SUPRASELLAR TUMORS

Suprasellar lesions span the range of pathology from benign to malignant. An understanding of the relevant regional neuroanatomy is essential for neurosurgical approaches in this area. In this section on suprasellar lesions, we briefly review craniopharyngiomas and pituitary adenomas in children and offer some insights into surgical considerations and approaches.

Craniopharyngioma

Craniopharyngioma represents 6% to 13% of all childhood brain tumors [23]. These tumors display a bimodal peak, with adults over the age of 65 years more frequently diagnosed whereas in children, these tumors present in the 5 to 14 year age group. Most pediatric cancer registries classify craniopharyngioma into tumors of benign or unspecified behavior [24,25]. Similarly, worldwide registries list the

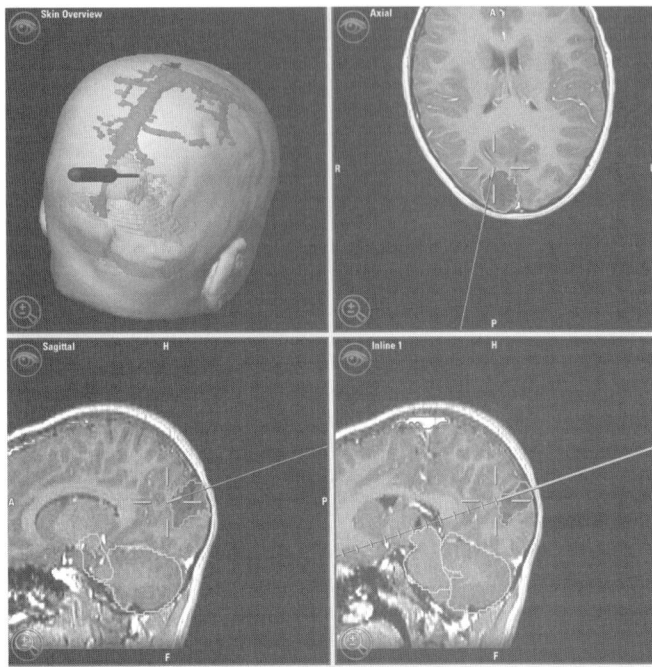

Figure 60.3 Utility of MEG demonstrated while linked to frameless stereotaxy in 8-year-old male with visual scintillations and right occipital tumor. The green squares to the right of the tumor mass (orange) represent the location of the interictal spike waves from the EEG. Using MEG, we can also map the visual evoked fields in the calcarine cortex, so as to attempt to preserve visual indices as best as possible. *See color insert.*

population incidence at approximately 1.4 cases per million children per year [23].

There are two predominant histopathological forms of craniopharyngioma. The adamantinous form is the typical pediatric variant, with the squamous papillary form more commonly seen in adults. Mixed or transitional forms have been reported but are rare in comparison [26]. The pathological differences between the two forms are well described in the literature [27–29].

The clinical presentation of children with craniopharyngioma can be divided into three categories: (1) Visual impairment due to chiasmal compression; (2) Hydrocephalus due to third ventricular obstruction; and (3) Endocrine deficits from disruption of the hypothalamic-pituitary axis [30]. The vast majority of children will present with headache and visual disturbances, including decreased acuity and bitemporal hemianopia in up to 70% of cases [24]. Two thirds of these children will experience resolution of these symptoms after surgery, and neuro-ophthalmological evaluation is therefore recommended. Typical signs and symptoms of raised intracranial pressure are found in 15% to 30% of patients at presentation and is more common in tumors with large solid or cystic components that extend to fill the third ventricle [31]. Most children do not present with symptoms of endocrinopathy yet up to 80% of children will have laboratory evidence of endocrine dysfunction at diagnosis. This is predominantly manifested in growth hormone deficiency (75% of cases), with gonadotropin and adrenocorticotropic hormone and strategy: The clinical condition of the patient, including rapidly deteriorating vision or level of consciousness from acute or severe hydrocephalus; the consistency of the tumor; and the goal of the attempted resection [30]. The personal experience of the neurosurgeon should not be underestimated. Those who operate on at least two pediatric craniopharyngioma cases per year have lower rates of operative morbidity and higher chances of achieving a gross total resection when desired [33].

Hydrocephalus

The optimal method of treating hydrocephalus is arguably to treat the tumor itself. In a large number of cases, however, it is not the tumor mass itself that causes third ventricular compression, rather the cystic component of tumor. Resultant ventriculomegaly allows uncomplicated access to the ventricular system and consequently to the cyst itself. We have increasingly employed neuroendoscopy to drain tumor cysts, create communications between the lateral ventricles by way of septostomy, and create a tract for easy placement of a permanent cerebrospinal fluid (CSF) diversion device or reservoir for cyst aspiration or injection. For patients *in extremis* from tumor-associated hydrocephalus, emergent CSF drainage either by external ventricular drainage or more commonly by shunt is recommended prior to embarking on direct surgical management of the tumor.

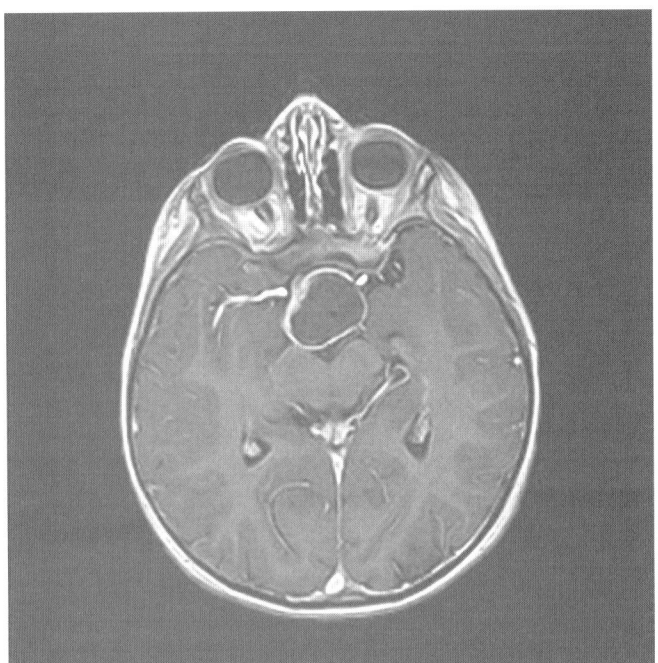

Figure 60.4 Three-year-old male with progressive visual loss and craniopharyngioma. Axial enhanced MRI showing cystic suprasellar lesion. Note relationship to intracranial carotid arteries and branches of the circle of Willis. The lesion compresses the optic chiasm. Treatment here consisted of instillation of bleomycin through an Ommaya reservoir for several months followed by neurosurgical removal of the lesion.

Surgical resection

The role of aggressive surgical resection in craniopharyngioma remains a subject of some controversy. Historically, pediatric neurosurgeons sought to achieve a cure by complete tumor resection [30,34,35]. Others, however, noticed that partial resection with postoperative radiotherapy provides similar rates of tumor control with better quality of life [36].

Surgical approaches to craniopharyngioma resection are well described elsewhere [37]. We have traditionally employed the unilateral subfrontal approach using a unilateral orbitotomy and an angled osteotomy that crosses the midline and provides the best exposure of the anterior cranial base and helps to minimize brain retraction. The anterior superior sagittal sinus close to the crista galli can be taken so as to facilitate exposure. Meticulous microneurosurgical techniques are essential for success in craniopharyngioma surgery. The cavitron for solid tumors and intraoperative neuronavigation are used in many cases. The subfrontal approach can be combined with an anterior interhemispheric approach for improved access to the sellar area. For craniopharyngiomas that invaginate into the third ventricle in a retrochiasmatic fashion, a translaminar terminalis approach is typically used (Figure 60.5). Other neurosurgical approaches that have been used for craniopharyngioma include pterional, subtemporal, transcallosal, and transcortical depending on the presentation of the cystic and solid tumor components.

In recent years, the use of transsphenoidal endoscopic approaches has exploded [38–42]. Patients with

thyroid stimulating hormone deficiency also causing significant morbidity [23].

MRI scan is the diagnostic imaging modality of choice. Three types of tumor are commonly found: primary solid, mainly cystic and thin-walled, and a mix of the two types. Similarly, relationship of the tumor to adjacent neural structures, including the cranial nerves and optic chiasm, and the nearby internal carotid arteries is crucial given the risk of tumor invasion (Figure 60.4). There is a suggestion that brain invasion, surrounding inflammatory reactions, adherence to nearby intracranial vessels and nerves, calcifications, and tumor recurrence are higher in the pediatric group; however, the impact of such radiographic findings on prognosis appear questionable [27–29,32]. Computed tomography scan is of value in diagnosing hydrocephalus and for readily identifiable calcifications, which may help distinguish craniopharyngioma from the large list of other lesions that may occupy the suprasellar space.

Surgical Considerations

The goals of surgical management in craniopharyngioma are multiple. Surgery aims to relieve raised intracranial pressure when present, reverse the symptoms of chiasmatic compression, and prevent tumor regrowth or progression. These goals must be balanced with maintenance of quality of life, including the preservation of pituitary and neurocognitive function. Several factors must be individualized to each patient before embarking on a surgical

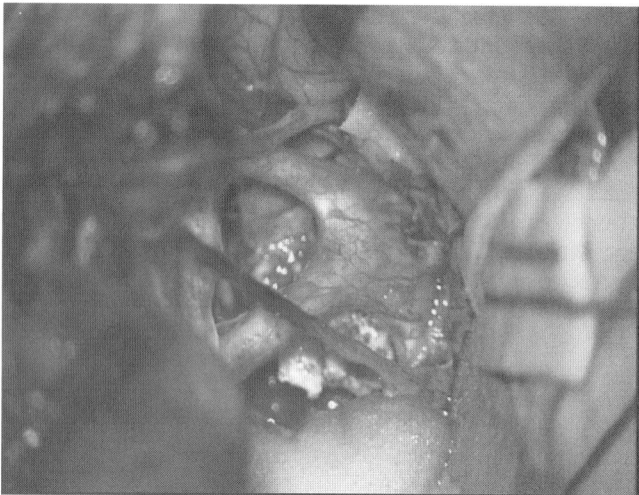

Figure 60.5 Subfrontal, trans-lamina terminalis approach to craniopharyngioma in a 10-year-old male presenting with left visual failure. Both olfactory nerves are seen coursing over the optic nerves. The lamina terminalis has been opened. Tumor is seen beneath the chiasm and the optic tracts bilaterally. The tumor is delivered from both the prechiasmatic and retrochiasmatic spaces using microneurosurgical techniques.

prechiasmatic lesions in which the diaphragma and sella are elevated are considered to be the best candidates for this procedure, as the subdiaphragmatic origin of the tumor allows resection by gentle retraction, and the diaphragma creates a barrier that separates tumor from brain and nearby neurovascular structures. In children, lack of pneumatization of the sphenoid sinus and a normal-sized sella can prove to be obstacles to performing transsphenoidal surgery [40]. Neuronavigation is useful in such cases. Despite earlier reports attesting to the limited tumor resection possible through endoscopy, several published reports have now confirmed the potential of this approach for craniopharyngioma [38–40].

Intracavitary Therapy

In patients with primarily cystic lesions, intracystic bleomycin may be used in conjunction with cyst aspiration by an Ommaya reservoir. Injections are carried out 2 to 3 times per week for several weeks, and cyst involution has been demonstrated. Blindness, perilesional edema, and death in one case have been reported [30]. Alpha-interferon and radioactive isotopes including ^{32}P and ^{90}Y have also been used as intracavitary therapy for craniopharyngioma. These modalities are helpful in cyst involution but not for prevention of solid tumor growth.

Radiation Therapy

The advent of conformal radiotherapy techniques have maintained tumor control while minimizing the adverse effects of radiation. Conformal external beam fractionated therapy has been the modality of choice in recent years. Standard treatment protocols deliver approximately 50Gy to the lesion over 30 to 35 fractions [30,36]. Gamma Knife stereotactic radiosurgery has been advocated by some, especially for patients receiving radiation in a delayed fashion. Lesions situated away from the optic chiasm are the best candidates given the low threshold for radiation damage to the chiasm. Marginal dose to the tumor is planned at 12Gy; lower doses do not appear to afford satisfactory long-term tumor control [30,36].

Postoperative Care

Multidisciplinary follow-up remains the mainstay of postoperative care in this group of patients. Neurocognitive, psychological, and social sequelae have been tied to aggressive attempts at surgical resection. The use of more conservative surgical approaches may mitigate these; however, such outcomes must be balanced with the cognitive impairments associated with radiotherapy. Postoperative endocrinopathy is common in those undergoing surgical resection, and endocrine hormone replacement must be provided. Hypothalamic dysfunction including obesity, narcolepsy, and severe behavioral disorders are common in those undergoing radical surgery. Selection of cases and the use of appropriate surgical technique is the key to avoiding this complication [26,28,43,44]. Finally, tumor recurrence, which is as high as 40% even after gross total resection, requires the pediatric neurosurgeon to revisit these issues over again.

Pituitary Adenoma

Pituitary adenomas in pediatric patients are a relatively rare entity, and account for approximately 6% of all intracranial tumors in adolescents [45–48]. A 25-year review at our institution revealed a 1.2% incidence out of all supratentorial lesions treated during that time period [49]. The majority of these cases occur in adolescence and given their low incidence, many are mistaken for craniopharyngioma. In contrast to adult lesions, where nonfunctioning adenomas represent up to 30% of tumors, the vast majority of pediatric pituitary adenomas are hormonally active, with nonfunctional lesions accounting for only 3% to 6% of lesions [50–52]. Prolactinomas are the most common form of tumor in pediatrics overall; however, its incidence peaks in adolescents over 12 years of age. Corticotropin secreting adenomas causing Cushing's disease and somatotroph adenomas are next in order of incidence [53].

Clinical presentation can be varied amongst age groups owing to the relative differences in tumor types; however, all present with a combination of disruption of growth or sexual maturation. Patients with adrenocorticotropic hormone releasing adenomas, most common in prepubescent children, often present with generalized weight gain and significant growth failure due to arrested skeletal development from hypercortisolemia. These adenomas are generally smaller than other tumor types [53]. Prolactinomas present with primary amenorrhea in females and hypogonadism in males. Although less common, prepubertal children may present with headache, visual disturbance, or growth failure. Galactorrhea may be found in select cases. The presentation of somatotrope adenomas varies on the state of the epiphyseal plate. Accelerated growth velocity is commonly observed in patients where fusion has not occurred; symptoms begin to reflect adult manifestations of acromegaly as plate fusion occurs. As these lesions often present as macroadenomas, headaches and visual disturbances from mass effect may also be observed [50].

Along with baseline endocrinological evaluation, MRI is the test of choice when investigating these patients. Adenomas absorb contrast at slower rates than surrounding normal pituitary tissue and usually appear hypointense. Deviation of the pituitary stalk, asymmetrical increases in glandular height, and extension to nearby structures may also be seen [50].

Surgical Considerations

It is in this group of patients where transsphenoidal surgery offers the greatest benefit over transcranial approaches, as significant reductions in morbidity and mortality have been observed. Sellar expansion is often seen with pituitary adenomas allowing for ease of transsphenoidal access. Perhaps most important in surgical management is patient selection. Medical management is advised as first-line treatment of prolactinomas, with surgery reserved for tumors insensitive to dopamine agonists.

Surgical excision is the optimal therapeutic strategy for all other functional adenomas and nonfunctional adenomas causing symptoms from mass effect. Adrenocorticotropic hormone secreting lesions display good results, with 90% success rates initially for noninvasive lesions (Figure 60.6). Radiation may be used at the time of recurrence although delayed hormone deficiency should be anticipated, with long-term cure rates reaching 60% to 80% [51]. Similar results have been observed with surgical removal of growth hormone secreting adenomas. Radiotherapy has also been administered in this group, with long-term control achieved in 60% to 80% of patients. This benefit is delayed by several years, however, and also carries significant risk to normal pituitary function [50,51,53].

Perioperative mortality is low, and most reports of death occur in a delayed fashion after surgery. Pituitary apoplexy has been reported as a cause of death in one patient two weeks after a second debulking operation; the pathological mechanism is unclear but may be related to hemorrhage into a devascularized portion of tumor after surgical interruption of blood supply [47]. Long-term pituitary function is often related to preoperative status, and proper surgical technique can preserve this postoperatively. Injury to the pituitary stalk should be avoided at all costs.

INTRAVENTRICULAR TUMORS

Approximately 10% of all brain tumors present in or near the ventricular system, and much like tumors of the pineal region, they are heterogeneous in pathology and prognosis [54,55]. Although some of these lesions are of high grade, and may be cured with aggressive surgical and adjuvant therapy, many are low grade and their inherent indolent nature creates unique diagnostic issues in children. Signs and symptoms are often caused by slowly developing hydrocephalus that is more easily diagnosed in older children presenting with typical headache or morning vomiting from raised intracranial pressure. In infants and nonverbal children, however, the only clues may be nonspecific: irritability, anhedonia, and macrocrania. Particular subtypes of intraventricular tumors present in certain ages and in specific locations within the ventricular system, and these two characteristics form a practical way by which these lesions can be classified [54,56–61]. In this section, we present a brief review of three types of lesions: tumors of the choroid plexus, central neurocytomas, and gliomas.

Choroid Plexus Tumors

Tumors of the choroid plexus account for less than 1% of all intracranial tumors [55]. Within the lateral ventricles, these tumors commonly occur in the trigone. Choroid plexus papillomas, largely benign lesions, are the most common tumor of the lateral ventricles with the majority of these presenting in the first 2 years of life. Older children and adolescents present in a fashion similar to adults, with a propensity for 4th ventricular lesions [62–64]. These patients present with marked ventriculomegaly and clinical manifestations of hydrocephalus. In the vast majority of cases, this occurs in the absence of CSF flow obstruction, implicating the overproduction of CSF as a major pathophysiological factor [65,66]. Obstructive hydrocephalus can occur with lesions preventing the flow of CSF through the foramen of Monro or aqueduct of Sylvius. Complicating

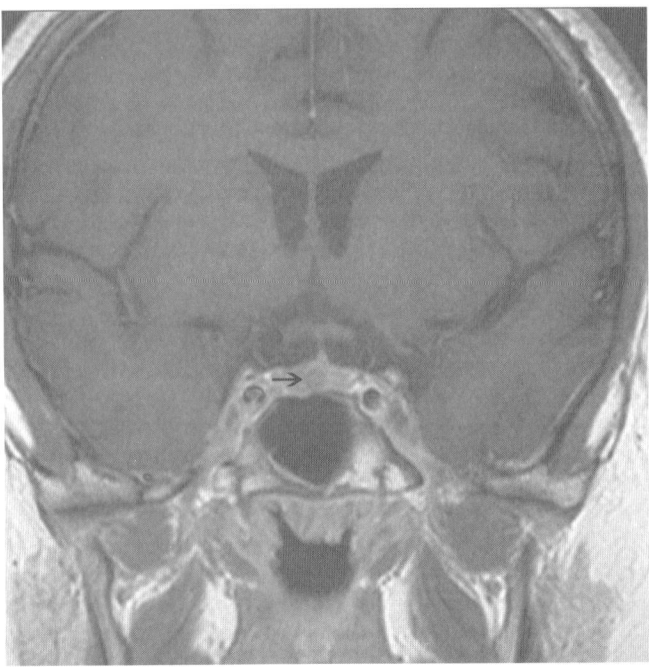

Figure 60.6 Gadolinium-enhanced coronal MRI through the pituitary gland in which a round lesion is found (arrow) to the right of midline in a 14-year-old female with Cushing disease. The lesion was removed transphenoidally, and a basophilic adenoma was found at histopathology.

this picture, many patients suffer from persistent hydrocephalus despite successful excision of the lesion. Further functional obstruction at the arachnoid granulations has been postulated with the mechanism being similar to that observed after head injury or subarachnoid hemorrhage [64]. Release of fibrinous material from the tumor is likely responsible, and the persistence of hydrocephalus with preoperative xanthochromia and CSF protein content has been correlated [67,68]. Complete surgical resection of these lesions is generally curative and adjuvant therapy is not required.

Choroid plexus carcinomas are less common and usually present in children 2 to 4 years of age. Pathological differentiation from papillomas is sometimes difficult, and keratin expression in carcinomas is a major distinguishing feature [55,67,69]. A higher risk of craniospinal metastasis, as well as the occasional case of systemic metastasis, is found in this group. They may be radiographically differentiated from papillomas by their heterogeneous enhancement, peritumoral edema, and subarachnoid dissemination. Long-term survival for patients with choroid plexus carcinomas relates to extent of resection as the role of radiation and/or chemotherapy is still unclear [64]. Some authors argue that, given the inability to completely resect many of these lesions, any observed survival benefit may owe to more favorable tumor biology and decreased vascularity [70]. In select cases, neoadjuvant chemotherapy following biopsy may improve the chances of obtaining a complete resection.

Surgical Considerations

The surgical management of choroid plexus tumors is complicated by unique issues. The young age of the patients coupled with the hypervascular nature of these lesions greatly increases the susceptibility of patients to hypovolemia and hemodynamic compromise. The need for invasive cardiovascular monitoring during surgical resection is well reported in the neuroanesthesia literature [71]. The pediatric neurosurgeon contemplating surgical resection should be prepared to deal with the following important issues.

Hypertrophied anterior and posterior choroidal arteries provide the primary supply to choroid plexus tumors (Figure 60.7). Generally speaking, the former supplies lesions in the atrium and temporal horns, and surgical opening of the choroidal fissure can provide proximal vascular pedicle control on approach to the lesion. The lateral posterior choroidal artery supplies a similar territory and can be isolated in a similar fashion. The medial posterior choroidal artery traverses the velum interpositum and sends branches to the third and lateral ventricles through the choroidal fissure and foramen of Monro. Surgeons should be aware that tumors may be supplied by enlarged branches of one or both choroidal arteries [72].

Surgical approaches should therefore be directed at early exposure and control of the vascular pedicle. Mobilization of large lesions is often difficult, and this can predispose to difficulties in vascular control and increase the need to perform a piecemeal resection. This can increase the risk of intraoperative hemorrhage, which

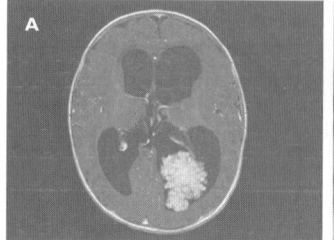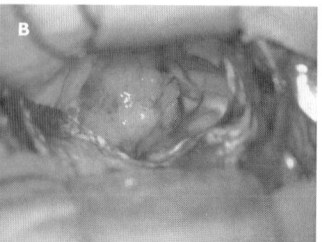

Figure 60.7 Six-month-old male with increasing head circumference, irritability, and vomiting. **(A)** Axial enhanced MRI shows left ventricular lesion with "frond"-like appearance. Note choroidal vessels feeding the tumor. The MRI scan is compatible with the diagnosis of choroid plexus papilloma. **(B)** Intraoperative photograph of ventricular anatomy and choroid plexus papilloma. These lesions are friable, vascular, and mobile. The neurosurgeon should identify the vascular pedicle first, eliminate the arterial supply by coagulation, and remove the lesion en bloc if possible.

in some cases can be massive, leading to significant coagulation derangements and intraoperative mortality [73,74]. Preoperative embolization has been attempted in selected cases; however, this is dependent on the size and number of tumor-feeding vessels [64].

The selection of surgical approach is determined by tumor location and vascular supply. Transcortical approaches provide access to all regions of the lateral ventricles but carry with them the risk of seizures; transcallosal approaches may mitigate these concerns in properly selected patients. Lesions in the posterior aspects of the ventricles may be approached through a superior parietal trajectory, similar to shunt catheter placement; however, middle temporal gyrus approaches provide excellent access to the ventricular system [72].

Postoperative CSF-related complications have been well described. Approximately 50% of patients may require CSF diversion [64,73]. Transcortical surgery predisposes to the formation of ventriculosubdural fistulae, and closure of the cortical incision may prevent this. Subdural-peritoneal shunting may need to be employed despite its relative long-term inefficiency.

Central Neurocytoma

Central neurocytomas are rare, usually benign neuronal tumors of the CNS, accounting for 0.25% to 0.5% of all primary brain tumors [75–78]. They are most common in young adults and are typically found intraventricularly near the foramina of Monro or septum pellucidum. This entity was first described by Hassoun et al. in 1982, and at that time, only the benign variety was recognized [79]. A more aggressive variant, labeled atypical neurocytoma, was reported in 1989 [80]. The pathological criteria for this is similar to other CNS neoplasms: MIB-1 labeling index of greater than or equal to 2% or atypical histological features including focal necrosis, vascular proliferation, and increased mitotic activity. Of these, an elevated MIB-1 level correlates with likelihood of recurrence [81–84]. The biological origins of this tumor continue to be debated: Yasargil has suggested that these tumors arise from a totipotent cell residing in the periventricular matrix, whereas others suggest origin from a neuronal cell mass in the subependymal zone [85].

Clinical presentation in children is primarily related to increased intracranial pressure, with headache and nausea and vomiting being the most common. Other presenting findings include memory deficits, visual loss, ataxia, seizures, and varying patterns of motor and sensory deficits. Intratumoral hemorrhage may be seen in select cases [85,86].

The optimal management of central neurocytoma remains in question although gross total resection, if feasible, followed by adjuvant radiotherapy likely provides the greatest degree of local control. In a large meta-analysis of 59 children, 100% of the cohort experienced local tumor control at 5 and 10 years after treatment with complete surgical resection and postoperative radiotherapy [87]. In the same series, incomplete resection with radiotherapy also provided 100% local control, with complete resection alone (86%) and incomplete resection alone not as favourable (60% at 5 years and 40% at 10 years). Similar outcomes were found in a study of adults and children, with no survival benefit provided by any particular modality [76]. Many therefore advocate reserving radiotherapy for children with recurrent lesions because of the risks of therapy at a young age and lack of survival benefit [87].

Thalamic Gliomas

Thalamic gliomas account for 2% to 5% of all brain tumors, with 40% of these in children under the age of 18 years [88–91]. Clinical presentation in these patients is highly variable including hemiparesis, sensory and visual field deficits, movement disorders, and symptomatic obstructive hydrocephalus from mass effect on the ventricular system. Diagnosis has in the past been made radiographically. Historically, survival has been poor with patients with the high-grade tumors not faring as well [92]. More recent studies have corroborated these findings, with the suggestion that bithalamic involvement is also an independent predictor of poor prognosis [88,90,91].

Radiotherapy has often been the mainstay of treatment in this disease, but recent advances in neuroanesthesia, neuroimaging, and intraoperative mapping allow for a more aggressive surgical approach. The predisposition to CSF outflow obstruction with progressive tumor growth makes the treatment of hydrocephalus, occurring in approximately 50% of patients, a real and sometimes emergent concern [90]. Selection of CSF diversion procedure must be individualized to patient and tumor anatomy. Large lesions occupying the third ventricle will not allow for entry of an endoscope and in these patients, ventriculoperitoneal shunting is the treatment of choice. Those with smaller, often unilateral tumors, may benefit from endoscopic third ventriculostomy (ETV) with successful control of intracranial pressure.

Surgical resection of these lesions is equally individualized, and the approaches to these tumors are chosen based on lesion location and nearby anatomy. A recent review of thalamic tumors has classified them into 3 groups: Unilateral thalamic tumors, thalamopeduncular lesions, and bithalamic tumors of which the first group is most common [90]. In unilateral lesions, the same review suggested that extent of resection directly correlated with improved survival without major morbidity. Neurosurgeons must be aware of critical structures in the vicinity before embarking on radical resection [93–97]. The choice of approach should be based on the location of the tumor within the thalamus, such that minimal manipulation and resection of normal brain is performed. Diffusely infiltrative lesions and bithalamic tumors remain best served by biopsy, either stereotactic or endoscopic, and directed adjuvant therapy. Proper patient selection has greatly improved perioperative mortality in the surgical management of thalamic tumors. Reports from the 1950s quoted up to 40% mortality, whereas 1% to 2% is now the norm [93,98].

The Role of Endoscopy in Intraventricular Tumors

The role of neuroendoscopy in the management of obstructive hydrocephalus secondary to intraventricular and pineal region tumors is well appreciated. ETV is the treatment of choice in treating hydrocephalus in pineal region lesions and has demonstrated success in selected intraventricular tumor cases [99,100]. Neuroendoscopic biopsy is also a viable option in a large number of cases and can provide tissue diagnosis that serves to direct further adjuvant therapy. First described by Fukushima in 1978, success rates in this regard are reported from 60% to 90% [101–106]. Although minimally invasive, the procedure is not risk free and overall complication rates lie between 8% and 20% [107]. Arguably hemorrhagic complications, including intraventricular or extra-axial hemorrhages, are most immediately concerning to the surgeon and occur in 1% to 10% of patients. This often occurs in the absence of intraoperative bleeding or coagulation defects. Subdural hygroma, CSF leak, and CSF infection are also reported and number approximately 5% each. When coupled with ETV, this technique provides a quick, minimally invasive method of managing intraventricular tumors.

The role of neuroendoscopy in the surgical resection of intraventricular tumors is less well studied, particularly in pediatrics. Technically, the ability to achieve a total resection requires developing an interface between the lesion and the adjacent white matter [101]. Aspiration is gently used to remove solid tumor material and in older series, the use of YAG laser has also been advocated [108]. Frameless stereotactic neuronavigation has now enabled ventricular cannulation with complete lesion resection in patients without hydrocephalus [109].

PINEAL REGION TUMORS

The surgical management of pineal region tumors in children begins with an understanding of the complexity of the neurovascular anatomy coupled with the heterogeneity of pathologies for lesions in this region. In this section, we discuss the classification of pineal region tumors and describe the surgical approaches that are frequently used.

Classification of Pineal Tumors

Pineal region tumors can be classified into four main groups, with each group consisting of certain subdivisions.

Each group comprises a range from benign to malignant and this distinction carries significant implications for therapy, both medical and surgical [110].

Germ Cell Tumors

This group of tumors accounts for less than 5% of CNS neoplasms and represents a highly diverse group. First classified in 1976 by Teilum, they differ in their degrees of differentiation with germinoma being the most undifferentiated. The nongerminomatous germ cell tumors consist of embryonal carcinoma, yolk sac tumours, choriocarcinoma, teratoma, and the mixed germ cell tumors. Differentiating between germinomatous and nongerminomatous germ cell tumors is key in offering optimal treatment to these patients.

Pineal Parenchymal Tumors

These tumours are intrinsic to the pineal gland itself and are of two types: pineoblastoma and pineocytoma. The former is a WHO grade IV primitive neuroectodermal tumor (PNET) and it possesses histopathological features similar to PNETs in other locations. They can metastasize to other regions of the CNS. By contrast, pineocytomas are slow growing WHO grade II lesions typically found in young adults. Unlike pineoblastoma, these patients fare well after surgical resection although metastasis is possible in rare cases.

Glial tumors

Glial cells of the adjacent thalamus anteriorly, and brainstem inferiorly, can give rise to gliomas of varying grades. Similarly, neoplastic transformation of nearby ependymal cells of the third ventricle can lead to growth of ependymomas.

Miscellaneous

A large variety of other tumors and nonneoplastic lesions are also found in this region. Meningioma, hemangioblastoma, choroid plexus lesions, adenocarcinoma, lymphoma, metastatic lesions, and benign pineal cysts are found here. One must also account for the possibility of vascular lesions including cavernomas, arteriovenous malformations, and vein of Galen malformations.

Management of Pineal Region Tumors

Standard preoperative evaluation consists of high resolution multiplanar MRI with and without contrast (Figure 60.8A). Images may be suggestive of a particular tumor type, but more useful from this modality is the anatomical relationship of the tumor to nearby structures and the degree of hydrocephalus with the potential for ETV to be discussed later. The preoperative evaluation of hormonal markers in the serum and CSF is integral to diagnosis. Elevated levels of beta human chorionic gonadotropin or alpha fetoprotein in either the CSF or serum are pathognomonic of a malignant nongerminomatous germ cell tumor. Patients may then be treated with radiotherapy and

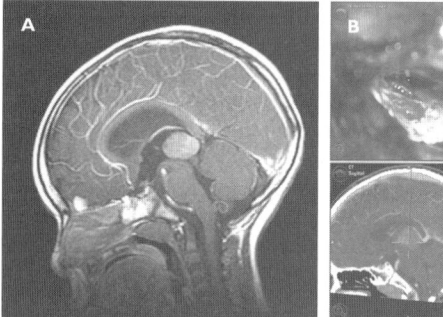
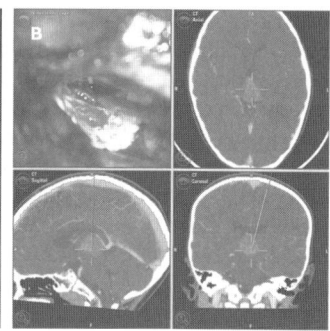

Figure 60.8 Three-year-old male with headache, vomiting, and Parinaud syndrome. **(A)** Gadolinium-enhanced sagittal MRI showing discrete lesion in the region of the pineal gland. There is obstructive hydrocephalus from occlusion of the aqueduct. The lesion was biopsied endoscopically at the time of ETV and proved to be a pineoblastoma. **(B)** Intraoperative photograph and neuronavigation screen saves show a posterior transcallosal approach and tumor being removed from between the two internal cerebral veins. In addition to the supracerebellar and occipital transtentorial approaches described in this chapter, the posterior transcallosal approach can be used in select instances.

chemotherapy without tissue diagnosis. In this group, the role of surgical resection and its impact on prognosis and outcome remains inconclusive [111]. In the face of normal markers, tissue diagnosis becomes imperative before further therapy can be offered. This can be obtained in conjunction with other necessary procedures.

Treatment of Hydrocephalus and Tissue Diagnosis

Obstructive hydrocephalus from pineal region tumors often produce visual symptoms from papilledema or a VIth nerve palsy due to raised intracranial pressure. The tumor's proximity to gaze centers in the midbrain also cause a variety of gaze palsies including Parinaud's syndrome.

ETV is now considered the treatment of choice for patients with pineal region tumors and obstructive hydrocephalus in whom treatment for hydrocephalus per se is required. In many cases, ETV can yield long-term shunt independence and avoid the inherent risks of shunt placement and the added theoretical risk of tumor metastasis [112–116]. At the time of ETV, a tumor specimen can be obtained as can CSF for tumor marker studies. Standard endoscopic biopsy forceps are used and hemostasis is achieved with combination of electrocautery and irrigation. Heavily encapsulated lesions and those completely covered by the ependymal lining of the ventricle can pose problems in obtaining an endoscopic biopsy and reversion to an open surgical biopsy may be necessary. In select cases, stereotactic biopsy provides a safe method by which tumor tissue can be obtained for histopathological analysis [111]. There is a small risk of hemorrhage with this procedure as well as the risk of not obtaining diagnostic tissue.

Microsurgical Approaches to the Pineal Region

Neurosurgery for pineal region tumors achieves three general goals: (1) Maximal resection of benign and low-grade lesions; (2) Cytoreduction prior to adjuvant therapy; (3) Second-look surgery after adjuvant therapy. A preferred approach is an infratentorial supracerebellar approach that provides a midline trajectory to the lesion while remaining beneath the veins of Galen and Rosenthal to minimize the risk of neurovascular compromise. The tentorium hinders visualization in the superior and lateral extremes of the operative field and as such, tumors with significant dorsal or lateral extension are likely better served by other approaches [117]. The sitting position is frequently used here, but the increased risk of air embolism and tension pneumocephalus must be remembered.

By contrast, the occipital transtentorial approach may provide a more extensive view of the pineal region owing to the reflection of the tentorium. Key considerations in this approach are the bridging veins, although few, from the medial occipital lobe to the transverse, straight, and sagittal sinuses; usually, gentle superolateral retraction can provide adequate interhemispheric exposure without venous sacrifice. The inferior cerebral veins should be preserved as edema and infarction of the occipital lobe has been reported. Tumors with significant dorsal extension and little to no contralateral extension are best served by this approach as visualization of the contralateral quadrigeminal plate and pulvinar is poor. Positioning for this approach usually places the patient in the 3/4 prone position providing the least chance of air embolism and minimal occipital lobe retraction [117,118]. Advances in neuronavigation have also greatly enhanced the surgeon's ability to maximally resect these lesions with minimal surgical morbidity (Figure 60.8B).

Postoperative complications are often transient, and most common are extraocular movement abnormalities, including upgaze and convergence, that usually improve over the first several days after surgery. Overall, surgical morbidity in this procedure is from 0% to 12% with mortality of 0% to 8%, with much of the latter owing to postoperative hemorrhage [111].

Outcomes

Treatment outcomes after surgery in this region are varied due to pathologic heterogeneity. Complete resection in benign lesions is curative, while the contribution of surgery for more malignant lesions has been in securing a tissue-proven diagnosis and treating the concomitant hydrocephalus. This is certainly true for germinoma where the role of surgical resection is minimal given that it remains exquisitely chemosensitive and radiosensitive [119,120]. Second-look surgery in the nongerminomatous germ cell tumors has proven beneficial following completion of radiation and chemotherapy. Debulking of residual masses in this fashion has yielded 90% 5-year survival rates with these remnants possibly representing more benign components not responsive to adjuvant therapy [121]. Attempted maximal surgical resection remains the initial strategy of choice in pineoblastoma, followed by radiotherapy or chemotherapy, despite the fact that its prognosis continues to be uniformly poor [111].

POSTERIOR FOSSA TUMORS

The posterior fossa tumor in children is one of the most complex, yet potentially most rewarding lesions for the pediatric neurosurgeon. Whereas historical reports of surgery in this location were fraught with high morbidity and mortality, contemporary neuroanesthesia, neuroimaging and navigation, and improvements in surgical technique have translated into better tumor resections and patient outcomes than were previously possible.

Medulloblastoma

Medulloblastoma is the most common malignant CNS tumor of childhood, and accounts for approximately 20% of all childhood intracranial tumors [122]. The term dates back to 1925 when Bailey and Cushing first coined it to describe distinct, midline, highly malignant cerebellar tumors [123]. Since then, the classification has changed many times, and the lesion is now designated by the WHO as a distinct embryonal tumor. The term PNET, often used interchangeably, is now reserved for pathologically similar lesions found outside the cerebellum [124]. There is a bimodal age distribution, with peaks in children occurring between 3 and 4 years, and between 8 and 9 years of age. Several familiar cancer syndromes have been associated with medulloblastoma including Gorlin syndrome, Rubenstein-Taybi syndrome, ataxia-telangiectasia, Turcot syndrome, Li-Fraumeni syndrome, neurofibromatosis, and tuberous sclerosis [122].

Most children with posterior fossa tumors present with unremitting headache, classically worse in the morning, vomiting, and lethargy. Cerebellar signs including truncal or limb ataxia, and dysmetria may occur although this is more common in older patients due to brainstem invasion and cerebellar hemispheric involvement. Infants, able to compensate for increased intracranial pressure due to cranial expansion, will often present with macrocephaly, a full anterior fontanelle, irritability, and sun setting.

MRI is the diagnostic test of choice, showing varying degrees of enhancement and can provide information on tumor location, brainstem invasion, ventricular extension, and subarachnoid spread (Figure 60.9). Similarly, MRI is the desired test for assessing potential metastasis to the spine. Preoperative MRI scanning of the entire neuraxis is recommended [122].

The optimal treatment of medulloblastoma is multi-modal. Surgery, the nuances of which will be discussed collectively later in this section, remains the initial strategy aimed at achieving cytoreduction prior to adjuvant therapy and at physically opening obstructed CSF pathways. Transvermian and telovelar approaches are commonly used, with the latter potentially decreasing the risk of postoperative posterior fossa syndrome [125]. Neuronavigation plays a limited role in these cases given the anatomical similarity and landmarks between patients. The extent of surgical resection and metastatic status forms the primary risk stratification scheme in this disease. Patients aged below 3 years with greater than 1.5 cm^3 residual disease or evidence of metastasis at diagnosis are considered high grade [126]. In patients more than 3 years old, 5-year

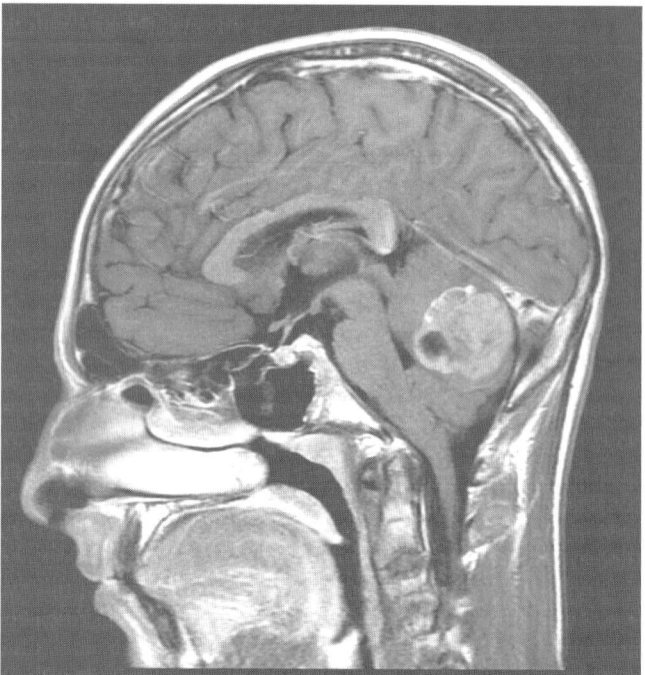

Figure 60.9 Fourteen-year-old male with progressive history of headache and vomiting. Gadolinium-enhanced sagittal MRI shows midline cerebellar tumor that enhances markedly with contrast. It was removed and proved to be a medulloblastoma.

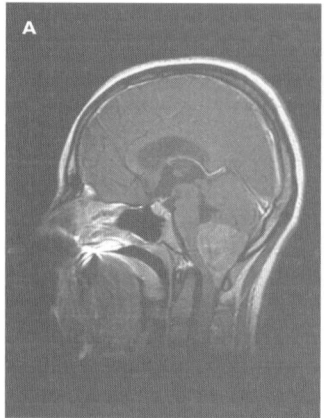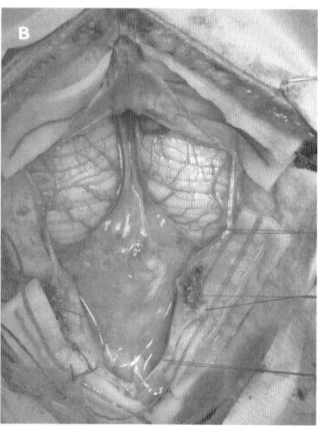

Figure 60.10 Eight-year-old female with protracted history of vomiting and headache. **(A)** Sagittal enhanced MRI scan shows homogeneously enhancing tumor in the midline, which descends down to and through the foramen magnum. **(B)** At surgery, the lesion was approached through a standard posterior fossa craniotomy, and removed. It was an ependymoma.

survival is still only 55%. By comparison, the average risk group with smaller residual tumors and no metastases fare much better with greater than 70% 5-year survival after maximal treatment with surgery, craniospinal irradiation, and chemotherapy [127]. This marks a great improvement over previous survival figures of 45% at 10 years with surgery and radiotherapy alone [128]. The use of high-dose chemotherapy and stem cell rescue has shown improved survival. Up to 85% of average risk and 70% of high-risk patients survive 5 years after diagnosis [129].

Ependymoma

Ependymomas make up approximately 5% to 10% of childhood brain tumors and are the third most common neoplasm after astrocytoma and medulloblastoma [130]. These lesions are comprised of cells from the ependymal and subependymal zones surrounding the ventricles, and in the posterior fossa, lesions arise from the roof or floor of the 4th ventricle. Lateral extension into the cerebellopontine angle through the foramina of Luschka, or into the cervical spinal canal via the foramen of Magendie is also observed. The latter may help differentiate these tumors from medulloblastoma. Ependymomas are usually well demarcated but brainstem infiltration can occur (Figure 60.10). Metastasis through the neuraxis via the CSF is well observed, and occasional extraneural spread has been reported [124,131,132]. The currently used WHO classification of ependymomas divides tumors into the benign cellular, papillary, clear cell and tanycytic ependymomas, anaplastic ependymomas, myxopapillary ependymomas, and subependymomas. The latter two are rare in children [133].

The management of ependymoma is primarily surgical. Tissue diagnosis, cytoreduction, relief of mass effect, and opening obstructed CSF pathways can all be achieved with surgery. Complete resection is the desired result. If there is one childhood brain tumor for which the role of complete resection has been shown time and again to play a critical role, it is ependymoma of the posterior fossa. The role of adjuvant therapy in this disease is reserved for high-grade lesions and consists of radiotherapy and/or chemotherapy. Five-year survival is variable from 30% to 70%, with those receiving radiotherapy possibly performing slightly better than those undergoing chemotherapy [133,134].

Cerebellar Astrocytoma

The cerebellar astrocytoma is the most common brain tumor in childhood, representing approximately 20% of tumors [135]. Most of these are low-grade, pilocytic astrocytomas. These lesions have equal gender distribution and generally peak in the middle of the first decade [136,137]. They have a typical radiographic appearance, usually with a large cystic component and mural nodule (Figure 60.11). There is variable enhancement of the cyst wall and the mural nodule. By definition, these are WHO grade I lesions and complete surgical resection is curative. Clinical presentation of these lesions is similar to other posterior fossa tumors. Headache and vomiting are the most common findings, followed by a mix of altered gait, visual disturbances, and in rare cases, coma due to obstructive hydrocephalus.

Surgical Considerations

Treatment of Hydrocephalus

Surgical management of children with posterior fossa tumors is somewhat analogous to the treatment of pineal region tumors: not only does the tumor need treatment but also does the consequent hydrocephalus. Historically,

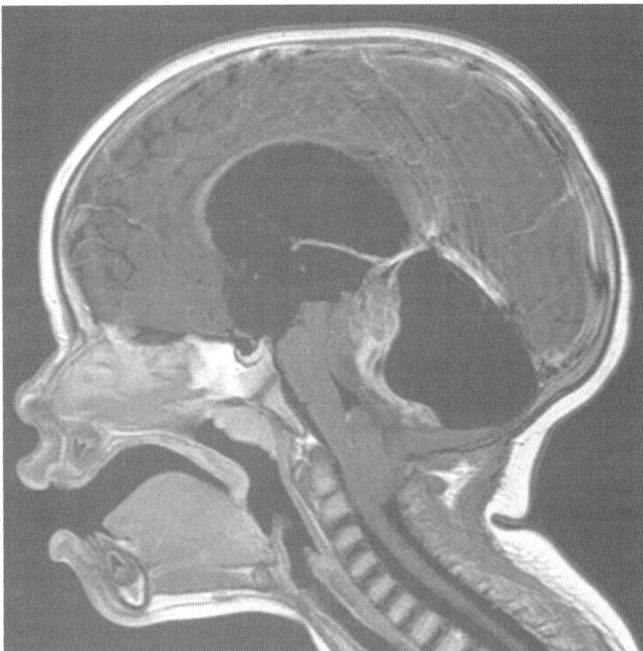

Figure 60.11 Three-year-old female with history of progressive ataxia, VIth nerve palsy, and vomiting. Sagittal-enhanced MRI shows large cystic lesion in the posterior fossa with an enhancing tumor within the cerebellum. The tumor was approached through a posterior fossa craniotomy and removed. It was a cystic cerebellar pilocytic astrocytoma.

patients with ventriculomegaly underwent preoperative CSF diversion by way of an external drain or shunt. Experience has shown that such a procedure is not benign. Shunts malfunction or become infected and rapid ventricular decompression can cause subdural hematoma formation. Rarely, shift of large posterior fossa lesions can lead to upward herniation with brainstem compression and hemorrhage [135]. Preoperative shunting is not routinely recommended unless the child is "in extremis" from raised intracranial pressure.

Perhaps even more important, studies have evaluated the need for postoperative CSF diversion after tumor resection. It appears that between 20% and 30% of patients will need placement of a permanent shunt [138–141]. Those of younger age, with midline tumors, those undergoing minimal or subtotal resection of medulloblastoma or ependymoma, and those developing CSF leak or infection are at an increased risk of shunt requirement [138,139,142].

The role of ETV in the treatment of hydrocephalus from posterior fossa lesions is still debated. It is generally accepted that, similar to preoperative shunting, preoperative ETV is not indicated due to the low risk of postoperative hydrocephalus. Uncontrolled retrospective studies suggest that ETV is beneficial in treating symptomatic hydrocephalus in this setting obviating the need for ventriculoperitoneal shunting [141,143].

Surgical Positioning

The prone position is typically used to access midline and hemispheric cerebellar tumors. Young patients can be placed face down on a well-padded horseshoe head holder, whereas older patients more than 5 years of age are placed in rigid pin fixation.

Surgical Technique

Access to the majority of posterior fossa lesions is obtained through the standard midline posterior fossa craniotomy or craniectomy. Exposure of the occipital bone is tailored to tumor location with increased dissection ipsilateral to hemispheric tumors. Careful exposure of C1 must also be performed, and injury to the vertebral artery can be avoided with subperiosteal dissection. The posterior arch of C1 and the occipital bone to the foramen magnum can then be removed. The dura is commonly opened in a Y fashion with the point placed just below the foramen magnum.

For cerebellar astrocytomas, a combination of ultrasonic aspiration and microdissection under magnification provides the optimal means of complete resection. However, the proximity of medulloblastoma and ependymoma to the IVth ventricle and brainstem mandates a slightly different approach. Tumors located in a more cephalad direction may still require a vermian incision for access. Those lesions found more caudally, and particularly those extending below the cerebellar tonsils, may be approached through a telovelar approach [125]. Medulloblastomas are generally friable and can be quickly aspirated with microsuction. A similar approach can be used to resect ependymomas taking care to protect cranial nerves from injury while ensuring maximal resection. Here, lower cranial nerve and brainstem neurophysiological monitoring can be very useful. Once exposed, the IVth ventricular floor should be protected to avoid damage to cranial nerve nuclei and the long tracts. The use of a dural graft such as bovine pericardium is recommended to achieve closure [135].

Traditional teaching has also recommended that posterior fossa craniectomy be performed to allow room for postoperative cerebellar swelling and thus prevent brainstem compression. Moreover, proponents of craniectomy have stated that there is significant risk to midline venous sinuses when using high speed drills to perform a craniotomy. In recent times, craniotomy has been used here. Decreased risk of CSF leak, pseudomeningocele formation, and need for wound reclosure were found in patients undergoing posterior fossa craniotomy [144,145]. No obvious physiological explanation exists for this; it is postulated that early reattachment of muscles to the replaced bone flap eliminates dead space into which CSF can otherwise leak [145]. Adult studies have also found that replacing the bone flap may decrease postoperative pain [146,147].

Posterior Fossa Syndrome and Mutism

The syndrome of posterior fossa mutism is sometimes seen after posterior fossa tumor resection in children. First described in 1985 by Rekate et al., descriptions in the literature now number several case reports [148]. The incidence of mutism is approximately 8% to 25% of children undergoing posterior fossa tumor resections [149]. The pathophysiology and anatomic basis of the syndrome remain unclear, with several anatomical sites proposed in its development. Involvement of the dentate nucleus has been implicated just as bilateral interruption of the dentatothalamocortical pathway. Finally, splitting of the vermis has been held responsible although this is likely one of many factors, as not all patients with vermian splitting develop mutism [150]. Other neurocognitive findings are prevalent in patients with posterior fossa syndrome including communication impairments of expressive and receptive language, mood lability, hypokinesis, hemiparesis, eye opening difficulties, and even lack of bowel and bladder control [149]. Rehabilitation is often focused at these deficits. The duration of the syndrome is variable and lasts 1 month on average although it can extend to 3 months.

CLINICAL PEARLS

The surgical management of brain tumors in children poses unique challenges to the treating neurosurgeon. As we have discussed in this chapter, the pathologic variance of brain tumors in children is significant. In addition, the age of the child is a significant factor in determining patient prognosis. We discuss some special considerations here.

Neonates and Infants

Although brain tumors in young children under 2 years of age are rare, they are the most common solid tumors in this age group (1.1/100000 live or stillborn infants) [151]. In descending order, the most common subtypes are astrocytomas, PNETs, ependymomas, and choroid plexus papillomas. Arguably the most important aspect of management is the formulation of an accurate diagnosis as the surgical strategy is based entirely on this. Preoperative MRI scanning, usually with tailored neuronavigation sequences, is the diagnostic test of choice.

The long-term consequences of administering radiotherapy in this young age group has encouraged neurosurgeons to pursue complete tumor removal where safely possible. Intraoperative blood loss is a real concern with aggressive resection and care must be taken from incision to closure to minimize bleeding, given the small physiologic blood volume. Carefully administered expert anesthesia is key to successfully performing these operations in young children.

Supratentorial Neoplasms

In supratentorial tumors, the key to surgical management is respecting normal anatomy while ensuring as complete a resection as possible. Functional MRI, MEG, positron-emission tomography scanning, neuronavigation, and electrocortical mapping are all used routinely in pediatric brain tumor surgery. The extent of resection correlates directly with outcome and survival.

Regarding intraventricular tumors, the neurosurgeon must have the utmost respect for the lesion's vascular supply. Surgical approaches should be directed at controlling the blood supply before attempting tumor resection.

Preventing large volume blood loss mitigates the need for massive transfusion as well as reducing the risk of postoperative hydrocephalus from fibrin-induced scarring. Despite meticulous surgical technique, up to 50% of patients still develop symptomatic hydrocephalus, and patients should be closely monitored for this complication.

Infratentorial Neoplasms

Gross total resection is usually the desired outcome, and several key aspects allow pediatric neurosurgeons to achieve this result with minimal morbidity. Positioning and well-administered anesthesia allow for a relaxed brain after exposure. Accurate placement of the dural incision avoids injury to the occipital sinuses and thus can prevent large volume blood loss. Symptomatic hydrocephalus is a prominent comorbidity and, for most patients, tumor resection provides the best treatment. In those 30% of patients in whom hydrocephalus persists, placement of a ventriculoperitoneal shunt likely provides the best management. Replacement of the bone flap provides a safe way to prevent CSF leak and pseudomeningocele formation and decreases postoperative pain. Posterior fossa craniotomy should be performed routinely.

CONCLUSIONS

We have provided a broad overview of surgery for brain tumors in children and discussed selected lesions in various anatomical regions as examples. Performing these operations can be a richly rewarding experience for the pediatric neurosurgeon; however, the operating surgeon must be aware of specific differences in children when compared to adults. Surgery in these patients provides tangible survival benefits yet further research is required to improve outcomes in this patient population.

ACKNOWLEDGMENTS

This work was supported by a grant from the Canadian Institutes of Health Research, the Wiley and Berman Funds for brain tumor research, and Brainchild. Dr. Rutka is a scientist of the Canadian Institutes of Health Research .

REFERENCES

1. Rickert CH, Paulus W. Epidemiology of central nervous system tumors in childhood and adolescence based on the new WHO classification. *Childs Nerv Syst.* 2001;17(9):503–511.
2. Tamber MS, Rutka JT. Pediatric supratentorial high-grade gliomas. *Neurosurg Focus.* 2003;14(2):e1.
3. Blümcke I, Wiestler OD. Gangliogliomas: an intriguing tumor entity associated with focal epilepsies. *J Neuropathol Exp Neurol.* 2002;61(7):575–584.
4. Luyken C, Blümcke I, Fimmers R, Urbach H, Wiestler OD, Schramm J. Supratentorial gangliogliomas: histopathologic grading and tumor recurrence in 184 patients with a median follow-up of 8 years. *Cancer.* 2004;101(1):146–155.
5. Luyken C, Blümcke I, Fimmers R, et al. The spectrum of long-term epilepsy-associated tumors: long-term seizure and tumor outcome and neurosurgical aspects. *Epilepsia.* 2003;44(6):822–830.

6. Schramm J, Kral T, Blümcke I, Elger CE. Surgery for neocortical temporal and frontal epilepsy. *Adv Neurol.* 2000;84:595–603.
7. Schramm J, Kral T, Grunwald T, Blümcke I. Surgical treatment for neocortical temporal lobe epilepsy: clinical and surgical aspects and seizure outcome. *J Neurosurg.* 2001;94(1):33–42.
8. Chan CH, Bittar RG, Davis GA, Kalnins RM, Fabinyi GC. Long-term seizure outcome following surgery for dysembryoplastic neuroepithelial tumor. *J Neurosurg.* 2006;104(1):62–69.
9. Nolan MA, Sakuta R, Chuang N, et al. Dysembryoplastic neuroepithelial tumors in childhood: long-term outcome and prognostic features. *Neurology.* 2004;62(12):2270–2276.
10. Gupta N, Berger MS. Brain mapping for hemispheric tumors in children. *Pediatr Neurosurg.* 2003;38(6):302–306.
11. Drake JM, Prudencio J, Holowaka S, Rutka JT, Hoffman HJ, Humphreys RP. Frameless stereotaxy in children. *Pediatr Neurosurg.* 1994;20(2):152–159.
12. Kremer P, Tronnier V, Steiner HH, et al. Intraoperative MRI for interventional neurosurgical procedures and tumor resection control in children. *Childs Nerv Syst.* 2006;22(7):674–678.
13. Ogawa S, Lee TM, Kay AR, Tank DW. Brain magnetic resonance imaging with contrast dependent on blood oxygenation. *Proc Natl Acad Sci U S A.* 1990;87(24):9868–9872.
14. Tharin S, Golby A. Functional brain mapping and its applications to neurosurgery. *Neurosurgery.* 2007;60(4 suppl 2):185–201; discussion 201.
15. Kotsoni E, Byrd D, Casey BJ. Special considerations for functional magnetic resonance imaging of pediatric populations. *J Magn Reson Imaging.* 2006;23(6):877–886.
16. Gallen CC, Bucholz R, Sobel DF. Intracranial neurosurgery guided by functional imaging. *Surg Neurol.* 1994;42(6):523–530.
17. Gallen CC, Schwartz BJ, Bucholz RD, et al. Presurgical localization of functional cortex using magnetic source imaging. *J Neurosurg.* 1995;82(6):988–994.
18. Kamada K, Takeuchi F, Kuriki S, Oshiro O, Houkin K, Abe H. Functional neurosurgical simulation with brain surface magnetic resonance images and magnetoencephalography. *Neurosurgery.* 1993;33(2):269–72; discussion 272.
19. McDonald JD, Chong BW, Lewine JD, et al. Integration of preoperative and intraoperative functional brain mapping in a frameless stereotactic environment for lesions near eloquent cortex. Technical note. *J Neurosurg.* 1999;90(3):591–598.
20. Rezai AR, Hund M, Kronberg E, et al. Introduction of magnetoencephalography to stereotactic techniques. *Stereotact Funct Neurosurg.* 1995;65(1–4):37–41.
21. Rezai AR, Hund M, Kronberg E, et al. The interactive use of magnetoencephalography in stereotactic image-guided neurosurgery. *Neurosurgery.* 1996;39(1):92–102.
22. Sutherling WW, Crandall PH, Darcey TM, Becker DP, Levesque MF, Barth DS. The magnetic and electric fields agree with intracranial localizations of somatosensory cortex. *Neurology.* 1988;38(11):1705–1714.
23. Garrè ML, Cama A. Craniopharyngioma: modern concepts in pathogenesis and treatment. *Curr Opin Pediatr.* 2007;19(4):471–479.
24. Bunin GR, Surawicz TS, Witman PA, Preston-Martin S, Davis F, Bruner JM. The descriptive epidemiology of craniopharyngioma. *Neurosurg Focus.* 1997;3(6):e1.
25. Haupt R, Magnani C, Pavanello M, Caruso S, Dama E, Garrè ML. Epidemiological aspects of craniopharyngioma. *J Pediatr Endocrinol Metab.* 2006;19 (suppl 1):289–293.
26. Puget S, Garnett M, Wray A, et al. Pediatric craniopharyngiomas: classification and treatment according to the degree of hypothalamic involvement. *J Neurosurg.* 2007;106(1 suppl):3–12.
27. Karavitaki N, Brufani C, Warner JT, et al. Craniopharyngiomas in children and adults: systematic analysis of 121 cases with long-term follow-up. *Clin Endocrinol (Oxf).* 2005;62(4):397–409.
28. Karavitaki N, Cudlip S, Adams CB, Wass JA. Craniopharyngiomas. *Endocr Rev.* 2006;27(4):371–397.
29. Sartoretti-Schefer S, Wichmann W, Aguzzi A, Valavanis A. MR differentiation of adamantinous and squamous-papillary craniopharyngiomas. *AJNR Am J Neuroradiol.* 1997;18(1):77–87.
30. Albright AL, Hadjipanayis CG, Lunsford LD, Kondziolka D, Pollack IF, Adelson PD. Individualized treatment of pediatric craniopharyngiomas. *Childs Nerv Syst.* 2005;21(8–9):649–654.
31. Zuccaro G. Radical resection of craniopharyngioma. *Childs Nerv Syst.* 2005;21(8–9):679–690.
32. Gupta DK, Ojha BK, Sarkar C, Mahapatra AK, Sharma BS, Mehta VS. Recurrence in pediatric craniopharyngiomas: analysis of clinical and histological features. *Childs Nerv Syst.* 2006;22(1):50–55.
33. Sanford RA. Craniopharyngioma: results of survey of the American Society of Pediatric Neurosurgery. *Pediatr Neurosurg.* 1994;21 (suppl 1):39–43.
34. Marchal JC, Klein O, Thouvenot P, Bernier V, Moret C, Chastagner P. Individualized treatment of craniopharyngioma in children: ways and means. *Childs Nerv Syst.* 2005;21(8–9):655–659.
35. Sainte-Rose C, Puget S, Wray A, et al. Craniopharyngioma: the pendulum of surgical management. *Childs Nerv Syst.* 2005;21(8–9):691–695.
36. Kalapurakal JA. Radiation therapy in the management of pediatric craniopharyngiomas–a review. *Childs Nerv Syst.* 2005;21(8–9):808–816.
37. Kennedy JD, Haines SJ. Review of skull base surgery approaches: with special reference to pediatric patients. *J Neurooncol.* 1994;20(3):291–312.
38. de Divitiis E, Cavallo LM, Cappabianca P, Esposito F. Extended endoscopic endonasal transsphenoidal approach for the removal of suprasellar tumors: Part 2. *Neurosurgery.* 2007;60(1):46–58; discussion 58.
39. Frank G, Pasquini E, Doglietto F, et al. The endoscopic extended transsphenoidal approach for craniopharyngiomas. *Neurosurgery.* 2006;59(1 suppl 1):ONS75–83; discussion ONS75.
40. Im SH, Wang KC, Kim SK, et al. Transsphenoidal microsurgery for pediatric craniopharyngioma: special considerations regarding indications and method. *Pediatr Neurosurg.* 2003;39(2):97–103.
41. Maira G, Anile C, Albanese A, Cabezas D, Pardi F, Vignati A. The role of transsphenoidal surgery in the treatment of craniopharyngiomas. *J Neurosurg.* 2004;100(3):445–451.
42. Teo C. Application of endoscopy to the surgical management of craniopharyngiomas. *Childs Nerv Syst.* 2005;21(8–9):696–700.
43. DeVile CJ, Grant DB, Hayward RD, Stanhope R. Growth and endocrine sequelae of craniopharyngioma. *Arch Dis Child.* 1996;75(2):108–114.
44. Poretti A, Grotzer MA, Ribi K, Schönle E, Boltshauser E. Outcome of craniopharyngioma in children: long-term complications and quality of life. *Dev Med Child Neurol.* 2004;46(4):220–229.
45. Chang CZ, Wang CJ, Howng SL. Pituitary adenomas in adolescence–ten-year experience and literature review. *Kaohsiung J Med Sci.* 1999;15(12):691–696.
46. Kane LA, Leinung MC, Scheithauer BW, et al. Pituitary adenomas in childhood and adolescence. *J Clin Endocrinol Metab.* 1994;79(4):1135–1140.
47. Mehrazin M. Pituitary tumors in children: clinical analysis of 21 cases. *Childs Nerv Syst.* 2007;23(4):391–398.
48. Singh SK, Aggarwal R. Pituitary adenomas in childhood. *Indian J Pediatr.* 2005;72(7):583–591.
49. Hoffman H. Pituitary adenomas. In: American Association of Neurological Surgeons, eds. *Pediatric Neurosurgery: Surgery of Developing Nervous System.* New York, NY: Grune & Stratton; 1982:493–499.
50. Lafferty AR, Chrousos GP. Pituitary tumors in children and adolescents. *J Clin Endocrinol Metab.* 1999;84(12):4317–4323.
51. Mindermann T, Wilson CB. Pediatric pituitary adenomas. *Neurosurgery.* 1995;36(2):259–268; discussion 269.
52. Partington MD, Davis DH, Laws ER Jr, Scheithauer BW. Pituitary adenomas in childhood and adolescence. Results of transsphenoidal surgery. *J Neurosurg.* 1994;80(2):209–216.
53. Kunwar S, Wilson CB. Pediatric pituitary adenomas. *J Clin Endocrinol Metab.* 1999;84(12):4385–4389.
54. Osborn A. In: Diagnostic Neuroradiology. St. Louis: Mosby; 1994:401–528.
55. Suh DY, Mapstone T. Pediatric supratentorial intraventricular tumors. *Neurosurg Focus.* 2001;10(6):E4.
56. Jelinek J, Smirniotopoulos JG, Parisi JE, Kanzer M. Lateral ventricular neoplasms of the brain: differential diagnosis based on clinical, CT, and MR findings. *AJR Am J Roentgenol.* 1990;155(2):365–372.
57. McConachie NS, Worthington BS, Cornford EJ, Balsitis M, Kerslake RW, Jaspan T. Review article: computed tomography and magnetic resonance in the diagnosis of intraventricular cerebral masses. *Br J Radiol.* 1994;67(795):223–243.
58. Morrison G, Sobel DF, Kelley WM, Norman D. Intraventricular mass lesions. *Radiology.* 1984;153(2):435–442.
59. Piepmeier JM. Tumors and approaches to the lateral ventricles. Introduction and overview. *J Neurooncol.* 1996;30(3):267–274.

60. Tien RD. Intraventricular mass lesions of the brain: CT and MR findings. *AJR Am J Roentgenol.* 1991;157(6):1283–1290.
61. Zuccaro G, Sosa F, Cuccia V, Lubieniecky F, Monges J. Lateral ventricle tumors in children: a series of 54 cases. *Childs Nerv Syst.* 1999;15(11–12):774–785.
62. Boyd MC, Steinbok P. Choroid plexus tumors: problems in diagnosis and management. *J Neurosurg.* 1987;66(6):800–805.
63. Levy ML, Goldfarb A, Hyder DJ, et al. Choroid plexus tumors in children: significance of stromal invasion. *Neurosurgery.* 2001;48(2):303–309.
64. Pencalet P, Sainte-Rose C, Lellouch-Tubiana A, et al. Papillomas and carcinomas of the choroid plexus in children. *J Neurosurg.* 1998;88(3):521–528.
65. Eisenberg HM, McComb JG, Lorenzo AV. Cerebrospinal fluid overproduction and hydrocephalus associated with choroid plexus papilloma. *J Neurosurg.* 1974;40(3):381–385.
66. Ghatak NR, McWhorter JM. Ultrastructural evidence for CSF production by a choroid plexus papilloma. *J Neurosurg.* 1976;45(4):409–415.
67. Ellenbogen RG, Winston KR, Kupsky WJ. Tumors of the choroid plexus in children. *Neurosurgery.* 1989;25(3):327–335.
68. Hawkins JC 3rd. Treatment of choroid plexus papillomas in children: a brief analysis of twenty years' experience. *Neurosurgery.* 1980;6(4):380–384.
69. Chow E, Reardon DA, Shah AB, et al. Pediatric choroid plexus neoplasms. *Int J Radiat Oncol Biol Phys.* 1999;44(2):249–254.
70. Greenberg ML. Chemotherapy of choroid plexus carcinoma. *Childs Nerv Syst.* 1999;15(10):571–577.
71. Piastra M, Di Rocco C, Tempera A, et al. Massive blood transfusion in choroid plexus tumor surgery: 10-years' experience. *J Clin Anesth.* 2007;19(3):192–197.
72. Ellenbogen RG, Scott RM. Choroid plexus tumors. In: Winn HR, Youmans JR, eds. *Youmans Neurological Surgery.* 5th ed. Philadelphia: W. B. Saunders; 2004:3612–3622.
73. Due-Tønnessen B, Helseth E, Skullerud K, Lundar T. Choroid plexus tumors in children and young adults: report of 16 consecutive cases. *Childs Nerv Syst.* 2001;17(4–5):252–256.
74. St Clair SK, Humphreys RP, Pillay PK, Hoffman HJ, Blaser SI, Becker LE. Current management of choroid plexus carcinoma in children. *Pediatr Neurosurg.* 1991;17(5):225–233.
75. Kim DG, Chi JG, Park SH, et al. Intraventricular neurocytoma: clinicopathological analysis of seven cases. *J Neurosurg.* 1992;76(5):759–765.
76. Leenstra JL, Rodriguez FJ, Frechette CM, et al. Central neurocytoma: management recommendations based on a 35-year experience. *Int J Radiat Oncol Biol Phys.* 2007;67(4):1145–1154.
77. Maiuri F, Spaziante R, De Caro ML, Cappabianca P, Giamundo A, Iaconetta G. Central neurocytoma: clinico-pathological study of 5 cases and review of the literature. *Clin Neurol Neurosurg.* 1995;97(3):219–228.
78. Yasargil MG, von Ammon K, von Deimling A, Valavanis A, Wichmann W, Wiestler OD. Central neurocytoma: histopathological variants and therapeutic approaches. *J Neurosurg.* 1992;76(1):32–37.
79. Hassoun J, Gambarelli D, Grisoli F, et al. Central neurocytoma. An electron-microscopic study of two cases. *Acta Neuropathol.* 1982;56(2):151–156.
80. Ferreol E, Sawaya R, de Courten-Myers GM. Primary cerebral neuroblastoma (neurocytoma) in adults. *J Neurooncol.* 1989;7(2):121–128.
81. Christov C, Adle-Biassette H, Le Guerinel C. Recurrent central neurocytoma with marked increase in MIB-1 labelling index. *Br J Neurosurg.* 1999;13(5):496–499.
82. Mackenzie IR. Central neurocytoma: histologic atypia, proliferation potential, and clinical outcome. *Cancer.* 1999;85(7):1606–1610.
83. Sharma MC, Rathore A, Karak AK, Sarkar C. A study of proliferative markers in central neurocytoma. *Pathology.* 1998;30(4):355–359.
84. Söylemezoglu F, Scheithauer BW, Esteve J, Kleihues P. Atypical central neurocytoma. *J Neuropathol Exp Neurol.* 1997;56(5):551–556.
85. Sharma MC, Deb P, Sharma S, Sarkar C. Neurocytoma: a comprehensive review. *Neurosurg Rev.* 2006;29(4):270–285; discussion 285.
86. Smoker WR, Townsend JJ, Reichman MV. Neurocytoma accompanied by intraventricular hemorrhage: case report and literature review. *AJNR Am J Neuroradiol.* 1991;12(4):765–770.
87. Rades D, Schild SE, Fehlauer F. Defining the best available treatment for neurocytomas in children. *Cancer.* 2004;101(11):2629–2632.
88. Di Rocco C, Iannelli A. Bilateral thalamic tumors in children. *Childs Nerv Syst.* 2002;18(8):440–444.
89. Fernandez C, Maues de Paula A, Colin C, et al. Thalamic gliomas in children: an extensive clinical, neuroradiological and pathological study of 14 cases. *Childs Nerv Syst.* 2006;22(12):1603–1610.
90. Puget S, Crimmins DW, Garnett MR, et al. Thalamic tumors in children: a reappraisal. *J Neurosurg.* 2007;106(5 suppl):354–362.
91. Reardon DA, Gajjar A, Sanford RA, et al. Bithalamic involvement predicts poor outcome among children with thalamic glial tumors. *Pediatr Neurosurg.* 1998;29(1):29–35.
92. Bernstein M, Hoffman HJ, Halliday WC, Hendrick EB, Humphreys RP. Thalamic tumors in children. Long-term follow-up and treatment guidelines. *J Neurosurg.* 1984;61(4):649–656.
93. Albright AL. Feasibility and advisability of resections of thalamic tumors in pediatric patients. *J Neurosurg.* 2004;100(5 suppl Pediatrics):468–472.
94. Drake JM, Joy M, Goldenberg A, Kreindler D. Computer- and robot-assisted resection of thalamic astrocytomas in children. *Neurosurgery.* 1991;29(1):27–33.
95. Kelly PJ. Stereotactic biopsy and resection of thalamic astrocytomas. *Neurosurgery.* 1989;25(2):185–194; discussion 194.
96. Ozek MM, Türe U. Surgical approach to thalamic tumors. *Childs Nerv Syst.* 2002;18(8):450–456.
97. Villarejo F, Amaya C, Pérez Díaz C, Pascual A, Alvarez Sastre C, Goyenechea F. Radical surgery of thalamic tumors in children. *Childs Nerv Syst.* 1994;10(2):111–114.
98. Arseni C. Tumors of the basal ganglia; their surgical treatment. *AMA Arch Neurol Psychiatry.* 1958;80(1):18–24.
99. Gaab MR, Schroeder HW. Neuroendoscopic approach to intraventricular lesions. *Neurosurg Focus.* 1999;6(4):e5.
100. Macarthur DC, Buxton N, Punt J, Vloeberghs M, Robertson IJ. The role of neuroendoscopy in the management of brain tumours. *Br J Neurosurg.* 2002;16(5):465–470.
101. Badie B, Brooks N, Souweidane MM. Endoscopic and minimally invasive microsurgical approaches for treating brain tumor patients. *J Neurooncol.* 2004;69(1–3):209–219.
102. Depreitere B, Dasi N, Rutka J, Dirks P, Drake J. Endoscopic biopsy for intraventricular tumors in children. *J Neurosurg.* 2007;106(5 suppl):340–346.
103. Fukushima T. Endoscopic biopsy of intraventricular tumors with the use of a ventriculofiberscope. *Neurosurgery.* 1978;2(2):110–113.
104. Fukushima T, Ishijima B, Hirakawa K, Nakamura N, Sano K. Ventriculofiberscope: a new technique for endoscopic diagnosis and operation. Technical note. *J Neurosurg.* 1973;38(2):251–256.
105. Macarthur DC, Buxton N, Vloeberghs M, Punt J. The effectiveness of neuroendoscopic interventions in children with brain tumours. *Childs Nerv Syst.* 2001;17(10):589–594.
106. Souweidane MM, Sandberg DI, Bilsky MH, Gutin PH. Endoscopic biopsy for tumors of the third ventricle. *Pediatr Neurosurg.* 2000;33(3):132–137.
107. Peretta P, Ragazzi P, Galarza M, et al. Complications and pitfalls of neuroendoscopic surgery in children. *J Neurosurg.* 2006;105(3 suppl):187–193.
108. Gaab MR, Schroeder HW. Neuroendoscopic approach to intraventricular lesions. *J Neurosurg.* 1998;88(3):496–505.
109. Souweidane MM. Endoscopic surgery for intraventricular brain tumors in patients without hydrocephalus. *Neurosurgery.* 2005;57(4 suppl):312–318; discussion 312.
110. Bruce JN. Pineal region tumors. In: Winn HR, Youmans JR, eds. *Youmans Neurological Surgery.* 5th ed. Philadelphia, PA: W. B. Saunders; 2004:1011–1130.
111. Bruce JN, Ogden AT. Surgical strategies for treating patients with pineal region tumors. *J Neurooncol.* 2004;69(1–3):221–236.
112. Pople IK, Athanasiou TC, Sandeman DR, Coakham HB. The role of endoscopic biopsy and third ventriculostomy in the management of pineal region tumours. *Br J Neurosurg.* 2001;15(4):305–311.
113. Ray P, Jallo GI, Kim RY, et al. Endoscopic third ventriculostomy for tumor-related hydrocephalus in a pediatric population. *Neurosurg Focus.* 2005;19(6):E8.
114. Roopesh Kumar SV, Mohanty A, Santosh V, et al. Endoscopic options in management of posterior third ventricular tumors. *Childs Nerv Syst.* 2007;23(10):1135–1145.
115. Teo C, Young R 2nd. Endoscopic management of hydrocephalus secondary to tumors of the posterior third ventricle. *Neurosurg Focus.* 1999;7(4):e2.

116. Yamini B, Refai D, Rubin CM, Frim DM. Initial endoscopic management of pineal region tumors and associated hydrocephalus: clinical series and literature review. *J Neurosurg.* 2004;100(5 suppl Pediatrics):437–441.
117. Yamamoto I. Pineal region tumor: surgical anatomy and approach. *J Neurooncol.* 2001;54(3):263–275.
118. Ausman JI, Malik GM, Dujovny M, Mann R. Three-quarter prone approach to the pineal-tentorial region. *Surg Neurol.* 1988;29(4):298–306.
119. Matsutani M, Sano K, Takakura K, et al. Primary intracranial germ cell tumors: a clinical analysis of 153 histologically verified cases. *J Neurosurg.* 1997;86(3):446–455.
120. Wolden SL, Wara WM, Larson DA, Prados MD, Edwards MS, Sneed PK. Radiation therapy for primary intracranial germ-cell tumors. *Int J Radiat Oncol Biol Phys.* 1995;32(4):943–949.
121. Kochi M, Itoyama Y, Shiraishi S, Kitamura I, Marubayashi T, Ushio Y. Successful treatment of intracranial nongerminomatous malignant germ cell tumors by administering neoadjuvant chemotherapy and radiotherapy before excision of residual tumors. *J Neurosurg.* 2003;99(1):106–114.
122. Kunscher LF, Lang FF. Medulloblastoma. In: Winn HR, Youmans JR, eds. *Youmans Neurological Surgery.* 5th ed. Philadelphia, PA: W. B. Saunders; 2004:1031–1042.
123. Rutka JT, Hoffman HJ. Medulloblastoma: a historical perspective and overview. *J Neurooncol.* 1996;29(1):1–7.
124. Kleihues P, Louis DN, Scheithauer BW, et al. The WHO classification of tumors of the nervous system. *J Neuropathol Exp Neurol.* 2002;61(3):215–225; discussion 226.
125. Ozgur BM, Berberian J, Aryan HE, Meltzer HS, Levy ML. The pathophysiologic mechanism of cerebellar mutism. *Surg Neurol.* 2006;66(1):18–25.
126. Albright AL, Wisoff JH, Zeltzer PM, Boyett JM, Rorke LB, Stanley P. Effects of medulloblastoma resections on outcome in children: a report from the Children's Cancer Group. *Neurosurgery.* 1996;38(2):265–271.
127. Gottardo NG, Gajjar A. Current therapy for medulloblastoma. *Curr Treat Options Neurol.* 2006;8(4):319–334.
128. Hughes EN, Shillito J, Sallan SE, Loeffler JS, Cassady JR, Tarbell NJ. Medulloblastoma at the joint center for radiation therapy between 1968 and 1984. The influence of radiation dose on the patterns of failure and survival. *Cancer.* 1988;61(10):1992–1998.
129. Gajjar A, Chintagumpala M, Ashley D, et al. Risk-adapted craniospinal radiotherapy followed by high-dose chemotherapy and stem-cell rescue in children with newly diagnosed medulloblastoma (St Jude Medulloblastoma-96): long-term results from a prospective, multicentre trial. *Lancet Oncol.* 2006;7(10):813–820.
130. Agaoglu FY, Ayan I, Dizdar Y, Kebudi R, Gorgun O, Darendeliler E. Ependymal tumors in childhood. *Pediatr Blood Cancer.* 2005;45(3):298–303.
131. Smyth MD, Horn BN, Russo C, Berger MS. Intracranial ependymomas of childhood: current management strategies. *Pediatr Neurosurg.* 2000;33(3):138–150.
132. West CR, Bruce DA, Duffner PK. Ependymomas. Factors in clinical and diagnostic staging. *Cancer.* 1985;56(7 suppl):1812–1816.
133. Teo C, Nakaji P, Symons P, Tobias V, Cohn R, Smee R. Ependymoma. *Childs Nerv Syst.* 2003;19(5–6):270–285.
134. van Veelen-Vincent ML, Pierre-Kahn A, Kalifa C, et al. Ependymoma in childhood: prognostic factors, extent of surgery, and adjuvant therapy. *J Neurosurg.* 2002;97(4):827–835.
135. Rutka J, Hoffman HJ, Duncan JA. Astrocytomas of the posterior fossa. In: Cohen A, ed. *Surgical Disorders of the Fourth Ventricle.* Cambridge, MA: Blackwell Science; 1996:189–208.
136. Ilgren EB, Stiller CA. Cerebellar astrocytomas. Clinical characteristics and prognostic indices. *J Neurooncol.* 1987;4(3):293–308.
137. Schneider JH Jr, Raffel C, McComb JG. Benign cerebellar astrocytomas of childhood. *Neurosurgery.* 1992;30(1):58–62; discussion 62.
138. Bognár L, Borgulya G, Benke P, Madarassy G. Analysis of CSF shunting procedure requirement in children with posterior fossa tumors. *Childs Nerv Syst.* 2003;19(5–6):332–336.
139. Culley DJ, Berger MS, Shaw D, Geyer R. An analysis of factors determining the need for ventriculoperitoneal shunts after posterior fossa tumor surgery in children. *Neurosurgery.* 1994;34(3):402–407; discussion 407.
140. Kumar V, Phipps K, Harkness W, Hayward RD. Ventriculo-peritoneal shunt requirement in children with posterior fossa tumours: an 11-year audit. *Br J Neurosurg.* 1996;10(5):467–470.
141. Sainte-Rose C, Cinalli G, Roux FE, et al. Management of hydrocephalus in pediatric patients with posterior fossa tumors: the role of endoscopic third ventriculostomy. *J Neurosurg.* 2001;95(5):791–797.
142. Papo I, Caruselli G, Luongo A. External ventricular drainage in the management of posterior fossa tumors in children and adolescents. *Neurosurgery.* 1982;10(1):13–15.
143. Ruggiero C, Cinalli G, Spennato P, et al. Endoscopic third ventriculostomy in the treatment of hydrocephalus in posterior fossa tumors in children. *Childs Nerv Syst.* 2004;20(11–12):828–833.
144. Gnanalingham KK, Lafuente J, Thompson D, Harkness W, Hayward R. Surgical procedures for posterior fossa tumors in children: does craniotomy lead to fewer complications than craniectomy? *J Neurosurg.* 2002;97(4):821–826.
145. Kurpad SN, Cohen AR. Posterior fossa craniotomy: an alternative to craniectomy. *Pediatr Neurosurg.* 1999;31(1):54–57.
146. Harner SG, Beatty CW, Ebersold MJ. Impact of cranioplasty on headache after acoustic neuroma removal. *Neurosurgery.* 1995;36(6):1097–1099; discussion 1099.
147. Schessel DA, Nedzelski JM, Rowed D, Feghali JG. Pain after surgery for acoustic neuroma. *Otolaryngol Head Neck Surg.* 1992;107(3):424–429.
148. Rekate HL, Grubb RL, Aram DM, Hahn JF, Ratcheson RA. Muteness of cerebellar origin. *Arch Neurol.* 1985;42(7):697–698.
149. Siffert J, Poussaint TY, Goumnerova LC, et al. Neurological dysfunction associated with postoperative cerebellar mutism. *J Neurooncol.* 2000;48(1):75–81.
150. Doxey D, Bruce D, Sklar F, Swift D, Shapiro K. Posterior fossa syndrome: identifiable risk factors and irreversible complications. *Pediatr Neurosurg.* 1999;31(3):131–136.
151. Lieberman DM, Berger MS. Brain tumors during the first 2 years of life. In: Albright AL, Pollack IF, Adelson PD, eds. *Operative Techniques in Pediatric Neurosurgery.* New York, NY: Thieme; 2001:125–130.

61 Brachial Plexus Tumors

Robert J. Spinner, Kimon Bekelis, and Kimberly K. Amrami

INTRODUCTION

Mass lesions affecting the brachial plexus can be difficult to diagnose and treat. Many of the challenges are related to their relative rarity and physicians' and surgeons' limited experience with them. Other challenges relate to their proximity to important structures (e.g., neurovascular elements, lung, spine, etc.) and the range of pathologies (i.e., benign and malignant). A variety of lesions exists, with different anticipated outcomes. The rarity of brachial plexus tumors makes the study of their epidemiologic features, through extensive case series, difficult. Only several subspecialty centers with many years of experience have addressed these issues in the literature. Management demands a knowledge of operative anatomy (and variations), pathoanatomy, and surgical approaches. Treatment must be individualized, and the role of multidisciplinary practice is often necessary. Referral of patients with complex lesions and atypical histologic features should be considered.

In this chapter, general principles for the management of brachial plexus tumors will be presented, concentrating on the most common lesions.

PREOPERATIVE EVALUATION

History

Patients typically present with a mass or a fullness that has grown in size. Whereas some patients may be asymptomatic, others may note local or radiating pain, experiencing paresthesias or dysesthesias when touching or bumping it, or with movement of the limb. Rarely do they notice weakness or other systemic symptoms. Occasionally, they may note dyspnea. A history of other lesions or family history of neurofibromatosis (NF) and so on should be sought.

Trying to distinguishing between benign and malignant lesions prospectively should be attempted, and an accurate history is the first step. Progressive, relatively rapid loss of function in a patient with severe pain would be worrisome for malignancy (especially in the context of a history of NF). In contrast, benign lesions typically grow more slowly and produce fewer or milder symptoms. While severe pain (including night pain) is a common feature of malignancy, the presence or absence of pain by itself is not a reliable means of differentiation between benign and malignant lesions. For example, malignant lesions can be painless, and benign lesions can be extremely painful.

Physical Examination

Physical examination should include careful assessment of the size, consistency, and location of the lesion [1]. Mobility of the mass in a side-to-side fashion but not up-down direction is consistent with a benign nerve sheath tumor. Although a hard, immobile lesion would be suspicious for a malignancy, a malignant peripheral nerve sheath tumor (MPNST) may still be mobile in a side-to-side fashion. Neurologic examination should document motor, sensory, and autonomic function. Motor testing is often normal with benign masses, even when they are large. Pulses should be assessed. Regardless of the size of mass, local pain or radiating paresthesias with percussion over the mass is frequently present. Stigmata of neurocutaneous syndromes and other mass lesions should be looked for. Identification of the symptomatic mass in some cases where numerous lesions are present may not be straightforward.

Electromyography/Nerve Conduction Study

Electromyography (EMG)/nerve conduction study can be helpful in determining, localizing, and quantifying neurologic deficit. Typically for benign nerve sheath tumors, preoperative electrophysiologic studies are normal or minimally abnormal. For dumbbell tumors, normal EMGs suggest that the root is nonfunctional [2]. Severe abnormalities are unusual for benign nerve sheath tumors (i.e., conventional schwannomas, neurofibromas) and would be more suggestive of another type of benign (e.g., perineurioma or inflammatory process) or malignant lesion.

Imaging

Imaging is a critical part of the preoperative evaluation. In our opinion, any mass lesion in the vicinity of the brachial plexus should be imaged. This can help avert an easily preventable error in management. We have cared for many patients who have been operated on for "simple" lymph nodes that were found to be benign nerve sheath tumors. Unfortunately, these tumors were resected along with segments of major nerves. Lymph nodes occurring in unusual locations (i.e., the anterior rather than the posterior triangle of the neck) should be imaged.

Radiography, computed tomography (CT), positron emission tomography (PET), and magnetic resonance imaging (MRI), all have a role in imaging the brachial plexus. Ultrasound is being used by some groups as well.

Radiography and computerized tomography may be helpful for evaluating primary bony lesions or secondary bony changes, for example, erosion. Three-dimensional reconstructions may be done when nerve compression contributing to brachial plexopathy is present. CT may provide some evaluation of muscle bulk and masses, but, in general, MRI is the preferred imaging method for the brachial plexus peripheral to the central cervical and thoracic spine due to its ability to distinguish different types of soft tissue (i.e., nerves, muscle, fat, masses) and to characterize pathology [3–8]. PET scanning, often coupled with CT, has become an important adjunct to imaging of the brachial plexus in selected cases. Advanced imaging modalities (i.e., high-resolution MRI, PET) are playing an increased role in surveillance, especially for some patients with NF [9–12].

MR imaging of the brachial plexus is complicated by its complex geometry and course from the cervical spine, through the neck and into the upper arm. There are also many air–tissue interfaces (lung/neck, neck surrounding air) that cause significant susceptibility artifacts that further challenge conventional imaging techniques. The relatively large fields of view required to image the entire plexus often lead to an overall lower-than-desirable spatial resolution unless high-field (3T) imaging is available and specialized receiver coils are used. In general imaging should be performed in three planes (axial, sagittal, and an oblique coronal that is angled along the plexus) using T1- and T2-weighted imaging with fat suppression. Ideally the T2-weighted sequence should be a fast-spin echo (T2 TR = 4000 ms, TE = 60 ms) with chemical fat suppression, but if there has been prior surgery, or susceptibility artifacts are extreme due to patient factors, then an inversion recovery sequence may be substituted, though generally with lower spatial resolution due to the increased time required for imaging. Postcontrast imaging can either be performed with T1-weighted spoiled gradient recalled sequences or with T1-weighted fast-spin echo. Fat suppression is required for either technique. Normal nerves will have signal intensity similar to normal skeletal muscle on T1 and T2 fast-spin echo imaging; slight hyperintensity compared with muscle on inversion recovery is often a normal finding. The normal brachial plexus does not enhance with contrast [3].

MRI can characterize some specific lesions within the brachial plexus; in other cases imaging findings may be indeterminate but still help to narrow the diagnostic possibilities [3–6]. Contrast enhancement is a basic requirement for imaging the brachial plexus. The only exceptions are patients with allergies to gadolinium or with compromised renal function or for those cases where follow-up examinations are being performed for a known entity and there is a prior examination with contrast for comparison. Knowledge of the complex anatomy of the brachial plexus and meticulous attention to MRI technique are both required for effective image interpretation. A description of common entities involving the brachial plexus and their imaging appearances follows.

MRI OF SPECIFIC LESIONS

Benign Peripheral Nerve Sheath Tumors

Benign neurogenic tumors such as schwannomas and neurofibromas commonly affect the brachial plexus; however, they may originate anywhere: from major neural elements or from tiny intramuscular twigs. These tumors have a very characteristic appearance on MRI. They are commonly very smoothly marginated, oval and, in some cases, the nerve of origin may be seen proximal and distal to the mass. They are isointense to muscle on T1-weighted imaging, very bright on T2, and generally avidly enhance after contrast material (Figure 61.1). They commonly have a central area of low signal on T2-weighted imaging, the so called "target"

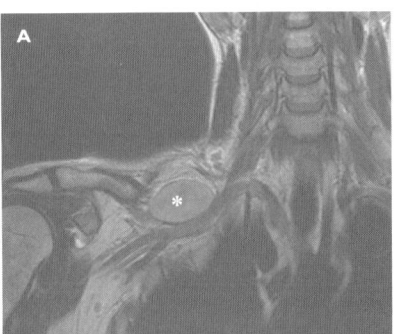
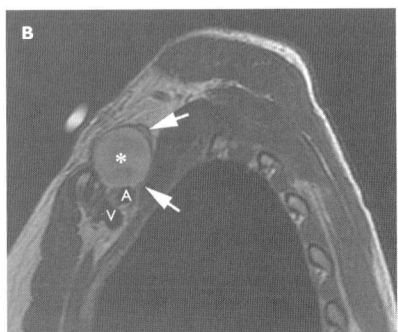
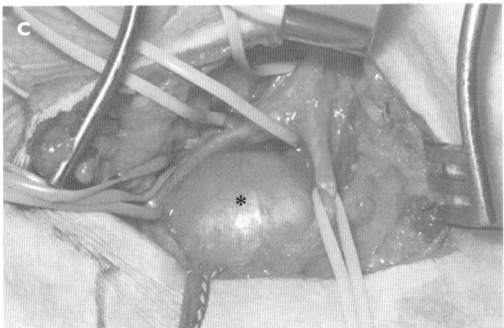

Figure 61.1 Schwannoma. **(A)** Coronal T2-weighted image shows the oval, hyperintense mass (asterisk) arising from the upper trunk of the brachial plexus. Signal intensity and pattern are consistent with a benign schwannoma. **(B)** Sagittal T2-weighted image shows the large, oval, retroclavicular mass (asterisk) that is displacing elements of the brachial plexus (arrows). A = subclavian artery; V = subclavian vein. **(C)** Through the right supraclavicular exposure, the upper trunk, anterior and posterior divisions, and suprascapular nerve have been mobilized in vasoloops. With the clavicle retracted inferiorly, the tumor (asterisk) could then be resected easily and safely at a fascicular level.

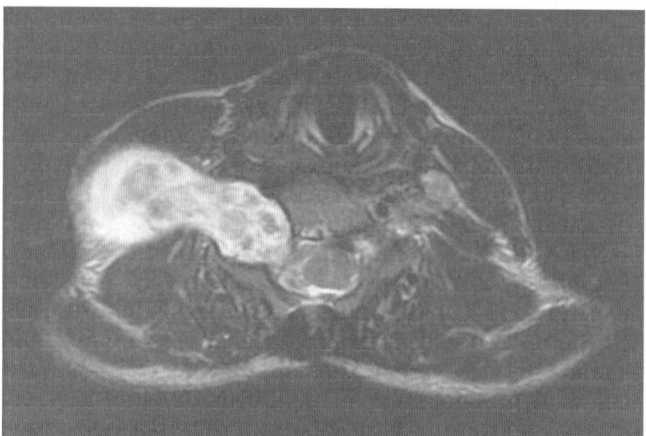

Figure 61.2 NF-2, large dumbbell schwannoma. Axial T2-weighted image with fat suppression at the level of the mid-cervical spine shows a heterogeneous, fusiform mass arising from the nerve root with central low signal consistent with a benign neurogenic tumor. Note the expansion of the neural foramen. Although the extensive tumor extended to the level of the axilla, the patient presented with a superficial neck mass.

sign that represents collagen at the center of the tumor (Figure 61.2). This area may not itself enhance after contrast. When the classic imaging features are present one may confidently diagnose these masses as benign. It is important to assess the lesions for any associated plexiform features such as more longitudinal or fusiform enlargement of the nerve and to prospectively report these features as treatment planning in these cases may be altered (Figure 61.3). Although plexiform lesions may occur by themselves, they may also be seen in combination with other more conventional histologies [13,14].

Perineurioma usually, but not always, involves a single nerve that often has segmental, fusiform enlargement. The size is variable and short-segment lesions may be subtle and difficult to localize on imaging without knowledge of the clinical findings. Perineurioma is isointense on T1 and hyperintense on T2 but, unlike inflammatory lesions, shows avid enhancement (Figure 61.4). It is also commonly associated with fatty atrophy and denervation in the affected muscles.

Benign Nonperipheral Nerve Sheath Tumors

Lipomas are very common around the brachial plexus and are easily identifiable by their similarity to subcutaneous fat on all imaging sequences (Figure 61.5). Ganglion cysts commonly are seen arising from the shoulder joint close to elements of the brachial plexus. Most are extraneural but may cause mass effect on the plexus and, therefore, lead to symptoms. Cysts are high in signal on T2-weighted imaging with no enhancement after contrast. Identifying the joint origin is critical and should be the focus of imaging in these cases. The most common scenario is a paralabral cyst arising from a labral (SLAP) tear at the shoulder that extends to the suprascapular notch to cause extrinsic compression on the suprascapular nerve (Figure 61.6). This should be distinguished from the much rarer intraneural ganglion cyst that

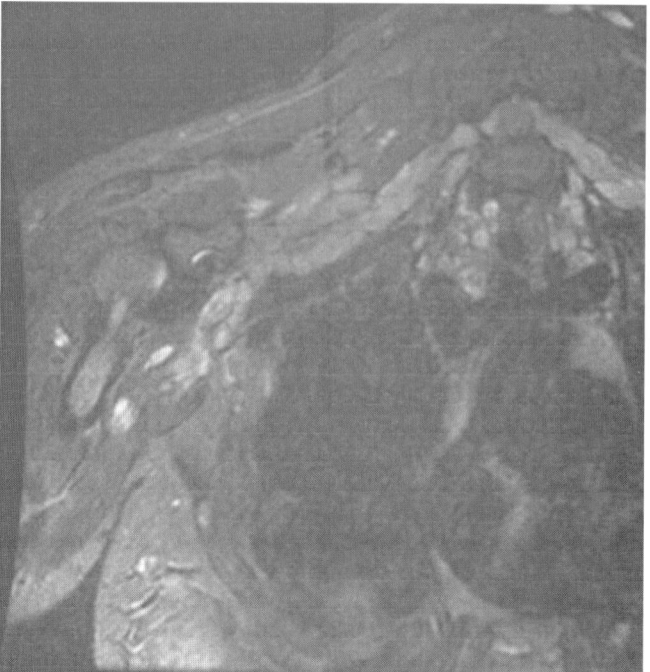

Figure 61.3 NF-1 related plexiform neurofibroma. Coronal T2-weighted STIR image shows innumerable hyperintense, continuous, fusiform plexiform masses involving the brachial plexus bilaterally consistent with plexiform neurofibromas.

can dissect along an articular branch from the shoulder to the plexus itself (Figure 61.7). These cysts are typical more tubular and have a course constrained by the nerve that is different from extraneural cysts [15]. As with the extraneural cysts, identification of the joint origin is an important finding on imaging that can assist in treatment planning.

Desmoid tumors will typically have low signal on T1-weighted imaging, low-to-intermediate signal on T2 compared with muscle, and will show prominent enhancement after gadolinium administration (Figure 61.8). Desmoids may cause mass effect on the brachial plexus but more commonly infiltrate or encase the nerves. Infiltration of the nerve can sometimes be appreciated on MRI by the indistinct and "feathered" margins of the mass around the nerve.

Other Benign Lesions Affecting Nerve

Inflammatory conditions such as chronic inflammatory demyelinating polyneuropathy (CIDP) may affect the brachial plexus either discretely or in association with other more generalized nerve involvement [3,16]. In CIDP, the nerves are usually very large and hyperintense on T2-weighted imaging. Unless the disease is very long standing, there is usually not associated muscle atrophy. The enhancement pattern in CIDP is very characteristic: the enlarged nerves do not enhance to any significant degree. On 3T it is sometimes possible to see very fine peripheral enhancement of the individual enlarged fascicles; this is nearly pathognomonic of CIDP. Other types of inflammatory processes such as Parsonage-Turner syndrome also have hyperintense nerves that do not enhance or enhance only mildly, but these are generally not very

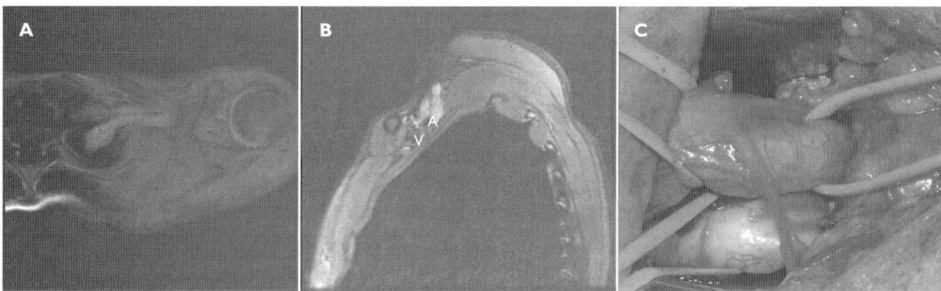

Figure 61.4 Perineurioma. **(A)** Axial T2-weighted image with fat suppression shows fusiform enlargement of the lower trunk of the brachial plexus. **(B)** Sagittal T2-weighted image with fat suppression shows the more distal, retroclavicular extent of the lesion that involves multiple nerves. A = subclavian artery; V = subclavian vein. **(C)** A left supraclavicular exposure demonstrated the enlarged upper and middle trunks. Phrenic nerve can be seen coursing obliquely after anterior scalene has been resected. Fascicular biopsy of the abnormal middle trunk revealed a perineurioma.

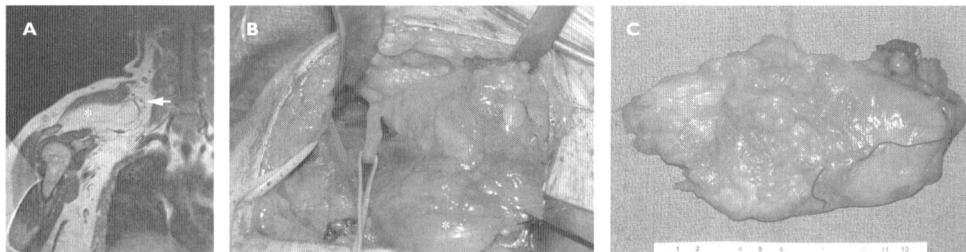

Figure 61.5 Recurrent extraneural lipoma. **(A)** Coronal T1-weighted MR image shows the large supra- and retroclavicular mass (asterisk) that is of the same signal intensity as subcutaneous fat, consistent with a benign lipoma. Note upward displacement of the trunks of upper and middle trucks of the brachial plexus (arrows). **(B)** The spinal accessory and long thoracic nerves (in vasoloops) were identified in order to facilitate tumor (asterisk) mobilization and resection. Other elements of the supraclavicular brachial plexus had been identified earlier in the dissection. **(C)** Resected mass.

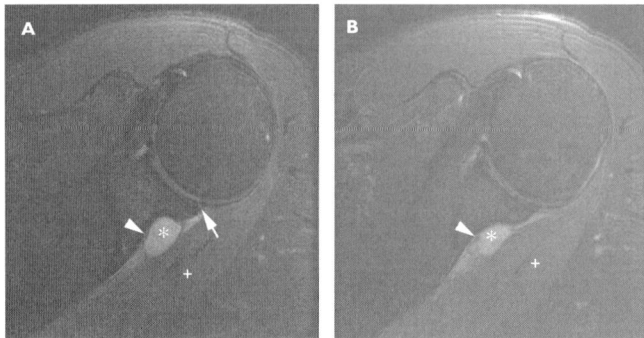

Figure 61.6 Paralabral cyst (extraneural ganglion) with suprascapular nerve compression **(A)** Axial fast-spin echo (FSE) T2-weighted image with fat suppression (3T) showing the labral tear (arrow) with posterior extension of the paralabral cyst (asterisk). Note mass effect within the suprascapular notch on the nerve (arrowhead). There is increased T2 signal within the infraspinatus muscle consistent with selective denervation (plus sign). **(B)** Axial FSE T2-weighted image slightly inferior to **A** shows the paralabral cyst (asterisk) within the suprascapular notch causing mass effect on the suprascapular nerve (arrowhead) and resultant infraspinatus atrophy (plus sign).

significantly enlarged, and subacute denervation changes (such as edema) are commonly present in the affected muscles. Rarely granulomatous diseases such as sarcoidosis may affect the brachial plexus. In this case, there may be mild enhancement of the nerves, and even some localized nodularity, but this is generally present when there is other evidence of sarcoidosis elsewhere that assists in making the diagnosis.

Malignant Peripheral Nerve and Nonperipheral Nerve Sheath Tumors

An MPNST should be suspected when imaging features such as irregular margins, large size, and areas of central nonenhancing necrosis are present (Figure 61.9). Malignant degeneration should be suspected when any atypical imaging features are present in a neurogenic tumor. PET imaging is an excellent complementary imaging modality to MRI that can help identify MPNSTs, though there is some overlap with hypercellular but benign lesions that may have increased metabolic activity.

Nonneurogenic, malignant, soft-tissue masses such as malignant fibrous histiocytoma or even lymphoma do not

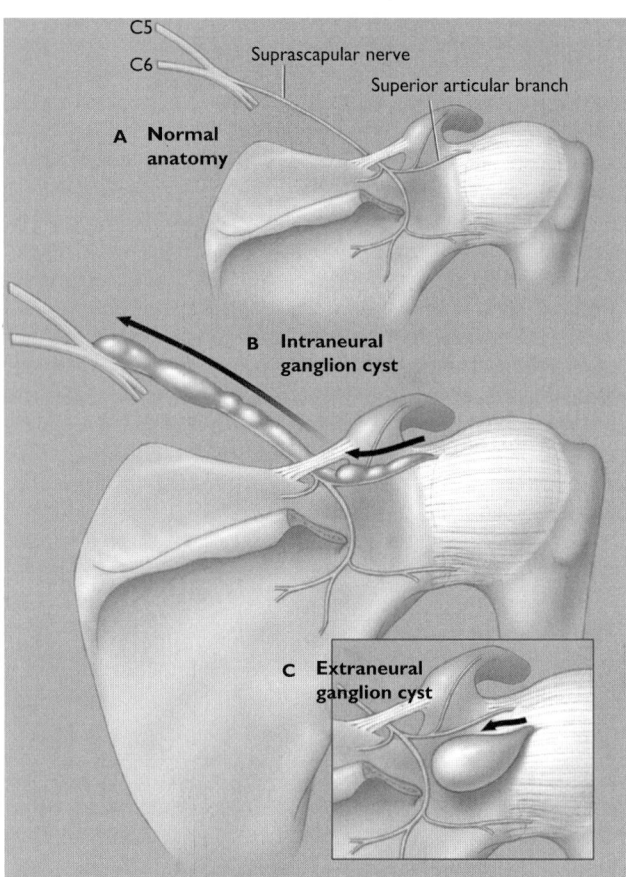

Figure 61.7 Suprascapular intraneural and extraneural ganglion cyst. **(A)** The anatomy of the suprascapular nerve and its relationship to the glenohumeral joint. **(B)** The formation of a suprascapular intraneural ganglion is from the glenohumeral joint and propagation occurs along its articular branch. **(C)** An extraneural ganglion (paralabral cyst) from the glenohumeral joint may compress the suprascapular nerve. With permission from Mayo Foundation for Medical Education and Research. All rights reserved.

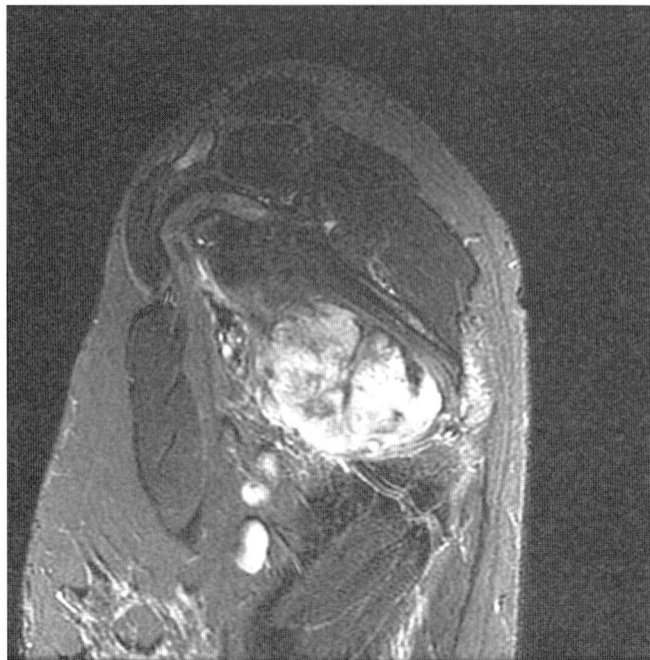

Figure 61.8 Desmoid tumor. Sagittal T2-weighted STIR image shows a large heterogeneous mass in the axilla that is infiltrating and encasing the brachial plexus, axillary artery, and vein. There has been prior surgery with some metallic artifact at the margins of the tumor. Signal characteristics are consistent with a desmoid.

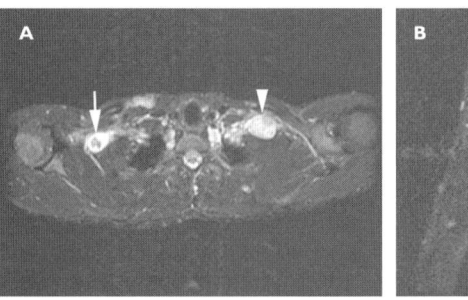 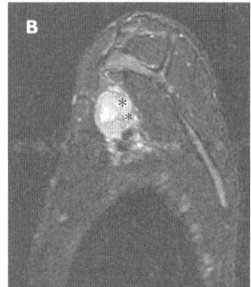

Figure 61.9 NF-related MPNST. This 25-year-old patient presented with radiating dysesthesias in the thumb. He had numerous NF-related tumors. **(A)** Axial STIR (short tau inversion recovery) image through the upper chest shows bilateral neurogenic tumors associated with the brachial plexus. The mass on the left (arrowhead) has typical imaging features of a benign neurofibroma. The lesion on the right (arrow) is indeterminate. **(B)** Sagittal STIR image showing the large mass on the right is associated with the lateral cord of the brachial plexus. The mass is very heterogeneous with eccentric areas of increased T2 signal (asterisks) that likely represent necrosis on this noncontrast study. This appearance, which is worrisome for malignant degeneration, was not appreciated on prospective review.

have a "typical" appearance and often require biopsy to characterize.

Lung cancer may affect the brachial plexus by direct extension from an apical Pancoast tumor; MRI will show the extent of involvement and other affected structures such as the subclavian artery and vein. Also, there are tumor extensions from other osseous tumors that involve the clavicle or shoulder girdle, such as chondrosarcoma or osteosarcoma. Ewing's sarcoma may also involve the brachial plexus primarily or via direct extension.

Involvement of the brachial plexus may occur in many types of malignancy but is most commonly seen with breast cancer [17] (Figure 61.10). Breast cancer to the plexus can be a difficult diagnostic dilemma, as postradiation fibrosis may have similar clinical and imaging findings. High-field (3T) imaging with optimum spatial resolution is preferred for this application, and contrast enhancement is an absolute requirement. Plexopathy from radiation fibrosis and breast cancer will both enhance, but fibrosis typically has smooth, consistent enhancement; breast cancer will often have more nodular or irregular enhancement. Both may be associated with soft-tissue masses but any such finding outside of the original radiation field or when radiation was not administered is very worrisome. PET is a very useful complement to the MRI and helps to improve both sensitivity and specificity for malignancy (Figure 61.11) [18]. Other malignancies involving the brachial plexus such as lymphoma may have more subtle findings such as mildly increased T2 signal, slightly enlarged nerves, and mild contrast enhancement.

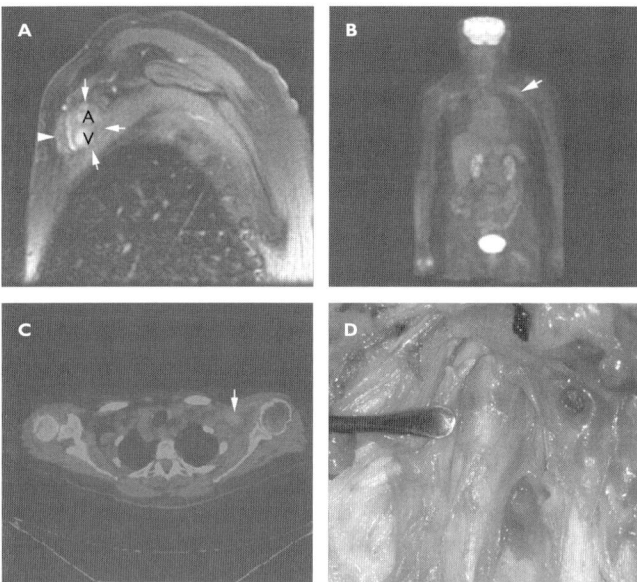

Figure 61.10 Infiltration of the brachial plexus by breast cancer. **(A)** Sagittal T1-weighted spoiled gradient recalled image with fat suppression after the administration of intravenous gadolinium shows the enhancing mass encasing the cords of the brachial plexus in the infraclavicular region (arrows). Note encasement of the axillary artery (A) and vein (V). **(B)** Coronal maximum-intensity projection from a PET scan shows avid, linear uptake in the left brachial plexus (arrow) consistent with breast cancer spread. **(C)**. Axial PET/CT fusion image shows avid uptake of tracer (arrow) in the left infraclavicular region, confirming the malignancy's hypermetabolic nature. **(D)** Exposure of the left infraclavicular brachial plexus was done. The probe points to the discolored area consistent with intraneural infiltration of the proximal portion of the lateral cord from breast cancer.

As with breast-cancer spread, these changes are best seen on high-field imaging where the inherent higher signal-to-noise ratio allows for greater spatial resolution and finer detail.

Percutaneous Biopsy

The role of image-guided biopsy is somewhat controversial. The role of biopsy is to establish a diagnosis preoperatively. While it can be performed in cases of mass lesions, it can not be done effectively in more infiltrative processes. The rationale for confirming a diagnosis in this manner is that it facilitates neoadjuvant therapy that can make operative intervention easier, safer, or achievable as well as help surgeons plan and counsel patients for surgical resection. The potential downsides of biopsy for routine use include the possibility of sampling error, neurologic complications (i.e., the development of motor or sensory abnormality and/or neuropathic pain), and operative scarring. Some have also considered the risk of seeding a malignancy along a track, though that has not been an issue at our institution. We perform image-guided percutaneous biopsies using either ultrasound or CT for guidance in patients in whom we are suspicious for malignant lesions. Prebiopsy imaging should be as complete as possible to best assess the lesion characteristics for effective sampling; that is, areas of tumor necrosis should be avoided, along with planning

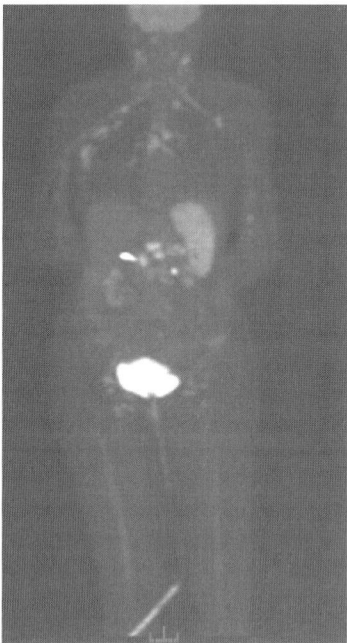

Figure 61.11 Neurolymphoma. This patient had a history of non-Hodgkin lymphoma but was thought to be in remission after treatment. The progressive neurologic deficits were thought to be due to the previous chemotherapy. Subtle MRI abnormalities were nonspecific. CSF was negative. Coronal maximum-intensity projection from an FDG PET examination shows prominent uptake in the brachial plexus and lumbosacral plexus and sciatic nerves bilaterally consistent with increased metabolism in this case of neurolymphoma. Sural biopsy confirmed the diagnosis.

an approach that will not contaminate unaffected compartments and compromise future resections.

THE DECISION ON WHOM TO OPERATE?

The decision on whom to operate is not always intuitively obvious. Masses that are symptomatic or of indeterminate nature or are concerning for malignancy (i.e., neurologic deficit, rapid increase in size, severe pain, changing imaging characteristics, especially when occurring in patients with NF-1) should be treated. In contrast, observation of small, stable lesions without associated neurologic deficit or compression on a vital structure is often appropriate. All too often, tumors fall in the gray zone, and many factors need to be considered. The management of peripheral-nerve tumors in NF patients (e.g., NF-1, NF-2, schwannomatosis) is even more complex. The diagnosis must consider the symptomatic nature and resectability of the lesion, the extent of disease, the size and growth curve of a lesion, and the age of the patient. There is a need for specific criteria for resection of asymptomatic lesions. Preoperative prediction of histology (conventional or plexiform neurofibroma or schwannoma and MPNST) is helpful in formulating a management strategy and gauging operative risks of resection or debulking. Whereas medical trials and protocols are being pursued by patients and investigators and will likely play an increasing role in the future, surgery at the current time remains the mainstay for definitive treatment.

Some groups are advocating radiosurgery for foraminal or paraspinal masses as a means of controlling disease; more data are necessary to support this treatment option.

Advantages of resection must be weighed against potential disadvantages. Advantages include obtaining definitive histology, resecting a mass rather than having to follow it serially, improving symptoms, ease of resection when the mass is smaller (compared to when it becomes larger), tendency of masses to grow with age (e.g., the increasing age in our society), the fact that larger masses are more likely to have more symptoms and signs, and also the earlier resection of a potentially unfavorable lesion. The major disadvantages include an operative procedure and its inherent risks, most notably, an impending neurologic deficit due the resection. This fact is particularly magnified when the patient was asymptomatic and the mass was stable and small.

Preoperative planning must take into account several factors: whether to biopsy, how to approach the procedure, the role of monitoring, and the potential for nerve grafting, and so on. Surgeons must fairly judge the ease of resection and the type of resection, especially in terms of the perceived pathology. Patients should be counseled regarding the risks/benefits of resection as well as the donor-site morbidity if nerve grafting is considered. Patients should be informed about the rare possibility of concomitant nerve reconstruction and the potential for secondary reconstruction (e.g., with tendon transfers, etc.) to augment function at a later date, if necessary. Patients and surgeons must have fair expectations about the intended resection. Still, even despite a thorough preoperative evaluation, occasionally unforeseen anatomic relationships or unfavorable pathologies are encountered that alter previous considerations.

OPERATIVE EVALUATION

Surgical Approach

Different operative approaches may be utilized for exposure. Standard anterior approaches include supraclavicular, infraclavicular, and/or axillary exposures. Other approaches may include a posterior subscapular [19], thoracotomy, laminectomy, and sternotomy. Often mobilization and retraction of the clavicle can provide adequate exposure. However, in select cases, especially for tumors in the retroclavicular space affecting divisions, a transclavicular approach may be helpful. The posterior subscapular approach may be useful for exposure of proximal or lower plexal elements or when extensive scarring is presented related to previous anterior surgery or radiation; it allows intra- and extraforaminal resection of benign tumors or wider resection for malignancy (i.e., where amputation would not have been effective) [19]. Often a single approach can be used. Other times more than one approach may be desirous, depending on the location and type of the tumor, surgeon's preference and familiarity. For example, combinations of procedures or staged procedures may be desirable when resecting dumbbell tumors.

Surgical Principles

Knowledge of anatomy, approaches, and principles is necessary [20]. Good lighting and immaculate hemostasis is critical. Tissues should be handled gently. Nerve stimulators may help confirm the anatomy, especially when the field is distorted. Proximal and distal control, when feasible, should be obtained. Neighboring nerves should be identified, mobilized, and protected. Neighboring vessels should also be anticipated and controlled. The main parent nerve should be preserved wherever possible. For benign nerve sheath tumors, resection at a fascicular level should be undertaken. For benign compressive lesions, the nerve(s) can often be preserved with careful dissection. For atypical lesions, we favor preoperative, percutaneous, or occasionally incisional biopsy. If a malignant lesion is diagnosed definitively, wide resection with negative margins is attempted. Prior to tumor resection, mapping of fascicles involved in a tumor is necessary and is aided by intraoperative stimulation and recording. During the tumor resection, the use of intraoperative electrophysiology is helpful whether to hear discharges during mobilization of the tumor or to map functioning (or nonfunctioning) fascicles during tumor resection [21–25]. Although operative loupes provide excellent magnification, the intraoperative microscope may be indicated in certain situations. In some cases, tumor can be removed in toto, other times in a piecemeal fashion. An ultrasonic surgical aspirator may be helpful for fibrotic tumors.

There is no substitute for experience, familiarity, and good judgment. These attributes can often, but not always, help avoid complications [21], such as those leading to neurologic, vascular, or pleural injury, chyle accumulation, nonunion, or mistreatment, which depends on the action taken on the basis of interpretation of incorrect frozen-section diagnosis.

Pathology

Routine microscopy is sometimes supplemented by special immunostains, electron microscopy, and cytogenetic analysis. Frozen-section interpretation is often helpful but not definitive. We wait for permanent sections interpreted by an experienced neuropathologist.

Large series by Dr. Kline's group [22,23,26,27] have carefully catalogued the variety of benign and malignant pathologies in the brachial plexus and their outcomes with tumors in this location compared to other sites. Others have made similar observations [26,28–31].

POSTOPERATIVE EVALUATION

Careful neurological examination is performed after operation to document function. We evaluate patients with benign lesions in whom complete resections were performed at 3 months and at 12 months postoperatively. In this group of patients we routinely obtain a postoperative MRI at 1 year. This serves as a baseline study. These patients are instructed to perform self-examinations and to return on a prn basis. In cases of a subtotal resection or after the first operation of a staged procedure, MRIs are obtained within a few days postoperatively. Patients with known residual tumor are followed closely for recurrence; patients who had large tumors or cellular schwannomas may be at increased risk of recurrence and should be followed closely.

Patients with malignant lesions benefit from a multidisciplinary approach. They frequently receive adjuvant radiation, chemo- or hormonal therapy. They are followed every 3 months after surgery.

MANAGEMENT OF SELECTED LESIONS AFFECTING THE BRACHIAL PLEXUS

Benign Peripheral Nerve Sheath Tumors

In general, the most common lesions include schwannomas and neurofibromas. These lesions may be solitary or be part of the spectrum of NF (NF-1, NF-2, schwannomatosis). They may be conventional or plexiform (schwannomas, neurofibromas), or solitary or multiple; sometimes they may occur segmentally in one portion of the body. In our experience, the most common solitary lesions are schwannomas. Both schwannomas and neurofibromas are either asymptomatic or mildly symptomatic with paresthesias. Neurologic assessment including EMG is generally normal.

These lesions can be resected safely in the majority of cases, when they are treated by experienced surgeons (Figure 61.12). The fact that these lesions can be resected while preserving the parent-nerve integrity is a relatively new development that was pioneered by David Kline [22,23,27]. Interfascicular dissection allows preservation of uninvolved fascicles. Identification of the proximal and distal poles of the tumor is an important step in resecting the tumor. Schwannomas can often be traced to a single entering/exiting fascicle and neurofibromas to several fascicles. This is not always the situation in larger tumors which may involve the majority of fascicles. Intraoperative recordings may help assess the functionality of the involved fascicles and guide safe resection of the tumor. Preservation of function can be achieved in approximately 80% of patients. In addition, pain is often eliminated or improved upon. Less favorable results may be seen in patients with larger tumors or in those whose lesions were previously biopsied or operated. Complete resection is often possible for tumors with conventional histologies. As combinations of conventional and plexiform lesions may occur, care should be taken in attempting complete resection when unfavorable findings, which may not have been anticipated on imaging preoperatively, are determined intraoperatively [13,14].

Syndromes (NF-1, NF-2, Segmental Forms of NF, Schwannomatosis)

The diagnostic criteria and clinical features for NF-1 and NF-2 are well known. Schwannomatosis, a more recently described entity, is becoming increasingly recognized and appears to be about as prevalent as NF-2. Its criteria are listed in Table 61.1 [32]. Like NF-2, schwannomatosis has conventional and plexiform schwannomas. Schwannomatosis results in peripheral, spinal, and intracranial schwannomas but differs from NF-2 in the absence of vestibular-nerve tumors [33]; in contrast, NF-1 frequently has conventional and plexiform neurofibromas affecting peripheral nerves. Like NF-2, the genetic locus of schwannomatosis is also on chromosome 22, but to a non-NF-2 gene. The majority of patients with schwannomatosis are sporadic. Rare familial forms of schwannomatosis have been described, with some recent evidence demonstrating that INI1, a tumor-suppressor gene, plays a role in the oncogenic mechanism in some familial cases [34]. Clinical testing for INI1 as well as NF-1 and NF-2 are commercially available.

The management of these syndromes is challenging and must be individualized [35]. In general, surgery is indicated for symptomatic lesions. More controversial is the role of surgery for asymptomatic lesions, especially those reaching several centimeters in size or those occurring in particular locations (i.e., areas of potential compression). On the whole outcomes for resection of conventional schwannomas in patients with NF-2 and schwannomatosis are more favorable than after resection of conventional neurofibromas in patients with NF-1. Plexiform lesions occurring in the brachial plexus should be considered cautiously in all cases. Though occasionally they may be debulked, often time, more extensive resection would certainly result in profound neurologic deficit. The management of patients with NF-1 is further complicated by the need to consider the potential for malignant transformation.

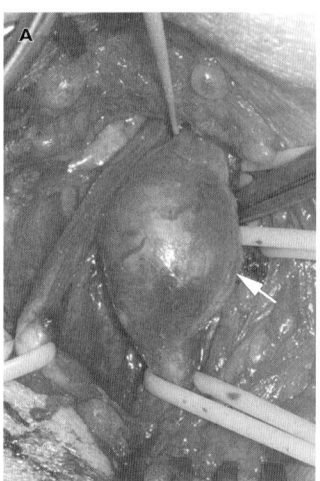 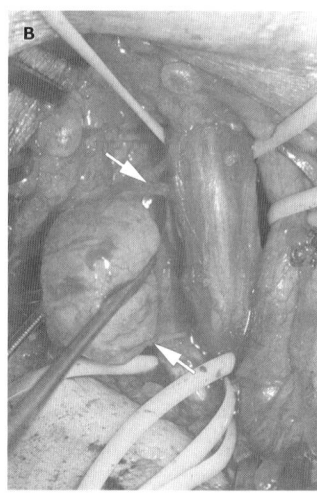

Figure 61.12 Median nerve schwannoma in axilla. (A) The nerve sheath tumor is located eccentrically within the nerve displacing its fascicles (arrow). Proximal and distal control of the median nerve (in vasoloops) facilitates the tumor resection. The medial antebrachial nerve is protected (in left vasoloop). (B). The entering and exiting fascicles (arrows) are shown. The brachial vein was protected.

Table 61.1 Criteria for Schwannomatosis

Definite schwannomatosis
    Two or more pathologically proven schwannomas, and
    Lack of radiographic evidence of vestibular nerve tumor at >18 years
Presumptive or probable schwannomatosis
    Two or more pathologically proven schwannomas, without symptoms of cranial nerve VIII dysfunction >30 years of age
    Two or more pathologically proven in an anatomically limited distribution (single limb or segment of the spine) without symptoms of cranial nerve VIII dysfunction at any age

From MacCollin et al [32].

Rapidly enlarging masses, especially those associated with pain, neurologic deficit, and/or changing imaging features should raise concerns for malignant transformation. This occurs in approximately 5% to 10% of patients with NF-1 and is more common in patients with larger, deeper lesions. Surveillance of patients with NF-1 is important. A large number of medical treatments are being investigated on protocol basis.

Hyperplastic Lesions

The most common hyperplastic lesions affecting the brachial plexus are intraneural perineuriomas and focal forms of CIPD. Though relatively rare, these lesions may affect the brachial plexus, leading to progressive neurologic deficits. The distinction of perineurioma from CIDP may be clinically difficult [3,16] but is critical to make. Although new patterns of MRI are emerging that distinguish these entities, careful histologic review of fascicular biopsy may be needed for definitive diagnosis. Nerve grafting has been reported in focal forms of intraneural perineuriomas [36]. In our experience, most of these present with longstanding lesions and lengthy lesions that would make this unrealistic; other forms of soft-tissue or bony reconstruction and reassurance can be offered. The nature of perineuriomas remains controversial, though some have recently demonstrated clonal expansion of intraneural and soft-tissue perineuriomas [37,38]. Patients with CIDP and other inflammatory conditions may respond to trials of intravenous steroids, immunoglobulins, or plasmapheresis.

Benign Lesions of Nonneural Sheath Origin

Intraneural Lesions

Intraneural ganglia

These non–neoplastic lesions consist of mucin within the epineurium of nerves. Over the past few years, they have been shown to be derived from a synovial joint via an articular branch that provides the neural pathway for propagation to extend into the parent nerve. Previously they were postulated to form de novo [15,39]. Cases of suprascapular intraneural ganglia have been reported derived from the glenohumeral joint. These lesions appear tubular as they are constrained by the nerve. Similar to the more common extraneural paralabral cysts they have been associated with labral tears (Figure 61.6). The joint-related origin of the intraneural cysts is important (Figure 61.7); if it is not recognized and treated, cyst persistence and the potential for recurrence exists.

Lipomatous Lesions of Nerve

Fatty tumors of nerve comprise a spectrum of pathologies ranging from fibrolipomatous hamartoma, a lesion of fat within nerve, to lipoma extrinsic to nerve compressing it. Fibrolipomatous hamartomas typically affect the median and digital nerves in the hand/palm region; in these cases, decompression of the carpal tunnel alone is typically performed in symptomatic adults. Rare cases of fibrolipomatous hamartomas may affect the brachial plexus [40]. The MRI appearance of this lesion is characteristic [41], even when it occurs in unusual sites, making biopsy unnecessary. Because of its rarity in proximal locations, the role of surgical debulking is unknown. Intraneural lipomas are adipose masses within nerve. They have a typical MRI appearance and can often be resected safely. Though rare, they are often found in the median nerve at the level of the wrist.

Extraneural Lesions

Benign lesions tend to displace nerves and may compress them. Such masses include soft-tissue lesions such as ganglia or lipomas, as well as bony masses (which may also result in nerve compression by edema [42]). Identification, protection, and preservation of neighboring nerves should be accomplished prior to tumor resection. Encapsulated benign masses seldom recur after resection. This is in contrast to interdigitating masses such as arborizing lipomas or desmoids, and the latter are well known to recur.

Desmoid Tumors

Desmoid tumors can involve the chest wall, axillary, infraclavicular, or supraclavicular areas. Though histologically benign and often slow-growing, they can act aggressively, encasing, or infiltrating the brachial plexus along its course. Distinction from fibrosarcomas is important. Desmoids do not transform into malignant lesions or metastasize. Currently their treatment is controversial. Because of the relationships of the mass to important neurovascular structures, attempts at gross total resection are often unsuccessful, especially with negative margins. Wide resection is typically impractical. Local recurrence rates are high. Radiation as well as hormonal and systemic cytotoxic chemotherapy is often attempted for local control, with or without surgical resection. There has been high morbidity associated with surgery. Pain and neurologic function not infrequently worsen after surgical intervention. When wide resection is not feasible, function-sparing resection is a viable option in combination with additional adjuvant therapy. The cost-benefit ratio must balance appropriateness and extent of surgical intervention [43–45]. Targeted therapeutics will likely play a role in determining who will benefit from trials with adjuvant therapies.

Malignant Peripheral Nerve Sheath Tumors

MPNSTs may be related to NF-1, radiation, or spontaneous onset. They usually present with increasing pain, tumor size, or decreasing function in relatively rapid fashion. Tumors typically are firm and fixed. Diagnosis may be difficult, especially in patients with NF. Physicians and surgeons must have a high index of suspicion on the basis of clinical and physical examination, as imaging is often inconclusive at differentiating benign from malignant lesions. All pathologic specimens should be interpreted by experienced neuropathologists. Care must be especially taken when interpreting limited biopsies either done percutaneously or with open biopsy. We make decisions after

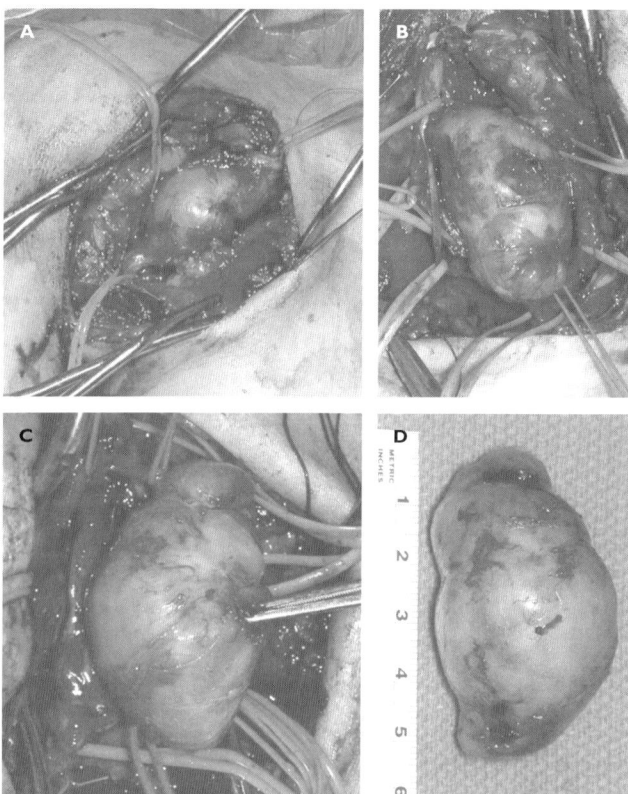

Figure 61.13 MPNST of the right lateral cord (MRIs in Figure 61.9). **(A)**. Proximal and distal control of the mass was obtained. **(B)** Branches were preserved in vasoloops. **(C)** Dissection at the poles of the tumor allowed identification of a single entering/exiting fascicular group. **(D)** Tumor was resected with negative margins obtained several centimeters proximally and distally at a fascicular level. Final pathology was consistent with an MPNST. He refused wide resection (nerve sacrificing) or amputation. He underwent radiation and chemotherapy postoperatively and has done well at 5-year follow-up.

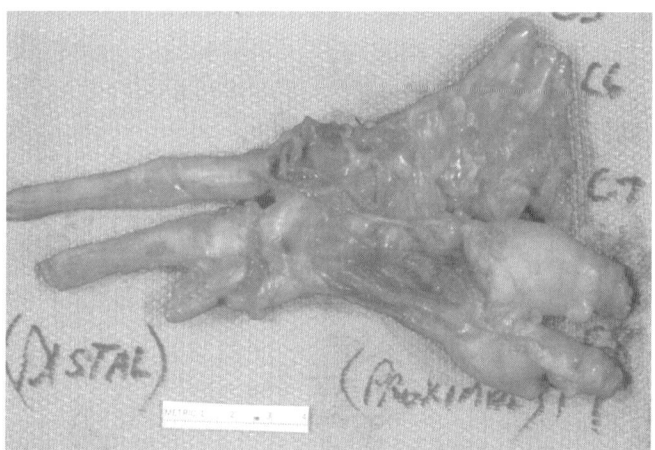

Figure 61.14 MPNST. Nerve sacrificing procedure.

permanent sections have been reviewed. For example, certain tumors such as cellular schwannomas can have a high mitotic index and can appear malignant at frozen section. Metastases should be sought prior to aggressive surgical treatment and work-up should include chest x-ray, CT chest/abdomen/pelvis, PET scan, and sometimes, bone scan.

There is no consensus as to the optimal treatment, though negative margins have been identified as being a good prognostic factor. Surgery may consist of subtotal resection, wide or en bloc resection, or amputation. Treatment must be individualized: depending on size and location of the mass, presence of metastases, patient's wishes, surgeon's preference, and so on. Although achieving a wide resection is the goal whenever possible, because of anatomic constraints, it is often not possible without causing neurovascular injury (Figures 61.13 and 61.14). Limb-sparing surgery is preferable to amputation/disarticulation; the latter being performed less now than several decades ago, but it is still done, particularly in cases with extensive or recurrent tumor, or when limb function is severely compromised. Frequently a mulitdisciplinary approach is utilized to assure complete resection. The resection of major nerves does not prevent limb salvage. Attempts at nerve grafting must be done realistically. Because of the long distances necessary for reinnervation, prolonged time for regeneration in patients often with limited survival, and the use of radiation, nerve grafting is frequently not indicated. Distal nerve transfers might be an option in select cases to expedite recovery and could be done away from irradiated operative fields. Poor prognostic factors have been associated with tumor size > 5 cm, high tumor grade, positive margins, proximal lesions where surgical margins are more difficult to achieve. Secondary tendon transfers or other reconstructive procedures could be considered to augment function.

Neoadjuvant treatment is performed at our institution in the hopes of decreasing size of the tumor prior to attempts at curative surgery. Adjuvant external beam radiation or brachytherapy is recommended often time in conjunction with pre- or post-operative chemotherapy. Surgery without adjuvant therapy is associated with high local recurrence rate. Radiation has been shown to help provide local control, delay recurrence but has not been shown to prolong survival.

Outcomes are guarded. There is a high mortality and morbidity despite very aggressive measures. At our institution, a 52% 5-year survival was reported for a large series of patients with MPNSTs. Survival rates for the brachial plexus have been lower, with mean survival of 2 to 3 years. In general, long-term survival rates have been relatively low; still there are reports of long-term survival. Surgery frequently helps pain. Palliative surgery in patients with metastatic disease may improve their quality of life [46–49].

Malignant Tumors of Nonneural Sheath Origin

On occasion, malignant lesions may compress or directly infiltrate neural elements of the brachial plexus. Primary lesions may result in symptoms from compression or direct spread; metastatic lesions may result from distant spread.

A number of these tumors may affect the brachial plexus. Apical lung carcinomas most often affect the brachial plexus (particularly the lower trunk) by direct extension; head and neck or thyroid carcinomas and bony lesions may act similarly. Of malignant lesions, breast cancer is the most common; metastatic lesions may occur including lymphoma, melanoma, bladder carcinoma, and so on.

The majority of patients present with pain and neurologic loss. Typically, diagnosis is delayed. Surgery may be necessary to obtain a diagnosis and guide treatment. Treatment should be individualized. Surgery may be indicated for mass lesions. For local spread of apical lung cancers, resections done together with thoracic surgeons can improve results and treat pain [50]. For the majority of infiltrative lesions, subtotal resection can typically only be performed. In such cases, we perform a targeted fascicular biopsy [51] and provide adjuvant radiation and chemotherapy. Adjuvant treatment by itself or in combination with surgery often improves pain that is frequently troublesome [52]; on occasion, it may also improve function to some degree. Unfortunately, many patients still succumb to their primary disease.

Distinction of brachial plexopathy due to breast cancer from radiation plexitis is difficult, and recurrent tumor and radiation plexitis can coexist. Occasionally, open fascicular biopsy may be necessary to help diagnose cancer; though a positive biopsy may be helpful for establishing a treatment plan, a negative biopsy still does not eliminate the possibility of unrecognized cancer. Patchy involvement by tumor (even in affected segments of nerve) makes definitive sampling problematic on limited biopsies done in efforts to avoid further neurologic deficit. These patients should be followed closely with serial imaging studies. On average, symptoms of radiation induced brachial plexopathy appear about 10 years after radiation. The findings of painless paralysis on examination, and fasciculations and myokymia on EMG favor radiation plexopathy. In contrast, spread from breast cancer often presents with more rapid, progressive onset and in those with a mass lesion [23]. Although surgery (e.g., neurolysis or local or distant flap coverage) has been recommended by some groups to improve function or retard deterioration, in our opinion, surgery for radiation plexopathy is reserved for patients with refractory pain. Function often deteriorates after neurolysis.

CONCLUSIONS

A number of pathologies may affect the brachial plexus. Recent advances have led to improvements in identification, diagnosis, and treatment of these entities. Because of the rarity of these pathologies, management often time should be done in tertiary care facilities.

REFERENCES

1. Lwu S, Midha R. Clinical examination of brachial and pelvic plexus tumors. *Neurosurg Focus.* 2007;22(6):E5.
2. Kim P, Ebersold MJ, Onofrio BM, Quast LM. Surgery of spinal nerve schwannoma. Risk of neurological deficit after resection of involved root. *J Neurosurg.* 1989;71(6):810–814.
3. Amrami KK, Port JD. Imaging the brachial plexus. *Hand Clin.* 2005;21(1):25–37.
4. Hyodoh K, Hyodoh H, Akiba H, et al. Brachial plexus: normal anatomy and pathological conditions. *Curr Probl Diagn Radiol.* 2002;31(5):179–188.
5. Kichari JR, Hussain SM, Den Hollander JC, Krestin GP. MR imaging of the brachial plexus: current imaging sequences, normal findings, and findings in a spectrum of focal lesions with MR-pathologic correlation. *Curr Probl Diagn Radiol.* 2003;32(2):88–101.
6. Filler AG, Kliot M, Howe FA, et al. Application of magnetic resonance neurography in the evaluation of patients with peripheral nerve pathology. *J Neurosurg.* 1996;85(2):299–309.
7. Grant GA, Britz GW, Goodkin R, Jarvik JG, Maravilla K, Kliot M. The utility of magnetic resonance imaging in evaluating peripheral nerve disorders. *Muscle Nerve.* 2002;25(3):314–331.
8. Singh T, Kliot M. Imaging of peripheral nerve tumors. *Neurosurg Focus.* 2007;22(6):E6.
9. Ferner RE, Lucas JD, O'Doherty MJ, et al. Evaluation of (18)fluorodeoxyglucose positron emission tomography ((18)FDG PET) in the detection of malignant peripheral nerve sheath tumours arising from within plexiform neurofibromas in neurofibromatosis 1. *J Neurol Neurosurg Psychiatr.* 2000;68(3):353–357.
10. Solomon SB, Semih Dogan A, Nicol TL, Campbell JN, Pomper MG. Positron emission tomography in the detection and management of sarcomatous transformation in neurofibromatosis. *Clin Nucl Med.* 2001;26(6):525–528.
11. Brenner W, Friedrich RE, Gawad KA, et al. Prognostic relevance of FDG PET in patients with neurofibromatosis type-1 and malignant peripheral nerve sheath tumours. *Eur J Nucl Med Mol Imaging.* 2006;33(4):428–432.
12. Bredella MA, Torriani M, Hornicek F, et al. Value of PET in the assessment of patients with neurofibromatosis type 1. *AJR Am J Roentgenol.* 2007;189(4):928–935.
13. White JB, Scheithauer BW, Amrami KK, Babovic-Vuksanovic D, Spinner RJ. Contiguous conventional and plexiform schwannomas. Report of two cases. *J Neurosurg.* 2006;104(2):319–324.
14. Spinner RJ, Scheithauer BW, Perry A, Amrami KK, Emnett R, Gutmann DH. Colocalized cellular schwannoma and plexiform neurofibroma in the absence of neurofibromatosis. Case report. *J Neurosurg.* 2007;107(2):435–439.
15. Spinner RJ, Amrami KK, Kliot M, Johnston SP, Casañas J. Suprascapular intraneural ganglia and glenohumeral joint connections. *J Neurosurg.* 2006;104(4):551–557.
16. Amrami KK, Felmlee JP, Spinner RJ. MRI of peripheral nerves. *Neurosurg Clin N Am.* 2008;19(4):559–72, vi.
17. Lingawi SS, Bilbey JH, Munk PL, et al. MR imaging of brachial plexopathy in breast cancer patients without palpable recurrence. *Skeletal Radiol.* 1999;28(6):318–323.
18. Lin M, Kilanowska J, Taper J, Chu J. Neurolymphomatosis—diagnosis and assessment of treatment response by FDG PET-CT. *Hematol Oncol.* 2008;26(1):43–45.
19. Dubuisson AS, Kline DG, Weinshel SS. Posterior subscapular approach to the brachial plexus. Report of 102 patients. *J Neurosurg.* 1993;79(3):319–330.
20. Tiel R, Kline D. Peripheral nerve tumors: surgical principles, approaches, and techniques. *Neurosurg Clin N Am.* 2004;15(2):167–175, vi.
21. Spinner RJ. Complication avoidance. *Neurosurg Clin N Am.* 2004;15(2):193–202, vii.
22. Ganju A, Roosen N, Kline DG, Tiel RL. Outcomes in a consecutive series of 111 surgically treated plexal tumors: a review of the experience at the Louisiana State University Health Sciences Center. *J Neurosurg.* 2001;95(1):51–60.
23. Kim DH, Midha R, Murovic J, Spinner RJ. *Kline and Hudson's Nerve Injuries: Operative Outcomes for Injuries, Entrapments, and Tumors.* Philadelphia: Elsevier; 2008.
24. Russell SM. Preserve the nerve: microsurgical resection of peripheral nerve sheath tumors. *Neurosurgery.* 2007;61(3 suppl):113–117; discussion 117.
25. Kwok K, Davis B, Kliot M. Resection of a benign brachial plexus nerve sheath tumor using intraoperative electrophysiological monitoring. *Neurosurgery.* 2007;60(4 suppl 2):316–320; discussion 320.
26. Huang JH, Zaghloul K, Zager EL. Surgical management of brachial plexus region tumors. *Surg Neurol.* 2004;61(4):372–378.
27. Das S, Ganju A, Tiel RL, Kline DG. Tumors of the brachial plexus. *Neurosurg Focus.* 2007;22(6):E26.
28. Knight DM, Birch R, Pringle J. Benign solitary schwannomas: a review of 234 cases. *J Bone Joint Surg Br.* 2007;89(3):382–387.

29. Gosk J, Rutowski R, Zimmer K, Rabczynski J. Brachial plexus tumours—own experience in diagnostics and surgical treatment. *Folia Neuropathol.* 2004;42(3):171–175.
30. Binder DK, Smith JS, Barbaro NM. Primary brachial plexus tumors: imaging, surgical, and pathological findings in 25 patients. *Neurosurg Focus.* 2004;16(5):E11.
31. Birch R, Bonney G, Wynn Parry CB. *Surgical Disorders of the Peripheral Nerves.* Edinburgh: Churchill Livingstone; 1998.
32. MacCollin M, Chiocca EA, Evans DG, et al. Diagnostic criteria for schwannomatosis. *Neurology.* 2005;64(11):1838–1845.
33. Westhout FD, Mathews M, Paré LS, Armstrong WB, Tully P, Linskey ME. Recognizing schwannomatosis and distinguishing it from neurofibromatosis type 1 or 2. *J Spinal Disord Tech.* 2007;20(4):329–332.
34. Hulsebos TJ, Plomp AS, Wolterman RA, Robanus-Maandag EC, Baas F, Wesseling P. Germline mutation of INI1/SMARCB1 in familial schwannomatosis. *Am J Hum Genet.* 2007;80(4):805–810.
35. Huang JH, Simon SL, Nagpal S, Nelson PT, Zager EL. Management of patients with schwannomatosis: report of six cases and review of the literature. *Surg Neurol.* 2004;62(4):353–361; discussion 361.
36. Gruen JP, Mitchell W, Kline DG. Resection and graft repair for localized hypertrophic neuropathy. *Neurosurgery.* 1998;43(1):78–83.
37. Emory TS, Scheithauer BW, Hirose T, Wood M, Onofrio BM, Jenkins RB. Intraneural perineurioma. A clonal neoplasm associated with abnormalities of chromosome 22. *Am J Clin Pathol.* 1995;103(6):696–704.
38. Giannini C, Scheithauer BW, Jenkins RB, et al. Soft-tissue perineurioma. Evidence for an abnormality of chromosome 22, criteria for diagnosis, and review of the literature. *Am J Surg Pathol.* 1997;21(2):164–173.
39. Spinner RJ, Amrami KK. Intraneural ganglion of the suprascapular nerve: Case report. *J Hand Surg Am.* 2006;31(10):1698–1699.
40. Golan JD, Jacques L. Nonneoplastic peripheral nerve tumors. *Neurosurg Clin N Am.* 2004;15(2):223–230.
41. Marom EM, Helms CA. Fibrolipomatous hamartoma: pathognomonic on MR imaging. *Skeletal Radiol.* 1999;28(5):260–264.
42. Angius D, Shaughnessy WJ, Amrami KK, Matsumoto JM, Spinner RJ. Infraclavicular brachial plexopathy secondary to coracoid osteoid osteoma. *J Surg Orthop Adv.* 2007;16(4):199–203.
43. Lillehei KO. Desmoid-type fibromatosis involving the brachial plexus: treatment options and assessment of c-KIT mutation. *J Neurosurg.* 2006;104:749–756.
44. Dafford K, Kim D, Nelson A, Kline D. Extraabdominal desmoid tumors. *Neurosurg Focus.* 2007;22(6):E21.
45. Seinfeld J, Kleinschmidt-DeMasters BK, Tayal S, Lillehei KO. Desmoid-type fibromatosis involving the brachial plexus. *Neurosurg Focus.* 2007;22(6):E22.
46. Wong WW, Hirose T, Scheithauer BW, Schild SE, Gunderson LL. Malignant peripheral nerve sheath tumor: analysis of treatment outcome. *Int J Radiat Oncol Biol Phys.* 1998;42(2):351–360.
47. Perrin RG, Guha A. Malignant peripheral nerve sheath tumors. *Neurosurg Clin N Am.* 2004;15(2):203–216.
48. Fuchs B, Spinner RJ, Rock MG. Malignant peripheral nerve sheath tumors: an update. *J Surg Orthop Adv.* 2005;14(4):168–174.
49. Gachiani J, Kim D, Nelson A, Kline D. Surgical management of malignant peripheral nerve sheath tumors. *Neurosurg Focus.* 2007;22(6):E13.
50. Davis GA, Knight S. Pancoast tumor resection with preservation of brachial plexus and hand function. *Neurosurg Focus.* 2007;22(6):E15.
51. Dyck PJB, Spinner RJ, Amrami KK, Klein CJ, Engelstad J, Dyck PJ. Targeted fascicular biopsy of proximal nerves with MRI abnormality usually diagnostically informative. *Neuromuscul Disord.* 2006;16(suppl 1):S97–98.
52. Gachiani J, Kim DH, Nelson A, Kline D. Management of metastatic tumors invading the peripheral nervous system. *Neurosurg Focus.* 2007;22(6):E14.

PART V: MEDICAL ONCOLOGY

62 General Principles

Karine Michaud

INTRODUCTION

This section focuses on the medical therapy of brain tumors and includes the use of antitumor agents as well as adjunctive agents in the management of patients. Historically, chemotherapeutic agents have been the mainstay of medical therapy; however, the increased knowledge of gliomagenesis has provided rational targets for treatment that are specific to the molecular and cytogenetic aberrations seen in tumors. In the following 11 chapters on Medical Oncology, we first review some general principles of medical therapy pertinent to brain tumors and subsequently emphasize disease-specific treatments.

GENERAL PRINCIPLES OF THERAPY

Blood-Brain Barrier

The existence of the blood-brain barrier (BBB) was first discovered by Paul Ehrlich (1854–1915), a German immunologist, more than 100 years ago when he found that intravenous dyes failed to stain certain regions of the brain and spinal cord [1]. At that time, he thought that the brain had a lesser affinity for the stains. His student Edwin Goldman showed in 1913 that if the dye was injected directly into the cerebrospinal fluid (CSF) the brain would become dyed, but the rest of the body would not. It then became clear that there was a barrier preventing compounds from easily traversing into the brain parenchyma. The actual concept of the BBB (then called the hematoencephalic barrier) was proposed by Lina Stern in 1921 [2]. But it is not until 1967 that Thomas Reese and Morris Karnofsky showed by electron microscopy that the endothelial cells (EC) of the brain capillaries and more precisely, the tight junctions (TJ) between those cells, were the anatomical basis of the BBB [3].

Neuronal network function is exquisitely sensitive to, and dependent on, specific neurotransmitter concentrations within the extracellular space. In addition, the CNS lacks lymphatic drainage, so passage of molecules or ions from the systemic circulation across the capillary wall would result in a net gain of water, possibly leading to an increase in intracranial pressure. The complex structure and function of the BBB act to protect the brain from toxic substances and help to control the neuronal environment by regulating the movement of biologically important molecules. Also, the BBB controls the homeostasis of the CSF that has a constant molecular and ionic composition that is different from the plasma. A BBB is present in 99% of the brain capillaries. Some areas of the brain called the circumventricular organs lack the BBB: These include the choroid plexus, median eminence, neurohypophysis, organum vasculosum of the lamina terminalis, pineal gland, subfornical organ, subcommissural organ, and area postrema. These organs need chemical or ionic exposure to systemic plasma composition to exert their function.

Anatomy and Physiology of the BBB

EC form the walls of the capillaries, the network of microvessels between the arterial and venous system. The capillaries in the human brain have an estimated total length of 650 km and a total surface area of 12 m². The differences between peripheral and brain endothelium are low pinocytic activity reflecting low level of transcellular transport, lack of fenestration, and high densities of mitochondria in the cytosol [4]. In the rest of the body, EC are connected by gap junctions, intercellular connexin hexamere channels that allow free passage of ions and small molecules from cell to cell. In the brain, EC are connected via TJ and adherens junctions (AJ) limiting paracellular diffusion. They make up an estimated 95% of the total surface area of the BBB [5].

AJ are cadherin dimer transmembrane-domain proteins belonging to a superfamily of cell-adhesion molecules [6]. E-cadherin mediates calcium-dependent cell adhesion by binding to actin via α- and β-catenin accessory proteins [7]. AJs are located near the basolateral side of the EC.

TJ seal EC just beneath apical surface and prevent paracellular passage of ions and molecules. A number of TJ proteins have been identified: claudins, occludins, and zonula occludens proteins—ZO-1, ZO-2, ZO-3. They are formed by different adhesive molecules that are linked inside the cell to cytoskeletal signaling proteins. Phosphorylation of the different cell-cell contact proteins is correlated to junctional complexity and transendothelial electrical resistance and is one of the known mechanisms of opening and closing of the TJ via rapid and reversible change in their architecture [8]. Cell-cell junctions are also regulated by constitutive factors induced by the neural microenvironment, particularly by factors released from astroglial cells [9].

Although EC are the main component of the BBB, other elements are important as well, such as glial endfeet, perivascular pericytes, and microglia. Astrocytes are involved in the embryologic development of the BBB as shown by isolated EC growing in vitro without the characteristics of the BBB. Astrocytes and their processes encompass more than 90% of endothelial capillaries and their endfeet are projected tightly around EC and serve to mediate communication between neurons and capillaries, particularly to mop excess potassium from the brain into the blood [10]. Pericytes are contractile cells that surround the brain capillaries and play a role in controlling growth of EC and influence capillary integrity by phagocytosis of compounds that have crossed the endothelial barrier [11].

Because of the TJ between the cells, molecules that need to cross the BBB must do so by transmembrane diffusion or via protein transporters. For transmembrane diffusion, the physical properties of the molecule is of paramount importance: lipid solubility, low molecular weight (less then 180 Da), and charge. Examples of transporters through the EC are GLUT-1 and GLUT-3 for glucose, and specific transporters for amino acids, neurotransmitters, and ions. Of importance in neuro-oncology is P-glycoprotein that is a transmembrane 170 kDa glycoprotein belonging to the superfamily of ATP-dependent efflux transport proteins. It is present at high concentration at the apical membrane of brain EC and is important in drug resistance. Multidrug resistance is another drug efflux transport system that prevents the accumulation of certain drugs in the CNS [12].

Pathology of the BBB in Brain Tumors

The capillary endothelium in brain tumors is abnormal and lacks BBB features. It highly expresses fenestrations, vesicular transport, gap junctions, and fragmented basal lamina. The combination of the above findings results in a highly increased permeability of the tumor vascular bed. This, in addition to the lack of lymphatics predispose the brain to development of cerebral edema. There are four ways for the tumor to disrupt the BBB: secretion of inducing agents that change the vessel phenotype, alteration of the extracellular milieu via their metabolism so that vessels change secondarily, physical impedance of factors needed by the capillaries to express their BBB features [13], and finally, stimulation of the proliferation of abnormal vessels by releasing angiogenic factors like vascular endothelial growth factor (VEGF). This regional breakdown in the BBB can be assessed by contrast imaging showing enhancement on CT or magnetic resonance imaging (MRI). The BBB breakdown is not limited to the margins of the tumor and is responsible for peritumoral vasogenic edema by extravasation of plasma proteins. The volume of peritumoral vasogenic edema depends on the rate of edema formation and the rate of reabsorption of extravasated fluid that is dependent on bulk flow, astrocytic cells, and capillaries. Tumor edema propagates by bulk flow rather than by simple diffusion. Thus, the pressure gradient between gray and white matter is sufficient to deviate the propagation of edema in the white matter that has a lesser resistance, resulting in the finger-like projections seen on imaging [14].

TREATMENT OF TUMORAL VASOGENIC EDEMA

Because patients' symptoms can be attributed to peritumoral edema, as well as the tumor itself, vasogenic edema treatment can have a dramatic effect on the patients' clinical status. Corticosteroids have been part of brain-tumor treatment since the 1960s and have significantly improved perioperative morbidity and mortality [15]. For acute management of high intracranial pressure, osmotherapy via hyperosmolar solutions is used.

Corticosteroids

The preferred compound is dexamethasone due to its low mineralocorticoid effect. The exact mechanism of steroids' action against vasogenic edema is still unclear. It is generally accepted that steroids decrease edema by limiting the permeability of the tumor capillaries to macromolecules. VEGF expression has been shown to be inhibited by dexamethasone in cultured glioma cells [16]. Although very effective, steroids are usually used for short term due to the long-term side effects [17].

Side effects of corticosteroids are summarized in Table 62.1. The importance of slow tapering of dexamethasone needs to be emphasized. Too rapid tapering could result in recurrence of cerebral edema and neurologic symptoms, depression, anorexia, muscle aches, and joint pains. Symptoms of adrenal insufficiency from suppression of hypothalamic-pituitary-adrenal axis can also occur. Consequently, long-term use of corticosteroids should be avoided if possible (Table 62.1).

To avoid potential adverse effects from steroid use, several antiinflammatory agents have been used.

Xerecept

XERECEPT® (corticorelin acetate injection) is a synthetic preparation of the natural human peptide corticotropin-releasing factor (CRF). Human CRF has significant anti-edema properties with potentially fewer side effects. It is currently in a phase III placebo-controlled, randomized clinical trial conducted at more than 20 sites in the United States and Canada and will include approximately 200 patients with peritumoral brain edema who require chronic treatment with steroids (dexamethasone). The primary endpoint of the study will be a 50% reduction in steroid use at the end of the 3-week treatment period.

Boswellic Acid

Boswellic acid is found in the resin of the plant *Boswellia serrate* and is well-known for its antiinflammatory effect. It is commonly used in treatment of Crohn disease, ulcerative colitis, bronchial asthma, endotoxin-induced hepatitis, and arthritis [18–21]. It is a selective

Table 62.1 Summary of Side Effects of Corticosteroids

System	Potential Side Effects
Cardiovascular and renal	- Hypertension
	- Sodium and water retention
	- Hypokalemic acidosis
CNS	- Progressive multifocal leukoencephalitis
	- Mental agitation/psychosis
	- Spinal-cord compression from spinal epidural lipomatosis
	- Pseudotumor cerebri
Endocrine	- Growth suppression in children
	- Secondary amenorrhea
	- Suppression hypothalamic-pituitary-adrenal axis
	- Cushingoid features (obesity, moon facies, buffalo hump, hirsutism)
GI	- Gastritis/steroid ulcers
	- Pancreatitis
	- Intestinal or sigmoid diverticular perforation
Cutaneous	By inhibition of fibroblasts
	- Impaired wound healing or wound breakdown
	- Subcutaneous tissue atrophy
Metabolic	- Glucose intolerance
	- Hyperosmolar nonketotic coma
	- Hyperlipidemia
Ophtalmologic	- Posterior subcapsular cataracts
	- Glaucoma
Musculoskeletal	- Avascular necrosis (prolonged administration)
	- Osteoporosis
	- Steroid myopathy
Infectious	- Immunosuppression
	- Possible reactivation of TB, chickenpox
Hematologic	- Hypercoagulopathy from inhibition of tissue plasminogen activator
	- Demargination of white blood cells
Miscellaneous	- Hiccups
	- Fetal adrenal hypoplasia

inhibitor of the 5-LOX,28 inhibiting the production of leukotrienes (such as LTB4), which are known to stimulate brain-tumor growth and increase brain edema [22]. In a study, patients with malignant glioma were given high-dose boswellic acid prior to craniotomy for tumor recurrence and were prohibited corticosteroids. After 7 days, boswellia achieved a mean 30% reduction in peritumoral edema, with marked improvement in clinical symptoms [23]. This study reports the effective dose of boswellic acid to be in the range of 1800 to 3200 mg/d. Two additional human studies have confirmed the anti-inflammatory effects of boswellia in brain-tumor patients [24,25]. Boswellia supplements have also been shown to be safe and effective in treating brain edema associated with radiation therapy, chemotherapy, and/or leukoencephalopathy [24].

Osmotherapy

Hyperosmolar solutions used for acute treatment of cerebral edema include mannitol, glycerol, and urea. The mechanism of action is the creation of an osmotic gradient between brain and blood, reducing extravasated fluid and intracranial pressure. Although very effective, the effect is temporary because an equilibrium is reached within a few hours. Also, there might be a rebound effect as solutes that have moved into the edematous tissue act to pull back water in the normal brain. Therefore, it should be used only as a temporary measure in critical situations (e.g., before surgical debulking).

Diuretics

Diuretic agents such as furosemide cause systemic dehydration but does not act on the existing pathologic process of edema formation. Therefore, it is ineffective as a single agent or as a long-term treatment of tumor-associated edema. It is typically used in combination with hyperosmolar agent as an acute temporizing measure.

Bevacizumab

Antiangiogenesis agents are popular in the treatment of highly vascularized tumor-like glioblastoma multiforme (GBM). Bevacizumab, a humanized monoclonal antibody against VEGF-A, in combination with irinotecan, has been shown in a phase II study to improve response rate and progression-free survival [26]. By the inhibition of VEGF, it normalizes the tumoral vasculature, restoring the blood-brain barrier and significantly decreases vasogenic edema. There is increasing evidence in the literature that bevacizumab improves quality of life (QOL) in GBM patients and also reduces the need for corticosteroids.

DELIVERY OF CHEMOTHERAPY TO THE BRAIN

Oral and intravenous accesses have been typically used for the delivery of therapeutic agents to the CNS. No one can ignore the importance of the BBB in limiting the delivery of biologically active compounds to the central nervous system (CNS). For a compound to easily reach the CNS, it must possess certain physical properties: low molecular weight, lack of ionization at physiological pH, and, more important, lipophilicity [6]. Only a small proportion of systemically administered agents will reach the CNS target via oral or intravenous administration, depending on their bioavailability. Examples of oral agents that readily cross the BBB include temozolomide, lomustine, procarbazine, and tamoxifen. Obviously easier to administer, oral therapy is complicated by different factors such as drug stability in gastric acid, absorption through gastric mucosa, inactivation by intestinal enzymes, hepatic metabolism, biliary excretion, and treatment-induced emesis [27]. Vincristine is an example of intravenous chemotherapeutic agent that does not cross readily the BBB [28]. As such, numerous drug-delivery strategies have been developed to bypass the BBB. They can be divided in four categories: manipulation of the drug to enhance delivery across the BBB, disruption of the BBB, the use of alternative routes for drug delivery [5], and overcoming drug resistance.

Drug Manipulation

For hydrophilic compounds to cross BBB without invasive routes, a way is to deliver them as lipophilic analog. Although appealing, the results in brain-tumor treatment have been deceiving. For example, lipophilic analogs of nitrosourea are less soluble in plasma and bind more readily to plasma proteins, lowering the drug concentration available in the CNS, and thereby decreasing its activity and increasing toxicity [5]. Another strategy to increase lipophilicity of a hydrophilic therapeutic agent is to surround it with a sphere of lipid in the form of a liposome. For a drug like irinotecan, the liposomal formulation has shown increased serum half-life, reduced liver concentrations, reduced side effects, and increased tumor concentration in a murine tumor model [29]. A phase 1 clinical trial is currently open in the United States. Vector/receptor-mediated delivery involves the conjugation of an active drug to a BBB receptor or transport vector to penetrate tumor cells. Gene therapy has been one area of focus, using vectors, often viruses, to insert immune-stimulating or drug susceptibility genes [30,31,32].

Osmotic Disruption of the BBB

Intracarotid injection of inert hypertonic solutions such as mannitol, arabinose, or urea has been used to disrupt the BBB. The mechanism of action is shrinkage of EC and opening of the BBB TJ for a temporary period, say a few hours, allowing delivery of macromolecules to the CNS [33]. Cellular messenger systems such as calcium influx and nitrous oxide as well as cytoskeletal changes contribute to this opening. The procedure involves general anesthesia followed by selective catheterization of the appropriate intracranial vessel and infusion of the hypertonic solution, with subsequent infusion of chemotherapeutic agent.

Animal studies suggest that this method increases drug delivery to the brain 10- to 100-fold over injection into the neck arteries without the osmotic solution [34]. Blood-brain barrier disruption has been used to treat hundreds of patients and is currently in phase I and II clinical trials at nine US institutions, as well as one in Canada and one in Israel. Osmotic reduction of the BBB seems to be effective in the treatment of primary non-AIDS CNS lymphoma [35]. Agents used include carboplatin, melphalan, and methotrexate.

Cereport RMP-7

The normal brain capillaries appear to be unaffected by vasoactive amines; however, brain tumor capillaries are sensitive, providing a potential selective opening of the BBB. The bradykinin B2 receptor agonist, lobradimil (Cereport® RMP-7), selectively increases permeability of the vasculature supplying brain tumors in both animal models and humans through bradykinin B2 receptors [36]. It has been used by intracarotid administration and shown to increase carboplatin level in a murine brain tumor model [37]. Phase I and II trials of lobradimil with carboplatin have been reported. There was minimal efficacy seen with this combination [38,39].

Intra-arterial Delivery

Intra-arterial delivery has the advantage of increasing the concentration of the drug in the CNS and minimizing the systemic exposure of the drug by reducing the dose. Selective catheterization of the appropriate intracranial vessel and direct infusion of the therapeutic agent is performed. The greatest advantage is seen in drugs where the first-pass extraction is significant (lipid-soluble drugs) and when the drug has a rapid systemic clearance [40]. Agents that have been used include carboplatin, methotrexate, melphalan, and cisplatin. Potential complications include neurologic (mainly from vascular complications), ophthalmologic, and otologic complications [41]. There is increased risk when the mass effect is significant and patients require 24-hour observation to assess potential side effects.

Intrathecal Delivery

Intrathecal or intraventricular delivery involves administration of therapeutic agents directly in the subarachnoid space either via a lumbar puncture or intraventricular catheter and reservoir system. The latter is the preferred approach because it is simpler, more convenient for the patient, and safer than repeated lumbar punctures. It also results in a more uniform distribution of the drug in the CSF space and produces the most consistent CSF levels. In up to 10% of lumbar punctures, the drug is delivered to the epidural space, even if there is CSF return after placement of the needle, and drug distribution has been shown to be better after drug delivery through a reservoir [42]. Theoretical advantages over the vascular delivery are as follows: It enables bypassing of the CSF-blood barrier, requires smaller doses, involves minimal protein binding, and decreases enzymatic activity, resulting in a longer half-life [5]. The disadvantages, however, of this form of delivery, are: slow rate of drug distribution; increase in intracranial pressure at the time of injection with limitation in volume that can be administered; the incidence of complications, including infections, hemorrhage, and neurotoxicity; and the relatively poor diffusion through brain parenchyma. The use of IT chemotherapy has not been associated with any benefit in the treatment of primary brain tumors or primary central nervous system lymphoma. Direct intermittent bolus injections of therapeutic substances within the brain through an Ommaya reservoir have failed to be effective mainly because of poor drug distribution. Intrathecal administration is still the mainstay of treatment for neoplastic meningitis. Agents used include methotrexate, cytarabine, thipenta, α-interferon, and depocyt [43]. A phase I study showed the safety and efficacy of intraventricular administration of rituximab (monoclonal CD20 antibody) in patients with recurrent CNS and intraocular lymphoma [44].

Intranasal Delivery

Intranasally delivered drugs are transported along the olfactory sensory neurons to yield significant concentrations in the CSF and olfactory bulb. The supratentorial brain is reached via the peripheral olfactory pathway, and the infratentorial brain is reached via the trigeminal pathway. This provides a practical, noninvasive, rapid, and simple method of delivery. The rich vasculature and highly permeable structure of the nasal mucosa greatly enhances drug absorption, and it avoids gastrointestinal (GI) and hepatic metabolism and reduces systemic exposure. Multiple agents are being studied for intranasal delivery: antiviral drugs, hormones, amines, vitamins, CSN depressants, stimulants, and so on [45]. Animal studies are ongoing to assess the intranasal delivery of chemotherapeutic agents.

Implantable Polymers

Surgically implanted polymers loaded with chemotherapy provide sustained delivery of the agent at the site of residual tumor. As opposed to the use of catheters with direct intratumoral injection, the polymers are not subject to clotting, and no maintenance is required. To effectively deliver drugs to the brain, several characteristics of the polymer are necessary: a biocompatible and biodegradable matrix, dependable and reproducible drug release, the ability to maintain the bioactivity of the therapeutic agent and ease of surgical handling. Gliadel wafers made of 3.8% BCNU in polyanhydride polymer were shown in a phase III clinical trial to increase the median survival from 23 to 31 weeks when compared with placebo in patients with recurrent gliomas [46–48].

Convection-Enhanced Delivery

In contrast to direct intracavitary delivery that relies on passive diffusion of drug, convection-enhanced delivery uses catheters to allow the delivery of various agents under continuous positive pressure, to evenly diffuse drug either directly into tumor or through the interstitial space of the brain around the resection cavity. The volume of distribution of the drug is influenced by a variety of factors: catheter placement, catheter shape, rate of infusion, volume of infusion, and physical properties of the injected agent (molecular weight, lipophilicity). Several agents have been tried in phase I and II trials; some of them show promising results, including transferrin-CRM107 and Cotara [49,50]. A phase III trial with Cintredekin Besudotox failed to demonstrate its superiority when compared to Gliadel wafers [51].

DRUG RESISTANCE AND SUSCEPTIBILITY

Drug resistance is frequent in brain tumors and can be either intrinsic or acquired. Multiple mechanisms have been described, the best characterized of which is P glycoprotein. As described previously, it is a transmembrane protein normally present on the luminal surface of brain capillaries EC and serves as an drug-efflux pump. It is also overexpressed on the surface on some cancer cells and contributes to multidrug resistance that is characterized by cross-resistance to several classes of chemotherapeutic agents [52]. The multidrug resistance-associated protein (MRP) is also expressed on the BBB, and MRP knockout mice are very sensitive to the neurotoxic effects of etoposide [53]. There are probably other unrecognized efflux pumps important in brain tumor resistance.

Other mechanisms of drug resistance involve the ability of tumor cells to repair deoxyribonucleic acid (DNA) damage produced by cytotoxic agents or to use a different metabolism pathway. O6-methylguanine-DNA-methyltransferase (MGMT or AGT) is a well-recognized DNA-repair protein that removes alkyl groups from the O6 position of guanine. This is a frequently methylated site by alkylating agents such as BCNU, CCNU, and Temozolomide. The epigenetic silencing of the MGMT DNA-repair gene by promoter methylation is associated with longer survival in patients with glioblastoma who receive alkylating agents and greater benefit from temozolomide [54]. In the age of targeted therapies, multiple molecular pathways have been studied and correlated to both prognosis and drug response. Epidermal growth factor receptor (EGFR) overexpression and presence of the mutated receptor EGFRvIII are bad prognosis indicators in GBM patients [55]. EGFRvIII sensitizes glioblastoma cells to EGFR kinase inhibitors, whereas PTEN loss confers resistance [56]. Some genetic markers are associated with greater sensitivity to therapeutic agents. Allelic loss of chromosome arms 1p and 19q is found in a substantial subpopulation of oligodendrogliomas, both low and high grade, and is associated with chemosensitivity and longer patient survival [57].

Mechanisms to Overcome Drug Resistance

P Glycoprotein/Multidrug-Resistance Reversal

Multiple drugs have been shown to bind to Pgp and competitively inhibit the membrane pump, thus resulting in higher intracellular concentrations and serve as modulator of multidrug resistance [58]. Examples are verapamil [59], cyclosporine [60], and cephalosporins [61]. Objective responses have been demonstrated in lymphoma [59], but Pgp modulation decreases the clearance of therapeutic agents and enhances their toxicities. In addition, the maximally tolerated dose of the Pgp modulators resulted in lower serum levels than the level needed to inhibit Pgp [62].

Inhibition of Repair Enzymes

MGMT (O(6)-methylguanine-DNA methyltransferase) or AGT (O(6)-alkylguanine-DNA transferase) is a DNA-repair protein that requires only a single turnover, so its ability to repair the methylated site on the O6 position of guanine is related to the number of MGMT molecules and the rate of protein resynthesis [63]. Its expression causes resistance to the antitumor effect of alkylating agents. Inhibition of AGT activity increased the sensitivity to nitrosourea [64]. O6-benzylguanine is a potent inactivator of AGT, acting as an alternate and specific, competitive, AGT-binding substrate, irreversibly inactivating AGT [65]. Early phase studies have combined temozolomide with O6-benzylguanine [66,67]. Protracted exposure to temozolomide leads to MGMT consumption and depletes the cell-repair mechanism that may overcome the resistance of the tumor to the chemotherapy [68]. Preclinical studies have demonstrated progressive depletion of MGMT, following prolonged exposure to temozolomide [69]. Clinical trials are currently ongoing to assess whether a more intense schedule of temozolomide will enhance its intrinsic cytotoxicity in malignant glioma.

MEASUREMENT OF EFFECTS

Assessment of response to treatment can be measured using survival time, tumor-response rate, progression-free survival, duration of objective response, and improvement of patient symptoms or QOL.

Imaging

Objective assessment of tumor response is complicated by the relative nonspecificity of MRI. This is particularly true not only with high-dose radiation therapy and brachytherapy but also with surgically implanted polymer-based chemotherapy or convection-enhanced delivery of therapeutic agents. Contrast-enhanced T1-weighted and T2-FLAIR images can be misleading in terms of tumor response or progression in the context of prior treatments and corticosteroids use. Steroids can alter the pattern of enhancement and the amount of vasogenic edema surrounding the tumor [70]. Typically in lymphoma, rapid radiographic responses with significant decrease in enhancement and mass effect can occur, following steroids administration [71]. Caution is advised in obtaining tissue diagnosis in those cases. Radionecrosis can be mistaken for tumor progression with increase in T2-FLAIR and enhancement volume. With antiangiogenesis agents such as bevacizumab, MRI responses are even more difficult to interpret, as there is change in enhancement but not in overall tumor burden. Objective criteria such as McDonald (50% volume reduction for response and 25% volume increase for progression) are useful in clinical-trial settings. However, they should be used with caution on a patient-to-patient basis because they may lead to a potential risk of discontinuing a treatment that is effective and delaying a change in a treatment that is not.

Biologic imaging such as perfusion, spectroscopy, and positron emission tomography imaging can assist with interpreting unclear anatomical changes. Perfusion can help determining the presence of neovascularization, more likely as a result of tumor progression. Spectroscopy can help differentiate between tumor versus radionecrosis on the basis of different chemical compositions of these two pathologic findings. There is, however, significant limitation in the use of spectroscopy in the location and size of the lesion to be studied. Ongoing studies are needed to validate the utility of these physiologic imaging techniques.

Clinical Evaluation

Because of the close radiographic follow-up in patients with brain tumors, it is rare that clinical decline or improvement will be the sole indicator of tumor progression or response. Nevertheless, a complete history and physical examination are important not only to evaluate neurological status but also to evaluate treatment tolerability. With the introduction of new agents that change our way of interpreting MRI (such as bevacizumab), clinical changes can be observed when subtle MRI changes, if any, are seen.

Although they are very important to assess, improvement of symptoms and QOL are rarely the primary endpoints of new therapeutic agent trials. The cognitive impairments of brain tumor patients are much more common than the physical disability [72], but for most clinical trials focus has continued to be on physical performance as measured by the Karnofsky Performance Status (KPS). Many of the challenges of assessing QOL relate to the difficulty in the validation of objective measures of various domains. Multiple tools have been used to evaluate QOL, including Spitzer Quality of Life Index, the Psychosocial Adjustment to Illness Scale, the Functional Living Index-Cancer, and the Ferrans and Powers Quality of Life Index [72].

Laboratory

Brain tumor patients represent a unique population in terms of drug metabolism because of the concurrent use of steroids and anticonvulsant therapy that both alter hepatic metabolism through various pathways, including cytochrome 450. Doses of different chemotherapeutic agents may need to be adjusted in the presence of these drugs, and toxicity may also differ. Regular laboratory assessments of organ function are mandatory to assess potential adverse effects.

TOXICITY OF CHEMOTHERAPY

Cytotoxic drugs have been shown to be beneficial for treating various histologic subtypes of primary brain tumors, including glioblastoma, oligodendroglioma, primitive

Table 62.2 General Side Effects of Chemotherapy

Category	Timing	Side Effects
Immediate	Within 24 hours	Nausea/vomiting
		Local tissue necrosis
		Phlebitis
		Anaphylaxis/skin rash
		Renal failure
Early	Days to weeks	Myelosuppression
		Alopecia
		Stomatitis
		Diarrhea
Delayed	Weeks to months	Anemia
		Aspermia
		Hepatocellular damage
		Hyperpigmentation
		Pulmonary fibrosis
Late	Months to years	Sterility/hypogonadism
		Premature menopause
		Secondary malignancies

Table 62.3 Drug Specific Side Effects of Chemotherapy Agents

Class	Agent	Toxicities
Alkylating	Temozolomide	Myelosupression, nausea, vomiting, constipation
	Carmustine	Myelosuppression, nausea, vomiting, pulmonary toxicity, secondary acute leukemia
	Lomustine	Myelosuppression, nausea, vomiting, delayed renal and pulmonary toxicity
Antimetabolites	Methotrexate	Neutropenia, mucositis, renal toxicity, hepatotoxicity, pulmonary toxicity
	5-Fluorouracil	Myelosuppression, stomatitis, diarrhea, rash, hand-foot syndrome, cardia toxicity
	Cytarabine	Leukopenia, thrombocytopenia, GI toxicity, conjunctivitis, keratitis, neurological toxicity
	Thioguanine	Myelosuppression, GI toxicity, hepatotoxicity
Vinca alkaloids	Vincristine	Neurological toxicity, constipation, hyponatremia, rash
Podophyllotoxins	Etoposide	Myelosuppression, allergic reaction, dermatological effects, hepatotoxicity
Antibiotics	Bleomycin	Anaphylaxis, mucositis, nausea, vomiting, pulmonary fibrosis, hyperpigmentation
Taxanes	Paclitaxel	Hypersensitivity reaction, myelosuppression, neurotoxicity, cardiac toxicity, alopecia
Topoisomerase I inhibitors	Irinotecan	Diarrhea, myelosuppression
Methylhydrazines	Procarbazine	Myelosuppression, nausea, vomiting, neurotoxicity, allergic reaction, azoospermia, infertility, monoamine oxidase drug reaction

neuroectodermal tumors, primary germ-cell tumors, and primary central nervous system lymphoma. The limitations of chemotherapy agents used include the inherent and acquired resistance of tumor cells to those agents, the inability to deliver adequate therapeutic concentration through the BBB, and, of course, the potential side effects and complications of those agents. Because of their ability to kill actively and rapidly dividing cells, these drugs can affect a wide array of organ systems: GI, bone marrow, lymphoid tissue, hair follicles, and germinal epithelium. Most of the side effects of chemotherapy are completely reversible, due to the capacity for stem-cell renewal, and other side effects can also be delayed, be they cumulative or dose dependent. Close monitoring is, therefore, crucial and supportive measures should be instituted prophylactically, for example, the use of antiemetic agents for chemotherapy-related emesis, and if needed, the use of colony stimulating growth factors for myelosuppression.

Several factors will influence the toxicity of chemotherapeutic treatment: patient's age, severity of the disease, number of previous treatments (including chemotherapy and radiotherapy), hepatic and renal function, and concomitant medication that may alter metabolism such as antiepileptic drugs.

The common side effects of chemotherapy can be divided in to four categories: immediate, early, delayed, and late (see Table 62.2). Specific toxicities related to chemotherapeutic agents commonly used in neuro-oncology are presented in Table 62.3.

REFERENCES

1. Ehrlich P. *Ueber die Beziehungen von chemister Constitution, Verteilung, und pharmacologische Wirkung.* New York: John Wiley, 567–595, 1906.
2. Vein AA. *Lina Stern: Science and Fate,* Department of Neurology, Leiden University Medical Centre, Leiden, The Netherlands.
3. Reese TS, Karnovsky MJ. Fine structural localization of a blood-brain barrier to exogenous peroxidase. *J. Cell Biol.* 1967;34:207–217.
4. Oldendorf WH, Cornford ME, Brown WJ. The large apparent work capability of the blood-brain barrier: a study of the mitochondrial content of capillary endothelial cells in brain and other tissues of the rat. *Ann Neurol.* 1977;1(5):409–417.
5. Misra A, Ganesh S, Shahiwala S. Drug delivery to the central nervous system: a review. *J Pharm Pharmaceut Sci.* 2003;6(2):252–273.
6. Takeichi M. Morphogenetic roles of classic cadherins. *Curr Opin Cell Biol.* 1995;7(5):619–627.
7. Abbruscato TJ, Davis TP. Protein expression of brain endothelial cell E-cadherin after hypoxia/aglycemia: influence of astrocyte contact. *Brain Res.* 1999;842(2):277–286.
8. Maher PA, Pasquale EB. Tyrosine phosphorylated proteins in different tissues during chick embryo development. *J Cell Biol.* 1988;106(5):1747–1755.
9. Stanness KA, Westrum LE, Fornaciari E, et al. Morphological and functional characterization of an in vitro blood-brain barrier model. *Brain Res.* 1997;771(2):329–342.
10. Stummer W, Betz AL, Shakui P, Keep RF. Blood-brain barrier taurine transport during osmotic stress and in focal cerebral ischemia. *J Cereb Blood Flow Metab.* 1995;15(5):852–859.
11. Farrell CR, Stewart PA, Farrell CL, Del Maestro RF. Pericytes in human cerebral microvasculature. *Anat Rec.* 1987;218(4):466–469.
12. Cordon-Cardo C, O'Brien JP, Casals D, et al. Multidrug-resistance gene (P-glycoprotein) is expressed by endothelial cells at blood-brain barrier sites. *Proc Natl Acad Sci USA.* 1989;86(2):695–698.
13. Stewart PA, Hayakawa K, Farrell CL, Del Maestro RF. Quantitative study of microvessel ultrastructure in human peritumoral brain tissue. Evidence for a blood-brain barrier defect. *J Neurosurg.* 1987;67(5):697–705.
14. Reulen HJ, Graham R, Spatz M, Klatzo I. Role of pressure gradients and bulk flow in dynamics of vasogenic brain edema. *J Neurosurg.* 1977;46(1):24–35.
15. Jelsma R, Bucy PC. The treatment of glioblastoma multiforme of the brain. *J Neurosurg.* 1967;27(5):388–400.
16. Bruce JN, Criscuolo GR, Merrill MJ, Moquin RR, Blacklock JB, Oldfield EH. Vascular permeability induced by protein product of malignant brain tumors: inhibition by dexamethasone. *J Neurosurg.* 1987;67(6):880–884.

17. Marshall LF, King J, Langfitt TW. The complications of high-dose corticosteroid therapy in neurosurgical patients: a prospective study. *Ann Neurol.* 1977;1(2):201–203.
18. Sharma ML, Bani S, Singh GB. Anti-arthritic activity of boswellic acids in bovine serum albumin (BSA)-induced arthritis. *Int. J. Immunopharmacol.* 1989;11:647–652.
19. Safayhi H, Mack T, Ammon HP. Protection by boswellic acids against galactosamine/endotoxin-induced hepatitis in mice. *Biochem. Pharmacol.* 1991;41:1536–1537.
20. Gupta I, Parihar A, Malhotra P, et al. Effects of Boswellia serrata gum resin in patients with ulcerative colitis. *Eur J Med Res.* 1997; 2:37–43.
21. Gupta I, Gupta V, Parihar A , et al. Effects of Boswellia serrata gum resin in patients with bronchial asthma: results of a double-blind, placebo-controlled, 6-week clinical study. *Eur J Med Res.* 1998;3(11):511–514.
22. Baba T, Chio CC, Black KL. The effect of 5-lipoxygenase inhibition on blood-brain barrier permeability in experimental brain tumors. *J Neurosurg.* 1992;77:403–406.
23. Boeker DK, Winking M. The role of boswellic acids in the therapy of malignant glioma. *Deutsches Aerzteblatt.* 1997;94:A1197-A1199.
24. Streffer JR, Bitzer M, Schabet M, Dichgans J, Weller M. Response of radiochemotherapy-associated cerebral edema to a phytotherapeutic agent, H15. *Neurology.* 2001;56(9):1219–1221.
25. Janssen G, Bode U, Breu H, Dohrn B, Engelbrecht V, Göbel U. Boswellic acids in the palliative therapy of children with progressive or relapsed brain tumors. *Klin Padiatr.* 2000;212(4):189–195.
26. Vredenburgh JJ, Desjardins A, Herndon JE, et al. Phase II trial of bevacizumab and irinotecan in recurrent malignant glioma. *Clin Cancer Res.* 2007;13(4):1253–1259.
27. DeMario MD, Ratain MJ. Oral chemotherapy: rationale and future directions. *J Clin Oncol.* 1998;16(7):2557–2567.
28. Jackson DV, Sethi VS, Spurr CL, McWhorter JM. Pharmacokinetics of vincristine in the cerebrospinal fluid of humans. *Cancer Res.* 1981;41(4):1466–1468.
29. Emerson DL. Liposomal delivery of camptothecins. *Pharm Sci Technol Today.* 2000;3(6):205–209.
30. Boviatsis EJ, Chase M, Wei MX, et al. Gene transfer into experimental brain tumors mediated by adenovirus, herpes simplex virus, and retro virus vectors. *Hum Gene Ther.* 1994:5:183–91.
31. Markert JM, Medlock MD, Rabkin SD, et al. Conditionally replicating herpes simplex virus mutant, G207 for the treatment of malignant glioma: results of a phase I trial. *Gene Ther.* 2000;7(10): 867–874.
32. Prados MD, McDermott M, Chang SM, et al. Treatment of progressive or recurrent glioblastoma multiforme in adults with herpes simplex virus thymidine kinase gene vector-producer cells followed by intravenous ganciclovir administration: a phase I/II multi-institutional trial. *J Neurooncol.* 2003;65(3):269–278.
33. Neuwelt EA, Dahlborg SA. Blood-brain barrier disruption in the treatment of brain tumors: clinical implication. In: Neuwelt EA, ed. *Implications of the Blood Brain Barrier and Its Manipulations: Clinical Aspects vol.2.* New York:Plenum Press; 1989:195–262 .
34. Miller G. Drug targeting: breaking down barriers. *Science.* 2002;297(5584):1116–1118.
35. Dahlborg SA, Henner WD, Crossen JR, et al. Non-AIDS primary CNS lymphoma: first example of a durable response in a primary brain tumor using enhanced chemotherapy delivery without cognitive loss and without radiotherapy. *Cancer J Sci Am.* 1996;2(3): 166–174.
36. Cloughesy TF, Black KL, Gobin YP, et al. Intra-arterial Cereport (RMP-7) and carboplatin: a dose escalation study for recurrent malignant gliomas. *Neurosurgery.* 1999;44(2):270–278; discussion 278.
37. Dean RL, Emerich DF, Hasler BP, Bartus RT. Cereport (RMP-7) increases carboplatin levels in brain tumors after pretreatment with dexamethasone. *Neuro-oncology.* 1999;1(4):268–274.
38. Packer RJ, Krailo M, Mehta M, et al. A phase I study of concurrent RMP-7 and carboplatin with radiation therapy for children with newly diagnosed brainstem gliomas. *Cancer.* 2005:104(9): 1968–1974.
39. Warren K, Jakacki R, Widemann B, et al. Phase II trial of intravenous lobradimil and carboplatin in childhood brain tumors: a report from the Children's Oncology Group. *Cancer Chemother Pharmacol.* 2006;58(3):343–347.
40. Fenstermacher JD, Cowles AL. Theoretic limitations of intracarotid infusions in brain tumor chemotherapy. *Cancer Treat Rep.* 1977;61(4):519–526.
41. Maiese K, Walker RW, Gargan R, Victor JD. Intra-arterial cisplatin–associated optic and otic toxicity. *Arch Neurol.* 1992;49(1):83–86.
42. Shapiro WR, Young DF, Mehta BM. Methotrexate: distribution in cerebrospinal fluid after intravenous, ventricular and lumbar injections. *N Engl J Med.* 1975;293(4):161–166.
43. Marc C. Neoplastic Meningitis. *J Clin Oncol.* 2005;23(15):3605–3613.
44. Rubenstein JL, Fridlyand J, Abrey L, et al. Phase I study of intraventricular administration of rituximab in patients with recurrent CNS and intraocular lymphoma. *J Clin Oncol.* 2007;25(11)1350–1356.
45. Talegaonkar S, Mishra PR. Intranasal delivery: an approach to bypass the blood brain barrier. *Indian J Pharmacol.* 2004;36(3) 140–147.
46. Brem H, Piantadosi S, Burger PC, et al. Placebo-controlled trial of safety and efficacy of intraoperative controlled delivery by biodegradable polymers of chemotherapy for recurrent gliomas. The Polymer-brain Tumor Treatment Group. *Lancet.* 1995;345: 1008–1012.
47. Westphal M, Hilt DC, Bortey E, et al. A phase 3 trial of local chemotherapy with biodegradable carmustine (BCNU) wafers (Gliadel wafers) in patients with primary malignant glioma. *Neuro-oncol* 2003;5:79–88.
48. Westphal M, Ram Z, Riddle V, Hilt D, Bortey E, on behalf of the Executive Committee of the Gliadel Study Group. Gliadel wafer in initial surgery for malignant glioma: long-term follow-up of a multicenter controlled trial. *Acta Neurochir (Wien)* 2006;148:269–275.
49. Hall WA, and Sherr GT. Convection-enhanced delivery: targeted toxin treatment of malignant glioma. *Neurosurg Focus.* 2006; 20(4):E10.
50. Vandergrift WA, Patel SJ. Convection-enhanced delivery of immunotoxins and radioisotopes for treatment of malignant gliomas. *Neurosurg Focus.* 2006;20(4):E13.
51. Kunwar S, Chang S, Westphal M, et al.; for the PRECISE Study Group. Phase III randomized trial of CED of IL13-PE38QQR vs Gliadel wafers for recurrent glioblastoma. *Neuro-oncol* 2010, Advance Access published on February 4, 2010; doi:10.1093/neuonc/nop054
52. Safa A. Multidrug Resistance. In: Schilsky R, Milano G, Ratain M, ed. *Principles of Antineoplasic Drug Development and Pharmacology.* New York: Marcel Dekker; 1996:457.
53. Lorico A, Rappa G, Finch RA, Yang D, Flavell RA, Sartorelli AC. Disruption of the murine MRP (multidrug resistance protein) gene leads to increased sensitivity to etoposide (VP-16) and increased levels of glutathione. *Cancer Res.* 1997;57(23):5238–5242.
54. Stupp R, Hegi ME, Diserens AC, et al. MGMT gene silencing and Benefit from Temozolomide in Glioblastoma. *N Engl J Med.* 2005;352:997–1003.
55. Heimberger AB, Hlatky R, Suki D, et al. Prognostic effect of epidermal growth factor receptor and EGFRvIII in glioblastoma multiforme patients. *Clin Cancer Res.* 2005;11(4):1462–1466.
56. Mellinghoff IK, Wang MY, Vivanco I, et al. Molecular determinants of the response of glioblastomas to EGFR kinase inhibitors. *N Engl J Med.* 2005;353(19):2012–2024.
57. Cairncross JG, Ueki K, Zlatescu MC, et al. Specific genetic predictors of chemotherapeutic response and survival in patients with anaplastic oligodendrogliomas. *J Natl Cancer Inst.* 1998;90(19): 1473–1479.
58. Kayes S. Reversal of multidrug resistance. *Cancer Treat Rev.* 1990;17(Suppl A):37–43.
59. Miller TP, Grogan TM, Dalton WS, Spier CM, Scheper RJ, Salmon SE. P-glycoprotein expression in malignant lymphoma and reversal of clinical drug resistance with chemotherapy plus high-dose verapamil. *J Clin Oncol.* 1991;9(1):17–24.
60. Twentyman PR, Fox NE, White DJ. Cyclosporin A and its analogues as modifiers of adriamycin and vincristine resistance in a multi-drug resistant human lung cancer cell line. *Br J Cancer.* 1987;56(1):55–57.
61. Gosland MP, Lum BL, Sikic BI. Reversal by cefoperazone of resistance to etoposide, doxorubicin, and vinblastine in multidrug resistant human sarcoma cells. *Cancer Res.* 1989;49:6901–6905.
62. Fisher GA, Sikic BI. Clinical studies with modulators of multidrug resistance. *Hematol Oncol Clin North Am.* 1995;9(2):363–382.
63. Gerson S, Liu L, Phillips W, et al. Drug resistance mediated by DNA repair: the paradigm of O6-akylguanine DNA alkyltranferase. *Proc Am Assoc Cancer Res.* 1994;35:699–700.

64. Bobola MS, Blank A, Berger MS, Silber JR. Contribution of O6-methylguanine-DNA methyltransferase to monofunctional alkylating-agent resistance in human brain tumor-derived cell lines. *Mol Carcinog.* 1995;13(2):70–80.
65. Pegg AE, Boosalis M, Samson L, et al. Mechanism of inactivation of human O6-alkylguanine-DNA alkyltransferase by O6-benzylguanine. *Biochemistry.* 1993;32(45):11998–12006.
66. Broniscer A, Gururangan S, MacDonald TJ, et al. Phase I trial of single-dose temozolomide and continuous administration of o6-benzylguanine in children with brain tumors: a pediatric brain tumor consortium report. *Clin Cancer Res.* 2007;13(22 Pt 1): 6712–6718.
67. Quinn JA, Desjardins A, Weingart J, et al. Phase I trial of temozolomide plus O6-benzylguanine for patients with recurrent or progressive malignant glioma. *J Clin Oncol.* 2005;23(28):7178–7187.
68. Tolcher AW, Gerson SL, Denis L, et al. Marked inactivation of O6-alkylguanine-DNA alkyltransferase activity with protracted temozolomide schedules. *Br J Cancer.* 2003;88(7):1004–1011.
69. Weller M, Steinbach JP, Wick W. Temozolomide: a milestone in the pharmacotherapy of brain tumors. *Future Oncol.* 2005;1(6):747–754.
70. Cairncross JG, Macdonald DR, Pexman JH, et al. Steroid-induced CT chages in patients with recurrent malignant glioma. *Neurology.* 1988;38:724–726.
71. DeAngelis LM, Yahalom J, Heinemann MH, Cirrincione C, Thaler HT, Krol G. Primary CNS lymphoma: combined treatment with chemotherapy and radiotherapy. *Neurology.* 1990;40(1):80–86.
72. Meyers CA. Neuropsychological deficits in brain tumor patients: Effect of location, chronicity, and treatment. *Cancer Bull.* 1986;38:30–32.

63 Medical Management of Suratentorial Gliomas in Adults

Jennifer L. Clarke, Douglas Edward Ney, Charles C. Shyu, and Andrew B. Lassman

INTRODUCTION

At any given time, approximately 80,000 residents of the United States live with primary malignant brain tumors, and new malignant brain tumors are diagnosed with an incidence of 7.3 per 100,000 person-years [1]. Approximately 190,000 individuals worldwide develop malignant brain tumors each year [1], of which the majority are gliomas [2,3]. While brain tumors represent only a small proportion of all cancers, they carry significant societal costs due to their devastating neurological symptoms and poor survival rates. In recent years, significant progress has been made toward understanding the environmental risk factors and patient behaviors that predispose to the development of a variety of common cancers. In contrast, there are no identifiable environmental causes for the vast majority of supratentorial gliomas. The only well-established risk factor for glioma is a history of ionizing radiation [4,5], but this accounts for a very small percentage of cases. Most malignant gliomas are sporadic, but approximately 5% occur in association with an identified familial cancer syndrome such as neurofibromatosis, tuberous sclerosis, or syndromes of Turcot, von Hippel-Linday, or Li-Fraumeni [6]. The lack of modifiable risk factors for glioma development means that they cannot be prevented through environmental or lifestyle measures, highlighting the importance of developing effective therapies to treat these tumors after they occur.

Therapy for gliomas has traditionally consisted of a combination of surgery, radiation, and chemotherapy, with the timing and aggressiveness of therapy guided by tumor grade and location. While surgery and radiation have long been shown to influence survival of high-grade gliomas, recurrence is nearly universal and mean survival time remains short, even in patients who receive optimum care. Many chemotherapy regimens have been used to supplement surgery and radiation, but it was only recently that a chemotherapeutic agent was unambiguously demonstrated to improve patient survival in a randomized controlled trial [7]. There are a variety of reasons that development of effective chemotherapeutic regimens for brain tumors has lagged behind that of systemic tumors. For example, the blood–brain barrier limits chemotherapy penetration to at least a subset of tumor cells. Potential drug interactions between definitive chemotherapeutic treatments and supportive treatments specific to patients with brain tumors (e.g., antiseizure medications or corticosteroids) can also complicate the treatment plan. Despite these hurdles, real progress is being made. This chapter will explore the current state of medical management of low-grade and malignant gliomas, as well as introduce areas of expected progress in the future.

LOW-GRADE GLIOMAS

Introduction

The term "low-grade glioma" (LGG) semantically refers to both World Health Organization (WHO) grade I and II tumors [6]. However, the WHO grade I gliomas, such as juvenile pilocytic astrocytomas, generally occur in the posterior fossa (infratentorial) in children and may be curable by surgical resection. The underlying molecular biology is distinct from supratentorial LGGs in adults. Accordingly, WHO grade I tumors are discussed elsewhere in this text and are not included in this section. In adults, therefore, the LGGs discussed here include the WHO grade II fibrillary astrocytomas, oligodendrogliomas, and oligoastrocytomas. LGGs are often called "benign" tumors, but they certainly do not behave benignly in the lay sense. Such tumors are only rarely if ever curable by surgical resection and almost invariably become more aggressive with time, likely resulting from the accumulation of oncogenic mutations.

LGGs typically demonstrate hyperintensity on T2/FLAIR weighted brain MR imaging and little or no contrast enhancement (Figure 63.1). Treatment remains controversial, with some neuro-oncologists advocating aggressive therapy at time of diagnosis and others preferring observation with treatment deferred until time of progression. Median survival associated with low-grade astrocytomas (LGAs) and low-grade oligodendrogliomas (LGOs) is approximately 5 and 10 years, respectively, with low-grade oligoastrocytomas (LGOAs) in between [3].

Definitive Therapy

Surgery

Surgical resection, although almost never curative, is critical for accurate diagnosis. Magnetic resonance

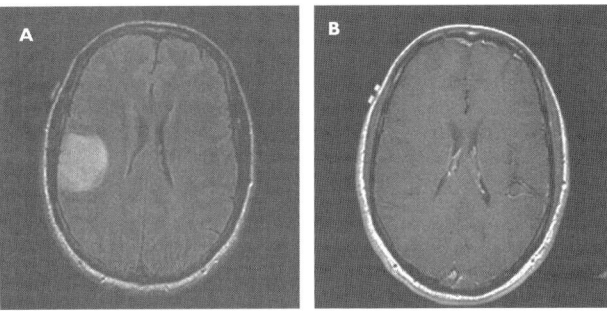

Figure 63.1 Low-grade glioma (LGG). Brain magnetic resonance imaging (MRI) from a patient who presented with seizures and was ultimately diagnosed by subtotal resection to have an LGG. **(A)** FLAIR sequence demonstrating hyperintensity relative to normal brain. **(B)** T1 image following gadolinium injection demonstrating subtle hypointensity and lack of contrast enhancement.

imaging (MRI) often suggests an LGG (Figure 63.1), but definitive diagnosis is dependent on pathology. In addition, larger resection reduces sampling bias, prompting most neuro-oncologists to recommend maximal safe surgical excision [8]. One study demonstrated that among patients who previously underwent a stereotactic biopsy, the pathologic diagnosis changed in up to 49% of patients following resection, and this change altered treatment in 33% [9]. No prospective randomized data exist to address whether larger resection improves survival, and none is likely to emerge. However, numerous series strongly support maximal surgical resection as best initial therapy to improve survival [10,11]. Finally, regardless of improved survival and accurate diagnosis, resection can improve seizure control, allowing decreases in anticonvulsant and corticosteroid dosing. Therefore, maximal safe surgical debulking is likely superior to biopsy for many reasons, although therapy must be individualized based on tumor location and risk of resection. It should also be noted that while most investigators advocate resection at diagnosis, others advocate deferral until clinical or radiographic progression among "low risk" patients (below) [12].

Radiotherapy

After surgical debulking, radiation therapy (RT) is the historic treatment of choice for LGGs. A detailed discussion of RT is found elsewhere in this text. While the question of optimal radiation dose for LGGs is largely settled, timing of therapy remains controversial and is an area of active clinical investigation. In practice, timing of RT is variable with some practitioners advocating treatment immediately after diagnosis and others preferring to reserve RT until disease progression.

Several phase III trials have examined the effect of various radiation doses on patient survival and quality of life. The European Organization for Research and Treatment of Cancer (EORTC) trial 22844 demonstrated neither an overall survival (OS) nor progression-free survival (PFS) benefit among 343 evaluable patients randomized to 45 or 59.4 Gy (median OS 6.6 vs. 6.6 years, 5-year OS 58% vs. 59%, 5-year PFS 47% vs. 50%, median PFS approximately 4.8 years in both as estimated from the published survival curve) [13]. Similar results were obtained from the North Central Cancer Treatment Group (NCCTG 86-72-51), Radiation Therapy Oncology Group (RTOG), and Eastern Cooperative Oncology Group (ECOG), which randomized 203 patients to either 50.4 or 64.8 Gy (50.4 Gy followed by a 14.4 Gy "boost") with no survival difference but increased toxicity with the higher dose [14]. Given the results of these trials, RT regimens for LGGs typically consist of 45 to 54 Gy delivered in 1.8 Gy fractions.

Optimum timing of RT remains controversial. EORTC trial 22845 randomized 311 patients to either RT (54 Gy in 6 weeks) at diagnosis or at progression [15]. Intent-to-treat analyses demonstrated that initial RT significantly prolonged PFS (median 5.3 vs. 3.4 years) but not OS (approximately 7.3 years in both arms). These conclusions remained valid following adjustment for patients who were ineligible on histologic (WHO grade I or III tumors) or clinical grounds, or who did not receive the intended treatment approach. If an OS benefit had been documented, the controversy over timing would have ended. Absent that, the critical and unresolved issue is whether one of these approaches offers patients superior quality of life despite a lack of impact on OS. In this setting, the question then becomes whether the PFS benefit of RT at time of diagnosis is worth the potential risks, such as RT-induced cognitive decline later [16,17]. Conversely, nonprogressing tumors should theoretically cause fewer neurologic symptoms than progressing tumors. For example, EORTC 22845 demonstrated a reduced incidence of seizures after 1 year among those who received initial (25%) rather than delayed (40%) RT ($p = .0329$) [15]. However, other key quality-of-life measures, such as neurocognitive assessments, were not collected. Until these issues are addressed, the timing for RT will remain debated when all LGGs are pooled. Recent work has instead focused on defining stratified "risk groups" and adjusting treatment accordingly.

In an effort to define patient subgroups with differing responses to RT, combined data from EORTC 22844 and 22845 were assessed for the prognostic value of clinical variables [18]. Patient age ≥40 years, largest tumor diameter ≥6 cm, tumor crossing midline, astrocytic dominant histology, and presence of neurologic deficits other than seizures were all significant negative prognostic factors. Median survival for patients with none versus all of these five risk "risk factors" was 9.2 and 0.7 years, respectively [18]. Of note, extent of resection was not identified as a prognostic factor in multivariate analyses, but tumor size (≥6 cm) and location (crossing midline) were prognostic, and these factors clearly affect resectability. Therefore, these data should not be interpreted as evidence against extent of resection as a prognostic factor. In addition, epilepsy was a positive prognostic factor, likely because patients with seizures rarely if ever had other neurologic impairments at diagnosis. Since these studies were analyzed, molecular studies have demonstrated that 1p19q codeletion is a clear prognostic factor as well, although the issue has not been studied as robustly for LGGs as it has been for anaplastic tumors [19–22].

RTOG 9802 was conceived to assess different treatment strategies based on clinically identified prognostic factors. It encompassed two substudies. The first (Arm 1) was a single arm phase II trial of observation for "low risk patients," defined in 9802 as age ≤40 years and treated with gross total resection as defined by the operating neurosurgeon. The second substudy addressed whether chemotherapy in addition to RT is superior to RT alone for "high risk patients" defined as age >40 or less than gross total resection. There were 111 "low risk" patients enrolled to Arm 1 who were periodically surveilled for progression by clinical and radiographic assessments. They did not undergo RT or chemotherapy until disease progression. The 5-year OS and PFS rates were 94% and 50%, respectively—significantly superior ($p = .0001$) than those for the "high risk" patients (regardless of RT or RT + chemotherapy below). However, tumor size (≥4 cm), astrocytoma dominant histology, and ≥1 cm of residual postoperative tumor (reviewed centrally on imaging) each significantly predicted early progression within the "low risk" cohort in multivariate analysis ($p = .05, .02,$ and $.0002$, respectively) [23]. Therefore, although observation may be a reasonable strategy among selected patient subsets, treatment should be considered for higher risk patients. In addition, this study demonstrated that age and extent of resection are not the only important clinical risk factors, as described later by Pignatti et al [18]. It also showed that postoperative imaging is critical for documentation of the extent of resection. An open question remains whether RT itself prolongs OS among patients with "high risk" LGGs. However, many neuro-oncologists advocate RT empirically for such patients, making the feasibility of a prospective randomized study doubtful.

Chemotherapy

The role of chemotherapy in the treatment of LGGs is even less clear than that of RT. This results, in part, from the traditional characterization of LGGs as chemoresistant because of their indolent growth pattern and low mitotic rate. For example, an early trial from the Southwest Oncology Group (SWOG) enrolled 54 eligible patients with incompletely resected WHO grade I ($n = 4$) or II ($n = 50$) gliomas from 1980 to 1985. Patients were randomized to RT (55 Gy) or RT + lomustine (CCNU) dosed 100 mg/m^2 every 6 weeks [24]. Median survival did not differ between the arms on initial analysis, but the trial was closed earlier because of poor accrual. In addition, the chemotherapy regimens used in these earlier studies were relatively toxic: 12% of patients treated with lomustine experienced severe or life-threatening hematologic toxicity versus 0% of those treated with RT alone [24]. On the surface, these results may limit enthusiasm for chemotherapy. However, survival trended toward a benefit for lomustine (median 7.4 vs. 4.5 years), and continued accrual may well have demonstrated a significant benefit from chemotherapy. Evaluation of the LGG chemotherapy literature as a whole is made more difficult by the fact that many studies included heterogeneous patient cohorts, with mixtures of tumor histologies, tumor grades, and prior treatment histories. Most prospective studies, for example, did not require rebiopsy at the time of disease progression, even after several years or in the setting of new enhancing disease, when malignant transformation is highly likely. Thus, it is difficult to determine the fraction of patients treated for continued low-grade histology rather than anaplastic tumors or even glioblastomas (GBMs) in some studies. Nonetheless, over the last decade, accumulating evidence supports a role for chemotherapy in LGGs, especially for LGOs or LGOAs.

PCV

Many older studies of chemotherapy for LGGs utilized the combination of procarbazine, lomustine, and vincristine known as PCV. Results of these studies are summarized in Table 63.1 [25–45]. Enthusiasm for PCV in LGGs derived in part from an early report of responses in 9 of 10 patients with recurrent anaplastic oligodendrogliomas (AOs) who initially presented with LGOs [25]. A number of other small case series and retrospective studies published during the same period reported response rates of 60%-67% in patients with LGOs or LGOAs in either the recurrent or newly diagnosed setting [26–28]. Long-term follow-up for some patients was also described [29]. Retrospective studies published more recently yielded similar results [30–31] with responses in 27%-81%, including patients without 1p19q codeletion with gliomatosis cerebri [31].

Prospective studies have analyzed various combinations regimens of PCV, with and without RT, for LGO and LGOA. An early phase II trial of 26 patients with recurrent LGO/LGOA treated with up to six cycles of PCV demonstrated responses in 62% [32]. Of note, six patients who developed late recurrence were rechallenged with PCV; one had a partial response and two had stable disease. Molecular analyses of archival tissue were not conducted, but time to progression was significantly longer among patients with "pure" oligodendrogliomas rather than mixed oligoastrocytomas, presumably a consequence of the high rate of 1p19q codeletion in pure tumors. Of note, contrast enhancing disease on imaging was common, implying undocumented malignant transformation. Therefore, this trial may have studied anaplastic tumors rather than LGGs in many cases. As mentioned in the preceding section on RT, RTOG 9802 tested whether the addition of up to six cycles of post-RT PCV improved outcome relative to RT (54 Gy) alone for "high risk" patients. In this phase III trial, "high risk" was defined as age >40 OR less than gross total resection. Initial analysis suggested no difference in OS but a trend toward improved PFS for the PCV arm [23]. Analysis of more mature data confirmed the lack of an OS benefit from the addition of PCV (median 7.5 years for RT, not reached for RT→PCV, $p = .33$), and the trend for the PFS benefit became stronger (median 4.4 years for RT, not reached for RT→PCV, $p = .06$) [33]. Clearly, longer follow-up is required for further survival analysis, as two-thirds of patients remain alive. 1p19q testing is planned but has not yet been performed in part

Table 63.1 Chemotherapy for Low-Grade Gliomas

Chemoregimen	Study Type	Histology	Newly Diagnosed or Recurrent Disease	No. of Patients	Response Rate (%)*	Notes	References
I-PCV	Pro	AO	Both	10	90	Subset of patients in AO study with prior LGO	Cairncross et al [25]
I-PCV and PCV	Retro	LGO	Both	10 (including addendum)	60		Mason et al [26]
PCV	Retro	LGO	New	5	60		Paleologos et al [27]
PCV	Retro	LGO, LGOA, 2 with gliomatosis	Recurrent	5	60		Stege et al [28]
PCV	Retro	LGO, LGOA, 9 with gliomatosis	New	16	81		Stege et al [28]
PCV	Retro	LGO	New	33	27	Median OS 10 years, 1-year PFS 90%, 5-year PFS 75%	Lebrun et al [29]
PCV	Pro	LGO, LGOA	Recurrent	26	62	1-year PFS approximately 80%	Soffietti et al [30]
I-PCV	Pro	LGO, LGOA	New	28	29–52	1-year PFS 91%, 1-year OS 100%, 5-year OS 89%	Buckner et al [31]
PCV and others	Retro	LGA	New	10	40		Frenay et al [32]
PCV	Retro	LGO, LGOA	New	12	58	1-year and 5-year OS 100%	Higuchi et al [32a]
TMZ	Pro	LGO, LGOA	Recurrent	28	25		van den Bent et al [33]
TMZ	Pro	LGO	Mix	28	61	Median PFS 31 months, 1-year PFS 89%	Levin et al [34]
PCV	Retro	LGO	Unknown	8	75		Levin et al [34]
TMZ	Pro	LGO, LGOA	Recurrent	60	31	1-year PFS 73%	Hoang-Xuan et al [35]
TMZ	Pro	LGO, LGOA, LGA	Recurrent	43	47	Median PFS 10 months, 1-year PFS 39%	Pace et al [36]
TMZ	Pro	LGO, LGOA, LGA	Recurrent	46	61	Median PFS 22 months, 1-year PFS 76%	Quinn et al [37]
TMZ	Pro	LGO, LGOA, LGA	New	30	10	1-year PFS and 1-year OS approximately 92%	Brada et al [38]
TMZ	Retro tissue	LGO, LGOA	Recurrent	149	53	Median PFS 28 months, median OS not reached, 1-year PFS 80%, 1-year OS 95%	Kaloshi et al [39], update of prior study [35]
TMZ	Retro	LGO, LGOA, LGA	New	68	57	Median PFS 28 months, 1-year PFS 77%	Everhard et al [40]
TMZ (alternate dosing)	Retro	LGO, LGOA, LGA, and LG not specified	Mix	25	24	Median PFS not reached, 1-year PFS 74%	Pouratian et al [41]
TMZ (alternate dosing)	Pro	LGO, LGOA, LGA	Recurrent	30	30	Median PFS 22 months, 1-year PFS 43%, median OS not reached, 1-year OS 97%	Tosoni et al [42]
PCV	Retro	LGO, LGOA, LGA gliomatosis	Mix	17	31	Median PFS and OS 16 and 26 months, eight tumors were WHO grade III or undetermined	Sanson et al [43]

Continued

Table 63.1 Continued

Chemoregimen	Study Type	Histology	Newly Diagnosed or Recurrent Disease	No. of Patients	Response Rate (%)*	Notes	References
TMZ	Retro	LGO, LGOA, LGA gliomatosis	Mix	46	24	Median PFS and OS 16 and 26 months, 15 tumors were not WHO grade III or undetermined, TMZ less toxic than PCV	Sanson et al [43]
TMZ	Retro	LGO, LGOA, LGA gliomatosis	Recurrent (at time of progression on PCV)	11	45	Median PFS 13 months, 1-year PFS 55%, median OS not reached	Levin et al [44]

AO, anaplastic oligodendroglioma; I-PCV, intense-PCV [25]; LGA, low-grade astrocytoma; LGO, low-grade oligodendroglioma; LGOA, low-grade oligoastrocytoma (mixed glioma); NA, not available(not reported or not reached); OS, overall survival; PCV, Procarbazine, lomustine (CCNU), and vincristine [45]; PFS, progression-free survival; Pro, prospective; retro, retrospective; TMZ, temozolomide.

Recurrent, disease that recurred or progressed during postoperative surveillance or during/following prior therapy.

*Includes complete and partial radiographic responses, although definitions of response are not uniform among trials with stricter definitions in more recent studies.

because this molecular prognostic factor was identified after the study opened to accrual.

In addition to treatment with chemotherapy alone, pre-RT PCV was assessed in another study. Patients with LGO or LGOA received RT within 10 weeks of completing chemotherapy or earlier if disease progression occurred during PCV [34]. The overall paradigm of PCV + RT, therefore, was similar to Arm 3 of RTOG 9802 (RT→PCV) but in the reverse order (PCV→RT). Central review demonstrated responses in up to 52% of patients. Codeletion of 1p and 19q was limited to patients with pure LGO rather than LGOA ($p = .009$) and inversely related to p53 expression. 1p19q codeletion did not correlate with response, possibly because of small sample size. However, other trials also report responses among LGG patients without 1p19q codeletion [31]. Therefore, it remains unclear whether molecular features should guide treatment decisions. As in other PCV trials, toxicity was substantial.

As a whole, these studies demonstrated that PCV commonly induces radiographic responses among LGOs and LGOAs, including those with intact 1p19q, but it remains unclear whether such treatment is associated with a survival advantage and/or improvement in quality of life in comparison with other therapies such as RT. This dilemma is analogous to the issue of up-front versus delayed RT for patients with "low risk" LGGs. Quality-of-life concerns are not trivial, especially as PCV is associated with substantial side effects. In addition, the long median survival for such patients, 13.5 years in one series [29], puts them at significant risk for late cognitive toxicity from RT [17], perhaps partially mitigating the up-front risks of chemotherapy. There is only one study that specifically addressed treatment of LGAs with up-front PCV chemotherapy [35]. In this retrospective analysis, 10 patients who underwent stereotactic biopsy did not receive RT because of safety concerns. Therefore, all were treated with PCV.

Efficacy appeared reasonable with three recurrences 4, 5, and 6 years, respectively, all of whom ultimately died. The other seven patients remained alive without progression at the time of report.

Temozolomide

In recent years, temozolomide (TMZ) has largely supplanted PCV as the treatment of choice for LGG both in clinical use and as the subject of clinical trials. It should be noted that TMZ has never been compared prospectively with PCV for efficacy in this setting, but its favorable safety profile and reports of efficacy in other glioma subtypes have led to its use as the de facto first-line chemotherapy for almost all adults with gliomas including LGGs.

As with PCV, the best evidence for the utility of TMZ among patients with LGGs comes from studies of oligodendroglial tumors. For example, EORTC 26972 enrolled patients with recurrent LGOs and LGOAs following PCV chemotherapy [36]. There were 28 patients treated with up to 12 cycles of TMZ; responses were observed in 25%, and the 6-month PFS was 29%. Treatment was well-tolerated overall. Similarly, RT-naïve patients with LGO were treated for clinical or radiographic progression in another small trial [37]. A subset of patients had previously received PCV, but the remainders were chemotherapy-naïve. Patients were treated with up to 24 cycles of TMZ. The objective response rate was 61%, and the 12-month PFS was 89%. Evaluation for 1p19q codeletion was undertaken in 15 patients, 10 of whom had codeletion. Of those 10 patients, nine manifested an objective response—a statistically significant correlation. A larger phase II trial of TMZ for progressive LGO or LGOA enrolled 60 patients [38]; responses were observed in 31%, and the 12-month PFS was 73%. Several prospective trials have also examined the efficacy of TMZ in progressive LGGs, including LGA in addition to LGO and LGOA. In two trials, one with 43 patients (29 with LGA) [36] and the other with 46 patients (16 with LGA) [40], median PFS was 10 and 22 months, respectively, for recurrent disease, with responses in 47% and 61%. The trial that enrolled more oligodendroglial tumors not surprisingly had superior PFS and response rate. Both of these cohorts included patients who had received prior treatment. In a trial that restricted entry to treatment-naïve patients, the 3-year PFS among 30 patients (17 with LGA) was 68% although some patients did not clearly have progressive disease at the time they began therapy [41].

Ongoing clinical trials promise to offer a better understanding of the efficacy of temozolomide for patients with LGG. RTOG 0424, modeled upon the PCV trial 9802, examines temozolomide therapy in "high risk" LGGs. RTOG 0424 defines high risk more strictly than 9802: patients with ≥3 of the risk factors (age ≥40 years, astrocytoma dominant histology, largest tumor diameter ≥6 cm, tumor crossing the midline, and neurologic deficit before surgery) identified in the analysis by Pignatti et al [18] of EORTC 22844 and 22845. The rationale relied on the median survival of 3.2 years for patients with 3 to 5 risk factors versus 7.7 years for those with 0 to 2 risk factors from EORTC 22844, validated with the data from 22845. Patients accrued to this single arm phase II trial received postoperative radiotherapy (54 Gy/30 fractions) and concurrent and adjuvant temozolomide [7]. The primary efficacy end point is OS at 3 years, with the hypothesized improvement from 54% using historical controls [18] to 65% on trial. Neurocognitive assessments are also collected to assess quantitatively the long-term toxicity of the regimen. Tissue analyses for O^6-methylguanine (O^6-MG)-DNA-methyltransferase (*MGMT*, detailed below) promoter methylation and 1p19q codeletion are also planned. Accrual was recently expanded and an interim analysis is ongoing (Paul D. Brown, personal communication). In addition, ECOG and the NCCTG initiated a randomized phase III study (E3F05) [42] to compare RT + TMZ with RT alone. However, unlike RTOG 0424, which will use historic controls, this study will include an RT (without chemotherapy) treatment arm. Eligibility criteria include age >40 AND clinically or radiographically progressive LGG. Neurocognitive assessments are incorporated along with 1p19q and MGMT tissue analyses. Such patients could be viewed as falling in between those with the highest risk required for RTOG 0424 eligibility (at least three among: age ≥40 years, diameter ≥6 cm, crossing midline, astrocytic histology, neurologic deficits) and lower risk observed on RTOG 9802 (age <40 AND gross total resection) for observation on RTOG 9802 (Minesh P. Mehta, personal communication). To definitively address the utility of chemotherapy (with TMZ) alone for newly diagnosed LGGs, EORTC and the National Cancer Institute of Canada (NCIC) are accruing to a phase III trial (EORTC 22033/26033, NCIC CE5) that randomizes patients to RT (50.5 Gy) or intensified TMZ (75 mg/m² days 1 to 21 of 28 × 12 cycles) [43]. Patients will be stratified for 1p19q status but those with LGA or intact 1p19q are not excluded. Quality of life and neurocognitive assessments are incorporated into the study design. Perhaps this trial will finally bring to an end the controversy over the efficacy of neoadjuvant chemotherapy for LGGs and the potential benefit to delaying the risk of neurocognitive toxicity from RT.

A variety of molecular markers have been evaluated as predictors of LGG tumor sensitivity to TMZ. Kaloshi et al [44] retrospectively reviewed molecular genetic data from an expansion of their previously reported cohort of LGG patients [38], and found an association between 1p19q codeletion and clinical outcome. The same group also retrospectively evaluated methylation of the *MGMT* promoter, and found methylation to be a good prognostic factor independent of 1p19q status [45]. Therefore, *MGMT* promoter methylation may predict TMZ sensitivity among all gliomas, as recent evidence from patients with GBMs demonstrates a similar correlation (below) [46]. Protracted regimens of TMZ are in use for LGG [47]. It is presently unknown, but widely theorized, that such alternate TMZ regimens may overcome MGMT mediated resistance in tumors with unmethylated *MGMT* promoters [48]. Notably, this theory also presupposes that MGMT activity is the relevant biologic mechanism by which *MGMT* promoter methylation affects chemosensitivity, although recent studies have suggested that the mechanism may be more complicated [49].

Other Chemotherapeutic Agents

There are scattered reports of the use of other chemotherapeutic agents for LGG, some of which have shown promise, but none of which have gained the acceptance of PCV or TMZ. Friedman assessed carboplatin in patients with LGO and radiographic evidence of tumor progression [50]. The preliminary report indicated good control of disease, with only one patient having had further progression at the time of publication; the remaining patients had ongoing disease control ranging between 6 and 22 months. Human fibroblast interferon (HFIF) was tested in patients with newly diagnosed LGA in a phase II trial, with a 5-year PFS rate of 65% and a median OS of 10.7 years [51]. High-dose methotrexate was assessed in eleven glioma patients, three of whom were felt to have LGA [52]. Two of the three survived only 6 months, but the third had survived 15 years from the first methotrexate treatment. Galanis et al [58] tested a combination of nitrogen mustard/vincristine/procarbazine (MOP) therapy in a variety of recurrent gliomas [53]. For LGGs, the median TTP was 20 weeks, and median OS was 51 weeks. Chamberlain evaluated irinotecan in 15 patients with recurrent LGO taking enzyme-inducing antiepileptic medications [54]. Toxicity was acceptable but there was minimal efficacy: median PFS and OS were 3 and 3.5 months, respectively. 2-Chlorodeoxyadenosine was ineffective in a mixed population of recurrent gliomas, with an overall median TTP of 3 months and median OS of 8 months. Although 33% of patients had LGGs, no specific efficacy data was provided by tumor grade [55]. Finally, intra-arterial carmustine (BCNU) was tested in patients at a Norwegian hospital [56] for patients with LGGs within the vascular supply from one of the internal carotid arteries; the treatment was not associated with prolonged survival.

Gliomatosis Cerebri

Treatment of gliomatosis is particularly challenging. Its characteristic diffuse infiltration of large areas of normal brain makes RT unappealing for fear of the cognitive effects of high-dose whole brain radiotherapy. As a result, there has been interest in the use of chemotherapy. Two retrospective studies were published in 2004, one from France with 63 patients [57] and the other from Israel with 11 patients [58]. The smaller study treated all patients with TMZ; the larger study encompassed 46 patients treated with TMZ and 17 with PCV. In all three groups of patients, the median PFS was 13 to 16 months. In the larger study, median OS was approximately 26 months; in the smaller study median OS had not been reached. Although prospective data should be collected for confirmation, it appears that chemotherapy with either TMZ or PCV is a reasonable alternative for initial treatment of gliomatosis cerebri; TMZ is likely the preferable choice because its superior toxicity profile allows for longer duration treatment in many patients. Others also reported efficacy of PCV in oligodendroglial gliomatosis cerebri [31].

A more recent follow-up to the 2004 French study examined molecular markers and response to chemotherapy in gliomatosis [59]. A cohort of 25 patients with gliomatosis cerebri who were treated with TMZ and had tissue available for analysis were evaluated; as might be expected from the data on anaplastic gliomas, patients with tumors containing the 1p19q codeletion were both more likely to respond to TMZ and to have improvement in PFS as well as OS relative to those without codeletion. However, again analogous to higher-grade tumors, there were patients without the codeletion who responded to chemotherapy. *MGMT* promoter methylation status was also evaluated, although analysis could not be accomplished in all patients; there was a trend toward improved PFS and OS in patients with methylation in the small cohort tested.

Conclusions

The optimal treatment of patients with LGGs remains controversial as there is no level 1 evidence addressing many of the pressing clinical issues. Even the question of whether initial therapy should consist of surgery or close observation remains debated, as suggested by Practice Guidelines from the National Comprehensive Cancer Network: "surgery is generally recommended, but serial observations are appropriate for some patients" [63]. Therefore, although general comments can be made regarding various options, ultimate decisions regarding therapeutic approach must stem from a comprehensive discussion of risks and benefits with the individual patient.

The bulk of available evidence supports improved outcome for maximal surgical resection rather than biopsy. In addition, more extensive resections lead to more accurate pathological diagnoses and provide tissue for molecular analysis. The implications of 1p19q and *MGMT* status in LGGs are just beginning to be understood, and in the future there will undoubtedly be more markers to inform prognosis and treatment decisions. When RT is administered, higher doses cause more toxicity without a survival benefit, and lower doses (e.g., 45–54 Gy) are standard. RT at time of LGG diagnosis seems to extend PFS without a clear impact on OS, so ongoing work is re-examining the issue of RT with an emphasis on quality-of-life measures and stratification by risk group. Chemotherapy is becoming more commonly used for LGGs. PCV and TMZ are both reasonable chemotherapy regimens, although the former is likely to be more toxic, and the latter is used more frequently despite lack of comparative data and unanswered questions about optimal dosing (standard, dose dense, dose intense, metronomic, protracted, etc.). Oligodendroglial tumors, particularly those with 1p19q codeletion, are thought to be especially sensitive to chemotherapy, but TMZ and PCV have been employed against LGGs of all subtypes.

Older patients (generally defined as ≥40 years, although recognizing that age is a continuous variable and 40 is an arbitrary cutoff point) [18] who are symptomatic from nonresectable large astrocytomas crossing the midline with neither 1p19q codeletion nor *MGMT* promoter methylation are at extremely high risk for short survival. Aggressive therapy for such patients with RT and/or chemotherapy may be undertaken, although it remains unclear whether such interventions immediately after diagnosis improve survival, and whether RT and chemotherapy should be used together (RTOG 0424, ECOG/NCCTG E3F05). In contrast, young epileptic patients (who are otherwise asymptomatic) with small, unilobar, pure oligodendrogliomas with 1p19q codeletion and *MGMT* promoter methylation who undergo gross total resection may live for a decade or more without disease progression. Deferring RT and chemotherapy in favor of surveillance by MRI and neurologic examination is a reasonable approach, and Arm 1 of RTOG 9802 (observation for patients under 40 with gross total resection) is predicated on the understanding that deferred RT for such "low risk" patients is a reasonable option. However, initiation of RT or chemotherapy postoperatively is also sound (EORTC 22845). When treatment is initiated, either at diagnosis or recurrence, chemotherapy may exert prolonged disease control, deferring the potential RT-induced neurocognitive toxicity. To address these questions regarding neoadjuvant chemotherapy and the potential benefit to delaying neurocognitive toxicity from RT, mature results from several studies (EORTC 22033/26033-NCIC CE5, E3F05, RTOG 0424, and RTOG 9802) are awaited.

HIGH-GRADE GLIOMAS

WHO grade III and IV tumors are often called high-grade gliomas or "malignant gliomas." Over 75% of gliomas are "malignant"[3]. Although they represent only 1.4% of all malignant cancers [1], they account for almost twice as many (2.4%) cancer deaths [1], reflecting their aggressive behavior. Notably, their malignancy derives from the intractable growth within the brain, usually at the same location, rather than from metastases to other organs. Such metastatic potential that helps to define malignancy in primary cancers of other organs (the "M" in TNM), while not unheard of, is distinctly unusual for gliomas. In addition, some patients with WHO grade III tumors may experience relatively long survival (e.g., young asymptomatic patients with completely resected pure oligodendrogliomas that harbor 1p19q codeletion and *MGMT* promoter methylation. Therefore, "malignant" gliomas are neither benign nor malignant in the traditional sense, although they certainly do become aggressive with time and are ultimately incurable in almost all patients with currently available therapies. Anaplastic astrocytomas (AAs), anaplastic oligodendrogliomas (AOs), and anaplastic oligoastrocytomas (AOAs, also called anaplastic mixed gliomas comprising elements of both), and GBM are the most common malignant gliomas in adults and are the subject of this chapter.

Older literature did not distinguish among histologic variants of malignant glioma in reporting treatment outcomes. However, the median survival differs among them, ranging from just over 1 year for patients with GBM treated in clinical trials to over 5 years for AO. Modern trials, recognizing these differences, often enroll patients with only one subtype or prespecify statistical subanalyses when enrolling all malignant gliomas.

Glioblastoma

GBM (or glioblastoma multiforme) [61] is the most common [3], and most aggressive, subtype of glioma (Figure 63.2). Typical symptoms include headache, cognitive changes, seizures, and/or focal neurological deficits such as weakness. MRI classically shows a ring-enhancing lesion surrounding a central area of necrosis on T1-weighted imaging, along with significant FLAIR hyperintensity surrounding the lesion representing vasogenic edema and non-enhancing tumor (Figure 63.2). Pseudopallisading necrosis is a histologic hallmark. In almost all cases, GBMs grow inexorably, eventually becoming refractory to all therapy. However, there are anecdotal reports of "cured" patients [62], and recent data demonstrate 5-year survival of almost 30% in patients with favorable prognostic factors (age <50 and high performance status) [63].

Surgery

Surgery has been and remains a critical component in the treatment of GBM. The survival benefit of resection was described over 80 years ago by Bailey and Cushing who observed that "in . . . 5 unoperated cases, average duration of life . . . was *3 months* . . . [and was] *12 months* for those surgically treated" (emphasis added) [64]. They were describing "spongioblastoma multiforme" corresponding to the modern designation of "glioblastoma multiforme" (Marc Rosenblum, personal communication). Results published 40 years later also appeared to confirm this observation, with patients undergoing "extensive resection" surviving longer than "partial resection" and in turn longer than "external decompression" presumably without any resection [65]. Several modern series also support the conclusion that extent of resection is an important determinant of survival [69]. Devaux et al [73] retrospectively studied patients with GBM who underwent resection and RT in comparison with those who underwent biopsy and RT [70]. Median survival for the resection group was 50.6 weeks, whereas those who underwent biopsy had a median survival of 33.0 weeks. Lacroix et al retrospectively analyzed results from over 400 patients and demonstrated that resection of at least 98% of tumor tissue significantly increased median

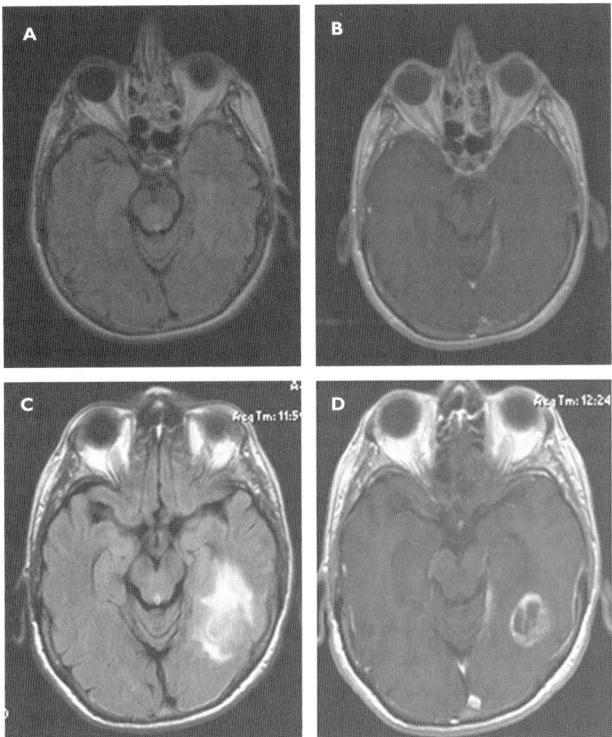

Figure 63.2 Glioblastoma (GBM). A seizure led to brain magnetic resonance imaging (MRI) scanning that was normal **(A)** FLAIR, **(B)** T1 image following gadolinium injection. Three months later a follow-up scan revealed mass characterized by edema and nonenhancing tumor **(C)** FLAIR surrounding an enhancing mass **(D)** typical of a GBM.

survival (13 vs. 8.8 months, $p < .0001$) [71]. Factors that limit extent of resection include tumor in areas of the brain considered eloquent, surgically inaccessible tumor locations, and other medical conditions that would otherwise make the patient a poor surgical candidate. Unfortunately, these same factors unavoidably generate potential bias in retrospective studies of the issue. Despite these limitations, maximal surgical resection is part of the currently accepted standard of care, certainly for patients <65 years old. As in LGGs, benefits of larger resection also include increased diagnostic accuracy and tissue for molecular profiling that may both prognosticate and guide therapy in the near future.

While surgery is an important part of the overall treatment paradigm for GBM, resection itself is not curative. In 1913, Ballance wrote: "No one in his senses has yet proposed to do a hemicerebrectomy for malignant disease in one cerebral hemisphere" [72]. Walter Dandy apparently disagreed, proclaiming "There is only one possible way of curing a patient with a brain tumor, and that is by complete removal" [73]. From the 1920s to 1950s, he and others attempted curative resection by removal of the entire right hemisphere [74,75]. Gliomas, however, have "infiltrating propensities" without clear demarcation from normal brain tissue, recognized as early as 1926 [64]. Therefore, recurrences were observed despite such hemispherectomies, and therapeutic efforts must include treatments with the potential to target both focal disease and microscopic tumor cells throughout the brain.

Radiotherapy

In its current form, RT for GBM is administered to the gross tumor volume and a margin of several centimeters. The benefits of radiation in high-grade gliomas have been clearly documented since the 1970s [76] and its use for "gliomata" dates back at least to 1925 [77]. Shapiro and Young in 1976 published a comparison of patients who received chemotherapy versus patients who received chemotherapy and RT [78]. The RT consisted of 4.5 Gy to the whole brain plus 1.5 Gy to the side of the tumor. They found an increased median survival of 44.5 weeks for the group that received both RT and chemotherapy (carmustine [BCNU] and vincristine) compared with 30 weeks for the group that received chemotherapy only. Cooperative group trials shortly thereafter demonstrated improved survival for RT with or without nitrosourea chemotherapy in comparison to best supportive care or nitrosourea alone. Median survival was 9 to 12 months when treatment included RT, and approximately one-half of that when RT was omitted [79–81]. Although there has been enthusiasm for radiosurgery in the past [82], its use in treatment of newly diagnosed GBM has been all but abandoned following negative randomized trials [83–85]. The current standard for RT is to deliver a total of approximately 60 Gy in 30 fractions. Many trials have explored different total radiation doses, fractionation, and delivery methods, although ~60 Gy in ~30 fractions remains the current standard. RT is discussed in more detail in a separate chapter.

Chemotherapy

Cytotoxic chemotherapy has been used for brain tumors for over 50 years [86]. Unlike surgical resection and RT, which have long been widely accepted as cornerstones of malignant glioma therapy, the merits of chemotherapy were debated until very recently. Early trials of cytotoxic agents suggested benefit, but no single randomized controlled trial demonstrated a statistically significant impact on survival. Efficacy was confirmed only by meta-analysis [87,88]. Not until the development of TMZ was the addition of chemotherapy to surgery and radiation unambiguously shown to prolong survival in patients with newly diagnosed GBM [7].

Nitrosoureas and other Chemotherapies

Early studies of the efficacy of various agents on malignant gliomas were disappointing. Benefits of chemotherapy, especially carmustine [79,80,89] or procarbazine [89], were small at best. However, it was noted that a subgroup of approximately 15% of patients survived at least two years, and some much longer [79,80]. Therefore, median survival was not improved by the addition of chemotherapy to radiation, but the "tail of the curve" flattened, improving the odds of prolonged survival from 5% or less to about 15%. Many clinicians, especially in the United States, advocated treatment of all patients because it would lead to definitive benefit for a fortunate few, whereas clinicians in Europe often advocated a more conservative approach. From these early studies, clinically important prognostic factors were identified, such as age, Karnofsky Performance Status [90], extent of resection, and histology (GBM vs. others). However, these were prognostic factors among all patients, rather than predictors of chemosensitivity in particular. A pooled analysis of two prospective Brain Tumor Study Group trials demonstrated improved survival with adjuvant nitrosourea chemotherapy that was independent of prognostic factors and not attributable to inclusion of AOs (which are more "chemosensitive" than other malignant glioma subtypes) [91]. The importance of *MGMT* promoter methylation in glioma sensitivity to alkylating agents such as carmustine was already known [92], but analysis of archival tissue for *MGMT* methylation status was neither widespread nor routine.

While the results of individual studies of chemotherapeutic agents did not show definitive survival advantage with chemotherapy, meta-analyses appeared to demonstrate a marginal benefit of chemotherapy. In 1993, Fine et al [87] studied 16 different clinical trials involving different chemotherapy agents, in an attempt to compare survival of patients who underwent RT alone versus patients who underwent RT and various nitrosoureas or other chemotherapy regimens. Results for over 3000 patients were considered, and the authors concluded that there was a survival advantage for patients with malignant gliomas who undergo adjuvant chemotherapy compared with those patients who undergo RT alone. Another meta-analysis by the Glioma Meta-analysis Trialists Group in 2002 sought to further clarify the issue of benefit of chemotherapy. It identified 19 randomized trials totaling 3004 patients with high-grade gliomas, also treated with a variety of chemotherapies. Their findings showed a statistically significant 2-month overall increase in median survival, as well as a 6% increase (40% to 46%) in 1-year survival with chemotherapy versus the groups with RT alone [88].

The most commonly used non-TMZ chemotherapies remain the nitrosoureas, especially carmustine, with procarbazine as an alternative [89]. Irinotecan is commonly administered with the targeted agent bevacizumab (below), but rarely as a monotherapy. The use of PCV has become less common following a large retrospective analysis that suggested no benefit but increased toxicity in comparison with carmustine monotherapy for patients with AA [93]. These therapies are now largely limited to use in recurrent GBM after RT and TMZ therapy.

Temozolomide

TMZ is an orally administered methylating agent with excellent bioavailability and blood–brain barrier penetration. In comparison with other DNA alkylating agents, TMZ is generally well-tolerated. Promising results in a single arm phase II study of recurrent AA [94] led to FDA approval for that indication. A follow-up study also demonstrated superiority to procarbazine in a randomized study of TMZ-naïve recurrent GBM [95]. This changed the standard treatment paradigm, as procarbazine was among the most commonly prescribed agents for recurrent disease at that time (with carmustine generally already used as part of the initial treatment strategy) [89,96]. Benefit in patients with newly diagnosed GBM was reported before [97], during [98], and both during and following RT [99] with reasonable safety.

The standard treatment of newly diagnosed GBM has included TMZ since the initial publication [7] of a phase III study of TMZ both during and following RT involving 573 patients conducted by the EORTC (22981/26981) and the NCIC (CE.3). TMZ during RT was dosed at 75 mg/m^2 daily, and following RT at 150 to 200 mg/m^2 for days 1 to 5 of 28 days (one cycle). Adjuvant treatment was administered for up to six cycles. The median improvement in survival was significant but modest: 14.6 months for RT alone and 12.1 months for RT with concurrent and adjuvant TMZ ($p < .001$). However, the benefit was sustained: the 2-year OS rate was 26.5% following RT + TMZ but only 10.7% following RT alone [7]. Long-term follow-up has also demonstrated prolonged benefit, with 3-year, 4-year, and 5-year OS rates of 16% versus 4%, 12% versus 3%, and 10% versus 2% (RT + TMZ vs. RT alone), respectively [63]. It is important to note that patients received prophylaxis for PCP pneumonia during the concurrent phase of therapy because of increased risk of such infection during that period, presumably related to lymphopenia.

Many active clinical trials are attempting to discover even more efficacious temozolomide-based regimens through a variety of different dosing schedules [100], or by combining temozolomide with other agents. An understanding of the mechanism of TMZ as well as proposed mechanisms of resistance to TMZ is important in conceptualizing these regimens. TMZ ultimately leads to cell death by methylating DNA at several sites including the O^6 position on guanine. This process can be reversed by the DNA repair enzyme O^6-alkylguanine DNA alkyltransferase (AGT or AGAT), which is encoded by the gene MGMT, and which is irreversibly inactivated in the process of DNA repair [101]. 1p19q codeletion is common in AOs [105, 106] but unusual in GBMs. Therefore, a companion study to the EORTC/NCIC phase III trial analyzed pretreatment archival tissue for other molecular correlates of outcome [46]. This study demonstrated that MGMT promoter methylation correlated with survival. The presumed explanation is that promoter methylation causes epigenetic silencing of AGT protein expression (commonly called MGMT for simplicity), reducing the ability of gliomas cells to thwart the methylation by TMZ. The effect of MGMT promoter methylation on median survival among those taking TMZ was striking: 23.4 months (methylated) versus 12.6 months (unmethylated), and the 2-year OS rate was 49% versus 15%. This difference was sustained: 4-year OS was 22.1% for patients with methylated promoter status who received RT and TMZ in comparison with 7.8% for RT alone (p=0.035) [102]. After 5 years of follow-up, MGMT promoter methylation status was the strongest prognostic factor for survival [63].

The mechanism by which MGMT promoter methylation status influences survival may be more complicated than initially appreciated. First, MGMT protein expression does not correlate with survival [49]. Although technical problems with immunohistochemistry could partially explain this discrepancy, it also suggests that the molecular biology remains incompletely understood. As further evidence, TMZ administration to patients who were later found to have tumors with unmethylated MGMT promoters also prolonged survival relative to patients treated with RT alone [7,63]. In addition, MGMT promoter methylation was associated with longer survival among patients who received RT alone (without TMZ) as initial therapy [108]. Thus, it appears that MGMT promoter methylation is a prognostic marker, conferring a survival advantage regardless of the therapy applied, in addition to serving as a predictive marker of TMZ sensitivity, further suggesting that the molecular mechanism is more complicated than presently understood. Several trials under development will use methylation status as an inclusion/exclusion criteria. However, outside of a clinical trial and absent superior alternatives, standard of care involves maximal surgical resection (with [104] or without [7] carmustine wafer placement detailed below) followed by RT with concurrent and adjuvant TMZ. This is true regardless of MGMT promoter methylation status [105]. The tolerability of TMZ [7] (including minimal effects on health-related quality of life [106]) reinforces this conclusion. However, the financial cost of TMZ administered during and following RT is substantial. Whether the potential benefit of TMZ in the setting of unmethylated MGMT promoter status warrants that financial burden is beyond the scope of this chapter. The poly(ADP-ribose) polymerase (PARP) system is another mechanism by which tumor cells repair the DNA damage induced by TMZ. While MGMT reverses methylation of the O^6 position on guanine, the PARP enzyme repairs methylation of several other sites, including N^7-guanine and N^3-adenine. The PARP system has, to date, been less well studied than MGMT, but it presents an attractive target for investigation, and may prove to have prognostic and/or therapeutic implications in the future [107].

In light of the mechanisms of temozolomide action and resistance discussed earlier, many of the avenues currently being investigated to improve temozolomide effectiveness are quite intuitive. First, a variety of alternative TMZ dosing regimens are being studied [100]. All patients in the EORTC/NCIC trial received both concurrent and adjuvant temozolomide [7]. However, it is unclear which phase of the chemotherapy is important or whether both are required. A planned trial with a double cross over design will seek to answer this question in patients with non-1p19q deleted anaplastic gliomas (EORTC 26053–22054 CATNON Intergroup trial), although application to GBMs would require extrapolation. There is evidence to suggest that TMZ is a radiation sensitizer [108], implying that the concurrent phase with RT is required for full effect, although not necessarily to the exclusion of adjuvant treatment. Moreover, a trial of 53 patients with GBM who received concurrent TMZ (at 50 mg/m^2) with RT but not adjuvant TMZ demonstrated a median OS of 19 months and 2-year OS of 29% [98]. This compares favorably with the results from the combined regimen (median OS 14.6 moths, 2-year OS 27%) [7,63]. Second, it is unknown whether TMZ intensification (using 75–100 mg/m^2 for days 1–21, 150 mg/m^2 for days 1–7 and 15–21, 50 mg/m^2 for days 1–28, or others) may prove superior to standard adjuvant dosing (150–200 mg/m^2 for days

1–5). Given that MGMT is irreversibly inactivated when it repairs methylation of O^6-guanine, there is reason to think that protracted dosing regimens may be able to overcome the MGMT DNA repair system and thus have greater efficacy [48]. Confirmation of this idea through a prospective trial, RTOG 0525/EORTC 26052–22053, is planned. That trial, which recently completed accrual of more than 1000 patients, randomized patients to either standard dose TMZ or a "dose-intense" regimen (75–100 mg/m^2 for days 1–21 of 28). More direct inhibition of DNA repair through the use of inhibitors of MGMT [109–112], or PARP [107] along with TMZ, may also prove useful. Third, the duration of post-RT adjuvant TMZ was set arbitrarily at six cycles in the NCIC-EORTC trial [7]. For patients who remain progression-free, it is possible that continued TMZ beyond six adjuvant cycles may improve outcome despite a potential risk of myelodysplasia/leukemia [113], although that remains highly controversial. Finally, the EORTC/NCIC trial excluded adults older than 70 years of age. Whether the treatment paradigm of concurrent and adjuvant TMZ with RT benefits these patients is unclear. Patients under 18 years of age were also excluded, and treatment of children is discussed in a separate chapter. Alternative strategies for treatment of the elderly are discussed below.

An unexpected observation in patients who receive concurrent RT and TMZ is that, for reasons that are unclear, the brain MRI may appear worse during the first few months after RT and then spontaneously improve. This phenomenon, called "pseudoprogression," is well known for patients with glioma who receive RT alone [114], and it may be more common among patients who receive concurrent TMZ occurring in 14%-67% of patients [115–118]. The wide range of reported incidence may result from differences in the definition of pseudoprogression. Nonetheless, it is probably fair to conclude that a substantial subset of patients with a post-RT MRI demonstrating disease progression may experience spontaneous improvement without a change in the planned therapy. In our experience, only surgical documentation accurately distinguished true progression from psuedoprogression, a conclusion also drawn by others [119]. Noninvasive imaging by positron emission tomography (PET), MR spectroscopy, and/or MR Perufsion is typically inadequate [120]. In patients without concurrent clinical worsening, it may be reasonable to continue adjuvant TMZ with close surveillance. Symptomatic patients may benefit from surgery, both therapeutically and diagnostically. However, this is an area of great controversy. *MGMT* promoter methylation may associate with pseudoprogression, but this requires validation by other studies [116]. There are also substantial implications for clinical trial design [121–123].

Chemotherapy as focal treatment

The use of chemotherapy as a focal treatment for residual macroscopic or microscopic disease in the postoperative cavity and surrounding tissue gained acceptance in the form of the Gliadel®. With this delivery method, concerns of medication delivery and the obstacle of the blood–brain barrier were circumvented. The wafers contain carmustine, which is released to the surrounding tissue as the wafers dissolve. Their efficacy was tested first for recurrent GBM, demonstrating a 2-month survival advantage for wafer therapy versus placebo (p = .02) [129]. A follow-up study evaluated wafer utility in patients with newly diagnosed malignant gliomas, again demonstrating a 2-month survival benefit [130]. Long-term follow-up demonstrated persistent benefits in survival after 2 and 3 years [131]. Of note, however, the advantage in the GBM subset did not achieve statistical significance. In addition, potential for side effects unique to chemotherapy wafers must be weighed against the reduced risk of systemic toxicity by avoidance of intravenous BCNU. Efficacy and toxicity of intracavitary versus systemically administered carmustine have not been compared. Nonetheless, Gliadel is an FDA-approved therapy during resection of recurrent GBM and newly diagnosed malignant gliomas.

Other locally delivered therapies have not proven useful. The PRECISE trial found no difference between patients randomized to Glaidel or convection enhanced delivery (CED) of IL-13 linked to *Pseudomonas* exotoxin [132]. Similarly, the TransMID trial for patients with recurrent GBM, which utilized transferrin linked to diphtheria toxin, was stopped early because of negative results [133].

GBM in the Elderly

There is no standard of care for patients over 70 years old with newly diagnosed GBM, despite the median age at diagnosis of 64 years [3]. Median survival for elderly patients is dismal. RT is associated with improved median OS when compared with supportive care [134]. However, the median duration of benefit (12.2) weeks is only about twice as long as the typical duration of RT. Abbreviated courses (40 Gy in 15 fractions over 3 weeks) of RT appear noninferior to standard schemes (60 Gy in 30 fractions over 6 weeks) [135]. The deleterious effects of brain RT on cognition may be pronounced for elderly patients. Therefore, several studies assessed the role of TMZ as first-line therapy without RT. In one phase II trial of 32 patients, responses were observed in 31%. Median OS and PFS were 6.4 and 5.0 months, respectively [136]. A retrospective comparison of elderly patients with malignant gliomas also suggested no survival difference between TMZ and RT [137].

The optimal approach remains unclear. High functioning patients in their early to mid-70s may benefit from combined RT and TMZ, and such treatment is a reasonable option [138]. Other patients, such as the very old or those with a KPS of 50 to 60, may not tolerate RT, and neoadjuvant TMZ is a rational approach for those in whom definitive therapy is appropriate. No consensus exists, and the exclusion of patients over 70 years from most large clinical trials suggests that none is likely to emerge. Ongoing European trials from the German and Nordic Neuro-Oncology groups may provide insight.

Recurrent GBM

Despite aggressive treatment with the best available initial therapy regimens, patients almost invariably suffer disease recurrence/progression. Typically, recurrent disease is observed at or adjacent to the site of the original tumor

[139] (although this is controversial following antiangiogenic therapies detailed below). Often, patients are asymptomatic and the recurrence is isolated to radiographic analyses. There is no standard of care for recurrent GBM at this time. The location may be amenable to reoperation. Generally, reirradiation is not applied because of concerns over neurotoxicity including radiation necrosis following 60 Gy of initial treatment. Chemotherapy is the mainstay of treatment for recurrent disease, but until recently there were few effective agents. TMZ can be considered in patients who are TMZ-naïve [98] or in whom TMZ was discontinued for reasons other than resistant tumor [140]. For patients with disease that has demonstrated resistance to TMZ, there is no standard regimen. Numerous phase II studies yielded unsatisfactory results. A pooled analysis of 225 patients enrolled to such trials has been used as the benchmark for the rate of ineffective therapy. The 6mPFS rate was 15% in this commonly cited analysis. Only 6% of patients responded, and median PFS and OS were 2 and 6 months, respectively [141]. Updated analysis yielded similar results with a 6mPFS of 9% in trials that excluded TMZ [142].

Nitrosoureas, or less commonly platinums, are often advocated [143]. Combinations of alkylators, such as carmustine with TMZ, appear to increase toxicity without a benefit [144]. Procarbazine is clearly inferior to TMZ among TMZ-naïve patients. For example, the 6mPFS rate for patients receiving procarbazine was 8% versus 21% for TMZ ($p = .008$) [98]. Others reported a similar 18% 6mPFS rate for TMZ [145]. However, most patients have already received TMZ as part of their initial therapy since publication of the EORTC/NCIC study by Stupp et al [7]. Presumably, procarbazine is inferior to carmustine as well based on indirect comparisons. For example, a recent phase II trial of 40 patients treated with carmustine administered systemically yielded a response rate of 15% and median PFS and OS of 3 and 7.5 months with a 6mPFS rate of 17.5% [146]. It remains unclear whether systemic carmustine is superior, inferior, or equivalent to Gliadel wafers. The potential for systemic toxicity of the former (e.g., fatigue, pulmonary fibrosis, and myelosuppression) must also be weighed against the potential for CNS toxicity from the latter (e.g., wound breakdown, CSF leak, infection, and difficulty interpreting brain imaging). Efforts at suppressing MGMT activity are also underway in an attempt to improve efficacy of alkylators [114–117].

Molecularly-Targeted Therapies

Efforts worldwide are underway to elucidate the molecular biology of GBM as a method to improve therapy. In brief, it is widely recognized that abnormalities in signaling pathways used by cells to control activities such as growth, division, and cell death contribute to the formation and behavior of glial tumors. The identification of abnormalities of epidermal growth factor receptor (EGFR), platelet derived growth factor receptor (PDGFR), vascular endothelial growth factor receptor (VEGFR), and other signaling pathways led to numerous trials of such molecularly targeted agents for recurrent GBM, and less frequently for newly diagnosed disease. Unfortunately, trials of such inhibitors of EGFR [147–152], PDGFR [153–155], and mTOR were all associated with 6mPFS rates and responses in <20% and 10% of patients with recurrent disease, respectively. Despite the disappointing results of these early trials, there remains a great deal of optimism that molecularly targeted therapies will prove effective in the treatment of GBM. An extensive review of molecularly targeted therapies is found elsewhere in this text. We will focus on the VEGF pathway as a model of this paradigm as well as discuss the direction of current and future trials of targeted therapies.

Since the 1970s, angiogenesis has been recognized as a key process in tumor growth and survival. Further, vascular proliferation is a pathological hallmark of GBM. Given this background, VEGF and its downstream signaling pathway have been the target of numerous agents in GBM and other cancers. The VEGF pathway agent that has been most extensively investigated is bevacizumab, a humanized monoclonal antibody that binds to VEGF and inhibits its ability to activate VEGFR.

The efficacy of bevacizumab was first demonstrated in colorectal cancer, where it was combined with irinotecan [156]. Drawing on this experience, similar regimens were evaluated in other cancers. Treatment of 21 patients with recurrent malignant gliomas (including 11 with GBM) induced responses in 43% and clinical improvement in others with radiographically stable disease [157]. This was followed by a single institution phase II study of 32 patients with malignant glioma demonstrating responses in 63% of patients [158]. Follow-up of those with GBMs demonstrated a 57% response rate, 46% 6mPFS rate, and 15.5-month median OS [159]. Retrospective series produced similar results [160]. A multicenter trial of 82 patients demonstrated responses in 38% (after central imaging review), 50% 6mPFS, and 8.7 month median OS [161]. The median OS (8.7 months, 95% CI 7.8–10.9) was clearly longer than historic controls (5.7 months, 95% CI 4.8–6.4) [141]. Although a randomized study comparing bevacizumab and irinotecan against other therapies has not been completed, these results are very encouraging. Similarly encouraging results have been observed with other VEGF-targeting agents including aflibercept (previously called VEGF-Trap) [162] and cediranib (previously called AZD2171) [163] as well as bevacizumab alone [164,165]. Reasonable safety and potential synergy with reirradiation for recurrent disease has also been reported, with an estimated 6mPFS rate of 76% in a pilot study [166]. Enthusiasm associated with agents such as bevacizumab has led to their use in the treatment of newly diagnosed GBM, typically as an addition to the standard regimen of RT with concurrent and adjuvant TMZ. One pilot study of 10 patients with GBM suggests that adding bevacizumab to RT and TMZ may improve median PFS (>8.8 months) [167] when indirectly compared with standard RT + TMZ (6.9 months) [7].

Anti-VEGF therapy is general well-tolerated. However, the potential toxicity is substantial and led to discontinuation of therapy in up to 31% of patients [158,159,164,165,167]. Adverse events included thromboembolic events (i.e., pulmonary embolus, ischemic, and hemorrhagic stroke), hypertension, reversible posterior leukoencephalopathy syndrome (PRES), heart failure, myelosuppression, sepsis, proteinuria, fatigue, gastrointestinal perforation, wound healing complications, and others. Deep venous thrombosis (DVT) was also reported, but up to 30% of patients with GBM develop DVT [168], and the contribution of bevacizumab is unclear for such venous thromboembolic events. Nonetheless, these toxicities were fatal in upto 10% of patients across the various studies [157–159,164,165]. For patients with recurrent disease with few alternatives outside of a clinical trial, the potential toxicity may be warranted. However, for patients with newly diagnosed disease, the risk of severe or even fatal toxicity is a serious consideration, especially in light of the observation that 49% of patients with tumors exhibiting *MGMT* promoter methylation were alive 2 years after standard treatment (RT + TMZ) [66]. It is conceivable that adding bevacizumab to the initial therapy for such patients may shorten rather than prolong survival because of either toxicity, or by changing the natural history of the disease toward a more invasive phenotype. Planned prospective trials of VEGF/VEGFR targeting agents will address this issue.

A variety of pressing questions about bevacizumab therapy remain unanswered. Among the most important is whether irinotecan is an important part of the regimen. Irinotecan was used with bevacizumab in the treatment of recurrent GBM because of the adoption of the regimen from the treatment of colon cancer [157]. However, irinotecan monotherapy has only minimal activity in treatment of recurrent GBM when compared with negative historic control data [141,159,169–171]. Bevacizumab alone appears to have noninferior efficacy to combined therapy with less toxicity in one trial; however, it should be noted that such a comparison was not part of the statistical design of the study [165]. Further studies of bevacizumab alone and in combination with irinotecan and other agents will be necessary to answer this question. Another area of uncertainty is how best to treat disease following progression on a bevacizumab containing regimen. For patients on a monotherapy, continuing bevacizumab but initiating TMZ or another agent is one approach; adding irinotecan appears to have very little efficacy in this setting [161,164,165]. For patients already receiving concurrent cytotoxic chemotherapy, such as with irinotecan, continuing the bevacizumab but switching the cytotoxic to an alternative agent does not appear particularly effective in observational series [172]. However, data suggest that discontinuing the bevacizumab altogether in favor of an alternate chemotherapy regimen without a direct VEGF/VEGFR inhibitor is equally discouraging [173]. Rapid deterioration often seen following discontinuation of bevacizumab could result from a "rebound" effect of increased edema. This effect has been observed in the setting of bevacizumab use for macular edema [174], although no similar data have been formally published for gliomas. It is also not clear if progression on bevacizumab implies failure of all VEGF/VEGFR inhibitors, or whether other drugs with a similar mechanism of action could provide "rescue." Therefore, changing VEGF/VEGFR targeting agents, either alone or in combination with other drugs, is one area of investigation [175]. It has also been proposed that treatment with VEGF/VEGFR inhibitors changes the natural history of the disease toward a more invasive and treatment resistant phenotype (Patrick Y. Wen, personal communication). A pattern of diffusely infiltrative, multifocal disease has been observed following progression on bevacizumab [160,176]. Therefore, it may be desirable to use bevacizumab for second or later GBM recurrence. New clinical trials will be required to answer these questions, and several are either ongoing or planned. Finally, imaging on bevacizumab trials is particularly difficult [127]. The agent itself directly affects cerebral vasculature and rapidly reduces contrast enhancement without necessarily reflecting true disease response, thus calling into question the validity of radiographic response rate and lack of radiographic progression at 6 months as end points for clinical trials. Whether response criteria must incorporate nonenhancing abnormality is an area of controversy at this time [127,128]. PET imaging with novel radiotracers, such as [^{18}F]-fluorothymidine (FLT), may also help predict bevacizumab response [177]. However, such imaging is not widely available.

Although questions of monotherapy versus combination therapy, response to treatment failure, and validity of response criteria have been discussed with an emphasis on antiangiogenic therapies in general and bevacizumab in specific, similar concerns apply to other novel targeted therapies [178]. Additionally, a great deal of recent work has focused on identifying a subset of patients who may respond to such agents based on analysis of pretreatment tissue. For example, expression of the most commonly found constitutively active mutant form of *EGFR*, variant III (EGFRvIII) in the setting of retained expression of phosphatase and tensin homologue deleted in chromosome 10 (PTEN) robustly predicted response to erlotinib or gefitinib in one study [179]. This result remains controversial and must be validated.

In summary, molecularly targeted agents such as bevacizumab will likely have a role in the standard management of patients with recurrent GBM and other malignant gliomas in the near future, and perhaps for newly diagnosed disease as well. However, when (at diagnosis, at first recurrence, at later recurrence) and how (alone, in combination with conventional chemotherapeutic agents, or in combination with other targeted therapies) such agents are best utilized remain unclear at this time, as does the optimal efficacy measurement.

Anaplastic Astrocytoma

After GBM, AAs are the most common malignant gliomas [3]. They are WHO grade III tumors [64], but are far less chemosensitive than the other less common WHO grade III tumor, AO. Median survival is approximately 2 to 4 years, and age and KPS are important prognostic factors as in other gliomas [3,180,181]. Deletion of 1p19q appears to confer a survival advantage for patients with AA as it does for patients with oligodendroglial tumors [19], However, 1p19q codeletion is distinctly unusual in AAs, and its presence may even suggest re-examination of the histologic diagnosis. Like GBMs, they may arise de novo, or less commonly from an LGA. The clinical manifestations are similar to those in patients with GBM and depend on tumor location. Radiographically, they generally exhibit contrast enhancement. However, it is usually less pronounced and more heterogeneous than in GBMs. Ring enhancement on imaging may represent a poor prognostic sign [181].

Definitive treatment

As in patients with GBM, maximal resection is important for both diagnostic and therapeutic purposes, and it is followed by RT as the current standard of care [63]. Results of a recent German study questioned whether chemotherapy could substitute for RT [182], but the trial design has been criticized [183], and most neuro-oncologists advocate RT after surgery. Utility of adjuvant treatment after RT is more controversial. Older clinical trials generally included patients with all malignant glioma subtypes [83]. As it became clear that optimal management of patients with low- and high-grade gliomas may differ, recent trials have focused either on LGGs or GBMs, excluding patients with AA. Trials that allow patients with AA to enroll typically do so as an exploratory end point without statistical power to make efficacy judgments, and often patients with AAs are enrolled as a small subset of patients with anaplastic gliomas of various histologies.

Data that exist on a benefit for post-RT chemotherapy have been conflicting. One randomized trial demonstrated that PCV produced no improvement in median OS (about 13 months) for 113 patients with AA treated with RT and PCV versus RT alone [184]. The results of that study were questioned because the medians were short relative to historic controls. However, as in early studies of all malignant gliomas, the tails of the curve suggested a benefit among long-term survivors, with a 5.5% improvement in 2-year OS following treatment with PCV. A retrospective study also cast doubt on the benefit of more aggressive therapy at diagnosis [180]. One study even suggested that more aggressive therapy was harmful [185]. In contrast, a later meta-analysis of high-grade glioma studies that included 706 patients with AA showed an improvement in 1-year (63% vs. 58%) and 2-year (37% vs. 31%) survival for patients who received RT + chemotherapy ($n = 400$) versus RT alone ($n = 306$) [91].

Among treatment regimens, in the pre-TMZ era the most commonly used agent was carmustine or PCV. One prospective study suggested that following RT, PCV improves OS in comparison with carmustine [186]. This trial enrolled GBMs and anaplastic gliomas, but the results only reached significance in the latter. This led to the adoption of PCV as the standard adjuvant chemotherapy regimen for anaplastic gliomas. However, that study was criticized for a number of potential biases [96]. In a retrospective analysis of 432 patients with AA, there was no difference in OS (approximately 3 years) between PCV ($n = 175$) and carmustine ($n = 257$). This conclusion remained valid following stratification by age, KPS, and extent of resection [96]. As PCV was certainly more toxic, there appeared to be no reason to advise PCV over carmustine. Among patients who do receive adjuvant chemotherapy at diagnosis, TMZ became the drug of choice after it became available for recurrent AA [97] because of its favorable toxicity profile relative to other regimens such as carmustine or PCV in use at the time. However, direct prospective comparisons of TMZ with other regimens in AA have not been performed. For example, after a phase I trial demonstrated unacceptable toxicity during combined treatment with TMZ and carmustine [187], a phase III trial comparing the two regimens was initiated (RTOG 9813) but was halted for poor accrual [188]. There was a retrospective analysis of outcome among 109 patients with newly diagnosed AA that found no difference between PCV and TMZ in either median PFS or OS [189]. Although not level 1 evidence, this supports the conclusion that TMZ is likely noninferior to PCV. As the data suggest equivalence of PCV and carmustine [96], there is also probably no advantage for carmustine over TMZ either. At this time, prospective randomized trials comparing regimens are probably not feasible because of both the widespread use and tolerability of TMZ, as well as the interest in evaluating more novel approaches.

Support for combining TMZ with RT for treatment of newly diagnosed AA rests on extrapolation of the efficacy data for newly diagnosed GBM [7]. A recent German trial casts doubt on that extrapolation, with neither a PFS nor OS benefit for TMZ concurrently with RT, although the dose was lower (50 mg/m^2 rather than 75 mg/m^2) and no adjuvant TMZ was administered [190]. However, evidence in GBMs suggests that the concurrent phase is the most important [113] and that 50 mg/m^2 is as effective as 75 mg/m^2 with less toxicity [191]. In addition, if one argues for benefit from adjuvant therapy, it is important to recall that the landmark GBM trial administered a maximum of six adjuvant TMZ cycles. Treatment for more than six cycles has been advocated after RT for GBM by some investigators [192]. However, the relatively short median survival for GBM means that it is the uncommon patient in whom this question becomes relevant, and opportunity for continued TMZ beyond 12 or at most 18 months without progression is distinctly unusual. However, for patients with AA, in whom median survival is at least 2 years in most studies and longer survival is common, administering TMZ at diagnosis and until progression could lead to many years of such continued therapy. Whether this increases the risk of myelosuppression is unknown but is a reason for caution [118]. Therefore, debate continues over the proper role of adjuvant chemotherapy for patients with newly diagnosed AA. The EORTC 26053–22054 CATNON Intergroup trial will evaluate efficacy of RT alone versus TMZ administered concurrently with RT, versus after RT, versus both with and after RT for patients with newly diagnosed anaplastic gliomas without 1p19q codeletion, of which AAs will likely represent the majority. However, data from this trial will take many years to mature.

For patients with recurrent AA who are TMZ-naïve, TMZ is an effective agent. In a phase II study open to patients with recurrent anaplasticgliomas, the response rate was 34%, 6mPFS rate was 49%, median PFS was 5.5 months, and median OS was 14.2 months among the AA subset [97]. A later study yielded similar results among patients with anaplastic gliomas of all histologies [145]. These results compare favorably with pooled results of eight negative phase II trials involving 150 patients with recurrent AA demonstrating a response rate of 14%, 6mPFS rate 31%, median PFS 3 months, median OS 10.8 months

[141]. For patients requiring surgery, Gliadel is an option for recurrent malignant gliomas in general, although data are lacking for treatment of AAs specifically as the majority of patients enrolled onto a placebo controlled trial had other high-grade histologies [129]. There have been numerous studies using other agents, including 13-*cis*-retinoic acid alone [193] or in combination with TMZ [194] as well as trials of cyclophosphamide [195] and irinotecan [196]. However, none of these agents has achieved widespread acceptance with most recurrent AAs treated with regimens extrapolated from experience with GBMs. For example, as in GBMs, the combination of bevacizumab and irinotecan [157,158] is reported to have substantial activity in recurrent anaplastic gliomas. However, as in most recurrent malignant glioma trials, accrual of patients with anaplastic gliomas is a secondary or exploratory end point not powered to provide robust statistical analysis of efficacy. In many patients with recurrent AA, it is logical to apply GBM data as there is often radiographic evidence (i.e., increased amount or intensity of contrast enhancement, increased mass effect, etc.) that the tumor has transformed into a GBM despite the absence of histologic proof. However, this extrapolation may not be appropriate for all patients.

Anaplastic Oligodendroglioma

Oligodendrogliomas (both low grade and anaplastic) are far less common than astrocytomas, accounting for 5% to 10% of all gliomas, with low-grade tumors approximately twice as common as anaplastic variants [3]. Extra-CNS metastases and leptomeningeal spread are rare, but perhaps more common than in patients with astrocytomas, especially among patients with long survival [197,198]. Although AO may present as a "de novo" tumor, they may also arise from low-grade tumors [47]. The importance of histology in predicting survival, longer among patients with oligodendroglial tumors than astrocytomas of the same WHO grade, has led to a shift in diagnosis toward oligodendroglioma or mixed oligoastrocytoma [199]. This trend has implications for patient management as the diagnosis of AA mandates treatment with RT in almost all cases, while neoadjuvant chemotherapy with deferred RT may be appropriate for some patients with AO or AOA as discussed below. Therefore, the treating physician must have confidence that the histologic sample is valid for diagnosis (a rationale for more extensive resection) and in the expertise of the pathologist. Even among a panel of experts, there is often diagnostic disagreement [200–204]. Codeletion of 1p and 19q [205] lends comfort to the diagnosis, but 1p19q codeletion occurs in the presence of nonclassic histology, and vice versa, demonstrating that molecular features are important but not to the exclusion of histology [200,202,204].

Several studies have demonstrated that 1p19q codeletion is both predictive of response to treatment and prognostic for improved survival [39,206,207]. Ino and colleagues [207] identified four distinct molecular subtypes of AO: those with 1p19q codeletion had a prolonged response to chemotherapy of over 2.6 years and survived longer than 10 years on average; those with 1p but neither 19q deletion nor other oncogenic abnormalities had an average response lasting 0.9 years and survived 5.9 years; those without 1p deletions but with *TP53* mutations had a shorter response interval of 0.6 years and OS of 5.9 years; those with neither 1p deletion nor *TP53* mutation but with the presence of other oncogenic mutations responded for only 0.4 years with OS of 1.3 years. Other investigators have confirmed these observations, making 1p19q status arguably the most important prognostic factor for oligodendrogliomas. In LGO with 1p19q codeletion, 5-year survival rates have been reported at 97% compared with 70% for those without deletions [208]. Median survival for LGOs in one study was 13.0 years for those with deletion versus 9.1 years for those without it [20]. AOs have a considerably worse prognosis than low-grade tumors; those with codeletion have a median OS of 6 to 7 years compared with 2 to 3 years for those without [207]. Furthermore, oligodendrogliomas with 1p19q codeletion may also exhibit more indolent behavior before treatment [209].

Definitive treatment

Surgery and Radiotherapy

As in other gliomas, resection of AOs is both diagnostic and therapeutic. Despite their potential chemo- and radiosensitivity, large trials for AOs demonstrated an association between extent of resection and survival [105,106]. Hence, maximal surgical resection is generally accepted as standard initial treatment. Early studies demonstrating the benefit of RT with or without chemotherapy (carmustine) in comparison to RT alone did not distinguish among histologic subtypes of high-grade gliomas [82]. Few addressed the utility of RT specifically in AOs [210,211]. Therefore, although RT is undisputed as an effective treatment modality for malignant gliomas in general, the risks of delayed toxicity are nontrivial for AO specifically, particularly in the subset of patients with 1p19q codeletion who may live decades or longer. Therefore, since the first reports of chemosensitivity 20 years ago, debate has centered on the optimal timing and type of chemotherapy. This controversy remains unresolved, as a recent survey of almost 100 neuro-oncology health-care providers demonstrated that treatment practices vary widely with no specific paradigm advised more than 33% of the time [212].

PCV Chemotherapy

Early chemotherapy studies for malignant gliomas demonstrated responses in a subset of patients treated with PCV [45,81,213,214]. In 1988, Cairncross and Macdonald first reported that eight consecutive patients with recurrent "malignant" oligodendrogliomas responded to chemotherapy, including PCV [45] in six and carmustine in one, and offered two additional cases in an addendum [215]. They concluded the likelihood of such an observation by chance alone was a statistical impossibility ($p < .00002–.00391$). Two years later, they reported anecdotal responses among patients with newly diagnosed AO [216]. Such responses to chemotherapy were previously uncommon in patients with gliomas, requiring quantitative criteria to allow strict interpretation of trial results with less subjectivity. Accordingly, radiographic response criteria based on brain MRI, updated from those of the early CT era [216], were published shortly thereafter [217], recognizing that corticosteroids can confound radiographic evaluation [218,219]. To confirm these responses observed retrospectively, a multicenter phase II prospective trial was opened in 1989 by the NCIC Clinical Trials Group for patients with newly diagnosed or recurrent AO (below). In the interim, others also published responses to PCV or to other chemotherapies among patients with low-grade and high-grade oligodendroglial tumors including those containing astrocytic elements (LGOA, AOA) [46,220]. The NCIC landmark phase II trial used an intensified PCV (I-PCV) schedule, and demonstrated durable responses (>16 months) in up to 75% of patients [25]. Follow-up studies also suggested about 70% of patients respond [221]. Of note, there were eight patients enrolled but deemed ineligible following central pathology review: two with non-AOs, two with AOAs, three with anaplastic gliomas of undetermined type, and one with radiation necrosis. Therefore, 24% of patients were ineligible based on histology alone, emphasizing the importance of central pathology review in conducting and interpreting clinical trials for AO or AOA.

Although responses in the NCIC study were often durable, patients were not cured when treated with PCV or I-PCV alone, requiring RT at recurrence or because of toxicity leading to discontinuation of the chemotherapy [221]. Therefore, RT remained the standard of care for newly diagnosed disease, and two phase III clinical trials were initiated to determine whether the addition of PCV to RT could improve outcome (Table 63.2). EORTC 26951 [106] randomized 368 patients with newly diagnosed AO or AOA to receive either RT (59.4 Gy) or RT followed by six cycles of adjuvant PCV. The addition of PCV prolonged median PFS from 1.1 to 1.9 years ($p = .0018$). However, there was no difference in OS of about 3 years in each group ($p = .23$). RTOG 9402 [105] evaluated potential benefit of neoadjuvant, intensive PCV. Of note, during accrual, others also published pre-RT PCV as an effective strategy [222], and in RTOG 9402, 289 patients with AO or AOA were randomly assigned to either RT alone or I-PCV for up to four cycles followed by RT. Again, median PFS was slightly but significantly ($p = .004$) longer in patients receiving I-PCV and RT (2.6 years) than RT alone (1.7 years). Second surgery after relapse was also more common in the RT group. However, OS was not different at just under 5 years for each group.

Table 63.2 Phase III Trials of RT and PCV versus RT Alone for Newly Diagnosed Anaplastic Oligodendroglial Tumors

	N	PFS (Median in Years)	OS (Median in Years)
RTOG 94021 [105]	249	$p = .004$	$p = .26$
I-PCV→RT	147	2.6	4.9
RT	142	1.7	4.7
EORTC 26951 [106]	368	$p = .0018$	$p = .23$
RT→PCV	185	1.9	3.4
RT	183	1.1	2.6

Although cross-trial comparisons are statistically dubious, PFS and OS appear shorter in the EORTC than in the RTOG trial. Differing definitions of "anaplastic" and fewer patients proportionally with tumors harboring 1p19q codeletion (25% vs. 46%) may explain the observed difference. It is important to note that in both trials approximately 80% of patients randomly assigned to RT "only" received chemotherapy at the time of disease recurrence. Accordingly, the lack of a difference between the two arms suggests that chemotherapy can be administered at diagnosis or recurrence with equivalent effects on OS for the entire group. Whether this applies to specific molecular subsets, such as those with or without 1p19q codeletion, awaits further maturity of the data. Additionally, there was increased toxicity in the PCV groups limiting its use. In fact, there was one treatment-related death from I-PCV [105]. Therefore, treatment with RT alone at diagnosis, reserving chemotherapy for recurrence, is also a reasonable strategy. Patients with recurrent AO following surgery and RT have shown a high response rate to subsequent PCV chemotherapy of 77% [223]. Standard dose TMZ has also been used in this context, producing a radiographic response rate of 62.6% and a 1-year PFS rate of 40% [224]. Accordingly, questions remain whether the prolongation of PFS warrants the potential toxicity of PCV (or any chemotherapy) at diagnosis in association with RT.

During accrual to both EORTC 26951 and RTOG 9402 the importance of 1p and then 1p19q codeletion in predicting patient outcome became apparent [207]. Both studies collected tissue for molecular analysis when available, and both demonstrated a significant benefit to 1p19q codeletion on PFS and OS [105,106]. It should be noted, however, that the PFS benefit from PCV was limited to the codeleted subset in RTOG 9402 [105]. This was not true for EORTC 26951 [106]. This discrepancy is unexplained but may result from the different order of RT and PCV in the two trials or perhaps from difference in dosing. *MGMT* promoter methylation status undoubtedly also influences outcome but has not been assessed for these trials. There is conflicting data regarding the correlation between *MGMT* promoter methylation and 1p19q status [225]. It should also be noted that median OS was not reached for patients with tumors harboring 1p19q codeletion who were treated with I-PCV then RT in RTOG 9402 [105]. Therefore, it remains plausible that extended follow-up may demonstrate a conditional survival advantage for those living beyond a specific time point [226], especially as the OS curves appear to separate approximately 4 years following treatment start. Confounding effects of follow-up treatment, including reoperation or other chemotherapies, will require exclusion before drawing any such conclusion.

Temozolomide Chemotherapy

Both RTOG 9402 and EORTC 26951 opened before TMZ became routinely available. Most clinicians now use upfront TMZ in place of PCV [212]. However, no formal comparison exists between PCV and TMZ for AO with the exception of a non-prespecified subset analysis in NOA-

04 discussed below [182] that may have been underpowered for this comparison [183]. The first report of TMZ, like PCV, related to treatment of recurrent disease. A single center trial enrolled 48 patients with recurrent AO or AOA who had failed prior PCV therapy [227]. Treatment with subsequent TMZ chemotherapy showed a response rate of 43.8% and a median PFS and OS of 6.7 and 10 months, respectively. A multicenter phase II trial, EORTC 26792, demonstrated a response rate of 25% [33]. As in other trials of oligodendroglial tumors, a substantial subset (4 of 24 evaluable patients) was deemed ineligible on histologic grounds following central review of pathology, which may explain, in part, the seemingly inferior results on multicenter trials employing such a strategy. The efficacy of TMZ in patients with recurrent disease following surgery and RT but who are PCV-naïve has also been assessed. In EORTC 26791, a single arm phase II study, such patients received standard dose TMZ. Objective responses were observed in 53% with a median TTP of 10.4 months for all patients [224]. However, PCV was the standard available chemotherapy for recurrent AO at that time. Therefore, patients with large lesions causing progressive neurologic symptoms were excluded, for fear of poor sensitivity to TMZ, and this may have positively biased results. Of note, 17% of patients who ultimately progressed on or after TMZ on EORTC 26791 later responded to PCV [228].

Patients with newly diagnosed AO also respond to TMZ. Preliminary results from a multicenter phase II trial using a dose-dense regimen of TMZ (150 mg/m^2 days 1–7 and 15–21 every 28 days) demonstrated responses in 50% of patients with measurable disease. Median PFS was 27 months, and median OS had not yet been reached [229]. An Israeli trial, in which 27 patients received standard dose TMZ, reported responses in 75% of patients and median TTP of 24 months. These results are particularly impressive because prior RT or chemotherapy (except TMZ) was allowed for treatment of a LGG [230]. A single arm phase II trial (RTOG 0131) of six pre-RT dose-dense TMZ cycles followed by concurrent RT and TMZ depending on response has completed accrual. Preliminary results demonstrate responses in 33% of evaluable patients and progression in only 10% of 29 patients during the first 6 months of treatment that compared favorably with the 20% rate for intensive PCV in RTOG 9402 [231]. Like PCV, numerous studies have demonstrated that 1p19q codeletion [232] increases TMZ sensitivity.

A large international retrospective study comparing various treatment strategies, including RT versus chemotherapy, is ongoing [233] and suggested efficacy of neoadjuvant PCV may be superior to TMZ in 1p19q codeleted cases. Recently presented phase III prospective data from the Neuro-oncology Working Group (NOA) of the German Cancer Society (NOA-04) demonstrated no survival disadvantage following two therapies (RT and chemotherapy) in either order [182]. It also suggested non-inferiority of PCV vs. TMZ. However, only 14.2% of patients in the German trial had AOs [182]. A phase III prospective trial comparing RT, TMZ, or RT with concurrent and adjuvant TMZ that also incorporates quality-of-life analyses is planned.

Summary

The optimal treatment strategy for oligodendrogliomas remains elusive and there is considerable treatment variability among neuro-oncologists [212]. Moreover, the relatively long survival for some patients with AO, like those with LGG, means that delayed RT-induced neurocognitive toxicity is a potential risk. Chemotherapy alone with the intent of deferring RT may be a reasonable treatment strategy in some patients, particularly those with tumors harboring a favorable molecular profile, such as deletion of 1p and 19q. However, despite data from three randomized phase III trials (EORTC 26951, RTOG 9402, NOA-04), the clinical application of 1p19q status to individual patient care remains controversial. For example, 80% of clinicians seek 1p19q data in patients with AO, but only 42% advocate treatment with chemotherapy alone (34% TMZ, 8% PCV) in such cases [212].

It is also of interest that the favorable toxicity profile and ease of administration for TMZ, regardless of dose schedule, have led most clinicians to routinely advocate TMZ in place of PCV [212] despite the absence of clear comparative data. This preference, among patients as well as physicians, is so robust that a prospective trial powered for comparison of the two regimens is of doubtful feasibility. Moreover, the prolonged accrual and observation period required for such a study (e.g., >10 years from study inception to publication of final results for EORTC 26951 and RTOG 9402) suggest that the question of superiority may become irrelevant as new and potentially superior agents become available. Therefore, no standard of care currently exists for AO.

AOA is often treated similarly to AO rather than AA, although most studies suggest outcome is between that for AO and AA. Neoadjuvant chemotherapy with TMZ (or PCV) is a reasonable strategy for asymptomatic patients with completely resected small pure AOs harboring 1p19q codeletion. However, the authors have also anecdotally observed unexpectedly rapid and dramatic disease progression in this setting. Conversely, older symptomatic patients with large incompletely resected AOAs with neither 1p19q codeletion nor MGMT promoter methylation are likely to behave more aggressively, and most investigators would advocate more aggressive therapy. Recommendations to individual patients should follow appropriate discussion of options, risks, and benefits and are difficult to standardize.

CONCLUSIONS

For patients with newly diagnosed GBM who are under 70 years old with high performance status, standard treatment is clear: maximal surgical resection (with or without Gliadel) followed by RT with concurrent TMZ followed by at least six cycles of adjuvant TMZ. For other histologies, however, the optimal therapy is unclear. Essentially no studies focus exclusively on oligoastrocytomas. Some advocate treatment of AOAs with 1p19q codeletion as if they were AOs and others as if they were AAs [234]. That is the basis of a pair of clinical trials (CATNON and CODEL) that will enroll patients with anaplastic gliomas of any subtype based on 1p19q status rather than histologic subtype. For patients with newly diagnosed AA, most advocate RT as in GBMs. However, the role of chemotherapy during or after RT is debated. LGGs also likely benefit from maximal surgical resection, but some argue for deferring even surgery in young asymptomatic patients. A number of risk factors have been identified that distinguish LGGs that will behave indolently from those that mimic GBMs in their aggressiveness. More aggressive therapy has traditionally been applied to the latter, although without clear evidence to support such an approach. Finally, for patients with AO, there is no consensus on optimal management, with RT, PCV, TMZ, and combinations thereof all reasonable approaches.

Most recent trials focus on small molecule inhibitors or other targeted therapeutics. They have been traditionally applied to treatment of recurrent malignant gliomas, with almost universal failure. However, knowledge gained yielded insight into the molecular biology of tumors and may allow tailoring therapy in the future to the subgroup of patients most likely to benefit.

REFERENCES

1. SEER (Surveillance Epidemiology and End Results): Cancer of the brain and other nervous system. 2004. http://seer.cancer.gov/statfacts/html/brain.html. Accessed August 15, 2008.
2. Chamberlain MC, Kormanik PA. Practical guidelines for the treatment of malignant gliomas. *West J Med.* 1998;168:114–120.
3. Central Brain Tumor Registry of the United States 2008 statistical report: primary brain tumors in the United States. 2008. http://www.cbtrus.org/. Accessed August 15, 2008.
4. Neglia JP, Robison LL, Stovall M, et al. New primary neoplasms of the central nervous system in survivors of childhood cancer: a report from the Childhood Cancer Survivor Study. *J Natl Cancer Inst.* 2006;98:1528–1537.
5. Fisher JL, Schwartzbaum JA, Wrensch M, Wiemels JL. Epidemiology of brain tumors. *Neurol Clin.* 2007;25:867–890, vii.
6. Farrell CJ, Plotkin SR. Genetic causes of brain tumors: neurofibromatosis, tuberous sclerosis, von Hippel-Lindau, and other syndromes. *Neurol Clin.* 2007;25:925–946, viii.
7. Stupp R, Mason WP, van den Bent MJ, et al. Radiotherapy plus concomitant and adjuvant temozolomide for glioblastoma. *N Engl J Med.* 2005;352:987–996.
8. Glantz MJ, Burger PC, Herndon JE 2nd, et al. Influence of the type of surgery on the histologic diagnosis in patients with anaplastic gliomas. *Neurology.* 1991;41:1741–1744.
9. Jackson RJ, Fuller GN, Abi-Said D, et al. Limitations of stereotactic biopsy in the initial management of gliomas. *Neuro-oncology.* 2001;3:193–200.
10. Keles GE, Lamborn KR, Berger MS. Low-grade hemispheric gliomas in adults: a critical review of extent of resection as a factor influencing outcome. *J Neurosurg.* 2001;95:735–745.
11. Smith JS, Chang EF, Lamborn KR, et al. Role of extent of resection in the long-term outcome of low-grade hemispheric gliomas. *J Clin Oncol.* 2008;26:1338–1345.
12. Bampoe J, Bernstein M. The role of surgery in low grade gliomas. *J Neurooncol.* 1999;42:259–269.
13. Karim AB, Maat B, Hatlevoll R, et al. A randomized trial on dose-response in radiation therapy of low-grade cerebral glioma: European Organization for Research and Treatment of Cancer (EORTC) Study 22844. *Int J Radiat Oncol Biol Phys.* 1996;36:549–556.
14. Shaw E, Arusell R, Scheithauer B, et al. Prospective randomized trial of low- versus high-dose radiation therapy in adults with supratentorial low-grade glioma: initial report of a North Central Cancer Treatment Group/Radiation Therapy Oncology Group/Eastern Cooperative Oncology Group study. *J Clin Oncol.* 2002;20:2267–2276.
15. van den Bent MJ, Afra D, de Witte O, et al. Long-term efficacy of early versus delayed radiotherapy for low-grade astrocytoma and oligodendroglioma in adults: the EORTC 22845 randomised trial. *Lancet.* 2005;366:985–990.
16. DeAngelis LM, Delattre JY, Posner JB. Radiation-induced dementia in patients cured of brain metastases. *Neurology.* 1989;39:789–796.
17. Douw L, Klein M, Fagel SS, et al. Cognitive and radiological effects of radiotherapy in patients with low-grade glioma: long-term follow-up. *Lancet Neurol.* 2009;8:810–818.
18. Pignatti F, van den Bent M, Curran D, et al. Prognostic factors for survival in adult patients with cerebral low-grade glioma. *J Clin Oncol.* 2002;20:2076–2084.
19. Iwamoto FM, Nicolardi L, Demopoulos A, et al. Clinical relevance of 1p and 19q deletion for patients with WHO grade 2 and 3 gliomas. *J Neurooncol.* 2008;88:293–298.
20. Jenkins RB, Blair H, Ballman KV, et al. A t(1;19)(q10;p10) mediates the combined deletions of 1p and 19q and predicts a better prognosis of patients with oligodendroglioma. *Cancer Res.* 2006;66:9852–9861.
21. Mariani L, Deiana G, Vassella E, et al. Loss of heterozygosity 1p36 and 19q13 is a prognostic factor for overall survival in patients with diffuse WHO grade 2 gliomas treated without chemotherapy. *J Clin Oncol.* 2006;24:4758–4763.
22. Kujas M, Lejeune J, Benouaich-Amiel A, et al. Chromosome 1p loss: a favorable prognostic factor in low-grade gliomas. *Ann Neurol.* 2005;58:322–326.
23. Shaw EG, Berkey B, Coons SW, et al. Initial report of Radiation Therapy Oncology Group (RTOG) 9802: prospective studies in adult low-grade glioma (LGG) [abstract]. *J Clin Oncol.* 2006;24:Abstract 1500.
24. Eyre HJ, Crowley JJ, Townsend JJ, et al. A randomized trial of radiotherapy versus radiotherapy plus CCNU for incompletely resected low-grade gliomas: a Southwest Oncology Group study. *J Neurosurg.* 1993;78:909–914.
25. Cairncross G, Macdonald D, Ludwin S, et al. Chemotherapy for anaplastic oligodendroglioma. National Cancer Institute of Canada Clinical Trials Group. *J Clin Oncol.* 1994;12:2013–2021.
26. Mason WP, Krol GS, DeAngelis LM. Low-grade oligodendroglioma responds to chemotherapy. *Neurology.* 1996;46:203–207.
27. Paleologos NA, Vick NA, Kachoris JP. Chemotherapy for low-grade oligodendrogliomas? *Ann Neurol.* 1994;36:294–295.
28. Stege EM, Kros JM, de Bruin HG, et al. Successful treatment of low-grade oligodendroglial tumors with a chemotherapy regimen of procarbazine, lomustine, and vincristine. *Cancer.* 2005;103:802–809.
29. Lebrun C, Fontaine D, Bourg V, et al. Treatment of newly diagnosed symptomatic pure low-grade oligodendrogliomas with PCV chemotherapy. *Eur J Neurol.* 2007;14:391–398.
30. Soffietti R, Rudà R, Bradac GB, Schiffer D. PCV chemotherapy for recurrent oligodendrogliomas and oligoastrocytomas. *Neurosurgery.* 1998;43:1066–1073.
31. Buckner JC, Gesme D Jr, O'Fallon JR, et al. Phase II trial of procarbazine, lomustine, and vincristine as initial therapy for patients with low-grade oligodendroglioma or oligoastrocytoma: efficacy and associations with chromosomal abnormalities. *J Clin Oncol.* 2003;21:251–255.
32. Frenay MP, Fontaine D, Vandenbos F, Lebrun C. First-line nitrosourea-based chemotherapy in symptomatic non-resectable supratentorial pure low-grade astrocytomas. *Eur J Neurol.* 2005;12:685–690.
32a. Higuchi Y, Iwadate Y, Yamaura A. Treatment of low-grade oligodendroglial tumors without radiotherapy. *Neurology.* 2004;63:2384–2386.
33. van den Bent MJ, Chinot O, Boogerd W, et al. Second-line chemotherapy with temozolomide in recurrent oligodendroglioma after PCV (procarbazine, lomustine and vincristine) chemotherapy: EORTC Brain Tumor Group phase II study 26972. *Ann Oncol.* 2003;14:599–602.
34. Levin N, Lavon I, Zelikovitsh B, et al. Progressive low-grade oligodendrogliomas: response to temozolomide and correlation between genetic profile and O6-methylguanine DNA methyltransferase protein expression. *Cancer.* 2006;106:1759–1765.
35. Hoang-Xuan K, Capelle L, Kujas M, et al. Temozolomide as initial treatment for adults with low-grade oligodendrogliomas or oligoastrocytomas and correlation with chromosome 1p deletions. *J Clin Oncol.* 2004;22:3133–3138.

36. Pace A, Vidiri A, Galiè E, et al. Temozolomide chemotherapy for progressive low-grade glioma: clinical benefits and radiological response. *Ann Oncol.* 2003;14:1722–1726.
37. Quinn JA, Reardon DA, Friedman AH, et al. Phase II trial of temozolomide in patients with progressive low-grade glioma. *J Clin Oncol.* 2003;21:646–651.
38. Brada M, Viviers L, Abson C, et al. Phase II study of primary temozolomide chemotherapy in patients with WHO grade II gliomas. *Ann Oncol.* 2003;14:1715–1721.
39. Kaloshi G, Benouaich-Amiel A, Diakite F, et al. Temozolomide for low-grade gliomas: predictive impact of 1p/19q loss on response and outcome. *Neurology.* 2007;68:1831–1836.
40. Everhard S, Kaloshi G, Crinière E, et al. MGMT methylation: a marker of response to temozolomide in low-grade gliomas. *Ann Neurol.* 2006;60:740–743.
41. Pouratian N, Gasco J, Sherman JH, Shaffrey ME, Schiff D. Toxicity and efficacy of protracted low dose temozolomide for the treatment of low grade gliomas. *J Neurooncol.* 2007;82:281–288.
42. Tosoni A, Franceschi E, Ermani M, et al. Temozolomide three weeks on and one week off as first line therapy for patients with recurrent or progressive low grade gliomas. *J Neurooncol.* 2008;89:179–185.
43. Sanson M, Cartalat-Carel S, Taillibert S, et al.; ANOCEF group. Initial chemotherapy in gliomatosis cerebri. *Neurology.* 2004;63:270–275.
44. Levin N, Gomori JM, Siegal T. Chemotherapy as initial treatment in gliomatosis cerebri: results with temozolomide. *Neurology.* 2004;63:354–356.
45. Levin VA, Edwards MS, Wright DC, et al. Modified procarbazine, CCNU, and vincristine (PCV 3) combination chemotherapy in the treatment of malignant brain tumors. *Cancer Treat Rep.* 1980;64:237–244.
46. Glass J, Hochberg FH, Gruber ML, Louis DN, Smith D, Rattner B. The treatment of oligodendrogliomas and mixed oligodendroglioma-astrocytomas with PCV chemotherapy. *J Neurosurg.* 1992;76:741–745.
47. Olson JD, Riedel E, DeAngelis LM. Long-term outcome of low-grade oligodendroglioma and mixed glioma. *Neurology.* 2000;54:1442–1448.
48. Shaw EG, Wang M, Coons S, et al. Final report of Radiation Therapy Oncology Group (RTOG) protocol 9802: radiation therapy (RT) versus RT + procarbazine, CCNU, and vincristine (PCV) chemotherapy for adult low-grade glioma (LGG) [abstract]. *J Clin Oncol.* 2008;26:Abstract 2006.
49. Schiff D, Brown PD, Giannini C. Outcome in adult low-grade glioma: the impact of prognostic factors and treatment. *Neurology.* 2007;69:1366–1373.
50. van den Bent MJ, Stupp R, Brandes AA, Lacombe D. Current and future trials of the EORTC brain tumor group. *Onkologie.* 2004;27:246–250.
51. Hegi ME, Diserens AC, Gorlia T, et al. MGMT gene silencing and benefit from temozolomide in glioblastoma. *N Engl J Med.* 2005;352:997–1003.
52. Kesari S, Schiff D, Drappatz J, et al. Phase II study of protracted daily temozolomide for low-grade gliomas in adults. *Clin Cancer Res.* 2009;15:330–337.
53. Tolcher AW, Gerson SL, Denis L, et al. Marked inactivation of O6-alkylguanine-DNA alkyltransferase activity with protracted temozolomide schedules. *Br J Cancer.* 2003;88:1004–1011.
54. Preusser M, Charles Janzer R, Felsberg J, et al. Anti-O6-methylguanine-methyltransferase (MGMT) immunohistochemistry in glioblastoma multiforme: observer variability and lack of association with patient survival impede its use as clinical biomarker. *Brain Pathol.* 2008;18:520–532.
55. Friedman HS, Lovell S, Rasheed K, Friedman AH. Treatment of adults with progressive oligodendroglioma with carboplatin (CBDCA): preliminary results. Writing Committee for The Brain Tumor Center at Duke. *Med Pediatr Oncol.* 1998;31:16–18.
56. Watanabe T, Katayama Y, Yoshino A, Komine C, Yokoyama T, Fukushima T. Treatment of low-grade diffuse astrocytomas by surgery and human fibroblast interferon without radiation therapy. *J Neurooncol.* 2003;61:171–176.
57. Djerassi I, Kim JS, Reggev A. Response of astrocytoma to high-dose methotrexate with citrovorum factor rescue. *Cancer.* 1985;55:2741–2747.
58. Galanis E, Buckner JC, Burch PA, et al. Phase II trial of nitrogen mustard, vincristine, and procarbazine in patients with recurrent glioma: North Central Cancer Treatment Group results. *J Clin Oncol.* 1998;16:2953–2958.
59. Chamberlain MC. Salvage chemotherapy with CPT-11 for recurrent oligodendrogliomas. *J Neurooncol.* 2002;59:157–163.
60. Rajkumar SV, Burch PA, Nair S, et al. Phase II North Central Cancer Treatment Group study of 2-cholorodeoxyadenosine in patients with recurrent glioma. *Am J Clin Oncol.* 1999;22:168–171.
61. Lote K, Egeland T, Hager B, et al. Survival, prognostic factors, and therapeutic efficacy in low-grade glioma: a retrospective study in 379 patients. *J Clin Oncol.* 1997;15:3129–3140.
62. Kaloshi G, Everhard S, Laigle-Donadey F, et al. Genetic markers predictive of chemosensitivity and outcome in gliomatosis cerebri. *Neurology.* 2008;70:590–595.
63. Central Nervous System Cancers (version 1). 2008. www.nccn.org. Accessed June 21, 2008.
64. Louis DN, Ohgaki H, Wiestler OD, Cavanee WK. *WHO Classification of Tumours of the Central Nervous System.* 4th ed. Lyon: International Agency for Research on Cancer; 2007.
65. Bucy PC, Oberhill HR, Siqueira EB, Zimmerman HM, Jelsma RK. Cerebral glioblastomas can be cured! *Neurosurgery.* 1985;16:714–717.
66. Stupp R, Hegi ME, Mason WP, et al. Effects of radiotherapy with concomitant and adjuvant temozolomide versus radiotherapy alone on survival in glioblastoma in a randomised phase III study: 5-year analysis of the EORTC-NCIC trial. *Lancet Oncol.* 2009;10:459–466.
67. Bailey P, Cushing H. *A Classification of the Tumors of the Glioma Group on a Histo-Genetic Basis with a Correlated Study of Prognosis.* Philadelphia: J.B. Lippincott Co.; 1926.
68. Jelsma RK, Bucy PC. The treatment of glioblastoma multiforme. *Trans Am Neurol Assoc.* 1967;92:90–93.
69. Stummer W, Pichlmeier U, Meinel T, Wiestler OD, Zanella F, Reulen HJ. Fluorescence-guided surgery with 5-aminolevulinic acid for resection of malignant glioma: a randomised controlled multicentre phase III trial. *Lancet Oncol.* 2006;7:392–401.
70. Laws ER, Parney IF, Huang W, et al. Survival following surgery and prognostic factors for recently diagnosed malignant glioma: data from the Glioma Outcomes Project. *J Neurosurg.* 2003;99:467–473.
71. Keles GE, Anderson B, Berger MS. The effect of extent of resection on time to tumor progression and survival in patients with glioblastoma multiforme of the cerebral hemisphere. *Surg Neurol.* 1999;52:371–379.
72. Vuorinen V, Hinkka S, Färkkilä M, Jääskeläinen J. Debulking or biopsy of malignant glioma in elderly people - a randomised study. *Acta Neurochir (Wien).* 2003;145:5–10.
73. Devaux BC, O'Fallon JR, Kelly PJ. Resection, biopsy, and survival in malignant glial neoplasms. A retrospective study of clinical parameters, therapy, and outcome. *J Neurosurg.* 1993;78:767–775.
74. Lacroix M, Abi-Said D, Fourney DR, et al. A multivariate analysis of 416 patients with glioblastoma multiforme: prognosis, extent of resection, and survival. *J Neurosurg.* 2001;95:190–198.
75. Ballance CA. Remarks on the treatment of brain tumour. *Lancet.* 1913;182:792–794.
76. Dandy WE. The treatment of brain tumors. *JAMA.* 1921;77:1853–1859.
77. Dandy WE. Removal of right cerebral hemisphere for certain tumors with hemiplegia. *JAMA.* 1928;90:823–825.
78. Gardner WJ, Karnosh LJ, McClure CC Jr, Gardner AK. Residual function following hemispherectomy for tumour and for infantile hemiplegia. *Brain.* 1955;78:487–502.
79. Andersen AP. Postoperative irradiation of glioblastomas. Results in a randomized series. *Acta Radiol Oncol Radiat Phys Biol.* 1978;17:475–484.
80. Bailey P. The results of roentgen therapy on brain tumors. *Am J Roentgenol Radium Ther.* 1925;13:48–53.
81. Shapiro WR, Young DF. Treatment of malignant glioma. A controlled study of chemotherapy and irradiation. *Arch Neurol.* 1976;33:494–450.
82. Walker MD, Alexander E Jr, Hunt WE, et al. Evaluation of BCNU and/or radiotherapy in the treatment of anaplastic gliomas. A cooperative clinical trial. *J Neurosurg.* 1978;49:333–343.
83. Walker MD, Green SB, Byar DP, et al. Randomized comparisons of radiotherapy and nitrosoureas for the treatment of malignant glioma after surgery. *N Engl J Med.* 1980;303:1323–1329.
84. Kristiansen K, Hagen S, Kollevold T, et al. Combined modality therapy of operated astrocytomas grade III and IV. Confirmation of the value of postoperative irradiation and lack of potentiation of bleomycin on survival time: a prospective multicenter trial of the Scandinavian Glioblastoma Study Group. *Cancer.* 1981;47:649–652.
85. Loeffler JS, Alexander E 3rd, Shea WM, et al. Radiosurgery as part of the initial management of patients with malignant gliomas. *J Clin Oncol.* 1992;10:1379–1385.

86. Souhami L, Seiferheld W, Brachman D, et al. Randomized comparison of stereotactic radiosurgery followed by conventional radiotherapy with carmustine to conventional radiotherapy with carmustine for patients with glioblastoma multiforme: report of Radiation Therapy Oncology Group 93–05 protocol. *Int J Radiat Oncol Biol Phys*. 2004;60:853–860.
87. Laperriere NJ, Leung PM, McKenzie S, et al. Randomized study of brachytherapy in the initial management of patients with malignant astrocytoma. *Int J Radiat Oncol Biol Phys*. 1998;41:1005–1011.
88. Shrieve DC, Alexander E 3rd, Wen PY, et al. Comparison of stereotactic radiosurgery and brachytherapy in the treatment of recurrent glioblastoma multiforme. *Neurosurgery*. 1995;36:275–282; discussion 282–274.
89. French JD, West PM, Von Amerongen FK, Magoun HW. Effects of intracarotid administration of nitrogen mustard on normal brain and brain tumors. *J Neurosurg*. 1952;9:378–389.
90. Fine HA, Dear KB, Loeffler JS, Black PM, Canellos GP. Meta-analysis of radiation therapy with and without adjuvant chemotherapy for malignant gliomas in adults. *Cancer*. 1993;71:2585–2597.
91. Stewart LA. Chemotherapy in adult high-grade glioma: a systematic review and meta-analysis of individual patient data from 12 randomised trials. *Lancet*. 2002;359:1011–1018.
92. Green SB, Byar DP, Walker MD, et al. Comparisons of carmustine, procarbazine, and high-dose methylprednisolone as additions to surgery and radiotherapy for the treatment of malignant glioma. *Cancer Treat Rep*. 1983;67:121–132.
93. Karnofsky DA, Abelmann WH, Carver LF, Burchenal JH. The use of the nitrogen mustards in the palliative treatment of carcinoma. With particular reference to bronchogenic carcinoma. *Cancer*. 1948;1:634–656.
94. DeAngelis LM, Burger PC, Green SB, Cairncross JG. Malignant glioma: who benefits from adjuvant chemotherapy? *Ann Neurol*. 1998;44:691–695.
95. Esteller M, Garcia-Foncillas J, Andion E, et al. Inactivation of the DNA-repair gene MGMT and the clinical response of gliomas to alkylating agents. *N Engl J Med*. 2000;343:1350–1354.
96. Prados MD, Scott C, Curran WJ Jr, Nelson DF, Leibel S, Kramer S. Procarbazine, lomustine, and vincristine (PCV) chemotherapy for anaplastic astrocytoma: A retrospective review of radiation therapy oncology group protocols comparing survival with carmustine or PCV adjuvant chemotherapy. *J Clin Oncol*. 1999;17:3389–3395.
97. Yung WK, Prados MD, Yaya-Tur R, et al. Multicenter phase II trial of temozolomide in patients with anaplastic astrocytoma or anaplastic oligoastrocytoma at first relapse. Temodal Brain Tumor Group. *J Clin Oncol*. 1999;17:2762–2771.
98. Yung WK, Albright RE, Olson J, et al. A phase II study of temozolomide vs. procarbazine in patients with glioblastoma multiforme at first relapse. *Br J Cancer*. 2000;83:588–593.
99. Gutin PH, Posner JB. Neuro-oncology: diagnosis and management of cerebral gliomas–past, present, and future. *Neurosurgery*. 2000;47:1–8.
100. Gilbert MR, Friedman HS, Kuttesch JF, et al. A phase II study of temozolomide in patients with newly diagnosed supratentorial malignant glioma before radiation therapy. *Neuro-oncology*. 2002;4:261–267.
101. Combs SE, Gutwein S, Schulz-Ertner D, et al. Temozolomide combined with irradiation as postoperative treatment of primary glioblastoma multiforme. Phase I/II study. *Strahlenther Onkol*. 2005;181:372–377.
102. Stupp R, Dietrich PY, Ostermann Kraljevic S, et al. Promising survival for patients with newly diagnosed glioblastoma multiforme treated with concomitant radiation plus temozolomide followed by adjuvant temozolomide. *J Clin Oncol*. 2002;20:1375–1382.
103. Wick W, Platten M, Weller M. New (alternative) temozolomide regimens for the treatment of glioma. *Neuro-oncology*. 2009;11:69–79.
104. Gerson SL. MGMT: its role in cancer aetiology and cancer therapeutics. *Nat Rev Cancer*. 2004;4:296–307.
105. Cairncross G, Berkey B, Shaw E, et al. Phase III trial of chemotherapy plus radiotherapy compared with radiotherapy alone for pure and mixed anaplastic oligodendroglioma: Intergroup Radiation Therapy Oncology Group Trial 9402. *J Clin Oncol*. 2006;24:2707–2714.
106. van den Bent MJ, Carpentier AF, Brandes AA, et al. Adjuvant procarbazine, lomustine, and vincristine improves progression-free survival but not overall survival in newly diagnosed anaplastic oligodendrogliomas and oligoastrocytomas: a randomized European Organisation for Research and Treatment of Cancer phase III trial. *J Clin Oncol*. 2006;24:2715–2722.
107. Mirimanoff R, Mason W, van den Bent M, et al. Is long-term survival in glioblastoma possible? Updated results of the EORTC/NCIC Phase III randomized trial on radiotherapy (RT) and concomitant and adjuvant temozolomide (TMZ) versus RT alone. *Int J Radiat Oncol Bio Phys*. 2007;69:S2.
108. Rivera AL, Pelloski CE, Gilbert MR, et al. MGMT promoter methylation is predictive of response to radiotherapy and prognostic in the absence of adjuvant alkylating chemotherapy for glioblastoma. *Neuro-oncology*. 2010;12:116–121.
109. La Rocca RV, Hodes J, Villanueva WG, et al. A phase II study of radiation with concomitant and then sequential temozolomide (TMZ) in patients with newly diagnosed supratentorial high grade malignant glioma who have undergone surgery with carmustine (BCNU) wafter insertion. [abstract TA-28]. *Neuro Oncol*. 2006;8:445.
110. Lassman AB, Holland EC. Incorporating molecular tools into clinical trials and treatment for gliomas? *Curr Opin Neurol*. 2007;20:708–711.
111. Taphoorn MJ, Stupp R, Coens C, et al. Health-related quality of life in patients with glioblastoma: a randomised controlled trial. *Lancet Oncol*. 2005;6:937–944.
112. Chalmers AJ. The potential role and application of PARP inhibitors in cancer treatment. *Br Med Bull*. 2009;89:23–40.
113. Chakravarti A, Erkkinen MG, Nestler U, et al. Temozolomide-mediated radiation enhancement in glioblastoma: a report on underlying mechanisms. *Clin Cancer Res*. 2006;12:4738–4746.
114. Quinn JA, Desjardins A, Weingart J, et al. Phase I trial of temozolomide plus O6-benzylguanine for patients with recurrent or progressive malignant glioma. *J Clin Oncol*. 2005;23:7178–7187.
115. Quinn JA, Jiang SX, Reardon DA, et al. Phase I trial of temozolomide plus O6-benzylguanine 5-day regimen with recurrent malignant glioma. *Neuro-oncology*. 2009;11:556–561.
116. Quinn JA, Jiang SX, Reardon DA, et al. Phase II trial of temozolomide plus o6-benzylguanine in adults with recurrent, temozolomide-resistant malignant glioma. *J Clin Oncol*. 2009;27:1262–1267.
117. Schold SC Jr, Kokkinakis DM, Chang SM, et al. O6-benzylguanine suppression of O6-alkylguanine-DNA alkyltransferase in anaplastic gliomas. *Neuro-oncology*. 2004;6:28–32.
118. Noronha V, Berliner N, Ballen KK, et al. Treatment-related myelodysplasia/AML in a patient with a history of breast cancer and an oligodendroglioma treated with temozolomide: case study and review of the literature. *Neuro-oncology*. 2006;8:280–283.
119. de Wit MC, de Bruin HG, Eijkenboom W, Sillevis Smitt PA, van den Bent MJ. Immediate post-radiotherapy changes in malignant glioma can mimic tumor progression. *Neurology*. 2004;63:535–537.
120. Chamberlain MC, Glantz MJ, Chalmers L, Van Horn A, Sloan AE. Early necrosis following concurrent Temodar and radiotherapy in patients with glioblastoma. *J Neurooncol*. 2007;82:81–83.
121. Brandes AA, Franceschi E, Tosoni A, et al. MGMT promoter methylation status can predict the incidence and outcome of pseudoprogression after concomitant radiochemotherapy in newly diagnosed glioblastoma patients. *J Clin Oncol*. 2008;26:2192–2197.
122. Clarke JL, Abrey LE, Karimi S, Lassman AB. Pseudoprogression (PsPr) after concurrent radiotherapy (RT) and temozolomide (TMZ) for newly diagnosed glioblastoma multiforme (GBM) [abstract 2025]. *J Clin Oncol*. 2008;26:2025.
123. Taal W, Brandsma D, de Bruin HG, et al. The incidence of pseudoprogression in a cohort of malignant glioma patients treated with chemo-radiation with temozolomide [abstract 2009] *J Clin Oncol*. 2007;25:2009.
124. Brandes AA, Tosoni A, Spagnolli F, et al. Disease progression or pseudoprogression after concomitant radiochemotherapy treatment: pitfalls in neurooncology. *Neuro-oncology*. 2008;10:361–367.
125. Robins HI, Lassman AB, Khuntia D. Therapeutic advances in malignant glioma: current status and future prospects. *Neuroimaging Clin N Am*. 2009;19:647–656.
126. Brandsma D, Stalpers L, Taal W, Sminia P, van den Bent MJ. Clinical features, mechanisms, and management of pseudoprogression in malignant gliomas. *Lancet Oncol*. 2008;9:453–461.
127. van den Bent MJ, Vogelbaum MA, Wen PY, Macdonald DR, Chang SM. End point assessment in gliomas: novel treatments limit usefulness of classical Macdonald's Criteria. *J Clin Oncol*. 2009;27:2905–2908.

128. Wen PY, Macdonald DR, Reardon DA, et al. Updated response assessment criteria for high-grade gliomas: response assessment in neuro-oncology working group. *J Clin Oncol*. 2010;28:1963–1972.
129. Brem H, Piantadosi S, Burger PC, et al. Placebo-controlled trial of safety and efficacy of intraoperative controlled delivery by biodegradable polymers of chemotherapy for recurrent gliomas. The Polymer-brain Tumor Treatment Group. *Lancet*. 1995;345:1008–1012.
130. Westphal M, Hilt DC, Bortey E, et al. A phase 3 trial of local chemotherapy with biodegradable carmustine (BCNU) wafers (Gliadel wafers) in patients with primary malignant glioma. *Neuro-oncology*. 2003;5:79–88.
131. Westphal M, Ram Z, Riddle V, Hilt D, Bortey E. Gliadel wafer in initial surgery for malignant glioma: long-term follow-up of a multicenter controlled trial. *Acta Neurochir (Wien)*. 2006;148:269–275; discussion 275.
132. Kunwar S, Westphal M, Medhorn M, et al. Results from PRECISE: a randomized phase 3 study in patients with first recurrent glioblastoma multiforme (GBM) comparing cinttredekin besudotox (CB) administered via convection-enhanced delivery (CED) with Gliadel wafers (GW) [abstract MA-61]. *Neuro Oncol*. 2007;9:531.
133. Celtic Pharma Terminates Transmid™ Trial KSB311R/CIII/001. 2008. www.celticpharma.com. Accessed August 10, 2008.
134. Keime-Guibert F, Chinot O, Taillandier L, et al. Radiotherapy for glioblastoma in the elderly. *N Engl J Med*. 2007;356:1527–1535.
135. Roa W, Brasher PM, Bauman G, et al. Abbreviated course of radiation therapy in older patients with glioblastoma multiforme: a prospective randomized clinical trial. *J Clin Oncol*. 2004;22:1583–1588.
136. Chinot OL, Barrie M, Frauger E, et al. Phase II study of temozolomide without radiotherapy in newly diagnosed glioblastoma multiforme in an elderly populations. *Cancer*. 2004;100:2208–2214.
137. Glantz M, Chamberlain M, Liu Q, Litofsky NS, Recht LD. Temozolomide as an alternative to irradiation for elderly patients with newly diagnosed malignant gliomas. *Cancer*. 2003;97:2262–2266.
138. Combs SE, Wagner J, Bischof M, et al. Postoperative treatment of primary glioblastoma multiforme with radiation and concomitant temozolomide in elderly patients. *Int J Radiat Oncol Biol Phys*. 2008;70:987–992.
139. Hochberg FH, Pruitt A. Assumptions in the radiotherapy of glioblastoma. *Neurology*. 1980;30:907–911.
140. Franceschi E, Omuro AM, Lassman AB, Demopoulos A, Nolan C, Abrey LE. Salvage temozolomide for prior temozolomide responders. *Cancer*. 2005;104:2473–2476.
141. Wong ET, Hess KR, Gleason MJ, et al. Outcomes and prognostic factors in recurrent glioma patients enrolled onto phase II clinical trials. *J Clin Oncol*. 1999;17:2572–2578.
142. Lamborn KR, Yung WK, Chang SM, et al. Progression-free survival: an important end point in evaluating therapy for recurrent high-grade gliomas. *Neuro-oncology*. 2008;10:162–170.
143. Huncharek M, Muscat J. Treatment of recurrent high grade astrocytoma; results of a systematic review of 1,415 patients. *Anticancer Res*. 1998;18:1303–1311.
144. Prados MD, Yung WK, Fine HA, et al. Phase 2 study of BCNU and temozolomide for recurrent glioblastoma multiforme: North American Brain Tumor Consortium study. *Neuro-oncology*. 2004;6:33–37.
145. Chang SM, Theodosopoulos P, Lamborn K, et al. Temozolomide in the treatment of recurrent malignant glioma. *Cancer*. 2004;100:605–611.
146. Brandes AA, Tosoni A, Amistà P, et al. How effective is BCNU in recurrent glioblastoma in the modern era? A phase II trial. *Neurology*. 2004;63:1281–1284.
147. Raizer JJ, Abrey LE, Lassman AB, et al. A phase II trial of erlotinib in patients with recurrent malignant gliomas and nonprogressive glioblastoma multiforme postradiation therapy. *Neuro-oncology*. 2010;12:95–103.
148. van den Bent MJ, Brandes AA, Rampling R, et al. Randomized phase II trial of erlotinib versus temozolomide or carmustine in recurrent glioblastoma: EORTC brain tumor group study 26034. *J Clin Oncol*. 2009;27:1268–1274.
149. Yung A, Vredenburgh J, Cloughesy T, et al. Erlotinib HCL for glioblastoma multiforme in first relapse, a phase II trial [abstract]. *J Clin Oncol*. 2004;22:1555.
150. Vogelbaum MA, Peerboom G, Stevens G, Barnett G, Brewer C. Phase II trial of the EGFR tyrosine kinase inhibitor erlotinib for single agent therapy of recurrent Glioblastoma Multiforme: interim results [abstract]. *J Clin Oncol*. 2004;22:1558.
151. Rich JN, Reardon DA, Peery T, et al. Phase II trial of gefitinib in recurrent glioblastoma. *J Clin Oncol*. 2004;22:133–142.
152. Lieberman FS, Cloughesy T, Malkin M, et al. Phase I-II study of ZD-1839 for recurrent malignant gliomas and meningiomas progressing after radiation therapy [abstract]. *J Clin Oncol*. 2003;22:105 (Abst 421).
153. Raymond E, Brandes AA, Dittrich C, et al. Phase II study of imatinib in patients with recurrent gliomas of various histologies: a European Organisation for Research and Treatment of Cancer Brain Tumor Group Study. *J Clin Oncol*. 2008;26:4659–4665.
154. Conrad C, Friedman H, Reardon D, et al. A phase I/II trial of single-agent PTK 787/ZK222584 (PTK/ZK), a novel, oral angiogenesis inhibitor, in patients with recurrent glioblastoma multiforme [abstract]. *J Clin Oncol*. 2004;22:1512.
155. Wen PY, Yung WK, Lamborn KR, et al. Phase I/II study of imatinib mesylate for recurrent malignant gliomas: North American Brain Tumor Consortium Study 99–08. *Clin Cancer Res*. 2006;12:4899–4907.
156. Hurwitz H, Fehrenbacher L, Novotny W, et al. Bevacizumab plus irinotecan, fluorouracil, and leucovorin for metastatic colorectal cancer. *N Engl J Med*. 2004;350:2335–2342.
157. Stark-Vance V. Bevacizumab and CPT-11 in the treatment of relapsed malignant glioma [abstract 342]. *Neuro-Oncol*. 2005;7:369.
158. Vredenburgh JJ, Desjardins A, Herndon JE 2nd, et al. Phase II trial of bevacizumab and irinotecan in recurrent malignant glioma. *Clin Cancer Res*. 2007;13:1253–1259.
159. Vredenburgh JJ, Desjardins A, Herndon JE 2nd, et al. Bevacizumab plus irinotecan in recurrent glioblastoma multiforme. *J Clin Oncol*. 2007;25:4722–4729.
160. Norden AD, Young GS, Setayesh K, et al. Bevacizumab for recurrent malignant gliomas: efficacy, toxicity, and patterns of recurrence. *Neurology*. 2008;70:779–787.
161. Cloughesy TF, Prados MD, Wen PY, et al. A phase II, randomized, non-comparative clinical trial of the effect of bevacizumab (BV) alone or in combination with irinotecan (CPT) on 6-month progression free survival (PFS6) in recurrent, treatment-refractory glioblastoma (GBM) [abstract 2010b, oral presentation update]. *J Clin Oncol*. 2008;26:Abstract 2010b.
162. de Groot JF, Wen PY, Lamborn K, et al. Phase II single arm trial of aflibercept in patients with recurrent temozolomide-resistant glioblastoma: NABTC 0601. [abstract 2020]. *J Clin Oncol*. 2008;26:2020.
163. Batchelor TT, Sorensen AG, di Tomaso E, et al. AZD2171, a pan-VEGF receptor tyrosine kinase inhibitor, normalizes tumor vasculature and alleviates edema in glioblastoma patients. *Cancer Cell*. 2007;11:83–95.
164. Kreisl TN, Kim L, Moore K, et al. Phase II trial of single-agent bevacizumab followed by bevacizumab plus irinotecan at tumor progression in recurrent glioblastoma. *J Clin Oncol*. 2009;27:740–745.
165. Friedman HS, Prados MD, Wen PY, et al. Bevacizumab alone and in combination with irinotecan in recurrent glioblastoma. *J Clin Oncol*. 2009;27:4733–4740.
166. Gutin PH, Iwamoto FM, Beal K, et al. Safety and efficacy of bevacizumab with hypofractionated stereotactic irradiation for recurrent malignant gliomas. *Int J Radiat Oncol Biol Phys*. 2009;75:156–163.
167. Lai A, Filka E, McGibbon B, et al. Phase II pilot study of bevacizumab in combination with temozolomide and regional radiation therapy for up-front treatment of patients with newly diagnosed glioblastoma multiforme: interim analysis of safety and tolerability. *Int J Radiat Oncol Biol Phys*. 2008;71:1372–1380.
168. Robins HI, O'Neill A, Gilbert M, et al. Effect of dalteparin and radiation on survival and thromboembolic events in glioblastoma multiforme: a phase II ECOG trial. *Cancer Chemother Pharmacol*. 2008;62:227–233.
169. Chamberlain MC. Salvage chemotherapy with CPT-11 for recurrent glioblastoma multiforme. *J Neurooncol*. 2002;56:183–188.
170. Friedman HS, Petros WP, Friedman AH, et al. Irinotecan therapy in adults with recurrent or progressive malignant glioma. *J Clin Oncol*. 1999;17(5):1516–1525.
171. Prados MD, Lamborn K, Yung WK, et al. A phase 2 trial of irinotecan (CPT-11) in patients with recurrent malignant glioma: a North American Brain Tumor Consortium study. *Neuro-oncology*. 2006;8:189–193.
172. Quant E, Norden AD, Drappatz J, et al. Role of a second chemotherapy in recurrent malignant glioma patients who progress

on a bevacizumab-containing regimen [abstract]. *J Clin Oncol.* 2008;26:Abstract 2008
173. Lassman AB, Iwamoto FM, Gutin PH, Abrey LE. Patterns of relapse and prognosis after bevacizumab (BEV) failure in recurrent glioblastoma (GBM) [abstract]. *J Clin Oncol.* 2008;26:Abstract 2028.
174. Matsumoto Y, Freund KB, Peiretti E, Cooney MJ, Ferrara DC, Yannuzzi LA. Rebound macular edema following bevacizumab (Avastin) therapy for retinal venous occlusive disease. *Retina (Philadelphia, Pa).* 2007;27:426–431.
175. Scott BJ, Quant EC, McNamara MB, Ryg PA, Batchelor TT, Wen PY. Bevacizumab salvage therapy following progression in high-grade glioma patients treated with VEGF receptor tyrosine kinase inhibitors. *Neuro-oncology.* 2010;12:603–607.
176. Iwamoto FM, Abrey LE, Beal K, et al. Patterns of relapse and prognosis after bevacizumab failure in recurrent glioblastoma. *Neurology.* 2009;73:1200–1206.
177. Chen W, Delaloye S, Silverman DH, et al. Predicting treatment response of malignant gliomas to bevacizumab and irinotecan by imaging proliferation with [18F] fluorothymidine positron emission tomography: a pilot study. *J Clin Oncol.* 2007;25:4714–4721.
178. Kreisl TN, Lassman AB, Mischel PS, et al. A pilot study of everolimus and gefitinib in the treatment of recurrent glioblastoma (GBM). *J Neurooncol.* 2009;92:99–105.
179. Mellinghoff IK, Wang MY, Vivanco I, et al. Molecular determinants of the response of glioblastomas to EGFR kinase inhibitors. *N Engl J Med.* 2005;353:2012–2024.
180. Prados MD, Gutin PH, Phillips TL, et al. Highly anaplastic astrocytoma: a review of 357 patients treated between 1977 and 1989. *Int J Radiat Oncol Biol Phys.* 1992;23:3–8.
181. Tortosa A, Viñolas N, Villà S, et al. Prognostic implication of clinical, radiologic, and pathologic features in patients with anaplastic gliomas. *Cancer.* 2003;97:1063–1071.
182. Wick W, Hartmann C, Engel C, et al. NOA-04 randomized phase III trial of sequential radiochemotherapy of anaplastic glioma with procarbazine, lomustine, and vincristine or temozolomide. *J Clin Oncol.* 2009;27:5874–5880.
183. DeAngelis LM. Anaplastic glioma: how to prognosticate outcome and choose a treatment strategy. [corrected]. *J Clin Oncol.* 2009;27:5861–5862.
184. Medical-Research-Council-Brain-Tumor-Working-Party. Randomized trial of procarbazine, lomustine, and vincristine in the adjuvant treatment of high-grade astrocytoma: a Medical Research Council trial. *J Clin Oncol.* 2001;19:509–518.
185. Laramore GE, Martz KL, Nelson JS, Griffin TW, Chang CH, Horton J. Radiation Therapy Oncology Group (RTOG) survival data on anaplastic astrocytomas of the brain: does a more aggressive form of treatment adversely impact survival? *Int J Radiat Oncol Biol Phys.* 1989;17:1351–1356.
186. Levin VA, Silver P, Hannigan J, et al. Superiority of post-radiotherapy adjuvant chemotherapy with CCNU, procarbazine, and vincristine (PCV) over BCNU for anaplastic gliomas: NCOG 6G61 final report. *Int J Radiat Oncol Biol Phys.* 1990;18:321–324.
187. Chang SM, Seiferheld W, Curran W, et al. Phase I study pilot arms of radiotherapy and carmustine with temozolomide for anaplastic astrocytoma (Radiation Therapy Oncology Group 9813): implications for studies testing initial treatment of brain tumors. *Int J Radiat Oncol Biol Phys.* 2004;59:1122–1126.
188. Stieber VW, Mehta MP. Advances in radiation therapy for brain tumors. *Neurol Clin.* 2007;25:1005–33, ix.
189. Brandes AA, Nicolardi L, Tosoni A, et al. Survival following adjuvant PCV or temozolomide for anaplastic astrocytoma. *Neuro-oncology.* 2006;8:253–260.
190. Combs SE, Nagy M, Edler L, et al. Comparative evaluation of radiochemotherapy with temozolomide versus standard-of-care postoperative radiation alone in patients with WHO grade III astrocytic tumors. *Radiother Oncol.* 2008;88:177–182.
191. Combs SE, Wagner J, Bischof M, et al. Radiochemotherapy in patients with primary glioblastoma comparing two temozolomide dose regimens. *Int J Radiat Oncol Biol Phys.* 2008;71:999–1005.
192. Franceschi E, Tosoni A, Brandes AA. Adjuvant temozolomide: how long and how much? *Expert Rev Anticancer Ther.* 2008;8:663–665.
193. Yung WK, Kyritsis AP, Gleason MJ, Levin VA. Treatment of recurrent malignant gliomas with high-dose 13-cis-retinoic acid. *Clin Cancer Res.* 1996;2:1931–1935.

194. Jaeckle KA, Hess KR, Yung WK, et al. Phase II evaluation of temozolomide and 13-cis-retinoic acid for the treatment of recurrent and progressive malignant glioma: a North American Brain Tumor Consortium study. *J Clin Oncol.* 2003;21:2305–2311.
195. Chamberlain MC, Tsao-Wei DD, Groshen S. Salvage chemotherapy with cyclophosphamide for recurrent temozolomide-refractory anaplastic astrocytoma. *Cancer.* 2006;106:172–179.
196. Chamberlain MC, Wei-Tsao DD, Blumenthal DT, Glantz MJ. Salvage chemotherapy with CPT-11 for recurrent temozolomide-refractory anaplastic astrocytoma. *Cancer.* 2008;112:2038–2045.
197. Macdonald DR, O'Brien RA, Gilbert JJ, Cairncross JG. Metastatic anaplastic oligodendroglioma. *Neurology.* 1989;39:1593–1596.
198. Cairncross JG, Macdonald DR, Ramsay DA. Aggressive oligodendroglioma: a chemosensitive tumor. *Neurosurgery.* 1992;31:78–82.
199. Burger PC. What is an oligodendroglioma? *Brain Pathol.* 2002;12:257–259.
200. Giannini C, Burger PC, Berkey BA, et al. Anaplastic oligodendroglial tumors: refining the correlation among histopathology, 1p 19q deletion and clinical outcome in Intergroup Radiation Therapy Oncology Group Trial 9402. *Brain Pathol.* 2008;18:360–369.
201. Giannini C, Scheithauer BW, Weaver AL, et al. Oligodendrogliomas: reproducibility and prognostic value of histologic diagnosis and grading. *J Neuropathol Exp Neurol.* 2001;60:248–262.
202. McDonald JM, See SJ, Tremont IW, et al. The prognostic impact of histology and 1p/19q status in anaplastic oligodendroglial tumors. *Cancer.* 2005;104:1468–1477.
203. Coons SW, Johnson PC, Scheithauer BW, Yates AJ, Pearl DK. Improving diagnostic accuracy and interobserver concordance in the classification and grading of primary gliomas. *Cancer.* 1997;79:1381–1393.
204. Kros J, Gorlia T, van den Bent M. Panel review of anaplastic oligodendroglioma from EORTC trial 26951: consensus in diagnosis, and influence of 1p/19q [abstract PA-16]. *Neuro Oncol.* 2007;9:545.
205. Cairncross JG, Ueki K, Zlatescu MC, et al. Specific genetic predictors of chemotherapeutic response and survival in patients with anaplastic oligodendrogliomas. *J Natl Cancer Inst.* 1998;90:1473–1479.
206. Smith JS, Perry A, Borell TJ, et al. Alterations of chromosome arms 1p and 19q as predictors of survival in oligodendrogliomas, astrocytomas, and mixed oligoastrocytomas. *J Clin Oncol.* 2000;18:636–645.
207. Ino Y, Betensky RA, Zlatescu MC, et al. Molecular subtypes of anaplastic oligodendroglioma: implications for patient management at diagnosis. *Clin Cancer Res.* 2001;7:839–845.
208. Felsberg J, Erkwoh A, Sabel MC, et al. Oligodendroglial tumors: refinement of candidate regions on chromosome arm 1p and correlation of 1p/19q status with survival. *Brain Pathol.* 2004;14:121–130.
209. van den Bent MJ, Looijenga LH, Langenberg K, et al. Chromosomal anomalies in oligodendroglial tumors are correlated with clinical features. *Cancer.* 2003;97(5):1276–1284.
210. Gannett DE, Wisbeck WM, Silbergeld DL, Berger MS. The role of postoperative irradiation in the treatment of oligodendroglioma. *Int J Radiat Oncol Biol Phys.* 1994;30:567–573.
211. Wallner KE, Gonzales M, Sheline GE. Treatment of oligodendrogliomas with or without postoperative irradiation. *J Neurosurg.* 1988;68:684–688.
212. Abrey LE, Louis DN, Paleologos N, et al. Survey of treatment recommendations for anaplastic oligodendroglioma. *Neuro-oncology.* 2007;9:314–318.
213. Shapiro WR, Young DF. Chemotherapy of malignant glioma with CCNU alone and CCNU combined with vincristine sulfate and procarbazine hydrochloride. *Trans Am Neurol Assoc.* 1976;101:217–220.
214. Gutin PH, Wilson CB, Kumar AR, et al. Phase II study of procarbazine, CCNU, and vincristine combination chemotherapy in the treatment of malignant brain tumors. *Cancer.* 1975;35:1398–1404.
215. Cairncross JG, Macdonald DR. Successful chemotherapy for recurrent malignant oligodendroglioma. *Ann Neurol.* 1988;23:360–364.
216. Macdonald DR, Gaspar LE, Cairncross JG. Successful chemotherapy for newly diagnosed aggressive oligodendroglioma. *Ann Neurol.* 1990;27:573–574.
217. Macdonald DR, Cascino TL, Schold SC Jr, Cairncross JG. Response criteria for phase II studies of supratentorial malignant glioma. *J Clin Oncol.* 1990;8:1277–1280.
218. Cairncross JG, Macdonald DR, Pexman JH, Ives FJ. Steroid-induced CT changes in patients with recurrent malignant glioma. *Neurology.* 1988;38:724–726.

219. Watling CJ, Lee DH, Macdonald DR, Cairncross JG. Corticosteroid-induced magnetic resonance imaging changes in patients with recurrent malignant glioma. *J Clin Oncol.* 1994;12:1886–1889.
220. Saarinen UM, Pihko H, Mäkipernaa A. High-dose thiotepa with autologous bone marrow rescue in recurrent malignant oligodendroglioma: a case report. *J Neurooncol.* 1990;9:57–61.
221. Paleologos NA, Macdonald DR, Vick NA, Cairncross JG. Neoadjuvant procarbazine, CCNU, and vincristine for anaplastic and aggressive oligodendroglioma. *Neurology.* 1999;53:1141–1143.
222. Streffer J, Schabet M, Bamberg M, et al. A role for preirradiation PCV chemotherapy for oligodendroglial brain tumors. *J Neurol.* 2000;247:297–302.
223. Brandes AA, Tosoni A, Vastola F, et al. Efficacy and feasibility of standard procarbazine, lomustine, and vincristine chemotherapy in anaplastic oligodendroglioma and oligoastrocytoma recurrent after radiotherapy. A Phase II study. *Cancer.* 2004;101: 2079–2085.
224. van den Bent MJ, Taphoorn MJ, Brandes AA, et al. Phase II study of first-line chemotherapy with temozolomide in recurrent oligodendroglial tumors: the European Organization for Research and Treatment of Cancer Brain Tumor Group Study 26971. *J Clin Oncol.* 2003;21:2525–2528.
225. van den Bent MJ. Anaplastic oligodendroglioma and oligoastrocytoma. *Neurol Clin.* 2007;25:1089–109, ix.
226. Cairncross JG, Wang M, Chang S, et al. A randomized trial of chemotherapy plus radiotherapy (RT) versus RT alone for anaplastic oligodendroglioma (RTOG 9402): the perspective of longer follow-up [abstract]. *Int J Radiat Oncol Biol Phys.* 2008;72:S7-S8.
227. Chinot OL, Honore S, Dufour H, et al. Safety and efficacy of temozolomide in patients with recurrent anaplastic oligodendrogliomas after standard radiotherapy and chemotherapy. *J Clin Oncol.* 2001;19:2449–2455.
228. Triebels VH, Taphoorn MJ, Brandes AA, et al. Salvage PCV chemotherapy for temozolomide-resistant oligodendrogliomas. *Neurology.* 2004;63:904–906.
229. Peereboom D, Brewer C, Schiff D, et al. Dose-intense temozolomide in patients with newly diagnosed pure and mixed anaplastic oligodendroglioma: phase II multicenter study [abstract TA-40]. *Neuro Oncol.* 2006;8:448.
230. Taliansky-Aronov A, Bokstein F, Lavon I, Siegal T. Temozolomide treatment for newly diagnosed anaplastic oligodendrogliomas: a clinical efficacy trial. *J Neurooncol.* 2006;79:153–157.
231. Vogelbaum MA, Berkey B, Peereboom D, et al. Phase II trial of pre-irradiation and concurrent temozolomide in patients with newly diagnosed anaplastic oligodendrogliomas and mixed anaplastic oligoastrocytomas: RTOG BR0131. *Neuro Oncol.* 2009;11: 167–175.
232. Chahlavi A, Kanner A, Peereboom D, Staugaitis SM, Elson P, Barnett G. Impact of chromosome 1p status in response of oligodendroglioma to temozolomide: preliminary results. *J Neurooncol.* 2003;61:267–273.
233. Lassman AB, Panageas KS, Iwamoto FM, et al. International retrospective study of 1000+ adults with anaplastic oligodendroglial tumors [Abstract 283]. *Neuro Oncol.* 2009;11:629.
234. Chamberlain MC, Chowdhary SA, Glantz MJ. Anaplastic astrocytomas: biology and treatment. *Expert Rev Neurother.* 2008;8:575–586.

64 Medical Management for Pediatric Gliomas

Sabine Mueller

INTRODUCTION

Astrocytomas are the most common childhood central nervous system (CNS) tumor representing approximately 40% to 50% of all pediatric tumors. The World Health Organization (WHO) classifies these tumors into low-grade (WHO grade I and II) and high-grade (WHO grade III and IV) astrocytomas [1]. These tumors demonstrate a wide range of histopathology including pilocytic and fibrillary astrocytomas, ependymoma, pleomorphic astrocytoma, dysembryoplastic neuroepithelial tumor, and desmoplastic infantile ganglioglioma. The clinical course follows the histological grade with low-grade tumors being less aggressive than high-grade tumors. For the majority of gliomas, the etiology is unknown but certain genetic syndromes like Neurofibromatosis 1 (NF1) or Li-Fraumeni syndrome have an increased risk of developing CNS tumors. Presenting symptoms depend upon the location, classification of the tumor, and age at presentation. The majority of pediatric CNS tumors are low-grade and only 20% of supratentorial tumors are high-grade gliomas, which is in contrast to the distribution in adults. Children also have a tendency to develop malignant gliomas within the brainstem, which is rarely seen in adults. Brainstem gliomas will be discussed in more detail elsewhere.

HIGH-GRADE GLIOMAS

Introduction

High-grade gliomas account for the minority of supratentorial tumors in the pediatric population. They are classically divided into anaplastic astrocytomas (AA) and glioblastoma multiforme (GBM). The 5-year survival ranges from 5% to 15% for GBM and 20% to 40% for AA. Their clinical course varies from the adult population; in particular pediatric high-grade astrocytomas have a better response to chemotherapy. In comparison to low-grade tumors, the onset of symptoms is more rapid and often these children present with signs of increased intracranial pressure. Only 30% of patients with high-grade gliomas, compared to more than 50% with low-grade gliomas, present with seizures. Histologically, these tumors resemble their adult counterpart but they exhibit distinct genetic properties. For example, pediatric gliomas show infrequently epidermal growth factor receptor amplification [2] or Phosphatase and Tensin homolog mutations [3] compared to adult GBMs. P53 is linked to poor outcome in the pediatric population. One study showed that patients with low p53 expression had a 5-year event-free survival (EFS) of 44% compared with 17% in patients with p53 overexpression, which also differs from GBMs in the adult population [4]. Despite these differences, we use knowledge gained from trials in the adult population to develop treatment modalities for pediatric patients. However, pediatric gliomas are a distinct disease entity and only better understanding of their genetic and biological characteristics will lead to improved therapies.

Management

Surgery

The first therapeutic step for these tumors remains surgical resection dependent on tumor location. Gross total resection (GTR) is preferred because the extent of resection is linked to survival [5–7]. If the tumor extends to the deep nuclei or other critical brain areas, often a stereotactic biopsy is performed first, to establish the diagnosis to direct further treatment.

Radiation and Chemotherapy

High-grade gliomas used to be treated with resection followed by radiation therapy to the tumor bed. In 1998, a hallmark study from the Children's Cancer Group (CCG), CCG-945, demonstrated that chemotherapy, consisting of nitrosourea, vincristine, and prednisone, in addition to surgical resection and radiation therapy, prolonged survival compared to resection and radiation therapy only. The authors demonstrated that 5-year EFS was 46% for patients, who received chemotherapy and radiation compared with 18% in patients who only received radiation therapy. Poor prognostic factors based on this study were tumor location involving the basal ganglia, surgery limited to biopsy, and pathologic tumor characteristics like mitosis and necrosis. Surprisingly, the effect of chemotherapy was strongest in patients with GBM. In this subgroup, 5-year EFS was 42% in the combined group compared to 6% in patients just receiving radiation therapy [8]. The response to conventional chemotherapy in this group was surprising given the low response rate in adult GBMs. However, another key lesson learned from this study was that one of the main pitfalls in assessing treatment efficacy in pediatric brain tumors is varying histological classification between reviewers [9]. Therefore, institutional or even multicenter trials with no neuropathological central review must be viewed with caution. A subsequent large phase III study involving more than 160 patients demonstrated that a more intense chemotherapy with the "8-in-one-day" regimen versus a three-drug regimen with lomustine, vincristine, and prednisone had no beneficial effect on survival but worse side effects. It is thought that the lower response in the more complex chemotherapy group is partially due to the suboptimum dose intensity of several components. This study confirmed that improved outcome is associated with histological grade, greater than 90% resection, and non-midline tumors. The EFS for patients treated with prednisone, vincristine, and lomustine was only 26% compared to 42% in the prior study from 1989 but nevertheless the combination regimen remains superior to radiation therapy only [7]. Since then, chemotherapy has been added to radiation therapy in different schedules, either in a "sandwich" protocol, in which chemotherapy is given prior to radiation therapy with the aim of obtaining maximal tumor reduction as well as after, concomitantly or as maintenance therapy. The German Society of Pediatric Oncology and Hematology conducted a phase III study, called the *HIT-91* study, which confirmed the extent of resection as a critical parameter for assessing prognosis. In this study, patients randomized to a sandwich therapy consisting of preradiation chemotherapy with ifosfamide, VP-16, methotrexate, cisplatin, and cytarabine followed by radiation therapy after surgery, had a significant better overall survival (OS) than patients treated with maintenance therapy, which started with radiation therapy followed by chemotherapy with lomustine, vincristine, and cisplatin. The median OS was 5.17 years for the sandwich arm compared to 1.94 years for the maintenance arm [5]. The authors also concluded that if resection exceeds 90% it is safe to postpone radiation therapy, whereas in patients with subtotal resection (STR) irradiation should be performed early in the treatment course. One limitation of this study was that pathology was not centrally reviewed. As mentioned above, the CCG-945 study showed that 28% of patients were misclassified by institutional review as high grade and revised by a consensus neuropathology review as low-grade tumors [10]. The favorable outcome observed in the *HIT-91* study might therefore be due to a larger number of patients with low-grade gliomas than indicated in the analysis. Because the "8-in-one-day" and other multiagent regimens failed, the approach to chemotherapy has shifted from increasing complexity to dose intensification. In the CCG-9933 study, the investigators compared three different alkylating agents administered in conjunction with etoposide (carboplatin/etoposide, ifosfamide/etoposide, and cyclophosphamide/etoposide) in patients with residual disease. Unfortunately, none of the three treatment arms showed beneficial effect toward survival [11]. Over the past years, multiple other phase II trials tested single agents like etoposide, cyclophosphamide, irinotectan, platinum compounds, procarbazine, and topotecan with marginal effect on OS. Because concomitant temozolamide (TMZ) and radiation therapy for adult patients with GBM led to prolonged survival, several studies have tested the efficacy of this drug in pediatric brain tumors. TMZ is of particular interest because it has excellent oral bioavailability and good penetration to the CNS. A phase I study of TMZ given over 5 days every 28 days in children led to treatment response in 2 out of 5 patients with high-grade glioma and stable disease in 1 patient [12]. This study also demonstrated that thrombocytopenia is the dose-limiting toxicity. Studies from the United Kingdom and France targeting heavily pretreated children with recurrent GBM and brainstem GBM with TMZ showed low response rates and similar toxicity profile [13]. The Children's Oncology group (COG) completed a phase II trial using the same regimen as published by Estlin et al. Out of 23 patients with high-grade astrocytomas, 1 patient showed partial response after 2 cycles but developed progressive disease after course 9. One patient experienced a transient response lasting less than 6 weeks after treatment start. Thus TMZ was not effective in this study for high-grade astrocytomas [14]. The enzyme O^6-methylguanine-DNA methyltransferase (MGMT) removes alkyl groups and several studies demonstrated that decreased MGMT expression or methylation of the MGMT promoter is associated with improved clinical response in adults [15-18]. In a retrospective analysis using methylation specific PCR and immunohistochemistry analysis in 24 children with relapsed high-grade gliomas, only DNA methylation status but not MGMT expression correlated with increased median EFS and OS [19]. These studies suggest that TMZ is less effective in pediatric high-grade astrocytomas relative to adults. Currently studies are ongoing using TMZ in combination with O6-benzylguanine. The recent experience from the German oncology group (HIT-gBM-c study) assessed the response in children with high-grade gliomas treated with standard fractionated radiation and simultaneous chemotherapy (cisplatin, etoposide, vincristine, ifosfamide) followed by maintenance chemotherapy (cisplatin, etoposide, ifosfamide and vincristine) and the histone deactelyase inhibitor valproic acid. The 5-year OS rate in patients with GTR was reported at 63% (± 12%) compared to 17% (± 10%) for the historical control group [20]. The optimal chemotherapeutical regimen for children with high-grade gliomas has not been established and therefore most patients are enrolled in clinical trials. A significant number of studies are underway testing newer agents that target specific molecular pathways for children with relapsed high-grade glioma. These are described in more detail below.

To date, multimodality treatment combining surgery, radiation, and chemotherapy is the standard approach for children with high-grade glioma older than 3 years of age, but further studies are needed to determine the best regimen. In the younger population, the main goal of therapy remains to delay the use of radiation therapy given its negative effect on neurocognitive development. Newer strategies with the goal to deliver radiation therapy more directed toward the target are essential to eliminate these side effects.

High-Grade Gliomas in Very Young Children

Introduction

Astrocytomas constitute approximately 30% of all CNS tumors in infants, of which 25% are high-grade gliomas. The main presenting symptom is macrocephaly, which is observed in more than 50% of cases. Over one third of patients will present with signs of increased intracranial pressure [21].

Management

To date there is no consensus about the best treatment modalities for these very young patients. The majority of patients undergo surgery after initial diagnosis. Over the past years, the main goal of postsurgical therapy is to delay the use of radiation therapy secondary to the known side effects affecting brain development. There is limited experience for young children. Two multi-institutional studies for children with newly diagnosed high-grade glioma showed that outcome at younger age was better even without the use of radiation therapy compared to older children [22,23]. The COG group showed that 39 children less than 24 month of age treated with "8-in-one-day" regimen had a PFS at 3 years follow-up of 36% and a 3-year survival of 44%. If analyzed for the different histological grades, AA had the expected more favorable outcome than GBM with PFS being 44% and 0% respectively [22]. Another study showed that 18 children with high-grade glioma less than 3 years of age treated with vincristine and cyclophosphamide after resection had a 5-year OS of 50% [23]. In this study, the extent of resection and pathology had no influence on outcome. Interestingly, infants less than 6 months of age faired better than older children.

Why this subpopulation has an apparent better response to chemotherapy than older children remains unclear. It might be due to a distinct genetic profile of these high-grade gliomas in the very young child. However, given the discordance amongst neuro-pathologists diagnosing high-grade gliomas in children, these results need to be interpreted with caution. Currently, children less than 3 years of age are treated with chemotherapy after resection with the goal to delay radiotherapy until at least 3 years of age.

Recurrent High-Grade Glioma

The prognosis for children with recurrent high-grade glioma remains poor. A standard of care for recurrent high-grade glioma does not exist. Treatment options at the time of relapse consist of surgery, radiation and chemotherapy and participation in clinical trials. In the CCG 945 trial, nearly all children who developed recurrent disease after surgery, chemotherapy, and radiation, died within 1 year. The outcome of children from the CCG 945 study who experienced relapse and were treated with conventional chemotherapy was compared with the outcome from patients from the CCG 9883 study, who received thiotepa and etoposide either alone or with carboplatin followed by autologous stem cell rescue. Patients treated with myeloablative therapy had a significant better outcome than children receiving conventional chemotherapy. Finlay et al. showed that using thiotepa and etoposide followed by autologous stem cell rescue showed long-term survival in 5 out of 18 patients with GBM. All 5 survivors had minimal residual disease at the time of chemotherapy, suggesting that this is a key factor for prognosis [24]. Bevacizumab, a monoclonal antibody against the vascular endothelial growth factor, has shown promise in treating adult high-grade gliomas and is approved by the FDA for adult patients with GBM. A recent study investigated the benefit of Bevacizumab in combination with Irinotecan in 12 pediatric patients with recurrent high-grade gliomas. Overall the regimen was tolerated quiet well. Two patients experienced a partial response and 4 patients were noted to have stable disease on magnetic resonance imaging (MRI). The PFS and OS were 2.25 and 6.25 month respectively [25].

Currently the COG is conducting a phase 2 study using cilengitide for progressive high-grade gliomas. Multiple phase I studies are currently carried out by the COG including Sorafenib, a Raf kinase and receptor kinase inhibitor; Sunitinib, a multi-targeted tyrosine kinase inhibitor; vascular epidermal growth factor (VEGF) Trap, a human soluble decoy receptor protein that binds VEGF and has been shown to block VEGF signaling; a aurora kinase inhibitor and a gamma-secretase inhibitor.

Future Direction for High-Grade Gliomas

The molecular pathways involved in adult high-grade gliomas are increasingly defined but it remains unknown if the same molecular events are involved in pediatric brain tumors. Growing body of evidence suggests that the molecular changes leading to the development of high-grade gliomas are distinct between children and adults. Therefore, the age of the targeted population needs to be taken into account when designing new drugs. Table 64.1 summarizes the key genetic alterations discovered in pediatric and adult gliomas.

Based on current knowledge, preclinical evaluation, and results from adult trials, a number of targeted therapies are currently being evaluated in pediatric brain tumors. Once the molecular biology of pediatric tumors is more defined, these approaches can be tailored more specifically to the pediatric population. Table 64.2 lists a number of targeted therapy trials conducted in children with brain tumors.

Unfortunately, adult trials using these agents as single drug regimens have been disappointing. Future designs of clinical trials will potentially involve the combination of key pathway inhibition and detailed molecular characterization of the tumors in order to be able to tailor therapy specifically toward the genetic modifications observed individually for each patient. Other areas currently explored to improve outcome are alternative delivery techniques like convection enhanced delivery, which will be discussed in more detail elsewhere.

Table 64.1 Summary of key molecular and genetic alterations in pediatric and adult high-grade gliomas

Genetic Alteration	Reference	Pediatric Gliomas (%)	Adult Gliomas (%)
EGFR amplification	Nakumara et al, 2007;	10% (1/44) AA; 11% (2/44) GBM	30–40
	Pollack et al, 2006;	2.6% (1/38) GMB	
	Raffel et al, 1999;	0% (0/15) GBM; 0% (0/17) AA	
	Bredel et al, 1999;	10% (2/19) GBM; 0% (0/6) AA	
	Cheng et al, 1999	0% (0/24) GBM + AA	
EGFR overexpression	Nakumara et al, 2007;	28% of AA and GBM	30–40
	Pollack et al, 2006;	36% (14/38) GBM	
	Ganigi et al, 2005;	25.9 % (13/54) GBM + AA	
	Bredel et al, 1999;	84% (16/19) GBM; 50% (3/6) AA	
	Surfe et al, 1995	11% (2/19) GBM +AA	
EGFRvIII expression	No data available		10–30
PDFGR amplification	Nakumara et al, 2007	0%	10–15
TP53 mutation	Nakumara et al, 2007;	30% AA; 33% GBM 30–35% (6/18 with 1/18 in pt < 6 years of age)	
	Ganigi et al, 2005;	53.7% (28/54) p53 overexpression GBM	
	Pollack et al 2002;	35% (41/115) overexpression; 33% (40/121) mutation GBM + AA	
	Cheng et al 1999;	38% (9/24) GBM + AA	
	Raffel et al, 1999;	20% (3/15) GBM; 24% (4/17) AA	
	Sure et al, 1995	25% (5/20) GBM	
Rb mutation	Ganigi et al, 2005;	7.4% (4/56) GBM	70–85
	Sung et al, 2000	< 25% GBM + AA	
PTEN mutation/deletion	Pollack et al, 2006;	13% (7/62) GBM deletion	20–30
	Cheng et al, 1999;	8% (2/24) GBM + AA	
	Raffel et al, 1999	20% (3/15) GBM, 6% (1/17) AA	
MGMT methylation	Donson et al, 2007	40% (4/10) GBM	45
Microsatellite instability	Alonso et al, 2001;	27% (12/45) GBM + AA	0–8
	Cheng et al, 1999	16% (4/24) GBM + AA	

Abbreviations: EGFR, epidermal growth factor receptor; PDGFR, platelet-derived growth factor receptor; MGMT, O^6-methylguanine–DNA methyltransferase.

Table 64.2 Summary of agents currently under investigation in clinical trials for children with high-grade gliomas.

Class of Agent	Drug	Type of Study	Type of Administration	Intracellular Target
EGFR inhibitors	Erlotinib	Phase I	Oral	EGFR
	Gefitinib	Phase I/II	Oral	EGFR
Farnesyltransferase inhibitors	Lonafarnib	Phase I	Oral	Farnesyltransferase
	Tipifarnib	Phase I/II	Oral	Farnesyltransferase
PDGFR inhibitors	Imatinib	Phase I/II	Oral	PDGFR
mTOR inhibitor	Temsirolimus	Phase I/II	Intravenous	PTEN/AKT pathway
	Everolimus		Oral	PTEN/Akt pathway
Antiangiogenic agents	Cilengitide	Phase I	Oral	$\alpha_v\beta_3$ Integrin receptor
	Lenalidomide	Phase I	Oral	TNG-α, VEGF
	Enzastaurine	Phase I	Oral	Proteinkinase Cβ
	Cediranib	Phase I	Oral	VEGFR 1,2,3
	Semaxanib	Phase I	IV	VEGFR-2
	Bevacizumab	Phase II	IV	VEGF Ab
MGMT inhibitor	O6-Benzylguanine and temozolamide			

LOW-GRADE GLIOMA

Introduction

Low-grade astrocytomas account for approximately 40% of all childhood CNS tumors. These tumors are often slow growing and have an indolent course, especially in patients with NF1. Despite histological similarities, low-grade gliomas display striking clinical heterogeneity depending where they are localized. Based on location, low-grade gliomas are generally divided into hemispheric, optic pathway, thalamic, and cerebellar lesions with distinct clinical features. Local progression, for example, is more common in young children with hypothalamic and thalamic lesions [26–28]. Histological low-grade gliomas are mainly classified into pilocytic astrocytomas (WHO grade I) and fibrillary astrocytomas (WHO grade II). Patients with pilocytic astrocytomas independent from location have a better outcome than patients with fibrillary astrocytomas. Depending on location, surgical resection is the mainstay of therapy and can lead to long-term survival of greater than 80%. Unsolved questions to date remain the timing as well as the desired extent of resection depending on location. Studies are ongoing to determine the ideal subsequent treatment with radiation therapy, chemotherapy, or a combination thereof.

Supratentorial Low-Grade Gliomas

Cerebral Low-Grade Glioma

Low-grade astrocytomas account for approximately 50% of hemispheric tumors and 8% to 20% of all pediatric low-grade gliomas in children, with a peak incidence between 8 to 12 years of age. The 5-year OS rate for patients with hemispheric low-grade gliomas ranges from 40% to 70% but a substantial number will have tumor recurrence necessitating multimodality treatment strategies. Therapies for inoperable, residual, or recurrent disease remain controversial and may include observation, second surgery, radiation, and/or chemotherapy. Because patients with low-grade gliomas have long-term survival chances, these patients must be considered having a chronic disease and treatment strategies need to focus on reducing treatment related morbidity.

Surgery

The mainstay of therapy today is surgical resection, either at diagnosis or relapse [29]. Children who underwent complete resection of their tumor had a superior outcome compared to patients who underwent STR [29,30]. Because malignant transformation of low-grade gliomas is rarely seen in the pediatric population, small residual tumors are often followed clinically with serial imaging. Repeat surgery for local recurrence is an important consideration. Furthermore, development of newer techniques like interstitial Iodine 125 radiosurgery alone or in combination with microsurgery might offer beneficial effects on outcome for tumors located in eloquent areas in this patient group [31].

Radiation Therapy

Early studies have shown that radiation therapy usually delays disease progression but many children will ultimately die from progressive disease [32]. Because radiation therapy might lead to severe neurocognitive, endocrine, and vascular sequalae, particularly in the younger population, recent trends have focused on the development of alternative strategies including chemotherapy to delay or avoid its use completely [33]. A subsequent analysis of the CCG-945 trial conducted for high-grade gliomas showed that 70 children were reclassified by central review with low-grade tumors. For these patients, the 5-year PFS was 38% for those treated with chemotherapy alone versus 68% for those treated with chemotherapy and radiation therapy. A more recent phase II study from St. Jude's hospital using conformal radiation radiation therapy for pediatric low-grade gliomas reported a 5-year EFS of 87% (± 4.4%) and a 10-year EFS of 74.3% (± 15.4%) [34]. Neuro-cognitive assessment of these children 5 years after radiation therapy demonstrated that children younger than 5 years of age had the greatest cognitive decline but that patients greater than 10 years fared quiet well [35]. Therefore despite its side effect, radiation therapy remains a valid option in these patients, especially in older children.

Chemotherapy

Chemotherapy protocols are under constant evolution and trials are ongoing to determine the best combination of agents. The first published series of children with low-grade glioma treated with chemotherapy was published in 1985. Since then, chemotherapy became an essential part of the treatment regimen for these tumors, mainly to delay radiation therapy for above-mentioned reasons. Because low-grade gliomas are a very heterogeneous group of tumors, it is difficult to compare the various trials performed. Since the introduction of carboplatin, multiple studies have shown moderate, to high partial, to complete response rates when used in combination with vincristine. In 1993, Packer et al. reported a radiographic response in 52% of patients with recurrent disease and 62% in newly diagnosed patients treated with vincristine and carboplatin [36]. Similar results were found in a larger study involving 78 patients with newly diagnosed tumors [37]. Interestingly, in the later study the authors showed that neither histopathological grade nor location affected the response rate, which is in contrast to other reports. The only prognostic factor found in this study was age, with children less than 5 years having a significantly better 3-year PFS. This is in contrast to multiple other studies showing that patients less than 1 year of age have a worse outcome [27,38]. Currently, vincristine in combination with carboplatin is the most commonly used multiagent chemotherapy for children with low-grade glioma and future trials will be judged against these results [39]. Because there is a high incidence of anaphylactic reactions to carboplatin and the long-term effects on overall health are unknown, there is a high demand for alternative agents. TMZ has been tested in pediatric low-grade gliomas with moderate success. Currently, studies are conducted using multiagent chemotherapy regimens like Irinotecan and Avastin, different radiation techniques like stereotactic conformal radiotherapy or proton beam therapy, as well as biological agents like Erlotinib, an epidermal growth factor receptor inhibitor, in combination with radiation therapy. Recently multiple reports have implicated BRAF in the molecular pathogenesis of pediatric low-grade gliomas and studies are on the way to test inhibitors of the MAP kinase signaling pathway [40,41]. Further discovery of molecular pathways involved in the development of low-grade tumors will enable the development of more specific agents with the goal to reduce side effects of current treatment strategies in this patient population.

Optic Pathway Glioma

Optic pathway gliomas are histopathologically characterized as low-grade astrocytomas with a majority being pilocytic astrocytomas (WHO grade I) [42,43]. They can arise anywhere along the optic nerve, chiasm, and hypothalamus and rarely extend along the visual pathways posterior. Most of these tumors occur early in life with a peak incidence of 8.8 years of age [44]. About 4% to 6% of all pediatric CNS tumors and 20% to 30% of all pediatric gliomas consist of optic pathway glioma, whereas the incidence in adults is only 2%. These tumors have a strong correlation with NF1. Studies suggest that up to 30% of patients with optic pathway glioma have stigmata of NF1 [44] and approximately 12% to 20% of patients with NF1 have signs of optic pathway glioma [45]. The discrepancy between these numbers is best explained by the fact that many NF1 patients are asymptomatic and therefore might never been diagnosed. The main diagnostic investigations include neuro-opthalmologic examination, endocrine evaluation, and MRI of the brain. Most of the tumors are diagnosed clinically on the basis of symptoms, age of patient, as well the radiographic appearance. For lesions involving the chiasm and hypothalamus, a broader differential diagnosis needs to be entertained. For example, germ cell tumors can present in a similar fashion in that age group. For these tumors, a biopsy is often required to ensure the right diagnosis unless the patient has a history of NF1 or the tumor involves the optic nerve or optic radiation. Management of patients with optic pathway glioma remains controversial and is based on an individual's disease course. The main challenge for the clinician remains to predict which tumors will follow a benign course and can be managed by observation only versus the more aggressive tumors that will need therapeutic intervention to assure the best possible outcome. Patients with optic pathway gliomas and minimally symptomatic disease can often be followed clinically with serial examination of their visual acuity and fields as well as periodic surveillance MRIs. To date, there is no consensus regarding the frequency of these examinations and it can vary from every 3 to 24 months [46]. Some studies argue that assessment of the visual system is sufficient to follow these patients and that MRI studies are not indicated in a patient with no sign of disease progression [46,47]. In general, optic pathway gliomas tend to be less aggressive in patients with NF1 and can often be observed without treatment initiation [48].

Surgical Intervention

The role of surgery in patients with optic pathway gliomas remains controversial. Most of the patients do not require a surgical biopsy unless atypical location or presentation warrants further investigation [49]. Consensus for surgical intervention exists for single nerve lesions, which cause disfiguring symptoms for patients. Also, if signs of increased intracranial pressure, mass effect, or hydrocephalus are present, surgery often is of benefit [50,51]. Patients with rapidly growing tumors, more frequently associated with hypothalamic and chiasmatic lesions, benefit from early surgery to preserve vision and reduction of mass effect [46].

Infants with optic pathway gliomas in the chiasm and hypothalamic area present more common with aggressive tumors and require surgical intervention early in their disease state. In younger patients, surgical intervention might be warranted to delay the use of more toxic therapies like chemotherapy or radiation [52]. One study showed that patients with NF1 have twice the recurrence rate than patients without NF1 after surgical resection, questioning the benefit of surgical intervention in this subset of patients [53].

Radiation Therapy

Radiation therapy plays a significant role in the management of optic pathway gliomas although current strategies favor to delay radiation in the younger patient. Radiation therapy is also discouraged in patients with NF1, mainly due to the development of neurovascular, endocrine, or neuropsychological side effects as well as the high risk of developing secondary malignancies [54]). One study by Singhal et al. showed that 3 out of 5 patients with NF1 and optic pathway glioma, who received radiation therapy for disease progression, developed a secondary CNS tumor, whereas none of the sporadic cases developed a secondary tumor [55]. On the other hand, fractionated stereotactic radiotherapy has been used in a cohort of 15 patients of whom 3 had NF1 and none of these patients developed endocrine abnormalities or secondary tumors. These patients had a 90% 5-year survival rate [56]. Further studies are required to further confirm this study and assure the beneficial effect of radiation therapy in this population. New techniques to reduce radiation toxicity are currently under development and will continue to improve outcome in these patients.

Chemotherapy

Chemotherapy has been shown to delay the need for radiation therapy and has become the mainstay of therapy for young children with optic pathway gliomas [57]. Combined therapy with carboplatin and vincristine has been effective in controlling progressive low-grade gliomas in patients less than 5 years of age [37,57]. Alkylating agents and multidrug regimens have been tried but carry the potential risk for the development of secondary malignancies, especially in NF1 patients. Failure of chemotherapy has historically been seen as an indication to initiate radiation therapy, but recent developments are directed toward chemotherapeutic salvage.

To date, the best therapy for progressive optic pathway gliomas after surgical resection is the combination of vincristine and carboplatin but novel chemotherapeutical agents are currently developed.

Cerebellar Astrocytomas

Cerebellar astrocytomas represent 12% to 17% of all pediatric brain tumors and 20% to 35% of all pediatric posterior fossa tumors [58,59]. Around 85% of these are pilocytic astrocytomas and classified as WHO grade I. The mean age of onset is 6.8 years. Typical presenting symptoms include headaches, ataxia, vomiting, visual symptoms like diplopia, and decreased level of arousal. Risk factors include prior radiation to the brain and a diagnosis of NF1. About 5% of patients with NF1 will develop cerebellar astrocytomas [60]. The natural history of these tumors consists of slow-growing lesions, which can cause progressive signs and symptoms related to hydrocephalus. Ultimately patients die from increasing mass effect and herniation if left untreated.

Surgical Intervention

When patients present with signs of increased intracranial pressure and are diagnosed with a posterior fossa mass, the first intervention often consists of steroids as well placement of an external ventricular shunt, if immediate relief of raised intracranial pressure is warranted based on the patient's clinical condition. In patients who are asymptomatic, GTR is the first treatment step. Only 10% to 40% of patients will require a permanent cerebrospinal fluid diversion procedure after resection [61]. If GTR is achieved, these patients are followed with surveillance MRIs. There is no agreement on frequency of these studies but most centers would monitor every 3 to 6 months in the 1st year and then annually for at least 3 to 4 years. If the tumor was classified as a grade 1 tumor, imaging surveillance can generally be aborted after 5 years. If there is any change in the clinical presentation, even years later, these patients need to be assessed for recurrence. In general, patients diagnosed with a grade 2 tumor are followed for longer periods of time with annual imaging. Cerebellar astrocytomas have a good prognosis after total resection, the outcome after STR is less well documented and ranges from 18% to 100% [62]. The management of these patients is particularly difficult because cerebellar astrocytomas do not always recur despite STR and no further treatment [63]. It has been speculated that growth arrest or spontaneous remission is due to either interruption of vascular supply or that remaining cells remained quiescent without dividing as a result of reduced concentrations of autocrine growth factors after surgical debulking [62].

Radiation Therapy

Radiation therapy after surgical resection remains controversial. The development of different radiation therapies like three-dimensional conformal radiotherapy and fractionated stereotactic radiotherapy might increase the delivery to the tumor field and reduce radiation to surrounding normal brain [64]. Tumor recurrence usually occurs locally at the primary side. Management after recurrence is controversial and consists of a combination of second surgery, radiation therapy, as well as chemotherapy depending on patient's age, presentation, as well physician's preference. The beneficial effect of chemotherapy for low-grade gliomas is discussed elsewhere.

A rare complication physicians treating children with cerebellar lesions should be aware of is cerebellar mutism. This normally occurs 24 hours to 6 days after surgical intervention and can last days up to 4 months [65]. Children stop speaking completely and then develop dysarthric speech, which improves over time. Some reports describe that patients have complete resolution, whereas others reported children with symptoms lasting more than 5 years [66]. No special treatment is available for these children but their parents should be warned about this complication and reassured given the general good prognosis.

Ependymomas

Ependymomas are localized mainly paraventricular with the majority of tumors occurring in the posterior fossa. They represent 5% to 10% of all pediatric brain tumors and 25% of all spinal cord tumors. It is the third most common pediatric brain tumor following astrocytomas and medulloblastomas. More than 50% of patients are under 5 years of age at time of diagnosis. Currently, ependymomas are classified by the WHO as either grade I (myxopapillary), grade II (cellular, papillary, clear cell and tancytic), and grade III (anaplastic) ependymomas. Unfortunately, the current classification system leaves room for individual interpretation and therefore clinical studies have failed to show a correlation between grade and overall outcome [29,67]. The difficulty on developing therapies and comparing trial is partially due to the high variability amongst neuropathologists, with reported discordance of 69% between central and local review [68,69]. Some studies have shown a 50% chance of recurrence even after 5 years with the majority of treatment failures occurring at the primary site. Spinal cord ependymomas are uncommon in younger patients [70] and overall have a better prognosis than ependymomas located within the brain, with 5-year OS of 70% to 100% [71].

Despite a multimodal therapy, outcome did not improve significantly over the last three decades, with less than 50% of patients surviving longer than 5 years, emphasizing the need for alternative treatment options [72]. Some series have shown that children less than 5 years of age have a worse prognosis than older children [73,74]. This phenomenon might be due to variable treatment regimens as suggested by the first baby pediatric oncology group study or be due to true biological differences between age groups.

Surgical Intervention

Outcome has been linked by multiple studies to the extent of surgical resection and in some studies to age. Patients with GTR and radiation have a 5-year PFS of 51% to 57% compared to a 5-year PFS of 0 to 26% for patients with STR and radiation therapy [29,75,76]. Patients undergoing GTR have a much better outcome than children with residual disease, providing some rational for "second look" surgery if the lesion is amenable for further resection [68]. A recent study completed by the COG (ACNS0121) assessed whether second surgery would increase surgical morbidity to an unacceptable level. The final analysis of this study has not been published but only 4 out 25 patients who underwent a second surgery had surgical complications. The staging work up should include MRI of the brain and spinal cord as well as cerebrospinal fluid cytology. Spinal seeding is most common in infratentorial high-grade ependymomas. Surgical intervention with the goal of GTR is the mainstay of initial therapy. Second-look surgery should be considered if patients have residual disease on follow-up MRIs.

Radiation Therapy

Postoperative radiation therapy is often used and is associated with improved tumor control. Due to the adverse effects of radiation on neurocognitive development studies have focused on the use of multiagent chemotherapy to delay radiation therapy. Few studies have shown that children with low-grade ependymomas have a good outcome despite foregoing radiation therapy [77–79]. A study from the United Kingdom Cancer study group and the International Society of Pediatric Oncology (UKCCSG/SIOP) treated children less than 3 years of age with combined adjuvant chemotherapy (carboplatin, vincristine, cyclophosphamide, cisplatin, methotrexate). Radiation therapy was reserved for patients with recurrent resistant disease. The authors reported a PFS of 69.5% at 3 years for children younger than 3 years of age. These findings are better than prior reports from the pediatric oncology group who treated patients from 1986 until 1990 with 12 or 24 months of chemotherapy prior to radiation with a disappointing 5-year PFS of 27% [80]. Also, the French oncology group reported only 22% 4-year PFS in 73 patients treated with chemotherapy only [81]. Researchers from St. Jude's hospital have shown in a phase II trial, using conformal radiotherapy in 88 children with ependymoma (55% < 3 years of age), a 3-year PFS was 69.5%. Serial neurocognitive evaluation demonstrated that there was no significant decline before and after radiation therapy independent from patient's age [82]. With the development of new radiation techniques, the effect on cognition and development might be reduced and therefore become a valid part in the treatment of these patients, independent of age. Currently studies are assessing these factors and include neurocognitive testing in the trial design.

Craniospinal irradiation introduced in 1975 for the treatment of ependymomas should be reserved for patients with evidence of spinal seeding and might be considered in patients with infratentorial anaplastic ependymomas. However, prophylactic spinal irradiation did not seem to modify outcome in multiple series [83–85]. Local relapse was confirmed to be the most significant component. Radiosurgery is a potential treatment option for patients with recurrent disease. In one study, local tumor control was achieved in 3 out of 5 patients treated for localized residual ependymoma [86].

Chemotherapy

The role of chemotherapy in the treatment of ependymomas remains controversial. Multiple agents like carboplatin, cisplatin, etoposide, idarubicin, ifosfamide, irinotectan, PCNU, and TMZ have been studied in phase II trials with modest response [87]. Multiagent strategies (e.g., lomustine, prednisone, and vincristine) [88] as well as high-dose chemotherapy with stem cell rescue have been disappointing [89,90] and cannot be recommended generally. The CCG 9921 study assessed the effect of two different chemotherapy regimens in children less than 3 years of age to estimate control intervals without irradiation. Chemotherapy consisted of induction chemotherapy with vincristine, cisplatin, etoposide, and cyclophosphamide or vincristine, carboplatin, ifosamide, and etoposide. Maintenance chemotherapy was the same in the two treatment arms and consisted of vincristine, etoposide, carboplatin, and cyclophosphamide. Radiation therapy was delayed in children with no residual or metastatic disease unless they progressed. A total of 74 patients with ependymoma were enrolled in this trial with 19% less than 1 year of age, 21% between 12 and 17 months and 39% less than 36 months of age. About 70% of these patients had no residual disease after surgery. There was no significant difference between the two treatment arms. Four patients showed complete response, three partial response, and six patients had stable disease after induction chemotherapy. The 1- and 5-year EFS were 72% and 32% respectively; 63% of the 5-year event-free survivors had not received radiation therapy and 83% of these patients had minimal residual disease. Except for incomplete resection, no other factor was prognostically significant [91]. One study using thiotepa, etoposide, and carboplatin with autologous stem cell rescue revealed that out of 15 children with recurrent disease 5 died of treatment complications and the rest of the patients had recurrent disease [92].

Currently the COG is conducting a multicenter trial to assess the response to post radiation chemotherapy with vincristine, cisplatin, etoposide and cyclophosphamide. The role of chemotherapy in patients with ependymoma remains uncertain, however preliminary support the role of chemotherapy in this population as outlined above.

Future Directions For Ependymomas

Little is known regarding the molecular pathways involved in the development of ependymomas compared with other brain tumors. The knowledge of the molecular characteristics will enable further development of new treatment strategies and should be one of the main focuses of ependymoma research. Recent studies identified radial glial cells as the potential cancer stem cells of ependymomas [93,94]. If the stem cell hypothesis holds true, it will be essential for further drug development in particular to address these cancer stem cells. One key player in ependymomas is the Notch signaling pathway, which might be a possible target for future drug development [93]. Trials are currently investigating the benefit of antiangiogenesis therapy with antibodies directed against VEGF in recurrent ependymomas.

REFERENCES

1. Kleihues P, Louis DN, Scheithauer BW, et al. The WHO classification of tumors of the nervous system. *J Neuropathol Exp Neurol.* 2002;61(3):215–225; discussion 226.
2. Bredel M, Pollack IF, Hamilton RL, James CD. Epidermal growth factor receptor expression and gene amplification in high-grade non-brainstem gliomas of childhood. *Clin Cancer Res.* 1999;5(7):1786–1792.
3. Nakamura M, Shimada K, Ishida E, et al. Molecular pathogenesis of pediatric astrocytic tumors. *Neuro-oncology.* 2007;9(2):113–123.
4. Pollack IF, Finkelstein SD, Woods J, et al. Expression of p53 and prognosis in children with malignant gliomas. *N Engl J Med.* 2002;346(6):420–427.
5. Wolff JE, Gnekow AK, Kortmann RD, et al. Preradiation chemotherapy for pediatric patients with high-grade glioma. *Cancer.* 2002;94(1):264–271.
6. Heideman RL, Kuttesch J Jr, Gajjar AJ, et al. Supratentorial malignant gliomas in childhood: a single institution perspective. *Cancer.* 1997;80(3):497–504.
7. Finlay JL, Boyett JM, Yates AJ, et al. Randomized phase III trial in childhood high-grade astrocytoma comparing vincristine, lomustine, and prednisone with the eight-drugs-in-1-day regimen. Childrens Cancer Group. *J Clin Oncol.* 1995;13(1):112–123.
8. Sposto R, Ertel IJ, Jenkin RD, et al. The effectiveness of chemotherapy for treatment of high grade astrocytoma in children: results of a

randomized trial. A report from the Childrens Cancer Study Group. *J Neurooncol.* 1989;7(2):165–177.
9. Pollack IF, Boyett JM, Yates AJ, et al. The influence of central review on outcome associations in childhood malignant gliomas: results from the CCG-945 experience. *Neuro-oncology.* 2003;5(3):197–207.
10. Finlay JL, Zacharoulis S. The treatment of high-grade gliomas and diffuse intrinsic pontine tumors of childhood and adolescence: a historical - and futuristic - perspective. *J Neurooncol.* 2005;75(3):253–266.
11. MacDonald TJ, Arenson EB, Ater J, et al. Phase II study of high-dose chemotherapy before radiation in children with newly diagnosed high-grade astrocytoma: final analysis of Children's Cancer Group Study 9933. *Cancer.* 2005;104(12):2862–2871.
12. Estlin EJ, Lashford L, Ablett S, et al. Phase I study of temozolomide in paediatric patients with advanced cancer. United Kingdom Children's Cancer Study Group. *Br J Cancer.* 1998;78(5):652–661.
13. Lashford LS, Thiesse P, Jouvet A, et al. Temozolomide in malignant gliomas of childhood: a United Kingdom Children's Cancer Study Group and French Society for Pediatric Oncology Intergroup Study. *J Clin Oncol.* 2002;20(24):4684–4691.
14. Nicholson HS, Kretschmar CS, Krailo M, et al. Phase 2 study of temozolomide in children and adolescents with recurrent central nervous system tumors: a report from the Children's Oncology Group. *Cancer.* 2007;110(7):1542–1550.
15. Esteller M, Garcia-Foncillas J, Andion E, et al. Inactivation of the DNA-repair gene MGMT and the clinical response of gliomas to alkylating agents. *N Engl J Med.* 2000;343:1350–1354.
16. Hegi ME, Diserens AC, Godard S, et al. Clinical trial substantiates the predictive value of O-6-methylguanine-DNA methyltransferase promoter methylation in glioblastoma patients treated with temozolomide. *Clin Cancer Res.* 2004;10:1871–1874.
17. Hegi ME, Diserens AC, Gorlia T, et al. MGMT gene silencing and benefit from temozolomide in glioblastoma. *N Engl J Med.* 2005;352:997–1003.
18. Brell M, Tortosa A, Verger E, et al. Prognostic significance of O6-methylguanine-DNA methyltransferase determined by promoter hypermethylation and immunohistochemical expression in anaplastic gliomas. *Clin Cancer Res.* 2005;11:5167–5174.
19. Schlosser S, Wagner S, Muhlisch J, et al. MGMT as a potential stratification marker in relapsed high-grade glioma of children: the HIT-GBM experience. *Pediatr Blood Cancer.* 2010;54:228–237.
20. Wolff JE, Driever PH, Erdlenbruch B, et al. Intensive chemotherapy improves survival in pediatric high-grade glioma after gross total resection: results of the HIT-GBM-C protocol. *Cancer.* 2010;116:705–712.
21. Larouche V, Huang A, Bartels U, Bouffet E. Tumors of the central nervous system in the first year of life. *Pediatr Blood Cancer.* 2007;49(7 suppl):1074–1082.
22. Geyer JR, Finlay JL, Boyett JM, et al. Survival of infants with malignant astrocytomas. A Report from the Childrens Cancer Group. *Cancer.* 1995;75(4):1045–1050.
23. Duffner PK, Krischer JP, Burger PC, et al. Treatment of infants with malignant gliomas: the Pediatric Oncology Group experience. *J Neurooncol.* 1996;28(2–3):245–256.
24. Finlay JL, Goldman S, Wong MC, et al. Pilot study of high-dose thiotepa and etoposide with autologous bone marrow rescue in children and young adults with recurrent CNS tumors. The Children's Cancer Group. *J Clin Oncol.* 1996;14(9):2495–2503.
25. Narayana A, Kunnakkat S, Chacko-Mathew J, et al. Bevacizumab in recurrent high-grade pediatric gliomas. *Neuro Oncol.* 2010
26. Gajjar A, Sanford RA, Heideman R, et al. Low-grade astrocytoma: a decade of experience at St. Jude Children's Research Hospital. *J Clin Oncol.* 1997;15(8):2792–2799.
27. Prados MD, Edwards MS, Rabbitt J, Lamborn K, Davis RL, Levin VA. Treatment of pediatric low-grade gliomas with a nitrosourea-based multiagent chemotherapy regimen. *J Neurooncol.* 1997;32(3):235–241.
28. Gururangan S, Cavazos CM, Ashley D, et al. Phase II study of carboplatin in children with progressive low-grade gliomas. *J Clin Oncol.* 2002;20(13):2951–2958.
29. Pollack IF, Claassen D, al-Shboul Q, Janosky JE, Deutsch M. Low-grade gliomas of the cerebral hemispheres in children: an analysis of 71 cases. *J Neurosurg.* 1995;82(4):536–547.
30. Berger MS, Deliganis AV, Dobbins J, Keles GE. The effect of extent of resection on recurrence in patients with low grade cerebral hemisphere gliomas. *Cancer.* 1994;74(6):1784–1791.
31. Peraud A, Goetz C, Siefert A, Tonn JC, Kreth FW. Interstitial iodine-125 radiosurgery alone or in combination with microsurgery for pediatric patients with eloquently located low-grade glioma: a pilot study. *Childs Nerv Syst.* 2007;23(1):39–46.
32. Guthrie BL, Laws ER Jr. Supratentorial low-grade gliomas. *Neurosurg Clin N Am.* 1990;1(1):37–48.
33. Grill J, Couanet D, Cappelli C, et al. Radiation-induced cerebral vasculopathy in children with neurofibromatosis and optic pathway glioma. *Ann Neurol.* 1999;45(3):393–396.
34. Merchant TE, Kun LE, Wu S, Xiong X, Sanford RA, Boop FA. Phase II trial of conformal radiation therapy for pediatric low-grade glioma. *J Clin Oncol.* 2009;27:3598–3604.
35. Merchant TE, Conklin HM, Wu S, Lustig RH, Xiong X. Late effects of conformal radiation therapy for pediatric patients with low-grade glioma: prospective evaluation of cognitive, endocrine, and hearing deficits. *J Clin Oncol.* 2009;27:3691–3697.
36. Packer RJ, Lange B, Ater J, et al. Carboplatin and vincristine for recurrent and newly diagnosed low-grade gliomas of childhood. *J Clin Oncol.* 1993;11(5):850–856.
37. Packer RJ, Ater J, Allen J, et al. Carboplatin and vincristine chemotherapy for children with newly diagnosed progressive low-grade gliomas. *J Neurosurg.* 1997;86(5):747–754.
38. Laithier V, Grill J, Le Deley MC, et al. Progression-free survival in children with optic pathway tumors: dependence on age and the quality of the response to chemotherapy-results of the first French prospective study for the French Society of Pediatric Oncology. *J Clin Oncol.* 2003;21(24):4572–4578.
39. Perilongo G. Considerations on the role of chemotherapy and modern radiotherapy in the treatment of childhood low-grade glioma. *J Neurooncol.* 2005;75(3):301–307.
40. Pfister S, Janzarik WG, Remke M, et al. BRAF gene duplication constitutes a mechanism of MAPK pathway activation in low-grade astrocytomas. *J Clin Invest.* 2008;118:1739–1749.
41. Jones DT, Kocialkowski S, Liu L, Pearson DM, Ichimura K, Collins VP. Oncogenic RAF1 rearrangement and a novel BRAF mutation as alternatives to KIAA1549:BRAF fusion in activating the MAPK pathway in pilocytic astrocytoma. *Oncogene.* 2009;28:2119–2123.
42. Guillamo JS, Créange A, Kalifa C, et al. Prognostic factors of CNS tumours in Neurofibromatosis 1 (NF1): a retrospective study of 104 patients. *Brain.* 2003;126(Pt 1):152–160.
43. Tow SL, Chandela S, Miller NR, Avellino AM. Long-term outcome in children with gliomas of the anterior visual pathway. *Pediatr Neurol.* 2003;28(4):262–270.
44. Dutton JJ. Gliomas of the anterior visual pathway. *Surv Ophthalmol.* 1994;38(5):427–452.
45. Listernick R, Charrow J, Greenwald M, Mets M. Natural history of optic pathway tumors in children with neurofibromatosis type 1: a longitudinal study. *J Pediatr.* 1994;125(1):63–66.
46. Listernick R, Ferner RE, Liu GT, Gutmann DH. Optic pathway gliomas in neurofibromatosis-1: controversies and recommendations. *Ann Neurol.* 2007;61(3):189–198.
47. Listernick R, Louis DN, Packer RJ, Gutmann DH. Optic pathway gliomas in children with neurofibromatosis 1: consensus statement from the NF1 Optic Pathway Glioma Task Force. *Ann Neurol.* 1997;41(2):143–149.
48. Listernick R, Darling C, Greenwald M, Strauss L, Charrow J. Optic pathway tumors in children: the effect of neurofibromatosis type 1 on clinical manifestations and natural history. *J Pediatr.* 1995;127(5):718–722.
49. Leonard JR, Perry A, Rubin JB, King AA, Chicoine MR, Gutmann DH. The role of surgical biopsy in the diagnosis of glioma in individuals with neurofibromatosis-1. *Neurology.* 2006;67(8):1509–1512.
50. Astrup J. Natural history and clinical management of optic pathway glioma. *Br J Neurosurg.* 2003;17(4):327–335.
51. Medlock MD, Scott RM. Optic chiasm astrocytomas of childhood. 2. Surgical management. *Pediatr Neurosurg.* 1997;27(3):129–136.
52. Wisoff JH, Abbott R, Epstein F. Surgical management of exophytic chiasmatic-hypothalamic tumors of childhood. *J Neurosurg.* 1990;73(5):661–667.
53. Alvord EC Jr, Lofton S. Gliomas of the optic nerve or chiasm. Outcome by patients' age, tumor site, and treatment. *J Neurosurg.* 1988;68(1):85–98.
54. Sharif S, Ferner R, Birch JM, et al. Second primary tumors in neurofibromatosis 1 patients treated for optic glioma: substantial risks after radiotherapy. *J Clin Oncol.* 2006;24(16):2570–2575.

55. Singhal S, Birch JM, Kerr B, Lashford L, Evans DG. Neurofibromatosis type 1 and sporadic optic gliomas. *Arch Dis Child.* 2002;87(1):65–70.
56. Combs SE, Schulz-Ertner D, Moschos D, Thilmann C, Huber PE, Debus J. Fractionated stereotactic radiotherapy of optic pathway gliomas: tolerance and long-term outcome. *Int J Radiat Oncol Biol Phys.* 2005;62(3):814–819.
57. Mahoney DH Jr, Cohen ME, Friedman HS, et al. Carboplatin is effective therapy for young children with progressive optic pathway tumors: a Pediatric Oncology Group phase II study. *Neuro-oncology.* 2000;2(4):213–220.
58. Dohrmann GJ, Farwell JR, Flannery JT. Astrocytomas in childhood: a population-based study. *Surg Neurol.* 1985;23(1):64–68.
59. Cochrane DD, Gustavsson B, Poskitt KP, Steinbok P, Kestle JR. The surgical and natural morbidity of aggressive resection for posterior fossa tumors in childhood. *Pediatr Neurosurg.* 1994;20(1):19–29.
60. Li J, Perry A, James CD, Gutmann DH. Cancer-related gene expression profiles in NF1-associated pilocytic astrocytomas. *Neurology.* 2001;56(7):885–890.
61. Imielinski BL, Kloc W, Wasilewski W, Liczbik W, Puzyrewski R, Karwacki Z. Posterior fossa tumors in children-indications for ventricular drainage and for V-P shunting. *Childs Nerv Syst.* 1998;14(6):227–229.
62. Palma L, Celli P, Mariottini A. Long-term follow-up of childhood cerebellar astrocytomas after incomplete resection with particular reference to arrested growth or spontaneous tumour regression. *Acta Neurochir (Wien).* 2004;146(6):581–588; discussion 588.
63. Schneider JH Jr, Raffel C, McComb JG. Benign cerebellar astrocytomas of childhood. *Neurosurgery.* 1992;30(1):58–62; discussion 62.
64. Nishihori T, Shirato H, Aoyama H, et al. Three-dimensional conformal radiotherapy for astrocytic tumors involving the eloquent area in children and young adults. *J Neurooncol.* 2002;60(2):177–183.
65. Ersahin Y, Mutluer S, Cagli S, Duman Y. Cerebellar mutism: report of seven cases and review of the literature. *Neurosurgery.* 1996;38(1):60–65;discussion 66.
66. Huber JF, Bradley K, Spiegler BJ, Dennis M. Long-term effects of transient cerebellar mutism after cerebellar astrocytoma or medulloblastoma tumor resection in childhood. *Childs Nerv Syst.* 2006;22(2):132–138.
67. Ross GW, Rubinstein LJ. Lack of histopathological correlation of malignant ependymomas with postoperative survival. *J Neurosurg.* 1989;70(1):31–36.
68. Bouffet E, Perilongo G, Canete A, Massimino M. Intracranial ependymomas in children: a critical review of prognostic factors and a plea for cooperation. *Med Pediatr Oncol.* 1998;30(6):319–329; discussion 329.
69. Robertson PL, Zeltzer PM, Boyett JM, et al. Survival and prognostic factors following radiation therapy and chemotherapy for ependymomas in children: a report of the Children's Cancer Group. *J Neurosurg.* 1998;88(4):695–703.
70. West CR, Bruce DA, Duffner PK. Ependymomas. Factors in clinical and diagnostic staging. *Cancer.* 1985;56(7 suppl):1812–1816.
71. Asai A, Hoshino T, Edwards MS, Davis RL. Predicting the recurrence of ependymomas from the bromodeoxyuridine labeling index. *Childs Nerv Syst.* 1992;8(5):273–278.
72. Grill J, Pascal C, Chantal K. Childhood ependymoma: a systematic review of treatment options and strategies. *Paediatr Drugs.* 2003;5(8):533–543.
73. Perilongo G, Massimino M, Sotti G, et al. Analyses of prognostic factors in a retrospective review of 92 children with ependymoma: Italian Pediatric Neuro-oncology Group. *Med Pediatr Oncol.* 1997;29(2):79–85.
74. Pollack IF, Gerszten PC, Martinez AJ, et al. Intracranial ependymomas of childhood: long-term outcome and prognostic factors. *Neurosurgery.* 1995;37(4):655–666; discussion 666–667.
75. Rousseau P, Habrand JL, Sarrazin D, et al. Treatment of intracranial ependymomas of children: review of a 15-year experience. *Int J Radiat Oncol Biol Phys.* 1994;28:381–386.
76. Horn B, Heideman R, Geyer R, et al. A multi-institutional retrospective study of intracranial ependymoma in children: identification of risk factors. *J Pediatr Hematol Oncol.* 1999;21:203–211.
77. Palma L, Celli P, Mariottini A, Zalaffi A, Schettini G. The importance of surgery in supratentorial ependymomas. Long-term survival in a series of 23 cases. *Childs Nerv Syst.* 2000;16(3):170–175.
78. Hukin J, Epstein F, Lefton D, Allen J. Treatment of intracranial ependymoma by surgery alone. *Pediatr Neurosurg.* 1998;29(1):40–45.
79. Healey EA, Barnes PD, Kupsky WJ, et al. The prognostic significance of postoperative residual tumor in ependymoma. *Neurosurgery.* 1991;28(5):666–71; discussion 671.
80. Duffner PK, Krischer JP, Sanford RA, et al. Prognostic factors in infants and very young children with intracranial ependymomas. *Pediatr Neurosurg.* 1998;28(4):215–222.
81. Grill J, Le Deley MC, Gambarelli D, et al. Postoperative chemotherapy without irradiation for ependymoma in children under 5 years of age: a multicenter trial of the French Society of Pediatric Oncology. *J Clin Oncol.* 2001;19(5):1288–1296.
82. Merchant TE, Mulhern RK, Krasin MJ, et al. Preliminary results from a phase II trial of conformal radiation therapy and evaluation of radiation-related CNS effects for pediatric patients with localized ependymoma. *J Clin Oncol.* 2004;22(15):3156–3162.
83. McLaughlin MP, Marcus RB Jr, Buatti JM, et al. Ependymoma: results, prognostic factors and treatment recommendations. *Int J Radiat Oncol Biol Phys.* 1998;40(4):845–850.
84. Schild SE, Nisi K, Scheithauer BW, et al. The results of radiotherapy for ependymomas: the Mayo Clinic experience. *Int J Radiat Oncol Biol Phys.* 1998;42(5):953–958.
85. Vanuytsel L, Brada M. The role of prophylactic spinal irradiation in localized intracranial ependymoma. *Int J Radiat Oncol Biol Phys.* 1991;21(3):825–830.
86. Aggarwal R, Yeung D, Kumar P, Muhlbauer M, Kun LE. Efficacy and feasibility of stereotactic radiosurgery in the primary management of unfavorable pediatric ependymoma. *Radiother Oncol.* 1997;43(3):269–273.
87. Hargrave DR, Zacharoulis S. Pediatric CNS tumors: current treatment and future directions. *Expert Rev Neurother.* 2007;7(8):1029–1042.
88. Evans AE, Anderson JR, Lefkowitz-Boudreaux IB, Finlay JL. Adjuvant chemotherapy of childhood posterior fossa ependymoma: craniospinal irradiation with or without adjuvant CCNU, vincristine, and prednisone: a Childrens Cancer Group study. *Med Pediatr Oncol.* 1996;27(1):8–14.
89. Zacharoulis S, Levy A, Chi SN, et al. Outcome for young children newly diagnosed with ependymoma, treated with intensive induction chemotherapy followed by myeloablative chemotherapy and autologous stem cell rescue. *Pediatr Blood Cancer.* 2007;49(1):34–40.
90. Grill J, Kalifa C. High dose chemotherapy for childhood ependymona. *J Neurooncol.* 1998;40(1):97.
91. Geyer JR, Sposto R, Jennings M, et al. Multiagent chemotherapy and deferred radiotherapy in infants with malignant brain tumors: a report from the Children's Cancer Group. *J Clin Oncol.* 2005;23(30):7621–7631.
92. Mason WP, Goldman S, Yates AJ, Boyett J, Li H, Finlay JL. Survival following intensive chemotherapy with bone marrow reconstitution for children with recurrent intracranial ependymoma-a report of the Children's Cancer Group. *J Neurooncol.* 1998;37(2):135–143.
93. Poppleton H, Gilbertson RJ. Stem cells of ependymoma. *Br J Cancer.* 2007;96(1):6–10.
94. Taylor MD, Poppleton H, Fuller C, et al. Radial glia cells are candidate stem cells of ependymoma. *Cancer Cell.* 2005;8(4):323–335.

65 Medical Management of Primitive Neuroectodermal Tumors

Sabine Mueller and Susan M. Chang

INTRODUCTION

Primitive neuroectodermal tumors (PNETs) are a heterogeneous group of tumors presenting normally in infancy and young childhood. PNETs occur in various locations but histologically are similar with the appearance of fairly uniform undifferentiated small blue cells. To date, there are multiple different classification systems available, which are either based on location and pattern of differentiation or are referred to as a single entity that can occur in different locations in the central nervous system (CNS). Undifferentiated neuroectodermal tumors of the cerebellum have historically been referred to as medulloblastomas. Tumors of identical histology in the pineal region are classified as pineoblastomas and cortical lesions as central neuroblastomas or cortical PNETs. For the purpose of this chapter, the latter group of tumors will be referred to as supratentorial PNETs (sPNETs), including pineoblastomas. To date, different molecular genetic aberrations in the tumor cells of medulloblastomas and sPNET were identified, supporting a different molecular pathway leading to these tumors despite a similar histological appearance [1–4].

The following chapter will discuss the management of pediatric PNET, including the role of surgery, radiation therapy as well as chemotherapy, and discuss future therapeutics. PNETs presenting in adulthood are discussed elsewhere.

INFRATENTORIAL PNET: MEDULLOBLASTOMA

Medulloblastoma is one of the most common pediatric brain tumor and accounts for 20% of all childhood CNS tumors and 40% of all cerebellar tumors. Peak incidence has a bimodal distribution and ranges from 3 to 4 years and 8 to 9 years. Approximately, 10% to 15% are diagnosed in infancy and will be discussed in more detail below. Most of the tumors are confined to the posterior fossa; however, 10% to 40% of patients with medulloblastoma have evidence of disseminated disease along the craniospinal axis, which is one of the most important predictor for outcome [5,6]. The clinical presentation consists of signs of increased intracranial pressure as well cerebellar signs like vomiting, headache, ataxia, and nausea. Over the years, prognosis for these patients has continued to improve with both progression-free survival and overall survival of up to 80% in the average risk group [7]. Unfortunately, cognitive side effects and other sequalae are common in children who survive given the toxicity of current treatment modalities available.

Medical Management of Medulloblastoma

Staging and Risk Stratification

In the management of patients with medulloblastoma, it is crucial to differentiate high-risk versus low-risk patients to tailor therapy appropriately and avoid unnecessary toxicity. Current staging classification requires cerebrospinal fluid (CSF) analysis and magnetic resonance imaging (MRI) of the brain and entire spine with gadolinium. In some series, over 30% of patients have evidence of disseminated disease at the time of presentation [8]. The CSF examination should occur at least 2 weeks after surgical intervention to avoid false positive results. It is best obtained from the lumbar region, which is more sensitive for detecting abnormal cells than obtaining CSF from a shunt [9]. To date, the evaluation of CSF as well as MRI of the spine is superior in detecting disseminated disease than either modality alone [10]. The Chang classification uses an intraoperative assessment based on tumor size and location combined with CSF analysis and myelography. M0 staging is assigned if there is no evidence of disseminated disease in the CSF, whereas M1 is assigned if CSF is positive for malignant cells. M2–3 denotes tumor seen on MRI, and M4 is assigned if there is extra-neuronal spread, which is more commonly seen in the very young child. This classification system has been modified over the years: pre- and postoperative imaging replaced the intraoperative assessment and other factors like age, tumor histology and molecular genetics have been shown to be of significant importance when determining the individual risk for each patient [8]. Currently, patients are divided into risk-adapted schemes based on age at presentation, the extent of residual disease, and presence of metastatic disease. Children less than 3 years of age, greater than 1.5 cm^2 residual disease after surgery, and/or evidence of metastasis are considered high risk, whereas patients greater than 3 years with minimal residual disease are classified as average risk group [11]. On a molecular level, improved outcome is associated with the expression of the neurotrophin-3 receptor (Trk C), beta-catenin, and activation of the Wnt/wingless pathway with loss of chromosome 6 [12–16]. Poor outcome is correlated with chromosome 17p loss, gain of chromosome 1q and 8q as well as *c-myc* expression, *erb2* receptor expression, high expression levels of eukaryotic translation elongation factor (EEF1D), ribosomal protein L30 (RPL30), ribosomal protein S20 (RPS20), survivin, and anaplastic histology [17–21]. Table 65.1 gives an overview of clinical and molecular markers associated with prognosis for patients with medulloblastoma.

Since the introduction of genomics and molecular profiling of tumors, few studies have shown that the most accurate outcome predictors are achieved by microarray gene expression analysis [3,22,23]. In an analysis of 55 patients with medulloblastoma, comparing gene expression patterns and clinical parameters like age, stage, and tumor subtype on the effect on survival, only expression profiles were statistically significant predictors. Interestingly, disseminated disease, which has been shown to be a poor prognostic factor, was not associated with poor outcome. The authors discussed this as an effect of a potentially too small sample size [11]. To date, these biological markers are not incorporated in any clinical management aspect. Past clinical trials have failed to successfully include molecular tumor analysis and therefore multiple opportunities have passed to achieve further insight into the molecular characteristics of these tumors. More recent trials from the Children's Oncology group and the European trial, HIT-SIOP PNET IV trial include a comprehensive molecular testing of the tumor specimens, which will hopefully lead to a better understanding and therefore improved treatments for these patients [24].

Surgery

Surgical resection remains the mainstay of therapy. The aim is to completely remove the tumor but avoiding significant morbidity. Multiple studies have linked survival to the extent of resection [25–27] although others did not confirm this observation [28,29]. Some patients might require a ventricular shunt or third ventriculostomy prior to resection of the tumor. One postsurgical complication characteristically developing after posterior fossa tumor resection is the cerebellar mutism syndrome also referred to as the posterior fossa syndrome. This entity starts typically within 1 to 2 days after surgery, persists for weeks to months, and consists of paucity of speech leading to mutism, hypotonia, ataxia, and emotional instability. In one large study of 450 children, 107 (24%) developed cerebellar mutism syndrome after surgery. Only brainstem involvement was predictive [30]. Another series analyzed 253 children of which 20 children developed cerebellar mutism syndrome. All of these cases had brainstem involvement [31]. Therefore, careful resection is warranted especially in children with brainstem involvement.

In summary, surgical resection remains the mainstay of therapy in patients with medulloblastoma. The goal is gross total resection as most studies support that outcome is linked to the extent of resection.

Radiation Therapy

In addition to surgical resection, adjuvant therapy with radiation has been the standard of care for patients older than 3 years of age. In young children, the associated morbidity forces the clinician to either delay the radiation treatment or forego it completely. The treatment for children less than 3 years of age will be discussed in more detail below. Standard treatment regimens included radiation of 54 to 55 Gy to the posterior fossa and 36 Gy to the craniospinal axis achieving 5-year survival rates of 60% to 70% [26,32]. One early study showed that the incidence of spinal metastasis is reduced by postoperative irradiation to 13% compared to 75% without subsequent radiation [33]. One prospective study of the Pediatric Oncology Group (POG) and Children's Cancer group (CCG) now merged to the Children's Oncology group randomized patients to receive either 23.4 or 36 Gy to the craniospinal axis in addition to 54 Gy to the posterior fossa without additional chemotherapy. The protocol was closed early, since 5-year event-free survival was reported to be 67% in the standard therapy arm versus 52% in the 23.4 Gy arm. Nevertheless, long-term follow-up of this study revealed that differences with time were less pronounced. The 8-year analysis of the event-free survival of a smaller cohort of eligible patients showed no statistical difference [32]. Currently, the type of radiation, target volume, and dosage is subject of debate. It has been the goal of many investigators to decrease the amount of radiation as well as the radiation field, which has been mainly achieved through the addition of chemotherapy.

Other radiation modalities like conformal radiation and intensity-modulated radiation therapy have the benefit of more targeted radiation to the tumor bed instead of the whole posterior fossa. Conformal techniques that allow treatment planning based on three-dimensional reconstructions using computed tomography or MRI have dramatically advanced the area of radiation oncology over the last years. An analysis of 32 patients with newly diagnosed medulloblastoma treated with conformal boost

Table 65.1 Summary of Clinical and Molecular Markers Associated with Poor and Favorable Outcome

	Poor Outcome	Favorable Outcome
Clinical parameters	Age <3 years	Age >3 years
	Residual disease >1.5 cm² after resection	Complete resection
	Metastasis	
Molecular markers	p17 chromosome loss	TRK C expression
	1q chromosome gain	Wnt/Wingles pathway activation and loss of chromosome 6
	8q chromosome gain	Beta-catenin expression
	C-myc expression	
	Erb2 receptor expression	
	P53 expression	
	Survivin expression	
	EEF1D, RPL30, RPS 20 expression	

to the tumor bed demonstrated that the relapse rate was similar to the ones reported using whole posterior fossa radiation [34]. A multi-institutional prospective trial using 23.4 Gy craniospinal irradiation followed by conformal posterior fossa (36 Gy) and primary site irradiation (55.8 Gy) and dose intensive chemotherapy for average risk medulloblastoma achieved similar disease control than irradiation of the complete posterior fossa [35]. Currently, prospective trials such as the HIT-SIOP PNET IV trial are underway comparing conformal with conventional whole posterior fossa radiation. Hyperfractionated craniospanial radiotherapy (HFRT) is another alternative compared to standard radiation therapy. Here, a lower dose of radiation per fraction is used, usually 1 to 1.1 Gy, and administered more than once daily. Decreasing the dose per fraction theoretically spares the delayed effects of radiation injury on healthy tissue more than it spares tumor cells, allowing for higher total doses to the tumor bed while maintaining smaller doses to the normal tissue [36]. Several phase-II studies have been published using HFRT for the treatment of medulloblastoma with mixed results [37–39]. The University of California, San Francisco, treated a total of 25 patients with medulloblastoma of which 16 patients had average risk factor profile. All patients were treated with 72 Gy to the primary tumor site except one who was treated with 70 Gy. All patients received 30 Gy to the neuroaxis, which was increased from a prior pilot study from 24 Gy secondary to a high rate of local treatment failure. Patients with poor risk features were treated with adjuvant chemotherapy using CCNU, cisplatin, and vincristine. The 5-year progression-free survival was only 49% and overall survival reported with 69%. The authors concluded that HFRT of 30 Gy to the neuroaxis is insufficient for patients with average risk medulloblastoma not receiving chemotherapy [38]. Other protocols have used adjuvant chemotherapy and HFRT also for average risk patients and achieving better outcomes. Based on the current studies, it remains unclear if HFRT has a beneficial effect on outcome in patients with medulloblastoma.

Proton beam therapy is another alternative to conventional radiation therapy. The benefit of using proton beams is the higher proportion of tumor versus normal tissue distribution. The advantage is based on the fact that there is no dose distal to the target for each proton beam path [40]. This technique is now investigated in treating pediatric CNS tumors, including medulloblastoma. Currently, there is a phase-II trial conducted at the Massachusetts General Hospital, Boston, to assess the efficacy and long-term cognitive outcome in patients receiving proton beam therapy to the posterior fossa and craniospinal axis.

Stereotactic radiation has been used for local tumor control in patients with recurrent or residual disease with mixed results [41–43]. As primary treatment modality, it seems less beneficial given the propensity of medulloblastomas for metastasis however local tumor control might be achieved. Treatment failure can occur due to subclinical craniospinal metastasis.

In summary, radiation therapy remains standard of care for most patients above 3 years of age presenting with medulloblastoma. The evolved standard for average risk medulloblastoma in North America includes postoperative craniospinal irradiation of 23.4 Gy, irradiation of the posterior fossa of 55.8 Gy followed by 12 months of chemotherapy. Different radiation modalities like conformal radiation, HFRT, and proton beam therapy are currently under investigation.

Chemotherapy

Since lowering the radiation dose has failed, multiple studies have investigated the role of chemotherapy in addition to radiation therapy for the treatment of medulloblastoma. A range of different chemotherapeutic agents has been used and is now standard of care in the management of children with medulloblastoma in all risk groups. Packer et al [7] reported on 65 children with nondisseminated disease, who were treated after surgery with low-dose craniospinal irradiation of 23.4 and 55.8 Gy to the posterior fossa with adjuvant vincristine, lomustine, and cisplatin. After a pilot study with 18 Gy to the craniospinal axis was completed and a higher relapse rate in the lower radiation dose was observed, the protocol was amended to the higher dose of 23.4 Gy. The progression free survival was 86% (± 4%) at 3 years and 79% (± 7%) at 5 years, which is similar to the results obtained with higher doses of craniospinal irradiation. This regimen remains the standard of therapy for low-risk medulloblastomas to date. Subsequently, a study from the St. Jude's hospital, Memphis, showed that irradiation to the posterior fossa can be more restricted. The protocol applied 23.4 Gy to the craniospinal axis, conformal radiation therapy to the posterior fossa of 36 Gy, and 55.8 Gy to the primary site leading to an overall mean reduction of 13% in the volume of the posterior fossa receiving doses greater than 55 Gy. Chemotherapy consisted of cyclophosphamide, cisplatin, and vincristine. Five year event-free survival was 83% (± 5.3%), which is similar to prior studies [44]. The goal for average-risk medulloblastoma is to avoid side effects and achieve still adequate survival. This is currently achieved by a combination of radiation therapy as well as multiagent chemotherapy. For high-risk medulloblastoma, the priority is to improve overall survival. Multiple studies have used different chemotherapy protocols in combination with surgery and radiation to improve survival with moderate success. Average event-free survival at 5 years for high-risk medulloblastoma ranges from 34% to 40% across studies [45]. Other avenues like myeloablative chemotherapy with stem cell rescue as well as intrathecal and intravenous methotrexate have been used for the treatment of high-risk medulloblastomas with various success [46,47]. Current trials are investigating different chemotherapy regimens in combination with autologous stem cell rescue (ASCR) and radiation therapy; intrathecal radioimmunotherapy as well as different radiation regimens in combination with chemotherapy, including HFRT as well as proton beam therapy.

In summary, chemotherapy plays a pivotal role in the treatment of patients with medulloblastoma. Adding chemotherapy to the treatment regimen enabled neuro-oncologists to lower the radiation dose and therefore limit significant side effects. The best regimen for each risk group still is under investigation.

Late Effects of Therapy

All treatment options currently used in young children with medulloblastoma have significant side effects, including hearing loss [48,49], cognitive decline [50], endocrine abnormalities [51], vascular complications [52] as well as secondary malignancies [53,54].

The pathophysiology of late CNS damage after radiation is not well understood. One part of this decline seems to be due to loss of white matter and/or failure to develop white matter appropriate for age. A longitudinal study showed a significant white matter volume decrease in patients undergoing treatment for medulloblastoma. The decrease was more rapid in patients receiving 36 Gy craniospinal axis irradiation, than in patients who only received 23.4 Gy [55]. Further studies established a relation between the volume of white matter, radiation dose, and IQ [56]. Given these findings, children should be undergoing neuropsychological assessment and specific cognitive-behavioral training long term. Current studies are limited to assess the benefit of pharmacotherapy. Stimulants like methylphenidate have been investigated in children with learning problems, which were presumed secondary to cancer treatment, with mixed results [57]. Environmental adaptations like extended time limits in school for completion of school tests, recording of classroom lectures for further review, and written handouts to decrease demand on copying might be very helpful for these patients. Centers treating children with brain tumors are encouraged to establish a structured school reentry program for their patients to help in the transition phase.

Endocrine abnormalities include hypothyroidism, adrenal insufficiency, hypogonadism, and short stature. Children need to be followed closely and potentially be substituted as needed. One retrospective analysis from the St. Jude's hospital, Memphis, evaluated 194 children less than 3 years of age with intracranial CNS tumors. Fifty-three (27%) developed a growth hormone deficiency, 36 (18.5%) precocious puberty, 31 (15.9%) adrenocorticotropic hormone deficiency, 8 (4.1%) diabetes insipidus, 7 (3.1%) delayed puberty, and 1 (0.5%) syndrome of inappropriate antidiuretic hormone hypersecretion. In this analysis, craniospinal irradiation was associated with a higher incidence of endocrinopathies compared to local radiation [58]. Children treated for brain tumors are also at higher risk to develop secondary malignancies. Among others, the use of alkylating agents and irradiation are causative agents for further malignancies.

In summary, children treated for brain tumors require long-term follow-up with specific attention to neurocognitive dysfunction, endocrinopathies, and secondary malignancies.

MEDULLOBLASTOMA IN THE VERY YOUNG CHILD

Medulloblastoma is one of the most common brain tumors in childhood and one third of the cases present in the first years of life. Management of these very young patients remains challenging as the immature brain is particularly susceptible to the toxicity of current treatment options. There is belief that medulloblastomas in the very young child have a more aggressive behavior and a higher incidence of metastasis at time of diagnosis, although data is limited. Evans et al [59] reported that 34% of children under the age of 4 years presented with disseminated disease compared to only 14% of children aged 4 years or older. Similar results were reported separately with 62% of children less than 5 years of age demonstrating metastatic disease versus 38% in children older than 5 years of age [60]. The impact of age on prognosis is difficult to assess as younger patients normally receive different treatment modalities than older children. In an attempt to delay or obviate radiation therapy, multiple studies have been performed using different chemotherapy regimens.

In the mid-80s, the POG conducted a trial (referred to as Baby-POG I) enrolling 102 children less than 3 years of age with brain tumors in which prolonged postoperative chemotherapy was given with an attempt to delay radiation therapy [61]. Prior to that, the treatment for infants and the very young children with CNS tumors consisted of surgery followed by radiation therapy. Given the poor outcomes and severe neurotoxicity of the treatment, some neuro-oncologist opted not to treat these patients at all. That changed when in 1985 van Eys et al [62] published their encouraging results using postoperative neoadjuvant chemotherapy. Two out of six children younger than 4 years of age with medulloblastoma treated with a postoperative course of MOPP (mechlorethamine, vincristin, procarbacine, and prednisone) remained in complete remission. The Baby-POG I study demonstrated a 5-year progression-free survival of 62 children less than 3 years of age with medulloblastoma of 31.8% ($\pm$ 8.3%) and a 5-year overall survival of 39.7 % ($\pm$ 6.9%) using a combination of cyclophosphamide, vincristine, cis-platinum, and etoposide. Radiation was delayed until age 3, and therefore children less than 2 years received chemotherapy for 2 years and children between the ages of 2 and 3 for 1 year followed by radiation. Dose reduction was given to children with no evidence of residual disease. Interestingly, there was no difference in survival by age at diagnosis. Thus, delay in radiation of 2 years versus 1 year had no impact on outcome. The main predictor for survival was extent of surgical resection. Twenty children undergoing gross total resection had a 5-year survival of 60% compared to 33 children with subtotal resection who had a 5-year survival of 32%. Thirteen children had no evidence of metastasis and received reduced radiation to the spinal axis of 24 and 50 Gy to the posterior fossa. The 5-year survival for this subset was 69%, which is comparable to outcomes for patients with good prognostic features given full-dose radiation [61]. Other studies investigated a similar approach. The CCG used the "8-in-one-day" regimen followed by either radiation after two cycles of chemotherapy versus craniospinal irradiation 1 year after diagnosis and completion of maintenance chemotherapy. Forty children with medulloblastoma were less than 18 month old. The 3-year progression-free survival was 22% ($\pm$ 6%). Thirty percent were alive and disease free with a mean follow-up of 72 month [63]. The poorer outcome in the "8-in-one-day" regimen might be explained by the less intensive chemotherapy regimen in this study compared to the Baby-POG I trial.

One of the largest trials for young children from the CCG (CCG 9921) reported on 92 children younger than 3 years of age, of which 61 patients had no evidence of metastasis by time of diagnosis. Children were treated with two different induction schemes followed by eight cycles of maintenance chemotherapy. Children with no residual tumor after induction therapy and no metastasis at diagnosis did not receive radiation therapy unless they had evidence of recurrence. The 5-year event-free survival in the nonmetastatic group was 41% in 38 patients with gross total resection and 26% in 23 patients with residual tumor. In patients with metastatic disease, the 5-year event-free survival was 25% (31 patients) [64]. The Head Start I study was designed to avoid radiotherapy. After gross total resection and induction chemotherapy with cisplatin, vincristine, etoposide, and cyclophosphamide, the patients underwent myeloablative consolidation chemotherapy with carboplatin, thiotepa, and etoposide and ASCR. Two-year event-free survival and overall survival was 38% and 62%, respectively [65]. The induction chemotherapy was intensified during the Head Start II protocol by addition of methotrexate, which showed promising results. In this study, nine children less than 3 years of age with disseminated medulloblastoma showed treatment response (eight with complete response and one child with partial response) [66]. The Head Start III protocol is currently investigating the role of oral etoposide and temozolamide. Other studies are currently exploring the role of systemic and intraventricular chemotherapy, systemic chemotherapy with local conformal radiotherapy, and high-dose chemotherapy followed by radiotherapy at relapse. Studies also now include standardized neuropsychological evaluations in comparison to questionnaires and parents interviews, which will be important in evaluating quality of life and long-term treatment side effects.

In summary, the optimal treatment for patients less than 3 years of age presenting with medulloblastoma has yet to be established. Promising results with intensified induction chemotherapy followed by high-dose chemotherapy with autologous stem cell transplantation might justify further evaluation of these regimens despite significant toxicity. Given the relatively low frequency of very young children with medulloblastoma, only international collaborations will lead to robust assessments of efficacy, quality of life, and neurocognitive outcomes of different treatment strategies.

SUPRATENTORIAL PRIMITIVE NEUROECTODERMAL TUMORS

sPNETs are referred to as a heterogeneous group of tumors occurring above the tentorium. To date, multiple pathological classification systems are available. Rubinstein classified PNETs based on their gross and histological features into six distinct types: medulloepithelioma, cerebral neuroblastomas, polar spongioblastoma, ependymoblastoma, pineoblastoma, and medulloblastoma. Each of these tumors is thought to have its own putative cell of origin [67]. Others suggested that the term PNET should be applied to a group of tumors occurring in infancy and early childhood, which are mainly composed of undifferentiated cells originating from one precursor cell independent of location [68]. The World Health Organization (WHO) classifies these tumors into central neuroblastomas (PNET with neuronal differentiation), ependymoblastomas (PNET with ependymal differentation), and PNET (tumors composed of at least >90% of undifferentiated cells, including pineoblastoma). Nevertheless, clinical studies have shown that there are important differences in clinical response to treatment among groups of patients with PNETs arising at different anatomic sites [69,70]. To date, this controversy persists as there is no reliable tumor marker, and therefore comparison between studies remains difficult.

sPNET are much less common than medulloblastoma and account for only 1% to 2.5% of all childhood tumors [71,72]. The mean age of onset falls within the first decade of life around 3 years of age. Patients with sPNETs present with nonspecific signs of increased intracranial pressure like vomiting, irritability, and lethargy. Older children might complain of headache, and seizures are not uncommon. Unlike medulloblastomas, which show a higher male predominance, there does not seem to be a sex difference. Overall, sPNETs have a worse outcome and respond less to therapy compared to medulloblastomas.

The following chapter will discuss treatment options for sPNET, including surgery, radiation therapy, and chemotherapy and a combination thereof.

Medical Management of sPNETs

Staging and Prognostic Factors

Patients newly diagnosed with sPNET should undergo gadolinium enhanced MRI of the brain and spine as well as cytological evaluation of the CSF as these tumors have a tendency to disseminate. Only less than 0.5% of patients with sPNETs present with metastasis outside the CSF and therefore bone marrow analysis or bone scans are typically not necessary [73]. Most commonly, the Chang classification system is used for staging, which is described in detail above. Some studies show a clear impact of the M-stage on overall survival. The CGC-921 study showed that 2 out of 3 (66%) patients with M1 pineoblastoma had progressive disease at 32 month, whereas only 4 out of 14 (29%) patient with M0 disease showed progression [74]. The PNET-3 study enrolled 68 patients with sPNET with a median age of 6.5 years. For 64 patients, the M-status was available. This trial confirmed that patients with M0/1 (55 patients) had a better overall survival (5-year overall survival 48.7%) than patients with M2/3 staging (9 patients; 5-year overall survival 36.4%). Other factors, which were associated with improved outcome, were tumor size and location. Patients with tumor size <5 cm had a significant better outcome than patients with tumors >5 cm. Patients with a pineal location showed improved outcome compared to hemispheric located tumors, although this observation did not reach statistically significant effect in a multivariante analysis [75]. Other studies confirmed that patients presenting with a pineal lesion have better outcome than patients with hemispheric lesions [74–76], however this remains controversial [73,77]. Younger age at disease onset is associated with poor prognosis in most studies [74,78,79]. Besides these clinical prognostic factors there is very little known about prognostic molecular markers in sPNETs.

Surgery

Surgical resection remains the mainstay of initial therapy in patients presenting with a sPNET. In some cases, the deep location of these tumors prohibits a gross total resection, but complete removal of the tumor has been associated with improved outcome [69,78]. Albright et al [80] showed that progression-free survival was longer in patients with non pineal sPNETs undergoing gross total resection compared to patients with subtotal resection. The CCG-921 trial showed a better trend regarding outcome for patients with residual disease less than 1.5 cm^2, which did not achieve statistical significance possible due to the small number of centrally reviewed patients. Reddy et al [69] assessed 22 patients with sPNET with a mean age of 10 years (range 3–10 years). The 5-year progression-free survival for patients who underwent gross total resection was 53% compared to 25% for those who underwent partial resection or biopsy ($p = 0.22$). Given the correlation of extent of resection and improved outcome in few series, some centers suggest second look surgery after initial chemotherapy or delayed surgical intervention if residual tumor is seen on imaging [81]. Others report significant mortality with aggressive surgery. Ashwal et al [82] described a mortality of 22%, and therefore some groups would recommend nonaggressive surgical intervention [83].

In summary, surgical resection remains standard of care for patients with sPNET. The available information is limited to date and further trials are indicated to readdress the role of aggressive surgery given the associated morbidity, but most centers will aim for a gross total resection whenever possible.

Radiation Therapy

Radiation therapy remains an important modality in the treatment of children with brain tumors, including sPNET. Dosing, timing, and target volume of radiation continues to be subject of debate. Studies assessing the benefit of radiotherapy in patients with sPNET are limited given the small incidence rate and the lack of multicenter conducted trials. Most of our knowledge comes from subset analysis of larger trials or retrospective studies and therefore often do not reach statistical significance. Few studies have shown improved overall survival for patients treated with radiotherapy in conjunction with surgery and chemotherapy but the significant associated morbidity limits its use, especially in the younger children. In 1990, the Society Francaise Oncologie Pediatrique (SFOP) initiated the "BB SFOP protocol." The goal of this study was to treat children less than 5 years of age with medulloblastoma and sPNET with postoperative conventional chemotherapy in order to delay radiation therapy. Twenty-three children were diagnosed by central review with sPNET and included in the analysis. The overall survival was documented at 1, 2, and 5 years with 48%, 29%, and 14%, respectively. The median survival time in all infants was only 12 months. The authors concluded that postoperative chemotherapy without radiation is not adequate for the treatment of children with sPNET [84]. The analysis of the German trials HIT 88/89 and HIT 91 revealed important information regarding the benefit of radiotherapy. A total of 63 children (median age 6.3 years with a range from 2.9 to 17.7 years) with sPNET were eligible for the analysis. All patients were treated with adjuvant chemotherapy. The progression-free survival rate for children treated with radiotherapy according to guidelines was 49.3% at 3 years. In contrast, children with major treatment violations regarding radiation therapy achieved a 3-year progression-free survival of only 6.7%. The authors found that doses to the neuroaxis of equal or greater than 35 Gy, dose to tumor region of equal or greater than 54 Gy, and volume of craniospinal irradiation had a significant impact on outcome and that early chemotherapy seems to be inferior compared to immediate radiation therapy [83]. Similar results have been reported by Tornesello et al [85]. Out of 12 patients with PNET, including high-risk medulloblastoma, 4 showed progressive disease while on high-dose chemotherapy. The authors concluded that pre-irradiation chemotherapy and therefore delayed radiation therapy resulted in an unacceptable rate of early progression. A recent retrospective analysis from Canada investigated outcome in 48 patients (median age 49.5 months) treated between 1995 and 2005. The 4-year survival was 37.7 (± 7.6%) years with a median follow-up of 42 months. Factors that increased survival were the use of radiation therapy and chemotherapy although multiple regression analysis found only radiation therapy to be independently associated with improved survival [73].

HFRT has been used in several studies. In 1993, Halperin et al [86] showed long-term survival in four out of five patients treated with chemotherapy and HFRT with 30.6 to 43.9 Gy followed by a tumor boost to a total dose of 50 to 63.7 Gy. Others used HFRT in conjunction with high-dose chemotherapy with moderate success [87]. Studies are difficult to compare given the differences in treatment protocols. Some protocols use radiation therapy as a single modality after surgery, and more often it is combined with different chemotherapy regimens. The different combinations make it very challenging to compare outcomes based on radiation dose and field.

In summary, for older children, the treatment for sPNET consists of surgical resection, followed by craniospinal irradiation and boost to the primary tumor side as well as adjuvant chemotherapy. The dose for craniospinal irradiation ranges from 23.4 to 36 Gy and the suggested tumor dose between 54 and 56 Gy. As outlined above, chemotherapy alone remains insufficient for the treatment of sPNET. Radiation therapy is associated with significant morbidity and therefore intensified chemotherapy regimens are currently explored with the goal to delay radiation therapy until 3 years of age.

Chemotherapy

The role of chemotherapy for patients with sPNET still has to be established. There have been several reports in the literature that sPNET respond to chemotherapy, but the timing of chemotherapy has been an unresolved issue [88–90]. To date, there is insufficient information available if chemotherapy improves outcome given the fact that there are limited case series published, in which patients were treated in a systematic fashion. The devastating side effects of radiation therapy led to multiple studies investigating different chemotherapy regimens to improve outcome, especially in the younger children. In the German prospective brain tumor trials HIT 88/89 and HIT 91, a total of 63 children were treated with a combination of surgery, radiation and chemotherapy. Patients were either randomized for preirradiation chemotherapy consisting of two cycles of ifosfamide, etoposide, methotrexate, cisplatin, and cytarabine (40 patients) or chemotherapy after irradiation consisting of eight cycles of cisplatin, vincristine, and lomustine (23 patients). Overall survival at 3 years was 48.4 % with a median follow-up of 31 months. The administration of chemotherapy had no significant correlation with survival. A subset analysis even showed that immediate radiation improved survival compared to preirradiation chemotherapy [83]. The "BB SFOP protocol" demonstrated that chemotherapy (seven courses of alternating cycles of carboplatin/procarbazine, etoposide/cisplatin, and vincristine/cyclophosphamide) alone is not sufficient to treat sPNET and that foregoing radiation therapy worsens outcome [84]. As part of the PNET-3 study, 68 patients with sPNET (mean age 6.5 years; range 2.9–16.6 years) were treated with either a combination of chemotherapy and radiation therapy (44 patients) or just radiation therapy (24 patients). Chemotherapy consisted of four cycles of alternating cycles of vincristine, etoposide, carboplatin and vincristine, etoposide, and cyclophosphamide. For the combination group, 3-year and 5-year overall survival was 52.3% (95% CI: 37.5–67.0) and 45% (95% CI: 30.2–59.8), respectively. The 24 patients treated only with radiation therapy showed a 3-year and 5-year survival of 58.3 % (95% CI: 38.6–71.1) and 54.2% (95% CI: 34.2–74.1), respectively. There was no statistically significant difference in overall survival according to treatment received [75].

High-dose chemotherapy with ASCR has also been studied in the treatment of sPNET. A combined analysis of patients enrolled in the CCG 9883 and Memorial Sloan-Kettering Cancer Center MSKCC-89-173 trials investigated this approach specifically for patients with recurrent sPNET. A total of 17 patients (median age 2.3 years with range of 6 month to 31.4 years) from 1989 to 1998 were analyzed. Initial treatment before relapse consisted of surgery in 16, chemotherapy in 14, and radiotherapy in 8 patients. Fourteen patients received additional treatment prior to myeloablative chemotherapy with ASCR and 11 patients showed minimal residual disease prior to therapy. The treatment consisted of a combination of thiotepa and etoposide with or without carboplatin. Ten patients experienced tumor relapse at a median of 160 days after ASCR (range 23–361 days) and died. All patients with pineoblastomas (eight patients) died, and five out of eight patients with hemispheric located sPNET remained alive with no recurrence. Other prognostic factors included surgery at time of relapse and radiotherapy after ASCR. The study showed that a subset of patients with recurrent cortical sPNET could be salvaged with myeloablative chemotherapy with ASCR in combination with surgery and radiation therapy [91]. The Head Start I and II investigated the role of intensive chemotherapy with ASCR in patients with newly diagnosed sPNET. Forty-three children with sPNET were treated from 1991 until 2002 in two serial studies (Head Start I and II as described above). The 5-year estimated overall survival was 49% (95% CI: 33–62). Sixty percent (12 out of 20) of the surviving patients remain alive without radiation exposure and 75% (15 out of 20) of survivors avoided craniospinal irradiation. This study supports the fact that a group of patients appear to be successfully treated with high-dose chemotherapy without the use of radiation. In this study, tumor location was the only significant prognostic factor with pineal tumor having much worse outcome than nonpineal tumors [77].

In summary, the role of chemotherapy in the treatment of sPNET remains unanswered. Changes in neurosurgical and radiation techniques might have improved outcome in more recent trials independent from the chemotherapeutical regimen used. There is a strong need for multicenter trials to address some of these questions in a systematic fashion.

FUTURE DIRECTIONS

Major advances have been accomplished over the last years in the diagnosis and treatment of PNET. However, there are still controversies regarding the treatment of these tumors. To date, multiagent chemotherapy is standard in the treatment of PNET, but the better outcome reported in current studies for average risk patients with medulloblastoma might be partially due to improved imaging technology leading to a better risk group stratification. Instead of relying on imaging as well as CSF studies, further characterization of the molecular signature determining low-risk versus high-risk tumors will hopefully improve comparability amongst trials. This information may also enable investigators to better classify patients and to determine who is in need for highly toxic therapies with the risk of severe long-term side effects and who is not. So far, the use of conventional therapies did not lead to satisfactory results, and it is essential to develop new therapeutics.

Few molecular pathways have been associated with the development of medulloblastomas, including the Sonic hedgehog (Shh) and NOTCH signaling pathway. The involvement of Shh in the pathogenesis of medulloblastoma was first discovered by mutation analysis of patients with Gorlin syndrome. This autosomal dominant condition results in multiple basal cell carcinomas at young age, jaw cysts, skeletal abnormalities, and palmar pits [92]. Patients with Gorlin syndrome are prone to develop medulloblastomas. The mutation is located on chromosome 9 in the gene Patched (PTCH) [93,94]. The gene product is known to be a receptor for the Shh family of proteins. Blockade of this pathway through cyclopamine, a natural occurring inhibitor of the Shh pathway as well as HhAntag-691, a small molecule inhibitor, have demonstrated in *in vitro* and *in vivo* models regression of tumors [95,96]. These studies are encouraging for the development of Shh antagonist for future trials. The NOTCH signaling pathway is highly conserved among species and controls multiple cell differentiation processes and is dysregulated in many different cancer types. A recent study showed that NOTCH blockade with a γ-secretase inhibitor GSI018 led to decreased growth in vitro as well as decreased ability to form xenografts. The authors suggest that inhibition of the NOTCH pathway leads to depletion of the cancer stem cells (CSC) making it a very attractive target for further therapeutic development [97]. The CSC hypothesis proposes that tumors are driven and maintained from a small portion of transformed stem cells. These cells have the capacity of self-renewal and therefore need to be targeted for successful treatment. A unique feature of these CSC is an innate resistance to radiation and chemotherapy drugs [98,99]. As we learn more about CSC, future therapeutic options may include specifically targeting these cells by inducing CSC differentiation, elimination as well as alteration of the tumor microenvironment leading potentially to loss of self-renewal of these cells.

REFERENCES

1. Russo C, Pellarin M, Tingby O, et al. Comparative genomic hybridization in patients with supratentorial and infratentorial primitive neuroectodermal tumors. *Cancer.* 1999;86(2):331–339.
2. Nicholson JC, Ross FM, Kohler JA, Ellison DW. Comparative genomic hybridization and histological variation in primitive neuroectodermal tumours. *Br J Cancer.* 1999;80(9):1322–1331.
3. Pomeroy SL, Tamayo P, Gaasenbeek M, et al. Prediction of central nervous system embryonal tumour outcome based on gene expression. *Nature.* 2002;415(6870):436–442.
4. Kagawa N, Maruno M, Suzuki T, et al. Detection of genetic and chromosomal aberrations in medulloblastomas and primitive neuroectodermal tumors with DNA microarrays. *Brain Tumor Pathol.* 2006;23(1):41–47.
5. Allen JC, Epstein F. Medulloblastoma and other primary malignant neuroectodermal tumors of the CNS. The effect of patients' age and extent of disease on prognosis. *J Neurosurg.* 1982;57(4):446–451.
6. Deutsch M. Medulloblastoma: staging and treatment outcome. *Int J Radiat Oncol Biol Phys.* 1988;14(6):1103–1107.
7. Packer RJ, Goldwein J, Nicholson HS, et al. Treatment of children with medulloblastomas with reduced-dose craniospinal radiation therapy and adjuvant chemotherapy: a Children's Cancer Group Study. *J Clin Oncol.* 1999;17(7):2127–2136.
8. Packer RJ, Rood BR, MacDonald TJ. Medulloblastoma: present concepts of stratification into risk groups. *Pediatr Neurosurg.* 2003;39(2):60–67.
9. Gajjar A, Fouladi M, Walter AW, et al. Comparison of lumbar and shunt cerebrospinal fluid specimens for cytologic detection of leptomeningeal disease in pediatric patients with brain tumors. *J Clin Oncol.* 1999;17(6):1825–1828.
10. Fouladi M, Gajjar A, Boyett JM, et al. Comparison of CSF cytology and spinal magnetic resonance imaging in the detection of leptomeningeal disease in pediatric medulloblastoma or primitive neuroectodermal tumor. *J Clin Oncol.* 1999;17(10):3234–3237.
11. Fernandez-Teijeiro A, Betensky RA, Sturla LM, Kim JY, Tamayo P, Pomeroy SL. Combining gene expression profiles and clinical parameters for risk stratification in medulloblastomas. *J Clin Oncol.* 2004;22(6):994–998.
12. Segal RA, Goumnerova LC, Kwon YK, Stiles CD, Pomeroy SL. Expression of the neurotrophin receptor TrkC is linked to a favorable outcome in medulloblastoma. *Proc Natl Acad Sci USA.* 1994;91(26):12867–12871.
13. Kim JY, Sutton ME, Lu DJ, et al. Activation of neurotrophin-3 receptor TrkC induces apoptosis in medulloblastomas. *Cancer Res.* 1999;59(3):711–719.
14. Grotzer MA, Janss AJ, Phillips PC, Trojanowski JQ. Neurotrophin receptor TrkC predicts good clinical outcome in medulloblastoma and other primitive neuroectodermal brain tumors. *Klin Padiatr.* 2000;212(4):196–199.
15. Ellison DW, Onilude OE, Lindsey JC, et al. beta-Catenin status predicts a favorable outcome in childhood medulloblastoma: the United Kingdom Children's Cancer Study Group Brain Tumour Committee. *J Clin Oncol.* 2005;23(31):7951–7957.
16. Clifford SC, Lusher ME, Lindsey JC, et al. Wnt/Wingless pathway activation and chromosome 6 loss characterize a distinct molecular sub-group of medulloblastomas associated with a favorable prognosis. *Cell Cycle.* 2006;5(22):2666–2670.
17. Herms J, Neidt I, Luscher B, et al. C-MYC expression in medulloblastoma and its prognostic value. *Int J Cancer.* 2000;89(5):395–402.
18. Gilbertson R, Wickramasinghe C, Hernan R, et al. Clinical and molecular stratification of disease risk in medulloblastoma. *Br J Cancer.* 2001;85(5):705–712.
19. Pizem J, Cort A, Zadravec-Zaletel L, Popovic M. Survivin is a negative prognostic marker in medulloblastoma. *Neuropathol Appl Neurobiol.* 2005;31(4):422–428.
20. De Bortoli M, Castellino RC, Lu XY, et al. Medulloblastoma outcome is adversely associated with overexpression of EEF1D, RPL30, and RPS20 on the long arm of chromosome 8. *BMC Cancer.* 2006;6:223.
21. Haberler C, Slavc I, Czech T, et al. Histopathological prognostic factors in medulloblastoma: high expression of survivin is related to unfavourable outcome. *Eur J Cancer.* 2006;42(17):2996–3003.
22. Golub TR, Slonim DK, Tamayo P, et al. Molecular classification of cancer: class discovery and class prediction by gene expression monitoring. *Science.* 1999;286(5439):531–537.
23. Ramaswamy S, Golub TR. DNA microarrays in clinical oncology. *J Clin Oncol.* 2002;20(7):1932–1941.
24. Gilbertson RJ, Gajjar A. Molecular biology of medulloblastoma: will it ever make a difference to clinical management? *J Neurooncol.* 2005;75(3):273–278.
25. Albright AL, Wisoff JH, Zeltzer PM, Boyett JM, Rorke LB, Stanley P. Effects of medulloblastoma resections on outcome in children: a report from the Children's Cancer Group. *Neurosurgery.* 1996;38(2):265–271.
26. Zeltzer PM, Boyett JM, Finlay JL, et al. Metastasis stage, adjuvant treatment, and residual tumor are prognostic factors for medulloblastoma in children: conclusions from the Children's Cancer Group 921 randomized phase III study. *J Clin Oncol.* 1999;17(3):832–845.
27. Grill J, Sainte-Rose C, Jouvet A, et al. Treatment of medulloblastoma with postoperative chemotherapy alone: an SFOP prospective trial in young children. *Lancet Oncol.* 2005;6(8):573–580.
28. Packer RJ, Sutton LN, Elterman R, et al. Outcome for children with medulloblastoma treated with radiation and cisplatin, CCNU, and vincristine chemotherapy. *J Neurosurg.* 1994;81(5):690–698.
29. Gajjar A, Sanford RA, Bhargava R, et al. Medulloblastoma with brain stem involvement: the impact of gross total resection on outcome. *Pediatr Neurosurg.* 1996;25(4):182–187.
30. Robertson PL, Muraszko KM, Holmes EJ, et al. Incidence and severity of postoperative cerebellar mutism syndrome in children with medulloblastoma: a prospective study by the Children's Oncology Group. *J Neurosurg.* 2006;105(6 suppl):444–451.
31. Doxey D, Bruce D, Sklar F, Swift D, Shapiro K. Posterior fossa syndrome: identifiable risk factors and irreversible complications. *Pediatr Neurosurg.* 1999;31(3):131–136.
32. Thomas PR, Deutsch M, Kepner JL, et al. Low-stage medulloblastoma: final analysis of trial comparing standard-dose with reduced-dose neuraxis irradiation. *J Clin Oncol.* 2000;18(16):3004–3011.
33. Hubbard JL, Scheithauer BW, Kispert DB, Carpenter SM, Wick MR, Laws ER Jr. Adult cerebellar medulloblastomas: the pathological, radiographic, and clinical disease spectrum. *J Neurosurg.* 1989;70(4):536–544.
34. Wolden SL, Dunkel IJ, Souweidane MM, et al. Patterns of failure using a conformal radiation therapy tumor bed boost for medulloblastoma. *J Clin Oncol.* 2003;21(16):3079–3083.
35. Merchant TE, Kun LE, Krasin MJ, et al. Multi-institution prospective trial of reduced-dose craniospinal irradiation (23.4 Gy) followed by conformal posterior fossa (36 Gy) and primary site irradiation (55.8 Gy) and dose-intensive chemotherapy for average-risk medulloblastoma. *Int J Radiat Oncol Biol Phys.* 2008;70(3):782–787.
36. Thames HD Jr, Withers HR, Peters LJ, Fletcher GH. Changes in early and late radiation responses with altered dose fractionation: implications for dose-survival relationships. *Int J Radiat Oncol Biol Phys.* 1982;8(2):219–226.

37. Marymont MH, Geohas J, Tomita T, Strauss L, Brand WN, Mittal BB. Hyperfractionated craniospinal radiation in medulloblastoma. *Pediatr Neurosurg.* 1996;24(4):178–184.
38. Prados MD, Edwards MS, Chang SM, et al. Hyperfractionated craniospinal radiation therapy for primitive neuroectodermal tumors: results of a Phase II study. *Int J Radiat Oncol Biol Phys.* 1999;43(2):279–285.
39. Allen JC, Donahue B, DaRosso R, Nirenberg A. Hyperfractionated craniospinal radiotherapy and adjuvant chemotherapy for children with newly diagnosed medulloblastoma and other primitive neuroectodermal tumors. *Int J Radiat Oncol Biol Phys.* 1996;36(5):1155–1161.
40. Kirsch DG, Tarbell NJ. New technologies in radiation therapy for pediatric brain tumors: the rationale for proton radiation therapy. *Pediatr Blood Cancer.* 2004;42(5):461–464.
41. Hodgson DC, Goumnerova LC, Loeffler JS, et al. Radiosurgery in the management of pediatric brain tumors. *Int J Radiat Oncol Biol Phys.* 2001;50(4):929–935.
42. Milker-Zabel S, Zabel A, Thilmann C, et al. Results of three-dimensional stereotactically-guided radiotherapy in recurrent medulloblastoma. *J Neurooncol.* 2002;60(3):227–233.
43. Abe M, Tokumaru S, Tabuchi K, Kida Y, Takagi M, Imamura J. Stereotactic radiation therapy with chemotherapy in the management of recurrent medulloblastomas. *Pediatr Neurosurg.* 2006;42(2):81–88.
44. Merchant TE, Kun LE, Krasin MJ, et al. Multi-institution prospective trial of reduced-dose craniospinal irradiation (23.4 Gy) followed by conformal posterior fossa (36 Gy) and primary site irradiation (55.8 Gy) and dose-intensive chemotherapy for average-risk medulloblastoma. *Int J Radiat Oncol Biol Phys.* 2008;70(3):782–787.
45. Taylor RE, Bailey CC, Robinson KJ, et al. Outcome for patients with metastatic (M2–3) medulloblastoma treated with SIOP/UKCCSG PNET-3 chemotherapy. *Eur J Cancer.* 2005;41(5):727–734.
46. Strother D, Ashley D, Kellie SJ, et al. Feasibility of four consecutive high-dose chemotherapy cycles with stem-cell rescue for patients with newly diagnosed medulloblastoma or supratentorial primitive neuroectodermal tumor after craniospinal radiotherapy: results of a collaborative study. *J Clin Oncol.* 2001;19(10):2696–2704.
47. Okada S, Hongo T, Sakaguchi K, Suzuki K, Nishizawa S, Ohzeki T. Pilot study of ifosfamide/carboplatin/etoposide (ICE) for peripheral blood stem cell mobilization in patients with high-risk or relapsed medulloblastoma. *Childs Nerv Syst.* 2007;23(4):407–413.
48. Plowman PN. Post-radiation sensorineuronal hearing loss. *Int J Radiat Oncol Biol Phys.* 2002;52(3):589–591.
49. Grau C, Overgaard J. Postirradiation sensorineural hearing loss: a common but ignored late radiation complication. *Int J Radiat Oncol Biol Phys.* 1996;36(2):515–517.
50. Mulhern RK, Kepner JL, Thomas PR, Armstrong FD, Friedman HS, Kun LE. Neuropsychologic functioning of survivors of childhood medulloblastoma randomized to receive conventional or reduced-dose craniospinal irradiation: a Pediatric Oncology Group study. *J Clin Oncol.* 1998;16(5):1723–1728.
51. Heikens J, Michiels EM, Behrendt H, Endert E, Bakker PJ, Fliers E. Long-term neuro-endocrine sequelae after treatment for childhood medulloblastoma. *Eur J Cancer.* 1998;34(10):1592–1597.
52. Maher CO, Raffel C. Early vasculopathy following radiation in a child with medulloblastoma. *Pediatr Neurosurg.* 2000;32(5):255–258.
53. Hope AJ, Mansur DB, Tu PH, Simpson JR. Metachronous secondary atypical meningioma and anaplastic astrocytoma after postoperative craniospinal irradiation for medulloblastoma. *Childs Nerv Syst.* 2006;22(9):1201–1207.
54. Starshak RJ. Radiation-induced meningioma in children: report of two cases and review of the literature. *Pediatr Radiol.* 1996;26(8):537–541.
55. Reddick WE, Mulhern RK, Elkin TD, Glass JO, Merchant TE, Langston JW. A hybrid neural network analysis of subtle brain volume differences in children surviving brain tumors. *Magn Reson Imaging.* 1998;16(4):413–421.
56. Reddick WE, White HA, Glass JO, et al. Developmental model relating white matter volume to neurocognitive deficits in pediatric brain tumor survivors. *Cancer.* 2003;97(10):2512–2519.
57. Mulhern RK, Merchant TE, Gajjar A, Reddick WE, Kun LE. Late neurocognitive sequelae in survivors of brain tumours in childhood. *Lancet Oncol.* 2004;5(7):399–408.
58. Fouladi M, Gilger E, Kocak M, et al. Intellectual and functional outcome of children 3 years old or younger who have CNS malignancies. *J Clin Oncol.* 2005;23(28):7152–7160.
59. Evans AE, Jenkin RD, Sposto R, et al. The treatment of medulloblastoma. Results of a prospective randomized trial of radiation therapy with and without CCNU, vincristine, and prednisone. *J Neurosurg.* 1990;72(4):572–582.
60. Rutkowski S, Bode U, Deinlein F, et al. Treatment of early childhood medulloblastoma by postoperative chemotherapy alone. *N Engl J Med.* 2005;352(10):978–986.
61. Duffner PK, Horowitz ME, Krischer JP, et al. Postoperative chemotherapy and delayed radiation in children less than three years of age with malignant brain tumors. *N Engl J Med.* 1993;328(24):1725–1731.
62. van Eys J, Cangir A, Coody D, Smith B. MOPP regimen as primary chemotherapy for brain tumors in infants. *J Neurooncol.* 1985;3(3):237–243.
63. Geyer JR, Zeltzer PM, Boyett JM, et al. Survival of infants with primitive neuroectodermal tumors or malignant ependymomas of the CNS treated with eight drugs in 1 day: a report from the Childrens Cancer Group. *J Clin Oncol.* 1994;12(8):1607–1615.
64. Geyer JR, Sposto R, Jennings M, et al. Multiagent chemotherapy and deferred radiotherapy in infants with malignant brain tumors: a report from the Children's Cancer Group. *J Clin Oncol.* 2005;23(30):7621–7631.
65. Mason WP, Grovas A, Halpern S, et al. Intensive chemotherapy and bone marrow rescue for young children with newly diagnosed malignant brain tumors. *J Clin Oncol.* 1998;16(1):210–221.
66. Chi SN, Gardner SL, Levy AS, et al. Feasibility and response to induction chemotherapy intensified with high-dose methotrexate for young children with newly diagnosed high-risk disseminated medulloblastoma. *J Clin Oncol.* 2004;22(24):4881–4887.
67. Rubinstein LJ. Embryonal central neuroepithelial tumors and their differentiating potential. A cytogenetic view of a complex neuro-oncological problem. *J Neurosurg.* 1985;62(6):795–805.
68. Rorke LB. The cerebellar medulloblastoma and its relationship to primitive neuroectodermal tumors. *J Neuropathol Exp Neurol.* 1983;42(1):1–15.
69. Reddy AT, Janss AJ, Phillips PC, Weiss HL, Packer RJ. Outcome for children with supratentorial primitive neuroectodermal tumors treated with surgery, radiation, and chemotherapy. *Cancer.* 2000;88(9):2189–2193.
70. Li MH, Bouffet E, Hawkins CE, Squire JA, Huang A. Molecular genetics of supratentorial primitive neuroectodermal tumors and pineoblastoma. *Neurosurg Focus.* 2005;19(5):E3.
71. Pollack IF. Brain tumors in children. *N Engl J Med.* 1994;331(22):1500–1507.
72. Michaelis J, Kaletsch U, Kaatsch P. [Epidemiology of childhood brain tumors]. *Zentralbl Neurochir.* 2000;61(2):80–87.
73. Johnston DL, Keene DL, Lafay-Cousin L, et al. Supratentorial primitive neuroectodermal tumors: a Canadian pediatric brain tumor consortium report. *J Neurooncol.* 2008;86(1):101–108.
74. Jakacki RI, Zeltzer PM, Boyett JM, et al. Survival and prognostic factors following radiation and/or chemotherapy for primitive neuroectodermal tumors of the pineal region in infants and children: a report of the Childrens Cancer Group. *J Clin Oncol.* 1995;13(6):1377–1383.
75. Pizer BL, Weston CL, Robinson KJ, et al. Analysis of patients with supratentorial primitive neuro-ectodermal tumours entered into the SIOP/UKCCSG PNET 3 study. *Eur J Cancer.* 2006;42(8):1120–1128.
76. Cohen BH, Zeltzer PM, Boyett JM, et al. Prognostic factors and treatment results for supratentorial primitive neuroectodermal tumors in children using radiation and chemotherapy: a Childrens Cancer Group randomized trial. *J Clin Oncol.* 1995;13(7):1687–1696.
77. Fangusaro J, Finlay J, Sposto R, et al. Intensive chemotherapy followed by consolidative myeloablative chemotherapy with autologous hematopoietic cell rescue (AuHCR) in young children with newly diagnosed supratentorial primitive neuroectodermal tumors (sPNETs): report of the Head Start I and II experience. *Pediatr Blood Cancer.* 2008;50(2):312–318.
78. Dirks PB, Harris L, Hoffman HJ, Humphreys RP, Drake JM, Rutka JT. Supratentorial primitive neuroectodermal tumors in children. *J Neurooncol.* 1996;29(1):75–84.
79. Hong TS, Mehta MP, Boyett JM, et al. Patterns of failure in supratentorial primitive neuroectodermal tumors treated in Children's Cancer Group Study 921, a phase III combined modality study. *Int J Radiat Oncol Biol Phys.* 2004;60(1):204–213.
80. Albright AL, Wisoff JH, Zeltzer P, et al. Prognostic factors in children with supratentorial (nonpineal) primitive neuroectodermal tumors.

A neurosurgical perspective from the Children's Cancer Group. *Pediatr Neurosurg.* 1995;22(1):1–7.
81. Foreman NK, Love S, Gill SS, Coakham HB. Second-look surgery for incompletely resected fourth ventricle ependymomas: technical case report. *Neurosurgery.* 1997;40(4):856–860; discussion 60.
82. Ashwal S, Hinshaw DB Jr, Bedros A. CNS primitive neuroectodermal tumors of childhood. *Med Pediatr Oncol.* 1984;12(3):180–188.
83. Timmermann B, Kortmann RD, Kuhl J, et al. Role of radiotherapy in the treatment of supratentorial primitive neuroectodermal tumors in childhood: results of the prospective German brain tumor trials HIT 88/89 and 91. *J Clin Oncol.* 2002;20(3):842–849.
84. Marec-Berard P, Jouvet A, Thiesse P, Kalifa C, Doz F, Frappaz D. Supratentorial embryonal tumors in children under 5 years of age: an SFOP study of treatment with postoperative chemotherapy alone. *Med Pediatr Oncol.* 2002;38(2):83–90.
85. Tornesello A, Mastrangelo S, Piciacchia D, et al. Progressive disease in children with medulloblastoma/PNET during preradiation chemotherapy. *J Neurooncol.* 1999;45(2):135–140.
86. Halperin EC, Friedman HS, Schold SC Jr, et al. Surgery, hyperfractionated craniospinal irradiation, and adjuvant chemotherapy in the management of supratentorial embryonal neuroepithelial neoplasms in children. *Surg Neurol.* 1993;40(4):278–283.
87. Massimino M, Gandola L, Spreafico F, et al. Supratentorial primitive neuroectodermal tumors (S-PNET) in children: a prospective experience with adjuvant intensive chemotherapy and hyperfractionated accelerated radiotherapy. *Int J Radiat Oncol Biol Phys.* 2006;64(4):1031–1037.
88. Lefkowitz IB, Packer RJ, Siegel KR, Sutton LN, Schut L, Evans AE. Results of treatment of children with recurrent medulloblastoma/primitive neuroectodermal tumors with lomustine, cisplatin, and vincristine. *Cancer.* 1990;65(3):412–417.
89. Gaynon PS, Ettinger LJ, Baum ES, Siegel SE, Krailo MD, Hammond GD. Carboplatin in childhood brain tumors. A Children's Cancer Study Group Phase II trial. *Cancer.* 1990;66(12):2465–2469.
90. Douek E, Kingston JE, Malpas JS, Plowman PN. Platinum-based chemotherapy for recurrent CNS tumours in young patients. *J Neurol Neurosurg Psychiatry.* 1991;54(8):722–725.
91. Broniscer A, Nicolaides TP, Dunkel IJ, et al. High-dose chemotherapy with autologous stem-cell rescue in the treatment of patients with recurrent non-cerebellar primitive neuroectodermal tumors. *Pediatr Blood Cancer.* 2004;42(3):261–267.
92. Gorlin RJ. Nevoid basal-cell carcinoma syndrome. *Medicine (Baltimore).* 1987;66(2):98–113.
93. Gailani MR, Bale SJ, Leffell DJ, et al. Developmental defects in Gorlin syndrome related to a putative tumor suppressor gene on chromosome 9. *Cell.* 1992;69(1):111–117.
94. Farndon PA, Del Mastro RG, Evans DG, Kilpatrick MW. Location of gene for Gorlin syndrome. *Lancet.* 1992;339(8793):581–582.
95. Berman DM, Karhadkar SS, Hallahan AR, et al. Medulloblastoma growth inhibition by hedgehog pathway blockade. *Science.* 2002;297(5586):1559–1561.
96. Romer JT, Kimura H, Magdaleno S, et al. Suppression of the Shh pathway using a small molecule inhibitor eliminates medulloblastoma in Ptc1(+/-)p53(-/-) mice. *Cancer Cell.* 2004;6(3):229–240.
97. Fan X, Matsui W, Khaki L, et al. Notch pathway inhibition depletes stem-like cells and blocks engraftment in embryonal brain tumors. *Cancer Res.* 2006;66(15):7445–7452.
98. Bao S, Wu Q, McLendon RE, et al. Glioma stem cells promote radioresistance by preferential activation of the DNA damage response. *Nature.* 2006;444(7120):756–760.
99. Dean M, Fojo T, Bates S. Tumour stem cells and drug resistance. *Nat Rev Cancer.* 2005;5(4):275–284.

66 Intracranial Meningiomas

Frank S. Lieberman

MENINGIOMA

Meningiomas comprise approximately 30% of all intracranial tumors, making this tumor type the most common nonglial intracranial tumor, with an annual incidence of approximately 4.5/100,000 [1]. The majority of meningiomas are well-circumscribed indolent tumors, and for many patients, surgical removal of the tumor produces long-term, tumor-free survival [2,3]. Meningiomas increase in incidence with age, with the most frequent age of diagnosis being middle age, and a female to male predominance of approximately 2:1 in most series. Only 2% of all meningiomas occur in childhood, and the diagnosis of meningioma in a child should prompt diagnostic evaluation for the presence of other stigmata suggesting familial tumor susceptibility syndromes, the most commonly associated with pediatric menigiomas being neurofibromatosis 2 (NF2) [4]. The majority of meningiomas are supratentorial tumors. A minority of meningiomas are clinically aggressive and may produce significant neurologic deficits and even death. The majority of clinically aggressive meningiomas are histologically grade 2 (atypical) or grade 3 (anaplastic), but even histologically low-grade meningiomas may behave more aggressively [2,3,5,6]. In the most recent epidemiologic survey using the World Health Organization (WHO) criteria for grading meningiomas (2007), atypical (grade 2) meningiomas constituted 4.7% to 7.2% of tumors and anaplastic tumors comprised 1.0% to 2.8% of the total [7,8]. Meningiomas appear to be more frequent in Afican Americans.

The outcome of treatment for the majority of patients with low-grade supratentorial meningiomas is good, and for this group of patients much of recent debate about optimal management pertains to the role of radiosurgical treatment modalities in patients who have tumors located in regions not easily amenable to surgery or as a possible more generally applicable alternative to surgery for small lesions [2,3]. Advances in neurosurgical techniques, including endoscopic techniques, allow for extensive cytoreduction of previously difficult to access skull base meningiomas [9–11]. Increasingly precise fractionated external beam radiotherapy (EBRT) techniques and radiosurgical approaches have expanded the role of radiotherapy [12–14].

Although outcomes for patients with low-grade, typical meningiomas amenable to complete surgical resection has been excellent for the decades of modern neurosurgery, the treatment of atypical and anaplastic tumors remains unsatisfactory [3]. Atypical and anaplastic meningiomas recur relentlessly after surgery and external beam radiation therapy, and have proven refractory to both single agent and combination cytotoxic chemotherapy regimens [15–17]. A diverse phase-2 clinical trial literature attests to the frustration of generations of investigators employing a variety of cytotoxic and biological response modifier drug therapies, and as of the writing of this review, there is no effective drug therapy for anaplastic meningiomas [2,3].

Despite the frequency of surgical resection, the understanding of the molecular biology of meningiomas is less advanced than for glial tumors, perhaps because the apparent benignity of the majority of tumors makes this area of investigation seem less urgent than for malignant gliomas or medulloblastoma. In addition, the development and preclinical evaluation of molecularly targeted therapeutic approaches for all grades of menignoma have been hampered by the lack of easily manipulated animal models that accurately reflect the human disease. However, recent insights into the molecular biology of menigiomas are leading to trials employing mechanistically based molecularly targeted agents [6,18,19]. Similar to the experience with gliomas, molecular neuropathology is being increasingly important in the diagnosis, categorizing, and treatment of meningiomas.

NEUROPATHOLOGY

Meningiomas arise from the meningeal coverings of the brain and spinal cord, and although the cell of origin is not definitively proven, meningioma cells cytologically resemble arachnoid cap cells. Arachnoid cap cells form the outer layer of the arachnoid matter.

The most commonly used pathologic diagnostic and grading system used in the United States and Canada is the WHO classification, which was most recently revised in 2007 [7,8]. In this schema, tumors are separated into three grades: benign (WHO grade 1), atypical (WHO grade 2), and malignant (WHO grade 3). The 2007 WHO grading system incorporates clinical pathologic correlation data indicating the relevance of histologic type as well as the presence of specific cytologic or histologic features

[8]. Grade 1 meningiomas comprise approximately 80% of the total. Beginning with the histological descriptions of Harvey Cushing and his disciples, variety of histologic subtypes have been described. The meningothelial, fibroblastic, transitional, angiomatous, microcystic, secretory, lymphoplasmacytic, meatpastic, and psammomatous variants are all considered compatible with WHO grade 1 [5–8]. Chordiod, clear cell, paiillary, and rhabdoid histologies, which are consistently associated with more aggressive biological behavior, including increased growth rate, increased risk of recurrence after resection, and increased metastasis, are graded as WHO 2.

Clear cell or chordoid meningiomas are graded as grade 2. In addition, tumors with the histologic appearance of a grade 1 tumor will be upgraded to grade 2 if they meet the following criteria: 4 or more mitotic cells per high-power field and/or 3 or more of increased cellularity, small cells, necrosis, prominent nucleoli, sheeting, and/or brain invasion. Papillary or rhaboid histology are defined as grade 3, as are tumors that demonstrate 20 or more mitotic cells per high-power field and/or malignant cytologic characteristics that resemble carcinoma, sarcoma, or melanoma.

How to interpret the impact of brain invasion on histologic grade has been controversial [5]. In the study of 116 cases referred to above, the median survival of patients whose tumors met the histologic criteria for grade 1, but showed brain invasion, had similar median survival to tumors that were histologically grade 2 [20]. Once the tumors reached the diagnostic threshold of grade 3 by other histologic criteria, the presence or absence of brain invasion did not seem to have an independent correlation with median survival.

Immunohistochemical profiling aids in the differentiation of anaplastic meningiomas from the carcinomas, sarcomas, or melanomas, which histologic variants of anaplastic meningiomas may resemble. The typical profile for meningiomas is at least focal positivity for epithelial membrane antigen (EMA) and vimentin, negative staining for cytokeratins, and weak or negative staining for S-100 protein. In addition, ultrastructural demonstration of interdigitating processes and intracellular junctions suggests meningioma in the setting where vimentin positivity is the only immunohistochemistry (IHC) characteristic [5].

The distinction between anaplastic meningioma and hemangiopericytoma is important because of the markedly different metastatic propensities and the difference in median survival between the two tumor types [5,21]. Anaplastic meningiomas have a median survival of approximately 2 years but infrequently metastasize outside the central nervous system, whereas hemangiopericytomas metastatize outside the central nervous system in 25% to 60% of cases but have a more favorable median survival of 5 to 12 years. The classic appearance of hemangiopericytoma is a staghorn pattern of vascular spaces with the tumor parenchyma. Hemangiopericytomas typically lack EMA antigen staining, manifest abundant intercellular reticulin, and ultrastructurally contain basal lamina like material. When these criteria are inconclusive, further IHC studies and microdissection-based genetic profiling may separate poorly differentiated anaplastic meningiomas from hemangiopericytomas. Strong expression of CD99 and bcl-2 protein are consistent with hemangiopericytoma rather than meningioma, while deletions of 1p32, 14q32, NF2, and 4.1B are common in anaplastic meningiomas but rare in hemangiopericytomas [21].

In a review of the histologic diagnostic markers employed in the grading of meningiomas, Cummins concluded that Ki-67 labeling index has been shown to correlate with tumor grade but that standard deviations within each grade are large enough to require caution in the use of labeling index as a criteria for establishing grade [5,22]. Although there are data indicating correlations between Ki-67 index and recurrence free survival in mengiomas after extent of resection was corrected for, a study of grade 1 meningiomas after radical resection did not demonstrate a significant correlation with Ki-67 labeling index and recurrence free survival [23–27]. Similarly, progesterone receptor (PR) expression has been correlated with tumors that demonstrated lower proliferation indices and better prognosis, and higher grade tumors are more frequently PR negative. However, it is unclear whether PR status by IHC is itself a discriminating factor regarding prognosis [28].

The relevance of brain invasion as a prognostic factor in both assigning grade and differentiating between subsets of tumors with different risk of recurrence within the same histologic grade is unclear. In a large retrospective study of 581 patients, Perry (1977) found brain invasion a predictor of shorter recurrence free survival. In that study, 43% of tumors were benign and 57% atypical [29]. Although brain invasion correlated with shorter recurrence free survival, the recurrence rate for invasive tumors was not significantly different from that of noninvasive tumors of equivalent grade. In a 2007 review of meningoma histopathology, Commins concluded that while invasion of soft tissue or bone by an otherwise benign meningioma does not affect grade, brain invasion by a benign appearing tumor results in a prognosis similar to that for atypical meningiomas [5]. A specific molecular signature for tumors demonstrating brain invasion has yet to be identified.

In a series of 74 patients, Yang et al reported that although brain invasion by atypical meningiomas was not associated with difference in survival, the survival benefit of adjuvant EBRT was seen in the subgroup with brain invasion [15].

MOLECULAR NEUROPATHOLOGY OF MENINGIOMAS

Although histologic grade of the tumor and extent of resection have been known as powerful predictors of risk of recurrence and time to progression for intracranial meningiomas, recurrance may occur in some patients with otherwise histologically typical benign meningiomas. Several studies suggest that histologically indistinguishable atypical meningiomas may segregate into different subgroups with different time to progression and overall survival [6,30–32]. For patients with medulloblastoma, the incorporation of genetic information relevant to the process of mutational or epigenetic processes involved in tumorigenesis and progression has improved the risk stratification and refined both clinical trial design and clinical decision making [33,34]. For gliomas, similarly, the presence of specific deletions of chromosome 1p and 19q subdivides anaplastic gliomas with varying degrees of oligodendroglial differention into different prognostic groups, and there is increasing evidence that glioblastomas segregate into different subtypes based on neuroectodermal verus mesenchymal differention profiles with microarray techniques [35,36]. Similar attempts to improve the predictive power of risk stratification using molecular genetic information are ongoing for meningiomas as well.

The application of genetic information to neuropathology of meningiomas has been evolving with the increasing application of high-throughput expression technologies and more recently with attention to potential epigenetic mechanisms of biologic variability in these tumors. Cytogenetic abnormalities in meningiomas have been well characterized, and comparative genomic hybridization studies as well as sequencing have identified a number of genes, and pathways, deregulated in meningiomas. The number and specific pattern of chromosomal loss or gains may correlate with specific histologic types and with WHO histologic grade. To date, expression microarrays have neither been able to robustly segregate tumors into groups consistent with histologic grade nor to differentiate robustly between different risk groups within a histologic grade. Nonetheless, microarray techniques have been informative in identifying gene copy number and transcript-level alterations which confirm the association of specific gene and pathway alterations with meningoma tumorigenesis and grade, and identify novel genes not previously implicated in meningiomas.

In a comprehensive review of the molecular pathogenesis of meningiomas, Perry noted that meningiomas were the first solid tumor to be associated with a characteristic cytogenetic abnormality, monosomy 22 [18]. The *NF2* gene appears to be the primary target and deletion or inactivating mutations of the *NF2* gene occur, as an early initiating event, in roughly half of sporadic meningiomas and the majority of NF2 associated meningiomas. Other loci on chromosome 22 may also be relevant to meningioma initiation and progression, including AP1B1, MN1, SMARCB1, IN11/hSNFS.

The product of the *NF2* gene, named merlin or schwannomin by the different groups who initially cloned the gene, is a 595 amino acid protein related to the protein 4.1 family, which includes exzrin, radaxin, and moesin [37,38]. This protein appears to have a role in control of cell growth and motility, and interacts with a number of transmembrane signaling proteins. Inactivation of other gene members of the protein 4.1 family has been indentified in meningiomas, including 4.1R and 4.1B (DAL-1) [18].

A number of cytogenetic alterations are associated with atypical or anaplastic grade of meningiomas and appear to be relevant to tumor progression [18]. Loss of chromosomal arms 1p, 6q, 9p, 10, 14q, and 18q have been described as well as gene amplifications or gains on 1q, 9q, 12q, 15q, 17q, and 20q. The relevant gene alterations on chromosome 9p21 include the *CDKN2A* (*p16INK4a*), *p14ARF*, and *CDKN2B* (*p15INK4B0*) genes, and loss or inactivation of these loci are found in approximately 2/3 of cases of atypical or anaplastic meningiomas [39]. In patients with anaplastic meningiomas, the presence of CDKN2A deletions correlates with shorter survival [40]. Mutations in phosphatase and tensin homolog (PTEN), common in malignant gliomas, are found only rarely in anaplastic meningiomas [18].

Perry has proposed a molecular model of meningioma tumorigenesis and progression. In this model, benign meningiomas are associated with loss of chromosome 22 with associated *NF2* gene loss or inactivation, 4.1B, 4.1R loss, and overexpression of PR. Atypical meningiomas manifest a more complex set of genetic changes: loss of 1p, 6q, 9p, 10, 14q, and 18q; gains of 1q, 9q, 12q, 15q, 17q, and 20q; the presence of dicentric or ring chromosomes; overexpression of telomerase and vascular endothelial growth factor (VEGF); and loss of PR expression. Amplification of 17q23 (PSK6) and loss of 9p correlate with anaplastic phenotype. Chromosome 14 loss seems to be associated with increased relapse rate in otherwise histologically benign tumors [41–43].

Maillo proposed a prognostic stratification scheme based on patient age, tumor grade, and presence of chromosome 14 losses. In a series reporting 26 atypical and 10 anaplastic meningomas, Krayenbuhl found significant differences between de nova tumors and those that had transformed from a lower grade [32]. For atypical meningomas, chromosomes 1, 14, and 22 demonstrated losses in 22% of transformed but in none of the de novo tumors. Similar patterns of chromosome cytogenetic change were seen in 71% of transformed anaplastic tumors but only 33% of de novo anaplastics. Monosomy 18 was seen only in transformed anaplastic tumors and monosomy or derivative chromosome 10 was overrepresented in the transformed versus de novo anaplastic group. In this study, de novo anaplastic tumors had a significantly longer survival (6.15 years vs. 1.95 years) than their transformed counterparts and a similar difference was seen for de novo versus transformed atypical tumors (5.36years vs. 1.95 years).

Numerous investigators in the past 5 years have begun to apply microarray-based gene profiling to the task of improving the understanding of those genetic changes that correlate with increased risk of progression. Wrobel et al [31] performed expression profiling of 30 meningiomas of different grades using cDNA arrays representing 2600 genes. Receiver operating characteristic analysis was used to identify genes showing differential expression between benign, atypical, and malignant meningiomas. Interestingly, 4 of the 10 genes showing highest expression in meningiomas had not previously been identified as relevant to meningioma pathogenesis or progression. These genes were *ANXA2*, *BAD*, *CCND1*, and *LIG1*. However, neither hierarchical clustering nor shrunken centroids analyses were able to identify classifiers for different meningioma grades. The investigators then employed an receiver operating characteristic analysis to identify single genes that were differentially expressed in the 17 atypical and anaplastic meningiomas compared to the 13 benign tumors. The differentially expressed genes had been previously identified by other techniques. Pathway analysis identified increased expression of insulin-like growth factor (IGF) pathway genes in benign tumors with losses on chromosome 10 or 14 and Wnt pathway genes in tumors with losses on chromosome 14.

In another microarray study, Wada et al were not able to find any critical correlation between pathologic diagnosis and type of genetic abnormality, though loss of chromosome 22q was seen in 10 transitional and 2/3 fibrous meningiomas but only 1/11 meningothelial meningomas [44]. In this study, *NF2* gene abnormalities was seen in only 5/29 tumors, substantially less frequent than in other studies, and the investigators suggest that this may indicate relative insensitivity of microarray techniques to point mutations or splicing errors.

In an interesting study employing both microarray and array comparative genomic hybridization (aCGH), Carvalho et al demonstrated that meningiomas of all three grades segregate into two molecular groups [30]. In pairwise comparisons between the three grades using significance analysis of microarray data 28 genes were found to be differentially expressed between grades 1 and 2 meningiomas; In contrast, 1212 genes were differentially expressed between grades 2 and 3. Unsupervised cluster analysis of the microarray data yielded a dendrogram with two main branches. All eight benign meningiomas segregrated to the left branch, and all eight malignant tumors to the right branch. Atypical meningiomas distributed in both branches. Of note, there were no specific histopathological criteria that distinguished the high- from low-proliferative atypical meningiomas.

In a clinical pathologic correlation study of 70 meningiomas, Maillo et al found numerical chromosomal abnormalities in 77% of tumors [41]. Chromosome 22 was the most frequently altered in the entire series, and chromosome y in males was also frequently altered. Multivariate analysis suggested that tumor grade, age, and chromosome 14 status were the best combination of independent variables for predicting RFS. In a study of 208 tumors by Mihaila et al, loss of heterozygosity (LOH) on chromosome 10 was seen in a high frequency of tumors of all three grades. To test the hypothesis that LOH at different allelic sites on chromosome 10 might allow for subclassifcation of tumors, the investigators determined LOH status at 11 different markers. LOH at D10S179 was highly associated with higher grade meningomas and when present in an apparently benign tumor may identify a more aggressive tumor. LOH at D10S209 and D102169 may predict shorter survival and higher risk of recurrence relative to tumors without LOH at these loci.

Telemerase activation is also implicated in tumor progression [18]. Activation of human telomerase reverse transcriptase (hTERT) was only found in 37% of benign meningiomas but up to 95% of grade 3 tumors. Activation of human telomerase reverse transcriptase is correlated with shorter progression free survival (PFS).

Gene expression profiling implicates that the Notch signaling pathway may be deregulated in meningiomas [31]. HES1, the Notch1 and 2 receptors, and ligand transcripts and proteins were expressed in tumors of all grades. Transducin-like enhancer protein 2 and transducin-like enhancer protein 3 were expressed only in higher grade meningiomas. Members of the Wnt and IGF signaling pathways have been associated with the losses in chromosome 10 and 14 in higher grade tumors. Epidermal growth factor receptor (EGFR) is widely expressed on meningoma cells and tumors, and autocrine production of TGFα and epidermal growth factor (EGF) are associated with aggressive growth [18,19,45–48]. PGFRB is activated in many meningiomas as well. Expression of somatastatin receptor by atypical and anaplastic meningiomas has led to clinical trials of octreotide for recurrent or progressive menigioma [49,50].

NEUROIMAGING OF MENINGOMAS

Intracranial meningiomas are typically extraaxial, contrast enhancing tumors on both computerized tomography (CT) scanning and magnetic resonance imaging (MRI). In order of decreasing frequency, meningiomas occur along the cerebral convexities, parafalcine, falx, sphenoid ridges, and posterior fossa. They may also be found in the tuberculum sella, olfactory grooves, tentorium, optic nerves, petrous ridges, and rarely as primary intraventricular tumors [51].

CT imaging of meningiomas typically demonstrates an isodense or hyperdense mass that enhance homogenously after contrast administration. Intratumoral calcifications are seen in 15% to 20% of cases and are more common in the transitional and fibroblastic subtypes [52]. Dense calcifications are suggestive of a psammomatous subtype, but these distinctions are not usually relevant to designing a treatment plan. Hyperostosis of underlying bone is seen in approximately 20% of meningiomas and does not clearly correlate with tumor grade or size [53].

MRI of intracranial meningiomas typically demonstrates an extra-axial mass, hyperintense on T2-weighted images, and PD sequences [53]. Typically, meningiomas homogenously enhance after gadolinium contrast and an extension of enhancement along the dural adjacent to tumor (the so called dural tail) is also typical. This tail is frequently a dural reaction to tumor rather than infiltrated meninges [54]. Other tumor types may show a dural tail, including lymphomas, schwannomas, and peripherally located gliomas with a meningeal reaction. The use of MRI to differentiate between tumor grades includes dynamic contrast MRI, for which the volume transfer constant is a discriminator. Malignant meningiomas tend to have higher signal intensities on diffusion-weighted images, and lower diffusion constants correlate with higher grade in some series [55]. The most typical feature of MRS of meningomas is the absence of an N-acetylaspartate peak and elevated choline/creatine ratios may be seen as well [56].

Differentiating hemangiopericytomas from malignant meningomas using neuroradiologic criteria is difficult to do with confidence [51]. Calcification is rare in hemangiopericytomas, which are frequently large, lobular, and heterogeneously hyperintense on CT [57–59]. Hemangiopericytomas are more frequently associated with lytic bone changes, unusual for menigiomas. The enhancement pattern tends to be more heterogeous than that of menigiomas. On MRI, these tumors are usually isointense on T1-weighted images and similarily heterogeneously isointense on T2 as well. Serpentine vascular flow voids are typical of hemangiopericytomas, and contrast enhancement is usually heterogeneous; there may be an associated dural tail, and usually there is significant perilesional edema.

TREATMENT OF MENINGIOMAS

Surgery

Surgical resection is the mainstay of therapy for meningiomas, with the goal of complete removal of gross tumor and microscopic tumor from underlying dural and soft tissue and bone [1,2]. Although a comprehensive review of operative technique are beyond the scope of this chapter, advances in neuroimaging, operative microscopy, and most recently in endoscopic techniques have expanded the scope of cytoreductive surgery for meningiomas [2,6,7,9–11]. For WHO grade 1 meningiomas, complete surgical resection by MRI and neuropathologic criteria is considered definite therapy, and the standard of practice is not to use adjuvant external beam or radiosurgery in this setting [60]. The Simpson grading system combines extent of resection with postoperative imaging to determine a score of 1 to 5. For patients with a Simpson grade 1 meningioma, the 10-year recurrence rate is 9% versus a 29% rate for grade 3. In one of the longer follow up studies, Jaaskelainen found a recurrence rate of 29% at 20 years after complete resection [61].

In patients with atypical or anaplastic meningiomas, complete surgical resection is not adequate therapy, with 5-year recurrence rates of 38% and 78%, respectively. In an institutional series of 40 atypical and 24 anaplastic meningiomas, Yang reported that extent of resection was not a prognostic factor in multivariate analysis of outcome for atypical meningiomas but was a favorable factor for anaplastic meningiomas [15].

The application of endoscopic techniques to skull base meningiomas is allowing for more aggressive cytoreductive operations with less perioperative morbidity [9–11]. For patients with recurrent tumors after radiation, this approach may allow the use of both cytotoxic and molecularly targeted systemic therapies in the setting of minimal residual disease.

Radiotherapy

Although, as noted above, even WHO grade 1 meningiomas after complete surgical resection do carry a risk of late recurrence, the use of adjuvant radiotherapy is usually reserved for subtotally resected grade 1 tumors and for atypical or anaplastic meningiomas regardless of extent of resection. In a 2007 review, the authors collated the results of 42 studies totallling 4585 patients [12].

This thoughtful review challenges the preconception that meningiomas are radioresistant tumors. In patients with medical contraindications to surgical resection, primary treatment with EBRT appears to produce excellent local control. In 1990, Glaholm reported experience in 186 patients, in which there was 47% disease free survival at 15 years, and a subsequent study reported on 59 patients undergoing treatment with a treatment plan designated as fractionated stereotactic radiotherapy in which there were no recurrences at 10 years after radiotherapy alone of large skull base meningiomas [62].

External beam radiation therapy (EBRT) appears to be the optimal management of optic nerve sheath meningiomas [12]. Narayan et al treated 14 patients with conformal EBRT and found no radiologic progression, with stable or improved visual acuity in 86% with median follow-up of 51.3 months [63]. Turbin et al found EBRT alone to be superior to surgery or surgery with subsequent EBRT at a median period of 8.3 years of follow-up [64]. Rogers identified eight studies comprising analysis of 75 eyes using highly conformal or fractionated stereotactic radiotherapy in which EBRT appears safe and effective [12].

Rogers collected 21 studies reported between 1983 and 2007 addressing the use of EBRT for treatment of meningiomas after varing extent of resection [12]. The introduction of image-based CT and subsequently MRI treatment planning techniques improved conformality and precision of targeting. If one defines modern treatment planning techniques as being available beginning in the mid-1990s, the 10-year PFS for modern versus nonimaged guided techniques is 98% versus 77% at 10 years. Mikler-Zabel et al reported the results of intensity modulated radiation therapy for complex skull base meningiomas [65]. Median target volume in this study was 81.4 ml and median total dose 57.6 Gy was given in 32 fractions. Overall control rate at a median of 4.4 years of follow up was 93.6%. Neurologic deficits improved after treatment in 39.4%. Tumor volume decreased in 20.2%, was stable in 73.4%, and progressed in 6.4%. The relatively small number of higher grade meningiomas precluded direct comparison, but WHO grade 2 tumors has recurrence free survivals of 89% and 77.8% at 3 and 5 years, respectively. The authors felt this compared favorably to their own experience with fractionated stereotactic radiotherapy [66].

Stereotactic radiosurgery (SRS) is being increasingly employed in the treatment of patients with meningiomas. Although there is ongoing controversy regarding the long-term efficacy and short-term safety of SRS versus surgery, several areas of consensus seem to be evolving. The choice of margin dose is a compromise between risk of radiotoxicity and diminished tumor control; most experienced centers now use margin doses ranging from 12 to 16 Gy [12]. The optimal radiosurgical situation is a tumor less than 3 to 4 cm in diameter, with distinct margins and sufficient distance from critical structures to allow for appropriate normal tissue dose restriction.

The radiosurgical group at University of Pittsburgh treated 1045 intracranial meningioma patients with Gamma Knife-based radiosurgery over a 20-year period. In 540 patients, the radiosurgery was the primary treatment, and in 151 radiosurgery was performed after prior resection and/or EBRT. Treatment planning was done using 3D conformal techniques with multiple isocenters. For the last decade, the margin dose is varied from 12 to 15 Gy depending on target volume. The mean optic chiasm dose in this series was 6.5 Gy. Of 384 evaluable patients treated with WHO grade 1 tumors, 172 tumors regressed, 186 were unchanged, and 26 had enlarged, for a tumor control rate of 93% at a median of 4 years. Follow-up of 8 and 10 years was available for 79 and 53 tumors, respectively, with a control rate at both intervals of 91%. For grade 1 meningiomas, the disease specific survival rates at 5, 10, and 15 years were 98.9%, 96.2%, and 96.2%, respectively. The corresponding tumor control rates were 97%, 87.2%, and 87.2%. Of 54 WHO grade 2 tumors, 16 regressed, 11 were unchanged, and 27 had enlarged, for a tumor control rate of 50% at a median of 2 years. For 29 grade 3 tumors, only 4 regressed, 1 was stable, and 24 enlarged, for a control rate of 17% at a median f/u of 15 m. For 536 tumors, SRS was performed as primary therapy without prior surgery or biopsy. In this group, the tumor control rate was 97% at a median f/u of 4 years, and for the subset with 8 and 10 year f/u the control rates were 94% and 95%. A complication related to radiosurgery was observed in 7.7% of patients at an average of 11 m. The morbidity rates for cavernous sinus and parasagital locations were 6.3% and 9.7%, respectively. Cranial nerve deficits developed in 12 patients with cavernous sinus tumors.

Kondziolka et al propose SRS as an effective and safe option for patients even when the tumor is considered amenable to surgical resection [13]. Referring to both Simpson's original series and a modern update by Pollack et al, these authors suggest that SRS provides better tumor control than resection for Simpson grade 2 and 3 to 4 lesions [67]. As the number of patients with long-term follow-up over 10 years are reported, the long-term tumor control for radiosurgery does not seem inferior to resection alone.

The role of SRS in the multimodality treatment of atypical and anaplastic meningiomas continues to evolve. The results reported by the University of Pittsburgh Medical Cente group demonstrate that SRS will not achieve durable tumor control. Stafford et al reported 5-year tumor control rates of 68% and 0% for atypical and anaplastic meningiomas, respectively. Kano reported 12 patients with high-grade meningiomas treated with Linac based SRS at Kyoto University Hospital between 1997 and 2002 [68]. The mean marginal dose was 18 Gy and mean tumor volume 4.4 cm. After a median f/u of 43 m, 13 lesions had progressed within the treatment field and 6 cases had progression outside of the treatment field. A marginal dose of greater than 20 Gy was associated with a lower risk of in-field progression, and a marginal dose of <20 Gy was significantly associated with a higher risk of in-field progression. For patients treated with marginal doses of 20 Gy, the 5-year PFS was 61% versus only 29% for patients treated with less than 20 Gy.

Drug Therapies

The development of effective drug treatments of meningiomas has been one of the most frustrating problems in adult neurooncology [2,3,19,69]. Despite the commitment of both major brain tumor clinical trials consortia through the 1990s, there is still controversy over the efficacy of any cytotoxic single agent or combination regimen for the treatment of any grade of meningoma. Effective drug discovery has lagged behind other brain tumors for several reasons. Establishing meningioma derived cell lines, xenografts, and autochonous models of the intracranial disease have been difficult. The recent application of molecular engineering techniques with viral vector immortization of meningoma derived cell lines is making preclinical studies more feasible [70]. The understanding of molecular pathways that could be relevant therapeutic targets is several years behind that for gliomas or medulloblastoma. Lastly, the heterogeneity of presentation, variation in practice patterns regarding timing of EBRT and use of SRS in the adjuvant or recurrent setting, and the relative rarity of atypical and anaplastic meningiomas even at major neurosurgical centers have compromised the ability to conduct phase-2 trials for these tumors. Nonetheless, as for gliomas, molecularly targeted strategies are beginning to enter the clinical trials repertoire, and with increasing understanding of the molecular underpinnings of differential response to specific regimens, the possibility of individualized molecularly targeted therapies for meningiomas appears to be a realistic goal [19].

Given the excellent prognosis for grade 1 meningiomas after resection and the consensus to the use of adjuvant external beam, as adjuvant treatment for higher Simpson grade WHO benign meningiomas, there is little role at present for adjuvant drug treatment trials for this histologic grade. In the absence of histopathologic or molecular criteria for identifying the small group of WHO grade 1 meningiomas that recur after radiation, adjuvant trials in this setting would be difficult to justify.

With the demonstration that meningiomas are frequently progesterone and estrogen receptor positive, a series of trials were conducted with estrogen or progesterone antagonists. After a small trial of megestrol acetate demonstrated no responses, and a pilot study of mifepriosne demonstrated minor objective responses in five patients, the Southwest Oncology Group conducted a trial of mifiprestone for unresectable meningiomas. This trial accrued 198 total patients of whom 160 were evaluable [66,71,72]. Median survival was not significantly different between the placebo and study arm (12 and 10 months, respectively). In a smaller phase-2 Southwest Oncology Group study with tamoxifen, 1 of 21 patients had a partial response, 2 had minor responses, and 6 had a time to progression of greater than 6 months.

The demonstration that recombinant interferon-α inhibited proliferation of meningioma cells in culture led to three small phase-2 trials of interferon for recurrent, unresectable meningiomas [3]. One patient had an objective response and 4 had stable disease for greater than 6 months [73].

In a study of 12 patients with three anaplastic meningiomas, five grade 1 and two grade 2 radiologic response by MRI was correlated with 11C-L-methionine positron emission tomography [74]. A reduction in uptake ratio was documented in 9/12 of the meningiomas, and three patients continued on drug for up to 8 years with stable disease. The mix of histologic grade and concomitant use of radiotherapy in some of the subjects compromise interpretation of the clinical activity, but the PET results suggest there is a physiologic effect of interferon therapy on meningiomas. The case report literature of meningiomas presenting or progressing while patients were treated with interferon-β for multiple sclerosis also suggests biological effects of this class of drugs on meningiomas [75].

In the mid-1990s, Schrell and colleagues reported first the in vitro cytotoxic effects of hydroxyurea on meningioma cells in culture and then clinical response of anaplastic meningiomas to single agent hydroxyurea in phase-2 trials [76–78]. A series of reports from this German group led to larger phase-2 trials conducted by Newton and Mason [79,80]. Radiologic responses were rare, somewhat disappointing after the earlier European reports, but the drug appeared to produce stabilization of disease, with median TTP of 20 to 30 m [69,70]. Temozolomide and irinotecan both failed to show activity in separate phase-2 trials [66,72].

The demonstration of overexpression of somatostatin receptors by meningiomas led to a phase-2 trial of long acting somatostatin analogue in 16 patients. PFS at 6 m was 44%, and 31% demonstrated a radiologic response [81]. This approach warrants further study. Recently, calcium channel antagonists have been demonstrated in vitro antiproliferative activity against meningioma cells in culture [82]. Phase-2 trial of this approach is underway.

Cytotoxic chemotherapy for recurrent atypical or anaplastic meningomas has been uniformly disappointing. In a review of the University of California, San Francisco, clinical trial experience, multiagent cytotoxic therapy of anaplastic meningioimas demonstrated no activity, with all patients having progressed at the first evaluation time point.

In a recent comprehensive review of preclinical and clinical trial data regarding potentially targetable pathways in meningioma, Norden summarizes the current state of clinical trials for molecularly targeted approaches [19]. Platelet derived growth factor (PDGF), EFG, VEGF, IGF, TGFβ, and their downstream signaling pathways are all implicated in meningioma neoplastic behavior.

PDGF ligands AA and BB and the PDGFr are expressed in the majority of meningiomas and expression levels may be higher in atypical and anaplastic tumors [47,48,83]. In an North American Brain Tumor Coalition phase-2 trial, imatinib was tested in patients with recurrent meningiomas [84]. Patients initially received 600 mg/day, increased to 800 mg/day in cycle two if there was no significant toxicity. Of 23 patients entered, 13 were grade 1, 5 grade 2, and 5 grade 3 meningiomas. The results of this trial were disappointing for imatinib as a single agent.

Of 19 evaluable patients, 10 progressed by the first interval MRI scan. Overall PFS was only 2 months. For benign meningiomas, PFS was 3 m and PFS 6 m 45%. For atypical and malignant meningiomas, PFS was 2 months and there were no patients with stable disease at 6 m. Although the combination of hydroxyurea, the most active cytotoxic agent against menigyuma, with imatinib has shown activity in a phase-2 trial in recurrent malignant glioma, imatinib containing regimens are not generating enthusiasm for further clinical trials.

EGFR is expressed in over 60% of meningiomas, though there may be an inverse correlation between receptor expression and grade [45,85]. In vitro studies indicate the potential relevance of autocrine stimulation by EGFR and TGFα to meningioma cell proliferation. Both erlatinib and gefitinib have been tested in small phase-2 trials by the North American Brain Tumor Coalition; only minor activity was seen for these drugs as single agents, but a small number of subjects in these trials demonstrated prolonged stable disease [86,87].

Downstream molecular targets may also be relevant. The RAF kinase inhibitor PD098059 reduces MAPK phosphorylation, antagonizes PDGF stimulation of proliferation, and inhibits meningioma cell proliferation in vitro [88]. Sorafinib, a RAFK inhibitor currently approved for treatment of renal cell cancer, may be a candidate for clinical trial in meningiomas. There is evidence that PI3K/AKT pathway is relevant to meningioma cell proliferation and that PI3K inhibitors antagonize the stimulatory effects of PDGFBB. PhosphAKT levels are higher in atypical and malignant meningiomas. Inhibitors of AKT and mTORR inhibitors may warrant evaluation [19].

Antiangiogenic drugs are being actively tested both as single agents and in combination with cytotoxics in a number of solid tumors, including malignant gliomas.

VEGF and VEGFr are expressed by most meningiomas, and expression levels seem to correlate with grade [89]. Multiagent TKI that target VEGFr as one of the targets includes ZD-6474, sunatinib, and sorafinib [19]. Phase-2 clinical trials with sunatinib and sorafinib are in progress.

REFERENCES

1. CBTRUS. Statistical report: primary brain tumors in the United States, 1998–2002. Hinsdale, IL: CBTRUS; 2005.
2. Grimm S, Raizer JJ. Meningiomas. *Curr Treat Options Neurol.* 2008;10(4):315–320.
3. Rockhill J, Mrugala M, Chamberlain MC. Intracranial meningiomas: an overview of diagnosis and treatment. *Neurosurg Focus.* 2007;23(4):E1.
4. Perry A, Dehner LP. Meningeal tumors of childhood and infancy. An update and literature review. *Brain Pathol.* 2003;13(3):386–408.
5. Commins DL, Atkinson RD, Burnett ME. Review of meningioma histopathology. *Neurosurg Focus.* 2007;23(4):E3.
6. Riemenschneider MJ, Perry A, Reifenberger G. Histological classification and molecular genetics of meningiomas. *Lancet Neurol.* 2006;5(12):1045–1054.
7. Louis DN, Scheithauer BW, Budka H, Von Deimling A, Kepes JJ. Meningiomas. In: Louis DN, et al, ed. *World Health Organization Classification of Tumours of the Central Nervous System.* Lyon, France: IARC; 2000:176–184.
8. Perry AL, Scheithauer BW, Budka H, Von Diemling A; Meningiomas. In: Louis DN, et al, ed. *World Health Organization Classification of Tumours of the Central Nervous System.* Lyon, France: IARC; 2007:164–172.
9. Schwartz TH, Fraser JF, Brown S, Tabaee A, Kacker A, Anand VK. Endoscopic cranial base surgery: classification of operative approaches. *Neurosurgery.* 2008;62(5):991–1002; discussion 5.
10. Gardner PA, Kassam AB, Thomas A, et al. Endoscopic endonasal resection of anterior cranial base meningiomas. *Neurosurgery.* 2008;63(1):36–52; discussion 4.
11. Prevedello DM, Kassam AB, Snyderman C, et al. Endoscopic cranial base surgery: ready for prime time? *Clin Neurosurg.* 2007;54:48–57.
12. Rogers L, Mehta M. Role of radiation therapy in treating intracranial meningiomas. *Neurosurg Focus.* 2007;23(4):E4.
13. Kondziolka D, Mathieu D, Lunsford LD, et al. Radiosurgery as definitive management of intracranial meningiomas. *Neurosurgery.* 2008;62(1):53–58; discussion 8–60.
14. Stafford SL, Pollock BE, Foote RL, et al. Meningioma radiosurgery: tumor control, outcomes, and complications among 190 consecutive patients. *Neurosurgery.* 2001;49(5):1029–1037; discussion 37–38.
15. Yang SY, Park CK, Park SH, Kim DG, Chung YS, Jung HW. Atypical and anaplastic meningiomas: prognostic implications of clinicopathological features. *J Neurol Neurosurg Psychiatry.* 2008;79(5):574–580.

16. Pearson BE, Markert JM, Fisher WS, et al. Hitting a moving target: evolution of a treatment paradigm for atypical meningiomas amid changing diagnostic criteria. *Neurosurg Focus.* 2008;24(5):E3.
17. Liu Y, Liu M, Li F, Wu C, Zhu S. Malignant meningiomas: a retrospective study of 22 cases. *Bull Cancer.* 2007;94(10):E27-E31.
18. Perry A, Gutmann DH, Reifenberger G. Molecular pathogenesis of meningiomas. *J Neurooncol.* 2004;70(2):183–202.
19. Norden AD, Drappatz J, Wen PY. Targeted drug therapy for meningiomas. *Neurosurg Focus.* 2007;23(4):E12.
20. Perry A, Scheithauer BW, Stafford SL, Lohse CM, Wollan PC. "Malignancy" in meningiomas: a clinicopathologic study of 116 patients, with grading implications. *Cancer.* 1999;85(9):2046–2056.
21. Rajaram V, Brat DJ, Perry A. Anaplastic meningioma versus meningeal hemangiopericytoma: immunohistochemical and genetic markers. *Hum Pathol.* 2004;35(11):1413–1418.
22. Modha A, Gutin PH. Diagnosis and treatment of atypical and anaplastic meningiomas: a review. *Neurosurgery.* 2005;57(3):538–550; discussion 50.
23. Bruna J, Brell M, Ferrer I, Gimenez-Bonafe P, Tortosa A. Ki-67 proliferative index predicts clinical outcome in patients with atypical or anaplastic meningioma. *Neuropathology.* 2007;27(2):114–120.
24. Nakasu S, Li DH, Okabe H, Nakajima M, Matsuda M. Significance of MIB-1 staining indices in meningiomas: comparison of two counting methods. *Am J Surg Pathol.* 2001;25(4):472–478.
25. Ho DM, Hsu CY, Ting LT, Chiang H. Histopathology and MIB-1 labeling index predicted recurrence of meningiomas: a proposal of diagnostic criteria for patients with atypical meningioma. *Cancer.* 2002;94(5):1538–1547.
26. Perry A, Stafford SL, Scheithauer BW, Suman VJ, Lohse CM. The prognostic significance of MIB-1, p53, and DNA flow cytometry in completely resected primary meningiomas. *Cancer.* 1998;82(11):2262–2269.
27. Roser F, Samii M, Ostertag H, Bellinzona M. The Ki-67 proliferation antigen in meningiomas. Experience in 600 cases. *Acta Neurochir (Wien).* 2004;146(1):37–44.
28. Roser F, Nakamura M, Bellinzona M, Rosahl SK, Ostertag H, Samii M. The prognostic value of progesterone receptor status in meningiomas. *J Clin Pathol.* 2004;57(10):1033–1037.
29. Perry A, Stafford SL, Scheithauer BW, Suman VJ, Lohse CM. Meningioma grading: an analysis of histologic parameters. *Am J Surg Pathol.* 1997;21(12):1455–1465.
30. Carvalho LH, Smirnov I, Baia GS, et al. Molecular signatures define two main classes of meningiomas. *Mol Cancer.* 2007;6:64.
31. Wrobel G, Roerig P, Kokocinski F, et al. Microarray-based gene expression profiling of benign, atypical and anaplastic meningiomas identifies novel genes associated with meningioma progression. *Int J Cancer.* 2005;114(2):249–256.
32. Krayenbuhl N, Pravdenkova S, Al-Mefty O. De novo versus transformed atypical and anaplastic meningiomas: comparisons of clinical course, cytogenetics, cytokinetics, and outcome. *Neurosurgery.* 2007;61(3):495–503; discussion 4.
33. Pomeroy SL, Tamayo P, Gaasenbeek M, et al. Prediction of central nervous system embryonal tumour outcome based on gene expression. *Nature.* 2002;415(6870):436–442.
34. Gajjar A, Hernan R, Kocak M, et al. Clinical, histopathologic, and molecular markers of prognosis: toward a new disease risk stratification system for medulloblastoma. *J Clin Oncol.* 2004;22(6):984–993.
35. Shirahata M, Iwao-Koizumi K, Saito S, et al. Gene expression-based molecular diagnostic system for malignant gliomas is superior to histological diagnosis. *Clin Cancer Res.* 2007;13(24):7341–7356.
36. Rivera AL, Pelloski CE, Sulman E, Aldape K. Prognostic and predictive markers in glioma and other neuroepithelial tumors. *Curr Probl Cancer.* 2008;32(3):97–123.
37. Trofatter JA, MacCollin MM, Rutter JL, et al. A novel moesin-, ezrin-, radixin-like gene is a candidate for the neurofibromatosis 2 tumor suppressor. *Cell.* 1993;75(4):826.
38. Rouleau GA, Merel P, Lutchman M, et al. Alteration in a new gene encoding a putative membrane-organizing protein causes neurofibromatosis type 2. *Nature.* 1993;363(6429):515–521.
39. Schnitt SJ, Vogel H. Meningiomas. Diagnostic value of immunoperoxidase staining for epithelial membrane antigen. *Am J Surg Pathol.* 1986;10(9):640–649.
40. Akat K, Mennel HD, Kremer P, Gassler N, Bleck CK, Kartenbeck J. Molecular characterization of desmosomes in meningiomas and arachnoidal tissue. *Acta Neuropathol.* 2003;106(4):337–347.
41. Maillo A, Orfao A, Sayagues JM, et al. New classification scheme for the prognostic stratification of meningioma on the basis of chromosome 14 abnormalities, patient age, and tumor histopathology. *J Clin Oncol.* 2003;21(17):3285–3295.
42. Cai DX, Banerjee R, Scheithauer BW, Lohse CM, Kleinschmidt-Demasters BK, Perry A. Chromosome 1p and 14q FISH analysis in clinicopathologic subsets of meningioma: diagnostic and prognostic implications. *J Neuropathol Exp Neurol.* 2001;60(6):628–636.
43. Tse JY, Ng HK, Lau KM, Lo KW, Poon WS, Huang DP. Loss of heterozygosity of chromosome 14q in low- and high-grade meningiomas. *Hum Pathol.* 1997;28(7):779–785.
44. Wada K, Maruno M, Suzuki T, et al. Chromosomal and genetic abnormalities in benign and malignant meningiomas using DNA microarray. *Neurol Res.* 2005;27(7):747–754.
45. Andersson U, Guo D, Malmer B, et al. Epidermal growth factor receptor family (EGFR, ErbB2–4) in gliomas and meningiomas. *Acta Neuropathol.* 2004;108(2):135–142.
46. Carroll RS, Black PM, Zhang J, et al. Expression and activation of epidermal growth factor receptors in meningiomas. *J Neurosurg.* 1997;87(2):315–323.
47. Maxwell M, Galanopoulos T, Hedley-Whyte ET, Black PM, Antoniades HN. Human meningiomas co-express platelet-derived growth factor (PDGF) and PDGF-receptor genes and their protein products. *Int J Cancer.* 1990;46(1):16–21.
48. Nagashima G, Asai J, Suzuki R, Fujimoto T. Different distribution of c-myc and MIB-1 positive cells in malignant meningiomas with reference to TGFs, PDGF, and PgR expression. *Brain Tumor Pathol.* 2001;18(1):1–5.
49. Arena S, Barbieri F, Thellung S, et al. Expression of somatostatin receptor mRNA in human meningiomas and their implication in in vitro antiproliferative activity. *J Neurooncol.* 2004;66(1–2):155–166.
50. Barresi V, Alafaci C, Salpietro F, Tuccari G. Sstr2A immunohistochemical expression in human meningiomas: is there a correlation with the histological grade, proliferation or microvessel density? *Oncol Rep.* 2008;20(3):485–492.
51. Christoforidis GA. *Meningeal Tumors. Handbook of Neuro-Oncology Neuroimaging.* London, England: Elsevier; 2008.
52. Buetow MP, Buetow PC, Smirniotopoulos JG. Typical, atypical, and misleading features in meningioma. *Radiographics.* 1991;11(6):1087–1106.
53. Engelhard HH. Progress in the diagnosis and treatment of patients with meningiomas. Part I: diagnostic imaging, preoperative embolization. *Surg Neurol.* 2001;55(2):89–101.
54. Nagele T, Petersen D, Klose U, Grodd W, Opitz H, Voigt K. The "dural tail" adjacent to meningiomas studied by dynamic contrast-enhanced MRI: a comparison with histopathology. *Neuroradiology.* 1994;36(4):303–307.
55. Yang S, Law M, Zagzag D, et al. Dynamic contrast-enhanced perfusion MR imaging measurements of endothelial permeability: differentiation between atypical and typical meningiomas. *AJNR Am J Neuroradiol.* 2003;24(8):1554–1559.
56. Jungling FD, Wakhloo AK, Hennig J. In vivo proton spectroscopy of meningioma after preoperative embolization. *Magn Reson Med.* 1993;30(2):155–160.
57. Chiechi MV, Smirniotopoulos JG, Mena H. Intracranial hemangiopericytomas: MR and CT features. *AJNR Am J Neuroradiol.* 1996;17(7):1365–1371.
58. Alen JF, Lobato RD, Gomez PA, et al. Intracranial hemangiopericytoma: study of 12 cases. *Acta Neurochir (Wien).* 2001;143(6):575–586.
59. Fountas KN, Kapsalaki E, Kassam M, et al. Management of intracranial meningeal hemangiopericytomas: outcome and experience. *Neurosurg Rev.* 2006;29(2):145–153.
60. Mirimanoff RO, Dosoretz DE, Linggood RM, Ojemann RG, Martuza RL. Meningioma: analysis of recurrence and progression following neurosurgical resection. *J Neurosurg.* 1985;62(1):18–24.
61. Glaholm J, Bloom HJ, Crow JH. The role of radiotherapy in the management of intracranial meningiomas: the Royal Marsden Hospital experience with 186 patients. *Int J Radiat Oncol Biol Phys.* 1990;18(4):755–761.

62. Debus J, Wuendrich M, Pirzkall A, et al. High efficacy of fractionated stereotactic radiotherapy of large base-of-skull meningiomas: long-term results. *J Clin Oncol.* 2001;19(15):3547–3553.
63. Narayan S, Cornblath WT, Sandler HM, Elner V, Hayman JA. Preliminary visual outcomes after three-dimensional conformal radiation therapy for optic nerve sheath meningioma. *Int J Radiat Oncol Biol Phys.* 2003;56(2):537–543.
64. Turbin RE, Thompson CR, Kennerdell JS, Cockerham KP, Kupersmith MJ. A long-term visual outcome comparison in patients with optic nerve sheath meningioma managed with observation, surgery, radiotherapy, or surgery and radiotherapy. *Ophthalmology.* 2002;109(5):890–899; discussion 9–900.
65. Milker-Zabel S, Zabel-du Bois A, Huber P, Schlegel W, Debus J. Intensity-modulated radiotherapy for complex-shaped meningioma of the skull base: long-term experience of a single institution. *Int J Radiat Oncol Biol Phys.* 2007;68(3):858–863.
66. Grunberg SM, Weiss MH, Spitz IM, et al. Treatment of unresectable meningiomas with the antiprogesterone agent mifepristone. *J Neurosurg.* 1991;74(6):861–866.
67. Pollock BE, Stafford SL, Utter A, Giannini C, Schreiner SA. Stereotactic radiosurgery provides equivalent tumor control to Simpson Grade 1 resection for patients with small- to medium-size meningiomas. *Int J Radiat Oncol Biol Phys.* 2003;55(4):1000–1005.
68. Kano H, Takahashi JA, Katsuki T, et al. Stereotactic radiosurgery for atypical and anaplastic meningiomas. *J Neurooncol.* 2007;84(1):41–47.
69. Chamberlain MC. Adjuvant combined modality therapy for malignant meningiomas. *J Neurosurg.* 1996;84(5):733–736.
70. Cargioli TG, Ugur HC, Ramakrishna N, Chan J, Black PM, Carroll RS. Establishment of an in vivo meningioma model with human telomerase reverse transcriptase. *Neurosurgery.* 2007;60(4):750–759; discussion 9–60.
71. Grunberg SMR, Townsend C, Ahmadi J, et al. Phase III double-blind randomized placebo controlled study of mifepristone (RU-486) for the treatment of unresectable meningioma. *Proc Am Soc Clin Oncol.* 2001;20.
72. Grunberg SM, Weiss MH. Lack of efficacy of megestrol acetate in the treatment of unresectable meningioma. *J Neurooncol.* 1990;8(1):61–65.
73. Kaba SE, DeMonte F, Bruner JM, et al. The treatment of recurrent unresectable and malignant meningiomas with interferon alpha-2B. *Neurosurgery.* 1997;40(2):271–275.
74. Muhr C, Gudjonsson O, Lilja A, Hartman M, Zhang ZJ, Langstrom B. Meningioma treated with interferon-alpha, evaluated with [(11)C]-L-methionine positron emission tomography. *Clin Cancer Res.* 2001;7(8):2269–2276.
75. Drevelegas A, Xinou E, Karacostas D, Parissis D, Karkavelas G, Milonas I. Meningioma growth and interferon beta-1b treated multiple sclerosis: coincidence or relationship? *Neuroradiology.* 2005;47(7):516–519.
76. Schrell UM, Rittig MG, Anders M, et al. Hydroxyurea for treatment of unresectable and recurrent meningiomas. I. Inhibition of primary human meningioma cells in culture and in meningioma transplants by induction of the apoptotic pathway. *J Neurosurg.* 1997;86(5):845–852.
77. Schrell UM, Rittig MG, Anders M, et al. Hydroxyurea for treatment of unresectable and recurrent meningiomas. II. Decrease in the size of meningiomas in patients treated with hydroxyurea. *J Neurosurg.* 1997;86(5):840–844.
78. Schrell UM, Rittig MG, Koch U, Marschalek R, Anders M. Hydroxyurea for treatment of unresectable meningiomas. *Lancet.* 1996;348(9031):888–889.
79. Newton HB, Scott SR, Volpi C. Hydroxyurea chemotherapy for meningiomas: enlarged cohort with extended follow-up. *Br J Neurosurg.* 2004;18(5):495–499.
80. Mason WP, Gentili F, Macdonald DR, Hariharan S, Cruz CR, Abrey LE. Stabilization of disease progression by hydroxyurea in patients with recurrent or unresectable meningioma. *J Neurosurg.* 2002;97(2):341–346.
81. Chamberlain MC, Glantz MJ, Fadul CE. Recurrent meningioma: salvage therapy with long-acting somatostatin analogue. *Neurology.* 2007;69(10):969–973.
82. Ragel BT, Couldwell WT, Wurster RD, Jensen RL. Chronic suppressive therapy with calcium channel antagonists for refractory meningiomas. *Neurosurg Focus.* 2007;23(4):E10.
83. Yang SY, Xu GM. Expression of PDGF and its receptor as well as their relationship to proliferating activity and apoptosis of meningiomas in human meningiomas. *J Clin Neurosci.* 2001;8(1):49–53.
84. Wen PY, Yung WK, Lamborn KR, et al. Phase I/II study of imatinib mesylate for recurrent malignant gliomas: North American brain tumor consortium study 99-08. *Clin Cancer Res.* 2006;12(16):4899–4907.
85. Smith JS, Lal A, Harmon-Smith M, Bollen AW, McDermott MW. Association between absence of epidermal growth factor receptor immunoreactivity and poor prognosis in patients with atypical meningioma. *J Neurosurg.* 2007;106(6):1034–1040.
86. Lieberman FS, Wen P, Abrey LE, et al. Phase I-II trial of ZD-1839 in recurrent malignant glioma and recurrent or progressive meningioma. An NABTC study, ASCO Proceedings 2003.
87. Raizer JJ, Abrey LE, Lassman AB, et al. A Phase II Trial of erlotinib in patients with non-progressive glioblastoma multiforme post radiation therapy, and recurrent malignant gliomas and meningiomas: a North American brain tumor consortium trial. *Neuro Oncol.* 2010 Jan;12(1):95–103.
88. Johnson MD, Woodard A, Kim P, Frexes-Steed M. Evidence for mitogen-associated protein kinase activation and transduction of mitogenic signals by platelet-derived growth factor in human meningioma cells. *J Neurosurg.* 2001;94(2):293–300.
89. Lamszus K, Lengler U, Schmidt NO, Stavrou D, Ergun S, Westphal M. Vascular endothelial growth factor, hepatocyte growth factor/scatter factor, basic fibroblast growth factor, and placenta growth factor in human meningiomas and their relation to angiogenesis and malignancy. *Neurosurgery.* 2000;46(4):938–947; discussion 47–48.

67 Medical Management for Brainstem Tumors

Sabine Mueller

INTRODUCTION

Brainstem gliomas are common in children and account for approximately 10% to 20% of all brain tumors [1,2]. Mean age at presentation is 7 to 9 years [3,4]. Brainstem gliomas are much less frequent in the adult population with estimated 2% of all adult gliomas. Before the era of modern imaging, brain stem gliomas were considered a homogenous group and generally classified as malignant tumors. Since the development of better imaging modalities, brainstem gliomas are currently classified into two broad categories, diffuse and focal tumors. Focal tumors are divided further into focal midbrain, dorsally exophytic, and cervicomedullary lesions. Brainstem gliomas associated with neurofibromatosis 1 (NF1) represent a particular entity with less aggressive behavior and will be discussed separately later.

BRAINSTEM GLIOMAS IN CHILDREN

Diffuse Brainstem Gliomas

Diffuse brainstem gliomas account for 58% to 75% of all pediatric brainstem tumors. They are characteristically malignant astrocytomas (World Health Organization [WHO] grade III and IV) although ependymoma, atypical teratoid/rhabdoid, and tuberculoma have been reported as well [5–7]. The long-term overall survival is very poor with only 6% to 10% of patients surviving beyond 2 years of age [8]. The classical clinical presentation consists of a triad of symptoms, including cranial neuropathies, long tract signs, and cerebellar findings. These tumors are diagnosed by magnetic resonance imaging (MRI) and rarely by tissue diagnosis unless an unusual presentation warrants further investigation. These tumors are classically localized in the pons, rarely enhance, and occupy greater than 50% of the pontine diameter [9]. The interpretation of MRI changes after treatment remains challenging. It is often impossible to distinguish between treatment-related changes versus disease progression. Despite various efforts to improve outcome in this population, the prognosis remains very poor.

Surgery

Surgical intervention has a limited role in the management of diffuse brainstem gliomas. MRI is generally sufficient to establish the diagnosis in most cases [10], and meaningful resection remains impossible due to the diffuse infiltration of the tumor in surrounding brainstem structures [11]. A biopsy can be performed safely if needed [12] but often does not alter the therapeutic approach [13]. In one series described by Sanford et al, 18 out of 33 children with diffuse pontine gliomas underwent biopsy. All except one child died with a reported median survival of 11.5 months. There was no difference in outcome based on pathology or whether the patient underwent a biopsy [7]. These findings were supported by a Children's Cancer Group study analyzing a total of 120 children with diffuse brainstem gliomas [10]. Of these, 45 children underwent biopsy with pathology available in 36 cases ranging from low-grade astrocytoma (13 cases) to anaplastic astrocytoma (20 cases) to glioblastoma multiforme (2 cases). One biopsy was nondiagnostic. Regardless of pathology or whether a biopsy was performed, all patients had a poor outcome [14,15]. As documented in the literature, the complication rate of stereotactic biopsy is low and therefore might be warranted to get a better understanding of the molecular biology of these tumors.

Radiation Therapy

Radiation therapy remains the standard of care for diffuse brainstem gliomas. To date radiation therapy remains the only therapeutic intervention leading to a significant reduction in tumor size and prolonging survival [16,17]. However, almost all children receiving radiation therapy invariably experience disease progression and die. There is no randomized trial available investigating radiation versus no treatment for diffuse brainstem gliomas. One study reviewing the outcome of 36 children with diffuse brainstem gliomas treated with radiation therapy (24 patients) to children not receiving any treatment (12 patients) based on parental decision revealed a median survival of 280 days in the treated group versus 140 days in the untreated group [18]. As radiation therapy seemed to have beneficial effects, numerous strategies assessed if higher radiation dose would lead to improved outcome. Multiple studies investigated the benefit of hyperfractionated radiation therapy for diffuse brainstem gliomas with disappointing results. A Pediatric Oncology Group (POG) study compared doses up to 7560 cGy and demonstrated that there was no significant survival benefit with higher doses of radiation therapy[19]. The Children's Cancer Group study using 7800 cGy found similar results[14]. Radiosensitizing agents like cisplatin have been tested with conventional versus hyperfractionated radiotherapy with no survival benefit for the latter group [20]. Agents like topotecan to increase radiosensitivity of these tumors have been evaluated in phase I/II trials with disappointing results as well [21,22].

The current standard of care for diffuse brainstem gliomas is conventional radiotherapy with a local field dose of 5400 to 6400 cGy, in 180 cGy daily fractions, 5 days a week. Despite radiotherapy survival remains dismal and innovative treatment strategies are needed.

Chemotherapy

The role of chemotherapy for diffuse brainstem gliomas remains controversial. A variety of different agents as single or multiagent regimens have been studied with minimal effect on survival [23]. One study compared the effect of irradiation with and without two different adjuvant chemotherapy regimens composed of carboplatin, etoposide, vincristine or cisplatin, cyclophosphamide, and vincristine. There was no significant improvement with the addition of either chemotherapy regimen [24]. Freemann et al [25] reported that children treated only with irradiation in the POG 8495 study had similar outcome compared to children treated with irradiation and cisplatin during the POG 9239 study. Marrow ablative chemotherapy with autologous stem cell rescue has been investigated in patients diagnosed with recurrent disease. Studies with thiotepa and busulfan or thiotepa and cyclophosphamide did not show any survival benefit compared to conventional radiotherapy and was associated with significant toxicities [26–28]. In contrast to these findings are studies showing moderate survival benefit when chemotherapy is added to the treatment regimen. An analysis of the Hirntumor-GBM database, which registers patients enrolled in the studies of the Pediatric Oncology and Hematology Society of the German language group, demonstrated that overall survival of patients treated with radiotherapy compared to radiotherapy and chemotherapy is 0.79 ($n = 17$; ± 0.11 year, confidence interval [CI] = 0.58–1.01) and 0.94 ($n = 88$; ± 0.08 years), respectively. This analysis also confirmed that radiotherapy is effective in the treatment of brainstem gliomas with an overall survival of 0.95 in irradiated patients ($n = 125$, ± 0.06 years CI = 0.84–1.07) versus 0.39 ($n = 21$, ± 0.19 years, CI = 0.01–0.72) in patients not undergoing radiotherapy [29]. Other prognostic factors included age, histological grade, and size of tumor. Children less than 4 years of age had better survival compared to older children. Small pontine lesions were also correlated with better outcome, which has been demonstrated by other studies as well [30]. Temozolamide has generated great excitement in the treatment of adult GBMs, but so far results from studies in the pediatric population are less promising [31]. Other agents like tamoxifen, an antiestrogenic drug used for the treatment of breast cancer, has been evaluated for the treatment of brainstem glioma. Studies have shown some beneficial effect in adult patients with GBM [32], but no benefit in survival has been reported in brainstem glioma in children [33,34]. An extensive review from Hargrave and Bouffet in 2006 summarizes the inconsistency between conducted clinical trials regarding eligibility criteria, definition, assessment of response or progression, statistical design, and endpoints. This review highlights the difficulty of assessing and comparing response rates of different chemotherapy regimens for the treatment of diffuse brainstem gliomas in children. However, despite this variability, no improvement in survival has been documented over the last 30 years [35]. As outcome has not been changed despite multiple different avenues investigated, these patients should be considered for phase-I trials whenever possible.

Future Directions for Brainstem Gliomas

Unlike for other brain tumors, brainstem gliomas are mainly diagnosed by imaging and therefore access to tissue to further investigate the genetic and molecular characteristics have been limited. The molecular pathways involved in the formation of brainstem gliomas are not well understood and therefore a rational approach to design new biological agents is limited. To date, new trials are often designed based on the knowledge from adult GBMs as these tumors are very well studied regarding their molecular characteristics. Currently, trials are ongoing investigating biological agents like inhibitors of the epidermal growth factor receptor, gefitinib or erlotinib, despite limited knowledge about the involvement of this pathway in diffuse brainstem gliomas. In a small, phase-I study using gefitinib in relapsed solid pediatric tumors, two out of three patients with brainstem glioma showed stable disease, but as one patient with ependymoma developed intratumoral hemorrhage, the study was closed for central nervous system tumors [36]. Gefitinib in combination with radiotherapy was studied in 20 patients with brainstem glioma and no treatment effect was noted [37]. Similar to the first study, five patients developed intratumoral hemorrhage, which might be an intrinsic problem of brainstem gliomas rather than treatment-related complication as shown later [38]. Inhibition of angiogenesis is another focus of current investigations. Recent studies suggest that cancer stem cells are dependent on the interaction with endothelial cells and the perivascular environment. The disruption of such a vascular niche for the tumor stem cells by an antiangiogenic therapy could result in increased response to conventional therapy by targeting these self-renewing cells. Bevacizumab might be one potential molecule attacking these stem cells [39]. Bevacizumab showed promising results in adult patient with high-grade glioma and is currently studied in pediatric brainstem gliomas [40]. Other antiangiogenic agents currently under investigation include the oral inhibitor of the vascular endothelial growth factor, AZD2171.

Another research area is the delivery of agents to the tumor, either by catheter-based technologies like convection-enhanced delivery or with use of small molecules interrupting the blood brain barrier. Few studies have investigated the use of molecules interrupting the blood brain barrier. The numbers are too small to draw a final conclusion, but it was alarming that in one study using RMP-7, a bradykinin analog, in combination with cisplatin and radiation therapy 3 out of 13 treated patients experienced disseminated disease [41]. Trials with convection-enhanced delivery are underway.

Focal Brainstem Tumors

Focal brainstem tumors are less common and only represent 5% to 25% of all brainstem tumors. These tumors are mainly benign tumors (WHO grade I or II) and diagnosed via imaging. These tumors have a much better prognosis compared to diffuse brainstem gliomas with greater than 80% 5-year survival rates. Mean age at presentation is 10 years, slightly older than patients presenting with diffuse brainstem tumors. Cranial nerves are less commonly involved and ataxia as well as long tract signs are the dominant symptoms. Based on their growth patterns, focal brainstem tumors are divided into dorsally exophytic, cervicomedullary, and midbrain tumors. Each is described in greater detail in the following sections.

Dorsally Exophytic Gliomas

Dorsally exophytic brainstem gliomas together with cervicomedullary gliomas comprise less than 20% of all brainstem tumors. The clinical presentation predominantly consists of headache and vomiting secondary to increased intracranial pressure. Papilledema and torticollis can be present on physical exam. Children less than 3 years of age can present with failure to thrive due to increased vomiting as their only presenting sign [2]. The onset of symptoms is often insidious and patients are diagnosed later in their disease course. MRI is generally diagnostic. These tumors enhance with gadolinium and can be difficult to distinguish from ependymomas or choroid plexus papillomas. Dorsally exophytic gliomas are generally benign tumors (WHO grade I and II) [42]. Long-term survival is common and children are generally able to resume normal activities.

Surgery

Surgery is the treatment of choice for dorsally exophytic gliomas with the goal of gross total resection (GTR). Residual tumor can be followed by serial imaging in 3 to 6 months intervals. Disease progression is seen in 25% to 30% of patients. Second-look surgery should be considered if additional treatment is indicated [43]. If the patient remains asymptomatic despite disease progression documented via imaging, observation with close follow-up is often the best option. Pollack et al reported 18 patients with dorsally exophytic brainstem gliomas. In this group, none of the patients had GTR. Residual disease was followed with imaging in 15 patients and 2 patients who underwent radiotherapy. Of these 15 patients, complete regression of the residual tumor was observed in 3, stable disease in 8, and progressive disease in 4 patients. Recurrence was managed by repeat resection or radiotherapy with long-term disease control [44]. Similar results were found by another study led by Khatib et al. In this study, 12 out of 51 patients were diagnosed with dorsally exophytic brainstem tumors. Of these, 50% underwent GTR and 50% subtotal resection. Two patients received either chemotherapy or radiation therapy after surgery. Of the 10 patients who had no additional postsurgical therapy, 7 remained stable and 3 showed disease progression, which were subsequently treated with radiation therapy leading to long-term survival. The one patient who was treated with chemotherapy after surgical resection died of acute myelogenous leukemia [42].

Adjuvant Radiation and Chemotherapy

Radiation therapy is only indicated in cases with disease progression and especially when second surgery cannot be performed safely. Only a few studies have assessed the benefit of radiotherapy in this patient population, but as outlined above, most patients respond to radiotherapy with long-term survival [42,44]. It remains a reasonable alternative for progressive or recurrence disease in the older population. The benefit of chemotherapy of low-grade gliomas is discussed in detail elsewhere.

In summary, dorsally exophytic gliomas are generally low-grade tumors with good prognosis and long-term survival of greater than 5 years. The mainstay of therapy remains surgical resection; and even with subtotal resection, the patients often require no further intervention. Radiation therapy is the most commonly used adjuvant therapy.

Cervicomedullary Gliomas

Cervicomedullary gliomas are similar to intramedullary spinal cord gliomas. They typically infiltrate the cervical spine and medulla and rarely extend above the pontomedullary junction. The presenting symptoms are very similar to those of the dorsally exophytic gliomas, with headache and vomiting being the most common symptom. Tumors involving the lower medulla may have lower cranial nerve deficits presenting with difficulty swallowing or speech problems. Dysfunction of medulla and spinal cord can be present. These signs can occur for several months to years prior to diagnosis [45]. MRI is the diagnostic test of choice. The most common pediatric tumors in this area are gliomas, medulloblastomas, and ependymomas [46]. The majority of the gliomas are low grade (WHO I and II), but 10% to 20% are high grade [45,47]. Fisher et al proposed that dorsally exophytic and cervicomedullary gliomas should be grouped under their histological classification of pilocystic astrocytoma rather than their MRI appearance [48].

Surgery

To date, the main treatment modality remains surgery. Biopsy is recommended if the clinical presentation or the radiographic appearance is atypical, otherwise maximal tumor resection is preferred. The amount of resection varies between studies. One study demonstrated that 30% (12 out of 39) of patients underwent GTR, whereas over 50% (20 out of 39) underwent less than 90% resection [49].

However, resection greater than 50% has been associated with increased long-term survival [50,51]. The surgical success is correlated with longer duration of symptoms as well as low-grade histology [45,47]. Surgical complications include damage to the lower cranial nerves resulting in gastrostomy, tracheostomy, and increased incidence of upper airway infections and pneumonia.

Adjuvant Radiation and Chemotherapy

Adjuvant therapy is mainly used for disease progression and recurrence. To date, there is very limited information on the benefit of radiotherapy or chemotherapy for these tumors and management is decided on a case-by-case basis by the treating physician and the family.

In summary, cervicomedullary gliomas are generally low-grade gliomas and treatment of choice is GTR whenever possible. Limited information is published on the benefit of radiotherapy and/or chemotherapy. Median survival is greater than 5 years.

Midbrain Tumors

Focal tectal or tegmental tumors are generally low-grade gliomas and represent 5% to 15% of all pediatric brainstem gliomas. They are well-circumscribed lesions on the MRI with clear borders. They generally occur in children but also manifest in adults. Median age at presentation is in the range from 6 to 14 years [52]. The classical presentation consists of symptoms of increased intracranial pressure like headache, vomiting, lethargy, and altered level of consciousness. The clinical course varies but generally symptoms are often present for few months. Tectal lesions are more commonly associated with Parinaud's syndrome, characterized by supranuclear paresis of upward gaze, convergence retraction nystagmus, and light-near dissociation of the pupils. Tegmental lesions, however, rarely present with hydrocephalus, and these patients more commonly present with motor weakness and ocular abnormalities. Focal midbrain tumors are rare in the adult population. Most patients are asymptomatic and are diagnosed incidentally. Some patients have signs of increased intracranial presssure and require a shunt procedure. Most series discussing focal midbrain tumors in adults would advocate for conservative management due to the benign nature of these tumors and follow these patients with serial imaging. Therapy should be reserved for patients who progress and includes surgery and radiation therapy as first line options [53,54].

Surgery

Most cases of focal midbrain tumors are managed conservatively and surgical intervention is mainly required for symptomatic relief of hydrocephalus [55–58]. Surgery is indicated when patients present with hydrocephalus due to aqueductal stenosis. Endoscopic third ventriculostomy is the procedure of choice to avoid shunt placement and associated morbidities like infection, overdrainage, and shunt insufficiency. Biopsies can be obtained during the same procedure for further diagnostic purposes but are generally not recommended unless clinical presentation and radiographic appearance are atypical. Careful follow-up with serial MRI is performed and open surgery mainly required when disease progression occurs. Studies report tumor progression in the range of 15% to 25% [52]. Radical surgical resection is possible in nonfiltrating midbrain tumors with low morbidity and no mortality in some series [59].

Adjuvant Radiation and Chemotherapy

Radiotherapy has been used in patients with disease progression. Studies have shown that routine use of radiation therapy does not influence survival and therefore should be reserved for patients with progressive disease [60]. The long-term benefit of radiation therapy has been poorly documented in the literature, but some studies suggest a favorable outcome after treatment. Pollack et al described 16 children with midbrain tumors. All patients underwent shunt procedures and were followed with repeated imaging. Four out of these 16 patients showed disease progression and subsequently underwent biopsy, which demonstrated in 3 out of 4 patient low-grade tumors and one case of anaplastic astrocytoma. All patients with disease progression received conventional radiotherapy and the patient with anaplastic astrocytoma also received focal stereotactic radiosurgery. All patients responded to treatment with three patients showing disease regression and one patient who had stable disease at a median follow-up time of 4.25 years [56]. Most centers would advocate for radiotherapy once there is clinical or radiographic evidence of disease progression [52,56,61]. It remains controversial whether a biopsy prior to radiation therapy is necessary. Chemotherapy is rarely necessary as most cases respond to conservative, surgical, or radiation therapy.

In summary, midbrain gliomas are mainly benign lesions. They often come to medical attention due to signs of increased intracranial pressure. Goal of surgical intervention is mainly the relief of hydrocephalus. Most cases can be followed conservatively with serial imaging as the tumor remains stable for many years [62]. In the event of tumor progression, surgical intervention and/or radiation therapy is recommended.

BRAINSTEM GLIOMAS AND NF I

Patients with NF1 have a tendency to develop astrocytic tumors, the most common being optic pathway gliomas, which are discussed elsewhere. They can also occur less frequently in the brainstem. Studies have shown that patients with NF1 have a better outcome than nonaffected children [63,64]. Brainstem tumors should not be confused with unspecific white matter changes, which are frequently found on MRIs in patients with NF1 of unknown clinical significance [64,65]. These unidentified bright objects are normally not associated with mass effect, edema, or contrast enhancement and tend to decrease in size overtime. To date, routine MRI in patients with NF1 is not recommended unless neurological exam warrants further investigations.

A recent study from the Children's hospital in Boston, the largest study published so far, identified 23 patients out of 125 with NF1 (18.4%) who presented with brainstem mass lesions. Eight out of these 23 patients received additional treatment with surgery, radiation therapy, or chemotherapy. Six of these patients received treatment for brainstem lesions, whereas two children received treatment for lesions other than brainstem. Of the patients who received treatment for the brainstem lesion, five out of six had stable disease. The neuroimaging characteristics did not differ between the treated versus untreated group. Reported outcome was favorable with 14/16 untreated and 6/23 treated patients being alive with stable or decreased disease burden on MRI at median follow-up of 67 months and 102 months, respectively. Only one patient previously untreated had disease progression. The authors concluded that brainstem lesions in patients with NF1 should be treated with caution and careful observation is warranted [66]. In contrast, a French study showed a less favorable outcome. Out of 104 patients with NF1 enrolled in the study, 43 patients presented with lesions outside the optic pathway, 21 (49%) located in the brainstem. Of these, 24 were asymptomatic and 19 had clinical correlates (13/33 children and 6/10 adults). Increased intracranial pressure was the most commonly presenting symptom for patients with brainstem lesions. Poor outcome was associated with location outside the optic pathway, diagnosis in adulthood, and symptoms at presentation. Of the 21 patients with brainstem gliomas, 3 children and 2 adults died during the study secondary to tumor progression [67]. Pollack et al reported on 21 patients with NF1 and brainstem lesions. In this series, 12 out of 21 patients had clinical symptoms related to the mass and 9 were asymptomatic. A total of 10/21 patients had either clinical ($n = 3$) or radiographic ($n = 7$) signs of disease progression. Of these 10 patients, 7 had stable disease or tumor regression without intervention with a median follow-up of 3.7 years. Only 4 out of 21 patients underwent tumor-specific therapy, including surgery and radiation therapy. The authors concluded that conservative management is indicated and only patients with a progressive clinical course should undergo therapeutic intervention. The treatment options remain the same as for non NF1 patients. For focal tumors, surgical resection is indicated. Radiotherapy needs to be considered with caution, as patients with NF1 have a higher risk developing radiation-induced malignancies [68].

In summary, most of the brainstem gliomas identified in NF1 patients remain asymptomatic and do not progress clinically without intervention. However, a few tumors, mainly those that show contrast enhancement and are diagnosed in adults, can progress and require further treatment. There is no consensus on the optimal therapy, and therapeutic options are mainly influenced by the appearance and localization of the tumor as outlined above.

BRAINSTEM GLIOMAS IN ADULTS

Adult brainstem gliomas are rare and account for less than 2% of adult gliomas. Few studies have shown that brainstem gliomas in adults are generally less aggressive compared to children [69–71]. Peak incidence is between the third and fourth decade of life [70,71]. In one study, most of the brainstem gliomas in adults were low grade with 80% (24/30) being either WHO grade I or II [70]. The French Association of Neuro-oncology (ANOCEF) published the largest cohort of adult brainstem gliomas to date and showed that favorable prognostic factors are: (1) age at disease onset < 40 years, (2) duration of symptoms > 3 months prior to diagnosis, (3) Karnofski Performance status > 70, (4) low-grade histology and (5) absence of contrast enhancement and signs of necrosis on MRI. Only the last three factors remained statistically significant after multivariate analysis [71]. In the French study, the overall median survival was 5.4 years and 3-year survival was 66%. MRI findings demonstrated diffuse infiltrating tumors in 50%, contrast enhancing focal mass lesion in 31%, isolated tectal tumors in 8%, and others in 11%. Histopathology revealed astrocytic gliomas (56%), oligodendrocytic and oligoastrocytic gliomas (25%), and unspecified gliomas (19%). The patients were classified based on prognostic factors and MRI findings in three main groups. Diffuse low-grade gliomas accounted for 46% (22 patients) with mean onset in third decade of life. Symptom duration was generally >3 month and histology revealed mainly low-grade gliomas (9/11). Radiation therapy significantly improved clinical status in 13 out of 21 patients. The median survival in this group was 7.3 years. Malignant brainstem tumors were found in 15 patients (31%). Of these, 10 patients (10/15) were older than 40 years of age and onset was rapid with altered performance status in 14/15. MRI showed contrast enhancement at diagnosis in all 15 patients, and necrosis was found in 2/3 of the patients. Histology showed high-grade gliomas (WHO III and IV) in all cases. The majority of tumors were therapy resistant with only two patients showing clinical and radiographic response to radiotherapy. Median survival was 11.2 months.

Focal tectal glioma was the third group identified. Only four patients (8%) were diagnosed with pure tectal tumors. These tumors have an indolent course and hydrocephalus was the main complication. All patients underwent radiotherapy and one patient had partial resection. Four patients survived > 5 years and three patients survived > 8 years. These results are similar to tectal tumors in the pediatric population [71].

It is interesting that the clinical presentation and radiographic appearance of diffuse low-grade gliomas in adults is similar to the presentation of diffuse pediatric brainstem gliomas; however, there is a radical difference in treatment response and survival. The malignant brainstem tumors in children have a similar clinical presentation and outcome as the supratentorial malignant gliomas.

As brainstem gliomas are very rare in adulthood and response to different therapy regimens is sparsely documented in the literature, treatment should be decided on an individual basis. The above mention classification might help to guide the treating physician.

REFERENCES

1. Albright AL, Price RA, Guthkelch AN. Brain stem gliomas of children. A clinicopathological study. *Cancer*. 1983;52(12):2313–2319.
2. Jallo GI, Biser-Rohrbaugh A, Freed D. Brainstem gliomas. *Childs Nerv Syst*. 2004;20(3):143–153.

3. Berger MS, Edwards MS, LaMasters D, Davis RL, Wilson CB. Pediatric brain stem tumors: radiographic, pathological, and clinical correlations. Neurosurgery. 1983;12(3):298–302.
4. Littman P, Jarrett P, Bilaniuk LT, et al. Pediatric brain stem gliomas. Cancer. 1980;45(11):2787–2792.
5. Chico-Ponce de Leon F, Perezpena-Diazconti M, Castro-Sierra E, et al. Stereotactically-guided biopsies of brainstem tumors. Childs Nerv Syst. 2003;19(5–6):305–310.
6. Zagzag D, Miller DC, Knopp E, et al. Primitive neuroectodermal tumors of the brainstem: investigation of seven cases. Pediatrics. 2000;106(5):1045–1053.
7. Sanford RA, Freeman CR, Burger P, Cohen ME. Prognostic criteria for experimental protocols in pediatric brainstem gliomas. Surg Neurol. 1988;30(4):276–280.
8. Freeman CR, Perilongo G. Chemotherapy for brain stem gliomas. Childs Nerv Syst. 1999;15(10):545–553.
9. Donaldson SS, Laningham F, Fisher PG. Advances toward an understanding of brainstem gliomas. J Clin Oncol. 2006;24(8):1266–1272.
10. Albright AL, Packer RJ, Zimmerman R, Rorke LB, Boyett J, Hammond GD. Magnetic resonance scans should replace biopsies for the diagnosis of diffuse brain stem gliomas: a report from the Children's Cancer Group. Neurosurgery. 1993;33(6):1026–1029; discussion 1029.
11. Epstein F, Constantini S. Practical decisions in the treatment of pediatric brain stem tumors. Pediatr Neurosurg. 1996;24(1):24–34.
12. Cartmill M, Punt J. Diffuse brain stem glioma. A review of stereotactic biopsies. Childs Nerv Syst. 1999;15(5):235–237; discussion 238.
13. Albright AL. Diffuse brainstem tumors: when is a biopsy necessary? Pediatr Neurosurg. 1996;24(5):252–255.
14. Packer RJ, Boyett JM, Zimmerman RA, et al. Outcome of children with brain stem gliomas after treatment with 7800 cGy of hyperfractionated radiotherapy. A Childrens Cancer Group Phase I/II Trial. Cancer. 1994;74(6):1827–1834.
15. Packer RJ, Boyett JM, Zimmerman RA, et al. Hyperfractionated radiation therapy (72 Gy) for children with brain stem gliomas. A Childrens Cancer Group Phase I/II Trial. Cancer. 1993;72(4):1414–1421.
16. Halperin EC, Wehn SM, Scott JW, Djang W, Oakes WJ, Friedman HS. Selection of a management strategy for pediatric brainstem tumors. Med Pediatr Oncol. 1989;17(2):117–126.
17. Freeman CR, Suissa S. Brain stem tumors in children: results of a survey of 62 patients treated with radiotherapy. Int J Radiat Oncol Biol Phys. 1986;12(10):1823–1828.
18. Langmoen IA, Lundar T, Storm-Mathisen I, Lie SO, Hovind KH. Management of pediatric pontine gliomas. Childs Nerv Syst. 1991;7(1):13–15.
19. Freeman CR, Krischer JP, Sanford RA, et al. Final results of a study of escalating doses of hyperfractionated radiotherapy in brain stem tumors in children: a Pediatric Oncology Group study. Int J Radiat Oncol Biol Phys. 1993;27(2):197–206.
20. Mandell LR, Kadota R, Freeman C, et al. There is no role for hyperfractionated radiotherapy in the management of children with newly diagnosed diffuse intrinsic brainstem tumors: results of a Pediatric Oncology Group phase III trial comparing conventional vs. hyperfractionated radiotherapy. Int J Radiat Oncol Biol Phys. 1999;43(5):959–964.
21. Sanghavi SN, Needle MN, Krailo MD, Geyer JR, Ater J, Mehta MP. A phase I study of topotecan as a radiosensitizer for brainstem glioma of childhood: first report of the Children's Cancer Group-0952. Neuro-oncology. 2003;5(1):8–13.
22. Bernier-Chastagner V, Grill J, Doz F, et al. Topotecan as a radiosensitizer in the treatment of children with malignant diffuse brainstem gliomas: results of a French Society of Paediatric Oncology Phase II Study. Cancer. 2005;104(12):2792–2797.
23. Walker DA, Punt JA, Sokal M. Clinical management of brain stem glioma. Arch Dis Child. 1999;80(6):558–564.
24. Jennings MT, Sposto R, Boyett JM, et al. Preradiation chemotherapy in primary high-risk brainstem tumors: phase II study CCG-9941 of the Children's Cancer Group. J Clin Oncol. 2002;20(16):3431–3437.
25. Freeman CR, Kepner J, Kun LE, et al. A detrimental effect of a combined chemotherapy-radiotherapy approach in children with diffuse intrinsic brain stem gliomas? Int J Radiat Oncol Biol Phys. 2000;47(3):561–564.
26. Finlay JL. The role of high-dose chemotherapy and stem cell rescue in the treatment of malignant brain tumors. Bone Marrow Transplant. 1996;18(suppl 3):S1-S5.
27. Dunkel IJ, O'Malley B, Finlay JL. Is there a role for high-dose chemotherapy with stem cell rescue for brain stem tumors of childhood? Pediatr Neurosurg. 1996;24(5):263–266.
28. Bouffet E, Raquin M, Doz F, et al. Radiotherapy followed by high dose busulfan and thiotepa: a prospective assessment of high dose chemotherapy in children with diffuse pontine gliomas. Cancer. 2000;88(3):685–692.
29. Wagner S, Warmuth-Metz M, Emser A, et al. Treatment options in childhood pontine gliomas. J Neurooncol. 2006;79(3):281–287.
30. Fischbein NJ, Prados MD, Wara W, Russo C, Edwards MS, Barkovich AJ. Radiologic classification of brain stem tumors: correlation of magnetic resonance imaging appearance with clinical outcome. Pediatr Neurosurg. 1996;24(1):9–23.
31. Broniscer A, Gururangan S, MacDonald TJ, et al. Phase I trial of single-dose temozolomide and continuous administration of o6-benzylguanine in children with brain tumors: a pediatric brain tumor consortium report. Clin Cancer Res. 2007;13(22 pt 1):6712–6718.
32. Couldwell WT, Hinton DR, Surnock AA, et al. Treatment of recurrent malignant gliomas with chronic oral high-dose tamoxifen. Clin Cancer Res. 1996;2(4):619–622.
33. Broniscer A, Leite CC, Lanchote VL, Machado TM, Cristófani LM. Radiation therapy and high-dose tamoxifen in the treatment of patients with diffuse brainstem gliomas: results of a Brazilian cooperative study. Brainstem Glioma Cooperative Group. J Clin Oncol. 2000;18(6):1246–1253.
34. Broniscer A, Iacono L, Chintagumpala M, et al. Role of temozolomide after radiotherapy for newly diagnosed diffuse brainstem glioma in children: results of a multiinstitutional study (SJHG-98). Cancer. 2005;103(1):133–139.
35. Hargrave D, Bartels U, Bouffet E. Diffuse brainstem glioma in children: critical review of clinical trials. Lancet Oncol. 2006;7(3):241–248.
36. Daw NC, Furman WL, Stewart CF, et al. Phase I and pharmacokinetic study of gefitinib in children with refractory solid tumors: a Children's Oncology Group Study. J Clin Oncol. 2005;23(25):6172–6180.
37. Freeman BB 3rd, Daw NC, Geyer JR, Furman WL, Stewart CF. Evaluation of gefitinib for treatment of refractory solid tumors and central nervous system malignancies in pediatric patients. Cancer Invest. 2006;24(3):310–317.
38. Broniscer A, Laningham FH, Kocak M, et al. Intratumoral hemorrhage among children with newly diagnosed, diffuse brainstem glioma. Cancer. 2006;106(6):1364–1371.
39. Folkins C, Man S, Xu P, Shaked Y, Hicklin DJ, Kerbel RS. Anticancer therapies combining antiangiogenic and tumor cell cytotoxic effects reduce the tumor stem-like cell fraction in glioma xenograft tumors. Cancer Res. 2007;67(8):3560–3564.
40. Vredenburgh JJ, Desjardins A, Herndon JE 2nd, et al. Phase II trial of bevacizumab and irinotecan in recurrent malignant glioma. Clin Cancer Res. 2007;13(4):1253–1259.
41. Packer RJ, Krailo M, Mehta M, et al. A Phase I study of concurrent RMP-7 and carboplatin with radiation therapy for children with newly diagnosed brainstem gliomas. Cancer. 2005;104(9):1968–1974.
42. Khatib ZA, Heideman RL, Kovnar EH, et al. Predominance of pilocytic histology in dorsally exophytic brain stem tumors. Pediatr Neurosurg. 1994;20(1):2–10.
43. Bowers DC, Krause TP, Aronson LJ, et al. Second surgery for recurrent pilocytic astrocytoma in children. Pediatr Neurosurg. 2001;34(5):229–234.
44. Pollack IF, Hoffman HJ, Humphreys RP, Becker L. The long-term outcome after surgical treatment of dorsally exophytic brain-stem gliomas. J Neurosurg. 1993;78(6):859–863.
45. Young Poussaint T, Yousuf N, Barnes PD, et al. Cervicomedullary astrocytomas of childhood: clinical and imaging follow-up. Pediatr Radiol. 1999;29(9):662–668.
46. Gilles FH, Sobel EL, Leviton A, et al. Temporal trends among childhood brain tumor biopsies. The Childhood Brain Tumor Consortium. J Neurooncol. 1992;13(2):137–149.
47. Epstein F, Wisoff J. Intra-axial tumors of the cervicomedullary junction. J Neurosurg. 1987;67(4):483–487.
48. Fisher PG, Breiter SN, Carson BS, et al. A clinicopathologic reappraisal of brain stem tumor classification. Identification of pilocystic astrocytoma and fibrillary astrocytoma as distinct entities. Cancer. 2000;89(7):1569–1576.

49. Weiner HL, Freed D, Woo HH, Rezai AR, Kim R, Epstein FJ. Intra-axial tumors of the cervicomedullary junction: surgical results and long-term outcome. *Pediatr Neurosurg.* 1997;27(1):12–18.
50. Abbott R, Shiminski-Maher T, Wisoff JH, Epstein FJ. Intrinsic tumors of the medulla: surgical complications. *Pediatr Neurosurg.* 1991;17(5):239–244.
51. Abbott R, Shiminski-Maher T, Epstein FJ. Intrinsic tumors of the medulla: predicting *outcome* after surgery. *Pediatr Neurosurg.* 1996;25(1):41–44.
52. Stark AM, Fritsch MJ, Claviez A, Dörner L, Mehdorn HM. Management of tectal glioma in childhood. *Pediatr Neurol.* 2005;33(1):33–38.
53. Yeh DD, Warnick RE, Ernst RJ. Management strategy for adult patients with dorsal midbrain gliomas. *Neurosurgery.* 2002;50(4):735–738; discussion 738.
54. Oka K, Kin Y, Go Y, et al. Neuroendoscopic approach to tectal tumors: a consecutive series. *J Neurosurg.* 1999;91(6):964–970.
55. Grant GA, Avellino AM, Loeser JD, Ellenbogen RG, Berger MS, Roberts TS. Management of intrinsic gliomas of the tectal plate in children. A ten-year review. *Pediatr Neurosurg.* 1999;31(4):170–176.
56. Pollack IF, Pang D, Albright AL. The long-term outcome in children with late-onset aqueductal stenosis resulting from benign intrinsic tectal tumors. *J Neurosurg.* 1994;80(4):681–688.
57. May PL, Blaser SI, Hoffman HJ, Humphreys RP, Harwood-Nash DC. Benign *intrinsic* tectal "tumors" in children. *J Neurosurg.* 1991;74(6):867–871.
58. Ternier J, Wray A, Puget S, Bodaert N, Zerah M, Sainte-Rose C. Tectal plate lesions in children. *J Neurosurg.* 2006;104(6 suppl):369–376.
59. Ramina R, Coelho Neto M, Fernandes YB, Borges G, Honorato DC, Arruda WO. Intrinsic tectal low grade astrocytomas: is surgical removal an alternative treatment? Long-term outcome of eight cases. *Arq Neuropsiquiatr.* 2005;63(1):40–45.
60. Hamilton MG, Lauryssen C, Hagen N. Focal midbrain glioma: long term survival in a cohort of 16 patients and the implications for management. *Can J Neurol Sci.* 1996;23(3):204–207.
61. Bowers DC, Georgiades C, Aronson LJ, et al. Tectal gliomas: natural history of an indolent lesion in pediatric patients. *Pediatr Neurosurg.* 2000;32(1):24–29.
62. Squires LA, Allen JC, Abbott R, Epstein FJ. Focal tectal tumors: management and prognosis. *Neurology.* 1994;44(5):953–956.
63. Listernick R, Charrow J, Greenwald M, Mets M. Natural history of optic pathway tumors in children with neurofibromatosis type 1: a longitudinal study. *J Pediatr.* 1994;125(1):63–66.
64. Sevick RJ, Barkovich AJ, Edwards MS, Koch T, Berg B, Lempert T. Evolution of white matter lesions in neurofibromatosis type 1: MR findings. *AJR Am J Roentgenol.* 1992;159(1):171–175.
65. Bognanno JR, Edwards MK, Lee TA, Dunn DW, Roos KL, Klatte EC. Cranial MR imaging in neurofibromatosis. *AJR Am J Roentgenol.* 1988;151(2):381–388.
66. Ullrich NJ, Raja AI, Irons MB, Kieran MW, Goumnerova L. Brainstem lesions in *neurofibromatosis* type 1. *Neurosurgery.* 2007;61(4):762–766; discussion 766.
67. Guillamo JS, Créange A, Kalifa C, et al. Prognostic factors of CNS tumours in *Neurofibromatosis* 1 (NF1): a retrospective study of 104 patients. *Brain.* 2003;126(Pt 1):152–160.
68. Pollack IF, Shultz B, Mulvihill JJ. The management of brainstem gliomas in patients with *neurofibromatosis* 1. *Neurology.* 1996;46(6):1652–1660.
69. Landolfi JC, Thaler HT, DeAngelis LM. Adult brainstem gliomas. *Neurology.* 1998;51(4):1136–1139.
70. Selvapandian S, Rajshekhar V, Chandy MJ. Brainstem glioma: comparative study of clinico-radiological presentation, pathology and outcome in children and adults. *Acta Neurochir (Wien).* 1999;141(7):721–726; discussion 726.
71. Guillamo JS, Monjour A, Taillandier L, et al. Brainstem gliomas in adults: prognostic factors and classification. *Brain.* 2001;124(pt 12):2528–2539.

68 Chemotherapy for Tumors of the Skull Base and Cranial Nerves

Jennifer L. Clarke and Andrew B. Lassman

INTRODUCTION

Several tumor types can affect the skull base or cranial nerves (Table 68.1). Skull base tumors present with a variety of neurologic complaints depending on the structures affected, including epistaxis, headache, diplopia, dysarthria, proptosis, hearing loss, facial weakness and/or numbness, anosmia, and essentially any other symptom arising from cranial nerve compression. In addition, such tumors can affect the cavernous sinus, compressing the cavernous carotid artery leading to cerebral infarction as a complication.

Metastases are probably the most common, as any primary malignancy that commonly spreads to bone can also spread to skull base. Meningiomas, schwannomas, and pituitary tumors are the most common primary tumors, and they are described in separate chapters. The remaining primary tumors are rare, with only limited data to guide therapy. Surgery and/or radiation therapy is typically the first-line treatment for these tumors. This chapter will focus on chemotherapy for this diverse group of tumors. As data are limited for primary skull base tumors, regimens are often borrowed from the sarcoma or head and neck cancer literature based on the histological overlap. Chemotherapeutics with reported efficacy in tumors of the skull base/peripheral nerves are shown in Table 68.2.

Table 68.1 Tumors Arising In or Affecting the Cranial Nerves and Skull Base

Metastases
Acoustic neuroma/schwannoma
Neurofibroma
Malignant peripheral nerve sheath tumor
   Meningioma[a]
   Pituitary tumors[b]
Chordoma
   Chondrosarcoma
   Other sarcomas
   Paraganglioma
   Esthesioneuroblastoma
   Other sinus tumors
   Malignant salivary gland tumors
   Epidermoid cyst

[a] See Chapters 10, 18, 66, 93.
[b] See Chapters 20, 34, 69, 96.

Table 68.2 Chemotherapeutics With Reported Efficacy

Tumor Type	Chemotherapeutics With Reported Efficacy
Chordoma	9-Nitro-camptothecin [1]
	Vincristine [2]
	Etoposide, cisplatin, vincristine, dacarbazine, cyclophosphamide, and doxorubicin [3]
	Ifosfamide [3]
	Isotretinoin and interferon [4]
	Thalidomide ± liposomal doxorubicin [4]
	Imatinib [5–9]
	Cetuximab, gefitinib [10]
	Razoxane (radiation sensitizer) [11]
Chondrosarcoma	Temozolomide [12]
	Ifosfamide, doxorubicin [13]
	Cisplatin, adriamycin [14]
	Razoxane (radiation sensitizer) [11]
Paraganglioma	Gemcitabine [15]
	Dacarbazine, fluorouracil [16]
	Temozolomide ± thalidomide [17,18]
	Carboplatin [19,20]
	Paclitaxel [21]
	Cyclophosphamide, doxorubicin and dacarbazine (CyADIC) ± vincristine (CyVADIC) [22–24]
	Cyclophosphamide, vincristine, dacarbazine [25–27]
	[131I]-MIBG [28–30]
	Octreotide [31]
Esthesioneuroblastoma	Etoposide, cisplatin [32]
	Platinum based regimen [33–36]
	Cyclophosphamaide based regimen [37–39]
	Cyclophosphamide, vincristine alternating with cisplatin, etoposide [40]
	Various [41]
	High-dose chemotherapy followed by stem cell rescue [42,43]
CNS metastases from esthesioneuroblastoma	Carboplatin, CCNU, vincristine [44,45]
	Intracavitary BCNU wafer [46]
	Temozolomide [47]
CNS metastases (leptomeningeal) from esthesioneuroblastoma	Intrathecal methotrexate, cytosine arabinoside, or thiotepa [44,45,48]
MPST	Cyclophosphamide, vincristine, doxorubicin, and imidazole carboxamide [49]
	Vincristine and cyclophosphamide [50]
	Ifosfamide, vincristine, and doxorubicin [51,52]
	Vincristine and doxorubicin [53]

CHORDOMA

Approximately 35% of chordomas occur in the clivus with the remainder in the sacrum or other vertebrae. The cell of origin is likely notochord, which may explain the most frequently affected sites (midline, axial skeleton). They are very uncommon tumors, and Surveillance Epidemiology and End Results (SEER) data from 1973 to 1975 among 400 cases across multiple locations demonstrates an age-adjusted incidence of 0.08 per 100,000 [54]. However, among all primary malignant tumors of bone, they are reported to account for up to 20% depending on the series and method of collection [55–59].

Patients with clival disease are typically younger than those with sacral disease, with a median age of 49 and 69, respectively, at presentation in the SEER data set [54]. Clival tumors occur in men and women at approximately equal rates, which differs from the male predominance seen when all tumors are grouped regardless of location [54]. Median survival in one study was 6.94 years, slightly longer for women (7.70 years) than men (6.42 years) [54].

Despite their benign appearance histologically, chordomas do metastasize to other organs, including liver, lung, and bone [60]. They also destroy bone during their relentless growth. They are generally chemoresistant. Surgery and radiation remain the mainstays of treatment although relentless local recurrence and, less often, metastasis remain the primary causes of death in this patient population. Most attempts at chemotherapy have been unsuccessful, but there are scattered anecdotes of success (Table 68.2).

Cytotoxic Chemotherapy

One phase II trial from the University of Michigan tested 9-nitro-camptothecin for advanced chordoma or soft-tissue sarcoma [1]. Among 15 patients with chordoma (of which four were clival), there was one partial response in a patient with metastases in the cerebellum and dura. Response continued until the patient discontinued therapy after 251 days because of toxicity. Overall, median time-to-progression for all chordomas was 9.9 weeks (range 4–36) and 6-month progression-free survival (PFS) was 33%.

Other agents with reported efficacy include vincristine [2]; a six-drug regimen combining etoposide, cisplatin, vincristine, dacarbazine, cyclophosphamide, and doxorubicin [3]; and ifosfamide [3]. All of these, however, are associated with substantial toxicity. One report described prolonged disease stabilization (1 year) associated with isotretinoin and interferon combination therapy, followed by radiation and then thalidomide, again with stabilization for a year [4].

Molecularly Targeted Agents

The most promising advance in medical treatment of chordoma has been the use of the platelet-derived growth factor receptor (PDGFR) and KIT inhibitor, imatinib. In a small series of six patients, all tumors exhibited PDGF-B ligand expression by RT-PCR, and the receptor (PDGFRB) was phosphorylated in four [5]. A follow-up study confirmed the molecular finding of PDGF signaling abnormalities in essentially all tumors, suggesting autocrine signaling through PDGFRB as well as less robust but clear abnormalities of PDGFRA and KIT [61]. Similar findings regarding PDGFR autocrine signaling were reported by others [62].

Partly based on the molecular data, imatinib 800 mg/day was administered to six patients with chordoma and induced responses or at least some benefit in all of them [5]. A follow-up report on these and 12 others demonstrated improvements in magnetic resonance imaging (MRI) and/or positron emission tomography (PET) (similar to gastrointestinal stromal tumor, or at least subjective improvement in the majority of patients, and relatively long PFS intervals (>1 year in surviving patients) [6]. These retrospective results led to a phase II multicenter prospective clinical trial in Europe [7]. The trial enrolled 55 patients, 15% with skull base disease, treated with imatinib 800 mg/day. All tumors expressed the imatinib target PDGFRB or its ligand PDGFB. There were 73% and 38% with stable disease or better at 6 months and 12 months, respectively, among 44 evaluable patients. Median PFS was 32 weeks, and 16% remained on therapy after 18 months. In addition, among six patients who progressed while on imatinib, cisplatin 25 mg/m^2/week was added and the imatinib dose reduced to 400 mg/day during combination therapy. PET responses were seen in four with subjective improvement and stable disease on CT/MRI, suggesting drug synergy [8].

Abnormalities of other receptor tyrosine kinases have also been reported. In a series of 17 chordomas, 10 primary tumors had sufficient tissue for immunohistochemical analysis [63]. There was a range of expression of HER2/neu (Erb-b2) from none (3), mild (1), moderate (2), and strong (4). Neither of two recurrent chordomas expressed HER2/neu. MET was expressed more consistently, with 7 of 10 primary and both recurrent tumors strongly staining; MET overexpression may be linked to gain at chromosome 7q amplification observed in 70% of chordomas in one series [64]. Epidermal growth factor receptor (EGFR) (Erb-b1/EGFR/HER1) was also expressed in all tumors, with strong staining in five of 10 primary chordomas and one of two recurrences. MET and EGFR expression appeared to correlate. One patient with an EGFR expressing chordoma metastatic to lung and lymph nodes was treated with a combination of EGFR inhibitors cetuximab 250 mg/m^2 weekly and gefitinib 250 mg daily [10]. The patient had a partial response that had persisted for 9 months as of the time of the report.

At this time, no prospective data exist from a trial involving EGFR-directed therapy, and it is not known whether other EGFR inhibitors, such as erlotinib or lapatinib, are effective. It is also not known how imatinib would compare with EGFR-directed therapies or with other PDGFR inhibitors such as dasatinib. It is also not known whether the combination of imatinib with a cytotoxic chemotherapy, such as cisplatin, is superior to imatinib alone although that is suggested by the efficacy of combination therapy in disease resistant to imatinib monotherapy. The low number of patients treated and the preliminary nature of the data make further conclusions difficult.

Radiation Sensitizers

As radiation is the mainstay of therapy, there have been efforts to combine radiation with other agents. A small study has been done looking at razoxane as a radiation sensitizer for chordoma and other tumors with intriguing results [11]. For example, among five chordomas treated with razoxane during radiotherapy, all had durable local control (≥5 years). However, without a control group it is difficult to compare this finding to other options including radiation alone.

CHONDROSARCOMA

Chondrosarcoma is presumedly derived from a mesenchymal/cartilaginous cell of origin. It is a relatively common tumor of bone, accounting for 11% to 26% of primary bone tumors depending on the series [58,65]. However, the skull base is a very unusual primary location, with chondrosarcomas accounting for only 0.1% of all head and neck cancers in the American College of Surgeons' National Cancer Data Base [65]. The rarity makes it difficult to comment accurately on true incidence. One clinical series of 14 cases suggested they are far more common in men (3.7:1), and they occur typically in younger patients than those with chordomas with the median age of 41 at diagnosis [66]. However, other studies suggested that the conventional histologic subtype, which comprise essentially all chondrosarcomas that occur in the skull base [67], occur slightly more commonly in women [68,69].

Most occur in the clivus [69]. Although chondrosarcomas are associated with several genetic syndromes, the majority are sporadic [68,69]. Survival is probably longer than for patients with skull base chordomas, with 5- and 10-year survival exceeding 90%. However, low numbers make comparisons statistically difficult [66]. Nonetheless, others have also made the same observation [69], lending it credence and emphasizing the importance of accurate histologic diagnosis.

Cytotoxic Chemotherapy

Surgery and radiation therapy again remain the mainstays of treatment although in many cases surgical control can be achieved without the need for radiation. There are scattered reports of responses to various chemotherapy regimens; one patient, for example, responded to 12 cycles of temozolomide [12]. However, a second patient who received temozolomide (albeit at a lower dose) as part of a phase II clinical trial progressed after two cycles [70]. Another report describes treatment of a woman with ifosfamide and doxorubicin with good response; she received five cycles and has remained without evidence of disease for more than 4 years [13]. There is also a report of a child treated with cisplatin and adriamycin for six cycles with response lasting at least 1 year [14].

Molecularly Targeted Agents

To date, molecularly targeted agents have not been evaluated in the treatment of skull base chondrosarcomas. However, there are reports of PDGFR and KIT abnormalities, as in chordomas [71], leading to consideration of treatment with PDGFR inhibitors such as imatinib or dasatinib.

Radiation sensitizers

Thirteen chondrosarcoma patients were treated in the study evaluating razoxane as described above. An objective response radiographically was seen in 75%, and the median duration of response was 22 months [11]. Of note, however, none of these patients had skull base disease.

PARAGANGLIOMA

Paraganglioma are rare neuroendocrine tumors in parasympathetic autonomic ganglia that likely arise from the chromaffin cells of the adrenal medulla (where they are called pheochromocytoma) or extra-adrenal paraganglionic sites. Whether they occur in the glomus jugulare, glomus vagale, glomus tympanicum, or the carotid body, they can involve the skull base. They can also extend intracranially to involve the clivus and compress brainstem or associated cranial nerves. Distinct from other tumors that become symptomatic mainly through local compression of critical neurologic structures, paragangliomas also rarely secrete catecholamines causing the cardiovascular symptoms typically associated with pheochromocytomas. Pathologic classification of these tumors has undergone revisions, and currently they are designated "neuroendocrine tumors" [67]. Tumors that initiate in the skull base typically involve middle ear structures (chemodectomas) and are in fact a common tumor of the middle ear [72]. In contrast with paragangliomas at other sites, glomus tumors are far more common in women than men, with median age of onset during middle age but with a wide range [72,73]. About 10% of patients have multiple lesions [73,74], and multiplicity is a particular feature among familial cases in which the incidence may reach 50% [73].

Paragangliomas are generally curable if gross total resection is possible although there are exceptions and they occasionally are aggressive and even metastasize [72,73,75]. Standard treatment is surgical, with radiation used as a second-line treatment. Chemotherapy may be used in recurrent or metastatic disease. Although no prospective trials have been reported specifically in paragangliomas, there are a few reports of advanced neuroendocrine tumors that may be applicable.

Cytotoxic Chemotherapy

A small trial tested gemcitabine monotherapy in 18 patients, 2 of whom had pheochromocytoma [15]. Median time on study was 3 months, with 75% of patients taken off treatment for progression of disease. Others have also reported that gemcitabine may have activity [76]. A second phase II trial evaluated the combination of dacarbazine and fluorouracil in 18 patients with advanced neuroendocrine tumors [16]. One half of the patients had carcinoid tumors; of those, only one responded objectively to treatment. Of the other half, those with noncarcinoid tumors, four had an objective response.

Another phase II trial evaluated temozolomide and thalidomide in combination in 29 patients, 3 of whom were pheochromocytomas or paragangliomas; 1 of the 3 had a response [17]. Temozolomide monotherapy was retrospectively analyzed in a group of 36 patients with advanced neuroendocrine tumors, one of which was a paraganglioma [18]. There were 10 partial responses although the patient with paraganglioma was not among them. Analysis for the DNA repair enzyme O^6-methylguanine-DNA methyhransferase (MGMT) was performed on a subset of tumors because MGMT promoter methylation may predict temozolomide efficacy in gliomas [77]. There was no clear correlation between MGMT immunoreactivity and response to treatment. However, immunohistochemistry is not the ideal method for assessing MGMT status [78].

There are reports of successful use of carboplatin [19,20] or paclitaxel [21] for paragangliomas. The combination of cyclophosphamide, doxorubicin, and dacarbazine, known as CyADIC, was administered to seven patients with paraganglioma; multiple partial responses were seen [22]. An additional paraganglioma case has also been reported, with good response [23]. The addition of vincristine to this combination (thus called CyVADIC) was administered to four patients in the same series [22] as well as in another case [24], with two of five total patients having objective responses and the other three demonstrating stable disease. Combination therapy with cyclophosphamide, vincristine, and dacarbazine (e.g., CyVADIC without the doxorubicin) has also been described in several case reports of pheochromocytoma [25–27].

Radioisotope Treatment

Adrenergic tissue typically takes up metaiodobenzylguanidine (MIBG), a molecule that resembles norepinephrine. It can be labeled with radioactive iodine to make [^{131}I]-MIBG, which can be used both in low doses for diagnostic purposes and in high doses for therapeutic purposes [28]. Five patients with malignant pheochromocytoma were with therapeutic intent, two of whom had clear objective response both anatomically and functionally (lower level of hormone secretion), whereas the other three remained stable.

[^{131}I]-MIBG has also been used in combination with chemotherapy although it is not well tolerated [29]. Very high-dose treatment with [^{131}I]-MIBG is also feasible although it is not clear that additional clinical benefit is gained over standard treatment doses [30]. Radioactive forms of the somatostatin analog, octreotide, can also be used for diagnostic scanning, taking advantage of somatostatin receptors on paragangliomas [79]. Therapeutic purposes have also been reported [31].

Molecularly Targeted Agents

One study suggests that RAF inhibitors inhibit pheochromocytoma cell growth in vitro [80]. Also of interest, lithium chloride inhibits growth of pheochromocytoma cells in vitro. The basis of this latter observation is presumably inhibition of glycogen synthase kinase 3 beta which, when active, may promote tumor growth [81]. These studies suggest that RAF and GSK3beta inhibitors may represent novel therapeutic strategies for pheochromocytomas and for paragangliomas by extension. However, human data are lacking.

ESTHESIONEUROBLASTOMA

Esthesioneuroblastoma, or olfactory neuroblastoma, is a rare neoplasm likely arising from the olfactory neuroepithelium [82,83], comprising 3% of nasal/paransal sinus tumors [84]. However, diagnostic difficulty and nomenclature controversies may lead to underreporting [85]. It is also important to note that esthesioneuroblastoma is not a member of the PNET class of tumors, a conclusion supported by the different immunohistochemical staining [86] and chromosomal alterations observed in the two entities [87].

There may be a very slight male predominance among patients with esthesioneuroblastoma [84,85]. There is a bimodal pattern of incidence peaks, in the 2nd to 3rd and 5th to 6th decades [84,88,89], although it varies widely with reports in the elderly as well as in children as young as 18 months [84]. Five-year survival rates of 45% to 81% have been reported in large series [82–85]. However, reports at the lower end of that range likely suffer from inclusion of patients with histologically similar but more aggressive tumor types, such that 70% may be a more accurate figure [83]. Nonetheless, the behavior of the disease can be extraordinarily heterogeneous, with some patients succumbing very rapidly and others remaining disease-free for more than 10 years. It should be noted that recurrences are observed following a prolonged period of quiescence, 10 years or more [82,83], requiring life-long vigilance. In contrast with other skull base tumors, esthesioneuroblastoma typically presents with symptoms referable to the nasal location, such as anosmia, epistaxis, or obstruction, rather than cranial neuropathies or other neurologic symptoms unless brain and/or leptomeningeal spread has occurred.

Staging is often performed according to the Kadish system [90] although other systems have been proposed as reviewed elsewhere [83,85,91,92]. Kadish stage A is confined to the nasal cavity, stage B extends into the paranasal sinus, and stage C extends beyond that, including involvement of the cribriform plate, the base of the skull, the orbit, or intracranially.

The first report of chemotherapy for esthesioneuroblastoma involved nitrogen mustard in combination with radiation for intrathoracic metastatic disease [93]. Since then, many newer agents have been developed although mustard derivatives such as lomustine (CCNU) and carmustine (BCNU) remain in use. There have been a number of different regimens with reported activity, and no paradigm is widely accepted as standard.

Cytotoxic chemotherapy

Kadish stage A or B disease is typically treated with surgery and postoperative radiation. In Kadish stage C disease, some advocate for the addition of chemotherapy, either in the neoadjuvant setting [33,94] or postradiation [37], while others reserve chemotherapy for salvage treatment [91,95]. Another approach focuses on grade rather than extent-of-disease, arguing for the addition of chemotherapy to the treatment of all high-grade tumors [41]. Different centers also employ different regimens, with successful therapy reported using cyclophosphamide, vincristine, and cisplatin, or cisplatin and etoposide [83].

Because of its rarity, reports are almost always retrospective in nature. One prospective trial enrolled 19 patients with neuroendocrine tumors of the sinonasal tract (10 patients with pure esthesioneuroblastoma and 9 with neuroendocrine carcinoma/mixed tumor) [32]. Following diagnostic resection or biopsy, all patients received two cycles of etoposide and cisplatin. If there was a response or if the tumor remained unresectable, they underwent a course of combined photon/proton radiation followed by two additional cycles of etoposide and cisplatin. If response was poor and the tumor appeared resectable, they underwent craniofacial resection followed by combined radiation and two additional cycles of chemotherapy as above. There were 13 responses (3 CR, 10 PR), five patients with stable disease, and one patient with progressive disease. Overall survival was 74% at 5 years. No difference in response was noted by histological type.

Platinum-based regimens, either in the recurrent setting [34] or up-front [33,35,36], and cyclophosphamide-based regimens [38,39]. have been most commonly used. One report describes a response to cyclophosphamide and vincristine alternating with cisplatin and etoposide although tumor recurred within 6 months of discontinuing therapy [40].

Aggressive chemotherapy with stem cell support has been attempted with some success. Twelve patients in Tokyo, diagnosed via biopsy, received 2 cycles of cyclophosphamide, doxorubicin, and vincristine with continuous infusion cisplatin and etoposide with collection of stem cells after the first or second cycle, followed by radiation. If residual disease remained, they underwent surgical resection [96]. Responses were seen in 75%; of those, four underwent autologous peripheral blood stem cell transplant (PBSCT), all of whom ultimately achieved a CR. A second group reports on eight patients with recurrent disease, either esthesioneuroblastoma or sinonasal undifferentiated carcinoma, who underwent intensive chemotherapy followed by autologous bone marrow transplant [42]. Five of the 8 patients had esthesioneuroblastoma; one was alive with no evidence of disease, one was alive with residual disease, and the other three died of tumor progression. Intra-arterial chemotherapy has also been reported to have activity. Heros and Hochberg reported a case of multiple recurrent esthesioneuroblastoma, following resistance to cyclophosphamide-based intravenous chemotherapy, treated for two cycles with intra-arterial cisplatin plus intravenous 5-fluorocytosine with transient clinical improvement [48]. In the authors' view, the risks associated with intra-arterial chemotherapy are not warranted without more data, especially in light of other available options administered either orally or intravenously.

Esthesioneuroblastoma can also spread to the central nervous system (CNS), either as parenchymal or leptomeningeal metastases or both. A patient with CNS metastases treated with six cycles of intra-arterial BCNU plus intravenous vincristine and oral procarbazine remained in CR at 24 months posttreatment [97]. Nonetheless, as above, the authors view other options as more palatable. For example, intracranial metastases have been treated via a variety of strategies, including carboplatin/lomustine/vincristine given to 6 patients on a bimonthly basis: four patients achieved a PR and two had progressive disease [44,45]. Park et al [46] reported the successful treatment of a single patient with carmustine (BCNU) eluting wafers (Gliadel, used for high-grade gliomas) within the surgical resection cavity after previously failing cisplatin/etoposide. Wick et al [47] treated one patient with intracranial metastatic disease successfully with temozolomide for 20 cycles after failure of multiple prior chemotherapy regimens. In the author's experience, temozolomide was of benefit in one patient in the management of CNS metastases (Figure 68.1). Intrathecal methotrexate, cytosine arabinoside, and thiotepa have all reported activity in leptomeningeal metastases from esthesioneuroblastoma [44,45,48].

Although it is clear that chemotherapy has some utility in the treatment of esthesioneuroblastoma, particularly in the case of advanced stage and/or high-grade disease, the role, regimen, and timing remain unclear. Additional prospective studies and more standardized treatment regimens are needed.

MALIGNANT PERIPHERAL NERVE SHEATH TUMORS

Schwannomas, acoustic neuromas, neurofibromas, and other peripheral nerve sheath tumors are typically benign and require only surgical management. However, malignant peripheral nerve sheath tumors (MPNSTs) can occur, though most often arising from neurofibromas, although some directly from a nerve. Rare cases of malignant schwannoma have been reported in the literature, although in the 2007 WHO Classification of Tumors of

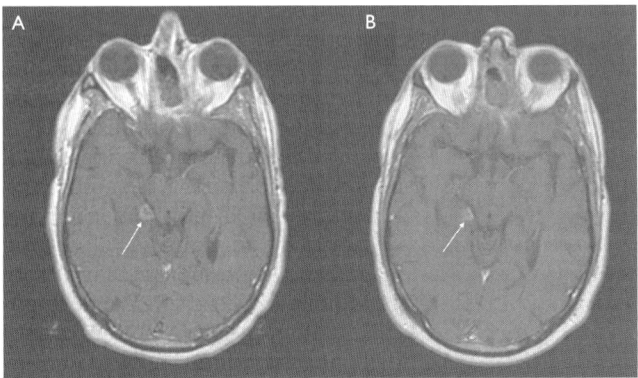

Figure 68.1 Metastasis (white arrow) from esthesioneuroblastoma before **(A)** and after **(B)** one cycle of temozolomide showing a minor response.

the CNS [98], the term malignant schwannoma is discouraged and these tumors are included under the category of MPNST. MPNSTs can occur anywhere in the body including in the skull base. There are a number of pathologic subtypes, and the interested reader is referred elsewhere for discussion [67].

There is a strong association with NF-1 in which approximately 5% of patients develop MPNSTs (compared with 0.001% in the general population) and patients are typically younger than those without NF-1 [99] over a wide age distribution. Analyzed another way, however, over one-half of patients with MPNSTs have NF-1 [98]. There is a slight female predominance (1.3:1) [99]. Radiation can be a predisposing factor but only after long latency. Complete surgical resection followed by radiation is the first-line treatment for focal MPNSTs. However, in the setting of either recurrence or metastatic disease, chemotherapy may be of use.

Cytotoxic chemotherapy

Little data regarding specific chemotherapy regimens are available; in general, regimens modeled after those used for sarcoma are advocated. Partly as a consequence, most reports do not distinguish presence or absence of skull base disease, and results discussed here include both settings. One report [49] describes two patients successfully treated with a combination of cyclophosphamide, vincristine, doxorubicin, and imidazole carboxamide [49]. Vincristine and cyclophosphamide were effective in another case [50] although follow-up was short. Ifosfamide, vincristine, and doxorubicin were partially effective in two other cases [51,52]. Vincristine and doxorubicin were tried in conjunction with radiation in another case report, with complete response for several months before distant metastases developed [53].

Interestingly, in the setting of bilateral (histologically benign) acoustic neuromas, chemotherapy was administered to a pair of patients in whom surgery was felt to present an unacceptable risk of deafness; a combination of cyclophosphamide, doxorubicin, and dacarbazine was used in both cases with stabilization of tumor size and progressive hearing loss [100].

Molecularly Targeted Agents

The association with NF-1 would suggest that drugs targeting RAS signaling may be of potential use but no such data yet exist. In addition, it is likely that alterations of p53 contribute as the "second hit" [101] to pathogenesis, but no therapeutic strategies have been reported to address it. PDGFR and KIT abnormalities were observed in a series of MPNSTs and corresponding plexiform neurofibromas [102]. Treatment of an MPNST cell line that also exhibited both types of abnormalities with imatinib inhibited cell growth and PDGFR phosphorylation [102]. Another series also suggested the presence of imatinib responsive PDGFR and KIT autocrine signaling and the presence of EGFR abnormalities in a subset of MPNSTs [103]. A subset of MPNSTs arising within neurofibromas also exhibited PDGF or PDGFR expression [104]. Whether treatment of patients with PDGFR or EGFR inhibitors would be helpful is unknown [9,43].

CONCLUSION

Tumors of the skull base and cranial nerves can be difficult to treat due to the difficulty of surgical resection, the significant morbidity that can be incurred due to the compression or invasion of critical structures, and the relative chemoresistance of many of the histological subtypes. However, the advent of new molecularly targeted agents holds out hope for more effective, better tolerated systemic treatments in the years to come. Multicenter clinical trials will continue to be an important method of evaluating novel therapies for these often rare tumors.

REFERENCES

1. Chugh R, Dunn R, Zalupski MM, et al. Phase II study of 9-nitro-camptothecin in patients with advanced chordoma or soft tissue sarcoma. *J Clin Oncol.* 2005;23:3597–3604.
2. Razis DV, Tsatsaronis A, Kyriazides I, Triantafyllou D. Chordoma of the cervical spine treated with vincristine sulfate. *J Med.* 1974;5:274–277.
3. Fleming GF, Heimann PS, Stephens JK, et al. Dedifferentiated chordoma. Response to aggressive chemotherapy in two cases. *Cancer.* 1993;72:714–718.
4. Schonegger K, Gelpi E, Prayer D, et al. Recurrent and metastatic clivus chordoma: systemic palliative therapy retards disease progression. *Anticancer Drugs.* 2005;16:1139–1143.
5. Casali PG, Messina A, Stacchiotti S, et al. Imatinib mesylate in chordoma. *Cancer.* 2004;101:2086–2097.
6. Casali PG, Stacchiotti SS, Messina AA, et al. Imatinib mesylate in 18 advanced chordoma patients [Abstract]. *J Clin Oncol, ASCO Ann Meeting Proc.* 2005;23.
7. Stacchiotti SS, Ferrari S, Ferraresi V, et al. Imatinib mesylate in advanced chordoma: a multicenter phase II study [Abstract]. *J Clin Oncol, ASCO Ann Meeting Proc Part I.* 2007;25.
8. Casali PG, Stacchiotti S, Sangalli C, Olmi P, Gronchi A. Chordoma. *Curr Opin Oncol.* 2007;19:367–370.
9. Casali PG, Stacchiotti SS, Grosso FF, et al. Adding cisplatin (CDDP) to imatinib (IM) re-establishes tumor response following secondary resistance to IM in advanced chordoma [Abstract]. *J Clin Oncol, ASCO Ann Meeting Proc Part I.* 2007;25.
10. Hof H, Welzel T, Debus J. Effectiveness of cetuximab/gefitinib in the therapy of a sacral chordoma. *Onkologie.* 2006;29:572–574.
11. Rhomberg W, Eiter H, Bohler F, Dertinger S. Combined radiotherapy and razoxane in the treatment of chondrosarcomas and chordomas. *Anticancer Res.* 2006;26:2407–2411.
12. Aksoy S, Abali H, Kilickap S, Guler N. Successful treatment of a chemoresistant tumor with temozolomide in an adult patient: report of a recurrent intracranial mesenchymal chondrosarcoma. *J Neurooncol.* 2005;71:333–334.
13. La Rocca RV, Morgan KW, Paris K, Baeker TR. Recurrent chondrosarcoma of the cranial base: a durable response to ifosfamide-doxorubicin chemotherapy. *J Neurooncol.* 1999;41:281–283.
14. Yoshimoto T, Sawamura Y, Ikeda J, Ishii N, Abe H. Successful chemoradiation therapy for high-grade skull base chondrosarcoma in a child. *Childs Nerv Syst.* 1995;11:250–253.
15. Kulke MH, Kim H, Clark JW, et al. A Phase II trial of gemcitabine for metastatic neuroendocrine tumors. *Cancer.* 2004;101:934–939.
16. Ollivier S, Fonck M, Becouarn Y, Brunet R. Dacarbazine, fluorouracil, and leucovorin in patients with advanced neuroendocrine tumors: a phase II trial. *Am J Clin Oncol.* 1998;21:237–240.
17. Kulke MH, Stuart K, Enzinger PC, et al. Phase II study of temozolomide and thalidomide in patients with metastatic neuroendocrine tumors. *J Clin Oncol.* 2006;24:401–406.

18. Ekeblad S, Sundin A, Janson ET, et al. Temozolomide as monotherapy is effective in treatment of advanced malignant neuroendocrine tumors. *Clin Cancer Res.* 2007;13:2986–2991.
19. Cairnduff F, Smith IE. Carboplatin chemotherapy for malignant paraganglioma. *Lancet.* 1986;2:982.
20. Jodrell DI, Smith IE. Carboplatin in the treatment of metastatic carcinoid tumours and paraganglioma: a phase II study. *Cancer Chemother Pharmacol.* 1990;26:62–64.
21. Kruijtzer CM, Beijnen JH, Swart M, Schellens JH. Successful treatment with paclitaxel of a patient with metastatic extra-adrenal pheochromocytoma (paraganglioma). A case report and review of the literature. *Cancer Chemother Pharmacol.* 2000;45:428–431.
22. Patel SR, Winchester DJ, Benjamin RS. A 15-year experience with chemotherapy of patients with paraganglioma. *Cancer.* 1995;76:1476–1480.
23. Argiris A, Mellott A, Spies S. PET scan assessment of chemotherapy response in metastatic paraganglioma. *Am J Clin Oncol.* 2003;26:563–566.
24. Nakane M, Takahashi S, Sekine I, et al. Successful treatment of malignant pheochromocytoma with combination chemotherapy containing anthracycline. *Ann Oncol.* 2003;14:1449–1451.
25. Siddiqui MZ, Von Eyben FE, Spanos G. High-voltage irradiation and combination chemotherapy for malignant pheochromocytoma. *Cancer.* 1988;62:686–690.
26. Senan S, Reed N, Connell J. Palliation of malignant phaeochromocytoma with combination chemotherapy. *Eur J Cancer.* 1992;28A:1006–1007.
27. Mertens WC, Grignon DJ, Romano W. Malignant paraganglioma with skeletal metastases and spinal cord compression: response and palliation with chemotherapy. *Clin Oncol (R Coll Radiol).* 1993;5:126–128.
28. Sisson JC, Shapiro B, Beierwaltes WH, et al. Radiopharmaceutical treatment of malignant pheochromocytoma. *J Nucl Med.* 1984;25:197–206.
29. Sisson JC, Shapiro B, Shulkin BL, Urba S, Zempel S, Spaulding S. Treatment of malignant pheochromocytomas with 131-I metaiodobenzylguanidine and chemotherapy. *Am J Clin Oncol.* 1999;22:364–370.
30. Rose B, Matthay KK, Price D, et al. High-dose 131I-metaiodobenzylguanidine therapy for 12 patients with malignant pheochromocytoma. *Cancer.* 2003;98:239–248.
31. Tonyukuk V, Emral R, Temizkan S, Sertcelik A, Erden I, Corapcioglu D. Case report: patient with multiple paragangliomas treated with long acting somatostatin analogue. *Endocr J.* 2003;50:507–513.
32. Fitzek MM, Thornton AF, Varvares M, et al. Neuroendocrine tumors of the sinonasal tract. Results of a prospective study incorporating chemotherapy, surgery, and combined proton-photon radiotherapy. *Cancer.* 2002;94:2623–2634.
33. Kim DW, Jo YH, Kim JH, et al. Neoadjuvant etoposide, ifosfamide, and cisplatin for the treatment of olfactory neuroblastoma. *Cancer.* 2004;101:2257–2260.
34. de Vos FY, Willemse PH, de Vries EG. Successful treatment of metastatic esthesioneuroblastoma. *Neth J Med.* 2003;61:414–416.
35. Eich HT, Hero B, Staar S, et al. Multimodality therapy including radiotherapy and chemotherapy improves event-free survival in stage C esthesioneuroblastoma. *Strahlenther Onkol.* 2003;179:233–240.
36. McLean JN, Nunley SR, Klass C, Moore C, Muller S, Johnstone PA. Combined modality therapy of esthesioneuroblastoma. *Otolaryngol Head Neck Surg.* 2007;136:998–1002.
37. Polin RS, Sheehan JP, Chenelle AG, et al. The role of preoperative adjuvant treatment in the management of esthesioneuroblastoma: the University of Virginia experience. *Neurosurgery.* 1998;42:1029–1037.
38. Wade PM Jr, Smith RE, Johns ME. Response of esthesioneuroblastoma to chemotherapy. Report of five cases and review of the literature. *Cancer.* 1984;53:1036–1041.
39. Newbill ET, Johns ME, Cantrell RW. Esthesioneuroblastoma: diagnosis and management. *South Med J.* 1985;78:275–282.
40. Goldsweig HG, Sundaresan N. Chemotherapy of recurrent esthesioneuroblastoma. Case report and review of the literature. *Am J Clin Oncol.* 1990;13:139–143.
41. McElroy EA Jr, Buckner JC, Lewis JE. Chemotherapy for advanced esthesioneuroblastoma: the Mayo clinic experience. *Neurosurgery.* 1998;42:1023–1027; discussion 7–8.
42. Stewart FM, Lazarus HM, Levine PA, Stewart KA, Tabbara IA, Spaulding CA. High-dose chemotherapy and autologous marrow transplantation for esthesioneuroblastoma and sinonasal undifferentiated carcinoma. *Am J Clin Oncol.* 1989;12:217–221.
43. Mishima K, Higashiyama S, Asai A, et al. Heparin-binding epidermal growth factor-like growth factor stimulates mitogenic signaling and is highly expressed in human malignant gliomas. *Acta Neuropathol (Berl).* 1998;96:322–328.
44. Chamberlain MC. Treatment of intracranial metastatic esthesioneuroblastoma. *Cancer.* 2002;95:243–248.
45. Chamberlain MC. Treatment of intracranial metastatic esthesioneuroblastoma. *J Clin Oncol.* 2002;20:357–358.
46. Park MC, Weaver CE Jr, Donahue JE, Sampath P. Intracavitary chemotherapy (Gliadel) for recurrent esthesioneuroblastoma: case report and review of the literature. *J Neurooncol.* 2006;77:47–51.
47. Wick W, Wick A, Kuker W, Dichgans J, Weller M. Intracranial metastatic esthesioneuroblastoma responsive to temozolomide. *J Neurooncol.* 2004;70:73–75.
48. Heros DO, Hochberg FH. Treatment of esthesioneuroblastoma with chemotherapy: a report of two cases. *J Neurooncol.* 1988;6:141–145.
49. Goldman RL, Jones SE, Heusinkveld RS. Combination chemotherapy of metastatic malignant schwannoma with vincristine, adriamycin, cyclophosphamide, and imidazole carboxamide: a case report. *Cancer.* 1977;39:1955–1958.
50. Valdes OS, Maurer HM. Combination therapy with vincristine sulfate (NSC-67574) and cyclophosphamide (NSC-26271) for generalized malignant schwannoma—a case report. *Cancer Chemother Rep.* 1970;54:65–68.
51. Athow AC, Kirkham N. Malignant parotid salivary gland peripheral nerve sheath tumour in a twelve-year-old girl. *J Laryngol Otol.* 1992;106:748–750.
52. Gallo A, Suriano M, Simonelli M, Ralli G, de Vincentiis M. Recurrent malignant schwannoma of the parapharyngeal space in neurofibromatosis type 1. *Ear Nose Throat J.* 2003;82:862–865.
53. Bruckner HW, Gorbaty M, Lipsztein R, Kranjac G, Lebwohl MG. Treatment of a large high-grade neurofibrosarcoma with concomitant vinblastine, doxorubicin, and radiotherapy. *Mt Sinai J Med.* 1992;59:429–432.
54. McMaster ML, Goldstein AM, Bromley CM, Ishibe N, Parry DM. Chordoma: incidence and survival patterns in the United States, 1973–1995. *Cancer Causes Control.* 2001;12:1–11.
55. Paavolainen P, Teppo L. Chordoma in Finland. *Acta Orthop Scand.* 1976;47:46–51.
56. Eriksson B, Gunterberg B, Kindblom LG. Chordoma. A clinicopathologic and prognostic study of a Swedish national series. *Acta Orthop Scand.* 1981;52:49–58.
57. Sundaresan N. Chordomas. *Clin Orthop Relat Res.* 1986;204:135–142.
58. Dorfman HD, Czerniak B. Bone cancers. *Cancer.* 1995;75:203–210.
59. Morita A, Sekhar LN, Wright DC. Current concepts in the management of tumors of the skull base. *Cancer Control.* 1998;5:138–149.
60. Muro K, Das S, Raizer JJ. Chordomas of the craniospinal axis: multimodality surgical, radiation and medical management strategies. *Expert Rev Neurother.* 2007;7:1295–1312.
61. Tamborini E, Miselli F, Negri T, et al. Molecular and biochemical analyses of platelet-derived growth factor receptor (PDGFR) B, PDGFRA, and KIT receptors in chordomas. *Clin Cancer Res.* 2006;12:6920–6928.
62. Orzan F, Terreni MR, Longoni M, et al. Expression study of the target receptor tyrosine kinase of Imatinib mesylate in skull base chordomas. *Oncol Rep.* 2007;18:249–252.
63. Weinberger PM, Yu Z, Kowalski D, et al. Differential expression of epidermal growth factor receptor, c-Met, and HER2/neu in chordoma compared with 17 other malignancies. *Arch Otolaryngol Head Neck Surg.* 2005;131:707–711.
64. Scheil S, Bruderlein S, Liehr T, et al. Genome-wide analysis of sixteen chordomas by comparative genomic hybridization and cytogenetics of the first human chordoma cell line, U-CH1. *Genes Chromosomes Cancer.* 2001;32:203–211.
65. Koch BB, Karnell LH, Hoffman HT, et al. National cancer database report on chondrosarcoma of the head and neck. *Head Neck.* 2000;22:408–425.
66. Gay E, Sekhar LN, Rubinstein E, et al. Chordomas and chondrosarcomas of the cranial base: results and follow-up of 60 patients. *Neurosurgery.* 1995;36:887–896; discussion 96–97.
67. McLendon RE, Rosenblum MK, Bigner DD, Russell DS, Rubinstein LJ. *Russell and Rubinstein's Pathology of Tumors of the Nervous System.* 7th ed. London: Hodder Arnold. Distributed in the United States of America by Oxford University Press; 2006.

68. Korten AG, ter Berg HJ, Spincemaille GH, van der Laan RT, Van de Wel AM. Intracranial chondrosarcoma: review of the literature and report of 15 cases. *J Neurol Neurosurg Psychiatry.* 1998;65:88–92.
69. Rosenberg AE, Nielsen GP, Keel SB, et al. Chondrosarcoma of the base of the skull: a clinicopathologic study of 200 cases with emphasis on its distinction from chordoma. *Am J Surg Pathol.* 1999;23:1370–1378.
70. Taub RR, Keohan MI, Plitsas MM, Scheinmann RR. Phase II study of temozolomide in advanced sarcomas [Abstract]. *Proc Annu Meet Am Assoc Cancer Res.* 2000;19.
71. Lagonigro MS, Tamborini E, Negri T, et al. PDGFRalpha, PDGFRbeta and KIT expression/activation in conventional chondrosarcoma. *J Pathol.* 2006;208:615–623.
72. Brown JS. Glomus jugulare tumors revisited: a ten-year statistical follow-up of 231 cases. *Laryngoscope.* 1985;95:284–288.
73. Jackson CG. Glomus tympanicum and glomus jugulare tumors. *Otolaryngol Clin North Am.* 2001;34:941–970, vii.
74. Spector GJ, Ciralsky R, Maisel RH, Ogura JH IV. Multiple glomus tumors in the head and neck. *Laryngoscope.* 1975;85:1066–1075.
75. Blades DA, Hardy RW, Cohen M. Cervical paraganglioma with subsequent intracranial and intraspinal metastases. Case report. *J Neurosurg.* 1991;75:320–323.
76. Pipas JM, Krywicki RF. Treatment of progressive metastatic glomus jugulare tumor (paraganglioma) with gemcitabine. *Neuro Oncol.* 2000;2:190–191.
77. Hegi ME, Diserens AC, Gorlia T, et al. MGMT gene silencing and benefit from temozolomide in glioblastoma. *N Engl J Med.* 2005;352:997–1003.
78. Preusser M, Janzer RC, Felsberg J, et al. Anti-O^6-methylguanine-methyltransferase (MGMT) immunohistochemistry in glioblastoma multiforme: observer variability and lack of association with patient survival impede its use as clinical biomarker. *Brain Pathol.* 2008;18:520–532.
79. Muros MA, Llamas-Elvira JM, Rodriguez A, et al. 111In-pentetreotide scintigraphy is superior to 123I-MIBG scintigraphy in the diagnosis and location of chemodectoma. *Nucl Med Commun.* 1998;19:735–742.
80. Kappes A, Vaccaro A, Kunnimalaiyaan M, Chen H. ZM336372, a Raf-1 activator, inhibits growth of pheochromocytoma cells. *J Surg Res.* 2006;133:42–45.
81. Kappes A, Vaccaro A, Kunnimalaiyaan M, Chen H. Lithium ions: a novel treatment for pheochromocytomas and paragangliomas. *Surgery.* 2007;141:161–165; discussion 5.
82. Bradley PJ, Jones NS, Robertson I. Diagnosis and management of esthesioneuroblastoma. *Curr Opin Otolaryngol Head Neck Surg.* 2003;11:112–118.
83. Dulguerov P, Allal AS, Calcaterra TC. Esthesioneuroblastoma: a meta-analysis and review. *Lancet Oncol.* 2001;2:683–690.
84. Broich G, Pagliari A, Ottaviani F. Esthesioneuroblastoma: a general review of the cases published since the discovery of the tumour in 1924. *Anticancer Res.* 1997;17:2683–2706.
85. Lund VJ, Howard D, Wei W, Spittle M. Olfactory neuroblastoma: past, present, and future? *Laryngoscope.* 2003;113:502–507.
86. Nelson RS, Perlman EJ, Askin FB. Is esthesioneuroblastoma a peripheral neuroectodermal tumor? *Hum Pathol.* 1995;26:639–641.
87. Mezzelani A, Tornielli S, Minoletti F, Pierotti MA, Sozzi G, Pilotti S. Esthesioneuroblastoma is not a member of the primitive peripheral neuroectodermal tumour-Ewing's group. *Br J Cancer.* 1999;81:586–591.
88. Dulguerov P, Calcaterra T. Esthesioneuroblastoma: the UCLA experience 1970–1990. *Laryngoscope.* 1992;102:843–849.
89. Morita A, Ebersold MJ, Olsen KD, Foote RL, Lewis JE, Quast LM. Esthesioneuroblastoma: prognosis and management. *Neurosurgery.* 1993;32:706–714; discussion 14–15.
90. Kadish S, Goodman M, Wang CC. Olfactory neuroblastoma. A clinical analysis of 17 cases. *Cancer.* 1976;37:1571–1576.
91. Constantinidis J, Steinhart H, Koch M, et al. Olfactory neuroblastoma: the University of Erlangen-Nuremberg experience 1975–2000. *Otolaryngol Head Neck Surg.* 2004;130:567–574.
92. Argiris A, Dutra J, Tseke P, Haines K. Esthesioneuroblastoma: the Northwestern University experience. *Laryngoscope.* 2003;113:155–160.
93. Mendeloff J. The olfactory neuroepithelial tumors; a review of the literature and report of six additional cases. *Cancer.* 1957;10:944–956.
94. Eden BV, Debo RF, Larner JM, et al. Esthesioneuroblastoma. Long-term outcome and patterns of failure—the University of Virginia experience. *Cancer.* 1994;73:2556–2562.
95. Diaz EM Jr, Kies MS. Chemotherapy for skull base cancers. *Otolaryngol Clin North Am.* 2001;34:1079–1085, viii.
96. Mishima Y, Nagasaki E, Terui Y, et al. Combination chemotherapy (cyclophosphamide, doxorubicin, and vincristine with continuous-infusion cisplatin and etoposide) and radiotherapy with stem cell support can be beneficial for adolescents and adults with estheisoneuroblastoma. *Cancer.* 2004;101:1437–1444.
97. Watne K, Hager B. Treatment of recurrent esthesioneuroblastoma with combined intra-arterial chemotherapy. A case report. *J Neurooncol.* 1987;5:47–50.
98. Louis DN, Ohgaki H, Wiestler OD, Cavanee WK. *WHO Classification of Tumours of the Central Nervous System.* 4th ed. Lyon: International Agency for Research on Cancer; 2007.
99. Ducatman BS, Scheithauer BW, Piepgras DG, Reiman HM, Ilstrup DM. Malignant peripheral nerve sheath tumors. A clinicopathologic study of 120 cases. *Cancer.* 1986;57:2006–2021.
100. Jahrsdoerfer RA, Benjamin RS. Chemotherapy of bilateral acoustic neuromas. *Otolaryngol Head Neck Surg.* 1988;98:273–282.
101. Knudson AG. Two genetic hits (more or less) to cancer. *Nat Rev Cancer.* 2001;1:157–162.
102. Holtkamp N, Okuducu AF, Mucha J, et al. Mutation and expression of PDGFRA and KIT in malignant peripheral nerve sheath tumors, and its implications for imatinib sensitivity. *Carcinogenesis.* 2006;27:664–671.
103. Aoki M, Batista O, Bellacosa A, Tsichlis P, Vogt PK. The akt kinase: molecular determinants of oncogenicity. *Proc Natl Acad Sci USA.* 1998;95:14950–14955.
104. Watanabe T, Oda Y, Tamiya S, Masuda K, Tsuneyoshi M. Malignant peripheral nerve sheath tumour arising within neurofibroma. An immunohistochemical analysis in the comparison between benign and malignant components. *J Clin Pathol.* 2001;54:631–636.

69 Tumors of the Pituitary and Sellar Region

Lewis S. Blevins, Jr. and Jessica Koch Devin

SELLAR MASSES

Pituitary adenomas comprise approximately 10% to 15% of all primary brain tumors in adults and 90% of all sellar lesions. It is estimated that 1 in 10,000 persons is diagnosed annually with a pituitary adenoma, though autopsy studies report its prevalence as high as 25% [1]. The remaining 10% of masses in the sellar region do not represent pituitary adenomas [2–4]. These nonadenomatous masses are of both pituitary and nonpituitary origin (Table 69.1). In many cases, accurate diagnosis of the sellar mass preoperatively is helpful as it may affect management. There are a number of clinical, biochemical, and imaging subtleties that may assist in the correct identification of the sellar lesion.

Unlike pituitary adenomas that have the capability of hormone oversecretion, nonadenomatous lesions of the sellar region commonly present with decreased pituitary function. This most commonly manifests as gonadotropin or growth hormone insufficiency, followed by thyroid and cortisol insufficiency. The hyperprolactinemia characteristic of these lesions is typically less than 200 ng/mL, whereas levels greater than this are most consistent with a prolactinoma. The elevation in prolactin in this setting is secondary to compression of the stalk or gland thus interfering with the transit of prolactin inhibitory factors. Finally, a diagnosis of diabetes insipidus should alert the clinician that a nonadenomatous sellar lesion may be compressing on the pituitary stalk or paraventricular region of the hypothalamus [5]. All sellar lesions of significant size may present with symptoms of mass effect such as visual compromise, cranial neuropathies, and headache.

Magnetic resonance imaging (MRI) has become the modality of choice to image the sellar and parasellar region. The ability to image the Sella from the sagittal view and the development of dynamic contrast-enhanced protocols has led to improved visualization of pathology, whereas computed tomography (CT) remains the most useful modality to evaluate neighboring bony anatomy as well as tumoral calcification. Angiography remains an important tool in the diagnosis of parasellar aneurysms [5].

In this chapter, we will provide an overview of nonadenomatous and adenomatous sellar masses. For each we will review the specific clinical signs and symptoms as well as distinguishing imaging and biochemical characteristics.

Nonadenomatous Pituitary-Derived Sellar Masses

Craniopharyngiomas

Craniopharyngiomas represent epithelial tumors that arise from the neoplastic transformation of embryonic squamous cell rests along the path of the craniopharyngeal duct that led from the stomodeal ectoderm to the evaginated Rathke's pouch [6]. Craniopharyngiomas are rare tumors comprising only 3% of all intracranial tumors; they represent 5.6% to 15% of all intracranial tumors in children, however, and are the most common tumors to involve the hypothalamic-pituitary region in this population [6,7]. A bimodal age distribution has been observed, with a peak incidence of the adamantinomatous type in children aged 5 to 14 years, whereas the papillary variety has been described in adults aged 50 to 74 years. The majority of the tumors are mixed cystic-solid with a suprasellar component and are well over 1 cm at the time of initial surgery [2].

The most common presenting symptoms in patients with craniopharyngiomas include headaches, nausea with vomiting, visual changes, growth failure in children, and hypogonadism in adults. The vast majority of patients exhibit at least one hormonal deficit, and diabetes insipidus may be present in up to one third at presentation. Whereas hormonal dysfunction is present in up to 90% of children upon presentation, visual symptoms are the primary complaint in adults [3]. CT may be particularly useful in children to detect tumoral calcifications and cystic components of the tumor, with the presence of suprasellar calcification being highly suspicious for the diagnosis. Both solid and cystic components are evident upon MRI and typically enhance following contrast administration [7].

The primary treatment of craniopharyngiomas remains surgical excision, which may be challenging given their size and adherence to vital nearby structures. The success of the surgery is dependent upon the size and location of the tumor, its invasiveness, and the aggressiveness and experience of the neurosurgeon. Recurrence following gross total resection is rare, whereas recurrence rates of up to 62% at 10 years are seen with partial resection [2]. When adjuvant radiation therapy is added to partial resection, the recurrence rates drop to 10% to 63% at 10 years [6]. There are, however, no currently published prospective

Table 69.1 Differential Diagnosis of Sellar Masses

Pituitary Derived Sellar Masses
Craniopharyngiomas
Rathke cleft cysts
Pituitary adenoma
Pituitary carcinoma
Pituitary astrocytoma (*pituicytoma*)
Granular cell tumors (*infundibuloma*)
Gangliocytoma (*mixed gangliocytoma-adenoma*)
Dermoid & epidermoid tumors
Nonpituitary Derived Sellar Masses
Meningiomas
Germ cell tumors (*teratoma, germinoma, embryonal cell, choriocarcinoma*)
Lymphoma
Glioma (*optic nerve, hypothalamic*)
Clival chordoma
Hypothalamic hamartoma
Schwannoma
Esthesioneuroblastoma
Metastases to the pituitary gland (*breast and lung*)
Other Sellar Lesions
Arachnoid cyst
Aneurysm
Inflammatory lesions (*sarcoidosis, hypophysitis, histiocytosis, giant cell*)
Infections lesions (*abscess, sphenoid mucocele*)

randomized studies to date evaluating the different forms of primary therapy [6].

The management of recurrent disease remains challenging. The success rate of a second surgical resection drops to less than 25% following reoperation, whereas perioperative morbidity increases [6]. Radiation therapy appears to be equally effective in patients receiving radiation therapy for recurrent tumor as in those who received it as adjuvant therapy following initial resection. Options for the management of recurrent cystic craniopharyngiomas include intracystic irradiation with β and γ-emitting isotopes. These therapies have been published with small groups of patients and appear to offer reduction and/or stabilization of craniopharyngiomas accompanied by low surgical morbidity. The long-term impact of this therapy on survival however remains to be assessed. Another modality, stereotactic radiosurgery, which delivers a single fraction of high-dose irradiation precisely to mapped targets while minimizing exposure to nearby structures, has the potential to achieve tumor control in patients with small foci of recurrent or residual disease [6].

Despite these therapeutic advances, long-term morbidity remains high in patients with craniopharyngiomas and largely involves endocrine, visual, hypothalamic, and cognitive sequelae attributed to damage by the invasive tumor or effects of the therapeutic interventions. Greater than 50% of patients exhibit three or more hormonal deficiencies following treatment. Hypothalamic damage often leads to obesity, behavioral issues, and may interfere with sense of thirst as well as sleep patterns [6]. Patients with a history of craniopharyngioma exhibit significantly higher standardized mortality ratios, attributed not only to their therapeutic interventions but also to increased cerebro- and cardiovascular disease as well as respiratory disease [8]. The optimal management of craniopharyngioma therefore remains challenging. The goals for primary and recurrent disease should not only focus on disease control but also on the minimization of associated morbidities and optimization of hormonal replacement therapies and quality of living.

Rathke Cleft Cysts

Rathke cleft cysts are common cystic tumors that form from the remnants of the squamous epithelium of Rathke's pouch and are estimated to occur in 13% to 22% of routinely examined pituitary glands [5]. These tumors can be seen at any age, but when symptomatic most often occur in adults 40 to 60 years of age [2].

These cystic tumors are seen as discrete lesions upon MRI imaging with variable enhancement intensity. Only the cyst wall enhances as a thin rim with contrast, which may help to differentiate the lesion from craniopharyngioma; calcifications are uncommon [2]. Rathke cleft cysts are primarily small and intrasellar, though up to one third may extend suprasellarly and thereby become symptomatic [3,5].

A high degree of suspicion for the diagnosis preoperatively is helpful because in many cases drainage of the cyst without full resection may be sufficient and results in a low rate of recurrence [3].

Pituicytomas

Pituicytomas represent low-grade glial tumors that arise from the pituicytes of the neurohypophysis; they are indistinguishable radiographically but histologically distinct from pilocytic astrocytomas by the presence of plump, spindle-shaped cells accompanied by a rich capillary network that are immunoreactive to vimentin, S-100, and neurospecific enolase antibodies [2,9]. The main differential diagnoses include granular cell tumors, schwannomas, and meningiomas [9].

The mean age of presentation of pituicytomas is 40 years with a male predominance. MRI imaging demonstrates a solid, well-circumscribed, uniformly hyperintense mass on T2-weighted imaging; its neurohypophyseal origin causes anterior displacement of the adenohypophysis. Despite this, diabetes insipidus is not a common presenting symptom and the clinical symptoms of pituicytoma remain nonspecific. Total resection via the transsphenoidal route is indicated and is usually curative [2].

Granular Cell Tumors

These benign tumors arising from the granular cell-type pituicytes of the neurohypophysis or infundibulum have also been termed choristomas, myoblastomas, and infundibulomas. Granular cell tumors represent the most common primary tumor of the neurohypophysis and present usually in the fifth decade with a female predominance. By the time of diagnosis most tumors are quite large; approximately 90% of patients present with visual symptoms and 50% demonstrate biochemical evidence of endocrinologic dysfunction. Headache is common [2].

Upon MRI imaging, the masses are isointense to gray matter on both T1- and T2-weighted sequences. Intense enhancement may be seen due to the high vascularity of the tumor. Nearly 50% of these tumors involve the suprasellar region [2]. The primary treatment is surgical resection. The surgical goal of tumor decompression has been advocated due to the benign nature and indolent growth along with their firm and vascular consistency. The role of adjuvant radiation therapy is yet to be defined [10].

Gangliocytomas

Gangliocytomas are rare tumors that consist of purely neuronal or mixed adenomatous and neuronal tissues and are found largely in adults with a female predominance. These tumors are most often (65%–76%) seen in association with adenomas, thus leading to the term mixed gangliocytoma-adenoma (MGA). MGAs are more likely to be hormonally active than pure gangliocytoma, with secretion of growth hormone being the most common followed by Cushing disease [2]. On MRI imaging, these tumors are indistinguishable from macroadenomas [3]. Treatment is surgical and medical therapy is indicated when residual hormonal hypersecretion is present.

Dermoid and Epidermoid Tumors

These congenital lesions represent slow-growing epithelial inclusion cysts that comprise less than 2% of all intracranial neoplasms [7]. These tumors present in the fourth to fifth decades with visual disturbances and endocrinologic dysfunction. Recurrent meningitis from leakage of cystic contents may indicate the diagnosis [3,11]. These cysts tend to be located in the sellar and parasellar regions and appear isointense to cerebrospinal fluid (CSF) on T1-weighted MRI imaging and do not enhance with contrast [3].

Nonpituitary Derived Sellar Masses

Meningiomas

Meningiomas account for 20% of all intracranial neoplasms; their incidence increases with age, with a peak incidence in adults of 60 to 70 years, and they are two times more common in females. Ten percent to 15% of meningiomas arise in the parasellar region from the tuberculum sella or the planum sphenoidale, whereas purely intrasellar meningiomas are rare with the majority arising from the diaphragma sella [2,3].

Intrasellar meningiomas may mimic pituitary adenomas in their presentation, with primary symptoms of headache, visual changes, and endocrinologic dysfunction [2]. Parasellar meningiomas most often present with severe visual disturbance manifested as progressive visual loss. An asymmetric variant of bitemporal hemianopsia is common. Visual symptoms can often be confused with retrobulbar neuritis; however, there is no pain upon eye movement and the visual loss is progressive rather than sudden. Optic atrophy is commonly seen upon examination and best correlates with loss of visual acuity [5].

Intrasellar meningiomas typically appear as hypo to isointense to gray matter on both T1- and T2-weighted sequences and show rapid homogeneous enhancement, whereas adenomas typically have more heterogeneous enhancement and enhance more slowly. Identification of the pituitary gland as separate from the sellar mass additionally differentiates an intrasellar meningioma from an adenoma, as does the findings of hyperostosis of the planum (particularly with tuberculum sellae meningiomas) and prominent vessels [2]. CT may be useful in detecting the hyperostosis, whereas arteriography may demonstrate the enlarged nutrient arteries. Parasellar meningiomas may exhibit a tapered extension of the dural base or "dural tail," which is suggestive of a meningioma but is not specific. The carotid artery may be narrowed in the event of cavernous sinus invasion, a rare finding with pituitary adenoma [3,7].

The opportunity to diagnose a meningioma preoperatively is fortunate, as a transcranial approach is usually preferred to a transsphenoidal procedure. Meningiomas can be highly vascular, thus predisposing them to intraoperative bleeding that may be easier to control from the transcranial approach. Duration of preoperative symptoms, patient age, and intact brain-tumor interface have been shown to significantly affect visual prognosis [12]. Radiotherapy may be useful in patients with cavernous sinus meningiomas and those with residual disease following debulking procedures.

Germ Cell Tumors

Intracranial germ cell tumors are rare, malignant, primarily midline, usually multifocal tumors that include teratomas, germinomas, embryonal cell carcinoma, choriocarcinoma, endodermal sinus (yolk sac) tumors, and mixed germ cell tumors. Germ cell tumors comprise only 0.1% to 0.2% of all primary brain neoplasms and present mainly in childhood, with a peak age of presentation of 10 to 12 years. Pure germinomas comprise two thirds of germ cell tumors, whereas nongerminomatous mixed germ cell tumors account for the majority of the remaining one third; pure germinomas occur at an older age than nongerminomatous tumors. The majority of tumors are found in the pineal or intra/suprasellar region, with a male predominance noted in the former and female in the latter [2].

Purely intrasellar germinomas are rare; suprasellar germinomas arise from the floor of the third ventricle or the infundibulum, presumably from totipent germ cells that have failed to migrate to the genital crest during embryogenesis. Patients most often present early in the course of disease with diabetes insipidus [5]. Hypopituitarism is seen in children and adults; precocious puberty may be observed as well. Normalization of endocrine function is rarely achieved following therapy [13]. Suprasellar tumors may cause headache and cranial nerve palsies [2]. Pineal tumors most commonly present with symptoms of increased intracranial pressure [14].

Serum tumor markers are uniquely useful in establishing the diagnosis of a germ cell tumor. Alpha-fetoprotein or β-human chorionic gonadotropin are expressed by a number of germ cell tumors; the presence of these markers in CSF or serum with evidence of an intracranial tumor is essentially diagnostic of a germ cell tumor [2]. Alpha-fetoprotein and high levels of β-human chorionic gonadotropin indicate a negative prognosis as they are specific to nongerminoma germ cell tumors. These markers can also serve as reliable indicators of disease response and progression with the appropriate radiographic and clinical correlation [13].

Once an intracranial germ cell tumor is identified, MRI of the entire craniospinal axis and sampling of the CSF for cytology are necessary, given the predilection for dissemination [2]. On MRI, germinomas tend to be a large homogeneous suprasellar mass, exhibit loss of the posterior bright spot, and rapidly enhance with contrast [3].

Preoperative diagnosis of pure germinomas is vital, as more then 90% can be effectively treated with radiation alone. Ten percent metastasize within the central nervous system; distant metastases to the lungs have been reported [3,5]. Prognosis for nongerminomatous lesions is not as favorable, with only 40% to 60% responding to radiation therapy alone [2]. Given that the prognosis of the tumors is most dependent upon the histological diagnosis and extent of disease, a tissue biopsy is recommended prior to the initiation of treatment. Radiation therapy for a localized tumor most often consists of radiation to the entire ventricular system with a boost to the focal tumor. Adjuvant surgical resection has not been shown to affect survival for patients with pure germinomas. For nongerminomatous germ cell tumors, however, gross total resection may be considered given the generally poor response to therapy [13].

Routine prophylactic craniospinal irradiation has previously been advocated for primary prevention of CSF dissemination in patients with germ cell tumors. This approach, however, is associated with significant morbidity, including axial growth arrest in children, marrow suppression, and radiation exposure to the gonads. Therefore craniospinal irradiation is most commonly reserved for patients with radiographic or cytologic evidence of CSF dissemination [13].

The benefits of chemotherapy for germ cell tumors remain uncertain; it is reserved for patients with non-germinomatous germ cell tumors and germinimonas not localized to the pineal or suprasellar region [13]. A combined chemo-radiotherapy regimen, which uses vincristine, etoposide, and carboplatin to induce tumor shrinkage thereby enabling lower doses of subsequent radiation therapy, has been advocated to improve disease-free survival while minimizing morbidity [14].

Lymphoma

Primary lymphoma of the sella is extremely rare, whereas primary CNS lymphoma represents up to 2% of all primary CNS malignancies. Lymphoma localized to the CNS is comprised mainly of non-Hodgkin type B-cell lymphoma. The incidence of lymphoma has nearly tripled in the United States since the 1980s, partially attributed to the increase in immunocompromised individuals [15]. The mean age of presentation is 30 to 40 years of age for immunocompromised individuals and 60 to 70 years of age for immunocompetent individuals [2]. Clinical signs and symptoms are nonspecific and mimic those of pituitary macroadenomas. Sellar lymphomas fail to exhibit any characteristic MRI findings. The majority of lesions present as homogenously or heterogeneously enhancing sellar masses [2].

Gliomas

Optic Nerve Glioma

Optic nerve gliomas comprise only 2% of orbital tumors in all ages. The presentation, however, differs somewhat in adults versus children. The disease in children is typically benign and slow growing. Multicentric disease is often seen in children with neurofibromatosis. The most common symptoms upon presentation in children include vision loss with proptosis and headaches. In adults the disease tends to be more aggressive. It begins with monocular blurring with retrobulbar pain and can progress rapidly to blindness. Visual field deficits in nonspecific patterns may be present. These lesions are distinctly hypointense on T1-weighted images and hyperintense on T2-weight images and homogeneously enhance with contrast. They often exhibit infiltration of the optic nerves tracts, and visual radiations [3,5].

The extent of treatment depends on the extent and location of disease. For localized tumor, surgical resection may be feasible. However, biopsy versus subtotal resection followed by radiotherapy is the preferred approach for bilateral disease. Chemotherapy, typically with carboplatin and vincristine, is preferred in very young children, to delay disease progression until radiation therapy or surgery may be more safely employed [16]. Endocrine dysfunction is the most commonly observed adverse effect of treatment for optic gliomas [17].

Hypothalamic Glioma

Hypothalamic glioma appears in children with the primary symptoms of diabetes insipidus and visual loss. Signs of hypothalamic dysfunction may be present, causing the characteristic "diencephalic syndrome" of strabismus, weight loss, and developmental delay [17]. Imaging characteristics are similar to that of optic nerve gliomas with the exception that the tumors typically arise from the anterior hypothalamus and invade the third ventricle, resulting in increased intracranial pressure [3,5].

Clival Chordoma

Chordomas arise from notochordal remnants within the clivus in approximately 40% of cases. They may additionally arise from other locations within the sellar/parasellar region. Chordomas present in adults between 30 and 50 years of age with a male predominance. Approximately one third of patients present with asymmetric involvement of the third, fourth, and/or sixth cranial nerve, thus diplopia is one of the most common presenting symptoms. Headaches, neck pain, and symptoms of nasopharyngeal congestion may occur, though endocrinologic dysfunction is rare [3,5].

Chordomas appear as destructive, infiltrative lesions in the clivus upon MRI imaging. Calcification is present in 50% of the lesions, and the pituitary gland can often be visualized as a distinct separate entity. The lesion appears heterogeneously hyperintense on T2-weighted images and enhances with contrast [7]. CT may be helpful in visualization of the bony destruction, as the sella floor is frequently thinned or destroyed. The location, extent of bony destruction, and separation from the pituitary gland generally allow differentiation of a chordoma from a pituitary adenoma [3,5].

Hypothalamic Hamartoma

Hamartoma represents a rare benign congenital heterotopia and represents the most common tumoral cause of central precocious puberty in children, likely secondary to secretion of LH-releasing hormone [7,18]. MRI and CT imaging shows a sellar or parasellar pedunculated mass in the area of the tuber cinereum. Hamartomas are isointense to the gray matter on both T1- and T2-weighted images and do not show contrast enhancement; they are distinct from the pituitary gland, generally noninvasive, and measure less than 1 to 2 cm and therefore exhibit little mass effect [3,7]. Treatment options for precocious puberty associated with hypothalamic hamartoma may include surgical excision or medical treatment with long-acting GnRH analogue or antagonists until puberty. Surgery is recommended in young children, whereas medical management is advocated more in children closer to puberty [18].

Schwannoma

Schwannomas most frequently present as intrathecal-intramedullary tumors of the spine, though intracranial schwannoma comprises approximately 8% of all primary intracranial tumors. Typically the tumor involves the vestibular portion of cranial nerve eight near to the cerebellopontine angle or in an intraparenchymal/intraventricular location as in association with neurofibromatosis type II; primary sellar schwannoma is rare [19].

Sellar schwannoma is often reported with suprasellar extension, presenting with a decrease in visual acuity and visual field defects. A significant number of patients present with endocrinologic dysfunction and mild elevation in prolactin, presumably secondary to compression of the infundibulum [19]. On imaging, schwanommas are hypointense on T1-weighted images and hyperintense on T2-weighted images and homogeneously enhance with contrast [7]. Though transsphenoidal surgical resection remains the treatment of choice, this may be challenging due to the tumor vascularity [19].

Esthesioneuroblastoma

Esthesioneuroblastoma is a neuroectodermal neoplasm believed to arise from olfactory receptors within the nasal mucosa. Intracranial extension is not uncommon, though primary sellar esthesioneuroblastoma is very rare. Rare tumors present with clinical symptoms and signs of hypercortisolism due to tumoral production and secretion of ACTH. Though these tumors are radiosensitive, primary surgical resection with adjuvant radiation therapy is favored [20].

Metastases

Metastases to the pituitary gland represent an uncommon complication of malignant disease and comprise less than 1% of surgically resected sellar masses. Breast, lung, and melanoma are the most common sites of primary disease. Typically, patients are within their sixth or seventh decade and present with diabetes insipidus. Most often metastases to the pituitary are seen in the setting of diffuse metastatic spread, though occasionally it has been reported as the first manifestation of an occult primary tumor such as metastatic melanoma [21].

The near universal presenting symptom of diabetes insipidus may be explained by predilection of metastases for the posterior lobe and infundibulum; modest elevation in prolactin level is additionally often seen. Bilateral hemianopsia as well as cranial neuropathies due to infiltration of the cavernous sinus may be present. Imaging characteristics are generally not sufficient to reliably distinguish metastases from pituitary adenoma, though a rapidly enlarging sellar mass and/or thickening of the infundibulum are frequently reported characteristics [3].

The preoperative diagnosis of metastatic disease is difficult. If meningeal spread has occurred, lumbar puncture may be diagnostic. Generally a history of a coexisting malignancy leads to the diagnosis, though this should be used with caution as previous series have indicated that in patients with metastatic disease a sellar lesion is twice as likely to represent an adenoma [21]. Total resection is challenging, as the tumors are generally highly vascular and often herald widespread metastases. Though resection is advocated for localized metastatic disease both to obtain a tissue diagnosis and alleviate symptoms, local radiation and/or the appropriate chemotherapy is most often recommended for initial treatment in patients with widespread metastases followed by initiation of pituitary hormone replacement therapy when appropriate. Age more than 65 years, a diagnosis of small cell lung cancer, and <1 year duration between cancer diagnosis and pituitary invasion are poor prognostic indicators [22].

Other Sellar Lesions

Arachnoid Cyst

Arachnoid cysts are believed to develop from penetration of subarachnoid space into the sella through a defect in the diaphragma sellae; they may also develop in the setting of postinfectious adhesive arachnoiditis [3]. Clinically, an arachnoid cyst mimics a nonfunctioning pituitary adenoma [23]. Radiographically they resemble Rathke cleft cysts with either an intrasellar or suprasellar location and appear as a distinct mass with CSF signal intensity [7]. Treatment consists of transsphenoidal surgical resection, which carries a risk of development of a CSF fistula [23].

Adenomatous Pituitary-Derived Sellar Masses

Pituitary adenomas arise from the glandular cells comprising the anterior pituitary gland. They may be classified according to their functional status (Table 69.2). A majority

Table 69.2 Pituitary Adenomas
Hormone-Inactive Aadenomas
Null cell adenomas
Silent hormone producing adenomas
Gonadotroph
ACTH
TSH
GH
Mixed
Hormone-Secreting Aadenomas
ACTH-secreting (Cushing disease)
GH-secreting (acromegaly
TSH-secreting (hyperthyroidism)
Prolactin-secreting (prolactinoma)
Plurihormonal

of the tumors are derived from nonfunctioning anterior pituitary cells or else from cells that produce gonadotropins. Less common tumors arise from growth hormone-secreting, ACTH-secreting, and thyrotropin (TSH)-secreting cells; most patients with tumors derived from these 3 cell types present with a clinical syndrome of hormone hypersecretion. Some of these tumors, however, are unable to produce biologically active peptide hormones and thus are felt to be clinically silent even though derived from a hormone producing cell. About 2% of patients have tumors that secrete more than one of the anterior pituitary hormones. Tumors may also be derived from stem cells and other pluripotent anterior pituitary cells.

Pituitary tumors may also be classified according to their size. Tumors with a maximum dimension of 1 cm or less are often referred to as microadenomas, whereas those greater than 1 cm in maximum diameter are referred to as macroadenomas. Tumors in excess of 4 cm are often referred to as giant adenomas. Large tumors may present with mass effects including headache, visual compromise due to optic chiasmal compression, diplopia due to cavernous sinus invasion and compression of one or more of the cranial nerves controlling eye movement, epistaxis, and even CSF rhinorrhea.

Cushing Disease

The term Cushing disease implies the presence of hypercortisolism due to an ACTH-secreting pituitary tumor. Most patients present with a multitude of clinical features that, collectively, are referred to as Cushing syndrome. These tumors account for 15% of all pituitary tumors and for about 65% of all causes of endogenous hypercortisolism. Eighty percent are microadenomas; about one third are 3 to 4 mm in size and often not recognized on MRI.

Transsphenoidal surgery is the initial treatment of choice for most patients with Cushing disease. The principal goals of surgery include complete resection of the ACTH-secreting pituitary tumor, resolution of the hypercortisolemic state and its associated morbidities, and restoration of the normal dynamic function of the hypothalamic-pituitary-adrenal axis. Published series demonstrate that remission following initial surgery can be expected in 70% to 90% of patients with Cushing disease caused by microadenomas [24–30]. Remission is seen in 50% to 65% of those patients with macroadenomas [26,30]. Recurrent hypercortisolism affects about 10% of patients with microadenomas and 30% of those with macroadenomas [26]. Some recurrences occur as late as a decade or more after an initially successful surgery.

Once a diagnosis of persistent or recurrent Cushing disease has been confirmed, one must consider treatment options in the context of the affected patient. Therapeutic strategies are directed at resolution of the hypercortisolism as well as control of the ACTH-secreting pituitary tumor. Additional goals of therapy include management of adverse consequences of therapy, such as hypopituitarism, and correction or control of the manifestations of hypercortisolim including hyperglycemia, hypertension, osteopenia, and the management of infections.

Repeat surgery should be considered for all patients with residual or recurrent Cushing disease. Approximately 50% to 75% of patients with microadenomas can be expected to enter remission following a second surgical procedure [26,31,32]. Success rates in those patients with macroadenomas are less encouraging but debulking procedures can result in overall improvement in cortisol levels and resultant morbidity of the disease.

Radiotherapy has been successfully employed in the management of patients with residual or recurrent Cushing disease. Remission can be expected in about 50% of adults and 80% of children who receive fractionated conventional radiotherapy. The time course to a beneficial response is such that only 50% of patients enter remission by 18 months after treatment. Normalization of cortisol secretion may be delayed by as much as 5 years [33–35]. Stereotactic radiosurgery, most commonly in the form of Gamma Knife® radiosurgery, has been increasingly employed in the management of patients with Cushing disease. Successful normalization of cortisol levels is achieved in 27% to 66% of adults [26–42]. The mean time to normalization of cortisol levels, however, is much shorter than with conventional radiotherapy, occurring on average in 6 to 8 months, with a reported range of 6 to 36 months [36–38,40,43,44,45]. Radiosurgery also appears to provide control of tumor burden in a majority of patients. Potential late sequelae of radiation therapy include hypopituitarism, radiation-induced optic neuropathy, temporal lobe necrosis, and secondary carcinogenesis [37,38].

Several steroid biosynthesis inhibitors can be employed in order to gain control of hypercortisolism in patients with Cushing disease. These drugs are often employed when surgery will be delayed by more than 4 to 8 weeks and while awaiting the beneficial effects of radiotherapy. We employ ketoconazole as first-line therapy [46]. This antifungal drug inhibits several of the cytochrome P450 enzymes required to synthesize cortisol. We typically initiate therapy with a dose of 200 mg twice daily. The dose is usually escalated as needed at 2- to 4-week intervals to a maximum of 400 mg four times daily in attempt to achieve normal urinary cortisol excretion rates. Metyrapone is useful, either alone or in combination with ketoconazole, when cortisol levels are refractory to treatment or the side effects of ketoconazole are intolerable [47]. Aminoglutethimide is also a useful agent but is becoming increasingly difficult to obtain by prescription. Mitotane, a congener of DDT, is a drug of last resort in patients with Cushing disease but can effectively lower cortisol levels [48]. Surveillance of urinary cortisol excretion rates at regular intervals is necessary in order to identify those who do not respond to treatment, those who suffer from breakthrough hypercortisolism, and also to detect hypocortisolism in those who may have responded to radiotherapy. Medical therapy should be discontinued for 6 weeks to permit reassessment of cortisol excretion rates in patients who have been treated with radiotherapy or repeat surgery when their serum or urine cortisol levels fall into the lower part of the respective normal ranges.

Laprascopic bilateral adrenalectomy is often employed as a last resort when all other therapeutic modalities have failed and the patient is in grave danger due to the consequences of hypercortisolism [49,50]. The operative mortality approaches 5% and as many as 20% of patients suffer from perioperative complications including deep vein thrombosis, delayed wound healing, bleeding disorders, and perioperative infections [51]. Nelson syndrome develops in a minority of patients following adrenalectomy and may require additional therapeutic intervention directed at the enlarging pituitary tumor.

Prolactinoma

Prolactinomas account for approximately 40% in of all pituitary tumors. Women often present with microadenomas and irregular or absent menses, infertility and, occasionally, galactorrhea. Men usually present with a decreased libido and erectile dysfunction as well as other symptoms and signs of testosterone deficiency and more often have macroadenomas. The goals of therapy of prolactinomas include normalization of the serum prolactin concentrations, which is usually accompanied by reversal of the associated hypogonadism and galactorrhea and control of tumor growth [52].

Normal prolactin producing pituitary cells and most prolactinomas express dopamine receptors on their cell surface membranes. Dopamine inhibits prolactin synthesis and secretion and decreases the size as well as proliferation of prolactin producing cells. Dopamine agonist drugs are commonly employed as first-line therapy in patients with hyperprolactinemia and those with prolactinomas. Bromocriptine has been commercially available for the management of hyperprolactinemia since the mid-1970s. A typical starting dose is 2.5 mg at bedtime. Effective doses range from 2.5 to 5 mg administered once daily at bedtime up to 30 mg daily administered in two to three divided doses [53]. Cabergoline, available since the late 1990s, is administered in doses ranging from 0.25 mg once weekly to 1.5 mg twice weekly and is probably a more effective and better tolerated therapeutic agent [54]. Side effects of dopamine agonist drugs include headache, nausea, vomiting, fatigue, orthostatic dizziness, and psychosis. High-dose cabergoline therapy in patients with Parkinson disease is associated with cardiac valvular abnormalities [55]. It is not clear whether similar abnormalities will result from long-term use in patients with hyperprolactinemia.

Prolactin levels normalize in roughly one-half to two thirds of patients with macroprolactinomas [53,54]. Levels typically fall to 90% of the baseline value in a majority of patients. Prolactin levels typically normalize in about 90% of patients with microadenomas [53,54]. Disturbances in gonadal function and galactorrhea resolve in a majority of patients who experience normalization of their prolactin concentrations with treatment. Patients with prolactinomas who have normal prolactin levels and radiographic evidence for complete disappearance of their pituitary tumor after 2 years of therapy might be candidates for discontinuation of dopamine agonist therapy. In those studies where patients have been followed between 2 and 5 years, the proportion of patients maintaining normal prolactin levels following discontinuation of successful dopamine agonist therapy ranges from 8% to 37% [56].

Some degree of regression in prolactinoma size in response to dopamine agonist therapy occurs in about three-quarters of patients treated with dopamine agonist drugs [52]. In one series of 27 men with macroadenomas, 46% experienced reduction in tumor size by 50% or more, 18% by 25% to 50%, and 36% of patients experienced some but less than 25% regression [57,58]. Tumor regression is usually evident within the 1st month of treatment but some patients may not experience significant reduction in tumor size for 6 to 12 months. Visual field deficits improve or resolve in roughly two thirds of patients [52].

Surgical resection is usually reserved for those patients with prolactinomas that have failed to respond to medical therapy, in the setting of pituitary apoplexy and mass effects, and when patients prefer surgery to lifelong medical therapy. Approximately 90% of patients with microadenomas can expect resolution of hyperprolactinemia [59]. The overall recurrence rate is estimated to be 10% to 15%. Success rates are lower in patients with macroadenomas, invasive tumors, and in the setting of marked suprasellar extension and, therefore, medical therapy is preferred in these instances.

Acromegaly

Growth hormone-secreting pituitary tumors account for 15% to 20% of all pituitary tumors. Approximately three quarters of patients present with macroadenomas. One or more component features of the clinical syndrome of acromegaly are apparent in a majority of the affected patients. The average delay in diagnosis from the time of onset of clinical features is roughly 7 years [60].

Surgery is still regarded as first-line therapy for patients with growth hormone secreting pituitary tumors. Revisions in the criteria for determination of the disease-free state over time have led to unreliability of reports of surgical success rates. In fact, some investigators now believe that acromegaly is incurable. Experienced neurosurgeons, however, expect to normalize growth hormone and IGF-I secretion in roughly 80% to 90% of patients with microadenomas, 30% to 60% of patients with macroadenomas, and only a small proportion of those patients with invasive disease and giant adenomas [61,62].

Radiotherapy can be a useful adjunct to surgery in the management of patients with residual and recurrent disease. Unfortunately, however, biochemical cure of acromegaly is achieved in only about 70% of patients at 7 to 10 years following the administration of conventional radiotherapy. Similar success rates can be achieved with Gamma Knife® radiosurgery, and the time course to normalization of growth hormone and IGF-I secretion appears to be much shorter [63,64].

A number of medical therapeutic agents are available to treat patients who have residual or recurrent acromegaly. These agents include dopamine agonist drugs, somatostatin analogues, and a growth hormone receptor antagonist. These drugs are also useful in patients who are not candidates for surgery and those who elect medical therapy instead of surgery when surgery is unlikely to render them disease free. The choice of agent depends in part on patient preference, tumor characteristics, urgency of need to lower growth hormone levels, comorbidities, and other factors.

Bromocriptine, a dopamine receptor agonist, normalizes growth hormone and IGF-I levels in roughly 15% of patients [65]. Effective doses range from 15 to 30 mg orally daily in divided doses. Cabergoline, a longer acting and more potent dopamine receptor agonist, normalizes IGF-I levels in 30% to 50% of affected patients [66]. Patients with tumors that secrete both growth hormone and prolactin seemed to be more likely to respond than patients whose tumors only secrete growth hormone. Effective doses of cabergoline range from 1.5 to 3 mg orally weekly in divided doses.

Somatostatin analogues are novel therapeutic agents that have dramatically altered the landscape and natural history of acromegaly. Octreotide for subcutaneous injection, the long-acting depot form of the drug (Octreotide LAR), and Lanreotide (Somatuline) depot are commercially available agents of this class approved by the U.S. Food and Drug Administration. These agents exert their effects on growth hormone secreting tumors by binding to somatostatin receptors expressed on cell surface membranes. Receptor activation inhibits growth hormone secretion and appears to have beneficial antiproliferative effects on growth hormone-secreting tumors [67]. Octreotide for subcutaneous injection is administered in a dose of 50 to 500 mcg every 8 hours [68]. Doses of Octreotide LAR range between 10 and 30 mg administered by deep intramuscular injection once monthly [69]. Lanreotide depot is administered subcutaneously in doses between 60 and 120 mg every 28 days [70]. The clinical efficacy of somatostatin analogues has been demonstrated in several studies [71]. Normalization of the growth hormone and IGF-I levels can be expected in 40% to 60% of patients. Acromegalic symptoms and signs, including sleep apnea, hypertension, acromegalic cardiomyopathy, impaired glucose tolerance, arthralgias, shoe size, and ring size, usually improve following successful lowering of the IGF-I levels. Side effects of somatostatin analogues are related to the ability of these agents to inhibit other endocrine and neuroendocrine systems. A reduction in gallbladder motility may lead to gallbladder sludge and gallstone formation. Hyperglycemia may result as a consequence of inhibition of insulin secretion by the pancreatic beta cells. Gastrointestinal discomfort, including diarrhea, abdominal pain, flatulence, constipation, and nausea may result from impaired intestinal motility and inhibition of various digestive processes and enzymes.

Pegvisomant, a growth hormone receptor antagonist, administered subcutaneously in doses between 10 and 40 mg can normalize IGF-I in up to 97% of patients [72]. This agent, a modified form of growth hormone produced by recombinant DNA technology, simply blocks the effects of growth hormone at the peripheral tissue level and does not have any particular antitumor activity. Side effects include abnormalities of liver function tests and local skin reactions.

TSH-Secreting Pituitary Tumors

TSH secreting pituitary tumors account for 1% to 5% of all pituitary tumors. Patients most commonly present with macroadenomas in the setting of TSH-dependent hyperthyroidism with goiter [73]. Surgical resection, though considered first-line therapy and useful in controlling tumor mass effects, does not usually result in remission of disease because of the aggressive nature of these tumors. There are insufficient data regarding the efficacy of radiotherapy in the management of patients with residual disease. Somatostatin analogs, in doses similar to those employed in acromegaly, normalize thyroid hormone levels in approximately three quarters of patients [74]. Beta-blockade is useful in controlling the symptoms of hyperthyroidism. Attempts to remove or to ablate the thyroid gland are often associated with rapid pituitary tumor growth, which is believed to occur due to the lack of negative feedback restraint of thyroid hormone on the pituitary tumor.

Endocrinologically Inactive Pituitary Adenomas

Endocrinologically inactive or so-called "nonfunctioning" pituitary tumors are a heterogeneous group of lesions including null-cell adenomas, silent hormone producing but not hormone secreting adenomas, and gonadotroph adenomas [75]. These lesions, by virtue of the fact that they do not produce hormones in excess resulting in a clinically recognizable syndrome, usually become macroadenomas and present with mass effects. Occasionally, these tumors are detected incidentally on radiologic imaging procedures performed for unrelated symptoms and complaints. There are no effective medical therapies for nonfunctioning and silent hormone producing tumors. Surgery is indicated to relieve mass effects, to control tumor growth, and occasionally to establish a diagnosis [76]. Adjuvant postoperative radiotherapy is reserved for patients who have progressive residual disease during a period of follow-up after surgery [77].

Pituitary Carcinoma

Pituitary carcinomas comprise only 0.2% of all pituitary-derived lesions. The majority of these lesions are recognized initially as invasive macroadenomas, with the majority being associated with ACTH or prolactin secretion. About one half of all reported cases were diagnosed postmortem in patients who had a history of aggressive pituitary tumors but had succumbed to other illnesses. It is hypothesized that pituitary carcinoma evolves from a macroadenoma over a long period of time through the accumulation of multiple genetic events. Histologic criteria are unable to reliably distinguish between carcinoma and adenoma; carcinomas unfortunately exhibit considerable variability with respect to proliferative markers. Instead, the criteria for classification of pituitary carcinoma includes identification of the primary tumor as a pituitary tumor by histology with evidence of craniospinal and/or systemic metastases and exclusion of an alternate primary tumor [78].

The treatment of pituitary carcinoma is similar to that of aggressive pituitary adenomas and may include surgery, radiation, and adjuvant medical therapy. While resection is rarely curative, it does provide symptomatic relief and helps to confirm the diagnosis. Radiotherapy may be helpful in temporary control of the primary lesion as well as bony and visceral metastases. Adjuvant medical therapy has been disappointing, with the majority of patients demonstrating resistance to treatment or early escape. The overall response to chemotherapy has been underreported and is disappointing, though observational data have suggested that patients with extra-CNS metastases may benefit from chemotherapy [78,79].

The current management options of pituitary carcinoma are therefore palliative and the prognosis dismal once metastases develop. Very high levels of hormone secretion, even following tumor resection, may indicate recurrent disease, the development of metastases, and/or the development of medication resistance. Corticotroph carcinomas and systemic metastases portend the worst survival [2]. It is estimated that less than 40% of patients are alive 1 year after discovery of metastases [78]. For this reason, an early diagnosis with aggressive initial surgical resection is essential [78].

REFERENCES

1. Jagannathan J, Kanter AS, Sheehan JP, Jane JA Jr, Laws ER Jr. Benign brain tumors: sellar/parasellar tumors. *Neurol Clin.* 2007;25(4):1231–1249, xi.
2. Huang BY, Castillo M. Nonadenomatous tumors of the pituitary and sella turcica. *Top Magn Reson Imaging.* 2005;16(4):289–299.
3. Freda PU, Post KD. Differential diagnosis of sellar masses. *Endocrinol Metab Clin North Am.* 1999;28(1):81–117, vi.
4. Sautner D, Saeger W, Lüdecke DK. Tumors of the sellar region mimicking pituitary adenomas. *Exp Clin Endocrinol.* 1993;101(5):283–289.
5. Post KD, McCormick PC, Bello JA. Differential diagnosis of pituitary tumors. *Endocrinol Metab Clin North Am.* 1987;16(3):609–645.
6. Karavitaki N, Cudlip S, Adams CB, Wass JA. Craniopharyngiomas. *Endocr Rev.* 2006;27(4):371–397.
7. Rennert J, Doerfler A. Imaging of sellar and parasellar lesions. *Clin Neurol Neurosurg.* 2007;109(2):111–124.
8. Tomlinson JW, Holden N, Hills RK, et al. Association between premature mortality and hypopituitarism. West Midlands Prospective Hypopituitary Study Group. *Lancet.* 2001;357(9254):425–431.
9. Figarella-Branger D, Dufour H, Fernandez C, Bouvier-Labit C, Grisoli F, Pellissier JF. Pituicytomas, a mis-diagnosed benign tumor of the neurohypophysis: report of three cases. *Acta Neuropathol.* 2002;104(3):313–319.
10. Cohen-Gadol AA, Pichelmann MA, Link MJ, et al. Granular cell tumor of the sellar and suprasellar region: clinicopathologic study of 11 cases and literature review. *Mayo Clin Proc.* 2003;78(5):567–573.
11. Landman RE, Wardlaw SL, McConnell RJ, Khandji AG, Bruce JN, Freda PU. Pituitary lymphoma presenting as fever of unknown origin. *J Clin Endocrinol Metab.* 2001;86(4):1470–1476.
12. Zevgaridis D, Medele RJ, Müller A, Hischa AC, Steiger HJ. Meningiomas of the sellar region presenting with visual impairment: impact of various prognostic factors on surgical outcome in 62 patients. *Acta Neurochir (Wien).* 2001;143(5):471–476.
13. Wolden SL, Wara WM, Larson DA, Prados MD, Edwards MS, Sneed PK. Radiation therapy for primary intracranial germ-cell tumors. *Int J Radiat Oncol Biol Phys.* 1995;32(4):943–949.
14. Janmohamed S, Grossman AB, Metcalfe K, et al. Suprasellar germ cell tumours: specific problems and the evolution of optimal management with a combined chemoradiotherapy regimen. *Clin Endocrinol (Oxf).* 2002;57(4):487–500.
15. Kaufmann TJ, Lopes MB, Laws ER Jr, Lipper MH. Primary sellar lymphoma: radiologic and pathologic findings in two patients. *AJNR Am J Neuroradiol.* 2002;23(3):364–367.
16. Bisson E, Khoshyomn S, Braff S, Maugans T. Hypothalamic-opticochiasmatic gliomas mimicking craniopharyngiomas. *Pediatr Neurosurg.* 2003;39(3):159–165.
17. Jahraus CD, Tarbell NJ. Optic pathway gliomas. *Pediatr Blood Cancer.* 2006;46(5):586–596.
18. Kizilkilic O, Yalcin O, Yildirim T, Sener L, Parmaksiz G, Erdogan B. Hypothalamic hamartoma associated with a craniopharyngeal canal. *AJNR Am J Neuroradiol.* 2005;26(1):65–67.
19. Perez MT, Farkas J, Padron S, Changus JE, Webster EL. Intrasellar and parasellar cellular schwannoma. *Ann Diagn Pathol.* 2004;8(3):142–150.
20. Sajko T, Rumboldt Z, Talan-Hranilovic J, Radic I, Gnjidic Z. Primary sellar esthesioneuroblastoma. *Acta Neurochir (Wien).* 2005;147(4):447–448; discussion 448.
21. McCutcheon IE, Waguespack SG, Fuller GN, Couldwell WT. Metastatic melanoma to the pituitary gland. *Can J Neurol Sci.* 2007;34(3):322–327.
22. Komninos J, Vlassopoulou V, Protopapa D, et al. Tumors metastatic to the pituitary gland: case report and literature review. *J Clin Endocrinol Metab.* 2004;89(2):574–580.
23. Dubuisson AS, Stevenaert A, Martin DH, Flandroy PP. Intrasellar arachnoid cysts. *Neurosurgery.* 2007;61(3):505–513; discussion 513.
24. Invitti C, Pecori Giraldi F, de Martin M, Cavagnini F. Diagnosis and management of Cushing's syndrome: results of an Italian multicentre study. Study Group of the Italian Society of Endocrinology on the Pathophysiology of the Hypothalamic-Pituitary-Adrenal Axis. *J Clin Endocrinol Metab.* 1999;84(2):440–448.
25. Bochicchio D, Losa M, Buchfelder M. Factors influencing the immediate and late outcome of Cushing's disease treated by transsphenoidal surgery: a retrospective study by the European Cushing's Disease Survey Group. *J Clin Endocrinol Metab.* 1995;80(11):3114–3120.
26. Blevins LS Jr, Christy JH, Khajavi M, Tindall GT. Outcomes of therapy for Cushing's disease due to adrenocorticotropin-secreting pituitary macroadenomas. *J Clin Endocrinol Metab.* 1998;83(1):63–67.
27. Mampalam TJ, Tyrrell JB, Wilson CB. Transsphenoidal microsurgery for Cushing disease. A report of 216 cases. *Ann Intern Med.* 1988;109(6):487–493.
28. Swearingen B, Biller BM, Barker FG 2nd, et al. Long-term mortality after transsphenoidal surgery for Cushing disease. *Ann Intern Med.* 1999;130(10):821–824.
29. Hammer GD, Tyrrell JB, Lamborn KR, et al. Transsphenoidal microsurgery for Cushing's disease: initial outcome and long-term results. *J Clin Endocrinol Metab.* 2004;89(12):6348–6357.
30. De Tommasi C, Vance ML, Okonkwo DO, Diallo A, Laws ER Jr. Surgical management of adrenocorticotropic hormone-secreting macroadenomas: outcome and challenges in patients with Cushing's disease or Nelson's syndrome. *J Neurosurg.* 2005;103(5):825–830.
31. Ram Z, Nieman LK, Cutler GB Jr, Chrousos GP, Doppman JL, Oldfield EH. Early repeat surgery for persistent Cushing's disease. *J Neurosurg.* 1994;80(1):37–45.
32. Locatelli M, Vance ML, Laws ER. Clinical review: the strategy of immediate reoperation for transsphenoidal surgery for Cushing's disease. *J Clin Endocrinol Metab.* 2005;90(9):5478–5482.
33. Mahmoud-Ahmed AS, Suh JH. Radiation therapy for Cushing's disease: a review. *Pituitary.* 2002;5(3):175–180.
34. Yoon SC, Suh TS, Jang HS, et al. Clinical results of 24 pituitary macroadenomas with linac-based stereotactic radiosurgery. *Int J Radiat Oncol Biol Phys.* 1998;41(4):849–853.
35. Estrada J, Boronat M, Mielgo M, et al. The long-term outcome of pituitary irradiation after unsuccessful transsphenoidal surgery in Cushing's disease. *N Engl J Med.* 1997;336(3):172–177.

36. Mitsumori M, Shrieve DC, Alexander E III, et al. Initial clinical results of LINAC-based stereotactic radiosurgery and stereotactic radiotherapy for pituitary adenomas. *Int J Radiat Oncol Biol Phys.* 1998;42(3):573–580.
37. Sheehan JM, Vance ML, Sheehan JP, Ellegala DB, Laws ER Jr. Radiosurgery for Cushing's disease after failed transsphenoidal surgery. *J Neurosurg.* 2000;93(5):738–742.
38. Degerblad M, Rähn T, Bergstrand G, Thorén M. Long-term results of stereotactic radiosurgery to the pituitary gland in Cushing's disease. *Acta Endocrinol.* 1986;112(3):310–314.
39. Hayashi M, Izawa M, Hiyama H, et al. Gamma Knife radiosurgery for pituitary adenomas. *Stereotact Funct Neurosurg.* 1999;72(suppl 1):111–118.
40. Kim SH, Huh R, Chang JW, Park YG, Chung SS. Gamma Knife radiosurgery for functioning pituitary adenomas. *Stereotact Funct Neurosurg.* 1999;72(suppl 1):101–110.
41. Kobayashi T, Kida Y, Mori Y. Gamma knife radiosurgery in the treatment of Cushing disease: long-term results. *J Neurosurg.* 2002;97(5 suppl):422–428.
42. Littley MD, Shalet SM, Beardwell CG, Ahmed SR, Sutton ML. Long-term follow-up of low-dose external pituitary irradiation for Cushing's disease. *Clin Endocrinol (Oxf).* 1990;33(4):445–455.
43. Morange-Ramos I, Régis J, Dufour H, et al. Short-term endocrinological results after gamma knife surgery of pituitary adenomas. *Stereotact Funct Neurosurg.* 1998;70(suppl 1):127–138.
44. Devin JK, Allen GS, Cmelak AJ, Duggan DM, Blevins LS. The efficacy of linear accelerator radiosurgery in the management of patients with Cushing's disease. *Stereotact Funct Neurosurg.* 2004;82(5–6):254–262.
45. Mokry M, Ramschak-Schwarzer S, Simbrunner J, Ganz JC, Pendl G. A six year experience with the postoperative radiosurgical management of pituitary adenomas. *Stereotact Funct Neurosurg.* 1999;72(suppl 1):88–100.
46. Sonino N, Boscaro M, Paoletta A, Mantero F, Ziliotto D. Ketoconazole treatment in Cushing's syndrome: experience in 34 patients. *Clin Endocrinol (Oxf).* 1991;35(4):347–352.
47. Verhelst JA, Trainer PJ, Howlett TA, et al. Short and long-term responses to metyrapone in the medical management of 91 patients with Cushing's syndrome. *Clin Endocrinol (Oxf).* 1991;35(2):169–178.
48. Luton JP, Mahoudeau JA, Bouchard P, et al. Treatment of Cushing's disease by O,p'DDD. Survey of 62 cases. *N Engl J Med.* 1979;300(9):459–464.
49. Favia G, Boscaro M, Lumachi F, D'Amico DF. Role of bilateral adrenalectomy in Cushing's disease. *World J Surg.* 1994;18(4):462–466.
50. O'Riordain DS, Farley DR, Young WF Jr, Grant CS, van Heerden JA. Long-term outcome of bilateral adrenalectomy in patients with Cushing's syndrome. *Surgery.* 1994;116(6):1088–1093; discussion 1093.
51. Jenkins P, Trainer P, Plowman PN, et al.. The long-term outcome after adrenalectomy and prophylactic pituitary radiotherapy in adrenocorticotropin-dependent Cushing's syndrome. *J Clin Endocrinol Metab.* 1994;79:165–171.
52. Gillam MP, Molitch ME, Lombardi G, Colao A. Advances in the treatment of prolactinomas. *Endocr Rev.* 2006;27(5):485–534.
53. Vance ML, Evans WS, Thorner MO. Drugs five years later. Bromocriptine. *Ann Intern Med.* 1984;100(1):78–91.
54. Verhelst J, Abs R, Maiter D, et al. Cabergoline in the treatment of hyperprolactinemia: a study in 455 patients. *J Clin Endocrinol Metab.* 1999;84(7):2518–2522.
55. Zanettini R, Antonini A, Gatto G, Gentile R, Tesei S, Pezzoli G. Valvular heart disease and the use of dopamine agonists for Parkinson's disease. *N Engl J Med.* 2007;356(1):39–46.
56. Schlechte J, Dolan K, Sherman B, Chapler F, Luciano A. The natural history of untreated hyperprolactinemia: a prospective analysis. *J Clin Endocrinol Metab.* 1989;68(2):412–418.
57. Molitch ME, Elton RL, Blackwell RE, et al. Bromocriptine as primary therapy for prolactin-secreting macroadenomas: results of a prospective multicenter study. *J Clin Endocrinol Metab.* 1985;60(4):698–705.
58. Bevan JS, Webster J, Burke CW, Scanlon MF. Dopamine agonists and pituitary tumor shrinkage. *Endocr Rev.* 1992;13(2):220–240.
59. Losa M, Mortini P, Barzaghi R, Gioia L, Giovanelli M. Surgical treatment of prolactin-secreting pituitary adenomas: early results and long-term outcome. *J Clin Endocrinol Metab.* 2002;87(7):3180–3186.
60. Ezzat S, Forster MJ, Berchtold P, Redelmeier DA, Boerlin V, Harris AG. Acromegaly. Clinical and biochemical features in 500 patients. *Medicine (Baltimore).* 1994;73(5):233–240.
61. De P, Rees DA, Davies N, et al. Transsphenoidal surgery for acromegaly in wales: results based on stringent criteria of remission. *J Clin Endocrinol Metab.* 2003;88(8):3567–3572.
62. Kreutzer J, Vance ML, Lopes MB, Laws ER Jr. Surgical management of GH-secreting pituitary adenomas: an outcome study using modern remission criteria. *J Clin Endocrinol Metab.* 2001;86(9):4072–4077.
63. Eastman RC, Gorden P, Glatstein E, Roth J. Radiation therapy of acromegaly. *Endocrinol Metab Clin North Am.* 1992;21(3):693–712.
64. Attanasio R, Epaminonda P, Motti E, et al. Gamma-knife radiosurgery in acromegaly: a 4-year follow-up study. *J Clin Endocrinol Metab.* 2003;88(7):3105–3112.
65. Jaffe CA, Barkan AL. Treatment of acromegaly with dopamine agonists. *Endocrinol Metab Clin North Am.* 1992;21(3):713–735.
66. Abs R, Verhelst J, Maiter D, et al. Cabergoline in the treatment of acromegaly: a study in 64 patients. *J Clin Endocrinol Metab.* 1998;83(2):374–378.
67. Bevan JS. Clinical review: The antitumoral effects of somatostatin analog therapy in acromegaly. *J Clin Endocrinol Metab.* 2005;90(3):1856–1863.
68. Ezzat S, Snyder PJ, Young WF, et al. Octreotide treatment of acromegaly. A randomized, multicenter study. *Ann Intern Med.* 1992;117(9):711–718.
69. Stewart PM, Kane KF, Stewart SE, Lancranjan I, Sheppard MC. Depot long-acting somatostatin analog (Sandostatin-LAR) is an effective treatment for acromegaly. *J Clin Endocrinol Metab.* 1995;80(11):3267–3272.
70. Caron P, Morange-Ramos I, Cogne M, Jaquet P. Three year follow-up of acromegalic patients treated with intramuscular slow-release lanreotide. *J Clin Endocrinol Metab.* 1997;82(1):18–22.
71. Freda PU. Somatostatin analogs in acromegaly. *J Clin Endocrinol Metab.* 2002;87(7):3013–3018.
72. Muller AF, Kopchick JJ, Flyvbjerg A, van der Lely AJ. Clinical review 166: Growth hormone receptor antagonists. *J Clin Endocrinol Metab.* 2004;89(4):1503–1511.
73. Brucker-Davis F, Oldfield EH, Skarulis MC, Doppman JL, Weintraub BD. Thyrotropin-secreting pituitary tumors: diagnostic criteria, thyroid hormone sensitivity, and treatment outcome in 25 patients followed at the National Institutes of Health. *J Clin Endocrinol Metab.* 1999;84(2):476–486.
74. Chanson P, Weintraub BD, Harris AG. Octreotide therapy for thyroid-stimulating hormone-secreting pituitary adenomas. A follow-up of 52 patients. *Ann Intern Med.* 1993;119(3):236–240.
75. Snyder PJ. Gonadotroph cell adenomas of the pituitary. *Endocr Rev.* 1985;6(4):552–563.
76. Ebersold MJ, Quast LM, Laws ER Jr, Scheithauer B, Randall RV. Long-term results in transsphenoidal removal of nonfunctioning pituitary adenomas. *J Neurosurg.* 1986;64(5):713–719.
77. Lillehei KO, Kirschman DL, Kleinschmidt-DeMasters BK, Ridgway EC. Reassessment of the role of radiation therapy in the treatment of endocrine-inactive pituitary macroadenomas. *Neurosurgery.* 1998;43(3):432–438; discussion 438–439.
78. Kaltsas GA, Nomikos P, Kontogeorgos G, Buchfelder M, Grossman AB. Clinical review: Diagnosis and management of pituitary carcinomas. *J Clin Endocrinol Metab.* 2005;90(5):3089–3099.
79. Scheithauer BW, Kurtkaya-Yapicier O, Kovacs KT, Young WF Jr, Lloyd RV. Pituitary carcinoma: a clinicopathological review. *Neurosurgery.* 2005;56(5):1066–1074; discussion 1066.

70 Medical Treatment of Spinal Cord Tumors

Karine Michaud

INTRODUCTION

This chapter focuses on medical treatment of different spinal cord tumors. The chapter is divided into three sections: extradural, intradural, and intramedullary lesion. Rarely is the medical treatment the mainstay of treatment of spinal lesions. Detailed medical treatment of specific systemic diseases is over the scope of this chapter. Specific pediatric considerations are outline in each section.

EXTRADURAL

Metastasis

The vast majority of extradural neoplasms in adults are metastatic. They are the results of hematogenous spread through the venous system of Batson's plexus into the vertebral elements of the spine. The spine is the most common site of skeletal metastatic involvement [1]. Conservatively, at least 30% of patients with systemic malignancies will develop spinal metastasis over the course of their disease [2]. Of the solid primary tumors, breast, lung, and prostate are the most prevalent, followed by renal, gastrointestinal, and thyroid tumors. Therapeutic decision making depends on several factors: the patient's general medical condition; the tumor type and its radiosensitivity; tumor stage, including the patient's life expectancy; previous therapy; neurological condition; time course of symptom onset; extent of spinal involvement, including issues of instability; and patient/ family wishes [3]. Surgery for one of the goals, namely, oncologic, stabilization, diagnostic, and/or radiotherapy, are the first-line of treatment for spine metastasis.

Pain Management

Pain is the initial symptom in 90% to 95% of patients with spinal metastasis [4]. Pain can be localized to the back in the area of involvement, radicular, myelopathic, or from mechanical instability. Obviously, the treatment of the metastasis constitutes the primary source of relief of the pain. Because inadequate pain relief has a significant effect on functional status and quality of life, it should be a priority in the treatment of those patients. A multimodalities approach should be undertaken, including systemic and local therapies such as radiation, nerve block, and surgery.

Analgesic therapy requires an ongoing assessment and adjustment of therapy. It is beneficial to involve pain specialists with cancer experience early in the course of the treatment. Anti-inflammatory agents are often used for mild pain. Opioids may be necessary with more significant pain. Sustained-released opioids allow for a more even pain control and can be supplemented by rapid-release agents for breakthrough pain. Neuropathic pain can be treated with anticonvulsants, such as gabapentin and pregabaline, and antidepressants, such as amitriptyline, desipramine, and nortriptyline. Epidural and intrathecal administration can be considered. Surgical treatment of pain such as cordotomy can also be considered in terminal/intractable cases. Steroids can improve pain relief and neurological function.

Biphosphonate Therapy

Biphosphonates are pyrophosphonates analogs that bind strongly to hydroxyapatite crystals in bone mineral, and, because their structure renders them resistant to enzyme degradation, they act principally by inhibiting bone resorption through osteoclast inhibition, although some effect on bone formation probably also occurs [5]. Agents such as pamidronate and zoledronate have been used to reduce bones metastasis-related complications such as development of pathological fractures, pain, spinal cord compression, hypercalcemia, and need for radiation and surgery [6]. There is also evidence that biphosphonates may have antiapoptotic and antiproliferative effects on macrophages and tumor cells [7].

Systemic Chemotherapy/Hormonal Therapy

With the exception of prostate, breast, and renal cell carcinoma, spinal metastases occur late in the course of the disease so patients are likely to have failed first- and second-line therapies, with progression of visceral and bone disease. Having failed the most effective systemic regimens, those patients are unlikely to have a good response to subsequent therapeutic trials. Breast and prostate cancer are particularly prone to respond to systemic treatment.

Primary Bone Lesions

Malignant

Primary malignant bone tumors are infrequent compared to metastasis. Treatment varies widely depending on the precise histologic type.

For plasmocytoma, multiple myeloma, and lymphoma, the primary treatment of spinal disease is nonsurgical. Surgery is usually reserved for diagnostic purposes; decompression in the case of acute, severe, and symptomatic compression of the spinal cord; or stabilization in case of spinal instability. Those lesions are exquisitely sensitive to radiotherapy, and this represents the primary treatment modality. Systemic chemotherapy is used to treat the primary disease.

Chordomas are benign histologically but malignant in behavior because of their local invasiveness, high recurrence rate, and potential for metastasis. The first line of treatment is aggressive surgical resection. Chordomas are typically radioresistant, and radiotherapy has a palliative role only [8]. The well-defined Bragg peak of protons allows planning with a sharp cutoff outside the target volume. This permits a higher dose of radiotherapy to be delivered to the tumor while avoiding excessive irradiation to radiosensitive structures [9].

Because of the relatively low proliferating rate of chordomas, chemotherapy is usually ineffective. There has been a report of responses for dedifferentiated chordomas with a combination of six drugs, including etoposide, cisplatin, vincristine, dacarbazine, cyclophosphamide, and doxorubicin [10].

Osteosarcoma is a rare tumor that affects the spine in only 3% of the cases. It affects mainly teenagers and young adults and the outcome remains poor despite aggressive treatment. To maximize chances of survival, aggressive surgical resection is the single most important factor. Neoadjuvant chemotherapy, usually methotrexate in combination with bleomycin, cyclophosphamide, dactnomyocin, and doxorubicin, should be used preoperatively [11]. Postoperative radiotherapy and chemotherapy should be given to attempt cure.

Spinal chondrosarcomas are often low-grade lesions with good prognosis. Radical surgical resection with wide margin is the mainstay of treatment. Radiotherapy has a palliative role only. Chemotherapy is reserved for dedifferentiated chondrosarcomas and regimens usually include doxorubicin, and cisplatin [12].

Pediatry

Ewing's sarcoma is the most common nonprimary malignant tumor involving the spine in children. Radical resection is difficult to obtain, and subtotal resection with decompression of neural structures is usually the goal of the initial surgery with a mind toward a second-look surgery after radiotherapy and chemotherapy. Chemotherapy commonly consists of vincristine, dactinomycin, cyclophosphamide, and doxorubicin [13,14].

Neuroblastoma is the most common extracranial malignancy in children. Treatment of neuroblastoma includes surgical decompression and multiagent chemotherapy. The role of radiotherapy is less clear because the results are inconsistent. Different combination of the following have been used: Cisplatin, cyclophosphamide, doxorubicin, etoposide, vincristine and topotecan [15].

Benign

Benign tumors of the spine include the following: osteoid osteoma, osteoblastoma, osteochondroma, hemangioma, aneurysmal bone cyst, giant cell tumor, and eosinophilic granuloma. For most benign spinal bone lesions, there is no medical treatment. Surveillance in most asymptomatic cases is recommended. Cure is usually amenable by total surgical resection.

Osteoid osteoma is a tumor of children and adolescent that usually presents with nonradiating back pain that is typically relieved by salicylates [16].

Eosinophilic granuloma is another benign tumor of the children and adolescents. It can be a solitary granuloma or part of a Langerhans cell histiocytosis complexes; either the acute Hand-Schuller-Christian disease or the subacute Letterer-Siwe disease. Conservative treatment is recommended for the unique granuloma. For systemic variants of histiocytosis, chemotherapy is used and various combination of prednisone, vincristine, vinblastin, methotrexate, VP-16, cyclophosphamide, or cyclosporine-A have been reported [17].

INTRADURAL-EXTRAMEDULLARY

Meningioma

The primary treatment of spinal meningiomas is surgical resection. Radiation therapy and radiosurgery have a limited role in benign meningioma. It should be reserved for tumor with atypical or malignant biologic behavior or in cases where repeat resection carries significant medical or surgical risks. Compared to other locations, the recurrence rate of spinal meningiomas is low [18]. Factors correlated to recurrence rate are older age, invasion of the arachnoid/pia mater, and histopathology. Chemotherapy has a limited role in treatment of spinal meningiomas and is usually reserved for recurrent malignant disease. Malignant and atypical meningiomas are rare in the spine. Medical treatment is extrapolated from cerebral meningiomas. Chemotherapy regimens used for malignant meningiomas include combinations of adriamycin and dacarbazine or ifosfamide and mesna, interferon alpha has also been reported [19]. There are reports of disease stabilization and even tumor response with hydroxyurea [20,21]. Targeted therapies are currently investigated.

Nerve Sheath Tumors of the Spine

Treatment of spinal schwanommas and benign neurofibromas is surgery. Association with neurofibromatosis 1 (NF1) and NF2 is well recognized. Prognosis of malignant nerve sheath tumors (MNSTs) involving the spine is uniformly poor and CNS seeding occurs early. En bloc resection aimed at cure is usually unobtainable because of the spinal cord proximity. Radiotherapy provides local control and may delay the onset of recurrence but has little effect on long-term survival rates. It is nevertheless recommended postoperatively [22].

Chemotherapy for adult soft tissue sarcomas is usually confined to the treatment of metastatic disease. Systemic spread, especially pulmonary metastasis, is a terminal event, and despite its limited efficacy, chemotherapy is indicated in this situation [23].

Malignant peripheral nerve sheath tumor (MPNST) appears to be of intermediate chemosensitivity. Options are single-agent doxorubicin or a combination of doxorubicin and ifosfamide with a partial response rate of 20% to 25% [24]. Dacarbazine has been shown to have activity against these tumors and was combined with doxorubicin in the CYVADIC chemotherapy regimen [25]. Very rare in children, MPNSTs have been consistently resistant to chemotherapy in case reports [26].

Targeted therapies are being investigated in the treatment of nerve sheath tumors. The NF1 heterozygote mast cell plays a significant role in the process of neurofibroma-related tumorigenesis, due in part to increased levels of stem cell factors in the local microenvironment, which promote hypermotility, hyperproliferation, and chemotaxis to the tumor microenvironment. Clinical trials using ketotifen fumarate, an antihistamine that helps to stabilize mast cells and prevent degranulation to inhibit mast cell function, showed subjective improvements in quality of life and decreased pruritus, pain, and tenderness. The effects on tumor size and growth were consistently positive although less uniform [27,28]. Thalidomide is an antiangiogenic agent that has been used in early clinical trial to treat MPNSTs [29]. Pirfenidone, an antifibrotic agent that inhibits fibroblast function by modulating the effect of growth-inducing cytokines, has been tested as a treatment for patients with NF1 and neurofibromas [30]. Erlotinib has been examined as a therapeutic approach for treatment of unresectable or metastatic MPNST and no demonstrable effect on progression was noted [31]. The receptor tyrosine kinase inhibitor STI571 (Gleveec) is a potent inhibitor of KIT and has been reported to result in dramatic tumor regressions in patients with gastrointestinals stromal tumors that appear to be durable [32]. Laboratory data have shown that it can inhibit cell invasion of MPNST in vitro [33]. Clinical studies are pending, but Gleevec seems like an interesting agent.

Ependymoma Myxopapillary

Maximal safe resection is recommended. Radiotherapy is debated in subtotal resection. Chemotherapy is reserved for recurrent unresectable disease that has already been exposed to radiotherapy. Case reports of etoposide, cisplatin, and tamoxifen have been reported with varying success [34,35].

Paraganglioma

Paragangliomas (chemodectomas) are tumors of the paraganglia and are composed of specialized neural crest cells arising in association with sympathetic ganglia. They frequently display an indolent course, often spanning a decade or more. They tend to be invasive and are associated with a high rate of local recurrence, especially after inadequate resection [36]. Patel et al. (1995) reviewed the 15-year experience with paragangliomas at M. D. Anderson Cancer Center and reported a 46% response rate with doxorubicin, dacarbazine, and cyclophosphamide-containing regimens. Solitary case reports have demonstrated activity for several agents, including carboplatin, cisplatin, etoposide, and gemcitabine [37–39] Yet another group reported no responses to a variety of chemotherapeutic regimens, including cyclophosphamide, cisplatin, doxorubicin, and dacarbazine in metastatic paragangliomas [40].

INTRAMEDULLARY

Ependymoma

Prognosis depends on extent of resection. Gross totally resected lesions with a clear plane are usually followed. Subtotally resected lesions have a high recurrence rate and therefore radiotherapy is recommended. In children, there is a concern about radiatotherapy and impact on children growth. The role of chemotherapy has not been well defined, and it is usually reserved for recurrent tumor in adults. About 50% of ependymomas occur in children less than 5 years old, who are more susceptible to the side effects of radiotherapy; chemotherapy in this patient population assumes a vital role [41]. Multiple agents and combinations have shown at least some degree of efficacy in intracranial ependymomas: carboplatin and etoposide, "8-in-1" ("8-in-1" refers to eight drugs in one day regimen, consisting of vincristine, carmustine, procarbazine, hydroxyurea, cisplatin, cytarabine, prednisone, and cyclophosphamide), carboplatin, ifosfamide, cyclophosphamide, and vincristine alternating with carboplatin and etoposide, and ICE [42–46]. Platinum-based chemotherapy regimens appear to result in higher response rates with lower rates of progression than nitrosourea-based regimens in recurrent tumors. Other regimens that do not include cisplatinum or nitrosourea appear to be even less effective [47]. Two reports on specific intramedullary ependymomas showed minimal response to Aziridinylbenzoquinone and Interferon-a2b [48,49].

Astrocytoma

Spinal astrocytoma are treated with maximal safe resection and adjuvant radiotherapy for residual or recurrent disease. There is no clear role for chemotherapy in adults. Studies regimens include "8-in-1," CCNU, and vincristine, carboplatin and vincristine, and PCV [50–53].

Hemangioblastoma

Radical resection is the mainstay of treatment. Asymptomatic lesions, particularly multiple lesions in the context of von Hippel-Lindau syndrome can be followed. The role of radiotherapy is not fully defined. There is no clear role for chemotherapy.

Sunitinib a multitargeted receptor tyrosine kinase (RTK) inhibitor (inhibiting PDGFR, VEGFR, and KIT) is currently studied in phase-II clinical trial in intracranial hemangioblastoma, hemangiopericytoma, and menigioma.

Metastasis

There have been reports in the literature of patients with intramedullary metastases treated with chemotherapy [54–57]. Most authors recommend chemotherapy if there is associated carcinomatous meningitis [58].

REFERENCES

1. Katagiri H, Takahashi M, Inagaki J, et al. Clinical results of nonsurgical treatment for spinal metastases. *Int J Radiat Oncol Biol Phys*. 1998;42(5):1127–1132.
2. Ortiz Gómez JA. The incidence of vertebral body metastases. *Int Orthop*. 1995;19(5):309–311.
3. Schuster JM, Grady MS. Medical management and adjuvant therapies in spinal metastatic disease. *Neurosurg Focus*. 2001;11(6):e3.
4. Bradley Jacobs W, Perrin RG. Evaluation and treatment of spinal metastases: an overview. *Neurosurg Focus*. 2001;11(6):e10.
5. Tsuchimoto M, Azuma Y, Higuchi O, et al. Alendronate modulates osteogenesis of human osteoblastic cells in vitro. *Jpn J Pharmacol*. 1994;66(1):25–33.
6. Berenson JR, Lichtenstein A, Porter L, et al. Efficacy of pamidronate in reducing skeletal events in patients with advanced multiple myeloma. Myeloma Aredia Study Group. *N Engl J Med*. 1996;334(8):488–493.
7. Senaratne SG, Pirianov G, Mansi JL, et al: Bisphosphonates induce apoptosis in human breast cancer cell lines. *Br J Cancer*. 2000;82:1459–1468.
8. Catton C, O Sulhvan B, Bell R, et al. Chordoma. long-term follow up after radical photon irradiation. *Radiother Oncol*. 1996;41:67–70.
9. The Proton Therapy Working Party. Proton therapy for base of skull chordoma: a report for the Royal College of Radiologists. *Clin Oncol*. 2000;12:75–79.
10. Fleming GF, Heimann PS, Stephens JK, et al. Dedifferentiated Chordoma: response to aggressive chemotherapy in two cases. *Cancer*. 1993;72(3):714–718.
11. Smeland S, Wiebe T, Böhling t, et al. Chemotherapy in osteosarcoma. The Scandinavian Sarcoma Group experience. *Acta Orthop Scand Suppl*. 2004;75(311):92–98.
12. Mitchell AD, Ayoub K, Mangham DC, et al. Experience in the treatment of dedifferentiated chondrosarcoma. *J Bone Joint Surg*. 2000;82:B55-B61.
13. Kissane JM, Askin FB, Foulkes M, et al. Ewing's Sarcoma of bone. *Hum Pathol*. 1983;14:773–779.
14. Zucker JM, Henry-Amar M, Sarrazin D, Blache R, Patte C, Schweisguth O. Intensive systemic chemotherapy in localized Ewing's sarcoma in childhood. A historical trial. *Cancer*. 1983;52(3):415–423.
15. Maris M. John. Recent Advances in Neuroblastoma. *N Engl J Med* 2010;362:2202–2211.
16. Raskas DS, Graziano GP, Herzenberg JE, Heidelberger KP, Hensinger RN. Osteoid osteoma and osteoblastoma of the spine. *J Spinal Disord*. 1992;5(2):204–211.
17. Donadieu J. Langerhans' cell histiocytosis. *Orphanet Encyclopedia*. May 2003;1–8.
18. Mirimanoff RO, Dosoretz DE, Linggood RM, Ojemann RG, Martuza RL. Meningioma: analysis of recurrence and progression following neurosurgical resection. *J Neurosurg*. 1985;62(1):18–24.
19. Kyritsis AR. Chemotherapy for meningiomas. *J Neuro-Oncol*. 1996;29:269–272.
20. Umh S, Rittig MG, Anders M, et al. Hydroxyurea for treatment of unresectable and recurrentmeningiomas. II. Decrease in the size of meningiomas in patients treated with hydroxyurea. *J Neurosurg*. 1997;86:840–844.
21. Newton BH. Hydroxyurea chemotherapy in the treatment of meningiomas. *Neurosurg Focus*. 2007;23(4):E11.
22. Ferner RE, Gutmann DH. International consensus statement on malignant peripheral nerve sheath tumors in neurofibromatosis. *Cancer Res*. 2002;62(5):1573–1577.
23. Angelov L, Davis A, O'Sullivan B, Bell R, Guha A. Neurogenic sarcomas: experience at the University of Toronto. *Neurosurgery*. 1998;43(1):56–64; discussion 64.
24. Santoro A, Tursz T, Mouridsen H, et al. Doxorubicin versus CYVADIC versus doxorubicin plus ifosfamide in first-line treatment of advanced soft tissue sarcomas: a randomized study of the European Organization for Research and Treatment of Cancer Soft Tissue and Bone Sarcoma Group. *J Clin Oncol*. 1995;13(7):1537–1545.
25. Bramwell V, Rouesse J, Steward W, et al. Adjuvant CYVADIC chemotherapy for adult soft tissue sarcoma–reduced local recurrence but no improvement in survival: a study of the European Organization for Research and Treatment of Cancer Soft Tissue and Bone Sarcoma Group. *J Clin Oncol*. 1994;12(6):1137–1149.
26. Yone K, Ijiri K, Hayashi K, et al. Primary malignant peripheral nerve sheath tumor of the cauda equina in a child case report. *Spinal Cord*. 2004;42(3):199–203.
27. Riccardi VM. A controlled multiphase trial of ketotifen to minimize neurofibroma-associated pain and itching. *Arch Dermatol*. 1993;129:577–581.
28. Riccardi VM. Mast-cell stabilization to decrease neurofibroma growth. Preliminary experience with ketotifen. *Arch Dermatol*. 1987;123(8):1011–1016.
29. Gupta A, Cohen BH, Ruggieri P, Packer RJ, Phillips PC. Phase I study of thalidomide for the treatment of plexiform neurofibroma in neurofibromatosis 1. *Neurology*. 2003;60(1):130–132.
30. Babovic-Vuksanovic D, Ballman K, Michels V, et al. Phase II trial of pirfenidone in adults with neurofibromatosis type 1. *Neurology*. 2006;67(10):1860–1862.
31. Kea A. Phase II study of erlotinib in metastatic or unresectable malignant peripheral nerve sheath tumors (MPNST). *J Clin Oncol*. 2006;24(18 Suppl):Abstract.
32. Oosterom AT, Judson IR, Verweij J, et al. STI571, an active drug in metastatic gastro-intestinal stromal tumors (GIST) an EORTC Phase I study. *Proc Am Soc Clin Oncol*. 2001;20:Abstract.
33. Aoki M, Nabeshima K, Koga K, et al. Imatinib mesylate inhibits cell invasion of malignant peripheral nerve sheath tumor induced by platelet-derived growth factor-BB. *Lab Invest*. 2007;87(8):767–779.
34. Madden JR, Fenton LZ, Weil M, Winston KR, Partington M, Foreman NK. Experience with tamoxifen/etoposide in the treatment of a child with myxopapillary ependymoma. *Med Pediatr Oncol*. 2001;37(1):67–69.
35. Schweitzer JS, Batzdorf U. Ependymoma of the cauda equina region: diagnosis, treatment, and outcome in 15 patients. *Neurosurgery*. 1992;30(2):202–207.
36. Patel SR, Winchester DJ, Benjamin RS. A fifteen year experience with chemotherapy of patients with paraganglioma. *Cancer*. 1995;76:1476–1480.
37. Cairnduff F, Smith IE. Carboplatin chemotherapy for malignant paraganglioma. *Lancet*. 1986;2(8513):982.
38. Mertens WC, Grignon DJ, Romano W. Malignant paraganglioma with skeletal metastases and spinal cord compression: response and palliation with chemotherapy. *Clin. Oncol*. 1993;5:126–128.
39. Pipas JM, Krywicki RF. Treatment of progressive metastatic glomus jugulare tumor (paraganglioma) with gemcitabine. *Neuro-oncology*. 2000;2(3):190–191.
40. Massey V, Wallner K. Treatment of metastatic chemodectoma. *Cancer*. 1992;69(3):790–792.
41. Casilda Balmaceda. Chemotherapy for intramedullary spinal cord tumors. *J Neuro-Oncol*. 2000;47:293–307.
42. Fouladi M, Baruchel S, Chan H, et al. Use of adjuvant ICE chemotherapy in the treatment of anaplastic ependymomas. *Childs Nerv Syst*. 1998;14(10):590–595.
43. Sexauer CL, Khan A, Burger PC, et al. Cisplatin in recurrent pediatric brain tumors. A POG Phase II study. A Pediatric Oncology Group Study. *Cancer*. 1985;56(7):1497–1501.
44. Gaynon PS, Ettinger U, Baum ES, Siegel SE, Krailo MD, Hominid GD: Carboplatin in childhood brain tumors. *Cancer*. 1990;66:2465–2469.
45. Chastagner P, Sommelet-Olive D, Kalifa C, et al. Phase II study of ifosfamide in childhood brain tumors: a report by the French Society of Pediatric Oncology (SFOP). *Med Pediatr Oncol*. 1993;21(1):49–53.

46. Duffner PK, Krischer JP, Burger PC, et al. Treatment of infants with malignant gliomas: the Pediatric Oncology Group experience. *J Neurooncol*. 1996;28(2–3):245–256.
47. Gornet MK, Buckner JC, Marks RS, Scheithauer BW, Erickson BJ. Chemotherapy for advanced CNS ependymoma. *J Neurooncol*. 1999;45(1):61–67.
48. Tan TC, Hancock CH, Mondora A, Hoffman N. Phase I study of aziridinylbenzoquinone (AZQ, NSC 182986) in children with cancer. *Cancer Res*. 1984;44:831–835.
49. Dorr RT, Salmon SE, Robertone A, Bonnem E. Phase I-II trial of interferon-alpha 2b by continuous subcutaneous infusion over 28 days. *J Interferon Res*. 1988;8(6):717–725.
50. Allen JV, Avivner S, Yates AJ, et al. Treatment of high-grade spinal cord astrocytoma of childhood with '8-in-1' chemotherapy and radiotherapy: a pilot study of CCG-945. *J Neurosurg*. 1998;88:215–220.
51. Packer RJ, Lange B, Ater J, et al. Carboplatin and vincristine for recurrent and newly diagnosed low-grade gliomas of childhood. *J Clin Oncol*. 1993;11(5):850–856.
52. Bouffet E, Amat D, Devaux Y, Desuzinges C. Chemotherapy for spinal cord astrocytoma. *Med Pediatr Oncol*. 1997;29(6):560–562.
53. Henson JW, Thornton AF, Louis DN. Spinal cord astrocytoma: response to PCV chemotherapy. *Neurology*. 2000;54(2):518–520.
54. Grem JL, Burgess J, Trump DL. Clinical features and natural history of intramedullary spinal cord metastasis. *Cancer*. 1985;56(9):2305–2314.
55. Ferroir JP, Cadranel J, Khalil A, Lebreton C, Contant S, Milleron B. [Intramedullary metastases of bronchogenic carcinoma. Two cases]. *Rev Neurol (Paris)*. 1998;154(2):166–169.
56. Connolly ES Jr, Winfree CJ, McCormick PC, Cruz M, Stein BM: Intramedullary spinal cord metastasis: report of three cases an review of the literature. *Surg Neurol*. 1996;46:329–337.
57. Dunne JW, Harper CG, Pamphlett R. Intramedullary spinal cord metastases: a clinical and pathological study of nine cases. *Q J Med*. 1986;61:1003–1020.
58. Schiff D, O'Neill BP. Intramedullary spinal cord metastases: clinical features and treatment outcome. *Neurology*. 1996;47:906–912.

71 Brain Metastases and Leptomeningeal Disease

Michelle E. Melisko

INCIDENCE

Brain metastases are the most common intracranial tumors in adults, occurring in approximately 10% to 30% of adult cancer patients [1,2]. Up to 170 000 new cases of brain metastases occur in the United States each year [3]. Brain metastases are most common among patients with lung cancer, which accounts for approximately one half of all brain metastases. Breast cancer, renal cell carcinoma, and melanoma are other malignancies commonly associated with brain metastases, but central nervous system (CNS) disease also occurs among patients with nearly all solid tumors including ovarian cancer, colon cancer, germ cell tumors, sarcomas, and carcinomas of unknown primary [4,5]. The incidence of brain metastases appears to be increasing among patients with metastatic disease who experience prolonged survival with improved control of systemic disease [6]. In addition, advances in technology and more frequent use of imaging modalities, such as magnetic resonance imaging (MRI), may detect smaller metastases in asymptomatic patients [7].

Among certain tumor types, particularly breast cancer, there have been a number of studies suggesting that subsets of patients may be at significantly higher risk of developing brain metastases. Early age at diagnosis, estrogen receptor (ER) negative disease, and presence of visceral disease have consistently been associated with an elevated risk of developing CNS disease among breast cancer patients [8–10]. Analysis of 664 patients with newly diagnosed breast cancer demonstrated that patients with tumors overexpressing the ErbB2 oncogene developed brain metastases four times more frequently than patients with non-ErbB2 overexpressing tumors [11].

At the time of diagnosis, approximately 10% of patient with small cell lung cancer (SCLC) present with brain metastases, and the percentage of patients with brain metastases increases to 50% to 80% after 2 years of survival [12,13]. Incidence of brain metastases is so high and has such an impact on outcomes among SCLC patients that prophylactic whole-brain radiation therapy (WBRT) has been tested in this population. A meta-analysis, and more recently, a randomized clinical trial have found that prophylactic cranial irradiation improved both overall survival and disease-free survival among patients with SCLC in complete remission [14,15].

Diagnosis and Prognosis

The diagnosis of brain metastasis is most commonly made during a radiologic examination ordered to investigate symptoms such as headache, dizziness, disturbances in vision, speech, or balance, or other focal neurologic deficits. One recent study found that approximately 70% of brain metastases are found in the cerebral hemispheres, 20% to 25% in the cerebellum, and 5% in the brainstem [16]. Brain metastases may be single or multifocal, and the prognosis, as well as appropriate treatment, is associated with the number, size, and location of brain metastases.

Retrospective studies have reported that the median survival of patients with brain metastases is less than 1 month if left untreated, 6 to 8 weeks if treated with steroids alone, and 3 to 6 months when treated with WBRT [17–20]. Single institution studies have shown that patients with a single brain metastasis amenable to treatment with surgery followed by radiation therapy have a significantly better prognosis, with median survival in the range of 10 to 18 months, or much longer in some cases [21]. Survival after the diagnosis of brain metastases depends on a number of factors, and a small number of patients may experience prolonged survival. For example, a retrospective review of 740 patients with brain metastases from various solid tumors identified 51 that survived 2 or more years from the time of diagnosis of the brain metastasis [22]. For all tumor types, the actuarial survival rate was 8.1% at 2 years, 4.8% at 3 years, and 2.4% at 5 years. At 2 years, patients with ovarian carcinoma had the highest survival rate (23.9%) and patients with SCLC had the lowest survival rate (1.7%). Multivariate analysis showed younger age, single metastasis, surgical resection, WBRT, and chemotherapy were associated with prolonged survival. Other studies have also identified features that predict for better survival including good performance status, age younger than 65 years, absence of extracranial metastases, or control of extracranial systemic disease.

A number of prognostic indices have been developed defining groups of patients with brain metastases in order to guide treatment decisions. The Radiation Therapy Oncology Group (RTOG) recursive partitioning analysis (RPA) describes three prognostic classes, defined by age, Karnofsky performance score (KPS), and disease status. RPA class 1 patients are younger (<65 years) and have higher KPS scores (≥70), no other sites of metastases with a controlled primary tumor, while RPA class 3 patients have a KPS <70, and RPA class 2 encompasses all other patients. The development and implementation of this index through analysis of outcomes of over 1200 patients in several RTOG trials revealed that median survival was 7.1 months for RPA class 1 patients, 4.2 months for RPA class 2 patients, and only 2.3 months for class 3 patients [23].

A new index, the Graded Prognostic Assessment (GPA), was recently shown to be as prognostic as the RPA as well as the least subjective, most quantitative, and easiest to use among a number of indices studied in the updated RTOG database [24]. The GPA is the sum of scores (0, 0.5, and 1.0) for four factors: age, KPS, extracranial metastases (none and present), and number of metastases (one, two to three, and more than three). The GPA was developed to improve upon several weaknesses of other indices, including the fact that control of extracranial disease is a somewhat subjective measure, and the absence of the inclusion of the number of brain metastases, which has been shown to be prognostic in other RTOG studies.

TREATMENT

Radiation Therapy

WBRT is the most frequently utilized treatment specific for brain metastases, particularly when the number or size of metastases precludes surgical resection or stereotactic radiosurgery (SRS). Between 50% to 80% of patients respond initially to WBRT [25–27]. Multiple studies have addressed the optimal WBRT regimen for patients with cerebral metastases. The RTOG has conducted a series of trials evaluating radiation dose, fractionation, and scheduling. Radiation doses of 20 to 40 Gy over periods of 2 to 4 weeks have been compared, and no significant differences have been observed in response rates or median survival [28–31].

Larger doses and accelerated fractionation (AF) have also been explored. The RTOG conducted a study comparing accelerated hyperfractionated (AH) radiotherapy (1.6 Gy twice a day) to a total dose of 54.4 Gy to an AF of 30 Gy in 10 daily fractions in patients with unresected brain metastasis [32]. The median survival time was 4.5 months in both arms and, in a multivariate model, only age, KPS, extent of metastatic disease (intracranial metastases only vs intra- and extracranial metastases), and status of primary (controlled vs uncontrolled) were statistically significant predictors of outcome. Therefore, this AH regimen to 54.4 Gy is generally not recommended for patients with intracranial metastatic disease.

Several studies in breast and lung cancer patients have explored short-course WBRT with 5 fractions of 4 Gy each [33,34]. The dose of 5 fractions of 4 Gy each resulted in survival and local control that was similar to longer programs of treatment and may be preferable for the majority of these patients because it is less time consuming and more convenient. Studies have shown that larger fractions over shorter periods of time may lead to faster neurologic improvement but may result in late radiation-associated toxicities such as dementia. Several studies have found the encephalopathic effects of 3 Gy or larger fractions had an onset of latency from 6 months to 3 years [35,36]. Based on the available data, the most common WBRT regimen has remained 30 Gy in 10 fractions. However, patients who have well-controlled systemic disease who are predicted to live longer than 6 months are frequently treated with smaller fraction size up to a total dose of 45 Gy over a longer period of time in order to avoid the possible long-term neurologic complications [20].

Surgical Resection Alone or with Radiotherapy

Selected patients with a single or a small number of brain metastases may be candidates for surgical resection, and in some cases such patients experience extended survival. Significant advances in microsurgical resection of brain tumors over the past 15 years have led to decreased morbidity and surgical mortality rates of less than 1% [37]. Unlike primary brain tumors, most metastatic lesions displace the brain tissue rather than infiltrate and intermix with functional tissue. However, most patients receive either WBRT or focal radiation to the tumor bed around the time of resection because surgery alone provides poor long-term local control with local recurrence rates for surgical resection alone of 46%, decreasing to 10% when WBRT is added postoperatively [21].

A number of trials have compared WBRT to surgical resection in patients with a single brain metastasis. In a prospective randomized trial of 48 patients, patients treated with surgery and WBRT had fewer local recurrences, better quality of life, and improved survival (40 weeks vs 15 weeks) than patients treated with WBRT alone [38]. These results were confirmed in another prospective randomized trial that showed prolonged survival (10 months vs 6 months) in patients who underwent surgery and WBRT compared to WBRT alone [39]. In contrast to these two studies, one randomized controlled trial of 84 patients with a single brain metastasis found no difference in survival between patients receiving radiation alone compared to patients who underwent surgery plus radiation (median survival 6.3 vs 5.6 months) [40]. Extracranial metastases were an important predictor of mortality, and this trial included a higher number of patients with disease outside the brain, perhaps explaining the lack of benefit from surgery in this patient population.

Retrospective studies have also concluded that surgery offers significant benefit. In a study of 70 breast cancer patients with brain metastases amenable to resection, median survival was 16 months [41]. In this series, median survival was not significantly different between patients with solitary vs multiple metastases (10.9 months and 14.8 months). While most of the patients in this series received WBRT after surgical resection, a small number underwent surgery when they experienced CNS recurrence or progression after previous WBRT. Another retrospective analysis was performed to evaluate the role of surgery followed by WBRT in the management of 46 patients with solitary and multiple brain metastases from a variety of solid tumors, with lung cancer as the primary site for 56% of the patients [42]. The median survival of all 46 patients was 11 months. Severe neurologic impairment at the time of diagnosis and the presence of multiple brain metastases were associated with a significantly poorer survival.

One of the most recent analyses addressing the role of surgery is a retrospective study of 208 patients with solid tumors who underwent surgical resection of one or more brain metastases [43]. The median survival from surgery was 8 months for all patients and 9 months for patients who did not undergo prior WBRT. There was no difference in survival between patients with a single metastasis versus two or three metastases (8 months vs 9 months). High KPS and RPA Class I assignment were associated with improved outcomes.

In summary, most studies evaluating surgery for patients with a single or even a small number of brain metastases suggest that surgical resection improves neurological symptoms and often conveys a survival advantage over radiation alone particularly in patients with a good performance status with either no extracranial metastases, or at least good control of systemic metastases.

Whole-Brain Radiation Therapy With or Without Radiosensitizers

A number of studies have examined the use of radiosensitizers in addition to WBRT for the treatment of unresectable brain metastases. Randomized trials have tested WBRT alone or in combination with lonidamine, metronidazole, misonidazole, and bromodeoxyuridine (BrdU) and found no difference in response rates or survival with the addition of any of these agents to radiation [44–47]. A small nonrandomized phase I/II study evaluated the safety and efficacy of celecoxib at a dose of 400 mg/day administered with concurrent WBRT consisting of a whole-brain dose of 32 Gy (20 fractions of 1.6 Gy twice daily) followed by a 22.4 Gy boost over evident lesions [48]. The overall response rate was 67% and the median survival time was 8.7 months. This median survival compares favorably to historical controls, but because this radiation dosing and fractionation is not commonly utilized, further investigation in a randomized trial is warranted to validate the clinical utility of this strategy.

Motexafin Gadolinium

More recently, several other agents have been tested in large, well-designed randomized clinical trials. Motexafin gadolinium (MGd) is a redox mediator that can sensitize tumor cells to ionizing radiation via formation of reactive oxygen species [49]. A randomized phase III randomized trial of WBRT with or without MGd was conducted in 401 patients with brain metastases from solid tumors (251 with non–small-cell lung cancer (NSCLC), 75 with breast cancer, and 75 with other cancers) [50]. Median survival was not significantly different in either treatment arm (5.2 months for MGd plus WBRT vs 4.9 months for WBRT alone). However, patients with lung cancer who were treated with MGd had improved memory and executive function and improved neurologic function [51].

Efaproxiral

Efaproxiral, another radiation enhancing agent, is a synthetic modifier of hemoglobin that decreases hemoglobin-oxygen binding affinity, facilitates the release of oxygen from hemoglobin, and thereby increases tissue pO_2. A phase III randomized trial with 538 patients with brain metastases from various solid tumors compared standard WBRT plus efaproxiral with supplemental oxygen to WBRT with supplemental oxygen. Median survival for patients of all tumor types who received WBRT and efaproxiral plus supplemental oxygen was 5.3 months versus 4.5 months for patients who received WBRT and supplemental oxygen alone. However, among breast cancer patients, survival was significantly prolonged in those who received efaproxiral with radiation and supplemental oxygen compared to those who received radiation and supplemental oxygen alone (9.3 months vs 4.57 months, $P = .006$) [52]. In the breast cancer subset, response rates were higher in the efaproxiral group than in the control group (71.7% vs 52.7%), as was increase in quality of life at 6 months measured by KPS and neurologic functioning score [53]. Based on the results of this subset analysis, another phase III multicenter, randomized trial of WBRT plus supplemental oxygen with or without efaproxiral was conducted in breast cancer patients with brain metastases not amenable to SRS. This study failed to achieve its primary endpoint and did not demonstrate an improvement in overall survival in patients receiving efaproxiral plus WBRT, compared with patients receiving WBRT alone [54]. Of the radiosensitizers reported in randomized trials, none is yet to show a survival benefit in the intended patient population as compared to WBRT alone, and therefore the use of radiosensitizers is not recommended outside of research studies.

Stereotactic Radiosurgery

SRS has emerged as an important modality in the primary treatment of low-volume brain metastases as well as the treatment of recurrent disease after surgery, WBRT, or prior SRS. SRS is a method of delivering a single high dose of radiation to a precisely defined volume of tumor tissue, with minimal delivery of radiation to surrounding brain tissue.

SRS has been studied as a single-treatment modality in several trials. Sneed et al. retrospectively reviewed the outcomes of patients with single or multiple brain metastases managed initially with SRS-alone ($n = 62$) versus SRS and WBRT ($n = 43$) [55]. Survival and local freedom from progression (FFP) were the same for SRS alone versus SRS plus WBRT (median survival 11.3 vs 11.1 months and 1-year local FFP by patient 71% vs 79%, respectively), but overall brain FFP was significantly worse for SRS alone versus SRS plus WBRT. However, salvage treatment after first failure in the brain was not significantly different for SRS alone versus SRS plus WBRT suggesting that the omission of WBRT in patients initially treated with SRS for up to 4 brain metastases did not compromise survival or intracranial control. Another study retrospectively compared the outcomes of 62 patients with cerebral metastases from breast cancer [56]. Ten patients received SRS alone (group 1), 13 patients were treated with WBRT and SRS as a focal boost (group 2), and 39 patients received WBRT and salvage SRS (group 3) for recurrent metastases at a later time point. Survival was increased in patients receiving

SRS only compared to WBRT and SRS as a focal boost, suggesting SRS alone is an effective treatment for patients with one to three brain metastases from breast cancer and salvage SRS is an effective therapy option after WBRT.

The results from these retrospective studies were reinforced by a prospective trial of 41 patients with brain metastases who were treated with SRS alone, achieving a local control rate of 76% and median survival of 10 months [57]. Fifty-six percent of patients experienced intracranial progression and then received salvage radiotherapy consisting of additional SRS in 22% of patients and WBRT in 29% of patients. This prospective study suggested that initial treatment of patients with SRS alone for four or less brain metastases may allow a significant proportion of patients to avoid WBRT.

Finally, a randomized trial was conducted in which 132 patients with one to four brain metastases, each less than 3 cm, received WBRT plus SRS ($n = 65$) or SRS alone ($n = 67$) [58]. The median survival time was 7.5 months in the WBRT plus SRS group and 8.0 months SRS alone ($P = .42$). The 12-month brain tumor recurrence was lower in the WBRT plus SRS group than the SRS-alone group (46.8% vs 76.4%, $P < .001$), and salvage brain treatment was less frequently required in the WBRT plus SRS group than with SRS alone. The authors of this study subsequently investigated the neurocognitive function of patients randomized on this trial. Neurocognitive function was evaluated at baseline in 110 patients using the Mini-Mental State Examination (MMSE). Of the 92 patients who underwent the follow-up MMSE, improvements of > or = 3 points in the MMSEs were observed in 9 WBRT plus SRS patients and 11 SRS-alone patients. Among patients who achieved a MMSE score of > or = 27 after treatment, the 12-, 24-, and 36-month actuarial free rate of a 3-point drop in the MMSE was 76.1%, 68.5%, and 14.7% in the WBRT plus SRS group and 59.3%, 51.9%, and 51.9% in the SRS-alone group, respectively. These data suggest that recurrences in the brain in patients receiving SRS alone may result in worsening neurocognitive function in the short-term, but for patients who survive up to 3 years after treatment, the long-term adverse effects of WBRT on neurocognitive function become evident and are not negligible.

At present, there is no standard guideline to suggest which patients could receive SRS alone, or which patients benefit from WBRT in combination with SRS. Often the decision depends on the treating institutions' bias as well as patient preference. Several groups, including the Eastern Cooperative Oncology Group, the North Central Cancer Cooperative Group, and the American College of Surgeons Oncology Group, are participating in a prospective randomized trial comparing WBRT plus SRS to SRS treatment alone in patients with one to three cerebral metastases, but no published results are available at this time [43].

Whole-Brain Radiotherapy Alone or With SRS

The addition of SRS to WBRT was superior to WBRT alone for patients with 2 to 4 brain metastases in a 27-patient randomized prospective clinical trial [59]. One-year local failure rates were 100% for WBRT alone versus 8% for WBRT with SRS. The study was stopped at an interim evaluation at 60% accrual because of the differences in local tumor control. The median survival rates were 7.5 months for WBRT and 11 months for WBRT and SRS, but this was not statistically significant due to the study being insufficiently powered after premature closure. Interestingly, survival did not depend on histology or number of tumors but was related to extent of extracranial disease. A subsequent study randomized 333 patients with 1 to 3 brain metastases to WBRT alone or WBRT and SRS [60]. This trial confirmed a survival advantage for the combination of WBRT and SRS in patients with solitary metastasis with improvement in median survival of 6.5 vs 4.9 months ($P = .039$). The study did not however demonstrate a survival benefit for WBRT and SRS in patients with two or three brain metastases. Interestingly, all patients treated with WBRT and SRS were more likely to have stable or improved performance scores at 6 months when compared to WBRT alone (43 vs 27%, $P = .03$).

Surgery Versus Stereotactic Radiosurgery

Prospective randomized trials directly comparing surgical resection to SRS have not been reported, and it is unlikely that such a trial will be successfully conducted due to patient and physician bias. However, several retrospective studies have been done to compare these treatment modalities. One retrospective study identified 13 patients treated by SRS with 62 patients treated by surgical resection [61]. Patients were matched by primary tumor histology, extent of systemic disease, KPS, time to brain metastases, number of brain metastases, and patient age and sex. The median survival was significantly longer for patients treated by surgery than with SRS (16.4 vs 7.5 months, respectively). This survival difference appeared to be due to a higher rate of mortality resulting from progression in the SRS-treated lesions and not due to development of new brain metastases or a difference in the rate of death from systemic disease. The authors conclude that surgery should remain the treatment of choice whenever possible and that SRS should be limited to surgically inaccessible metastatic tumors or patients in poor medical condition.

Another retrospective review compared 74 patients with a solitary brain metastasis who underwent surgical resection to 23 patients with a solitary brain metastasis who underwent SRS [62]. There were no significant differences between the groups in terms of age, gender, systemic disease type or status, or percentage of patients who received WBRT. There was no significant difference in patient survival with a 1-year survival rate of 56% for the SRS patients and 62% for the surgery patients. In contrast to the previous series, local tumor control was significantly better in the SRS group (no local recurrences) compared to 19 local recurrences (58%) in the surgery group.

Systemic Chemotherapy Alone or in Combination With WBRT

There is a relative paucity of clinical studies, particularly randomized trials, of single agents or combination chemotherapy regimens for the treatment of brain metastases from solid tumors. Studies from decades ago tested chemotherapy regimens that are not frequently utilized in cancer management today. Also, many of these trials predate the use of MRI in the diagnosis and follow-up of brain metastases, making evaluation of response rates described in these trials difficult to compare to those in trials conducted more recently. Nevertheless, multiple studies have reported reasonable anticancer activity with various systemic chemotherapy regimens given to patients either as initial treatment for brain metastases or as a salvage treatment after failure of radiation (see Table 71.1). A variety of regimens have also been tested in combination with WBRT to evaluate safety and to see if response rates and survival can be improved compared to treatment with WBRT alone (see Table 71.2).

Temozolomide

Temozolomide (TMZ) is an alkylating agent that can achieve therapeutic levels in the brain as a result of its low molecular weight and lipid solubility. The concentration of TMZ measured in the cerebrospinal fluid (CSF) is ~30% to 40% of that measured in plasma [93]. In patients with brain metastases from solid tumors, including breast and NSCLC, treatment with TMZ has resulted in short-term disease stabilization in 17% to 41% of patients, but partial responses (PR) have been largely limited to patients with NSCLC [63,64]. TMZ was given at a dose of $150/mg/m^2$ for 5 days in 28-day cycles to 41 patients with recurrent brain metastases after WBRT [63]. Of the 34 patients assessed for radiologic response at 8 weeks, there were two PR, both in patients with NSCLC. Among the breast cancer patients, there were no responders, but four patients (40%) had stable disease (SD). Median survival for the whole group was 6.6 months. In another study, TMZ was tested in 27 heavily pretreated patients with recurrent brain metastases NSCLC or SCLC cancer, breast cancer (4 patients), or other solid tumors [64]. One PR was observed in a patient with NSCLC, and 4 patients (17%) showed disease stabilization. Overall median survival was 4.5 months and median time to progression was 3 months.

The combination of TMZ and capecitabine in escalating doses was evaluated in 24 patients with brain metastases from breast cancer [65]. Fourteen patients had newly diagnosed brain metastases and 10 patients had recurrent brain metastases. One complete response (CR) and 3 PRs in the brain were observed, with 2 PRs occurring in patients who had received prior radiation. Eleven additional

Table 71.1 Summary of Chemotherapies Tested for Brain Metastases from Solid Tumors

Regimen	Tumor Type	Cases	Responses	Median Survival
TMZ [63]	Solid tumors	41	2 PR (NSCLC)	6.6 months
TMZ [64]	Solid tumors	24	1 PR	4.5 months
Capecitabine/TMZ [65]	Breast	24	1 CR, 3 PR	Not reported
High dose Cisplatin [66]	NSCLC	24	2CR, 3PR	Not reported
Cisplatin/Etoposide [67]	Breast	22	5 CR, 7 PR	58 weeks
Cisplatin/Etoposide [68]	Breast (B) NSCLC, melanoma (M)	116	7 CR, 14 PR (B); 3 CR, 10 PR (NSCLC)	31 weeks (B); 32 weeks (NSCLC); 17 weeks (M)
Cisplatin/Etoposide [69]	Solid tumors	14	1 CR, 1 PR	6 months
Carboplatin/Etoposide [70]	Lung	30	3 CR, 4 PR (SCLC); 3 PR (NSCLC)	23 weeks (SCLC); 30 weeks (NSCLC)
Cisplatin/Teniposide [71]	NSCLC	23	3 CR, 5 PR	21 weeks
Carboplatin [72]	Ovarian	3	3	16 months
Lom/Carbo/Vrl/5-FU [73]	Breast and NSCLC	6	3 PR	Not reported
Topotecan [74]	Breast	24	1 CR, 5 PR	6.25 months
CFP [75]	Breast	52	27[a]	Rosner grouped data
CFPMV [75]	Breast	35	19[a]	CR → 39.5 months
MVP [75]	Breast	7	3[a]	PR → 10.5 months
AC [75]	Breast	6	1[a]	SD → 6.5 months
CAF [76]	Breast	2	1 PR, 1CR	6.75 months
CMF [76]	Breast	20	1 CR, 9 PR	6.25 months
High dose etoposide [77]	SCLC	23	10	Not reported
CAVE [78]	SCLC	14	1 CR, 8 PR	34 weeks
Teniposide [79]	SCLC	80	26	Not reported
Etoposide [80]	Lung	19	2 (SCLC); 4 (NSCLC)	10 weeks
TPDC-FuHu [81]	Solid tumors	115	NSCLC (52% PR+SD); SCLC (66% PR+SD); Breast (60% PR+SD); Melanoma (22% PR+SD)	Not reported

Regimens: AC, adriamycin, cyclophosphamide; CAF, Cyclophosphamide, adriamycin, 5-fluorouracil; CAVE, cyclophosphamide, adriamycin, vincristine, etoposide; CFP, cyclophosphamide, 5-fluorouracil, prednisone; CFPMV, cyclophosphamide, 5-fluorouracil, prednisone, methotrexate, vincristine; Cis/Etop, cisplatin, etoposide; CMF, cyclophosphamide, methotrexate, 5-fluorouracil; Lom/Carbo/Vrl/5-FU, lomustine, carboplatin, vinorelbine, 5-fluorouracil; MVP, methotrexate, vincristine, prednisone; TMZ, temozolomide; TPDC-FuHu, thioguanine, procarbazine, dibromodulcitol, CCNU, fluorouracil, and hydroxyurea

[a] Responses determined by radionuclide scan prior to 1977 and by CT scan after 1977

Table 71.2 Radiation with Concurrent Chemotherapy

Author, Year	Chemotherapy	Patient Number	Tumor Type	Response Rates	Survival
Huang, 2007 [82]	Gemcitabine	16	Lung	NR	NR
Maravayas, 2005 [83]	Gemcitabine	36	Solid tumors	NR	NR
Mirmiran, 2007 [84]	Topotecan	9	Solid Tumors	11%	14.6 weeks
Kocher, 2005 [85]	Topotecan	47, 26 eval	Solid tumors	58% (T)	20.4 weeks
Gruschow, 2002 [86]	Topotecan	20, 13 eval	Solid tumors	46%(T)	20 weeks(T)
Kouvaris, 2007 [87]	Temozolomide	33	Solid Tumors	58%	12 months
Antanadou, 2002 [88]	Temozolomide	45	Solid tumors	67% (XRT) 96% (TMZ+XRT)	NR
Ushio, 1991 [89]	Chloroethylnitrosoureas or chlorethylnitrosureas plus tegafur	100, 88 eval	Lung	36%(XRT) 69% (C) 74% (C+T)	27 weeks (XRT) 30.5 weeks (C) 29 weeks (C+T)
Lange, 1990 [90]	Ifosfamide + Carmustine	61	Breast	65%	8 months
Hidalgo, 1987 [91]	Intracarotid Cisplatin Intravenous Cisplatin	9 5	Solid tumors	89% (ICC) 100% (IVC)	NR
Stewart, 1983 [92]	Cisplatin	18	Melanoma	8% (C)	NR

Table includes published series only.

patients experienced either a minor response or SD, suggesting that this combination may merit further investigation as an alternative to or in combination with WBRT for the treatment of multiple brain metastases.

TMZ has also been tested in combination with concurrent radiation therapy for previously untreated brain metastases [88]. Fifty-two patients with brain metastases were randomized to receive TMZ at a dose of 75 mg/m^2/day concurrent with 40-Gy radiation for 4 weeks versus WBRT alone. After completing radiation, patients randomized to TMZ continued to receive this drug at a dose of 200mg/m^2/day for 5 days in 28-day cycles. Response rates were significantly higher in the group receiving TMZ with WBRT. Forty-five patients were evaluated for response by CT or MRI scan 2 months after completion of their radiation. In the TMZ plus radiation group, 9 CRs, 14 PRs, and 1 SD were observed compared to 7 CRs, 7 PRs, and 5 SD with RT alone. Medial survival was slightly prolonged in the TMZ + WBRT group versus the WBRT group (8.6 vs 7.0 months), but this was not statistically significant.

Platinum Agents Alone or in Combination

Platinum concentrations have been studied in autopsy tumor samples obtained from patients who had received cisplatin antemortem. Concentrations in brain metastases were similar to platinum concentrations in other extrahepatic tumors suggesting that these agents may penetrate the blood-brain barrier (BBB) and have activity in brain metastases [94].

Cisplatin at a dose of 200 mg/m^2 divided over 5 days was tested in 24 patients with brain metastases from lung carcinoma [66]. Two CR and 3 PR were achieved but toxicities included partial deafness, renal toxicity, and severe myelotoxicity.

Twenty-two patients with brain metastases from breast carcinoma were treated with a combination of cisplatin (100 mg/m^2 day 1) and etoposide (100 mg/m^2 days 4, 6, 8) every 3 weeks [67]. Five patients (23%) achieved a CR while seven patients (32%) obtained a PR for an overall response rate of 55%. Median duration of survival was 58 weeks. The combination of cisplatin and etoposide at the same doses as above was then tested prospectively in 116 patients (56 breast cancer, 43 NSCLC, and 8 melanoma) previously untreated with radiation [68]. Seven breast cancer patients and 3 NSCLC patients achieved a CR, and PR was observed in 14 breast cancer patients and 10 NSCLC patients. No responses were observed in patients with melanoma. The CR plus PR rate was 30%. The median survival was 31 weeks for breast cancer, 32 weeks for NSCLC, and 17 weeks for melanoma patients. Another trial of 14 patients with brain metastases from solid tumors (lung, breast, colon, and stomach) tested cisplatin, 40 mg/m^2/day and etoposide, 150 mg/m^2/day, for 3 days every 3 weeks [69]. One CR occurred in a patient with poorly differentiated lung cancer and one PR was observed in a breast cancer patient. The overall response rate was 14%, with a median survival of 6 months. Twenty-three patients with brain metastases from NSCLC were treated with cisplatin (100 mg/m^2, day 1) and teniposide (80 mg/m^2, days 1, 3 and 5) every 3 weeks [71]. The response rate of brain metastases was 35%. Three patients achieved CR and five patients had a PR. The median survival was 21 weeks and 45 weeks for responding patients. The combination of carboplatin (300 mg/m^2 every 4 weeks) with etoposide (120 mg/m^2 days 1–3 every 4 weeks) was tested in 30 patients with brain metastases from lung cancer (12 SCLC, 18 NSCLC) [70]. Complete response occurred among 3 patients with SCLC and 7 PR were observed (4 SCLC, 3 NSCLC). Overall survival was 23 weeks in SCLC patients and 29.8 weeks in NSCLC 29.8 patients.

Additional small series have described CNS responses in ovarian cancer patients with brain metastases treated with single agent carboplatin, and in breast and NSCLC patients with brain metastases treated with a regimen of lomustine, carboplatin, vinorelbine, leucovorin, and fluorouracil [72,73].

Topotecan

Topotecan, a camptothecin derivative and inhibitor of topoisomerase I, has been observed to penetrate the intact BBB with some efficiency [95]. Topotecan was investigated as a primary treatment for brain metastases in 24 breast cancer patients who had not received prior radiation therapy [74]. Topotecan was administered at a dose of 1.5 mg/m² per day for 5 days every 3 weeks. One patient experienced a CR, 5 patients had a PR, and median survival was 6.3 months.

Topotecan given as a 21-day continuous infusion of 0.4 to 0.6 mg/m²/day was tested in combination with WBRT (40 Gy) in 20 patients [86]. Four CR and 2 PR were observed, and median survival was 5 months. A similar study tested topotecan at 0.4 to 0.6 mg/m²/day with concurrent WBRT (30 Gy in 10 fractions) in 9 patients with brain metastases from solid tumors [84]. A single PR was observed and median survival was 102 days. In a third study, topotecan was administered a range of doses (0.5 mg/m²/day × 5 doses up to 0.6 mg/m²/day × 12 doses) prior to WBRT (36 Gy/3-Gy fractions) in 47 patients with previously untreated brain metastases [85]. Overall response rate was 58% with 5 CR and 5 PR, and median survival was 5.1 months. Taken together, these studies do not indicate that addition of topotecan to WBRT results in significant improvements in responses in the CNS or overall survival compared to historical controls receiving WBRT alone. However, in patients who have rapidly progressing systemic disease and need treatment for this during radiation, topotecan may be a reasonable option.

Other Regimens

A variety of other chemotherapy regimens have been evaluated for activity against brain metastases, and the choice of these regimens appears to be more related to their efficacy against the primary tumor type rather than their ability to penetrate the BBB. Systemic chemotherapy was evaluated in 100 consecutive patients with symptomatic brain metastases documented by radionuclide brain scan (technetium 99 pertechnetate) or CT scan between 1970 and 1985 [75]. Patients were treated with cyclophosphamide, 5-flourouracil, and prednisone (CFP); CFP plus methotrexate (M) and vincristine (V); MV plus prednisone (MVP); or doxorubicin plus cyclophosphamide. Overall, 52% of patients achieved objective responses in brain metastases to primary chemotherapy. 35 patients went on to receive second-line chemotherapy after not responding to an initial regimen, and 37% of these patients experienced further response. 8 patients received third-line chemotherapy, and 4 of these patients responded. The overall median survival from the time of initiation of chemotherapy for all 100 patients was 5.5 months. However, the median survival for complete responders was 39.5 months (range, 6–62 months) and for partial responders was 10.5 months (range, 3–78 months).

Another prospective, nonrandomized study evaluated systemic chemotherapy of brain metastases in 22 breast cancer patients between 1987 and 1990 [76]. Twenty patients were treated with cyclophosphamide/methotrexate/5-fluorouracil (CMF) and 2 with cyclophosphamide/doxorubicin/5-fluorouracil (CAF). Seven patients had previously been treated for brain metastases with surgery or radiation therapy. CT scans after two cycles of chemotherapy showed a CR in 2 patients and PR in 10 patients. Median survival was 25 weeks for all patients, but was 66 weeks in patients who responded to chemotherapy.

A number of chemotherapies including single agent etoposide, teniposide, and the combination of cyclophosphamide, adriamycin, vincristine, and etoposide (CAVE) have been tested for brain metastases in patients with SCLC [77–79]. Response rates ranged from 33% for teniposide alone to 82% for CAVE. Since SCLC is generally considered an extremely chemosensitive disease, it is very reasonable to consider chemotherapy as a primary therapy for patients who are not candidates for SRS and who would like to avoid WBRT or as salvage therapy for patients with SCLC who already received WBRT for prophylaxis or treatment of previously diagnosed brain metastases.

Small Molecule Tyrosine Kinase Inhibitors

Gefitinib and Erlotinib

Gefitinib and erlotinib are orally active inhibitors of the epidermal growth factor receptor (EGFR or ErbB1) tyrosine kinase. Multiple case reports have described responses to gefitinib in patient with brain metastases from NCSLC (see Table 71.3). Despite the numerous responses in the CNS reported with gefitinib, it appears the drug is not entirely protective. In retrospective study of 139 patients with NSCLC treated with gefitinib, 15% achieved a PR systemically, with the CNS as the initial site of disease recurrence in 7 (33%) patients and the lung in 9 (43%) patients [105]. The CNS was a frequent site of disease recurrence in patients with NSCLC after an initial response to gefitinib, regardless of disease control in the lungs. The authors suggest that intrinsic resistance of metastatic clones, incomplete

Table 71.3 Published Case Reports of Gefitinib Responses in Brain Metastases

Author, Year	Cases	Responses	Comments	Survival
Ceresoli, 2004 [96]	37 (18 with previous XRT)	4 PR 7 SD	PFS 3 months	Not reported
Hotta, 2004 [97]	14	1 CR, 5PR	Response duration 7.7 months	9.1 months
Ishida, 2004 [98]	2	2	No prior tx	Not reported
Namba, 2004 [99]	15	9	Response duration 8.7 months	8.3 months
Roggero, 2005 [100]	1	1		Not reported
Stemmler, 2005 [101]	1	1		Not reported
Nichi, 2006 [102]	2	2		3–4 years
Shimato, 2006 [103]	8	3	Responses assoc with EGFR mutations	Not reported
Wu, 2007 [104]	40	32%	PFS 9 months	15 months

CNS penetration of the drug, and longer survival are possible explanations for this high incidence of recurrence in the CNS.

Similar to gefitinib, several case reports have described complete responses in brain metastases in a patient with NSCLC treated with erlotinib [106,107]. One report describes a patient with NSCLC with progressive brain metastases after WBRT whose brain metastases responded both initially and on re-treatment with erlotinib, but whose extracranial disease remained erlotinib-resistant throughout. This suggests that there may be a role for erlotnib for the treatment of brain metastases in NSCLC even if the patient experienced systemicprogression on the drug in the past.

Lapatinib

Lapatinib is an orally available dual tyrosine kinase inhibitor (TKI) that specifically inhibits the EGFR and the HER2/neu (or ErbB2) receptor. Clinical studies with lapatinib in women with ErbB2+ metastatic breast cancer have shown activity both as first-line therapy and for patients who have relapsed on trastuzumab [108,109]. Case reports of significant shrinkage of ErbB2+ breast cancer brain metastases were noted early in the clinical development of lapatinib, prompting prospective investigation of lapatinib in this setting. A phase II trial evaluated objective response in the brain to 750 mg of lapatinib twice daily in 39 women with ErbB2+ breast cancer who had developed CNS disease during trastuzumab therapy, and in most of whom [38,39] CNS disease had progressed after prior radiotherapy [110]. Two patients achieved a PR (5%) in the CNS by standard criteria, with 8 patients progression-free in the CNS at 16 weeks. The median time to progression was 3 months and median overall survival was 6.6 months. Data have also been published recently from a larger phase II study of lapatinib for brain metastases in patients with ErbB2+ breast cancer following trastuzumab treatment and radiotherapy [111]. This study enrolled 242 patients and objective responses in the CNS were observed in 6% of patients. In an exploratory analysis, 21% of patients experienced a ≥20% volumetric reduction in their CNS lesions.

Evidence for the activity of lapatinib against ErbB2+ brain metastases has also emerged from the phase III study of lapatinib plus capecitabine versus capecitabine monotherapy in 324 women with ErbB2+ breast cancer that had progressed following trastuzumab-based therapy [112]. In this study, new or progressive CNS metastases occurred in a smaller number of women in the combination therapy group than in the monotherapy group (4 vs 11) although the difference did not reach statistical significance. With this accumulating anecdotal data to suggest that lapatinib crosses the BBB, this agent may play a role in future prophylactic strategies in patients with ErbB2-overexpressing breast cancer who are at risk for CNS progression.

Conclusions

Brain metastases are a serious and increasing problem in patients with nearly all solid tumor types. As outcomes continue to improve, particularly in breast, colorectal, and lung cancer, brain metastases and other forms of CNS disease are likely to become a dominant management issue in these patients. With heightened awareness of the problem, appropriate imaging, and more mainstream use of SRS, patients may be treated at a point when they have minimal burden of disease in the CNS, likely leading to less toxicity and longer survival. In addition, further testing of novel chemotherapies and biological therapies that have the potential to cross the BBB are imperative to prevent this devastating complication of cancer in the future.

LEPTOMENINGEAL DISEASE

Leptomeningeal metastases (LMM), leptomeningeal carcinomatosis, and leptomeningeal disease (LMD) all refer to a condition where malignant cells from another primary tumor site infiltrate the leptomeninges, almost always resulting in progressive neurologic dysfunction, and often death. Breast and lung cancer are the most frequent primary sites leading to LMD [113]. Autopsy studies suggest that meningeal metastases may be present in as many as 18% of patients with metastatic disease [114]. Although clinically evident, LMD is often a late-stage complication of metastatic cancer, the diagnosis may be increasing due to more frequent use of and advances in MRI and PET imaging [115,116]. Furthermore, the underlying incidence may be increasing due to improvements in survival in patients with controlled systemic metastatic disease [117].

Presentation and Diagnosis

Patients with LMD may present with a variety of neurologic symptoms including headache, gait disturbance, vision loss, or other nonspecific symptoms such as nausea and vomiting or pain. The diagnosis of LMD is usually established by the detection of malignant cells in the CSF or by the presence of enhancing tumor nodules on cranial or spinal MRI. Prior to the routine use of MRI, patients were usually diagnosed only after they developed neurologic deficits due to impingement on cranial nerves or nerves exiting the spinal cord. Although a positive CSF cytology is considered the gold standard to confirm the diagnosis of LMD, many patients with clinical findings suspicious for LMD do not have malignant cells detected in their CSF, at least on initial examination. Routine cytologic examination alone appears inadequate to diagnose LMD, with approximately 50% of cases confirmed as positive in the first lumbar puncture (LP), but up to 85% to 90% after multiple LPs [113]. Other techniques, including immunohistochemistry for cytotokeratin positive cells, measurement of the vascular endothelial growth factor (VEGF), and other tumor markers including carcinoembryonic antigen (CEA) and CA 15–3 have been tested to attempt to improve the sensitivity of making the diagnosis of LMD [118–120].

Palliative Treatments—Steroids, Shunting, Radiation

Steroids are often initiated to decrease inflammation at sites of nerve root impingement and also to decrease cerebral edema. For patients presenting with hydrocephalus, ventriculoperitoneal shunting for relief of increased intracranial pressure may be the first step in treatment. Craniospinal irradiation (CSI) is one option to treat LMD [121], particularly in cases where CSF flow is disturbed, or when bulky disease-causing neurologic deficits are seen on imaging. The presence of bulky disease that impedes flow of CSF affects the feasibility and efficacy of other treatment options and also increases symptoms and side effects from treatment. Irradiation of the entire craniospinal axis is quite toxic and often results in significant bone marrow suppression that subsequently delays or prevents patients from receiving further chemotherapy for their systemic metastatic disease. Radiation to the lumbar-sacral region may be indicated to palliate symptoms of cauda equina syndrome including low back pain, leg weakness, or anal sphincter dysfunction. Similarly, radiation to the base of skull may be appropriate in patients with cranial neuropathies.

Intrathecal Chemotherapy for LMD

Most systemically administered cytotoxic agents are only minimally effective in the treatment of LMD due to their poor penetration into the CSF due to the BBB and blood-CSF barrier. Even in LMD, where it is believed that there is some breakdown of these barriers, CSF exposure to most cytotoxic agents is less than 10% of the plasma concentration [122]. Administration of chemotherapy directly into the CSF (intrathecal chemotherapy) either via repeated LP or intraventricularly (IVT) via an Ommaya reservoir bypasses the blood-CSF barrier, maximizing drug exposure to tumor cells in the CSF and the meninges.

Intrathecal (IT) chemotherapy with methotrexate (MTX), cytarabine (Ara-C), and thiotepa (TT) has been studied in small series with variable results [123–127]. MTX is usually administered at a dose of 12 mg twice a week initially, with the frequency of dosing decreasing after 4 to 6 weeks of treatment or after there has been a documented cytologic response. A clinical trial randomized 59 patients with solid tumor malignancies (primarily breast and lung cancer) to IT MTX (10 mg) or TT (10 mg) twice weekly [127]. Median survival for patients receiving MTX was 15.9 weeks and 14.1 weeks for patients treated with TT. Shorter survival was predicted by progressive systemic disease, poor performance status, and significant cranial nerve palsies. Mucositis and neurologic complications were more common in patients who received MTX.

Intraventricular cytosine arabinoside (IVT Ara-C) 100 mg initially given three times weekly and then less frequently was evaluated in 10 breast cancer patients newly diagnosed with LMD [124]. Two patients had PR lasting 9 and 40 weeks, and two other patients had SD. Median survival was 30 weeks. Side effects included meningismus, nausea, vomiting, and myelosuppression. The efficacy of DepoCyt, a slow-release formulation of Ara-C that maintains cytotoxic concentrations of free Ara-C in the CSF for >14 days following a single injection, was evaluated in 110 patients with LMD from solid tumors [128]. Patients received DepoCyt 50 mg either IVT or via LP every 2 weeks for 1 month of induction therapy, and then received further consolidation therapy if they had not experienced neurologic progression. Median time to neurologic progression was 55 days and median overall survival was 95 days. Headache and arachnoiditis were the most significant adverse effects.

A study comparing the efficacy of intrathecal MTX alone to the combination of MTX, Ara-C, and TT reported a higher cytological response rate in the combination group than in the MTX alone group (38.5 vs 13.8%), and patients who received combination treatment had a median survival of 18.6 weeks compared to 10.4 weeks in the MTX-only arm [123]. In contrast, one study in 13 breast cancer patients with LMD showed no objective responses or improvement in neurologic symptoms with IT chemotherapy consisting of alternating doses of MTX, Ara-C, TT, and hydrocortisone with folinic acid support [129].

Systemic Therapy Options

Several systemic chemotherapy regimens have been studied for the treatment of solid tumor LMD. Rapid infusion of high-dose intravenous MTX (HD IV MTX) has been shown to penetrate the BBB and has reported activity in LMD [130]. A retrospective review described the outcomes of 32 patients (most with breast cancer) treated with HD IV MTX (3.5 g/m^2) for CNS parenchymal or LMM. Among 14 patients with isolated LMD, five (36%) improved, two (14%) remained stable and seven (50%) progressed. Among the nine patients with both parenchymal and LMM, one (11%) improved in both areas; two (22%) were stable in both areas, and six (67%) progressed in one or both areas. Myelosuppression and elevated serum hepatic transaminases were the most common acute toxicities.

TMZ, an orally administered alkylating agent that is able to cross the BBB and has shown activity in primary and recurrent brain tumors and brain metastases from lung cancer and melanoma, was tested in 10 patients with LMD at a dose of 75 mg/m^2 daily 6 continuous weeks, followed by a 4-week break [131]. Two patients had SD through 2 cycles, but progressed during the 4-week chemotherapy break, suggesting that alternate dosing schedules or more continuous therapy may be necessary for this agent to have persistent activity.

At least one randomized trial has compared systemic chemotherapy to IT chemotherapy in breast cancer patients with LMD [132]. Neurological improvement or stabilization was observed in 59% of the IT and in 67% of the non-IT group, with median time to progression of 23 weeks (IT) and 24 weeks (non-IT). Median survival of IT patients was 18.3 weeks and 30.3 weeks for non-IT patients. The authors concluded that standard systemic chemotherapy with involved field radiation therapy for LMD from breast cancer was associated with less neurotoxicity than IT chemotherapy and did not compromise survival.

Rare case reports have documented clinical responses and stabilization of LMD with systemic therapies including letrozole, tamoxifen, and megestrol acetate in breast cancer and the small molecule TKI, gefitinib, in NSCLC [133–135]. Ongoing studies with other small molecule TKIs that target EGFR, HER2/neu, and VEGF pathways and based on their size have the potential to cross the BBB, may elucidate the role of these agents in the treatment of CNS metastases including LMD.

REFERENCES

1. Posner JB, Chernik NL. Intracranial metastases from systemic cancer. *Adv Neurol.* 1978;19:579–592.
2. Loeffler JS, Patchell RA, Sawaya R. Treatment of metastatic cancer. In: Devita VT, Hellman S, Rosenberg SA, eds. *Cancer: Principles and Practice of Oncology.* 5th ed. Philadelphia, PA: Lippincott-Raven;1997:2523.
3. Lassman AB, DeAngelis LM. Brain metastases. *Neurol clin.* 2003;21(1):1–23, vii.
4. Barnholtz-Sloan JS, Sloan AE, Davis FG, Vigneau FD, Lai P, Sawaya RE. Incidence proportions of brain metastases in patients diagnosed (1973 to 2001) in the Metropolitan Detroit Cancer Surveillance System. *J Clin Oncol.* 2004;22(14):2865–2872.
5. Schouten LJ, Rutten J, Huveneers HA, Twijnstra A. Incidence of brain metastases in a cohort of patients with carcinoma of the breast, colon, kidney, and lung and melanoma. *Cancer.* 2002;94(10):2698–2705.
6. Sundermeyer ML, Meropol NJ, Rogatko A, Wang H, Cohen SJ. Changing patterns of bone and brain metastases in patients with colorectal cancer. *Clin Colorectal Cancer.* 2005;5(2):108–113.
7. Yuh WT, Tali ET, Nguyen HD, Simonson TM, Mayr NA, Fisher DJ. The effect of contrast dose, imaging time, and lesion size in the MR detection of intracerebral metastasis. *AJNR Am J Neuroradiol.* 1995;16(2):373–380.
8. Hicks DG, Short SM, Prescott NL, et al. Breast cancers with brain metastases are more likely to be estrogen receptor negative, express the basal cytokeratin CK5/6, and overexpress HER2 or EGFR. *Am J Surg Pathol.* 2006;30(9):1097–1104.
9. Slimane K, Andre F, Delaloge S, et al. Risk factors for brain relapse in patients with metastatic breast cancer. *Ann Oncol.* 2004;15(11):1640–1644.
10. Tham YL, Sexton K, Kramer R, Hilsenbeck S, Elledge R. Primary breast cancer phenotypes associated with propensity for central nervous system metastases. *Cancer.* 2006;15;107(4):696–704.
11. Gabos Z, Sinha R, Hanson J, et al. Prognostic significance of human epidermal growth factor receptor positivity for the development of brain metastasis after newly diagnosed breast cancer. *J Clin Oncol.* 2006;24(36):5658–5663.
12. Nugent JL, Bunn PA Jr, Matthews MJ, et al. CNS metastases in small cell bronchogenic carcinoma: increasing frequency and changing pattern with lengthening survival. *Cancer.* 1979;44(5):1885–1893.
13. Postmus PE, Smit EF. Chemotherapy for brain metastases of lung cancer: a review. *Ann Oncol.* 1999;10(7):753–759.
14. Auperin A, Arriagada R, Pignon JP, et al. Prophylactic cranial irradiation for patients with small-cell lung cancer in complete remission. Prophylactic Cranial Irradiation Overview Collaborative Group. *N Engl J Med.* 1999;341(7):476–484.
15. Slotman B, Faivre-Finn C, Kramer G, et al. Prophylactic cranial irradiation in extensive small-cell lung cancer. *N Engl J Med.* 2007;357(7):664–672.
16. Ghia A, Tome WA, Thomas S, et al. Distribution of brain metastases in relation to the hippocampus: implications for neurocognitive functional preservation. *Int J Radiat Oncol Biol Phys.* 2007;68(4):971–977.
17. Weissman DE. Glucocorticoid treatment for brain metastases and epidural spinal cord compression: a review. *J Clin Oncol.* 1988;6(3):543–551.
18. Posner JB. Management of central nervous system metastases. *Semin Oncol.* 1977;4(1):81–91.
19. Lock M, Chow E, Pond GR, et al. Prognostic factors in brain metastases: can we determine patients who do not benefit from whole-brain radiotherapy? *Clin Oncol (R Coll Radiol).* 2004;16(5):332–338.
20. Sneed PK, Larson DA, Wara WM. Radiotherapy for cerebral metastases. *Neurosurg Clin N Am.* 1996;7(3):505–515.
21. Patchell RA, Tibbs PA, Regine WF, et al. Postoperative radiotherapy in the treatment of single metastases to the brain: a randomized trial. *JAMA.* 1998;280(17):1485–1489.
22. Hall WA, Djalilian HR, Nussbaum ES, Cho KH. Long-term survival with metastatic cancer to the brain. *Med Oncol.* 2000;17(4):279–286.
23. Gaspar L, Scott C, Rotman M, et al. Recursive partitioning analysis (RPA) of prognostic factors in three Radiation Therapy Oncology Group (RTOG) brain metastases trials. *Int J Radiat Oncol Biol Phys.* 1997;37(4):745–751.
24. Sperduto PW, Berkey B, Gaspar LE, Mehta M, Curran W. A new prognostic index and comparison to three other indices for patients with brain metastases: an analysis of 1,960 patients in the RTOG database. *Int J Radiat Oncol Biol Phys.* 2008;1;70(2):510–514.
25. Mahmoud-Ahmed AS, Suh JH, Lee SY, Crownover RL, Barnett GH. Results of whole brain radiotherapy in patients with brain metastases from breast cancer: a retrospective study. *Int J Radiat Oncol Biol Phys.* 2002;54(3):810–817.
26. Li B, Yu J, Suntharalingam M, et al. Comparison of three treatment options for single brain metastasis from lung cancer. *Int J Cancer.* 2000;90(1):37–45.
27. Khuntia D, Brown P, Li J, Mehta MP. Whole-brain radiotherapy in the management of brain metastasis. *J Clin Oncol.* 2006;24(8):1295–1304.
28. Haie-Meder C, Pellae-Cosset B, Laplanche A, et al. Results of a randomized clinical trial comparing two radiation schedules in the palliative treatment of brain metastases. *Radiother Oncol.* 1993;26(2):111–116.
29. Gelber RD, Larson M, Borgelt BB, Kramer S. Equivalence of radiation schedules for the palliative treatment of brain metastases in patients with favorable prognosis. *Cancer.* 1981;48(8):1749–1753.
30. Borgelt B, Gelber R, Larson M, Hendrickson F, Griffin T, Roth R. Ultra-rapid high dose irradiation schedules for the palliation of brain metastases: final results of the first two studies by the Radiation Therapy Oncology Group. *Int J Radiat Oncol Biol Phys.* 1981;7(12):1633–1638.
31. Borgelt B, Gelber R, Kramer S, et al. The palliation of brain metastases: final results of the first two studies by the Radiation Therapy Oncology Group. *Int J Radiat Oncol Biol Phys.* 1980;6(1):1–9.
32. Murray KJ, Scott C, Greenberg HM, et al. A randomized phase III study of accelerated hyperfractionation versus standard in patients with unresected brain metastases: a report of the Radiation Therapy Oncology Group (RTOG) 9104. *Int J Radiat Oncol Biol Phys.* 1997;39(3):571–574.
33. Rades D, Schild SE, Lohynska R, Veninga T, Stalpers LJ, Dunst J. Two radiation regimens and prognostic factors for brain metastases in nonsmall cell lung cancer patients. *Cancer.* 2007;110(5):1077–1082.
34. Rades D, Lohynska R, Veninga T, Stalpers LJ, Schild SE. Evaluation of 2 whole-brain radiotherapy schedules and prognostic factors for brain metastases in breast cancer patients. *Cancer.* 2007;110(11):2587–2592.
35. DeAngelis LM, Delattre JY, Posner JB. Radiation-induced dementia in patients cured of brain metastases. *Neurology.* 1989;39(6):789–796.
36. Pavy JJ, Denekamp J, Letschert J, et al; EORTC Late Effects Working Group. Late effects toxicity scoring: the SOMA scale. *Radiother Oncol.* 1995;35(1):11–15.
37. Sawaya R, Hammoud M, Schoppa D, et al. Neurosurgical outcomes in a modern series of 400 craniotomies for treatment of parenchymal tumors. *Neurosurgery.* 1998;42(5):1044–1055; discussion 55–56.
38. Patchell RA, Tibbs PA, Walsh JW, et al. A randomized trial of surgery in the treatment of single metastases to the brain. *N Engl J Med.* 1990;322(8):494–500.
39. Vecht CJ, Haaxma-Reiche H, Noordijk EM, et al. Treatment of single brain metastasis: radiotherapy alone or combined with neurosurgery? *Ann Neurol.* 1993;33(6):583–590.
40. Mintz AH, Kestle J, Rathbone MP, et al. A randomized trial to assess the efficacy of surgery in addition to radiotherapy in patients with a single cerebral metastasis. *Cancer.* 1996;78(7):1470–1476.
41. Wronski M, Arbit E, McCormick B. Surgical treatment of 70 patients with brain metastases from breast carcinoma. *Cancer.* 1997;80(9):1746–1754.
42. Hazuka MB, Burleson WD, Stroud DN, Leonard CE, Lillehei KO, Kinzie JJ. Multiple brain metastases are associated with poor survival in patients treated with surgery and radiotherapy. *J Clin Oncol.* 1993;11(2):369–373.
43. Paek SH, Audu PB, Sperling MR, Cho J, Andrews DW. Reevaluation of surgery for the treatment of brain metastases: review of 208 patients with single or multiple brain metastases treated at one institution with modern neurosurgical techniques. *Neurosurgery.* 2005;56(5):1021–1034; discussion 1021–1034.
44. Phillips TL, Scott CB, Leibel SA, Rotman M, Weigensberg IJ. Results of a randomized comparison of radiotherapy and bromodeoxyuridine with radiotherapy alone for brain metastases: report of RTOG trial 89-05. *Int J Radiat Oncol Biol Phys.* 1995;33(2):339–348.
45. Komarnicky LT, Phillips TL, Martz K, Asbell S, Isaacson S, Urtasun R. A randomized phase III protocol for the evaluation of misonidazole combined with radiation in the treatment of patients with brain metastases (RTOG-7916). *Int J Radiat Oncol Biol Phys.* 1991;20(1):53–58.
46. DeAngelis LM, Currie VE, Kim JH, et al. The combined use of radiation therapy and lonidamine in the treatment of brain metastases. *J Neurooncol.* 1989;7(3):241–247.
47. Eyre HJ, Ohlsen JD, Frank J, et al. Randomized trial of radiotherapy versus radiotherapy plus metronidazole for the treatment metastatic

cancer to brain. a Southwest Oncology Group study. *J Neurooncol.* 1984;2(4):325–330.
48. Cerchietti LC, Bonomi MR, Navigante AH, Castro MA, Cabalar ME, Roth BM. Phase I/II study of selective cyclooxygenase-2 inhibitor celecoxib as a radiation sensitizer in patients with unresectable brain metastases. *J Neurooncol.* 2005;71(1):73–81.
49. Magda D, Lepp C, Gerasimchuk N, et al. Redox cycling by motexafin gadolinium enhances cellular response to ionizing radiation by forming reactive oxygen species. *Int J Radiat Oncol Biol Phys.* 2001;51(4):1025–1036.
50. Mehta MP, Rodrigus P, Terhaard CH, et al. Survival and neurologic outcomes in a randomized trial of motexafin gadolinium and whole-brain radiation therapy in brain metastases. *J Clin Oncol.* 2003;21(13):2529–2536.
51. Meyers CA, Smith JA, Bezjak A, et al. Neurocognitive function and progression in patients with brain metastases treated with whole-brain radiation and motexafin gadolinium: results of a randomized phase III trial. *J Clin Oncol.* 2004;22(1):157–165.
52. Suh JH, Stea B, Nabid A, et al. Phase III study of efaproxiral as an adjunct to whole-brain radiation therapy for brain metastases. *J Clin Oncol.* 2006;24(1):106–114.
53. Suh J, Stea BD, Kresl JJ, et al. Results from a subgroup analysis of patients with metastatic breast cancer (MBC) in a phase 3, randomized, open-label, comparative study of standard whole brain radiation therapy (WBRT) with supplemental oxygen, with or without RSR13, in patients with brain metastases. *Breast Cancer Res Treat.* 2003;82:Abstr 175.
54. Salmaggi A, Silvani A, Boiardi A. Brain metastases in patients receiving trastuzumab for breast cancer. *Neurol Sci.* 2007;28(1):1.
55. Sneed PK, Lamborn KR, Forstner JM, et al. Radiosurgery for brain metastases: is whole brain radiotherapy necessary? *Int J Radiat Oncol Biol Phys.* 1999;43(3):549–558.
56. Combs SE, Schulz-Ertner D, Thilmann C, Edler L, Debus J. Treatment of cerebral metastases from breast cancer with stereotactic radiosurgery. *Strahlenther Onkol.* 2004;180(9):590–596.
57. Chitapanarux I, Goss B, Vongtama R, et al. Prospective study of stereotactic radiosurgery without whole brain radiotherapy in patients with four or less brain metastases: incidence of intracranial progression and salvage radiotherapy. *J Neurooncol.* 2003;61(2):143–149.
58. Aoyama H, Shirato H, Tago M, et al. Stereotactic radiosurgery plus whole-brain radiation therapy vs stereotactic radiosurgery alone for treatment of brain metastases: a randomized controlled trial. *JAMA.* 2006;295(21):2483–2491.
59. Kondziolka D, Patel A, Lunsford LD, Kassam A, Flickinger JC. Stereotactic radiosurgery plus whole brain radiotherapy versus radiotherapy alone for patients with multiple brain metastases. *Int J Radiat Oncol Biol Phys.* 1999;45(2):427–434.
60. Andrews DW, Scott CB, Sperduto PW, et al. Whole brain radiation therapy with or without stereotactic radiosurgery boost for patients with one to three brain metastases: phase III results of the RTOG 9508 randomised trial. *Lancet.* 2004;363(9422):1665–1672.
61. Bindal AK, Bindal RK, Hess KR, et al. Surgery versus radiosurgery in the treatment of brain metastasis. *J Neurosurg.* 1996;84(5):748–754.
62. O'Neill BP, Iturria NJ, Link MJ, Pollock BE, Ballman KV, O'Fallon JR. A comparison of surgical resection and stereotactic radiosurgery in the treatment of solitary brain metastases. *Int J Radiat Oncol Biol Phys.* 2003;55(5):1169–1176.
63. Abrey LE, Olson JD, Raizer JJ, et al. A phase II trial of temozolomide for patients with recurrent or progressive brain metastases. *J Neurooncol.* 2001;53(3):259–265.
64. Christodoulou C, Bafaloukos D, Kosmidis P, et al. Phase II study of temozolomide in heavily pretreated cancer patients with brain metastases. *Ann Oncol.* 2001;12(2):249–254.
65. Rivera E, Meyers C, Groves M, et al. Phase I study of capecitabine in combination with temozolomide in the treatment of patients with brain metastases from breast carcinoma. *Cancer.* 2006;107(6):1348–1354.
66. Kleisbauer JP, Guerin JC, Arnaud A, Poirier R, Vesco D. Chemotherapy with high-dose cisplatin in brain metastasis of lung cancers [in French]. *Bulletin du cancer.* 1990;77(7):661–665.
67. Cocconi G, Lottici R, Bisagni G, et al. Combination therapy with platinum and etoposide of brain metastases from breast carcinoma. *Cancer Invest.* 1990;8(3–4):327–334.
68. Franciosi V, Cocconi G, Michiara M, et al. Front-line chemotherapy with cisplatin and etoposide for patients with brain metastases from breast carcinoma, nonsmall cell lung carcinoma, or malignant melanoma: a prospective study. *Cancer.* 1999;85(7):1599–1605.
69. Vinolas N, Graus F, Mellado B, Caralt L, Estape J. Phase II trial of cisplatinum and etoposide in brain metastases of solid tumors. *J Neurooncol.* 1997;35(2):145–148.
70. Malacarne P, Santini A, Maestri A. Response of brain metastases from lung cancer to systemic chemotherapy with carboplatin and etoposide. *Oncology.* 1996;53(3):210–213.
71. Minotti V, Crino L, Meacci ML, et al. Chemotherapy with cisplatin and teniposide for cerebral metastases in non-small cell lung cancer. *Lung Cancer.* 1998;20(2):93–98.
72. Cooper KG, Kitchener HC, Parkin DE. Cerebral metastases from epithelial ovarian carcinoma treated with carboplatin. *Gynecol Oncol.* 1994;55(2):318–323.
73. Colleoni M, Graiff C, Nelli P, et al. Activity of combination chemotherapy in brain metastases from breast and lung adenocarcinoma. *Am J Clin Oncol.* 1997;20(3):303–307.
74. Oberhoff C, Kieback DG, Wurstlein R, et al. Topotecan chemotherapy in patients with breast cancer and brain metastases: results of a pilot study. *Onkologie.* 2001;24(3):256–260.
75. Rosner D, Nemoto T, Lane WW. Chemotherapy induces regression of brain metastases in breast carcinoma. *Cancer.* 1986;58(4):832–839.
76. Boogerd W, Dalesio O, Bais EM, van der Sande JJ. Response of brain metastases from breast cancer to systemic chemotherapy. *Cancer.* 1992;69(4):972–980.
77. Postmus PE, Haaxma-Reiche H, Sleijfer DT, Kirkpatrick A, McVie JG, Kleisbauer JP. High dose etoposide for brain metastases of small cell lung cancer. A phase II study. The EORTC Lung Cancer Cooperative Group. *Br J Cancer.* 1989;59(2):254–256.
78. Lee JS, Murphy WK, Glisson BS, Dhingra HM, Holoye PY, Hong WK. Primary chemotherapy of brain metastasis in small-cell lung cancer. *J Clin Oncol.* 1989;7(7):916–922.
79. Postmus PE, Smit EF, Haaxma-Reiche H, et al. Teniposide for brain metastases of small-cell lung cancer: a phase II study. European Organization for Research and Treatment of Cancer Lung Cancer Cooperative Group. *J Clin Oncol.* 1995;13(3):660–665.
80. Kleisbauer JP, Vesco D, Orehek J, et al. Treatment of brain metastases of lung cancer with high doses of etoposide (VP16-213). Cooperative study from the Groupe Franais Pneumo-Cancerologie. *Eur J Cancer Clin Oncol.* 1988;24(2):131–135.
81. Kaba SE, Kyritsis AP, Hess K, et al. TPDC-FuHu chemotherapy for the treatment of recurrent metastatic brain tumors. *J Clin Oncol.* 1997;15(3):1063–1070.
82. Huang YJ, Wu YL, Xie SX, Yang JJ, Huang YS, Liao RQ. Weekly gemcitabine as a radiosensitiser for the treatment of brain metastases in patients with non-small cell lung cancer: phase I trial. *Chin Med J.* 2007;120(6):458–462.
83. Maraveyas A, Sgouros J, Upadhyay S, Abdel-Hamid AH, Holmes M, Lind M. Gemcitabine twice weekly as a radiosensitiser for the treatment of brain metastases in patients with carcinoma: a phase I study. *Br J Cancer.* 2005;92(5):815–819.
84. Mirmiran A, McClay E, Spear MA. Phase I/II study of IV topotecan in combination with whole brain radiation for the treatment of brain metastases. *Med Oncol.* 2007;24(2):147–153.
85. Kocher M, Eich HT, Semrau R, Guner SA, Muller RP. Phase I/II trial of simultaneous whole-brain irradiation and dose-escalating topotecan for brain metastases. *Strahlenther Onkol.* 2005;181(1):20–25.
86. Gruschow K, Klautke G, Fietkau R. Phase I/II clinical trial of concurrent radiochemotherapy in combination with topotecan for the treatment of brain metastases. *Eur J Cancer.* 2002;38(3):367–374.
87. Kouvaris JR, Miliadou A, Kouloulias VE, et al. Phase II study of temozolomide and concomitant whole-brain radiotherapy in patients with brain metastases from solid tumors. *Onkologie.* 2007;30(7):361–366.
88. Antonadou D, Paraskevaidis M, Sarris G, et al. Phase II randomized trial of temozolomide and concurrent radiotherapy in patients with brain metastases. *J Clin Oncol.* 2002;20(17):3644–3650.
89. Ushio Y, Arita N, Hayakawa T, et al. Chemotherapy of brain metastases from lung carcinoma: a controlled randomized study. *Neurosurgery.* 1991;28(2):201–205.
90. Lange OF, Scheef W, Haase KD. Palliative radio-chemotherapy with ifosfamide and BCNU for breast cancer patients with cerebral metastases. A 5-year experience. *Cancer Chemother Pharmacol.* 1990;26(suppl):S78-S80.

91. Hidalgo V, Dy C, Fernandez Hidalgo O, Calvo FA. Simultaneous radiotherapy and cis-platinum for the treatment of brain metastases. A pilot study. *Am J Clin Oncol.* 1987;10(3):205–209.
92. Stewart DJ, Feun LG, Maor M, et al. Weekly Cisplatin during cranial irradiation for malignant melanoma metastatic to brain. *J Neurooncol.* 1983;1(1):49–51.
93. Newlands ES, Stevens MF, Wedge SR, Wheelhouse RT, Brock C. Temozolomide: a review of its discovery, chemical properties, pre-clinical development and clinical trials. *Cancer Treat Rev.* 1997;23(1):35–61.
94. Stewart DJ, Mikhael NZ, Nair RC, et al. Platinum concentrations in human autopsy tumor samples. *Am J Clin Oncol.* 1988;11(2):152–158.
95. Lamond JP, Mehta MP, Boothman DA. The potential of topoisomerase I inhibitors in the treatment of CNS malignancies: report of a synergistic effect between topotecan and radiation. *J Neurooncol.* 1996;30(1):1–6.
96. Ceresoli GL, Cappuzzo F, Gregorc V, Bartolini S, Crino L, Villa E. Gefitinib in patients with brain metastases from non-small-cell lung cancer: a prospective trial. *Ann Oncol.* 2004;15(7):1042–1047.
97. Hotta K, Kiura K, Ueoka H, et al. Effect of gefitinib ('Iressa', ZD1839) on brain metastases in patients with advanced non-small-cell lung cancer. *Lung Cancer.* 2004;46(2):255–261.
98. Ishida A, Kanoh K, Nishisaka T, et al. Gefitinib as a first line of therapy in non-small cell lung cancer with brain metastases. *Intern Med.* 2004;43(8):718–720.
99. Namba Y, Kijima T, Yokota S, et al. Gefitinib in patients with brain metastases from non-small-cell lung cancer: review of 15 clinical cases. *Clin Lung Cancer.* 2004;6(2):123–128.
100. Roggero E, Busi G, Palumbo A, Pedrazzini A. Gefitinib ('Iressa', ZD1839) is active against brain metastases in a 77 year old patient. *J Neurooncol.* 2005;71(3):277–280.
101. Stemmler HJ, Weigert O, Krych M, Schoenberg SO, Ostermann H, Hiddemann W. Brain metastases in metastatic non-small cell lung cancer responding to single-agent gefitinib: a case report. *Anticancer Drugs.* 2005;16(7):747–749.
102. Nishi N, Kawai S, Yonezawa T, Fujimoto K, Masui K. Effect of gefitinib on brain metastases from non-small cell lung cancer. *Neurol Med Chir (Tokyo).* 2006;46(10):504–507.
103. Shimato S, Mitsudomi T, Kosaka T, et al. EGFR mutations in patients with brain metastases from lung cancer: association with the efficacy of gefitinib. *Neuro-oncol.* 2006;8(2):137–144.
104. Wu C, Li YL, Wang ZM, Li Z, Zhang TX, Wei Z. Gefitinib as palliative therapy for lung adenocarcinoma metastatic to the brain. *Lung Cancer.* 2007;57(3):359–364.
105. Omuro AM, Kris MG, Miller VA, et al. High incidence of disease recurrence in the brain and leptomeninges in patients with nonsmall cell lung carcinoma after response to gefitinib. *Cancer.* 2005;103(11):2344–2348.
106. Fekrazad MH, Ravindranathan M, Jones DV Jr. Response of intracranial metastases to erlotinib therapy. *J Clin Oncol.* 2007;25(31):5024–5026.
107. Lai CS, Boshoff C, Falzon M, Lee SM. Complete response to erlotinib treatment in brain metastases from recurrent NSCLC. *Thorax.* 2006;61(1):91.
108. Blackwell KL, Burstein H, Pegram M, et al. Determining relevant biomarkers from tissue and serum that may predict response to single agent lapatinib in trastuzumab refractory metastatic breast cancer. *Proc Am Soc Clin Oncol.* 2005;23(16S):Abstr 3004.
109. Gomez HL, Chavez MA, Doval DC, et al. A phase II, randomized trial using the small molecule tyrosine kinase inhibitor lapatinib as a first-line treatment in patients with FISH positive advanced or metastatic breast cancer. *Proc Am Soc Clin Oncol.* 2005;23(16S):Abstr 3064.
110. Lin NU, Carey LA, Liu MC, et al. Phase II trial of lapatinib for brain metastases in patients with HER2+ breast cancer. *Proc Am Soc Clin Oncol.* 2006;24(18S suppl):Abstr 503.
111. Lin NU, Diéras V, Paul D, et al. Multicenter phase II study of lapatinib in patients with brain metastases from HER2-positive breast cancer. *Clin Cancer Res.* 2009;15(4):1452–1459.
112. Geyer CE, Forster J, Lindquist D, et al. Lapatinib plus capecitabine for HER2-positive advanced breast cancer. *N Engl J Med.* 2006;355(26):2733–2743.
113. Wasserstrom WR, Glass JP, Posner JB. Diagnosis and treatment of leptomeningeal metastases from solid tumors: experience with 90 patients. *Cancer.* 1982;49:759–772.
114. Yap HY, Yap BS, Tashima CK, DiStefano A, Blumenschein GR. Meningeal carcinomatosis in breast cancer. *Cancer.* 1978;42:283–286.
115. Chamberlain MC, Sandy AD, Press GA. Leptomeningeal metastasis: a comparison of gadolinium-enhanced MR and contrast-enhanced CT of the brain. *Neurology.* 1990;40:435–438.
116. Padma MV, Jacobs M, Kraus G, Collins M, Dunigan K, Mantil J. 11C-methionine PET imaging of leptomeningeal metastases from primary breast cancer--a case report. *J Neurooncol.* 2001;55:39–44.
117. Aisner J, Aisner SC, Ostrow S, Govindan S, Mummert K, Wiernik P. Meningeal carcinomatosis from small cell carcinoma of the lung. Consequence of improved survival. *Acta cytologica.* 1979;23:292–299.
118. Yap BS, Yap HY, Fritsche HA, Blumenschein G, Bodey GP. CSF carcinoembryonic antigen in meningeal carcinomatosis from breast cancer. *JAMA.* 1980;244:1601–1603.
119. Garson JA, Coakham HB, Kemshead JT, et al. The role of monoclonal antibodies in brain tumour diagnosis and cerebrospinal fluid (CSF) cytology. *J Neurooncol.* 1985;3:165–171.
120. Herrlinger U, Wiendl H, Renninger M, Forschler H, Dichgans J, Weller M. Vascular endothelial growth factor (VEGF) in leptomeningeal metastasis: diagnostic and prognostic value. *Br J Cancer.* 2004;91:219–224.
121. Hermann B, Hultenschmidt B, Sautter-Bihl ML. Radiotherapy of the neuroaxis for palliative treatment of leptomeningeal carcinomatosis. *Strahlenther Onkol.* 2001;177:195–199.
122. Taillibert S, Laigle-Donadey F, Chodkiewicz C, Sanson M, Hoang-Xuan K, Delattre JY. Leptomeningeal metastases from solid malignancy: a review. *J Neurooncol.* 2005;75:85–99.
123. Kim DY, Lee KW, Yun T, et al. Comparison of intrathecal chemotherapy for leptomeningeal carcinomatosis of a solid tumor: methotrexate alone versus methotrexate in combination with cytosine arabinoside and hydrocortisone. *Jpn J Clin Oncol.* 2003;33:608–612.
124. Esteva FJ, Soh LT, Holmes FA, et al. Phase II trial and pharmacokinetic evaluation of cytosine arabinoside for leptomeningeal metastases from breast cancer. *Cancer Chemother Pharmacol.* 2000;46:382–386.
125. Chamberlain MC, Kormanik P. Leptomeningeal metastasis. *J Neurosurg.* 1997;86:576–577.
126. Hara H, Igarashi A, Yano Y, Yashiro T, Ueno E, Aiyoshi Y. Interventricular methotrexate therapy for carcinomatous meningitis due to breast cancer: a case with leukoencephalopathy. *Breast Cancer.* 2000;7:247–251.
127. Grossman SA, Finkelstein DM, Ruckdeschel JC, Trump DL, Moynihan T, Ettinger DS. Randomized prospective comparison of intraventricular methotrexate and thiotepa in patients with previously untreated neoplastic meningitis. Eastern Cooperative Oncology Group. *J Clin Oncol.* 1993;11:561–569.
128. Jaeckle KA, Batchelor T, O'Day SJ, et al. An open label trial of sustained-release cytarabine (DepoCyt) for the intrathecal treatment of solid tumor neoplastic meningitis. *J Neurooncol.* 2002;57:231–239.
129. Orlando L, Curigliano G, Colleoni M, et al. Intrathecal chemotherapy in carcinomatous meningitis from breast cancer. *Anticancer Res.* 2002;22:3057–3059.
130. Lassman AB, Abrey LE, Shah GG, et al. Systemic high-dose intravenous methotrexate for central nervous system metastases. *J Neurooncol.* 2006;78(3):255–260.
131. Davis T, Fadul C, Glantz M, et al. Pilot phase II trial of temozolomide for leptomeningeal metastases: Preliminary report. *Proc Am Soc Clin Oncol.* 2003;22:115:(Abstr 460).
132. Boogerd W, van den Bent MJ, Koehler PJ, et al. The relevance of intraventricular chemotherapy for leptomeningeal metastasis in breast cancer: a randomised study. *Eur J Cancer.* 2004;40:2726–2733.
133. Ozdogan M, Samur M, Bozcuk HS, et al. Durable remission of leptomeningeal metastasis of breast cancer with letrozole: a case report and implications of biomarkers on treatment selection. *Jpn J Clin Oncol.* 2003;33:229–231.
134. Sakai M, Ishikawa S, Ito H, et al. Carcinomatous meningitis from non-small-cell lung cancer responding to gefitinib. *Int J Clin Oncol.* 2006;11:243–245.
135. Boogerd W, Dorresteijn LD, van Der Sande JJ, de Gast GC, Bruning PF. Response of leptomeningeal metastases from breast cancer to hormonal therapy. *Neurology.* 2000;55:117–119.

72 Primary Central Nervous System Lymphoma

Cigall Kadoch and James L. Rubenstein

INTRODUCTION

Primary central nervous system lymphoma (PCNSL) is a rare variant of non-Hodgkin lymphoma (NHL), representing 1% to 2% of all cases of NHL [1]. PCNSL is defined as lymphoma presenting in the brain, spinal cord, leptomeninges, or within the orbits and which is restricted entirely to the central nervous system (CNS). The disease presents unique prognostic and treatment considerations among primary brain tumors, and the therapeutic arsenal used in PCNSL is distinct from systemic NHL.

Over the past three decades, the incidence of PCNSL has increased in parallel with a rise in the number of cases of systemic NHL. PCNSL now accounts for 3.1% of all primary brain tumors in the United States. At present, this rise cannot be completely explained by the HIV epidemic and does not appear to be a consequence of advances in diagnostic techniques [2,3]. Among immunocompetent patients with PCNSL, there is a slight male predominance (3:2 ratio of males to female), while in the AIDS population, 90% are men.

Greater than 90% of PCNSL cases in the immunocompetent patient population exhibit the pathologic characteristics of diffuse large B-cell lymphoma (DLBCL); the remainder includes other B-cell histologies such as immunoblastic and lymphoblastic B-cell lymphoma, Burkitt and Burkitt-like lymphoma as well as T-cell lymphomas. Both B- and T-cell variants are histologically identical to their systemic counterparts; however, PCNSL is associated with a worse prognosis than other localized extranodal lymphomas.

Despite recent advances in treatment, nearly all patients with PCNSL relapse or exhibit refractory disease requiring salvage therapy, which to date remains unsatisfactory (Figure 72.1).

CLINICAL FEATURES AND PRESENTATION

While PCNSL can affect all ages, the peak incidence is in the sixth decade, with a mean age of 55 years in immunocompetent patients; for the immunocompromised PCNSL patients, the mean age of diagnosis is 30 years. The absence of systemic tumor confirms the primary nature of this disease. If lymphoma is found concomitantly outside the CNS, the diagnosis is not PCNSL but rather stage IV NHL with CNS involvement.

PCNSL may disrupt virtually any aspect of normal CNS function, depending on the location(s) of the tumor. Greater than 50% of patients present with focal neurologic deficits such as hemiparesis or aphasia; 35% exhibit alteration in cognition, behavior, or personality; 11% present with seizure; and 32% present with headache, hydrocephalus, nausea, vomiting, and papilledema as a manifestation of increased intracranial pressure. PCNSL most commonly involves the cerebral hemispheres, followed by the basal ganglia, corpus callosum, and cerebellum. Rarely, these tumors arise in deep brain structures such as the brainstem and spinal cord. PCNSL tumors are typically in contact with cerebrospinal fluid spaces [1]. In 20% to 40% of immunocompetent patients, multiple lesions are observed at initial diagnosis; nearly 100% of AIDS patients present with multifocal lesions.

Approximately, 10% to 20% of patients present with intraocular lymphoma (IOL) manifest by ocular floaters, blurred vision, and clumped cellular infiltrates detected on slit-lamp examination. It is often difficult to distinguish IOL from vitreitis/uveitis. Fewer than 10% of patients exhibit spinal dissemination marked by cauda equina syndrome, back pain, or radiculopathy. It is useful to obtain information relating to truncal anesthesias, bladder problems, or nonspecific pain in order to appropriately evaluate these symptoms.

DIAGNOSIS AND CLINICAL EVALUATION

Gadolinium-enhanced magnetic resonance imaging (MRI) is the standard imaging modality used to facilitate the diagnostic work-up of PCNSL. Usually, PCNSL is hypointense on T1-weighted images and hypo to isointense on T2-imaging with intense homogeneous contrast enhancement due to the diffuse nature and poorly defined borders of these lesions. Necrotic centers often characterize the lesions following corticosteroid therapy. The majority of radiographic lesions are supratentorial and exhibit periventricular localization as demonstrated by neuroimaging. Significant peritumoral edema is less frequently observed in PCNSL compared with high-grade gliomas or brain metastases. In AIDS-related PCNSL, lesions are usually less homogenous with peripheral areas of enhancement surrounding necrotic centers, thus appearing as ring-enhancing on T-1 weighted imaging. Approximately, one

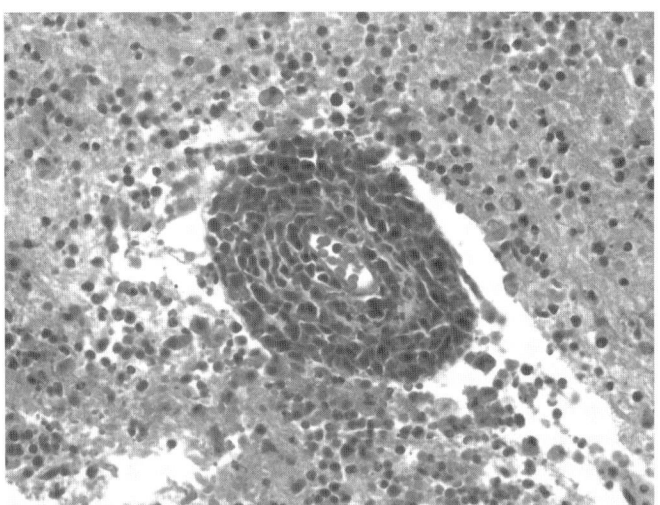

Figure 72.1 Perivascular growth pattern of a B-cell primary CNS lymphoma Hematoxylin Eosin at 400× magnification. See color insert.

third of immunocompromised patients have masses that do not enhance following contrast administration. PCNSL lesions are unifocal in approximately 60% of cases and multifocal in 20% to 40% of cases by MRI. More than 90% of AIDS patients have multifocal PCNSL on radiographic imaging [4,5]. There is a significant tendency for PCNSL tumors at relapse to progress within the leptomeninges [6]. This manifestation of biologic invasiveness is a significant factor in terms of therapeutic management as PCNSL is virtually always refractory to surgical resection or focal radiotherapy. Magnetic resonance spectroscopy identifies lesions with decreased levels of N-acetyl-aspartate and increased ratios (>3:1) of choline to creatinine. Because of the high intrinsic metabolic activity of the brain, PET imaging is rarely used to facilitate diagnosis of PCNSL.

When NHL presents with only neurologic signs and symptoms, and a pathologic diagnosis of NHL is established by detection of tumor within the CNS, in 90% of cases the diagnosis is PCNSL. Nevertheless, a thorough staging work-up is requisite to definitively rule out systemic disease and to define the extent of CNS involvement. This process requires careful evaluation of distinct compartments within the CNS axis. An MRI with contrast is needed to evaluate brain and spine; an ophthalmologic evaluation, including slit-lamp exam, is mandated to evaluate possible concomitant intravitreous disease. Lumbar puncture is appropriate in all patients (unless contraindicated because of increased intracranial pressure), not only to facilitate diagnosis but also to assess for evidence of leptomeningeal involvement. MRI of the total spine with gadolinium is necessary in patients with suspicion for leptomeningeal dissemination. In addition, staging bone marrow biopsy as well as CT scan of the chest, abdomen, and pelvis should be performed.

Because approximately 30% of testicular lymphomas metastasize to the brain, a testicular examination is indicated to rule out concomitant testicular lymphoma. HIV antibody testing is indicated in all patients with suspicion for CNS lymphoma, as HIV-associated lymphoma has different implications in terms of therapy and prognosis. As with systemic NHL, a serum lactate dehydrogenase (LDH) measurement informs prognosis. Approximately, 10% of patients who present with a tentative diagnosis of PCNSL will ultimately be found to have occult systemic NHL on rigorous systemic staging evaluation, which includes bone marrow biopsy. In addition, there is recent preliminary evidence that the identification of clonally rearranged immunoglobulin-heavy chain (IgH) genes, identified by polymerase chain reaction, may be useful as biomarkers for the identification of subclinical disease in bone marrow [7,8].

Establishing a diagnosis of PCNSL may be a significant challenge in the patient who presents with neurologic symptoms and suspicious findings on radiographic imaging. The differential diagnosis may be broad, given the nonspecific findings on neuroimaging, and often includes glioma, metastatic malignancy, vasculitis, sarcoid, infection, or multiple sclerosis. There is often significant diagnostic latency in the presentation of PCNSL—in particular, in immunocompetent patients in whom the disease may present with a smoldering course. A critical problem in the initial diagnostic work-up of patients with PCNSL is the common practice of administering glucocorticoids as an early intervention to attenuate or reverse progressive neurologic decline at first presentation, before diagnosis. Because glucocorticoids usually induce tumor regression, likely through induction of apoptosis, administration of steroids such as dexamethasone before diagnosis increases risk for a nondiagnostic specimen at initial work-up. The rate of complete response to single-agent glucocorticoids may be as high as 20% [9]. The ideal approach, therefore, is to withhold corticosteroids prior to biopsy unless there is active clinical decompensation mandating this intervention before diagnosis.

Stereotactic biopsy is the preferred method for obtaining a tissue diagnosis in patients suspected of having PCNSL. There is up to a 4% risk of significant intracranial hemorrhage associated with stereotactic biopsy [10]. In addition, stereotactic biopsy is associated with an 8% to 9% rate of diagnostic failure, defined as a biopsy in which a definitive histological diagnosis is not achieved based on the tissue obtained [11]. Unlike malignant gliomas, aggressive surgical resection in PCNSL has no proven therapeutic value, unless immediate surgical decompression is required because of impending herniation or critical neurologic deterioration. Failed stereotactic biopsies are frequently associated with antecedent use of glucocorticoids or absent intraoperative pathological examination [12].

In subsets of patients who present with signs and symptoms of IOL, pathologic diagnosis of lymphoma may be obtained by vitreal biopsy after detection of a suspicious intraocular infiltrate by slit lamp, fluorescein angiography, or ocular ultrasound. Another means of establishing tissue diagnosis is by evaluation of the cerebrospinal fluid: 10% to 20% of patients with PCNSL present with overt leptomeningeal lymphoma. In these patients, diagnostic information may be achieved via lumbar puncture with cytologic analysis and/or flow cytometric analysis to identify kappa or lambda light chain restriction in lymphoma cells. Pathologic diagnosis of either leptomeningeal or brain parenchymal lymphoma are essentially equivalent to establish the diagnosis of PCSNL and have identical prognostic and therapeutic implications. IOL may exist as an independent entity, with an approximate 80% risk of eventual CNS dissemination; because the intraocular compartment is a chemotherapeutic sanctuary site, the diagnosis of IOL raises an independent set of therapeutic concerns.

Recent evidence suggests that diagnostic brain biopsy may be obviated in selected cases in the setting of suspected AIDS-associated PCNSL. The association between Epstein-Barr virus (EBV) infection and AIDS-related PCNSL is well established, and the detection of EBV DNA in CSF by polymerase chain reaction has been shown to be a useful biomarker with specificity in excess of 95%. Because single photon emission computed tomography (SPECT) is also able to differentiate between cerebral lymphoma and nonneoplastic lesions in patients with AIDS such as toxoplasmosis, concordant positive SPECT and EBV DNA polymerase chain reaction results appear to obviate the need for brain biopsy and may facilitate immediate clinical intervention in the treatment of AIDS-associated PCNSL [13]. Positron emission tomography has also been shown to facilitate distinction between CNS lymphoma and cerebral toxoplasmosis in AIDS patients with contrast-enhancing lesions [14]. Unfortunately, there is, at present, no established CSF marker to facilitate the noninvasive diagnosis of PCNSL arising in immunocompetent patients, and definitive diagnosis is usually dependent upon histopathologic analysis.

Because the diagnosis of CNS lymphoma is often delayed as lesions may not be amenable to brain biopsy or because of lesional response to steroids, the detailed proteomic evaluation of the CSF is under investigation as a novel approach to identify specific protein biomarkers that may distinguish lymphomatous lesions within the brain from inflammatory lesions with similar radiographic appearance. The utilization of such biomarkers may complement neuroimaging to facilitate early and noninvasive diagnosis as well as clinical monitoring [15].

RISK FACTORS FOR DISEASE DEVELOPMENT AND CLINICAL PROGNOSTIC FACTORS FOR OUTCOME

Risk factors for the development of PCNSL are similar to those associated with other types of NHL, namely, chronic inflammation and stimulation of the immune system. Profound immunodeficiency associated with AIDS, the Wiskott-Aldrich syndrome, immunoglobulin-A deficiency syndrome, and severe combined immunodeficiency (SCID), or even more subtle immunodeficiency states such as those associated with rheumatoid arthritis and systemic lupus erythematosus, clearly represent predisposing factors to the development of PCNSL. In AIDS, PCNSL tends to be a manifestation of advanced disease and is associated with a CD4 count of less than 50 cells/mm3 [16,4].

Two major prognostic schemes have recently been proposed for newly diagnosed patients with PCNSL. In 2003, Ferreri, on behalf of the International Extranodal Lymphoma Study Group (IELSG), proposed a disease-specific prognostic score based upon five variables: age, PS, LDH serum level, CSF protein concentration, and involvement of deep regions of the brain. Age greater than 60 years, ECOG performance status greater than one, elevated serum LDH level, elevated CSF protein concentration, and involvement of deep regions of the brain (periventricular regions, basal ganglia, brainstem, and/or cerebellum) were significantly and independently associated with a worse survival. Each of these five factors, when considered as discrete variables added together, constitute the prognostic score according to this system. Each variable was assigned a value of either 0, if favorable, or 1, if unfavorable. The cumulative prognostic score was then tested in 105 assessable PCNSL patients for which complete data for all five variables were available. The 2-year overall survival (OS) was 80%, 48%, and 15% ($P = 0.00001$) for patients with zero to one, two to three, and four to five unfavorable features, respectively [17]. The prognostic value of this score was validated by analysis of PCNSL patients who were treated with high-dose methotrexate-based chemotherapy. Neither the histologic subtype of NHL (large cell vs. nonlarge cell) nor the presence of leptomeningeal or ocular disease had an impact on survival in PCNSL. The only treatment-related variable that has been shown to reproducibly impact survival is the use of high-dose systemic methotrexate-containing regimens [18]. Use of intrathecal chemotherapy, high-dose cytarabine, and the use of anthracyclines did not impact survival in multivariate analysis. This analysis, which was based upon the evaluation of 378 PCNSL patients treated at 23 cancer centers in 5 different countries, includes variables related to tumor aggressiveness such as extension and site of disease.

Memorial-Sloan-Kettering Cancer Center has proposed a simpler prognostic model based upon clinical variables of age and Karnovsky performance status, which was developed on the basis of a retrospective analysis of 282 patients who were treated on RTOG studies [19]. It is currently undetermined whether the inclusion of all five prognostic biomarkers proposed by the IELSG provides greater accuracy or whether the discrepancies in these two schemas is based on the fact that European versus American PCNSL are treated with significantly different therapeutic regimens.

PATHOLOGY AND PROGNOSIS IN PCNSL

At least 95% of PCNSL are B-cell neoplasms that express the B-cell marker CD20. A central puzzle in the pathogenesis of PCNSL is what accounts for the presentation of lymphoma within the brain, an organ devoid of resident lymphocytes under normal circumstances. In addition, while the lymphoma spreads aggressively within the CNS, these tumors rarely metastasize elsewhere in the body. At least two hypotheses may explain this phenomena: one is that lymphoma represents the malignant transformation of an inflammatory process that has developed *in situ* within the CNS. A second is that malignant B-lymphocytes acquire selective adhesion receptors for ligands expressed by the brain, for example, the cerebral vascular endothelium. However, to date, no unique adhesion receptors have been identified that distinguish CNS lymphomas from systemic lymphoma. A recent study identified CXCL13, a lymphoid chemokine involved in B-cell compartmental homing within secondary lymphoid organs in PCNSL tumors, suggesting that this chemokine may influence CNS localization [20]. Indeed, high expression of CXCL13 was also confirmed at the RNA level by gene expression profile analysis [21]. However, vascular expression of CXCL13 could not be demonstrated, suggesting that expression of this chemokine alone does not contribute to CNS tropism of lymphoma. A recent gene expression profile analysis of brain lymphomas that compared the transcriptome of PCNSL with nodal large B-cell NHL identified several hundred genes with significant differential expression between PCNSL and its systemic counterpart. Interleukin-4 (IL-4), a B-cell growth factor, was also demonstrated to be ectopically expressed both by the tumor vasculature as well as by the lymphoma cells in PCNSL. The study proposed that IL-4 elaborated by the tumor microenvironment may facilitate lymphoma survival signaling and stimulate a favorable tumor microenvironment, perhaps facilitating lymphoma survival and CNS tropism. In support of this hypothesis was the observation that tumors with high expression of activated STAT-6, a transcriptional mediator of IL-4 signaling, exhibited significantly shorter survival among patients treated with high-dose, methotrexate-containing regimens compared with tumors with lower expression of activated STAT-6 [22].

The vast majority of PCNSL in immunocompetent individuals are large B-cell neoplasms that express the transcription factor BCL-6 as well as the oncogene BCL-2 [23]. Molecular genetic studies have revealed that the p14 ARF gene and p16INK4a gene are frequently inactivated by either homozygous deletion or by hypermethylation in approximately 56% of cases of PCNSL [24]. In addition to BCL-6 protein expression, genetic evidence supports the notion that primary CNS lymphomas originate from germinal centers, given shared genetic properties, including a high frequency of mutations in the immunoglobulin variable gene region [25]. The notion that PCNSL are related to germinal center large B-cell lymphomas is, in a sense, paradoxical given that the prognosis for patients diagnosed with PCNSL is significantly worse than the prognosis of patients with most cases of limited stage, aggressive NHL. This concept is in disagreement with the data that germinal center large cell lymphomas are associated with a favorable prognosis relative to the activated B-cell type [26]. Recent gene expression profile data of PCNSL tumors obtained from immunocompetent patients not only provide evidence for germinal center ontogeny but also demonstrate that PCNSL express features of both germinal center as well as activated B-cell lymphomas and thus represent a unique histogenetic time slot of B-cell tumorigenesis [21,27,28]. In AIDS, the majority of PCNSL are EBV-driven neoplasms of either Burkitt's or large-cell histology.

In the latter, PCNSL arises from EBV infection of B-lymphocytes, which proliferate unchecked forming neoplasms in the immunoprivilaged environment of the CNS. PCNSL in this setting is observed mainly in patients afflicted with HIV or congenital immunodeficiency syndromes as well as patients who are status-post organ transplantation.

THERAPY OF PCNSL

Immunocompetent PCNSL

Untreated, most patients with PCNSL succumb to this aggressive neoplasm within 3 months of diagnosis. Treatments for this disease are in evolution and the optimal therapy for PCNSL has yet to be defined. However, a number of therapeutic principles have emerged with the accumulation of formal clinical experience and with the perspective of multicenter phase-II clinical trials in PCNSL.

In the past 5 to 10 years, clinical investigators have recognized that, unlike the vast majority of patients with malignant gliomas, long-term lymphoma-free survival is possible in PCNSL, with 5-year rates of overall survival approaching 30% to 40% [29]. Overview of multiple clinical series demonstrates, however, that approximately 20% of patients exhibit primary refractory disease to chemotherapeutic interventions within the first 6 months of therapy and succumb to tumor progression.

Glucocorticoids

Glucocorticoids are a cornerstone of treatment in PCNSL given their direct lymphocytoxic effects as well as their ability to reduce tumor-associated edema. There is evidence that the oncolytic effect of glucocorticoids may be more marked in PCNSL than in systemic lymphomas, with single-agent response rates approaching 70% in lymphomas which involve the brain [9]. As above, a common problem is that initial complete responses yielded by glucocorticoids may increase the risk for nondiagnostic biopsies, resulting in significant delays both in diagnosis as well as in the initiation of definitive therapy.

Radiation Therapy

PCNSL is a radiation-sensitive disease: response rates to whole-brain irradiation exceed 90% and rates of complete response are approximately 60%. Whole-brain irradiation therapy has historically been a cornerstone of the therapeutic management of PCNSL and extends survival compared with no therapy; median survival with radiation alone is between 12 and 18 months [30]. Approaches using focal irradiation are not used because of the multifocal, highly infiltrative nature of this tumor. There also is currently no data to support the use of a radiation boost to the tumor bed [31]. Total radiation dose may also be a significant factor given the data of Bessel et al, which compared outcomes in patients who received identical chemotherapy programs followed by whole-brain irradiation at 4500 cGy versus 3060 cGy. Reduction in the dose of radiation from 4500 to 3060 cGy was associated with a significantly increased risk of relapse and lower overall survival [32]. For this reason, the standard dose of whole-brain irradiation is generally still considered to be between 4000 cGy and 4500 cGy.

There is, however, recent preliminary evidence to support the use of lower dose whole-brain irradiation (2340 cGy) in patients who achieve a complete remission to induction based upon combination methotrexate, rituximab plus procarbazine [33]. There is no evidence that craniospinal axis irradiation provides meaningful therapeutic benefit unless there is evidence of spinal dissemination or meningeal drop metastases. It is important to note that spinal cord irradiation may ultimately compromise therapeutic options because of radiation-induced bone marrow suppression [4].

Chemotherapy

Conventional therapy for systemic large B-cell lymphoma includes combination chemotherapy, usually with cyclophosphamide, doxorubicin, vincristine, and prednisone (CHOP). Multicenter studies of CHOP (or of CHO with dexamethasone substituting for prednisone) followed by cranial radiation demonstrate that these agents are ineffective for PCNSL and do not improve survival over whole-brain irradiation alone [34,35]. The biological basis for the differential sensitivity may relate to the blood-brain barrier: the majority of compounds in the CHOP regimen penetrate poorly into the CNS due to the specific molecular characteristics of the CNS vasculature, including the unique expression of tight junctions. Another possible contributing factor are molecular distinctions between PCNSL and systemic lymphomas, which potentially are responsible for differential chemotherapeutic sensitivity [27].

Intravenous administration of methotrexate at ≥ 1 gm/m^2 yields cytotoxic levels in the CSF (> 1 micromolar) [36] in patients with brain tumors. Canellos and colleagues in the 1970s were among the first to describe dramatic antilymphoma effects in recurrent primary and secondary CNS lymphomas with the use of high dose methotrexate monotherapy [37,38]. Bokstein et al provided evidence that the rate of complete response to high-dose intravenous methotrexate for metastatic NHL within the brain was twofold higher than the rate of response for systemic lymphoma in the same patients [39]. As above, the use of high-dose methotrexate has emerged in multivariate analyses as the most important treatment-related prognostic variable in PCNSL.

Combined-Modality Therapy

Combined-modality therapy for PCNSL was developed in the 1980s by investigators at Memorial Sloan-Kettering Cancer Center. This approach involved methotrexate administered both by intrathecal injection through an Ommaya reservoir as well as high-dose intravenous injection at doses equal to or greater than 1 gm/m^2 body surface area, in combination with the alkylating agent procarbazine plus the vinca alkaloid, vincristine. Repeat administration of combination chemotherapy preceded the initiation of whole-brain irradiation. High-dose intravenous cytarabine was administered at the completion of irradiation. This combined-modality approach resulted in prolongation of survival with median overall survival of 42 months and 5-year survival of 22.3 months, significantly better than the 3% to 5% rate of 5-year survival that results with the use of whole-brain irradiation without pretreatment chemotherapy [29].

The problem of treatment-related neurotoxicity in PCNSL has become a central issue in the consideration of treatment planning for these patients. The use of whole-brain irradiation has been associated with at least 80% rate of delayed neurotoxicity, characterized by a syndrome of progressive dementia, gait ataxia, and urinary incontinence, presenting with an average latency of 13 months in patients aged 60 or greater [29]. Neurotoxicity associated with the combination of whole-brain irradiation plus high-dose methotrexate is associated with diffuse white matter disease and cortical-subcortical atrophy. Autopsy data have demonstrated white matter damage with gliosis, small vessel thickening, and demyelination [20]. Because the use of chemotherapy alone in PCNSL patients has not been associated with a high rate of profound neurotoxicity, there is great interest in the implementation of more effective chemotherapy regimens that eliminate the use of whole-brain irradiation.

Evaluation of late neurotoxicity in PCNSL patients was formally evaluated by an EORTC study (European Organization for Research and Treatment of Cancer), which focused on combined-modality therapy involving high-dose methotrexate followed by whole-brain irradiation. This evaluation included extensive neuropsychological assessments, including quality-of-life measures in 19 patients. The average age of patients in this study was 44 years. Results were compared with age- and sex-matched control subjects with systemic hematologic malignancies who received similar types of chemotherapy regimens as well as radiotherapy that did not involve the brain. Significant cognitive impairment was found in 63% of patients with PCNSL compared to only 11% of control subjects. Only 42% of surviving PCNSL patients resumed work compared to 81% of control subjects. The conclusions of this formal neurocognitive evaluation therefore extend the conclusions of Abrey et al in that significant cognitive impairment was commonly detected in patients younger than 60 years who were treated with combined-modality therapy involving whole-brain irradiation [40].

The regimen developed at Memorial Sloan-Kettering that involves high-dose methotrexate, procarbazine, and vincristine followed by whole-brain irradiation was recently studied in a multicenter evaluation involving the RTOG in 102 immunocompetent patients with PCNSL. The rate of complete response to preirradiation chemotherapy (methotrexate, procarbazine and vincristine) was 58%; the median overall survival was 36.9 months. Fifteen percent of patients ($n = 12$) exhibited delayed neurologic toxicity; eight of these died, thus confirming the potential for severe neurotoxicity with combined modality therapy [29,41]. No prospective neuropsychological testing was performed, and the 15% incidence of neurotoxicity reported was clearly a minimum estimate.

Intrathecal Methotrexate

The role of intrathecal chemotherapy during the induction chemotherapy for PCNSL is also a significant consideration under debate. A recent study of high-dose intravenous methotrexate that evaluated matched CSF and serum pharmacokinetic data demonstrated that cytotoxic CSF and serum MTX concentrations were maintained much longer after intravenous administration compared with intrathecal dosing of methotrexate. Outcomes in 16 patients who received high-dose intravenous methotrexate at 8 gm/m^2 over 4 hours for solid tumor neoplastic meningitis malignancies were retrospectively compared to a reference group of patients treated only with intrathecal methotrexate. The median survival in the group treated with high-dose methotrexate was significantly longer than the group treated with intrathecal methotrexate 13.8 months versus 2.3 months (P = 0.003) [36]. Two retrospective studies suggest that PCNSL patients do not benefit from additional intrathecal chemotherapy through an Ommaya reservoir if they receive high-dose intravenous methotrexate. There is, at present, no evidence to support the routine administration of intrathecal methotrexate in newly diagnosed PCNSL patients who receive intensive high-dose methotrexate therapy exceeding a dose of at least 1 gm/m^2 body surface area [42].

Moreover, complications of intrathecal chemotherapy include neurotoxicity, chemical meningitis, and infection of the Ommaya reservoir. Ommaya reservoir infection occurs commonly in cancer patients treated with cytotoxic chemotherapy, affecting 19% of patients in one recent trial [43]. This serious complication can lead to considerable morbidity, including disruption of treatment schedules. At present, many neuro-oncologists therefore restrict the use of intrathecal chemotherapy to patients with positive CSF cytology.

High-Dose Methotrexate

In parallel with the development of combined-modality therapy for PCNSL, clinical investigators at Massachusetts General Hospital performed evaluations of intensive intravenous methotrexate monotherapy with deferral of radiotherapy until progression. Methotrexate at 8 gm/m^2 was given every 2 weeks until complete response followed by four more cycles every 2 weeks then monthly methotrexate treatments through 1 year of therapy. The initial responses in 31 patients were promising, with an overall rate of response of 100% and a complete response rate of 65%. The treatment was demonstrated to be well tolerated with a minimal rate of myelosuppression and mucositis. Quality-of-life assessment in 11 long-term survivors was similar to normative groups and there was no evidence of delayed encephalopathy related to methotrexate exposure [44]. This pilot experience led to a recent multicenter study of intensive high-dose methotrexate (8 gm/m^2) administered every 2 weeks through the New Approaches to Brain Tumor Therapy Consortium (NABTT) [45]. The rate of complete response to high-dose methotrexate in the multicenter study was 52%; no delayed neurotoxicity was detected in this multicenter study. Median progression-free survival was 12.8 months.

A similar trial of high-dose methotrexate monotherapy, performed in Germany, demonstrated weaker activity of high-dose methotrexate monotherapy in the induction treatment of PCNSL. Only 30% of 37 patients achieved a CR and 38% had progressive disease while on treatment. After 4 years of follow-up, the rate of leukoencephalopathy in patients who survived more than 12 months was 58% for the group that received salvage therapy with whole-brain irradiation and only 10% for the patients who did not receive whole-brain irradiation [46,47].

Because there is evidence that the blood-brain barrier may contribute to resistance to chemotherapeutic agents and to therapeutic failure in brain tumors, there has been considerable interest in developing methods to disrupt the tight junctions and specializations of CNS endothelia that normally restrict entry of macromolecules into the brain. One approach has been to use osmotic agents to disrupt the blood-brain barrier followed by intra-arterial or intravenous chemotherapy. The experience with 74 PCNSL patients treated with osmotic blood-brain barrier disruption followed by intra-arterial methotrexate, intravenous cyclophosphamide, and either oral procarbazine or intravenous or intra-arterial etoposide was recently described by McAllister et al. The estimated 5-year survival in this group was 42% over a 15-year period. The rate of complete response was 65%, and the estimated median survival was 40.7 months. While each disruption procedure requires general anesthesia and is associated with significant acute toxicities, including stroke and seizure, comprehensive neuropsychological testing performed in 36 patients who achieved a durable CR (>1 year) revealed no evidence of cognitive loss in those patients who ultimately did not receive whole-brain irradiation [48].

AUTOLOGOUS STEM-CELL TRANSPLANT

Because high-dose chemotherapy with the support of autologous stem-cell transplantation (ASCT) is an effective treatment for a subset of patients with high-risk or relapsed systemic NHL [49], this strategy is being evaluated in PCNSL, both to maximize the potential benefit of chemotherapy and to avoid the toxicity of whole-brain irradiation in patients with newly diagnosed PCNSL. Abrey et al were among the first to conduct a trial involving ASCT in this disease. These investigators used high-dose methotrexate and cytarabine as induction therapy followed by BEAM (carmustine, etoposide, cytarabine and melphalan) as the preparative regimen without whole-brain irradiation. Fourteen of 28 patients enrolled exhibited sufficient response to induction to ultimately warrant ASCT. Median progression-free survival for transplanted patients was only 9.3 months; 8 of 14 patients who received ASCT developed progressive disease at a median of 2.3 months after transplantation [50].

While these results demonstrate that ASCT is feasible for patients with PCNSL, the unacceptable rate of early relapse in the study using the BEAM combination raises the question of whether other preparative regimens may exhibit greater disease control in PCNSL. Soussain et al used a conditioning regimen consisting of busulfan, thiotepa, and cyclophosphamide in 22 patients with recurrent (10 patients) or refractory (12 patients) PCNSL and/or ocular lymphoma. Transplantation was associated with a 53%

rate of 3-year event-free survival and 20% rate of relapse in this heavily pretreated population. Patients over 60 years suffered a 71% rate of treatment-related mortality. An unexpected aspect of this study was the efficacy of combination high-dose cytarabine plus etoposide as salvage therapy before ASCT. Combination high-dose cytarabine plus etoposide resulted in 12 responses (8 complete) among 14 treated patients [51]. A recent successor study performed by this French group confirms their preliminary data regarding the efficacy of intensive chemotherapy plus autologous stem cell transplant in patients with recurrent disease [52].

Several principles have thus emerged with respect to therapeutic options for patients with PCNSL. One, an accumulation of evidence demonstrates that long-term survival and cure is now possible in PCNSL. While approximately 20% of patients exhibit early refractory disease in response to cytotoxic therapy, a significant fraction of these patients (between 20%–30%) exhibit durable responses and long-term survival with simple high-dose methotrexate-based chemotherapy without receipt of whole-brain irradiation [45]. In addition, there is increasing evidence that augmentation of high-dose methotrexate with other chemotherapeutic and/or biologic agents may result in durable responses for a greater fraction of patients with acceptable toxicity [53,54–58,59] (Table 72.1).

Immunotherapy

Management of relapsed or refractory disease is an area of active clinical study. A number of agents are under investigation, including the anti-CD20 monoclonal antibody rituximab. Rituximab is the first monoclonal antibody to receive FDA approval in the treatment of cancer. CD20 is a cell-surface protein that is expressed exclusively on mature B cells and is not expressed by neurons or by glia. Rituximab is a chimeric human IgG1 in which the CD20-binding region was derived by genetic engineering from a mouse monoclonal antibody.

While rituximab has activity as a single agent in the treatment of relapsed large cell lymphoma, there is an accumulation of data demonstrating synergistic interaction with chemotherapy. Randomized data generated by the Groupe d'Etude des Lymphomes de l'Adulte (GELA) comparing CHOP chemotherapy plus rituximab versus CHOP alone in 399 elderly patients with systemic, non-CNS diffuse large-B-cell lymphoma revealed that the rate of complete response was significantly higher in the group that received CHOP plus rituximab than in the group that received CHOP alone (76% vs. 63%, $P = 0.005$). The addition of rituximab to standard CHOP chemotherapy also significantly reduced the risk of treatment failure and death [60].

This data is likely relevant to PCNSL as large B-cell lymphoma is the most common lymphoma histology to present in the brain [60]. For this reason, a number of studies are exploring use of rituximab in this disease, both as a single agent and in combination with chemotherapy [55,61]. One of the limitations of the systemic administration of rituximab, however, is that only approximately 0.1% of this monoclonal antibody appears to penetrate the

Table 72.1 Recent Therapeutic Trials in Primary CNS Lymphoma

Study	No. of Patients	Regimen	Response Rate (%) (CR and PR)	Median PFS (mo)	Median OS (mo)
Radiotherapy alone					
Nelson et al [31]	41	40 Gy WBRT with 20 Gy boost	NA*	NA	12.2
Chemoradiotherapy					
Abrey et al [29]	52	MPV (MTX 3.5 g/m^2) cytarabine (3 g/m^2) IT MTX +/- 45 Gy WBRT	94	NA	60
DeAngelis et al [41]	102	MPV (MTX 2.5 g/m^2) + IT MTX + 36–45 Gy WBRT	94	24	36.9
Poortmans et al [56]	52	MTX (3 g/m^2) teniposide/camustine + IT MTX + IT cytarabine + 30 Gy WBRT with 10 Gy boost	81	NA	46
Omuro et al [57]	17	MTX 1 g/m^2) thiotepa/procarbazine + IT MTX+ 41.4 Gy WBRT with 14.4 boost	88	18	32
Shah et al [33]	30	Rituximab + MPV + WBRT (45 Gy vs 23.4 Gy for patients in CR)	9300%	57	67
Multidrug chemotherapy without radiotherapy					
Abrey et al [29]	22	MPV (MTX 3.5 g/m^2), cytarabine (3 g/m^2), IT MTX	NA	NA	33
Pels et al [43]	65	MTX (5 g/m^2) + cytarabine (3 g/m^2) + ifosfamide/vinca alkaloids/cyclophosphamide IT MTX + IT cytarabine	71	21	50
Hoang-Xuan et al [58]	50	MTX (1 g/m^2) + lomustine/procarbazine + IT MTX + IT cytarabine	71	21	50
Issa et al [55]	23	MTR (MTX 8 g/m^2) + temozolomide + rituximab + cytarabine-etoposide consolidation	73	NA	NA
MTX single agent					
Batchelor et al [45]	25	MTX (8 g/m^2)	74	12.8	22.8+
Herrlinger et al [46,47]	37	MTX (8 g/m^2)	35.1	10	25

Adapted from DeAngelis and Iwamoto [59].

Abbreviations: IT, intrathecal; MPV, methotrexate, procarbazine, vincristine; MTR, methotrexate, temozolomide, rituximab; MTX, methotrexate; NA, not available; OS, overall survival; PFS, progression-free survival; WBRT, whole-brain radiotherapy.

intact blood-brain barrier to enter the cerebrospinal fluid [62]. While anecdotal responses in the CNS have been described after the systemic administration of rituximab, retrospective analysis of the GELA data demonstrated that systemic administration of rituximab did not affect the rate of CNS relapse in this population of patients [63]. For these reasons, there is, at present, interest in the evaluation of the intrathecal administration of rituximab, both in the treatment of PCNSL as well as in the prophylaxis against CNS dissemination of non-Hodgkin's lymphoma [64–66]. A recent phase-I study of intraventricular administration of rituximab in patients with refractory PCNSL provided preliminary evidence for the safety as well as therapeutic efficacy against recurrent CNS lymphoma involving the leptomeninges, brain, and intraocular comparments [67].

Other Investigational Therapy

A number of other chemotherapeutic agents that have been shown to have activity in the treatment of PCNSL are under clinical investigation. One example is the alkylating agent temozolomide, a congener of dacarbazine (DTIC), initially approved for the treatment of malignant glioma. Temozolomide is administered orally and exhibits excellent CNS penetrance as well as a favorable side effect profile. Its use is associated with improvements in health-related quality of life in brain tumor patients [68]. There is increasing evidence that temozolomide has activity in PCNSL, both at diagnosis and at relapse with response rates on the order of 26% [69]. The administration of temozolomide in combination with rituximab is also under investigation [61]. At the University of California, San Francisco (UCSF), the combination of high-dose methotrexate plus temozolomide and intravenous rituximab is currently being investigated as an intensive induction regimen followed by high-dose cytarabine plus etoposide as consolidation [55]. This UCSF regimen is also being evaluated through the national consortium CALGB.

Another chemotherapeutic agent being studied in PCNSL is the topoisomerase I inhibitor topotecan, a derivative of camptothecan. Fischer et al treated 16 immunocompetent patients with refractory or relapsed PCNSL: six of these patients exhibited responses, four of which were complete [70].

Leptomeningeal dissemination of NHL represents a common pathway of relapse and dissemination, both in PCNSL as well as systemic disease. Standard treatment of lymphomatous meningitis consists of radiation to sites of radiographically visible disease and the intrathecal administration of chemotherapy with either cytarabine or methotrexate. A randomized evaluation of intrathecal administration of the long-acting form of cytarabine, Depocyt, in the treatment of lymphomatous meningitis demonstrated its favorable response rate (71%) compared with free cytarabine (15%) [71]. Arachnoiditis associated with the intrathecal administration of depocyt appears to be common and may be ameliorated by the concomitant administration of dexamethasone [72].

Intraventricular administration of chemotherapy drugs such as cytarabine or methotrexate using an Ommaya reservoir device is sometimes favored in neoplastic meningitis because of evidence suggesting more reliable efficacy compared to intrathecal administration of drugs by lumbar puncture [73]. Ommaya reservoir placement requires a neurosurgical procedure and is associated with an approximate 10% risk of complications such as infection [74]. Therefore, the decision to place such a device needs to be balanced with respect to probability of benefit and expectation for long-term survival. A significant and avoidable complication may occur when there is tumor-associated obstruction in the ventricular system; delayed clearance of chemotherapy drugs from the cerebral ventricles can result in severe neurotoxicitiy. For this reason, a radionuclide CSF flow study may be indicated to evaluate the patency of the ventricular outflow system before administration of cytotoxic agents using an Ommaya reservoir [75].

AIDS-Related PCNSL

AIDS-associated PCNSL has, until recently, been associated with a dismal prognosis and a median survival of only 3 months [4]. The standard approach in treating AIDS-associated PCNSL has been to use whole-brain irradiation, largely because of concern that patients with this condition have significant comorbidities that contradindicate the use of chemotherapy. A pilot study described by Jacomet et al demonstrated encouraging results with the use of high-dose intravenous methotrexate at 3 gm/m^2 every 14 days in AIDS-related PCNSL: 7 out of 15 patients exhibited complete responses with a median overall survival of 290 days. The treatment was well tolerated and the median Karnofsky performance score improved from 50 to 80. Similar results have not been achieved using whole-brain irradiation monotherapy in this population [76]. There is also significant evidence that highly active antiretroviral therapy (HAART) has resulted in a decreased incidence of AIDS-related PCNSL [77], and the use of HAART is associated with a survival benefit in this disease [78].

PRIMARY IOL

Primary IOL is characterized by invasion of malignant lymphoid cells in the retina, vitreous, and/or optic nerve head. In 80% of cases, the disease is bilateral. IOL complicates up to 20% of cases of primary CNS lymphoma, and 60% to 80% of patients who present with primary IOL will develop primary CNS lymphoma within 2 years. IOL is a distinct entity from systemic lymphomas that metastasize via the circulation to the uvea and/or develop *de novo* in the external eye (conjunctiva, lacrimal gland, or orbit).

Treatment options for IOL are limited because of the blood-ocular barrier resulting from tight junctions between vascular endothelial cells and pigmented epithelial cells of the anterior uvea and retina. While both intravenous methotrexate and intravenous cytarabine are able to penetrate the blood-ocular barrier and have activity in IOL [79,80], responses with these agents are variable. Radiotherapy alone has long been used to treat patients with isolated ocular lymphoma [81]. Radiation-associated ocular toxicities include retinopathy, visual loss, and cataracts. In addition, radiotherapy to the eye cannot be repeated should tumor relapse in the irradiated eye. For this reason, intravitreal administration of methotrexate is being evaluated on an experimental basis for isolated and recurrent ocular disease. Intravitreal methotrexate yields therapeutic concentrations in the vitreous humor for up to 5 days, significantly longer than after intravenous administration. Intravitreal injection of rituximab, an anti-CD20 monoclonal antibody, is also being investigated in this disease [82,83].

One approach to treatment of the ocular involvement of PCNSL is combined-modality therapy with systemic high-dose methotrexate-based chemotherapy and with radiation to the ocular globes [84]. Recurrence of IOL alone may be treated with intravitreal methotrexate as a single agent at some centers. There is evidence that intrathecal rituximab also has activity in recurrent ocular lymphoma [65,67].

REFERENCES

1. Hochberg FH, Baehring JM, Hochberg EP. Primary CNS lymphoma. *Nat Clin Pract Neurol*. 2007;3(1):24–35.
2. Olson JE, Janney CA, Rao RD, et al. The continuing increase in the incidence of primary central nervous system non-Hodgkin lymphoma: a surveillance, epidemiology, and end results analysis. *Cancer*. 2002;95(7):1504–1510.
3. Corn BW, Marcus SM, Topham A, Hauck W, Curran W. Will primary central nervous system lymphoma be the most frequent brain tumor diagnosed in the year 2000? *Cancer*. 1997;79(12):2409–2413.
4. Fine HA, Mayer RJ. Primary central nervous system lymphoma. *Ann Intern Med*. 1993;119:1093–1104.
5. Cha S, Knopp EA, Johnson G, Wetzel SG, Litt AW, Zagzag D. Intracranial mass lesions: dynamic contrast-enhanced susceptibility-weighted echo-planar perfusion MR imaging. *Radiology*. 2002;223(1):11–29.
6. Chamberlain MC, Kormanik P, Glantz M. Recurrent primary central nervous system lymphoma complicated by lymphomatous meningitis. *Oncol Rep*. 1998;5(2):521–525.
7. O'Neill BP, Dinapoli RP, Kurtin PJ, Habermann T. Occult systemic non-Hodgkin's lymphoma (NHL) in patients initially diagnosed as primary central nervous system lymphoma (PCNSL): how much staging is enough? *J Neurooncol*. 1995;25(1):67–71.
8. Jahnke K, Hummel M, Korfel A, et al. Detection of subclinical systemic disease in primary CNS lymphoma by polymerase chain reaction of the rearranged immunoglobulin heavy-chain genes. *J Clin Oncol*. 2006;24(29):4754–4757.
9. Weller M. Glucocorticoid treatment of primary CNS lymphoma. *J Neurooncol*. 1999;43(3):237–239.
10. Kulkarni AV, Guha A, Lozano A, Bernstein, M. Incidence of silent hemorrhage and delayed deterioration after stereotactic brain biopsy. *J Neurosurg*. 1998;89(1):31–35.
11. Soo TM, Bernstein M, Provias J, Tasker R, Lozano A, Guha A. Failed stereotactic biopsy in a series of 518 cases. *Stereotact Funct Neurosurg*. 1995;64(4):183–196.
12. Bernstein M, Berger MS. *Neuro-Oncology: The Essentials*. New York, NY: Thieme Medical Publishers; 2000: 122–134.
13. Antinori A, De Rossi G, Ammassari A, et al. Value of combined approach with thallium-201 single-photon emission computed tomography and Epstein-Barr virus DNA polymerase chain reaction in CSF for the diagnosis of AIDS-related primary CNS lymphoma. *J Clin Oncol*. 1999;17(2):554–560.
14. Pierce MA, Johnson MD, Maciunas RJ,et al. Evaluating contrast-enhancing brain lesions in patients with AIDS by using positron emission tomography. *Ann Intern Med*. 1995;123(8):594–598.
15. Roy S, Josephson SA, Fridlyand J, et al. Protein biomarker identification in the CSF of patients with CNS lymphoma. *J Clin Oncol*. 2008;26(1):96–105.
16. Levine A. Acquired immunodeficiency syndrome-related lymphoma. *Blood*. 1992;80(1):8–20.
17. Ferreri AJ, Blay JY, Reni M, et al. Prognostic scoring system for primary CNS lymphomas: the International Extranodal Lymphoma Study Group experience. *J Clin Oncol*. 2003;21(2):266–272.
18. Blay JY, Conroy TCC, Thyss A, et al. High-dose methotrexate for the treatment of primary cerebral lymphomas: analysis of survival and late neurologic toxicity in a retrospective series. *J Clin Oncol*. 1998;16(3):864–871.
19. Abrey LE, Ben-Porat L, Panageas KS, et al. Primary central nervous system lymphoma: the Memorial Sloan-Kettering Cancer Center prognostic model. *J Clin Oncol*. 2006;24(36):5711–5715.
20. Smith JR, Braziel RM, Paoletti S, Lipp M, Uguccioni M, Rosenbaum J. Expression of B-cell-attracting chemokine 1 (CXCL13) by malignant lymphocytes and vascular endothelium in primary central nervous system lymphoma. *Blood*. 2003;101(3):815–821.
21. Tun HW, Personnet D, Baskerville KA, et al. Pathway analysis of primary central nervous system lymphoma. *Blood*. 2008;111(6):3200–3210.
22. Rubenstein JL, Fridlyand J, Shen A, et al. Gene expression and angiotropism in primary CNS lymphoma. *Blood*. 2006;107(9):3716–3723.
23. Braaten KM, Betansky RA, de Leval L, et al. BCL-6 expression predicts improved survival in patients with primary central nervous system lymphoma. *Clin Cancer Res*. 2003;9(3):1063–1069.
24. Nakamura M, Sakaki T, Hashimoto H, et al. Frequent alterations of the p14(ARF) and p16(INK4a) genes in primary central nervous system lymphomas. *Cancer Res*. 2001;61(17):6335–6339.
25. Larocca LM, Capello D, Rinelli A, et al. The molecular and phenotypic profile of primary central nervous system lymphoma identifies distinct categories of the disease and is consistent with histogenetic derivation from germinal center-related B cells. *Blood*. 1998;92(3):1011–1019.
26. Alizadeh AE, Davis M, Ma R, et al. Distinct types of diffuse large B-cell lymphoma identified by gene expression profiling. *Nature*. 2000;403(6769):503–511.
27. Rubenstein JL, Shen A, Fridlyand J, et al. Gene expression profile analysis of primary cns lymphoma: class distinction and outcome prediction. *Proc Am Assoc Cancer Res*. 2004;45:4433.
28. Camilleri-Broet S, Crinière E, Broët P, et al. A uniform activated B-cell-like immunophenotype might explain the poor prognosis of primary central nervous system lymphomas: analysis of 83 cases. *Blood*. 2006;107(1):190–196.
29. Abrey LE, DeAngelis LM, Yahalom J. Long-term survival in primary CNS lymphoma. *J Clin Oncol*. 1998;16(3):859–863.
30. Deangelis L. Current management of primary central nervous system lymphoma. *Oncology*. 1995;9(1)::63–71.
31. Nelson DF, Martz KL, Bonner H, et al. Non-Hodgkin's lymphoma of the brain: can high dose, large volume radiation therapy improve survival? Report on a prospective trial by the Radiation Therapy Oncology Group (RTOG): RTOG 83. *Int J Radiat Oncol Biol Phys*. 1992;23(1):9–17.
32. Bessell EM, Lopez-Guillermo A, Villa S, et al. Importance of radiotherapy in the outcome of patients with primary CNS lymphoma: an analysis of the CHOD/BVAM regimen followed by two different radiotherapy treatments. *J Clin Oncol*. 2002;20(1):231–236.
33. Shah GD, Yahalom J, Correa DD, et al. Combined immunochemotherapy with reduced whole-brain radiotherapy for newly diagnosed primary CNS lymphoma. *J Clin Oncol*. 2007;25(30):4730–4735.
34. Schultz C, Scott C, Sherman W, et al. Preirradiation chemotherapy with cyclophosphamide, doxorubicin, vincristine, and dexamethasone for primary CNS lymphomas: initial report of radiation therapy oncology group protocol 88–06. *J Clin Oncol*. 1996;14(2):556–564.
35. O'Neill BP, O'Fallon JR, Earle JD, Colgan JP, Brown LD, Krigel R. Primary central nervous system non-Hodgkin's lymphoma: survival advantages with combined initial therapy? *Int J Radiat Oncol Biol Phys*. 1995;33(3):663–673.
36. Glantz MJ, Cole BF, Recht L, et al. High-dose intravenous methotrexate for patients with nonleukemic leptomeningeal cancer: is intrathecal chemotherapy necessary? *J Clin Oncol*. 1998;16(4):1561–1567.
37. Ervin T, Canellos GP. Successful treatment of recurrent primary central nervous system lymphoma with high-dose methotrexate. *Cancer*. 1980;45(7):1556–1557.

38. Skarin AT, Zuckerman KS, Pitman SW, et al. High-dose methotrexate with folinic acid in the treatment of advanced non-Hodgkin lymphoma including CNS involvement. *Blood.* 1977;50(6):1039–1047.
39. Bokstein F, Lossos A, Lossos IS, Siegal T. Central nervous system relapse of systemic non-Hodgkin's lymphoma: results of treatment based on high-dose methotrexate combination chemotherapy. *Leuk Lymphoma.* 2002;43(3):587–593.
40. Harder H, Holtel H, Bromberg JE, et al. Cognitive status and quality of life after treatment for primary CNS lymphoma. *Neurology.* 2004;62(4):544–547.
41. DeAngelis LM, Seiferheld W, Schold SC, Fisher B, Schultz CJ; Radiation Therapy Oncology Group Study 93–10. Combination chemotherapy and radiotherapy for primary entral nervous system lymphoma: Radiation Therapy Oncology Group Study 93–10. *J Clin Oncol.* 2002;20(24):4643–4648.
42. Khan RB, Shi W, Thaler HT, DeAngelis LM, Abrey L. Is intrathecal methotrexate necessary in the treatment of primary CNS lymphoma? *J Neurooncol.* 2002;58(2):175–178.
43. Pels, H, Schmidt-Wolf IG, Glasmacher A, et al. Primary central nervous system lymphoma: results of a pilot and phase II study of systemic and intraventricular chemotherapy with deferred radiotherapy. *J Clin Oncol.* 2003;21(24):4489–4495.
44. Guha-Thakurta N, Damek D, Pollack C, Hochberg F. Intravenous methotrexate as initial treatment for primary central nervous system lymphoma: response to therapy and quality of life of patients. *J Neurooncol.* 1999;43(3):259–268.
45. Batchelor T, Carson K, O'Neill A, et al. Treatment of primary CNS lymphoma with methotrexate and deferred radiotherapy: a report of NABTT 96–07. *J Clin Oncol.* 2003;21(6):1044–1049.
46. Herrlinger U, Küker W, Uhl M, et al. NOA-03 trial of high-dose methotrexate in primary central nervous system lymphoma: final report. *Ann Neurol.* 2005;57(6):843–847.
47. Herrlinger U, Schabet M, Brugger W, et al. German Cancer Society Neuro-Oncology Working Group NOA-03 multicenter trial of single-agent high-dose methotrexate for primary central nervous system lymphoma. *Ann Neurol.* 2002;51(2):247–252.
48. McAllister LD, Doolittle ND, Guastadisegni PE, et al. Cognitive outcomes and long-term follow-up results after enhanced chemotherapy delivery for primary central nervous system lymphoma. *Neurosurgery.* 2000;46(1):51–60.
49. Van Besien K, Ha CS, Murphy S, et al. Risk factors, treatment and outcome of central nervous recurrence in adults with intermediate-grade and immunoblastic lymphoma. *Blood.* 1998;91(4):1174–1184.
50. Abrey LE, Moskowitz C, Mason WP, et al. Intensive methotrexate and cytarabine followed by high-dose chemotherapy with autologous stem-cell rescue in patients with newly diagnosed primary CNS lymphoma: an intent-to-treat analysis. *J Clin Oncol.* 2003;21(22):4151–4156.
51. Soussain C, Suzan F, Hoang-Xuan K, et al. Results of intensive chemotherapy followed by hematopoietic stem-cell rescue in 22 patients with refractory or recurrent primary CNS lymphoma or intraocular lymphoma. *J Clin Oncol.* 2001;19(3):742–749.
52. Soussain C, Hoang-Xuan K, Taillandier L, et al. Intensive chemotherapy followed by hematopoietic stem-cell rescue for refractory and recurrent primary CNS and intraocular lymphoma: Societe Francaise de Greffe de Moelle Osseuse-Therapie Cellulaire. *J Clin Oncol.* 2008;26(15):2512–2518.
53. Sandor V, Stark-Vancs V, Pearson D, et al. Phase II trial of chemotherapy alone for primary CNS and intraocular lymphoma. *J Clin Oncol.* 1998;16(9):3000–3006.
54. Pels H, Schmidt-Wolf IG, Glasmacher A, et al. Primary central nervous system lymphoma: results of a pilot and phase II study of systemic and intraventricular chemotherapy with deferred radiotherapy. *J Clin Oncol.* 2003;21(24):4489–4495.
55. Issa S, Shen A, Karch J, et al. Treatment of primary CNS lymphoma with induction high-dose methotrexate, temozloomide, rituximab followed by consolidation cytarabine/etoposide: a pilot study with biomarker analysis. Proceedings of the American Society of Hematology, 2007.
56. Poortmans PM, Kluin-Nelemans HC, Haaxma-Reiche H, et al. High-dose methotrexate-based chemotherapy followed by consolidating radiotherapy in non-AIDS-related primary central nervous system lymphoma: European Organization for Research and Treatment of Cancer Lymphoma Group Phase II Trial 20962. *J Clin Oncol.* 2003;21(24):4483–4488.
57. Omuro AM, DeAngelis LM, Yahalom J, Abrey LE. Chemoradiotherapy for primary CNS lymphoma: an intent-to-treat analysis with complete follow-up. *Neurology.* 2005;64(1):69–74.
58. Hoang-Xuan K, Taillandier L, Chinot O, et al. Chemotherapy alone as initial treatment for primary CNS lymphoma in patients older than 60 years: a multicenter phase II study (26952) of the European Organization for Research and Treatment of Cancer Brain Tumor Group. *J Clin Oncol.* 2003;21(14):2726–2731.
59. Deangelis LM, Iwamoto FM. An update on therapy of primary central nervous system lymphoma. *Hematology Am Soc Hematol Educ Program.* 2006:311–316.
60. Coiffier B, Lepage E, Briere J, et al. CHOP chemotherapy plus rituximab compared with CHOP alone in elderly patients with diffuse large-B-cell lymphoma. *N Engl J Med.* 2002;346(4):235–242.
61. Wong ET, Tishler R, Barron L, Wu JK. Immunochemotherapy with rituximab and temozolomide for central nervous system lymphomas. *Cancer.* 2004;101(1):139–145.
62. Rubenstein JL, Combs D, Rosenberg J, et al. Rituximab therapy for CNS lymphomas: targeting the leptomeningeal compartment. *Blood.* 2003;101(2):466–468.
63. Feugier P, Virion JM, Tilly H, et al. Incidence and risk factors for central nervous system occurrence in elderly patients with diffuse large-B-cell lymphoma: influence of rituximab. *Ann Oncol.* 2004;15(1):129–133.
64. Schulz H, Pels H, Schmidt-Wolf I, Zeelen, U Germing, U, Engert A. Intraventricular treatment of relapsed central nervous system lymphoma with the anti-CD20 antibody rituximab. *Haematologica.* 2004;89(6):753–754.
65. Rubenstein JL, Shen A, Abrey L, et al. Results from a phase I study of intraventricular administration of rituximab in patients with recurrent lymphomatous meningitis. *Proceedings of the American Society of Clinical Oncology #6593,* 2004.
66. van de Glind G, de Graaf S, Klein C, Cornelissen M, Maecker B, Loeffen J. Intrathecal rituximab treatment for pediatric post-transplant lymphoproliferative disorder of the central nervous system. *Pediatr Blood Cancer.* 2008;50(4):886–888.
67. Rubenstein JL, Fridlyand J, Abrey L, et al. Phase I study of intraventricular administration of rituximab in patients with recurrent CNS and intraocular lymphoma. *J Clin Oncol.* 2007;25(11):1350–1356.
68. Osoba D, Brada M, Yung WK, Prados M. Health-related quality of life in patients treated with temozolomide versus procarbazine for recurrent glioblastoma multiforme. 2000;18(7):1481–1491.
69. Reni M, Mason W, Zaja F, et al. Salvage chemotherapy with temozolomide in primary CNS lymphomas: preliminary results of a phase II trial. *Eur J Cancer.* 2004;40(11):1682–1688.
70. Fischer L, Thiel E, Klasen HA, Kirchen H, Jahnke K, Korfel A. Response of relapsed or refractory primary central nervous system lymphoma (PCNSL) to topotecan. *Neurology.* 2004;25;62(10):1885–1887.
71. Glantz MJ, LaFollette SJ, Shapiro KA, et al. Randomized trial of a slow-release versus a standard formulation of cytarabine for the intrathecal treatment of lymphomatous meningitis. *J Clin Oncol.* 1999;(10):3110–3116.
72. Bomgaars L, Geyer JR, Franklin J, et al. Phase I trial of intrathecal liposomal cytarabine in children with neoplastic meningitis. *J Clin Oncol.* 2004;22(19):3916–3921.
73. Bleyer WA, Poplack DG. Intraventricular versus intralumbar methotrexate for central-nervous-system leukemia: prolonged remission with the Ommaya reservoir. *Med Pediatr Oncol.* 1979;6(3):207–213.
74. Sandberg DI, Bilsky MH, Souweidane MM, Bzdil J, Gutin P. Ommaya reservoirs for the treatment of leptomeningeal metastases. *Neurosurgery.* 2000;47(1):49–54.
75. Mason WP, Yeh SD, DeAngelis L. 111Indium-diethylenetriamine pentaacetic acid cerebrospinal fluid flow studies predict distribution of intrathecally administered chemotherapy and outcome in patients with leptomeningeal metastases. *Neurology.* 1998;50(2):438–444.
76. Jacomet C, Girard PM, Lebrette MG, Farese VL, Monfort L, Rozenbaum W. Intravenous methotrexate for primary central nervous system non-Hodgkin's lymphoma in AIDS. *AIDS.* 1997;11(14):1725–1730.
77. Inungu J, Melendez MF, Montgomery J. AIDS-related primary brain lymphoma in Michigan, January 1990 to December 2000. *AIDS Patient Care STDS.* 2002;16(3):107–112.

78. Skiest D, Crosby C. Survival is prolonged by highly active antiretroviral therapy in AIDS patients with primary central nervous system lymphoma. *AIDS*. 2003;17(12):1787–1793.
79. Baumann MA, Ritch PS, Hande KR, Williams GA, Topping TM, Anderson T. Treatment of intraocular lymphoma with high-dose Ara-C. *Cancer*. 1986;57(7):1273–1275.
80. Batchelor TT, Kolak G, Ciordia R, Foster CS, Henson J. High-dose methotrexate for intraocular lymphoma. *Clin Cancer Res*. 2003;9(2):711–715.
81. Margolis L, Fraser R, Lichter A, Char D. The role of radiation therapy in the management of ocular reticulum cell sarcoma. *Cancer*. 1980;45(4):688–692.
82. Kim H, Csaky KG, Chan CC, et al. The pharmacokinetics of rituximab following an intravitreal injection. *Exp Eye Res*. 2006;82(5):760–766.
83. Kitzmann AS, Pulido JS, Mohney BG, et al. Intraocular use of rituximab. *Eye*. 2007;21(12):1524–1527.
84. Hormigo A, DeAngelis L. Primary ocular lymphoma: clinical features, diagnosis, and treatment. *Clin Lymphoma*. 2003;4(1):22–29.

73 Medical Treatment of Primary Central Nervous System Germ Cell Tumors

Raymond Liu

INTRODUCTION

Intracranial germ cell tumors are uncommon malignancies in the central nervous system (CNS) and make up less than 5% of brain tumors [1]. Because of midline migration patterns, intracranial germ cell tumors are most commonly found in the suprasellar or pineal region. When found in the suprasellar region, germ cell tumors may affect hypothalamic/pituitary or visual function. In contrast, hydrocephalus or Parinaud syndrome may be apparent when germ cell tumors are located in the pineal region.

The evaluation of germ cell tumors includes monitoring of serum and cerebrospinal fluid tumor markers such as alpha fetoprotein (AFP) and beta-human chorionic gonadotropin (B-HCG) and staging with MRI of the spine. Elevations in AFP indicate a nongerminomatous component [2]. High serum levels of tumor markers, especially in the setting of negative cerebrospinal fluid levels, should prompt evaluation for the presence of a germ cell tumor outside the CNS.

Because of their midline location, germ cell tumors can be difficult to approach surgically. Therefore, there is a clear role for radiation and chemotherapy in this group of diseases. Chemotherapy regimens have been chosen based on clinical trials developed in germ cell tumors outside the CNS [3,4]. Also based on experience in systemic germ cell tumors, second look surgeries may be warranted in those with negative markers but with residual radiographic abnormalities after chemotherapy [5]. The treatment of germinomas and nongerminomatous germ cell tumors differ, and so they will be discussed separately.

GERMINOMAS

Germinomas make up 50% to 65% of all intracranial germ cell tumors [6]. Pure germinomas do not secrete B-HCG or AFP, although about 5% of germinomas contain syncytiotrophoblastic giant cells that can secrete HCG [7]. The prognostic implications remain debated in this subgroup of germinomas [8,9].

Germinomas are sensitive to radiation therapy with long-term survival rates of 70% to 100% with radiotherapy alone [2,9,10]. There is some concern however, especially in the pediatric population, that there may be long-term cognitive and neuroendocrine sequelae from this therapy [11–13]. Because of the potential long-term side effects of radiotherapy, studies have tried to establish the role of chemotherapy in germinomas.

Germinomas are also sensitive to chemotherapy, although chemotherapy alone is not considered curative for many patients [14]. This was seen in the First International CNS Germ Cell Tumor Study Group trial, where 45 patients with germinomas received four cycles of carboplatin, etoposide, and bleomycin followed by two additional cycles of chemotherapy in complete responders [15]. In this trial, 84% of the germinoma patients were able to achieve a complete response with chemotherapy alone. However, of the 55 germ cell tumor patients who achieved a complete response with chemotherapy alone, 28 patients relapsed with a median time of 18 months from diagnosis, and 20 of these 28 patients had germinomas. To improve on the responsiveness of germ cell tumors to chemotherapy, the Second International CNS Germ Cell Tumor Study Group protocol was initiated [16]. In this protocol, intensive cisplatin was substituted for carboplatin, and high-dose cyclophosphamide was added to the chemotherapy regimen. Furthermore, additional cycles of chemotherapy were given to those patients achieving complete responses. Unfortunately, this regimen was associated with significant toxicity with treatment-related mortality involving 4 of 19 germinoma patients in the study. To further examine whether chemotherapy alone can be successful at treating germinomas, a retrospective study examined treatment patterns in 117 germinoma patients [17]. Seventy-one of the patients received radiation alone, nine received chemotherapy alone, and 37 received combined therapy; 10-year overall survivals were 97%, 89%, and 92% respectively. Patients treated with chemotherapy alone did show earlier recurrence and a higher overall tumor recurrence rate [17]. Despite the data showing higher relapse rates with those treated with chemotherapy alone, some continue to advocate for upfront chemotherapy alone, with radiotherapy to be reserved in relapse settings [18].

Other studies have attempted to use chemotherapy prior to radiotherapy to reduce the irradiated dose and volume. Most of these studies have enrolled a small number of patients and have used platinum-based regimens such as cisplatin and etoposide followed by radiotherapy [19,20]. For example, one study enrolling 27 germinoma patients instituted etoposide and cisplatin chemotherapy followed by 24 Gy radiation, with 5-year overall survival at 100% and relapse-free survival at 86% for germinomas [19]. Other regimens tested with radiation include cisplatin and etoposide alternating with vincristine and cyclophosphamide [8], etoposide and carboplatin alternating with etoposide and ifosfamide [21], cyclophosphamide alone or in combination with vinblastine, bleomycin, and cisplatin [22], and carboplatin alone [23]. In yet another small prospective study, solitary germinomas were treated with cisplatin and etoposide, and disseminated germinomas were treated with ifosfamide, cisplatin, and etoposide [24]. Twenty-four Gray of radiation was used with craniospinal ports reserved for three patients with dissemination. Ninety-four percent were alive without recurrence at a median follow-up duration of 24 months, and the one patient who experienced a recurrence had a B-HCG-secreting germinoma and underwent successful salvage therapy. Because of the encouraging outcomes of these smaller studies, the Children's Oncology Group (COG) has initiated a trial COG-ACNS0232, to prospectively randomize germinoma patients to standard-dose radiation only or to two to four cycles of carboplatin and etoposide followed by reduced-dose radiotherapy treatment based on a risk-adapted approach [25].

In the salvage setting, radiation therapy may be used in areas that have not received definitive radiation previously [26, 27]. There is also a clear role for chemotherapy, and the regimens used are similar to those used in the upfront setting [15,28,29]. High-dose chemotherapy, in the setting of autologous stem-cell transplant, is feasible as tested in several small trials, but its role in the treatment of germinomas is not clearly defined [30,31].

In summary, radiation therapy is curative in many cases of pure germinomas but may result in potential long-term neurocognitive sequelae. Chemotherapy alone is likely inadequate for initial therapy given the high incidence of recurrence. Ongoing trials are examining the role of sequential or combined chemotherapy and radiotherapy regimens in germinomas.

NONGERMINOMATOUS GERM CELL TUMORS

Nongerminomatous germ cell tumors are composed of several histological types, including embryonal carcinoma, yolk sac tumors, choriocarcinomas, and teratomas. Mixed tumors that contain multiple histological types are common in nongerminomatous germ cell tumors [32]. Unlike pure germinomas, nongerminomatous germ cell tumors are not as responsive to radiation therapy, with 20% to 45% 5-year survival with radiation alone [6,33,34]. Therefore, there is a relatively important role for chemotherapy in nongerminomatous germ cell tumors in comparison to germinomas.

Several chemotherapy regimens have been studied. Like germinomas, early studies in intracranial nongerminomatous germ cell tumors focused on platinum agents, mostly cisplatin and etoposide [28,35,36]. Alkylating agents such as cyclophosphamide may also have some activity [15,22,37]. Early European experience with nongerminomatous germ cell tumors used cisplatin, etoposide, bleomycin followed by radiation and ifosfamide, cisplatin, and vinblastine. Fourteen patients treated in this fashion obtained a 5-year survival rate of 80% [37]. Carboplatin regimens have similar response rates to cisplatin-containing regimens [15,37–39]. The First International CNS Germ Cell Tumor Study Group trial was initiated to examine the effect of carboplatin, etoposide, and bleomycin chemotherapy on outcomes in germ cell tumors [15]. Twenty-six patients with nongerminomatous germ cell tumors were enrolled in the study. Like the germinoma patients in the study, those nongerminomatous germ cell tumor patients treated with upfront chemotherapy had a high response rate, with complete responses in 78% of patients. However, 13 of these 26 patients had experienced progression or relapse, and salvage radiation was not generally effective in this population [15]. The follow-up Second International CNS Germ Cell Tumor Study Group protocol substituted intensive cisplatin for carboplatin, added high-dose cyclophosphamide, and gave additional cycles of chemotherapy to patients who achieved complete responses [40]. There was a 94% response rate of 17 patients assessable for response, with 75% survival at 5 years. Eleven of the patients had relapsed with a median follow-up of 6.3 years.

Multimodality therapy may further improve survival rates. As with germinomas, platinum-based regimens are often used, followed by radiotherapy. Cisplatin and etoposide [20], cisplatin and cyclophosphamide [8], or cisplatin, etoposide, and ifosfamide followed by radiotherapy are typical regimens used in small patient series [19]. A study of 18 patients undergoing cisplatin and VP-16 chemotherapy following surgery, followed by radiation therapy, then followed by vinblastine, bleomycin, VP-16, and carboplatin chemotherapy was well-tolerated and was associated with 4-year survival rates of 74% [38]. Unfortunately, survival after treatment failure was brief in this study. In an attempt to develop a risk-adapted approach to multimodal therapy in the treatment of nongerminomatous germ cell tumors, the COG has initiated a protocol (ACNS0122) for nongerminomatous germ cell tumors, which uses carboplatin and etoposide alternating with ifosfamide and etoposide. Those in complete remission or those with some response and normal tumor markers will complete radiation therapy. Those with stable disease or partial response, with abnormal tumor markers, will undergo consolidation with thiotepa and etoposide followed by autologous stem-cell rescue and radiation therapy. In salvage settings, radiotherapy may be used, although its effectiveness in this setting is limited in comparison to germinomas [15]. Other potential salvage therapies include high-dose chemotherapy with autologous transplant [30,40–43].

In summary, in contrast to pure germinomas, radiotherapy alone does not provide adequate tumor control in most nongerminomatous germ cell tumors. A combined modality approach is often used with chemotherapy, followed by radiation. Better treatments options are necessary for nongerminomatous germ cell tumors, especially in the salvage setting.

REFERENCES

1. Jellinger K. Primary intracranial germ cell tumours. *Acta Neuropathol*. 1973;25(4):291–306.
2. Wolden SL, Wara WM, Larson DA, Prados MD, Edwards MS, Sneed PK. Radiation therapy for primary intracranial germ-cell tumors. *Int J Radiat Oncol Biol Phys*. 1995;32(4):943–949.
3. Peckham MJ, Horwich A, Hendry WF. Advanced seminoma: treatment with cis-platinum-based combination chemotherapy or carboplatin (JM8). *Br J Cancer*. 1985;52(1):7–13.
4. Einhorn LH. General Motors Cancer Research Prizewinners laureates lectures. Charles F. Kettering Prize. Clinical trials in testicular cancer. *Cancer*. 1993;71(10):3182–3184.
5. Aprikian AG, Herr HW, Bajorin DF, Bosl GJ. Resection of postchemotherapy residual masses and limited retroperitoneal lymphadenectomy in patients with metastatic testicular nonseminomatous germ cell tumors. *Cancer*. 1994;74(4):1329–1334.
6. Jennings MT, Gelman R, Hochberg F. Intracranial germ-cell tumors: natural history and pathogenesis. *J Neurosurg*. 1985;63(2):155–167.
7. Matsutani M, Sano K, Takakura K, et al. Primary intracranial germ cell tumors: a clinical analysis of 153 histologically verified cases. *J Neurosurg*. 1997;86(3):446–455.
8. Ogino H, Shibamoto Y, Takanaka T, et al. CNS germinoma with elevated serum human chorionic gonadotropin level: clinical characteristics and treatment outcome. *Int J Radiat Oncol Biol phys*. 2005;62:803–808.
9. Ogawa K, Shikama N, Toita T, et al. Long-term results of radiotherapy for intracranial germinoma: a multi-institutional retrospective review of 126 patients. *Int J Radiat Oncol Biol Phys*. 2004;58(3):705–713.
10. Huh SJ, Shin KH, Kim IH, Ahn YC, Ha SW, Park CI. Radiotherapy of intracranial germinomas. *Radiother Oncol*. 1996;38(1):19–23.
11. Syndikus I, Tait D, Ashley S, Jannoun L. Long-term follow-up of young children with brain tumors after irradiation. *Int J Radiat Oncol Biol Phys*. 1994;30(4):781–787.
12. Oka H, Kawano N, Tanaka T, et al. Long-term functional outcome of suprasellar germinomas: usefulness and limitations of radiotherapy. *J Neurooncol*. 1998;40(2):185–190.
13. Sands SA, Kellie SJ, Davidow AL, et al. Long-term quality of life and neuropsychologic functioning for patients with CNS germ-cell tumors: from the First International CNS Germ-Cell Tumor Study. *Neuro-oncology*. 2001;3(3):174–183.
14. Osuka S, Tsuboi K, Takano S, et al. Long-term outcome of patients with intracranial germinoma. *J Neurooncol*. 2007;83(1):71–79.
15. Balmaceda C, Heller G, Rosenblum M, et al. Chemotherapy without irradiation–a novel approach for newly diagnosed CNS germ cell tumors: results of an international cooperative trial. The First International Central Nervous System Germ Cell Tumor Study. *J Clin Oncol*. 1996;14(11):2908–2915.
16. Kellie SJ, Boyce H, Dunkel IJ, et al. Intensive cisplatin and cyclophosphamide-based chemotherapy without radiotherapy for intracranial germinomas: failure of a primary chemotherapy approach. *Pediatr Blood Cancer*. 2004;43(2):126–133.
17. Shim KW, Kim TG, Suh CO, et al. Treatment failure in intracranial primary germinomas. *Childs Nerv Syst*. 2007;23(10):1155–1161.
18. Ueba T, Yamashita K, Fujisawa I, et al. Long-term follow-up of 5 patients with intracranial germinoma initially treated by chemotherapy alone. *Acta Neurochir (Wien)*. 2007;149(9):897–902; discussion 902.
19. Aoyama H, Shirato H, Ikeda J, Fujieda K, Miyasaka K, Sawamura Y. Induction chemotherapy followed by low-dose involved-field radiotherapy for intracranial germ cell tumors. *J Clin Oncol*. 2002;20(3):857–865.
20. Buckner JC, Peethambaram PP, Smithson WA, et al. Phase II trial of primary chemotherapy followed by reduced-dose radiation for CNS germ cell tumors. *J Clin Oncol*. 1999;17(3):933–940.
21. Bouffet E, Baranzelli MC, Patte C, et al. Combined treatment modality for intracranial germinomas: results of a multicentre SFOP experience. Société Française d'Oncologie Pédiatrique. *Br J Cancer*. 1999;79(7–8):1199–1204.
22. Allen JC, Kim JH, Packer RJ. Neoadjuvant chemotherapy for newly diagnosed germ-cell tumors of the central nervous system. *J Neurosurg*. 1987;67(1):65–70.
23. Allen JC, DaRosso RC, Donahue B, Nirenberg A. A phase II trial of preirradiation carboplatin in newly diagnosed germinoma of the central nervous system. *Cancer*. 1994;74(3):940–944.
24. Sawamura Y, Shirato H, Ikeda J, et al. Induction chemotherapy followed by reduced-volume radiation therapy for newly diagnosed central nervous system germinoma. *J Neurosurg*. 1998;88(1):66–72.
25. Marcus KJ. Intracranial germinomas: can we improve upon our success? *Pediatr Blood Cancer*. 2006;47(1):2–3.
26. Merchant TE, Davis BJ, Sheldon JM, Leibel SA. Radiation therapy for relapsed CNS germinoma after primary chemotherapy. *J Clin Oncol*. 1998;16(1):204–209.
27. Shibamoto Y, Sasai K, Kokubo M, Hiraoka M. Salvage radiation therapy for intracranial germinoma recurring after primary chemotherapy. *J Neurooncol*. 1999;44(2):181–185.
28. Yoshida J, Sugita K, Kobayashi T, et al. Prognosis of intracranial germ cell tumours: effectiveness of chemotherapy with cisplatin and etoposide (CDDP and VP-16). *Acta Neurochir (Wien)*. 1993;120(3–4):111–117.
29. Bamberg M, Kortmann RD, Calaminus G, et al. Radiation therapy for intracranial germinoma: results of the German cooperative prospective trials MAKEI 83/86/89. *J Clin Oncol*. 1999;17(8):2585–2592.
30. Modak S, Gardner S, Dunkel IJ, et al. Thiotepa-based high-dose chemotherapy with autologous stem-cell rescue in patients with recurrent or progressive CNS germ cell tumors. *J Clin Oncol*. 2004;22(10):1934–1943.
31. Mahoney DH Jr, Strother D, Camitta B, et al. High-dose melphalan and cyclophosphamide with autologous bone marrow rescue for recurrent/progressive malignant brain tumors in children: a pilot pediatric oncology group study. *J Clin Oncol*. 1996;14(2):382–388.
32. Bjornsson J, Scheithauer BW, Okazaki H, Leech RW. Intracranial germ cell tumors: pathobiological and immunohistochemical aspects of 70 cases. *J Neuropathol Exp Neurol*. 1985;44(1):32–46.
33. Dearnaley DP, A'Hern RP, Whittaker S, Bloom HJ. Pineal and CNS germ cell tumors: Royal Marsden Hospital experience 1962–1987. *Int J Radiat Oncol Biol Phys*. 1990;18(4):773–781.
34. Hoffman HJ, Otsubo H, Hendrick EB, et al. Intracranial germ-cell tumors in children. *J Neurosurg*. 1991;74(4):545–551.
35. Kobayashi T, Yoshida J, Ishiyama J, Noda S, Kito A, Kida Y. Combination chemotherapy with cisplatin and etoposide for malignant intracranial germ-cell tumors. An experimental and clinical study. *J Neurosurg*. 1989;70(5):676–681.
36. Itoyama Y, Kochi M, Kuratsu J, et al. Treatment of intracranial non-germinomatous malignant germ cell tumors producing alpha-fetoprotein. *Neurosurgery*. 1995;36(3):459–64; discussion 464.
37. Calaminus G, Bamberg M, Baranzelli MC, et al. Intracranial germ cell tumors: a comprehensive update of the European data. *Neuropediatrics*. 1994;25(1):26–32.
38. Robertson PL, DaRosso RC, Allen JC. Improved prognosis of intracranial non-germinoma germ cell tumors with multimodality therapy. *J Neurooncol*. 1997;32(1):71–80.
39. Baranzelli MC, Patte C, Bouffet E, et al. An attempt to treat pediatric intracranial alphaFP and betaHCG secreting germ cell tumors with chemotherapy alone. SFOP experience with 18 cases. Société Française d'Oncologie Pédiatrique. *J Neurooncol*. 1998;37(3):229–239.
40. Kellie SJ, Boyce H, Dunkel IJ, et al. Primary chemotherapy for intracranial nongerminomatous germ cell tumors: results of the second international CNS germ cell study group protocol. *J Clin Oncol*. 2004;22(5):846–853.
41. Graham ML, Herndon JE II, Casey JR, et al. High-dose chemotherapy with autologous stem-cell rescue in patients with recurrent and high-risk pediatric brain tumors. *J Clin Oncol*. 1997;15(5):1814–1823.
42. Tada T, Takizawa T, Nakazato F, et al. Treatment of intracranial nongerminomatous germ-cell tumor by high-dose chemotherapy and autologous stem-cell rescue. *J Neurooncol*. 1999;44(1):71–76.
43. Jahnke K, Kraemer DF, Knight KR, et al. Intraarterial chemotherapy and osmotic blood-brain barrier disruption for patients with embryonal and germ cell tumors of the central nervous system. *Cancer*. 2008;112(3):581–588.

74 Medical Management for Choroid Plexus Tumors

Sabine Mueller and Susan M. Chang

INTRODUCTION

Choroid plexus tumors are derived from the epithelium of the choroid plexus within the ventricular system. Mean age at presentation is 3.5 years; therefore, choroid plexus tumors are considered pediatric malignancies, but they can occur in adults as well. They represent 0.4% to 0.6% of all brain tumors at all ages but constitute 2% to 4% of tumors occurring in children, with 10% to 20% manifesting in the first year of life [1,2]. Choroid plexus tumors are divided into three distinct types: the indolent choroid plexus papilloma (CPP), atypical CPP, and the more aggressive choroid plexus carcinoma (CPC). The clinical presentation varies depending on the localization of the tumor and the age of the patient. Infants often present with macrocephaly due to underlying hydrocephalus. Older children present with signs of increased intracranial pressure. Choroid-plexus tumors are mainly localized within the lateral ventricles, but studies have shown that caudal lesions are found more commonly with advancing age [3]. CPC is more commonly found in the younger population (median age 2 years), whereas CPP present at a significantly older age (median age 6 years) [4]. In a meta-analysis from Wolff et al looking at a total of 566 patients, median age at presentation was 1.5 years, 1.5 years, 22.5 years, and 33.5 years in the groups of tumors localized to the lateral ventricle, third ventricle, fourth ventricle, and cerebellopontine angle, respectively. CPC is more commonly found in the lateral ventricles, whereas CPP is found more often in the cerebellopontine angle [3]. Survival is correlated with histology and 1-, 5-, and 10-year survival rate for CPP reported at 90%, 81%, and 77% versus 71%, 41%, and 35% for CPC, respectively. There is a higher incidence of metastasis in patients presenting with CPC, with an overall incidence rate of 12% [3]. Diagnosis is mainly established via imaging and histopathology.

MANAGEMENT

Surgery

Surgical resection is the mainstay of therapy. Surgical interventions are necessary for diagnostic purposes, CSF shunting procedures in patients with hydrocephalus and complete tumor removal when possible. Most patients do not require a permanent shunt after the tumor is removed [1]. Patients presenting with hydrocephalus are therefore often managed with a temporary extraventricular drain. Gross total resection (GTR) is the goal of surgery, which is challenging because these tumors are highly vascularized and hence have a tendency to bleed. These tumors are large in size and often invade adjacent brain. Studies have shown that outcome is linked to the degree of resection. The previously mentioned meta-analysis of 566 patients showed that patients with CPP had a 10-year survival rate of 85% when undergoing GTR versus only 56% with subtotal resection (STR). One-year survival rate was 50% for patients only undergoing biopsy. Patients with CPC had a 2-year survival rate of 72% versus 34% for those with GTR and incomplete resection, respectively [3]. These findings are supported by a retrospective analysis of all reported cases in the English literature of CPC from 1985 until 2000. The authors found that of 75 identified cases, 37 underwent a GTR versus 38 patients who had a STR. For patients after GTR, survival was documented as 84% compared with 18% for patients who underwent STR [5]. This study also supported the role of adjuvant therapy in patients who first underwent a STR. Seven patients underwent adjuvant therapy after STR, followed by a second surgery allowing GTR. All seven patients were alive and disease free by the time of publication [5]. One other study suggests that adjuvant therapy reduces the peritumoral vascularity and hence limits the often observed significant bleeding and, therefore, allows for more complete resection during surgery [6].

In summary, the goal of surgery is complete resection whenever possible, and second surgery is indicated if after adjuvant therapy GTR can be achieved safely.

Radiation Therapy

The role of radiotherapy in the treatment of choroid-plexus tumors remains controversial. The peak incidence of these tumors is in young children and infants, a population group that is highly susceptible to the negative consequences of radiation. In up to 30% of cases cerebrospinal metastasis is present. This warrants radiation-field extension to the whole neuroaxis, which unfortunately increases the potential of severe adverse side effects [7], but several studies have documented the beneficial effect of postoperative radiation for CPC [3,4,8]. Wolff et al showed in his meta-analysis that patients with CPC who received radiation did better than those without radiation regardless of the extent of resection. Another analysis showed that 5-year survival was 47.4% (±6.5%) in patients receiving radiation therapy versus 25.2% (±4.3%) without radiotherapy [4]. Duffner et al reported on 14 cases that received radiation therapy; 5 out of 7 patients with GTR had long-term survival, whereas only 1 out of 7 patients with STR achieved 5-year survival, which suggests that the degree of resection is important for the beneficial response to radiotherapy [9]. Another series reported 4 patients with STR who received radiotherapy, but no long-term survival was achieved [6].

In general, postoperative radiation is recommended in children older than 3 years of age, though no clinical trial has been conducted regarding the benefit of radiotherapy.

Chemotherapy

The role of chemotherapy in choroid-plexus tumors has been controversial. There are several reports of small series and individual cases suggesting an effect of chemotherapy in patients with STR, whereas the role of chemotherapy in patients undergoing GTR is more questionable. A recent meta-analysis summarized a total of 857 cases of choroid-plexus tumors until 2004. Of these 495 (57.8%) had a CPP, 347 (40.5%) had a CPC, and 15 patients were diagnosed with atypical CPP. Information about chemotherapy and survival was evaluated for 230 patients with CPC. Of these, 104 patients (45.2%) had chemotherapy and 126 patients (54.8%) had no chemotherapy. Of the 104 patients, 34.6% also received radiotherapy. Overall survival was better in patients receiving chemotherapy (5-year survival 46.4 ± 6.1%) than those not receiving chemotherapy (5-year survival 27.6 ± 4.8%), regardless of radiotherapy. Patients with STR receiving chemotherapy had a significantly longer median survival (2.75 years ± 0.85) compared to patients not treated with chemotherapy (0.58 years ± 0.1). Patients after GTR had no apparent benefit from chemotherapy. Further subanalysis revealed that patients after incomplete resection had the best 2-year overall survival with combined radiochemotherapy (63%), compared to chemotherapy only (45%), radiotherapy alone (32%), or no further treatment (15%) [4]. The authors concluded that patients after STR and older than 3 years of age should undergo radiochemotherapy for adjuvant therapy. In a separate study, Duffner et al reported the results from the pediatric oncology group who treated 8 patients prospectively with chemotherapy to delay radiation therapy. Of these 8 patients, 4 had residual disease; 1 had partial response to chemotherapy for 24 months and was subsequently irradiated, resulting in long-term survival. The other 3 patients with STR progressed on chemotherapy and received subsequently radiotherapy [9]. The role of adjuvant treatment after GTR is not well understood. Packer et al reported 5 patients with CPC who underwent GTR. Of these, 4 patients remained progression free, with only 1 patient receiving radiotherapy [10]. Ellenbogen et al described similar results in 4 patients with CPC after GTR who had no recurrence at a median follow-up of 9.8 years with, only 1 patient receiving radiotherapy [1].

For patients with CPP, surgery appears to be the most important treatment modality. To date, there is no published evidence yet, that adjuvant therapy has a beneficial effect on survival [3].

REFERENCES

1. Ellenbogen RG, Winston KR, Kupsky WJ. Tumors of the choroid plexus in children. *Neurosurgery*. 1989;25(3):327–335.
2. Ho DM, Wong TT, Liu HC. Choroid plexus tumors in childhood. Histopathologic study and clinico-pathological correlation. *Childs Nerv Syst*. 1991;7(8):437–441.
3. Wolff JE, Sajedi M, Brant R, Coppes MJ, Egeler RM. Choroid plexus tumours. *Br J Cancer*. 2002;87(10):1086–1091.
4. Wrede B, Liu P, Wolff JE. Chemotherapy improves the survival of patients with choroid plexus carcinoma: a meta-analysis of individual cases with choroid plexus tumors. *J Neurooncol*. 2007;85(3):345–351.
5. Fitzpatrick LK, Aronson LJ, Cohen KJ. Is there a requirement for adjuvant therapy for choroid plexus carcinoma that has been completely resected? *J Neurooncol*. 2002;57(2):123–126.
6. St Clair SK, Humphreys RP, Pillay PK, Hoffman HJ, Blaser SI, Becker LE. Current management of choroid plexus carcinoma in children. *Pediatr Neurosurg*. 1991;17(5):225–233.
7. Greenberg ML. Chemotherapy of choroid plexus carcinoma. *Childs Nerv Syst*. 1999;15(10):571–577.
8. Wolff JE, Sajedi M, Coppes MJ, Anderson RA, Egeler RM. Radiation therapy and survival in choroid plexus carcinoma. *Lancet*. 1999;353(9170):2126.
9. Duffner PK, Kun LE, Burger PC, et al. Postoperative chemotherapy and delayed radiation in infants and very young children with choroid plexus carcinomas. The Pediatric Oncology Group. *Pediatr Neurosurg*. 1995;22(4):189–196.
10. Packer RJ, Perilongo G, Johnson D, et al. Choroid plexus carcinoma of childhood. *Cancer*. 1992;69(2):580–585.

75 General Principles of Targeted Therapies

Nicholas Butowski

MECHANISM OF ACTION OF TARGETED AGENTS

Until recently, cancer treatments like surgery, radiotherapy, and cytotoxic chemotherapy, although sometimes effective, have been relatively nonspecific in their actions. Traditional chemotherapy consists of cytotoxic drugs that affect rapidly dividing cells such as those found not only in cancer but also cells in normal tissues such as hair, bone marrow, and gastrointestinal epithelium. As a result, most patients taking cytotoxic agents experience the classic toxicities of alopecia, gastrointestinal upset, and myelosuppression. By contrast to cytotoxic agents that are "targeted," chemotherapeutic agents "target" molecular alterations in cell-signaling pathways [1]. These agents arose from advances in molecular cancer biology that have shown us that the transformation into cancer involves the mutation or amplification of oncogenes and/or loss of tumor-suppressor genes leading to abnormalities in the signaling pathways of cells that in turn result in unregulated cell proliferation, angiogenesis, and invasion. The molecular targets of these agents are at times found in normal tissue; consequently, targeted agents may produce side effects, but these toxicities may be reasonably dissimilar from those seen with cytotoxic agents, as they depend on the target hit and resulting specific disruption in normal cell function. It is also possible that targeted agents may be more effective in patients whose cancer possesses the specific target, amount of target or variant of the target—a principle that has expanded the idea of individually tailored treatment.

There are many molecular pathways "targeted" in the treatment of cancer, but common pathways involve those of epidermal growth factor receptor (EGFR, also known as HER1) and vascular endothelial growth factor (VEGF) [2]. See other relevant chapters in this text for more in-depth information on other molecular pathways involved in targeted therapy. These pathways, which often give cancer cells a gain of function as a consequence of overexpression or gene alteration, can be inhibited at multiple levels by (a) neutralizing signaling molecules or ligands (molecules that bind to specific growth receptors on cells), (b) binding blocking receptor-binding sites (preventing ligand binding), (c) blocking cell-cycle proteins or receptor signaling within a tumor cell, and (d) interfering with downstream-pathway molecular signals such as modulators of apoptosis.

TYPES OF TARGETED AGENTS

The main categories of targeted agents include small-molecule inhibitors (SMI) and monoclonal antibodies (mAbs). However, gene therapy and immunotherapy may also be included as categories. SMIs usually have small molecular weights and can enter cells directly and interfere with the intracellular signaling of tyrosine kinases (these are called tyrosine kinase inhibitors or TKI) or with downstream intracellular molecules [3,4]. Tyrosine kinases, such as EGFR or VEGF, initiate cell signaling pathways that may lead to cell growth, proliferation, migration, and angiogenesis in normal or cancer tissue. SMIs can inhibit a single target or multiple targets simultaneously and are usually administered orally and are generally metabolized by the liver, which may result in interactions with several medicines, including coumadin, macrolide antibiotics, and enzyme-inducing antiepileptic drugs. For more information on SMI, approaches for cancer in general, and specifically for brain tumors, you can refer to several recently published review articles or to other pertinent chapters in this text book [3–9].

mAbs were first created in the 1970s, using the technique of somatic-cell hybridization [10]. In early trials, these mAbs of murine origin led to the production of human anti-mouse antibodies. To avoid this immunogenicity and increase the activity of the new mAbs, new chimeric and humanized mAbs were generated by biotechnology. mAbs usually have larger molecular weights than SMIs and target extracellular molecules and exert their anticancer effects through a variety of mechanisms: by recruiting host immune functions to attack the target cell; binding to ligands or receptors, thereby interrupting cancer-cell pathways; or carrying a lethal or radioactive toxin to the target cell [11]. mAbs are given intravenously because their protein structure would be denatured in the gastrointestinal tract, if given orally. mAbs also do not undergo hepatic metabolism and are not subject to significant drug interactions. For more information on mAbs approaches for cancer therapy in general and specifically for brain tumors, you can refer to several recently published review articles [11–13]

Gene therapy uses nucleic acids as drugs to express or knock out a specific gene in a target cell. An appropriate delivery or vector system is what delivers these therapeutic genes. Viral and nonviral delivery systems are being studied, though the majority of gene therapy protocols are based on viral delivery systems, with the most popular being vectors from adenovirus and herpes simplex virus. For more information on gene therapy approaches for cancer in general and specifically for brain tumors, you can refer to several recently published review articles [6,7,14–17].

Immunotherapy entails manipulation or enhancement of the immune system to attack and kill tumor cells. Such therapies generally focus on one of three strategies: (a) establishing a systemic cellular antitumor immune response via antitumor immunization (vaccination), (b) local cytokine-focused approaches to bolster nascent immune responses, (c) passive immune-based targeting of chemotherapy or toxins by conjugation to mAbs directed against tumor cells. For more information on immunotherapy approaches for cancer in general and specifically for brain tumors, you can refer to several recently published review articles [7,8,18].

TARGETED THERAPY FOR BRAIN TUMORS

A first step in the process of developing targeted therapy is identification of highly prevalent or specific targets that are promoters of oncogenesis. Because of their significant molecular and genetic heterogeneity, there has been a wide interest in a variety of targets in brain tumors and in multiples forms of cancer. However, there has been particular interest on inhibitors targeting receptor tyrosine kinases such as EGFR, platelet-derived growth factor receptor, and VEGF receptor, as well as signal transduction inhibitors targeting mTOR, farnesyltransferase, and Raf kinase [2,6].

After identifying a target, the development of agents that "hit" or affect the target and restore normal cell function is a process that needs to be continuously reassessed on the basis of laboratory, animal, and clinical trial data. Thus far, brain tumors studies of single-targeted agents have reported modest activity, with response rates of 0% to 15% and no improvement of 6M-PFS [19]. These frustrating results are likely due to the fact that gliomas have coactivation of multiple tyrosine kinases as well as redundant molecular-signaling pathways, thereby limiting the efficacy of a single agent. In addition, many of the molecularly targeted agents have poor penetration across the blood-brain barrier. Current strategies to increase the efficacy of targeted agents include the use of multitargeted agents, combinations of targeted agents, and combinations of targeted agents with radiotherapy and chemotherapy. Many reviews on this topic have been written and can be obtained for further information [2,9,12,19].

CLINICAL TRIALS FOR TARGETED AGENTS

Because of their novel mechanisms of action and the fact that they may have different side effects compared with traditional chemotherapy, targeted agents need to be studied in innovatively designed and conducted clinical trials that incorporate new approaches to determine optimal dosing, patient adherence, and efficacy. The traditional paradigm of dose selection based on maximum tolerable toxicity may not apply to novel therapies that target cell-signaling pathways or the cellular environment. Unlike cytotoxic agents, which act on DNA, these novel therapies have different targets such as membrane receptors, signaling pathways, and proteins, or factors important in cell-cycle regulation or in angiogenesis. As such, in laboratory models these agents seem to inhibit tumor progression rather than cause tumor regression. Novel agents also seem to be more selective and less toxic to normal tissue. Considering these points, the dose of the targeted agent needed to achieve tumor inhibition may not be the one that produces significant organ toxicity. Therefore, although the goal of phase I trials of targeted agents remains the basis for recommended phase II dose, this dose is likely to be determined by biological endpoints and not necessarily by the maximum-tolerated dose (MTD). Biological endpoints are associated with a desired biological effect such as inhibition of an enzyme or immunological change, but not necessarily with a specific toxicity and may actually be reached below the MTD. In addition, the toxic effects of molecular agents may be achieved through different mechanisms than the therapeutic effect and hence may not parallel one another at all.

Until such alternative endpoints are validated, phase I trials of novel agents incorporating multiple endpoints may be the most practical approach. For example, a useful design may be to define the recommended phase II dose on the basis of the MTD and the maximum target-inhibition dose. Taking into account that many targeted agents may require longer-term treatment than the relatively short-term treatment of cytotoxic agents, the definition of tolerable toxicity may need to be adjusted. In order to limit the intensity of daily toxicity, there may be more impetus to discover a therapeutic dose below the MTD level. In this vein, concurrent pharmacokinetic and pharmacodynamic studies with molecularly targeted agents may prove important in assessing the time that inhibitory concentrations are sustained for a given schedule and how this may correspond with response and efficacy in subsequent trials.

In terms of phase II trials, one must consider that molecular agents may prevent tumor growth without shrinking the tumor, and as such response measured as tumor regression is not an appropriate endpoint for these agents. Possible endpoints for molecularly targeted agents include time to tumor progression, change in tumor markers, measures of target inhibition, and metabolic imaging. Time to progression is a well-described endpoint in the literature, where benefit is measured by comparison with a historical cohort treated with the standard of care. Ideally, the only difference between the control and treatment group is the treatment itself. Selection bias may unduly make such comparison invalid as groups often differ in comparability of such factors as response assessment, ancillary care, and patient characteristics. One way to minimize selection bias is to use groups evaluated at the same institution. Change in tumor markers is an appealing endpoint, but the technique is unproven and not widely employed in brain-tumor therapy for lack of a marker to measure. If a marker did exist, physicians must be certain that the drug itself does not directly lower the level by protein degradation independent of tumor burden. Measures of target inhibition require a definitive cause and effect relationship between the novel agent, the targeted molecule, and tumor growth. As the current level of understanding of these relationships is inadequate, such targeting has yet to be shown to be clinically effective.

CONCLUSIONS

Neuro-oncology has emerged from the empirical era where systemic therapy was given to all patients, irrespective of any particular tumor features, and to the targeted therapy era where efforts are ongoing to determine a molecular profile of each patient's tumor, in the hope of selecting those patients who will benefit most from specific, molecularly based treatments. The use of biomarkers for identifying which patients are most likely to respond to a given agent remains an active area of research but requires validation. Also, there are high economic costs associated with development and production of targeted agents and the relevant biomarker assays. Vigilant and deliberate understanding of the underlying biology and accurate patient selection will assist in avoiding unnecessary costs.

REFERENCES

1. Abou-Jawde R, Choueiri T, Alemany C, Mekhail T. An overview of targeted treatments in cancer. *Clin Ther.* 2003;25(8):2121–2137.
2. Lukas RV, Boire A, Nicholas MK. Emerging therapies for malignant glioma. *Expert Rev Anticancer Ther.* 2007;7(12 suppl):S29-S36.
3. Arora A, Scholar EM. Role of tyrosine kinase inhibitors in cancer therapy. *J Pharmacol Exp Ther.* 2005;315(3):971–979.
4. Traxler P. Tyrosine kinases as targets in cancer therapy—successes and failures. *Expert Opin Ther Targets.* 2003;7(2):215–234.
5. Dear R, Wilcken N, Shannon J. Beyond chemotherapy—demystifying the new 'targeted' cancer treatments. *Aust Fam Physician.* 2008;37(1–2):45–49.
6. Kanzawa T, Ito H, Kondo Y, Kondo S. Current and future gene therapy for malignant gliomas. *J Biomed Biotechnol.* 2003;2003(1):25–34.
7. Selznick LA, Shamji MF, Fecci P, Gromeier M, Friedman AH, Sampson J. Molecular strategies for the treatment of malignant glioma–genes, viruses, and vaccines. *Neurosurg Rev.* 2008;31(2):141–155; discussion 155.
8. Gale DM. Molecular targets in cancer therapy. *Semin Oncol Nurs.* 2003;19(3):193–205.
9. Kalyn R. Overview of targeted therapies in oncology. *J Oncol Pharm Pract.* 2007;13(4):199–205.
10. Köhler G, Milstein C. Continuous cultures of fused cells secreting antibody of predefined specificity. *Nature.* 1975;256(5517):495–497.
11. Oldham RK, Dillman RO. Monoclonal antibodies in cancer therapy: 25 years of progress. *J Clin Oncol.* 2008;26(11):1774–1777.
12. Newton HB. Small-molecule and antibody approaches to molecular chemotherapy of primary brain tumors. *Curr Opin Investig Drugs.* 2007;8(12):1009–1021.
13. Gerber DE. Targeted therapies: a new generation of cancer treatments. *Am Fam Physician.* 2008;77(3):311–319.
14. King GD, Curtin JF, Candolfi M, Kroeger K, Lowenstein PR, Castro MG. Gene therapy and targeted toxins for glioma. *Curr Gene Ther.* 2005;5(6):535–557.
15. Cutter JL, Kurozumi K, Chiocca EA, Kaur B. Gene therapeutics: the future of brain tumor therapy? *Expert Rev Anticancer Ther.* 2006;6(7):1053–1064.
16. Aghi M, Chiocca EA. Gene therapy for glioblastoma. *Neurosurg Focus.* 2006;20(4):E18.
17. Benítez JA, Domínguez-Monzón G, Segovia J. Conventional and gene therapy strategies for the treatment of brain tumors. *Curr Med Chem.* 2008;15(8):729–742.
18. Fenstermaker RA, Ciesielski MJ. Immunotherapeutic strategies for malignant glioma. *Cancer Control.* 2004;11(3):181–191.
19. Sathornsumetee S, Reardon DA, Desjardins A, Quinn JA, Vredenburgh JJ, Rich JN. Molecularly targeted therapy for malignant glioma. *Cancer.* 2007;110(1):13–24.

General Principles of Angiogenesis

Nicholas Butowski

ANGIOGENESIS

In 1971, Folkman hypothesized that inhibition of angiogenesis, the formation of new blood vessels, would be an effective anticancer therapy [1]. His theory was confirmed in 2004 when bevacizumab, a monoclonal antibody against vascular endothelial growth factor (VEGF), was approved by the FDA for the treatment of metastatic colorectal cancer in combination with cytotoxic chemotherapy. Now, there are several antiangiogenic agents in clinical trials for different types of cancer including brain cancer.

Tumoral angiogenesis is a critical process in cancer growth and may occur in a number of different ways. It is widely accepted that initial tumor growth occurs by co-option of preexisting vessels which causes tumor cells to migrate along blood vessels thereby compressing them which leads to reduced perfusion and hypoxia. Hypoxia and mutations in cancer cells lead to outright angiogenesis via secretion of proteic angiogenic factors such as VEGF, platelet-derived growth factor (PDGF), and basic and acidic fibroblast growth factor (FGF), among others [2]. VEGF is an endothelial cell-specific mitogen which promotes the growth, proliferation, and migration and survival of vascular endothelial cells derived from arteries, veins, and lymphatics. VEGF also stimulates the recruitment of bone marrow–derived endothelial progenitor cells to the new vasculature and increases vascular permeability [2]. Each of these steps involves several molecular step and alterations that can be potentially targeted therapeutically [3].

At least seven VEGF isoforms (VEGF-A to F) exist. VEGF-A is a key proangiogenic factor because of its specificity to endothelial cells and the multitude of responses it can elicit. VEGF-B not only plays a role in vasculogenesis but also activates invasive enzymes on endothelial cells. VEGF-C is most commonly associated with lymphangiogensis. VEGF-D, E, and F have roles that are less well defined but involved angiogenesis and endothelial cell mitosis [4]. Overexpression of VEGF-A occurs in response to hypoxia and numerous growth factors such as PDGF and FGF. The main receptors involved in relaying VEGF-A signaling are VEGFR-1 and VEGFR-2. The best studied receptor is VEGFR-2, a potent tyrosine kinase that mediates endothelial cell signaling through the activation of Ras/Raf/MEK/MAPK, PI3K/Akt, and protein kinase C-beta. Gliomas, especially GBM, are highly vascularized tumors and overexpress VEGF-A. Furthermore, several molecular abnormalities found in GBM promote angiogenesis including mutations in the PI3K/Akt and protein kinase C-beta pathways. In addition, VEGFR is upregulated in glioma endothelium suggesting a paracrine response [5]. There have been several recent reviews of the molecular pathways involved in angiogenesis in brain tumors which can be read for further information [6–9].

Several strategies for targeting VEGF exist including anti-VEGF-A and VEGFR-2 monoclonal antibodies, antisense oligonucletides, and VEGFR TKI. TKI may have broad spectrum activity against many tyrosine kinases, and their activity may reflect other targets than VEGFR. Testing these agents has been challenging because they have called for new paradigms and novel clinical trial design. Challenges include defining the optimal dose of the drugs that do not cause much apparent toxicity during the first months of treatment. At the clinical level, evidence is emerging that circulating endothelial cells (CEC) kinetics and viability might correlate with clinical outcomes in cancer patients who undergo antiangiogenic treatment which may serve as a surrogate marker for monitoring antiangiogenic treatment and drug activity and could help to determine the optimal biological dose of antiangiogenic drugs [10,11]. Other difficulties include determining whether these agents should be used in combination with cytotoxic chemotherapy or radiotherapy and what molecular markers might predict response [12].

Other possible antiangiogenic approaches include metronomic chemotherapy or designing agents that target other molecules involved in angiogenesis. With metronomic chemotherapy, traditional cytotoxic chemotherapy is given at a continuous low dose disrupting rapidly proliferating tumor endothelium and preventing tumor growth [13,14]. Other potential targets having to do with angiogenesis include angiopoietin which is an endothelial cell-specific molecule, its receptor TIE-2, and integrins which are also functional receptors of angiopoietin. The complex interplay between the different types of angiopoietin and their receptors is still being studied, but these pathways may be involved in how tumors overcome anti-VEGF/VEGFR agents and thus represent an exciting area of research [4].

Antiangiogenic Therapies [15,16]

Different approaches to disrupting tumor-induced angiogenesis include tyrosine kinase inhibitor, monoclonal antibodies, small-molecule inhibitors, and transcription inhibitors [9]. However, monoclonal antibody and tyrosine kinase inhibitors are the most used drug classes currently being investigated in clinical trials.

Targeting of VEGF limits solid cancer growth by preventing angiogenesis and promoting apoptosis. Targeting of VEGF may also transiently "normalize" the abnormal structure and function of tumor vasculature to make it more efficient for oxygen and concurrent cytotoxic or targeted drug delivery. It is theorized that antiangiogenic agents may lower interstitial pressure by normalizing blood vessels thereby improving the delivery of chemotherapy at certain time points and if the agents are dosed in appropriate time in relation to one another [17]. Reviews of this topic in cancer and in brain tumors have been recently published [6,7,18,19].

Antiangiogenic Escape Mechanisms and Treatment Strategies

Tumors can compensate for the therapy-induced VEGF blockade through one or more escape mechanisms [20–22]. Escape mechanisms include (1) upregulation of VEGF, (2) contribution of VEGF by host stroma, (3) hyperactivation of alternate signaling pathways, (4) co-option of existing blood vessels that are less susceptible to VEGF blockade, (5) transformation of the tumor vasculature to a more mature, less VEGF-dependent phenotype, (6) genetic selection for tumor cells exhibiting increased resistance to both hypoxia and chemotherapy [21]. Whatever the escape mechanism may be, it does appear that antiangiogenic therapy may be altering the natural history of tumors by selecting for increased invasion. There has been some published reports in systemic cancers that treatment with antiangiogenic agents stimulates invasion and metastasis [16]. Thus, it may be necessary to simultaneously inhibit tumor angiogenesis and invasion in order to prevent the tumor's ability to resist antiangiogenic therapy. Several strategies are currently being studied, and there is some evidence that inhibiting EGFR may make tumors more angiogenesis dependent and thus more susceptible to VEGF inhibitors [23]. Therefore targeting both VEGF and EGFR at the same time is being explored as a way to circumvent anti-VEGF escape mechanisms. Also, inhibition of the PI3K/Akt pathway, which is critical to glioma angiogenesis and invasion, may be another viable strategy. Last, using multitargeted kinase inhibitors which can inhibit multiple cell signaling pathways may be more effective at controlling angiogenesis, invasion, and growth. Drugs like sunitinib (VEGFR-2, PDGFR, c-Kit, Flt-3 inhibitor) or sorafenib (VEGFR, PDGFR, Raf, c-Kit, and Flt-3) are being studied in GBM.

There is discussion and some empiric evidence that anti-VEGF therapy may induce a cytostatic effect characterized by a reduction in tumor vascular density. This fact begs the question of whether patients can benefit from continuation of anti-VEGF treatment in the context of disease progression. Research has shown that tumor vasculature can regrow aggressively soon after anti-VEGF therapy is discontinued. Therefore discontinuing therapy in the face of tumor growth could initiate even more rapid disease progression. Similarly, continuing anti-VEGF therapy may provide survival and quality-of-life benefits even in the absence of tumor response [24]. There may be patients who have tumor progression resulting from chemotherapy resistance rather than anti-VEGF evasion though the opposite is also possible and leaves the treating physician with two distinct treatment problems.

Toxicites Associated With Antiangiogenic Therapy

In general, targeting VEGF can also lead to effects on normal blood vessels resulting in bleeding, thrombosis, hypertension, and proteinuria [25]. Fatigue is also a very common toxicity experienced by patients treated with antiangiogenic agents [6]. Delayed incision or wound healing has also been commonly reported. As most antiangiogenic agents have been used only for the past few years, unanticipated long-term toxicities such as cardiomyopathy are of some concern.

VARIOUS ANTIANGIOGENIC AGENTS CURRENTLY BEING RESEARCHED IN BRAIN TUMORS

Bevacizumab

Bevacizumab (Avastin®; Genetech Inc., South San Francisco, CA) was developed by Genentech and is marketed in the United States by Genentech and elsewhere by Roche under the brand name Avastin. In 2004, the FDA approved bevacizumab, a humanized mAb against VEGF, as the first antiangiogenic therapy to be used in combination with irinotecan and 5-FU-based chemotherapy in previously untreated metastatic colorectal cancer [26–28]. Bevacizumab is usually given intravenously every 14 days and is not affected by enzyme-inducing antiepileptic drugs (EIAEDs). In colon cancer, it is given in combination with 5-FU, leucovorin, and oxaliplatin or irinotecan. Bevacizumab has also demonstrated activity in renal cell cancer and ovarian cancer when used as a single agent and in lung cancer and breast cancer when combined with chemotherapy [29,30].

Several adverse side effects have been reported with bevacizumab [31]. The main observed toxicities include hypertension, proteinuria, mild to moderate hemorrhage, wound-healing complications, and thromboembolic events. Bowel perforation has also rarely been reported [32,33]. The FDA updated the label on the drug on September 25, 2006 to note rare cases of reversible posterior leukoencephalopathy syndrome and nasal septum perforation [34,35]. A variety of dosing schemes have been investigated in solid cancers, but no consensus has been reached on the optimal bevacizumab regimen [28,36].

There is a growing amount of published information regarding bevacizumab's potential role in brain tumor patients and any adverse effects unique to this patient population. A recently published phase II study used bevacizumab in combination with irinotecan for patients with recurrent grade III or IV gliomas [37,38]. Patients with evidence of intracranial hemorrhage on initial brain magnetic resonance imaging were excluded. No central nervous system hemorrhages occurred, but three patients developed deep venous thromboses or pulmonary emboli, and one patient had an arterial ischemic stroke Patients received bevacizumab and irinotecan iv every 2 weeks of a 6-week cycle. Bevacizumab was administered at 10 mg/kg. Radiographic responses were noted in 63% of patients, but improvements in PFS and OS were less impressive (GBM patients: median PFS 20 weeks; median OS 10 months; $n = 23$). This dramatic radiographic response rate versus more modest improvements in OS and PFS raise the question that the observed radiographic response was secondary to decreased vascular permeability and edema rather than to a real antitumor effect. An updated phase II study from the same group of GBM patients showed a response rate of 57% and 6M-PFS of 46%. A retrospective study evaluated whether expression of the components of the VEGF pathway and hypoxic response were predictive of radiographic response and survival benefit in this updated phase-II study [39]; only tumor expression levels of VEGF were associated with radiographic response and no marker was predictive of survival benefit.

A randomized phase-II trial in which recurrent GBM patients were assigned bevacizumab alone or in combination with irinotecan has recently completed accrual with results pending. A phase-II study of avastin in combination with temozolomide (TMZ) and radiotherapy (RT) in newly diagnosed GBM patients recently reported preliminary toxicity results on 10 patients [40]. This trial added avastin to upfront RT and TMZ based on the theory that an antiangiogenic agent such as avastin may normalize blood vessels and thus reduce hypoxia and counteract the effects of radiation-induced VEGF secretion from tumor cells while increasing the amount of TMZ reaching the tumor [40,41]. The analysis did not reveal any serious unexpected toxicities except optic neuropathy in one patient, the etiology of which was unclear. An interim PFS of 8.8 months was also reported and the study is ongoing.

Another recent study examined bevacizumab's potential role in reducing radiation necrosis of the brain [42]. The study reported significant positive changes observed in the imaging studies of 8 patients with radiation necrosis. The authors attributed the response to the normalization of the blood–brain barrier attained by decreasing the levels of VEGF through the use of bevacizumab. They did not comment on adverse affects.

Clinical trials continue with avastin in combination with cytotoxic and or targeted agents both in newly diagnosed and recurrent brain tumor patients. These trials may also provide information on whether metronomic dosing of traditional chemotherapy is a better option for combination use with avastin and whether avastin and similar agents alter the recurrence pattern for high-grade gliomas [36,43]. In addition, studies using imaging techniques such as PET scanning are being performed in order to ascertain which patients may benefit the most from treatment with avastin and whether such imaging can be used to predict survival [44,45].

Enzastaurin

Enzastaurin (Eli Lilly Indianapolis, IN) is a potent, selective, oral serine-threonine kinase inhibitor of PKCβ with potent antiproliferative, proapoptotic, and antiangiogenic activities. It is manufactured by Eli Lilly and Company. EIAEDs decrease enzastaurin exposure. Enzastaurin studies in human patients have used oral doses ranging from 20 to 700 mg [46,47]. Although no MTD was identified up to 700 mg/day, 525 mg was chosen as the recommended dose based on bioavailability data when the drug is used alone and not with other agents with overlapping toxicity profiles. The most commonly reported toxicities were fatigue and reddish discoloration of urine and feces (enzastaurin is red in color).

ENZ disrupts the phosphotransferase activity of conventional and novel PKC isoforms via an interaction at the ATP binding site and displays selectivity in inhibiting the beta isoform [48]. The PKC family of enzymes is essential to numerous functions in cancer cells including cell growth, proliferation, and apoptosis thus making ENZ an appealing anticancer agent [49–51]. The beta isoform of PKC also lies in the signal cascade of VEGF, upregulated in most GBMs with concomitant overexpression of VEGFR [52]; inhibition of this pathway by ENZ leads to a block in tumor angiogenesis in addition to growth, and thus ENZ is considered an antiangiogenic agent. PKC activity is also thought to regulate Akt, a protein that has antiapoptotic effects and is involved in cell proliferation in GBM [53–55]. Thus, inhibition of the Akt pathway may lead to decreased growth and increased cell death.

Preclinical research on ENZ illustrates that it inhibits the pathways that GBMs need for angiogenesis, invasion, and proliferation. Moreover, preclinical data demonstrate that ENZ enhances the efficacy of RT by preventing unwanted proinvasive and angiogenic effects and also enhances TMZ-induced cell death in GBM cell lines [55,56]. Clinical studies in healthy volunteers and patients with solid tumors showed that ENZ was well tolerated at doses that achieved a biologically active serum and cerebrospinal fluid concentration. Results from a phase-II study using ENZ in patients with recurrent GBM demonstrated that it was also well tolerated in this patient population and suggested significant antitumor activity (personal communication). However, a multicentered phase-III trial of enzastaurin versus lomustine (Study Evaluating Enzastaurin in Recurrent Glioblastoma [STEERING] trial) was prematurely terminated as enzastaurin failed to demonstrate interim survival benefit.

Several trials in brain tumors are ongoing at the time this chapter was written but results are not published yet and thus information regarding toxicity or efficacy is not available. A phase-II single-arm trial of enzastaurin as single-agent therapy in patients with recurrent high-grade glioma is being conducted by the NCI. Patients receive oral enzastaurin 525 mg in capsules once daily. Each cycle of therapy consists of daily administration of enzastaurin for 6 weeks with no breaks between cycles. The UCSF neuro-oncology group is conducting a phase-I/II study of enzastaurin plus temozolomide during and following radiation therapy in patients with newly diagnosed GBM.

Enzastaurin is administered daily during radiation and during adjuvant cycles without interruption. There were two planned phase-I dosing cohorts based on enzastaurin dosing: 250 mg/day and 500 mg/day. Twelve patients enrolled in phase I (2 cohorts of 6 patients). There were no dose limiting toxicities (DLTs) in the 6 patients of Cohort 1 dosed at 250 mg ENZ. In the second cohort at 500 mg ENZ, 2 of 6 patients experienced a DLT; one grade-IV and one grade-III thrmbocytopenia. The patient with the grade-III DLT recovered in less than 28 days and reinitiated adjuvant TMZ and reduced-dose ENZ at 250 mg/day. The other patient recovered after 28 days but discontinued treatment. Phase II began accrual in 9/07 with a dose of ENZ at 250 mg/day. The same UCSF ENZ study will also determine whether pretreatment molecular profiles relative to the targets of ENZ and TMZ are predictive of outcome. It will also explore how physiological imaging contributes to the evaluation of these patients.

Thalidomide

Thalidomide (Celegene Corp; Summit, NJ) is a sedative and anti-inflammatory medication and is thought to have anti-angiogenesis properties mediated in part through by VEGF and FGF inhibition [57,58]. Thalidomide was developed by German pharmaceutical company Grünenthal and was chiefly sold and prescribed during the late 1950s to pregnant women as an antiemetic. Unfortunately, inadequate tests were performed to assess the drug's safety, with resulting devastating results for the children of women who had taken thalidomide during their pregnancies. From 1956 to 1962, approximately 10,000 children were born with severe malformations, including phocomelia, because their mothers had taken thalidomide during pregnancy [59]. Despite these results, researchers continued to work with the drug, and Celegene Corp. now manufactures thalidomide for a number of indications. In 2006, the FDA granted accelerated approval for thalidomide in combination with dexamethasone for the treatment of newly diagnosed multiple myeloma [60,61]. Thalidomide is also being investigated for treating prostate cancer, glioblastoma, lymphoma, arachnoiditis, Behçet's disease, and Crohn's disease.

Thalidomide has been used in several different brain tumor clinical trials [62–69]. It has been used alone or in conjunction with other agents in both adults and children and with patients with newly diagnosed brain tumors as well as recurrent tumors. Unfortunately, while most trials indicated that thalidomide was relatively well tolerated, it is unclear whether there is an added advantage to using thalidomide for patients with brain tumors. In recurrent GBM, overall survival rates were approximately 7 months. In two separate studies of newly diagnosed GBM, thalidomide was used with TMZ and radiotherapy but there was no survival advantage compared to TMZ alone [65,66]. Lenalidomide, a potent analogue of thalidomide, has shown significant activity in several hematologic malignancies, and studies have explored its tolerability and activity in patients with primary central nervous system tumors but there is no published efficacy data to date [70].

The doses of thalidomide used in trials ranged from 200 mg orally once a day to a maximum of 1200 mg/day. Adverse effects appear to be dose dependent with higher doses leading to a higher incidence of fatigue, peripheral neuropathy, and constipation [57,59,66,71]. Apart from its infamous tendency to induce birth defects and peripheral neuropathy, the main side effects of thalidomide include fatigue and constipation. It is also associated with an increased risk of deep-vein thrombosis especially when combined with dexamethasone. Higher doses can lead to pulmonary edema, atelectasis, aspiration pneumonia, and refractory hypotension.

Sorafenib

Sorafenib (Nexavar®; Bayer Pharmaceuticals Corporation, West Haven, CT) is a multitargeted kinase inhibitor approved by the FDA in 2005 as a second-line agent for advanced renal cell carcinoma after cytokine failure [72–74]. It is a small molecular inhibitor of Raf kinase, PDGF, and VEGF receptor kinase (VEGFR).

Side effects of sorafenib include rash, diarrhea, and hypertension. The most common skin irritations were rash and hand–foot skin reaction, which generally appeared during the first 6 weeks of treatment [74–76]. Management of dermatologic reactions may include topical therapies for symptomatic relief [77]; Temporary treatment interruption, dose reduction, or discontinuation may be required. Treatment-related hypertension during therapy is usually mild and managed with standard antihypertensive therapy. There is also a small risk of hemorrhage and cardiac ischemia associated with sorafenib use.

There are no published results of sorafenib's use in brain tumors. However, based on preclinical data, the North American Brain Tumor Consotium (NABTC) has an ongoing phase I/II of sorafenib in combination with erlotinib, tipifarnib, or temsirolimus in patients with recurrent GBM [78,79].

Sunitinib

Sunitinib (Sutent®; Pfizer Inc., New York) was developed by SUGEN, a South San Francisco biotechnology company which later merged into Pfizer in 2003. Sunitinib is a multitargeted kinase inhibitor, approved by the FDA in 2006 for patients with gastrointestinal stromal tumors (GIST) previously treated with imatinib and for advanced renal cell carcinoma as first-line treatment [80]. Sunitinib inhibits signaling through multiple receptor tyrosine kinases, including PDGFR and VEGFR [81,82]. GIST is driven by a mutationally activated kit kinase, and this is also inhibited by Sunitinib [80]. Notable side effects included diarrhea, hypertension, skin discoloration, mucositis, fatigue, and hypothyroidism. Neutropenia, thrombocytopenia, and decreases in left ventricular ejection fraction have also been seen with sunitinib [81–83]. Trials using sunitinib in brain tumor patients are in the planning stages.

Preclinically, sutnitinib demonstrated a potent inhibition of angiogenesis and meaningful prolongation of survival of mice bearing intracerebral GBM [84]. The hoped-for antiproliferative effects via the PDGFR pathway and anti-invasive effects via Src were not seen in *in vivo* studies. Brain tumor clinical trials with this agent are in the planning stages.

AZD2171

AZD2171 (AstraZeneca; London) is a new oral pan-VEGFR, PDGFR, and c-Kit inhibitor produced by AstraZeneca [85,86]. It is in initial stages of testing in recurrent GBM patients. Toxicity has yet to be fully documented. A recent study evaluated its use in 16 patients with recurrent GBM and demonstrated an immediate and significant radiographic normalizing effect with reduced blood vessel permeability and associated tumor-associated edema [87]. This same study also showed decreased blood vessel size was maintained for 28 days after administration of AZD2171. This result indicates that the concurrent use of cytotoxic therapies at the onset of concurrent antiangiogenic therapy may be most beneficial as its use falls within the presumed best window of opportunity. Otherwise, concurrent use of cytotoxic agents outside this window may suffer from decreased delivery of the drug to the tumor due to reduced blood supply. The study did not comment on survival. Trials with AZD2171 are ongoing.

SUMMARY

The expanding amount of information on cell signaling pathways, oncogenes and tumor suppressor genes, and tumoral angiogenesis is critical to developing new molecular-based and antiangiogenic approaches to brain tumors and cancer therapy. Appropriate evaluation of the efficacy of these novel agents requires the neuro-oncology community to continually redefine clinical trial design and strategy. Antiangiogenic agents are not necessarily cytotoxic and may require different methods to evaluate appropriate dose, effectiveness, response, or stability. New protocol designs may require tissue sampling or surrogate markers indicating molecular changes. Also, as the molecular pathogenesis of brain tumors has not been linked to a single genetic defect or target, a single molecular or antiangiogenic agent is not expected to be an effective treatment. Thus, these novel agents may need to be studied in tandem with cytotoxic agents or other novel agents, which will require a combination of clinical trial designs to properly determine patient benefit.

REFERENCES

1. Folkman J. Tumor angiogenesis: therapeutic implications. *N Engl J Med*. 1971;285(21):1182–1186.
2. Hicklin DJ, Ellis LM. Role of the vascular endothelial growth factor pathway in tumor growth and angiogenesis. *J Clin Oncol*. 2005;23(5):1011–1027.
3. Duda DG, Batchelor TT, Willett CG, Jain RK. VEGF-targeted cancer therapy strategies: current progress, hurdles and future prospects. *Trends Mol Med*. 2007;13(6):223–230.
4. Khosravi Shahi P, Fernández Pineda I. Tumoral angiogenesis: review of the literature. *Cancer Invest*. 2008;26(1):104–108.
5. Plate KH, Breier G, Weich HA, Mennel HD, Risau W. Vascular endothelial growth factor and glioma angiogenesis: coordinate induction of VEGF receptors, distribution of VEGF protein and possible *in vivo* regulatory mechanisms. *Int J Cancer*. 1994;59(4):520–529.
6. Jain RK, di Tomaso E, Duda DG, Loeffler JS, Sorensen AG, Batchelor TT. Angiogenesis in brain tumours. *Nat Rev Neurosci*. 2007;8(8):610–622.
7. Sathornsumetee S, Rich JN. Antiangiogenic therapy in malignant glioma: promise and challenge. *Curr Pharm Des*. 2007;13(35):3545–3558.
8. Tuettenberg J, Friedel C, Vajkoczy P. Angiogenesis in malignant glioma–a target for antitumor therapy? *Crit Rev Oncol Hematol*. 2006;59(3):181–193.
9. Veeravagu A, Hsu AR, Cai W, Hou LC, Tse VC, Chen X. Vascular endothelial growth factor and vascular endothelial growth factor receptor inhibitors as anti-angiogenic agents in cancer therapy. *Recent Pat Anticancer Drug Discov*. 2007;2(1):59–71.
10. Duda DG, Cohen KS, Scadden DT, Jain RK. A protocol for phenotypic detection and enumeration of circulating endothelial cells and circulating progenitor cells in human blood. *Nat Protoc*. 2007;2(4):805–810.
11. Bertolini F, Shaked Y, Mancuso P, Kerbel RS. The multifaceted circulating endothelial cell in cancer: towards marker and target identification. *Nat Rev Cancer*. 2006;6(11):835–845.
12. Duda DG, Jain RK, Willett CG. Antiangiogenics: the potential role of integrating this novel treatment modality with chemoradiation for solid cancers. *J Clin Oncol*. 2007;25(26):4033–4042.
13. Kesari S, Schiff D, Doherty L, et al. Phase II study of metronomic chemotherapy for recurrent malignant gliomas in adults. *Neuro-oncology*. 2007;9(3):354–363.
14. Miller KD, Sweeney CJ, Sledge GW Jr. Redefining the target: chemotherapeutics as antiangiogenics. *J Clin Oncol*. 2001;19(4):1195–1206.
15. Herbst RS. Therapeutic options to target angiogenesis in human malignancies. *Expert Opin Emerg Drugs*. 2006;11(4):635–650.
16. Shojaei F, Ferrara N. Antiangiogenic therapy for cancer: an update. *Cancer J*. 2007;13(6):345–348.
17. Jain RK. Normalization of tumor vasculature: an emerging concept in antiangiogenic therapy. *Science*. 2005;307(5706):58–62.
18. Gerstner ER, Duda DG, di Tomaso E, Sorensen G, Jain RK, Batchelor TT. Antiangiogenic agents for the treatment of glioblastoma. *Expert Opin Investig Drugs*. 2007;16(12):1895–1908.
19. Puduvalli VK. Inhibition of angiogenesis as a therapeutic strategy against brain tumors. *Cancer Treat Res*. 2004;117:307–336.
20. Chi A, Norden AD, Wen PY. Inhibition of angiogenesis and invasion in malignant gliomas. *Expert Rev Anticancer Ther*. 2007;7(11):1537–1560.
21. Casanovas O, Hicklin DJ, Bergers G, Hanahan D. Drug resistance by evasion of antiangiogenic targeting of VEGF signaling in late-stage pancreatic islet tumors. *Cancer Cell*. 2005;8(4):299–309.
22. Cristini V, Frieboes HB, Gatenby R, Caserta S, Ferrari M, Sinek J. Morphologic instability and cancer invasion. *Clin Cancer Res*. 2005;11(19 Pt 1):6772–6779.
23. Petit V, Nussbaumer U, Dossenbach C, Affolter M. Downstream-of-FGFR is a fibroblast growth factor-specific scaffolding protein and recruits Corkscrew upon receptor activation. *Mol Cell Biol*. 2004;24(9):3769–3781.
24. Grothey A. Does bevacizumab improve survival in patients with metastatic colorectal cancer treated with chemotherapy? *Nat Clin Pract Oncol*. 2006;3(1):22–23.
25. Tandle A, Libutti SK. Antiangiogenic therapy: targeting vascular endothelial growth factor and its receptors. *Clin Adv Hematol Oncol*. 2003;1(1):41–48.
26. Ellis LM. Bevacizumab. *Nat Rev Drug Discov*. 2005;suppl:S8–S9.
27. Ferrara N, Hillan KJ, Novotny W. Bevacizumab (Avastin), a humanized anti-VEGF monoclonal antibody for cancer therapy. *Biochem Biophys Res Commun*. 2005;333(2):328–335.
28. Shih T, Lindley C. Bevacizumab: an angiogenesis inhibitor for the treatment of solid malignancies. *Clin Ther*. 2006;28(11):1779–1802.
29. Micha JP, Goldstein BH, Rettenmaier MA, et al. A phase II study of outpatient first-line paclitaxel, carboplatin, and bevacizumab for advanced-stage epithelial ovarian, peritoneal, and fallopian tube cancer. *Int J Gynecol Cancer*. 2007;17(4):771–776.
30. Ramaswamy B, Elias AD, Kelbick NT, et al. Phase II trial of bevacizumab in combination with weekly docetaxel in metastatic breast cancer patients. *Clin Cancer Res*. 2006;12(10):3124–3129.
31. Sanborn RE, Sandler AB. The safety of bevacizumab. *Expert Opin Drug Saf*. 2006;5(2):289–301.
32. Gordon MS, Cunningham D. Managing patients treated with bevacizumab combination therapy. *Oncology*. 2005;69(suppl 3):25–33.

33. Hurwitz H, Saini S. Bevacizumab in the treatment of metastatic colorectal cancer: safety profile and management of adverse events. *Semin Oncol.* 2006;33(5 suppl 10):S26–S34.
34. Allen JA, Adlakha A, Bergethon PR. Reversible posterior leukoencephalopathy syndrome after bevacizumab/FOLFIRI regimen for metastatic colon cancer. *Arch Neurol.* 2006;63(10):1475–1478.
35. Glusker P, Recht L, Lane B. Reversible posterior leukoencephalopathy syndrome and bevacizumab. *N Engl J Med.* 2006;354(9):980–2; discussion 980.
36. Bergsland E, Dickler MN. Maximizing the potential of bevacizumab in cancer treatment. *Oncologist.* 2004;9(suppl 1):36–42.
37. Vredenburgh JJ, Desjardins A, Herndon JE 2nd, et al. Phase II trial of bevacizumab and irinotecan in recurrent malignant glioma. *Clin Cancer Res.* 2007;13(4):1253–1259.
38. Vredenburgh JJ, Desjardins A, Herndon JE 2nd, et al. Bevacizumab plus irinotecan in recurrent glioblastoma multiforme. *J Clin Oncol.* 2007;25(30):4722–4729.
39. Sathornsumetee S, Cao Y, Marcello JE, et al. Tumor angiogenic and hypoxic profiles predict radiographic response and survival in malignant astrocytoma patients treated with bevacizumab and irinotecan. *J Clin Oncol.* 2008;26(2):271–278.
40. Lai A. et al. Phase II pilot study of bevacizumab in combination with temozolomide and regional radiation therapy for up-front treatment of patients with newly diagnosed glioblastoma multiforme: interim analysis of safety and tolerability. *Int J Radiat Oncol Biol Phys*, 2008.
41. Hovinga KE, Stalpers LJ, van Bree C, et al. Radiation-enhanced vascular endothelial growth factor (VEGF) secretion in glioblastoma multiforme cell lines–a clue to radioresistance? *J Neurooncol.* 2005;74(2):99–103.
42. Gonzalez J, Kumar AJ, Conrad CA, Levin VA. Effect of bevacizumab on radiation necrosis of the brain. *Int J Radiat Oncol Biol Phys.* 2007;67(2):323–326.
43. Norden AD, Young GS, Setayesh K, et al. Bevacizumab for recurrent malignant gliomas: efficacy, toxicity, and patterns of recurrence. *Neurology.* 2008;70(10):779–787.
44. Chen W, Delaloye S, Silverman DH, et al. Predicting treatment response of malignant gliomas to bevacizumab and irinotecan by imaging proliferation with [18F] fluorothymidine positron emission tomography: a pilot study. *J Clin Oncol.* 2007;25(30):4714–4721.
45. Chamberlain MC. MRI in patients with high-grade gliomas treated with bevacizumab and chemotherapy. *Neurology.* 2006;67(11):2089; author reply 2089.
46. Carducci MA, Musib L, Kies MS, et al. Phase I dose escalation and pharmacokinetic study of enzastaurin, an oral protein kinase C beta inhibitor, in patients with advanced cancer. *J Clin Oncol.* 2006;24(25):4092–4099.
47. Robertson MJ, Kahl BS, Vose JM, et al. Phase II study of enzastaurin, a protein kinase C beta inhibitor, in patients with relapsed or refractory diffuse large B-cell lymphoma. *J Clin Oncol.* 2007;25(13):1741–1746.
48. Teicher BA, Alvarez E, Mendelsohn LG, Ara G, Menon K, Ways DK. Enzymatic rationale and preclinical support for a potent protein kinase C beta inhibitor in cancer therapy. *Adv Enzyme Regul.* 1999;39:313–327.
49. Gescher A. Analogs of staurosporine: potential anticancer drugs? *Gen Pharmacol.* 1998;31(5):721–728.
50. Jarvis WD, Grant S. Protein kinase C targeting in antineoplastic treatment strategies. *Invest New Drugs.* 1999;17(3):227–240.
51. Parker PJ. Inhibition of protein kinase C–do we, can we, and should we? *Pharmacol Ther.* 1999;82(2–3):263–267.
52. Chan AS, Leung SY, Wong MP, et al. Expression of vascular endothelial growth factor and its receptors in the anaplastic progression of astrocytoma, oligodendroglioma, and ependymoma. *Am J Surg Pathol.* 1998;22(7):816–826.
53. Kawakami Y, Nishimoto H, Kitaura J, et al. Protein kinase C betaII regulates Akt phosphorylation on Ser-473 in a cell type- and stimulus-specific fashion. *J Biol Chem.* 2004;279(46):47720–47725.
54. Aeder SE, Martin PM, Soh JW, Hussaini IM. PKC-eta mediates glioblastoma cell proliferation through the Akt and mTOR signaling pathways. *Oncogene.* 2004;23(56):9062–9069.
55. Graff JR, McNulty AM, Hanna KR, et al. The protein kinase Cbeta-selective inhibitor, Enzastaurin (LY317615.HCl), suppresses signaling through the AKT pathway, induces apoptosis, and suppresses growth of human colon cancer and glioblastoma xenografts. *Cancer Res.* 2005;65(16):7462–7469.
56. Tabatabai G, Frank B, Wick A, et al. Synergistic antiglioma activity of radiotherapy and enzastaurin. *Ann Neurol.* 2007;61(2):153–161.
57. Diggle GE. Thalidomide: 40 years on. *Int J Clin Pract.* 2001;55(9):627–631.
58. D'Amato RJ, Loughnan MS, Flynn E, Folkman J. Thalidomide is an inhibitor of angiogenesis. *Proc Natl Acad Sci USA.* 1994;91(9):4082–4085.
59. Laffitte E. [The revival of thalidomide: an old drug with new indications]. *Rev Prat.* 2006;56(18):1977–1983.
60. Harousseau JL. Thalidomide in multiple myeloma: past, present and future. *Future Oncol.* 2006;2(5):577–589.
61. Bernardeschi P, Giustarini G, Montenora I, et al. Thalidomide plus monthly high-dose dexamethasone in chemorefractory myeloma. Results of a phase II clinical study. *In Vivo.* 2006;20(6A):719–720.
62. Marx GM, Pavlakis N, McCowatt S, et al. Phase II study of thalidomide in the treatment of recurrent glioblastoma multiforme. *J Neurooncol.* 2001;54(1):31–38.
63. Short SC, Traish D, Dowe A, Hines F, Gore M, Brada M. Thalidomide as an anti-angiogenic agent in relapsed gliomas. *J Neurooncol.* 2001;51(1):41–45.
64. Fine HA, Wen PY, Maher EA, et al. Phase II trial of thalidomide and carmustine for patients with recurrent high-grade gliomas. *J Clin Oncol.* 2003;21(12):2299–2304.
65. Baumann F, Bjeljac M, Kollias SS, et al. Combined thalidomide and temozolomide treatment in patients with glioblastoma multiforme. *J Neurooncol.* 2004;67(1–2):191–200.
66. Chang SM, Lamborn KR, Malec M, et al. Phase II study of temozolomide and thalidomide with radiation therapy for newly diagnosed glioblastoma multiforme. *Int J Radiat Oncol Biol Phys.* 2004;60(2):353–357.
67. Groves MD, Puduvalli VK, Chang SM, et al. A North American brain tumor consortium (NABTC 99–04) phase II trial of temozolomide plus thalidomide for recurrent glioblastoma multiforme. *J Neurooncol.* 2007;81(3):271–277.
68. Turner CD, Chi S, Marcus KJ, et al. Phase II study of thalidomide and radiation in children with newly diagnosed brain stem gliomas and glioblastoma multiforme. *J Neurooncol.* 2007;82(1):95–101.
69. Zustovich F, Cartei G, Ceravolo R, et al. A phase I study of cisplatin, temozolomide and thalidomide in patients with malignant brain tumors. *Anticancer Res.* 2007;27(2):1019–1024.
70. Fine HA, Kim L, Albert PS, et al. A phase I trial of lenalidomide in patients with recurrent primary central nervous system tumors. *Clin Cancer Res.* 2007;13(23):7101–7106.
71. Wu JJ, Huang DB, Pang KR, Hsu S, Tyring SK. Thalidomide: dermatological indications, mechanisms of action and side-effects. *Br J Dermatol.* 2005;153(2):254–273.
72. Hahn O, Stadler W. Sorafenib. *Curr Opin Oncol.* 2006;18(6):615–621.
73. Kane RC, Farrell AT, Saber H, et al. Sorafenib for the treatment of advanced renal cell carcinoma. *Clin Cancer Res.* 2006;12(24):7271–7278.
74. Rini BI. Sorafenib. *Expert Opin Pharmacother.* 2006;7(4):453–461.
75. Strumberg D, Richly H, Hilger RA, et al. Phase I clinical and pharmacokinetic study of the Novel Raf kinase and vascular endothelial growth factor receptor inhibitor BAY 43-9006 in patients with advanced refractory solid tumors. *J Clin Oncol.* 2005;23(5):965–972.
76. Awada A, Hendlisz A, Gil T, et al. Phase I safety and pharmacokinetics of BAY 43-9006 administered for 21 days on/7 days off in patients with advanced, refractory solid tumours. *Br J Cancer.* 2005;92(10):1855–1861.
77. Alexandrescu DT, Vaillant JG, Dasanu CA. Effect of treatment with a colloidal oatmeal lotion on the acneform eruption induced by epidermal growth factor receptor and multiple tyrosine-kinase inhibitors. *Clin Exp Dermatol* 2007;32(1):71–74.
78. Jane EP, Premkumar DR, Pollack IF. Coadministration of sorafenib with rottlerin potently inhibits cell proliferation and migration in human malignant glioma cells. *J Pharmacol Exp Ther.* 2006;319(3):1070–1080.
79. Newton HB. Small-molecule and antibody approaches to molecular chemotherapy of primary brain tumors. *Curr Opin Investig Drugs.* 2007;8(12):1009–1021.
80. Goodman VL, Rock EP, Dagher R, et al. Approval summary: sunitinib for the treatment of imatinib refractory or intolerant gastrointestinal stromal tumors and advanced renal cell carcinoma. *Clin Cancer Res.* 2007;13(5):1367–1373.

81. Faivre S, Delbaldo C, Vera K, et al. Safety, pharmacokinetic, and antitumor activity of SU11248, a novel oral multitarget tyrosine kinase inhibitor, in patients with cancer. *J Clin Oncol*. 2006;24(1):25–35.
82. Izzedine H, Buhaescu I, Rixe O, Deray G. Sunitinib malate. *Cancer Chemother Pharmacol*. 2007;60(3):357–364.
83. Cabebe E, Wakelee H. Sunitinib: a newly approved small-molecule inhibitor of angiogenesis. *Drugs Today*. 2006;42(6):387–398.
84. de Boüard S, Herlin P, Christensen JG, et al. Antiangiogenic and anti-invasive effects of sunitinib on experimental human glioblastoma. *Neuro-oncology*. 2007;9(4):412–423.
85. Brandsma D, van den Bent MJ. Molecular targeted therapies and chemotherapy in malignant gliomas. *Curr Opin Oncol*. 2007;19(6):598–605.
86. Drevs J, Siegert P, Medinger M, et al. Phase I clinical study of AZD2171, an oral vascular endothelial growth factor signaling inhibitor, in patients with advanced solid tumors. *J Clin Oncol*. 2007;25(21):3045–3054.
87. Batchelor TT, Sorensen AG, di Tomaso E, et al. AZD2171, a pan-VEGF receptor tyrosine kinase inhibitor, normalizes tumor vasculature and alleviates edema in glioblastoma patients. *Cancer Cell*. 2007;11(1):83–95.

77 Inhibitors of Signal Transduction Pathways in Malignant Glioma Therapy

Andrew D. Norden and Patrick Y. Wen

INTRODUCTION

Most human cancers result from aberrations in cell signal transduction pathways. There is growing evidence that targeted molecular drugs that specifically inhibit these signaling pathways have potential therapeutic applications in the treatment of cancer [1,2]. The first generation of trials of targeted molecular therapies has been completed in malignant gliomas (MG). As with the majority of solid tumors, results from many of these trials have been disappointing, with response rates of 10% to 15% or less and no significant prolongation of survival [3]. A recent exception is combination therapy with the humanized monoclonal antibody against vascular endothelial growth factor (VEGF), bevacizumab (Avastin), and irinotecan. Results from a randomized phase-II trial demonstrated a promising 6-month progression-free survival (6M-PFS) of 51% [4]. This chapter summarizes the current status of targeted molecular therapies in adult MG.

TARGETED MOLECULAR AGENTS FOR MALIGNANT GLIOMAS

Ongoing research efforts are elucidating the molecular changes that occur in MG [5–12]. These tumors show a stepwise progression of genetic changes involving overexpression of proto-oncogenes and loss of tumor suppressor genes (Figure 77.1). Low-grade astrocytomas (WHO Grade II) tend to have inactivating mutations of *TP53*, loss of heterozygosity (LOH) of 17p, and overexpression of platelet-derived growth factor (PDGF) and PDGF receptors (PDGFR). Progression to anaplastic astrocytoma (WHO Grade III) is associated with inactivation of the p16-Rb pathway, LOH of 19q, and cyclin-dependent kinase 4 (CDK4) amplification, while further progression to a secondary glioblastoma (GBM; WHO Grade IV) is associated with loss of chromosome 10 and other changes. Primary GBMs, which arise *de novo*, often have amplification, mutation, or overexpression of the epidermal growth factor receptor (EGFR) and mouse double minute 2 (mdm2); mutations of *PTEN* (phosphatase and tensin homologue deleted on chromosome 10); and loss of a portion or all of chromosome 10 [12]. Molecular profiling studies using a variety of techniques [13–16] have assisted in identifying genes that are important in tumor progression [16–18]. In addition, morphologically indistinguishable MGs can be differentiated into molecular subtypes that may eventually be used for identifying potential therapeutic targets [19], stratifying patients in clinical studies [20], and determining prognosis [16,21].

Targeted molecular agents have shown promising therapeutic potential in several systemic cancers [22]. The prototypical targeted molecular agent is imatinib mesylate (Gleevec), a small molecule inhibitor of the Abl, c-Kit, and PDGFR tyrosine kinases. It has significant antitumor activity in chronic myelogenous leukemia (CML) by inhibiting Abl [23] and in gastrointestinal stromal tumors (GIST) by inhibiting c-Kit [24]. The success of imatinib (Gleevec) in CML and GIST demonstrates the potential of these agents in tumors with well-defined molecular targets. Although the complexity of the molecular abnormalities in MGs and the redundancy of the signaling pathways make it unlikely that single agents will achieve the same success as imatinib (Gleevec), there has been significant interest in this approach. Data from several of the first-generation trials evaluating targeted molecular agents in MGs have reached maturity. In general, these agents have been well tolerated, but only a minority of patients have benefited thus far [25].

Epidermal Growth Factor Receptor Inhibitors

The EGFR is an especially attractive therapeutic target in GBM [26]. EGFR is overexpressed in over 60% of GBMs, and the gene amplified in over 40% to 50% of primary GBMs[550–60]. Of tumors with EGFR amplification, 50% to 60% also have a constitutively active mutant with deletion of exons 2–7 (EGFRvIII). Other missense mutations in the EGFR extracellular domain may also be important [27]. Overactivity of the EGFR pathway results in cell proliferation, increased tumor invasiveness, motility, angiogenesis, and apoptosis inhibition. Several small-molecule inhibitors of the EGFR are being evaluated in MGs (Table 77.1). These agents are well tolerated, but responses tend to be limited and short lived. Two phase-II studies of gefitinib (Iressa) [28,29] produced no radiographic responses, while a third study produced responses in 13% of patients but no prolongation of 6M-PFS [30]. In preliminary results

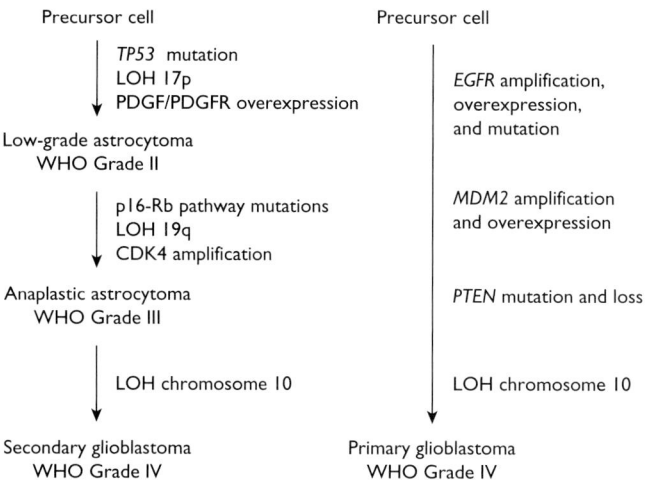

Figure 77.1 Stepwise molecular changes observed in malignant gliomas. Abbreviations: epidermal growth factor receptor (EGFR), loss of heterozygosity (LOH), mouse double minute 2 (MDM2), phoshastase and tensin homologue deleted on chromosome 10 (PTEN), platelet-derived growth factor (PDGF). (Adapted with permission from Tysnes BB, Mahesparan R. Biological mechanisms of glioma invasion and potential therapeutic targets. J Neurooncol. 2001;53:129–147.)

from phase-II studies of erlotinib (Tarceva), 0% to 25% of patients achieved partial responses [31–33]. When given as monotherapy, neither agent has resulted in prolongation of 6M-PFS. There appears to be little or no correlation between EGFR expression in the tumors and response. In addition, when given at conventional doses, EGFR inhibitors may not have a consistent impact on EGFR activity in vivo, as assessed by EGFR phosphorylation status [34]. Tumors with the EGFRvIII mutant and intact PTEN [35], and tumors with low phosphorylated protein kinase B/Akt levels [36,37] may be more likely to respond to EGFR inhibitors. These studies suggest that single agent EGFR inhibitors are most likely to be effective when phosphatidylinositol 3-kinase (PI3K)/Akt pathway signaling is attenuated. However, preliminary results from other studies have failed to confirm an increased response rate to EGFR inhibitors in tumors with the EGFRvIII mutant and intact PTEN [38]. The activating EGFR mutations found in non–small cell lung cancer (NSCLC) that increase the sensitivity of these tumors to EGFR inhibitors are not present in GBMs [34,39,40], although a small subset have missense mutations in the extracellular domain [4127]. Trials are underway to confirm that molecular markers such as EGFRvIII, PTEN, and Akt may be used to identify a subset of GBM patients with an increased likelihood of response to EGFR inhibitors.

Also ongoing are studies in which EGFR inhibitors are given in conjunction with temozolomide (TMZ) and radiation therapy (RT) for patients with newly diagnosed MG. Studies with other EGFR inhibitors, including lapatinib (GW-572016), a dual EGFR and ErbB2 inhibitor, more potent irreversible EGFR inihibitors such as BIBW 2992, the dual EGFR and VEGF receptor (VEGFR) inhibitors AEE788 and vandetanib (ZD6474; Zactima), and the humanized monoclonal antibody against EGFR, nimotuzumab (TheraCIM h-R3), are also in progress. CDX-110, an intradermally administered peptide vaccine against EGFRvIII that has a favorable toxicity profile and early evidence of efficacy [41], is undergoing evaluation as adjuvant therapy in combination with temozolomide in patients with newly diagnosed GBMs. Finally, combinations of EGFR inhibitors with other targeted therapies including inhibitors of the mammalian target of rapamycin (mTOR) and VEGFR are being evaluated. Combination therapy will be discussed in greater detail below.

Platelet-Derived Growth Factor Receptor Inhibitors

There is increasing evidence that overexpression and activation of PDGFRs may contribute to the transformed phenotype of MGs [42]. PDGF A and B and PDGFR α and β are frequently overexpressed in MGs, potentially resulting in autocrine or paracrine loops that drive cell proliferation. Imatinib (Gleevec), an inhibitor of PDGFR α and β, significantly inhibited the growth of GBM cell lines in vitro and in vivo in orthotopic glioma models [43]. These data suggest that inhibition of PDGF/PDGFR autocrine loops with imatinib (Gleevec) may be of therapeutic value in patients with MGs. The North American Brain Tumor Consortium (NABTC) and the European Organization for Research and Treatment of Cancer (EORTC) conducted phase-II trials of imatinib in patients with recurrent MGs. Minimal activity was observed; the response rates ranged from 0% to 6% and 6M-PFS from 3% to 16% [44–46]. Imatinib has also been evaluated in combination with hydroxyurea, a ribonucleotide reductase inhibitor. Initial phase-II studies in patients with recurrent MG showed modest radiographic response rates of 9% to 10% and 6M-PFS of 24% to 27% [47,48]. However, a recent large multicenter trial of imatinib and hydroxyurea in recurrent GBMs failed to show improvement in 6M-PFS [49]. Studies with more potent PDGFR inhibitors and agents with improved central nervous system (CNS) penetration such as MLN518, dasatinib, and pazopanib (GW786034) are underway (Table 77.1). In contrast to the disappointing results with imatinib (Gleevec) monotherapy or imatinib (Gleevec) with hydroxyurea, the combination of imatinib (Gleevec) with other targeted molecular agents may have greater potential and will be discussed later.

Farnesyltransferase Inhibitors

Signal transduction from activated tyrosine kinases such as EGFR and PDGFR is mediated in part by the Ras/Raf/mitogen-activated protein (MAP) kinase pathway (Figure 77.2). Activation of Ras requires localization to the intracellular surface of the cell membrane [50]. This subcellular localization is dependent on the addition of a hydrophobic farnesyl moiety to the Ras protein, catalyzed by the enzyme farnesyltransferase. In addition to blocking the mitogenic function of Ras, farnesyltransferase inhibitors (FTI) prevent the posttranslational modification and function of other farnesylated proteins that may be important in MG such as RhoB, centromere binding proteins, lamin B,

Table 77.1 *Selected Investigational Targeted Molecular Agents for Malignant Glioma Therapy*

Class/Agent	Alternative Name(s)	Mechanism(s)
Integrin Inhibitor		
Cilengitide	EMD 121974	αvβ3 and αvβ5 integrin inhibitor
c-Met (HGF/SF) Inhibitor		
AMG-102		HGF/SF antibody
XL184		c-Met, VEGFR inhibitor
EGFR Inhibitors		
AEE788		EGFR, VEGFR inhibitor
BIBW2992		EGFR inhibitor
Cetuximab	Erbitux	EGFR antibody
Erlotinib	OSI-774, Tarceva	EGFR inhibitor
Gefitinib	ZD1839, Iressa	EGFR inhibitor
Lapatinib	GW-572016	EGFR, HER2 inhibitor
Nimotuzumab	TheraCIM	EGFR antibody
Vandetanib	ZD6474, Zactima	EGFR, VEGFR inhibitor
Farnesyltransferase Inhibitors		
Lonafarnib	SCH 66336, Sarasar	FT inhibitor
Tipifarnib	R115777, Zarnestra	FT inhibitor
Histone Deacetylase Inhibitors		
Depsipeptide		HDAC inhibitor
Voronistat	SAHA	HDAC inhibitor
Valproic acid	Depakote	HDAC inhibitor
HSP-90 Inhibitor		
17AAG		HSP-90 inhibitor
AT13387		HSP-90 Inhibitor
mTOR Inhibitors		
Deforolimus	AP23573	mTOR inhibitor
Everolimus	RAD001	mTOR inhibitor
Sirolimus	Rapamycin, Rapamune	mTOR inhibitor
Temsirolimus	CCI-779, Torisel	mTOR inhibitor
PDGFR Inhibitors		
Dasatinib	Sprycel	PDGFR, Src, c-Kit, ephrin A inhibitor
Imatinib mesylate	Gleevec	
MLN518		PDGFR, c-Kit inhibitor
Pazopanib	GW786034	PDGFR, VEGFR, c-Kit inhibitor
Sunitinib	Sutent	PDGFR, VEGFR, c-Kit inhibitor
Vatalanib	PTK787	PDGFR, VEGFR inhibitor
PKC β2 Inhibitor		
Enzastaurin	LY31761	PKC β2 inhibitor
PI3K Inhibitors		
BEZ235		PI3K inhibitor, mTOR
PX-866		PI3K inhibitor
XL765		PI3K inhibitor, mTOR
Proteasome Inhibitor		
Bortezomib	Velcade	Proteasome inhibitor
Raf Inhibitor		
Sorafenib	BAY 43–9006, Nexavar	Raf, VEGFR, PDGFR inhibitor
VEGF Inhibitors		
Bevacizumab	Avastin	VEGF antibody
VEGF Trap	Aflibercept	VEGF soluble decoy receptor
VEGFR Inhibitors		
AEE788		VEGFR, EGFR inhibitor
Cediranib	AZD2171, Recentin	VEGFR inhibitor
Pazopanib	GW786034	VEGFR, PDGFR, c-Kit inhibitor
Sorafenib	BAY 43–9006, Nexavar	Raf, VEGFR, PDGFR inhibitor
Sunitinib	Sutent	PDGFR, VEGFR, c-Kit inhibitor
Vandetanib	ZD6474; Zactima	VEGFR, EGFR inhibitor
Vatalanib	PTK787	PDGFR, VEGFR inhibitor
XL184		VEGFR, c-Met inhibitor

Abbreviations: 17AAG, 17-allylamino-17-demethoxygeldanamycin; EGFR, epidermal growth factor receptor; FT, farnesyltransferase; HDAC, histone deacetylase; HGF/SF, hepatocyte growth factor/scatter factor; mTOR, mammalian target of rapamycin; PI3K, phosphatidylinositol 3-kinase; PDGFR, platelet-derived growth factor receptor; PKC β2, protein kinase C β2; SAHA, suberoylanilide hydroxamic acid; VEGFR, vascular endothelial growth factor receptor.

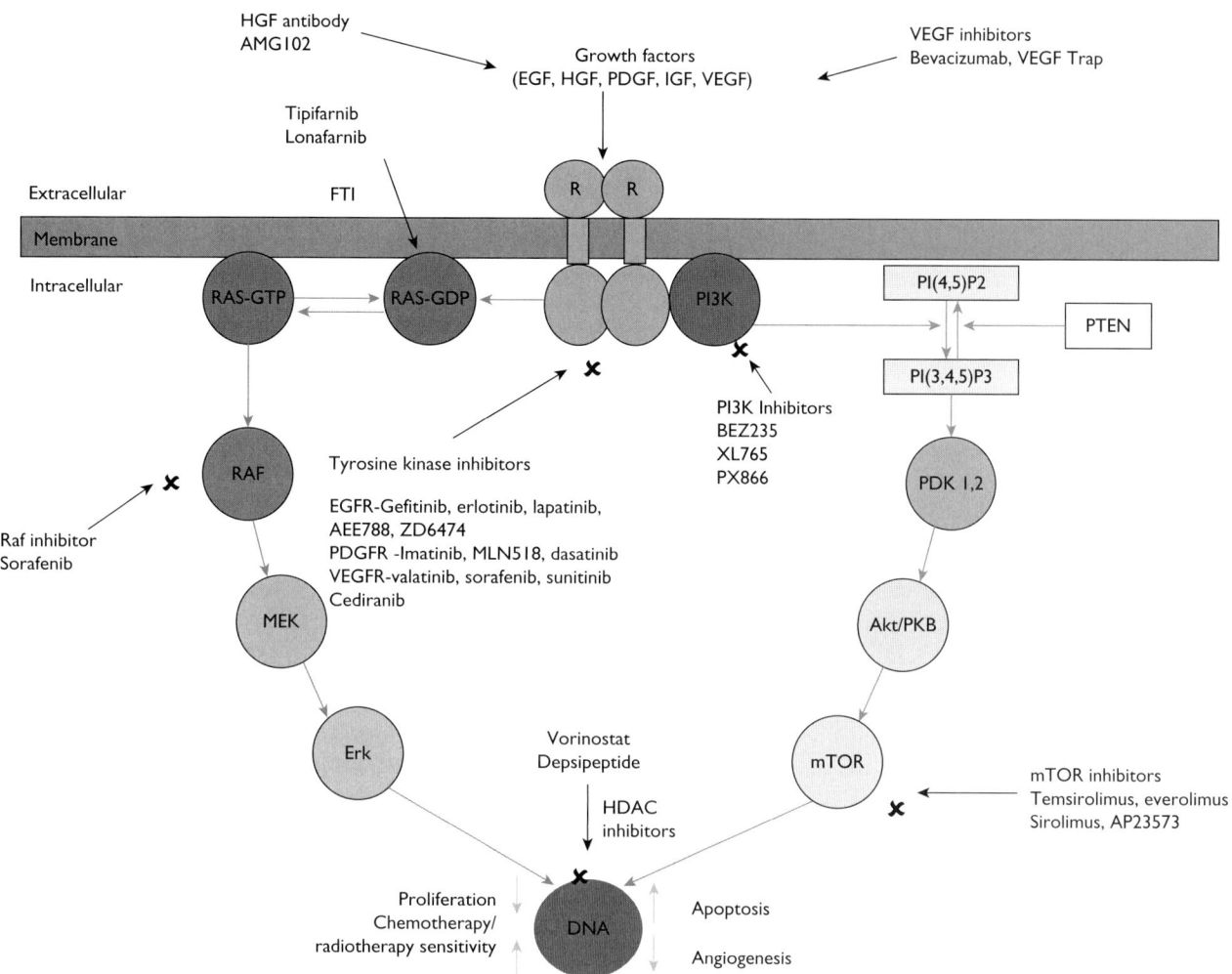

Figure 77.2 Major growth factor receptor signaling pathways in malignant gliomas with sites of action of targeted molecular drugs. Abbreviations: deoxyribonucleic acid (DNA), epidermal growth factor (EGF), extracellular signal-regulated kinase (ERK), farnesyltransferase inhibitor (FTI), guanosine diphosphate (GDP), guanosine triphosphate (GTP), histone deacetylase (HDAC), insulin-like growth factor (IGF), mitogen-activated protein kinase kinase (MEK), mammalian target of rapamycin (mTOR), platelet-derived growth factor (PDGF), phosphoinositide-dependent protein kinase-1 and -2 (PDK-1,2), phosphatidylinositol triphosphate (PI(3,4,5)P$_3$), phosphatidylinositol bisphosphate (PI(4,5)P$_2$), phosphoinositol 3-kinase (PI3K), protein kinase B (PKB), phoshatase and tensin homologue deleted on chromosome 10 (PTEN), vascular endothelial growth factor (VEGF). Adapted with permission from ref. [25].

and protein tyrosine phosphatase. Though Ras mutations are not observed in MG, Ras activation is a critical step in signaling from several receptor tyrosine kinases (RTK). FTI-induced Ras blockade inhibits proliferation of glioma cells in vitro [51] and in vivo [52]. Two FTIs are currently being evaluated in MGs, tipifarnib (R115777, Zarnestra) and lonafarnib (SCH 66336, Sarasar). The NABTC recently completed a phase-I/II study of tipifarnib in recurrent MGs [53,54]. Modest activity was observed with a response rate of 7.5% in GBM patients; the 6M-PFS was 16.7% in patients not receiving enzyme-inducing antiepileptic drugs (EIAED), compared to 6.5% in patients receiving EIAED. A recent phase-I/II study from M. D. Anderson Cancer Center enrolled patients with recurrent GBM who were TMZ-naïve. Patients were treated with a dose-dense TMZ regimen and tipifarnib (Zarnestra). Though the regimen resulted in high rates of myelosuppression, the 6M-PFS was a promising 31% [55]. A phase-I study from Duke University combined lonarfarnib (Sarasar) with TMZ for patients with stable or recurrent MG [56]. Toxicity was minimal, and there was at least one partial responder. A phase-I study combining tipifarnib (Zarnestra) with RT and TMZ was recently completed by the NABTC.

Mammalian Target of Rapamycin Inhibitors

Activation of RTKs such as EGFR and PDGFR results in increased signaling through the PI3K/Akt pathway, which leads to activation of a serine-threonine kinase known as mTOR (Figure 77.2) [57]. Downstream targets include p70S6 kinase and hypoxia inducible factor-1α (HIF-1α), which mTOR activates, and the eukaryotic initiation factor 4E-binding protein-1 (4E-BP1), which mTOR inhibits. These molecules have diverse effects including ribosome biogenesis, hypoxic adaptation, and protein translation, respectively [58]. In MGs, tyrosine kinase receptor overexpression and mutation or deletion of *PTEN* stimulate increased PI3K/Akt signaling (Figure 77.2) [5,8]. Since mTOR plays a central role in this important pathway, mTOR inhibitors have been evaluated as therapeutic agents against MG. Several mTOR inhibitors are undergoing evaluation including sirolimus (rapamycin, Rapamune), temsirolimus (CCI-779, Torisel), everolimus (RAD001), and deforolimus (AP23573).

Temsirolimus (Torisel) is an ester of the immunosuppressive agent sirolimus (Rapamune). Temsirolimus (Torisel) binding to the immunophilin FK-506 binding protein 12 (FKBP12) forms a complex that inhibits mTOR. The NABTC conducted a phase-II study of temsirolimus (Torisel) in recurrent GBM. Single agent activity was limited with a 5% partial response rate and only 2.5% 6M-PFS [59]. In another phase-II study of temsirolimus (Torisel) for patients with recurrent MGs conducted by the North Central Cancer Treatment Group (NCCTG), the drug was moderately well tolerated. Minor responses were seen in 36% of patients and 6M-PFS was 7.8% [60]. Patients with p70S6 kinase in baseline tumor samples were more likely to benefit from treatment. These results suggest that mTOR inhibitors have only modest single agent activity against MG.

Phosphatidylinositol-3 Kinase Inhibitors

As described above, the PI3K/Akt pathway is a critical signal transduction pathway that regulates functions such as cell metabolism, growth, proliferation, and survival [61]. Besides mTOR, which is activated by PI3K signaling, important downstream targets of the PI3K pathway that have a potential role in tumorigenesis include Bcl-2-antagonist of cell death (BAD), a proapoptotic protein, and forkhead (FOXO) family transcription factors, which facilitate apoptosis and limit cell cycle entry; both BAD and FOXO are inhibited by PI3K signaling [61]. *PTEN* is a tumor suppressor gene located at 10q23 whose protein product functions as a phosphatidylinositol trisphosphate (PIP_3) phosphatase. By opposing the action of PI3K which phosphorylate phosphatidylinositol bisphosphate (PIP_2) to make PIP_3, PTEN acts as a negative regulator of PI3K signaling. In addition to PTEN loss which is common in MGs, PI3K mutations are observed in a minority of cases [62–64]. Activation of PI3K signaling is often observed in MGs and appears to correlate with tumor histology and survival [65]. Inhibitors of PI3K itself and Akt are currently in preclinical development [66–69]. PI3K inhibitors entering clinical trials for recurrent MG soon include XL765 (Exelixis), BEZ-235 (Novartis), and PX-866 (Prolx).

Vascular Endothelial Growth Factor and Vascular Endothelial Growth Factor Receptor Inhibitors

Inhibitors of VEGF and VEGFR are among the most promising agents in MGs, with the potential not only to inhibit angiogenesis but also to decrease peritumoral edema. These agents are discussed in detail in the chapter on angiogenesis (see Chapter 76). Recent data indicate that bevacizumab (Avastin), a humanized monoclonal antibody against VEGF, is active against recurrent MG [4,70–73]. In a randomized, multicenter phase-II study, patients with recurrent GBM in first or second relapse received bevacizumab (Avastin) with or without irinotecan (Camptosar) [4]. Response rate was 21.2% and 6M-PFS was 35.6% for patients treated with bevacizumab (Avastin) alone, and response rate was 34.1% and 6M-PFS was 51.0% for patients treated with the combination of bevacizumab and irinotecan. Treatment was well tolerated with a CNS hemorrhage rate of 1.2% to 1.3%. Another anti-VEGF agent under investigation is aflibercept (VEGF-Trap), a highly potent soluble decoy receptor for VEGF [74]. Trials of VEGFR inhibitors such as cediranib (AZD2171, Recentin), sorafenib (Nexavar), vandetanib (ZD6474, Zactima), AEE788, pazopanib (GW786034), and sunitinib (Sutent) are ongoing. In a preliminary analysis of the first 16 patients treated with cediranib in a phase-II trial in patients with recurrent GBM, there was a partial response rate of 56% and median PFS of 111 days [75]. Preclinical data [76–78] and early clinical observations [79] suggest that antiangiogenic therapies may promote an infiltrative tumor growth pattern in a subset of patients [80]. Research in this area is ongoing, but if these observations are confirmed, strategies to inhibit tumor invasion will assume even greater importance.

Protein Kinase C Inhibitors

Protein kinase C-β (PKC-β) plays an important role in VEGF pathway signaling, making it an attractive therapeutic target [81]. Enzastaurin (LY317615) is a potent inhibitor of PKC-β2 that also suppresses PI3K/Akt pathway signaling [81]. Promising activity was observed in a phase-II trial of enzastaurin in patients with recurrent MG; 23% of 87 evaluable patients had radiographic responses, and 7% had stable disease [82]. The drug was generally well tolerated, although 7 patients, all of whom were receiving anticoagulant medications, developed intratumoral hemorrhages. Based on these encouraging results, a phase-III study randomizing patients with recurrent GBM to enzastaurin or lomustine (CCNU) was initiated. However, the study was closed at interim analysis because of lack of efficacy. Despite the lack of single-agent efficacy, enzastaurin may have synergistic effects with RT [83], and trials of the agent in conjunction with RT and TMZ for newly diagnosed GBM patients are in progress.

Cyclooxygenase Inhibitors

Cyclooxygenase-1 (COX-1) and -2 (COX-2) are involved in cancer cell survival, growth, and angiogenesis, suggesting that COX inhibitors may have antitumor activity. COX-2 expression is upregulated in gliomas [84], and high COX-2 expression correlates with increasing histological grade and poor survival [85,86]. Several trials combining COX-2 inhibitors, such as celecoxib, with chemotherapy, RT, or antiangiogenic agents have been conducted.

Preliminary results fail to show any clear benefit with the addition of COX-2 inhibitors [87]. The initial enthusiasm for this class of drugs has been tempered by evidence indicating that they are associated with cardiovascular complications [88].

Matrix Metalloproteinase and Integrin Inhibitors

Invasion of brain parenchyma by tumor cells impedes our ability to eradicate gliomas with standard treatments [89]. Tumor-secreted matrix metalloproteinases (MMPs) allow invading tumor cells to attach to extracellular matrix (ECM) and disrupt the ECM components and subsequently invade into the surrounding region [90]. Studies with MMP inhibitors alone have been disappointing, but combinations of these agents with chemotherapy have shown activity. Despite promising results from a phase-II trial of TMZ and the MMP inhibitor marimastat in patients with recurrent GBM [91], marimastat proved no better than placebo in a randomized, double-blind trial of 162 patients with GBM following surgery and RT [92].

Integrins $\alpha v\beta 3$ and $\alpha v\beta 5$ play critical roles in angiogenesis and invasion. They are present on endothelial cells and promote endothelial cell invasion and viability. Cilengitide (EMD 121974) is a cyclic pentapeptide that targets the RGD sequence on vitronectin and acts as a specific inhibitor of both $\alpha v\beta 3$ and $\alpha v\beta 5$ integrins, potentially inhibiting angiogenesis and invasion. Preclinical studies indicate that cilengitide has activity against αv integrin-expressing MGs [93]. The New Approaches to Brain Tumor Therapy (NABTT) consortium conducted a phase-I trial of cilengitide in recurrent MGs and reported that it was well tolerated [94]. Doses up to 2400 mg/m^2 twice weekly were administered without the maximal tolerated dose (MTD) being reached. There were 2 complete responses, 3 partial responses, and 4 stable disease in 51 evaluable patients. Several larger phase-II studies of this drug in patients with recurrent MG are in progress [95]. In one phase-II trial, 2000 mg/m^2 of cilengitide appeared to be slightly more effective than 500 mg/m^2 [95]. Promising results were observed in a phase-II study in which 52 patients with newly diagnosed GBM were treated with cilengitide in conjunction with RT and TMZ [96]. The 6M-PFS rate was 69%, and the 6-month overall survival rate was greater than 90%. This benefit was primarily in patients with hypermethylation of the promoter of the repair enzyme O^6-methylguanine-DNA-methyltransferase (MGMT). The EORTC is planning further studies with cilengitide in this subgroup of patients.

Histone Deacetylase Inhibitors

Cellular DNA exists as chromatin, a form in which DNA is tightly bound to histone proteins, creating structural elements called nucleosomes. Modulation of chromatin structure by histone acetylation is an important mechanism by which the cell regulates transcription. Histone acetylation typically promotes a relaxed chromatin structure that permits transcription. Enzymes known as histone acetyltransferases (HATs) add acetyl groups, and histone deacetylases (HDACs) remove them. HDACs therefore function as inhibitors of transcription, but their effects are more complex than this suggests because HDACs act upon many nonhistone targets that are involved in cell growth and apoptosis [97]. By a variety of mechanisms, HDAC inhibitors can induce growth arrest, terminal differentiation, and apoptosis of tumor cells [97]. Vorinostat (suberoylanilide hydroxamic acid [SAHA]) is a HDAC inhibitor that has potent antitumor activity in preclinical GBM models and adequately penetrates the blood-brain barrier (BBB) [98]. This class of drugs may also have synergistic activity with RT [99] and chemotherapeutic agents such as temozolomide [100]. Vorinostat and other HDAC inhibitors such as depsipeptide and valproic acid are being evaluated in recurrent MG. In a recent NCCTG phase-II trial in recurrent GBM, vorinostat resulted in a 15% 6M-PFS rate [101]. Treatment was well tolerated, and findings from a surgical cohort suggest that target pathways were inhibited in tumor specimens. The NABTC is currently completing a phase-I study of vorinostat with TMZ (NABTC 04–03) and a joint NABTC/NCCTG phase-I/II trial of vorinostat with RT and temozolomide in newly diagnosed GBM patients (NABTC 08–01) is planned.

Proteasome Inhibitors

Proteasomes are ubiquitous protease complexes involved in aspects of cell biology such as protein homeostasis, cell cycle progression, apoptosis, and inflammation, and they may mediate resistance to antineoplastic therapy. Inhibiting proteasome activity results in apoptosis and increased sensitivity to chemotherapy and RT [102].

Bortezomib (Velcade), a recently approved proteasome inhibitor for treatment of multiple myeloma, has cytotoxic effects on glioma cell lines *in vitro* [103]. Bortezomib also indirectly inhibits nuclear factor-kappa B (NFκB), an important mediator of resistance to chemotherapy [104]. This provides sound rationale for combining it with other cytotoxic agents. phase-I results using bortezomib as monotherapy in recurrent MG [105] and combined with RT and TMZ in newly diagnosed GBM [106] have been reported. Treatment is generally well tolerated, and some responses were observed. There is synergistic activity with the HDAC inhibitor vorinostat, and the NCCTG is conducting a trial evaluating this combination. The poor penetration of this drug across the BBB may limit its usefulness.

IMPROVING THE EFFICACY OF TARGETED MOLECULAR AGENTS

Though targeted molecular agents are safe and well tolerated in the majority of patients, most of these drugs have not had a marked impact on survival. For the second generation of clinical trials, a variety of strategies are being implemented to improve outcomes. These including optimizing target selection, developing more reliable animal models, using drugs or combinations of drugs that simultaneously inhibit multiple targets, and combining targeted molecular agents with cytotoxic chemotherapy, RT, or both.

Optimizing Target Selection

As a result of molecular profiling [15,107], advanced statistical techniques [108], network analysis [109], and correlative studies in clinical trials [35,110,111], novel targets that drive glioma growth and prevent tumor cell death are emerging at an unprecedented pace. For example, functional network analysis suggests that myc, integrin signaling pathways, and NFκB may be particularly important therapeutic targets [15,112,113]. Though effective myc inhibitors are not currently available, agents such as sulfasalazine and bortezomib inhibit NFκB directly or indirectly and may have therapeutic potential in gliomas, in combination with other agents.

Because of the marked heterogeneity and relatively low prevalence of individual molecular changes in MGs, determining which molecules to target is challenging and requires frequent reassessment at the preclinical and clinical levels [114]. Potential therapeutic targets in preclinical and early clinical development include insulin-like growth factor binding protein 2 [115], insulin-like growth factor 2 [116], hepatocyte growth factor/scatter factor and its receptor, c-Met [117,118], fibroblast growth factor receptor [75], transforming growth factor β receptors [119], Raf [120], Mek [121], heat shock protein 90 (Hsp90) [122], several ephrin ligands and receptors [123–125], integrin-linked kinase [126], Src kinase [127], focal adhesion kinase [128], anaplastic lymphoma kinase [129], hypoxia-inducible factor 1α [130], cyclins and CDKs [131], checkpoint kinase [132], antiapoptotic proteins (Bcl-2 and Bcl-X) [133], inhibitors of apoptosis proteins (IAPs) [134,135], C-X-C chemokine receptor 4 (CXCR4) [136,137], and cannabinoid receptors [138]. Ongoing research efforts will determine which of these targets lead to the next major phase of targeted molecular drug development.

Adding to the challenge of optimal target selection is recent data supporting the glioma stem cell as the cell of origin for MGs [139,140]. These cells appear also to have a crucial role in maintenance of gliomas. Some excellent review articles have discussed the glioma stem cell hypothesis in detail [141–143]. Initial studies suggest that glioma stem cells are highly resistant to chemotherapy [144] and RT [132]. Molecular analyses of the stem cell subpopulation of glioma cells may identify unique targets such as Notch and sonic hedgehog and suggest novel therapeutic approaches [143]. In addition to conventional antineoplastic treatments such as chemotherapy and RT, stem cells may be amenable to differentiation therapy, in which they are forced to terminally differentiate and give up their self-renewing phenotype [143]. Because stem cells produce VEGF [145] and reside within a perivascular niche [146], antiangiogenic therapy may also represent a powerful therapeutic tool.

Creating Reliable Animal Models

An important obstacle in the development of effective targeted agents against MGs has been the lack of predictive animal models. Older xenograft models produced by implanting human glioma cell lines into the brains of immunodeficient mice or rats do not accurately recapitulate the histologic and genetic features of human gliomas [147,148]. In recent years, a number of mouse glioma models have been generated that better reflect the major genetic abnormalities in human tumors [148,149]. These models may help characterize the important molecular mechanisms driving glioma growth and perhaps allow targeted agents to be evaluated more effectively.

One promising tumor model uses serially transplanted GBM xenograft lines established by subcutaneous injection of patient tumor tissue in the flanks of nude mice [150]. When tumor cells from short-term cultures are injected into the brains of nude mice, the resulting tumors retain the molecular changes of the original tumor such as EGFR and PDGFR amplification. Other current models involve genetically engineered mice [149]. For example, the nestin tv-a mouse expresses the retroviral receptor, tv-a, under the control of the nestin promoter. When the mouse is infected with avian retrovirus A encoding PDGF, it develops high-grade and low-grade gliomas with features characteristic of human tumors [149]. Xenograft models using human glioma stem cells maintained in EGF and fibroblast growth factor without exposure to culture medium also appear to retain the genotype of the original tumor [148]. Magnetic resonance imaging techniques accurately distinguish between histologic subtypes and may be utilized to evaluate response to therapy [151]. Models such as these may be more reliable than the traditional xenograft models.

Addressing Multiple Targets Simultaneously

Given the marked molecular heterogeneity of MGs, the limited success of monotherapy with targeted agents is not surprising. While there may be small subsets of patients whose tumors are driven by activating mutations of a single protein kinase that may be amenable to treatment with a single targeted molecular agent, for most tumors multiple target inhibition may be more effective. Recent data demonstrate that multiple RTK are coactivated in GBM cell lines and primary cultures; in addition, inhibition of multiple RTK targets is required to abrogate PI3K signaling, glioma cell survival, and anchorage-independent growth, even in tumor cells that have lost PTEN [152]. In this study, all the GBM lines had activation of EGFR and coactivation of a total of 3–11 RTKs. These findings provide a compelling rationale for combination therapy using single agents that inhibit multiple targets (so-called "dirty drugs") or multiple agents that inhibit complementary pathways.

Agents that Inhibit Multiple Targets

The original promise of targeted molecular agents was that they would serve as "magic bullets," inhibiting single biological targets and reducing the risk of systemic complications [153]. However, it became clear that many of the targeted molecular drugs were less specific than initially thought. For example, imatinib mesylate (Gleevec) inhibits not only Abl but also c-Kit and PDGFR. The ability of imatinib (Gleevec) to inhibit c-Kit explains its marked efficacy against GIST [154]. A number of multitargeted drugs are currently undergoing phase-I and phase-II evaluation in MGs including sunitinib maleate (Sutent), vatalanib (PTK 787/ZK222584), and pazopanib (GW786034), which inhibit VEGFR, PDGFR, and c-Kit; dasatinib (BMS-354825), which inhibits VEGFR, PDGFR, c-Kit, Src, and ephrin A2; MLN 518 which inhibits c-Kit, PDGFR, FLT3, and CSF-1R; sorafenib (Nexavar), which inhibits Raf, VEGFR, and PDGFR; vandetanib (Zactima) and AEE788, which inhibit EGFR and VEGFR; and XL184 which inhibits VEGFR and c-Met. The theoretical disadvantage of drugs that impact multiple targets is that they may produce more adverse effects.

Hsp90, mentioned briefly above in the section on "Optimizing Target Selection," is a molecular chaperone protein required for the conformational maturation and stability of a variety of client proteins involved in cell growth and survival [155]. Several of these proteins are important in MG cells, including EGFR, Akt, Raf, Met, p53, and CDK4. 17-allylamino-17-demethoxygeldanamycin (17AAG) is an Hsp90 inhibitor that appears to inhibit multiple relevant targets. Preclinical studies suggest that this class of drugs has activity in gliomas alone [156,157] or in combination with RT [158]. Many Hsp90 inhibitors are in early stages of development and may have therapeutic potential in GBMs.

The effects of multitargeted drugs on tumor cells are significantly more complex than the effects of drugs against single targets. There is growing interest in using network biology to model the effects of these drugs on the molecular constituents of tumor cells [159]. Such models may improve predictions of drug efficacy and adverse effects [153].

Combinations of Targeted Molecular Agents

Combining targeted agents directed against complementary molecular pathways is an alternative approach to monotherapy with multitargeted drugs (Table 77.2). Regimens may be designed to inhibit multiple receptors, parallel signaling pathways, or several nodes in the same signaling pathway. Since the most common molecular changes in gliomas are EGFR amplification or overexpression and PTEN loss, particular interest has focused on the combination of EGFR inhibitors and mTOR inhibitors [160,161]. Trials of erlotinib (Tarceva) and temsirolimus (Torisel; NABTC 04–02) [162], gefitinib (Iressa) and sirolimus [161], gefitinib and everolimus (RAD001) [163] or AEE788 are in progress.

Some trials are investigating combinations of monotargeted and multitargeted agents. NABTC 05–02 is a three-arm study examining the combination of sorafenib (Nexavar), an inhibitor of VEGFR, PDGFR, and Raf with either temsirolimus (Torisel), tipifarnib (R115777, Zarnestra), or erlotinib (Tarceva), using a novel sequential design to accelerate accrual. The NCCTG and NABTT are also evaluating some of these combinations. Researchers at Duke University are combining hydroxyurea, imatinib (Gleevec), which inhibits PDGFR and c-Kit, and the VEGFR/PDGFR inhibitor vatalanib. A multicenter phase-I/II trial of combination therapy with the EGFR and Her2 inhibitor lapatinib (Tykerb) and pazopanib, an inhibitor of VEGFR, PDGFR, and c-Kit recently completed accrual. There is emerging evidence that insulin-like growth factor-1 (IGF-1) inhibitors may synergize with other tyrosine kinase inhibitors and therefore represent a promising therapeutic approach [164–166]. There is also accumulating evidence that combinations of targeted molecular agents with drugs that promote apoptosis may result in enhanced antitumor effects [167].

Trials involving agents which inhibit parallel pathways are of great interest. For example, NABTC 05–02 includes one arm that will combine sorafenib (Nexavar), a multitargeted Raf inhibitor, with the mTOR inhibitor temsirolimus (Torisel). Raf is a critical component of the MAP kinase pathway, while mTOR occupies an essential position in PI3K signaling (Figure 77.2). NABTC 05–02 is also an example of a trial that targets several elements of the same signaling pathway, with two different combination regimens that attack the Ras/Raf/MAP kinase pathway, erlotinib (Tarceva) with sorafenib (Nexavar) and tipifarnib (Zarnestra) with sorafenib (Nexavar). In the future, potentially attractive combinations of drugs include those inhibiting Akt or PI3K with components of the MAP kinase pathway or Hsp90 [122]; inhibiting IGFR with other tyrosine kinases; and inhibiting tyrosine kinases with cell cycle components, NFκB, or IAPs.

As the molecular biology of gliomas and targeted therapies is elucidated, new ideas for combination therapies emerge. For example, recent data indicate that mTOR functions as part of two different complexes, mTOR complexes 1 and 2 (mTORC1, mTORC2). The downstream effects of mTOR described earlier appear to depend primarily on mTORC1 activation. Though a detailed mechanism remains to be determined, mTORC2 is required for maximal activation of Akt. The identification of multiple positive and negative regulatory interactions between Akt and mTOR indicates that the signaling axis is more complex than was originally thought [58]. There is a concern that specific inhibitors of mTORC1 such as sirolimus (Rapamune) and its analogs may result in the unintended activation of a feedback loop that promotes Akt activity. This suggests that combination therapy with mTOR and PI3K/Akt inhibitors may be a useful approach [168]. Similarly, the concern mentioned earlier that aggressive inhibition of angiogenesis using anti-VEGF antibodies and inhibitors of VEGR may promote infiltrative tumor growth leads to the hypothesis that antiangiogenic therapies and anti-invasion therapies may act synergistically against MGs [79].

While combinations of targeted agents are a promising approach, the initial enthusiasm has been tempered by the realization that some of these combinations are poorly tolerated. For example, combinations of EGFR inhibitors with mTOR inhibitors have been associated with a high incidence of dermatologic toxicity and mucositis [162]. An important challenge in developing more effective targeted therapies is to define combinations with acceptable toxicity profiles. It will also be important to improve our ability to manage dose-limiting toxicities such as rash and mucositis in the same way that anemia and neutropenia are now routinely managed in patients on conventional chemotherapies.

Table 77.2 Selected Ongoing Trials of Combinations of Targeted Molecular Agents for Recurrent Malignant Gliomas

Agents	Targets	Site / Consortium
AEE788 and everolimus (RAD001)	EGFR and mTOR	UCLA
Bevacizumab (Avastin) and enzastaurin (LY31761)	VEGF and PKC β2	NCI
Erlotinib (Tarceva) and sirolimus (Rapamune)	EGFR and mTOR	UCLA
Erlotinib (Tarceva) and sorafenib (Nexavar)	EGFR, PDGFR, Raf, VEGFR	NABTC, NABTT
Erlotinib (Tarceva) and temsirolimus (Torisel)	EGFR and mTOR	NABTC
Gefitinib (Iressa) and everolimus (RAD001)	EGFR and mTOR	MSKCC
Hydroxyurea, imatinib (Gleevec), and vatalanib (PTK787)	PDGFR, c-Kit, VEGFR	Duke University
Lapatinib (Tykerb) and pazopanib	EGFR, Her2, c-Kit, PDGFR, VEGFR	Multiple sites
Sorafenib (Nexavar) and temsirolimus (Torisel)	PDGFR, Raf, VEGFR, mTOR	NABTC, NCCTG
Sorafenib (Nexavar) and tipifarnib (Zarnestra)	PDGFR, Raf, VEGFR, FT	NABTC
Tamoxifen and bortezomib (Velcade)	PKC, proteasome	NCI
Vandetanib (ZD6474; Zactima) and sirolimus	VEGFR, EGFR, mTOR	DF/HCC
Vandetanib (ZD6474; Zactima), imatinib, and hydroxyurea	VEGFR, EGFR, PDGFR	Duke
Vorinostat and bortezomib	HDAC and proteosome	NCCTG

Abbreviations: DF/HCC, Dana-Farber/Harvard Cancer Center; EGFR, epidermal growth factor receptor; FT, farnesyltransferase; mTOR, mammalian target of rapamycin; MSKCC, Memorial Sloan-Kettering Cancer Center; NCI, National Cancer Institute; NABTC, North American Brain Tumor Consortium; NABTT, New Approaches to Brain Tumor Therapy; NCCTG, North Central Cancer Treatment Group; PDGFR, platelet-derived growth factor receptor; PKC β2, protein kinase C-β2; UCLA, University of California-Los Angeles; VEGFR, vascular endothelial growth factor receptor.

With the increasing availability of targeted agents, the number of potential combinations has risen exponentially such that only a small fraction of these combinations can be evaluated in clinical trials. Preclinical studies, molecular profiling, and network analysis will assume increasingly important roles in selecting the most promising combinations to take to clinical trials. Identifying the most effective and tolerable combinations of targeted agents will be an important focus of research in MGs over the next several years.

Combining Targeted Molecular Agents With RT

In an effort to improve the efficacy of targeted molecular agents, there is extensive interest in combining these novel therapies with standard treatments such as RT and chemotherapy (Table 77.3) [158,169–171]. Enhancing tumor radiation sensitivity has been a long-standing goal in cancer therapy, but early experience with radiosensitizing agents for MG was disappointing. Preclinical studies suggest that radiation sensitivity can be regulated by growth factors (EGFR, IGFR), signal transduction pathways (Ras/Raf/MAP kinase, PI3K/Akt), cell cycle and DNA repair enzymes (PARP, ATM, Chk1, Rad 51), and apoptosis-related proteins (Fas, Bcl-2) [158]. Many of these can be inhibited by targeted molecular agents.

There is increasing evidence that EGFR signaling contributes to radiation resistance in MGs and that EGFR inhibitors may increase the sensitivity of tumor cells to RT [172–174]. Based on these data, a number of clinical trials of EGFR inhibitors in combination with RT or RT and TMZ have been conducted. In RTOG 0211, gefitinib was combined with RT alone in newly diagnosed glioblastomas and did not improve survival [175]. In a recent phase-II study of erlotinib combined with RT and temozolomide conducted at the University of California, San Francisco (UCSF), the median survival of 84 weeks was superior to historic controls treated with other agents [176]. There is also evidence that inhibition of other molecular targets enhances the effects of RT. Imatinib (Gleevec), a PDGFR inhibitor, increased radiosensitivity in mouse GBM models [177]. The FTI, tipifarnib (Zarnestra), may sensitize gliomas cells to RT by a mechanism that involves HDJ-2, a co-chaperone of heat shock protein 70 [178,179]. mTOR inhibitors may promote radiosensitization by enhancing radiation damage to tumor vasculature [180]. Molecular agents directed against other targets including Akt [67], PI3K [67], Hsp90 [181], COX-2 [182], PKC [183], and HDAC [99,184,185] may also increase radiation sensitivity of MG cells.

There is evidence that angiogenesis inhibitors may enhance radiation sensitivity as well [186], perhaps as a result of direct effects on endothelial cells [187], inhibition of VEGF produced by tumor cells, or due to normalization of tumor vasculature with improved oxygenation and reduced interstitial pressure [188]. Particular interest has focused on the use of VEGFR inhibitors. Winkler et al. demonstrated that VEGFR2 blockade creates a "normalization window" during which gliomas are more sensitive to RT [189]. Vandetanib (Zactima), an inhibitor of VEGFR and EGFR which enhances the antitumor effects of RT in GBM *in vitro* and *in vivo*, is a particularly attractive therapeutic agent [190,191]. A multicenter trial of this drug in newly diagnosed GBM in combination with RT and TMZ is in progress. Some of the other angiogenesis inhibitors that are being evaluated with RT include cediranib (AZD2171, Recentin), vatalanib (PTK787), sorafenib (Nexavar), enzastaurin (LY317615), bevacizumab (Avastin), and aflibercept (VEGF-Trap).

Combining Targeted Molecular Agents With Chemotherapy

The combination of targeted agents with chemotherapy is another area of significant interest (Table 77.3). In other cancers, the experience with this approach has

Table 77.3 Selected Ongoing Trials of Targeted Molecular Agents With Radiation or Chemotherapy

Agents	Targets	Phase	Site / Consortium
Trials for Newly Diagnosed Glioblastoma			
Aflibercept (VEGF-Trap), TMZ, and RT	VEGF	I	NABTC
Bevacizumab (Avastin), TMZ, and RT	VEGF	II	UCLA
Bevacizumab (Avastin), RT, TMZ, and Irinotecan	VEGF	II	Duke
Bevacizumab (Avastin), erlotinib (Tarceva), and TMZ	VEGF, EGFR	II	UCSF
Cilengitide (EMD 121974), TMZ, and RT	Integrins	II	NABTT, EORTC
Enzastaurin (LY31761), TMZ, and RT	PKC β2	I/II	UCSF
Erlotinib (Tarceva), TMZ, and RT	EGFR	II	UCSF, Cleveland Clinic
Everolimus (RAD001), TMZ, and RT	mTOR	I/II	NCCTG
Gefitinib and RT	EGFR	I/II	RTOG
Temsirolimus (Torisel), TMZ, and RT	mTOR	I	NCCTG
Tipifarnib (Zarnestra), TMZ, and RT	FT	I	NABTC
Valproic acid (Depakote), TMZ, and RT	HDAC	II	NCI
Vandetanib (ZD6474; Zactima), TMZ, and RT	EGFR, VEGFR	I/II	MGH and DFBWCC
Vatalanib (PTK787), TMZ, and RT	VEGFR, PDGFR	I	MGH and DFBWCC, EORTC
Vorinostat (SAHA) and TMZ	HDAC	I	NABTC
Vorinostat (SAHA), TMZ, and RT	HDAC	I/II	NABTC and NCCTG
Trials for Recurrent Malignant Glioma			
Bevacizumab (Avastin) and CPT-11 following bevacizumab (Avastin) failure	VEGF	II	NCI
Bevacizumab (Avastin) and metronomic TMZ	VEGF	II	Duke University
Bevacizumab (Avastin), erlotinib (Tarceva), and TMZ	VEGF, EGFR	II	UCSF
Bortezomib and TMZ	Proteasome	I	CHCCC
Cediranib (AZD2171, Recentin) and lomustine	VEGFR	I	MGH, DFBWCC
Enzastaurin (LY31761) and carboplatin	PKC β2	I	NCI
Enzastaurin (LY31761) and TMZ	PKC β2	I	EORTC
Imatinib (Gleevec), vatalanib (PTK787), and hydroxyurea	PDGFR, c-Kit, VEGFR	I	Duke University
Imatinib (Gleevec) and TMZ	PDGFR	I	Duke University
Lonafarnib (Sarasar) and TMZ	FT	I	EORTC, MDACC
Tipifarnib (Zarnestra) and TMZ	FT	I/II	MDACC
Vorinostat (SAHA), isotretinoin, and carboplatin	HDAC	I/II	MDACC

Abbreviations: CHCCC, City of Hope Comprehensive Cancer Center; DFBWCC, Dana-Farber/Brigham and Women's Cancer Center; EORTC, European Organization for Research and Treatment of Cancer; EGFR, epidermal growth factor receptor; FT, farnesyltransferase; HDAC, histone deacetylase; mTOR, mammalian target of rapamycin; MGH, Massachusetts General Hospital; MSKCC, Memorial Sloan-Kettering Cancer Center; NCI, National Cancer Institute; NABTC, North American Brain Tumor Consortium; NABTT, New Approaches to Brain Tumor Therapy consortium; NCCTG, North Central Cancer Treatment Group; PDGFR, platelet-derived growth factor receptor; PKC β2, protein kinase C-β2; RT, radiation therapy; RTOG, Radiation Therapy Oncology Group; SAHA, suberoylanilide hydroxamic acid; TMZ, temozolomide; UCLA, Univeristy of California-Los Angeles; UCSF, University of California-San Francisco; VEGFR, vascular endothelial growth factor receptor.

been inconsistent. Combinations such as bevacizumab (Avastin) with irinotecan (Camptosar) in colon cancer [192] or with paclitaxel and carboplatin in non–small cell lung cancer (NSCLC) [193] have increased survival, but trials of gefitinib (Iressa) and erlotinib (Tarceva) with chemotherapy in NSCLC have been largely unsuccessful [194]. This raises the possibility that drugs such as EGFR inhibitors which induce cell cycle arrest may reduce the efficacy of certain cytotoxic agents. Many trials of targeted molecular agents combined with TMZ in MG are currently underway. Preliminary results suggest that the combinations of FTIs with TMZ [55,56] may be associated with increased antitumor activity. Early studies of imatinib with hydroxyurea [48] showed promising activity, but a recent multicenter phase-III trial comparing imatinib and hydroxyurea versus hydroxyurea alone failed to confirm a benefit [49].

Temozolomide, the most widely used chemotherapeutic agent for MG, is an alkylating agent that methylates the O^6 and N^7 positions of guanine, resulting in DNA adducts that are subsequently processed by the mismatch repair system. The O^6-methylguanine adducts are repaired by the enzyme O^6-methylguanine-DNA-methyltransferase (MGMT). Thus, the level of MGMT activity confers a variable degree of TMZ resistance. The MGMT inactivator O^6-benzylguanine (O^6BG) is currently under clinical investigation as a potential chemotherapy-sensitizing agent [195], although there appears to be significant myelotoxicity. Another MGMT inhibitor, O^6-(4-bromothenyl)-guanine (PaTrin-2), not only has potential advantages over O^6BG in terms of higher activity against wild-type MGMT and oral formulation but also causes myelotoxicity [196,197]. Poly(ADP-ribose) polymerase (PARP) is involved in repair of N^7 methylation. PARP inhibitors such as BSI-201, GPI 15427, INO1001, AG14361, ABT-888, and AGO14699 may have a role in combination therapy with TMZ and radiotherapy [198,199].

Other Approaches

A major factor reducing the effectiveness of targeted agents in MG is the limited penetration of these agents across the BBB and blood-tumor barrier (BTB), resulting in insufficient concentrations within the tumor to inhibit the molecular targets of interest. This may be particularly problematic for monoclonal antibodies and antisense oligonucleotides, which are excluded because of their high molecular weight and hydrophilic nature. Drug efflux transporters such as P-glycoprotein, breast cancer-resistance protein (BCRP, also known as ABCG2), and other ATP-binding cassette transporters also appear to play an important role in limiting drug penetration [200–203]. Optimizing BBB penetration of targeted molecular agents is an area of active investigation. Local methods of drug delivery are being evaluated. Examples include biodegradable polymer wafer placement into the surgical cavity [204], convention-enhanced delivery, in which a drug is slowly infused under positive pressure through catheters placed stereotactically into the brain parenchyma surrounding the surgical cavity [205], nanoparticles, and stem cells.

An important obstacle to the development of targeted molecular therapies for MG is the difficulty of obtaining tumor tissue in brain tumor patients as compared to patients with other cancers. Nonetheless an increasing number of trials are incorporating molecular analyses of tumor specimens [20,35]. Tissue studies allow researchers to assay drug penetration, degree of target inhibition *in vivo*, and resistance mechanisms. This information will facilitate the rational design of future trials and hopefully result in more rapid development of effective therapies. Emerging neuroimaging technologies may eventually permit some of these analyses to be performed noninvasively, which would allow physicians to modify treatment regimens at the earliest sign of failure [206].

An important focus of research is to identify the subgroups of MG patients who respond to specific drugs in the same way that NSCLC patients with activating EGFR mutations have been shown to respond to EGFR inhibitors [207]. Studies that include molecular profiling, proteomics, and network analysis are expected to be fruitful. To date, the strongest evidence suggests that GBMs with the EGFRvIII mutant and intact PTEN are more likely to respond to EGFR inhibitors [35], while the presence of phosphorylated Akt is a negative predictor of response [37]. As described earlier, these findings remain to be confirmed in larger, prospective trials.

CONCLUSIONS

The first generation of studies of targeted molecular therapies in MGs focused on inhibitors of EGFR, PDGFR, VEGF/VEGFR, farnesyltransferase, and mTOR. Although these agents were generally well tolerated, low response rates are reported, and a definitive survival benefit remains to be demonstrated. Recent experience with bevacizumab (Avastin) and irinotecan (Camptosar) suggests that this combination may be the most active regimen in recurrent MG, with a 6M-PFS rate of 51% [4]. Thus far, attempts to correlate genotype to response have been largely unsuccessful. MGs that express EGFRvIII and retain PTEN may be more likely to respond to EGFR inhibitors [35], while the presence of phosphorylated Akt predicts against response [37]. An emerging understanding of the molecular pathophysiology of MG will assist in effective target selection. Combination therapies are more likely to succeed than monotherapies [152], and rigorous preclinical testing is needed to identify combinations of drugs and targets that are most likely to be effective and least toxic. Clinical trials that incorporate tumor tissue and molecular endpoints may also be helpful in understanding why certain drugs succeed or fail in individual tumors [20].

Although the initial results have been less dramatic than expected, targeted molecular agents hold tremendous promise. The recent progress in understanding the biology of microRNAs suggests that RNAi may also have therapeutic potential in inhibiting signal transduction pathways. There is reason for optimism that the ultimate goal of selecting effective targeted molecular therapies based on a patient's tumor genotype will eventually be realized.

ADDENDUM

Recent data from the Tumor Cancer Genome Atlas (TCGA) project showed that mutations in the *IDH1* gene occur in approximately 12% of GBM and a substantially higher proportion of secondary GBM [208]. A subsequent study found that *IDH1* or *IDH2* mutations occur in the majority of grade II and III gliomas and secondary GBM. Tumors with such mutations lack isocitrate dehydrogenase enzyme activity and are associated with better outcomes than those with wild-type *IDH* genes [209]. These mutations identify an important prognostic subclass of gliomas; whether they can be used for predictive purposes in tailoring therapy remains to be determined.

ACKNOWLEDGMENT

We gratefully acknowledge the support of the Sam Longo Brain Tumor Research Fund.

REFERENCES

1. Adjei AA, Hidalgo M. Intracellular signal transduction pathway proteins as targets for cancer therapy. *J Clin Oncol*. 2005;23(23):5386–5403.
2. Sebolt-Leopold JS, English JM. Mechanisms of drug inhibition of signalling molecules. *Nature*. 2006;441(7092):457–462.
3. Kesari S, Ramakrishna N, Sauvageot C, Stiles CD, Wen PY. Targeted molecular therapy of malignant gliomas. *Curr Oncol Rep*. 2006;8(1):58–70.
4. Cloughesy T, Prados M, Wen P, et al. A Phase II, Randomized, noncomparative clinical trial of bevacizumab alone or in combination with CPT-11 prolongs 6-month PFS in recurrent, treatment-refractory glioblastoma. Society for Neuro-Oncology 12th Annual Meeting, 2007.
5. Furnari FB, Fenton T, Bachoo RM, et al. Malignant astrocytic glioma: genetics, biology, and paths to treatment. *Genes Dev*. 2007;21(21):2683–2710.
6. Maher EA, Brennan C, Wen PY, et al. Marked genomic differences characterize primary and secondary glioblastoma subtypes and identify two distinct molecular and clinical secondary glioblastoma entities. *Cancer Res*. 2006;66(23):11502–11513.
7. Newton HB. Molecular neuro-oncology and development of targeted therapeutic strategies for brain tumors. Part 1: Growth factor and Ras signaling pathways. *Expert Rev Anticancer Ther*. 2003;3(5):595–614.
8. Newton HB. Molecular neuro-oncology and development of targeted therapeutic strategies for brain tumors. Part 2: PI3K/Akt/PTEN, mTOR, SHH/PTCH and angiogenesis. *Expert Rev Anticancer Ther*. 2004;4(1):105–128.

9. Newton HB. Molecular neuro-oncology and the development of targeted therapeutic strategies for brain tumors. Part 4: p53 signaling pathway. *Expert Rev Anticancer Ther*. 2005;5(1):177–191.
10. Newton HB. Molecular neuro-oncology and the development of targeted therapeutic strategies for brain tumors. Part 5: apoptosis and cell cycle. *Expert Rev Anticancer Ther*. 2005;5(2):355–378.
11. Louis DN, Ohgaki H, Wiestler OD, et al. The 2007 WHO classification of tumours of the central nervous system. *Acta Neuropathol*. 2007;114(2):97–109.
12. Ohgaki H, Kleihues P. Genetic pathways to primary and secondary glioblastoma. *Am J Pathol*. 2007;170(5):1445–1453.
13. Chakravarti A, Tyndall E, Palanichamy K, Mehta M, Aldape K, Loeffler J. Impact of molecular profiling on clinical trial design for glioblastoma. *Curr Oncol Rep*. 2007;9(1):71–79.
14. Kunitz A, Wolter M, van den Boom J, et al. DNA hypermethylation and aberrant expression of the EMP3 gene at 19q13.3 in Human Gliomas. *Brain Pathol*. 2007;17(4):363–370.
15. Tso CL, Freije WA, Day A, et al. Distinct transcription profiles of primary and secondary glioblastoma subgroups. *Cancer Res*. 2006;66(1):159–167.
16. Phillips HS, Kharbanda S, Chen R, et al. Molecular subclasses of high-grade glioma predict prognosis, delineate a pattern of disease progression, and resemble stages in neurogenesis. *Cancer Cell*. 2006;9(3):157–173.
17. van den Boom J, Wolter M, Blaschke B, Knobbe CB, Reifenberger G. Identification of novel genes associated with astrocytoma progression using suppression subtractive hybridization and real-time reverse transcription-polymerase chain reaction. *Int J Cancer*. 2006;119(10):2330–2338.
18. van den Boom J, Wolter M, Kuick R, et al. Characterization of gene expression profiles associated with glioma progression using oligonucleotide-based microarray analysis and real-time reverse transcription-polymerase chain reaction. *Am J Pathol*. 2003;163(3):1033–1043.
19. Shai R, Shi T, Kremen TJ, et al. Gene expression profiling identifies molecular subtypes of gliomas. *Oncogene*. 2003;22(31):4918–4923.
20. Lassman AB, Holland EC. Incorporating molecular tools into clinical trials and treatment for gliomas? *Curr Opin Neurol*. 2007;20(6):708–711.
21. Pelloski CE, Ballman KV, Furth AF, et al. Epidermal growth factor receptor variant III status defines clinically distinct subtypes of glioblastoma. *J Clin Oncol*. 2007;25(16):2288–2294.
22. Rosa DD, Ismael G, Lago LD, Awada A. Molecular-targeted therapies: lessons from years of clinical development. *Cancer Treat Rev*. 2008;34(1):61–80.
23. Druker BJ, Talpaz M, Resta DJ, et al. Efficacy and safety of a specific inhibitor of the BCR-ABL tyrosine kinase in chronic myeloid leukemia. *N Engl J Med*. 2001;344(14):1031–1037.
24. Demetri GD, van Oosterom AT, Garrett CR, et al. Efficacy and safety of sunitinib in patients with advanced gastrointestinal stromal tumour after failure of imatinib: a randomised controlled trial. *Lancet*. 2006;368(9544):1329–1338.
25. Wen PY, Kesari S, Drappatz J. Malignant gliomas: strategies to increase the effectiveness of targeted molecular treatment. *Expert Rev Anticancer Ther*. 2006;6(5):733–754.
26. Nakamura JL. The epidermal growth factor receptor in malignant gliomas: pathogenesis and therapeutic implications. *Expert Opin Ther Targets*. 2007;11(4):463–472.
27. Lee JC, Vivanco I, Beroukhim R, et al. Epidermal growth factor receptor activation in glioblastoma through novel missense mutations in the extracellular domain. *PLoS Med*. 2006;3(12):e485.
28. Franceschi E, Cavallo G, Lonardi S, et al. Gefitinib in patients with progressive high-grade gliomas: a multicentre phase II study by Gruppo Italiano Cooperativo di Neuro-Oncologia (GICNO). *Br J Cancer*. 2007;96(7):1047–1051.
29. Rich JN, Reardon DA, Peery T, et al. Phase II trial of gefitinib in recurrent glioblastoma. *J Clin Oncol*. 2004;22(1):133–142.
30. Lieberman F, Cloughesy T, Fine H, et al. NABTC phase I/II trial of ZD-1839 for recurrent malignant gliomas and unresectable meningiomas. In: Proceedings of the American Society of Clinical Oncology; 2004.Clin Oncol.2004:Abstract 1510.
31. Raizer JJ. HER1/EGFR tyrosine kinase inhibitors for the treatment of glioblastoma multiforme. *J Neurooncol*. 2005;74(1):77–86.
32. Vogelbaum M, Peereboom D, Stevens G, Barnett G, Brewer C. Phase II trial of the EGFR tyrosine kinase inhibitor erlotinib for single agent therapy of recurrent Glioblastoma Multiforme: Interim results. In: Proceedings of the American Society of Clinical Oncology; 2004: Journal of Clinical Oncology; 2004. Abstract 1558.
33. Raizer J, Abrey L, Wen P, et al. A phase II trial of erlotinib (OSI-774) in patients (pts) with recurrent malignant gliomas (MG) not on EIAEDs. In: Proceedings of the American Society of Clinical Oncology; 2004. *J Clin Oncol*. 2004:Abstract 1502.
34. Lassman AB, Rossi MR, Raizer JJ, et al. Molecular study of malignant gliomas treated with epidermal growth factor receptor inhibitors: tissue analysis from North American Brain Tumor Consortium Trials 01–03 and 00–01. *Clin Cancer Res*. 2005;11(21):7841–7850.
35. Mellinghoff IK, Wang MY, Vivanco I, et al. Molecular determinants of the response of glioblastomas to EGFR kinase inhibitors. *N Engl J Med*. 2005;353(19):2012–2024.
36. Haas-Kogan DA, Prados MD, Lamborn KR, Tihan T, Berger MS, Stokoe D. Biomarkers to predict response to epidermal growth factor receptor inhibitors. *Cell Cycle*. 2005;4(10):1369–1372.
37. Haas-Kogan DA, Prados MD, Tihan T, et al. Epidermal growth factor receptor, protein kinase B/Akt, and glioma response to erlotinib. *J Natl Cancer Inst*. 2005;97(12):880–887.
38. Van den Bent M, Brandes A, Rampling R, et al. Randomized phase II trial of erlotinib versus temozolomide or BCNU in recurrrent glioblastoma multiforme. *Neuro-Oncol*. 2007;9:522 (MA-27).
39. Marie Y, Carpentier AF, Omuro AM, et al. EGFR tyrosine kinase domain mutations in human gliomas. *Neurology*. 2005;64(8):1444–1445.
40. Barber TD, Vogelstein B, Kinzler KW, Velculescu VE. Somatic mutations of EGFR in colorectal cancers and glioblastomas. *N Engl J Med*. 2004;351(27):2883.
41. Heimberger AB, Hussain SF, Aldape K, et al. Tumor-specific peptide vaccination in newly-diagnosed patients with GBM. *J Clin Oncol*. 2006;24:2529.
42. Guha A, Dashner K, Black PM, Wagner JA, Stiles CD. Expression of PDGF and PDGF receptors in human astrocytoma operation specimens supports the existence of an autocrine loop. *Int J Cancer*. 1995;60(2):168–173.
43. Kilic T, Alberta JA, Zdunek PR, et al. Intracranial inhibition of platelet-derived growth factor-mediated glioblastoma cell growth by an orally active kinase inhibitor of the 2-phenylaminopyrimidine class. *Cancer Res*. 2000;60(18):5143–5150.
44. Raymond E, Brandes A, Van Oosterom A, et al. Multicentre phase II study of imatinib mesylate in patients with recurrent glioblastoma: An EORTC: NDDG/BTG Intergroup Study. *J Clin Oncol*. 2004;22:1501.
45. van den Bent M, Brandes A, Frenay M, et al. Multicentre phase II study of Imatinib Mesylate (Gleevec®) in patients with recurrent anaplastic oligodendroglioma (AOD)/mixed oligoastrocytoma (MOA) and anaplastic astrocytoma (AA)/low grade astrocytoma (LGA): An EORTC New Drug Development Group (NDDG) and Brain Tumor Group (BTG) study. *J Clin Oncol*. 2005;23:1517.
46. Wen PY, Yung WK, Lamborn KR, et al. Phase I/II study of imatinib mesylate for recurrent malignant gliomas: North American Brain Tumor Consortium Study 99-08. *Clin Cancer Res*. 2006;12(16):4899–4907.
47. Desjardins A, Quinn JA, Vredenburgh JJ, et al. Phase II study of imatinib mesylate and hydroxyurea for recurrent grade III malignant gliomas. *J Neurooncol*. 2007;83(1):53–60.
48. Reardon DA, Egorin MJ, Quinn JA, et al. Phase II study of imatinib mesylate plus hydroxyurea in adults with recurrent glioblastoma multiforme. *J Clin Oncol*. 2005;23(36):9359–9368.
49. Dresemann G, Rosenthal M, Hoffken K, et al. Imatinib plus hydroxyurea versus hydroxyurea monotherapy in progressive glioblastoma-an international open label randomized phase III study (AMBROSIA). *Neuro-Oncology*. 2007;9:519.
50. Adjei AA. Farnesyltransferase inhibitors. *Cancer Chemother Biol Response Modif*. 2005;22:123–133.
51. Guha A, Feldkamp MM, Lau N, Boss G, Pawson A. Proliferation of human malignant astrocytomas is dependent on Ras activation. *Oncogene*. 1997;15(23):2755–2765.
52. Kurimoto M, Hirashima Y, Hamada H, et al. *In vitro* and *in vivo* growth inhibition of human malignant astrocytoma cells by the farnesyltransferase inhibitor B1620. *J Neurooncol*. 2003;61(2):103–112.

53. Cloughesy TF, Kuhn J, Robins HI, et al. Phase I trial of tipifarnib in patients with recurrent malignant glioma taking enzyme-inducing antiepileptic drugs: a North American Brain Tumor Consortium Study. J Clin Oncol. 2005;23(27):6647–6656.
54. Cloughesy TF, Wen PY, Robins HI, et al. Phase II trial of tipifarnib in patients with recurrent malignant glioma either receiving or not receiving enzyme-inducing antiepileptic drugs: a North American Brain Tumor Consortium Study. J Clin Oncol. 2006;24(22):3651–3656.
55. Gilbert M, Gaupp P, Ictech S, et al. A phase I/II study of temozolomide and the farnesyltransferase inhibitor, tipifarnib in recurrent glioblastoma. Neuro-Oncol. 2007;9:524.
56. Desjardins A, Sathornsumetee S, Reardon D, et al. A phase I trial of the addition of the farnesyl transferase inhibitor SCH 66336 to temozolomide for patients with grade 3 or 4 malignant gliomas. Neuro-Oncol. 2007;9:524.
57. Mita MM, Mita A, Rowinsky EK. The molecular target of rapamycin (mTOR) as a therapeutic target against cancer. Cancer Biol Ther. 2003;2(4 Suppl 1):S169–S177.
58. Chiang GG, Abraham RT. Targeting the mTOR signaling network in cancer. Trends Mol Med. 2007;13(10):433–442.
59. Chang SM, Wen P, Cloughesy T, et al.; North American Brain Tumor Consortium and the National Cancer Institute. Phase II study of CCI-779 in patients with recurrent glioblastoma multiforme. Invest New Drugs. 2005;23(4):357–361.
60. Galanis E, Buckner JC, Maurer MJ, et al.; North Central Cancer Treatment Group. Phase II trial of temsirolimus (CCI-779) in recurrent glioblastoma multiforme: a North Central Cancer Treatment Group Study. J Clin Oncol. 2005;23(23):5294–5304.
61. Engelman JA, Luo J, Cantley LC. The evolution of phosphatidylinositol 3-kinases as regulators of growth and metabolism. Nat Rev Genet. 2006;7(8):606–619.
62. Gallia GL, Rand V, Siu IM, et al. PIK3CA gene mutations in pediatric and adult glioblastoma multiforme. Mol Cancer Res. 2006;4(10):709–714.
63. Hartmann C, Bartels G, Gehlhaar C, Holtkamp N, von Deimling A. PIK3CA mutations in glioblastoma multiforme. Acta Neuropathol. 2005;109(6):639–642.
64. Mizoguchi M, Nutt CL, Mohapatra G, Louis DN. Genetic alterations of phosphoinositide 3-kinase subunit genes in human glioblastomas. Brain Pathol. 2004;14(4):372–377.
65. Chakravarti A, Zhai G, Suzuki Y, et al. The prognostic significance of phosphatidylinositol 3-kinase pathway activation in human gliomas. J Clin Oncol. 2004;22(10):1926–1933.
66. Fan QW, Weiss WA. Isoform specific inhibitors of PI3 kinase in glioma. Cell Cycle. 2006;5(20):2301–2305.
67. Kao GD, Jiang Z, Fernandes AM, Gupta AK, Maity A. Inhibition of phosphatidylinositol-3-OH kinase/Akt signaling impairs DNA repair in glioblastoma cells following ionizing radiation. J Biol Chem. 2007;282(29):21206–21212.
68. Koul D, Shen R, Bergh S, et al. Inhibition of Akt survival pathway by a small-molecule inhibitor in human glioblastoma. Mol Cancer Ther. 2006;5(3):637–644.
69. Su JD, Mayo LD, Donner DB, Durden DL. PTEN and phosphatidylinositol 3'-kinase inhibitors up-regulate p53 and block tumor-induced angiogenesis: evidence for an effect on the tumor and endothelial compartment. Cancer Res. 2003;63(13):3585–3592.
70. Pope WB, Lai A, Nghiemphu P, Mischel P, Cloughesy TF. MRI in patients with high-grade gliomas treated with bevacizumab and chemotherapy. Neurology. 2006;66(8):1258–1260.
71. Stark Vance V. Bevacizumab (Avastin®) and CPT-11 (Camptosar®) in the Treatment of Relapsed Malignant Glioma. Neuro-oncol. 2005;7:369.
72. Vredenburgh JJ, Desjardins A, Herndon JE 2nd, et al. Phase II trial of bevacizumab and irinotecan in recurrent malignant glioma. Clin Cancer Res. 2007;13(4):1253–1259.
73. Vredenburgh JJ, Desjardins A, Herndon JE, et al. Bevacizumab, a monoclonal antibody to vascular endothelial growth factor (VEGF), and irinotecan for treatment of malignant gliomas. J Clin Oncol. 2006;24:1506.
74. Holash J, Davis S, Papadopoulos N, et al. VEGF-Trap: a VEGF blocker with potent antitumor effects. Proc Natl Acad Sci USA. 2002;99(17):11393–11398.
75. Batchelor TT, Sorensen AG, di Tomaso E, et al. AZD2171, a pan-VEGF receptor tyrosine kinase inhibitor, normalizes tumor vasculature and alleviates edema in glioblastoma patients. Cancer Cell. 2007;11(1):83–95.
76. Kunkel P, Ulbricht U, Bohlen P, et al. Inhibition of glioma angiogenesis and growth in vivo by systemic treatment with a monoclonal antibody against vascular endothelial growth factor receptor-2. Cancer Res. 2001;61(18):6624–6628.
77. Lamszus K, Kunkel P, Westphal M. Invasion as limitation to anti-angiogenic glioma therapy. Acta Neurochir Suppl. 2003;88:169–177.
78. Rubenstein JL, Kim J, Ozawa T, et al. Anti-VEGF antibody treatment of glioblastoma prolongs survival but results in increased vascular cooption. Neoplasia. 2000;2(4):306–314.
79. Norden AD, Young GS, Setayesh K, et al. Bevacizumab for recurrent malignant gliomas: efficacy, toxicity, and patterns of recurrence. Neurology. 2008;70(10):779–787.
80. Chi A, Norden AD, Wen PY. Inhibition of angiogenesis and invasion in malignant gliomas. Expert Rev Anticancer Ther. 2007;7(11):1537–1560.
81. Graff JR, McNulty AM, Hanna KR, et al. The protein kinase Cbeta-selective inhibitor, Enzastaurin (LY317615.HCl), suppresses signalingthrough the AKT pathway, induces apoptosis, and suppresses growth of human colon cancer and glioblastoma xenografts. Cancer Res. 2005;65(16):7462–7469.
82. Fine HA, Kim L, Royce C, et al. Results from phase II trial of Enzastaurin (LY317615) in patients with recurrent high grade gliomas. J Clin Oncol. 2005;23:1504.
83. Tabatabai G, Frank B, Wick A, et al. Synergistic antiglioma activity of radiotherapy and enzastaurin. Ann Neurol. 2007;61(2):153–161.
84. Joki T, Heese O, Nikas DC, et al. Expression of cyclooxygenase 2 (COX-2) in human malignant glioma and in vitro inhibition by a specific COX-2 inhibitor, NS-398. Cancer Res. 2000;60(17):4926–4931.
85. Perdiki M, Korkolopoulou P, Thymara I, et al. Cyclooxygenase-2 expression in astrocytomas. Relationship with microvascular parameters, angiogenic factors expression and survival. Mol Cell Biochem. 2007;295(1–2):75–83.
86. Shono T, Tofilon PJ, Bruner JM, Owolabi O, Lang FF. Cyclooxygenase-2 expression in human gliomas: prognostic significance and molecular correlations. Cancer Res. 2001;61(11):4375–4381.
87. Kesari S, Schiff D, Henson JW, et al. Phase II study of temozolomide, thalidomide, and celecoxib for newly diagnosed glioblastoma in adults. Neuro-oncology. 2008;10(3):300–308.
88. Brophy JM. Celecoxib and cardiovascular risks. Expert Opin Drug Saf. 2005;4(6):1005–1015.
89. Lefranc F, Brotchi J, Kiss R. Possible future issues in the treatment of glioblastomas: special emphasis on cell migration and the resistance of migrating glioblastoma cells to apoptosis. J Clin Oncol. 2005;23(10):2411–2422.
90. Rao JS. Molecular mechanisms of glioma invasiveness: the role of proteases. Nat Rev Cancer. 2003;3(7):489–501.
91. Groves MD, Puduvalli VK, Hess KR, et al. Phase II trial of temozolomide plus the matrix metalloproteinase inhibitor, marimastat, in recurrent and progressive glioblastoma multiforme. J Clin Oncol. 2002;20(5):1383–1388.
92. Levin VA, Phuphanich S, Yung WK, et al. Randomized, double-blind, placebo-controlled trial of marimastat in glioblastoma multiforme patients following surgery and irradiation. J Neurooncol. 2006;78(3):295–302.
93. Taga T, Suzuki A, Gonzalez-Gomez I, et al. alpha v-Integrin antagonist EMD 121974 induces apoptosis in brain tumor cells growing on vitronectin and tenascin. Int J Cancer. 2002;98(5):690–697.
94. Nabors LB, Mikkelsen T, Rosenfeld SS, et al. Phase I and correlative biology study of cilengitide in patients with recurrent malignant glioma. J Clin Oncol. 2007;25(13):1651–1657.
95. Reardon D, Fink K, Nabors L, et al. An update of the phase IIa trial of cilengitide (EMD121974) single-agent therapy in patients with recurrent glioblastoma: EMD 121974–009. Neuro-Oncol. 2007;9:517.
96. Stupp R, Goldbrunner R, Neyns B, et al. Mature results of a phase I/IIa trial of the integrin inhibitor cilengitide (EMD121974) added to standard concomitant and adjuvant temozolomide and radiotherapy for newly diagnosed glioblastoma. Neuro-Oncol. 2007;9:517.
97. Xu WS, Parmigiani RB, Marks PA. Histone deacetylase inhibitors: molecular mechanisms of action. Oncogene. 2007;26(37):5541–5552.

98. Yin D, Ong JM, Hu J, et al. Suberoylanilide hydroxamic acid, a histone deacetylase inhibitor: effects on gene expression and growth of glioma cells *in vitro* and in vivo. *Clin Cancer Res.* 2007;13(3):1045–1052.
99. Chinnaiyan P, Vallabhaneni G, Armstrong E, Huang SM, Harari PM. Modulation of radiation response by histone deacetylase inhibition. *Int J Radiat Oncol Biol Phys.* 2005;62(1):223–229.
100. Kim MS, Blake M, Baek JH, Kohlhagen G, Pommier Y, Carrier F. Inhibition of histone deacetylase increases cytotoxicity to anticancer drugs targeting DNA. *Cancer Res.* 2003;63(21):7291–7300.
101. Galanis E, Jaeckle KA, Maurer MJ, et al. NCCTG phase II trial of vorinostat (suberoylanilide hydroxamic acid) in recurrent glioblastoma multiforme. *J Clin Oncol.* 2007;25:2004.
102. Mani A, Gelmann EP. The ubiquitin-proteasome pathway and its role in cancer. *J Clin Oncol.* 2005;23(21):4776–4789.
103. Yin D, Zhou H, Kumagai T, et al. Proteasome inhibitor PS-341 causes cell growth arrest and apoptosis in human glioblastoma multiforme (GBM). *Oncogene.* 2005;24(3):344–354.
104. Nakanishi C, Toi M. Nuclear factor-kappaB inhibitors as sensitizers to anticancer drugs. *Nat Rev Cancer.* 2005;5(4):297–309.
105. Phuphanich S, Supko J, Carson KA, et al. Phase I trial of bortezomib in adults with recurrent malignant glioma. *J Clin Oncol.* 2006;24:1567.
106. Dicker A, Werner-Wasik M, Machtay M, et al. A phase I trial using the proteasome inhibitor bortezomib and concurrent temazolomide and radiotherapy for high grade gliomas. *J Clin Oncol.* 2007;25:2061.
107. Mischel PS, Cloughesy TF, Nelson SF. DNA-microarray analysis of brain cancer: molecular classification for therapy. *Nat Rev Neurosci.* 2004;5(10):782–792.
108. Beroukhim R, Getz G, Nghiemphu L, et al. Assessing the significance of chromosomal aberrations in cancer: methodology and application to glioma. *Proc Natl Acad Sci USA.* 2007;104(50):20007–20012.
109. Rual JF, Venkatesan K, Hao T, et al. Towards a proteome-scale map of the human protein-protein interaction network. *Nature.* 2005;437(7062):1173–1178.
110. Carlson MR, Pope WB, Horvath S, et al. Relationship between survival and edema in malignant gliomas: role of vascular endothelial growth factor and neuronal pentraxin 2. *Clin Cancer Res.* 2007;13(9):2592–2598.
111. Hegi ME, Diserens AC, Gorlia T, et al. MGMT gene silencing and benefit from temozolomide in glioblastoma. *N Engl J Med.* 2005;352(10):997–1003.
112. Bredel M, Bredel C, Juric D, et al. Tumor necrosis factor-alpha-induced protein 3 as a putative regulator of nuclear factor-kappaB-mediated resistance to O6-alkylating agents in human glioblastomas. *J Clin Oncol.* 2006;24(2):274–287.
113. Bredel M, Bredel C, Juric D, et al. Functional network analysis reveals extended gliomagenesis pathway maps and three novel MYC-interacting genes in human gliomas. *Cancer Res.* 2005;65(19):8679–8689.
114. Omuro AM, Faivre S, Raymond E. Lessons learned in the development of targeted therapy for malignant gliomas. *Mol Cancer Ther.* 2007;6(7):1909–1919.
115. Dunlap SM, Celestino J, Wang H, et al. Insulin-like growth factor binding protein 2 promotes glioma development and progression. *Proc Natl Acad Sci USA.* 2007;104(28):11736–11741.
116. Soroceanu L, Kharbanda S, Chen R, et al. Identification of IGF2 signaling through phosphoinositide-3-kinase regulatory subunit 3 as a growth-promoting axis in glioblastoma. *Proc Natl Acad Sci USA.* 2007;104(9):3466–3471.
117. Abounader R, Laterra J. Scatter factor/hepatocyte growth factor in brain tumor growth and angiogenesis. *Neuro-oncology.* 2005;7(4):436–451.
118. Martens T, Schmidt NO, Eckerich C, et al. A novel one-armed anti-c-Met antibody inhibits glioblastoma growth in vivo. *Clin Cancer Res.* 2006;12(20 Pt 1):6144–6152.
119. Wick W, Naumann U, Weller M. Transforming growth factor-beta: a molecular target for the future therapy of glioblastoma. *Curr Pharm Des.* 2006;12(3):341–349.
120. Hjelmeland AB, Lattimore KP, Fee BE, et al. The combination of novel low molecular weight inhibitors of RAF (LBT613) and target of rapamycin (RAD001) decreases glioma proliferation and invasion. *Mol Cancer Ther.* 2007;6(9):2449–2457.
121. Sebolt-Leopold JS, Herrera R. Targeting the mitogen-activated protein kinase cascade to treat cancer. *Nat Rev Cancer.* 2004;4(12):937–947.
122. Premkumar DR, Arnold B, Jane EP, Pollack IF. Synergistic interaction between 17-AAG and phosphatidylinositol 3-kinase inhibition in human malignant glioma cells. *Mol Carcinog.* 2006;45(1):47–59.
123. Nakada M, Drake KL, Nakada S, Niska JA, Berens ME. Ephrin-B3 ligand promotes glioma invasion through activation of Rac1. *Cancer Res.* 2006;66(17):8492–8500.
124. Nakada M, Niska JA, Miyamori H, et al. The phosphorylation of EphB2 receptor regulates migration and invasion of human glioma cells. *Cancer Res.* 2004;64(9):3179–3185.
125. Wykosky J, Gibo DM, Stanton C, Debinski W. EphA2 as a novel molecular marker and target in glioblastoma multiforme. *Mol Cancer Res.* 2005;3(10):541–551.
126. Koul D, Shen R, Bergh S, et al. Targeting integrin-linked kinase inhibits Akt signaling pathways and decreases tumor progression of human glioblastoma. *Mol Cancer Ther.* 2005;4(11):1681–1688.
127. Lund CV, Nguyen MT, Owens GC, et al. Reduced glioma infiltration in Src-deficient mice. *J Neurooncol.* 2006;78(1):19–29.
128. Liu TJ, LaFortune T, Honda T, et al. Inhibition of both focal adhesion kinase and insulin-like growth factor-I receptor kinase suppresses glioma proliferation *in vitro* and in vivo. *Mol Cancer Ther.* 2007;6(4):1357–1367.
129. Pulford K, Lamant L, Espinos E, et al. The emerging normal and disease-related roles of anaplastic lymphoma kinase. *Cell Mol Life Sci.* 2004;61(23):2939–2953.
130. Gillespie DL, Whang K, Ragel BT, Flynn JR, Kelly DA, Jensen RL. Silencing of hypoxia inducible factor-1alpha by RNA interference attenuates human glioma cell growth in vivo. *Clin Cancer Res.* 2007;13(8):2441–2448.
131. Shapiro GI. Cyclin-dependent kinase pathways as targets for cancer treatment. *J Clin Oncol.* 2006;24(11):1770–1783.
132. Bao S, Wu Q, McLendon RE, et al. Glioma stem cells promote radioresistance by preferential activation of the DNA damage response. *Nature.* 2006;444(7120):756–760.
133. Liu X, Chen N, Wang X, et al. Apoptosis and proliferation markers in diffusely infiltrating astrocytomas: profiling of 17 molecules. *J Neuropathol Exp Neurol.* 2006;65(9):905–913.
134. Ghobrial IM, Witzig TE, Adjei AA. Targeting apoptosis pathways in cancer therapy. *CA Cancer J Clin.* 2005;55(3):178–194.
135. Liston P, Fong WG, Korneluk RG. The inhibitors of apoptosis: there is more to life than Bcl2. *Oncogene.* 2003;22(53):8568–8580.
136. Bian XW, Yang SX, Chen JH, et al. Preferential expression of chemokine receptor CXCR4 by highly malignant human gliomas and its association with poor patient survival. *Neurosurgery.* 2007;61(3):570–578; discussion 578.
137. Rubin JB, Kung AL, Klein RS, et al. A small-molecule antagonist of CXCR4 inhibits intracranial growth of primary brain tumors. *Proc Natl Acad Sci USA.* 2003;100(23):13513–13518.
138. Parolaro D, Massi P. Cannabinoids as potential new therapy for the treatment of gliomas. *Expert Rev Neurother.* 2008;8(1):37–49.
139. Galli R, Binda E, Orfanelli U, et al. Isolation and characterization of tumorigenic, stem-like neural precursors from human glioblastoma. *Cancer Res.* 2004;64(19):7011–7021.
140. Singh SK, Hawkins C, Clarke ID, et al. Identification of human brain tumour initiating cells. *Nature.* 2004;432(7015):396–401.
141. Sanai N, Alvarez-Buylla A, Berger MS. Neural stem cells and the origin of gliomas. *N Engl J Med.* 2005;353(8):811–822.
142. Vescovi AL, Galli R, Reynolds BA. Brain tumour stem cells. *Nat Rev Cancer.* 2006;6(6):425–436.
143. Lee da Y, Gutmann DH. Cancer stem cells and brain tumors: uprooting the bad seeds. *Expert Rev Anticancer Ther.* 2007;7(11):1581–1590.
144. Liu G, Yuan X, Zeng Z, et al. Analysis of gene expression and chemoresistance of CD133+ cancer stem cells in glioblastoma. *Mol Cancer.* 2006;5:67.
145. Bao S, Wu Q, Sathornsumetee S, et al. Stem cell-like glioma cells promote tumor angiogenesis through vascular endothelial growth factor. *Cancer Res.* 2006;66(16):7843–7848.
146. Calabrese C, Poppleton H, Kocak M, et al. A perivascular niche for brain tumor stem cells. *Cancer Cell.* 2007;11(1):69–82.
147. Li A, Walling J, Kotliarov Y, et al. Genomic changes and gene expression profiles reveal that established glioma cell lines are

poorly representative of primary human gliomas. *Mol Cancer Res.* 2008;6(1):21–30.
148. Lee J, Kotliarova S, Kotliarov Y, et al. Tumor stem cells derived from glioblastomas cultured in bFGF and EGF more closely mirror the phenotype and genotype of primary tumors than do serum-cultured cell lines. *Cancer Cell.* 2006;9(5):391–403.
149. Fomchenko EI, Holland EC. Mouse models of brain tumors and their applications in preclinical trials. *Clin Cancer Res.* 2006;12(18):5288–5297.
150. Giannini C, Sarkaria JN, Saito A, et al. Patient tumor EGFR and PDGFRA gene amplifications retained in an invasive intracranial xenograft model of glioblastoma multiforme. *Neuro-oncology.* 2005;7(2):164–176.
151. McConville P, Hambardzumyan D, Moody JB, et al. Magnetic resonance imaging determination of tumor grade and early response to temozolomide in a genetically engineered mouse model of glioma. *Clin Cancer Res.* 2007;13(10):2897–2904.
152. Stommel JM, Kimmelman AC, Ying H, et al. Coactivation of receptor tyrosine kinases affects the response of tumor cells to targeted therapies. *Science.* 2007;318(5848):287–290.
153. Frantz S. Drug discovery: playing dirty. *Nature.* 2005;437(7061): 942–943.
154. Demetri GD, von Mehren M, Blanke CD, et al. Efficacy and safety of imatinib mesylate in advanced gastrointestinal stromal tumors. *N Engl J Med.* 2002;347(7):472–480.
155. Whitesell L, Lindquist SL. HSP90 and the chaperoning of cancer. *Nat Rev Cancer.* 2005;5(10):761–772.
156. Newcomb EW, Lukyanov Y, Schnee T, et al. The geldanamycin analogue 17-allylamino-17-demethoxygeldanamycin inhibits the growth of GL261 glioma cells *in vitro* and in vivo. *Anticancer Drugs.* 2007;18(8):875–882.
157. Yang J, Yang JM, Iannone M, Shih WJ, Lin Y, Hait WN. Disruption of the EF-2 kinase/Hsp90 protein complex: a possible mechanism to inhibit glioblastoma by geldanamycin. *Cancer Res.* 2001;61(10):4010–4016.
158. Camphausen K, Tofilon PJ. Combining radiation and molecular targeting in cancer therapy. *Cancer Biol Ther.* 2004;3(3):247–250.
159. Barabási AL, Oltvai ZN. Network biology: understanding the cell's functional organization. *Nat Rev Genet.* 2004;5(2):101–113.
160. Doherty L, Gigas DC, Kesari S, et al. Pilot study of the combination of EGFR and mTOR inhibitors in recurrent malignant gliomas. *Neurology.* 2006;67(1):156–158.
161. Reardon DA, Quinn JA, Vredenburgh JJ, et al. Phase 1 trial of gefitinib plus sirolimus in adults with recurrent malignant glioma. *Clin Cancer Res.* 2006;12(3 Pt 1):860–868.
162. Wen P, Chang S, Kuhn J, et al. Phase I study of erlotinib (Tarceva) and temsirolimus (CCI-779) for patients with recurrent malignant gliomas (NABTC 04–02). In: Society for Neuro-Oncology Eleventh Annual Meeting; 2006: Neuro-Oncology; 2006. p. 454; Abstract TA65.
163. Nguyen TD, Lassman AB, Lis E, et al. A pilot study to assess the tolerability and efficacy of RAD-001 (everolimus) with gefitinib in patients with recurrent glioblastoma multiforme *Neuro-Oncology.* 2006;8:447, TA 39.
164. Camirand A, Zakikhani M, Young F, Pollak M. Inhibition of insulin-like growth factor-1 receptor signaling enhances growth-inhibitory and proapoptotic effects of gefitinib (Iressa) in human breast cancer cells. *Breast Cancer Res.* 2005;7(4):R570-R579.
165. Lu D, Zhang H, Ludwig D, et al. Simultaneous blockade of both the epidermal growth factor receptor and the insulin-like growth factor receptor signaling pathways in cancer cells with a fully human recombinant bispecific antibody. *J Biol Chem.* 2004;279(4): 2856–2865.
166. Steinbach JP, Eisenmann C, Klumpp A, Weller M. Co-inhibition of epidermal growth factor receptor and type 1 insulin-like growth factor receptor synergistically sensitizes human malignant glioma cells to CD95L-induced apoptosis. *Biochem Biophys Res Commun.* 2004;321(3):524–530.
167. Ziegler DS, Kung AL, Kieran MW. Anti-apoptosis mechanisms in malignant gliomas. *J Clin Oncol.* 2008;26(3):493–500.
168. Hay N. The Akt-mTOR tango and its relevance to cancer. *Cancer Cell.* 2005;8(3):179–183.
169. Bentzen SM, Harari PM, Bernier J. Exploitable mechanisms for combining drugs with radiation: concepts, achievements and future directions. *Nat Clin Pract Oncol.* 2007;4(3):172–180.
170. Chinnaiyan P, Allen GW, Harari PM. Radiation and new molecular agents, part II: targeting HDAC, HSP90, IGF-1R, PI3K, and Ras. *Semin Radiat Oncol.* 2006;16(1):59–64.
171. Zhang M, Chakravarti A. Novel radiation-enhancing agents in malignant gliomas. *Semin Radiat Oncol.* 2006;16(1):29–37.
172. Chakravarti A, Dicker A, Mehta M. The contribution of epidermal growth factor receptor (EGFR) signaling pathway to radioresistance in human gliomas: a review of preclinical and correlative clinical data. *Int J Radiat Oncol Biol Phys.* 2004;58(3):927–931.
173. Contessa JN, Abell A, Valerie K, Lin PS, Schmidt-Ullrich RK. ErbB receptor tyrosine kinase network inhibition radiosensitizes carcinoma cells. *Int J Radiat Oncol Biol Phys.* 2006;65(3):851–858.
174. Sartor CI. Mechanisms of disease: Radiosensitization by epidermal growth factor receptor inhibitors. *Nat Clin Pract Oncol.* 2004;1(2):80–87.
175. Chakravarti A, Berkey B, Robins HI, et al. An update of phase II results from RTOG 0211: A phase I /II study of gefitinib with radiotherapy in newly-diagnosed glioblastoma multiforme. *Neuro-Oncol.* 2006;8:439, TA-08.
176. Prados M, DeBoer R, Chang SM, et al. Phase II study of tarceva plus temodar during and following radiotherapy in patients newly-diagnosed with glioblastoma or gliosarcoma. *Neuro-Oncol.* 2007;9:528; MA-50.
177. Geng L, Shinohara ET, Kim D, et al. STI571 (Gleevec) improves tumor growth delay and survival in irradiated mouse models of glioblastoma. *Int J Radiat Oncol Biol Phys.* 2006;64(1):263–271.
178. Wang CC, Liao YP, Mischel PS, Iwamoto KS, Cacalano NA, McBride WH. HDJ-2 as a target for radiosensitization of glioblastoma multiforme cells by the farnesyltransferase inhibitor R115777 and the role of the p53/p21 pathway. *Cancer Res.* 2006;66(13):6756–6762.
179. Delmas C, Heliez C, Cohen-Jonathan E, et al. Farnesyltransferase inhibitor, R115777, reverses the resistance of human glioma cell lines to ionizing radiation. *Int J Cancer.* 2002;100(1):43–48.
180. Eshleman JS, Carlson BL, Mladek AC, Kastner BD, Shide KL, Sarkaria JN. Inhibition of the mammalian target of rapamycin sensitizes U87 xenografts to fractionated radiation therapy. *Cancer Res.* 2002;62(24):7291–7297.
181. Bull EE, Dote H, Brady KJ, et al. Enhanced tumor cell radiosensitivity and abrogation of G2 and S phase arrest by the Hsp90 inhibitor 17-(dimethylaminoethylamino)-17-demethoxygeldanamycin. *Clin Cancer Res.* 2004;10(23):8077–8084.
182. Kuipers GK, Slotman BJ, Wedekind LE, et al. Radiosensitization of human glioma cells by cyclooxygenase-2 (COX-2) inhibition: independent on COX-2 expression and dependent on the COX-2 inhibitor and sequence of administration. *Int J Radiat Biol.* 2007;83(10):677–685.
183. Martin PM, Hussaini IM. PKC eta as a therapeutic target in glioblastoma multiforme. *Expert Opin Ther Targets.* 2005;9(2): 299–313.
184. Camphausen K, Burgan W, Cerra M, et al. Enhanced radiation-induced cell killing and prolongation of gammaH2AX foci expression by the histone deacetylase inhibitor MS-275. *Cancer Res.* 2004;64(1):316–321.
185. Kim JH, Shin JH, Kim IH. Susceptibility and radiosensitization of human glioblastoma cells to trichostatin A, a histone deacetylase inhibitor. *Int J Radiat Oncol Biol Phys.* 2004;59(4):1174–1180.
186. Citrin D, Ménard C, Camphausen K. Combining radiotherapy and angiogenesis inhibitors: clinical trial design. *Int J Radiat Oncol Biol Phys.* 2006;64(1):15–25.
187. Geng L, Donnelly E, McMahon G, et al. Inhibition of vascular endothelial growth factor receptor signaling leads to reversal of tumor resistance to radiotherapy. *Cancer Res.* 2001;61(6):2413–2419.
188. Jain RK, di Tomaso E, Duda DG, Loeffler JS, Sorensen AG, Batchelor TT. Angiogenesis in brain tumours. *Nat Rev Neurosci.* 2007;8(8):610–622.
189. Winkler F, Kozin SV, Tong RT, et al. Kinetics of vascular normalization by VEGFR2 blockade governs brain tumor response to radiation: role of oxygenation, angiopoietin-1, and matrix metalloproteinases. *Cancer Cell.* 2004;6(6):553–563.
190. Damiano V, Melisi D, Bianco C, et al. Cooperative antitumor effect of multitargeted kinase inhibitor ZD6474 and ionizing radiation in glioblastoma. *Clin Cancer Res.* 2005;11(15):5639–5644.
191. Frederick B, Gustafson D, Bianco C, Ciardiello F, Dimery I, Raben D. ZD6474, an inhibitor of VEGFR and EGFR tyrosine kinase

activity in combination with radiotherapy. *Int J Radiat Oncol Biol Phys.* 2006;64(1):33–37.
192. Hurwitz H, Fehrenbacher L, Novotny W, et al. Bevacizumab plus irinotecan, fluorouracil, and leucovorin for metastatic colorectal cancer. *N Engl J Med.* 2004;350(23):2335–2342.
193. Sandler A, Gray R, Perry MC, et al. Paclitaxel-carboplatin alone or with bevacizumab for non-small-cell lung cancer. *N Engl J Med.* 2006;355(24):2542–2550.
194. Herbst RS, Prager D, Hermann R, et al.; TRIBUTE Investigator Group. TRIBUTE: a phase III trial of erlotinib hydrochloride (OSI-774) combined with carboplatin and paclitaxel chemotherapy in advanced non-small-cell lung cancer. *J Clin Oncol.* 2005;23(25):5892–5899.
195. Quinn JA, Desjardins A, Weingart J, et al. Phase I trial of temozolomide plus O6-benzylguanine for patients with recurrent or progressive malignant glioma. *J Clin Oncol.* 2005;23(28):7178–7187.
196. Barvaux VA, Ranson M, Brown R, McElhinney RS, McMurry TB, Margison GP. Dual repair modulation reverses Temozolomide resistance in vitro. *Mol Cancer Ther.* 2004;3(2):123–127.
197. Woolford LB, Southgate TD, Margison GP, Milsom MD, Fairbairn LJ. The P140K mutant of human O(6)-methylguanine-DNA-methyltransferase (MGMT) confers resistance *in vitro* and *in vivo* to temozolomide in combination with the novel MGMT inactivator O(6)-(4-bromothenyl)guanine. *J Gene Med.* 2006;8(1):29–34.
198. Cheng CL, Johnson SP, Keir ST, et al. Poly(ADP-ribose) polymerase-1 inhibition reverses temozolomide resistance in a DNA mismatch repair-deficient malignant glioma xenograft. *Mol Cancer Ther.* 2005;4(9):1364–1368.
199. Donawho CK, Luo Y, Luo Y, et al. ABT-888, an orally active poly(ADP-ribose) polymerase inhibitor that potentiates DNA-damaging agents in preclinical tumor models. *Clin Cancer Res.* 2007;13(9):2728–2737.
200. Breedveld P, Beijnen JH, Schellens JH. Use of P-glycoprotein and BCRP inhibitors to improve oral bioavailability and CNS penetration of anticancer drugs. *Trends Pharmacol Sci.* 2006;27(1):17–24.
201. Löscher W, Potschka H. Drug resistance in brain diseases and the role of drug efflux transporters. *Nat Rev Neurosci.* 2005;6(8):591–602.
202. Löscher W, Potschka H. Role of drug efflux transporters in the brain for drug disposition and treatment of brain diseases. *Prog Neurobiol.* 2005;76(1):22–76.
203. Löscher W, Potschka H. Blood-brain barrier active efflux transporters: ATP-binding cassette gene family. *NeuroRx.* 2005;2(1):86–98.
204. Lawson HC, Sampath P, Bohan E, et al. Interstitial chemotherapy for malignant gliomas: the Johns Hopkins experience. *J Neurooncol.* 2007;83(1):61–70.
205. Vogelbaum MA, Sampson JH, Kunwar S, et al. Convection-enhanced delivery of cintredekin besudotox (interleukin-13-PE38QQR) followed by radiation therapy with and without temozolomide in newly diagnosed malignant gliomas: phase 1 study of final safety results. *Neurosurgery.* 2007;61(5):1031–1037; discussion 1037.
206. Jacobs AH, Kracht LW, Gossmann A, et al. Imaging in neurooncology. *NeuroRx.* 2005;2(2):333–347.
207. Lynch TJ, Bell DW, Sordella R, et al. Activating mutations in the epidermal growth factor receptor underlying responsiveness of non-small-cell lung cancer to gefitinib. *N Engl J Med.* 2004;350(21):2129–2139.
208. Parsons DW, Jones S, Zhang X, et al. An integrated genomic analysis of human glioblastoma multiforme. *Science* 2008;321:1807–1812.
209. Yan H, Parsons DW, Jin G, et al. IDH1 and IDH2 mutations in gliomas. *N Engl J Med.* 2009;360(8):765–773.

78 Biologics

Sith Sathornsumetee, John Howard Sampson, and David A. Reardon

GENERAL PRINCIPLES

Malignant brain tumors are associated with high mortality despite current multidisciplinary treatments. Recent understanding of the genetic and molecular alterations in brain tumors has shed lights on identifying new therapeutic targets and thus developing novel treatment venues. "Biologics" are among new therapeutics for human cancers. As nonspecific cytotoxic modalities such as radiation and chemotherapy for brain tumors remain palliative at best, and many typically are associated with local and systemic toxicities, biological therapeutics have been increasingly developed to deliver more specific tumor cytotoxicity by targeting or modifying biological processes while minimizing toxicities. Biologics include immunotherapy, gene therapy, and virotherapy.

IMMUNOTHERAPY

Understanding basic tumor immunology is essential for designing immunotherapeutic strategies for brain tumors. Immunity is the basic biological process in humans against potentially harmful microbes, macromolecules, and unregulated cell growth. Immunity can be classified into two types, innate immunity and adaptive immunity. Innate immunity provides an immediate first-line defense against threats such as micro-organisms, and it is mediated by inflammatory cytokines, complement, polymorphonuclear leukocytes, macrophages, and natural killer (NK) cells. These effector cells can quickly identify threats through nonspecific pattern recognition. In contrast, adaptive immune response mediated by lymphocytes is highly specific and unique to each nonself antigen. T lymphocytes are the primary effectors in adaptive immunity and activation requires two signals: T-cells receptors binding to antigen presented on major histocompatibility complexes (MHC) and a costimulatory second signal. Two classes of MHC molecules include (1) MHC class I molecules expressed on the surface of all nucleated cells presenting antigenic peptides to CD8+ (cytotoxic) T cells and (2) MHC class II molecules expressed on the surface of antigen-presenting cells (APCs) presenting antigens to CD4+ T cells. APCs are an important link between adaptive and innate immunities. Dendritic cells (DCs) are prototypic, professional APCs, which internalize peptides in the periphery and then travel to lymph nodes, where they present antigenic peptides in the context of both MHC class I and MHC class II to T cells. In addition, APCs also provide costimulatory signals through B7–1 and B7–2 required for T-cell activation. Without costimulatory second signals, T cells become tolerant to antigen. Following appropriate antigen presentation, T cells undergo clonal proliferation, which is further stimulated by cytokines such as interleukin (IL)-2 and interferon-γ.

Adaptive immunity can be classified into humoral and cell-mediated immunity. The humoral immune response is mediated by B-cells through signals from Th2-CD4+ T cells with the support of IL-4, IL-5, and IL-10. Humoral immunity functions primarily through antibodies that bind soluble and cell surface molecules and then induce phagocytosis, complement-mediated cytotoxicity and other pathways leading to cell lysis. Antigen-specific antibodies are secreted by plasma cells, which derive from B-cells. Cell-mediated immunity is orchestrated by Th1-CD4+ T cells, CD8+ T cells, and macrophages with the support from IL-2, IFN-γ, and IL-12. Cytotoxic T-cells induce cell lysis after they encounter nonself antigen presented on MHC class I of APCs. In addition, cell-mediated immunity also activates innate effectors, including macrophages, by IFN-γ to help destroy nonself antigens. Once nonself antigens are eliminated, these effectors undergo apoptosis and leave only long-term memory lymphocytes to react if these nonself antigens are encountered again. Recently, regulatory (CD4+CD25+) T cells (T regs) have emerged as important immune modulatory cells. T regs play an important role in maintaining peripheral immune homeostasis by suppressing autoreactive and pathogen-specific T cells and turning off the immune response after pathogen clearance. However, in cancer, T regs may play a critical role in immune tolerance. Removal of T regs can suppress CD4+ T-cell proliferative defects and can induce tumor rejection in a murine glioma model [1].

Antitumor immune responses are generally ineffective as cancer cells share a common characteristic of evasion of immune surveillance [2]. In addition, localization in the immune privileged central nervous system (CNS) further diminishes detection of brain tumors by the immune system. The immune privileged status of the CNS derives from several factors, including the presence of blood-brain barrier, low levels of leukocyte adhesion molecules, the absence of a well-established lymphatic system, and the presence of anti-inflammatory cytokines such as transforming growth factor (TGF)-β. Nonetheless, several lines of evidence suggest that immune responses can occur in the CNS. Many brain tumors display immune cell (such as CD4+ and CD8+ T cells) infiltrates [3]. Tumor-infiltrating lymphocytes (TIL) isolated from tumors can elicit tumor-specific cytotoxicity following appropriate in vitro stimulation. Taken together, these findings support the existence of antigen-specific antitumor immune responses. However, such antitumor immune responses are generally not effective in cancer (tumor immune escape) due to failure of antigen presentation and failure to elicit effective immune responses. Several factors contribute to "immune escape," including MHC downregulation, lack of costimulatory signals of APCs, evolving tumor-associated antigen heterogeneity, secretion of immunosuppressive factors, increased T regs fraction, and low levels of tumor-associated antigen expression [4]. Strategies have been developed to overcome immune escape of tumors, including synthetic molecules that mimic pathogen invasion at the tumor site to optimize DC activation with subsequent triggering of cancer cell death, multiple specific antigen immunotherapy, and inhibition of immunosuppressive factors and T regs [5].

Immunotherapy may represent a new therapeutic venue for brain tumors. Cancer immunotherapy involves manipulation or enhancement of the immune system to detect and eliminate tumors [6]. Immunotherapeutic approaches can be simply classified into cell-mediated (active and adoptive) immunotherapy and humoral-mediated immunotherapy. Cell-mediated active immunotherapy can confer long-term immunity, whereas passive immunotherapy approaches, such as antibody and cytokine transfers, may only provide immediate effect without long-term immunity.

Cell-Mediated Immunotherapy

Although the CNS is considered an immune privileged site, several lines of evidence suggest that activation of immune responses can occur in the CNS [7,8]. Therefore, treatment aimed to enhance antitumor immune responses in the brain may represent a new promising therapeutic strategy for malignant glioma patients; however, immunotherapy for malignant gliomas is not straightforward as these tumors exhibit potent immunosuppressive properties such as secretion of TGF-ß and IL-10. In fact, many malignant glioma patients develop lymphopenia [1], decreased T-cell responsiveness and antibody production, and impaired function of APCs. Cell-mediated immunotherapy may include adoptive cellular immunotherapy and active immunotherapy (vaccination).

Adoptive Cellular Immunotherapy

Immune cells can be isolated from a patient, expanded in vitro, and then readministered back (adoptive transfer) to the patient to elicit antitumor immune responses. Initial studies using intratumoral [9] or intrathecal [10] injection of autologous immune cells, either alone or in combination with interferon, were unsuccessful [11]. Later studies using lymphokine-activated killer (LAK) cells isolated from peripheral blood, activated with IL-2, and administered into the resection cavity following tumor debulking was associated with promising survival outcome but with significant toxicities, including aseptic meningitis and increased intracranial pressure [12–14]. Another approach involves intratumoral infusion of autologous TILs with concurrent IL-2 infusion [15]. However, TILs did not demonstrate antitumor activity, probably due to the immunosuppressive environment associated with malignant glioma tumors [16]. Recently, adoptive transfer of TILS in the context of induced lymphopenia has resulted in profound immunologic and clinical antitumor responses [17]. An alternative of T-cell therapies is to use allogenic T cells for graft versus tumor effect; however, a pilot clinical study failed to confirm encouraging efficacy observed in preclinical studies [18,19].

Another adoptive cellular transfer strategy involves patient immunization with irradiated tumor cells plus adjuvant granulocyte-macrophage colony stimulating factor (GM-CSF), following which T cells harvested from draining lymph nodes are expanded and activated in vitro and then readministered back to the patient. A phase-I trial of this approach among 10 patients with recurrent malignant glioma demonstrated a 30% radiographic response rate [20]. A phase-II study in patients with newly diagnosed malignant glioma is ongoing.

Active Immunotherapy (Vaccination)

Active antitumor immunization (vaccination) has been evaluated extensively in malignant gliomas. An efficient tumor-specific T-cell response requires antigen presentation by professional APCs such as DCs. One of the most promising active immunotherapy approaches employs DCs primed with tumor antigen in vitro to process exogenous tumor antigens and present them on MHC class I and MHC class II molecules to both CD8+ and CD4+ T cells, respectively, in order to elicit antitumor immune response. DCs can also activate NK cells and induce humoral immunity by activation of B-cells. Strategies to antigen-prime DCs include either fusion with MHC-matched glioma cells or pulsing DCs with either apoptotic tumor cells, total tumor lysate, tumor-specific peptides, or tumor RNA [21]. Preclinical studies demonstrate that glioma antigen-pulsed DCs can prime CD8+ cytotoxic T lymphocytes (CTL) to induce a specific cytotoxic response [22,23]. A phase-I trial of glioma cell lysate-pulsed DCs demonstrated a significant CTL infiltrate in 50% of treated patients [24]. Furthermore, the median survival was 133 weeks and treatment was well tolerated without serious adverse events. Another phase I/II study of tumor lysate-pulsed DCs vaccination in Japanese patients with recurrent malignant glioma demonstrated safety and a median survival of 480 days [25]. As tumor lysate-pulsed DCs are not entirely tumor specific and may have cross reactivity with normal neurons and glial cells, a strategy to use tumor-specific antigens has been developed. At present, EGFR-vIII is probably the only tumor-specific antigen exploited as immunotherapy in patients with malignant glioma. EGFR-vIII has a deletion of exons 2 to 7 causing a defect in the extracellular ligand binding domain and constitutive activation in a ligand-independent manner [26]. A peptide consisting of the mutated segment of EGFR-vIII (Pep-3) has demonstrated efficacy in both in vitro and in vivo preclinical studies of malignant glioma. Preliminary results from a phase-II trial in newly diagnosed EGFR-vIII-positive glioblastoma multiforme (GBM) showed a median time-to-progression (TTP) of 12 months, which is highly encouraging in comparison to a 7.1 month TTP among historical matched controls [27].

Recently, cytomegalovirus (CMV) was identified in malignant glioma without infecting surrounding normal brain, which may represent a new tumor-specific target [3,28]. In addition, EGFR has been demonstrated as a cellular binding site for CMV entry into tumor cells [29]. Clinical development of CMV-specific DC vaccines or T-cell adoptive immunotherapy is in progress.

Humoral-Mediated Immunotherapy

Passive Antibody Transfer

Monoclonal antibodies are multivalent proteins with high affinity and selectivity to antigenic epitopes. Antitumor effects of antibodies can be mediated by antibody-dependent complement-mediated cytotoxicity, antibody-dependent cell-mediated cytotoxicity, direct induction of tumor cell apoptosis, inhibition of protein-protein interactions, and neutralizing angiogenic growth factors such as vascular endothelial growth factor (VEGF) by bevacizumab (Avastin, Genentech, South San Francisco, CA, USA) [30]. Furthermore, monoclonal antibodies can be armed with radioisotopes, drugs, or toxins. An example of radiolabeled monoclonal antibody therapy in brain tumors may include ^{131}I-labeled monoclonal antibody against tenascin (^{131}I-m81C6; Neuradiab; Bradmer Pharmaceuticals, Toronto, Canada). Tenascin is commonly expressed in high-grade gliomas but not in normal brain. Preclinical studies of ^{131}I-m81C6 demonstrated significant tumor growth delay and regression in athymic mice bearing subcutaneous human glioma xenografts and prolongation of median survival of athymic rats bearing intracranial tumors [31,32]. Intracavitary administration of ^{131}I-m81C6 has demonstrated promising survival benefit with median survivals of 79.4 weeks in newly diagnosed GBM and 64 weeks in recurrent GBM [33,34]. Treatment was generally well tolerated, with 27% of patients developing reversible hematologic toxicity and 15% developing histologically confirmed, treatment-related neurologic toxicity. A multicenter, phase-III trial randomizing newly diagnosed GBM patients to standard XRT plus temozolomide (TMZ) or this approach plus ^{131}I-m81C6 has been approved by the FDA and initiated accrual in 2008. Another technique to enhance tenascin targeting involves a three-step delivery approach, including intravenous delivery of biotinylated antitenascin antibody followed by secondary delivery of avidin/streptavidin and completed with tertiary delivery of ^{90}Y-DOTA-biotin [35]. A phase-II study exploiting this technique in malignant glioma demonstrated promising survival benefit (28 months for GBM and 56 months for WHO grade III gliomas) [36].

In brain tumors, most monoclonal antibodies are delivered locally to tumor or resection cavity as systemic administration may not achieve adequate delivery due to restriction by the blood-brain barrier. Modulation of blood-barrier integrity may overcome this challenge. A phase-II trial of blood-brain barrier disruption with mannitol followed by chemotherapy and trastuzumab (Herceptin, Genentech), a human epidermal growth factor receptor (HER)-2 monoclonal antibody, is ongoing in HER-2 positive breast cancer patients with brain metastases. In addition, monoclonal antibodies that can function on the abluminal side of blood vessels (such as a neutralizing monoclonal antibody to VEGF, bevacizumab) without a need to traverse the blood-brain barrier may be effective in the treatment of brain tumors. The dramatic antiangiogenic and antitumor effects of bevacizumab in malignant gliomas are discussed in other chapters.

Ligand-Toxin Conjugates

Glioma cells commonly express several high-affinity cell surface receptors at greater density than normal surrounding brain cells. The ligands for these receptors can be engineered to specifically deliver toxins or radioisotopes to permit specific tumor cytotoxicity upon binding and internalization. Most current immunotoxins are derived from plant, fungal, or bacterial toxins. Several agents based on this approach are summarized in Table 78.1, which include TGF-α conjugated with mutated pseudomonas toxin (TP-38, IVAX, Miami, FL & Teva Pharmaceuticals, North Wales, PA) that binds epidermal growth factor receptor (EGFR) [8]; transferrin-CRM107 (TransMID, Xenova, Berkshire, UK), a transferrin-diphtheria conjugate [37]; ^{131}I-TM-601 (TransMolecular, Cambridge, MA), a radiolabeled chlorotoxin [38]; IL-4-conjugated pseudomonas exotoxin [39] and IL-13 conjugated with pseudomonas exotoxin (IL13-PE38QQR, cintredekin besudotox [CB], NeoPharm, IL, USA) [40]. Among these ligand-conjugated toxins, IL13-PE38QQR has undergone phase-III clinical trial evaluation.

The majority of malignant glioma cell lines and xenografts express the IL-13 receptor alpha-2 (IL-13Rα2). In addition, IL-13Rα2 represents a good therapeutic target as it is expressed higher in malignant glioma than in low-grade glioma and normal glial cells. CB is a recombinant cytotoxin consisting of human IL-13 and a truncated form of *Pseudomonas aeruginosa* exotoxin A (PE38QQR). IL13-PE38QQR mediates cytotoxicity by enzymatic inhibition of protein synthesis and apoptosis leading to cell death.

Table 78.1 Ligand-Toxin Conjugates Evaluated in Clinical Trials for Brain Tumor Patients

Agent	Toxin	Target
TP-38	Pseudomonas exotoxin	EGFR
Transferrin-CRM107	Diphtheria exotoxin	EGFR
^{131}I-TM-601	Radiolabeled chlorotoxin	Chloride channel
IL-4-pseudomonas toxin	Pseudomonas exotoxin	IL-4 receptor
IL13-PE38QQR (cintredekin besudotox)	Pseudomonas exotoxin	IL-13 receptor

Most ligand-toxin conjugates are delivered intratumorally or peritumorally, thus increased tumor interstitial pressure may limit distribution of therapeutic toxins. Convection-enhanced delivery (CED) is a novel technique of local drug delivery that may overcome this challenge by using a "pressure gradient" concept of infusing small volumes at continuous high pressures over periods of hours to days into the tumor or resection cavity through a stereotactically placed catheter [41]. CED of ligand-toxin conjugates, including CB, has shown promise in preclinical and early clinical studies.

Three phase-I trials evaluated CED of CB following surgical resection in 51 patients with recurrent malignant glioma. The maximal tolerated intraparenchymal concentration of CB was 0.5 μg/ml and tumor necrosis was observed at this concentration. Infusion durations of up to 6 days were well tolerated. Treatment was generally well tolerated and adverse events were limited to the CNS. Through these trials, it was determined that optimal postoperative catheter placement is critical to achieve adequate drug distribution, which may subsequently dictate patient outcome. The median overall survival for GBM patients was 42.7 weeks and 55.6 weeks for patients who had optimally positioned catheters. This encouraging benefit led to a randomized phase-III trial of CB delivered by CED versus carmustine wafer (Gliadel®) following surgical resection (PRECISE study) for patients with recurrent malignant glioma. Unfortunately, this trial failed to demonstrate a survival advantage of CB over carmustine wafer. Recent data suggests that one possible explanation for the disappointing results of this trial includes lower rates of IL-13Rα2 expression among primary GBM tumors than originally anticipated. Specifically, a recent analysis revealed that an increased expression of IL-13Rα2 gene relative to non-neoplastic brain was observed in only 36 of 81 (44%) and 8 of 17 (47%) GBM samples assessed by microarray and quantitative real-time reverse transcription polymerase chain reaction, respectively [42]. In addition, recent studies that included co-infusion of ^{123}I-labeled human serum albumin during CED revealed that standard CED approaches to date achieve limited volumes of distribution in that most catheters failed to achieve adequate intraparenchymal distribution of therapeutics [43,44].

GENE THERAPY

The first clinical trial of gene therapy in cancer was reported in 1990 by Rosenberg and colleagues [45]. In this study, TILs genetically modified by retroviral gene transduction were administered in malignant melanoma patients with success. Since then, there have been a large number of clinical studies using gene therapy for treatment of cancers. At present, cancers are the most common disease for which gene therapy is being evaluated. Recent advances in the discovery of genetic aberrations in malignant brain tumors, particularly malignant glioma, the most common primary brain tumor in adults, has stimulated not only the development of molecularly targeted therapies but also "gene therapy" to reverse or modify genetic abnormalities underlying malignancy. Gliomas are locally invasive cancers that rarely metastasize; hence, they represent a great candidate for local treatment such as gene therapy. Local administration of such therapeutics may enhance efficacy and limit systemic toxicity.

Gene therapy constitutes biological techniques that deliver selected genetic material into cells or tissue with therapeutic intent. In order to transfer genetic material into human cells or tissue, three factors, including vector, transgene, and delivery, are required. In general, viral vectors can deliver genes to cells with higher efficiencies compared to nonviral gene transfer techniques, including direct in vivo DNA injection or local delivery of cationic lipids.

Nonviral Vectors

Nonviral vectors have advantages of low immunogenicity and toxicity and long-term stability. Cationic liposomes have been used to deliver the suicidal gene Herpes simplex virus-thymidine kinase (HSV-TK) to GBM patients by CED in a phase-I/II trial. Treatment was generally well tolerated without serious adverse events. In two of eight patients, more than 50% reduction of tumor volume was observed [46]. Positron-emission tomography (PET) can be used to monitor HSV-TK gene expression and treatment effect. Another pilot study exploited cationic liposomes to deliver the human interferon-β gene into patients with malignant glioma. Four of five patients displayed transgene expression and an antitumor effect was observed following treatment [47]. In addition, pegylated immunoliposomes containing plasmid encoding a short hairpin RNA directed against human EGFR mRNA with monoclonal antibodies have demonstrated preclinical efficacy in animal models of glioma [48].

VIRUSES

Anticancer effects have been observed following both viral infection and live virus vaccination, particularly in hematologic malignancies such as leukemia or lymphoma. In addition, viruses can be used as a vector to deliver a specific gene for cancer therapy. Viral vectors are simply classified into two types: replication-defective and replication-competent (oncolytic) viruses. (Table 78.2) Replication-defective viruses cannot grow in cells due to a defective replication genome, but they can deliver an anticancer gene to elicit tumor cytotoxicity. Replication-defective viruses may include retrovirus, adenovirus, adeno-associated virus (AAV), and herpes simplex virus type 1 (HSV-1). Replication-competent or oncolytic viruses can selectively grow in cancer cells but not normal cells. Oncolytic viruses include genetically engineered ("armed") viruses—such as herpes simplex virus, adenovirus, and measles—and nonengineered viruses—such as Newcastle disease virus and reovirus. The advantages of oncolytic viruses are an increase in volume of distribution and induction of tumor-specific immunity and antivascular effects, whereas disadvantages may include toxicity due to loss of selective replication and potential immunogenicity.

Table 78.2 Viral Vectors Used in Gene Therapy for Brain Tumors

Viral Vectors	Characteristics	Advantages	Disadvantages
Retrovirus	Low transgene capacity	Persistent gene expression	Low transduction efficiency
	Infects dividing cells	Low toxicity	Insertional mutagenesis
	Low immunogenicity		
Lentivirus	Infects both dividing and quiescent cells	Long-term, stable gene expression	Insertional mutagenesis
	Low immunogenicity	Low toxicity	
HSV-1	High transgene capacity	Persistent gene expression	Neurovirulence
	High immunogenicity	Capability of multiple transgene expression	Pre-existent immunity to HSV
	Neurotropism	Available anti-HSV agents	Relative difficulty with large genome manipulation
		Available in oncolytic strains	
Adenovirus	High cloning capacity	High viral titers	Short-term transgene expression
	Infects both dividing and quiescent cells	Available in oncolytic strains	
	High immunogenicity		Potential neurovirulence
AAV	Low transgene capacity	Persistent gene expression	Low viral titers
	Site-specific integration	Effective tumor penetration	Low transgene capacity
	Infects both dividing and quiescent cells		
	Low immunogenicity		

Replication-Competent (Oncolytic) Viruses

As replication-defective viruses have limitations of inadequate delivery, low transgene expression, and short-term efficacy, replication-competent (oncolytic) viruses have been developed to selectively replicate and kill cancer cells [49]. While cancer cells undergo cytolysis, virus particles are released, which then infect and kill other cells in successive rounds. Several approaches to increase the tumor selectivity of oncolytic viruses include utilizing attenuated viruses that preferentially infect tumor cells, the inactivation of viral genes required for replication in normal cells, or engineering viruses to include tumor-specific promoter containing genes necessary for replication. Preclinical studies have demonstrated promising efficacy of oncolytic viruses and have translated into several clinical trials [50] as summarized in Table 78.3.

Oncolytic HSV-1

HSV-1 is a neurotropic DNA virus with a relatively large genome. Wild-type HSV-1 is pathogenic and can cause severe encephalitis in normal individuals. Advantages of using HSV-1 as a vector for gene therapy are high transgene capacity and stability, high viral titers, neuro- and glio-tropism, and the availability of anti-HSV agents. Disadvantages may include difficulty to manipulate the relatively large viral genome, preexisting human immunity, and potential neurovirulence of HSV-1. In 1991, Martuza et al first reported the feasibility of genetically engineered HSV as oncolytic therapy in a preclinical model of glioma [58]. This HSV was modified to have deletion of thymidine kinase, an enzyme essential for DNA replication in nondividing cells. A preclinical study demonstrated that thymidine kinase-deleted HSV can replicate within and kill glial tumor cells. However, it has not been developed into clinical studies as there is a concern of neurovirulence such as encephalitis that cannot be treated with anti-HSV treatment due to the lack of thymidine kinase domain.

Subsequently, the G207 strain of HSV was developed. G207 is a double-mutated HSV-1 that has homozygous deletions of the $\gamma_1 34.5$ neurovirulence gene and the ribunucleotide reductase (RR) gene. G207 retains susceptibility to ganciclovir as the thymidine kinase gene is intact. Preclinical studies demonstrated safety and efficacy in both subcutaneous and intracranial xenograft models of gliomas [59]. A phase-I clinical study with G207 in recurrent malignant glioma patients demonstrated safety without dose-limiting toxicities, when administered intratumorally [51]. The therapeutic benefits of oncolytic HSV-1 depend on the extent of both intratumoral viral replication and induction of host antitumor immune responses. A second-generation HSV-1 vector, G47delta, was developed by manipulating genetic elements of G207. G47delta is associated with better cytopathic effect in vitro and better antitumor efficacy in both immuno-competent and -incompetent animals, while preserving safety in the brain of HSV-1-sensitive mice. A clinical trial of G47delta in progressive GBM is underway. In addition, G47delta is also suited as a backbone vector for expressing foreign molecules.

Another mutant, HSV1716, has deletions of only $\gamma_1 34.5$ genes. HSV1716 has undergone evaluation in three phase-I clinical trials for malignant gliomas with demonstrable safety. In addition, these studies demonstrated proof of principle for this approach as resected tumor following intratumoral viral injection revealed an increased number of therapeutic virus particles, confirming in vivo replication in human glioma [54].

Oncolytic Adenovirus

Adenoviruses are nonenveloped DNA viruses capable of infecting both proliferating and quiescent cells. While adenoviruses can infect tumor cells and produce new viral progeny to infect additional cells in the tumor mass, they have minimal pathogenic potential. ONYX-015 is an adenovirus that has a deletion of E1B-55K protein, which inactivates host cell p53 protein. ONYX-015 has been evaluated in several phase-I/II studies alone or in combination with radiation or chemotherapy in a variety of cancers. Preclinical studies revealed antitumor activity of ONYX-015 independent of p53 status

Table 78.3 Summary of Oncolytic Virotherapy in Malignant Glioma

Virus	Route	Study	Tumor Response Toxicity	Median Survival (months)	Ref.
G207 HSV ($\alpha_1$34.5-, RR-null)	Intratumoral	Phase I; recurrent GBM (15), AA (4)	38% response; 2 long-term survivors Mild neurologic symptoms	6	51
HSV1716 (γ34.5-null)	Intratumoral	Phase I; recurrent GBM (8), AA (1)	5 patients with SD 1 patient alive after 13 months Mild neurologic symptoms	9	52
HSV1716	Intratumoral; followed by resection	Phase I/II; recurrent GBM (10) & AA (1), newly diagnosed GBM (1)	1 CR and 3 PR No significant toxicity	11.3	53
HSV1716	Injection into resection cavity after debulking	Phase I; newly diagnosed GBM (6), recurrent GBM (4), AA (1), AO (1)	1 PR and 1 SD No significant toxicity	6.5	54
ONYX-015 (E1B-55K deleted adenovirus)	Injection into resection cavity after debulking	Phase I; recurrent GBM (17), AA (6), AO (1)	1 SD 3 patients alive after 19 months No significant toxicity	6.2	55
NDV	Intracutaneous	Phase I, newly diagnosed GBM (11)	No significant toxicity	11	56
NDV-HUJ	Intravenous	Phase I/II, recurrent GBM (11)	1 CR Low-grade fever	Not reported	57
Reovirus (Reolysin)	Intratumoral	Phase I/II; recurrent MG (n = 44)	Ongoing	a	a
Measles virus with CEA	Intratumoral and injection into resection cavity	Phase I; recurrent GBM (n = 40)	Ongoing	a	a
Poliovirus	—	Phase I- planned in recurrent MG	—	—	—

a Source: www.clinicaltrials.gov

of glioma xenografts [60]. A phase-I trial of ONYX-015 demonstrated safety and tolerability; however, no radiographic responses were observed [55]. The median survival was 6.2 months.

Measles Virus

Measles virus is an RNA virus in the Paramyxoviridae family. Glioblastoma cells overexpress the measles virus receptor CD46, which allows for preferential tumor targeting. Measles virus derivative has been engineered to overexpress the human carcinoembryonic antigen (CEA), and infection of glioma cells results in a characteristic cytopathic effect followed by apoptotic cell death and prolongation of survival in subcutaneous and orthotopic tumor models. In addition, this oncolytic measles virus has synergistic effect with radiation therapy in preclinical models of glioblastoma [61]. A phase-I trial of measles virus derivative producing CEA in patients with recurrent GBM is ongoing.

Newcastle Disease Virus

Newcastle disease virus (NDV) is a highly contagious, single-stranded RNA avian paramyxovirus. Human exposure (e.g., in poultry farmers) to the virus can cause conjunctivitis or flu-like illness. Attenuated NDV can selectively kill tumor cells with limited toxicities to normal tissue. NDVs have been evaluated in the treatment for GBM [57,62]. The HUJ strain underwent evaluation in a phase-I/II trial in 11 patients with GBM [63]. The first part of this trial included an intrapatient dose escalation phase, followed by maintenance therapy among nonprogressive patients. Intravenous NDV-HUJ was well tolerated. NDV-HUJ was recovered from blood, saliva, urine samples, and one tumor biopsy. One patient achieved a complete response lasting 3 months. In addition, the NDV has been used in a phase-II study of active immunization in 23 GBM patients by using patient's tumor cell culture infected with NDV that was inactivated by gamma irradiation. There were no serious side effects. The median survival was significantly improved when compared to that of the control group.

In addition, NDV can function as an immunomodulator to increase the immunogenicity of glioblastoma cells. Following vaccination with tumor cells cultured and infected with NDV, patients demonstrated enhanced activation of CTL, compared to that of noninfected tumor cells. Treatment was well tolerated and demonstrated prolongation of survival [64].

Poliovirus

Poliovirus is a nonenveloped RNA virus with inherent neurotropism. CD155 is a cellular poliovirus receptor that is highly expressed in malignant glioma [65]. A recombinant poliovirus (PV-RIPO) was developed by exchanging the internal ribosome entry site element of poliovirus with that of human rhinovirus type 2. This recombinant poliovirus has excellent tumor cytolytic activity, while normal neurons are not significantly affected. PV-RIPO failed to cause poliomyelitis in CD155 transgenic mice and in monkeys. Preclinical studies of PV-RIPO demonstrated both in vitro and in vivo antitumor effect with regression of intracranial glioma xenografts in 72% of treated mice. A phase-I clinical trial of poliovirus in patients with recurrent malignant glioma is planned.

Replication-Defective Viruses

Retroviral Vectors

Retroviruses are RNA viruses that are capable of integrating into the host cell genome by transcribing DNA from their RNA template using virally encoded reverse transcriptase. The integrated viral DNA is transcribed and then translated to form the viral proteins. Retroviral vectors are constructed by replacing the viral protein coding regions with the gene of interest, which makes these vectors replication incompetent [66]. Vector plasmid constructs containing long-terminal repeats (LTRs), the packaging sequence ψ, and the transgene of interest are transfected into vector-producing cells (usually NIH-3T3 fibroblasts). Retroviral vectors can then be harvested from the medium of vector-producing cells. Advantages of retroviral vectors are the ability to stably integrate into the host genome, particularly in dividing cells, that is, tumor cells, and the absence of viral protein expression. Potential disadvantages may include a risk of insertional mutagenesis to host cells and low transduction efficiency. Insertional mutagenesis may be eliminated through suicidal HSV-thymidine kinase (TK) gene following ganciclovir treatment. Inefficient transduction in human is perhaps due to rapid inactivation of vectors by complement and lack of dissemination of viruses away from the injection sites.

Lentiviral Vectors

Lentivirus is a slow virus of retroviridae family, characterized by a long incubation period. Lentiviral infection has advantages over other viral vectors, including high-efficiency infection of dividing and nondividing cells, long-term stable expression of a transgene, and low immunogenicity. In addition, lentiviruses can be designed to block specific genes using RNA interference system. A recent preclinical study demonstrated promising anti-glioma activity of lentiviral vectors pseudotyped with glycoproteins of lymphocytic choriomeningitis [67]. In addition, lentivirus can be used to mediate small interfering RNA (siRNA) deletion of target genes in malignant glioma [68].

Adenoviral Vectors

Whereas some adenoviruses are replication-competent as described above, others are replication-defective and can be used to deliver specific transgenes of interest. Unlike retrovirus that required vector-producing cells, adenoviruses can be administered directly into target sites with high titer. The adenoviral genome is divided into four early gene regions, E1 through E4 and late genes, which primarily encode viral structural proteins. Upon infection, the E1 gene products are expressed and then transcriptionally activate other genes leading to viral replication. Removing E1 therefore results in a replication-defective adenoviral particle. Genes of interest can be cloned into the deleted E1 region. However, recombinant E1 deleted adenovirus must be produced in cell lines such as 293 cells engineered to express the E1 gene. The advantages of adenoviruses include high cloning capacities, high viral titers, and the ability to infect both proliferating and quiescent cells. Thus, adenoviruses may be effective in tumors with low mitotic index. Disadvantages of adenoviral vectors include neurovirulence of wild-type virus and immunogenicity. While adenoviruses are associated with immunogenicity that can result in transient inflammatory response in the brain, these humoral and cellular immune responses may contribute to antitumor activity.

Adeno-Associated Virus Vectors

AAV is a nonpathogenic parvovirus that requires other helper viruses (such as adenovirus) to replicate in human cells. It is a nonenveloped, single-stranded DNA virus that can integrate into the host genome. Advantages of recombinant AAV vectors include lack of pathogenicity and immunogenicity, ability to infect both proliferating and quiescent cells, and site-specific integration that can mediate long-term transgene expression in tissues. Disadvantages may include low viral titers and low transgene capacity. Newer generation recombinant AAV vectors pseudotyped with capsids derived from AAV serotypes 7 and 8 are associated with increased gene transfer efficiency in a murine model of orthotopic human glioma xenografts [69].

Transgene Strategies

Prodrug-Suicidal Gene Therapy

The most common transgene strategy utilized in malignant glioma is HSV-TK/ganciclovir system. Ganciclovir is a synthetic analogue of 2'-deoxy-guanosine that is used for the treatment of herpes virus (particularly CMV) infection as it has preferential activity against viral TK over human nucleoside kinase. Tumor cells are transfected with the HSV-TK gene phosphorylate ganciclovir. Ganciclovir monophosphate is subsequently bis- and tri-phosphorylated by cellular kinases and is then incorporated into the DNA of replicating cells, blocking the cell cycle and inducing apoptosis. Cells that are transfected and exposed to ganciclovir can also kill adjacent, untransfected cells by the so-called *bystander effect*. This effect requires cell-to-cell contact mediated by transfer of toxic metabolites and stimulation of tumor-infiltrating T lymphocytes and NK cells [70]. Preclinical studies have demonstrated survival benefit of intratumoral injection of HSV-TK retroviral vectors with intraperitoneal ganciclovir administration in murine models of malignant glioma.

A total of nine phase-I/II trials of retroviral vector-mediated HSV-TK gene transfer in patients with recurrent GBM demonstrated complete or partial responses of 13% with minor responses or stable disease in 18% (Table 78.4). Responses were usually observed at the recurrent site, where intratumoral injection of retroviral vector-producing cells was performed [74]. However, in most cases, treatment involved injection into resection cavity following tumor resection, thus response to treatment was difficult to assess. A subsequent phase-III trial of retroviral vector-mediated HSV-TK gene therapy after tumor debulking for newly diagnosed GBM demonstrated no survival benefit

Table 78.4 Summary of Selected Viral Vector-Mediated Gene Therapy Clinical Trials in Malignant Gliomas

Gene Therapy System	Study Design	Treatment Response	Median Survival	Related Toxicity	Ref.
Retroviral-HSV-TK/GCV: 10^9 VPC	Phase I, recurrent GBM (n = 12)	1 CR 3 PR	8.1 months	Increased seizures	71
Retroviral-HSV-TK/GCV: 10^8 VPC/ml, 10 ml	Phase I/II, recurrent GBM (n = 48)	7 responders (MRI-progression-free > 6 months)	8.6 months	None	72
Retroviral-HSV-TK/GCV: 10^8 VPC/ml, 10 ml, repeated on day 7	Phase I/II, recurrent GBM (n = 30)	–	8.4 months	Serious adverse event in 16 patients	73
Retroviral-HSV-TK/GCV: 10^8 VPC/ml, 9.1 ml	Phase III, newly diagnosed GBM with radiation (n = 248)	–	12 months	None	74
Retrovirus-HSV-TK/GCV: 10^9 VPC/ml Adenovirus-HSV-TK/GCV: 3×10^{10} pfu/10 ml	Phase I/II, recurrent GBM (n = 7 for retrovirus group; n = 12 for adenovirus group)	–	7 months 14 months	Low-grade fever; increased seizures	75
Adenovirus-HSV-TK/GCV: 3×10^{10} pfu/10 ml	Phase IIb, newly diagnosed/ recurrent GBM (n = 36)	Extension of survival 80%	14.4 months	Local edema	76
Adenovirus-HSV-TK/GCV	Phase I, recurrent GBM (n = 13)	3 responders (survival > 25 months)	4 months	Confusion; seizures; hyponatremia	77
Adenovirus-p53	Phase I, recurrent malignant gliomas (n = 15)	5 responders (MRI-progression-free > 6 months)	10 months	Mild headache; fatigue; low-grade fever	78

of gene therapy over radiation therapy alone [74]. In addition, some patients in the gene therapy arm developed side effects such as intracranial hemorrhage and thromboembolic events. Serum from patients on the gene therapy arm displayed cytokine changes consistent with Th-1 inflammatory response.

Fourteen patients were evaluated in a clinical study designed to evaluate the efficacy and toxicity of an HSV-TK/ganciclovir gene therapy system using retroviral vector-producing cells versus adenoviruses [75]. Both vectors were deemed to be safe and well tolerated. However, the survival of patients in adenovirus group was significantly longer than that of retrovirus group. (Table 78.4) Therefore, adenoviral vectors have become more popular and have generally replaced retroviral vector-producing cells for use in malignant glioma treatment. Several clinical studies using adenoviral vectors-mediated gene therapy have been completed in malignant glioma [75,76,78–80]. A randomized, controlled study of adenovirus-HSV/TK gene therapy following tumor resection versus tumor resection (with radiation therapy in newly diagnosed cases) in 36 patients with malignant glioma demonstrated significant survival benefit from gene therapy with the median survival time increased from 37.7 to 62.4 weeks [76]. Further clinical development of adenovirus-HSV/TK gene therapy is ongoing.

Gene Replacement Strategy

Another distinct transgene approach includes restoration of defective genes in gliomas. *TP53* tumor suppressor gene mutations are pathogenetic abnormalities found in low-grade astrocytoma and "secondary" glioblastomas. Prelinical studies of wild-type *TP53* replacement were associated with antitumor efficacy in both in vitro and in vivo models of glioma. A phase-I study of intratumoral *TP53* adenoviral vector-mediated gene injection followed by gross total resection demonstrated safety and tolerability but no evidence of efficacy. The maximal tolerated dose was not reached and no systemic dissemination of viruses was observed. P53 was found in transduced tumor cells, but such cells were identified at only a short distance from the injection site [78].

STRATEGIES TO ENHANCE EFFICACY OF GENE THERAPY AND VIROTHERAPY FOR BRAIN TUMORS

Preclinical studies of oncolytic virotherapy and gene therapy have demonstrated promising antitumor activity that has prompted clinical trial evaluation. Several phase-I/II clinical studies using this approach have shown safety and tolerability with encouraging efficacy; however, there has not been a phase-III trial to date to confirm antitumor activity. Several strategies have been developed to improve effectiveness of gene and virus therapies for brain tumor patients [81].

Strategies to improve retroviral transduction efficiency include (1) the use of engineered replication-defective HSV-1 or adenovirus to deliver retrovirus packaging sequences and transgenes to tumor cells as described above and (2) to engineer replication-competent retroviruses that confer higher transduction efficiency without affecting surrounding normal tissue [82].

Oncolytic viruses can replicate and cause cytotoxicity to tumor cells. The effectiveness can be enhanced by several approaches, including incorporation of therapeutic transgenes or advanced engineering of viral vectors, such as double deletions of E1A and E1B in adenovirus that can induce regression in malignant glioma xenografts [83]. Deletion of *ICP47* in HSV-1 can improve antigen presentation [84]. Tumor selectivity may be improved with glioma-selective promoters to facilitate expression of transgenes.

An oncolytic HSV-1 mutant *ICP34.5* under control of a nestin promoter increased survival of symptomatic mice with intracranial glioma xenografts [85]. Enhancement of adenovirus delivery to tumor cells may be achieved with antibody-mediated redirection to overexpressed receptors on glioma cells. This approach may include incorporation of the integrin-binding (RGD) motif, which has demonstrated regression of glioma xenografts in 90% of treated animals [86].

Cell-based gene delivery has gained popularity for use in gene therapy in human diseases, including cancers. Bone marrow-derived stem/progenitor cells [87], neural stem cells [88], endothelial progenitor cells [89], and mesenchymal stem cells [90] have been exploited to deliver cytotoxic genes to brain tumors as they exhibit tumor tropism ("homing"), immune tolerance, and tumor-killing properties.

In addition to advanced gene delivery technique, strategies that can improve efficacy of gene therapy in brain tumors include selection and optimization of transgenes and prodrugs. Growth factor receptors, intracellular signaling molecules, immune modulators, apoptotic modulators, inhibitors of angiogenesis, and invasion may represent novel transgene candidates for tumor delivery by gene therapy approaches. Roles of these molecules in pathogenesis and maintenance of brain tumor are described in other chapters. A new ganciclovir formulation may improve the bioavailability of HSV-TK/ganciclovir delivery system [91], whereas TK can be optimized to have increased enzymatic activity [92]. Furthermore, the timing of gene and drug delivery also represents an important factor [93]. New prodrug systems include rat cytochrome P450/cyclophosphamide, carboxylase/CPT11, and uracil phosphoribosyl transferase/5-fluorouracil (UPRT/5-FU). Combination of prodrug systems such as UPRT/5-FU and TK-ganciclovir may be more effective than either prodrug alone [94].

Other advances in molecular biology, genetics, and imaging may improve effectiveness of gene therapy in brain tumors. Animal models that recapitulate diffuse infiltrative, genetically heterogeneous, human gliomas may serve as preclinical models for reliable therapeutic evaluation. A systematic approach by genomic or network analyses may identify promising targets that can be used in gene therapy or immunotherapy. Moreover, given the existence of intra- and interpatient genetic heterogeneities of gliomas, gene expression analysis may identify specific aberrant proteins/antigens in each individual patient, which may subsequently lead to "personalized" gene therapy or immunotherapy. Noninvasive imaging techniques that can follow viruses and/or a transgene may prove useful as a pharmacodynamic marker to monitor treatment effect and to identify biomarkers of response or resistance. New surgical techniques such as 3D-neuronavigational system and convention-enhanced delivery may improve precision, dispersal, and efficiency of target gene delivery.

MULTIMODAL BIOLOGIC THERAPY

As we have learned from the history of cancer treatment with either chemotherapy or novel targeted therapeutics, it is unlikely that single agent monotherapy will provide remarkable response and survival benefit [63]. Genetic heterogeneity of tumor, redundant and overlapping signal transduction pathways, intrinsic or acquired resistance to therapeutics, and limited drug delivery to the tumor are among several mechanisms underlying therapeutic failure in malignant glioma. Combination therapy and multimodality treatment should have a higher chance of success as they disrupt several targets simultaneously. This paradigm can also apply to gene therapy, virotherapy, and immunotherapy [95]. A polygene therapy approach, including delivery of suicide, cytokine, and antiangiogenic genes may achieve better antitumor efficacy. As reported in other systemic cancers, virotherapy may be more efficacious when combined with chemotherapy and/or radiotherapy.

Immunotherapy with Chemotherapy and Radiation

Several lines of evidence have supported the use of chemotherapy to enhance efficacy of immunotherapy. Combination of low-dose TMZ—a standard chemotherapy in malignant glioma—followed by vaccination with TAT-survivin-pulsed DCs enhanced T-cell responses specific for survivin and improved survival rate, as compared with DCs alone or TMZ alone in a murine model of glioma [96]. Furthermore, a recent clinical study suggested that DC vaccination followed by chemotherapy was associated with prolonged survival [97]. The mechanism of TMZ enhancing immunotherapy efficacy may involve the suppression of regulatory (CD4+CD25+) T cells. In addition, migration of regulatory T cells is in part mediated by CCL2 secreted by glioblastoma, which can be blocked by TMZ or carmustine [98]. Interestingly, a pilot clinical study is ongoing with daclizumab (a monoclonal antibody against CD25) after therapeutic TMZ-induced lymphopenia in the context of vaccinating newly diagnosed adult GBM patients with CMV pp65-lysosomal-associated membrane protein (LAMP) mRNA-loaded DCs with autolymphocyte therapy. In addition to synergistic activity with chemotherapy, immunotherapy can be augmented by radiation as demonstrated in cancer cell vaccines associated with GM-CSF, IL-4, and IL-12 secretion in a murine glioma model [99].

Immunogene Therapy

Escape from immune surveillance is one of the hallmarks of cancers. Immunogene therapy entails genetic manipulation to enhance antitumor immune response. This process may include transfer of proinflammatory cytokine genes, anti-inflammatory cytokine gene inhibitors, and tumor antigen genes or costimulatory molecules to optimize antigen presentation [100]. Gene therapy is an attractive option to deliver cytokines as direct administration of cytokines may be limited by short half-life and local toxicity. A variety of cytokines have been studied in brain tumors, which may include IL-2, IL-4, IL-12, interferons (IFNs), tumor necrosis factor (TNF)-α, and GM-CSF. Methods of cytokine gene delivery include viral and nonviral vectors, and cell-based therapeutics. A recent clinical trial demonstrated safety and encouraging activity of B7-2/GM-CSF gene therapy to increase T-cell costimulation in six glioma patients [101]. In addition, immunogene approaches can be used to improve effectiveness of the HSV-TK/ganciclovir system. Combined delivery of HSV-TK/ganciclovir with human IL-2 gene by retroviral vector to increase antitumor immune response has been evaluated in recurrent GBM patients [102,103]. Treatment was generally well tolerated, although two fatal cases of pulmonary embolism were reported. Response was observed in 50% of patients who had increased plasma Th-1 cytokines, particularly IFN-γ and TNF-α. Post-treatment tumor biopsies revealed tumor necrosis around the injection site and abundant infiltration of activated T cells and macrophages [103].

Vaccination of whole tumor lysate can be potentiated by transducing irradiated tumor cells with GM-CSF. DC therapy may be improved by simultaneous transduction of tumor cells with cytokines such as IFN-β. Several challenges in cytokine gene therapy include identification of the cytokine expression levels in an optimal range for effectiveness and genetic heterogeneity of tumors that leads to emerging resistant cells. Further understanding of the complex interaction between tumors and the immune system may lead to novel immunogene therapeutic approaches.

REFERENCES

1. Fecci PE, Mitchell DA, Whitesides JF, et al. Increased regulatory T-cell fraction amidst a diminished CD4 compartment explains cellular immune defects in patients with malignant glioma. *Cancer Res.* 2006;66:3294–3302.
2. Swann JB, Smyth MJ. Immune surveillance of tumors. *J Clin Invest.* 2007;117(5):1137–1146.
3. Sabatier J, Uro-Coste E, Pommepuy I, et al. Detection of human cytomegalovirus genome and gene products in central nervous system tumours. *Br J Cancer.* 2005;92(4):747–750.
4. Mantovani A, Romero P, Palucka AK, Marincola FM. Tumour immunity: effector response to tumour and role of the microenvironment. *Lancet.* 2008;371(9614):771–783.
5. Jiang X, Lu X, Liu R, Zhang F, Zhao H. HLA Tetramer Based Artificial Antigen-Presenting Cells Efficiently Stimulate CTLs Specific for Malignant Glioma. *Clin Cancer Res.* 2007;13(24):7329–7334.
6. Carpentier AF, Meng Y. Recent advances in immunotherapy for human glioma. *Curr Opin Oncol.* 2006;18(6):631–636.
7. Bullard DE, Gillespie GY, Mahaley MS, Bigner DD. Immunobiology of human gliomas. *Semin Oncol.* 1986;13(1):94–109.
8. Sampson JH, Akabani G, Archer GE, et al. Intracerebral infusion of an EGFR-targeted toxin in recurrent malignant brain tumors. *Neuro-oncology.* 2008;10(3):320–329.
9. Young H, Kaplan A, Regelson W. Immunotherapy with autologous white cell infusions ("lymphocytes") in the treatment of recurrrent glioblastoma multiforme: a preliminary report. *Cancer.* 1977;40(3):1037–1044.
10. Neuwelt EA, Clark K, Kirkpatrick JB, Toben H. Clinical studies of intrathecal autologous lymphocyte infusions in patients with malignant glioma: a toxicity study. *Ann Neurol.* 1978;4(4):307–312.
11. Vaquero J, Martínez R, Ramiro J, Salazar FG, Barbolla L, Regidor C. Immunotherapy of glioblastoma with intratumoural administration of autologous lymphocytes and human lymphoblastoid interferon. A further clinical study. *Acta Neurochir (Wien).* 1991;109(1–2):42–45.
12. Hayes RL, Koslow M, Hiesiger EM, et al. Improved long term survival after intracavitary interleukin-2 and lymphokine-activated killer cells for adults with recurrent malignant glioma. *Cancer.* 1995;76(5):840–852.
13. Barba D, Saris SC, Holder C, Rosenberg SA, Oldfield EH. Intratumoral LAK cell and interleukin-2 therapy of human gliomas. *J Neurosurg.* 1989;70(2):175–182.
14. Sankhla SK, Nadkarni JS, Bhagwati SN. Adoptive immunotherapy using lymphokine-activated killer (LAK) cells and interleukin-2 for recurrent malignant primary brain tumors. *J Neurooncol.* 1996;27(2):133–140.
15. Merchant RE, Grant AJ, Merchant LH, Young HF. Adoptive immunotherapy for recurrent glioblastoma multiforme using lymphokine activated killer cells and recombinant interleukin-2. *Cancer.* 1988;62(4):665–671.
16. Quattrocchi KB, Miller CH, Cush S, et al. Pilot study of local autologous tumor infiltrating lymphocytes for the treatment of recurrent malignant gliomas. *J Neurooncol.* 1999;45(2):141–157.
17. Rosenberg SA, Restifo NP, Yang JC, Morgan RA, Dudley ME. Adoptive cell transfer: a clinical path to effective cancer immunotherapy. *Nat Rev Cancer.* 2008;8(4):299–308.
18. Kruse CA, Cepeda L, Owens B, Johnson SD, Stears J, Lillehei KO. Treatment of recurrent glioma with intracavitary alloreactive cytotoxic T lymphocytes and interleukin-2. *Cancer Immunol Immunother.* 1997;45(2):77–87.
19. Kruse CA, Schiltz PM, Bellgrau D, Kong Q, Kleinschmidt-DeMasters BK. Intracranial administrations of single or multiple source allogeneic cytotoxic T lymphocytes: chronic therapy for primary brain tumors. *J Neurooncol.* 1994;19(2):161–168.
20. Plautz GE, Miller DW, Barnett GH, et al. T cell adoptive immunotherapy of newly diagnosed gliomas. *Clin Cancer Res.* 2000;6(6):2209–2218.
21. de Vleeschouwer S, Rapp M, Sorg RV, et al. Dendritic cell vaccination in patients with malignant gliomas: current status and future directions. *Neurosurgery.* 2006;59(5):988–999; discussioin 999.
22. Heimberger AB, Crotty LE, Archer GE, et al. Bone marrow-derived dendritic cells pulsed with tumor homogenate induce immunity against syngeneic intracerebral glioma. *J Neuroimmunol.* 2000;103(1):16–25.
23. Liau LM, Black KL, Prins RM, et al. Treatment of intracranial gliomas with bone marrow-derived dendritic cells pulsed with tumor antigens. *J Neurosurg.* 1999;90(6):1115–1124.
24. Yu JS, Liu G, Ying H, Yong WH, Black KL, Wheeler CJ. Vaccination with tumor lysate-pulsed dendritic cells elicits antigen-specific, cytotoxic T-cells in patients with malignant glioma. *Cancer Res.* 2004;64(14):4973–4979.
25. Yamanaka R, Homma J, Yajima N, et al. Clinical evaluation of dendritic cell vaccination for patients with recurrent glioma: results of a clinical phase I/II trial. *Clin Cancer Res.* 2005;11(11):4160–4167.
26. Kuan CT, Wikstrand CJ, Bigner DD. EGF mutant receptor vIII as a molecular target in cancer therapy. *Endocr Relat Cancer.* 2001;8(2):83–96.
27. Heimberger AB, Hussain SF, Aldape K, et al. Tumor-specific peptide vaccination in newly-diagnosed patients with GBM. *J Clin Oncol.* 2006;24:2529.
28. Cobbs CS, Harkins L, Samanta M, et al. Human cytomegalovirus infection and expression in human malignant glioma. *Cancer Res.* 2002;62(12):3347–3350.
29. Wang X, Huong SM, Chiu ML, Raab-Traub N, Huang ES. Epidermal growth factor receptor is a cellular receptor for human cytomegalovirus. *Nature.* 2003;424(6947):456–461.
30. Sharkey RM, Goldenberg DM. Targeted therapy of cancer: new prospects for antibodies and immunoconjugates. *CA Cancer J Clin.* 2006;56(4):226–243.
31. Colapinto EV, Lee YS, Humphrey PA, et al. The localisation of radiolabelled murine monoclonal antibody 81C6 and its Fab fragment in human glioma xenografts in athymic mice. *Br J Neurosurg.* 1988;2(2):179–191.
32. Lee YS, Bullard DE, Zalutsky MR, et al. Therapeutic efficacy of antiglioma mesenchymal extracellular matrix 131I-radiolabeled murine monoclonal antibody in a human glioma xenograft model. *Cancer Res.* 1988;48(3):559–566.
33. Reardon DA, Akabani G, Coleman RE, et al. Phase II trial of murine (131)I-labeled antitenascin monoclonal antibody 81C6 administered into surgically created resection cavities of patients with newly diagnosed malignant gliomas. *J Clin Oncol.* 2002;20(5):1389–1397.
34. Reardon DA, Akabani G, Coleman RE, et al. Salvage radioimmunotherapy with murine iodine-131-labeled antitenascin monoclonal antibody 81C6 for patients with recurrent primary and metastatic malignant brain tumors: phase II study results. *J Clin Oncol.* 2006;24(1):115–122.
35. Paganelli G, Grana C, Chinol M, et al. Antibody-guided three-step therapy for high grade glioma with yttrium-90 biotin. *Eur J Nucl Med.* 1999;26(4):348–357.

36. Grana C, Chinol M, Robertson C, et al. Pretargeted adjuvant radioimmunotherapy with yttrium-90-biotin in malignant glioma patients: a pilot study. *Br J Cancer*. 2002;86(2):207–212.
37. Weaver M, Laske DW. Transferrin receptor ligand-targeted toxin conjugate (Tf-CRM107) for therapy of malignant gliomas. *J Neurooncol*. 2003;65(1):3–13.
38. Mamelak AN, Rosenfeld S, Bucholz R, et al. Phase I single-dose study of intracavitary-administered iodine-131-TM-601 in adults with recurrent high-grade glioma. *J Clin Oncol*. 2006;24(22):3644–3650.
39. Weber F, Asher A, Bucholz R, et al. Safety, tolerability, and tumor response of IL4-Pseudomonas exotoxin (NBI-3001) in patients with recurrent malignant glioma. *J Neurooncol*. 2003;64(1–2):125–137.
40. Kunwar S, Prados MD, Chang SM, et al.; Cintredekin Besudotox Intraparenchymal Study Group. Direct intracerebral delivery of cintredekin besudotox (IL13-PE38QQR) in recurrent malignant glioma: a report by the Cintredekin Besudotox Intraparenchymal Study Group. *J Clin Oncol*. 2007;25(7):837–844.
41. Vogelbaum MA, Sampson JH, Kunwar S, et al. Convection-enhanced delivery of cintredekin besudotox (interleukin-13-PE38QQR) followed by radiation therapy with and without temozolomide in newly diagnosed malignant gliomas: phase 1 study of final safety results. *Neurosurgery*. 2007;61(5):1031–1037; discussion 1037.
42. Jarboe JS, Johnson KR, Choi Y, Lonser RR, Park JK. Expression of interleukin-13 receptor alpha2 in glioblastoma multiforme: implications for targeted therapies. *Cancer Res*. 2007;67(17):7983–7986.
43. Sampson JH, Brady ML, Petry NA, et al. Intracerebral infusate distribution by convection-enhanced delivery in humans with malignant gliomas: descriptive effects of target anatomy and catheter positioning. *Neurosurgery*. 2007;60(2 Suppl 1):ONS89–ONS98; discussion ONS98.
44. Sampson JH, Raghavan R, Provenzale JM, et al. Induction of hyperintense signal on T2-weighted MR images correlates with infusion distribution from intracerebral convection-enhanced delivery of a tumor-targeted cytotoxin. *AJR Am J Roentgenol*. 2007;188(3):703–709.
45. Rosenberg SA, Aebersold P, Cornetta K, et al. Gene transfer into humans–immunotherapy of patients with advanced melanoma, using tumor-infiltrating lymphocytes modified by retroviral gene transduction. *N Engl J Med*. 1990;323(9):570–578.
46. Voges J, Reszka R, Gossmann A, et al. Imaging-guided convection-enhanced delivery and gene therapy of glioblastoma. *Ann Neurol*. 2003;54(4):479–487.
47. Yoshida J, Mizuno M, Fujii M, et al. Human gene therapy for malignant gliomas (glioblastoma multiforme and anaplastic astrocytoma) by in vivo transduction with human interferon beta gene using cationic liposomes. *Hum Gene Ther*. 2004;15(1):77–86.
48. Zhang Y, Zhang YF, Bryant J, Charles A, Boado RJ, Pardridge WM. Intravenous RNA interference gene therapy targeting the human epidermal growth factor receptor prolongs survival in intracranial brain cancer. *Clin Cancer Res*. 2004;10(11):3667–3677.
49. Barzon L, Zanusso M, Colombo F, Palù G. Clinical trials of gene therapy, virotherapy, and immunotherapy for malignant gliomas. *Cancer Gene Ther*. 2006;13(6):539–554.
50. Liu TC, Kirn D. Systemic efficacy with oncolytic virus therapeutics: clinical proof-of-concept and future directions. *Cancer Res*. 2007;67(2):429–432.
51. Markert JM, Medlock MD, Rabkin SD, et al. Conditionally replicating herpes simplex virus mutant, G207 for the treatment of malignant glioma: results of a phase I trial. *Gene Ther*. 2000;7(10):867–874.
52. Rampling R, Cruickshank G, Papanastassiou V, et al. Toxicity evaluation of replication-competent herpes simplex virus (ICP 34.5 null mutant 1716) in patients with recurrent malignant glioma. *Gene Ther*. 2000;7(10):859–866.
53. Harrow S, Papanastassiou V, Harland J, et al. HSV1716 injection into the brain adjacent to tumour following surgical resection of high-grade glioma: safety data and long-term survival. *Gene Ther*. 2004;11(22):1648–1658.
54. Papanastassiou V, Rampling R, Fraser M, et al. The potential for efficacy of the modified (ICP 34.5(-)) herpes simplex virus HSV1716 following intratumoural injection into human malignant glioma: a proof of principle study. *Gene Ther*. 2002;9(6):398–406.
55. Chiocca EA, Abbed KM, Tatter S, et al. A phase I open-label, dose-escalation, multi-institutional trial of injection with an E1B-Attenuated adenovirus, ONYX-015, into the peritumoral region of recurrent malignant gliomas, in the adjuvant setting. *Mol Ther*. 2004;10(5):958–966.
56. Schneider T, Gerhards R, Kirches E, Firsching R. Preliminary results of active specific immunization with modified tumor cell vaccine in glioblastoma multiforme. *J Neurooncol*. 2001;53(1):39–46.
57. Freeman AI, Zakay-Rones Z, Gomori JM, et al. Phase I/II trial of intravenous NDV-HUJ oncolytic virus in recurrent glioblastoma multiforme. *Mol Ther*. 2006;13(1):221–228.
58. Martuza RL, Malick A, Markert JM, Ruffner KL, Coen DM. Experimental therapy of human glioma by means of a genetically engineered virus mutant. *Science*. 1991;252(5007):854–856.
59. Hunter WD, Martuza RL, Feigenbaum F, et al. Attenuated, replication-competent herpes simplex virus type 1 mutant G207: safety evaluation of intracerebral injection in nonhuman primates. *J Virol*. 1999;73(8):6319–6326.
60. Geoerger B, Grill J, Opolon P, et al. Oncolytic activity of the E1B-55 kDa-deleted adenovirus ONYX-015 is independent of cellular p53 status in human malignant glioma xenografts. *Cancer Res*. 2002;62(3):764–772.
61. Liu C, Sarkaria JN, Petell CA, et al. Combination of measles virus virotherapy and radiation therapy has synergistic activity in the treatment of glioblastoma multiforme. *Clin Cancer Res*. 2007;13(23):7155–7165.
62. Csatary LK, Bakács T. Use of Newcastle disease virus vaccine (MTH-68/H) in a patient with high-grade glioblastoma. *JAMA*. 1999;281(17):1588–1589.
63. Sathornsumetee S, Reardon DA, Desjardins A, Quinn JA, Vredenburgh JJ, Rich JN. Molecularly targeted therapy for malignant glioma. *Cancer*. 2007;110(1):13–24.
64. Steiner HH, Bonsanto MM, Beckhove P, et al. Antitumor vaccination of patients with glioblastoma multiforme: a pilot study to assess feasibility, safety, and clinical benefit. *J Clin Oncol*. 2004;22(21):4272–4281.
65. Gromeier M, Lachmann S, Rosenfeld MR, Gutin PH, Wimmer E. Intergeneric poliovirus recombinants for the treatment of malignant glioma. *Proc Natl Acad Sci USA*. 2000;97(12):6803–6808.
66. Culver KW, Ram Z, Wallbridge S, Ishii H, Oldfield EH, Blaese RM. In vivo gene transfer with retroviral vector-producer cells for treatment of experimental brain tumors. *Science*. 1992;256(5063):1550–1552.
67. Miletic H, Fischer YH, Giroglou T, et al. Normal brain cells contribute to the bystander effect in suicide gene therapy of malignant glioma. *Clin Cancer Res*. 2007;13(22 Pt 1):6761–6768.
68. Zhao P, Wang C, Fu Z, et al. Lentiviral vector mediated siRNA knockdown of hTERT results in diminished capacity in invasiveness and in vivo growth of human glioma cells in a telomere length-independent manner. *Int J Oncol*. 2007;31(2):361–368.
69. Harding TC, Dickinson PJ, Roberts BN, et al. Enhanced gene transfer efficiency in the murine striatum and an orthotopic glioblastoma tumor model, using AAV-7- and AAV-8-pseudotyped vectors. *Hum Gene Ther*. 2006;17(8):807–820.
70. Barba D, Hardin J, Sadelain M, Gage FH. Development of anti-tumor immunity following thymidine kinase-mediated killing of experimental brain tumors. *Proc Natl Acad Sci USA*. 1994;91(10):4348–4352.
71. Ram Z, Culver KW, Oshiro EM, et al. Therapy of malignant brain tumors by intratumoral implantation of retroviral vector-producing cells. *Nat Med*. 1997;3(12):1354–1361.
72. Shand N, Weber F, Mariani L, et al. A phase 1–2 clinical trial of gene therapy for recurrent glioblastoma multiforme by tumor transduction with the herpes simplex thymidine kinase gene followed by ganciclovir. GLI328 European-Canadian Study Group. *Hum Gene Ther*. 1999;10(14):2325–2335.
73. Prados MD, McDermott M, Chang SM, et al. Treatment of progressive or recurrent glioblastoma multiforme in adults with herpes simplex virus thymidine kinase gene vector-producer cells followed by intravenous ganciclovir administration: a phase I/II multi-institutional trial. *J Neurooncol*. 2003;65(3):269–278.
74. Rainov NG. A phase III clinical evaluation of herpes simplex virus type 1 thymidine kinase and ganciclovir gene therapy as an adjuvant to surgical resection and radiation in adults with previously untreated glioblastoma multiforme. *Hum Gene Ther*. 2000;11(17):2389–2401.
75. Sandmair AM, Loimas S, Puranen P, et al. Thymidine kinase gene therapy for human malignant glioma, using replication-deficient retroviruses or adenoviruses. *Hum Gene Ther*. 2000;11(16):2197–2205.
76. Immonen A, Vapalahti M, Tyynelä K, et al. AdvHSV-tk gene therapy with intravenous ganciclovir improves survival in human malignant glioma: a randomised, controlled study. *Mol Ther*. 2004;10(5):967–972.
77. Trask TW, Trask RP, Aguilar-Cordova E, et al. Phase I study of adenoviral delivery of the HSV-tk gene and ganciclovir

administration in patients with current malignant brain tumors. *Mol Ther.* 2000;1(2):195–203.
78. Lang FF, Bruner JM, Fuller GN, et al. Phase I trial of adenovirus-mediated p53 gene therapy for recurrent glioma: biological and clinical results. *J Clin Oncol.* 2003;21(13):2508–2518.
79. Germano IM, Fable J, Gultekin SH, Silvers A. Adenovirus/herpes simplex-thymidine kinase/ganciclovir complex: preliminary results of a phase I trial in patients with recurrent malignant gliomas. *J Neurooncol.* 2003;65(3):279–289.
80. Smitt PS, Driesse M, Wolbers J, Kros M, Avezaat C. Treatment of relapsed malignant glioma with an adenoviral vector containing the herpes simplex thymidine kinase gene followed by ganciclovir. *Mol Ther.* 2003;7(6):851–858.
81. Lawler SE, Peruzzi PP, Chiocca EA. Genetic strategies for brain tumor therapy. *Cancer Gene Ther.* 2006;13(3):225–233.
82. Wang WJ, Tai CK, Kasahara N, Chen TC. Highly efficient and tumor-restricted gene transfer to malignant gliomas by replication-competent retroviral vectors. *Hum Gene Ther.* 2003;14(2):117–127.
83. Gomez-Manzano C, Balague C, Alemany R, et al. A novel E1A-E1B mutant adenovirus induces glioma regression in vivo. *Oncogene.* 2004;23(10):1821–1828.
84. Todo T, Martuza RL, Rabkin SD, Johnson PA. Oncolytic herpes simplex virus vector with enhanced MHC class I presentation and tumor cell killing. *Proc Natl Acad Sci USA.* 2001;98(11):6396–6401.
85. Kambara H, Okano H, Chiocca EA, Saeki Y. An oncolytic HSV-1 mutant expressing ICP34.5 under control of a nestin promoter increases survival of animals even when symptomatic from a brain tumor. *Cancer Res.* 2005;65(7):2832–2839.
86. Lamfers ML, Grill J, Dirven CM, et al. Potential of the conditionally replicative adenovirus Ad5-Delta24RGD in the treatment of malignant gliomas and its enhanced effect with radiotherapy. *Cancer Res.* 2002;62(20):5736–5742.
87. Lee J, Elkahloun AG, Messina SA, et al. Cellular and genetic characterization of human adult bone marrow-derived neural stem-like cells: a potential antiglioma cellular vector. *Cancer Res.* 2003;63(24):8877–8889.
88. Brown AB, Yang W, Schmidt NO, et al. Intravascular delivery of neural stem cell lines to target intracranial and extracranial tumors of neural and non-neural origin. *Hum Gene Ther.* 2003;14(18):1777–1785.
89. Moore XL, Lu J, Sun L, Zhu CJ, Tan P, Wong MC. Endothelial progenitor cells' "homing" specificity to brain tumors. *Gene Ther.* 2004;11(10):811–818.
90. Nakamura K, Ito Y, Kawano Y, et al. Antitumor effect of genetically engineered mesenchymal stem cells in a rat glioma model. *Gene Ther.* 2004;11(14):1155–1164.
91. Miura F, Moriuchi S, Maeda M, et al. Sustained release of low-dose ganciclovir from a silicone formulation prolonged the survival of rats with gliosarcomas under herpes simplex virus thymidine kinase suicide gene therapy. *Gene Ther.* 2002;9(24):1653–1658.
92. Wiewrodt R, Amin K, Kiefer M, et al. Adenovirus-mediated gene transfer of enhanced Herpes simplex virus thymidine kinase mutants improves prodrug-mediated tumor cell killing. *Cancer Gene Ther.* 2003;10(5):353–364.
93. Tyynelä K, Sandmair AM, Turunen M, et al. Adenovirus-mediated herpes simplex virus thymidine kinase gene therapy in BT4C rat glioma model. *Cancer Gene Ther.* 2002;9(11):917–924.
94. Desaknai S, Lumniczky K, Esik O, Hamada H, Safrany G. Local tumour irradiation enhances the anti-tumour effect of a double-suicide gene therapy system in a murine glioma model. *J Gene Med.* 2003;5(5):377–385.
95. Selznick LA, Shamji MF, Fecci P, Gromeier M, Friedman AH, Sampson J. Molecular strategies for the treatment of malignant glioma–genes, viruses, and vaccines. *Neurosurg Rev.* 2008;31(2):141–155; discussion 155.
96. Kim CH, Woo SJ, Park JS, et al. Enhanced antitumour immunity by combined use of temozolomide and TAT-survivin pulsed dendritic cells in a murine glioma. *Immunology.* 2007;122(4):615–622.
97. Wheeler CJ, Das A, Liu G, Yu JS, Black KL. Clinical responsiveness of glioblastoma multiforme to chemotherapy after vaccination. *Clin Cancer Res.* 2004;10(16):5316–5326.
98. Jordan JT, Sun W, Hussain SF, DeAngulo G, Prabhu SS, Heimberger AB. Preferential migration of regulatory T cells mediated by glioma-secreted chemokines can be blocked with chemotherapy. *Cancer Immunol Immunother.* 2008;57(1):123–131.
99. Lumniczky K, Desaknai S, Mangel L, et al. Local tumor irradiation augments the antitumor effect of cytokine-producing autologous cancer cell vaccines in a murine glioma model. *Cancer Gene Ther.* 2002;9(1):44–52.
100. Cheuk AT, Mufti GJ, Guinn BA. Role of 4–1BB:4–1BB ligand in cancer immunotherapy. *Cancer Gene Ther.* 2004;11(3):215–226.
101. Parney IF, Chang LJ, Farr-Jones MA, Hao C, Smylie M, Petruk KC. Technical hurdles in a pilot clinical trial of combined B7–2 and GM-CSF immunogene therapy for glioblastomas and melanomas. *J Neurooncol.* 2006;78(1):71–80.
102. Colombo F, Barzon L, Franchin E, et al. Combined HSV-TK/IL-2 gene therapy in patients with recurrent glioblastoma multiforme: biological and clinical results. *Cancer Gene Ther.* 2005;12(10):835–848.
103. Palù G, Cavaggioni A, Calvi P, et al. Gene therapy of glioblastoma multiforme via combined expression of suicide and cytokine genes: a pilot study in humans. *Gene Ther.* 1999;6(3):330–337.

79 Other Therapies

Daniela A. Bota and David A. Reardon

INTRODUCTION

Primary brain tumors continue to remain one of the major challenges in the world of oncology. There are about 18,500 new cases diagnosed every year in the United States, and currently 350,000 people are affected by this severe disease [1]. The most common of these tumors (50%) are of glial origin and high grade (glioblastoma multiforme [GBM] and anaplastic astrocytoma).

Although the outcome of the protean group of brain tumors is highly variable, the most common is disability and death. The standard of care established for malignant gliomas consists of surgery, radiotherapy, and chemotherapy with the alkylating agent temozolomide, and it has led to an overall survival (OS) of 14.6 months [2]. The need to develop more effective treatments remains paramount to improve outcome.

Modern research in the field of neuro-oncology follows general oncology trends, focusing on the development of targeted treatments to specific molecular mechanisms involved in abnormal signaling and resistance to apoptosis. Two important classes of new agents are retinoids and histone deacetylase (HDAC) inhibitors.

RETINOIC ACIDS (RETINOIDS)

Background

Retinoic acids (RAs) are essential molecules involved in development during embryogenesis [3] as well as in mature adults by regulating cell growth, differentiation, and death [4–6]. The action of RAs is mediated by their nuclear retinoid (RARα, β, and γ) and rexinoid (RXRα, β, and γ) receptors, which form active heterodimers responsible for the mediation of RAs cellular mechanisms. These receptors belong to the steroid/thyroid hormone receptor family and regulate the expression of multiple target genes [7], establishing genetic networks that are essentials for embryological development [3]. RAs are especially important in the brain by regulating organogenesis [4] and organ homeostasis.

Pharmacology and Preclinical Data

Retinoids are derivates of dietary vitamin A and provitamin β-carotene of plants. After uptake in the intestinal tract, retinol is esterified to retinyl esters and stored in the liver. A small proportion of the plasma retinol is converted to all-*trans* retinoic acid (ATRA), which functions as the main signaling retinoid in the body. 13-*cis*-retinoic acid is a metabolite of ATRA [8]. Numerous synthetic retinoids are also available, which have selective effects on the six types of retinoid receptors [9] and are able to exert apoptotic activity that is not mediated by retinoid receptors [10].

Vitamin A, as well as its derivatives, is fat soluble and transported in plasma linked with binding proteins. Both ATRA and 13-*cis*-retinoic acid have good water solubility, which make them excellent candidates for the treatment of brain tumors, owing to their ability to diffuse efficiently through water-soluble phases as well as hydrophobic membranes such as the blood-brain barrier [11,12].

ATRA has the capacity to induce cell cycle arrest and apoptosis in many types of malignant cells such as leukemia [13], melanoma [14], and pancreatic [15] and gastric malignancies [16]. ATRA inhibits human glioma cell proliferation and migration and induces apoptosis [17]. In medulloblastoma, ATRA induces cell growth arrest by decreasing the expression of cyclin D1 and C-myc, which regulate cell cycle transition [18]. In the clinic, ATRA has become part of the standard of treatment for promyelocytic leukemia [19].

13-*cis*-retinoic acid binds to all three subtypes of RA receptors. In malignant glioma cell cultures, it induces astrocytic differentiation as well as apoptosis and cell death [20] and in combination with interferon-α2a enhances radiosensitization [21]. 13-*cis*-retinoic acid has shown promising activity in combination with the HDAC inhibitor suberoylanilide hydroxamic acid (SAHA) in preclinical models of medulloblastoma [22]. 13-*cis*-retinoic acid significantly improves event-free survival in patients with high-risk neuroblastoma [23], and it is the standard treatment for oral cancer prevention in patients with leukoplakia [24].

Fenretinide (4-hydroxyphenyl-retinamide) is a synthetic retinoid with activity against numerous tumor types [25–27]. Its mechanism of action is different from the classical retinoids, as it induces apoptosis by generating free radicals and by activating the ceramide pathway by both retinoid receptor-dependent and -independent pathways [28]. Fenretinide is more potent than 13-*cis*-retinoic acid in inducing cell death at equimolar concentrations in malignant glioma cell models [29] and can cross the blood-brain barrier in animal studies [30], which supports its use in therapeutic trials for patients with brain tumors. Fenretinide also induces apoptotic cell death in human medulloblastoma cells [31]. In clinical trials, fenretinide has shown efficacy in preventing a second breast malignancy in premenopausal females [32].

Clinical Experience with RAs in Malignant Gliomas

Based on highly encouraging preclinical data, a variety of RAs have been tested for newly diagnosed and recurrent malignant gliomas as well as for maintenance therapy for patients who have achieved complete response after completing radiation and chemotherapy. Initial studies, conducted using RAs as monotherapy, were associated with limited success. However, more recent studies, using RAs in combination therapy with different chemotherapeutic agents, are showing promise for the treatment of malignant gliomas. The use of RAs in the treatment of other primary adult brain tumors is unclear because of limited data. However, encouraging anecdotal cases have been reported including long-term survival in a patient with a relapsing malignant meningioma treated with a combination of 13-cis-retinoic acid and BCNU [33] and another patient with resolution of a recurrent malignant ganglioglioma after treatment with 13-cis-retinoic acid [34].

Newly Diagnosed Malignant Glioma

Three clinical trials (two in adults and one in pediatric patients) have used 13-cis-retinoic acid for patients with newly diagnosed malignant glioma.

The first study is a three-institution, phase II trial that enrolled a total of 40 patients with GBM ($n = 36$) and anaplastic astrocytoma ($n = 4$) [35]. The patients received a combination of 13-cis-retinoic acid (1 mg/kg 4 times a day, 5 days a week) and interferon-$\alpha 2\alpha$ (3–6 million IU sq 4 times a day, 3 days a week) during delivery of focal brain radiation (59.4 Gy over 7 weeks) and for 9 weeks after the completion of radiation therapy, for a total of 16 weeks. The median OS was 9.3 months, and the 1-year survival rate was 42%, which is inferior to the survival data from the current standard regimen using temozolomide during and after radiation [2]. The most significant toxicities seen in this study were severe rash, including Stevens-Johnson syndrome in two patients who were also receiving phenytoin, elevated serum triglycerides, fatigue, and malaise.

The second study was conducted at the University of California San Francisco and enrolled 61 patients with newly diagnosed GBM [36]. The treatment regimen consisted of a combination of 13-cis-retinoic acid administered at 50 mg/m^2 twice a day for 3 weeks every 4 weeks during and after radiation and temozolomide dosed at 75 mg/m^2/day during radiation therapy, followed by 150 to 200 mg/m^2/day for 5 days every 28 days for 1 year after radiation therapy or until disease progression. Focal beam radiation was administered to a total of 60 Gy over 6 weeks. In this study, the 6-month progression-free survival (PFS) was 38%, and the 1-year PFS was 15%, which suggested no therapeutic advantage of adding 13-cis-retinoic acid to the initial treatment of patients with GBM. No grade 5 adverse events were reported, and the most common side effects were myelosuppression, fatigue, and nausea/vomiting.

In the pediatric population, a small phase II clinical trial ($n = 12$) studied the regimen of concurrent radiotherapy with temozolomide followed by adjuvant temozolomide and 13-cis-retinoic acid in patients with diffuse intrinsic pontine glioma. The median time to progression was 10 months, the 1-year PFS was 41.7%, and the 1-year OS was 58% ± 14.2%. The results are encouraging, and a large clinical trial is underway [37].

Recurrent Malignant Glioma

Three different retinoids were studied for the treatment of relapsed malignant glioma: 13-cis-retinoic acid, ATRA, and fenretinide.

(a) 13-cis-retinoic acid activity in recurrent gliomas was evaluated as monotherapy and as combination therapy with temozolomide and with celecoxib, respectively.

The monotherapy phase II trial enrolled patients with recurrent malignant glioma ($n = 50$), who received 13-cis-retinoic acid at a dose of 60 to 100 mg/m^2/day for 3 weeks, followed by a week of rest [38]. The median time to progression was 16 weeks, and the median survival for GBM was 58 weeks. A more recent retrospective study from the same institution analyzed the effectiveness of 13-cis-retinoic acid in patients with recurrent GBM ($n = 85$) [39]. Reported PFS was 10 weeks, and the 6-month PFS was 19%, comparable with other classical chemotherapy drugs. Grade 3 or 4 toxicities developed in 16% of the patients, and one patient died of pancreatitis.

The North American Brain Tumor Consortium evaluated the combination of 13-cis-retinoic acid plus temozolomide in adult patients with malignant glioma who failed first-line chemotherapy [40]. Treatment consisted of temozolomide 150 to 200 mg/m^2/day days 1 to 5 and 13-cis-retinoic acid 100 mg/m^2/day days 1 to 21 every 28 days. The combination showed very promising activity, with 6-month PFS of 43% (32% for glioblastoma and 50% for anaplastic astrocytoma) and a median OS of 47 weeks.

The combination of celecoxib and 13-cis-retinoic acid in the treatment of recurrent GBM was less effective, with a median PFS of 8 weeks and a 6-month PFS of 19% [41]. Based on the single-agent studies, adding celecoxib did not improve patient outcome versus 13-cis-retinoic acid alone.

(b) Three phase II clinical trials evaluated the efficacy of ATRA as a single agent in adult patients with recurrent malignant glioma.

MD Anderson conducted a phase II study including 36 patients with recurrent glioma who were treated with 120 mg or 150 mg/m^2/day of ATRA as a single agent. The higher dose was associated with more side effects, mainly severe headaches, which resolved with dose reduction, but did not show superior efficacy compared with the lower dose. The median time to progression was 8 weeks and suggests that ATRA has no activity as a single agent in the treatment of recurrent gliomas [42].

The Radiation Therapy Oncology Group (RTOG) has also completed a single-agent ATRA trial for patients with recurrent malignant glioma (RTOG91–13). Most common toxicities seen were dry skin, cheilitis, anemia, and headaches. The response rate was 12%, confirming the minimal efficacy of ATRA as monotherapy in this disease setting.

A small study had also addressed the effect of combining ATRA with cytosine arabinoside in relapsing malignant gliomas [43]. All nine patients were treated with ATRA at 90 mg/day and six patients also received cytosine arabinoside (4 g/course, 1 to 9 courses every 4 weeks). All four responding patients received the combination therapy, with a median time to progression of 9 months. This stabilization was associated with the appearance of intratumoral calcifications visualized on repeated computed tomography scans.

(c) Fenretinide as single agent was evaluated in a multicenter, phase II clinical trial conducted by the North American Brain Tumor Consortium (NSC 374551) [44]. Forty-five patients with recurrent anaplastic glioma ($n = 21$) and recurrent GBM ($n = 23$) received fenretinide dosed at either 600 or 900 mg/m^2 twice daily on days 1 to 7 and 22 to 28 in 6-week cycles. The median PFS was reported as 6 weeks for both anaplastic glioma and GBM groups, and the study was closed after the first analysis because of the lack of activity. Only grades 1 and 2 toxicities were reported.

Maintenance Therapy for Patients with Stable Disease after Discontinuing Chemotherapy

One of the Most Challenging tasks in neuro-oncology is the prevention of tumor relapse for patients with high-grade glioma who have completed planned therapy without disease progression. The retinoids inhibit tumor growth and proliferation in vitro [17] and in vivo [45], which justified the use of 13-*cis*-retinoic acid in a clinical trial aiming to prevent malignant glioma recurrence. A phase II study using 13-*cis*-retinoic acid as maintenance therapy enrolled 23 patients with histologically confirmed grade III ($n = 13$) and grade IV ($n = 10$) gliomas, who showed complete response to treatment (surgery, radiation, chemotherapy) based on Macdonald criteria (no residual gadolinium enhancing lesions) [46]. The patients were treated with 13-*cis*-retinoic acid 60 mg/m^2 (days 1–21 of 28-day cycles), with dose escalation up to 100 mg/m^2 if well tolerated or until tumor recurrence. The treatment was tolerated very well for up to 149 weeks, with moderate dermatological symptoms such as dryness of skin and mucous membranes and ocular symptoms (xerophthalmia and conjunctivitis). Median time to progression was 41 weeks. The median OS was 74 weeks after the inclusion in the protocol (63 weeks for GBM) and 133 weeks from the initial diagnosis (114 weeks for GBM). These results are very encouraging, but a two-arm controlled clinical trial is needed to confirm 13-*cis*-retinoic acid efficacy in preventing malignant glioma relapse.

Current Clinical Trials

Based on the previous published studies showing modest activity of retinoids in multiple-drugs regimens among recurrent malignant gliomas, additional combination therapies are currently being investigated. Four clinical trials are actively enrolling patients looking at the following treatment regimens: temozolomide, thiotepa, and carboplatin with autologous stem cell rescue followed by 13-*cis*-retinoic acid; temozolomide and radiation therapy followed by temozolomide and RA; procarbazine and isotretinoin; and vorinostat and isotretinoin. The results of these studies will guide future decisions regarding the incorporation of retinoids into multimodality regimens for malignant glioma.

Summary

RAs have been extensively studied in preclinical malignant glioma models with encouraging results. However, combinations using 13-*cis*-retinoic acid and interferon-2α or temozolomide for newly diagnosed malignant glioma, as well as 13-*cis*-retinoic acid and celecoxib in recurrent glioblastoma, did not show superior efficacy compared with the currently accepted treatment paradigm for this disease. Clinical trials using different retinoids as single agents for the treatment of recurrent malignant gliomas also failed to show significant clinical benefit. Most encouraging results were obtained by combining 13-*cis*-retinoic acid and temozolomide for recurrent patients, supporting the use of this combination in clinical practice. The use of 13-*cis*-retinoic acid to delay malignant glioma recurrence after completing standard therapy is also promising but awaits confirmation in a controlled clinical trial. The results of currently enrolling studies will shed more light on the optimal use of this promising class of agents in clinical practice.

HDAC INHIBITORS

Background

Histone proteins are responsible for organizing the DNA structure into nucleosomes, which represent the principal protein-nucleic acid complex found in chromatin and which are involved in regulation of gene expression [47]. Chromatin architecture is modulated by acetylation of these histones, which, in turn, affect gene expression [48]. The opposing activities of histone acetyltransferases (HATs) and HDACs closely regulate these processes [49]. HATs transfer acetyl groups to amino-terminal lysine residues in histones, which lead to local expansion of chromatin and increased accessibility of regulatory proteins to DNA [50]. Conversely, HDACs catalyze the removal of acetyl groups, leading to chromatin condensation and transcriptional repression [51].

Epigenetic changes, defined by DNA methylation patterns and associated posttranslational modifications of nuclear histones, have recently been implicated in cancer pathogenesis [52]. Several distinct families of HAT proteins have altered activity in cancer, including the GCN5/PCAF, p300/CBP, and MYST families [50]. For example, missense mutations of p300 have been identified in colorectal and breast cancer as well as 80% of GBM. Similarly, altered expression of HDACs, which comprise 18 family members and are divided into four classes, have been reported in several malignancies, including breast, colon, prostate, gastric, and cervical cancer. In addition, more than 50 nonhistone proteins have been identified that are HDAC substrates, including several regulators of cell proliferation, migration, and survival [53]. Consequently, there has been considerable interest in the development of HDAC inhibitors.

There are many classes of HDAC inhibitors that include short-chain fatty acids such as valproic acid and 4-phenylbutyrate, hydroxamic acids such as SAHA (vorinostat), pyroxamide, TSA, oxamflatin and CHAPs, cyclic tetrapeptides (trapoxin, apicidin, and depsipeptide), and benzamides (MS-275) [52].

Pharmacology and Preclinical Data

HDAC inhibitors can release transcriptional repression of tumor suppressor genes as well as genes involved in cell cycle progression and differentiation. They have also been shown to cause growth arrest and death in a variety of cancer models [54] as well as to inhibit angiogenesis by altering vascular endothelial growth factor signaling [55].

Preclinical studies demonstrate potent antitumor activity of HDAC inhibitors against primary central nervous system tumors including medulloblastoma [56] and malignant gliomas [57–59]. In malignant glioma lines, treatment with HDAC inhibitors alone resulted in a dose-response increase in the G2/M cell-phase arrest, apoptosis induction, increased expression of the cyclin-dependent kinase inhibitor p21, and decreased progrowth signals [59], while in combination with radiotherapy, a synergistic effect in increasing the level of DNA double strands breaks and inhibition of cell proliferation is seen [60].

Moreover, many HADC inhibitors are able to disrupt cellular redox state, to regulate p53 expression, as well as disrupt the hsp90 chaperone function—a crucial mechanism for tumor resistance to apoptosis [61]. Furthermore, HDAC inhibitors are synergistic with multiple classes of chemotherapy including etoposide, camptothecin, cisplatin, doxorubicin, 5-FU, and cyclophosphamide [27]. SAHA and TSA are also able to dramatically reduce cell viability and promote apoptosis in multiple-drug-resistant cell lines, with makes HDAC inhibitors uniquely suited for treatment of recurrent disease [62].

Many HDAC inhibitors such as SAHA (vorinostat), AN-9, and MS-275 are able to cross the blood-brain barrier in animal models, inhibit xenograft growth, and increase histone (H_3, H_4) acetylation [61], which makes these drugs very promising agents for clinical testing in patients with brain tumor.

Clinical Experience with HDAC Inhibitors in Malignant Gliomas

SAHA (vorinostat) is the first HDAC inhibitor FDA approved for the treatment of cancer, namely, for patients with cutaneous T-cell lymphoma [63], and is currently being studied in clinical trials for recurrent GBM. An interim analysis of a single-agent phase II study was recently presented, at which time 68 patients were actively enrolled [64]. The vorinostat dose was 200 mg twice a day for 14 days every 3 weeks. The most common toxicities were fatigue, diarrhea, and thrombocytopenia. The trial met the prospectively defined primary efficacy endpoint at the planned interim analysis with 5 of the first 22 patients (23%) being progression-free at 6 months. The final results of this trial are eagerly awaited.

The North American Brain Tumor Consortium is conducting a phase I study of vorinostat in combination with temozolomide in patients with malignant gliomas, and preliminary results are available [65]. All patients received temozolomide at a dose of 150 mg/m²/day on days 1 to 5 every 28 days. Variable doses of vorinostat were administered, and the maximum tolerated dose of vorinostat in combination with temozolomide was identified as 300 mg daily on days 1 to 14 every 28 days.

Current Clinical Trials

Three clinical trials are actively researching the use of HDAC inhibitors for the treatment of malignant gliomas. The first is recruiting patients with newly diagnosed GBM for a phase II trial studying the efficacy of adding valproic acid to standard treatment with temozolomide and radiation. In the recurrent setting, separate clinical trials are evaluating the combinations of valproic acid and etoposide for patients with progressive, relapsed, or refractory neuronal tumors and brain metastases (phase I), and of vorinostat, isotretinoin, and carboplatin in adults with recurrent GBM (phase I/II), respectively. More HDAC inhibitors are in various stages of preclinical development for brain tumors and are planned to enter clinical trials in the near future.

Summary

HDAC inhibitors represent a new class of targeted anticancer agents. Several drugs from this class show promising activity in preclinical models of malignant glioma, and preliminary results of vorinostat trials are encouraging. Additional preclinical studies to evaluate how to optimize these agents when administered with chemotherapy, radiotherapy, or other molecularly targeted therapies will be highly informative. In addition, results of ongoing clinical trials will provide critical insight into the role of HDAC inhibitors in the treatment of malignant glioma.

REFERENCES

1. CBTRUS. *Primary Brain Tumors in the United States. Statistical Report 1997–2001.* Chicago: Central Brain Tumor Registry of the United States; 2004–2005.
2. Stupp R, Mason WP, van den Bent MJ, et al.; European Organisation for Research and Treatment of Cancer Brain Tumor and Radiotherapy Groups; National Cancer Institute of Canada Clinical Trials Group. Radiotherapy plus concomitant and adjuvant temozolomide for glioblastoma. *N Engl J Med.* 2005;352(10):987–996.
3. Niederreither K, Subbarayan V, Dollé P, Chambon P. Embryonic retinoic acid synthesis is essential for early mouse post-implantation development. *Nat Genet.* 1999;21(4):444–448.

4. Krezel W, Ghyselinck N, Samad TA, et al. Impaired locomotion and dopamine signaling in retinoid receptor mutant mice. *Science*. 1998;279(5352):863–867.
5. Massaro GD, Massaro D. Retinoic acid treatment partially rescues failed septation in rats and in mice. *Am J Physiol Lung Cell Mol Physiol*. 2000;278(5):L955-L960.
6. Massaro GD, Massaro D, Chan WY, et al. Retinoic acid receptor-beta: an endogenous inhibitor of the perinatal formation of pulmonary alveoli. *Physiol Genomics*. 2000;4(1):51–57.
7. Blomhoff R, Blomhoff HK. Overview of retinoid metabolism and function. *J Neurobiol*. 2006;66(7):606–630.
8. Arnhold T, Tzimas G, Wittfoht W, Plonait S, Nau H. Identification of 9-cis-retinoic acid, 9,13-di-cis-retinoic acid, and 14-hydroxy-4,14-retro-retinol in human plasma after liver consumption. *Life Sci*. 1996;59:PL169-PL177.
9. Bourguet W, Vivat V, Wurtz JM, Chambon P, Gronemeyer H, Moras D. Crystal structure of a heterodimeric complex of RAR and RXR ligand-binding domains. *Mol Cell*. 2000;5(2):289–298.
10. de Lera AR, Bourguet W, Altucci L, Gronemeyer H. Design of selective nuclear receptor modulators: RAR and RXR as a case study. *Nat Rev Drug Discov*. 2007;6(10):811–820.
11. Lin HS, Leong WW, Yang JA, Lee P, Chan SY, Ho PC. Biopharmaceutics of 13-cis-retinoic acid (isotretinoin) formulated with modified beta-cyclodextrins. *Int J Pharm*. 2007;341(1–2):238–245.
12. Szuts EZ, Harosi FI. Solubility of retinoids in water. *Arch Biochem Biophys*. 1991;287(2):297–304.
13. Zhang JW, Wang JY, Chen SJ, Chen Z. Mechanisms of all-trans retinoic acid-induced differentiation of acute promyelocytic leukemia cells. *J Biosci*. 2000;25(3):275–284.
14. Jacob K, Wach F, Holzapfel U, et al. In vitro modulation of human melanoma cell invasion and proliferation by all-trans-retinoic acid. *Melanoma Res*. 1998;8(3):211–219.
15. Guo J, Xiao B, Lou Y, et al. Antitumor effects of all-trans-retinoic acid on cultured human pancreatic cancer cells. *J Gastroenterol Hepatol*. 2006;21(2):443–448.
16. Zhang JP, Chen XY, Li JS. Effects of all-trans-retinoic on human gastric cancer cells BGC-823. *J Dig Dis*. 2007;8(1):29–34.
17. Bouterfa H, Picht T, Kess D, et al. Retinoids inhibit human glioma cell proliferation and migration in primary cell cultures but not in established cell lines. *Neurosurgery*. 2000;46(2):419–430.
18. Chang Q, Chen Z, You J, et al. All-trans-retinoic acid induces cell growth arrest in a human medulloblastoma cell line. *J Neurooncol*. 2007;84(3):263–267.
19. Lazzarino M, Regazzi MB, Corso A. Clinical relevance of all-trans retinoic acid pharmacokinetics and its modulation in acute promyelocytic leukemia. *Leuk Lymphoma*. 1996;23(5–6):539–543.
20. Das A, Banik NL, Ray SK. Retinoids induced astrocytic differentiation with down regulation of telomerase activity and enhanced sensitivity to taxol for apoptosis in human glioblastoma T98G and U87MG cells. *J Neurooncol*. 2008;87(1):9–22.
21. Malone C, Schiltz PM, Nayak SK, Shea MW, Dillman RO. Combination interferon-alpha2a and 13-cis-retinoic acid enhances radiosensitization of human malignant glioma cells in vitro. *Clin Cancer Res*. 1999;5(2):417–423.
22. Spiller SE, Ditzler SH, Pullar BJ, Olson JM. Response of preclinical medulloblastoma models to combination therapy with 13-cis retinoic acid and suberoylanilide hydroxamic acid (SAHA). *J Neurooncol*. 2008;87(2):133–141.
23. Matthay KK, Villablanca JG, Seeger RC, et al. Treatment of high-risk neuroblastoma with intensive chemotherapy, radiotherapy, autologous bone marrow transplantation, and 13-cis-retinoic acid. Children's Cancer Group. *N Engl J Med*. 1999;341(16):1165–1173.
24. Scardina GA, Carini F, Maresi E, Valenza V, Messina P. Evaluation of the clinical and histological effectiveness of isotretinoin in the therapy of oral leukoplakia: ten years of experience: is management still up to date and effective? *Methods Find Exp Clin Pharmacol*. 2006;28(2):115–119.
25. Bu P, Wan YJ. Fenretinide-induced apoptosis of Huh-7 hepatocellular carcinoma is retinoic acid receptor beta dependent. *BMC Cancer*. 2007;7:236.
26. Kadara H, Lacroix L, Lotan D, Lotan R. Induction of endoplasmic reticulum stress by the pro-apoptotic retinoid N-(4-hydroxyphenyl)retinamide via a reactive oxygen species-dependent mechanism in human head and neck cancer cells. *Cancer Biol Ther*. 2007;6(5):705–711.
27. Kim MS, Blake M, Baek JH, Kohlhagen G, Pommier Y, Carrier F. Inhibition of histone deacetylase increases cytotoxicity to anticancer drugs targeting DNA. *Cancer Res*. 2003;63(21):7291–7300.
28. Wu JM, DiPietrantonio AM, Hsieh TC. Mechanism of fenretinide (4-HPR)-induced cell death. *Apoptosis*. 2001;6(5):377–388.
29. Puduvalli VK, Saito Y, Xu R, Kouraklis GP, Levin VA, Kyritsis AP. Fenretinide activates caspases and induces apoptosis in gliomas. *Clin Cancer Res*. 1999;5(8):2230–2235.
30. Le Doze F, Debruyne D, Albessard F, Barre L, Defer GL. Pharmacokinetics of all-trans retinoic acid, 13-cis retinoic acid, and fenretinide in plasma and brain of Rat. *Drug Metab Dispos*. 2000;28(2):205–208.
31. Damodar Reddy C, Guttapalli A, Adamson PC, et al. Anticancer effects of fenretinide in human medulloblastoma. *Cancer Lett*. 2006;231(2):262–269.
32. Veronesi U, Mariani L, Decensi A, et al. Fifteen-year results of a randomized phase III trial of fenretinide to prevent second breast cancer. *Ann Oncol*. 2006;17(7):1065–1071.
33. Westarp ME, Westarp MP, Grundl W, Biesalski H, Kornhuber HH. Improving medical approaches to primary CNS malignancies--retinoid therapy and more. *Med Hypotheses*. 1993;41(3):267–276.
34. Kaba SE, Langford LA, Yung WK, Kyritsis AP. Resolution of recurrent malignant ganglioglioma after treatment with cis-retinoic acid. *J Neurooncol*. 1996;30(1):55–60.
35. Dillman RO, Shea WM, Tai DF, et al. Interferon-alpha2a and 13-cis-retinoic acid with radiation treatment for high-grade glioma. *Neuro-oncology*. 2001;3(1):35–41.
36. Butowski N, Prados MD, Lamborn KR, et al. A phase II study of concurrent temozolomide and cis-retinoic acid with radiation for adult patients with newly diagnosed supratentorial glioblastoma. *Int J Radiat Oncol Biol Phys*. 2005;61(5):1454–1459.
37. Sirachainan N, Pakasakama S, Visudithbhan A, et al. Concurrent radiotherapy with temozolomide followed by adjuvant temozolomide and cis-retinoic acid in children with diffuse intrinsic pontine glioma. *Neuro-oncology*. 2008;10(4):577–582.
38. Yung WK, Kyritsis AP, Gleason MJ, Levin VA. Treatment of recurrent malignant gliomas with high-dose 13-cis-retinoic acid. *Clin Cancer Res*. 1996;2(12):1931–1935.
39. See SJ, Levin VA, Yung WK, Hess KR, Groves MD. 13-cis-retinoic acid in the treatment of recurrent glioblastoma multiforme. *Neuro-oncology*. 2004;6(3):253–258.
40. Jaeckle KA, Hess KR, Yung WK, et al.; North American Brain Tumor Consortium. Phase II evaluation of temozolomide and 13-cis-retinoic acid for the treatment of recurrent and progressive malignant glioma: a North American Brain Tumor Consortium study. *J Clin Oncol*. 2003;21(12):2305–2311.
41. Levin VA, Giglio P, Puduvalli VK, et al. Combination chemotherapy with 13-cis-retinoic acid and celecoxib in the treatment of glioblastoma multiforme. *J Neurooncol*. 2006;78(1):85–90.
42. Kaba SE, Kyritsis AP, Conrad C, et al. The treatment of recurrent cerebral gliomas with all-trans-retinoic acid (tretinoin). *J Neurooncol*. 1997;34(2):145–151.
43. Defer GL, Adle-Biassette H, Ricolfi F, et al. All-trans retinoic acid in relapsing malignant gliomas: clinical and radiological stabilization associated with the appearance of intratumoral calcifications. *J Neurooncol*. 1997;34(2):169–177.
44. Puduvalli VK, Yung WK, Hess KR, et al.; North American Brain Tumor Consortium. Phase II study of fenretinide (NSC 374551) in adults with recurrent malignant gliomas: A North American Brain Tumor Consortium study. *J Clin Oncol*. 2004;22(21):4282–4289.
45. Rodts GE Jr, Black KL. Trans retinoic acid inhibits in vivo tumour growth of C6 glioma in rats: effect negatively influenced by nerve growth factor. *Neurol Res*. 1994;16(3):184–186.
46. Macdonald DR, Cascino TL, Schold SC Jr, Cairncross JG. Response criteria for phase II studies of supratentorial malignant glioma. *J Clin Oncol*. 1990;8(7):1277–1280.
47. Kornberg RD, Lorch Y. Twenty-five years of the nucleosome, fundamental particle of the eukaryote chromosome. *Cell*. 1999;98(3):285–294.
48. Davie JR. Covalent modifications of histones: expression from chromatin templates. *Curr Opin Genet Dev*. 1998;8(2):173–178.

49. Kim DH, Kim M, Kwon HJ. Histone deacetylase in carcinogenesis and its inhibitors as anti-cancer agents. *J Biochem Mol Biol.* 2003;36(1):110–119.
50. Acharya MR, Sparreboom A, Venitz J, Figg WD. Rational development of histone deacetylase inhibitors as anticancer agents: a review. *Mol Pharmacol.* 2005;68(4):917–932.
51. Kouzarides T. Histone acetylases and deacetylases in cell proliferation. *Curr Opin Genet Dev.* 1999;9(1):40–48.
52. Marks P, Rifkind RA, Richon VM, Breslow R, Miller T, Kelly WK. Histone deacetylases and cancer: causes and therapies. *Nat Rev Cancer.* 2001;1(3):194–202.
53. Marks PA, Rifkind RA, Richon VM, Breslow R. Inhibitors of histone deacetylase are potentially effective anticancer agents. *Clin Cancer Res.* 2001;7(4):759–760.
54. Marks PA, Breslow R. Dimethyl sulfoxide to vorinostat: development of this histone deacetylase inhibitor as an anticancer drug. *Nat Biotechnol.* 2007;25(1):84–90.
55. Deroanne CF, Bonjean K, Servotte S, et al. Histone deacetylases inhibitors as anti-angiogenic agents altering vascular endothelial growth factor signaling. *Oncogene.* 2002;21(3):427–436.
56. Sonnemann J, Kumar KS, Heesch S, et al. Histone deacetylase inhibitors induce cell death and enhance the susceptibility to ionizing radiation, etoposide, and TRAIL in medulloblastoma cells. *Int J Oncol.* 2006;28(3):755–766.
57. Chinnaiyan P, Vallabhaneni G, Armstrong E, Huang SM, Harari PM. Modulation of radiation response by histone deacetylase inhibition. *Int J Radiat Oncol Biol Phys.* 2005;62(1):223–229.
58. Eyüpoglu IY, Hahnen E, Buslei R, et al. Suberoylanilide hydroxamic acid (SAHA) has potent anti-glioma properties in vitro, ex vivo and in vivo. *J Neurochem.* 2005;93(4):992–999.
59. Yin D, Ong JM, Hu J, et al. Suberoylanilide hydroxamic acid, a histone deacetylase inhibitor: effects on gene expression and growth of glioma cells *in vitro* and in vivo. *Clin Cancer Res.* 2007;13(3):1045–1052.
60. Entin-Meer M, Yang X, VandenBerg SR, et al. *In vivo* efficacy of a novel histone deacetylase inhibitor in combination with radiation for the treatment of gliomas. *Neuro-oncology.* 2007;9(2):82–88.
61. Eyüpoglu IY, Hahnen E, Tränkle C, et al. Experimental therapy of malignant gliomas using the inhibitor of histone deacetylase MS-275. *Mol Cancer Ther.* 2006;5(5):1248–1255.
62. Castro-Galache MD, Ferragut JA, Barbera VM, et al. Susceptibility of multidrug resistance tumor cells to apoptosis induction by histone deacetylase inhibitors. *Int J Cancer.* 2003;104(5):579–586.
63. Mann BS, Johnson JR, Cohen MH, Justice R, Pazdur R. FDA approval summary: vorinostat for treatment of advanced primary cutaneous T-cell lymphoma. *Oncologist.* 2007;12(10):1247–1252.
64. Galanis E, Jaeckle KA, Maurer MJ, et al. N047B: NCCTG phase II trial of vorinostat (suberoylanilide hydroxamic acid) in recurrent glioblastoma multiforme (GBM). 2007 ASCO Annual Meeting Proceedings Part I. *J Clin Oncol.* 2007;25:2004.
65. Wen P, Puduvalli VK, Kuhn J, et al. Phase I study of vorinostat (suberoylanilide hydroxamic acid [SAHA]) in combination with temozolomide in patients with malignant gliomas (NABTC 04–03). Twelfth Annual Meeting of the Society for Neuro-Oncology 2007:518.

80 Alternative Therapies

Raymond Liu

INTRODUCTION

The National Center for Complementary and Alternative Medicine (NCCAM) defines complementary and alternative medicine (CAM) as "a group of diverse medical and health care systems, practices, and products that are not presently considered to be part of conventional medicine [1]." Therefore, CAM covers a broad realm of modalities that supplement conventional medicines.

The five main modalities of CAM, as proposed by the NCCAM, are as follows: alternative medical systems (i.e., Chinese medicine, Ayurveda, homeopathy, naturopathy, etc.), mind-body modalities (i.e., meditation, prayer, etc.), biologically based modalities (herbal products, dietary supplements, etc.), manipulative and body-based therapies (i.e., massage, etc.), and energy-based modalities (i.e., Qigong, Reishi, etc.). Although these categories provide some organization to the vast array of CAM therapies, many of the individual treatments classified as CAM may cross over several of these modalities. For example, Chinese medicine may employ herbal products as well as energy-based Qigong. Qigong is energy based, but elements of Qigong employed in Tai Chi are also considered mind-body therapy.

Patients with brain tumors seek alternative therapies for many reasons. They may be attempting to prevent the occurrence of a brain tumor or to improve tumor control. In addition, patients are seeking additional modalities for symptom management, either from the tumor itself or treatment-related effects. Also, patients may seek CAM to decrease their sense of helplessness and to improve their sense of control over their illness [2–4].

CAM IN PATIENTS WITH BRAIN TUMOR

The literature on CAM in patients with brain tumor has been mostly descriptive in nature. In studies, measured use of CAM therapies by patients with brain tumor ranges from 24% to 34% [3–5]. The most common type of alternative therapy used is biologically based therapy. Cost of CAM therapies range from $55 to $69 a month, although there may be underreporting of actual costs [3,4].

A prospective study of CAM use in the primary brain tumor population at MD Andersen was performed by Armstrong et al [3]. This group reported that 34% of patients use CAM; 74% of these patients reported that their physicians were unaware of their CAM use, and 88% expressed satisfaction that the CAM was helpful and contributed to tumor shrinkage. Analysis of data revealed that a higher performance status was the only factor significantly related to the use of CAM.

Another CAM study in patients with brain tumor reported on data collected from the Glioma Outcomes Project [5]. In this study, 32.3% of patients with high-grade glioma were users of complementary and alternative practices and products. Users tended to be female, younger, and with higher education, similar to figures reported for the general cancer population [6]. At enrollment, those who used complementary and alternative practices and products had higher mean scores in quality of life. The patients were recruited from 51 hospitals, from both academic centers and the community. However, only patients with high-grade glioma were enrolled, and missing data were significant.

A third study of patients who visited a cancer center in Southern Alberta, Canada, found CAM use to be around 24%. Patients who used CAM were younger but, in contrast to the preceding studies, tended to have lower quality of life. Together, these studies suggest that CAM use among patients with brain tumor is common and likely underreported.

BIOLOGICALLY BASED THERAPIES

The largest body of literature of CAM in patients with brain tumor is related to biologically based therapies. Melatonin, cannabis, and nutritional supplements have been tested, but mostly in the preclinical setting. These CAM interventions have not been rigorously tested, and potential interactions with conventional therapies have not been well studied. The major barriers that remain before these types of compounds can be recommended for clinical use are standardization of supplement formulation, determining the physiological dosing of these compounds necessary for effect, and testing these compounds in large-scale clinical trials. The National Institutes of Health Office of Dietary Supplements (ods.od.nih.gov) and the US Food and Drug Administration Office for Food Safety and Applied Nutrition (cfsan.fda.gov) are potential resources for more information on biologically based therapies used in the United States.

Melatonin

Melatonin is a hormone made nocturnally in the human pineal gland, which acts to promote sleep and regulates circadian rhythms. Melatonin is generally well tolerated, with few reported side effects at doses that ranged from 1 to 36 mg [7]. Melatonin can inhibit glioma cell growth in cell culture [8,9], but few clinical studies have been performed on its use. A single randomized study of 30 patients with glioblastoma receiving radiotherapy has been performed. One-year survival was 43% in those randomized to receive 20 mg/day of melatonin by mouth compared with 6% in those who received radiotherapy alone [10]. Larger trials are needed to establish whether melatonin has antitumor effects. Given melatonin's effect on circadian rhythms, those with sleep disturbance would be an ideal population to test such an intervention.

Marijuana

The plant from which marijuana is derived is cannabis. Data supporting the use of cannabis in patients with brain tumor are mostly preclinical. Potential pathways of glioma inhibition by cannabis include promotion of apoptotic death [11,12] and regulation of tumor angiogenesis [13]. Down-regulation of metalloproteinases-1 inhibitors may also play a role [14]. In addition, cannabinoid receptors are expressed in glioma stem cells, and cannabinoid stimulation can induce cell differentiation and inhibit gliomagenesis [15]. Cannabinoid administration to mice with glioma xenografts has been reported to cause regression of gliomas [16].

The only reported clinical data on cannabis in patients with brain tumor so far is a phase I trial demonstrating the safety of direct intratumoral injection of tetrahydrocannabinol, one of the main active ingredients in cannabis, in patients with recurrent glioblastoma [17]. The effectiveness of cannabis in controlling glioma growth and the methods of administration of active ingredients have not been determined in clinical trials. However, because of marijuana's purported benefit in improving nausea and vomiting, it would be an ideal agent to test in conjunction with other therapies that may induce emesis.

Nutritional Supplements

There are many categories of commonly used nutritional supplements, such as phytoestrogens (i.e., soy), polysaccharide peptides (i.e., mushroom extracts), fatty acids (i.e., primrose oil, fish oil), flavonoids, antioxidants, and antiinflammatory agents. Because in most cases, no formal clinical studies have been performed on supplements and supplements are not regulated by the US Food and Drug Administration in the same way as pharmaceutical products, limited clinical information about formulation and dosing is available. In addition, potential interactions with conventional therapies have not been well studied with these agents. More standardization and research is needed to help define the roles of these supplements in patients with brain tumor.

Nutritional Supplements/Phytoestrogens

Phytoestrogens are plant-derived chemicals that have antioxidative and estrogenic properties. They can be categorized as isoflavones (genistein, daidzein, biochanin A, formononetin), lignins (matairesinol, secoisolariciresinol), and coumestans (coumestrol). Phytoestrogens can be found in soy, lentil, and beans. Some epidemiological evidence exists that phytoestrogen intake [18], in particular the isoflavone daidzein, may be associated with a decreased incidence of gliomas [19]. No prospective clinical trials have been performed to confirm the epidemiological findings. However, preclinical data have been generated on the effect of the isoflavone genistein on glioblastoma cell culture growth. In particular, there is a synergistic effect of genistein and bischloroethyl-nitrosourea on glioblastoma cells [20]. Genestein is thought to have multiple potential actions, including inhibition of epidermal growth factor receptor, inhibition of angiogenesis, inhibition of topoisomerase II, and inhibition of matrix metalloprotease-2 [21].

Nutritional Supplements/Polysaccharide peptides

Krestin (PSK) is a commonly used polysaccharide peptide in Japan for different cancers and comes from the extract of the mushroom *Coriolus versicolor*. Another extract from the *Coriolus versicolor* mushroom called PSP is more commonly used in China. PSK/PSP extract has purported antioxidant and immune properties, with in vivo as well as in vitro activation of natural killer cells and lymphocytes [22,23]. A clinical study from Japan has been performed with polysaccharide peptides in combination with chemotherapy, but no conclusions can be drawn given the small sample size and lack of a control population [24].

Nutritional Supplements/Fatty acids

Unsaturated fatty acids have been studied in gliomas. Gamma-linolenic acid (GLA) found in primrose oil has been the most extensively examined, although mostly in the preclinical setting. The literature on GLA in brain tumors has been recently reviewed [25]. GLA can suppress the expression of Bcl-2 and ras, enhance p53 activity, and form lipid peroxides owing to increased free-radical generation in tumor cells. GLA has also been shown to selectively kill rat astrocytoma cells and enhance the cytotoxic action of radiation because of its incorporation into the cell membrane [26]. In cell culture, GLA also increased apoptosis in several different human glioma cell lines [27]. GLA has been injected intratumorally in patients with glioma, but definitive conclusions cannot be made given that all three studies were underpowered and lacked a control population [28–30].

Unsaturated fatty acids such as eicosapentaenoic acid and docosahexanoic acid found in fish oil have been less studied in gliomas [25]. In neuroblastoma cell cultures, docosahexanoic acid was able to induce time- and dose-dependent cell death [31]. In glioblastoma cell lines, docosahexanoic acid has improved the cytotoxicity of doxorubicin [32].

In contrast to unsaturated fatty acids, saturated fatty acids may actually stimulate tumor growth in cell culture. For example, palmitate (fatty acid found in butter, cheese, and milk) may induce glioma cell growth through Acyl-Co-A synthetase [33].

Nutritional Supplements/Vitamin D

The purported mechanism of action of vitamin D and its analogues is in promoting redifferentiation of malignant cells. Effects of vitamin D on glioblastoma cell lines [34–38] and gene expression of rat C6.9 glioma cells undergoing apoptosis from vitamin D have been examined [39]. In addition, the role of vitamin D analogue alfacalcidiol (10alpha-hydroxycholecalciferol) was examined in a case series of 11 patients with malignant glioma, in conjunction with either VM26 and CCNU, or fotemustine. In this study, three patients responded to combined chemotherapy and vitamin D [40]. As vitamin D was not tested separately, it is not possible to determine if responses were secondary to chemotherapy alone. Clearly, more rigorous studies into different vitamin D analogues and their effect on gliomas are needed prior to widespread use of this strategy. Monitoring of serum calcium should be performed if testing this supplement.

Nutritional Supplements/Flavonoids

Flavonoids are plant compounds that are thought to have multiple properties including antioxidant, antiinflammatory, and antiangiogenesis properties (see Table 80.1). No studies to date have been performed on patients with brain tumor with these compounds, although there have been preclinical experiments.

Nutritional Supplements/Antioxidants

Epidemiological evidence on antioxidant intake and the risk of adult gliomas is discouraging—the two prospective studies that have examined intake of fruit, vegetables, and carotenoids have not shown a correlation between dietary intake of antioxidants and glioma risk [48,49]. Carotenoids such as lycopene are examples of antioxidants that have also been examined in preclinical settings [50] and in one small study of patients with newly diagnosed high-grade glioma [51]. The study comparing placebo to lycopene with radiation and concurrent paclitaxel chemotherapy in high-grade gliomas showed a trend toward improved response rates and time to progression with lycopene use, but further studies are needed to validate this finding [51].

Nutritional Supplements/Antiinflammatory Agents

Boswellic acids are obtained from extracts of gum resin and are thought to have antiinflammatory properties [52]. They have also been shown in cell cultures to induce apoptosis [53,54] and in rat models to inhibit glioma growth [55], although they do not appear to improve survival in one study of patients with glioblastoma [54].

Nutritional Supplements/Selenium

The role of selenium supplementation has been studied in brain tumors. In cell culture, selenium can reduce tumor growth and induce apoptosis [56–58]. Potential mechanisms of action include inhibition of protein kinase C [59], angiogenesis [60], or regulation of cellular immune responses [61]. Selenium supplementation may improve survival in rat glioma models [62]. Selenium supplementation also appears well tolerated in patients with brain tumor [63,64], but adequately powered and controlled studies remain lacking.

Miscellaneous Supplements

Several other supplements are commercially available and have been tested in cell culture and/or limited animal experiments, but they have not been formally tested in patients with brain tumor (Table 80.2).

Dietary Restriction

Although addition of supplements to conventional therapy is popular, reduction of intake has also been considered. Moderate dietary restriction has been studied in mouse models and may contribute to decreased tumor growth in these models [92,93]. In another mouse model experiment, dietary restriction designed to reduce plasma glucose levels reduced brain tumor growth [94]. The mechanism of action of caloric restriction may be in its effect on angiogenesis and/or induction of apoptosis. An attempt to maintain a ketogenic diet was reported in two pediatric patients with advanced malignant astrocytic tumors [95], but no formal investigations have been undertaken in patients with brain tumor.

Copper Depletion

The role of copper depletion has been studied in patients with brain tumor. Copper levels in some brain tumors may be elevated compared with normal [96,97]. In vivo experiments

Table 80.1 Some Flavonoids, Proposed Mechanism of Action(s), and Level of Evidence in Brain Tumor Patients

Flavonoid	Proposed Mechanism of Action(s)	Level of Evidence in Brain Tumors
Apigenin	Antiangiogenesis	Cell culture data but minimal effect in vivo [41]
Chrysin	Antiinflammatory, induction of apoptosis, anti-oxidant, block cell-cycle progression	Cell culture [42]
Kaempherol	Induction of apoptosis	Cell culture [43]
Silibinin, i.e., milk thistle	Induction of apoptosis, EGFR inhibitor	Cell culture [44,45]
Quercetin	Induction of apoptosis	Cell culture [46,47]

Abbreviation: EGFR, epidermal growth factor receptor.

Table 80.2 Miscellaneous Supplements, Proposed Mechanism of Action(s), and Level of Evidence in the Brain Tumor Population

Supplement (Active Ingredient)	Proposed Mechanism of Action(s)	Level of Evidence in Brain Tumors
Angelica sinesis roots (unknown)	Induction of apoptosis	Cell culture, in vivo [65]
Broccoli (sulphoraphane)	Induction of apoptosis	Cell culture [66]
Garlic (organosulfur compounds)	Induction of apoptosis	Cell culture [67,68]
Goldenseal (Berberine)	Radiation sensitizer	Cell culture, in vivo [75–78]
Grapes and berries (Resveratrol)	Induction of apoptosis, anti-angiogenesis, antioxidant, anti-inflammatory	Cell culture, in vivo [79–84]
Green tea (epigallocatechin-3-galate—EGCG)	Anti-angiogenesis, radio-sensitizer, antimatrix metalloproteinase, PDGF inhibition	Cell culture [69–74]
Pineapple stems (Bromelian)	Reduction of tumor cell adhesion, migration and invasion	Cell culture [85]
Shark liver oil (Alkylglycerols)	Inhibiting invasion	Cell culture [86]
Triterpenoids (oleanolic acid, ursolic acid)	Induction of apoptosis, anti-inflammatory	Cell culture [87]
Tumeric (Curcumin)	Antiangiogenesis, cell-cycle arrest	Cell culture [88–91]

Abbreviation: PDGF, platelet derived growth factor.

suggest that copper may be important for tumor angiogenesis and invasion [98–101]. Copper depletion and penicillamine was tested as an antiangiogenesis strategy in a small group of patients with newly diagnosed glioblastoma [102]. Unfortunately, the study did not show improvement in survival compared with historical controls.

ALTERNATIVE MEDICAL SYSTEMS

Alternative medical systems are whole medical systems that employ multiple modalities to complement standard medical care. For example, traditional Chinese medicine may employ biologically based therapies (i.e., mushroom extracts, etc.) as well as energy-based therapies (i.e., acupuncture, etc.) and integrate these therapies into standard medical care. Research into these systems of care is currently still focused on individual components of integrative care rather than whole systems of care. Challenges to researching these whole systems remain, as treatment under these systems is often nonstandardized and highly individualized.

MIND-BODY THERAPIES

Typical mind-body modalities include hypnosis, guided imagery, meditation, yoga, biofeedback, Tai Chi, and cognitive-behavioral therapies. Literature on these therapies has been focused on the purported connection between the mind and other autonomous systems such as immune function, the endocrine system, and autonomic functioning. The placebo effect is thought to be a result of such a connection [103]. In patients with cancer, the effect of behavioral therapies has been reviewed [104]. Behavioral therapies may be effective in controlling anticipatory nausea and vomiting [105] and in decreasing levels of anxiety. Hypnotic therapy in particular may have a role in managing cancer-related pain [104]. No particular studies with these types of behavioral interventions have addressed patients with brain tumors directly.

NCCAM also designates other therapies such as prayer, mental healing, art, music, or dance as mind-body CAM, although no research has particularly addressed the role that these therapies play in the treatment of brain tumors. Intercessory prayer has been studied and is discussed under energy-based therapies.

NCCAM no longer designates support groups as a mind-body CAM, as it is well integrated into conventional care. This highlights one of the difficulties with studying CAM, as definitions of alternative therapies change as some practices become more mainstream and more widely accepted by the medical community.

BODY-BASED THERAPIES

Body-based therapies employ the use of physical manipulation of tissues to obtain a desired effect. Examples of body-based therapies include massage and chiropractic and osteopathic manipulation. Limited preclinical models have addressed the mechanism of actions of body-based therapies. However, their effect may be mediated through effects on the nervous system [106,107].

Little is known about the utilization or effectiveness of body-based therapies in patients with brain tumors. One study of caregivers of patients with brain tumors showed that most caregivers would like to receive more information about stress-reduction programs including body-based therapies such as massage [108].

Literature on the effectiveness of aromatherapy and massage for palliation of symptoms in patients with cancer has been reviewed [109]. There was limited evidence to support the use of massage on reducing anxiety in the short term, with no clear evidence to any additional benefit of aromatherapy to massage. A recent randomized controlled trial on aromatherapy massage in patients with cancer noted a potential short-term benefit of the intervention on psychological well-being [110]. The study showed an improvement in clinical anxiety and/or depression compared with usual care at 6 weeks postintervention which did not remain significant 10 weeks after the intervention. In another small study, aromatherapy massage was reported to subjectively promote relaxation in a population of eight patients with brain tumors, but it did not improve psychological well-being as measured by the Hospital Anxiety and Depression Scale [111].

ENERGY-BASED THERAPIES

NCCAM divides energy therapies into two types of energy: veritable and putative. Veritable energies use electromagnetic waves or mechanical vibrations for treatment and are measurable and reproducible. In contrast, putative energy fields (biofields) are unmeasurable with conventional instruments but are purportedly detectable by practitioners in the field. Examples of veritable energy therapy include light therapy or magnetic waves. Examples of putative energy fields include Reiki, Johrei, Qigong, therapeutic touch, acupuncture, and intercessory prayer.

Research in veritable energies in brain tumors has recently focused on alternating electric fields. It is postulated that "tumor-treating fields"—low-intensity intermediate frequency electric fields—inhibit cell growth via an antimicrotubule mechanism in cell culture and animal tumor models [112,113]. Ten patients with glioblastoma were also tested with the "tumor-treating fields" and the therapy was well tolerated [113]. A phase III trial has been initiated in patients with recurrent or progressive glioblastoma, randomizing patients to treatment with tumor-treating electric fields (NovoTTF-100a/Novocure) versus best standard of care.

Limited research in veritable energy therapy has also been performed. One small study found an increase in cell proliferation of normal brain cells when treated with Qigong, which became nonsignificant when retested with a larger sample size [114]. Studies using Johrei on glioblastoma multiforme cell culture compared with controls [115], and on primary human glial cells exposed to radiation [116], showed no effect.

Intercessory prayer has been researched in the brain tumor population. Pilot research suggests that patients with brain tumor and their spouses are in need of existential support [117]. Furthermore, small studies have supported the concept of a relationship between distant intentionality and brain function [118–121]. Unfortunately, studies on intercessory prayer have been poorly designed and underpowered. Furthermore, a recent Cochrane collaboration review on the use of intercessory prayer in alleviating ill health confirmed no consistent benefit of prayer in health outcomes [122]. In relation to patients with brain tumor, data from an NCCAM-sponsored randomized double-blind controlled study on the efficacy of distant healing in glioblastoma treatment suggest that anonymous distant healing does not provide a survival advantage for patients with newly diagnosed glioblastomas (unpublished data). In studying the role of intercessory prayer, fundamental questions remain on the timing and "dose" of prayer and finding adequate control populations. There are also questions about whether existential matters can truly be studied using traditional clinical protocols.

Although evidence for an antitumor effect is lacking, some energy therapies may improve symptom control. For example, a National Institutes of Health consensus statement in 1997 did note that there is sufficient evidence that needle acupuncture can treat adult postoperative and chemotherapy-induced nausea and vomiting [123]. The mechanism of action of this effect has not been fully elucidated.

CONCLUSIONS

The use of CAMs in patients with brain tumor is common and understudied. Biologically based therapies are the most commonly used CAM intervention by patients with brain tumor in the United States. High-quality evidence is lacking for most of these interventions, and further research and standardization is imperative to advance our understanding of this field.

There are many challenges that make it difficult to advance CAM research [124]. Previous literature has used different definitions of what constitutes CAM, which has led to wildly different estimates of actual CAM use among patients with cancer. In addition, there is no standardization for the actual interventions, and preclinical and clinical data for the interventions are often lacking. Furthermore, appropriate quality control and monitoring procedures during intervention studies are necessary to continue to advance the field. It is becoming increasingly important to develop a better understanding of these alternative therapies as the complexity of standard medical interventions increases and the potential for interactions between CAM and conventional medicine rises. Further standardization, followed by stronger preclinical data informing well-conducted clinical research, is needed to advance our understanding of this field.

REFERENCES

1. What is CAM? National Institutes of Health, 2007. http://nccam.nih.gov/health/whatiscam/. Accessed September 25, 2007.
2. Paltiel O, Avitzour M, Peretz T, et al. Determinants of the use of complementary therapies by patients with cancer. *J Clin Oncol.* 2001;19(9):2439–2448.
3. Armstrong T, Cohen MZ, Hess KR, et al. Complementary and alternative medicine use and quality of life in patients with primary brain tumors. *J Pain Symptom Manage.* 2006;32(2):148–154.
4. Verhoef MJ, Hagen N, Pelletier G, Forsyth P. Alternative therapy use in neurologic diseases: use in brain tumor patients. *Neurology.* 1999;52(3):617–622.
5. Fox S, Laws ER Jr, Anderson F Jr, Farace E. Complementary therapy use and quality of life in persons with high-grade gliomas. *J Neurosci Nurs.* 2006;38(4):212–220.
6. Mao JJ, Farrar JT, Xie SX, Bowman MA, Armstrong K. Use of complementary and alternative medicine and prayer among a national sample of cancer survivors compared to other populations without cancer. *Complement Ther Med.* 2007;15(1):21–29.
7. Morera AL, Henry M, de La Varga M. [Safety in melatonin use]. *Actas Esp Psiquiatr.* 2001;29(5):334–337.
8. Martín V, Herrera F, Carrera-Gonzalez P, et al. Intracellular signaling pathways involved in the cell growth inhibition of glioma cells by melatonin. *Cancer Res.* 2006;66(2):1081–1088.
9. González A, Martínez-Campa C, Mediavilla MD, Alonso-González C, Sánchez-Barceló EJ, Cos S. Inhibitory effects of pharmacological doses of melatonin on aromatase activity and expression in rat glioma cells. *Br J Cancer.* 2007;97(6):755–760.
10. Lissoni P, Meregalli S, Nosetto L, et al. Increased survival time in brain glioblastomas by a radioneuroendocrine strategy with radiotherapy plus melatonin compared to radiotherapy alone. *Oncology.* 1996;53(1):43–46.
11. Carracedo A, Gironella M, Lorente M, et al. Cannabinoids induce apoptosis of pancreatic tumor cells via endoplasmic reticulum stress-related genes. *Cancer Res.* 2006;66(13):6748–6755.
12. McAllister SD, Chan C, Taft RJ, et al. Cannabinoids selectively inhibit proliferation and induce death of cultured human glioblastoma multiforme cells. *J Neurooncol.* 2005;74(1):31–40.
13. Pisanti S, Borselli C, Oliviero O, Laezza C, Gazzerro P, Bifulco M. Antiangiogenic activity of the endocannabinoid anandamide: correlation to its tumor-suppressor efficacy. *J Cell Physiol.* 2007;211(2):495–503.

14. Blázquez C, Carracedo A, Salazar M, et al. Down-regulation of tissue inhibitor of metalloproteinases-1 in gliomas: a new marker of cannabinoid antitumoral activity? *Neuropharmacology.* 2008;54(1):235–243.
15. Aguado T, Carracedo A, Julien B, et al. Cannabinoids induce glioma stem-like cell differentiation and inhibit gliomagenesis. *J Biol Chem.* 2007;282(9):6854–6862.
16. Galve-Roperh I, Sánchez C, Cortés ML, Gómez del Pulgar T, Izquierdo M, Guzmán M. Anti-tumoral action of cannabinoids: involvement of sustained ceramide accumulation and extracellular signal-regulated kinase activation. *Nat Med.* 2000;6(3):313–319.
17. Guzmán M, Duarte MJ, Blázquez C, et al. A pilot clinical study of Delta9-tetrahydrocannabinol in patients with recurrent glioblastoma multiforme. *Br J Cancer.* 2006;95(2):197–203.
18. Chen H, Ward MH, Tucker KL, et al. Diet and risk of adult glioma in eastern Nebraska, United States. *Cancer Causes Control.* 2002;13(7):647–655.
19. Tedeschi-Blok N, Lee M, Sison JD, Miike R, Wrensch M. Inverse association of antioxidant and phytoestrogen nutrient intake with adult glioma in the San Francisco Bay Area: a case-control study. *BMC Cancer.* 2006;6:148.
20. Khoshyomn S, Nathan D, Manske GC, Osler TM, Penar PL. Synergistic effect of genistein and BCNU on growth inhibition and cytotoxicity of glioblastoma cells. *J Neurooncol.* 2002;57(3):193–200.
21. Puli S, Lai JC, Bhushan A. Inhibition of matrix degrading enzymes and invasion in human glioblastoma (U87MG) cells by isoflavones. *J Neurooncol.* 2006;79(2):135–142.
22. Fisher M, Yang LX. Anticancer effects and mechanisms of polysaccharide-K (PSK): implications of cancer immunotherapy. *Anticancer Res.* 2002;22(3):1737–1754.
23. Mao XW, Green LM, Gridley DS. Evaluation of polysaccharopeptide effects against C6 glioma in combination with radiation. *Oncology.* 2001;61(3):243–253.
24. Kaneko S, Abe H, Aida T, et al. [Evaluation of radiation immunochemotherapy in the treatment of malignant glioma. Combined use of ACNU, VCR and PS-K]. *Hokkaido Igaku Zasshi.* 1983;58(6):622–630.
25. Das UN. Gamma-linolenic acid therapy of human glioma-a review of in vitro, in vivo, and clinical studies. *Med Sci Monit.* 2007;13(7):RA119–31.
26. Vartak S, McCaw R, Davis CS, Robbins ME, Spector AA. Gamma-linolenic acid (GLA) is cytotoxic to 36B10 malignant rat astrocytoma cells but not to 'normal' rat astrocytes. *Br J Cancer.* 1998;77(10):1612–1620.
27. Bell HS, Wharton SB, Leaver HA, Whittle IR. Effects of N-6 essential fatty acids on glioma invasion and growth: experimental studies with glioma spheroids in collagen gels. *J Neurosurg.* 1999;91(6):989–996.
28. Das UN, Prasad VV, Reddy DR. Local application of gamma-linolenic acid in the treatment of human gliomas. *Cancer Lett.* 1995;94(2):147–155.
29. Bakshi A, Mukherjee D, Bakshi A, Banerji AK, Das UN. Gamma-linolenic acid therapy of human gliomas. *Nutrition.* 2003;19(4):305–309.
30. Naidu MR, Das UN, Kishan A. Intratumoral gamma-linoleic acid therapy of human gliomas. *Prostaglandins Leukot Essent Fatty Acids.* 1992;45(3):181–184.
31. Lindskog M, Gleissman H, Ponthan F, Castro J, Kogner P, Johnsen JI. Neuroblastoma cell death in response to docosahexaenoic acid: sensitization to chemotherapy and arsenic-induced oxidative stress. *Int J Cancer.* 2006;118(10):2584–2593.
32. Rudra PK, Krokan HE. Cell-specific enhancement of doxorubicin toxicity in human tumour cells by docosahexaenoic acid. *Anticancer Res.* 2001;21(1A):29–38.
33. Yamashita Y, Kumabe T, Cho YY, et al. Fatty acid induced glioma cell growth is mediated by the acyl-CoA synthetase 5 gene located on chromosome 10q25.1-q25.2, a region frequently deleted in malignant gliomas. *Oncogene.* 2000;19(51):5919–5925.
34. Magrassi L, Butti G, Pezzotta S, Infuso L, Milanesi G. Effects of vitamin D and retinoic acid on human glioblastoma cell lines. *Acta Neurochir (Wien).* 1995;133(3–4):184–190.
35. Naveilhan P, Berger F, Haddad K, et al. Induction of glioma cell death by 1,25(OH)2 vitamin D3: towards an endocrine therapy of brain tumors? *J Neurosci Res.* 1994;37(2):271–277.
36. Zou J, Landy H, Feun L, et al. Correlation of a unique 220-kDa protein with vitamin D sensitivity in glioma cells. *Biochem Pharmacol.* 2000;60(9):1361–1365.
37. Baudet C, Chevalier G, Chassevent A, et al. 1,25-Dihydroxyvitamin D3 induces programmed cell death in a rat glioma cell line. *J Neurosci Res.* 1996;46(5):540–550.
38. Baudet C, Chevalier G, Naveilhan P, Binderup L, Brachet P, Wion D. Cytotoxic effects of 1 alpha,25-dihydroxyvitamin D3 and synthetic vitamin D3 analogues on a glioma cell line. *Cancer Lett.* 1996;100(1–2):3–10.
39. Baudet C, Perret E, Delpech B, et al. Differentially expressed genes in C6.9 glioma cells during vitamin D-induced cell death program. *Cell Death Differ.* 1998;5(1):116–125.
40. Trouillas P, Honnorat J, Bret P, Jouvet A, Gerard JP. Redifferentiation therapy in brain tumors: long-lasting complete regression of glioblastomas and an anaplastic astrocytoma under long term 1-alpha-hydroxycholecalciferol. *J Neurooncol.* 2001;51(1):57–66.
41. Engelmann C, Blot E, Panis Y, et al. Apigenin-strong cytostatic and anti-angiogenic action *in vitro* contrasted by lack of efficacy in vivo. *Phytomedicine.* 2002;9(6):489–495.
42. Weng MS, Ho YS, Lin JK. Chrysin induces G1 phase cell cycle arrest in C6 glioma cells through inducing p21Waf1/Cip1 expression: involvement of p38 mitogen-activated protein kinase. *Biochem Pharmacol.* 2005;69(12):1815–1827.
43. Sharma V, Joseph C, Ghosh S, Agarwal A, Mishra MK, Sen E. Kaempferol induces apoptosis in glioblastoma cells through oxidative stress. *Mol Cancer Ther.* 2007;6(9):2544–2553.
44. Son YG, Kim EH, Kim JY, et al. Silibinin sensitizes human glioma cells to TRAIL-mediated apoptosis via DR5 up-regulation and down-regulation of c-FLIP and survivin. *Cancer Res.* 2007;67(17):8274–8284.
45. Qi L, Singh RP, Lu Y, et al. Epidermal growth factor receptor mediates silibinin-induced cytotoxicity in a rat glioma cell line. *Cancer Biol Ther.* 2003;2(5):526–531.
46. Chen TJ, Jeng JY, Lin CW, Wu CY, Chen YC. Quercetin inhibition of ROS-dependent and -independent apoptosis in rat glioma C6 cells. *Toxicology.* 2006;223(1–2):113–126.
47. Braganhol E, Zamin LL, Canedo AD, et al. Antiproliferative effect of quercetin in the human U138MG glioma cell line. *Anticancer Drugs.* 2006;17(6):663–671.
48. Holick CN, Giovannucci EL, Rosner B, Stampfer MJ, Michaud DS. Prospective study of intake of fruit, vegetables, and carotenoids and the risk of adult glioma. *Am J Clin Nutr.* 2007;85(3):877–886.
49. Mills PK, Preston-Martin S, Annegers JF, Beeson WL, Phillips RL, Fraser GE. Risk factors for tumors of the brain and cranial meninges in Seventh-Day Adventists. *Neuroepidemiology.* 1989;8(5):266–275.
50. Wang CJ, Chou MY, Lin JK. Inhibition of growth and development of the transplantable C-6 glioma cells inoculated in rats by retinoids and carotenoids. *Cancer Lett.* 1989;48(2):135–142.
51. Puri T, Julka K, HGoyal S, Nair O, Sharma DN, Rath GK. Role of natural lycopene and phytonutrients along with radiotherapy and chemotherapy in high grade gliomas. *J Clin Oncol,* 2005 *ASCO Annual Meeting Proc.* 23, No 16S (June 1 Supplement), 2005: 1561.
52. Streffer JR, Bitzer M, Schabet M, Dichgans J, Weller M. Response of radiochemotherapy-associated cerebral edema to a phytotherapeutic agent, H15. *Neurology.* 2001;56(9):1219–1221.
53. Glaser T, Winter S, Groscurth P, et al. Boswellic acids and malignant glioma: induction of apoptosis but no modulation of drug sensitivity. *Br J Cancer.* 1999;80(5–6):756–765.
54. Winking M, Nestler U, Oertel M, et al. Boswellic acids fail to inhibit tumour growth in malignant glioma treatment. In: Deutsche Gesellschaft für Neurochirurgie (DGNC); 2004.
55. Winking M, Sarikaya S, Rahmanian A, Jödicke A, Böker DK. Boswellic acids inhibit glioma growth: a new treatment option? *J Neurooncol.* 2000;46(2):97–103.
56. Zhang Z, Miyatake S, Saiki M, et al. Selenium and glutathione peroxidase mRNA in rat glioma. *Biol Trace Elem Res.* 2000;73(1):67–76.
57. Sundaram N, Pahwa AK, Ard MD, Lin N, Perkins E, Bowles AP Jr. Selenium causes growth inhibition and apoptosis in human brain tumor cell lines. *J Neurooncol.* 2000;46(2):125–133.
58. Zhu Z, Kimura M, Itokawa Y, et al. Apoptosis induced by selenium in human glioma cell lines. *Biol Trace Elem Res.* 1996;54(2):123–134.
59. Gopalakrishna R, Gundimeda U. Protein kinase C as a molecular target for cancer prevention by selenocompounds. *Nutr Cancer.* 2001;40(1):55–63.
60. Lu J, Jiang C. Antiangiogenic activity of selenium in cancer chemoprevention: metabolite-specific effects. *Nutr Cancer.* 2001;40(1):64–73.

61. Kiremidjian-Schumacher L, Roy M, Wishe HI, Cohen MW, Stotzky G. Regulation of cellular immune responses by selenium. *Biol Trace Elem Res*. 1992;33:23–35.
62. Zhang ZH, Kimura M, Itokawa Y. Inhibitory effect of selenium and change of glutathione peroxidase activity on rat glioma. *Biol Trace Elem Res*. 1996;55(1–2):31–38.
63. Philipov P, Tzatchev K. Selenium in the treatment of patients with brain gliomas. A pilot study. *Zentralbl Neurochir*. 1990;51(3):145–146.
64. Pakdaman A. Symptomatic treatment of brain tumor patients with sodium selenite, oxygen, and other supportive measures. *Biol Trace Elem Res*. 1998;62(1–2):1–6.
65. Tsai NM, Lin SZ, Lee CC, et al. The antitumor effects of Angelica sinensis on malignant brain tumors *in vitro* and in vivo. *Clin Cancer Res*. 2005;11(9):3475–3484.
66. Karmakar S, Weinberg MS, Banik NL, Patel SJ, Ray SK. Activation of multiple molecular mechanisms for apoptosis in human malignant glioblastoma T98G and U87MG cells treated with sulforaphane. *Neuroscience*. 2006;141(3):1265–1280.
67. Das A, Banik NL, Ray SK. Garlic compounds generate reactive oxygen species leading to activation of stress kinases and cysteine proteases for apoptosis in human glioblastoma T98G and U87MG cells. *Cancer*. 2007;110(5):1083–1095.
68. Karmakar S, Banik NL, Patel SJ, Ray SK. Garlic compounds induced calpain and intrinsic caspase cascade for apoptosis in human malignant neuroblastoma SH-SY5Y cells. *Apoptosis*. 2007;12(4):671–684.
69. Yokoyama S, Hirano H, Wakimaru N, Sarker KP, Kuratsu J. Inhibitory effect of epigallocatechin-gallate on brain tumor cell lines in vitro. *Neuro-oncology*. 2001;3(1):22–28.
70. McLaughlin N, Annabi B, Bouzeghrane M, et al. The Survivin-mediated radioresistant phenotype of glioblastomas is regulated by RhoA and inhibited by the green tea polyphenol (-)-epigallocatechin-3-gallate. *Brain Res*. 2006;1071(1):1–9.
71. Pilorget A, Berthet V, Luis J, Moghrabi A, Annabi B, Béliveau R. Medulloblastoma cell invasion is inhibited by green tea (-)epigallocatechin-3-gallate. *J Cell Biochem*. 2003;90(4):745–755.
72. Annabi B, Lachambre MP, Bousquet-Gagnon N, Page M, Gingras D, Beliveau R. Green tea polyphenol (-)-epigallocatechin 3-gallate inhibits MMP-2 secretion and MT1-MMP-driven migration in glioblastoma cells. *Biochim Biophys Acta*. 2002;1542(1–3):209–220.
73. Ahn HY, Hadizadeh KR, Seul C, Yun YP, Vetter H, Sachinidis A. Epigallocathechin-3 gallate selectively inhibits the PDGF-BB-induced intracellular signaling transduction pathway in vascular smooth muscle cells and inhibits transformation of sis-transfected NIH 3T3 fibroblasts and human glioblastoma cells (A172). *Mol Biol Cell*. 1999;10(4):1093–1104.
74. Sachinidis A, Seul C, Seewald S, Ahn H, Ko Y, Vetter H. Green tea compounds inhibit tyrosine phosphorylation of PDGF beta-receptor and transformation of A172 human glioblastoma. *FEBS Lett*. 2000;471(1):51–55.
75. Yount G, Qian Y, Moore D, et al. Berberine sensitizes human glioma cells, but not normal glial cells, to ionizing radiation in vitro. *J Exp Ther Oncol*. 2004;4(2):137–143.
76. Sanders MM, Liu AA, Li TK, et al. Selective cytotoxicity of topoisomerase-directed protoberberines against glioblastoma cells. *Biochem Pharmacol*. 1998;56(9):1157–1166.
77. Chen KT, Hao DM, Liu ZX, Chen YC, You ZS. Effect of berberine alone or in combination with argon ion laser treatment on 9L rat glioma cell line. *Chin Med J*. 1994;107(11):808–812.
78. Zhang RX, Dougherty DV, Rosenblum ML. Laboratory studies of berberine used alone and in combination with 1,3-bis(2-chloroethyl)-1-nitrosourea to treat malignant brain tumors. *Chin Med J*. 1990;103(8):658–665.
79. Quincozes-Santos A, Andreazza AC, Nardin P, Funchal C, Gonçalves CA, Gottfried C. Resveratrol attenuates oxidative-induced DNA damage in C6 Glioma cells. *Neurotoxicology*. 2007;28(4):886–891.
80. Zhang W, Fei Z, Zhen HN, Zhang JN, Zhang X. Resveratrol inhibits cell growth and induces apoptosis of rat C6 glioma cells. *J Neurooncol*. 2007;81(3):231–240.
81. Jiang H, Zhang L, Kuo J, et al. Resveratrol-induced apoptotic death in human U251 glioma cells. *Mol Cancer Ther*. 2005;4(4):554–561.
82. Chen JC, Chen Y, Lin JH, Wu JM, Tseng SH. Resveratrol suppresses angiogenesis in gliomas: evaluation by color Doppler ultrasound. *Anticancer Res*. 2006;26(2A):1237–1245.
83. Tseng SH, Lin SM, Chen JC, et al. Resveratrol suppresses the angiogenesis and tumor growth of gliomas in rats. *Clin Cancer Res*. 2004;10(6):2190–2202.
84. Chen Y, Tseng SH, Lai HS, Chen WJ. Resveratrol-induced cellular apoptosis and cell cycle arrest in neuroblastoma cells and antitumor effects on neuroblastoma in mice. *Surgery*. 2004;136(1):57–66.
85. Tysnes BB, Maurer HR, Porwol T, Probst B, Bjerkvig R, Hoover F. Bromelain reversibly inhibits invasive properties of glioma cells. *Neoplasia*. 2001;3(6):469–479.
86. Engebraaten O, Bjerkvig R, Berens ME. Effect of alkyl-lysophospholipid on glioblastoma cell invasion into fetal rat brain tissue in vitro. *Cancer Res*. 1991;51(6):1713–1719.
87. Gao X, Deeb D, Jiang H, Liu Y, Dulchavsky SA, Gautam SC. Synthetic triterpenoids inhibit growth and induce apoptosis in human glioblastoma and neuroblastoma cells through inhibition of prosurvival Akt, NF-kappaB and Notch1 signaling. *J Neurooncol*. 2007;84(2):147–157.
88. Dhandapani KM, Mahesh VB, Brann DW. Curcumin suppresses growth and chemoresistance of human glioblastoma cells via AP-1 and NFkappaB transcription factors. *J Neurochem*. 2007;102(2):522–538.
89. Liu E, Wu J, Cao W, et al. Curcumin induces G2/M cell cycle arrest in a p53-dependent manner and upregulates ING4 expression in human glioma. *J Neurooncol*. 2007;85(3):263–270.
90. Aoki H, Takada Y, Kondo S, Sawaya R, Aggarwal BB, Kondo Y. Evidence that curcumin suppresses the growth of malignant gliomas *in vitro* and *in vivo* through induction of autophagy: role of Akt and extracellular signal-regulated kinase signaling pathways. *Mol Pharmacol*. 2007;72(1):29–39.
91. Gao X, Deeb D, Jiang H, Liu YB, Dulchavsky SA, Gautam SC. Curcumin differentially sensitizes malignant glioma cells to TRAIL/Apo2L-mediated apoptosis through activation of procaspases and release of cytochrome c from mitochondria. *J Exp Ther Oncol*. 2005;5(1):39–48.
92. Mukherjee P, Abate LE, Seyfried TN. Antiangiogenic and proapoptotic effects of dietary restriction on experimental mouse and human brain tumors. *Clin Cancer Res*. 2004;10(16):5622–5629.
93. Mukherjee P, El-Abbadi MM, Kasperzyk JL, Ranes MK, Seyfried TN. Dietary restriction reduces angiogenesis and growth in an orthotopic mouse brain tumour model. *Br J Cancer*. 2002;86(10):1615–1621.
94. Seyfried TN, Sanderson TM, El-Abbadi MM, McGowan R, Mukherjee P. Role of glucose and ketone bodies in the metabolic control of experimental brain cancer. *Br J Cancer*. 2003;89(7):1375–1382.
95. Nebeling LC, Miraldi F, Shurin SB, Lerner E. Effects of a ketogenic diet on tumor metabolism and nutritional status in pediatric oncology patients: two case reports. *J Am Coll Nutr*. 1995;14(2):202–208.
96. Turecký L, Kalina P, Uhlíková E, Námerová S, Krizko J. Serum ceruloplasmin and copper levels in patients with primary brain tumors. *Klin Wochenschr*. 1984;62(4):187–189.
97. Yoshida D, Ikeda Y, Nakazawa S. Quantitative analysis of copper, zinc and copper/zinc ratio in selected human brain tumors. *J Neurooncol*. 1993;16(2):109–115.
98. Brem SS, Zagzag D, Tsanaclis AM, Gately S, Elkouby MP, Brien SE. Inhibition of angiogenesis and tumor growth in the brain. Suppression of endothelial cell turnover by penicillamine and the depletion of copper, an angiogenic cofactor. *Am J Pathol*. 1990;137(5):1121–1142.
99. Yoshida D, Ikeda Y, Nakazawa S. Copper chelation inhibits tumor angiogenesis in the experimental 9L gliosarcoma model. *Neurosurgery*. 1995;37(2):287–92; discussion 292.
100. Yoshida D, Ikeda Y, Nakazawa S. Suppression of tumor growth in experimental 9L gliosarcoma model by copper depletion. *Neurol Med Chir (Tokyo)*. 1995;35(3):133–135.
101. Yoshida D, Ikeda Y, Nakazawa S. Suppression of 9L gliosarcoma growth by copper depletion with copper-deficient diet and D-penicillamine. *J Neurooncol*. 1993;17(2):91–97.
102. Brem S, Grossman SA, Carson KA, et al.; New Approaches to Brain Tumor Therapy CNS Consortium. Phase 2 trial of copper depletion and penicillamine as antiangiogenesis therapy of glioblastoma. *Neuro-oncology*. 2005;7(3):246–253.
103. Mind-body medicine: an overview. nccam.nih.gov/health/backgrounds/mindbody.htm. Accessed December 21, 2007.
104. Mundy EA, DuHamel KN, Montgomery GH. The efficacy of behavioral interventions for cancer treatment-related side effects. *Semin Clin Neuropsychiatry*. 2003;8(4):253–275.

105. Figueroa-Moseley C, Jean-Pierre P, Roscoe JA, et al. Behavioral interventions in treating anticipatory nausea and vomiting. *J Natl Compr Canc Netw.* 2007;5(1):44–50.
106. Pickar JG. Neurophysiological effects of spinal manipulation. *Spine J.* 2002;2(5):357–371.
107. Lund I, Ge Y, Yu LC, et al. Repeated massage-like stimulation induces long-term effects on nociception: contribution of oxytocinergic mechanisms. *Eur J Neurosci.* 2002;16(2):330–338.
108. Keir ST. Levels of stress and intervention preferences of caregivers of brain tumor patients. *Cancer Nurs.* 2007;30(6):E33-E39.
109. Fellowes D, Barnes K, Wilkinson S. Aromatherapy and massage for symptom relief in patients with cancer. *Cochrane Database Syst Rev.* 2004;2:CD002287.
110. Wilkinson SM, Love SB, Westcombe AM, et al. Effectiveness of aromatherapy massage in the management of anxiety and depression in patients with cancer: a multicenter randomized controlled trial. *J Clin Oncol.* 2007;25(5):532–539.
111. Hadfield N. The role of aromatherapy massage in reducing anxiety in patients with malignant brain tumours. *Int J Palliat Nurs.* 2001;7(6):279–285.
112. Kirson ED, Gurvich Z, Schneiderman R, et al. Disruption of cancer cell replication by alternating electric fields. *Cancer Res.* 2004;64(9):3288–3295.
113. Kirson ED, Dbalý V, Tovarys F, et al. Alternating electric fields arrest cell proliferation in animal tumor models and human brain tumors. *Proc Natl Acad Sci USA.* 2007;104(24):10152–10157.
114. Yount G, Solfvin J, Moore D, et al. *In vitro* test of external Qigong. *BMC Complement Altern Med.* 2004;4:5.
115. Taft R, Moore D, Yount G. Time-lapse analysis of potential cellular responsiveness to Johrei, a Japanese healing technique. *BMC Complement Altern Med.* 2005;5:2.
116. Hall Z, Luu T, Moore D, Yount G. Radiation response of cultured human cells is unaffected by johrei. *Evid Based Complement Alternat Med.* 2007;4(2):191–194.
117. Strang S, Strang P, Ternestedt BM. Existential support in brain tumour patients and their spouses. *Support Care Cancer.* 2001;9(8):625–633.
118. Achterberg J, Cooke K, Richards T, Standish LJ, Kozak L, Lake J. Evidence for correlations between distant intentionality and brain function in recipients: a functional magnetic resonance imaging analysis. *J Altern Complement Med.* 2005;11(6):965–971.
119. Standish LJ, Johnson LC, Kozak L, Richards T. Evidence of correlated functional magnetic resonance imaging signals between distant human brains. *Altern Ther Health Med.* 2003;9(1):128, 122–125.
120. Standish LJ, Kozak L, Johnson LC, Richards T. Electroencephalographic evidence of correlated event-related signals between the brains of spatially and sensory isolated human subjects. *J Altern Complement Med.* 2004;10(2):307–314.
121. Richards TL, Kozak L, Johnson LC, Standish LJ. Replicable functional magnetic resonance imaging evidence of correlated brain signals between physically and sensory isolated subjects. *J Altern Complement Med.* 2005;11(6):955–963.
122. Roberts L, Ahmed I, Hall S. Intercessory prayer for the alleviation of ill health. *Cochrane Database Systematic Rev.* 2007;1:CD000368.
123. Acupuncture. NIH Consensus Statement Online 2007 November 3–5. 1997. Accessed December 17, 2007, at Statement can be accessed directly at: http://consensus.nih.gov/1997/1997Acupuncture107html.htm
124. Buchanan DR, White JD, O'Mara AM, Kelaghan JW, Smith WB, Minasian LM. Research-design issues in cancer-symptom-management trials using complementary and alternative medicine: lessons from the National Cancer Institute Community Clinical Oncology Program experience. *J Clin Oncol.* 2005;23(27):6682–6689.

PART VI: RADIATION THERAPY

81 Introduction to Radiation Therapy

Tod W. Speer and Deepak Khuntia

INTRODUCTION

It has been longer than a century since the discovery of x-rays by Conrad Roentgen. Although the mainstay for treating central nervous system (CNS) tumors is surgery, most glial tumors exhibit anatomic and pathological correlates of invasion [1–3], limiting complete surgical extirpation. Therefore, radiotherapy, whether by external beam techniques, brachytherapy, or a more targeted approach, remains a vital adjunct to surgery in the management of CNS malignancies.

Unfortunately, with the exception of adjuvant temozolomide chemotherapy [1], little progress has been made over the last 20 years for survival improvement in glioblastoma multiforme (GBM). Approximately one half of the 18,000 newly diagnosed CNS neoplasms in the United States are glioblastoma [2], and the majority will die from their disease in less than 2 years. This underscores the need for new and effective therapies. Most likely, the next-generation "breakthrough therapy" will consist of a culmination of improved imaging, surgery, radiation delivery technique, radiation sensitization, chemotherapy, targeting agents, and the understanding and utilization of molecular profiling [4].

If one considers the failure of recent dose escalation attempts utilizing external beam radiotherapy (EBRT) when treating glioma, perhaps a targeted radionuclide therapy (TRT) approach will be of considerable merit. TRT potentially allows for the most conformal, intensity-modulated, and guided radiation therapy known. The potential for dose escalation, with this form of therapy, is promising. Phase I and II studies are currently being explored, in spite of previously failed phase II trials [5].

The objective of this chapter is to provide an overview of the radiation physics, radiobiology, and the various radiation delivery mechanisms used to treat CNS tumors.

THE BASIC PHYSICS OF RADIATION THERAPY

Although a thorough description of the radiation physics is beyond the scope of this book, here we will discuss basic principles guiding the use of modern technology in radiation oncology.

Structure of Matter

The types of radiation used with therapeutic intent include photons, electrons, and heavy particles (such as protons and neutrons). In the past, photons created via the decay of radioactive isotopes (i.e., Co-60) were the primary source of therapeutic photons. Now, the mainstay of therapy is a linear accelerator (Figure 81.1) that can generate high-energy electrons and, from the electrons, create high-energy photons.

X-Rays

X-rays were first discovered by Wilhelm Conrad Roentgen in 1895, which was then followed by the discovery of radioactivity 3 years later by the Curies [6]. Roentgen's classic x-rays are generated from electrons hitting the nucleus of matter or other electrons. If the incident electron has high enough energy, it can interact with a free orbital electron, causing an ionization to occur, which yields a characteristic x-ray when an outer orbital electron moves closer to the nucleus in the vacated inner shell. If the characteristic x-ray interacts with another orbital electron, that electron can leave the atom and is known as an Auger electron. The second-method x-rays are generated through a process known as "Bremsstrahlung." Bremsstrahlung, or breaking energy, was discovered by Nikola Tesla in 1897 and refers to the generation of x-rays that is released when an electron changes its path as a result of interacting with the electric field of another atom (Figure 81.2). The resultant photon can then interact with tissue to create fast electrons that eventually cause DNA damage and is described later (Figure 81.3).

Radioactivity

There are various modes of radioactive decay that will be summarized here. Alpha particle decay occurs with very high atomic number elements. The coulombic forces of repulsion are so large that they become so significant that they are able to overcome the nuclear forces that bind the nucleons together. The unstable nucleus emits a heavy particle made up of two protons and two neutrons.

In beta particle decay, there is an ejection of a positron or an electron, depending on the energy involved and

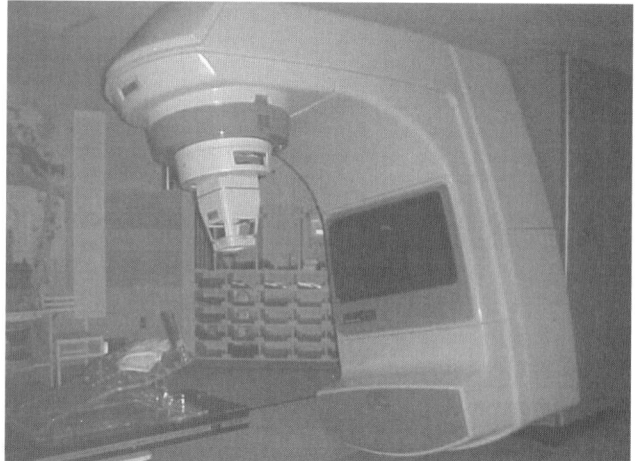

Figure 81.1 Standard linear accelerator capable of delivery both megavoltage photons and electrons.

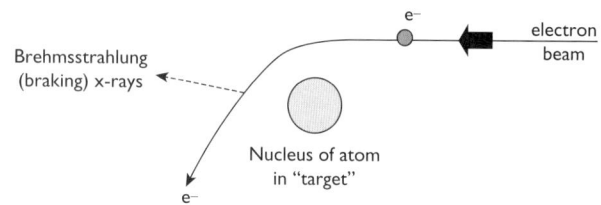

Figure 81.2 Process of bremsstrahlung or "breaking energy," the primary method in which x-rays are created.

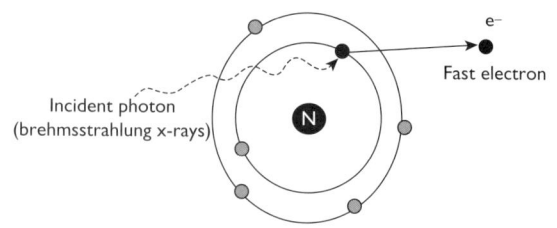

Figure 81.3 Photons interaction within tissue creates fast electrons responsible for DNA damage.

neutron to proton ratio (n/p) required to maintain a stable atom. Neither beta plus or beta minus decay occurs inside the nucleus, but they are created at the instant of the decay process. With *beta minus* decay, the n/p is high and the resultant decay of a neutron yields a proton, an electron, and an antineutrino. With *beta plus* decay, the n/p is low and, to maintain nuclear stability, a proton is decayed to a neutron, a positron and a neutrino. Positron emission tomography imaging is an example of beta plus decay. If there is insufficient energy in the system for beta plus decay, an inner-shell electron can be consumed by the nucleus, resulting in the formation of a neutron in a process known as *electron capture*. Therefore, the number of protons decreases by one, but neutrons increase by one to maintain a stable atom.

Internal conversion occurs when there is extra energy within the nucleus where a photon (γ ray) is ejected that interacts with the orbiting electrons. This can lead to an ejection of an electron in orbit (Auger electron), with a corresponding release of a characteristic x-ray as an outer shell electron is brought into lower energy shell.

Fission reactions occur when certain high-Z nuclei are bombarded by neutrons. The nucleus, after absorbing the neutron, divides into the nucleus of lower atomic number as well as additional neutrons. The decay of U-235 is a classic example where several neutrons are emitted that can then cause more fission reactions resulting in a chain reaction. Fusion is the reverse of fission. Low-mass nuclei are combined to produce one nucleus. This is done by heating low-Z nuclei to a very high temperature to overcome repulsive coulomb forces. Because the total mass of the product is less than the total mass of the reactants, energy is released in the process.

Interaction of Photons with Matter

Photons interact with matter in three main ways. The first is through coherent scattering. In this interaction, there is no change in energy, just a change in direction as the photon interacts with matter. These are very small angles of directional change in lower energy, high-Z materials. This becomes an important issue with diagnostic imaging where energies are lower.

The photoelectric effect is produced when a photon interacts with a tightly bound electron (usually K or L shell) resulting in ejection of this "photoelectron" along with the creation of a characteristic x-ray as a higher shell electron drops to an inner-shell electron in the process. This is an important phenomenon in low-energy (orthovoltage, for example) therapy. The probability of a photoelectric interaction is proportional to Z^3 and inversely proportional to E^3. This discovery earned Albert Einstein the Noble Prize in Physics in 1921.

Compton scattering is an incredibly important interaction in modern-day radiation oncology with megavoltage treatment machines. In this interaction, a photon interacts with an atomic electron in the outermost shell (so no vacancy is produced). This results in a scattered photon and a Compton electron. This interaction can occur between 25 KeV and 25 MV. Typical linear accelerators run in the 6- to 20-MV range. Radiation delivery devices, including a description of heavy particles, will be discussed later.

GENERAL RADIOBIOLOGICAL PRINCIPLES

There are three general methods to deliver therapeutic radiation to patients with a malignant disease. The first method consists of local/regional therapy from an external source, such as the radiation generated from kilovoltage units, teletherapy γ ray units (cobalt-60), linear accelerators, nuclear reactors (neutrons), or cyclotrons (protons). The second method consists of the local implantation (permanent or temporary) of sealed sources, termed brachytherapy. The third method is the local, compartmental, or systemic delivery of unsealed sources. The unsealed sources may be unconjugated (i.e., ^{153}Sm, ^{131}I) or conjugated to a delivery construct (i.e., ibritumomab tiuxetan, Zevalin; tositumomab, Bexxar).

An x-ray or photon is a form of electromagnetic radiation that is produced extranuclearly, typically by accelerating electrons into a high atomic mass material, such as tungsten. This process will produce x-rays as the electrons rapidly decelerate, in a process called "bremsstrahlung" or "braking radiation." [7–11] This is the basic premise by which modern accelerators operate. A γ ray is electromagnetic radiation that is emitted from a radioactive isotope. Both forms of radiation can be described by wave and particle theory.

When radiation interacts with biological material, excitation or ionization may occur. If the imparted energy does not exceed a certain threshold, an electron in the material will only be raised to a higher energy state and not ejected. This is termed excitation. Ionization occurs when the imparted energy is great enough to cause ejection of one or more orbital electrons from an atom or molecule in the material. The energy released in an ionization event is 33 eV [12]. The radiation causing the ionization is hence termed ionizing radiation. Ionizing radiation can be either electromagnetic (photons or γ rays) or particulate (electrons, α particles, neutrons, protons, heavy charged particles). The particulate radiation is generally considered directly ionizing, and electromagnetic radiation is generally considered indirectly ionizing. Directly ionizing radiation interacts with and "directly" alters the molecular structure of the biologically important molecule or target, such as an α particle, causing a DNA double strand break. Indirectly ionizing radiation interacts with the target molecule through intermediary products, such as a photon producing free radicals that will subsequently interact with DNA. As ionizing radiation interacts with biological material, the resulting ionizing events are distributed along the path of the incident photon or particulate radiation. If the ionizing events are separated by relatively large distances in space, the radiation is termed "sparsely ionizing." If the ionizing events are geometrically very close, the radiation is termed "densely ionizing" (Figure 81.4). The amount of energy that is deposited per unit length is termed the linear energy transfer (LET), and it is usually defined by keV per μm (Table 81.1). Because these different types of radiation cause different biological effects, a means for comparison was developed and called the relative biological effectiveness (RBE). Classically, the RBE is defined as the ratio of the dose of a known, standard radiation (250 kVp x-rays) to the dose of a "test" radiation that results in the same biological end point.

Many targets have been proposed as the recipient cause of the biological impact of radiation. These include DNA, lipids and proteins, cell membrane [13], mitochondria [14], and microvasculature [15]. It is largely asserted that it is the interaction of ionizing radiation with the cell DNA that leads to the terminal event. Using a polonium-tipped microneedle, α particle radiation (range, 25–35 μm from needle tip) was directed to different regions of a cell. When doses as high as 100,000 cGy were directed at large portions of the cytoplasm only (and within 2–3 μm of the nucleus), there was no negative impact on subsequent cell proliferation. However, with an α particle fluence of 0.3 to 3.0 particles/μm², penetrating only 1 to 2 μm into the nucleus, 92% of the cells either died or had a significantly diminished reproductive integrity. The conclusion was that it only takes a few α particles to traverse several cubic micrometers into the nucleus (location of the DNA) for the negative impact on cell survival to occur [16]. Thus, it would appear that DNA is a very sensitive target for the effects of ionizing radiation. The consequences of this interaction of radiation with the cell nucleus or DNA may result in the cell undergoing quiescence, apoptosis, mitotic catastrophe, replicative senescence, accelerated senescence, treatment induced senescence, terminal differentiation, terminal growth arrest, or necrosis [17–20].

If the log surviving fraction of cells is plotted against the dose of radiation delivered in a single fraction, a cell survival curve is generated. Because radiation will kill an equal proportion of cells per dose (not equal number), a component of the cell survival/dose relation is logarithmic. As a result, the following becomes evident. If 3 Gy will inactivate 50% of the cells, then increasing the dose to 6 Gy, 9 Gy, and 12 Gy will result in a 25%, 12.5%, and 6.25% surviving fraction, respectively. For prokaryotic systems, such as bacteria, this log surviving fraction versus dose results in a straight line (Figure 81.5). Quite simply, this represents an exponential cell kill with a linear increase in dose. Eukaryotic (mammalian cells) systems differ from bacteria cells in that there is a "shoulder" on the initial cell

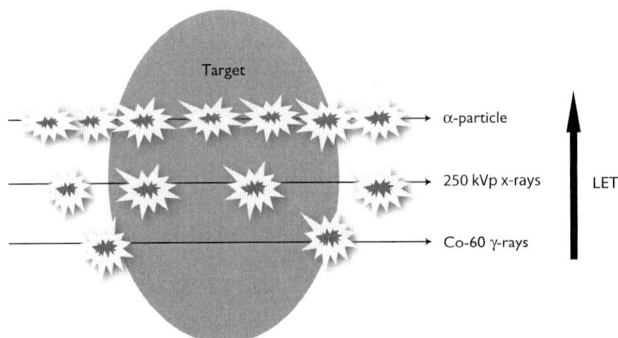

Figure 81.4 Schematic representation of an ionization track produced by different types of radiation with increasing linear energy transfer (LET). Closely spaced ionization events represent densely ionizing radiation (as opposed to sparsely ionizing radiation). In general, radiation with a higher LET will have a higher relative biological effectiveness.

Table 81.1 Radiation Modalities

Type of Radiation	LET (keV/μm)[a]
60Co γ rays	0.2–0.3
250 kVp x-rays	2.0
Protons[b]	0.5–5.0
Neutrons[b]	12–150
α particles[b]	100–150
Heavy charged ions[b]	100–2500

[a] As defined by the International Commission of Radiological Protection.

Units: LET = L = dE/dl (dE is the average energy locally delivered to the biological medium by the radiation, when traversing the distance, dl).

[b] Range of energies.

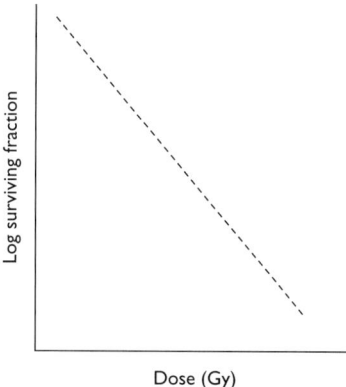

Figure 81.5 Cell survival curve for a prokaryotic system representing an exponential cell kill with a linear increase in dose.

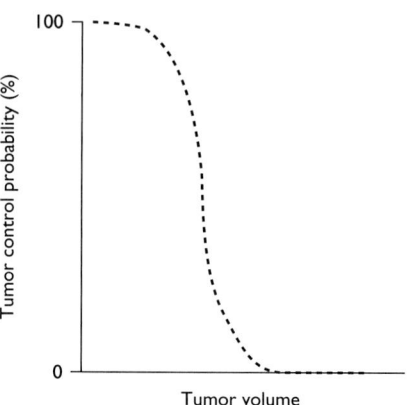

Figure 81.6 Relation between tumor control and volume of tumor (number of clonogens), for a given dose of radiation.

survival curve, at lower doses. This represents a region of reduced efficiency in cell killing. Another important concept, all parameters being equal, is that larger tumors simply require larger doses of radiation for tumor control probability (Figure 81.6). If one considers a large tumor with 10,000 clonogens (cells capable of continued replication) versus a smaller tumor with 100 clonogens and applies the aforementioned logarithmic cell-kill concept, it takes more radiation to reach a <1 surviving clonogen number in the larger tumor as opposed to the smaller tumor. Less than one surviving clonogen should translate into 100% tumor control probability.

For mammalian cells, when dose (Gy) is plotted on the abscissa for single fractions of radiation and log surviving fraction is plotted on the ordinate, the resulting cell survival curve appears different than the typical straight line of prokaryotic systems. Qualitatively, the curve can be described as having a shoulder in the low-dose region. At higher doses, the curve changes into a straight line; however, there are data to support that some cell survival curves continue to curve or bend "downward," even in the range of high doses per fraction.

Several models have been developed to explain the observed findings of the response of eukaryotic cells to radiation. Almost all models and theory can account for the actual shape of the curve, but it is exceedingly difficult to actually know which model truly represents the biological and molecular mechanisms of the interaction of radiation and cells in vivo. Therefore, a few brief comments, about two prevailing radiobiology models used to try and explain mammalian cell survival curves, are warranted.

The multitarget model (Figure 81.7) assumes that the radiation damage must accumulate before the resulting effect becomes evident. This dose-response relation can be mathematically described by $S = e - D/D_0$, where S is the surviving fraction of cells after a given dose (D), and D_0 represents the dose that reduces the cell population to 0.37 (1/e) of a value on the exponential (straight) region of the cell survival curve [21]. The initial slope, D_1, results from single-event cell kill, and the final slope, D_0, results from multievent cell kill. The extrapolation number, "n," and the quasithreshold, D_q, measure the width of the shoulder of the curve. If "n" is large, the shoulder is broad and the cells

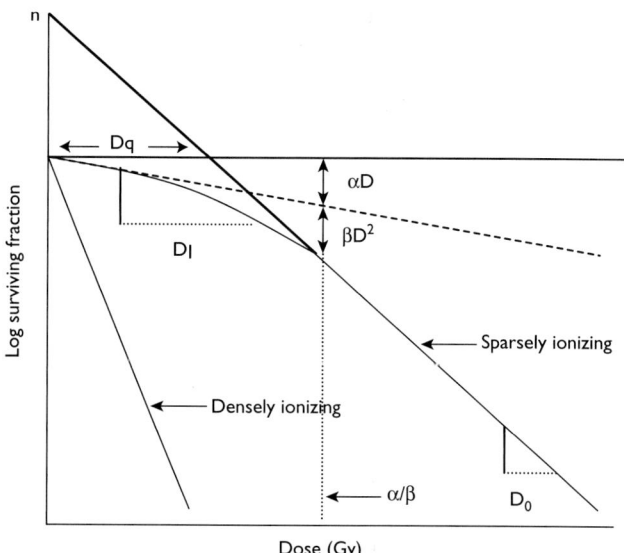

Figure 81.7 Mammalian cell survival curve for densely and sparsely ionizing radiation. D_q and n define the width of the shoulder region. D_1 is the initial slope where cell killing is proportional to dose (αD). D_0 represents the final slope where cell killing is proportional to the dose squared (βD^2). The α/β ratio for the cell population is defined when the linear (αD) component of cell killing is equal to the quadratic (βD^2). See *color insert*.

tend to be more resistant to radiation in this dose range. Hence, more radiation is required to result in the same proportion of cells killed as would result on the straight portion of the curve (compare slopes of D_1 and D_0). The quasithreshold represents a dose range below which there is no impact on cell survival. Because there truly is no such threshold, it is termed "quasi" or an "almost" threshold [12]. For densely ionizing radiation, the cell survival curve is a straight line.

The linear-quadratic (LQ) model was developed to try and better explain continuously bending cell survival curve, rather than the initial shoulder and straight line of the multitarget model. A problem with the multitarget model is that it predicts an initial cell-kill slope of zero (no cell kill) at very low doses, and this is simply not the case, as typified in experiments using increased fractionation or low-dose-rate treatment approaches [21]. The accumulation of damage or "sublesions" in cells [22], often referred to as sublethal damage, was proposed to account for some of these observations. The LQ model assumes that there are two components to cell kill: α, being proportional to dose (initial slope; linear cell kill described by a single-hit process), and β, being proportional to the square of the dose (final slope; quadratic cell kill described by a two-hit process), which can be expressed as $S = e^{-\alpha D - \beta D^2}$ [23].

These coefficients are felt to represent nonrepairable (α) and repairable (β) components of cell damage [10]. In this expression, S is the fraction of surviving cells after dose, D, whereas α and β are constants for a given cell line. The α/β ratio is the ratio of the linear to quadratic component of cell killing. When both components are equal, the α/β ratio is defined as a dose in Gy. This ratio helps describe the shape of a cell survival curve as well as the response to fractionated radiation. If the α/β is >1 or <1, then the α or β component to cell-killing predominates, respectively.

The goal of radiation oncology is to maximize dose to the tumor while sparing as much normal tissue as possible. To fully utilize radiation as an effective treatment modality, an understanding of early- and late-responding tissues is necessary. Early-responding tissues typically exhibit high cell propagation rates. Relevant examples would include skin, hair follicles, and mucosa. Radiation damage will become apparent in these tissues within weeks after the initial radiation exposure. Late-responding tissues exhibit low or no cell propagation rates. Relevant examples would include brain, spinal cord, kidneys, and peripheral nerves. Radiation damage will become apparent in these tissues only after months or years after the initial radiation exposure. It should be noted that there does not appear to be a direct relationship between the acute side effects induced in the irradiated tissue and the subsequent development of late complications. Additionally, acute radiation reactions tend to respond to therapeutic interventions, whereas late complications tend to be more difficult to manage and often will not respond significantly to current interventions. Increasing tumor control and lowering complications results in a larger therapeutic ratio or gain. Concerning the delivery of radiation, the therapeutic ratio can be maximized by (1) decreasing the volume of normal tissue being irradiated (conformal techniques, intensity-modulated radiation therapy [IMRT], proton therapy, four-dimensional planning), (2) combined modality approaches (combining surgery, chemotherapy, biologics, targeting agents and radiopharmaceuticals with radiation), and (3) modification of the delivery of radiation to exploit radiobiology properties (fractionation, duration of treatment, dose rate, and type of radiation [photons, protons, charged particles, neutrons]). The following section will focus on the modification of the delivery of radiation, namely, fractionation, treatment time considerations, and dose rate.

Standard fractionation, in the United States, can be characterized as delivering 1.8 to 2.0 Gy fractions, 5 days per week. Fractionation evolved early in the history of radiobiology with the understanding that there was sparing of late-responding tissues relative to the tumor, compared with high-dose single-fraction regimens. Because the shoulder region of the cell survival curve is repeated with each fraction, the overall dose must be increased to help offset this "less effective" radiation (a dose region where it is less likely that sublethal damage will accumulate). A deviation from the standard fractionation schedule is termed "altered fractionation." [24] The three most common altered fractionation schedules are hyperfractionation, accelerated fractionation, and hypofractionation. Hyperfractionation consists of using more than one fraction per day. The daily dose is less than that used in standard fractionation (i.e., 110–160 cGy, bid). The overall dose is higher than conventional overall doses owing to the lower daily dose. It is felt that this regimen will improve local control and potentially spare late-responding tissues. Accelerated fractionation consists of shortening the overall treatment time, using standard daily doses (1.8–2.0 Gy), and keeping the overall dose similar to standard fractionation schedules. Hypofractionation is the delivery of daily doses larger than 2 Gy, shorter overall treatment times, and lower overall doses.

There appears to be a reproducible difference in how early- and late-responding tissues react to fractionated radiation. Early-responding tissue has less of an ability to recover between fractions of radiation, compared with late-responding tissue. As a result, fractionation tends to diminish potential complications in late-responding tissue while remaining relatively effective against tumors and early-responding tissue. The relation of the impact of fractionated radiation on early- and late-responding tissue may also be described in terms of the α/β ratio. Early-responding tissues (and tumor) are assigned high values for the α/β ratio, usually in the 7 to 20 Gy range, with 10 Gy being a typical value. Late-responding tissue has an α/β ratio of 1 to 5 Gy [25].

Thus, the α/β ratio may be used to quantify the effects of different fractionation regimens on early- and late-responding tissues. Of course, if tumors and late-responding tissues exist as representing a spectrum of α/β ratios, then local control and toxicity data may be variable and unpredictable. It may be too difficult to consistently apply specific α/β ratios to tissues when other differences such as tumor hypoxia, tumor volume, repopulation, and patient-specific variables may prevail. In fact, there is some evidence that prostate cancer may have an α/β ratio similar to late-responding tissue [26].

Another radiobiology principle that is intimately related to overall treatment time and fractionation is the concept of repopulation. Repopulation represents the proliferation of clonogens within the tumor (or stem cells within normal tissue) during fractionated radiotherapy. This process will diminish the effectiveness of radiotherapy by eventually increasing the number of clonogens that need to be sterilized, during the radiation therapy course. The initiation of repopulation appears to be stimulated by a cytotoxic event (injury) and represents a complex relation between growth fraction and cell cycle kinetics. Repopulation is not felt to begin immediately, but after a several week delay from the beginning of radiotherapy [27,28]. Repopulation becomes "accelerated" when the tumor doubling time is shorter during therapy than the doubling time prior to the initiation of therapy. In fact, it has been estimated than 0.6 Gy per day is lost because of repopulation in head and neck squamous cell carcinoma [28]. Because of accelerated repopulation, treatment breaks or protraction of a radiation course can have a significant negative impact on tumor control. Altered fractionation programs, therefore, have been designed to ultimately shorten the overall treatment time with an attempt to abrogate the negative impact of accelerated repopulation (note: hyperfractionation uses an overall similar treatment time but the final dose is increased, thus ultimately resulting in a shorter treatment time for the larger end dose).

Dose rate is another important determinant of the biological response to irradiation. When the dose rate is lowered, the impact on cell kill is lessened. The dose-rate effect seems to result from the repair of sublethal damage. As the dose rate is lowered, the ability of a cell to repair the damage increases. The resulting cell survival curve becomes "shallower" or, in other terms, D_0 decreases. In comparison with high-dose-rate single-fraction irradiation, continuous low-dose-rate irradiation can be thought of as approaching an infinite number of fractions. The resulting cell survival curve would be expected to have no shoulder and to be shallow. The dose-rate effect is most pronounced between 1 and 100 cGy/minute [12]. At these low-dose rates, some cell lines will actually exhibit an increase in cell kill compared with higher dose rates. This is felt to be secondary to the cells being "blocked" in G2, a more radiosensitive portion of the cell cycle. This phenomenon is termed the inverse dose-rate effect.

It has been known for many decades that molecular oxygen is one of the most powerful agents for enhancing the effects of ionizing radiation. Early studies revealed that 150 to 200 μm was the maximum range that oxygen would diffuse from a blood vessel and into the tissue. These distances were confirmed by histopathological analysis of tumors [29]. Thus, it was inferred that tumor cells could represent a spectrum of cells ranging from fully anoxic (greater distances from blood vessels in areas of necrosis) to fully oxic (close proximity to blood vessels). Intermediate regions, therefore, could potentially harbor hypoxic, radioresistant, viable, and clonogenic cells. Subsequently, it has been extensively confirmed by in vitro and in vivo studies that hypoxic cells are more radioresistant than well-oxygenated cells [30–32]. In an effort to measure the benefit of oxygen as a dose-modifying agent, the oxygen enhancement ration (OER) has been developed. The OER is defined as the ratio of the dose required to achieve the same end point (i.e., cell survival) under hypoxic conditions to that under oxic or aerobic conditions. Typical values are 2.5 to 3.0 for large fractions of sparsely ionizing radiation and 1.0 for high LET irradiation [21].

Because of the benefit of oxygenation, a single fraction of sparsely ionizing radiation will preferentially spare hypoxic regions of the tumor from cell killing. As a result, multiple fractions of radiation would be expected to slowly increase the hypoxic cell fraction within a tumor, rendering it relatively incurable with a large number of hypoxic and radioresistant cells remaining at the end of therapy. It has been shown, however, that this is not the case and that the hypoxic fraction of cells within a tumor remains relatively constant [33]. This occurs because of the process of reoxygenation, which returns the proportion of hypoxic cells back to the level that existed prior to each fraction. If the time between fractions is sufficient to allow for reoxygenation, then tumor hypoxia should potentially have a minimal impact on tumor control probability.

RADIATION DELIVERY MECHANISM

Brachytherapy

Radiotherapy remains the most effective adjuvant therapy for treating CNS malignancies. The Brain Tumor Study Group confirmed a survival benefit of EBRT, following surgery for patients with malignant glioma, in the landmark 1978 publication [34]. The radiotherapy arm of this study revealed a significant improvement in median survival, from 14 weeks (surgery only) to 36 weeks (surgery and radiotherapy; $P = 0.001$). It is quite clear that dose escalation with EBRT in excess of 60 Gy has had no significant impact on survival [35–37] and often exceeds normal tissue tolerance. In fact, it has been shown that there is typically no incidence of CNS necrosis with external beam doses < 57 Gy compared with 18% incidence of CNS necrosis with external beam doses > 64.8 Gy [36]. Considering that most recurrences of high-grade gliomas are local [38,39], there has been a more recent emphasis on focal radiation techniques such as radiosurgery and brachytherapy. The obvious goal is to safely dose escalate by increasing the radiation dose to the high-risk portion of the CNS and minimize normal tissue exposure, hence, increasing the therapeutic ratio. However, because of the infiltrating nature of these tumors, local targeting with a more focal radiation technique appears to be a formidable task.

Brachytherapy for CNS tumors has a long history dating back to the first treatment of a glioma reported in 1914 [40]. This somewhat cumbersome, freehand, treatment technique was soon surpassed by the less invasive delivery of radiotherapy using "teletherapy machines." During this time period, there was also the concurrent development of stereotactic localization devices (frame based and frameless). This, coupled with the improved availability and an increase in choice of radioisotopes, resulted in a resurgence of interest in CNS brachytherapy throughout the 1970s and 1980s. Encouraging initial single-institution experiences seemed to indicate a survival advantage for selected patients treated with stereotactic guided brachytherapy [41,42]. However, because of the invasive nature of the procedure, the potential for hemorrhage, infection, necrosis, and frequent need for reoperation, there was reasonable concern for restraint. Criticism, claiming "patient selection" as the cause for the initial favorable results, was often levied [43]. The answer came from two Phase III trials [44,45] published in 1998 and 2002. Although different in design, each study used a combination of EBRT and a stereotactic guided temporary ^{125}I implant. The conclusion of each study was that there was no statistically significant survival benefit for the patients receiving the brachytherapy. As a result, there has been a rather marked decrease in the utilization of brachytherapy for primary and recurrent CNS malignancies over the ensuing years [46]. This is not to say, however, that brachytherapy is no longer a viable option for certain clinical situations involving brain tumors [47]. There appears to be a strong potential for a dose-effect relationship when reviewing external beam [48] and brachytherapy [49] data. When this concept is taken in context with improved imaging modalities, the potential therapeutic ratio enhancement of brachytherapy due to improved radiobiology, and the fact that radioisotopes are more cytotoxic than commonly used chemotherapy agents [50] and that there are new and intriguing radionuclide delivery techniques, further preclinical and clinical investigation is certainly warranted.

The intrigue of utilizing brachytherapy in CNS malignancies is largely due to the potential normal tissue sparing from low-dose-rate irradiation and the inverse-square law. Commonly used radioisotopes for CNS brachytherapy are shown in Table 81.2. Selection of the isotope often depends on availability, half-life, activity, energy, dose rate, and shielding requirements that potentially impact upon exposure risk to health care personal. A select group of patients with cystic lesions or craniopharyngiomas may benefit from the direct instillation of colloidal ^{32}P, ^{90}Y, or ^{198}Au [51–55]. This technique will deliver between 20,000 and 40,000 cGy to the cyst wall, assuming a uniform dispersion of the radionuclide within the cystic structure. It has been estimated that the dose will often be less than the actual calculated dose because of the phenomenon of "plating." [56]

A review of the CNS brachytherapy literature reveals that ^{125}I is the most commonly used encapsulated or sealed source isotope. This is mainly due to its availability, low half-value layer, and low exposure rate constant. Personal near the patient can actually acquire shielding from a standard lead apron [47]. ^{125}I decays by electron capture. This process results in an excited state of ^{125}Te, which then spontaneously decays to a stable ground state, emitting a 35.5-keV photon. Also, because of electron capture and internal conversion, characteristic x-rays are produced with energies between 27 and 35 keV. All electron emissions and photons (with energies < 5 keV) are filtered by the titanium capsule [11]. Typically, permanent ^{125}I implants are planned with dose rates in the range of 3 to 8 cGy/h, whereas temporary ^{125}I implants are planned with dose rates in the range of 40 to 70 cGy/h [47]. Some have concluded that the preferred stereotactic implant is a temporary procedure, utilizes ^{125}I at a dose rate of 10 cGy/h, and prescribes a reference dose of 60 Gy to the margin of the tumor. With this approach, "toxic vasogenic edema" has virtually been eliminated in this particular series of patients [57]. With the advent of remote after-loading technology, different isotopes such as ^{192}Ir [58–62], ^{252}Cf [63], and ^{60}Co [64] have been employed.

Patient selection for brachytherapy is critical. Although there are slight variations between institutions, it is generally accepted that patients should have solitary, well-demarcated lesions that are typically <6 cm in maximum dimension. There should not be any involvement of the leptomeningies, corpus callosum, or evidence of subependymal spread [41,44,45,65]. A high performance status (KPS ≥ 70) is desirable, and some institutions exclude patients with involvement of their speech center because of "quality of life" issues [42]. As a result of this selective triage for brachytherapy candidates, only 10 to 30% of all patients with high-grade gliomas will be eligible for the procedure [43,66].

The typical CNS brachytherapy program consists of an attempt at maximal surgical debulking of the tumor, implantation of radioactive sources or delivery device (catheters or balloon), and EBRT [67,68]. The EBRT is variably sequenced [44,45,69], some institutions have incorporated hyperthermia [70,71], and most will utilize chemotherapy at some point in the treatment process [44,45,72]. Interstitial CNS brachytherapy can be broadly classified as either "open" (craniotomy and source placement) or "closed" (stereotactic source placement). The open technique involves layering of permanent, titanium-encapsulated radioactive seeds, connected with suture, into the resection cavity. Alternatively, the seeds can be placed directly into the adjacent tissue of the resection cavity. In all cases, the seeds are fixed in place with an application of fibrin glue, cyanoacrylate, or a tissue adhesive [73,74]. A permutation of the open technique involves placement of a balloon catheter (Gliasite, Cytyc Surgical Products) into the resection cavity, which is then after-loaded via a subcutaneous port [58,75–77]. The balloon is instilled with an organically

Table 81.2 Common Brachytherapy Isotopes

Isotope	Half-Life	Typical Dose rate (cGy/h)	Energy (MeV)	Decay/Product	Exposure Rate Constant (Γ)
^{60}Co	5.263 yr	> 1000	1.25	$\beta \rightarrow \beta, \gamma$	13.07
^{252}Cf	2.645 yr	> 350	2.3	$\alpha \rightarrow n$	—
^{125}I[a]	60.2 d	3–8 (permanent) 40–70 (temporary)	0.027–0.035	EC $\rightarrow$ x	1.46
^{192}Ir	74.2 d	80–100 (LDR) 120–360 (HDR)	0.38	EC, $\beta \rightarrow \beta, \gamma$	4.69
^{198}Au[b]	2.7 d	—	0.412	$\beta \rightarrow \beta, \gamma$	2.38
^{32}P[c]	14.28 d	—	1.7	$\beta \rightarrow \beta$	—
^{90}Y[c]	2.67 d	—	2.3	$\beta \rightarrow \beta$	—

[a] Seeds or organically bound aqueous solution
[b] Seeds and colloidal preparation (for cystic lesions)
[c] Colloidal preparation (for cystic lesions)

$\Gamma = R \times cm^2 \times mCi^{-1} \times h^{-1}$

Notes: β, beta particle; γ, gamma irradiation; n, neutron; EC, electron capture; x, characteristic x-rays.

bound aqueous solution of ^{125}I (Iotrex). The closed technique involves the placement of temporary or permanent radioactive sources using a computed tomography (CT)- or magnetic resonance imaging (MRI)-guided stereotactic localization [42,65]. Often, a template is attached to the stereotactic frame to aide with catheter spacing. The initial, outer catheters are secured to the scalp. After appropriate dosimetric calculations, a smaller caliber catheter, containing the radioactive sources, is placed within the larger initial catheter. This array is left in place so that the calculated dose is delivered to the tumor volume. Most implants are adequately performed by using two to ten catheters, each containing two to six seeds [47]. When the treatment is complete, all catheters are removed en block in the operating room or at bedside.

The majority of CNS brachytherapy studies are retrospective or are of phase I and II design. Of course, all of these studies are subject to the possibility of selection bias [78]. It has been shown that patients with GBM, eligible for brachytherapy, exhibit improved median survivals compared with those who are ineligible (13.9 months vs. 5.8 months, $P = 0.0001$), when they are treated in the same manner, with surgery, EBRT, and chemotherapy [43]. Conversely, using the Radiation Therapy Oncology Group recursive partitioning analysis, it has been shown that patients with malignant glioma experience a survival benefit from a ^{125}I implant that is not purely based on selection bias [68].

In general, the median survival for patients receiving either a temporary or permanent ^{125}I brachytherapy implant as part of their initial therapy is 6 to 23 months [42,44,45,57,65,68,69,79] for GBM and 31 to 39.3 months [65,69,79] for anaplastic astrocytoma (AA). For recurrent lesions, the median survivals are 11.7 to 16 months [65,73,74] for GBM and 13 to 17 months [65,74] for AA. When the data are combined (GBM and AA), the median survival is 6 to 11.5 months [42,72,80–82] (53). The results for high-dose rate after loading techniques with ^{192}Ir, ^{252}Cf, and ^{60}Co are disappointingly similar with median survivals of 6 to 17 months for GBM and AA [61,63,64].

As previously mentioned, there have been two prospective randomized clinical trial using CNS brachytherapy as a portion of the initial management of CNS glioma. The first study was performed by Princess Margaret Hospital (PMH) and the University of Toronto and was published in 1998 [44]. The second study, performed by the Brain Tumor Cooperative Group (BTCG; the National Institutes of Health [NIH] trial 87–01), was published in 2002 [45].

The PMH study accrued patients from 1986 to 1996. A temporary stereotactic ^{125}I implant was utilized after EBRT. A total of 140 patients, diagnosed with a supratentorial malignant astrocytoma (gliosarcoma in two patients), were randomized either to EBRT (50 Gy/25 fractions; 69 patients) or EBRT (50 Gy/25 fractions; 71 patients), followed by the brachytherapy procedure (60 Gy minimum peripheral tumor dose at 70 cGy/h). Patients were selected with a KPS ≥ 70 and maximum tumor size ≤ 6 cm. There could be no involvement of the corpus callosum. Of note, one patient in the EBRT arm actually received an implant and eight patients in the EBRT plus implant arm did not receive an implant (five disease progression, two myocardial infarction, one pulmonary emboli; 11%). The study was analyzed on an "intention-to-treat" basis, and the median survival for the EBRT vs. EBRT plus implant arm was 13.2 months vs. 13.8 months ($P = 0.49$). If only the patients who received the implant as part of their therapy were analyzed (63 patients), their median survival was 15.7 months. In all fairness, for this type of comparison, patients should also be excluded from the analysis of the EBRT arm during the same time period, owing to progression of disease or death from various comorbidities. Although this particular information was not reported in the study, the survival in this group of patients would also, most likely, improve. Regardless, this represents a subset analysis and was not an intended end point. There was a 15% (15/63) significant complication rate attributed to the implant. Overall, 26% of the patients received chemotherapy at the time of relapse (all received oral CCNU, two patients received intravenous carmustine, and two patients received PCV). A partial or subtotal excision was accomplished as the initial surgery in 86% of the patients, and reoperation was aggressively performed in 32% of the patients. Both these surgical events were equally distributed between both treatment arms. Analysis of the pattern of failure revealed a 93% failure at the original site in the EBRT arm vs. 82% in the implant arm.

The BTCG accrued patients from 1987 to 1994 and also used a temporary stereotactic ^{125}I implant (60 Gy at 40 cGy/h, prescribed to enclose the enhancing tumor). In this study, the EBRT (60.2 Gy/35 fractions) was delivered after the implant. The randomization was to implant plus EBRT plus BCNU (133 patients) vs. EBRT plus BCNU (137 patients). The patients were equally stratified by age, KPS (≥50), gender, histology (85% GBM, 10% AA, 3% anaplastic oligodendroglioma, 2% malignant mixed glioma), and date of operation. Anatomic exclusion criterion included a tumor that crossed midline, multicentric tumors, and lack of contrast enhancement (target) following initial surgery. Because the implant was performed prior to the EBRT, all patients received the intended brachytherapy procedure. The median survival in the EBRT plus implant plus BCNU vs. EBRT plus BCNU arm was 17.02 months vs. 14.7 months ($P = 0.101$).

Although not significantly impacting upon survival, brachytherapy does seem to alter the recurrence pattern in some studies [44,83], although this is not a uniform finding [65,84]. Considering that radiotherapy remains the most effective adjuvant treatment, it is not unreasonable to consider further dose escalation, and perhaps a favorable alteration of the therapeutic ratio, by employing an approach such as TRT.

External Beam Radiation

Classic external beam radiation is delivered in either two- or three-dimensional treatments. Prior to the advent of CT simulation and modern treatment planning software, radiation was delivered using two-dimensional techniques. Typically, two-dimensional radiation was set up using fluoroscopy using a clinical anatomical decision-making process. This is accomplished with two to four orthogonal radiation beam fields on an x-ray simulator with bony anatomy providing the bulk of the guidance. Tissues not needing treatment were identified on plain films, and lead or cerrobend (a much lighter and pliant alloy) blocks, and more recently with multileaf collimators, are designed to protect the normal structures by blocking the incident radiation beam. Bony anatomy visualized on plain radiographs was the primary method of determining field placement, and generally this meant using orthogonal and occasionally oblique or vertex fields. The uncertainty in target determination with this rudimentary method mandated the incorporation of error as a significant element in the radiation field design, generally resulting in large volumes being irradiated. As CT technology emerged, it became possible to incorporate three-dimensional cross-sectional data into treatment planning systems not only to delineate targets accurately (both normal structures and tumor) but also to calculate radiation doses efficiently from multiple beams from multiple directions and block out normal tissue more effectively, yielding a more "conformal" three-dimensional radiation plan. CT reconstruction allows one to display beam's eye view, which allows visualization from the perspective of the axis of the radiation source, irrespective of the direction of beam entry. With the advent of three-dimensional conformal radiation, radiation oncologists are able to quantify radiation doses to the normal structures and modify the beam to maximize dose to the target while limiting dose to the normal structures. Consequently, the "error margins" are reduced, and there is more accurate "shielding" of normal structures to improve the safety profile of radiation. Graphically, these data are represented on a dose-volume histogram, an analysis that yields information pertinent to the adequacy of tumor dose, as well as the ability to maintain normal tissue doses below known and safe thresholds (Figure 81.8) [85]. This type of radiation delivery is the most common treatment used for primary brain tumors, although the use

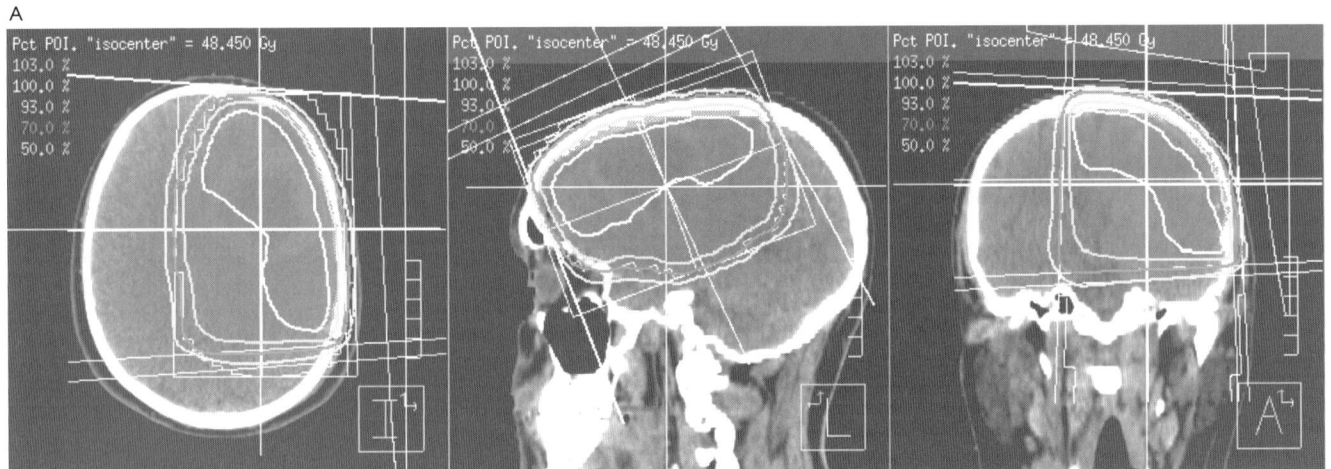

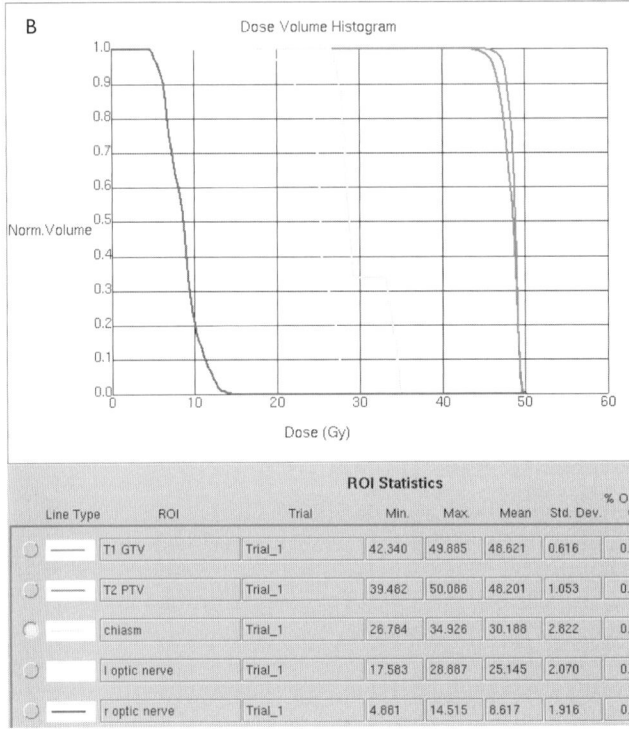

Figure 81.8 (**A**) Typical 3D conformal plan for a GBM. (**B**) Dose-volume histogram (DVH) showing the dose and volume related to the different structures within the treatment plan. *See color insert.*

of IMRT is increasing. Both three-dimensional and IMRT involve considerably more effort and resources to delineate target and normal structures as well as the requirement for precision during delivery. Because of the more rapid dose fall off with these technologies (especially IMRT), special mobilization and image guidance is necessary to optimize delivery. The major hypothesized benefits are a reduction in the dose to normal structures as well as the potential for dose escalation.

IMRT was developed in the late 1980s and became widely available in the mid 1990s. This technology allows the radiation beam to be subdivided into a very large number of optimized beamlets from multiple different directions, each with a unique "intensity" of radiation, mimicking the patient anatomy in the path of the beamlet, allowing significantly improved radiation dose distributions, both to tumor and normal tissues. With IMRT, dose distributions can be shaped three-dimensionally in concave or convex configurations, resulting in a dramatic reduction of high doses of radiation to normal structures near the target. Additionally, IMRT allows for "differential" doses to be deposited within a target, such that a component at higher risk of recurrence can be irradiated to a higher dose, while the rest of the target is being treated to a conventional dose.

Because of the rapid fall off of dose, patient immobilization and daily setup verification is critical. Slight motion or setup error will result in a geographic miss, and in the worst-case scenario, the high dose is deposited in the critical structure designated for avoidance. Fortunately, the brain moves minimally, and standard craniofacial immobilization devices yield relatively high daily setup accuracy (Figure 81.9). Another possible feature of IMRT is dose-escalating within a target, also known as a simultaneous integrated boost. This is ideal in situations as this allows a higher dose per fraction to the target, while giving a lower dose per fraction to normal structures. However, the potential for late injury with high dose per fraction to normal tissue does exist, further emphasizing the need for treatment delivery accuracy [86]. Because IMRT dose distributions are highly complex, it is not unusual to see unanticipated toxicities in low-dose areas such as alopecia or mucositis in the exit beam regions. Finally, because of the potentially larger volume receiving low doses of radiation, it is conceivable that the risk of second malignancies may be higher, over several decades. Because this often takes years or even decades to develop and there has not been sufficient time since the adoption of IMRT, it remains difficult to quantify this hypothetical risk [87].

IMRT has several potential benefits in specific CNS tumors, and medulloblastoma represents a good example. Children with medulloblastoma are frequently treated with a multimodality approach including surgery, cisplatin-based chemotherapy, and radiation. Both chemotherapy and radiotherapy can significantly contribute to ototoxicity. IMRT allows sparing of the auditory apparatus, while still maintaining full dose to the target. Huang and colleagues were able to show a reduction in cochlear dose from 54.2 to 36.7 Gy and a reduction of grade 3 or 4 hearing loss from 64% to 13% with the use of IMRT compared with conventional radiation therapy [88].

As mentioned earlier, daily setup immobilization and verification of the setup accuracy is critically important for IMRT. Image-guided radiation therapy (IGRT), the technique of using imaging technology at the time of each treatment to verify accurate positioning, has become a significant part of IMRT delivery. Several types of IGRT systems include cone-beam CT, megavoltage CT (e.g., helical tomotherapy), ultrasound guidance for prostate cancer, CT-on-Rails, CALYPSO fiducial monitoring, or the use of electronic portal imaging devices. Advances in IGRT allow us to selectively boost dose to some targets while selectively sparing normal structures more aggressively. An example of this approach has been presented by Gutiérrez and colleagues for the case of selective boosting of brain metastases to twice the whole brain dose while reducing the dose to the hippocampi to a 20% of the whole brain dose, leading to a dose differential between target structures and normal tissue structures of 10 [89]. This is achieved using helical tomotherapy, a prototypical IMRT-IGRT system with the expectation that reduction of hippocampal dose will prevent neurocognitive decline in patients receiving whole brain radiation therapy (Figure 81.10) [90,91]. Prospective studies evaluating this approach are currently under investigation.

Stereotactic Radiosurgery and Fractionated Stereotactic Radiotherapy

Radiosurgery was described in 1951 by Lars Leksell, a neurosurgeon at the Karolinska Institute in Stockholm [92]. The first gamma knife (GK) treatment was conducted in 1968 [93]. Because of its prohibitive cost and limited availability, the spread of this technology was stagnant for decades. As linac-based radiosurgery systems and improved imaging technology developed, interest in stereotactic radiosurgery (SRS) dramatically increased. Most major cancer centers

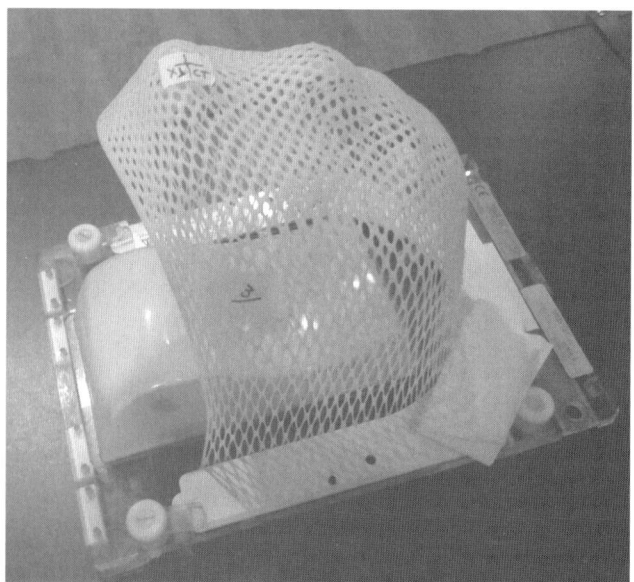

Figure 81.9 Typical aquaplast immobilization device for a patient receiving external beam radiation therapy for a brain tumor.

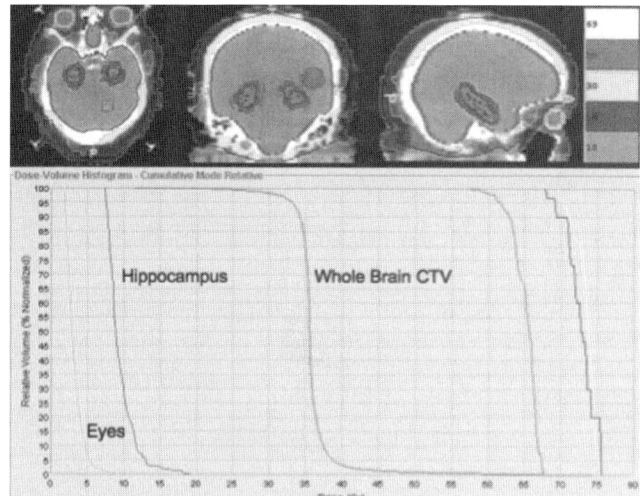

Figure 81.10 Tomotherapy plan showing sparing of the hippocampus while escalating doses to the metastatic tumors. This is done in an effort to simultaneously improving local control while sparing neurcognition. *See color insert.*

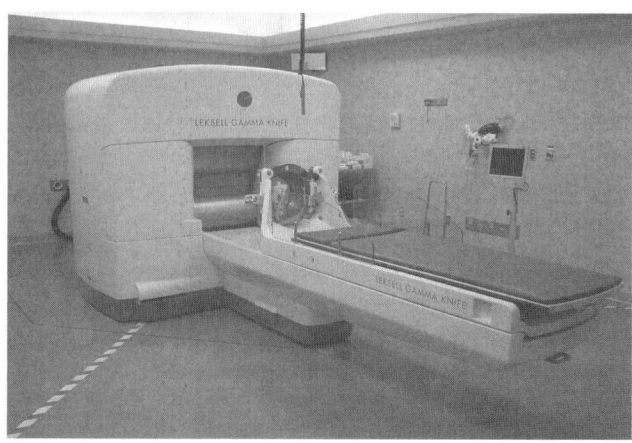

Figure 81.11 Gamma knife model C equipped with the Automatic Positioning System (APS).

in the United States now have the capability of delivering some forms of SRS.

Radiosurgery differs from the conventional fractionated radiotherapy in several ways. Traditionally, radiosurgery implies a single treatment, whereas conventional radiation therapy involves multiple treatments. Additionally, in conventional fractionation regimens, normal brain tissue adjacent to the target receives near full dose of radiation. Because normal brain parenchyma is relatively unforgiving in regards to late toxicity, the ability of radiosurgery to treat with high-dose gradients adjacent to a nonmobile target makes its use in the brain ideal. The use of a very large number of beams ensures that no single beam on its own contributes significant dose, and this minimizes dose to normal tissues in its path. To optimize tight gradients, tumors treated with SRS are generally under 4 cm.

A variety of commercial hardware systems are available for SRS. Radiosurgery can be performed using various devices, including the GK (Figure 81.11), particle beam devices, or modified linear accelerators (such as Cyberknife, Tomotherapy, Novalis, etc.) (Table 81.3). With technological advances in software and hardware, there is no clear advantage of one technology over the other [94]. Because the linear accelerator-based units can serve to treat non-radiosurgery patients during its "down time," these units have become more popular, especially where limited numbers of patients would be treated with SRS and vault size is at a premium [94].

Radiosurgery and neurosurgical approaches are often complementary, but there are important differences. Radiosurgery does not require a craniotomy and is generally done as an outpatient procedure. In a cost-effectiveness/cost-utility analysis, Mehta and colleagues showed that the average cost per week of survival for single brain metastasis was $310 for radiotherapy, $524 for resection plus radiation, and only $270 for radiosurgery plus whole brain radiation [95]. Other advantages include lower postoperative risks for bleeding, lower risks for anesthesia complications and infection, and also rapid recovery times. Patients who are working prior to treatment can often return to work within 1 to 2 days. More importantly, medically unfit patients or patients with neurosurgically inaccessible lesions can often be treated with radiosurgery.

The delivery of radiosurgery is complex, and a multidisciplinary approach involving neurosurgery, radiation oncology, and medical physics is essential for a quality program. This allows for coordination of care, improved quality of care, reduction in practice variation, and improved patient satisfaction [96].

Neutron Capture Therapy

Neutron capture therapy (NCT) is defined as the activation of a stable nuclide, by neutrons, resulting in the subsequent release of ionizing radiation. Tumor cells are initially loaded with the stable nuclide. When the nuclide has cleared from the blood and normal tissues (assuming preferential uptake in malignant tissue), neutrons from an external source are then used to activate the nuclide and produce a targeted cytotoxic event in the tumor. At least in theory, this form of treatment represents a true form of "binary therapy." A binary system consists of two nontoxic components. Each component by itself is harmless. When combined, however, cell death will ensue [97–111]. NCT has been proposed for ^{10}B, ^{157}Gd [112], and ^{235}U [113]. Neutron sources are typically external and are produced by nuclear reactors [114] in the form of thermal neutrons (E_n < 0.5 eV), epithermal neutrons (E_n < 10 keV), or mixed thermal and epithermal neutron beams [115]. Epithermal neutron beams are attractive because the neutrons lose energy and fall into the thermal range as they traverse tissue. This allows for greater depth of penetration when compared with nearly pure thermal neutron beams. In fact, a standard epithermal reactor beam will result in peak thermalization of the neutrons at approximately 2 cm below the skull surface. Regardless, beam contamination with photons and fast neutrons continue to be a problem. Accelerator-based neutron sources are being developed [116]. These systems produce the neutron beam

Table 81.3 Neutron Capture Various Nuclides

Device	Description
CT-on-Rails (Siemens, Concord, CA)	Unit that incorporates a kilovoltage CT scanner with a linear accelerator. Patient is scanned on CT for image guidance. The table is then rotated 180 degrees and patient is treated on the adjacent linear accelerator. This allows additional certainty in target localization.
Tomotherapy HI-ART (Tomotherapy Inc, Middleton, WI)	This unit incorporates a megavoltage CT scanner as a delivery device. Unlike CT-on-Rails, this unit not only can scan the patient prior to treatment for target delineation but also is able to deliver radiation. There is a high degree of beam modulation (leafs adjust at 300 cm per second which is much higher than any other delivery device) which allows for very conformal radiation dose delivery.
Volumetric arc therapy	Volumetric modulated arc therapy is a new way of delivering IMRT, which combines 3D volumetric imaging with arc treatment delivery. This technique allows for IGRT with significantly reduced treatment times. Currently, volumetric arc technology is available through Elekta (VMAT, Stockholm, Sweden) and Varian (Rapid Arc, Palo Alto, CA)
Gamma knife (Elekta, Stockholm, Sweden)	Dedicated stereotactic radiosurgery unit primarily used to treat lesions in the brain. Co-60 is the radiation source used in gamma knife. This technology has had the longest track-record of radiosurgery in the brain.
CyberKnife (Accuray, Sunnyvale, CA)	This is a linac-based radiosurgery unit that includes a 6 MV linear accelerator mounted onto a robot that allows radiation to be delivered with sub-millimeter accuracy in virtually any direction. There are on board image detectors for target delineation.
Novalis (Brainlab, Feldkirchen, Germany)	This radiosurgery system utilizes a 120 mini multileaf collimator (2.5 m) to modulate the beam, which is mounted on a standard Varian linear accelerator. On board detectors are used to ensure reproducible setup. Often, a frameless radiosugery delivery is incorporated.
MRI guided therapy machines	Multiple MR guided machines are under development. The Renaissance RT system (ViewRay, Inc, Gainsville, FL) will have an onboard 0.3 Tesla open MRI with real time image guidance and/or dose guidance during treatment delivery. This system will be capable of delivering IMRT, intensity modulated radiosurgery, 3D conformal photon beam therapy employing three treatment heads that are spaced apart by 120 degrees with Co-60 sources.

by accelerating protons into a ^{7}Li target. Internal neutron sources, using ^{252}Cf brachytherapy, have been suggested for boron neutron capture therapy (BNCT) [117]. This form of NCT, however, has not reached the clinical setting for CNS malignancies. Currently, all clinical data have been generated using boron as the capture agent. Natural boron consists of 80% ^{11}B and 20% ^{10}B (61). ^{10}B is the nuclide with the large neutron capture cross-section. It is generally accepted that the intracellular ^{10}B concentration must be ≥20 μg/g tumor [118] or ~10^9 ^{10}B atoms per cell [119]. This concentration must be achieved in ≥90% of the tumor cells [120] for NCT to be successful. It has been calculated that a thermal neutron fluence of 10^{12} to 10^{13} n/cm^2 is necessary to sustain the BNCT reaction [121]. BNCT involves the nuclear reaction ^{10}B + ^{1}n → ^{7}Li + ^{4}He. The concept was first proposed in 1936 [122]. The reaction is based on the ability of ^{10}B to react with thermal neutrons (0.025 eV). The reaction occurs with a high probability and has a nuclear cross section of 3838 barns [123]. A barn is defined as 10^{-24} cm^2. The larger the barn number, the greater the probability of a reaction or capture event. In general, the probability for neutron capture is high for low-energy (thermal) neutrons and low for high-energy (fast) neutrons, for a given nucleus. The cross section of ^{10}B can be contrasted to the fission reaction of ^{235}U which has a cross section of 583 barns and a fission product release energy of 200.0 MeV [113]. Interestingly, ^{157}Gd has a cross section of 255,000 barns (Table 81.4), but the reaction must be located in the nucleus, owing to the short range (0–150 nm) of the Auger and Coster-Kronig electrons, for cellular damage to occur. BNCT liberates an α particle and a recoiling lithium nucleus with an energy of 2.79 MeV (6% probability) or an α particle and lithium nucleus with an energy of 2.31 MeV (94% probability) plus a lithium nucleus and γ with an energy of 0.48 MeV [118]. The α particle and Li nucleus are of high LET and are responsible for the cytotoxic effect. The resulting γ radiation has minimal local biological impact but may contribute to the whole-body dose. Additionally, the γ radiation may serve as a means to measure dose, as the γ emission will be concentrated in a region of local ^{10}B concentration, in a neutron activated treatment area. The path length of the high LET particles is between 5 and 9 μm, approximately one cell diameter [118]. The obvious goal of BNCT is to supply a selective cytotoxic treatment to the malignancy, while sparing normal tissues. Weighted doses between 60 and 70 Gy can be reasonably delivered with BNCT in approximately 1 hour as opposed to 6 to 7 weeks with standard external beam photon therapy [122–124].

Initial studies using BNCT to treat GBM were performed at the Brookhaven National Laboratory (BNL) in 1951 [125], using isotopically enriched borax [126]. Another series of patients ($n = 17$) were treated at BNL [126–128] between 1959 and 1961 and ($n = 18$) at the Massachusetts Institute of Technology (MIT) [126,128–130] between 1959 and 1961 [131]. These trials concluded in 1961, and the results have been analyzed [132]. The disappointing results seemed to be primarily due to lack of specificity of the boron agents for the tumor (tumor:blood ratio < 1), high blood boron concentrations (leading to vascular injury), and the inability of thermal neutrons to reach deep seated tumors (>6 cm depth). These problems often resulted in severe skin reactions and damage to normal tissues. BNCT was thus discontinued in the United States. In the late 1960s, BNCT was initiated in Japan [133,134] under the guidance of Dr. Hatanaka [118,135]. Dr. Hatanaka learned the pioneering procedure to lessen scalp and bone dose by surgically reflecting these structures at the time of neutron treatment. The Japanese approach, therefore, was to use sodium mercaptoundecahydrododecaborate, $Na_2B_{12}H_{11}SH$ (BSH), as the neutron capture agent [135]. Of note, BSH is generally not found to cross the blood-brain barrier (BBB), although a CNS malignancy will cause BBB disruption because of local invasion [131], hence allowing some accumulation of BSH. BSH can be contrasted to p-boronophenylalanine, another commonly used neutron

Table 81.4 Neutron Capture of Various Nuclides

Nuclide	Cross Section (Barns)	Reaction	Path Length	Energy (MeV)
^{1}H	0.33	$^1H+n \rightarrow {}^2H+\gamma^{(a)}$	—	2.22
^{14}N	1.75	$^{14}N+n \rightarrow {}^{14}C+{}^1H$	10–11 µm	0.626
^{10}B	3838	$^{10}B+n \rightarrow {}^7Li+{}^4He$	5–9 µm	2.79
^{157}Gd	255,000	$^{157}Gd+n \rightarrow {}^{158}Gd+\gamma^{(b)}$	0–150 nm	7.94
^{235}U	583	$^{235}U+n \rightarrow {}^{86}Kr+{}^{136}Xe^{(c)}$	11–18 µm	200.00

(a) Radiative capture
(b) Auger Cascade
(c) Many possible fission products

capture agent, which does cross the BBB [131]. In the Japanese series, BSH was initially given intra-arterially and eventually intravenously. The tumors were maximally surgically debulked. During the actual neutron treatment, a skin and bone flap was raised so as to avoid excessive radiation damage, as reported in the early BNL and MIT experiences. As the technique evolved, a silastic sphere was placed into the resection cavity in an attempt to further improve upon the depth of penetration of the thermal neutron beam. Eventually, BNCT trials resumed in the United States and Europe, and epithermal neutron beams were used to increase neutron depth of penetration and decrease the dose to the scalp, thus abrogating the need for a skin and bone flap. More recent trials in Japan have initiated BNCT with epithermal beams [136].

Favorable initial reports with long-term survivors [134,137] led to a renewed interest of BNCT in many countries. However, an analysis of patients from the United States, treated in these Japanese series, was performed [138]. A matched cohort of patients with high-grade glioma, treated by conventional therapy, was compared with the 12 remaining patients treated by BNCT in Japan. There was no significant difference in survival between the two groups.

The results from more recent BNCT trials performed in the United States, Japan, Finland, Sweden, the Netherlands, and the Czech Republic have been extensively reviewed. In general, the results appear to support a baseline level of efficacy comparable with standard therapy (Table 81.5). It appears that further research is warranted. Clinical investigations continue in the United States, Japan, Europe, and Argentina. Areas of active research include improved neutron sources (accelerator-based neutron production and reliable collimation), more targeted boron delivery agents, new neutron capture agents, better dosimetry, improved neutron beams and dose components (lowering of fast neutron and photon contamination of the primary beam as well as lessening of the proton and gamma dose to normal tissue from the interaction of neutrons with hydrogen and nitrogen), combined modality approaches (photons and neutrons), fractionation of the neutron beam, and the overwhelming need for randomized trials. If BNCT can become more targeted, the delivery of neutron irradiation moved from the realm "unfriendly" nuclear reactors to hospital environments and favorable randomized results reported, then perhaps this form of therapy has a chance to survive.

Protons and Heavy Particles

As mentioned earlier, photons and electrons are the primary therapeutic radiation modalities. Photons are massless and electrons have a mass of a mere 9.1×10^{-31} kg. This is in sharp contrast to protons and neutrons and other heavy particles whose mass is in excess of 1.6×10^{-27} kg. Particle beam radiotherapy is used to describe therapy utilizing protons, neutrons, α particles, or heavier particles such as carbon ions. Further, they are characterized as either high or low LET, depending on the amount of energy deposited over a given distance. Standard photon and electron beams are considered low LET in the range of 0.2 to 2 keV/µ as opposed to fast neutrons which have a 10- to 100-fold higher LET. Protons and α particles have low LET like photons and electrons, whereas carbon ions have high LET properties. The RBE is defined as the ratio of the dose of Cobalt-60 radiation to the dose of any other type of radiation that produces the same biological endpoint and is related to the LET. For photons and electrons, the RBE is 1. Protons and α particles are slightly higher at 1.1 to 1.2. Fast neutrons and other high LET particles can be between three and eight.

Fast neutron therapy has been used since the 1930s to treat cancers [139]. About 30,000 patients have been treated with this technology. However, because of the associated late side effects, the expense associated with creating neutron delivery systems, and advances in other radiation technology, interest in and access to neutron centers is limited, with only five operating centers worldwide (three in the United States) Areas where neutrons have shown potential benefits include salivary gland tumors (specifically adenoid cystic carcinoma) [140–142], squamous cell carcinomas of the head and neck [143,144], non-small cell lung cancer [145], prostate cancer [146–148], and sarcomas [149].

Recently, charged particle therapy, especially proton beam therapy, has gained interest in the radiation oncology community. With protons, and other charged particles, energy is deployed rapidly in a narrow range, at the end of its path length as the particle slows. This phenomenon is the "Bragg Peak" and has the advantage of delivering radiation with a rapid fall with little exit dose (Figure 81.12). The concerns over spraying low doses of radiation to normal tissues, as seen with IMRT, is less of a concern with protons because they stop at a given depth which depends on their initial energy.

Traditional proton accelerators are bulky and expensive. Newer devices are currently in development,

Table 81.5 BNC for Malignant Glioma and Other Brain Tumors

Facility (Year)	Beam/Fraction/Number of Fields/Dose	Neutron Capture Agent	Patients (n)	Median Survival (months)	Reference
Japan; multiple[a] (1968–1995)	Thermal Neutrons[b]/1/1/ 10.4–11.3 Gy	BSH (60–80 mg/kg)	n = 149; GBMF = 64; AA = 39	GBMF = 21.33 AA = 60.36	88
The Netherlands; Petten Irradiation facility (1997–2002)	Epithermal Neutrons/4/1–2/8.6–11.4 Gy	BSH (100 mg/kg)	n = 26; GBMF = 26	No data; Phase I dose-searching	90, 57, 91
Finland; FiRI(1999–2001 P-01; 2001 P-03)	Epithermal Neutrons/1/2/ 25–29 Gy (W)[c]	BPA (290–400 mg/kg P-01; 290 mg/kg P-03)	n = 21; GBMF = 18, P-01; GBMF = 3, P-03	61 % one year OAS	92
Sweden; Studsvik Medical AB (2001–2002)	Epithermal Neutrons/1/2/ 8.0–15.5 Gy (W)[d]	BPA (900 mg/kg)[e]	n = 17; GBMF = 17	GBMF = 18[f]	57, 93
Czech Republic; LVR-15 (2001)	Thermal Neutrons/1/1/ < 14.2 Gy (W)	BSH (100 mg/kg)	n = 5; GBMF = 5	Less than conventional therapy	57, 94
USA, Harvard-MIT; MITR-II, M67 (1996–1999)[g]	Epithermal Neutrons/ 1–2/1–3/8.8–14.2 Gy[h]	BPA (250–350 mg/kg)	n = 22; GBMF = 20[i]	All patients = 13	57, 95, 96, 97
USA, BNL, BMRR (1994–1999)	Epithermal Neutrons/ 1/1–3/8.9–15.9 Gy-Eq	BPA (250–330 mg/kg)	n = 53; GBMF = 53	1 field = 14.8 2 field = 12.1 3 field = 11.9	98, 99

Abbreviations: AA, anaplastic astrocytoma; BNL, Brookhaven National Laboratory; BSH, mercaptoundecahydrododecaborate; BPA, p-boronophenylalanine; GBMF, glioblastoma multiforme.

[a] Hitachi training (HTR); Japan Atomic Research Institute (JJR-3); Musashi Institute of Technology (MulTR); Kyoto University (KUR); Japan Atomic Research Inst (JRR-2).

[b] Skin and bone flap removed during the irradiation process; silastic covered sphere or tube placed in resection cavity.

[c] Weighted dose.

[d] Estimated peak normal brain dose.

[e] Infusion of BPA performed over 6 hours.

[f] No prior therapy other than surgery.

[g] Only US facility treating with BNCT.

[h] RBE-Gy (sum of the physical dose for each component in the neutron beam, weighted by its RBE).

[i] Two patients with melanoma.

including a single-room compact proton solution. Tomotherapy proton therapy system (Compact Particle Acceleration Corp, Madison, WI) represents a dramatic departure from all current systems, both in terms of proton generation as well as delivery. The Tomotherapy proton therapy system is based on the concept of distal edge tracking or distal gradient tracking using rotational delivery to deliver intensity-modulated proton therapy. To accelerate protons to a maximal energy of 200 MeV, a dielectric wall linear accelerator will be employed. The system will impart a lower neutron dose to patients, because neutrons are not produced in the aperture and range compensators; however, neutrons will still be produced in the patient. Pretreatment image guidance will be accomplished employing a conventional kVCT scanner mounted to the back of the unit.

Heavy ions, such as carbon, neon, nitrogen, argon, and silicon, are also being investigated. These have the advantage of protons with the rapid fall off (Bragg Peak) and also possess a higher RBE, similar to that of fast neutrons. There are three units worldwide (HIMAC and HARIMAC in Japan and GSI in Germany), and these centers are carbon ion facilities. Efficacy using heavy ions is currently being evaluated, and no centers currently exist in the United States.

Charged particle therapy has been investigated in a variety of disease sites. With prices exceeding $100 million per unit for full-size units, the cost benefit ratio remains to be accurately described as efficacy data are still maturing. Diseases that have potential benefits with charged particles include uveal melanomas [150], optic pathway gliomas [151], skull-based tumors [152], pituitary adenomas [153], acoustic neuromas [154], nasopharynx and paranasal sinuses [155,156], spinal cord tumors [157,158], prostate cancer [159,160], lung cancer [161–164], gastrointestinal malignancies [165–167], and pediatric cancers [168–170].

Targeted Radionuclide Radiotherapy

Currently, the most cytotoxic agents known are α, β, and the low-energy (Auger) electron-emitting radionuclides. It has been estimated that one gram of unconjugated ^{210}Po would be lethal to as many as 10 million humans (http://en.wikipedia.org/wiki/polonium). On a molar basis, ^{111}In is 85, 200, and 300 times more cytotoxic than the commonly used chemotherapy agents, paclitaxel, methotrexate, and adriamycin, respectively [171].

The properties of commonly employed radionuclides for TRT are shown in Table 81.6 [172–175]. TRT is a treatment modality that employs the conjugation or bonding of a radionuclide to a delivery construct that has a high avidity for the specific tumor cell or target. Based on the path length, the LET, and the decay properties, it is generally accepted that Auger or low-energy electron emitters are best suited to sterilize single cells, α emitters for cell clusters or preangiogenic micrometastases, and β emitters for bulkier lesions. Cell-kill modeling indicates that the ideal location for Auger electron emitters is in the cell nucleus and α emitters on the cell surface or in the cytoplasm. Beta emitters largely exert their toxicity through the "cross-fire" effect [176].

Typically, the delivery construct consists of an intact antibody, an antibody fragment, or an affinity ligand (Table 81.7). The size of the construct has significant ramifications concerning biodistribution, excretion, and tumor penetration [177]. Ultimately, the larger antibodies will remain bound to solid tumors to a greater extent than antibody fragments. Unfortunately, the longer biological half-life of intact antibodies will lead to increased dose to normal tissues, most notably, the bone marrow. The route of delivery for such constructs, as applied to CNS malignancies, can be systemic, intracavitary, intracompartmental, or intratumoral. Additionally, there appears to be several ways by which the therapeutic ratio of TRT can be enhanced. These include fractionation, pretargeting, protection of normal tissues, and a combined modality approach with chemotherapy and EBRT. Although TRT has been utilized for treating neuroblastoma, brain metastasis, and meningeal disease, this section will refer to its specific clinical application as it applies to treating grade III and IV astrocytoma.

The perfect antigenic target would be highly expressed on the tumor cell (tumor specific) and not expressed within normal tissue or secreted or "shed" systemically. If internalization occurs, then an α- or low-energy electron emitter should be considered as the therapeutic radionuclide. In reality, the best targets tend to be excessively expressed in the malignant tissue and minimally expressed in benign tissue. To date, the most commonly identified antigenic targets for CNS malignancies are the epidermal growth factor receptor (EGFR), neural cell adhesion molecule (NCAM), tenascin, placental alkaline phosphatase, and phosphatidyl inositide. The EGFR is variably amplified in malignant tissue and is also present in benign tissue. NCAM is present on both benign and malignant glioma cells, and tenascin is an extracellular glycoprotein ubiquitously expressed by glioma. A comprehensive review of clinical trials using TRT to treat malignant glioma is listed in Table 81.8.

Most of the trials to date are of "dose searching pilot" or phase I design. The evolution of the trials has seen the delivery route move from systemic (intra-arterial or intravenous) to local instillation of the TRT agent into a surgically created resection cavity (SCRC). Even though the BBB is often disrupted by a rapidly growing CNS

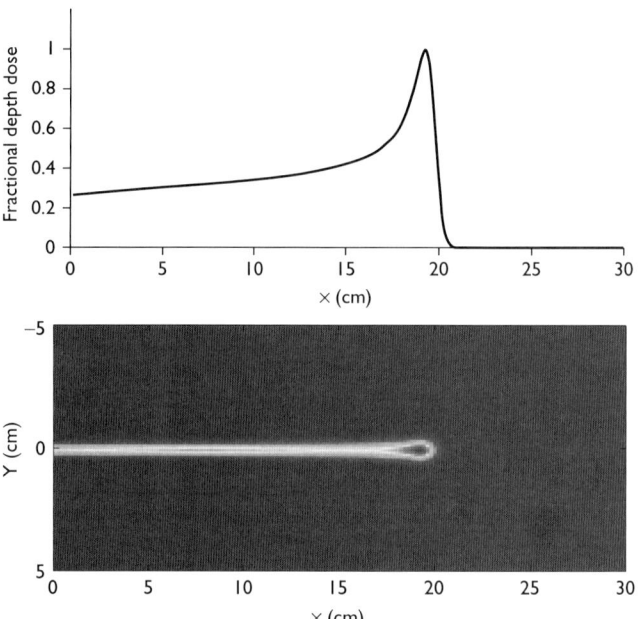

Figure 81.12 Fractional depth dose in water of a 170 MeV proton beam having a full width half maximum of 8mm. There is a rapid rise and then a fall off with little exit dose (Bragg Peak.) The associated proton pencil beam is shown below the fractional depth dose curve. (Courtesy of Wolfgang Tomè) See color insert.

Table 81.6 Commonly Used Radionuclides for TRT

Radionuclide	Physical Half-life	E max (MeV)	Maximum Range in Tissue	LET (keV/μm)	Approximate Cell Diameters
β-Emitters		β-Particle		0.2	
^{90}Y	2.7 days	2.30	12.0 mm		400–1100
^{131}I	8.0 days	0.81	2.0 mm		10–230
^{177}Lu	6.7 days	0.50	1.5 mm		4–180
^{186}Re	3.8 days	1.10	3.6 mm		
^{188}Re	17.0 hours	2.10	11.0 mm		200–1000
^{67}Cu	2.6 days	0.60	2.8 mm		5–210
α-Emitters		α-Particle		80	
^{213}Bi	45.7 minutes	5.87	70–100 μm		7–10
^{211}At	7.2 hours	5.87	55–60 μm		5–6
Low-energy electron emitters		Low-energy electron		4–26	
^{125}I	60.1 days	0.35	2–500 nm		1
^{67}Ga	3.3 days	0.18	2–500 nm		1
^{111}In	2.83 days	0.04–0.2	2–500 nm		1

Table 81.7 Targeting Construct

Targeting Construct	Size (kDa)
IgG	150
CH2-deletion	125
Minibody	100
F(ab')$_2$	100
Fab'	50
scFv	25
Affibodies	6–7
Peptides	1–2

malignancy, this phenomenon is not well defined, and 150-kDa antibodies would still not likely cross, to a significant degree, although there does appear to be an element of nonspecific uptake [178]. As a result, studies using the systemic approach often deliver EBRT in conjunction with TRT. It has been well documented that EBRT will cause an increase in the permeability of the BBB and increased vascular leakage [179–181]. Regardless, it has been disappointingly estimated that only 0.001 to 0.01% of the systemically delivered antibody will penetrate each gram of solid tumor [182]. Furthermore, biopsy data have revealed that a single systemic injection of radiolabled anti-EGFR antibody will deliver only 0.02% of the injected activity per gram of tumor, resulting in a dose of only 100 to 200 cGy [178].

Direct instillation of the TRT agent into the SCRC is an attractive alternative to the systemic approach. Unlike other malignant sites where the potential for systemic spread mandates a systemic approach, this is not the case for malignant gliomas. The local approach is accomplished by injecting or instilling the TRT agent directly into the SCRC via an Ommaya or Rickam catheter. Preliminary dosimetry is performed to ensure localization within the surgical bed and that no direct communication with the ventricular system has occurred. Institutions using this technique have utilized murine, chimeric, or humanized monoclonal antibodies attached to ^{131}I, ^{90}Y, ^{188}Re, and ^{211}At. Other important treatment variances include fractionation, pretargeting, and a combined modality approach using EBRT and chemotherapy. The success of direct instillation into the SCRC will depend on meaningful penetration of the TRT agent into the local brain parenchyma such that the monoclonal antibodies (or targeting construct) can bind to areas of microscopic extension of malignant cells at some distance from the SCRC margin. It is still unknown as to what impact the healing process/inflammation at the surgical margin has on the success of antibody penetration. Also, it is well known that binding site barrier phenomena, interstitial tumor pressure, aberrant tumor vasculature, and a recusant extracellular tumor matrix will significantly impede antibody penetration.

Hopkins obtained biopsy data from three patients with glioma who received two to three cycles of either ^{131}I or ^{90}Y-ERIC-1 (anti-NCAM antibody), directly instilled into an SCRC [183]. Relevant assumptions were that the SCRCs were spherical, the radionuclide was spread evenly around the resection margin, 100% of the TRT agent was bound to its target, and diffusion into the resection margin was uniform. It was shown that "modest" diffusion occurred and the process was exponential. The peak dose occurred between 0.16 and 0.18 cm beyond the resection margin and 4.4 to 5.8% of the peak dose was delivered to a depth of 2 cm. Of note, NCAM is expressed on benign and malignant cells, and perhaps a more tumor-specific antigen would allow for greater depth of penetration. Certainly, smaller targeting constructs have been shown to penetrate to a greater depth in brain parenchyma, compared with intact antibodies [184]. Using the same antibody, radiolabeled with ^{131}I and instilled into an SCRC, Papanatassiou [182] showed that diffusion occurred from 0.5 to 1.0 cm (SPECT). Additionally, the range of binding of antibody to the target was 8 to 80%. Because the R_{95} (thickness of tissue where 95% of the β energy is deposited) for ^{131}I is only 0.992 mm, it was concluded that a more optimal radionuclide would potentially be ^{90}Y with an R_{95} of 5.94 mm [185]. Assuming a 2 cm SCRC and 100% binding, as much as 351 Gy could be delivered to the tumor with a single instillation of 18.2 mCi of ^{90}Y-ERIC-1. This calculation resulted in an impressive minimum tumor/whole brain dose ratio of 140:1.

Using ^{131}I-81C6 (anti-tenascin monoclonal antibody), dose-limiting toxicity was reached with a single injection (fraction) of 80 mCi for leptomeningeal disease (intrathecal delivery), 100 mCi for heavily pretreated and recurrent glioma (into SCRC), and 120 mCi for de novo glioma (into SCRC), also receiving EBRT and chemotherapy [186]. Using a standard, fixed, mCi dose, a wide range of absorbed doses (18–186 Gy) will be delivered to a depth of 2 cm beyond the SCRC margin [187]. On further analysis, an optimal dose of 44 Gy to 2 cm beyond SCRC was identified. Doses < 44 Gy resulted in increased recurrence rates and doses > 44 Gy resulted in a higher rate of necrosis. A trend toward a significant improvement in median survival was shown for patients receiving 40 to 48 Gy vs. <40 Gy [188]. Refining the technique further, it was shown that 20/21 patients could be successfully dosed to 44 Gy by varying the initial injection activity and considering the volume of the SCRC [189]. Zalutsky showed that a high LET, α-emitting radioconjugate (^{211}At-81C6) could be safely delivered in a small cohort of patients with glioma [190].

The median survival for TRT for treating glioma appears extremely favorable when compared with other treatment approaches. For de novo lesions, the median survival range is 50.9 to 57.6 months (three studies not reaching median survival at the time of the report) for AA and 13.4 to 35.5 months for GBM. For recurrent lesions, the median survival range is 13.0 to 52.0 months (one study not reaching median survival at the time of the report) for AA and 14.0 to 25.0 months for GBM. Further improvements can be expected as this field matures and phase II and III data are generated. Unlike brachytherapy, there appears to be a very low rate of CNS toxicity and a minimal need for surgical intervention for removal of necrotic regions. Areas of active research include variable sized targeting agents, utilization of fully human constructs, clinically appropriate radionuclides, antibody "cocktails," combined modality approaches, BBB disruption, and exploration of the type of delivery route.

In summary, tumors of the brain have several challenges that need to be overcome. Often, surgery is

Table 81.8 Targeted Radionuclide Trials

Study/Inst./ Published date (Ref.)	Design/ Cohort Years	Nuclide-Antibody/ Type	Antigen or Target/ Antigen Tested on Tumor	Tumor Type = No. of Pats/ Presentation/ KPS	Route	Activity per fraction/ No. of fractions	Other Therapies	MTD/DLT	BBB Disruption via EBRT	Type of surgery/ Residual	Pretargeting/ HAMA	RFN	POF	Median Survival (months)
Epenetos/ London/ 1985 [146]	Case Report/ 1984	131I-9A/ murine	EGFR/Yes	GBM = 1/R/No; stated	IA	45 mCi/1	Prior S and EBRT (70 Gy)	ND/None	No	None/ Enlarging mass	No/No data	0%	No data	Improved symptoms and partial response via CT
Kalofonos/ London/1989 [133]	Phase I/ No data	131I-EGFR1, 131I-H17E2/ murine	EGFR, PLAP/ Yes	GBM = 5 AA = 3 BSG = 2/R/ Not stated	IA (n = 5) IV (n = 5)	40–140 mCi/1	Prior S (80%), EBRT (100%), C (10%)	ND/None	No	Not stated/ No data	No/ 1/10 (10%)	No data	No data	40% clinical and 30% CT improvement
Brady/ Philadelphia/ 1990 [147]	Phase I–II/ No data	125I-425/ murine	EGFR/ No	GBM = 4 AA = 6 LGG = 3 ACA = 1 Unknown = 1/ R/Not stated	IA (1)	8–75 mCi/ ≥2 11/15 patients	Prior S (100%), EBRT (100%)	50 mCi/ Neurologic	No	Not stated/ No data	No/No data	1/15 (7%)	No data	GBM & AA = 5.5 (relapse free interval)
Papanastassiou/ UK/1993 [137]	Pilot Study/ No data	131I-ERIC-1/ murine	NCAM/ No	Glioma = 7/R = 6, DN = 1/ Not stated	SCRC or intracystic via O/R	36–59 mCi/1	Prior S (100%)	59 mCi/ Neurologic	No	Gross total resection/ No data	No/No data	1/7 (14%)	No data	No data
Hopkins/ UK/1995 (140)	Pilot Study/ 1992–1993	90y-ERIC-1/ murine	NCAM/ No	GBM = 10 AA = 4 LGG = 1 R/ Not stated	SCRC or Intratumor via O/R	11–25 mCi/1–3	Prior S (100%), EBRT (100%)	ND/None	No	Gross Total resection/no excessive tumor	No/No data	No data	No data	All = 6
Bigner/ Duke/1998 [148]	Phase I/ 1992–1996	131I-81C6/ murine	Tenascin/ Yes	GBM = 26 AA = 3 AO = 2 Epen = 1 MM = 2/R/ KPS≥50	SCRC via O/R	20–120 mCi/ 1	Prior S (100%), EBRT (73%), C (55%)	100 mCi/ Neurologic	No	SCRC/ Tumor ≤ 1 cm from SCRC margin	No/17/30 (57%)	0%	34% Noncontiguous; 91%≤2 cm of SCRC	GBM = 14 All = 15
Riva/Cesena/ 1999 [149]	Phase I & 2/1990–1997	131I-BC-2, BC-4/ murine	Tenascin/ Yes	GBM = 91 AA = 10 LGG = 2 AO = 7, O = 1/ R & DN/ KPS≥60	SCRC via O/R	5–75 mCi/3–6 (2)	S (100%), EBRT (100%), C (54%)	70 mCi/CNS edema at ≥MTD	No	Maximum debulking/ 52<2 cm³, 39>3 cm³	No/(59%) (3)	3/111 (2.7%)	83.5% Local, 16.4% distant	GBM = 19 AA=46 AO = 23 O = 31

Continued

Table 81.8 Continued

Study/Inst./ Published date (Ref.)	Design/ Cohort Years	Nuclide-Antibody/ Type	Antigen or Target/ Antigen Tested on Tumor	Tumor Type = No. of Pats/ Presentation/ KPS	Route	Activity per fraction/ No. of fractions	Other Therapies	MTD/DLT	BBB Disruption via EBRT	Type of surgery/ Residual	Pretargeting/ HAMA	RFN	POF	Median Survival (months)
Cokgor/ Duke/2000 [150]	Phase I/ 1993–1998	131I-81C6/ murine	Tenascin/ Yes	GBM = 32 AA = 3 AO = 5 O = 2/DN/ KPS≥50	SCRC via O/R	20–180 mCi/1	S (100%), EBRT 1 month after 131I-81C6	120 mCi/ Neurologic	No	Gross total resection/≤1 cm tumor	N0/34/38 (89%)	1/42 (2.4%)	No data	GBM = 17.3 All = 19.8
Pagnelli/ Milan/2001 [151]	Phase I/ No data	90Y-BC4/ murine	Tenascin/ No Data	GBM = 16 AA = 8/R/ KPS≥60	SCRC via O/R	15–30 mCi/2(4)	Prior S (100%), EBRT (100%)	30 mCi/ Neurologic (5)	No	Surgical debulking/ No data	Yes/No data	0%	No data	GBM = 20 AA = 52
Ppperl/ Munich/ 2002 [152]	Phase I/ No data	131I-BC-4/ murine	Tenascin/ No data	GBM = 8 AA = 4/DN/ KPS>70	SCRC via O/R	30 mCi (6)/1–5	S (100%), EBRT (100%)	ND/None	Yes	Surgical debulking/ No data	No/ 8/12 (67%)	No data	No data	All = 18.5
Emrich/ Drexel/2002 [153]	Phase II/ 1987–1997	125I-425/ murine (7)	EGFR/ No data	GBM = 118 AA = 55/DN/ KPS = 80	IV or IA	140 mCi (8)/3 (9)	S (100%), EBRT (100%), C (32%)	50 mCi/None	Yes	Surgical debulking (10)/No data	No/ No HAMA (11)	No data	No data	GB = 13.4 AA = 50.9
Grana/ EIO/2002 [154]	Phase II/ 1994–1997	90Y-BC4/ murine	Tenascin/ Yes	GBM = 20 AA = 17 (12)/DN/ KPS>70	IV (13)	59 mCi per m²/1	S (100%), EBRT (100%), C (24%)	ND/None	Yes	Absence of gross disease after surgery/ No data	Yes/(20%) (14)	0%	No data	Control GBM = 8 AA = 33 Treatment GBM = 35.5 AA = NR (15)
Wygoda/ Poland/2002 [155]	Phase III/ No data	125I-425/ murine	EGFR/ No	GBM = 8 AA = 4 (16)/DN/ Not stated	IV (17)	50 mCi/3	S (100%), EBRT (100%), C (0%)	None/None	Yes	Macroscopic radical surgery/ No data	No/No data	0%	No data	Control All = 3/4 Treatment All = 5/7 (18)
Reardon/ Duke/2002 [141]	Phase II/ 1996–2000	131I-81C6/ murine	Tenascin/ Yes	GBM = 27 AA = 4 AO = 2/DN/ KPS≥70	SCRC via O/R	120 mCi/1	S (100%), EBRT one month after 131I-81C6	Previously done/ Neurologic	No	Gross total resection/ ≤1 cm tumor	No/27/30 (90%)	1/33 (3%)	No data	GBM = 19.9 All = 21.7
Goetz/ Munich & Cesena/2003 [156]	Phase I/ 1995-publication	90Y & 131I-BC4/ murine	Tenascin/ Yes	GBM = 24 AA = 13/DN/ KPS≥70	SCRC via O/R	30 mCi/ 2.96 (19)	S (100%), EBRT (100%), C (0%)	ND/None (20)	Yes	Surgical debulking/ minimal (21)	No/8/12 (67%)	0%	No data	GBM = 17 AA = NR (22)
Bartolomei/ Milan/2004 [157]	Phase II/ No data	90Y-BC4/ murine	Tenascin/ No data	GBM = 73/R/ KPS≥70, Group A = 38 Group B = 35 (23)	SCRC via O/R	10–25 mCi/2–7	Prior S (100%), EBRT (100%). C (41%)	ND/None	No	Surgical debulking/ No data	Yes/No data	3/73 (4%) (24)	No data	Group A 17.5 Group B 25.0 (25)
Boiardi/ Milan/2005 [158]	Phase I/ 1999–2001	90Y-BC4/ murine	Tenascin/ No data	GBM = 25/R/ KPS>60	SCRC via O/R	5–25 mCi/ 2 (26)	Prior S (100%), EBRT (100%), C (100%)	None/None (27)	No	Partial resection/ 75% had tumor >2 cm	Yes/No data	0%	No data	18 month OAS = 42%

Study/Location/Year [Ref]	Phase/Dates	Antibody/Internalizing	Target/Internalizing	Patients	Route	Dose (mCi)/Cycles	Prior Treatment	BBB disruption	Surgical debulking	HAMA	Pattern of Failure	Median Survival (months)
Mamelak/Los Angeles/2006 [139]	Phase I/No data	^{131}I-TM-601 (28)/Synthetic peptide	Phosphatidyl inositide	GBM = 17 AA = 1/R/ KPS≥60	SCRC via O/R	10 mCi/1	Prior S (100%), EBRT (100%), C (100%)	ND/None	No	Surgical debulking No data	0%	No data	All = 6.75
Reardon/Duke/2006 [142]	Phase II/1996–2003	^{131}I-81C6/murine	Tenascin/No data	GBM = 33 AA = 6 AO = 2 GS = 1 M = 1/R/ KPS≥60	SCRC via O/R	100 mCi (29)/1	Prior S (100%), EBRT (93%), C (53%)	100 mCi/None (30)	No	Maximum debulking/ ≤1 cm tumor	No/27/34 (79%)	0% (31)	2/43 (5%) Failed in opposite hemisphere	GBM/GS = 16.0 AA/AO = 24.75
Reardon/Duke/2006 [159]	Phase I/1999–2002	^{131}I-81C6/chimeric	Tenascin/Yes	GBM = 38 AA = 7 AO = 2/R & DN/ KPS≥60	SCRC via O/R	<80 mCi-120(32) mCi/1	80 mCi Hematologic and neurologic	No	SCRC/Little or no residual	No/19/41 (46%)	0%	14/47 (30%) Distant failure	Stratum A and B GBM = 21.5 AA = 57.6 Stratum C GBM = 12.2 AA = NR
Wygoda/Poland 2006 [160]	Phase III/No data	^{125}I-425/murine	EGFR/No	GBM = 12 AA = 6/DN/ Zubrod 0–2	IV	52 mCi/3	(33)	None/None	Yes	Maximum debulking <2 mL or no residual	No/No data	0%	Treatment 8/8 (100%) local Standard 9/9 (100%) local	Treatment All = 14 Standard All = 13, $P = 0.23$
Casaco/Cuba/2007 [161]	Phase I/No data	^{188}Re-h-R3/humanized	EGFR/No data	GBM = 8 AA = 3/R/ Not stated	Intratumor	10–15 mCi/1	Not stated	10 mCi/ neurologic	Not stated	No data/No data	No data	No data	No data
Reardon/Duke/2008 [144]	Phase II/2002–2004	^{131}I-81C6/murine	Tenascin/Yes	GBM = 15 AA = 6/DN/ KPS≥60 (34)	SCRC via O/R	25–150 mCi (35)/1	S (100%), EBRT (95%), C (95%) (36)	Previously done/ mild & limited	Yes (3/20 patients)	Gross total resection/≤1 cm tumor	No/17/17 (100%)	1/20 (5%) distant, 19/20 (95%) local	GBM = 22.6 AA = NR
Zalutsky/Duke/2008 [145]	Phase I/1998–2001	^{211}At-81C6/chimeric	Tenascin/Yes	GBM = 14 AA = 1 AO = 3/R/ KPS>70	SCRC via O/R	1.9–9.2 mCi/1	Prior S (100%), EBRT (100%), C (44%)	None/None	No	Gross total resection/ ≤1 cm tumor	No/5/15 (33%)	0%	Local in all but one case	GBM = 13.5 AA = 13.0 AO = 29

Abbreviations: AA, anaplastic astrocytoma; ACA, metastatic adenocarcinoma; AO, anaplastic oligodendroglioma; BBB, blood-brain barrier; BSG, brain stem glioma; C, chemotherapy; DLT, dose limiting toxicity; DN, de novo at presentation; EBRT, external beam radiotherapy; EGFR, epidermal growth factor receptor; EIO, European Institute of Oncology; Epen, ependymoma; GBM, glioblastoma multiforme; GS, gliosarcoma; HAMA, human anti-mouse antibody; IA, intra-arterial; IV, intravenous; LGG, low grade glioma; M, metastatic lesion; MM, malignant melanoma; MTD, maximum tolerated dose; NCAM, neural cell adhesion molecule; ND, not determined; NR, median survival not reached; O, oligodendroglioma; O/R, Ommaya or Rickam catheter; PLAP, placental alkaline phosphatase; POF, pattern of failure; R, recurrent presentation; RFN, reoperation for necrosis; S, surgery; SCRC, surgically created resection cavity.

Antibody delivered via internal carotid or vertebral artery system after cannulation of femoral artery.

Patients had multiple cycles (every 30–60 days) for 3 cycles, then repeated after 4–6 months (3 cycles, n = 24; 4 cycles, n = 18; 5 cycles, n = 10; 6 cycles, n = 6).

Largest HAMA titer in those receiving ≥3 cycles.

Each fraction 8–10 weeks apart.

Three patients' infection at catheter site.

Average dose.

Internalizing antibody.

Mean cumulative dose.

Once per week x 3; 50 mCi/dose, IV or IA.

30/55 (55%) debulking for AA; 93/118 (79%) debulking for GBMF.

No HAMA with ≤ 3 doses of targeted radionuclide.

Table 81.8 Continued

Control group, n = 18, S + EBRT +/- C, only; Treatment group, n = 19, S + EBRT + ^{90}Y-BC4 +/- C.

Targeted radionuclide delivered one month after EBRT.

90% anti-streptavidin antibodies; 70% anti-avidin antibodies.

Significant survival advantage for treatment vs. control group for GBMF ($P = 0.014$) and AA ($P = 0.002$).

GBMF; EBRT + ^{125}I-425, n = 5, EBRT only, n = 3. AA; EBRT +^{125}I-425, n = 2, EBRT only, n = 2.

Targeted radionuclide therapy initiated during 4th week of EBRT and repeated at one week intervals for 3 fractions.

Crude survival.

Patients at Cesena received ^{90}Y-BC4 and ^{131}I-BC4 in unspecified dose schedule; 30 mCi/fraction ^{131}I-BC4 used in Munich; mean number of fractions 2.96/patient, maximum of 8, given every 6–8 weeks.

Two patients developed skin necrosis, at injection site on scalp, requiring surgical closure.

No or "small" enhancement on MRI.

AA 5 year survival = 85%.

Group A = ^{90}Y-BC4 alone; Group B =^{90}Y-BC4 + Temodar.

All 3 patients still had viable tumor with necrosis.

Significant survival advantage for Group B vs. Group A ($P < 0.01$).

All patients were treated with ^{90}Y-BC4 (2 cycles, 10 weeks apart), PCV chemotherapy, mitoxantrone via O/R at 4 mg every 20 days.

No toxicity from targeted radionuclide therapy; 44% of patients experienced grade 3–4 hematologic toxicity secondary to PCV chemotherapy; 5 cases had O/R removed secondary to local decubitous or asceptic osteitis.

TM-601 is a synthetic 36 amino acid peptide (chlorotoxin), derived from scorpion venum. TM-601 binds to phosphatidyl inositide on the lamellipodia of tumor cells.

Average dose to 2 cm rim of tissue of SCRC = 46 Gy; range = 18–186 Gy; 58% of the patients received chemotherapy after ^{131}I-8IC6.

One patient experienced irreversible neurotoxicity (grade 2 hemiparesis worsened to grade 3); 23% developed reversible acute hematologic toxicity.

6/43 (14%) had a stereotactic biopsy showing gliosis and necrosis.

Patients divided onto stratum A (newly diagnosed and treated; SCRC and catheter→^{131}I-8IC6→EBRT→chemotherapy for 1 year), stratum B (newly diagnosed and prior EBRT; initial S→EBRT→SCRC and catheter→^{131}I-8IC6→chemotherapy for 1 year), stratum C (recurrent disease; SCRC and catheter→^{131}I-8IC6→chemotherapy for 1 year); The dose to a 2 cm margin of the SCRC was A = 32 Gy, B = 45 Gy, C = 40 Gy.

Treatment group (S + EBRT + 125I-425; n = 8); Standard therapy group (S + EBRT; n = 10)

One patient excluded from study due to subgaleal leak (therefore, n = 20).

Injected activity, into the SCRC, ranged from 25–150 mCi. This was done in order to deliver a uniform dose of 44Gy ±10% to a 2 cm rim of the SCRC. This was achieved in 20/21 (95%) patients.

17/20 patients were treated with S+^{131}I-8IC6→EBRT + C; 3/20 patients were treated with S+EBRT→^{131}I-8IC6 + C.

unattainable or incomplete. Systemic agents are often impenetrable because of the BBB. As a result, radiation therapy has been a mainstay treatment for decades. New advances, including IGRT and particle beam therapy, offer the hope of reduce toxicity and potentially improved efficacy. As our knowledge of the behavior and localization of tumor growth improves and our precision in radiation delivery enhances, it is the hope that we can further improve the outcomes seen in tumors of the brain.

REFERENCES

1. Stupp R, Mason WP, van den Bent MJ, et al. European Organisation for Research and Treatment of Cancer Brain Tumor and Radiotherapy Groups; National Cancer Institute of Canada Clinical Trials Group. Radiotherapy plus concomitant and adjuvant temozolomide for glioblastoma. *N Engl J Med.* 2005;352(10):987–996.
2. Robins HI, Chang S, Butowski N, Mehta M. Therapeutic advances for glioblastoma multiforme: current status and future prospects. *Curr Oncol Rep.* 2007;9(1):66–70.
3. Giese A, Westphal M. Glioma invasion in the central nervous system. *Neurosurgery.* 1996;39(2):235–50; discussion 250.
4. Chakravarti A, Tyndall E, Palanichamy K, Mehta M, Aldape K, Loeffler J. Impact of molecular profiling on clinical trial design for glioblastoma. *Curr Oncol Rep.* 2007;9(1):71–79.
5. Perry JR. Bias, benefit, or both: evaluating new glioma therapies. *Neurosurg Focus.* 1998;4(6):e9.
6. Daniel TM. Wilhelm Conrad Rötgen and the advent of thoracic radiology. *Int J Tuberc Lung Dis.* 2006;10(11):1212–1214.
7. Perez C, Halperin E, Brady L, eds. *Principle and Practice of Radiation Oncology.* 4thed. Philadelphia: Lippincott Willimas & Wilkins; 2004.
8. Bedford JS, Dewey WC. Radiation Research Society. 1952–2002. Historical and current highlights in radiation biology: has anything important been learned by irradiating cells? *Radiat Res.* 2002;158(3):251–291.
9. Willers H, Beck-Bornholdt HP. Origins of radiotherapy and radiobiology: separation of the influence of dose per fraction and overall treatment time on normal tissue damage by Reisner and Miescher in the 1930s. *Radiother Oncol.* 1996;38(2):171–173.
10. Fowler JF. Development of radiobiology for oncology-a personal view. *Phys Med Biol.* 2006;51(13):R263-R286.
11. Khan FM. *The Physics of Radiation Therapy.* Baltimore: Williams and Wilkens; 1984.
12. Hall EJ. *Radiobiology for the Radiologist.* 3rd ed. New York: Lippincott; 1988.
13. Kolesnick R, Fuks Z. Radiation and ceramide-induced apoptosis. *Oncogene.* 2003;22(37):5897–5906.
14. Taneja N, Tjalkens R, Philbert MA, Rehemtulla A. Irradiation of mitochondria initiates apoptosis in a cell free system. *Oncogene.* 2001;20(2):167–177.
15. Garcia-Barros M, Paris F, Cordon-Cardo C, et al. Tumor response to radiotherapy regulated by endothelial cell apoptosis. *Science.* 2003;300(5622):1155–1159.
16. Munro TR. The relative radiosensitivity of the nucleus and cytoplasm of Chinese hamster fibroblasts. *Radiat Res.* 1970;42(3):451–470.
17. Rainaldi G, Romano R, Indovina P, et al. Metabolomics using 1H-NMR of apoptosis and Necrosis in HL60 leukemia cells: differences between the two types of cell death and independence from the stimulus of apoptosis used. *Radiat Res.* 2008;169(2):170–180.
18. Jänicke RU, Engels IH, Dunkern T, Kaina B, Schulze-Osthoff K, Porter AG. Ionizing radiation but not anticancer drugs causes cell cycle arrest and failure to activate the mitochondrial death pathway in MCF-7 breast carcinoma cells. *Oncogene.* 2001;20(36):5043–5053.
19. Roninson IB. Tumor cell senescence in cancer treatment. *Cancer Res.* 2003;63(11):2705–2715.
20. Chang BD, Broude EV, Dokmanovic M, et al. A senescence-like phenotype distinguishes tumor cells that undergo terminal proliferation arrest after exposure to anticancer agents. *Cancer Res.* 1999;59(15):3761–3767.
21. Zeman EM. Biologic basis of radiation oncology. In: Tepper Ga, ed. *Clinical Radiation Oncology.* New York: Churchill-Livingston; 2007.
22. Obaturov GM. [Kellerer-Rossi dual action theory]. *Radiobiologiia.* 1977;17(5):764–771.
23. Hall E. *Radiobiology for the Radiologist.* 5th ed: Lippincott Williams and Wilkins; 2000.
24. Mendenhall WM, Riggs CE, Amdur RJ, Hinerman RW, Villaret DB. Altered fractionation and/or adjuvant chemotherapy in definitive irradiation of squamous cell carcinoma of the head and neck. *Laryngoscope.* 2003;113(3):546–551.
25. Willers H, Held KD. Introduction to clinical radiation biology. *Hematol Oncol Clin North Am.* 2006;20(1):1–24.
26. Fowler J, Chappell R, Ritter M. Is alpha/beta for prostate tumors really low? *Int J Radiat Oncol Biol Phys.* 2001;50(4):1021–1031.
27. Fowler JF. Non-standard fractionation in radiotherapy. *Int J Radiat Oncol Biol Phys.* 1984;10(5):755–759.
28. Withers HR, Taylor JM, Maciejewski B. The hazard of accelerated tumor clonogen repopulation during radiotherapy. *Acta Oncol.* 1988;27(2):131–146.
29. Thomlinson RH, Gray LH. The histological structure of some human lung cancers and the possible implications for radiotherapy. *Br J Cancer.* 1955;9(4):539–549.
30. Powers WE, Tolmach LJ. Demonstration of an anoxic component in a mouse tumor-cell population by in vivo assay of survival following irradiation. *Radiology.* 1964;83:328–336.
31. Moulder JE, Rockwell S. Hypoxic fractions of solid tumors: experimental techniques, methods of analysis, and a survey of existing data. *Int J Radiat Oncol Biol Phys.* 1984;10(5):695–712.
32. Carlson DJ, Stewart RD, Semenenko VA. Effects of oxygen on intrinsic radiation sensitivity: A test of the relationship between aerobic and hypoxic linear-quadratic (LQ) model parameters. *Med Phys.* 2006;33(9):3105–3115.
33. Van Putten LM, Kallman RF. Oxygenation status of a transplantable tumor during fractionated radiation therapy. *J Natl Cancer Inst.* 1968;40(3):441–451.
34. Walker MD, Alexander E Jr, Hunt WE, et al. Evaluation of BCNU and/or radiotherapy in the treatment of anaplastic gliomas. A cooperative clinical trial. *J Neurosurg.* 1978;49(3):333–343.
35. Walker MD, Green SB, Byar DP, et al. Randomized comparisons of radiotherapy and nitrosoureas for the treatment of malignant glioma after surgery. *N Engl J Med.* 1980;303(23):1323–1329.
36. Marks JE, Wong J. The risk of cerebral radionecrosis in relation to dose, time and fractionation. A follow-up study. *Prog Exp Tumor Res.* 1985;29:210–218.
37. Bleehen NM, Stenning SP. A Medical Research Council trial of two radiotherapy doses in the treatment of grades 3 and 4 astrocytoma. The Medical Research Council Brain Tumour Working Party. *Br J Cancer.* 1991;64(4):769–774.
38. Hochberg FH, Pruitt A. Assumptions in the radiotherapy of glioblastoma. *Neurology.* 1980;30(9):907–911.
39. Wallner KE, Galicich JH, Krol G, Arbit E, Malkin MG. Patterns of failure following treatment for glioblastoma multiforme and anaplastic astrocytoma. *Int J Radiat Oncol Biol Phys.* 1989;16(6):1405–1409.
40. Gupta VK. Brachytherapy-past present and future. *J Med Phys.* 1995;20:31–38.
41. Gutin PH, Phillips TL, Wara WM, et al. Brachytherapy of recurrent malignant brain tumors with removable high-activity iodine-125 sources. *J Neurosurg.* 1984;60(1):61–68.
42. Malkin MG. Interstitial brachytherapy of malignant gliomas: the Memorial Sloan-Kettering Cancer Center experience. *Recent Results Cancer Res.* 1994;135):117–125.
43. Florell RC, Macdonald DR, Irish WD, et al. Selection bias, survival, and brachytherapy for glioma. *J Neurosurg.* 1992;76(2):179–183.
44. Laperriere NJ, Leung PM, McKenzie S, et al. Randomized study of brachytherapy in the initial management of patients with malignant astrocytoma. *Int J Radiat Oncol Biol Phys.* 1998;41(5):1005–1011.
45. Selker RG, Shapiro WR, Burger P, et al.; Brain Tumor Cooperative Group. The Brain Tumor Cooperative Group NIH Trial 87–01: a randomized comparison of surgery, external radiotherapy, and carmustine versus surgery, interstitial radiotherapy boost, external radiation therapy, and carmustine. *Neurosurgery.* 2002;51(2):343–55; discussion 355.
46. McDermott MW, Berger MS, Kunwar S, Parsa AT, Sneed PK, Larson DA. Stereotactic radiosurgery and interstitial brachytherapy for glial neoplasms. *J Neurooncol.* 2004;69(1–3):83–100.
47. Vitaz TW, Warnke PC, Tabar V, Gutin PH. Brachytherapy for brain tumors. *J Neurooncol.* 2005;73(1):71–86.

48. Walker MD, Strike TA, Sheline GE. An analysis of dose-effect relationship in the radiotherapy of malignant gliomas. *Int J Radiat Oncol Biol Phys*. 1979;5(10):1725–1731.
49. Sneed PK, Lamborn KR, Larson DA, et al. Demonstration of brachytherapy boost dose-response relationships in glioblastoma multiforme. *Int J Radiat Oncol Biol Phys*. 1996;35(1):37–44.
50. Bailey KE, Costantini DL, Cai Z, et al. Epidermal growth factor receptor inhibition modulates the nuclear localization and cytotoxicity of the Auger electron emitting radiopharmaceutical 111In-DTPA human epidermal growth factor. *J Nucl Med*. 2007;48(9):1562–1570.
51. Hood TW, Shapiro B, Taren JA. Treatment of cystic astrocytomas with intracavitary phosphorus 32. *Acta Neurochir Suppl (Wien)*. 1987;39:34–37.
52. Lunsford LD, Gumerman L, Levine G. Stereotactic intracavitary irradiation of cystic neoplasms of the brain. *Appl Neurophysiol*. 1985;48(1–6):146–150.
53. Zeng J, Patterson BW, Klein S, et al. Whole body leptin kinetics and renal metabolism in vivo. *Am J Physiol*. 1997;273(6 Pt 1):E1102-E1106.
54. Kobayashi T, Kageyama N, Ohara K. Internal irradiation for cystic craniopharyngioma. *J Neurosurg*. 1981;55(6):896–903.
55. Tian Z, Liu Z, Wang Y. [Stereotactic intratumoral irradiation of huge craniopharyngioma]. *Zhonghua Zhong Liu Za Zhi*. 1996;18(3):234–236.
56. Fig LM, Shapiro B, Taren J. Distribution of [32P]-chromic phosphate colloid in cystic brain tumors. *Stereotact Funct Neurosurg*. 1992;59(1–4):166–168.
57. Ostertag CB. Interstitial implant radiosurgery of brain tumors: radiobiology, indications, and results. *Recent Results Cancer Res*. 1994;135:105–116.
58. Johannesen TB, Watne K, Lote K, et al. Intracavity fractionated balloon brachytherapy in glioblastoma. *Acta Neurochir (Wien)*. 1999;141(2):127–133.
59. Micheletti E, La Face B, Feroldi P, et al. High-dose-rate brachytherapy for poor-prognosis, high-grade glioma: (phase II) preliminary results. *Tumori*. 1996;82(4):339–344.
60. Matsumoto K, Nakagawa M, Higashi H, et al. Preliminary results of interstitial 192Ir brachytherapy for malignant gliomas. *Neurol Med Chir (Tokyo)*. 1992;32(10):739–746.
61. Chun M, McKeough P, Wu A, Kasdon D, Heros D, Chang H. Interstitial iridium-192 implantation for malignant brain tumours. Part II: Clinical experience. *Br J Radiol*. 1989;62(734):158–162.
62. Kolotas C, Birn G, Baltas D, Rogge B, Ulrich P, Zamboglou N. CT guided interstitial high dose rate brachytherapy for recurrent malignant gliomas. *Br J Radiol*. 1999;72(860):805–808.
63. Patchell RA, Yaes RJ, Beach L, et al. A phase I trial of neutron brachytherapy for the treatment of malignant gliomas. *Br J Radiol*. 1997;70(839):1162–1168.
64. Kumar PP, Good RR, Jones EO, Patil AA, Leibrock LG, McComb RD. Survival of patients with glioblastoma multiforme treated by intraoperative high-activity cobalt 60 endocurietherapy. *Cancer*. 1989;64(7):1409–1413.
65. Scharfen CO, Sneed PK, Wara WM, et al. High activity iodine-125 interstitial implant for gliomas. *Int J Radiat Oncol Biol Phys*. 1992;24(4):583–591.
66. Bernstein M, Laperriere N. Indications for brachytherapy for brain tumours. *Acta Neurochir Suppl*. 1995;63:25–28.
67. Chin HW, Lefkowitz DM, Eisenberg RL. Treatment options in high-grade brain tumors: brain brachytherapy. *Radiographics*. 1992;12(4):721–729.
68. Videtic GM, Gaspar LE, Zamorano L, Stitt LW, Fontanesi J, Levin KJ. Implant volume as a prognostic variable in brachytherapy decision-making for malignant gliomas stratified by the RTOG recursive partitioning analysis. *Int J Radiat Oncol Biol Phys*. 2001;51(4):963–968.
69. Fernandez PM, Zamorano L, Yakar D, Gaspar L, Warmelink C. Permanent iodine-125 implants in the up-front treatment of malignant gliomas. *Neurosurgery*. 1995;36(3):467–473.
70. Stea B, Kittelson J, Cassady JR, et al. Treatment of malignant gliomas with interstitial irradiation and hyperthermia. *Int J Radiat Oncol Biol Phys*. 1992;24(4):657–667.
71. Sneed PK, Stauffer PR, Gutin PH, et al. Interstitial irradiation and hyperthermia for the treatment of recurrent malignant brain tumors. *Neurosurgery*. 1991;28(2):206–215.
72. Chamberlain MC, Barba D, Kormanik P, Berson AM, Saunders WM, Shea MC. Concurrent cisplatin therapy and iodine 125 brachytherapy for recurrent malignant brain tumors. *Arch Neurol*. 1995;52(2):162–167.
73. Patel S, Breneman JC, Warnick RE, et al. Permanent iodine-125 interstitial implants for the treatment of recurrent glioblastoma multiforme. *Neurosurgery*. 2000;46(5):1123–1128; discussion 1128.
74. Halligan JB, Stelzer KJ, Rostomily RC, Spence AM, Griffin TW, Berger MS. Operation and permanent low activity 125I brachytheraphy for recurrent high-grade astrocytomas. *Int J Radiat Oncol Biol Phys*. 1996;35(3):541–547.
75. Dempsey JF, Williams JA, Stubbs JB, Patrick TJ, Williamson JF. Dosimetric properties of a novel brachytherapy balloon applicator for the treatment of malignant brain-tumor resection-cavity margins. *Int J Radiat Oncol Biol Phys*. 1998;42(2):421–429.
76. Chan TA, Weingart JD, Parisi M, et al. Treatment of recurrent glioblastoma multiforme with GliaSite brachytherapy. *Int J Radiat Oncol Biol Phys*. 2005;62(4):1133–1139.
77. Gabayan AJ, Green SB, Sanan A, et al. GliaSite brachytherapy for treatment of recurrent malignant gliomas: a retrospective multi-institutional analysis. *Neurosurgery*. 2006;58(4):701–709; discussion 701.
78. Haines SJ. Moving targets and ghosts of the past: outcome measurement in brain tumour therapy. *J Clin Neurosci*. 2002;9(2):109–112.
79. Gutin PH, Prados MD, Phillips TL, et al. External irradiation followed by an interstitial high activity iodine-125 implant "boost" in the initial treatment of malignant gliomas: NCOG study 6G-82-2. *Int J Radiat Oncol Biol Phys*. 1991;21(3):601–606.
80. Kitchen ND, Hughes SW, Taub NA, Sofat A, Beaney RP, Thomas DG. Survival following interstitial brachytherapy for recurrent malignant glioma. *J Neurooncol*. 1994;18(1):33–39.
81. Bernstein M, Laperriere N, Glen J, Leung P, Thomason C, Landon AE. Brachytherapy for recurrent malignant astrocytoma. *Int J Radiat Oncol Biol Phys*. 1994;30(5):1213–1217.
82. Ryken TC, Hitchon PW, VanGilder JC, Wen BC, Jani S. Interstitial brachytherapy versus cytoreductive surgery in recurrent malignant glioma. *Stereotact Funct Neurosurg*. 1994;63(1–4):241–245.
83. Wen PY, Alexander E III, Black PM, et al. Long term results of stereotactic brachytherapy used in the initial treatment of patients with glioblastomas. *Cancer*. 1994;73(12):3029–3036.
84. Agbi CB, Bernstein M, Laperriere N, Leung P, Lumley M. Patterns of recurrence of malignant astrocytoma following stereotactic interstitial brachytherapy with iodine-125 implants. *Int J Radiat Oncol Biol Phys*. 1992;23(2):321–326.
85. Emami B, Lyman J, Brown A, et al. Tolerance of normal tissue to therapeutic irradiation. *Int J Radiat Oncol Biol Phys*. 1991;21(1):109–122.
86. Mohan R, Wu Q, Manning M, Schmidt-Ullrich R. Radiobiological considerations in the design of fractionation strategies for intensity-modulated radiation therapy of head and neck cancers. *Int J Radiat Oncol Biol Phys*. 2000;46(3):619–630.
87. Hall EJ. Intensity-modulated radiation therapy, protons, and the risk of second cancers. *Int J Radiat Oncol Biol Phys*. 2006;65(1):1–7.
88. Huang E, Teh BS, Strother DR, et al. Intensity-modulated radiation therapy for pediatric medulloblastoma: early report on the reduction of ototoxicity. *Int J Radiat Oncol Biol Phys*. 2002;52(3):599–605.
89. Gutiérrez AN, Westerly DC, Tomé WA, et al. Whole brain radiotherapy with hippocampal avoidance and simultaneously integrated brain metastases boost: a planning study. *Int J Radiat Oncol Biol Phys*. 2007;69(2):589–597.
90. Roman DD, Sperduto PW. Neuropsychological effects of cranial radiation: current knowledge and future directions. *Int J Radiat Oncol Biol Phys*. 1995;31(4):983–998.
91. Mizumatsu S, Monje ML, Morhardt DR, Rola R, Palmer TD, Fike JR. Extreme sensitivity of adult neurogenesis to low doses of X-irradiation. *Cancer Res*. 2003;63(14):4021–4027.
92. LEKSELL L. The stereotaxic method and radiosurgery of the brain. *Acta Chir Scand*. 1951;102(4):316–319.
93. Leksell L. [Trigeminal neuralgia. Some neurophysiologic aspects and a new method of therapy]. *Lakartidningen*. 1971;68(45):5145–5148.
94. Stieber VW, Bourland JD, Tome WA, Mehta MP. Gentlemen (and ladies), choose your weapons: Gamma knife vs. linear accelerator radiosurgery. *Technol Cancer Res Treat*. 2003;2(2):79–86.
95. Mehta M, Noyes W, Craig B, et al. A cost-effectiveness and cost-utility analysis of radiosurgery vs. resection for single-brain metastases. *Int J Radiat Oncol Biol Phys*. 1997;39(2):445–454.

96. Larson DA, Bova F, Eisert D, et al. Current radiosurgery practice: results of an ASTRO survey. Task Force on Stereotactic Radiosurgery, American Society for Therapeutic Radiology and Oncology. Int J Radiat Oncol Biol Phys. 1994;28(2):523–526.
97. Shaw E, Scott C, Souhami L, et al. Single dose radiosurgical treatment of recurrent previously irradiated primary brain tumors and brain metastases: final report of RTOG protocol 90–05. Int J Radiat Oncol Biol Phys. 2000;47(2):291–298.
98. Andrews DW, Scott CB, Sperduto PW, et al. Whole brain radiation therapy with or without stereotactic radiosurgery boost for patients with one to three brain metastases: phase III results of the RTOG 9508 randomised trial. Lancet. 2004;363(9422):1665–1672.
99. Souhami L, Seiferheld W, Brachman D, et al. Randomized comparison of stereotactic radiosurgery followed by conventional radiotherapy with carmustine to conventional radiotherapy with carmustine for patients with glioblastoma multiforme: report of Radiation Therapy Oncology Group 93–05 protocol. Int J Radiat Oncol Biol Phys. 2004;60(3):853–860.
100. Sanghavi SN, Miranpuri SS, Chappell R, et al. Radiosurgery for patients with brain metastases: a multi-institutional analysis, stratified by the RTOG recursive partitioning analysis method. Int J Radiat Oncol Biol Phys. 2001;51(2):426–434.
101. Stafford SL, Pollock BE, Foote RL, et al. Meningioma radiosurgery: tumor control, outcomes, and complications among 190 consecutive patients. Neurosurgery. 2001;49(5):1029–1037; discussion 1037.
102. Kondziolka D, Niranjan A, Lunsford LD, Flickinger JC. Stereotactic radiosurgery for meningiomas. Neurosurg Clin N Am. 1999;10(2):317–325.
103. Lee JY, Niranjan A, McInerney J, Kondziolka D, Flickinger JC, Lunsford LD. Stereotactic radiosurgery providing long-term tumor control of cavernous sinus meningiomas. J Neurosurg. 2002;97(1):65–72.
104. Rogers L, Mehta M. Role of radiation therapy in treating intracranial meningiomas. Neurosurg Focus. 2007;23(4):E4.
105. Flickinger JC, Kondziolka D, Niranjan A, Maitz A, Voynov G, Lunsford LD. Acoustic neuroma radiosurgery with marginal tumor doses of 12 to 13 Gy. Int J Radiat Oncol Biol Phys. 2004;60(1):225–230.
106. Pollock BE, Lunsford LD, Kondziolka D, et al. Outcome analysis of acoustic neuroma management: a comparison of microsurgery and stereotactic radiosurgery. Neurosurgery. 1995;36(1):215–224; discussion 224.
107. Régis J. [New developments in the management of vestibular schwannomas in the modern era of radiosurgery]. Neurochirurgie. 2004;50(2–3 Pt 2):156–158.
108. Sheehan JP, Kondziolka D, Flickinger J, Lunsford LD. Radiosurgery for residual or recurrent nonfunctioning pituitary adenoma. J Neurosurg. 2002;97(5 Suppl):408–414.
109. Friedman WA. Radiosurgery versus surgery for arteriovenous malformations: the case for radiosurgery. Clin Neurosurg. 1999;45:18–20.
110. Maesawa S, Salame C, Flickinger JC, Pirris S, Kondziolka D, Lunsford LD. Clinical outcomes after stereotactic radiosurgery for idiopathic trigeminal neuralgia. J Neurosurg. 2001;94(1):14–20.
111. Crossley EL, Ziolkowski EJ, Coderre JA, Rendina LM. Boronated DNA-binding compounds as potential agents for boron neutron capture therapy. Mini Rev Med Chem. 2007;7(3):303–313.
112. De Stasio G, Rajesh D, Casalbore P, et al. Are gadolinium contrast agents suitable for gadolinium neutron capture therapy? Neurol Res. 2005;27(4):387–398.
113. Hainfeld JF. Uranium-loaded apoferritin with antibodies attached: molecular design for uranium neutron-capture therapy. Proc Natl Acad Sci USA. 1992;89(22):11064–11068.
114. Harling OK, Riley KJ. Fission reactor neutron sources for neutron capture therapy–a critical review. J Neurooncol. 2003;62(1–2):7–17.
115. Kageji T, Nagahiro S, Matsuzaki K, et al. Boron neutron capture therapy using mixed epithermal and thermal neutron beams in patients with malignant glioma-correlation between radiation dose and radiation injury and clinical outcome. Int J Radiat Oncol Biol Phys. 2006;65(5):1446–1455.
116. Blue TE, Yanch JC. Accelerator-based epithermal neutron sources for boron neutron capture therapy of brain tumors. J Neurooncol. 2003;62(1–2):19–31.
117. Rivard MJ, Zamenhof RG. Moderated 252Cf neutron energy spectra in brain tissue and calculated boron neutron capture dose. Appl Radiat Isot. 2004;61(5):753–757.
118. Barth RF, Coderre JA, Vicente MG, Blue TE. Boron neutron capture therapy of cancer: current status and future prospects. Clin Cancer Res. 2005;11(11):3987–4002.
119. Tolpin EI, Wellum GR, Dohan FC Jr, Kornblith PL, Zamenhof RG. Boron neutron capture therapy of cerebral gliomas. II. Utilization of the blood-brain barrier and tumor-specific antigens for the selective concentration of boron in gliomas. Oncology. 1975;32(5–6):223–246.
120. Fowler JF, Kinsella TJ. The limiting radiosensitisation of tumours by S-phase sensitisers. Br J Cancer Suppl. 1996;27:S294-S296.
121. Barth RF, Soloway AH, Fairchild RG, Brugger RM. Boron neutron capture therapy for cancer. Realities and prospects. Cancer. 1992;70(12):2995–3007.
122. Locher GL. Biological effects and therapeutic possibilities of neutrons. Am J Roentgenol Radium Ther. 1936;36:1–13.
123. Beddoe AH. Boron neutron capture therapy. Br J Radiol. 1997;70(835):665–667.
124. Barth RF, Joensuu H. Boron neutron capture therapy for the treatment of glioblastomas and extracranial tumours: as effective, more effective or less effective than photon irradiation? Radiother Oncol. 2007;82(2):119–122.
125. Diaz AZ. Assessment of the results from the phase I/II boron neutron capture therapy trials at the Brookhaven National Laboratory from a clinician's point of view. J Neurooncol. 2003;62(1–2):101–109.
126. Palmer MR, Goorley JT, Kiger WS, et al. Treatment planning and dosimetry for the Harvard-MIT Phase I clinical trial of cranial neutron capture therapy. Int J Radiat Oncol Biol Phys. 2002;53(5):1361–1379.
127. Farr LE, Sweet WH, Robertson JS, et al. Neutron capture therapy with boron in the treatment of glioblastoma multiforme. Am J Roentgenol Radium Ther Nucl Med. 1954;71(2):279–293.
128. Goodwin JT, Farr LE, Sweet WH, Robertson JS. Pathological study of eight patients with glioblastoma multiforme treated by neutron-capture therapy using boron 10. Cancer. 1955;8(3):601–615.
129. Asbury AK, Ojemann RG, Nielsen SL, Sweet WH. Neuropathologic study of fourteen cases of malignant brain tumor treated by boron-10 slow neutron capture radiation. J Neuropathol Exp Neurol. 1972;31(2):278–303.
130. Sweet WH. Practical problems in the past in the use of boron-neutron capture therapy in the treatment of glioblastoma multiforme. In: Proceedings of the First International Symposium on Neutron Capture Therapy; Brookhaven: Brookhaven National Laboratory; 1983:376–378.
131. Carlsson J, Forssell-Aronsson E, Glimelius B; Swedish Cancer Society Investigation Group. Radiation therapy through activation of stable nuclides. Acta Oncol. 2002;41(7–8):629–634.
132. Slatkin DN. A history of boron neutron capture therapy of brain tumours. Postulation of a brain radiation dose tolerance limit. Brain. 1991;114 (Pt 4):1609–1629.
133. Hatanaka H, Moritani M, Camillo M. Possible alteration of the blood-brain barrier by boron-neutron capture therapy. Acta Oncol. 1991;30(3):375–378.
134. Hatanaka H, Nakagawa Y. Clinical results of long-surviving brain tumor patients who underwent boron neutron capture therapy. Int J Radiat Oncol Biol Phys. 1994;28(5):1061–1066.
135. Soloway AH, Hatanaka H, Davis MA. Penetration of brain and brain tumor. VII. Tumor-binding sulfhydryl boron compounds. J Med Chem. 1967;10(4):714–717.
136. Miyatake SI, Kajimoto Y. Clinical results of modified BNCT for malignant glioma using two boron. In: World Conference on Neutron Capture Therapy, Boston, MA; 2004:61.
137. Nakagawa Y, Hatanaka H. Boron neutron capture therapy. Clinical brain tumor studies. J Neurooncol. 1997;33(1–2):105–115.
138. Laramore GE, Spence AM. Boron neutron capture therapy (BNCT) for high-grade gliomas of the brain: a cautionary note. Int J Radiat Oncol Biol Phys. 1996;36(1):241–246.
139. STONE RS. Neutron therapy and specific ionization. Am J Roentgenol Radium Ther. 1948;59(6):771–785.
140. Douglas JG, Lee S, Laramore GE, Austin-Seymour M, Koh W, Griffin TW. Neutron radiotherapy for the treatment of locally advanced major salivary gland tumors. Head Neck. 1999;21(3):255–263.
141. Douglas JG, Laramore GE, Austin-Seymour M, Koh W, Stelzer K, Griffin TW. Treatment of locally advanced adenoid cystic carcinoma

of the head and neck with neutron radiotherapy. *Int J Radiat Oncol Biol Phys.* 2000;46(3):551–557.
142. Laramore GE, Krall JM, Griffin TW, et al. Neutron versus photon irradiation for unresectable salivary gland tumors: final report of an RTOG-MRC randomized clinical trial. Radiation Therapy Oncology Group. Medical Research Council. *Int J Radiat Oncol Biol Phys.* 1993;27(2):235–240.
143. Griffin TW, Davis R, Laramore GE, Hussey DH, Hendrickson FR, Rodriguez-Antunez A. Fast neutron irradiation of metastatic cervical adenopathy: the results of a randomized RTOG study. *Int J Radiat Oncol Biol Phys.* 1983;9(9):1267–1270.
144. Griffin TW, Pajak TF, Maor MH, et al. Mixed neutron/photon irradiation of unresectable squamous cell carcinomas of the head and neck: the final report of a randomized cooperative trial. *Int J Radiat Oncol Biol Phys.* 1989;17(5):959–965.
145. Koh WJ, Krall JM, Peters LJ, et al. Neutron vs. photon radiation therapy for inoperable regional non-small cell lung cancer: results of a multicenter randomized trial. *Int J Radiat Oncol Biol Phys.* 1993;27(3):499–505.
146. Laramore GE, Krall JM, Thomas FJ, et al. Fast neutron radiotherapy for locally advanced prostate cancer. Final report of Radiation Therapy Oncology Group randomized clinical trial. *Am J Clin Oncol.* 1993;16(2):164–167.
147. Fleurette F, Charvet-Protat S. [Proton and neutron radiation in cancer treatment: clinical and economic outcomes]. *Bull Cancer Radiother.* 1996;83:223s-227s.
148. Forman JD, Shamsa F, Maughan RL, Duclos M, Orton C. Comparison of hyperfractionated conformal photon with conformal mixed neutron/photon irradiation in locally advanced prostate cancer. *Bull Cancer Radiother.* 1996;83:101s-105s.
149. Laramore GE, Griffith JT, Boespflug M, et al. Fast neutron radiotherapy for sarcomas of soft tissue, bone, and cartilage. *Am J Clin Oncol.* 1989;12(4):320–326.
150. Gragoudas E, Li W, Goitein M, Lane AM, Munzenrider JE, Egan KM. Evidence-based estimates of outcome in patients irradiated for intraocular melanoma. *Arch Ophthalmol.* 2002;120(12):1665–1671.
151. Fuss M, Hug EB, Schaefer RA, et al. Proton radiation therapy (PRT) for pediatric optic pathway gliomas: comparison with 3D planned conventional photons and a standard photon technique. *Int J Radiat Oncol Biol Phys.* 1999;45(5):1117–1126.
152. Munzenrider JE, Liebsch NJ. Proton therapy for tumors of the skull base. *Strahlenther Onkol.* 1999;175(Suppl 2):57–63.
153. Ronson BB, Schulte RW, Han KP, Loredo LN, Slater JM, Slater JD. Fractionated proton beam irradiation of pituitary adenomas. *Int J Radiat Oncol Biol Phys.* 2006;64(2):425–434.
154. Harsh GR, Thornton AF, Chapman PH, Bussiere MR, Rabinov JD, Loeffler JS. Proton beam stereotactic radiosurgery of vestibular schwannomas. *Int J Radiat Oncol Biol Phys.* 2002;54(1):35–44.
155. Fitzek MM, Thornton AF, Varvares M, et al. Neuroendocrine tumors of the sinonasal tract. Results of a prospective study incorporating chemotherapy, surgery, and combined proton-photon radiotherapy. *Cancer.* 2002;94(10):2623–2634.
156. Lin R, Slater JD, Yonemoto LT, et al. Nasopharyngeal carcinoma: repeat treatment with conformal proton therapy–dose-volume histogram analysis. *Radiology.* 1999;213(2):489–494.
157. Nowakowski VA, Castro JR, Petti PL, et al. Charged particle radiotherapy of paraspinal tumors. *Int J Radiat Oncol Biol Phys.* 1992;22(2):295–303.
158. Hug EB, Fitzek MM, Liebsch NJ, Munzenrider JE. Locally challenging osteo- and chondrogenic tumors of the axial skeleton: results of combined proton and photon radiation therapy using three-dimensional treatment planning. *Int J Radiat Oncol Biol Phys.* 1995;31(3):467–476.
159. Shipley WU, Verhey LJ, Munzenrider JE, et al. Advanced prostate cancer: the results of a randomized comparative trial of high dose irradiation boosting with conformal protons compared with conventional dose irradiation using photons alone. *Int J Radiat Oncol Biol Phys.* 1995;32(1):3–12.
160. Benk VA, Adams JA, Shipley WU, et al. Late rectal bleeding following combined X-ray and proton high dose irradiation for patients with stages T3-T4 prostate carcinoma. *Int J Radiat Oncol Biol Phys.* 1993;26(3):551–557.
161. Bush DA, Slater JD, Shin BB, Cheek G, Miller DW, Slater JM. Hypofractionated proton beam radiotherapy for stage I lung cancer. *Chest.* 2004;126(4):1198–1203.
162. Bonnet RB, Bush D, Cheek GA, et al. Effects of proton and combined proton/photon beam radiation on pulmonary function in patients with resectable but medically inoperable non-small cell lung cancer. *Chest.* 2001;120(6):1803–1810.
163. Moyers MF, Miller DW, Bush DA, Slater JD. Methodologies and tools for proton beam design for lung tumors. *Int J Radiat Oncol Biol Phys.* 2001;49(5):1429–1438.
164. Bush DA, Slater JD, Bonnet R, et al. Proton-beam radiotherapy for early-stage lung cancer. *Chest.* 1999;116(5):1313–1319.
165. Chiba T, Tokuuye K, Matsuzaki Y, et al. Proton beam therapy for hepatocellular carcinoma: a retrospective review of 162 patients. *Clin Cancer Res.* 2005;11(10):3799–3805.
166. Matsuzaki Y, Osuga T, Chiba T, et al. New, effective treatment using proton irradiation for unresectable hepatocellular carcinoma. *Intern Med.* 1995;34(4):302–304.
167. Bush DA, Hillebrand DJ, Slater JM, Slater JD. High-dose proton beam radiotherapy of hepatocellular carcinoma: preliminary results of a phase II trial. *Gastroenterology.* 2004;127(5 Suppl 1): S189-S193.
168. Levin WP, Kooy H, Loeffler JS, DeLaney TF. Proton beam therapy. *Br J Cancer.* 2005;93(8):849–854.
169. Hug EB, Sweeney RA, Nurre PM, Holloway KC, Slater JD, Munzenrider JE. Proton radiotherapy in management of pediatric base of skull tumors. *Int J Radiat Oncol Biol Phys.* 2002;52(4):1017–1024.
170. Hug EB, Slater JD. Proton radiation therapy for pediatric malignancies: status report. *Strahlenther Onkol.* 1999;175 (Suppl 2): 89–91.
171. Chen P, Mrkobrada M, Vallis KA, et al. Comparative antiproliferative effects of (111)In-DTPA-hEGF, chemotherapeutic agents and gamma-radiation on EGFR-positive breast cancer cells. *Nucl Med Biol.* 2002;29(6):693–699.
172. Ercan MT, Caglar M. Therapeutic radiopharmaceuticals. *Curr Pharm Des.* 2000;6(11):1085–1121.
173. Kassis AI, Adelstein SJ. Radiobiologic principles in radionuclide therapy. *J Nucl Med.* 2005;46 (Suppl 1):4S-12S.
174. Goldenberg DM, Sharkey RM, Paganelli G, Barbet J, Chatal JF. Antibody pretargeting advances cancer radioimmunodetection and radioimmunotherapy. *J Clin Oncol.* 2006;24(5):823–834.
175. Sharkey RM, Goldenberg DM. Targeted therapy of cancer: new prospects for antibodies and immunoconjugates. *CA Cancer J Clin.* 2006;56(4):226–243.
176. Karagiannis TC. Comparison of different classes of radionuclides for potential use in radioimmunotherapy. *Hell J Nucl Med.* 2007;10(2):82–88.
177. Wong JY. Basic immunology of antibody targeted radiotherapy. *Int J Radiat Oncol Biol Phys.* 2006;66(2 Suppl):S8-S14.
178. Kalofonos HP, Pawlikowska TR, Hemingway A, et al. Antibody guided diagnosis and therapy of brain gliomas using radiolabeled monoclonal antibodies against epidermal growth factor receptor and placental alkaline phosphatase. *J Nucl Med.* 1989;30(10):1636–1645.
179. Qin DX, Zheng R, Tang J, Li JX, Hu YH. Influence of radiation on the blood-brain barrier and optimum time of chemotherapy. *Int J Radiat Oncol Biol Phys.* 1990;19(6):1507–1510.
180. Quang TS, Brady LW. Radioimmunotherapy as a novel treatment regimen: 125I-labeled monoclonal antibody 425 in the treatment of high-grade brain gliomas. *Int J Radiat Oncol Biol Phys.* 2004;58(3):972–975.
181. Cao Y, Tsien CI, Shen Z, et al. Use of magnetic resonance imaging to assess blood-brain/blood-glioma barrier opening during conformal radiotherapy. *J Clin Oncol.* 2005;23(18):4127–4136.
182. Papanastassiou V, Pizer BL, Coakham HB, Bullimore J, Zananiri T, Kemshead JT. Treatment of recurrent and cystic malignant gliomas by a single intracavity injection of 131I monoclonal antibody: feasibility, pharmacokinetics and dosimetry. *Br J Cancer.* 1993;67(1): 144–151.
183. Hopkins K, Chandler C, Eatough J, Moss T, Kemshead JT. Direct injection of 90Y MoAbs into glioma tumor resection cavities leads to limited diffusion of the radioimmunoconjugates into normal brain parenchyma: a model to estimate absorbed radiation dose. *Int J Radiat Oncol Biol Phys.* 1998;40(4):835–844.
184. Mamelak AN, Rosenfeld S, Bucholz R, et al. Phase I single-dose study of intracavitary-administered iodine-131-TM-601 in adults with recurrent high-grade glioma. *J Clin Oncol.* 2006;24(22):3644–3650.
185. Hopkins K, Chandler C, Bullimore J, Sandeman D, Coakham H, Kemshead JT. A pilot study of the treatment of patients with

recurrent malignant gliomas with intratumoral yttrium-90 radioimmunoconjugates. *Radiother Oncol*. 1995;34(2):121–131.
186. Reardon DA, Akabani G, Coleman RE, et al. Phase II trial of murine (131)I-labeled antitenascin monoclonal antibody 81C6 administered into surgically created resection cavities of patients with newly diagnosed malignant gliomas. *J Clin Oncol*. 2002;20(5):1389–1397.
187. Reardon DA, Akabani G, Coleman RE, et al. Salvage radioimmunotherapy with murine iodine-131-labeled antitenascin monoclonal antibody 81C6 for patients with recurrent primary and metastatic malignant brain tumors: phase II study results. *J Clin Oncol*. 2006;24(1):115–122.
188. Akabani G, Reardon DA, Coleman RE, et al. Dosimetry and radiographic analysis of 131I-labeled anti-tenascin 81C6 murine monoclonal antibody in newly diagnosed patients with malignant gliomas: a phase II study. *J Nucl Med*. 2005;46(6):1042–1051.
189. Reardon DA, Zalutsky MR, Akabani G, et al. A pilot study: 131I-antitenascin monoclonal antibody 81c6 to deliver a 44-Gy resection cavity boost. *Neuro-oncology*. 2008;10(2):182–189.
190. Zalutsky MR, Reardon DA, Akabani G, et al. Clinical experience with alpha-particle emitting 211At: treatment of recurrent brain tumor patients with 211At-labeled chimeric antitenascin monoclonal antibody 81C6. *J Nucl Med*. 2008;49(1):30–38.

82 Radiation for Glioblastoma

Samuel T. Chao and John H. Suh

Glioblastoma (GBM) is the most common primary brain tumor, and unfortunately, the most malignant. In the United States, it represents 7,000 or 40% of the 18,000 primary brain tumors diagnosed each year. Given the aggressive nature of this tumor and poor outcomes, a number of clinical trials and treatment approaches have been investigated. Common to these various trials and treatment approaches, the use of radiation therapy has been important in the management of this tumor. Today, treatment typically involves external beam radiation therapy with concurrent temozolomide followed by adjuvant temozolomide.

RADIATION IS THE STANDARD TREATMENT IN THE UPFRONT SETTING

Radiation has been the mainstay of treatment for GBM. These tumors tend to diffusely infiltrate normal brain beyond the gross tumor and recur locally. Given its focal nature and typical localized failure pattern, radiation is an ideal modality to focus treatment to the areas of highest risk.

The Brain Tumor Study Group (BTSG) conducted three protocols from 1966 to 1975 assessing the use of radiation in the treatment of malignant gliomas. BTSG 6901 assessed the role of chemotherapy and/or radiation compared to best supportive care. The median survival improved from 14 to approximately 35 weeks with the addition of radiation [1]. Chemotherapy alone (carmustine [BCNU]), showed a slight improvement over best supportive care with a median survival of 18.5 weeks, but was inferior to the radiation arm. The addition of BCNU to radiation did not improve outcomes. Another study, BTSG 7201, randomized patients to receive one of four regimens: semustine (MeCCNU), radiation alone, BCNU plus radiation, or MeCCNU plus radiation [2]. Again, this study showed that radiation, either alone or in combination with chemotherapy, improved survival over chemotherapy alone. On the basis of these studies, which are summarized in Table 82.1, radiation became an upfront standard in the management of malignant gliomas. Several other randomized trials have reinforced the role of radiotherapy.

RADIATION DOSE

A retrospective data review by Walker et al [3] of 621 patients enrolled onto three BTSG studies from 1966 to

Table 82.1 Early Brain Tumor Study Group Studies

	Median Survival (Weeks)	p-Value
BTSG 6901[1]		
Best supportive care	14	
BCNU	18.5	0.119
Radiation	35	0.001
Radiation + BCNU	34.5	0.001
BTSG 7201[2]		
MeCCNU	31	
Radiation	37	0.003
Radiation + BCNU	49	<0.001
Radiation + MeCCNU	43	<0.001

Table 82.2 Dose-Response to Radiation-Based on Three BTSG Studies [3]

	No RT	≤45 Gy	50 Gy	55 Gy	60 Gy
Median Survival (weeks)	18	13.5	28	36	42
P-value		0.346	<0.001	<0.001	<0.001

1975 assessed median survival stratified by dose. Patients who did not receive radiation had a median survival of 18 weeks, whereas patients receiving 60 Gy of radiation survived a median of 42 weeks ($P < 0.001$). Table 82.2 shows the effect of dose on survival.

Doses beyond 60 Gy have been studied as well. Dose escalation can be achieved using different modalities: fractionated radiation boost, brachytherapy, or stereotactic radiosurgery (SRS). Early studies did suggest an increase in survival with the addition of a boost of 15 to 20 Gy in addition to the standard 50 to 60 Gy, but with increased risk for radiation necrosis [4]. The Radiation Therapy Oncology Group (RTOG) and Eastern Cooperative Oncology Group performed a study randomizing 626 patients into 4 arms: (1) 60 Gy whole-brain radiation therapy (WBRT), (2) 60 Gy WBRT + 10 Gy partial brain boost, (3) 60 Gy WBRT + BCNU, (4) 60 Gy + lomustine (CCNU) + dacarbazine (DTIC) [5]. In this study, survival among the various groups, including those that received a 10 Gy boost, were equivalent. Since then, 60 Gy has remained the standard radiation dose for RTOG studies.

Further dose escalation, using an intensity-modulated radiation therapy (IMRT) boost has been studied at the University of Michigan [6]. Patients were treated with a

2.5 cm margin around the gross tumor volume (GTV) to 44 Gy, then to 60 Gy with a margin of 1.5 cm around the GTV. A 30 Gy boost was delivered to the GTV plus a 0.5 cm margin, for a total tumor dose of 90 Gy. The goal was improved local control. In 78% of the patients, 95% of the recurrence volume was in the 90 Gy region, showing that failures continue to occur locally despite higher doses, of course, one cannot rule out the possibility that intact tumor cells from the lower dose zones might have migrated into the high dose zone. Median survival was comparable with other studies at 11.7 months.

Another means to increase the dose of radiation locally, but spare the normal brain tissue, involves the use of brachytherapy. Retrospective data showed this technique to be promising [7]. The addition of I-125 improved median survival from 17.9 months in RTOG Class III patients to 28 months. Survival in Class IV and V patients improved as well. Unfortunately, prospective studies failed to support these encouraging results. The Brain Tumor Cooperative Group randomized patients to 60.2 Gy in 35 fractions with BCNU or 60.2 Gy in 35 fractions with BCNU and temporary I-125 brachytherapy for an additional 60 Gy [8]. Median survival was 68.1 weeks in the I-125 group versus 58.5 weeks in the group without brachytherapy ($p = 0.101$). The Princess Margaret Hospital performed a similar study randomizing patients to 50 Gy in 25 fractions versus 50 Gy in 25 fractions with I-125 seeds for an additional 60 Gy [9]. Again, no benefit was seen. Patients undergoing brachytherapy survived a median of 13.8 months versus 13.2 months for those not receiving brachytherapy ($p = 0.49$). Table 82.3 summarizes these results.

The University of California, San Francisco, was able to show a benefit to brachytherapy with the addition of hyperthermia [10]. Hyperthermia is a means to achieve additional cell kill by targeting cells in the S-phase, which are resistant to radiation, but sensitive to heat. Also, it inhibits sublethal repair and improves reoxygenation, thus improving the efficacy of radiation. In this study, hyperthermia was applied 30 minutes before and after implant. Patients receiving hyperthermia had a median survival of 85 weeks versus 76 weeks for brachytherapy alone ($p = 0.02$). Further studies have not been performed, and given the results from the other prospective brachytherapy studies, upfront brachytherapy has been abandoned for the most part.

Another method to achieve dose escalation is using SRS. A number of retrospective studies showed benefit with the addition of SRS boost [11,12]. The RTOG performed a study randomizing 203 patients to 60 Gy of fractionated radiation with BCNU versus 60 Gy with BCNU and upfront SRS (RTOG 93–05) [13]. Dosing for SRS was determined in part by the results of an earlier RTOG study which showed that 24 Gy can be given safely to tumors 2 cm or less [14]. For tumor measuring 2 to 3 cm, 18 Gy was the recommended dose, and for tumors 3 to 4 cm in diameter, the recommended dose was 15 Gy. Similar to the results seen with brachytherapy, the results from RTOG 93–05 were disappointing. The median survival was approximately 13.5 months in the SRS arm versus 13.6 in the standard treatment group ($p = 0.57$). There was no difference in 2- or 3-year survival rates. Based largely on this study, the American Society for Therapeutic Radiology and Oncology issued a consensus statement that there is no benefit to up-front SRS boost for malignant gliomas [15].

Alternative dose-fractionation regimens also have been investigated with the hope that by hyperfractionating radiation through twice-a-day treatments, higher doses of radiation may be achieved, which may have an advantage in suppressing the growth of rapidly dividing cells and preventing repopulation. RTOG 83–02 investigated various hyperfractionated dose regimens for malignant gliomas and found that 72 Gy given in 1.2 Gy per fraction delivered twice a day resulted in the best median survival with reasonable toxicity [16]. This led to a Phase III study randomizing patients to 72 Gy given in fractions of 1.2 Gy twice daily versus 60 Gy over 30 fractions given daily (RTOG 90–06) [17]. BCNU was given in both arms. This study failed to show a benefit from altered fractionation. In fact in patients who were less than 50 years old, those receiving the standard fractionation had a median survival of 15.7 months versus 12.2 months for those who were in the hyperfractionation arm ($p = 0.02$).

Additional dose beyond 60 Gy, irrespective of the delivery method, has failed to show benefit and 60 Gy has remained the standard in the treatment of GBMs.

RADIATION VOLUMES

Another consideration regarding radiation is the treatment volume or margins. This is still an area of controversy, and is a factor in considering the ideal treatment modality, 3D conformal therapy versus IMRT. Historically, margins have been employed to cover potential microscopic disease beyond the visualized area of disease. Typically, this is 2 cm around the gross tumor [18,19]. The development of better imaging and more sophisticated radiation delivery have led to variations on the appropriate treatment margins.

Partial brain radiation is standard as there is no benefit to whole-brain radiation in terms of survival or local control [20]. In addition, it is known that 90% of the recurrences occur within 2 cm of the known primary tumor. Thus, a 2 to 3 cm margin is typically used when radiating GBMs.

Each study group has defined treatment margins differently. The RTOG had previously used a block margin of 2 cm around the clinical target volume (CTV), defined as the

Table 82.3 Brachytherapy for GBM

	Median Survival (Weeks)	p-Value
Brain Tumor Cooperative Group [8]		
60.2 Gy	58.5	
60.2 Gy + I-125 (60 Gy)	68.1	0.101
Princess Margaret [9]		
50 Gy	57.2	
50 Gy + I-125 (60 Gy)	59.8	0.49
UCSF [10]		
59.4 Gy + I-125 (60 Gy)	76.0	
59.4 Gy + I-125 (60 Gy) + hyperthermia	85.0	0.02

T2 or fluid attenuated inversion recovery (FLAIR) change, for the first 46 Gy [13]. The T2/FLAIR change or edema is thought to represent microscopic disease, although this can also represent mass effect or surgical changes. For the remaining 14 Gy, a block margin of 2.5 cm is added around the GTV, defined as the area of enhancement and resection bed. For the RTOG 0525 study, which is assessing a dose intensive regimen of temozolomide, the margin definitions became more rigorous with a 2 cm dosimetric margin around the CTV for the first 46 Gy and 2.5 cm around the GTV for the last 14 Gy. A dosimetric margin requires more planning and ensures full dose within the margin, whereas a block margin requires dose buildup within that margin so that only a portion of what is in the field receives full dose. Usually an 8 mm margin is incorporated beyond the dosimetric margin to create the block margin.

The definition chosen by the European Organization for the Research and Treatment of Cancer (EORTC) is a "single-phase" treatment volume where a 2 to 3 cm margin is added to the GTV, defined similarly as the area of enhancement and the tumor bed, to form the CTV [21]. An additional margin of 0.5 to 0.7 cm is added beyond the CTV to create the prescribed treatment volume (PTV) for setup errors. This is a similar volume used by MD Anderson as part of their standard treatment.

Table 82.4 and Figure 82.1 illustrate the differences between these volumes.

Arguably, there is no difference between the various volumes. In a study at MD Anderson, there was no difference in control rates whether using the larger RTOG definition or the smaller EORTC and MD Anderson definition [22]. The variation in volume definition, however, can potentially create controversy when comparing data from different study groups. Also, it may complicate the development of international studies as the United States and European groups have differing opinions on how to define these volumes.

In addition, other institutions are using more modern imaging techniques to better define these volumes. At University of California, San Francisco, magnetic resonance imaging (MRI) spectroscopy has been studied to help define whether there could be an effect on volume [23]. Using edema to delineate microscopic disease is imperfect since surgical changes or mass effect can also cause edema. Imaging that is more specific to tumor may better limit the volume and identify areas of disease not seen using traditional imaging. Further investigation with MRI spectroscopy is underway. Similarly, the University of Michigan is investigating the use of 11C-methionine positron emission tomography to define their volume [24]. Certainly, improved imaging techniques, which may incorporate molecular imaging, may change how we define these volumes in the future.

IMRT has not been standard among study groups because of the lack of prospective studies incorporating this technique. Some centers have used IMRT under study as a means to hypofractionate or deliver more radiation centrally, but limit peripheral doses. Preliminary studies delivering radiation over 2 or 4 weeks without concurrent chemotherapy show this technique to be comparable to a full 6 weeks of treatment [25,26]. Radiation can be given safely and effectively in a shorter period of time with this technique. IMRT using standard fractionation is being incorporated into current studies, including studies from the New Approaches to Brain Tumor Therapy (NABTT), Consortium and the new RTOG study, 0825. NABTT uses a 5 mm margin for CTV and a 5 mm margin for PTV for both the initial and boost volume. Although this may better spare normal tissue and allow for a more homogeneous dose within the treatment volume [27], use of this treatment modality is controversial. The rapid dose falloff beyond the PTV may theoretically spare microscopic disease. Until more studies are done to evaluate the appropriate margins around IMRT, widespread use is cautioned.

SIMULATION

Currently, computerized tomography (CT)-based simulation is typically used. A thermoplastic mask is used for head immobilization and contrast is often given, even though MRI fusion is planned for volume delineation. It is known that the GBM may progress after postoperative images have been acquired for volume delineation. Contrast used in simulation may help identify progression following surgery.

After CT simulation, fusion of the MRI scan, if available, is performed to better identify the tumor/tumor bed and critical structures. Figure 82.2 is an example of CT and MRI fusion. Critical structures typically included are lenses, eyes, optic nerve, optic chiasm, pituitary, hypothalamus, cochleas, and brainstem.

Magnetic resonance simulators have been used at various institutions, but are not currently commonplace. They have the advantage of avoiding some of the inaccuracies associated with MRI fusion, including interval tumor progression or brain shift, and poor fusion.

Table 82.4 Volume Definitions

	RTOG (old)	**RTOG (new)**	**EORTC**	**NABTT**
Initial Dose	46 Gy	46 Gy	60 Gy	46 Gy
Initial Margin	2 cm block	2 cm dosimetric to PTV	2–3 cm dosimetric to PTV	1 cm dosimetric to PTV
Initial Volume Definition	T2/FLAIR	T2/FLAIR	T1 + Contrast	T2/FLAIR
Boost	+	+	–	+
Boost Dose	14 Gy	14 Gy		14 Gy
Boost Margin	2.5 cm block	2.5 cm dosimetric to PTV		1 cm dosimetric to PTV
Boost Volume Definition	T1 + Contrast	T1 + Contrast		T1 + Contrast
IMRT Allowed	No	No	No	Yes
Final Dose	60 Gy	60 Gy	60 Gy	60 Gy

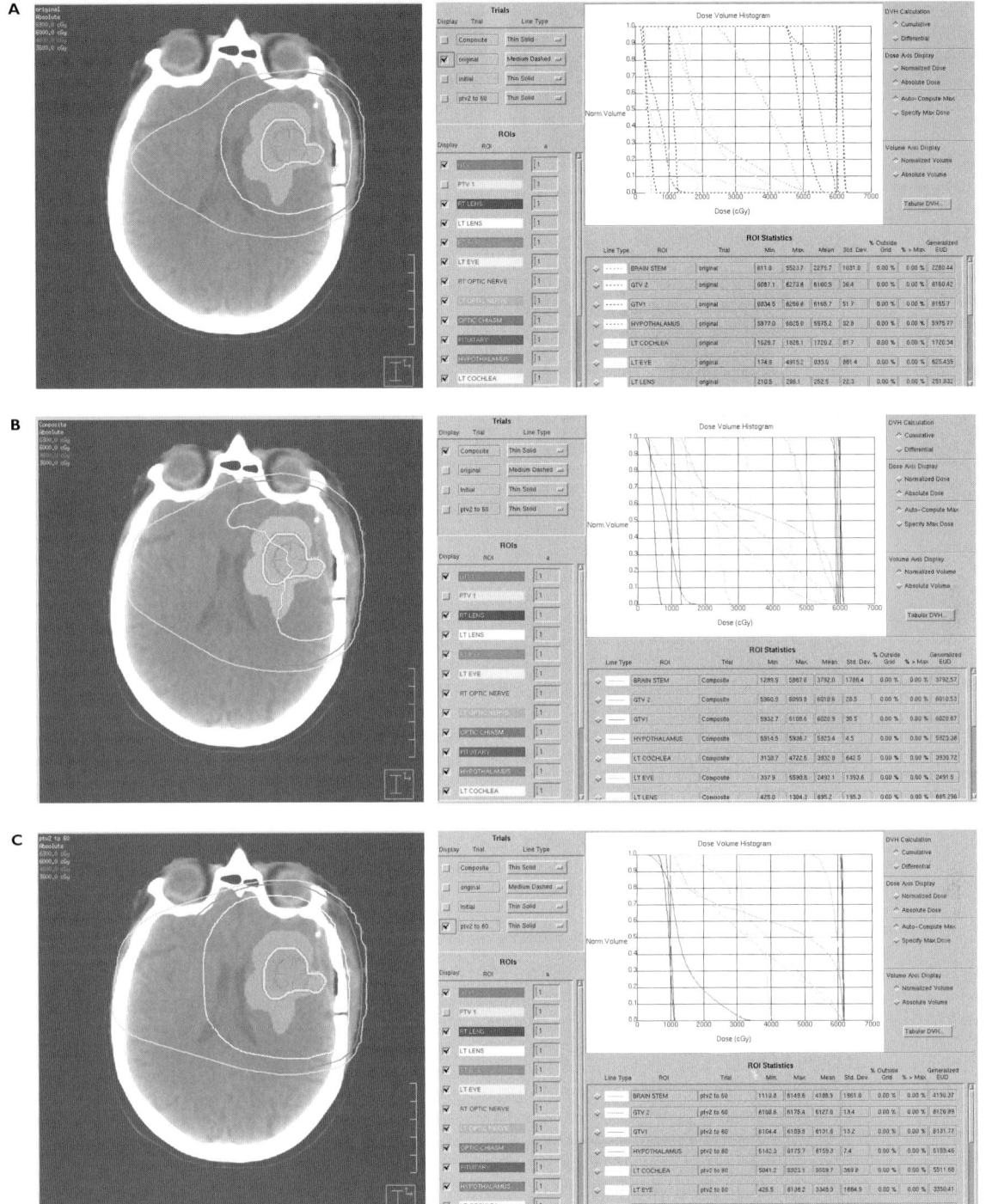

Figure 82.1 Comparison of dose plans for different volume definitions. (A) Dose plan using block margins per older RTOG studies. (B) Dose plan using dosimetric margins per RTOG 0525. (C) Dose plan using EORTC volume definition. *See color insert.*

DOSE-LIMITING STRUCTURES

Given the poor outcomes associated with this disease, tumor coverage is often not sacrificed to limit the dose to critical structures. However, with improved outcomes and subsets of patients living 5 years or more, reducing late toxicity may need to be considered. Table 82.5 lists the dose limitations for various structures used by the RTOG 0525 study. It is important to note that under the protocol

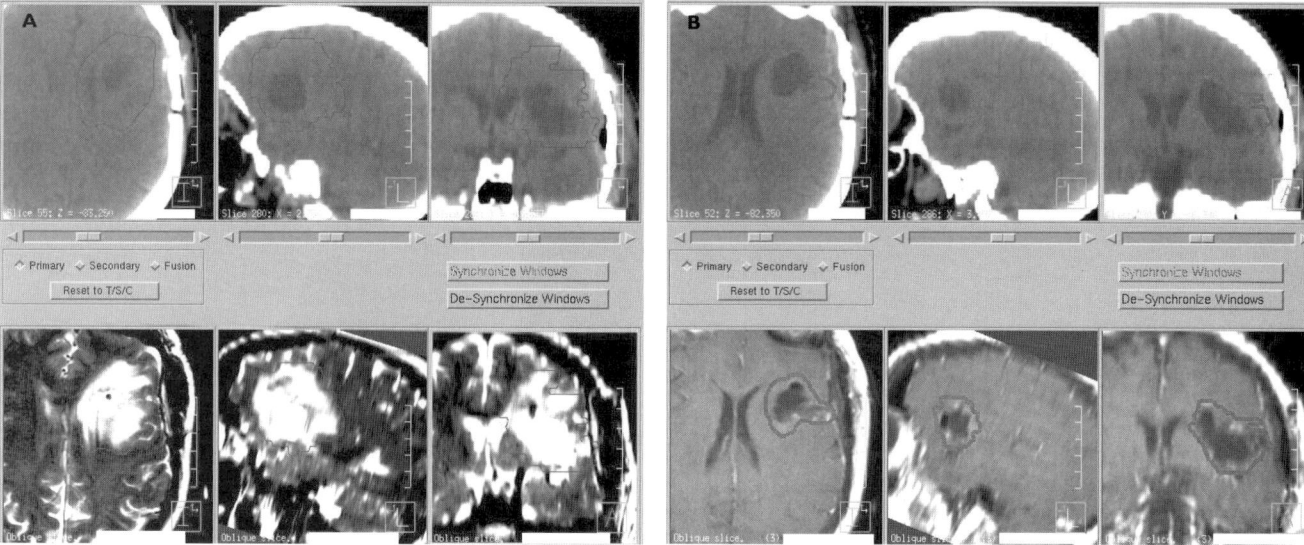

Figure 82.2 Example of MRI fusion. **(A)** MRI fusion for initial volume. **(B)** MRI fusion for boost volume. *See color insert.*

Table 82.5 Dose Limitation to Critical Structures

Structure	Dose Limit
Optic Chiasm/Optic Nerve	54 Gy
Retina	50 Gy
Brainstem	60 Gy
Lens	Shielded from direct beam
Cervical Spine	Shielded from direct beam

Table 82.6 Acute and Long-Term Toxicities

Likely (greater than 10%)	Scalp redness or soreness; Hair loss which may be temporary or permanent; Fatigue; Lethargy; Temporary aggravation of brain tumor symptoms such as headaches, seizures, or weakness
Less likely (less than 10%)	Mental slowing; Ear/ear canal reactions possibly resulting in short-term hearing loss; Cataracts; Behavioral change; Nausea; Vomiting; Temporary worsening of existing neurological deficits; Endocrine problems related to changes in the pituitary gland; Dry mouth/altered taste; Severe local damage to normal brain tissue, a condition called necrosis; Dizziness; Seizures
Rare but serious (less than 1%)	Optic injury with possibility of blindness; Permanent hearing loss; Depression

guidelines, higher doses can be given to these structures since compromise of tumor coverage is not allowed.

As in the RTOG 0525 study, clinical judgment may be used to exclude these sensitive structures from the PTV. Also, one may exclude regions where natural barriers would preclude microscopic tumor extension, including the cerebellum, contralateral hemisphere, directly across from the tentorium cerebri, and ventricles.

TOXICITY

Typical acute effects include erythema, dry skin, hair loss, and fatigue. Temporary loss of smell and serous otitis are also common. Occasionally, there is an increase in brain tumor symptoms due to edema and this may include headaches, nausea, vomiting, worsening weakness, or seizures. This may be managed with corticosteroids. The lowest effective dose of dexamethasone is typically used.

Long-term toxicities include neurocognitive deficits, endocrine dysfunction, and radiation necrosis. Other possible long-term toxicities may also include permanent hearing changes, visual damage, cataracts, and radiation-induced neoplasms. These are rare as many do not survive long enough to develop these symptoms. Table 82.6 summarizes some of the toxicities associated with radiation.

Radiation injury can be classified based on the temporal relationship to the radiation treatment [28]. Acute injury occurs during or shortly after radiation and is characterized by edema. Up to 12 weeks, early delayed injury occurs and is characterized by FLAIR and T2 changes. Late injury or radiation necrosis occurs several months to several years after radiation. The incidence of radiation necrosis in GBM following 60 Gy of radiation is very difficult to determine, but estimated to be 5 % by extrapolating data from the treatment of lower grade brain tumors [29]. Radiation necrosis can be difficult to diagnose as MRI findings are very similar to recurrence [30]. Treatment can be challenging. Steroid therapy is the upfront treatment of choice, however in some cases, it is difficult to wean off of steroids. In such cases, treatment options include hyperbaric oxygen [31], cyclooxygenase-2 inhibitors [32], bevacizumab [33], or surgical resection.

GBM IN ELDERLY/POOR PERFORMANCE PATIENTS

Radiation is beneficial in elderly patients. In a randomized study comparing best supportive care to radiation,

radiation improves survival [34]. This study randomized 81 patients aged 70 or older to 50 Gy of radiation or no radiation. Those receiving radiation had a median survival of 29.1 weeks versus 16.9 weeks for those receiving only supportive care ($p = 0.002$). No chemotherapy was given.

The dose scheme used, however, may not have an effect on outcomes. In a prospective study of 100 patients aged 60 years or over, patients were randomized to 60 Gy in 30 fractions versus 40 Gy in 15 fractions [35]. The median survival was 5.1 months for standard radiation compared to 5.6 months for the shorter course ($p = 0.57$); there was no difference in median overall survival. Again, no chemotherapy was given in this study. As such, the RTOG 0525 study does allow elderly patients to enroll into the study with the presumption that the elderly may benefit from aggressive treatment incorporating chemotherapy. Similarly, other studies are underway to determine whether chemotherapy can benefit this subset. Temozolomide alone, without radiation, is being investigated for the elderly [36].

In poor performance status patients, typically those with a Karnofsky performance status <60, a hypofractionated course of radiation is very reasonable [37,38]. A palliative dose regimen of 30 Gy in 10 fractions or 37.5 Gy in 15 fractions to the whole brain, or a hypofractionated course of focal radiation to 40 to 45 Gy in 15 fractions is given to expedite the completion of treatment. Unfortunately, these patients often do poorly with a median survival of approximately 7 months.

RADIATION SENSITIZERS

Motexafin gadolinium (Xcytrin®, Pharmacyclics Inc., Sunnyvale, CA), previously known as gadolinium texaphyrin or Gd-Tex, is a redox mediator that selectively targets tumor cells [39]. It catalyzes the oxidation of reducing metabolites, thus allowing for the generation of reactive oxygen species and fixation of damage by radiation. Animal studies have demonstrated selective uptake in tumor cells and enhancement of radiation responsiveness [40,41]. A Phase I study of this drug in GBM found that the maximum tolerated dose was 5 mg/kg/day, given daily for 2 weeks then three times per week until the completion of radiation [42]. Temozolomide was not given in this study. With temozolomide now being standard in the treatment of GBMs, RTOG 0513, a Phase I/II study of this drug with concurrent temozolomide, has just been completed.

RADIATION RETREATMENT

Re-irradiation for GBMs has been studied for both local and distant recurrence. Given the potential toxicities from high total doses of radiation, this is often given stereotactically. The University of Michigan reviewed their series of 20 patients who received repeat radiation for their GBMs [43]. The median dose used was 36 Gy (range: 30.6–50.4). Median survival was 9 months. Another study from Germany employed a hypofractionated, stereotactic approach in 14 patients with GBM [44]. The treatment margins were tight with 1 to 3 mm PTV expansion. Median dose was 30 Gy and median dose per fraction was 5 Gy. Median survival for the GBM subset was 7.9 months.

A larger series of patients were reviewed by the University of Heidelberg [45]. This series of 53 patients were re-irradiated to median dose of 36 Gy using a median fraction size of 2 Gy per fraction. A 1 cm margin was used and radiation was delivered stereotactically. There were no Common Toxicity Criteria Grade 3 or 4 toxicities. Median survival following re-irradiation was 8 months.

The University of Wisconsin is currently investigating low-dose rate radiation to retreat these tumors [46]. This approach takes advantage of the inverse dose rate effect where the radiation blocks cells from cycling through the G_2M phase, and the ongoing radiation in G_2M phase, which is the most sensitive phase to radiation, allows for increased cell kill. The technique at University of Wisconsin involves 0.2 Gy pulses delivered 3 minutes apart since conventional linear accelerators cannot deliver continuous low-dose rate radiation at this time. In one case study, 50 Gy at 2 Gy per fraction was delivered. This patient had good local control with no evidence of necrosis. He ultimately died 6 months later due to progression along the craniospinal axis outside of the treatment field. From 1999 to 2007, 99 patients were treated in this fashion, 31% of whom survived 6 months or more [47].

FOLLOW-UP

Typically, patients are followed with an MRI scan 4 weeks after completion of their chemoradiation, and every 2 to 3 months thereafter. One area of controversy is pseudoprogression [48]. One may see worsening FLAIR or T1 contrast changes soon after the completion of radiation, which may resolve if followed long enough rather than changing the planned treatment course. Pseudoprogression has yet to be properly defined. It is controversial how to image pseudoprogression and distinguish this from tumor growth. Its cause is unknown, although it is being seen more frequently with the use of more aggressive upfront treatment. Presumably, there are acute treatment-related changes including blood-brain barrier disruption and edema. As such, when following GBM patients, pseudoprogression must be considered as part of the differential diagnosis.

FUTURE DIRECTIONS

Radiation has been and will continue to be an essential component in the multimodality treatment of GBMs. Future directions will likely incorporate better molecular imaging techniques to define and follow areas of disease, and a better understanding of the biology of this tumor. In addition, the use of heavy particles, which have higher biological activity, should be investigated in these "hard to treat" tumors. Preliminary studies have been done in Japan using carbon ions, but more research is needed [49]. Radioimmunotherapy with I-125-EGFR MAb 425 has been investigated and is also promising with a median survival of 20.4 months when added to radiation and temozolomide [50]. Future studies are needed to define its role and the role of other radioimmunotherapies in the management of GBMs.

Various agents, some with radiosensitizing properties such as motexafin gadolinium, are currently being studied. The best "radiosensitizer" to date, temozolomide, has become standard in the treatment of GBMs [21]. Agents to improve the efficacy of temozolomide are being developed and assessed.

ACKNOWLEDGMENT

We would like to thank Nicky Pavelecky, Alwyn Reuther, and Shlomo Koyfman for their help with this chapter.

REFERENCES

1. Walker MD, Alexander E Jr, Hunt WE, et al. Evaluation of BCNU and/or radiotherapy in the treatment of anaplastic gliomas. A cooperative clinical trial. *J Neurosurg.* 1978;49(3):333–343.
2. Walker MD, Green SB, Byar DP, et al. Randomized comparisons of radiotherapy and nitrosoureas for the treatment of malignant glioma after surgery. *N Engl J Med.* 1980;303(23):1323–1329.
3. Walker MD, Strike TA, Sheline GE. An analysis of dose-effect relationship in the radiotherapy of malignant gliomas. *Int J Radiat Oncol Biol Phys.* 1979;5(10):1725–1731.
4. Salazar OM, Rubin P, McDonald JV, Feldstein ML. High dose radiation therapy in the treatment of glioblastoma multiforme: a preliminary report. *Int J Radiat Oncol Biol Phys.* 1976;1(7–8):717–727.
5. Nelson DF, Diener-West M, Horton J, Chang CH, Schoenfeld D, Nelson JS. Combined modality approach to treatment of malignant gliomas–re-evaluation of RTOG 7401/ECOG 1374 with long-term follow-up: a joint study of the Radiation Therapy Oncology Group and the Eastern Cooperative Oncology Group. *NCI Monogr.* 1988;6:279–284.
6. Chan JL, Lee SW, Fraass BA, et al. Survival and failure patterns of high-grade gliomas after three-dimensional conformal radiotherapy. *J Clin Oncol.* 2002;20(6):1635–1642.
7. Videtic GM, Gaspar LE, Zamorano L, et al. Use of the RTOG recursive partitioning analysis to validate the benefit of iodine-125 implants in the primary treatment of malignant gliomas. *Int J Radiat Oncol Biol Phys.* 1999;45(3):687–692.
8. Selker RG, Shapiro WR, Burger P, et al.; Brain Tumor Cooperative Group. The Brain Tumor Cooperative Group NIH Trial 87-01: a randomized comparison of surgery, external radiotherapy, and carmustine versus surgery, interstitial radiotherapy boost, external radiation therapy, and carmustine. *Neurosurgery.* 2002;51(2):343–355; discussion 355.
9. Laperriere NJ, Leung PM, McKenzie S, et al. Randomized study of brachytherapy in the initial management of patients with malignant astrocytoma. *Int J Radiat Oncol Biol Phys.* 1998;41(5):1005–1011.
10. Sneed PK, Stauffer PR, McDermott MW, et al. Survival benefit of hyperthermia in a prospective randomized trial of brachytherapy boost +/- hyperthermia for glioblastoma multiforme. *Int J Radiat Oncol Biol Phys.* 1998;40(2):287–295.
11. Shrieve DC, Alexander E 3rd, Black PM, et al. Treatment of patients with primary glioblastoma multiforme with standard postoperative radiotherapy and radiosurgical boost: prognostic factors and long-term outcome. *J Neurosurg.* 1999;90(1):72–77.
12. Nwokedi EC, DiBiase SJ, Jabbour S, Herman J, Amin P, Chin LS. Gamma knife stereotactic radiosurgery for patients with glioblastoma multiforme. *Neurosurgery.* 2002;50(1):41–46; discussion 46.
13. Souhami L, Seiferheld W, Brachman D, et al. Randomized comparison of stereotactic radiosurgery followed by conventional radiotherapy with carmustine to conventional radiotherapy with carmustine for patients with glioblastoma multiforme: report of Radiation Therapy Oncology Group 93-05 protocol. *Int J Radiat Oncol Biol Phys.* 2004;60(3):853–860.
14. Shaw E, Scott C, Souhami L, et al. Single dose radiosurgical treatment of recurrent previously irradiated primary brain tumors and brain metastases: final report of RTOG protocol 90-05. *Int J Radiat Oncol Biol Phys.* 2000;47(2):291–298.
15. Tsao MN, Mehta MP, Whelan TJ, et al. The American Society for Therapeutic Radiology and Oncology (ASTRO) evidence-based review of the role of radiosurgery for malignant glioma. *Int J Radiat Oncol Biol Phys.* 2005;63(1):47–55.
16. Werner-Wasik M, Scott CB, Nelson DF, et al. Final report of a phase I/II trial of hyperfractionated and accelerated hyperfractionated radiation therapy with carmustine for adults with supratentorial malignant gliomas. Radiation Therapy Oncology Group Study 83-02. *Cancer.* 1996;77(8):1535–1543.
17. Curran W, Scott C, Yung W, et al. No survival benefit of hyperfractionated radiotherapy (RT) to 72.0 Gy & carmustine versus standard RT & carmustine for malignant glioma patients: preliminary results of RTOG 90–06. *Proc Am Soc Clin Oncol.* 1996;1S:154.
18. Hochberg FH, Pruitt A. Assumptions in the radiotherapy of glioblastoma. *Neurology.* 1980;30(9):907–911.
19. Wallner KE, Galicich JH, Krol G, Arbit E, Malkin MG. Patterns of failure following treatment for glioblastoma multiforme and anaplastic astrocytoma. *Int J Radiat Oncol Biol Phys.* 1989;16(6):1405–1409.
20. Shibamoto Y, Yamashita J, Takahashi M, Yamasaki T, Kikuchi H, Abe M. Supratentorial malignant glioma: an analysis of radiation therapy in 178 cases. *Radiother Oncol.* 1990;18(1):9–17.
21. Stupp R, Mason WP, van den Bent MJ, et al. European Organisation for Research and Treatment of Cancer Brain Tumor and Radiotherapy Groups; National Cancer Institute of Canada Clinical Trials Group. Radiotherapy plus concomitant and adjuvant temozolomide for glioblastoma. *N Engl J Med.* 2005;352(10):987–996.
22. Chang EL, Akyurek S, Avalos T, et al. Evaluation of peritumoral edema in the delineation of radiotherapy clinical target volumes for glioblastoma. *Int J Radiat Oncol Biol Phys.* 2007;68(1):144–150.
23. Park I, Tamai G, Lee MC, et al. Patterns of recurrence analysis in newly diagnosed glioblastoma multiforme after three-dimensional conformal radiation therapy with respect to pre-radiation therapy magnetic resonance spectroscopic findings. *Int J Radiat Oncol Biol Phys.* 2007;69(2):381–389.
24. Lee IH, Cao Y, Junck L, et al. Patterns of failure in primary GBM following high-dose radiation therapy and concurrent temozolomide, indicating a potential role for methionine-PET in GTV definition. *Int J Radiat Oncol Biol Phys.* 2007; 69(3S):S102.
25. Floyd NS, Woo SY, Teh BS, et al. Hypofractionated intensity-modulated radiotherapy for primary glioblastoma multiforme. *Int J Radiat Oncol Biol Phys.* 2004;58(3):721–726.
26. Sultanem K, Patrocinio H, Lambert C, et al. The use of hypofractionated intensity-modulated irradiation in the treatment of glioblastoma multiforme: preliminary results of a prospective trial. *Int J Radiat Oncol Biol Phys.* 2004;58(1):247–252.
27. Hermanto U, Frija EK, Lii MJ, Chang EL, Mahajan A, Woo SY. Intensity-modulated radiotherapy (IMRT) and conventional three-dimensional conformal radiotherapy for high-grade gliomas: does IMRT increase the integral dose to normal brain? *Int J Radiat Oncol Biol Phys.* 2007;67(4):1135–1144.
28. Sheline GE, Wara WM, Smith V. Therapeutic irradiation and brain injury. *Int J Radiat Oncol Biol Phys.* 1980;6(9):1215–1228.
29. Shaw E, Arusell R, Scheithauer B, et al. Prospective randomized trial of low- versus high-dose radiation therapy in adults with supratentorial low-grade glioma: initial report of a North Central Cancer Treatment Group/Radiation Therapy Oncology Group/Eastern Cooperative Oncology Group study. *J Clin Oncol.* 2002;20(9):2267–2276.
30. Mullins ME, Barest GD, Schaefer PW, Hochberg FH, Gonzalez RG, Lev MH. Radiation necrosis versus glioma recurrence: conventional MR imaging clues to diagnosis. *AJNR Am J Neuroradiol.* 2005;26(8):1967–1972.
31. Leber KA, Eder HG, Kovac H, Anegg U, Pendl G. Treatment of cerebral radionecrosis by hyperbaric oxygen therapy. *Stereotact Funct Neurosurg.* 1998;70 (suppl 1):229–236.
32. Khan RB, Krasin MJ, Kasow K, Leung W. Cyclooxygenase-2 inhibition to treat radiation-induced brain necrosis and edema. *J Pediatr Hematol Oncol.* 2004;26(4):253–255.
33. Gonzalez J, Kumar AJ, Conrad CA, Levin VA. Effect of bevacizumab on radiation necrosis of the brain. *Int J Radiat Oncol Biol Phys.* 2007;67(2):323–326.
34. Keime-Guibert F, Chinot O, Taillandier L, et al.; Association of French-Speaking Neuro-Oncologists. Radiotherapy for glioblastoma in the elderly. *N Engl J Med.* 2007;356(15):1527–1535.
35. Roa W, Brasher PM, Bauman G, et al. Abbreviated course of radiation therapy in older patients with glioblastoma multiforme: a prospective randomized clinical trial. *J Clin Oncol.* 2004;22(9):1583–1588.
36. Chamberlain MC, Chalmers L. A pilot study of primary temozolomide chemotherapy and deferred radiotherapy in elderly patients with glioblastoma. *J Neurooncol.* 2007;82(2):207–209.

37. Bauman GS, Gaspar LE, Fisher BJ, Halperin EC, Macdonald DR, Cairncross JG. A prospective study of short-course radiotherapy in poor prognosis glioblastoma multiforme. *Int J Radiat Oncol Biol Phys.* 1994;29(4):835–839.
38. Chang EL, Yi W, Allen PK, Levin VA, Sawaya RE, Maor MH. Hypofractionated radiotherapy for elderly or younger low-performance status glioblastoma patients: outcome and prognostic factors. *Int J Radiat Oncol Biol Phys.* 2003;56(2):519–528.
39. Carde P, Timmerman R, Mehta MP, et al. Multicenter phase Ib/II trial of the radiation enhancer motexafin gadolinium in patients with brain metastases. *J Clin Oncol.* 2001;19(7):2074–2083.
40. Miller RA, Woodburn K, Fan Q, Renschler MF, Sessler JL, Koutcher JA. In vivo animal studies with gadolinium (III) texaphyrin as a radiation enhancer. *Int J Radiat Oncol Biol Phys.* 1999;45(4):981–989.
41. Xu S, Zakian K, Thaler H, et al. Effects of Motexafin gadolinium on tumor metabolism and radiation sensitivity. *Int J Radiat Oncol Biol Phys.* 2001;49(5):1381–1390.
42. Ford JM, Seiferheld W, Alger JR, et al. Results of the phase I dose-escalating study of motexafin gadolinium with standard radiotherapy in patients with glioblastoma multiforme. *Int J Radiat Oncol Biol Phys.* 2007;69(3):831–838.
43. Kim HK, Thornton AF, Greenberg HS, Page MA, Junck L, Sandler HM. Results of re-irradiation of primary intracranial neoplasms with three-dimensional conformal therapy. *Am J Clin Oncol.* 1997;20(4):358–363.
44. Vordermark D, Kölbl O, Ruprecht K, Vince GH, Bratengeier K, Flentje M. Hypofractionated stereotactic re-irradiation: treatment option in recurrent malignant glioma. *BMC Cancer.* 2005;5:55.
45. Combs SE, Gutwein S, Thilmann Ch, Huber P, Debus J, Schulz-Ertner D. Stereotactically guided fractionated re-irradiation in recurrent glioblastoma multiforme. *J Neurooncol.* 2005;74(2):167–171.
46. Cannon GM, Tomé WA, Robins HI, Howard SP. Pulsed reduced dose-rate radiotherapy: case report: a novel re-treatment strategy in the management of recurrent glioblastoma multiforme. *J Neurooncol.* 2007;83(3):307–311.
47. Tome WA, Atkinson J, Robins HI, et al. Pulsed reduced dose-rate radiotherapy: a novel re-treatment strategy in the management of large volume recurrent glioma. *Int J Radiat Oncol Biol Phys.* 2007;69(3S):S241–242.
48. Mason WP, Maestro RD, Eisenstat D, et al.; Canadian GBM Recommendations Committee. Canadian recommendations for the treatment of glioblastoma multiforme. *Curr Oncol.* 2007;14(3):110–117.
49. Mizoe JE, Tsujii H, Hasegawa A, et al. Organizing Committee of the Central Nervous System Tumor Working Group. Phase I/II clinical trial of carbon ion radiotherapy for malignant gliomas: combined X-ray radiotherapy, chemotherapy, and carbon ion radiotherapy. *Int J Radiat Oncol Biol Phys.* 2007;69(2):390–396.
50. Li L, Quang TS, Gracely EJ, et al. Radioimmunotherapy and temozolomide in the treatment of glioblastoma multiforme: a 20 year experience. *Int J Radiat Oncol Biol Phys.* 2007; 69(3S):S48.

83 Anaplastic Glioma

Malika L. Siker and Minesh P. Mehta

Anaplastic gliomas constitute approximately 25% of high-grade gliomas in adults, occurring typically in patients during youth to middle adulthood. Anaplastic gliomas may be of astrocytic, oligodendrocytic, or mixed lineage and correspond to World Health Organization (WHO) Grade III with nuclear atypia and increased mitotic activity [1]. They may arise primarily (*de novo*) or secondarily from a lower-grade precursor. Despite being aggressive, invasive tumors, they usually do not demonstrate necrosis or neovascularization. They display distinct clinical and biologic heterogeneity, which is also reflected on imaging, where lesions may show enhancement and necrosis similar to glioblastoma (GBM, WHO grade IV) or appear non-enhancing like WHO grade II gliomas.

For patients with anaplastic astrocytoma, median survival is approximately 3 years following diagnosis. Important prognostic factors include age at diagnosis, Karnofsky Performance Score (KPS), extent of resection, and mental status as determined by the Radiation Therapy Oncology Group (RTOG) recursive partitioning analysis (RPA), a statistical tool that allows for patients to be categorized into groups with similar outcomes through the identification of significant prognostic factors [2]. RTOG RPA classified patients with anaplastic astrocytoma into three prognostic groups based on these factors on a retrospective review of trials evaluating patients with malignant gliomas (Table 83.1).

Patients with anaplastic oligodendroglioma have a better prognosis with a median survival of 5 to 7 years [3,4]. With the advent of molecular genetics, patients with chromosome changes characterized by the loss of heterozygosity at 1p and 19q have emerged as an important subgroup that has shown improved outcomes as discussed in more detail below. Age at diagnosis, location and extent of resection, performance status, and the presence of chromosomal deletions are predictive of survival [3]. Patients with mixed histologies, anaplastic oligoastrocytoma, have a variable prognosis depending on dominant histological cell type and other prognostic factors [5].

IMPORTANCE OF MOLECULAR GENETICS

Alterations involving 1p and 19q have been found to be a significant prognostic factor and potential predictor of response to treatment, allowing further division of anaplastic oligodendrogliomas into two separate groups. Loss of heterozygosity at these alleles is thought to be an early genetic alteration in the transformation and progression of oligodendrogliomas. Combined codeletions at 1p and 19q have been found to occur in 63% of patients with oligodendroglioma and 52% of patients with mixed oligoastrocytoma, although this finding is rare in patients with astrocytomas (8%–11%) [6]. Deletions in 1p and 19q have been associated with longer progression-free survival and chemo- and radiosensitivity in uncontrolled studies [6–9].

Two prospective clinical trials have evaluated the importance of 1p and 19q deletions in patients treated for anaplastic gliomas (Table 83.2). They found that the combined loss of 1p and 19q is a strong favorable prognostic factor. The European Organisation for Research and Treatment of Cancer (EORTC) trial 26951 randomized 368 patients with anaplastic oligodendroglioma or oligoastrocytoma to receive radiotherapy alone or radiotherapy followed by procarbazine, lomustine, and vincristine (PCV) chemotherapy [4]. The status of 1p and 19q was determined and the presence of chromosomal deletions was balanced between the treatment groups. Combined loss of 1p and 19q was found in 25% of patients ($n = 78$). At median follow-up of approximately 60 months, patients with a combined loss of 1p and 19q were found to have significantly longer overall survival irrespective of treatment compared to those who were not codeleted (median survival not reached vs approximately 2 years). However, treatment with radiotherapy plus PCV did not improve outcome compared to radiotherapy alone even in this favorable subgroup as shown in Table 83.2 (69.5% vs 50.2% 5-year progression-free survival and 74% vs 74.7% 5-year overall survival). Codeletions of 1p and 19q were found to be the most important predictor of outcome (hazard ratio 0.27).

Table 83.1 RTOG Recursive Partitioning Analysis for Patients with Anaplastic Astrocytoma

Class	Features
I	Age <50, normal mental status
II	Age ≥50, KPS 70 to 100, and at least 3 months from the time of first symptoms to initiation treatment
III	Age <50, abnormal mental status

Table 83.2 Phase III Trials Examining Median Progression-Free Survival (a) and Median Overall Survival (b) in 1p19q Status and Response to Chemoradiotherapy in Patients with Anaplastic Oligodendroglioma/Oligoastrocytoma

Study	CRT with 1p19 del	95% CI	CRT minus 1p19q del	95% CI	RT with 1p19 del	95% CI	RT minus 1p19q del	95% CI
Median Progression-Free Survival								
RTOG 9402 [3]	NR	—	1.4 years	0.9–2.6	2.6 years	1.5–4.1	1.0 years	0.6–1.9
EORTC 26951 [4]	NR	—	15.3 months	11.9–23	62.2 months	43.4–NR	9.9 months	7.1–14.9
Median Overall Survival								
RTOG 9402 [3]	NR	—	2.7 years	2.0–5.5	6.6 years	5.4–NA	2.8 years	1.9–4.4
EORTC 26951 [4]	NR	—	25.2 months	19.9–42.6	NR	—	21.4	17.6–30

CI, confidence interval; CRT, chemoradiotherapy; del, deletion; NR, not reached; RT, radiotherapy.

The second trial, RTOG 9402, assessed 1p and 19q status in 206 of 289 enrolled patients (71%) with anaplastic oligodendroglioma/oligoastrocytoma randomized to receive chemotherapy with PCV followed by radiotherapy or radiotherapy alone [3]. Combined loss of 1p and 19q was present in 43% of patients in the PCV plus radiotherapy arm and in 50% in the radiotherapy alone arm. At median follow-up of 5.1 years, combined loss of 1p and 19q resulted in a longer median survival time of greater than 7 years versus 2.8 years ($p < 0.001$). There was no effect of tumor genotype on overall survival by treatment. The addition of PCV to radiotherapy did not improve survival for any patient subgroup (Table 83.2). In contrast to EORTC 26951, there was a lower risk of progression in patients with 1p and 19q deletions after treatment with PCV plus radiotherapy compared to radiotherapy alone, providing indirect evidence that allelic loss of 1p and 19q may be predictive for chemotherapy response (not reached vs 2.6 years, $p = 0.001$).

Indirect evidence of this relationship was again suggested in the updated results of RTOG 9402 that were recently presented [10]. At median follow-up of 6.9 years, patients with 1p and 19q codeletions were again found to have a significantly improved overall survival (8.7 vs 2.7 years, $p < 0.0001$). Additionally, longer progression-free survival was observed in patients with codeletions at 1p and 19q treated with PCV followed by radiotherapy compared to radiotherapy alone, suggesting potential predictive significance to response to chemotherapy. Longer follow-up is awaited to determine overall survival in these subgroups. Nevertheless, patients with 1p and 19q deletions represent a unique biologic subgroup that should be considered separately in future trials examining patients with anaplastic oligodendrogliomas.

The enzyme O^6-methylguanine-DNA methyltransferase (MGMT) has emerged as a potentially important regulator in the response to chemotherapy. Alkylating agents act by adding a methyl group at specific sites of DNA, triggering apoptosis and cytotoxicity if left unrepaired. MGMT is a suicide enzyme that removes this methyl group at the O^6 position of guanine, a key lesion created by temozolomide. In this process, MGMT becomes irreversibly methylated and must be regenerated for further activity. Increased MGMT is thought to blunt the therapeutic effects of alkylating agents and lead to increased resistance [11]. The loss of function of this gene is most often due to epigenetic changes, specifically promoter methylation [12]. Epigenetic silencing of the *MGMT* gene through promoter methylation has been found to lead to increased overall survival and better response to treatment with temozolomide and bischloroethylnitrosourea (BCNU) in patients with gliomas [12–14]. In EORTC 22981/26981, a large phase III trial investigating the use of chemoradiotherapy with temozolomide compared to radiotherapy alone in patients with GBM, patients with methylated *MGMT* promoter regions were found to have significantly improved survival (18.2 vs 12.2 months, $p < 0.001$) [15]. When treatment assignment was considered, only patients with *MGMT* promoter methylation demonstrated an improvement in survival with the addition of chemoradiotherapy compared to radiotherapy alone, suggesting a prognostic and predictive significance.

The importance of *MGMT* promoter methylation in patients with anaplastic glioma has not been adequately studied and only conflicting data on small numbers of patients are found in the literature. Incidence of *MGMT* promoter methylation has ranged from 12% to 42% in patients with anaplastic gliomas compared to 45% found in patients with GBM in EORTC 22981/26981 [11,12,14,15]. Further studies are needed to clarify the significance of *MGMT* promoter methylation in patients with anaplastic glioma.

TREATMENT APPROACH

Historically, the majority of trials examining patients with anaplastic gliomas are general series on malignant or high-grade gliomas that include patients with GBM, a more aggressive and biologically distinct tumor that occurs more commonly. Patients with anaplastic gliomas comprise the minority of patients in these trials. Treatment of patients with anaplastic gliomas has traditionally been extrapolated from the results of these trials despite the unique clinical and pathologic characteristics of anaplastic gliomas. As more trials investigate solely patients with anaplastic gliomas, specialized treatment guidelines will be established.

The current standard of care for patients with anaplastic gliomas is maximal surgical resection followed by adjuvant radiotherapy. This was first examined in a historic trial by Walker et al [16] which showed that patients with anaplastic glioma randomized to received radiotherapy had improved survival compared to patients receiving best supportive care, chemotherapy with BCNU alone, and radiotherapy plus BCNU. Further rationale for this approach and established radiotherapy techniques are based on trials that included all patients with malignant gliomas and are described further in the previous section, Glioblastoma. Treatment with radiotherapy in terms of volume and dose is the same as for GBM. Despite several subsequent trials that have examined the addition of chemotherapy in patients with anaplastic glioma, the role of chemotherapy in these patients remains controversial. The use of treatment modifiers such as radiation and chemotherapy sensitizers is also investigational.

CHEMOTHERAPY

The addition of chemotherapy to maximal surgical resection followed by radiotherapy has long been contentious in patients with malignant gliomas. Despite many prospective trials showing equivocal results compared to standard therapy, a meta-analysis by Stewart et al [17] examining 12 randomized trials including patients with malignant gliomas treated with radiotherapy plus chemotherapy showed a small significant long-term survival benefit with the addition of chemotherapy that was equivalent to an increase in 1-year survival of 6%, from 40% to 46%, and a 2-month increase in median survival. Although this meta-analysis suggested a small survival advantage, less than 30% of the included patients had anaplastic gliomas. Furthermore, the marginal survival advantage shown in this study given the additional toxicity associated with adjuvant chemotherapy has not led to universal acceptance of this approach.

With the seminal trial EORTC 22981/26981 by Stupp et al [18] demonstrating a significant survival benefit in patients with GBM treated with concomitant and adjuvant temozolomide following maximal surgical resection and radiotherapy, the use of chemotherapy in patients with GBM has become the standard of care. The applicability of this regimen for patients with anaplastic gliomas has been the subject of further debate. Ironically, GBM had historically been considered chemoresistant while anaplastic gliomas had been believed to be more chemosensitive. The results of this trial have given rise to a paradigm shift in favor of chemoradiotherapy for all malignant gliomas despite the lack of evidence showing a benefit in patients with anaplastic gliomas specifically. The results of subsequent prospective trials have begun to elucidate the role of chemotherapy in patients with anaplastic gliomas, but clear guidelines from the results of prospective randomized trials are awaited.

Anaplastic Astrocytoma

Adjuvant treatment with chemotherapy following radiotherapy has not been universally adopted for patients with anaplastic astrocytoma due to conflicting data in the literature. The addition of chemotherapy, best agents, and timing of treatment have all been debated. PCV chemotherapy was initially considered the standard regimen for proponents of adjuvant chemotherapy with the results of a trial by Levin et al [19]. Patients with malignant gliomas were randomized to radiotherapy with adjuvant chemotherapy with BCNU or PCV. While improved survival was found in all patients administered PCV compared to BCNU, the difference was only statistically significant for patients with anaplastic glioma. Opponents of this approach cited a retrospective review of RTOG protocols published almost a decade later by Prados et al [20] showing contradictory results. The outcome of 432 patients with newly diagnosed anaplastic astrocytoma treated with radiotherapy and either BCNU or PCV adjuvant chemotherapy was reviewed with no statistically significant difference in survival detected.

Further investigation into the benefit of the addition of adjuvant PCV after standard treatment was conducted by a prospective phase III trial by the United Kingdom Medical Research Council [21]. In this trial, 674 patients with malignant glioma were randomized after maximal surgical resection to radiotherapy alone or radiotherapy followed by PCV. Seventeen percent (117 patients) had anaplastic astrocytoma. Survival was found to be statistically equivalent in both treatment arms and in all subgroups, including histology. However, the median survival in the anaplastic astrocytoma subgroup, 13 to 15 months, was substantially lower than the expected survival rate of 2 to 3 years in previous trials, leading to a debate over the applicability of these results.

Another recently published trial by Hildebrand et al [22] further examined the use of adjuvant chemotherapy in patients with anaplastic astrocytomas. It is the only trial including solely patients with anaplastic astrocytoma with radiotherapy alone as a control arm. This trial was a continuation of a previous phase III trial that found a significant survival benefit in patients with malignant glioma treated with radiotherapy plus concurrent dibromodulcitol (DBD) and adjuvant DBD and BCNU compared to radiotherapy alone (13 vs 10.4 months, $p = 0.044$) [23]. On further review, investigators noted that survival in patients with anaplastic astrocytoma was improved to a greater extent compared with patients with GBM but the number of patients with anaplastic astrocytoma was too small to reach statistical significance. The trial was reopened to accrue only patients with anaplastic astrocytoma, and 193 patients were randomized to receive radiotherapy alone or radiotherapy with concurrent and adjuvant BCNU/DBD. It was closed early due to decreasing accrual rate, short of the intended 212 patients. Although there was a trend toward improved survival, it was not found to be statistically significant (23.9 vs 27.3 months, $p = 0.111$).

Another trial examining chemoradiotherapy in patients with anaplastic gliomas was performed by Levin et al [24]. The safety and outcomes of patients treated with accelerated fractionated radiotherapy with carboplatin followed by PCV was examined in a phase II trial. A total of 90 patients (76.7% with anaplastic astrocytoma) were enrolled and median survival for all patients was 28.1 months, and 28.7 months for patients with anaplastic astrocytoma.

Serious neurologic deterioration and/or dementia resulted in 10% patients. Authors concluded that while excessive central nervous system toxicity from this intense regimen may have been a major contributing factor to the inferior median survival found, patients with treatment-induced necrosis had a significantly longer survival compared with those without any radiologic or histologic evidence of necrosis.

Temozolomide, which has been shown to significantly prolong survival in patients with GBM in a phase III trial by Stupp et al [18] has shown activity in patients with recurrent anaplastic astrocytoma. In a phase II trial by Yung et al [25], 162 patients with anaplastic astrocytoma were treated with temozolomide at first relapse. The 6-month progression-free survival was 46% and overall survival was 13.6 months. The objective response rate was 35% (complete response 8%, partial response 27%). The results of this trial suggest that temozolomide has antitumor activity with an acceptable safety profile for recurrent anaplastic astrocytoma. However, Combs et al [26] retrospectively compared outcomes of patients treated with radiotherapy alone vs radiotherapy with temozolomide. No difference in survival was detected. Another trial examined this agent given in a dose-dense schedule with good activity [27]. Balmaceda et al [28] reported the results of a study of 28 patients treated with twice daily temozolomide with recurrent anaplastic astrocytoma as part of a multi-institutional phase II dose escalation trial for malignant gliomas and found median progression-free survival of 5.8 months and median overall survival of 14.6 months without increasing toxicity, suggesting that increasing dose may be achieved without adding significant toxicity. Overall response rate was 46%. Other agents examined in recurrent anaplastic astrocytoma including cyclophosphamide and CPT-11 have shown modest efficacy [29,30]. While these agents may be promising, future prospective trials are needed to define their role in these patients.

To assess the benefit of temozolomide as adjuvant chemotherapy after radiotherapy in patients with anaplastic astrocytoma, RTOG 9813 was initiated and is now closed. Patients were randomized to radiotherapy plus adjuvant BCNU or temozolomide. This trial did not use the continuous concomitant dosing regimen with temozolomide during radiotherapy as examined in EORTC 22981/26981. Approximately 180 patients have been enrolled, and results from RTOG 9813 are needed to further elucidate the role of temozolomide in the treatment of anaplastic astrocytoma.

In summary, no prospective, randomized trials exist showing a benefit with the addition of chemotherapy to standard therapy of maximal surgical resection followed by radiotherapy. While some trials suggest a benefit, improvements have been modest and not statistically significant. PCV chemotherapy with or without other agents has been the regimen most frequently examined. With the results of Stupp et al showing significantly improved survival in patients with GBM treated with chemoradiotherapy, temozolomide has emerged as a potentially promising treatment for anaplastic gliomas and has shown activity in early clinical trials. Larger phase III trials examining patients with anaplastic astrocytoma alone are needed to better define treatment guidelines.

Anaplastic Oligodendroglioma/Oligoastrocytoma

Because of the high rates of radiographic response to PCV in several early clinical studies, anaplastic oligodendroglioma and oligoastrocytoma gained the reputation of being exquisitely chemosensitive [31,32]. These results prompted two large randomized trials, RTOG 9402 and EORTC 26951, to determine if sequential combination of radiotherapy and chemotherapy provided a therapeutic benefit over radiotherapy alone (Table 83.3). The results of these trials have produced more controversy, showing significantly improved progression-free survival without an increase in overall survival in patients treated with sequential chemoradiotherapy compared to radiotherapy alone with chemotherapy reserved for salvage. As median follow-up increases in these trials, forthcoming data may help resolve this impasse. An update of RTOG 9402 was recently presented and now suggests a significant improvement in survival in patients treated with sequential chemoradiotherapy; these results have very small patient numbers at long follow-up periods and remain preliminary at this point.

EORTC 26951 examined the potential benefit of radiotherapy followed by adjuvant PCV chemotherapy. In this phase III trial reported by van den Bent et al [4], 368 patients with newly diagnosed anaplastic oligodendroglioma or oligoastrocytoma were randomized to receive either radiotherapy alone with chemotherapy reserved for salvage or

Table 83.3 Phase III Trials Examining Chemoradiotherapy in Patients with Anaplastic Oligodendroglioma/Oligoastrocytoma and 1p19 Status

Study	Treatment arms	N	MOS	p Value	PFS	p Value	Grade 3/4 toxicity
RTOG 9402 [3]	RT alone	142	4.7 years	0.26	2.6 years	0.004	5%
	PCV + RT	147	4.9 years		1.7 years		65%
			at 3 years		at 3 years		
EORTC 26951 [4]	RT alone	183	30.6 months	0.23	13.2 months	0.0018	NR
	RT + PCV	185	40.3 months		23.0 months		NR
			at 60 months		at 60 months		

MOS, median overall survival; N, number of patients; NR, not reported; PCV, CCNU, procarbazine, and vincristine; PFS, progression free Survival; RT, radiotherapy.

with radiotherapy followed by up to 6 cycles of adjuvant PCV. At a median follow-up of 5 years, progression-free survival was significantly improved in patients receiving radiotherapy plus adjuvant PCV compared to radiotherapy alone (23 vs 13.2 months, $p = 0.0018$). However, overall survival was not found to be statistically equivalent in patients treated with chemoradiotherapy compared to radiotherapy alone with median survival of 40.3 months and 30.6 months respectively ($p = 0.23$).

The second trial, RTOG 9402 reported by Cairncross et al [3], confirmed these results. Investigators randomized 289 patients with newly diagnosed anaplastic oligodendroglioma or oligoastrocytoma to radiotherapy alone with chemotherapy reserved for salvage or neoadjuvant PCV followed by radiotherapy. At median follow-up of 5.1 years, no statistically significant difference is survival was detected with median survival of 4.9 years in patients treated with chemoradiotherapy compared to 4.7 years in patients treated with radiotherapy alone ($p = 0.26$). Similar to EORTC 26951, progression-free survival was significantly longer in the group treated with PCV followed by radiotherapy compared to radiotherapy alone (2.6 vs 1.7 years, $p = 0.008$). Grade 3/4 toxicity was observed more frequently in patients receiving neoadjuvant PCV (65%), resulting in one death.

An update of RTOG 9402 was recently presented and indicates that more time may be needed for an improvement in survival to manifest [10]. At median follow-up of 6.9 years, the unadjusted estimated for 5-year overall survival remains statistically equivalent for patients treated with chemoradiotherapy compared to radiotherapy alone (49 vs 46%, $p = 0.1$). However, after adjusting for patient-specific risk factors, overall survival was significantly longer with the addition of neoadjuvant PCV. A significant improvement in estimated 5-year progression-free survival persisted for unadjusted and adjusted patient groups.

The effect of salvage therapy in patients treated in the radiotherapy alone arms of the RTOG 9402 and EORTC 26951 trials has been offered as a possible explanation for the lack of a statistically significant survival benefit observed in these trials. In RTOG 9402, 57% of patients treated with radiotherapy alone received salvage chemotherapy with PCV or temozolomide at recurrence. In addition, 43% of patients treated with radiotherapy alone were treated with second surgery at recurrence compared to 20% in the PCV plus radiotherapy arm. In EORTC 26951, salvage PCV was given at recurrence to 65% of patients in the radiotherapy-only arm and 11% in the radiotherapy and adjuvant PCV arm. Salvage with any type of chemotherapy was used in 82% of patients in the radiotherapy-alone arm compared to 55% in the radiotherapy plus PCV arm. These differences might have favorably influenced the overall survival in the radiotherapy-alone arm, illustrating that while initial treatment with sequential chemoradiotherapy does not prolong life compared to radiotherapy alone, the potential impact of salvage chemotherapy cannot be ignored. With the high percentage of patients receiving salvage therapy, this trial may be interpreted as assessing the benefit of early or delayed chemotherapy.

Although an improvement in survival with chemoradiotherapy remains unclear, the PCV regimen was shown to have a high rate of toxicity. Therefore, development of a better-tolerated regimen may change the treatment approach by shifting the "risk to benefit" ratio. Temozolomide, which has demonstrated a good toxicity profile in large randomized trials, is a potential agent. Recent studies have examined the use of this agent in patients with anaplastic oligodendrogliomas, producing high response rates. Chinot et al [33] administered temozolomide to 48 patients with anaplastic oligodendroglioma or oligoastrocytoma who had previously failed PCV chemotherapy. Objective response rate was found to be 43.8% (complete response 16.7%, partial response 27.1%) with overall survival at 10 months. Grade 3 thrombocytopenia occurred in 6.3% patients. Newly diagnosed patients with anaplastic oligodendroglioma were found to have a response rate of 75% with a median time to tumor progression of 24 months with few grade 3/4 toxicities in a trial including 20 pateints by Taliansky-Aronov et al [34].

Another strategy from RTOG 0131, reported by Vogelbaum et al [35], examined neoadjuvant temozolomide followed by radiotherapy in patients with newly diagnosed anaplastic oligodendroglioma or oligoastrocytoma. In this phase II trial, 40 patients received temozolomide 6 months before radiotherapy. Of the 27 patients available for review, objective response rate was 33.3% (complete response 3.7%, partial response 29.6%). The 6-month progression rate was 10.3% with acceptable toxicity. Response to temozolomide has also been shown to be significantly associated to loss of 1p in a small retrospective study [36].

The results of 24 patients with recurrent anaplastic oligodendroglioma treated with twice daily temozolomide as part of a multi-institutional phase II dose escalation trial for recurrent malignant gliomas [28]. Overall response rate was 46%. Median progression-free survival was found to be 7.7 months and median overall survival was 18 months without increased toxicity. Brandes et al [9] examined the results of 67 patients with anaplastic oligodendroglioma ($n = 39$) and anaplastic oligoastrocytoma ($n = 28$) treated with temozolomide and found an overall response rate of 46.3% that was significantly higher in patients with anaplastic oligodendroglioma compared to oligoastroctyoma (61.5% vs 25%, $p = 0.003$). Furthermore, codeletions at 1p and 19q have been suggested as markers for response to treatment with temozolomide in uncontrolled studies [9,37]. While these trials suggest good activity, the use of temozolomide in these patients remains investigational.

Despite its putative reputation as a chemosensitive tumor due to dramatic responses seen on imaging following chemotherapy in early clinical trials, large, prospective, randomized trials have not yet definitively shown an improvement in survival with the addition of chemotherapy to standard therapy of maximal resection followed by radiotherapy. Reasons for this current stalemate include the effect of salvage therapy in the control arms of these trials and the long survival of these patients, suggesting that longer follow-up is needed to demonstrate a significant survival advantage as shown by the updated results of RTOG 9402. It is also important to consider that the PCV regimen was associated with substantial toxicity in these trials. Temozolomide has shown good activity with little toxicity, but has not yet been evaluated in phase III trials in patients with anaplastic oligodendrogliomas. The updated results of RTOG 9402 and EORTC 26951 and further prospective randomized trials are needed to provide the needed data to define standard treatment for patients with anaplastic oligodendrogliomas.

RADIOTHERAPY AND CHEMOTHERAPY MODIFIERS

Radiotherapy and chemotherapy modifiers are designed to enhance the efficacy of treatment in tumors with no added toxicity to normal tissue and have been investigated in clinical trials in patients with anaplastic gliomas with mixed results. Bromodeoxyuridine (BUdR) is a halogenated pyrimidine that functions as a substitue for thymidine during DNA synthesis and has been evaluated as a radiosensitizer. In a phase III prospective randomized trial, Prados et al [38] sought to investigate the addition of BUdR in an anticipated 293 patients with anaplastic astrocytoma randomized to receive conventional radiotherapy plus PCV chemotherapy with or without BUdR given as an infusion during each week of radiotherapy. The study was closed before full accrual based on an interim analysis that predicted no survival advantage for the BUdR arm. In the remaining 190 patients that were eligible for analysis, there was no survival benefit found with the addition of BUdR.

Difluoromethylornithine (DFMO), an inhibitor of ornithine decarboxylase, is a potential chemosenitizer that works by increasing the intracellular accumulation of polyamine cations that lead to the conformal stabilization of DNA. The addition of DFMO to PCV in adjuvant treatment of anaplastic gliomas was evaluated in a phase III trial by Levin et al [39] Patients were randomized to PCV alone or PCV plus DFMO, following radiotherapy. Of the 228 evaluable patients, the majority had anaplastic astrocytoma compared to oligodendroglioma/oligoastrocytoma (78.1% and 17.5%, respectively). While the hazard function showed a significant difference in survival over the first 2 years of the study (hazard ratio 0.53, $p = 0.02$), this did not continue after 2 years (hazard ratio 1.06, $p = 0.84$). Differences in overall survival and progression-free survival were not found to be significant. The use of radiotherapy and chemical modifiers remains investigational.

RE-IRRADIATION

Despite best available treatment, the majority of patients develop local progression within or near the site of initial disease within 5 years or less [40]. Re-irradiation of recurrent anaplastic gliomas after standard treatment of maximal safe resection followed by radiotherapy has been historically contraindicated due to the increased risk of radionecrosis. However, newer techniques using conformal external beam radiotherapy, brachytherapy, and stereotactic radiosurgery have been shown to be safe in carefully selected patients as seen in Table 83.4.

CONCLUSION

Anaplastic gliomas are aggressive, invasive tumors that demonstrate clinical and biologic heterogeneity depending on cell type, astrocytic, oligodendrocytic, or mixed. Molecular genetics has become increasingly important with codeletions at 1p19q emerging as an important prognostic and potentially predictive factor for patients with anaplastic oligodendroglioma. Standard treatment includes maximal surgical resection followed by adjuvant radiotherapy. The addition of chemotherapy has not been universally adopted due to conflicting data regarding outcome and concern for additional toxicity with the regimens studied thus far in patients with anaplastic glioma. Proponents of chemoradiotherapy extrapolate the results of EORTC 22981/26981 that showed a significant benefit with addition of concurrent and adjuvant temozolomide to radiotherapy in patients with GBM and point out the improved survival of patients with anaplastic oligodendrogliomas treated with PCV [18]. However, several trials have failed to show a survival benefit in patients with anaplastic gliomas treated with chemotherapy.[3,4,21,22] Radiation and chemotherapy modifiers have not shown to improve

Table 83.4 Results of Re-irradiation for Patients with Recurrent Anaplastic Gliomas

Study	Retreatment Modality	Patient Number and Histology	Median Survival (Months)
Bauman et al [40]	Conventional EBRT	11 GBM and AG	2.8
Kim et al [41]	3-D EBRT	7 GBM/7 AG	7.0
Voynov et al [42]	IMRT	5 GBM/5 AG	10.1
Sneed et al [43]	Brachytherapy	45 AG	12.3
Gabayan et al [44]	Brachytherapy	15 AG	10.0
Tatter et al [45]	Brachytherapy	21 GBM and AG	12.7
Sanghavi et al [46]	Radiosurgery	30 GBM and AG	8.0
Cho et al [47]	Radiosurgery	27 GBM/19 AG	11.0
Kondziolka et al [48]	Radiosurgery	23 AG	31.0
Cho et al [47]	FSRT	15 GBM/10 AG	12.0
Vordermark et al [49]	FSRT	5 AG	15.4
Shepherd et al [50]	FSRT	29 GBM and AG	11.0
Combs et al [51]	FSRT	42 AG	16.0

AG, anaplastic glioma; EBRT, external beam radiation therapy; FSRT, fractionated stereotactic radiation therapy; GBM, glioblastoma; IMRT, intensity-modulated radiation therapy.

outcomes in prospective randomized trials. Future directions include treatment with temozolomide but no phase III trials have been completed in patients with anaplastic gliomas. Further studies are needed before the addition of chemotherapy is considered standard of care.

REFERENCES

1. Kleihues P, Cavenee WK. *Pathology and Genetics of Tumours of the Nervous System.* Lyon: IARC Press; 2000.
2. Curran WJ Jr, Scott CB, Horton J, et al. Recursive partitioning analysis of prognostic factors in three Radiation Therapy Oncology Group malignant glioma trials. *J Natl Cancer Inst.* 1993;85(9):704–710.
3. Cairncross G, Berkey B, Shaw E, et al.; Intergroup Radiation Therapy Oncology Group Trial 9402. Phase III trial of chemotherapy plus radiotherapy compared with radiotherapy alone for pure and mixed anaplastic oligodendroglioma: Intergroup Radiation Therapy Oncology Group Trial 9402. *J Clin Oncol.* 2006;24(18):2707–2714.
4. van den Bent MJ, Carpentier AF, Brandes AA, et al. Adjuvant procarbazine, lomustine, and vincristine improves progression-free survival but not overall survival in newly diagnosed anaplastic oligodendrogliomas and oligoastrocytomas: a randomized European Organisation for Research and Treatment of Cancer phase III trial. *J Clin Oncol.* 2006;24(18):2715–2722.
5. Donahue B, Scott CB, Nelson JS, et al. Influence of an oligodendroglial component on the survival of patients with anaplastic astrocytomas: a report of Radiation Therapy Oncology Group 83–02. *Int J Radiat Oncol Biol Phys.* 1997;38(5):911–914.
6. Smith JS, Perry A, Borell TJ, et al. Alterations of chromosome arms 1p and 19q as predictors of survival in oligodendrogliomas, astrocytomas, and mixed oligoastrocytomas. *J Clin Oncol.* 2000;18(3):636–645.
7. Cairncross JG, Ueki K, Zlatescu MC, et al. Specific genetic predictors of chemotherapeutic response and survival in patients with anaplastic oligodendrogliomas. *J Natl Cancer Inst.* 1998;90(19):1473–1479.
8. Bauman GS, Ino Y, Ueki K, et al. Allelic loss of chromosome 1p and radiotherapy plus chemotherapy in patients with oligodendrogliomas. *Int J Radiat Oncol Biol Phys.* 2000;48(3):825–830.
9. Brandes AA, Tosoni A, Cavallo G, et al.; GICNO. Correlations between O6-methylguanine DNA methyltransferase promoter methylation status, 1p and 19q deletions, and response to temozolomide in anaplastic and recurrent oligodendroglioma: a prospective GICNO study. *J Clin Oncol.* 2006;24(29):4746–4753.
10. Cairncross G, Wang M, Chang SM, et al. A Randomized Trial of Chemotherapy Plus Radiotherapy (RT) versus RT alone for Anaplastic Oligodendroglioma (RTOG 9402): The Perspective of Longer Follow-Up. *Int J Radiat Oncol Biol Phys.* 2008;72:S7-S8.
11. Jaeckle KA, Eyre HJ, Townsend JJ, et al. Correlation of tumor O6 methylguanine-DNA methyltransferase levels with survival of malignant astrocytoma patients treated with bis-chloroethylnitrosourea: a Southwest Oncology Group study. *J Clin Oncol.* 1998;16(10):3310–3315.
12. Esteller M, Garcia-Foncillas J, Andion E, et al. Inactivation of the DNA-repair gene MGMT and the clinical response of gliomas to alkylating agents. *N Engl J Med.* 2000;343(19):1350–1354.
13. Hegi ME, Diserens AC, Godard S, et al. Clinical trial substantiates the predictive value of O-6-methylguanine-DNA methyltransferase promoter methylation in glioblastoma patients treated with temozolomide. *Clin Cancer Res.* 2004;10(6):1871–1874.
14. Paz MF, Yaya-Tur R, Rojas-Marcos I, et al. CpG island hypermethylation of the DNA repair enzyme methyltransferase predicts response to temozolomide in primary gliomas. *Clin Cancer Res.* 2004;10(15):4933–4938.
15. Hegi ME, Diserens AC, Gorlia T, et al. MGMT gene silencing and benefit from temozolomide in glioblastoma. *N Engl J Med.* 2005;352(10):997–1003.
16. Walker MD, Alexander E Jr, Hunt WE, et al. Evaluation of BCNU and/or radiotherapy in the treatment of anaplastic gliomas. A cooperative clinical trial. *J Neurosurg.* 1978;49(3):333–343.
17. Stewart LA. Chemotherapy in adult high-grade glioma: a systematic review and meta-analysis of individual patient data from 12 randomised trials. *Lancet.* 2002;359(9311):1011–1018.
18. Stupp R, Mason WP, van den Bent MJ, et al.; European Organisation for Research and Treatment of Cancer Brain Tumor and Radiotherapy Groups; National Cancer Institute of Canada Clinical Trials Group. Radiotherapy plus concomitant and adjuvant temozolomide for glioblastoma. *N Engl J Med.* 2005;352(10):987–996.
19. Levin VA, Silver P, Hannigan J, et al. Superiority of post-radiotherapy adjuvant chemotherapy with CCNU, procarbazine, and vincristine (PCV) over BCNU for anaplastic gliomas: NCOG 6G61 final report. *Int J Radiat Oncol Biol Phys.* 1990;18(2):321–324.
20. Prados MD, Scott C, Curran WJ Jr, Nelson DF, Leibel S, Kramer S. Procarbazine, lomustine, and vincristine (PCV) chemotherapy for anaplastic astrocytoma: A retrospective review of radiation therapy oncology group protocols comparing survival with carmustine or PCV adjuvant chemotherapy. *J Clin Oncol.* 1999;17(11):3389–3395.
21. Medical Research Council Brain Tumor Working Party. Randomized trial of procarbazine, lomustine, and vincristine in the adjuvant treatment of high-grade astrocytoma: a Medical Research Council trial. *J Clin Oncol.* 2001;19:509–518.
22. Hildebrand J, Gorlia T, Kros JM, et al.; EORTC Brain Tumour Group investigators. Adjuvant dibromodulcitol and BCNU chemotherapy in anaplastic astrocytoma: results of a randomised European Organisation for Research and Treatment of Cancer phase III study (EORTC study 26882). *Eur J Cancer.* 2008;44(9):1210–1216.
23. Hildebrand J, Sahmoud T, Mignolet F, Brucher JM, Afra D. Adjuvant therapy with dibromodulcitol and BCNU increases survival of adults with malignant gliomas. EORTC Brain Tumor Group. *Neurology.* 1994;44(8):1479–1483.
24. Levin VA, Yung WK, Bruner J, et al. Phase II study of accelerated fractionation radiation therapy with carboplatin followed by PCV chemotherapy for the treatment of anaplastic gliomas. *Int J Radiat Oncol Biol Phys.* 2002;53(1):58–66.
25. Yung WK, Prados MD, Yaya-Tur R, et al. Multicenter phase II trial of temozolomide in patients with anaplastic astrocytoma or anaplastic oligoastrocytoma at first relapse. Temodal Brain Tumor Group. *J Clin Oncol.* 1999;17(9):2762–2771.
26. Combs SE, Nagy M, Edler L, et al. Comparative evaluation of radiochemotherapy with temozolomide versus standard-of-care postoperative radiation alone in patients with WHO grade III astrocytic tumors. *Radiother Oncol.* 2008;88(2):177–182.
27. Neyns B, Chaskis C, Joosens E, et al. A multicenter cohort study of dose-dense temozolomide (21 of 28 days) for the treatment of recurrent anaplastic astrocytoma or oligoastrocytoma. *Cancer Invest.* 2008;26(3):269–277.
28. Balmaceda C, Peereboom D, Pannullo S, et al. Multi-institutional phase II study of temozolomide administered twice daily in the treatment of recurrent high-grade gliomas. *Cancer.* 2008;112(5):1139–1146.
29. Chamberlain MC, Tsao-Wei DD, Groshen S. Salvage chemotherapy with cyclophosphamide for recurrent temozolomide-refractory anaplastic astrocytoma. *Cancer.* 2006;106(1):172–179.
30. Chamberlain MC, Wei-Tsao DD, Blumenthal DT, Glantz MJ. Salvage chemotherapy with CPT-11 for recurrent temozolomide-refractory anaplastic astrocytoma. *Cancer.* 2008;112(9):2038–2045.
31. Cairncross JG, Macdonald DR. Successful chemotherapy for recurrent malignant oligodendroglioma. *Ann Neurol.* 1988;23(4):360–364.
32. Kim L, Hochberg FH, Thornton AF, et al. Procarbazine, lomustine, and vincristine (PCV) chemotherapy for grade III and grade IV oligoastrocytomas. *J Neurosurg.* 1996;85(4):602–607.
33. Chinot OL, Honore S, Dufour H, et al. Safety and efficacy of temozolomide in patients with recurrent anaplastic oligodendrogliomas after standard radiotherapy and chemotherapy. *J Clin Oncol.* 2001;19(9):2449–2455.
34. Taliansky-Aronov A, Bokstein F, Lavon I, Siegal T. Temozolomide treatment for newly diagnosed anaplastic oligodendrogliomas: a clinical efficacy trial. *J Neurooncol.* 2006;79(2):153–157.
35. Vogelbaum MA, Berkey B, Peereboom D, al. e. RTOG 0131: Phase II Trial of pre-irradiation and concurrent temozolomide in patients with newly diagnosed anaplastic oligodendrogliomas and mixed anaplastic oligodendrogliomas. *Proc Am Soc Clin Oncol.* 2005;23:1520.
36. Chahlavi A, Kanner A, Peereboom D, Staugaitis SM, Elson P, Barnett G. Impact of chromosome 1p status in response of oligodendroglioma to temozolomide: preliminary results. *J Neurooncol.* 2003;61(3):267–273.

37. Kouwenhoven MC, Kros JM, French PJ, et al. 1p/19q loss within oligodendroglioma is predictive for response to first line temozolomide but not to salvage treatment. *Eur J Cancer.* 2006;42(15):2499–2503.
38. Prados MD, Seiferheld W, Sandler HM, et al. Phase III randomized study of radiotherapy plus procarbazine, lomustine, and vincristine with or without BUdR for treatment of anaplastic astrocytoma: final report of RTOG 9404. *Int J Radiat Oncol Biol Phys.* 2004;58(4):1147–1152.
39. Levin VA, Hess KR, Choucair A, et al. Phase III randomized study of postradiotherapy chemotherapy with combination alpha-difluoromethylornithine-PCV versus PCV for anaplastic gliomas. *Clin Cancer Res.* 2003;9(3):981–990.
40. Bauman GS, Sneed PK, Wara WM, et al. Reirradiation of primary CNS tumors. *Int J Radiat Oncol Biol Phys.* 1996;36(2):433–441.
41. Kim HK, Thornton AF, Greenberg HS, Page MA, Junck L, Sandler HM. Results of re-irradiation of primary intracranial neoplasms with three-dimensional conformal therapy. *Am J Clin Oncol.* 1997;20(4):358–363.
42. Voynov G, Kaufman S, Hong T, Pinkerton A, Simon R, Dowsett R. Treatment of recurrent malignant gliomas with stereotactic intensity modulated radiation therapy. *Am J Clin Oncol.* 2002;25(6):606–611.
43. Sneed PK, McDermott MW, Gutin PH. Interstitial brachytherapy procedures for brain tumors. *Semin Surg Oncol.* 1997;13(3):157–166.
44. Gabayan AJ, Green SB, Sanan A, et al. GliaSite brachytherapy for treatment of recurrent malignant gliomas: a retrospective multi-institutional analysis. *Neurosurgery.* 2006;58(4):701–709; discussion 701.
45. Tatter SB, Shaw EG, Rosenblum ML, et al.; New Approaches to Brain Tumor Therapy Central Nervous System Consortium. An inflatable balloon catheter and liquid 125I radiation source (GliaSite Radiation Therapy System) for treatment of recurrent malignant glioma: multicenter safety and feasibility trial. *J Neurosurg.* 2003;99(2):297–303.
46. Sanghavi S, Skrupsky R, Badie B, Robins HI, Tome WA, Mehta M. Recurrent malignant gliomas treated witih radiosurgery. *J Radiosurgery.* 1999;2:119–125.
47. Cho KH, Hall WA, Gerbi BJ, Higgins PD, McGuire WA, Clark HB. Single dose versus fractionated stereotactic radiotherapy for recurrent high-grade gliomas. *Int J Radiat Oncol Biol Phys.* 1999;45(5):1133–1141.
48. Kondziolka D, Flickinger JC, Bissonette DJ, Bozik M, Lunsford LD. Survival benefit of stereotactic radiosurgery for patients with malignant glial neoplasms. *Neurosurgery.* 1997;41(4):776–783; discussion 783.
49. Vordermark D, Kölbl O, Ruprecht K, Vince GH, Bratengeier K, Flentje M. Hypofractionated stereotactic re-irradiation: treatment option in recurrent malignant glioma. *BMC Cancer.* 2005;5:55.
50. Shepherd SF, Laing RW, Cosgrove VP, et al. Hypofractionated stereotactic radiotherapy in the management of recurrent glioma. *Int J Radiat Oncol Biol Phys.* 1997;37(2):393–398.
51. Combs SE, Thilmann C, Edler L, Debus J, Schulz-Ertner D. Efficacy of fractionated stereotactic reirradiation in recurrent gliomas: long-term results in 172 patients treated in a single institution. *J Clin Oncol.* 2005;23(34):8863–8869.

84 Low-Grade Glioma Radiation Therapy

Nadia N. Issa Laack and Paul D. Brown

INTRODUCTION

Low-grade gliomas (LGGs) are a diverse group of rare central nervous system tumors that occur primarily in children and young adults. Prognosis varies widely and depends largely on age at presentation and pathological type. Treatment of LGG is one of the most controversial topics in neuro-oncology. This controversy is due in part to the variability in natural history and the potential toxicities of treatment. The extent of surgery, timing of radiotherapy, and role of chemotherapy are hotly debated. In this chapter we will summarize the natural history and controversies between different treatment strategies for patients with LGG.

Approximately 2000 new cases of LGG are diagnosed in the United States each year [1,2]. Median age at diagnosis is 37 years. LGG tend to occur in the hemispheres of young adults and in brainstem of young children (<18) [3].

Median age at diagnosis for pilocytic astrocytoma is 14 years. Pilocytic astrocytomas typically arise within the visual system, hypothalamus, 3rd ventricle, cerebellum, and rarely cerebral hemispheres [4,5–7].

Etiological factors for LGGs are largely unknown. Low-grade astrocytomas have been associated with neurofibromatosis type 1 and 2 [8,9]. Tuberous sclerosis has also been linked more directly to the development of subependymal giant cell astrocytoma, an uncommon pathological type of low-grade astrocytoma [9–13].

The most common molecular genetic alterations present in LGG are seen at the p arm of chromosome 17, which is where the tumor suppressor gene *TP53* resides, and loss of heterozygosity (LOH) of chromosomes 1p and 19q. Interestingly, they are mutually exclusive with only rare cases showing coexistence of both mutations [14]. Low-grade astrocytomas are associated with alterations in TP53 or its protein, p53, which is seen in 50% to 88% of fibrillary or gemistocytic astrocytomas [15]. In contrast, LOH 1p/19p is the most frequent abnormality in oligodendrogliomas (55–81%), and rare in astrocytomas (<10%) [16]. Mixed tumors have intermediate incidence of TP53 mutations [15] or LOH 1p/19q [16].

PATHOLOGY

The most commonly accepted classification system is the World Health Organization (WHO) classification of primary central nervous system tumors as it applies to LGGs [17]. Table 84.1 lists the WHO classification for neuroepithelial tumors [17]. LGGs can be classified broadly into three groups: oligodendrogliomas, oligoastrocytomas, and astrocytic tumors. Astrocytic tumors can be further classified into diffuse, pilocytic, and a few rare variants. The diffusely infiltrative low-grade astrocytomas are the most common (70%) and include the fibrillary, protoplasmic, and gemistocytic types [18]. These tumors expand and distort brain architecture, and tumor cells are often seen several centimeters away from the bulk of the tumor [19]. Because of this infiltration, diffuse astrocytomas are usually poorly circumscribed. Diffuse astrocytomas are associated with a more unfavorable natural history as nearly 80% of diffuse astrocytomas will eventually undergo malignant transformation [20].

The pilocytic astrocytomas (WHO grade I) comprise nearly all the remainder of the cerebral astrocytomas. Pleomorphic xanthoastrocytomas (WHO grade II) [21,22], subependymal giant cell astrocytomas (WHO grade I) [11,12], and pilomyxoid astrocytomas (WHO grade II) are rare variants that comprise the remaining astrocytomas [17].

Oligodendrogliomas form a distinct class that ontologically arises from the O2A progenitor cells in the white matter. These pluripotent cells can differentiate into either type II (fibrillary) astrocytomas or oligodendrogliomas. Among diffuse LGGs, pure oligodendroglioma and astrocytoma are relatively easy to define and diagnose. The diagnosis of oligoastrocytoma is more problematic and less reproducible [17,23–25]. Nevertheless, histological classification is of paramount importance in determining prognosis. Median survival for pure oligodendroglioma is 9.5 years, mixed oligoastrocytomas 8.2 years, and only 5.1 years for pure astrocytomas (Table 84.2) [26].

Grade is also an important pathological prognostic factor in LGG. The most widely used and accepted grading system today is the WHO (see Table 84.1) [17], which is based on classic morphological criteria.

PROGNOSTIC FACTORS

Clinical Prognostic Factors

Several clinical variables contribute significantly to outcome in LGG. The most important clinical variables with prognostic significance for poor overall survival (OS) are the following: age (>40 years), tumor diameter (≥6 cm), tumor crossing midline, neurological deficit, and astrocytic histology [25].

Advancing age is most consistently confirmed as a poor prognostic factor [23,27,28]. For example, studies in pediatric LGG document a low incidence of malignant transformation, typically around 10%, even for diffuse grade II astrocytomas [29]. This is in stark contrast to adult tumors in which as many as 50% to 90% are expected to transform [30,31]. Although clearly a biological difference between tumors acquired in childhood relative to adults exists, there is likely a continuum in the biological behavior rather than a sharp age cut-off, which is consistent with the improved clinical outcomes for younger adult patients.

Increasing tumor size is generally accepted as a marker of poor prognosis [23,27,28,32–35]. Larger tumors are less likely to be operable [25,26] and may be at an increased risk of malignant transformation [36], both of which contribute to the poor survival in these patients.

Contrast enhancement has been proposed as a possible prognostic factor. As a greater percentage of high-grade gliomas display contrast enhancement than LGGs, the presence of enhancement might indicate a focus of histologically under-sampled anaplasia in a tumor with a LGG component. Although a large retrospective study suggested that enhancement was an unfavorable prognostic factor [26,28], prospective studies have not confirmed this [23,37].

Seizures, especially in the absence of other neurological symptoms, are associated with a better prognosis in patients with LGG [3,31,38]. Seizures are more common in younger patients, those with good performance status, and with slowly growing tumors so the prognostic effect diminishes somewhat (although still significant) on multivariate analysis [39,40].

Molecular Prognostic Factors

Although alterations in p53 are felt to be important in tumorigenesis, it is also believed that the loss of p53 function in low-grade astrocytomas could be a predisposing factor for the accumulation of genetic damage leading to the progression of low-grade astrocytoma to glioblastoma [41]. Positive TP53 mutation, mutant p53 protein, and the inactivation of wild-type p53 protein have been found to be an independent unfavorable predictor of survival, progression-free survival (PFS), and time to malignant transformation [42–44]. Allelic loss on the p arm of chromosome 19 is seen more often in patients with high-grade than LGGs and may also harbor a tumor suppressor gene important in the malignant transformation of low-grade to high-grade astrocytomas [45].

Oligodendrogliomas are distinctive for characteristic chromosomal translocations resulting in LOH of chromosome 1p/19q. Up to 80% of oligodendrogliomas show concurrent deletion of chromosomal arms 1p and 19q [16,46,47]. LOH of chromosome 1p and 19q is associated with superior prognosis [48]. In one study, patients with LOH 1p/19q had a median survival of 11.9 years compared to 8.1 years for those without it [49]. Oligoastrocytomas appear to be genetically heterogeneous with two fundamental genetic subsets, one genetically related to oligodendrogliomas and the other to astrocytomas [50,51]. Oligoastrocytomas show either the characteristic combined loss of 1p/19q seen in oligodendrogliomas or TP53 mutations. Prognosis in mixed histology cases mirrors the genetic alterations. Patients with chromosome 1p/19q deletions have a more favorable prognosis and natural history approximating oligodendrogliomas; whereas tumors without LOH 1p/19q tend to behave more similar to astrocytomas [51].

O^6–methylguanine–DNA methyltransferase (MGMT) is a DNA-repair enzyme that removes alkyl groups from the O^6 position of guanine in DNA and therefore repairs damage induced by alkylating agents (e.g., BCNU, temozolomide). Promoter methylation results in epigenetic silencing and thereby decreased MGMT expression which is associated with longer survival in patients with glioblastoma who receive alkylating agents [52]. Recent data suggest MGMT may have a similar role in LGG.

Table 84.1 WHO Classification and Grading of Low-Grade Gliomas

	WHO Grade
Astrocytic tumors	
Subependymal giant cell astrocytoma	I
Pilocytic astrocytoma	I
Pilomyxoid astrocytoma	II
Diffuse astrocytoma	II
Pleomorphic xanthoastrocytoma	II
Oligodendroglial tumors	
Oligodendroglioma	II
Oligoastrocytic tumors	
Oligoastrocytoma	II

Data from Louis et al [17].

Table 84.2 Survival of Supratentorial Gliomas, Mayo Clinic Experience

	Histologic Type			
Survival	Pilocytic	Oligodendroglioma	Oligoastrocytoma	Astrocytoma
Median (years)	–	9.5	8.2	5.1
5 years (%)	95	70	69	51
10 years (%)	79	45	44	30
15 years (%)	79	41	25	18
20 years (%)	75	25	18	11

Data from Brown et al [7], Shaw et al [18], Schomas et al [26], and Stüer et al [107].

Oligodendrogliomas are considered to be the most chemosensitive of the LGG and have been reported to have higher rates of MGMT promoter silencing and decreased MGMT expression [53–56]. Evidence is also accumulating for a link between LOH 1p/19q and MGMT promoter hypermethylation. Several studies suggest that approximately 85% of 1p/19q-deleted oligodendrogliomas have MGMT promoter hypermethylation [54–56], and oligodendrogliomas with the highest levels of MGMT expression are generally 1p-intact [57,58]. MGMT promoter hypermethylation is also seen in 30% to 50% of low-grade astrocytomas, yet less than 10% of astrocytomas are 1p/19q deleted [59]. Further study is necessary to elucidate other potential mechanisms of MGMT promoter silencing in LGG.

As understanding of the molecular and cellular biological characterization of LGG increases, it is expected we will better predict which patients are more likely to require earlier and more aggressive therapy and which patients may be observed initially, withholding treatment until the time of disease progression.

RADIOLOGICAL FEATURES

On computed tomography (CT), the typical low-grade astrocytoma is lobar in location, involves the frontal or temporal lobes, is larger than 5 cm in diameter, and is nonenhancing or minimally enhancing with the administration of intravenous contrast material. Because of the infiltrative nature of low-grade astrocytomas, the CT appearance of a typical nonenhancing tumor is a poorly defined area of low attenuation (Figure 84.1).

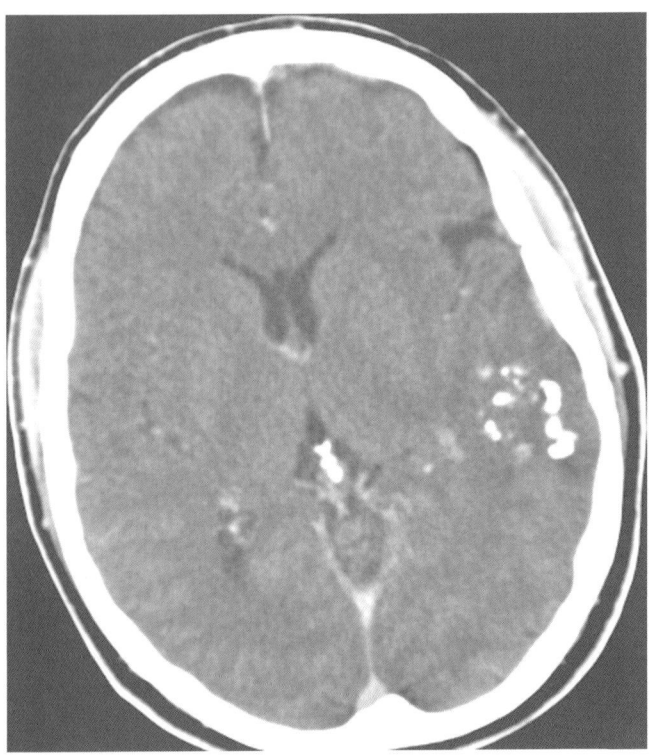

Figure 84.1 CT of left temporal lobe grade II oligodendroglioma with calcifications

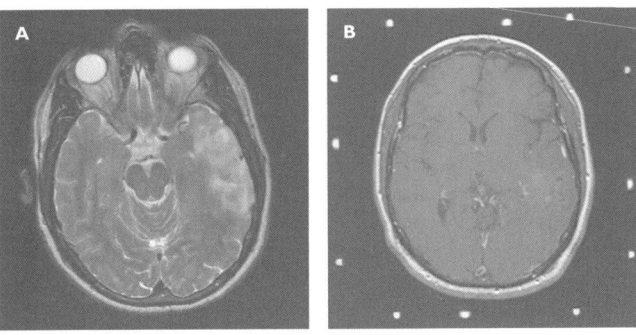

Figure 84.2 **(A)** T2 fat-suppressed MR images of left temporal lobe grade II oligodendroglioma. **(B)** T1 with gadolinium MR images of left temporal lobe grade II oligodendroglioma

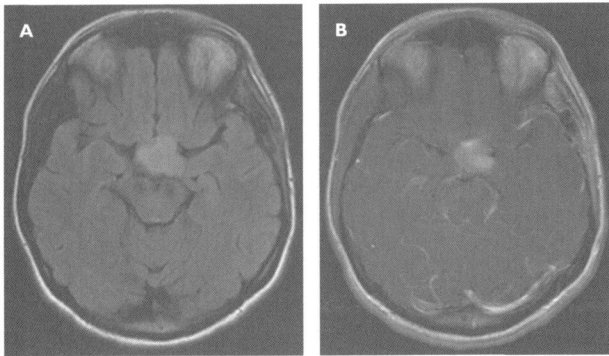

Figure 84.3 **(A)** T2 FLAIR MR images of juvenile pilocytic astrocytoma. **(B)** T1 with gadolinium MR images of juvenile pilocytic astrocytoma

Magnetic resonance imaging (MRI) (Figure 84.2) is the diagnostic imaging method of choice for LGG. Both T2- and T1-weighted images (without and with contrast) provide anatomical detail that is useful in defining the extent of the tumor and for surgical and radiation therapy (RT) treatment planning. Generally, the MRI scan defines a larger area of increased signal on T2-weighted images for diffuse LGG in comparison with CT. In addition, histological studies have found microscopic tumor cells extending several centimeters beyond the MRI-defined abnormality. Although most LGG do not enhance, approximately one-third of diffuse LGG show gadolinium enhancement on MRI. Enhancing areas on MRI are more solid on histological examination, whereas the areas of T2 hyperintensity correspond to regions of intact brain parenchyma infiltrated by tumor cells [19].

Pilocytic astrocytomas have a distinctive imaging pattern. MRI scan appearance is that of a well-circumscribed area of contrast enhancement in the absence of surrounding low-attenuation change or edema (Figure 84.3). This is consistent with the pathological finding of an extremely vascular, but well-demarcated solid tumor embedded in normal surrounding brain parenchyma [19,60].

CLINICAL PRESENTATION

The most common presenting symptom for patients with LGG is seizure, occurring in 65% of patients. Focal seizures are more common than generalized ones [61]. Headache and weakness occur in approximately one-third of patients. The median duration from onset of symptoms to diagnosis is between 6 and 17 months, with a range of 1 day to 17 years. About one-half of patients with LGG have a normal neurological examination. The most common presenting sign is sensory or motor deficit occurring in 42% of patients [26,27,61].

TREATMENT OPTIONS

Observation

The combination of relatively favorable natural history of the disease, the lack of proven benefit for invasive interventions such as surgical resection or RT, and the potential morbidities of treatment have lead some neuro-oncologists to favor observation as initial management for patients with LGG [34,62–65]. Despite the relatively favorable survival observed in certain subsets of patients with LGG, the natural history of all pathological types of supratentorial LGGs is significantly worse than that of an age- and sex-matched control population, for which the expected long-term survival is greater than 95% (Figure 84.4) [66,67]. On the basis of this observation, some have argued that all such patients should undergo maximally safe surgical resection followed by postoperative radiotherapy [68], although a survival benefit for treatment, either with aggressive surgery or RT, even though suggested by the retrospective literature [26,69], has not been demonstrated in prospective clinical trials.

The Radiation Therapy Oncology Group (RTOG) phase II observation portion of protocol 9802 prospectively observed 111 "low-risk" (defined as age <40 years and gross total resection [GTR]) LGG patients [37]. The 2- and 5-year PFS rates were 93% and 78% for oligodendrogliomas (or oligo-dominant mixed oligoastrocytomas) less than 4 cm compared to 67% and 34% for diffuse astrocytomas (or astro-dominant mixed oligoastrocytomas) 4 cm or greater. Even in this "low-risk" group of patients, nearly 60% of astrocytomas greater than 4 cm progressed within 3 years from GTR [70]. These data suggest observation is a reasonable strategy for some subsets of younger patients after a GTR of a LGG, but postoperative adjuvant treatment should still be considered for some "low-risk" patients (i.e., large, diffuse astrocytomas).

Observation (or "late" radiotherapy, delayed until the time of progression) was also assessed by the European Organization for Research and Treatment of Cancer (EORTC). In a Phase III randomized trial (EORTC 22845), 311 adults with supratentorial LGGs of all histological types (excluding pilocytic astrocytomas) were randomized to either observation with radiotherapy at progression or initial RT using 54 Gy to localized treatment fields [71,72]. With follow-up just over 7 years, postoperative RT significantly prolonged PFS (median 5.4 vs 3.7 years) without affecting OS (median 7.4 vs 7.2 years) [25,71–73]. These data suggest that observation is a reasonable strategy in adults with asymptomatic supratentorial LGG.

Surgery

As the morbidity of stereotactic biopsy has improved, pathological confirmation is nearly always recommended for suspected LGG to establish tissue diagnosis for prognostic and treatment purposes. With molecular markers available to guide treatment decisions, histological confirmation and examination has become more important.

Table 84.3 Prospective Neurocognitive Trials (with Baseline Testing) of Low-Grade Neoplasms

Author	Histology (Number Receiving RT)	Radiation Total Dose/ Fraction Size (Gray)	Mean Follow-up (year)	Extensive Neurocognitive Assessment at Each Evaluation	Neurotoxicity After RT
Glosser et al [108]	Chordoma, chondrosarcoma (17)	Proton RT median 68.4 CGE/1.8 CGE	4	Yes	No; mild decline in psychomotor speed with high doses
Vigliani et al [94]	LGG, AA (17)	Focal RT 54/1.8	4	Yes	No; transient decline in RcT
Armstrong et al [93]	LGG, pituitary, pineal, meningioma (26)	Focal RT Mean 54.6/1.8–2.0	3	Yes	No; mild decline in visual memory after 5 years
Brown [24]	LGG (203)	Focal RT 50.4/1.8 or 64.8/1.8	7.4 (median)	No (MMSE and NFS)	5.3% with MMSE decline at 5 years
Torres et al [95]	Meningioma, LGG, GBM, ependymoma, adenoma (15)	Focal RT Mean 54/1.8	2	Yes	No; decline in memory and attention only if tumor progression
Laack et al [37]	LGG (20)	Focal RT 50.4/28 or 64.8/33	3	Yes	No; mild decline in 64.8 Gy arm in immediate verbal memory, learning, and spatial problem solving

Abbreviations: AA, anaplastic astrocytoma; GBM, glioblastoma multiforme; LGG, low-grade glioma; MMSE, Folstein Mini-Mental State Examination; NFS, neurologic function scores; RT, radiotherapy.

With permission from Gunderson LL, Tepper JE, eds. Clinical Radiation Oncology, 2nd edn. Philadelphia: Elsevier Churchill Livingstone; 2006:509.

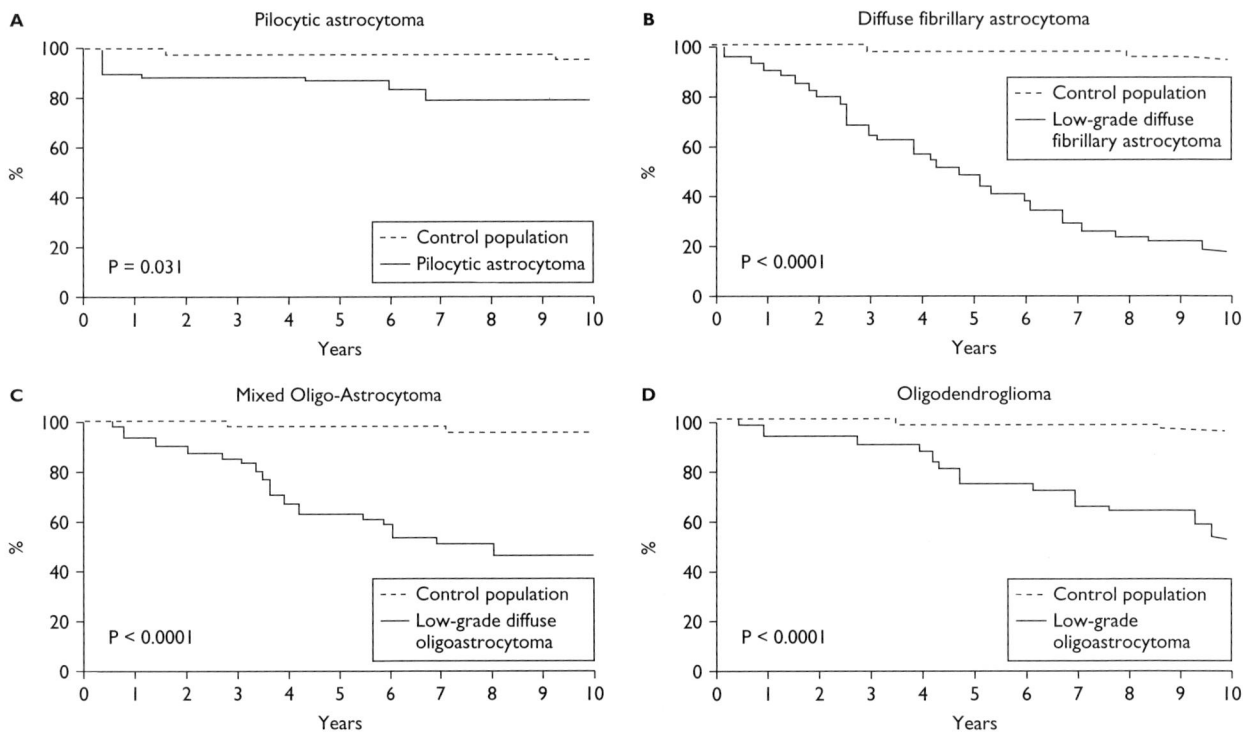

Figure 84.4 Survival curves for patients with the various subtypes of low-grade glioma compared with curves for an age- and sex-matched control population. (A) pilocytic astrocytoma. (B) diffuse fibrillary astrocytoma. (C) mixed oligo-astrocytoma. (D) oligodendroglioma. With permission from Gunderson LL, Tepper JE, eds. Clinical Radiation Oncology, 2nd edn. Philadelphia: Elsevier Churchill Livingstone; 2006:500.

The primary controversy currently in regards to surgery is the extent of resection that should be attempted in patients who may be relatively asymptomatic from their disease. There are no randomized trials that have specifically compared "up-front" surgery with a more conservative approach of delaying surgery. Although not randomized, two prospective studies did show a correlation with aggressive surgery (GTR or near GTR) and improved prognosis [23,35]. Additionally, a report from Brigham and Women's Hospital utilizing intraoperative MRI found that patients undergoing STR experienced 1.4 and 4.9 times the risk of recurrence and death, respectively, compared to GTR [74]. Another recent account from University of California, San Francisco outlined the use of MRI volumetric analysis to assess extent of resection and correlated extent of resection of ≥90% with improved OS and PFS outcomes [75]. It is expected, however, that surgery will more often be possible in patients with smaller, more peripheral tumors, and as such may not be an independent prognostic factor.

Most retrospective surgical series show a significant improvement in PFS and often OS in patients who are able to undergo more extensive surgical resection [26,27,32,38,39,69,76–84]. For example, in a recent Mayo Clinic series with long-term follow-up (13.2 years), patients who underwent GTR or near-total resection had a 10-year OS of 57%, compared to only 30% in patients undergoing less aggressive surgery [26]. However, GTR is often not possible without significant risk of neurological injury due to location or the infiltrative nature of tumor. As expected, the Mayo Clinic series confirmed that aggressive surgeries were more likely to have occurred in patients with more favorable tumor characteristics, such as size <5 cm, lack of enhancement on CT scan, and lack of sensory-motor symptoms [26]. It is suspected that the improved outcomes with more aggressive surgery is at least in part accounted for by the more favorable tumor characteristics at presentation. However, postoperative tumor size has also been shown to be independently predictive, suggesting a role for more aggressive surgery [27,70].

Therefore, controversy remains regarding the role of surgery in the initial management of patients. Nonetheless, due to the overall weight of both retrospective and prospective data, many neurosurgeons currently favor a maximally safe resection as a reasonable initial approach [23,25,35,74,75,85–88].

Radiotherapy

Timing of radiotherapy continues to be an area of intense debate for patients with LGG. Although the previously reviewed, prospective, randomized trial, EORTC 22845, addressed this question and demonstrated a PFS but not an OS benefit for early radiotherapy [72,73], the effect of the benefit in PFS in unknown since this study did not include detailed quality of life and neurocognitive measures, and therefore the question of radiotherapy timing cannot be definitively answered. In contrast to the findings of the EORTC, recent results from a large series (314 patients) of LGG patients with long-term follow-up (median 13.2 years) at the Mayo Clinic suggest that an OS benefit may exist for adjuvant radiotherapy, especially in patients with subtotal or minimal resection. Ten-year OS for patients with biopsy or subtotal resection followed by immediate radiotherapy was 34%, compared to only 11% for subtotal resection or biopsy alone. OS at 10 years for patients undergoing aggressive surgical resection with or without adjuvant radiotherapy was 57%. The difference in findings between the Mayo Clinic study and the prospective EORTC trial may be due to the large number of patients with aggressive (>90% GTR) surgical resection in the EORTC trial (44% compared to only 23% in the Mayo Clinic series), which resulted in a higher risk population in the Mayo series. Presumably these patients were more likely to benefit from early radiotherapy. These results are retrospective and need confirmation in prospective trials; however, these data suggest that although delayed radiotherapy is a reasonable strategy in adults with asymptomatic supratentorial LGG, especially with GTR, patients with more limited resection may benefit from early radiotherapy.

Besides delaying the time to tumor recurrence, radiation has several other potential beneficial effects such as symptom control in up to 80% of cases [89]. For example, 19 of 25 patients with medically intractable epilepsy due to LGG who were treated with RT achieved a significant reduction (>50% decrease) in seizure frequency [90]. In EORTC 22845, there were no differences in seizure frequency at baseline, but by 1 year there were significantly more seizures in the observation group (41%) than the irradiated group (25%) [71].

Radiotherapy dose has also been studied in two prospective randomized clinical trials. In one trial 50.4 Gy was compared with 64.8 Gy [23] and the other trial [35] compared 45 Gy and 59.4 Gy. Neither studies found differences in PFS or OS between the different dose arms but did find increased toxicity with higher doses. Therefore, total radiation doses of 45 to 54 Gy utilizing local fields are considered standard for LGGs.

Because of its proven benefits, radiotherapy is an accepted, widely utilized modality in the treatment of LGG. However, much of the controversy surrounding the use of radiotherapy stems over concerns over long-term toxicity of radiotherapy. Primary late effects that have been documented after radiotherapy include radiation necrosis, endocrinopathies, and neurocognitive dysfunction. Radiation necrosis is relatively rare, occurring in approximately 2% of patients with moderate dose focal radiotherapy [23]. Symptoms depend on the location of the necrosis within the brain. Diagnosis often requires surgical intervention as imaging of necrosis cannot easily be discriminated from recurrent tumor [91]. Treatment is usually conservative with a slow oral steroid taper for patients who are symptomatic. Occasionally, aggressive surgical resection is necessary to terminate the progression of the necrosis [92].

Because several retrospective studies have found increased neurocognitive deficits after cranial radiotherapy, the possible deleterious effects of radiotherapy on cognitive function are of great concern. However, the majority of these studies are flawed by issues such as outdated techniques (e.g., whole brain radiotherapy), large radiation fraction sizes (>2 Gy), difficulty of controlling for other variables known to influence cognitive performance such as tumor progression, surgery, chemotherapy, or anti-epileptics [24], and most importantly, lack of baseline neurocognitive testing since the brain tumor itself is often the primary cause of cognitive difficulties [92]. When prospective studies with extensive neuropsychological testing (up to 6 years after radiotherapy) along with baseline evaluation have been conducted, significant neurocognitive deterioration has *not* been found when compared to either baseline [37,93] or to a cohort of patients with low-grade brain neoplasms not treated with radiotherapy [94,95]. Another large LGG cohort study found that although LGG patients performed worse on neurocognitive tests than controls, the tumor itself, antiepileptic drugs, and radiation fractions >200 cGy were felt to be the primary cause of any detectable neurocognitive deficit [96,97]. Table 84.3 summarizes the prospective neurocognitive studies with baseline evaluations in patients with low-grade brain tumors. Overall, the weight of evidence suggests a low incidence of neurocognitive difficulties after focal, conventionally fractionated (1.8–2 Gy) radiotherapy using modern techniques to deliver moderate dose (45–54 Gy) in adults. For most patients, and especially patients with higher-risk features, radiotherapy's beneficial effect upon the primary cause of cognitive deficits, the tumor, outweighs potential detrimental cognitive effects [24,37].

Chemotherapy in Combination with Radiotherapy

Chemotherapy has emerged as an important treatment modality in LGG over the past decade. Initial investigations drew upon success with the combination of procarbazine, CCNU, and vincristine (PCV) in anaplastic oligodendrogliomas and focused upon low-grade oligodendrogliomas and oligoastrocytomas [24,98–100]. Because of these preliminary data, the RTOG conducted a phase III, randomized trial (RTOG 9802) comparing RT alone to PCV and RT in high-risk LGG. PCV was poorly tolerated and no improvement in PFS or OS was documented [49]. PCV continues to find utility in the recurrent setting.

Recently, attention has shifted to the oral alkylating agent temozolomide (TMZ), which has a superior tolerability profile to PCV. Several studies have demonstrated that TMZ produces objective shrinkage in 31% to 62% of LGGs [57,58,101–105]. The median duration of tumor response or stabilization ranges from 10 to 31 months for recurrent LGGs and may exceed 3 years in patients previously untreated with radiotherapy [104]. Several small studies suggest that favorable responses are not limited to tumors with oligodendroglial components, although two studies suggest oligodendroglial tumors with 1p deletion are more likely to shrink with TMZ than 1p-intact tumors [57,58]. Maximum tumor shrinkage may take 12 to 15 months [58,104]. Currently the RTOG is examining the combination of radiotherapy and TMZ in high-risk LGG patients. The EORTC is conducting a phase III trial comparing 12 cycles of TMZ to RT for LGG patients >40 years of age with either symptomatic disease or radiological evidence of progression.

RECURRENT DISEASE

LGG typically recur within 2 cm of the original tumor [23,69]. Leptomeningeal failure also has been rarely reported. In one pediatric series of intracranial LGGs, the incidence of leptomeningeal failure was 4% [106].

Treatment options for tumor recurrence include surgery, external beam radiation, brachytherapy, radiosurgery, intraoperative electron radiation, and chemotherapy depending on the treatment modality used at diagnosis and the location of the recurrence.

In general, survival after tumor recurrence is poor. Between 50% and 90% of tumors will undergo malignant transformation. Patients whose disease progressed after treatment with surgery and postoperative RT have a median survival time of approximately 1 year [26,38]. Longer median survival is seen in patients who recur without malignant transformation (median 16–60 months) [27,107,108].

CONCLUSIONS

LGGs are a heterogenous group of central nervous system neoplasms, whose natural history depends primarily on pathological type and patient age. Despite historically being considered "benign," most of these tumors behave in an aggressive manner, and are the primary cause of death in this otherwise young cohort of patients. Radiotherapy has proven benefit in improving PFS and symptom control. The effects of radiotherapy on quality of life and neurocognitive outcomes are the focus of ongoing studies. The role of chemotherapy remains to be determined. Translational research, including studies of proliferation, cytogenetics, and molecular genetics, will provide much needed insight for the next generation of biologically based therapies.

REFERENCES

1. Levin VA, Gutin PH, Leibel S. Neoplasms of the central nervous system. In: DeVita V, Hellman J, Rosenberg S, eds. *Cancer: Principles and Practice of Oncology*. Philadelphia: JB Lippincott; 1993.
2. Okazaki H. Neoplastic and related lesions. In: Okazaki H, ed. *Fundamentals of Neuropathology*. New York, NY: Igaku-Shoin; 1983.
3. Laws ER Jr, Taylor WF, Clifton MB, Okazaki H. Neurosurgical management of low-grade astrocytoma of the cerebral hemispheres. *J Neurosurg*. 1984;61(4):665–673.
4. Hayostek CJ, Shaw EG, Scheithauer B, et al. Astrocytomas of the cerebellum. A comparative clinicopathologic study of pilocytic and diffuse astrocytomas. *Cancer*. 1993;72(3):856–869.
5. Forsyth PA, Shaw EG, Scheithauer BW, O'Fallon JR, Layton DD Jr, Katzmann JA. Supratentorial pilocytic astrocytomas. A clinicopathologic, prognostic, and flow cytometric study of 51 patients. *Cancer*. 1993;72(4):1335–1342.
6. Garcia DM, Fulling KH. Juvenile pilocytic astrocytoma of the cerebrum in adults. A distinctive neoplasm with favorable prognosis. *J Neurosurg*. 1985;63(3):382–386.
7. Brown PD, Buckner JC, O'Fallon JR, et al. Adult patients with supratentorial pilocytic astrocytomas: a prospective multicenter clinical trial. *Int J Radiat Oncol Biol Phys*. 2004;58(4):1153–1160.
8. Blatt J, Jaffe R, Deutsch M, Adkins JC. Neurofibromatosis and childhood tumors. *Cancer*. 1986;57(6):1225–1229.
9. Kleihues P, Ohgaki H. Genetics of glioma progression and the definition of primary and secondary glioblastoma. *Brain Pathol*. 1997;7:1131.
10. Cooper JR. Brain tumors in hereditary multiple system hamartomatosis (tuberous sclerosis). *J Neurosurg*. 1971;34(2 pt 1):194–202.
11. Kapp JP, Paulson GW, Odom GL. Brain tumors with tuberous sclerosis. *J Neurosurg*. 1967;26(2):191–202.
12. Chow CW, Klug GL, Lewis EA. Subependymal giant-cell astrocytoma in children. An unusual discrepancy between histological and clinical features. *J Neurosurg*. 1988;68(6):880–883.
13. Shepherd CW, Scheithauer BW, Gomez MR, Altermatt HJ, Katzmann JA. Subependymal giant cell astrocytoma: a clinical, pathological, and flow cytometric study. *Neurosurgery*. 1991;28(6):864–868.
14. Ohgaki H, Kleihues P. Population-based studies on incidence, survival rates, and genetic alterations in astrocytic and oligodendroglial gliomas. *J Neuropathol Exp Neurol*. 2005;64(6):479–489.
15. Kitange GJ, Templeton KL, Jenkins RB. Recent advances in the molecular genetics of primary gliomas. *Curr Opin Oncol*. 2003;15(3):197–203.
16. Jenkins RB, Blair H, Ballman KV, et al. A t(1;19)(q10;p10) mediates the combined deletions of 1p and 19q and predicts a better prognosis of patients with oligodendroglioma. *Cancer Res*. 2006;66(20):9852–9861.
17. Louis DN, Ohgaki H, Wiestler OD, et al. The 2007 WHO classification of tumours of the central nervous system. *Acta Neuropathol*. 2007;114(2):97–109.
18. Shaw EG, Scheithauer BW, O'Fallon JR. Supratentorial gliomas: a comparative study by grade and histologic type. *J Neurooncol*. 1997;31(3):273–278.
19. Kelly PJ, Daumas-Duport C, Scheithauer BW, Kall BA, Kispert DB. Stereotactic histologic correlations of computed tomography- and magnetic resonance imaging-defined abnormalities in patients with glial neoplasms. *Mayo Clin Proc*. 1987;62(6):450–459.
20. Soffietti R, Chiò A, Giordana MT, Vasario E, Schiffer D. Prognostic factors in well-differentiated cerebral astrocytomas in the adult. *Neurosurgery*. 1989;24(5):686–692.
21. Heyerdahl Strøm E, Skullerud K. Pleomorphic xanthoastrocytoma: report of 5 cases. *Clin Neuropathol*. 1983;2(4):188–191.
22. Whittle IR, Gordon A, Misra BK, Shaw JF, Steers AJ. Pleomorphic xanthoastrocytoma. Report of four cases. *J Neurosurg*. 1989;70(3):463–468.
23. Shaw E, Arusell R, Scheithauer B, et al. Prospective randomized trial of low- versus high-dose radiation therapy in adults with supratentorial low-grade glioma: initial report of a North Central Cancer Treatment Group/Radiation Therapy Oncology Group/Eastern Cooperative Oncology Group study. *J Clin Oncol*. 2002;20(9):2267–2276.
24. Buckner JC, Gesme D Jr, O'Fallon JR, et al. Phase II trial of procarbazine, lomustine, and vincristine as initial therapy for patients with low-grade oligodendroglioma or oligoastrocytoma: efficacy and associations with chromosomal abnormalities. *J Clin Oncol*. 2003;21(2):251–255.
25. Pignatti F, van den Bent M, Curran D, et al. Prognostic factors for survival in adult patients with cerebral low-grade glioma. *J Clin Oncol*. 2002;20(8):2076–2084.
26. Schomas DA, Laack NN, Rao RD, et al. Intracranial low-grade gliomas in adults: 30-year experience with long-term follow-up at Mayo Clinic. *Neuro-Oncology* 2009;11:437–445.
27. Leighton C, Fisher B, Bauman G, et al. Supratentorial low-grade glioma in adults: an analysis of prognostic factors and timing of radiation. *J Clin Oncol*. 1997;15(4):1294–1301.
28. Lote K, Stenwig AE, Skullerud K, Hirschberg H. Prevalence and prognostic significance of epilepsy in patients with gliomas. *Eur J Cancer*. 1998;34(1):98–102.
29. Broniscer A, Baker SJ, West AN, et al. Clinical and molecular characteristics of malignant transformation of low-grade glioma in children. *J Clin Oncol*. 2007;25(6):682–689.
30. Vertosick FT Jr, Selker RG, Arena VC. Survival of patients with well-differentiated astrocytomas diagnosed in the era of computed tomography. *Neurosurgery*. 1991;28(4):496–501.
31. McCormack BM, Miller DC, Budzilovich GN, Voorhees GJ, Ransohoff J. Treatment and survival of low-grade astrocytoma in adults--1977–1988. *Neurosurgery*. 1992;31:636–42; discussion 42.
32. Shibamoto Y, Kitakabu Y, Takahashi M, et al. Supratentorial low-grade astrocytoma. Correlation of computed tomography findings with effect of radiation therapy and prognostic variables. *Cancer*. 1993;72(1):190–195.
33. Miralbell R, Balart J, Matias-Guiu X, Molet J, Ariza A, Craven-Bartle J. Radiotherapy for supratentorial low-grade gliomas: results and prognostic factors with special focus on tumour volume parameters. *Radiother Oncol*. 1993;27(2):112–116.
34. Recht LD, Lew R, Smith TW. Suspected low-grade glioma: is deferring treatment safe? *Ann Neurol*. 1992;31(4):431–436.
35. Karim AB, Maat B, Hatlevoll R, et al. A randomized trial on dose-response in radiation therapy of low-grade cerebral glioma: European Organization for Research and Treatment of Cancer (EORTC) Study 22844. *Int J Radiat Oncol Biol Phys*. 1996;36(3):549–556.

36. Berger MS, Deliganis AV, Dobbins J, Keles GE. The effect of extent of resection on recurrence in patients with low grade cerebral hemisphere gliomas. *Cancer.* 1994;74(6):1784–1791.
37. Laack NN, Brown PD, Ivnik RJ, et al. Cognitive function after radiotherapy for supratentorial low-grade glioma: a North Central Cancer Treatment Group prospective study. *Int J Radiat Oncol Biol Phys.* 2005;63(4):1175–1183.
38. North CA, North RB, Epstein JA, Piantadosi S, Wharam MD. Low-grade cerebral astrocytomas. Survival and quality of life after radiation therapy. *Cancer.* 1990;66(1):6–14.
39. Reichenthal E, Feldman Z, Cohen ML, Loven D, Zucker G. Hemispheric supratentorial low-grade astrocytoma. *Neurochirurgia (Stuttg).* 1992;35(1):18–22.
40. Rudoler S, Corn BW, Werner-Wasik M, et al. Patterns of tumor progression after radiotherapy for low-grade gliomas: analysis from the computed tomography/magnetic resonance imaging era. *Am J Clin Oncol.* 1998;21(1):23–27.
41. Osoba D. Lessons learned from measuring health-related quality of life in oncology. *J Clin Oncol.* 1994;12(3):608–616.
42. Ständer M, Peraud A, Leroch B, Kreth FW. Prognostic impact of TP53 mutation status for adult patients with supratentorial World Health Organization Grade II astrocytoma or oligoastrocytoma: a long-term analysis. *Cancer.* 2004;101(5):1028–1035.
43. Chozick BS, Pezzullo JC, Epstein MH, Finch PW. Prognostic implications of p53 overexpression in supratentorial astrocytic tumors. *Neurosurgery.* 1994;35(5):831–7; discussion 837.
44. Hagel C, Krog B, Laas R, Stavrou DK. Prognostic relevance of TP53 mutations, p53 protein, Ki-67 index and conventional histological grading in oligodendrogliomas. *J Exp Clin Cancer Res.* 1999;18(3):305–309.
45. Ritland SR, Ganju V, Jenkins RB. Region-specific loss of heterozygosity on chromosome 19 is related to the morphologic type of human glioma. *Genes Chromosomes Cancer.* 1995;12(4):277–282.
46. Reifenberger G, Louis DN. Oligodendroglioma: toward molecular definitions in diagnostic neuro-oncology. *J Neuropathol Exp Neurol.* 2003;62(2):111–126.
47. Jeuken JW, von Deimling A, Wesseling P. Molecular pathogenesis of oligodendroglial tumors. *J Neurooncol.* 2004;70(2):161–181.
48. Jenkins RB, Blair H, Ballman KV, et al. At (1;19)(q10;p10) mediates the combined deletions of 1p and 19q and predicts a better prognosis of patients with oligodendroglioma. Cancer Res 2006;66(20):9852–9861.
49. Cairncross G, Berkey B, Shaw E, et al. Phase III trial of chemotherapy plus radiotherapy compared with radiotherapy alone for pure and mixed anaplastic oligodendroglioma: Intergroup Radiation Therapy Oncology Group Trial 9402. *J Clin Oncol.* 2006;24(18):2707–2714.
50. Maintz D, Fiedler K, Koopmann J, et al. Molecular genetic evidence for subtypes of oligoastrocytomas. *J Neuropathol Exp Neurol.* 1997;56(10):1098–1104.
51. Mueller W, Hartmann C, Hoffmann A, et al. Genetic signature of oligoastrocytomas correlates with tumor location and denotes distinct molecular subsets. *Am J Pathol.* 2002;161(1):313–319.
52. Hegi ME, Diserens AC, Gorlia T, et al. MGMT gene silencing and benefit from temozolomide in glioblastoma. *N Engl J Med.* 2005;352(10):997–1003.
53. Eoli M, Bissola L, Bruzzone MG, et al. Reclassification of oligoastrocytomas by loss of heterozygosity studies. *Int J Cancer.* 2006;119(1):84–90.
54. Möllemann M, Wolter M, Felsberg J, Collins VP, Reifenberger G. Frequent promoter hypermethylation and low expression of the MGMT gene in oligodendroglial tumors. *Int J Cancer.* 2005;113(3):379–385.
55. Dong SM, Pang JC, Poon WS, et al. Concurrent hypermethylation of multiple genes is associated with grade of oligodendroglial tumors. *J Neuropathol Exp Neurol.* 2001;60(8):808–816.
56. Alonso ME, Bello MJ, Gonzalez-Gomez P, et al. Aberrant promoter methylation of multiple genes in oligodendrogliomas and ependymomas. *Cancer Genet Cytogenet.* 2003;144(2):134–142.
57. Levin N, Lavon I, Zelikovitsh B, et al. Progressive low-grade oligodendrogliomas: response to temozolomide and correlation between genetic profile and O6-methylguanine DNA methyltransferase protein expression. *Cancer.* 2006;106(8):1759–1765.
58. Hoang-Xuan K, Capelle L, Kujas M, et al. Temozolomide as initial treatment for adults with low-grade oligodendrogliomas or oligoastrocytomas and correlation with chromosome 1p deletions. *J Clin Oncol.* 2004;22(15):3133–3138.
59. Komine C, Watanabe T, Katayama Y, Yoshino A, Yokoyama T, Fukushima T. Promoter hypermethylation of the DNA repair gene O6-methylguanine-DNA methyltransferase is an independent predictor of shortened progression free survival in patients with low-grade diffuse astrocytomas. *Brain Pathol.* 2003;13(2):176–184.
60. Daumas-Duport C, Scheithauer BW, Kelly PJ. A histologic and cytologic method for the spatial definition of gliomas. *Mayo Clin Proc.* 1987;62(6):435–449.
61. Liigant A, Haldre S, Oun A, et al. Seizure disorders in patients with brain tumors. *Eur Neurol.* 2001;45(1):46–51.
62. Surma-aho O, Niemelä M, Vilkki J, et al. Adverse long-term effects of brain radiotherapy in adult low-grade glioma patients. *Neurology.* 2001;56(10):1285–1290.
63. Hammack JE, Shaw EG, Ivnik RJ, Arusell R, Novotny P, O'Fallon JR. Neurocognitive function in patients receiving radiation therapy (rt) for supratentorial low grade glioma (lgg): a North Central Cancer Treatment Group (NCCTG) prospective study. (Abstract no. 299). *Proc Am Soc Clin Oncol.* 1995;14:151.
64. Cairncross JG, Laperriere NJ. Low-grade glioma. To treat or not to treat? *Arch Neurol.* 1989;46(11):1238–1239.
65. Morantz RA. Radiation therapy in the treatment of cerebral astrocytoma. *Neurosurgery.* 1987;20(6):975–982.
66. Shaw EG. The low-grade glioma debate: evidence defending the position of early radiation therapy. *Clin Neurosurg.* 1995;42:488–494.
67. Horrax G. Benign (favorable) types of brain tumor; the and results (up to twenty years), with statistics of mortality and useful survival. *N Engl J Med.* 1954;250(23):981–984.
68. Shaw EG. Low-grade gliomas: to treat or not to treat? A radiation oncologist's viewpoint. *Arch Neurol.* 1990;47(10):1138–1140.
69. Shaw EG, Daumas-Duport C, Scheithauer BW, et al. Radiation therapy in the management of low-grade supratentorial astrocytomas. *J Neurosurg.* 1989;70(6):853–861.
70. Shaw E, Berkey B, Coons S, et al. Update of an RTOG prospective study of observation in completely resected adult low-grade glioma. *Neuro Oncol.* 2006;8(4):452.
71. Stupp R, Mason WP, van den Bent MJ, et al. Radiotherapy plus concomitant and adjuvant temozolomide for glioblastoma. *N Engl J Med.* 2005;352(10):987–996.
72. van den Bent MJ, Afra D, de Witte O, et al. Long-term efficacy of early versus delayed radiotherapy for low-grade astrocytoma and oligodendroglioma in adults: the EORTC 22845 randomised trial. *Lancet.* 2005;366(9490):985–990.
73. Karim AB, Afra D, Cornu P, et al. Randomized trial on the efficacy of radiotherapy for cerebral low-grade glioma in the adult: European Organization for Research and Treatment of Cancer Study 22845 with the Medical Research Council study BR04: an interim analysis. *Int J Radiat Oncol Biol Phys.* 2002;52(2):316–324.
74. Claus EB, Horlacher A, Hsu L, et al. Survival rates in patients with low-grade glioma after intraoperative magnetic resonance image guidance. *Cancer.* 2005;103(6):1227–1233.
75. Smith JS, Chang EF, Lamborn KR, et al. The role of extent of resection in the long-term outcome of low-grade hemispheric gliomas. *Neuro Oncol.* 2007;9:599–600.
76. Westergaard L, Gjerris F, Klinken L. Prognostic parameters in benign astrocytomas. *Acta Neurochir (Wien).* 1993;123(1–2):1–7.
77. Janny P, Cure H, Mohr M, et al. Low grade supratentorial astrocytomas. Management and prognostic factors. *Cancer.* 1994;73(7):1937–1945.
78. Philippon JH, Clemenceau SH, Fauchon FH, Foncin JF. Supratentorial low-grade astrocytomas in adults. *Neurosurgery.* 1993;32(4):554–559.
79. Lote K, Egeland T, Hager B, et al. Survival, prognostic factors, and therapeutic efficacy in low-grade glioma: a retrospective study in 379 patients. *J Clin Oncol.* 1997;15(9):3129–3140.
80. Piepmeier JM. Observations on the current treatment of low-grade astrocytic tumors of the cerebral hemispheres. *J Neurosurg.* 1987;67(2):177–181.
81. Scerrati M, Roselli R, Iacoangeli M, Pompucci A, Rossi GF. Prognostic factors in low grade (WHO grade II) gliomas of the cerebral hemispheres: the role of surgery. *J Neurol Neurosurg Psychiatr.* 1996;61(3):291–296.
82. Nicolato A, Gerosa MA, Fina P, Iuzzolino P, Giorgiutti F, Bricolo A. Prognostic factors in low-grade supratentorial astrocytomas: a uni-multivariate statistical analysis in 76 surgically treated adult patients. *Surg Neurol.* 1995;44(3):208–21; discussion 221.

83. Piepmeier J, Christopher S, Spencer D, et al. Variations in the natural history and survival of patients with supratentorial low-grade astrocytomas. *Neurosurgery*. 1996;38(5):872–8; discussion 878.
84. Bahary JP, Villemure JG, Choi S, et al. Low-grade pure and mixed cerebral astrocytomas treated in the CT scan era. *J Neurooncol*. 1996;27(2):173–177.
85. Keles GE, Lamborn KR, Berger MS. Low-grade hemispheric gliomas in adults: a critical review of extent of resection as a factor influencing outcome. *J Neurosurg*. 2001;95(5):735–745.
86. Berben D. Follow-up of post-operative irradiation for low-grade gliomas. *Neuro Oncol*. 2006;8:335–6.
87. Hanzély Z, Polgár C, Fodor J, et al. Role of early radiotherapy in the treatment of supratentorial WHO Grade II astrocytomas: long-term results of 97 patients. *J Neurooncol*. 2003;63(3):305–312.
88. Winger MJ, Macdonald DR, Cairncross JG. Supratentorial anaplastic gliomas in adults. The prognostic importance of extent of resection and prior low-grade glioma. *J Neurosurg*. 1989;71(4):487–493.
89. Kortmann RD, Jeremic B, Weller M, Lutterbach J, Paulsen F, Bamberg M. Immediate postoperative radiotherapy or "watch and wait" in the management of adult low-grade glioma? *Strahlenther Onkol*. 2004;180(7):408–418.
90. Soffietti R, Costanza A, Laguzzi E, Nobile M, Rudà R. Radiotherapy and chemotherapy of brain metastases. *J Neurooncol*. 2005;75(1):31–42.
91. Francavilla TL, Miletich RS, Di Chiro G, Patronas NJ, Rizzoli HV, Wright DC. Positron emission tomography in the detection of malignant degeneration of low-grade gliomas. *Neurosurgery*. 1989;24(1):1–5.
92. Laack NN, Brown PD. Cognitive sequelae of brain radiation in adults. *Semin Oncol*. 2004;31(5):702–713.
93. Armstrong CL, Hunter JV, Ledakis GE, et al. Late cognitive and radiographic changes related to radiotherapy: initial prospective findings. *Neurology*. 2002;59(1):40–48.
94. Vigliani MC, Sichez N, Poisson M, Delattre JY. A prospective study of cognitive functions following conventional radiotherapy for supratentorial gliomas in young adults: 4-year results. *Int J Radiat Oncol Biol Phys*. 1996;35(3):527–533.
95. Torres IJ, Mundt AJ, Sweeney PJ, et al. A longitudinal neuropsychological study of partial brain radiation in adults with brain tumors. *Neurology*. 2003;60(7):1113–1118.
96. Klein M, Heimans JJ, Aaronson NK, et al. Effect of radiotherapy and other treatment-related factors on mid-term to long-term cognitive sequelae in low-grade gliomas: a comparative study. *Lancet*. 2002;360(9343):1361–1368.
97. Klein M, van der Ploeg HM, Taphoorn MJ, et al. The prognostic value of neurobehavioral functioning in high-grade glioma. *Neuro Oncol*. 2002;4S:S53.
98. Mason WP, Krol GS, DeAngelis LM. Low-grade oligodendroglioma responds to chemotherapy. *Neurology*. 1996;46(1):203–207.
99. Soffietti R, Rudà R, Bradac GB, Schiffer D. PCV chemotherapy for recurrent oligodendrogliomas and oligoastrocytomas. *Neurosurgery*. 1998;43(5):1066–1073.
100. Stege EM, Kros JM, de Bruin HG, et al. Successful treatment of low-grade oligodendroglial tumors with a chemotherapy regimen of procarbazine, lomustine, and vincristine. *Cancer*. 2005;103(4):802–809.
101. Pace A, Vidiri A, Galiè E, et al. Temozolomide chemotherapy for progressive low-grade glioma: clinical benefits and radiological response. *Ann Oncol*. 2003;14(12):1722–1726.
102. Quinn JA, Reardon DA, Friedman AH, et al. Phase II trial of temozolomide in patients with progressive low-grade glioma. *J Clin Oncol*. 2003;21(4):646–651.
103. Pouratian N, Gasco J, Sherman JH, Shaffrey ME, Schiff D. Toxicity and efficacy of protracted low dose temozolomide for the treatment of low grade gliomas. *J Neurooncol*. 2006;8:450.
104. Brada M, Viviers L, Abson C, et al. Phase II study of primary temozolomide chemotherapy in patients with WHO grade II gliomas. *Ann Oncol*. 2003;14(12):1715–1721.
105. van den Bent MJ, Looijenga LH, Langenberg K, et al. Chromosomal anomalies in oligodendroglial tumors are correlated with clinical features. *Cancer*. 2003;97(5):1276–1284.
106. Civitello LA, Packer RJ, Rorke LB, Siegel K, Sutton LN, Schut L. Leptomeningeal dissemination of low-grade gliomas in childhood. *Neurology*. 1988;38(4):562–566.
107. Stüer C, Vilz B, Majores M, Becker A, Schramm J, Simon M. Frequent recurrence and progression in pilocytic astrocytoma in adults. *Cancer*. 2007;110(12):2799–2808.
108. Glosser G, McManus P, Munzenrider J, et al. Neuropsychological function in adults after high dose fractionated radiation therapy of skull base tumors. *Int J Radiat Oncol Biol Phys*. 1997;38(2):231–239.

85 Ganglioglioma

John C. Breneman

GANGLIOMAS

Overview and Natural History

Ganglioma is composed of cells of both glial and neuronal origin. The entity was originally described by Perkins in 1926 [1] and comprises approximately 6% of primary brain tumors [2]. Though these tumors occur in all age groups, they are most common in the pediatric and young adult population with a mean age at presentation in the teens to early 20s [2,3]. Some authors report a slight male predominance [3,4]. The majority of tumors (approximately 80%) arise in the temporal lobes with most of the remainder occurring in the frontal lobes [3,5]. Midbrain, infratentorial, and spinal presentations occur but are rare. The great majority of patients present with a long-standing seizure disorder which, in some cases, predates diagnosis by 10 or more years [3]. Gangliogliomas generally behave in an indolent manner though there is a subset which are clinically aggressive—a behavior which correlates with the histologic grade of the glial component of the tumor [6–8].

Pathology

Ganglioglioma consists of dysplastic neurons and neoplastic glial cells [9]. The glial component contains astrocytic cells surrounded by a reticulin network and often has a pilocytic appearance. The neuronal component is composed of large multipolar neurons that have synaptophysin immunoreactivity. Electron microscopic studies suggest a neural crest origin [10]. Most lesions have very low proliferative indices and are classified as WHO grade I or II, but up to 30% of cases may contain a high-grade glial component [6,11].

Expression of CD34 helps to distinguish ganglioglioma from oligodendroglioma or dysembryoplastic neuroepithelial tumor (DNT) with which they are sometimes confused [5]. Variants of ganglioglioma include Lhermitte-Duclos which occurs in the cerebellum and is associated with a PTEN germline mutation [9], and papillary glioneuronal tumor which occurs almost exclusively adjacent to the lateral ventricles and has a consistently excellent prognosis [12–14]. Gangliogliomas are histologically and clinically distinct from the similarly named desmoplastic infantile ganglioglioma (DIG).

Radiographic Appearance

The radiologic appearance of ganglioglioma is often heterogenous with mixed solid and cystic components and frequent calcifications [2,15]. Lesions are typically well circumscribed with low signal on T1-weighted MRI, high signal on T2 MRI and varying degrees of contrast enhancement, which may be present even in well-differentiated tumors [14,16] (Figure 85.1). FDG-PET is usually hypo- or isometabolic [4].

Treatment and Outcomes

The treatment of choice for ganglioglioma is surgical resection. Complete resection results in long-term disease-

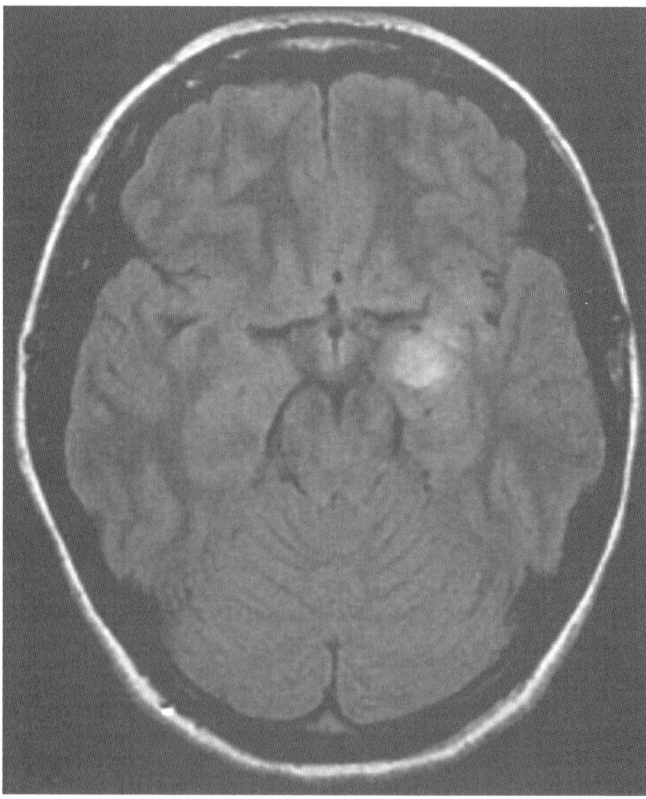

Figure 85.1 Appearance of left medial temporal ganglioglioma on an axial FLAIR MRI sequence. A foci of contrast enhancement within this lesion is also visible on T1 images.

free survival in 80% or more of patients [3,6,7,16–22] and is often curative of the epileptic symptoms associated with these tumors [22,23]. A high-grade glial component predicts a substantially greater risk of relapse and death with reported survival rates of under 50% [6,7,24,25]. Subtotal resection is associated with a higher risk of recurrence in some, but not all, reported series with relapse rates of 8% to 25% [3,4,6,25]. Other features that have correlated with increased risk of relapse include age greater than 30 years [6,24], short duration of preoperative symptoms [24], male gender [6], and location other than supratentorial [3,18].

Radiotherapy is indicated for adjuvant treatment of ganglioglioma with malignant features. In addition, radiotherapy has been used for tumors with recurrence after previous resection and subtotally resected lesions, especially in anatomic locations where recurrence could cause excessive morbidity [26,27]. However, the efficacy of radiotherapy in these circumstances is unclear [6]. Liauw recommends 54 Gy for patients in which recurrence would cause significant neurologic sequelae or would be difficult to salvage with further surgery [27]. Fisher suggests adjuvant radiotherapy for those with bulky residual tumor and tumors located in the midbrain or brainstem [17]. Others have reported excellent outcomes after subtotal resection without further intervention [3,6,28].

Radiotherapy techniques parallel those used for pure glial tumors. Though lesions often appear well demarcated on imaging studies, microscopic clusters of tumor cells in adjacent, normal-appearing brain region are often seen pathologically [5], and radiotherapy target volumes should include the radiographically defined tumor with a 1- to 2-cm margin. Highly conformal techniques sparing brain outside the target volume may be especially useful given the extended survival that many patients enjoy. There is no dose response evident, but most authors have used doses of at least 50 Gy for low-grade tumors and 60 Gy for high-grade lesions. Some have used stereotactic radiosurgery in selected patients with small, well-demarcated lesions [4,27]. Radiotherapy has been reported to result in malignant transformation [29–31] though not all authors have noted this correlation [25], and malignant transformation has been described in tumors after surgical treatment only [4,32]. Chemotherapy has been used in small numbers of patients, but its efficacy is unknown [2,21,27].

REFERENCES

1. Perkins OC. Gangliogliomas. *Arch Pathol Lab Med.* 1926;2:11–17.
2. Demierre B, Stichnoth FA, Hori A, Spoerri O. Intracerebral ganglioglioma. *J Neurosurg.* 1986;65:177–182.
3. Luyken C, Blumcke I, Fimmers R, Urbach H, Wiestler OD, Schramm J. Supratentorial gangliogliomas: histopathologic grading and tumor recurrence in 184 patients with a median follow-up of 8 years. *Cancer.* 2004;101:146–155.
4. Im SH, Chung CK, Cho BK, et al. Intracranial ganglioglioma: preoperative characteristics and oncologic outcome after surgery. *J Neurooncol.* 2002;59:173–183.
5. Blumcke I, Wiestler OD. Gangliogliomas: an intriguing tumor entity associated with focal epilepsies. *J Neuropathol Exp Neurol.* 2002;61:575–584.
6. Rumana CS, Valadka AB, Contant CF. Prognostic factors in supratentorial ganglioglioma. *Acta Neurochir (Wien).* 1999;141:63–68; discussion 8–9.
7. Hakim R, Loeffler JS, Anthony DC, Black PM. Gangliogliomas in adults. *Cancer.* 1997;79:127–131.
8. Matsuzaki K, Uno M, Kageji T, Hirose T, Nagahiro S. Anaplastic ganglioglioma of the cerebellopontine angle. Case report. *Neurol Med Chir (Tokyo).* 2005;45:591–595.
9. Kleihues P, Cavenee WK, eds. *Pathology and Genetics of Tumours of the Nervous System.* Lyon, France: IARC Press; 2000.
10. Miller DC, Lang FF, Epstein FJ. Central nervous system gangliogliomas. Part 1: pathology. *J Neurosurg.* 1993;79:859–866.
11. Wolf HK, Muller MB, Spanle M, Zentner J, Schramm J, Wiestler OD. Ganglioglioma: a detailed histopathological and immunohistochemical analysis of 61 cases. *Acta Neuropathol (Berl).* 1994;88:166–173.
12. Dim DC, Lingamfelter DC, Taboada EM, Fiorella RM. Papillary glioneuronal tumor: a case report and review of the literature. *Hum Pathol.* 2006;37:914–918.
13. Komori T, Scheithauer BW, Anthony DC, et al. Papillary glioneuronal tumor: a new variant of mixed neuronal-glial neoplasm. *Am J Surg Pathol.* 1998;22:1171–1183.
14. Epelbaum S, Kujas M, Van Effenterre R, Poirier J. Two cases of papillary glioneuronal tumours. *Br J Neurosurg.* 2006;20:90–93.
15. Matsumoto K, Tamiya T, Ono Y, Furuta T, Asari S, Ohmoto T. Cerebral gangliogliomas: clinical characteristics, CT and MRI. *Acta Neurochir (Wien).* 1999;141:135–141.
16. Ildan F, Tuna M, Gocer IA, Erman T, Cetinalp E. Intracerebral ganglioglioma: clinical and radiological study of eleven surgically treated cases with follow-up. *Neurosurg Rev.* 2001;24:114–118.
17. Fisher BJ, Leighton CC, Vujovic O, Macdonald DR, Stitt L. Results of a policy of surveillance alone after surgical management of pediatric low grade gliomas. *Int J Radiat Oncol Biol Phys.* 2001;51:704–710.
18. Lang FF, Epstein FJ, Ransohoff J, et al. Central nervous system gangliogliomas. Part 2: clinical outcome. *J Neurosurg.* 1993;79:867–873.
19. Chintagumpala MM, Armstrong D, Miki S, et al. Mixed neuronal-glial tumors (gangliogliomas) in children. *Pediatr Neurosurg.* 1996;24:306–313.
20. Park CK, Chung CK, Choe GY, Wang KC, Cho BK, Kim HJ. Intramedullary spinal cord ganglioglioma: a report of five cases. *Acta Neurochir (Wien).* 2000;142:547–552.
21. Silver JM, Rawlings CE III, Rossitch E Jr, Zeidman SM, Friedman AH. Ganglioglioma: a clinical study with long-term follow-up. *Surg Neurol.* 1991;35:261–266.
22. Johnson JH Jr, Hariharan S, Berman J, et al. Clinical outcome of pediatric gangliogliomas: ninety-nine cases over 20 years. *Pediatr Neurosurg.* 1997;27:203–207.
23. Zentner J, Wolf HK, Ostertun B, et al. Gangliogliomas: clinical, radiological, and histopathological findings in 51 patients. *J Neurol Neurosurg Psychiatry.* 1994;57:1497–1502.
24. Krouwer HG, Davis RL, McDermott MW, Hoshino T, Prados MD. Gangliogliomas: a clinicopathological study of 25 cases and review of the literature. *J Neurooncol.* 1993;17:139–154.
25. Selch MT, Goy BW, Lee SP, et al. Gangliogliomas: experience with 34 patients and review of the literature. *Am J Clin Oncol.* 1998;21:557–564.
26. Ulutin HC, Onguru O, Pak Y. Postoperative radiotherapy for ganglioglioma; report of three cases and review of the literature. *Minim Invasive Neurosurg.* 2002;45:224–227.
27. Liauw SL, Byer JE, Yachnis AT, Amdur RJ, Mendenhall WM. Radiotherapy after subtotally resected or recurrent ganglioglioma. *Int J Radiat Oncol Biol Phys.* 2007;67:244–247.
28. Celli P, Scarpinati M, Nardacci B, Cervoni L, Cantore GP. Gangliogliomas of the cerebral hemispheres. Report of 14 cases with long-term follow-up and review of the literature. *Acta Neurochir (Wien).* 1993;125:52–57.
29. Hayashi Y, Iwato M, Hasegawa M, Tachibana O, von Deimling A, Yamashita J. Malignant transformation of a gangliocytoma/ganglioglioma into a glioblastoma multiforme: a molecular genetic analysis. Case report. *J Neurosurg.* 2001;95:138–142.
30. Jay V, Squire J, Becker LE, Humphreys R. Malignant transformation in a ganglioglioma with anaplastic neuronal and astrocytic components. Report of a case with flow cytometric and cytogenetic analysis. *Cancer.* 1994;73:2862–2868.
31. Rumana CS, Valadka AB. Radiation therapy and malignant degeneration of benign supratentorial gangliogliomas. *Neurosurgery.* 1998;42:1038–1043.
32. Kim NR, Wang KC, Bang JS, et al. Glioblastomatous transformation of ganglioglioma: case report with reference to molecular genetic and flow cytometric analysis. *Pathol Int.* 2003;53:874–882.

86 Optic Pathway Glioma

Bernadine R. Donahue

INTRODUCTION AND EPIDEMIOLOGY

Optic pathway glioma (OPG) is a unique subset of intracranial low-grade gliomas accounting for 5% of all childhood brain tumors [1]. In 1833, Wishart reported the case of an intrinsic tumor of the optic nerve in a 13-year-old girl [2], with the incidence marking the early part of the twentieth century to be the period during which these tumors began to be described and classified by pathologists [3,4]. OPG is a tumor of childhood, predominantly arising within the first 5 years of life: 25% present before the age of 1.5 years and 50% present before the age of 5 years [5–7].

Optic-pathway tumors may be associated with neurofibromatosis type I (NF1); approximately 30% of all OPG occur in this setting [8]. In children whose tumors involve only the optic nerve itself, there is a 50% to 75% chance that NF1 is present. This is contrary in the case of lesions that arise from the chiasm in which no more than 20% are associated with NF1. The disease may be more indolent in children with NF1. In this subset of patients, the tumors rarely grow after the age of 6 [9]. Many children with NF1 who undergo surveillance imaging have radiographically identified OPG, but such children never develop visual symptoms [10,11]. However, NF1-associated OPG may be less localized and, thus, have a higher propensity to recur after surgery [12,13].

PATHOLOGY AND RADIOGRAPHIC FINDINGS

Histologically, the vast majority of OPG are low-grade glial neoplasms [14,15]. Approximately two-thirds of OPG cases were reported to be presenting pilocytic astrocytomas and one-quarter presenting WHO grade II astrocytomas. The remaining histologies include gangliogliomas, hamartomas, or germ-cell tumors; high-grade glial neoplasms are rare.

Macroscopically, OPG can be classified on the basis of the anatomic structure of the optic pathway from which they arise. Tumors may arise from the optic nerve (the intraorbital and/or intracranial portion with or without extension to the chiasm), the chiasm itself, or involve both the chiasm and hypothalamus with or without posterior extension to the optic tracts (see Figures 86.1 and 86.2). The latter is the most common [16,17]. In general, lesions that extend to or involve the hypothalamus tend to be somewhat more aggressive than those that are confined to the visual pathway.

Radiographically, the lesions are best imaged by MRI. OPG tend to be solid tumors that are hypointense on T1, hyperintense on T2, and, like most pilocytic astrocytomas, brightly enhance with gadolinium. Cystic tumors have been described [18]. Diffusion-weighted imaging has been helpful in patients with NF1 in differentiating tumor from other lesions commonly seen in patients with NF1 such as myelin disorders and hamartomas [19].

CLINICAL PRESENTATION

The most common presentation is visual impairment with a loss of visual acuity [1]. Proptosis, strabismus, nystagmus, and optic atrophy are other clinical signs that may

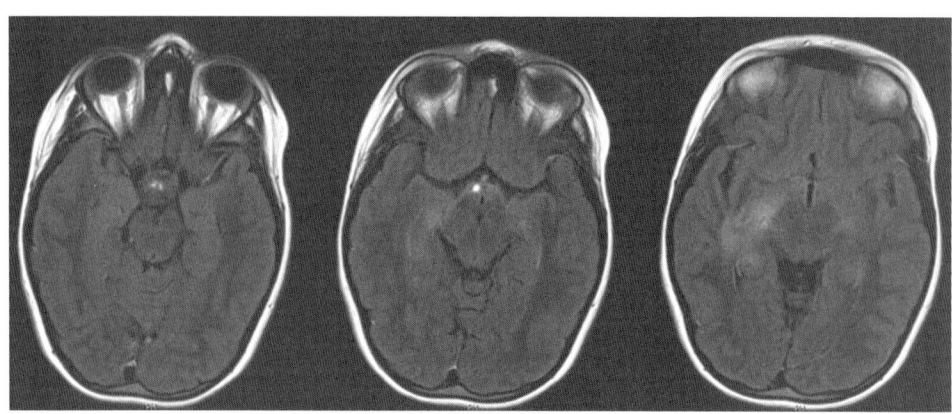

Figure 86.1 OPG with posterior extension and infiltrative appearance on FLAIR MRI.

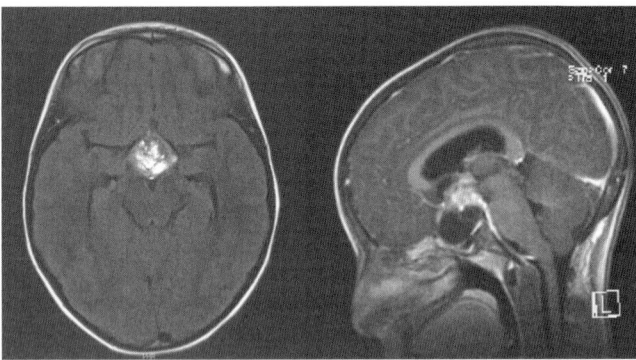

Figure 86.2 Axial and sagittal MRI of OPG arising from the chiasm.

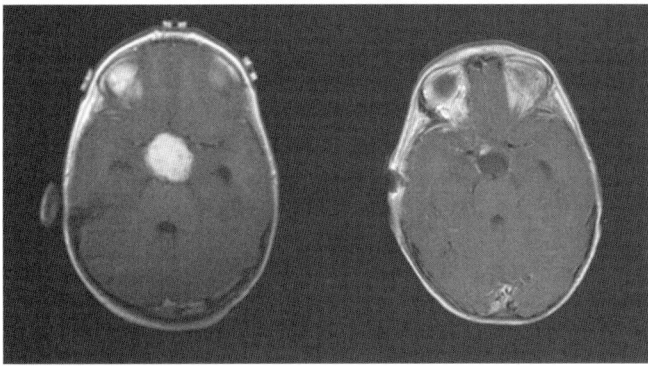

Figure 86.3 Pre- and postoperative appearance of a chiasmatic pilocytic astrocytoma.

be found [20]. Tumors that involve the diencephalon may present with the diencephalic syndrome charcterized by hyperactivity, cheerful disposition, and failure to thrive with weight loss despite adequate nutritional intake; this is most often seen in infants and very young children [21]. Young children with OPG may also be diagnosed when they are evaluated for pendular nystagmus, the need to bring objects close to the face, or fear of ambulating. Progressive growth of OPG can cause anterior pituitary deficiencies and precocious puberty. Hydrocephalus can result from occlusion of the third ventricle or the Foramen of Monro. These tumors, like other low-grade glial neoplasms, can metastasize, albeit rarely (see chapter on *Adult and Pediatric Pilocytic Astrocytoma*).

TREATMENT AND OUTCOME

Surgery, radiation therapy, and chemotherapy have all been utilized in the treatment of OPG. However, in many situations "watchful waiting" with surveillance MRI and scheduled ophthamologic exams is the best approach. It is clear that the nature of these tumors can be indolent, and cases of spontaneous regression have been recognized [22]. However, it is also widely acknowledged that, despite a potentially more indolent course in NF1, OPG progresses in 75% to 85% of children, usually within 2 years of the diagnosis [1]. Given that overall survival is unaffected by the initial therapeutic approach, one of the necessary and critical components of caring for children with OPG is knowing when to intervene and then choosing the intervention that is most appropriate for the location of the tumor, the age of the child, and the severity of the symptoms.

Surgery

Surgery may be utilized in the setting of OPG for biopsy, definitive resection, or decompression. Biopsy for tissue diagnosis may be indicated in the setting of an unusual radiographic appearance that raises the question of a nonsecretory germ-cell tumor or a high-grade neoplasm. Surgery is the treatment of choice for unilateral optic-nerve tumors, particularly if there is potentially disfiguring proptosis and if there is no useful vision. Despite the loss of vision with this approach, the long-term outcome following complete surgical removal of an optic-nerve tumor is quite good with low recurrence rates of 5% [16] and a reported 10-year survival of >90% [17].

Unlike the most anteriorly located tumors, the most posteriorly located tumors, that is, those with extension to the optic tracts or optic radiations, or those with infiltration to the lateral geniculate body, are not particularly suitable for a surgical approach and are usually managed on the basis of clinical and radiographic findings.

Some surgical series have suggested a role for local excision in selected presentations of the "middle" tumors, that is, those arising from the chiasm/hypothalamus without posterior extension (see Figure 86.3) [15,23–25]. Experience from New York University demonstrated that tumors can be operated on in this area with relative safety in terms of further visual compromise [15]. In this series utilizing an "aggressive" surgical approach, 50% of patients remained stable, that is, without the need for further intervention for 3 to 5 years. Advocates of such an approach note that surgery, particularly for young children, avoids or delays chemotherapy and radiation, which is important, considering that both of them cause toxicities. However, this approach is not without neurodevelopmental and/or endocrine toxicities, and other authors advocate for a more conservative approach [26].

Chemotherapy

Similar to the approach in infant CNS tumors, chemotherapy was introduced in the 1980s as treatment for OPG, primarily to delay radiation and its associated sequela in young children. In 1985, a preliminary experience using chemotherapy for optic chiasm glioma was published [27]. Packer's original approach employed vincristine and actinomycin-D in children younger than 5 years of age, and an objective response was seen in 25% of the children thus studied. The median time to progression was 3 years [28]. Ultimately, 60% of children required radiation therapy. Subsequently, Packer went on to develop an 18-month regimen of carboplatin and vincristine that resulted in a nearly 3-year freedom from progression (70%) [29,30]. The efficacy of this regimen appeared to be age dependent: children younger than 5 years had a 75% progression-free survival, whereas the survival rate for older children was 39%. The presence of neurofibromatosis did not affect the progression-free survival rate. This also appeared to be true in a phase II POG trial evaluating the efficacy of carboplatin for progressive OPG, although the study was not designed for formal comparison of outcome between NF1 and non-NF1 patients [31].

The group from UCSF explored a 5-drug regimen (6-thioguanine, procarbazine, dibromodulcitol, CCNU, and vincristine) that showed similar results [32,33]. The French Society of Pediatric Oncology enrolled 85 children with progressive OPG on a prospective trial using alternating courses of carboplatin/procarbazine, etoposide/cisplatin, and vincristine/cyclophosphamide [34]. The 5-year progression-free survival was 34%, the 5-year radiotherapy-free survival was 61%, and the 5-year overall survival as 89%. However, rigorous assessment of visual function was difficult in this study, given the young age of the children, and retention of useful vision did not appear to be a primary endpoint.

Currently, the most commonly used regimen is the "standard" of carboplatin and vincristine; however, the results of studies comparing this to other chemotherapy regimens is pending. COG A9952 compared the regimen of procarbazine, 6-thioguanine, CCNU, and vincristine to carboplatin and vincristine in a randomized phase III study for children younger than 10 years of age. Patients on this study had low-grade astrocytoma that was progressive following initial surgical excision or incompletely resected and requiring immediate treatment due to a risk of neurologic impairment with progression. Patients with chiasmatic lesions with contiguous extension of tumor into other regions of the visual pathways were eligible for study without histopathological confirmation, and all NF patients were eligible, provided progression was documented radiographically. Another COG trial, ACNS0223, evaluated the feasibility of carboplatin, vincristine, and temozolomide in children younger than 10 years of age with progressive and/or symptomatic low-grade gliomas. Children with optic pathway tumors were eligible if there was evidence of progressive disease on MRI and/or symptoms of deteriorating vision, progressive hypothalamic/pituitary dysfunction, diencephalic syndrome, or precocious puberty. Results from both these recent COG trials are pending.

Radiation Therapy

Radiation therapy has been utilized in the treatment of OPGs for many years [35–38]. Several single institution studies published after the advent of CT scanning report 10 year progression-free survival rates in excess of 80% [7,17,39–42]. In these series, one-quarter to one-third of patients experienced improvement in vision, and approximately 50% showed some radiographic regression, which can occur over years after treatment. Cystic degeneration of tumor has been described as occurring 6 months after RT [7]. This can be manifested clinically by a worsening in vision, if there is a resultant pressure effect; it may require management with steroids, or in severe instances, surgical decompression.

The doses and fields used for OPG are similar to those described in the chapter *Adult and Pediatric Pilocytic Astrocytoma*, with the important caveat that tumor must be distinguished from other commonly encountered T2 radiographic abnormalities, particularly along the optic tracts, in patients with neurofibromatosis. In addition, when there is optic nerve involvement, the nerve up to its junction with the posterior globe must be included in the target volume. Again, as with pilocytic astrocytomas, various types of conformal techniques are acceptable. Combs et al [43] reported the updated experience from Heidelberg with fractionated stereotactic radiotherapy (1.8 Gy fractions to a total dose of 52.2 Gy) in 15 patients with optic-pathway gliomas . Vision improved in 6 patients after RT and remained stable in 7 patients after RT. The 5-year progression-free survival was 72%, and the 5-year overall survival was 90%.

Late effects are an important concern when RT is used. Neurocognitive sequelae are particularly of concern, given the young age of most children with OPG [42,44], and may be of particular concern in children with neurofibromatosis [45]. However, it is not only the tumor but surgery itself can lead to neuropsychological deficits [46,47]. Endocrine impairment can also result from RT; growth-hormone deficiency is the most frequently described adverse effect post-RT [48]. Late vascular effects include moyamoya syndrome, characterized by obliteration of vessels at the circle of Willis; there is a particularly high incidence (18%) in young children with NF1 [42,49]. Second malignancies have been reported [17,24] and require long-term follow-up after radiation therapy. This is of particular concern in NF1 patients, for whom a relative risk (at 3.0) of second nervous system tumors, following RT for OPG, has been reported [50].

The indications for RT may be somewhat open to discussion, but in general RT should be considered for children aged more than 5 years (or perhaps 10 years) who have substantial visual or neurologic deficits at presentation or who have evidence of clinical or radiographic progression. Most younger children initially are treated with chemotherapy, and radiation is reserved for progression. A comprehensive treatment algorithm addressing the use of RT for OPG can be found in Jahraus' review of optic gliomas [20].

REFERENCES

1. Halperin EC, Constine LS, Tarbell NJ, Kun LE, (eds). *Pediatric Radiation Oncology*. 4th ed. Philadelphia, PA: Lippincott, Williams and Wilkins; 2005:50–54.
2. Wishart JH. Case of extirpation of the eye-ball. *Edin Med Surg J.* 1833;40:274–276.
3. Parsons JH. *The Pathology of the Eye*. London: Hodder and Stoughton; 1905:693–715.
4. Parsons JH. *Diseases of the Eye*. 9th ed. New York: Macmillan; 1938:646–649.
5. Wong JY, Uhl V, Wara WM, et al. Optic gliomas. A reanalysis of the University of California, San Francisco experience. *Cancer.* 1987;60(8):1847–1855.

6. Janss AJ, Grundy R, Cnaan A, et al. Optic pathway and hypothalamic/chiasmic gliomas in children younger than age 5 years with 6-year follow-up. *Cancer.* 1995;75(4):1051–1059.
7. Tao ML, Barnes PD, Billett AL, et al. Childhood optic chiasm gliomas: radiographic response following radiotherapy and long-term clinical outcome. *Int J Radiat Oncol Biol Phys.* 1997;39:579–587.
8. Listernick R, Louis DN, Packer RJ, et al. Optic pathway gliomas in children with neurofibromatosis, type I: consensus statement from the NF1 Optic Pathway Glioma Task Force. *Ann Neurology.* 1997;41(2):143–149.
9. Grill J, Lathier V, Rodriguez D, et al. When do children with optic pathway tumors need treatment? An oncological perspective in 106 patients treated in a single centre. *Eur J Pediatr.* 2000;159:692–696.
10. Listernick R, Charrow J, Greenwald MJ, et al. Optic gliomas in children with neurofibromatosis type 1. *J Pediatr.* 1989;114:788–792.
11. Rosser T, Packer RJ. Intracranial neoplasms in children with neurofibromatosis 1. *J Child Neurol.* 2002;17:630–637.
12. Tenny RT, Laws ER, Younge BR, et al. The neurosurgical management of optic glioma: results in 104 patients. *J Neurosurg.* 1982;57:452–458.
13. Deliganis AV, Geyer JR, Berger MS. Prognostic significance of type 1 neurofibromatosis (von Recklinghausen disease) in childhood optic glioma. *Neurosurg.* 1996;38:1114–1119.
14. Bilgic S, Erbengi A, Tinaztepe B, et al. Optic glioma of childhood: clinical, histopathological, and histochemical observations. *Br J Ophthalmol.* 1989;73:832–837.
15. Wisoff JH, Abbott R, Epstein F. Surgical management of exophytic chiasmatic-hypothalamic tumors of childhood. *J Neurosurg.* 1990;73(5):661–667.
16. Alvord EC, Lofton S. Gliomas of the optic nerves or chiasm. Outcome by patients' age, tumor site, and treatment. *J Neurosurg.* 1988;68(1):85–98.
17. Jenkin D, Angyalfi S, Becker L, et al. Optic glioma in children: surveillance, resection, or irradiation? *Int J Radiat Oncol Biol Phys.* 1993;25(2):215–225.
18. Gower DJ, Pollay M, Shuman RM, et al. Cystic optic glioma. *Neurosurg.* 1990;26:133–136.
19. Sener RN. Diffusion MRI in neurofibromatosis type 1: ADC evaluations of the optic pathways, and comparison with normal individuals. *Comput Med Imaging Graph.* 2002;26:59–64.
20. Jahraus CD, Tarbell NJ. Optic pathway gliomas. *Pediatr Blood Cancer.* 2006;46:586–596.
21. Gropman AL, Packer RJ, Nicholson HS, et al. Treatment of diencephalic syndrome with chemotherapy. *Cancer.* 1998;83:166–172.
22. Schmandt SM, Packer RJ, Vezina LG, et al. Spontaneous regression of low-grade astrocytomas in childhood. *Pediatr Neurosurg.* 2000;32(3):132–136.
23. Hoffman HJ, Soloniuk DS, Humphreys RP, et al. Management and outcome of low-grade astrocytomas of the midline in children: a retrospective review. *Neurosurgery.* 1993;33(6):964–971.
24. Hoffman HJ, Humphreys RP, Drake JM, et al. Optic pathway/hypothalamic gliomas—a dilemma in management. *Pediatr Neurosurg.* 1993;19(4):186–195.
25. Medlock MD, Scott RM. Optic chiasm astrocytomas of childhood. 2. Surgical management. *Pediatr Neurosurg.* 1997;27(3):129–136.
26. Sutton LN, Molloy PT, Sernyak H, et al. Long-term outcome of hypothalamic/chiasmatic astrocytomas in children treated with conservative surgery. *J Neurosurg.* 1995;83(4):583–589.
27. Rosenstock JG, Packer RJ, Bilaniuk L, et al. Chiasmatic optic glioma treated with chemotherapy. A preliminary report. *J Neurosurg.* 1985;63:862–866.
28. Packer RJ, Sutton LN, Bilaniuk L, et al. Treatment of chiasmatic/hypothalamic gliomas of childhood with chemotherapy: an update. *Ann Neurol.* 1988;23(1):79–85.
29. Packer RJ, Lange B, Ater J, et al. Carboplatin and vincristine for recurrent and newly diagnosed low-grade gliomas of childhood. *J Clin Oncol.* 1993;11:850–856.
30. Packer RJ, Ater J, Allen J, et al. Carboplatin and vincristine for children with newly diagnosed progressive low-grade gliomas. *J Neurosurg.* 1997;86:747–754.
31. Mahoney DH, Cohen ME, Friedman HS, et al. Carboplatin is effective therapy for young children with progressive optic pathway tumors: a pediatric oncology group phase II study. *Neuro-Oncology.* 2000;2:213–220.
32. Petronio J, Edwards MSB, Prados M, et al. Management of chiasmal and hypothalamic gliomas of infancy and childhood with chemotherapy. *J Neurosurg.* 1991;74:701–708.
33. Prados MD, Edwards MSB, Rabbitt J, et al. Treatment of pediatric low-grade gliomas with a nitrosourea-based multiagent chemotherapy regimen. *J Neuro Oncol.* 1997;32:235–241.
34. Laithier V, Grill J, Le Deley M-C, et al. Progression-free survival in children with optic pathway tumors: dependence on age and the quality of the response to chemotherapy—results of the first French prospective study for the French Society of Pediatric Oncology. *J Clin Oncol.* 2003;21:4572–4578.
35. Taveras JM, Mount LA, Wood EH. The value of radiation therapy in the management of glioma of the optic nerves and chiasm. *Radiology.* 1956;66:518–528.
36. Montgomery AB, Griffin T, Parker RG, et al. Optic nerve glioma: the role of radiation therapy. *Cancer.* 1977;40:2079–2080.
37. Dosoretz DE, Blitzer PH, Wang CC, et al. Management of glioma of the optic nerve and/or chiasm: an analysis of 20 cases. *Cancer.* 1980;45:1467–1471.
38. Danoff BF, Kramer S, Thompson N. The radiotherapeutic management of optic nerve gliomas in children. *Int J Radiation Oncol Biol Phys.* 1980;6:45–50.
39. Pierce SM, Barnes PD, Loeffler JS, et al. Definitive radiation therapy in the management of symptomatic patients with optic glioma. *Cancer.* 1990;65:45–52.
40. Kovalic JJ, Grigsby PW, Shepard MJ, et al. Radiation therapy for gliomas of the optic nerve and chiasm. *Int J Radiat Oncol Biol Phys.* 1990;18:927–932.
41. Bataini JP, Delanian S, Ponvert D. Chiasmal gliomas: results of irradiation management in 57 patients and review of the literature. *Int J Radiat Oncol Biol Phys.* 1991;21(3):615–623.
42. Cappelli C, Grill J, Raquin M, et al. Long-term follow-up of 69 patients treated for optic pathway tumors before the chemotherapy era. *Arch Dis Child.* 1998;79(4):334–338.
43. Combs SE, Schulz-Ertner D, Moschos D, et al. Fractionated stereotactic radiotherapy of optic pathway gliomas: tolerance and long-term outcome. *Int J Radiat Oncol Biol Phys.* 2005;62(3):814–819.
44. Lacaze E, Kieffer V, Streri A, et al. Neuropsychological outcome in children with optic pathway tumors when first-line treatment is chemotherapy. *Br J Cancer.* 2003;89:2038–2044.
45. Chadderton RD, West CG, Schuller S, et al. Radiotherapy in the treatment of low-grade astrocytomas II. The physical and cognitive sequelae. *Chil Nerv Sys.* 1995;11:443–448.
46. Carpentieri SC, Waber DP, Pomeroy SL et al. Neuropsychological functioning after surgery in children treated for brain tumor. *Neurosurg.* 2003;52:1348–1357.
47. Fouladi M, Wallace D, Langston JW, et al. Survival and functional outcome of children with hypothalamic/chiasmatic tumors. *Cancer.* 2003;97:1084–1092.
48. Brauner R, Malandry F, Rappaport R, et al. Growth and endocrine disorders in optic glioma. *Eur J Pediatr.* 1990;149:825–828.
49. Kestle JRW, Hoffman HJ, Mock ASR. Moyamoya phenomenon after radiation for optic glioma. *J Neurosurg.* 1993;79:32–35.
50. Sharif S, Ferner R, Birch JM, et al. Second primary tumors in Neurofibromatosis 1 patients treated for optic glioma: substantial risks after radiotherapy. *J Clin Oncol.* 2006;24:2570–2575.

87 The Current Role for Radiation Therapy in Pediatric Grade II–IV (Non-JPA) Gliomas

Sameer Keole and Daniel J. Indelicato

INTRODUCTION

Gliomas, also called astrocytomas, have two distinct subsets: low-grade gliomas (LGGs), which encompass grade I and II astrocytomas, and high-grade gliomas (HGGs), which encompass grade III and IV astrocytomas. Grade I astrocytomas, also called juvenile pilocytic astrocytomas, are discussed in another chapter. Grade III astrocytomas are also called anaplastic astrocytomas (AAs) and grade IV astrocytomas are also called glioblastoma multiforme (GBM).

The role of radiation therapy (RT) in pediatric grade II astrocytomas is evolving, and there is a paucity of data that focuses on these tumors exclusively; most data incorporate all LGGs including juvenile pilocytic astrocytomas. Adult grade II data do not support the use of up-front RT in either gross total resection (GTR) or near GTR [1]. In pediatric HGG, the role of RT is fairly straightforward and its use is routine. In all pediatric central nervous system (CNS) tumors, especially those in patients less than 3 years of age, the use of RT needs to be carefully evaluated on an individual basis. Currently, the use of RT in younger patients is discouraged in the treatment of LGG, unless there is a clear indication of tumor progression, the lesion is unresectable, and chemotherapy is failing to halt progression.

REVIEW OF DATA IN PEDIATRIC GRADE II ASTROCYTOMAS

There is almost no data on pediatric LGG that exclusively focus on grade II astrocytoma. While the standard approach after gross total resection (GTR) is to withhold RT, this issue is not as clear in the setting of incomplete or subtotal resection (<GTR). The University of California, San Francisco (UCSF) experience [2] is one of the few studies that focused on pediatric grade II astrocytoma. In this 90-patient retrospective review, the authors specifically investigated the role of RT in patients with <GTR who were older than 3 years of age. The extent of resection was the only variable that statistically improved outcome. They were unable to attribute a benefit in progression-free survival (PFS) or overall survival (OS) by adding "early RT."

A modern series from the Harvard programs documented the use of stereotactic fractionated RT in a variety of settings, including for patients with symptomatic or progressive LGG ≤5 cm in maximum dimension. Using modern RT techniques for LGG demonstrated an excellent 5-year PFS and OS of 82.5% and 97.8%, respectively. At 8 years, PFS was 65% and OS was 82%, confirming that the indolent nature of these tumors requires long-term observation both for late effects and for tumor control durability [3].

Beyond pediatric settings, some randomized trials have investigated the role of RT in adult grade II astrocytomas. This data is frequently applied to the pediatric population; therefore, the pediatric radiation oncologist should be familiar with these trials. The EORTC 22844 was a dose-finding trial in which 45 versus 59.4 Gy was tested in patients with LGG who had grade I or II astrocytoma. Surgery was either minimal (<50%), debulking (50–89%), or almost total removal (>90%). Grade I astrocytomas that were GTRs were not included. Patients who received the higher dose did not exhibit an improved outcome (PFS or OS) [4]. The EORTC 22845 was a trial testing if "early RT" was superior to RT given at salvage. In this trial, high-risk patients (defined as patients >40 years old or with <GTR) were randomized to 54 Gy versus no RT. Low-risk patients (patients <40 years old with GTR) were not eligible because their standard treatment was observation without RT. The EORTC 22845 found that early RT conferred a PFS advantage but not an OS advantage. However, 65% of the patients in the observation arm did end up receiving RT at progression [1]. A corollary paper from this trial found that certain subsets of high-risk LGG patients may benefit from RT, specifically those patients with large tumors (>6 cm), tumors crossing the midline, pure astrocytomas (lacking an oligodendroglial component), and presenting with neurological symptoms before surgery [5]. It remains to be seen, however, if any of these factors can be applied to the pediatric population. Finally, a retrospective series from Mayo Clinic documented improved survival when RT doses >53 Gy were used [6].

There is limited documentation of successful institutional experiences with interstitial brachytherapy, specifically iodine-125. This technique is not readily available in most RT clinics, but when used, proper patient selection is critical and tumors should be <4 cm and well circumscribed [7,8].

For pediatric grade II astrocytomas, the available data suggest that the use of postoperative (post-op) RT is not indicated in those who have undergone GTR. Patients who have <GTR can also be observed, although some believe early RT may still provide a local control benefit [9]. In patients who have had progressive disease, chemotherapy should be considered if the patient is less than 10 years old and should definitely be administered if the patient is less than 5 years old. Radiation can be considered as first-line salvage therapy (instead of chemotherapy) in patients older than 10 years. The appropriate RT dose for grade II astrocytoma is between 45 and 54 Gy.

REVIEW OF DATA IN PEDIATRIC HGGS

Although the molecular characteristics of HGG in children may differ from their adult counterparts, both groups share a poor clinical outcome. As mentioned previously, the role of RT in HGG has been firmly established for decades as a means of improving survival time; however, OS, when judged at longer endpoints (e.g., 5 years), remains dismal [10]. Tumors that demonstrate an oligodendroglial component may be more responsive to chemotherapy and/or RT [11,12]. Historically, AA has shown a 20% to 40% 5-year OS, whereas GBM has shown a 5% to 15% 5-year OS [13–15].

The role of dose escalation with standard (photon) RT has been explored, and there appears to be no clear benefit to doses above 60 Gy [16–18]. In fact, in AA, there may be a detriment to outcome in the long-term survivors as toxicities in this subset may outweigh the benefits [19]. In a phase II trial from Massachusetts General Hospital, AA patients had a median survival time of 20 months with a dose of 90 cobalt gray equivalent using combined photon–proton irradiation with accelerated fractionation. Three-year OS, however, was still poor at 18% [20].

As in all gliomas, the extent of resection in HGG appears to be the factor most influential in long-term outcome, including survival. For GBM, when >90% of the tumor can be resected, the 5-year PFS is 35%, whereas when <90% is resected, this number drops to 17%. This PFS ratio remains double for AA as well (5-year PFS of 44% vs 22% for >90% vs <90% resection) [21,22].

There are limited published outcomes regarding the effect of delaying RT in younger children, although the data available suggests that this is a reasonable approach. The landmark "Baby POG" study included 18 patients <3 years old with HGG. These patients were treated with post-op chemotherapy and delayed RT. Five-year OS was 50%, and four children were able to avoid RT altogether [23]. A more recent French series reported on 21 patients <5 years old with HGG who received upfront chemotherapy after maximal resection with RT reserved for recurrence or progression. Five-year PFS was 35% and 5-year OS was 59% [24]. These two trials demonstrate that HGG in the very young may have a different clinical behavior than HGG in older pediatric patients and adults.

In summary, post-op RT is indicated in all patients with HGG who are older than 3 years of age, although there is at least one series that could advocate using age 5 as the minimum age [24,25]. The appropriate RT dose is between 54 and 60 Gy depending on a combination of factors, including nearby critical structures and patient age.

SIMULATION

Simulation consists of three parts: (1) patient positioning; (2) patient immobilization; and (3) computed tomography (CT) scanning [26].

Patient positioning and immobilization in pediatrics depend heavily upon the requirement for daily anesthesia and compliance with instructions. Patients are usually simulated supine with the neck neutral. For immobilization, some type of customized positioning device for the head is preferred. This positioning device can either be placed on a standard treatment table or integrated into a customized tabletop design.

Immobilization devices include thermoplastic mask systems and stereotactic fixation systems based on an individual dental cast or optical guidance. These systems have been shown to have an accuracy below 2 mm for daily setup [27,28]. Alternatively, a thermoplastic mask can also be used with excellent daily reproducibility and accuracy [29].

In pediatric patients requiring anesthesia, it may be difficult to use an oral stereotactic system, and so a thermoplastic mask system is preferred. Minimal disruption of mask integrity is necessary in case it needs to be cut to gain airway access. At the University of Florida, patients requiring anesthesia are considered for fiducial marker placement within the outer table of the skull. This process requires that four noncolinear titanium screws be placed by a neurosurgeon. The patient is simulated with the screws in place. Before each daily treatment, orthogonal imaging is done, the screws are marked, and then software autoregisters the coordinates and determines all position shifts required for that day's treatment.

CT scan acquisition should encompass the entire brain, and the AAPM TG-66 report recommends that at least 5 cm beyond the target volume be scanned. With a modern CT scanner, each axial cut can be as little as 1 mm, and the scan can still be done quickly. Smaller axial cuts (1–3 mm) allow for better contouring by reducing volume averaging and generate superior digital radiographic reconstructions.

TREATMENT PLANNING

Treatment planning refers to a complex process, but for this discussion, it will refer to the act of gross tumor volume (GTV), clinical target volume (CTV), and planning target volume (PTV) delineation. Per ICRU 50, which was intended for three-dimensional treatment planning, GTV refers to visible tumor, CTV refers to a region of potential microscopic tumor spread, and PTV refers to a region accommodating geometric uncertainties [30].

In CNS malignancies, the GTV is best defined by combining the CT dataset with a fusion-quality magnetic resonance imaging (MRI) scan. A fusion-quality MRI scan is not universally defined, but at the University of Florida, we order an MRI scan (either T1 with contrast or T2) of 1 mm axial thickness. An MRI scan with the slices separated more than 3 mm can be difficult to align accurately. Most commercial planning systems can fuse image datasets. Relying on CT planning alone for intracranial CNS malignancies has been shown to miss as much as 72% of the GTV [31]. In addition, image fusion results in significantly less interobserver variations in tumor definition [32].

For LGGs, the GTV includes all tumor and cysts visualized on the MRI. The MRI should be obtained as close to the time of treatment planning as possible, ideally within 30 days of the first treatment. This timing is crucial because the most frequent indication for RT in LGG is disease progression after either chemotherapy or observation. CTV in the MRI fusion era is commonly a 5 mm expansion with anatomic limitations, meaning that the expansion is not uniform and rigid boundaries to spread are respected and not included. For example, a tumor adjacent to bone will not be expanded *through* the bone for the CTV expansion. PTV is a uniform expansion of 2 to 5 mm, depending on the accuracy of setup. The specific expansion needs to be determined by each institution. As described previously, the use of a stereotactic system (e.g., dental anatomy or optical guidance) would permit the use of smaller margins. The expansion from CTV to PTV is uniform without respect to anatomy.

The stereotactic RT series from Marcus et al actually bypassed the GTV to CTV expansion in some cases, with the rationale that many LGGs are not locally infiltrative and therefore may not require this margin. In the same series, the margin for PTV was as little as 2 mm using modern localization techniques. They did not find marginal failures to be a problem. It should be noted that 35 of the 50 patients in the series had grade I astrocytomas, while the remaining 15 had grade II astrocytomas [3].

For HGG, the GTV will include all tissues initially involved with disease and the entire residual tumor as defined by the contrast-enhanced preoperative and post-op MRI scans. Ideally, both image sets should be fused to the CT dataset for planning. There are two GTV volumes: the first volume (commonly called GTV1) includes the enhancing and nonenhancing areas of the tumor; the second volume (commonly called GTV2) includes the residual tumor seen on the post-op MRI. There is no GTV2 if the resection was a GTR. The CTV expansion for each GTV can vary so that, when constructing CTV1 and CTV2, a common practice is to use a 2 cm anatomically confined expansion for GTV1 and a 1 cm anatomically confined expansion for GTV2. As with LGGs, the PTV expansion is a uniform expansion, usually ranging from 2 to 5 mm, and is institution specific.

In the current COG HGG protocol, the PTV1 dose is 54 Gy and the PTV2 dose is 5.4 Gy. Therefore, if the surgery is a GTR, there is no PTV2 and the final dose is 54 Gy. In all other cases, the target dose is 59.4 Gy, with accommodations made for critical structures.

TOXICITY

The therapeutic ratio of adjuvant RT for HGG is clear, with little debate that the benefits outweigh the risks in all but the youngest patients. In the LGG population, the decision is not as straightforward: while a significant percentage of patients have indications for adjuvant radiation, the side effects and potential complications of treatment prompt many oncologists to delay or forgo radiation. This topic is an area of active controversy. Although recent data highlights the neurocognitive effects associated with chemotherapy alone, this section will focus on the neurotoxicity and other treatment-related sequelae observed in LGG patients treated with RT ± chemotherapy.

A number of retrospective studies have asserted that radiation, through alterations of both white matter and microvasculature [33], is the major contributor to the wide range of neurological symptoms observed in patients with brain tumors. These studies have been criticized on the basis of numerous methodological and therapeutic shortcomings [34–41], but nonetheless carry great influence among oncologists due to their breadth. Another limitation includes the fact that with a few exceptions [42], these retrospective studies do not specifically address pediatric patients, who face additional challenges due to unique developmental issues.

Regardless of the population, the main difficulty in assessing neurotoxicity is that the neuropsychological symptoms related to LGG can overlap with side effects attributed to treatment. For example, in a rigorous prospective long-term study including adult patients with LGG who never received RT, Klein et al documented a higher rate of depression, fatigue, stress, memory loss, distractibility, and speech problems in patients with LGG compared to unaffected controls [39]. In a similar study limited to pediatric patients, North et al found that 40% of children with LGG who had never been treated with RT were cognitively impaired [43].

Longitudinal prospective studies have attempted to isolate the effect of RT by performing an extensive battery of psychometric tests at baseline (before RT) and at subsequent intervals for as long as 5 years after completing RT [44–46]. By evaluating cognitive function as it changed over time, these studies allowed patients to serve as their own controls. In each cohort examined, patients underwent various neurocognitive assessments before receiving between 50.4 and 64.8 Gy focal radiation at 1.8 to 2 Gy/fx. Each study found cognitive function to be generally stable—and in some cases, improved [46]—following RT. This data has lead authors to conclude that if moderate-dose RT is delivered in a focal manner for adult LGG, the neurocognitive toxicity of treatment is minimal and acceptable [39,46–48]. Whether LGG or HGG, recurrent or progressive brain tumors ultimately provide the largest source of neuropsychological disability.

Radiation necrosis following treatment for LGG is less controversial than neurotoxicity. The incidence falls between 1% to 3% [43,49–52]. and is probably dependant on total dose [53] and fraction size [54]. Acute toxic effects of RT, including mild headache, skin reactions, otitis, and occasional nausea and vomiting, are also well recognized and widely accepted. These acute reactions rarely become severe enough to necessitate a change in treatment. For example, in the 154 LGG patients who received focal RT in the EORTC 22845 trial, only six had treatment interruptions caused by acute toxicity [1]. Approximately 20% of patients experience peritumoral edema in the weeks following treatment, but this usually passes in 6 to 12 months without clinical sequelae [55,56].

Because of the perceived impact of brain radiation on CNS development and the risk of second malignancies, chemotherapy has become the adjuvant treatment of choice for children with LGG younger than 10 years old. In many infants or children with unresectable midline tumors, chemotherapy may be the only treatment. The toxicity of radiation in children with LGG has been comprehensively reviewed in a recent article by Kortmann et al [57]; however, most of the toxicity data cited in that publication and elsewhere comes from a historical series where children were treated with large-field radiation [42,58,59]. Consistent with adult data [35], recent experience suggests that focal irradiation may be less detrimental [60–64]. In one study by Merchant et al, 35 pediatric LGG patients treated with conformal irradiation did not demonstrate significant IQ deficits as noted with 30 months of follow-up [65]. The effectiveness and toxicity of conformal radiation in patients with LGG is systematically being examined in a current phase II COG study (ACNS0221). With 20-year survival rates now exceeding 80% in children with LGG, survivors face an elevated risk of second malignancies disproportionate to their adult counterparts [57]. Presumably, limiting field sizes will reduce this risk as well. In particular, children with neurofibromatosis have an elevated risk of neurocognitive dysfunction at baseline, but this seems to become disproportionately elevated following RT [42,66,67]. Neurofibromatosis has also been associated with a baseline increase in second malignancies.

Endocrine dysfunction, radiation vasculopathy, and optic neuropathy are side effects specific to tumor location that occur in both adults and pediatric patients with LGG and are primarily associated with midline tumors, such as optic pathway gliomas. In much of the literature to date, the causative relationship between the tumor, surgery, radiation, and chemotherapy cannot be discerned. Regardless, endocrine dysfunction is common (up to 80% in patients with optic pathway gliomas) and can have a dramatic impact on development if not recognized early in children. Pierce et al observed a 74% incidence of treatment-related endocrinopathy, with growth hormone most frequently affected [68]. Radiation vasculopathy is characterized by atheromatous changes and basilar or carotid artery stenosis predisposing a patient to infarction. The incidence has been reported to be 19% overall, with a higher prevalence observed in neurofibromatosis patients [69]. Fortunately, with conventional doses and fractionation, optic neuropathy is rare (1.6%) following RT for LGG [57,70,71]. This is important as most optic pathway tumors cannot be completely removed with surgery and thus have indication for RT ± chemotherapy.

FUTURE DIRECTIONS

The future of RT in pediatric CNS tumors, including gliomas, will continue to focus on refining indications, implementing new treatment modalities, and further improving treatment delivery.

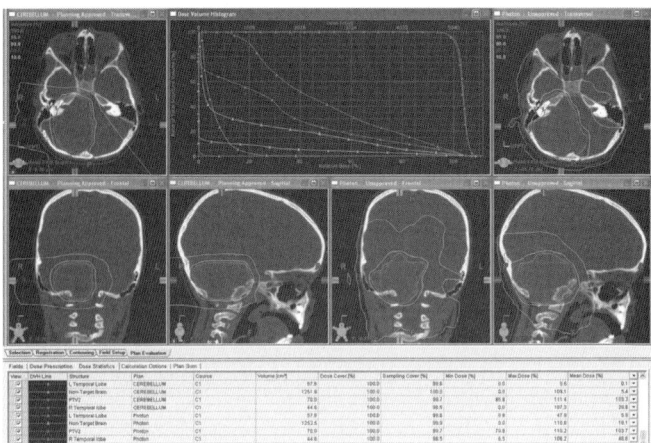

Figure 87.1 Dosimetric comparison of proton therapy and IMRT for a patient with LGG of the posterior fossa treated at the University of Florida Proton Therapy Institute. *See color insert.*

The initial role of RT in HGG for children older than 3 years seems to be relatively entrenched at this time. Likewise, today's limited role of RT in pediatric grade II astrocytomas is relatively consistent, but new technology shows promise in reducing the late toxicity of RT and thereby offers an increased therapeutic ratio in LGG. These results will presumably lead to expanded use of RT and new challenges. For example, treatment delivery through intensity-modulated RT improves tumor conformality while decreasing the dose to specified nontarget structures [72,73]. Techniques such as "conformal avoidance" can then be used to avoid these structures safely [74]. We are learning which parts of the brain may be more sensitive to RT effects, but many techniques are still under investigation.

Proton therapy is another new modality becoming more available within the United States and across the globe. Through the unique physical characteristics of protons, this form of RT has the ability to give both excellent tumor coverage while significantly decreasing dose to the nontarget brain (Figure 87.1). This decade alone has seen the development of three new sites for proton therapy (Indiana University; MD Anderson Cancer Center, Houston; and the University of Florida, Jacksonville). Before the end of the decade, additional centers are expected at the University of Pennsylvania and in Oklahoma City. There are also prospects of a single-room proton system, which, if built, would significantly increase the potential scope of proton therapy. Limited availability at this time keeps this technology from becoming a standard of care.

REFERENCES

1. van den Bent MJ, Afra D, de Witte O, et al. Long-term efficacy of early versus delayed radiotherapy for low-grade astrocytoma and oligodendroglioma in adults: the EORTC 22845 randomised trial. *Lancet.* 2005;366(9490):985–990.
2. Mishra KK, Puri DR, Missett BT, et al. The role of up-front radiation therapy for incompletely resected pediatric WHO grade II low-grade gliomas. *Neuro-oncology.* 2006;8(2):166–174.

3. Marcus KJ, Goumnerova L, Billett AL, et al. Stereotactic radiotherapy for localized low-grade gliomas in children: final results of a prospective trial. *Int J Radiat Oncol Biol Phys*. 2005;61(2):374–379.
4. Karim AB, Maat B, Hatlevoll R, et al. A randomized trial on dose-response in radiation therapy of low-grade cerebral glioma: European Organization for Research and Treatment of Cancer (EORTC) Study 22844. *Int J Radiat Oncol Biol Phys*. 1996;36(3):549–556.
5. Pignatti F, van den Bent M, Curran D, et al. Prognostic factors for survival in adult patients with cerebral low-grade glioma. *J Clin Oncol*. 2002;20(8):2076–2084.
6. Shaw EG, Daumas-Duport C, Scheithauer BW, et al. Radiation therapy in the management of low-grade supratentorial astrocytomas. *J Neurosurg*. 1989;70(6):853–861.
7. Peraud A, Goetz C, Siefert A, Tonn JC, Kreth FW. Interstitial iodine-125 radiosurgery alone or in combination with microsurgery for pediatric patients with eloquently located low-grade glioma: a pilot study. *Childs Nerv Syst*. 2007;23(1):39–46.
8. Chuba PJ, Zamarano L, Hamre M, et al. Permanent I-125 brain stem implants in children. *Childs Nerv Syst*. 1998;14(10):570–577.
9. Fisher BJ, Leighton CC, Vujovic O, Macdonald DR, Stitt L. Results of a policy of surveillance alone after surgical management of pediatric low grade gliomas. *Int J Radiat Oncol Biol Phys*. 2001;51(3):704–710.
10. Gorlia T, van den Bent MJ, Hegi ME, et al. Nomograms for predicting survival of patients with newly diagnosed glioblastoma: prognostic factor analysis of EORTC and NCIC trial 26981–22981/CE.3. *Lancet Oncol*. 2008;9(1):29–38.
11. van den Bent MJ. Anaplastic oligodendroglioma and oligoastrocytoma. *Neurol Clin*. 2007;25(4):1089–109, ix.
12. Donahue B, Scott CB, Nelson JS, et al. Influence of an oligodendroglial component on the survival of patients with anaplastic astrocytomas: a report of Radiation Therapy Oncology Group 83–02. *Int J Radiat Oncol Biol Phys*. 1997;38(5):911–914.
13. Marchese MJ, Chang CH. Malignant astrocytic gliomas in children. *Cancer*. 1990;65(12):2771–2778.
14. Phuphanich S, Edwards MS, Levin VA, et al. Supratentorial malignant gliomas of childhood. Results of treatment with radiation therapy and chemotherapy. *J Neurosurg*. 1984;60(3):495–499.
15. Sposto R, Ertel IJ, Jenkin RD, et al. The effectiveness of chemotherapy for treatment of high grade astrocytoma in children: results of a randomized trial. A report from the Childrens Cancer Study Group. *J Neurooncol*. 1989;7(2):165–177.
16. Graf R, Hildebrandt B, Tilly W, et al. Dose-escalated conformal radiotherapy of glioblastomas – results of a retrospective comparison applying radiation doses of 60 and 70 Gy. *Onkologie*. 2005;28(6–7):325–330.
17. Fulton DS, Urtasun RC, Scott-Brown I, et al. Increasing radiation dose intensity using hyperfractionation in patients with malignant glioma. Final report of a prospective phase I-II dose response study. *J Neurooncol*. 1992;14(1):63–72.
18. Walker MD, Strike TA, Sheline GE. An analysis of dose-effect relationship in the radiotherapy of malignant gliomas. *Int J Radiat Oncol Biol Phys*. 1979;5(10):1725–1731.
19. Werner-Wasik M, Scott CB, Nelson DF, et al. Final report of a phase I/II trial of hyperfractionated and accelerated hyperfractionated radiation therapy with carmustine for adults with supratentorial malignant gliomas. Radiation Therapy Oncology Group Study 83–02. *Cancer*. 1996;77(8):1535–1543.
20. Fitzek MM, Thornton AF, Rabinov JD, et al. Accelerated fractionated proton/photon irradiation to 90 cobalt gray equivalent for glioblastoma multiforme: results of a phase II prospective trial. *J Neurosurg*. 1999;91(2):251–260.
21. Campbell JW, Pollack IF, Martinez AJ, Shultz B. High-grade astrocytomas in children: radiologically complete resection is associated with an excellent long-term prognosis. *Neurosurgery*. 1996;38(2):258–264.
22. Wisoff JH, Boyett JM, Berger MS, et al. Current neurosurgical management and the impact of the extent of resection in the treatment of malignant gliomas of childhood: a report of the Children's Cancer Group trial no. CCG-945. *J Neurosurg*. 1998;89(1):52–59.
23. Duffner PK, Krischer JP, Burger PC, et al. Treatment of infants with malignant gliomas: the Pediatric Oncology Group experience. *J Neurooncol*. 1996;28(2–3):245–256.
24. Dufour C, Grill J, Lellouch-Tubiana A, et al. High-grade glioma in children under 5 years of age: a chemotherapy only approach with the BBSFOP protocol. *Eur J Cancer*. 2006;42(17):2939–2945.
25. Broniscer A. Past, present, and future strategies in the treatment of high-grade glioma in children. *Cancer Invest*. 2006;24(1):77–81.
26. Mutic S, Palta JR, Butker EK, et al. Quality assurance for computed-tomography simulators and the computed-tomography-simulation process: report of the AAPM Radiation Therapy Committee Task Group No. 66. *Med Phys*. 2003;30(10):2762–2792.
27. Sweeney RA, Bale R, Auberger T, et al. A simple and non-invasive vacuum mouthpiece-based head fixation system for high precision radiotherapy. *Strahlenther Onkol*. 2001;177(1):43–47.
28. Tomé WA, Meeks SL, McNutt TR, et al. Optically guided intensity modulated radiotherapy. *Radiother Oncol*. 2001;61(1):33–44.
29. Fuss M, Salter BJ, Cheek D, Sadeghi A, Hevezi JM, Herman TS. Repositioning accuracy of a commercially available thermoplastic mask system. *Radiother Oncol*. 2004;71(3):339–345.
30. ICRU. *International Commission on Radiation Units and Measurements 62: Prescribing, Recording, and Reporting Photon Beam Therapy*. Bethesda, MD: ICRU; 1999. Supplement to ICRU Report 50.
31. Lattanzi JP, Fein DA, McNeeley SW, Shaer AH, Movsas B, Hanks GE. Computed tomography-magnetic resonance image fusion: a clinical evaluation of an innovative approach for improved tumor localization in primary central nervous system lesions. *Radiat Oncol Investig*. 1997;5(4):195–205.
32. Aoyama H, Shirato H, Nishioka T, et al. Magnetic resonance imaging system for three-dimensional conformal radiotherapy and its impact on gross tumor volume delineation of central nervous system tumors. *Int J Radiat Oncol Biol Phys*. 2001;50(3):821–827.
33. Belka C, Budach W, Kortmann RD, Bamberg M. Radiation induced CNS toxicity-molecular and cellular mechanisms. *Br J Cancer*. 2001;85(9):1233–1239.
34. Surma-aho O, Niemelä M, Vilkki J, et al. Adverse long-term effects of brain radiotherapy in adult low-grade glioma patients. *Neurology*. 2001;56(10):1285–1290.
35. Kleinberg L, Wallner K, Malkin MG. Good performance status of long-term disease-free survivors of intracranial gliomas. *Int J Radiat Oncol Biol Phys*. 1993;26(1):129–133.
36. Gregor A, Cull A, Traynor E, Stewart M, Lander F, Love S. Neuropsychometric evaluation of long-term survivors of adult brain tumours: relationship with tumour and treatment parameters. *Radiother Oncol*. 1996;41(1):55–59.
37. Curnes JT, Laster DW, Ball MR, Moody DM, Witcofski RL. MRI of radiation injury to the brain. *AJR Am J Roentgenol*. 1986;147(1):119–124.
38. Scheibel RS, Meyers CA, Levin VA. Cognitive dysfunction following surgery for intracerebral glioma: influence of histopathology, lesion location, and treatment. *J Neurooncol*. 1996;30(1):61–69.
39. Klein M, Heimans JJ, Aaronson NK, et al. Effect of radiotherapy and other treatment-related factors on mid-term to long-term cognitive sequelae in low-grade gliomas: a comparative study. *Lancet*. 2002;360(9343):1361–1368.
40. Imperato JP, Paleologos NA, Vick NA. Effects of treatment on long-term survivors with malignant astrocytomas. *Ann Neurol*. 1990;28(6):818–822.
41. Laack NN, Brown PD. Cognitive sequelae of brain radiation in adults. *Semin Oncol*. 2004;31(5):702–713.
42. Chadderton RD, West CG, Schuller S, et al. Radiotherapy in the treatment of low-grade astrocytomas. II. The physical and cognitive sequelae. *Childs Nerv Syst*. 1995;11(8):443–448.
43. North CA, North RB, Epstein JA, Piantadosi S, Wharam MD. Low-grade cerebral astrocytomas. Survival and quality of life after radiation therapy. *Cancer*. 1990;66(1):6–14.
44. Armstrong C, Mollman J, Corn BW, Alavi J, Grossman M. Effects of radiation therapy on adult brain behavior: evidence for a rebound phenomenon in a phase 1 trial. *Neurology*. 1993;43(10):1961–1965.
45. Armstrong CL, Hunter JV, Ledakis GE, et al. Late cognitive and radiographic changes related to radiotherapy: initial prospective findings. *Neurology*. 2002;59(1):40–48.
46. Laack NN, Brown PD, Ivnik RJ, et al. Cognitive function after radiotherapy for supratentorial low-grade glioma: a North Central Cancer Treatment Group prospective study. *Int J Radiat Oncol Biol Phys*. 2005;63(4):1175–1183.
47. Taphoorn MJ, Schiphorst AK, Snoek FJ, et al. Cognitive functions and quality of life in patients with low-grade gliomas: the impact of radiotherapy. *Ann Neurol*. 1994;36(1):48–54.
48. Gunderson LL, Tepper JE. *Low-Grade Gliomas. Clinical Radiation Oncology*. 2nd ed. Philadelphia, PA: Churchill Livingstone; 2006.
49. Miralbell R, Balart J, Matias-Guiu X, Molet J, Ariza A, Craven-Bartle J. Radiotherapy for supratentorial low-grade gliomas: results and

prognostic factors with special focus on tumour volume parameters. *Radiother Oncol.* 1993;27(2):112–116.
50. Piepmeier JM, Christopher S. Low-grade gliomas: introduction and overview. *J Neurooncol.* 1997;34(1):1–3.
51. Shaw EG, Scheithauer BW, Gilbertson DT, et al. Postoperative radiotherapy of supratentorial low-grade gliomas. *Int J Radiat Oncol Biol Phys.* 1989;16(3):663–668.
52. Janny P, Cure H, Mohr M, et al. Low grade supratentorial astrocytomas. Management and prognostic factors. *Cancer.* 1994;73(7):1937–1945.
53. Shaw E, Arusell R, Scheithauer B, et al. Prospective randomized trial of low- versus high-dose radiation therapy in adults with supratentorial low-grade glioma: initial report of a North Central Cancer Treatment Group/Radiation Therapy Oncology Group/Eastern Cooperative Oncology Group study. *J Clin Oncol.* 2002;20(9):2267–2276.
54. Grabb PA, Lunsford LD, Albright AL, Kondziolka D, Flickinger JC. Stereotactic radiosurgery for glial neoplasms of childhood. *Neurosurgery.* 1996;38(4):696–701; discussion 701.
55. Sung DI. Suprasellar tumors in children: a review of clinical manifestations and managements. *Cancer.* 1982;50(7):1420–1425.
56. Freeman CR, Souhami L, Caron JL, et al. Stereotactic external beam irradiation in previously untreated brain tumors in children and adolescents. *Med Pediatr Oncol.* 1994;22(3):173–180.
57. Kortmann RD, Timmermann B, Taylor RE, et al. Current and future strategies in radiotherapy of childhood low-grade glioma of the brain. Part II: Treatment-related late toxicity. *Strahlenther Onkol.* 2003;179(9):585–597.
58. al-Mefty O, Kersh JE, Routh A, Smith RR. The long-term side effects of radiation therapy for benign brain tumors in adults. *J Neurosurg.* 1990;73(4):502–512.
59. Barr RD, Simpson T, Whitton A, Rush B, Furlong W, Feeny DH. Health-related quality of life in survivors of tumours of the central nervous system in childhood–a preference-based approach to measurement in a cross-sectional study. *Eur J Cancer.* 1999;35(2):248–255.
60. Freeman CR, Farmer JP, Montes J. Low-grade astrocytomas in children: evolving management strategies. *Int J Radiat Oncol Biol Phys.* 1998;41(5):979–987.
61. Steen RG, Koury B S M, Granja CI, et al. Effect of ionizing radiation on the human brain: white matter and gray matter T1 in pediatric brain tumor patients treated with conformal radiation therapy. *Int J Radiat Oncol Biol Phys.* 2001;49(1):79–91.
62. Debus J, Kocagoncu KO, Hoss A, Wenz F, Wannenmacher M. Fractionated stereotactic radiotherapy (FSRT) for optic glioma. *Int J Radiat Oncol Biol Phys.* 1999;44(2):243–248.
63. Hug EB, Muenter MW, Archambeau JO, et al. Conformal proton radiation therapy for pediatric low-grade astrocytomas. *Strahlenther Onkol.* 2002;178(1):10–17.
64. Saran FH, Baumert BG, Khoo VS, et al. Stereotactically guided conformal radiotherapy for progressive low-grade gliomas of childhood. *Int J Radiat Oncol Biol Phys.* 2002;53(1):43–51.
65. Merchant TE, Goloubeva O, Kiehna EN et al. Neurocognitive effects of radiation therapy. *Int J Radiat Oncol Biol Phys.* 2001;51:136.
66. Tao ML, Barnes PD, Billett AL, et al. Childhood optic chiasm gliomas: radiographic response following radiotherapy and long-term clinical outcome. *Int J Radiat Oncol Biol Phys.* 1997;39(3):579–587.
67. Cappelli C, Grill J, Raquin M, et al. Long-term follow up of 69 patients treated for optic pathway tumours before the chemotherapy era. *Arch Dis Child.* 1998;79(4):334–338.
68. Pierce SM, Barnes PD, Loeffler JS, McGinn C, Tarbell NJ. Definitive radiation therapy in the management of symptomatic patients with optic glioma. Survival and long-term effects. *Cancer.* 1990;65(1):45–52.
69. Grill J, Couanet D, Cappelli C, et al. Radiation-induced cerebral vasculopathy in children with neurofibromatosis and optic pathway glioma. *Ann Neurol.* 1999;45(3):393–396.
70. Aristizabal S, Caldwell WL, Avila J. The relationship of time-dose fractionation factors to complications in the treatment of pituitary tumors by irradiation. *Int J Radiat Oncol Biol Phys.* 1977;2(7–8):667–673.
71. Becker G, Kocher M, Kortmann RD, et al. Radiation therapy in the multimodal treatment approach of pituitary adenoma. *Strahlenther Onkol.* 2002;178(4):173–186.
72. Merchant TE, Kiehna EN, Li C, et al. Modeling radiation dosimetry to predict cognitive outcomes in pediatric patients with CNS embryonal tumors including medulloblastoma. *Int J Radiat Oncol Biol Phys.* 2006;65(1):210–221.
73. Bradbury J. New targets identified for preventing cognitive decline after cranial irradiation. *Lancet Oncol.* 2002;3(9):521.
74. Ghia A, Tomé WA, Thomas S, et al. Distribution of brain metastases in relation to the hippocampus: implications for neurocognitive functional preservation. *Int J Radiat Oncol Biol Phys.* 2007;68(4):971–977.

# 88 Medulloblastoma and Primitive Neuroectodermal Tumors

John C. Breneman

INTRODUCTION

The outlook for patients with medulloblastoma has improved significantly over the past several decades. Overall survival of children diagnosed in the 1950s and 1960s was less than 35%, with 25% succumbing to operative mortality [1]. Advances in surgical and radiotherapeutic technology, along with the introduction of chemotherapy into treatment regimens, have since doubled this survival rate with approximately 70% of patients now attaining long-term survival.

Medulloblastoma is usually recognized as a subset of neoplasms termed primitive neuroectodermal tumors (PNETs) [2]. PNETs arising in the posterior fossa are called medulloblastoma, and those that arise elsewhere in the brain are termed supratentorial PNET (though many authors retain the term pineoblastoma for PNETs of the pineal region). Medulloblastoma represents the great majority of PNETs with supratentorial PNET accounting for only about 15% of tumors. Primary spinal PNET is rare [3].

Medulloblastoma is primarily a disease of the young with a mean age at diagnosis of 9 years and 70% of tumors occurring before the age of 16 years [4]. It accounts for as many as 30% of all childhood brain tumors [5]. Although medulloblastoma occurs in adults, it is rare after the age of 40 years. There is an approximately 3:2 male to female distribution, and the incidence is higher in Caucasians than in Blacks.

Approximately three-fourths of medulloblastomas arise in the vermis of the cerebellum. Lateralization to the cerebellar hemispheres correlates with increasing patient age. Dissemination of medulloblastoma occurs primarily via the cerebrospinal fluid (CSF) and can be detected at diagnosis in approximately 20% of patients. However, patterns of treatment failure indicate a much higher incidence of subclinical involvement of the CSF, and any treatment strategy must incorporate cytotoxic therapy to the entire neuroaxis. Historically, most medulloblastoma treatment failures occurred in the posterior fossa. More recently, however, patterns of failure have shifted with the majority of failures now including at least a component of supratentorial or spine recurrence [6,7].

EVALUATION

Maximal surgical resection establishes the diagnosis and is the first component of treatment for PNET. Imaging of the entire neuroaxis with magnetic resonance imaging (MRI) is required, along with cytologic examination of the spinal CSF. Ideally, these evaluations are done preoperatively because of artifactual changes that can be induced by the surgical procedure. If done postoperatively, scanning and lumbar puncture should not be performed sooner than 2 weeks after surgery to minimize false-positive findings. Patients who have not had adequate staging have inferior outcomes, probably due to undertreatment of their disease [6].

RISK GROUPS

For purposes of establishing prognosis and guiding treatment, patients with PNET are categorized as either "average risk" or "high risk." High-risk features are generally agreed to include residual tumor of greater than 1.5 cm^2 on a postoperative MRI scan, leptomeningeal tumor dissemination, or supratentorial tumor location [8–10]. High-risk features are reported in 30% to 54% of patients [11,12]. Children under the age of 3 years also have inferior outcomes independent of these risk factors, but are usually considered separately due to significant differences in treatment approaches for this age group.

A TNM staging known as the Chang system has been described, but is not commonly used as it has limited prognostic value, especially with regard to T stage [9,10,12]. The M stage (Table 88.1) does have prognostic significance, however, with M1 patients typically faring better than M2–4 [10,13]. Additionally, large cell anaplastic histology and glial differentiation are associated with inferior survival [6,7,14] as are low trkC and elevated Ki-67, ERBB2 protein and c-myc mRNA expression [15–18]. These biologic and molecular risk factors are beginning to be incorporated into risk-based treatment algorithms.

EVOLUTION OF RADIOTHERAPY TREATMENT—CLINICAL TRIALS

Prior to the 1980s, medulloblastoma was treated rather uniformly using maximal surgical resection followed by radiotherapy to the craniospinal axis with the addition of single-agent chemotherapy [19]. Radiotherapy doses of 30 to 40 Gy to the spine and 50 Gy to the posterior fossa were typical. Today, surgery followed by craniospinal irradiation

Table 88.1 M Staging of PNET Tumors

M0:	No evidence of subarachnoid or hematogenous metastasis
M1:	Microscopic tumor cells in CSF
M2:	Gross nodular intracranial seeding distant from the primary site
M3a:	Gross nodular spinal seeding without intracranial seeding
M3b:	Gross nodular intracranial and spinal seeding
M4:	Extraneural metastasis

(CSI) with a supplemental boost to the primary tumor site remains the backbone of treatment for medulloblastoma. However, numerous modifications to this approach have been explored, driven by two factors—the desire to reduce the morbidity often associated with CSI, and the wish to improve cure rates by adding multiagent chemotherapy to the treatment regimens. A number of clinical trials have been conducted in Europe and North America testing various schemes of radiotherapy doses and treatment volumes, along with a variety of chemotherapy combinations and timings (Table 88.2). Radiotherapy study questions usually involve attempts to reduce the dose or volume of radiation or the use of altered fractionation schemes. Chemotherapy questions address the efficacy of different drug combinations and intensities and the timing of chemotherapy relative to radiotherapy. Much has been learned from these trials, though some caution must be exercised when attempting to make inter-trial comparisons. In particular, the methods of staging patients and the definition of risk groups often differ among studies. The following sections summarize outcomes of the major trials by risk group and treatment strategy.

Average Risk Patients

Reduced Dose Radiotherapy Trials

The successful use of reduced dose radiotherapy for average-risk medulloblastoma is intimately linked to the addition of adjuvant chemotherapy to the treatment regimen. Although early single-institution pilot studies suggested that CSI dose as the sole treatment modality could be decreased for average-risk patients without compromising survival [20,21,] cooperative group trials that reduced the dose of CSI in the absence of effective adjuvant chemotherapy were associated with inferior outcomes. The Children's Cancer Group (CCG) and Pediatric Oncology Group (POG) conducted a joint study, CCG 923/POG 8631, which randomized average-risk patients to receive 36 versus 23.4 Gy CSI with all receiving 54 Gy to the posterior fossa. No chemotherapy was given. The trial closed early after interim analysis revealed increased failures in the reduced CSI dose arm, and 5-year event-free survival (EFS) was 52% in the reduced dose CSI arm versus 67% in the standard dose arm [22]. Subsequent reduced dose radiotherapy trials, summarized in the following section, added chemotherapy to reduced dose radiotherapy with greater success. In particular, the CCG 9892 and Children's Oncology Group (COG) A9961 studies discussed below yielded 5-year progression-free survival (PFS) of approximately 80%, defining the current standard of care for average-risk medulloblastoma in North America [6,12].

Attempts are being made to further reduce the CSI dose to 18 Gy in selected patients. A pilot study of 10 children with average-risk medulloblastoma reported 70% PFS at 6 years with 18 Gy CSI and 50.4 to 55.8 Gy to the posterior fossa given concurrently with vincristine, followed by vincristine, CCNU, and cisplatin [23]. The current COG average-risk medulloblastoma study is investigating in a prospective randomized trial the efficacy of reduced CSI dose of 18 Gy together with adjuvant chemotherapy in children less than 8 years of age.

Neoadjuvant Chemotherapy Trials

Several studies have examined preradiotherapy (neoadjuvant) chemotherapy for patients with average-risk medulloblastoma, often in conjunction with a decreased CSI dose. The SIOP II trial accrued patients from 1984 to 1989 and was designed with a double randomization. Patients were randomized to receive or not receive neoadjuvant procarbazine, vincristine, and methotrexate and also to receive either 35 or 25 Gy CSI. All patients were given a boost to the posterior fossa. No advantage was seen for the addition of chemotherapy in this study, and in fact, the cohort receiving chemotherapy followed by reduced dose CSI had inferior outcomes with only a 42% 5-year EFS—a result attributed to the choice of suboptimal chemotherapy and the delay in radiotherapy from the neoadjuvant treatment [24]. Survival for other cohorts was 55% to 68%.

Neoadjuvant chemotherapy with "eight drugs in 1 day" for two cycles was tested nonrandomly in the French M7 study, which accrued patients from 1985 to 1988. Study outcome was tainted by inadequate staging and problems with radiotherapy quality control. However, 5-year EFS for average-risk patients was a respectable 74% [11].

The German HIT 91 trial, conducted between 1991 and 1997, tested the timing of adjuvant chemotherapy relative to radiotherapy in both average- and high-risk patients. The study randomized children to neoadjuvant chemotherapy with ifosfamide, etoposide, cisplatin, cytarabine, and high-dose methotrexate versus postradiotherapy chemotherapy with CCNU, cisplatin, and vincristine. Radiotherapy with a CSI dose of 35.2 Gy and posterior fossa dose of 55.2 Gy was given [13]. Neoadjuvant chemotherapy was associated with increased myelotoxicity and treatment delays during radiotherapy. Three-year EFS for patients with M1 disease or better was 65% for neoadjuvant chemotherapy versus 78% for post-XRT chemotherapy, suggesting a detriment to the delays associated with the neoadjuvant arm.

The French Society of Pediatric Oncology conducted a nonrandomized study between 1991 and 1998 using neoadjuvant "eight drugs in 1 day" followed by etoposide and carboplatin. A reduced dose of CSI with 25 Gy was used. Five-year EFS was 65% [25].

The best outcomes for neoadjuvant chemotherapy in average-risk medulloblastoma were obtained in the PNET-3 trial [26]. This study, which accrued patients from 1992 to 2003, is the only randomized trial to show a benefit for chemotherapy in average-risk patients. Standard radiotherapy

Table 88.2 Selected Medulloblastoma Clinical Trials

Trial	No. of Patients	Risk Groups	Dates of Accrual	Randomized	Pre-XRT Chemo	Post-XRT Chemo	XRT Dose/Volume/Fractionation	Major Findings
CCG/RTOG [46]	233	Both	1975–1981	Yes		X		Improved survival for M+ patients treated with chemo
SIOP I [28]	286	Both	1975–1980	Yes		X		Early survival advantage for chemo lost with further follow-up
POG 7909 [29]	71	Both	1979–1986	Yes		X		Trend toward improved survival with chemo
CHOP Multicenter [47]	63	High	1983–1993	No		X	X	67% 5 year PFS for M+ patients.
SIOP II (MED84) [24]	135	High	1984–1989	Yes	X	X		No advantage to neo-adjuvant chemo
SIOP II (MED84) [24]	229	Average	1984–1989	Yes	X		X	Inferior outcome for neo-adjuvant chemo with reduced dose CSI
French M7 [11]	68	Both	1985–1988	No	X	X		7-year DFS 62% in average risk and 57% in high risk patients
CCG 921 [10]	203	High	1986–1992	Yes	X	X		Inferior survival with neo-adjuvant chemo compared to post-radiotherapy chemo
CCG 923/POG 8631 [22]	81	Average	1986–1990	Yes			X	Inferior survival for 23.4 Gy CSI without chemo.
POG 8695 [40]	30	High	1986–1990	No	X			23% of patients progressed during neo-adjuvant chemo. 40% 2 yr PFS.
HIT 88/89 [27]	94	Both	1987–1991	No	X		X	5-year EFS 57% for all patient groups
CCG 9892 [101]	65	Average	1990–1994	No		X	X	5-year PFS of 79%
POG 9031 [42]	210	High	1990–1996	Yes	X	X		No advantage to neo-adjuvant chemo. 5 yr EFS of 68% for all patients
HIT 91 [13]	137	Both	1991–1997	Yes	X	X		Inferior survival with neo-adjuvant chemo for average risk patients
SFOP [25]	136	Average	1991–1998	No	X		X	5-year PFS of 72%
PNET-3 [43]	68	High	1992–2000	No	X			5-year PFS 35%
PNET 3 [26]	179	Average	1992–2003	Yes	X			Improved survival for patients treated with chemo
SFOP [44]	115	High	1993–1999	No	X	X		5-year EFS 50%
CCG 9931 [45]	127	High	1994–1997	No	X		X	43 patients did not complete therapy primarily due to progression or toxicity
COG A9961 [6]	379	Average	1996–2000	Yes		X	X	5-year EFS 83%. No difference between two different post-radiation chemo regimens.
St. Jude-96 [7]	48	High	1996–2003	No		X		5-year EFS 70%
St. Jude-96 [7]	86	Average	1996–2003	No		X	X	5-year EFS 83%
M-SFOP [31]	48	Average	1998–2001	No			X	3-year PFS 81% without chemo
COG 99701 [48]	57	High	1998–2004	No		X		CSI, carboplatin and vincristine can be administered concurrently

doses were used, with half of patients randomly assigned to receive neoadjuvant vincristine, etoposide, carboplatin, and cyclophosphamide. A significant difference in 5-year EFS in favor of the chemotherapy arm was demonstrated (74% vs 60%) though the results are somewhat confounded by the inclusion of some patients who would now be considered as "high risk."

In general, chemotherapy given in the neoadjuvant setting has been associated with lower survivals than when given postradiotherapy, perhaps due to a deleterious effect of delaying radiotherapy [10,24,27]. Therefore, postradiotherapy chemotherapy has become the preferred treatment strategy in children with average-risk medulloblastoma.

Postradiotherapy Chemotherapy Trials

Postradiotherapy chemotherapy has the advantage of allowing radiotherapy to begin immediately following surgery and is subject to less risk of treatment delays due to complications from neoadjuvant therapy. One of the earliest adjuvant chemotherapy trials was the SIOP I study, conducted from 1975 to 1980. This study included both average- and high-risk patients and used standard radiotherapy doses given concurrently with vincristine, with patients randomized to receive or not receive postradiotherapy chemotherapy using vincristine and CCNU. The trial closed early due to an initial advantage for patients given adjuvant chemotherapy. However, with additional follow-up, this advantage was lost, and ultimately no survival difference was seen between the two treatment arms [28].

The POG 7909 trial accrued patients from 1979 to 1986 [29]. All patients with medulloblastoma were eligible, regardless of risk factors. Radiotherapy was given after surgery using 35 to 40 Gy CSI with posterior fossa boost to 54 Gy. Patients were randomized to receive or not receive postradiation chemotherapy with nitrogen mustard, vincristine, prednisone, and procarbazine (MOPP). A nonsignificant trend toward better survival was observed in the chemotherapy group with 5-year survival of 74% versus 56%.

The CCG studied postradiotherapy chemotherapy in a phase II study, CCG 9892, for average-risk patients. Reduced dose CSI with 23.4 Gy concurrent with vincristine was given, followed by CCNU, vincristine, and cisplatin. This study accrued patients from 1990 to 1994 and achieved one of the highest survival rates reported in a multi-institution trial with a 5-year PFS of 79% [12].

The excellent results from the CCG 9892 trial led to a follow-up study, COG A9961, testing two different postradiotherapy chemotherapy regimens. This study, which accrued from 1996 to 2000, used the same radiotherapy with 23.4 Gy CSI and posterior fossa boost followed by a randomization of CCG 9892 chemotherapy versus cyclophosphamide, cisplatin, and vincristine [6]. Though no difference was seen between the two chemotherapy regimens, the overall EFS at 5 years of 81% established the strategy of reduced dose CSI plus postoperative chemotherapy as the standard of care for average-risk medulloblastoma in North America.

Subsequently, these excellent results have been confirmed by another multi-institution trial. In a St Jude-based study, children with average-risk medulloblastoma were treated with 23.4 Gy CSI with a boost to 55.8 Gy to the primary site. Following radiotherapy, patients received high-dose cytoxan, cisplatin, and vincristine with stem cell rescue. Five-year EFS was 83% [7].

Reduced Radiotherapy Volume Trials

An attempt to decrease radiotherapy toxicity by excluding the supratentorial brain from the CSI resulted in an unacceptable failure rate [30]. However, there has been success in reducing the volume of the posterior fossa boost field in patients with average-risk disease. Decreasing the boost volume from the entire posterior fossa to the tumor bed plus a margin has been accomplished without compromising survival in a number of single-institution studies [31–34]. The current COG average-risk medulloblastoma trial is studying this prospectively and includes a randomization to boost only the tumor bed versus the entire posterior fossa.

Hyperfractionated Radiotherapy Trials

Hyperfractionated radiotherapy for medulloblastoma has been used both to decrease radiotherapy side effects [31,35,36] and to improve tumor control [36–38]. The recently reported M-SFOP 98 study used a hyperfractionated radiotherapy regimen without adjuvant chemotherapy. Patients received twice-daily treatment with 36 Gy CSI in 36 fractions and conformal boost to the tumor bed to a total dose of 68 Gy in 68 fractions. Three-year PFS was 81%, and though only 2-year neurocognitive follow-up is available, no decrease in intelligence has yet been observed [31]. Ongoing European studies are comparing the above hyperfractionated radiotherapy regimen to a conventionally fractionated regimen of 23.4 Gy CSI and 55.8 Gy to the posterior fossa, with all patients receiving post-XRT vincristine, cisplatin, and CCNU.

Current Standard of Care

Outside of the investigational setting, current standard of care for average-risk medulloblastoma in children older than 3 years consists of surgery followed by 23.4 Gy CSI given concurrently with vincristine weekly and a 30.6 Gy boost to the posterior fossa. Postradiotherapy chemotherapy using various combinations of drugs such as vincristine, cisplatin, carboplatin, CCNU and cyclophosphamide is then given. Long-term survival of approximately 80% of patients is expected with this approach. Though the addition of chemotherapy to the treatment of medulloblastoma carries additional long-term consequences [39,] it is likely that the radiotherapy dose reduction it allows is a favorable compromise, at least in the pediatric population.

High-Risk Patients

Long-term survival for patients with high-risk PNET is only about 50% and patients who are M+ fare even more poorly. Therefore, aggressive treatment regimens are required. These almost always consist of multimodality treatment programs with maximal surgery, followed by a combination of radiotherapy and chemotherapy.

Neoadjuvant Chemotherapy Trials

Neoadjuvant (pre-radiotherapy) chemotherapy has been extensively investigated for high-risk PNET. The SIOP II trial, conducted between 1984 and 1989, randomized patients to receive or not receive neoadjuvant procarbazine, vincristine, and methotrexate. All patients received postradiotherapy vincristine and CCNU. No benefit was demonstrated for neoadjuvant chemotherapy and 5-year EFS was 54% [24].

The French M7 trial accrued from 1985 to 1988. High-risk patients were nonrandomly assigned to two cycles of neoadjuvant "eight drugs in 1 day" chemotherapy and four additional cycles of the same chemotherapy following completion of radiotherapy [11]. A somewhat nonstandard radiotherapy regimen was used with patients receiving 30 to 36 Gy to the spine, 27 Gy to the brain, and 50 to 55 Gy to the posterior fossa. Five-year disease free survival (DFS) was 57%.

A similar chemotherapy regimen was used in the CCG 921 study conducted between 1986 and 1982. It compared "eight drugs in 1 day" given both before and after radiotherapy to a regimen of concurrent radiotherapy and vincristine followed by vincristine, CCNU, and prednisone (VCP). Radiotherapy for all patients consisted of 36 Gy CSI and 54 Gy to the primary site. PFS for the neoadjuvant arm was significantly inferior with a 5-year PFS of 47% versus 64% for post-XRT VCP [10]. Potential reasons cited for the suboptimal results with neoadjuvant chemotherapy arm include the delay in XRT administration, lack of concurrent vincristine with the XRT, and lesser vincristine dose intensity.

POG 8695 was a phase II study conducted between 1986 and 1990. It used neoadjuvant vincristine, cisplatin, and cyclophosphamide followed by 36 Gy CSI with 54 Gy to the primary site and additional boosts to sites of metastatic tumor [40]. A response rate of 43% to the neoadjuvant therapy was seen. However, 7 of 36 patients had progressive disease during chemotherapy, again raising concerns regarding the consequences of delayed radiotherapy.

The HIT 88/89 German phase II feasibility study accrued patients from 1987 to 1991. Two cycles of neoadjuvant procarbazine, ifosfamide, etoposide, methotrexate, cisplatin, and cytarabine were given postoperatively. Subsequently, radiotherapy was given using 35.2 Gy CSI and posterior fossa boost to 55.2 Gy beginning a mean of 23 weeks after surgery [27]. Five-year PFS was 33% with most failures occurring outside the posterior fossa. Objective response to the neoadjuvant chemotherapy was predictive for better survival, though 14% of patients experienced tumor progression during chemotherapy. This study was followed by HIT 91, which was active between 1991 and 1997 [13]. HIT 91 was a randomized trial comparing the HIT 88/89 neoadjuvant chemotherapy to post-radiation chemotherapy with vincristine, CCNU, and cisplatin. No difference was seen between the neoadjuvant and postradiation chemotherapy arms, with a relapse-free survival at 30 months of 30% for patients with M2 or M3 disease.

POG 9031 was a randomized study conducted between 1990 and 1996. Radiotherapy consisted of 35.2 to 40 Gy CSI plus a boost, followed by vincristine and cyclophosphamide chemotherapy [41]. In addition, half were randomized to receive neoadjuvant cisplatin and etoposide with the other half receiving the same chemotherapy after radiotherapy. Overall, 5-year EFS was a very respectable 68%, with no difference between the two groups [42].

The PNET-3 study for high-risk medulloblastoma accrued patients between 1992 and 2000. This nonrandomized trial used four cycles of neoadjuvant vincristine, etoposide, carboplatin, and cyclophosphamide, followed by 35 Gy CSI with posterior fossa boost to 55 Gy [43]. Five-year EFS was 35%, which was significantly less than the contemporary POG 9031 study. Possible explanations for this difference include the higher CSI dose and more effective chemotherapy regimen used in the POG trial.

The French SFOP conducted a phase II study using "eight drugs in 1 day" plus etoposide and carboplatin given both before and after CSI [44]. Dose to the supratentorial brain was 30 to 36 Gy with dose to the spine of 36 Gy plus boosts when appropriate. This study accrued from 1993 to 1999 and achieved a 5-year EFS of 50%.

CCG 9931 was conducted between 1994 and 1997. It was a phase I/II study using neoadjuvant cyclophosphamide, vincristine, etoposide, cisplatin, and carboplatin, followed by hyperfractionated radiotherapy given as 1 Gy bid using 40 Gy CSI and 72 Gy to the primary site [45]. Although 127 patients were entered onto the study, only 84 were able to complete therapy, primarily due to disease progression during neoadjuvant chemotherapy and/or toxicity. Additionally, 3-year EFS was disappointing with only 46% of M0 patients and 38% of M+ patients free of disease.

It is difficult to evaluate the role of preoperative chemotherapy for high-risk PNET from these trials. The advantage of delivering chemotherapy to an unirradiated tumor may be negated by the delay in radiotherapy it causes. The encouraging results of the POG 9031 study suggest that escalating doses of radiotherapy may be one of the most important factors for improving survival in these high-risk patients.

Postradiotherapy Chemotherapy Trials

The CCG and the Radiation Therapy Oncology Group (RTOG) conducted a study of postradiotherapy chemotherapy beginning in 1975. This trial used radiotherapy doses of 35 to 40 Gy CSI with 15 to 20 Gy boost to the primary tumor and gross metastatic deposits. Patients were then randomized to receive or not receive post-XRT CCNU, vincristine, and prednisone. The trial included patients with both average- and high-risk disease, and overall, there was no survival difference between the two arms. However, in the subgroup of patients with high-risk features, adjuvant chemotherapy significantly improved survival from 0% to 46% [46]. Similarly, the SIOP I trial conducted from 1975 to 1980 used concurrent radiotherapy and vincristine, followed by adjuvant CCNU and vincristine. A survival benefit was observed for patients with high-risk features who received adjuvant chemotherapy [28].

A multi-institution study conducted from 1983 to 1993 used a regimen of concurrent radiotherapy and vincristine, followed by adjuvant cisplatin, CCNU, and vincristine. Overall 5-year PFS was an impressive 83% and even those with M2 and M3 disease had a 5-year PFS of 67% [47].

Another multicenter trial used 36 to 39.6 Gy CSI with boost to 55.8 Gy followed by dose-intense cyclophosphamide, cisplatin, and vincristine with stem-cell rescue [7]. In addition, some patients received neoadjuvant topotecan. Five-year EFS was 70% for all high-risk patients and 66% for those with metastatic disease.

Concurrent Radiotherapy and Chemotherapy Trials

The COG conducted a phase I/II trial from 1998 to 2004 using 36 Gy CSI concurrent with vincristine and carboplatin, followed by maintenance therapy with vincristine and cyclophosphamide plus/minus cisplatin. The 4-year EFS of 66% for the initial cohort of 57 patients was promising for this group of patients [48]. On the basis of this data, the COG is currently conducting a trial using vincristine and 36 Gy CSI plus boost with or without concurrent carboplatin, followed by vincristine, cyclophosphamide, and cisplatin plus/minus isoretionoin.

Hyperfractionated Radiotherapy Trials

Results of hyperfractionated XRT for high-risk PNET have largely been disappointing [38,45,] though this may be due in part to factors such as delays in beginning radiotherapy due to neoadjuvant chemotherapy, as occurred in the CCG 9931 trial mentioned earlier [45]. Currently, hyperfractionation is being studied in the United Kingdom CNS 2006 trial, which uses hyperfractionated accelerated radiotherapy together with cisplatin, CCNU, and vincristine chemotherapy.

Hyperfractionation introduces additional logistic and technical difficulties for the radiotherapy team, especially in the children who require anesthesia. Multiple-daily anesthesia with the required restrictions on food intake limits the feasibility of this approach [8].

Radiotherapy Dose Escalation Trials

No randomized studies investigating radiotherapy dose escalation for the treatment of high-risk PNET have been conducted. However, some of the best outcomes in this patient group used treatment regimens, which included radiotherapy doses of up to 40 Gy CSI [7,42]. The encouraging results of these studies with 5-year EFS as high as 70% may be due, in part, to their aggressive radiotherapy regimen.

Current Standard of Care

A current standard for treatment for high-risk PNET has not been defined. Most regimens use high doses of CSI (36–40 Gy) with primary site boost to a total of 55.8 to 59.4 Gy and boosts to 45 to 50 Gy for gross spinal disease. Intensive chemotherapy is given, usually following radiotherapy, though some approaches use concurrent or pre-radiotherapy chemotherapy. Five-year survivals for high-risk patients are typically 50% to 60%, with the worst prognoses seen in patients with extensive metastatic disease.

RADIOTHERAPY TECHNIQUE

CSI has been the standard radiotherapy technique for treatment of newly diagnosed medulloblastoma for more than 50 years [49]. Attempts to decrease the volume of tissue receiving radiotherapy have shown consistently inferior results [30,50,51]. CSI is one of the most technically demanding radiotherapy treatments that is performed. It requires a high level of clinical physics support and a radiation therapist staff who are experienced in the delivery of this treatment. Improved outcomes have been documented for centers that perform CSI frequently compared to those with less experience [28]. Conversely, inferior results are seen when radiotherapy technique is incorrectly implemented [13,25,52–54].

Megavoltage radiotherapy equipment is required, with sufficient source-to-patient distances to generate the large radiation field sizes that are needed. Immobilization devices such as head masks and vac-lock body shells are often necessary to minimize day-to-day variation in patient position and prevent movement during treatment. Additionally, anesthesia support is frequently needed, given the young age of the affected patient population.

CSI radiotherapy fields are designed to encompass the meninges of the entire brain and spine caudally to the bottom of the thecal sac. Following completion of CSI, a boost is delivered to the area of the primary tumor and, if possible, to the areas of metastases. In the case of medulloblastoma, the boost traditionally covers the entire posterior fossa, though studies suggest that smaller, individually tailored boost fields may be efficacious and have the benefit of greater normal tissue sparing [31–34]. For supratentorial PNET, the boost encompasses the tumor bed plus a margin of 1 to 2 cm. Though these treatment fields can be devised using two-dimensional (2D) simulation techniques, CT-based treatment planning helps insure coverage of all pertinent anatomic areas and should be considered standard of care.

Treatment Volumes—Gross Tumor Volume and Clinical Target Volume

Craniospinal Irradiation

Craniospinal irradiation (CSI) encompasses subclinical tumor spread in the central nervous system (CNS). Therefore, the concept of gross tumor volume (GTV) is not applicable for simulation of these fields. Rather, the CTV is defined as all of the leptomeninges of the CNS. As mentioned earlier, CT-based treatment planning is superior to older 2D treatment planning techniques, especially for defining coverage of areas such as the cribiform plate and floor of the temporal lobes, which can be difficult to appreciate with 2D planning.

Several aspects of the clinical target volume (CTV) definition for CSI deserve special mention. Treatment must include the meninges of nerves, such as the optic nerve, as they exit the brain [8]. As previously noted, the cribiform plate must be included in the treatment volume. This area may lie between the eyes, especially in younger children [8], and may be difficult or impossible to adequately treat while shielding the lens of the eye (Figure 88.1). Therefore, in some patients, cataract may be a necessary complication of medulloblastoma treatment. Fortunately, this is an easily correctable condition for most patients. In the spine, there is wide variation in the inferior border of the thecal sac, which can range from L5 to S3. Spine MRI is required to correctly place this field border for the individual patient [55]. The lateral borders of the spinal portion of the CTV should cover the extension of the meninges along the nerve roots, usually corresponding to the intervertebral foramina [8]. Therefore, the inferior portion of the spine field is typically wider than the superior portion, though inclusion laterally of the sacroiliac joints is not necessary [55].

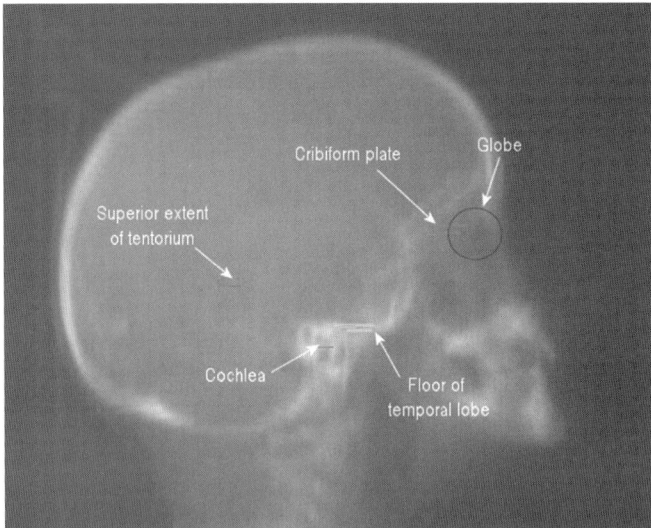

Figure 88.1 This lateral skull film is digitally reconstructed from a treatment planning CT scan. Note the positions of the cribiform plate and superior aspect of the posterior fossa, which can be easily identified on the CT planning study. See color insert.

Boost Fields

The GTV for boost fields is the residual tumor, if any, as defined on MRI done within 48 h of surgery. For medulloblastoma, the boost CTV has traditionally been the entire posterior fossa defined as extending superiorly from the foramen magnum to the most superior aspect of the tentorium. However, there is growing evidence that a smaller CTV defined as the post-op GTV and/or operative cavity plus 1.5 or 2 cm may be adequate [31–34]. The validity of this approach is currently being tested in a prospective randomized trial being conducted by the COG. CTV for boosts of metastatic disease is typically 0.5 to 1 cm beyond the GTV.

Craniospinal Irradiation Techniques

A variety of approaches have been described for delivery of CSI [56]. The most frequently described techniques include photon irradiation in the prone position, photon irradiation in the supine position, electron beam radiotherapy, intensity-modulated radiotherapy (IMRT), and proton beam. The technique chosen typically depends upon the technical capabilities and experience of the treating institution and physician.

Photon Irradiation in the Prone Position

This has been the most common CSI technique for the last several decades. Though still popular, it is gradually being supplanted by supine positioning. The chief advantage of the prone technique is the ability to directly visualize the join between the cranial and spinal fields. However, the prone position is often uncomfortable for the patient, difficult to reproduce, and can introduce additional challenges for the anesthesiologist if sedation is necessary.

Like most CSI techniques, prone photon irradiation uses parallel opposed lateral fields to treat the brain and one or two PA fields to treat the spine. The patient is first placed in the prone position with arms by his/her side. The head is immobilized in extension so that the exit dose from the spine field does not pass through the oral cavity, and a small cushion is placed under the ankles for patient comfort. A treatment planning CT is then performed from the top of the head to below the level of S3. Care must be taken in acquiring and setting the window and level of the planning CT scan. Slice thickness of no more than 5 mm should be used (3 mm thickness is useful in the brain), and bone windows are helpful so as not to underestimate the peripheral extent of the meninges [57]. During the subsequent virtual simulation, the spine fields are usually created first. With extended treatment distances, most linear accelerators can create field lengths of 50 to 55 cm, which accommodate the majority of children with medulloblastoma. Taller children and adults may require two matched PA fields separated by an appropriate gap on the skin surface to create maximum dose homogeneity at the depth of the spinal cord. The lateral borders of the spine field are shaped to encompass the CTV as defined earlier. The superior extent of the spine field should be placed as cranial as possible without exiting through the mouth.

Next, the brain fields are created to encompass the intracranial contents. Placement of the field isocenter at the boney canthus of the orbits eliminates radiation divergence into the eyes and provides a reproducible landmark for treatment setup each day. The collimator for the cranial fields is swiveled so as to match the angle of divergence of the spine field. This angle of divergence is calculated as the arc tangent of half the length of the spine field divided by the source-to-skin distance (SSD) of the spine field (the angle of the treatment couch can be adjusted in an analogous way to correct for the divergence of the cranial fields), and the inferior border of the brain fields is directly abutted to the superior border of the spine field.

Each day during treatment setup, the join between the brain and spine fields is verified by direct visualization. During the course of radiotherapy, the physical location of this match between the brain and spine fields (together with the join between spine fields if more than one spine field is used) is moved three or four times to minimize dose heterogeneity at the joint [58]. This can be accomplished by increasing the length of the cranial fields by 1 to 2 cm and leaving the isocenter placement and collimator swivel unchanged. The spine field is then moved caudally to match the new location of the inferior border of the cranial field, blocking its most caudal extent to maintain the desired inferior border. A tissue compensator is often necessary to achieve dose homogeneity in the spine, depending on the degree of kyphosis and lordosis present.

Photon Irradiation in the Supine Position

As previously mentioned, CSI in the supine position has several advantages compared to that in the prone position. Its major drawback is the difficulty in visually verifying the join between the brain and spine fields. However, methods to verify and reproduce this field matching have been described, and the technique is now in routine use at a number of centers [59–63]. Other than verification of the match line, simulation and treatment setup are analogous to those described earlier for supine CSI (Figure 88.2). Placement of

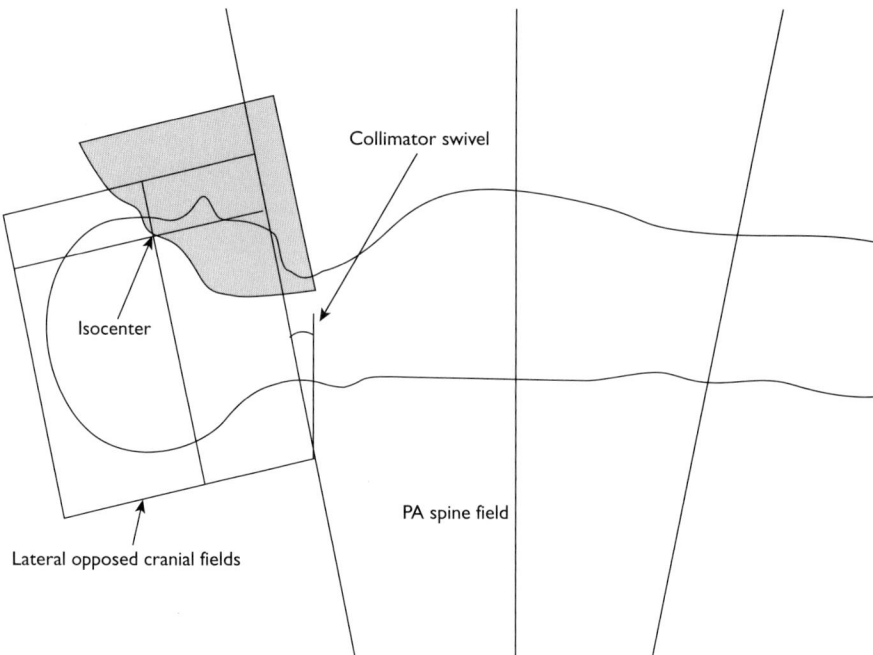

Figure 88.2 Three-field CSI technique in the prone position.

the patient's head in extension to control exit dose of the spine remains important and is aided by the ability to use conventional supine head immobilization techniques.

Intensity-Modulated Radiotherapy

IMRT techniques for the spine and boost portions of CSI have been described using techniques such as multiple posterior oblique fields [64] and helical tomotherapy [65–67]. Dosimetric analyses have shown advantages in normal organ sparing without significantly increasing integral dose for carefully designed plans [64,68]. In particular, decreased doses to the cochlea, pituitary, temporal lobes, and mediastinum can be achieved as compared to conventional radiotherapy techniques.

Protons

Proton radiotherapy with its Bragg peak effect has potential advantages over photon radiotherapy for the spinal portion of CSI. A PA proton beam can be created to deliver dose to the spinal meninges with almost complete sparing of ventral structures [68–71](Figure 88.3). As the availability of proton radiotherapy increases, it will likely assume a greater role in the treatment of PNET.

Electrons

The use of high-energy electrons to treat the spine has been described [72]. Similar to protons, electrons have an advantage of lower exit dose into the body. However, significant concerns exist regarding dose homogeneity of this modality because of the varying depth of the spinal cord along its length and the presence of bone proximal to the CTV. With the increasing availability of spine IMRT and proton therapy, this treatment has been largely abandoned.

Boost Fields

The boost field to the posterior fossa is best performed with the patient in the supine position, where the head can be more easily immobilized. Older techniques of parallel opposed treatment fields have been replaced by noncoplanar conformal or IMRT techniques to better spare the cochlea, pituitary, and medial temporal lobes [31,73–75](Figure 88.4).

Dose

In the commonly used photon techniques, radiation dose to the brain is prescribed to the midplane of the head, and dose to the spine from the PA spine fields are prescribed to the ventral surface of the spinal cord. For average-risk patients, a CSI dose of 23.4 Gy followed by chemotherapy has become the standard of care [37]. For high-risk patients, CSI doses of at least 36 Gy are necessary [7,42,76]. In patients with M2 or M3 disease, 4000 cGy to the CSI combined with chemotherapy and radiotherapy boosts to bulk disease have given 5-year EFS of up to 70% [7]. The dose of radiation to the primary tumor site, including the contribution from CSI, is typically 54 to 59.4 Gy, with the greater doses used in high-risk patients with bulky disease.

Radiotherapy/Chemotherapy Interactions

Vincristine given concurrently with radiotherapy is commonly used in medulloblastoma treatment protocols, though in vitro studies show no synergistic value to this approach [77]. Newer treatment regimens use other agents, such as carboplatin, concurrently, and pilot data suggest that this is tolerated reasonably well [48]. However, attention to the consequences of acute toxicity of combined modality approaches is required as significant negative impact on survival has been reported when the duration of radiotherapy exceeds 45 to 50 days [78,79].

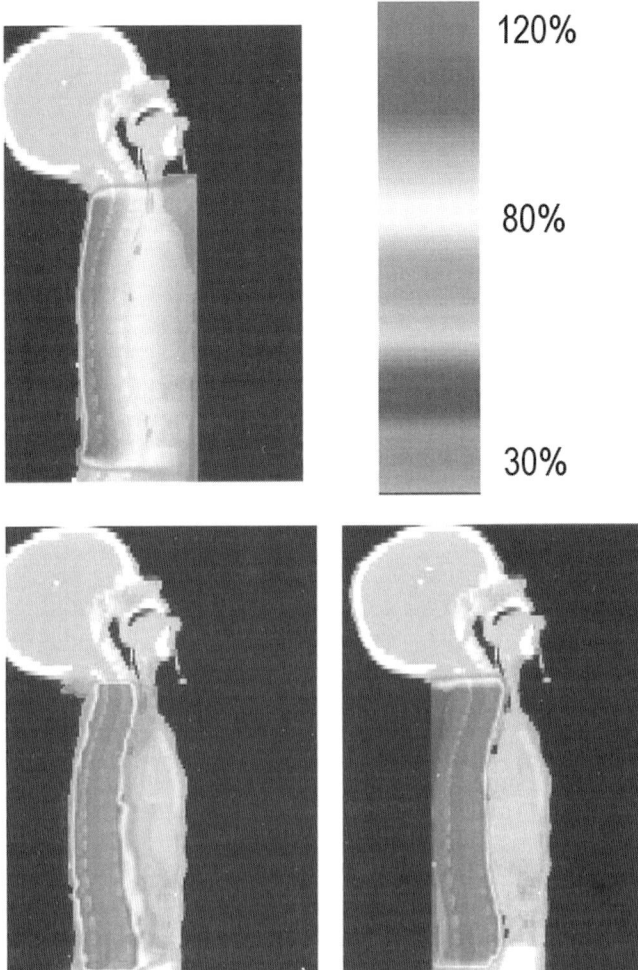

Figure 88.3 Comparisons of x-rays (upper left), IMRT (lower left), and proton (lower right) isodoses for CSI. Reprinted from Int J Rad Oncol Biol Phys, Vol 58:3, St. Clair WH, Adams JA, Bues M, et al., Advantage of protons compared to conventional x-ray or IMRT in the treatment of a pediatric patient with medulloblastoma, 731. © 2004 with permission from Elsevier. *See color insert.*

Many clinicians prefer a patient's hemoglobin level to be greater than 10 gm/dl at the time of radiotherapy to avoid hypoxic resistance of tumor cells. However, the efficacy of this practice has not been confirmed [80].

ADULT MEDULLOBLASTOMA

For purposes of analysis, many authors classify PNET in patients 16 years and older as adult medulloblastoma. Clinical presentation and natural history in the adult are similar to those seen in younger children, though as previously mentioned, lateralization of the primary to the cerebellar hemispheres increases with increasing patient age. Also, while most relapses in children occur within 3 years of treatment, up to 30% of relapses in adults occur more than 5 years after treatment [81,82].

Most reports indicate outcomes for adult medulloblastoma that are similar to those reported in children [83,84] though, in contrast to children, a benefit for the addition of

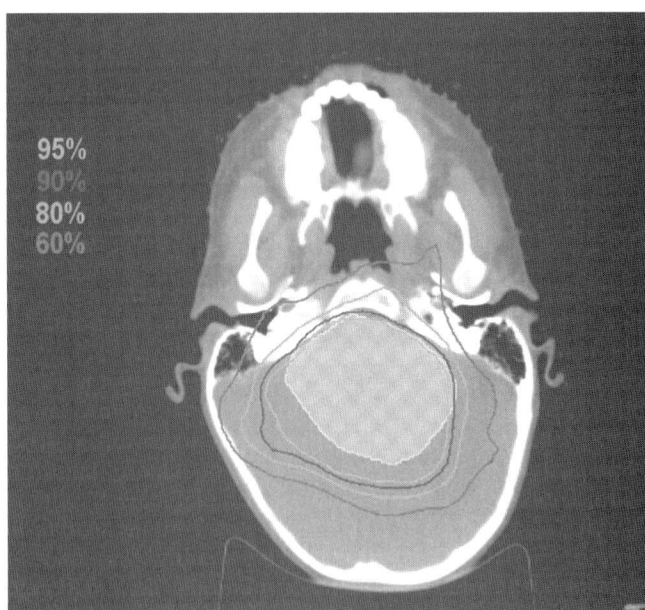

Figure 88.4 Isodose distribution for boost of the primary site in a child with medulloblastoma. Use of IMRT allows sparing of the cochlea and lateral temporal lobes. *See color insert.*

chemotherapy in adults has not been convincingly demonstrated. Abacioglu et al reported on 30 adult patients treated with CSI, with some patients also receiving chemotherapy. EFS was 50% at 8 years, and M stage and delay in starting radiotherapy were adverse prognostic factors. There was no survival advantage when chemotherapy was added to the treatment regimen [82].

A large, European multicenter retrospective study reported 156 adult patients over 18 years of age treated primarily with radiotherapy [85]. Five and 10-year EFS of 61% and 48% was observed. Again, no benefit was reported for patients who received chemotherapy.

Herrlinger et al [86] reported 26 adult patients with medulloblastoma. Survival was 79% and 56% at 5 and 10 years, respectively, with a nonsignificant trend toward improved outcome in the 20 patients who also received chemotherapy.

Selek et al [87] reported 36 patients with medulloblastoma over the age of 16 years. All patients received CSI of 30 to 36 Gy and 54 Gy to the primary site. Only six patients received chemotherapy. Five-year EFS was 92% for average-risk patients and 75% for high-risk patients.

Radiotherapy techniques and doses for adult medulloblastoma are similar to those used in children, except that two adjacent spinal fields are often necessary because of the adult patients' height. Though chemotherapy is probably indicated for high-risk patients, there is no clear role for chemotherapy in adults with average-risk disease, and given the potential long-term risks of this treatment [39] many prefer to use radiotherapy as the sole modality for average-risk adult patients.

SUPRATENTORIAL PNET

Supratentorial primary sites occur in 15% to 20% of patients. Patients with this tumor presentation are recognized as having an inferior prognosis and are classified in the high-risk category [88–91]. Radiotherapy treatment principles are similar to medulloblastoma of the posterior fossa and consist of initial CSI to doses of 36 to 40 Gy, followed by a boost to the primary site to a total dose of at least 54 Gy. Chemotherapy is used for all patients. As in classic medulloblastoma, M stage appears to be an important prognostic factor. Extent of surgical resection is less clearly prognostic in this group, but may still be important [91,92]. Pineal primary site may have a better prognosis compared to other supratentorial sites [91].

Local relapse is a much more significant failure pattern in supratentorial PNET as compared to medulloblastoma. For example, analysis of failure patterns in the CCG 921 study for high-risk patients showed 42% local failures for M0 supratentorial tumors compared to only 18% for infratentorial tumors when doses of 45 to 54 Gy were given to the primary site [90]. This prompted an escalation of the boost doses to 72 Gy with hyperfractionation in the follow-up CCG 9931 study. Radiotherapy dose to the primary site less than 54 Gy has been associated with increased local failure rates [93]. PFS rates at 5 years range from 49% to 52% for patients with M0 disease and from 0% to 29% for M+ patients [88,90,91].

INFANT MEDULLOBLASTOMA

It is widely recognized that very young children with medulloblastoma have inferior outcomes compared to older patients [28,46,94]. This may be due to several factors including the use of less aggressive radiotherapy, advanced disease stage at diagnosis, or inherently poor biology [10,46]. In spite of this poorer prognosis, the significant morbidity caused by CSI in young children has generated great interest in minimizing or eliminating radiotherapy for this patient population [95].

Beginning in 1986, the POG treated children under the age of 3 years with primary chemotherapy consisting of vincristine and cyclophosphamide alternating with cisplatin and etoposide [96]. Response-based radiotherapy was delivered after 1 or 2 years of chemotherapy, depending upon the age of the child at the time of diagnosis. Fifty-three children with medulloblastoma were enrolled. Overall two-year PFS was discouraging at 34% and was best for those children who were able to undergo resection of all visible tumors.

The CCG 921 study treated 65 children with high-risk PNET under the age of 18 months using "eight drugs in 1 day" chemotherapy for eight cycles. Radiotherapy was optional and was administered to only nine patients prior to disease progression [50]. Three-year PFS was just 22% for posterior fossa PNET tumors, though survival for those children who had complete resection and no metastatic disease was slightly better at 30%. Sixteen of 19 progression-free survivors did not receive radiotherapy. Local recurrence of tumor was the predominate failure pattern [51].

A follow-up study, CCG-9921, randomized children age less than 3 years to one of two chemotherapy regimens, reserving radiotherapy for patients with incomplete response or metastatic disease [97]. Five-year EFS was only 32% though radiotherapy was avoided in 75% of patients. Similar results were obtained in a SFOP trial conducted from 1990 to 2002. In this study, children less than 5 years old were treated with chemotherapy only [98]. Five-year PFS was 29% for M0 patients with completely resected tumors.

In two German trials, HIT-SKK87 and HIT-SKK92, outcome with chemotherapy only for infants with supratentorial PNET was poor with the majority of patients failing at the original tumor site. Only one child survived without receiving radiotherapy [99], and in the current HIT2000 trial, all children receive craniospinal radiotherapy.

Recent treatment protocols for infants have achieved better results using more effective and intensive chemotherapy regimens. Rutkowski et al [100] reported 5-year PFS of 82% in young children with complete resection of medulloblastoma who were treated with chemotherapy only, including intraventricular methotrexate. The current COG infant medulloblastoma study uses a regimen of induction chemotherapy, followed by attempted second surgery and high-dose chemotherapy consolidation with stem-cell rescue.

COMPLICATIONS OF RADIOTHERAPY

Acute Side Effects

Acute side effects of radiotherapy are primarily a consequence of CSI. Boost field radiotherapy is usually well tolerated. Side effects can occur at any time during radiotherapy and may persist for 2 to 6 weeks following completion of treatment. These include myelosuppression, alopecia, serous otitis media, nausea, change in taste, esophagitis, abdominal cramping, diarrhea, and fatigue. All of these effects can be more severe or protracted when neoadjuvant or concurrent chemotherapy is used. Supportive treatment of these symptoms is very important to avoid unnecessary interruptions in radiotherapy, which have been associated with inferior outcomes [78,79].

Late Complications

Late complications of radiotherapy for medulloblastoma are a significant concern because of the large tissue volume that is treated and the young age of the typical patient. Many of the most significant complications of radiotherapy are due to effects on growing tissue.

One of the most concerning sequelae is the potential for harming cognitive function. The detrimental effects of radiotherapy on the developing brain have been well documented and include deficits in fine motor, cognitive, and memory functions [101]. Decreases in intelligence quotient (IQ) scores after treatment are related to multiple factors, including the volume of brain treated, the dose of radiation used, the patient's baseline IQ, the use of chemotherapy, and the age at the time of treatment [102]. Some data also suggests that radiation-induced neurocognitive deficits may be greater in females [103].

In particular, age less than 7 years and whole-brain radiotherapy dose of 36 Gy or more have been associated with significant declines in IQ. Long-term survivors with this combination of risk factors may have declines of as many as 30 to 40 points below expected norms [101,103,104]. Reducing the whole-brain radiation dose from 36 to 23.4

Gy can significantly ameliorate declines in IQ, especially in younger children [102,105]. In one study of children treated with 23.4 Gy CSI together with chemotherapy, the average decline in IQ after 4 years was 17.4 points overall and 20.8 points in children less than 7 years [103]. Additional reductions in CSI dose may reduce neurocognitive risks even further. In a small pilot series, decreasing CSI dose to 18 Gy produced little, if any, cognitive deficits—even in young children [23].

Short stature of children treated with CSI is common and can be caused by a reduction of growth hormone production [106], together with a direct effect on growing bones in the spine. Routine replacement of growth hormone deficiencies in recent years has lessened this effect [107,] though survivors of medulloblastoma still often show discrepancies in seated versus standing height. Neuroendocrine sequelae also include the possibility of premature sexual development and thyroid dysfunction [108].

Other late effects of radiotherapy can include primary hypothyroidism, cataract, restrictive lung disease, and secondary malignancies [109–111]. Radiotherapy also likely contributes to sensorineural hearing loss associated with cisplatin chemotherapy. Hyperfractionation may decrease the risk of some of these complications [35,112].

The addition of chemotherapy to CSI has been reported to significantly increase the severity of many of these late effects, including a general decline in quality-of-life assessments [39,113,114].

RE-TREATMENT OF MEDULLOBLASTOMA

Recurrence of medulloblastoma has historically been associated with very poor outcomes and few survivors [115]. More recently, however, the use of lower CSI doses during initial treatment and availability of aggressive high-dose salvage chemotherapy have provided the opportunity for salvage of treatment failures in some patients [37,50].

Repeat limited-field radiotherapy, including radiosurgery techniques, in combination with chemotherapy has provided meaningful extension of survival and improvement in quality of life for selected patients [116,117]. Ridola et al [118] reported a 5-year survival of 69% in children who had localized tumor recurrence after primary chemotherapy when treated with repeat surgery, high-dose chemotherapy with stem-cell support, and radiotherapy to the posterior fossa.

REFERENCES

1. Bloom HJ, Wallace EN, Henk JM. The treatment and prognosis of medulloblastoma in children. A study of 82 verified cases. *Am J Roentgenol Radium Ther Nucl Med*. 1969;105(1):43–62.
2. Kleihues P, Cavenee WK. *Pathology and Genetics of Tumours of the Nervous System*. World Health Organization classification of tumours. Lyon: IARC Press, 2000.
3. Jain A, Jalali R, Nadkarni TD, Sharma S. Primary intramedullary primitive neuroectodermal tumor of the cervical spinal cord. Case report. *J Neurosurg Spine*. 2006;4(6):497–502.
4. Roberts RO, Lynch CF, Jones MP, Hart MN. Medulloblastoma: a population-based study of 532 cases. *J Neuropathol Exp Neurol*. 1991;50(2):134–144.
5. Freeman CR, Taylor RE, Kortmann RD, Carrie C. Radiotherapy for medulloblastoma in children: a perspective on current international clinical research efforts. *Med Pediatr Oncol*. 2002;39(2):99–108.
6. Packer RJ, Gajjar A, Vezina G, et al. Phase III study of craniospinal radiation therapy followed by adjuvant chemotherapy for newly diagnosed average-risk medulloblastoma. *J Clin Oncol*. 2006;24(25):4202–4208.
7. Gajjar A, Chintagumpala M, Ashley D, et al. Risk-adapted craniospinal radiotherapy followed by high-dose chemotherapy and stem-cell rescue in children with newly diagnosed medulloblastoma (St Jude Medulloblastoma-96): long-term results from a prospective, multicentre trial. *Lancet Oncol*. 2006;7(10):813–820.
8. Taylor RE. United Kingdom Children's Cancer Study Group (UKCCSG) radiotherapy and brain tumour groups: medulloblastoma/PNET and craniospinal radiotherapy (CSRT): report of a workshop held in Leeds, 30 June 1999. *Clin Oncol (R Coll Radiol)*. 2001;13(1):58–64.
9. Albright AL, Wisoff JH, Zeltzer PM, Boyett JM, Rorke LB, Stanley P. Effects of medulloblastoma resections on outcome in children: a report from the Children's Cancer Group. *Neurosurgery*. 1996;38(2):265–271.
10. Zeltzer PM, Boyett JM, Finlay JL, et al. Metastasis stage, adjuvant treatment, and residual tumor are prognostic factors for medulloblastoma in children: conclusions from the Children's Cancer Group 921 randomized phase III study. *J Clin Oncol*. 1999;17(3):832–845.
11. Gentet JC, Bouffet E, Doz F, et al. Preirradiation chemotherapy including "eight drugs in 1 day" regimen and high-dose methotrexate in childhood medulloblastoma: results of the M7 French Cooperative Study. *J Neurosurg*. 1995;82(4):608–614.
12. Packer RJ, Goldwein J, Nicholson HS, et al. Treatment of children with medulloblastomas with reduced-dose craniospinal radiation therapy and adjuvant chemotherapy: A Children's Cancer Group Study. *J Clin Oncol*. 1999;17(7):2127–2136.
13. Kortmann RD, Kühl J, Timmermann B, et al. Postoperative neoadjuvant chemotherapy before radiotherapy as compared to immediate radiotherapy followed by maintenance chemotherapy in the treatment of medulloblastoma in childhood: results of the German prospective randomized trial HIT '91. *Int J Radiat Oncol Biol Phys*. 2000;46(2):269–279.
14. Janss AJ, Yachnis AT, Silber JH, et al. Glial differentiation predicts poor clinical outcome in primitive neuroectodermal brain tumors. *Ann Neurol*. 1996;39(4):481–489.
15. Gajjar A, Hernan R, Kocak M, et al. Clinical, histopathologic, and molecular markers of prognosis: toward a new disease risk stratification system for medulloblastoma. *J Clin Oncol*. 2004;22(6):984–993.
16. Rutkowski S, von Bueren A, von Hoff K, et al. Prognostic relevance of clinical and biological risk factors in childhood medulloblastoma: results of patients treated in the prospective multicenter trial HIT'91. *Clin Cancer Res*. 2007;13(9):2651–2657.
17. Grotzer MA, Janss AJ, Fung K, et al. TrkC expression predicts good clinical outcome in primitive neuroectodermal brain tumors. *J Clin Oncol*. 2000;18(5):1027–1035.
18. Grotzer MA, Geoerger B, Janss AJ, Zhao H, Rorke LB, Phillips PC. Prognostic significance of Ki-67 (MIB-1) proliferation index in childhood primitive neuroectodermal tumors of the central nervous system. *Med Pediatr Oncol*. 2001;36(2):268–273.
19. Mazza C, Pasqualin A, Da Pian R, Donati E. Treatment of medulloblastoma in children: long-term results following surgery, radiotherapy and chemotherapy. *Acta Neurochir (Wien)*. 1981;57(3–4):163–175.
20. Tomita T, McLone DG. Medulloblastoma in childhood: results of radical resection and low-dose neuraxis radiation therapy. *J Neurosurg*. 1986;64(2):238–242.
21. Halberg FE, Wara WM, Fippin LF, et al. Low-dose craniospinal radiation therapy for medulloblastoma. *Int J Radiat Oncol Biol Phys*. 1991;20(4):651–654.
22. Thomas PR, Deutsch M, Kepner JL, et al. Low-stage medulloblastoma: final analysis of trial comparing standard-dose with reduced-dose neuraxis irradiation. *J Clin Oncol*. 2000;18(16):3004–3011.
23. Goldwein JW, Radcliffe J, Johnson J, et al. Updated results of a pilot study of low dose craniospinal irradiation plus chemotherapy for children under five with cerebellar primitive neuroectodermal tumors (medulloblastoma). *Int J Radiat Oncol Biol Phys*. 1996;34(4):899–904.
24. Bailey CC, Gnekow A, Wellek S, et al. Prospective randomised trial of chemotherapy given before radiotherapy in childhood medulloblastoma. International Society of Paediatric Oncology (SIOP) and the (German) Society of Paediatric Oncology (GPO): SIOP II. *Med Pediatr Oncol*. 1995;25(3):166–178.

25. Oyharcabal-Bourden V, Kalifa C, Gentet JC, et al. Standard-risk medulloblastoma treated by adjuvant chemotherapy followed by reduced-dose craniospinal radiation therapy: a French Society of Pediatric Oncology Study. *J Clin Oncol*. 2005;23(21):4726–4734.
26. Taylor RE, Bailey CC, Robinson K, et al.; International Society of Paediatric Oncology; United Kingdom Children's Cancer Study Group. Results of a randomized study of preradiation chemotherapy versus radiotherapy alone for nonmetastatic medulloblastoma: The International Society of Paediatric Oncology/United Kingdom Children's Cancer Study Group PNET-3 Study. *J Clin Oncol*. 2003;21(8):1581–1591.
27. Kühl J, Müller HL, Berthold F, et al. Preradiation chemotherapy of children and young adults with malignant brain tumors: results of the German pilot trial HIT'88/'89. *Klin Padiatr*. 1998;210(4):227–233.
28. Tait DM, Thornton-Jones H, Bloom HJ, Lemerle J, Morris-Jones P. Adjuvant chemotherapy for medulloblastoma: the first multi-centre control trial of the International Society of Paediatric Oncology (SIOP I). *Eur J Cancer*. 1990;26(4):464–469.
29. Krischer JP, Ragab AH, Kun L, et al. Nitrogen mustard, vincristine, procarbazine, and prednisone as adjuvant chemotherapy in the treatment of medulloblastoma. A Pediatric Oncology Group study. *J Neurosurg*. 1991;74(6):905–909.
30. Bouffet E, Bernard JL, Frappaz D, et al. M4 protocol for cerebellar medulloblastoma: supratentorial radiotherapy may not be avoided. *Int J Radiat Oncol Biol Phys*. 1992;24(1):79–85.
31. Carrie C, Muracciole X, Gomez F, et al.; French Society of Pediatric Oncology. Conformal radiotherapy, reduced boost volume, hyperfractionated radiotherapy, and online quality control in standard-risk medulloblastoma without chemotherapy: results of the French M-SFOP 98 protocol. *Int J Radiat Oncol Biol Phys*. 2005;63(3):711–716.
32. Merchant TE, Happersett L, Finlay JL, Leibel SA. Preliminary results of conformal radiation therapy for medulloblastoma. *Neuro-oncology*. 1999;1(3):177–187.
33. Fukunaga-Johnson N, Lee JH, Sandler HM, Robertson P, McNeil E, Goldwein JW. Patterns of failure following treatment for medulloblastoma: is it necessary to treat the entire posterior fossa? *Int J Radiat Oncol Biol Phys*. 1998;42(1):143–146.
34. Wolden SL, Dunkel IJ, Souweidane MM, et al. Patterns of failure using a conformal radiation therapy tumor bed boost for medulloblastoma. *J Clin Oncol*. 2003;21(16):3079–3083.
35. Ricardi U, Corrias A, Einaudi S, et al. Thyroid dysfunction as a late effect in childhood medulloblastoma: a comparison of hyperfractionated versus conventionally fractionated craniospinal radiotherapy. *Int J Radiat Oncol Biol Phys*. 2001;50(5):1287–1294.
36. Marymont MH, Geohas J, Tomita T, Strauss L, Brand WN, Mittal BB. Hyperfractionated craniospinal radiation in medulloblastoma. *Pediatr Neurosurg*. 1996;24(4):178–184.
37. Prados MD, Edwards MS, Chang SM, et al. Hyperfractionated craniospinal radiation therapy for primitive neuroectodermal tumors: results of a Phase II study. *Int J Radiat Oncol Biol Phys*. 1999;43(2):279–285.
38. Allen JC, Donahue B, DaRosso R, Nirenberg A. Hyperfractionated craniospinal radiotherapy and adjuvant chemotherapy for children with newly diagnosed medulloblastoma and other primitive neuroectodermal tumors. *Int J Radiat Oncol Biol Phys*. 1996;36(5):1155–1161.
39. Bull KS, Spoudeas HA, Yadegarfar G, Kennedy CR; CCLG. Reduction of health status 7 years after addition of chemotherapy to craniospinal irradiation for medulloblastoma: a follow-up study in PNET 3 trial survivors on behalf of the CCLG (formerly UKCCSG). *J Clin Oncol*. 2007;25(27):4239–4245.
40. Mosijczuk AD, Nigro MA, Thomas PR, et al. Preradiation chemotherapy in advanced medulloblastoma. A Pediatric Oncology Group pilot study. *Cancer*. 1993;72(9):2755–2762.
41. Yock TI, Friedman HS, Kun L, Kepner JL, Barnes P, Tarbell NJ. Response to pre-radiation chemotherapy is predictive of improved survival in high risk medulloblastoma: results from Pediatric Oncology Group (POG 9031). *Int J Radiat Oncol Biol Phys*. 2001;51:120–121.
42. Miralbell R, Fitzgerald TJ, Laurie F, et al. Radiotherapy in pediatric medulloblastoma: quality assessment of Pediatric Oncology Group Trial 9031. *Int J Radiat Oncol Biol Phys*. 2006;64(5):1325–1330.
43. Taylor RE, Bailey CC, Robinson KJ, et al. Outcome for patients with metastatic (M2-3) medulloblastoma treated with SIOP/UKCCSG PNET-3 chemotherapy. *Eur J Cancer*. 2005;41(5):727–734.
44. Verlooy J, Mosseri V, Bracard S, et al. Treatment of high risk medulloblastomas in children above the age of 3 years: a SFOP study. *Eur J Cancer*. 2006;42(17):3004–3014.
45. Allen J, Prados MB, Donahue B, et al. A phase I/II study for newly diagnosed high risk PNET consisting of neoadjuvant chemotherapy (CHT) followed by hyperfractionated radiotherapy (RT): preliminary results of CCG protocol 9931. *Neuro Oncol*. 2000;2:247.
46. Evans AE, Jenkin RD, Sposto R, et al. The treatment of medulloblastoma. Results of a prospective randomized trial of radiation therapy with and without CCNU, vincristine, and prednisone. *J Neurosurg*. 1990;72(4):572–582.
47. Packer RJ, Sutton LN, Elterman R, et al. Outcome for children with medulloblastoma treated with radiation and cisplatin, CCNU, and vincristine chemotherapy. *J Neurosurg*. 1994;81(5):690–698.
48. Jakacki RI, Burger PC, Zhou T, et al. Outcome for metastatic (M+) medulloblastoma (MB) treated with carboplatin during caniospinal radiotherapy (CSRT) followed by cyclophosphamide (CPM) and vincristine (VCR): preliminary results of COG 99701. *J Clin Oncol*. 2007;25:2018.
49. PATERSON E, FARR RF. Cerebellar medulloblastoma: treatment by irradiation of the whole central nervous system. *Acta radiol*. 1953;39(4):323–336.
50. Geyer JR, Zeltzer PM, Boyett JM, et al. Survival of infants with primitive neuroectodermal tumors or malignant ependymomas of the CNS treated with eight drugs in 1 day: a report from the Childrens Cancer Group. *J Clin Oncol*. 1994;12(8):1607–1615.
51. Hong TS, Mehta MP, Boyett JM, Donahue B, Rorke LB, Zeltzer PM. Patterns of treatment failure in infants with primitive neuroectodermal tumors who were treated on CCG-921: a phase III combined modality study. *Pediatr Blood Cancer*. 2005;45(5):676–682.
52. Miralbell R, Bleher A, Huguenin P, et al. Pediatric medulloblastoma: radiation treatment technique and patterns of failure. *Int J Radiat Oncol Biol Phys*. 1997;37(3):523–529.
53. Carrie C, Alapetite C, Mere P, et al. Quality control of radiotherapeutic treatment of medulloblastoma in a multicentric study: the contribution of radiotherapy technique to tumour relapse. The French Medulloblastoma Group. *Radiother Oncol*. 1992;24(2):77–81.
54. Taylor RE, Bailey CC, Robinson KJ, et al.; United Kingdom Children's Cancer Study Group Brain Tumour Committee; International Society of Paediatric Oncology. Impact of radiotherapy parameters on outcome in the International Society of Paediatric Oncology/United Kingdom Children's Cancer Study Group PNET-3 study of preradiotherapy chemotherapy for M0-M1 medulloblastoma. *Int J Radiat Oncol Biol Phys*. 2004;58(4):1184–1193.
55. Halperin EC. Concerning the inferior portion of the spinal radiotherapy field for malignancies that disseminate via the cerebrospinal fluid. *Int J Radiat Oncol Biol Phys*. 1993;26(2):357–362.
56. Urie M, FitzGerald TJ, Followill D, Laurie F, Marcus R, Michalski J. Current calibration, treatment, and treatment planning techniques among institutions participating in the Children's Oncology Group. *Int J Radiat Oncol Biol Phys*. 2003;55(1):245–260.
57. Coles CE, Hoole AC, Harden SV, et al. Quantitative assessment of inter-clinician variability of target volume delineation for medulloblastoma: quality assurance for the SIOP PNET 4 trial protocol. *Radiother Oncol*. 2003;69(2):189–194.
58. Kiltie AE, Povall JM, Taylor RE. The need for the moving junction in craniospinal irradiation. *Br J Radiol*. 2000;73(870):650–654.
59. Michalski JM, Klein EE, Gerber R. Method to plan, administer, and verify supine craniospinal irradiation. *J Appl Clin Med Phys*. 2002;3(4):310–316.
60. Hawkins RB. A simple method of radiation treatment of craniospinal fields with patient supine. *Int J Radiat Oncol Biol Phys*. 2001;49(1):261–264.
61. Bauman G, Wong E, Trenka K, Scott D. A simple technique for craniospinal radiotherapy in the supine position. *Radiother Oncol*. 2006;80(3):394.
62. Rades D, Holtzhauer R, Baumann R, Leuwer M, Karstens JH. Craniospinal axis irradiation in children. Treatment in supine position including field verification as a prerequisite for anesthesia without intubation. *Strahlenther Onkol*. 1999;175(8):409–412.
63. Thomadsen B, Mehta M, Howard S, Das R. Craniospinal treatment with the patient supine. *Med Dosim*. 2003;28(1):35–38.
64. Parker W, Filion E, Roberge D, Freeman CR. Intensity-modulated radiotherapy for craniospinal irradiation: target volume considerations, dose constraints, and competing risks. *Int J Radiat Oncol Biol Phys*. 2007;69(1):251–257.
65. Bauman G, Yartsev S, Coad T, Fisher B, Kron T. Helical tomotherapy for craniospinal radiation. *Br J Radiol*. 2005;78(930):548–552.

66. Cao D, Holmes TW, Afghan MK, Shepard DM. Comparison of plan quality provided by intensity-modulated arc therapy and helical tomotherapy. *Int J Radiat Oncol Biol Phys.* 2007;69(1):240–250.
67. Penagaricano JA, Yan Y, Corry P, Moros E, Ratanatharathorn V. Retrospective evaluation of pediatric cranio-spinal axis irradiation plans with the Hi-ART tomotherapy system. *Technol Cancer Res Treat.* 2007;6(4):355–360.
68. St Clair WH, Adams JA, Bues M, et al. Advantage of protons compared to conventional X-ray or IMRT in the treatment of a pediatric patient with medulloblastoma. *Int J Radiat Oncol Biol Phys.* 2004;58(3):727–734.
69. DeLaney TF. Clinical proton radiation therapy research at the Francis H. Burr Proton Therapy Center. *Technol Cancer Res Treat.* 2007;6(4 Suppl):61–66.
70. Krejcarek SC, Grant PE, Henson JW, Tarbell NJ, Yock TI. Physiologic and radiographic evidence of the distal edge of the proton beam in craniospinal irradiation. *Int J Radiat Oncol Biol Phys.* 2007;68(3):646–649.
71. Lundkvist J, Ekman M, Ericsson SR, Jönsson B, Glimelius B. Proton therapy of cancer: potential clinical advantages and cost-effectiveness. *Acta Oncol.* 2005;44(8):850–861.
72. Dewit L, Van Dam J, Rijnders A, van de Velde G, Ang KK, van der Schueren E. A modified radiotherapy technique in the treatment of medulloblastoma. *Int J Radiat Oncol Biol Phys.* 1984;10(2):231–241.
73. Paulino AC, Narayana A, Mohideen MN, Jeswani S. Posterior fossa boost in medulloblastoma: an analysis of dose to surrounding structures using 3-dimensional (conformal) radiotherapy. *Int J Radiat Oncol Biol Phys.* 2000;46(2):281–286.
74. Huang E, Teh BS, Strother DR, et al. Intensity-modulated radiation therapy for pediatric medulloblastoma: early report on the reduction of ototoxicity. *Int J Radiat Oncol Biol Phys.* 2002;52(3):599–605.
75. Fukunaga-Johnson N, Sandler HM, Marsh R, Martel MK. The use of 3D conformal radiotherapy (3D CRT) to spare the cochlea in patients with medulloblastoma. *Int J Radiat Oncol Biol Phys.* 1998;41(1):77–82.
76. Strother D, Ashley D, Kellie SJ, et al. Feasibility of four consecutive high-dose chemotherapy cycles with stem-cell rescue for patients with newly diagnosed medulloblastoma or supratentorial primitive neuroectodermal tumor after craniospinal radiotherapy: results of a collaborative study. *J Clin Oncol.* 2001;19(10):2696–2704.
77. Kumar KS, Sonnemann J, Hong le TT, et al. Histone deacetylase inhibitors, but not vincristine, cooperate with radiotherapy to induce cell death in medulloblastoma. *Anticancer Res.* 2007;27(1A):465–470.
78. del Charco JO, Bolek TW, McCollough WM, et al. Medulloblastoma: time-dose relationship based on a 30-year review. *Int J Radiat Oncol Biol Phys.* 1998;42(1):147–154.
79. Paulino AC, Wen BC, Mayr NA, et al. Protracted radiotherapy treatment duration in medulloblastoma. *Am J Clin Oncol.* 2003;26(1):55–59.
80. Chow E, Danjoux CE, Pataki I, Franssen E, Jenkin RD. Effect of hemoglobin on radiotherapy response in children with medulloblastoma: should patients with a low hemoglobin be transfused? *Med Pediatr Oncol.* 1999;32(5):395–397.
81. Chan AW, Tarbell NJ, Black PM, et al. Adult medulloblastoma: prognostic factors and patterns of relapse. *Neurosurgery.* 2000;47(3):623–631; discussion 631.
82. Abacioglu U, Uzel O, Sengoz M, Turkan S, Ober A. Medulloblastoma in adults: treatment results and prognostic factors. *Int J Radiat Oncol Biol Phys.* 2002;54(3):855–860.
83. Prados MD, Warnick RE, Wara WM, Larson DA, Lamborn K, Wilson CB. Medulloblastoma in adults. *Int J Radiat Oncol Biol Phys.* 1995;32(4):1145–1152.
84. Le QT, Weil MD, Wara WM, et al. Adult medulloblastoma: an analysis of survival and prognostic factors. *Cancer J Sci Am.* 1997;3(4):238–245.
85. Carrie C, Lasset C, Alapetite C, et al. Multivariate analysis of prognostic factors in adult patients with medulloblastoma. Retrospective study of 156 patients. *Cancer.* 1994;74(8):2352–2360.
86. Herrlinger U, Steinbrecher A, Rieger J, et al. Adult medulloblastoma: prognostic factors and response to therapy at diagnosis and at relapse. *J Neurol.* 2005;252(3):291–299.
87. Selek U, Zorlu F, Hurmuz P, et al. Craniospinal radiotherapy in adult medulloblastoma. *Strahlenther Onkol.* 2007;183(5):236–240.
88. Reddy AT, Janss AJ, Phillips PC, Weiss HL, Packer RJ. Outcome for children with supratentorial primitive neuroectodermal tumors treated with surgery, radiation, and chemotherapy. *Cancer.* 2000;88(9):2189–2193.
89. Paulino AC, Melian E. Medulloblastoma and supratentorial primitive neuroectodermal tumors: an institutional experience. *Cancer.* 1999;86(1):142–148.
90. Hong TS, Mehta MP, Boyett JM, et al. Patterns of failure in supratentorial primitive neuroectodermal tumors treated in Children's Cancer Group Study 921, a phase III combined modality study. *Int J Radiat Oncol Biol Phys.* 2004;60(1):204–213.
91. Cohen BH, Zeltzer PM, Boyett JM, et al. Prognostic factors and treatment results for supratentorial primitive neuroectodermal tumors in children using radiation and chemotherapy: a Childrens Cancer Group randomized trial. *J Clin Oncol.* 1995;13(7):1687–1696.
92. Albright AL, Wisoff JH, Zeltzer P, et al. Prognostic factors in children with supratentorial (nonpineal) primitive neuroectodermal tumors. A neurosurgical perspective from the Children's Cancer Group. *Pediatr Neurosurg.* 1995;22(1):1–7.
93. Timmermann B, Kortmann RD, Kühl J, et al. Role of radiotherapy in the treatment of supratentorial primitive neuroectodermal tumors in childhood: results of the prospective German brain tumor trials HIT 88/89 and 91. *J Clin Oncol.* 2002;20(3):842–849.
94. Pezzotta S, Cordero di Montezemolo L, Knerich R, et al. CNS-85 trial: a cooperative pediatric CNS tumor study–results of treatment of medulloblastoma patients. *Childs Nerv Syst.* 1996;12(2):87–96.
95. Kretschmar CS, Tarbell NJ, Kupsky W, et al. Pre-irradiation chemotherapy for infants and children with medulloblastoma: a preliminary report. *J Neurosurg.* 1989;71(6):820–825.
96. Duffner PK, Horowitz ME, Krischer JP, et al. Postoperative chemotherapy and delayed radiation in children less than three years of age with malignant brain tumors. *N Engl J Med.* 1993;328(24):1725–1731.
97. Geyer JR, Sposto R, Jennings M, et al.; Children's Cancer Group. Multiagent chemotherapy and deferred radiotherapy in infants with malignant brain tumors: a report from the Children's Cancer Group. *J Clin Oncol.* 2005;23(30):7621–7631.
98. Grill J, Sainte-Rose C, Jouvet A, et al.; French Society of Paediatric Oncology. Treatment of medulloblastoma with postoperative chemotherapy alone: an SFOP prospective trial in young children. *Lancet Oncol.* 2005;6(8):573–580.
99. Timmermann B, Kortmann RD, Kühl J, et al. Role of radiotherapy in supratentorial primitive neuroectodermal tumor in young children: results of the German HIT-SKK87 and HIT-SKK92 trials. *J Clin Oncol.* 2006;24(10):1554–1560.
100. Rutkowski S, Bode U, Deinlein F, et al. Treatment of early childhood medulloblastoma by postoperative chemotherapy alone. *N Engl J Med.* 2005;352(10):978–986.
101. Packer RJ, Sutton LN, Atkins TE, et al. A prospective study of cognitive function in children receiving whole-brain radiotherapy and chemotherapy: 2-year results. *J Neurosurg.* 1989;70(5):707–713.
102. Silber JH, Radcliffe J, Peckham V, et al. Whole-brain irradiation and decline in intelligence: the influence of dose and age on IQ score. *J Clin Oncol.* 1992;10(9):1390–1396.
103. Ris MD, Packer R, Goldwein J, Jones-Wallace D, Boyett JM. Intellectual outcome after reduced-dose radiation therapy plus adjuvant chemotherapy for medulloblastoma: a Children's Cancer Group study. *J Clin Oncol.* 2001;19(15):3470–3476.
104. Radcliffe J, Bunin GR, Sutton LN, Goldwein JW, Phillips PC. Cognitive deficits in long-term survivors of childhood medulloblastoma and other noncortical tumors: age-dependent effects of whole brain radiation. *Int J Dev Neurosci.* 1994;12(4):327–334.
105. Mulhern RK, Kepner JL, Thomas PR, Armstrong FD, Friedman HS, Kun LE. Neuropsychologic functioning of survivors of childhood medulloblastoma randomized to receive conventional or reduced-dose craniospinal irradiation: a Pediatric Oncology Group study. *J Clin Oncol.* 1998;16(5):1723–1728.
106. Packer RJ, Meadows AT, Rorke LB, Goldwein JL, D'Angio G. Long-term sequelae of cancer treatment on the central nervous system in childhood. *Med Pediatr Oncol.* 1987;15(5):241–253.
107. Packer RJ, Boyett JM, Janss AJ, et al. Growth hormone replacement therapy in children with medulloblastoma: use and effect on tumor control. *J Clin Oncol.* 2001;19(2):480–487.
108. Sklar CA, Constine LS. Chronic neuroendocrinological sequelae of radiation therapy. *Int J Radiat Oncol Biol Phys.* 1995;31(5):1113–1121.

109. Pasqualini T, Diez B, Domene H, et al. Long-term endocrine sequelae after surgery, radiotherapy, and chemotherapy in children with medulloblastoma. *Cancer.* 1987;59(4):801–806.
110. Jakacki RI, Schramm CM, Donahue BR, Haas F, Allen JC. Restrictive lung disease following treatment for malignant brain tumors: a potential late effect of craniospinal irradiation. *J Clin Oncol.* 1995;13(6):1478–1485.
111. Cohen MS, Kushner MJ, Dell S. Frontal lobe astrocytoma following radiotherapy for medulloblastoma. *Neurology.* 1981;31(5):616–619.
112. Chin D, Sklar C, Donahue B, et al. Thyroid dysfunction as a late effect in survivors of pediatric medulloblastoma/primitive neuroectodermal tumors: a comparison of hyperfractionated versus conventional radiotherapy. *Cancer.* 1997;80(4):798–804.
113. Goldstein AM, Yuen J, Tucker MA. Second cancers after medulloblastoma: population-based results from the United States and Sweden. *Cancer Causes Control.* 1997;8(6):865–871.
114. Stavrou T, Bromley CM, Nicholson HS, et al. Prognostic factors and secondary malignancies in childhood medulloblastoma. *J Pediatr Hematol Oncol.* 2001;23(7):431–436.
115. Torres CF, Rebsamen S, Silber JH, et al. Surveillance scanning of children with medulloblastoma. *N Engl J Med.* 1994;330(13):892–895.
116. Gannett DE, Hill D, Hamilton AJ, Stea B. Paclitaxel as a radiosensitizer combined with fractionated stereotactic radiotherapy in the treatment of recurrent medulloblastoma. *Am J Clin Oncol.* 1997;20(3):233–236.
117. Milker-Zabel S, Zabel A, Thilmann C, et al. Results of three-dimensional stereotactically-guided radiotherapy in recurrent medulloblastoma. *J Neurooncol.* 2002;60(3):227–233.
118. Ridola V, Grill J, Doz F, et al. High-dose chemotherapy with autologous stem cell rescue followed by posterior fossa irradiation for local medulloblastoma recurrence or progression after conventional chemotherapy. *Cancer.* 2007;110(1):156–163.

89 Adult and Pediatric Pilocytic Astrocytoma

Bernadine R. Donahue

INTRODUCTION AND EPIDEMIOLOGY

Pilocytic astrocytoma (PA) is a tumor of the central nervous system that falls within the category of low-grade gliomas. In 1931, Cushing described the entity of cystic cerebellar astrocytoma and recognized the relatively "benign" nature of such lesions [1]. There are approximately 1500 cases of PA per year in the United States [2], and the worldwide incidence has been estimated to be 4.8 per million per year [3]. PA is predominantly a tumor of childhood and presents within the first 2 decades of life; hence, the designation *juvenile* PA. PA accounts for 20% of all primary brain tumors in children under 15 years of age but only 2% of all brain tumors [2].

PATHOLOGY AND RADIOGRAPHIC FINDINGS

The WHO system categorizes PAs as Grade I astrocytoma [4]. PA consists of astrocytes forming a glioma matrix with intermixed Rosenthal fibers [5]. These bipolar astrocytes are elongated and organized in a parallel array of glial fibers leading to what has been described as a "hairlike" appearance. Eosinophilic material composed of degenerating astrocytes, that is, so-called "Rosenthal fibers," are present throughout. Microcysts are another common feature of PA. Cellularity and mitotic activity are usually low, and vascular proliferation and necrosis may be present. However, unlike infiltrating gliomas, these findings are not indicative of anaplasia. Tumor cells stain positive for glial fibrillary acid protein and microtubule-associated protein 2. The low-grade histologic features of PA are retained even in settings of recurrent or disseminated disease. Rarely, PA may undergo frank malignant transformation, a change characterized by high mitotic rate, microvascular proliferation, and palisading necrosis. A subset of lesions previously classified as PA, pilomyxoid astrocytoma, appears to have a more aggressive biologic behavior, and as such, will not be addressed here [6].

Macroscopically, PA usually has a visible cystic component and a smaller solid component frequently referred to as a "mural nodule." Despite the well-circumscribed appearance grossly, infiltration into surrounding brain tissue has been documented histopathologically [7]. PA can be imaged radiographically with both computed tomography and magnetic resonance imaging (MRI). On noncontrast computed tomography, the cysts are hypodense and the solid portions are isodense or hypodense. Calcifications can be seen but are not typical. On MRI, these lesions are typically well circumscribed with vivid enhancement of the solid component [8,9]. The cyst wall may or may not enhance, and it has been controversial as to whether the cyst wall is neoplastic. Classically, it was thought that it was not; however, biopsy and resection specimens have shown neoplastic cells [10]. On perfusion imaging, PA have been reported to have low relative cerebral blood volume (<1.50) as would be expected in a low-grade neoplasm [11].

CLINICAL PRESENTATION

PA has a predilection for the posterior fossa but can also occur along the optic nerves, within the cerebral hemispheres, and as dorsally exophytic brain stem tumors. The clinical manifestations will vary depending on the anatomic location. Tumors that are located in the posterior fossa may present with headache, nausea, vomiting, ataxia, or other cerebellar findings. PA is typically a localized disease and rarely metastasizes. However, multifocal presentation and dissemination have been described [12–14]. A series from New York University and Beth Israel Medical Center reported 13 children with leptomeningeal dissemination at diagnosis in a cohort of more than 500 children with low-grade neoplasms [15]. Five of these 13 children had PA, and in four of the five children the primary tumor was noncerebellar in origin. The true incidence of dissemination may actually be higher, as this series spanned the years 1983 to 1997, and MRI imaging of the spine was not available for the first several years. In addition, the incidence may be higher as imaging of the spinal axis is not routinely done in the setting of a low-grade neoplasm.

TREATMENT AND OUTCOME

Surgery has been the mainstay of treatment for the vast majority of low-grade gliomas of childhood including PA. Radiation therapy and chemotherapy also are utilized in the treatment of PA. In some situations, observation may be the most appropriate intervention.

Completely Resected PA

Gross total excision of PA offers the potential for cure [16–18]. PAs, particularly those located in the cerebellum, are usually more amenable to gross total resection than the other types of low-grade gliomas. Cyst fenestration and resection of the tumor nodule is usually performed. Some surgeons advocate resection of the entire cyst, particularly when the wall of the cyst enhances strongly. In cystic cerebellar tumors, frequently only the mural nodule is resected [19]. In many institutions, a second surgery to achieve a gross total excision is strongly considered [20].

Completely resected PA is associated with excellent survival [20–22]. In a series from the Mayo Clinic, 16 patients who underwent gross total or radical subtotal resection had a 100% 10-year survival [23]. Results from larger cohorts of patients have shown similar good survival rates of >90% at 10 years and >80% at 20 years [3]. CCG9891/POG 9130, a prospective study of children with low-grade gliomas, reported a 95% 5-year progression-free survival in children with totally resected PA [24].

Incompletely Resected PA

Observation

Radical resection may not always be feasible for PA; some arising from the optic pathway, deep thalamic region, basal ganglia, and brainstem may be considered surgically inaccessible. Long-term survival can occur even in the setting of incompletely resected PA. A proportion of incompletely resected PA can behave indolently, and spontaneous regression of residual disease has been described [25–27]. Surveillance MRI every 6 months for the first 3 years has been recommended [28].

Given the favorable outcome, the decision to proceed with postoperative treatment must be made on an individual basis. The prospective nonrandomized CCG9891/POG9130 low-grade astrocytoma study was conducted from 1991 through 1996 and included children with PA [29]. That study specified that tumors which had been "radically resected," defined as >95% resection and <1.5 cc residual, would be observed. Tumors that were less than radically resected were to be observed or irradiated at the discretion of the treating physician. More than 700 children with low-grade astrocytoma were accrued to this study, including close to 400 patients with PA. The extent of resection appears to have a marked influence on the progression-free survival with a 5-year progression-free survival rate, for all eligible patients on study, of 90% in the setting of gross total resection versus 45% to 65% with any volume of residual disease. The overall progression-free survival for patients with PA appears to be >75%; however, long-term results based on histology, location, and extent of resection are still pending. Given the young age of most patients with PA and the potential toxicity of postoperative treatment, close observation with serial imaging in patients with incompletely resected PA and neurologic stability is a reasonable approach. It would be anticipated that many of these children will have stable disease for years and, hopefully, can be treated successfully at the time of progression. Long-term results of the prospective study should help clarify this.

Radiation Therapy

The use of postoperative radiotherapy (RT) in incompletely resected PA is controversial [19,30]. Radiation therapy may be appropriate, depending on neurological signs or symptoms caused by residual tumor, the potential for neurological deficit resulting from growth of residual tumor, and the feasibility of a second surgical excision. Several single institution series have reported the outcome following subtotal excision and radiation therapy in the treatment of PA [20–22,31]. However, much of the published data are somewhat difficult to interpret given inclusion of patients treated over many decades, advances in imaging and surgery, and the variability in treatment at time of recurrence. In the series reported by Wallner et al, the 10- and 20-year progression-free survival rates in the setting of incompletely resected PA treated with postoperative radiation therapy were 74% and 41%, respectively [21]. Unfortunately, many of the single institution series are limited by small numbers and lack of a control group of patients with incompletely resected, nonirradiated PA. The series from the Mayo Clinic did report that the 5-year survival rate for patients who had less than total resection and who were not irradiated was 50%, compared with 85% for those who had less than total resection and received postoperative irradiation ($p = 0.08$) [31]. However, the comparison is limited by the small number of patients treated with surgery alone.

Attempts have been made to identify prognostic factors which predict for recurrence, and several of the aforementioned series suggest a greater risk in solid rather than cystic tumors, in tumors that extend to the peduncle, and in tumors that have markers of increased proliferative activity, for example, high MIB-1 labeling index [32–35]. However, the clinical utility of these factors remains questionable, and the role of postoperative RT for asymptomatic residual disease remains unclear.

Radiation therapy can be used in the setting of residual symptomatic or progressive disease in older children and adults, particularly when re-resection is not feasible. When radiation therapy is used, doses of 50 to 54 Gy are administered in 1.8 Gy fractions. There is no evidence that higher doses are necessary [36,37]. Radiation therapy is usually delivered with one of several conformal techniques, including 3D conformal, intensity-modulated radiation therapy, fractionated stereotactic radiation therapy, and protons. Given that PAs are usually well demarcated on MRI and there is incentive to reduce toxicity in children by limiting the volume of normal tissue irradiated, margins are generally "tight." Typically, for PAs, the planning target volume includes the gross tumor as imaged on MR (including the cysts), plus a 1 cm anatomically limited margin (the margin may vary based upon institutional setup and technique of treatment).

Outcomes in modern series of low-grade gliomas utilizing conformal techniques indicate 5-year progression-free survivals in the range of 80% to 90% [38–40]. A publication from St. Jude Children's Research Hospital in which

MR registration for treatment planning and 3 to 5 mm planning target volume margins were utilized, reported a 5-year event-free survival of 89% for WHO I tumors [40]. An open COG trial for low-grade gliomas, ACNS 0221, is evaluating conformal RT in patients with progressive or symptomatic low-grade gliomas (children under 10 years of age, though, must have received at least one prior course of chemotherapy).

Early reports of functional outcomes after radiation therapy with conformal techniques are encouraging with limited side effects [40]. The risk of second malignancy or transformation into an anaplastic tumor after RT remains [39], although it is interesting to note that a series from UCLA identified a 10% rate of anaplastic transformation following surgery alone [41].

Chemotherapy

The intent of chemotherapy is to achieve disease control in young children for as long as possible, thereby avoiding or at least deferring the need for radiation therapy. The majority of the literature addressing the role of chemotherapy in low-grade astrocytoma deals with optic gliomas, and few publications exclusively deal with the role of chemotherapy for PA [42]. Packer's initial experience with carboplatin included 13 patients with histologic confirmation of pilocytic histology [43], and most cooperative group pediatric protocols evaluating the role of chemotherapy in low-grade gliomas include children with PA. Extrapolation of the experience with optic gliomas would lead to an expected 3-year progression-free survival of 75% for children less than 5 years of age and nearly 40% for children older than 5 years of age [44–46]. COG A9952 compared the regimen of procarbazine, 6-thioguanine, CCNU, and vincristine to the "standard" regimen of carboplatin and vincristine in a randomized Phase-III study for patients under 10 years of age with low-grade astrocytoma which was progressive following initial surgical excision or incompletely resected and requiring immediate treatment because of a risk of neurologic impairment with progression. A recent COG trial (ACNS0223) has evaluated the feasibility of carboplatin, vincristine, and temozolomide in children <10 years of age with progressive and/or symptomatic low-grade gliomas. Both of these trials included patient with PA, and results are pending.

ADULT PA

PA is a rare tumor in adults, and when it does occur, it had been thought to have a relatively benign course. The median age at presentation is in the early 30s [47], and the most common symptom is headache [48]. Many studies have suggested that in adults, PA is more likely to be supratentorial in location (involving the temporal and parietal lobes than in childhood [47,48]. An early series (1950–1981) from Barnes Hospital reported on seven adults with supratentorial PA all of whom were treated with excision; three also received postoperative RT [49]. Six of the seven were alive at a median follow-up of 9 years (one died of necrosis). A series from the United Kingdom reported 10 cases of adult PA all of whom were alive after surgery (one received postoperative RT) [48]. However, in this series, tumors were equally distributed between the supra- and infratentorial spaces.

Brown et al reported the results of a prospective NCCTG/RTOG trial in 20 adults with supratentorial PA treated between 1986 and 1994 [47]. Patients who had subtotal or gross total resection were observed; patients with biopsy only were treated with postoperative RT with a dose of 50.4 Gy in 28 fractions delivered to the tumor volume and edema. Eleven patients underwent complete resection, six had incomplete resections, and three had biopsy only. At a median follow-up of 10 years, the 5-year progression-free and overall survival rates were 95%. One of the 17 patients who was observed experienced disease progression, but on retrospective review it appeared that only a "minimal" subtotal resection had been performed; this patient was salvaged with RT. One patient who had biopsy and postoperative RT died of unknown causes. Neurologic function remained high in the patients on this study. In general, adults with PAs appear to have a favorable prognosis with regard to survival and neurologic function. A recent series from Germany described 45 patients over the age of 16 years who underwent surgery for primary or recurrent PA [50]. In this series,18% of patients died from disease at a mean follow-up of greater than 6 years; however, slightly more than a quarter of the patients in this series had pathologic features of increased proliferation or anaplasia.

REFERENCES

1. Cushing H. Experiences with the cerebellar astrocytomas: a critical review of 76 cases. *Surg Gynecol Obstet*. 1931;52:129–191.
2. CBTRUS. Statistical report: Primary brain tumors in the United States, 1998–2002. www.cbtrus.org. Accessed January 7, 2008.
3. Burkhard C, Di Patre PL, Schuler D, et al. A population-based study of the incidence and survival rates in patients with pilocytic astrocytoma. *J Neurosurg*. 2003;98;1170–1174.
4. Kleihues P, Burger PC, Scheithaur BW et al. *World Health Organization International Histological Classification of Tumours: Histological Typing of Tumours of the Central Nervous System*. 2nd ed. New York, NY: Springer-Verlag, Berlin and Heidelberg; 1993.
5. Bigner DD, McLendon RE, Bruner JM. *Russel and Rubenstein's Pathology of Tumors of the Nervous System*. 6th ed. London: Arnold; 1998.
6. Tihan T, Fisher PG, Kepner JL, et al. Pediatric astrocytomas with monomorphus pilomyxoid features and less favorable outcome. *J Neuropathol Exp Neurol*. 1999;58(10):1061–1068.
7. Coakley KJ, Huston J, Scheithauer B, et al. Pilocytic Astrocytomas: well-demarcated magnetic resonance appearance despite frequent infiltration histologically. *Mayo Clin Proc*. 1995;70:747–751.
8. Lee YY, Van Tassel P, Bruner JM, et al. Juvenile pilocytic astrocytomas: CT and MR characteristics. *AJNR*. 1989;10:363–370.
9. Strong JA, Hatten HP Jr, Brown MT, et al. Pilocytic astrocytoma: correlation between the initial imaging features and clinical aggressiveness. *AJR Am J Roentgenol*. 1993;161:369–372.
10. Campbell JW, Pollack IF. Cerebellar astrocytomas in children. *J Neurooncol*. 1996;28(2–3):223–231.
11. Grand SD, Kremer S, Tropres IM, et al. Perfusion-sensitive MRI of pilocytic astrocytomas: initial results. *Neuroradiology*. 2007;49:545–550.
12. Mamelak AN, Prados MD, Obana WG et al. Treatment options and prognosis for multicentric juvenile pilocytic astrocytoma. *J Neurosurg*. 1994;81(1):24–30.
13. Pollack IF, Hurtt M, Pang D, et al. Dissemination of low grade intracranial astrocytomas in children. *Cancer*. 1994;73(11):2671–2673.
14. Gajjar A, Bhargava R, Jenkins JJ, et al. Low-grade astrocytoma with neuraxis dissemination at diagnosis. *J Neurosurg*. 1995;83(1):67–71.

15. Hukin J, Siffert J, Cohen H, et al. Leptomeningeal dissemination at diagnosis of pediatric low-grade neuroepithelial tumors. *Neuro Oncology*. 2003;5(3):188–196.
16. Laws, ER, Taylor WF, Clifton MB, et al. Neurosurgical management of low-grade astrocytoma of the cerebral hemispheres. *J Neurosurg*. 1984;61:665–673.
17. Palma L, Guidetti B. Cystic pilocytic astrocytomas of the cerebral hemispheres. Surgical experience with 51 cases and long-term results. *J Neurosurg*. 1985;62:811–815.
18. Hirsch JF, Sainte Rose C, Pierre-Kahn A, et al. Benign astrocytic and oligodendrocytic tumors of the cerebral hemispheres in children. *J Neurosurg*. 1989;70:568–572.
19. Watson GA, Kadota RP, Wisoff JH. Multidisciplinary management of pediatric low-grade gliomas. *Semin Radiat Oncol*. 2001;11(2):152–162.
20. Gajjar A, Sanford RA, Heidman R, et al. Low-grade astrocytomas: a decade of experience at St. Jude Children's Research Hospital. *J Clin Oncol*. 1997;15:2792–2799.
21. Wallner KE, Gonzales MF, Edwards MS, et al. Treatment results of juvenile pilocytic astrocytoma. *J Neurosurg*. 1988;69(2):171–176.
22. Larson DA, Wara MW, Edwards MS: Management of childhood cerebellar astrocytoma. *Int J Radiat Oncol Biol Phys*. 1990;18:971–973.
23. Forsyth PA, Shaw EG, Scheithauer BW, et al. Supratentorial pilocytic astrocytomas. A clinicopathologic, prognostic, and flow cytometric study of 51 patients. *Cancer*. 1993;72:1335–1342.
24. Wisoff JH, Sanford R, Holmes E, et al. Impact of surgical resection on low-grade gliomas of childhood: a report from the CCC9891/POG9130 low grade astrocytoma study. Paper presented at: The International Society for Pediatric Neuro-oncology; June 9–12, 2002; Porto, Portugal.
25. Smoots D, Russell Geyer J, Lieberman DM, et al. Predicting disease progression in childhood cerebellar astrocytoma. *Childs Nerv Syst*. 1998;14:636–648.
26. Due-Tonnessen BJ, Helseth E, Scheie D, et al. Long term outcome after resection of benign cerebellar astrocytomas in children and young adults (0–19 years): report of 110 consecutive cases. *Pediatr Neurosurg*. 2002;37:71–80.
27. Gunny RS, Hayward RD, Phipps KM, et al. Spontaneous regression of residual low-grade cerebellar pilocytic astrocytomas in children. *Pediatr Radiol*. 2005;35(11):1086–1091.
28. Saunders DE, Phipps KP, Wade AM, et al. Surveillance imaging strategies following surgery and/or radiotherapy for childhood cerebellar low-grade astrocytoma. *J Neurosurg*. 2005;102(2 suppl):172–178.
29. Shaw E, Wisoff J. Prospective clinical trials of intracranial low-grade glioma in adults and children. *Neuro Oncology*. 2003;5(3):153–160.
30. Freeman CR, Farmer JP, Mentes J. Low-grade astrocytomas in children: evolving management strategies. *Int J Radiat Oncol Biol Phys*. 1998;41:979–987.
31. Shaw EG, Daumas-Duport C, Scheithauer BW, et al. Radiation therapy in the management of low-grade supratentorial astrocytomas. *J Neurosurg*. 1989;70(6):853–861.
32. Ilgren EB, Stiller CA. Cerebellar Astrocytomas. Clinical characteristics and prognostic indices. *J Neurooncol*. 1987;4(3):293–308.
33. Schneider JH, Raffel C, McComb JG. Benign cerebellar astrocytomas of childhood. *Neurosurgery*. 1992;30(1):58–62.
34. Desai KI, Nadkarni TD, Muzumdar DP, et al. Prognostic factors for cerebellar astrocytomas in children: a study of 102 cases. *Pediatr Neurosurg*. 2001;35(6):311–317.
35. Bowers DC, Gargan L, Kapur P, et al. Study of the MIB-1 labeling index as a predictor of tumor progression in pilocytic astrocytomas in children and adolescents. *J Clin Oncol*. 2003;21(15):2968–2973.
36. Karim AB, Maat B, Hatlevoll R, et al. A randomized trial on dose-response in radiation therapy of low-grade cerebral glioma (EORTC Study 22844). *Int J Radiat Oncol Biol Phys*. 1999;36:549–556.
37. Fisher BJ, Leighton CC, Vujovic O, Macdonald DR, Stitt L. Results of a policy of surveillance alone after surgical management of pediatric low grade gliomas. *Int J Radiat Oncol Biol Phys*. 2001;51(3):704–710.
38. Hug EB, Muenter MW, Archambeau JO, et al. Conformal proton radiation therapy for pediatric low-grade astrocytomas. *Strahlenther Onkol*. 2002;178:10–17.
39. Marcus KJ, Goumnerora L, Billet AL, et al. Stereotactic radiotherapy for localized low-grade gliomas in children: final results of a prospective trial. *Int J Radiat Oncol Biol Phys*. 2005; 61(2):374–379.
40. Merchant TE, Kun LE, Gajjar A, et al. A phase II trial of conformal radiation therapy for pediatric low-grade glioma: 5-year disease control and functional outcomes. *Int J Radiat Oncol Biol Phys*. 2007;69(suppl 3):60(Abst).
41. Krieger MD, Gonzalez-Gomez I, Levy ML, et al. Recurrence patterns and anaplastic change in a long-term study of pilocytic astrocytomas. *Pediatr Neurosurg*. 1997;27(1):1–11.
42. Lesser GJ. Chemotherapy of low-grade gliomas. *Semin Radiat Oncol*. 2001; 11(2):138–144.
43. Packer RJ, Sutton LN, Bilaniuk LT, et al. Treatment of chiasmatic/hypothalamic gliomas of childhood with chemotherapy: an update. *Annals Neurol*. 1988;23:79–85.
44. Packer RJ, Ater J, Allen J, et al. Carboplatin and vincristine chemotherapy for children with newly diagnosed progressive low-grade gliomas. *J Neurosurg*. 1997;86(5):747–754.
45. Prados MD, Edwards MS, Rabbitt J, et al. Treatment of pediatric low-grade gliomas with a nitrosourea-based multiagent chemotherapy regimen. *J Neurooncol*. 1997;32(3):235–241.
46. Packer RJ. Chemotherapy: low-grade gliomas of the hypothalamus and thalamus. *Pediatr Neurosurg*. 2000;32(50):259–263.
47. Brown PD, Buckner JC, O'Fallon JR, et al. Adult patients with supratentorial pilocytic astrocytomas: a prospective multicenter clinical trial. *Int J Radiat Oncol Biol Phys*. 2004;58:1153–1160.
48. Bell D, Chitnavis BP, Al-Sarraj S, et al. Pilocytic astrocytoma of the adult- clinical features, radiological features and management. *Br J Neurosurg*. 2004;18:613–616.
49. Garcia DM, Fulling KH. Juvenile pilocytic astrocytoma of the cerebrum in adults. A distinctive neoplasm with favorable prognosis. *J Neurosurg*. 1985;63:382–386.
50. Stuer C, Vilz B, Majores M, et al. Frequent recurrence and progression in pilocytic astrocytoma in adults. *Cancer*. 2007;110:2799–2808.

90 Ependymoma (Intracranial)

Lisa Hazard and C. Leland Rogers

INTRODUCTION

Percival Bailey first described ependymomas as a separate clinicopathologic entity in 1926 [1].Since that time, several studies have corroborated the existence of this distinct, although rare, glioma subtype. There are <200 cases diagnosed annually in the United States [2,3]. Ependymomas can arise from the ependymal cells lining the ventricles of the brain, from ependymal rests within the cerebral hemispheres, or from the vestigial central canal of the spinal cord [4]. This chapter is limited to the discussion of intracranial ependymomas.

HISTOLOGY AND GRADING

The World Health Organization classifies ependymomas as grade I (subependymoma and myxopapillary), grade II (differentiated ependymoma and its variants: cellular, papillary, clear cell, and tanycytic), and grade III (anaplastic) [5]. Subependymomas are low grade and usually display an indolent clinical course [6], usually discovered incidentally on imaging or at autopsy [7,8]. Myxopapillary ependymomas occur in the spine, typically in the conus-cauda-filum terminale region, and have rarely been found intracranially [9,10]. Grade I lesions will not be specifically addressed in this chapter.

Microscopically, ependymomas are highly cellular. A classic feature is the ependymal rosette in which polarized cells form a circle with an extracellular lumen, a finding which is not, however, as common as a pseudorosette in which such polarized cells encircle a blood vessel [11,12]. Histologic characteristics of high-grade tumors include marked cellularity, mitotic activity, endothelial proliferation, and necrosis [13]. Reliable and reproducible differentiation between high- and low-grade ependymomas is difficult to achieve, and predicting behavior on the basis of histologic appearance remains problematic [13–15].

EPIDEMIOLOGY

Ependymomas account for about 1.7% of all childhood cancers [16–18] and about 5% to 10% of intracranial childhood cancers [11,16,18–20], whereas they account for 1% to 5% of intracranial neoplasms in adults [11,20,21]. The incidence is about 2.2 per million children [2,22] and 2.7 per million adults [23].

In a Surveillance, Epidemiology, and End Results (SEER) study, children with infratentorial tumors had a mean age at diagnosis of 5 years versus 8 years for those who had supratentorial tumors, although this difference did not reach statistical significance [23]. The mean age was about 45 years in adults, regardless of location in the brain. As found in the SEER study and as reported by others, there may be a slight male predominance (55%–60%) [15,24].

LOCATION

About two-thirds of intracranial ependymomas are infratentorial [25–27]. Among infratentorial primaries, about 80% are intraventricular. In contrast, fewer supratentorial ependymomas are intraventricular (9%–30%) [11,25,28]. Infratentorial ependymomas most commonly arise from the fourth ventricle: 60% from the floor, 30% from the lateral walls, and 10% from the roof [3].

IMAGING

Preoperative computed tomography (CT) or magnetic resonance imaging (MRI) findings may suggest ependymoma, but imaging characteristics alone are not sufficient to establish the diagnosis, and biopsy confirmation is mandatory. On CT or MRI, enhancement is typically prominent, and cysts and calcification are common. A cystic component is identified in 40% to 85% of ependymomas [6,11,25,29,30]. Specifically on CT scans, these tumors can demonstrate calcifications (40%–80%), ranging from small punctate foci to dense calcifications occupying most of the tumor [6,29,31]. The soft tissue component on CT imaging is commonly isodense or slightly hyperdense compared with white matter, and the majority (about 80%) exhibit enhancement [6]. In the series by Furie and Provenzale [6], ependymomas that did not exhibit enhancement on CT were densely calcified and lacked a noncalcified soft tissue component. In this and other reports, patterns of enhancement can vary [6,27,29].

On MRI, the soft tissue component is typically isointense or hypointense on T1 and hyperintense on T2

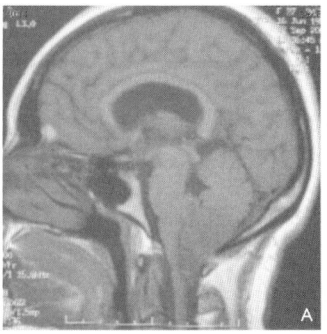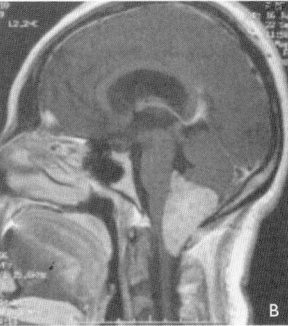

Figure 90.1 Panel A shows posterior fossa ependymoma in a T1 sagittal MRI scan of the brain, pre-contrast. Panel B shows the same ependymoma post-contrast.

compared with white matter [6]. Furie and Provenzale found that 72% of supratentorial tumors and 95% of infratentorial tumors exhibited heterogenous enhancement. In general, MRI is superior to CT in defining the tumor extent of ependymomas [6]. Figure 90.1 depicts a posterior fossa ependymoma on MRI.

PRESENTING SIGNS AND SYMPTOMS

Both supratentorial and infratentorial tumors can cause symptoms of increased intracranial pressure, including headaches, nausea, vomiting, and ataxia. Infratentorial tumors are particularly prone to ventricular obstruction. With posterior fossa primaries, owing to proximity to the brainstem, cranial nerve deficits can also occur. Supratentorial tumors can result in seizures and focal neurologic deficits [26,28].

Spinal cord metastases are uncommon at presentation, with an incidence ranging from 0% to 15% in the literature [32–35]. In a review of the literature by McLaughlin et al [12], spinal metastases were reported in 29 of 268 tumors (8%) and were more common for intraventricular tumors (11%) compared with extraventricular tumors (3%), p = 0.005. For infratentorial tumors, high-grade histology was associated with a greater incidence of spinal metastasis compared with low-grade histology (19% vs 7%, p = 0.05). In this same review, the incidence of spinal metastases with supratentorial tumors was 3% irrespective of grade. Schild et al [13] also reported that high-grade histology correlated with increased risk for spinal dissemination at presentation (20% with high-grade tumors versus 6% with low-grade tumors).

TREATMENT

Surgery

Treatment of intracranial ependymomas begins with maximal safe resection. Complete resection is associated with improvement in local control and survival in most studies (Table 90.1) [14,15,36–41]. In a recent prospective multi-institutional study, gross total resection was achieved in 82% of patients and near total resection in 11% [36]. Likely because of improvements in surgical technique over time,

Table 90.1 Effect of Resection on Outcome

Institute (N)	GTR	OS(%)	EFS(%)	LC(%)
Pittsburgh [39] (37)	GTR	80	68	
	STR	22[a]	9	
Pediatric Oncology Group [15] (83)	GTR	57	70	
	STR		20[a]	
Washington University [14] (60)	GTR	84	58	
	STR	66[b]		
University of Iowa [37] (49)	GTR	69	69	75
	STR			49[a]
Institute Gustave Roussy [41] (80)	GTR	75	51	
	STR	41[a]	26[a]	
University of Pennsylvania [42] (51)	GTR	30	46	
	STR			
Mayo Clinic [43] (33)	GTR	62	61	
	STR			
Italy [38] (92)	GTR	70[c]	33[c]	
	STR	57[a,c]	10[a,c]	
Barrow Neurological Institute [40] (45)	GTR + RT	83[c]		100[c]
	GTR	67[c]		50[c]
	STR	43[b,c]		35[a,c]
Germany (55)	GTR	92[d]	57[e]	
	STR	56[d]	30[e]	
Multi-Institutional [68] (22)	GTR	100[d]		82[d]
	STR	60[a,d]		40[a,d]
St Judes [36] (153)	GTR	93	82	16[f]
	STR	52[a]	41[a]	

[a] significant (p<0.05)
[b] trend towards significance (p = 0.05–0.10)
[c] 10 year data
[d] 3 year data
[e] Estimated from figure
[f] LC was superior with GTR compared with STR, but LC in each group was not reported separately

Abbreviations: EFS, event-free survival; GTR, gross total resection, LC, local control; N, number; OS, overall survival; STR, subtotal resection.

recent series have documented higher rates of gross total resection [14,37,38,41–43].

Radiation Therapy after Gross Total Resection

Retrospective series evaluating outcomes with or without radiation therapy are summarized in Table 90.2. Although most of these demonstrated improvements in outcome with the addition of radiation to surgery, these series are small and retrospective, with a heterogeneous population treated over decades, during which time both surgical and radiation techniques have improved [20,39,41]. Studies using gross total resection alone are small, and definite conclusions are difficult to draw [2,20,28,44,45]. Rogers et al [40] evaluated patients treated at the Barrow Neurological Institute in Phoenix, Arizona, from 1983 to 2002. During that period, some but not all physicians at their institute adopted a preference for the omission of radiation after gross total resection. Gross total resection was achieved in 32 of 45 patients (71%). Of the 32 patients with gross total resection, 13 (41%) received postoperative radiation therapy. Ten-year local control was 50% with gross total resection alone compared with 100% with gross total resection plus radiation (p = 0.018). Ten-year cause-specific and overall survival numerically favored gross

Table 90.2 Retrospective Studies Evaluating the Use of Radiation

Institute	Treatment	N	5-year OS (%)	5-year EFS (%)	LC (%)	%GTR
Norway [20]	RT	16	38	NR	NR	17
	No RT	28	15[a]	NR	NR	
Institute Gustave Roussy [41]	RT	65	63	45	NR	48
	No RT	15	23[a]	0[a]	NR	
Italy [38]	RT	74	58[b]	38[b]	NR	60
	No RT	16	52[b]	20[a,b]	NR	
Barrow Neurological Institute [40]	GTR and RT	14	83[b]	NR	100	100
	STR and RT	12	43[b]	NR	36	0
	GTR no RT	19	67[b]	NR	50[a]	100
Surveillance Epidemiology and End Results [46]	Infratentorial					
	RT	116	57	NR	NR	NR
	No RT	68	48[a]	NR	NR	
	Supratentorial					
	RT	65	54	NR	NR	NR
	No RT	38	68	NR	NR	

[a] $p<0.05$ no RT compared with RTNR

[b] 10 year overall survival.

Abbreviations: EFS, event-free survial; GTR, gross total resection; LC, local control; N, number; OS, overall survival; RT, radiation therapy; STR, subtotal resection.

total resection plus radiation but did not reach statistical significance. Given the potential morbidity associated with local recurrence and the low rate of late complications from radiation therapy observed in this study, the authors favored the use of postoperative radiation therapy after gross total resection.

Hukin et al [44] treated 10 patients with gross total resection without postoperative radiation therapy in a prospective trial, and seven remained disease free at a median follow-up of 48 months. Of the three who had a recurrence, two were salvaged with surgery and radiation therapy. An ongoing prospective study by the Children's Oncology Group (COG) (ACNS 0121) uses observation after gross total resection alone for nonanaplastic supratentorial ependymoma. All patients with infratentorial and/or anaplastic ependymomas undergo postoperative radiation regardless of the extent of resection.

Radiation after Subtotal Resection

The role of radiation after subtotal resection is generally not disputed. Although randomized data do not exist, retrospective data support the use of radiation therapy. A SEER multivariate analysis of 635 patients reported that the use of radiotherapy was associated with improved survival after surgery in children with infratentorial but not supratentorial tumors [46].

Radiation Dose

Most retrospective studies have shown doses >45 Gy to be superior to lower doses [32,42,47–54]. Garrett and Simpson [47] reported that 5 of 18 patients (28%) treated with doses ≤45 Gy were alive at the last follow-up, whereas 49 of 73 patients (67%) who received a higher dose were living. Stuben et al [48] showed superior progression-free survival with doses >45 Gy. Shaw et al found improved local control with doses >50 Gy and recommended 55 Gy after either a gross total or subtotal resection [13]. In disseminated disease, dose to the craniospinal axis is generally 36 Gy, followed by boost to the primary site to a total dose of 54–60 Gy [55,56].

Stereotactic Radiosurgery

Even with aggressive resection, and with conventional radiation therapy using the published dose fractionation schemes, local failure remains an obstacle to cure in some patients. Although leptomeningeal dissemination can occur, it is relatively uncommon for this to develop in the absence of local relapse [7,19,36,57–63]. Thus, more aggressive local measures, such as radiosurgery, have been proposed [62]. Radiosurgery has only been studied in small series [57–61], largely composed of patients with small-volume gross residual disease after surgery or with recurrent ependymoma. Kano et al [60] recently reported 39 patients with recurrent ependymoma treated with radiosurgery to a median dose of 15 Gy. All patients had prior external beam radiation. With a median follow-up of 15 months, local control at the treated site was 73%, and 5-year progression-free survival was 46%. Adverse events occurred in three patients (8%) and included radiation necrosis in two patients and ipsilateral facial paralysis in one. Stafford et al [58] reported similar results in their series. Data regarding the role of radiosurgery as a boost after external beam radiation therapy for patients with postoperative gross residual disease are limited, but is intriguing given that local recurrence remains the principal mode of failure, and warrants further investigation [14,57].

Altered Fractionation

A Pediatric Oncology Group study (POG 9132) evaluated hyperfractionation using 69.6 Gy in 58 fractions delivered twice daily [62]. In comparison with an earlier POG study (8532) using standard fractionation, event-free survival was superior after hyperfractionation in patients who underwent subtotal resection (4-year event-free survival of 50% and 24%, respectively). However, a separate prospective study from Italy failed to show a benefit with hyperfractionation, and altered fractionation is not considered the standard [63].

Radiation Therapy–Overall Treatment Time

A series by Paulino and Wen [56] using 54 Gy standard fractionation showed that radiation therapy duration <50 days yielded a 10-year local control rate of 66%, whereas treatment duration of ≥50 days yielded a 10-year local control rate of 36% (p = 0.01), lending possible support to shorter treatment duration. In this series, the majority of patients who had treatment duration >50 days received craniospinal radiation, and treatment delay was due to myelosuppression. These findings could suggest that accelerated repopulation of tumor clonogens may play a role in radioresistance for ependymomas.

Radiation Therapy Field Size

Current recommendations for radiation field size are local radiation in nondisseminated disease and craniospinal irradiation (CSI) in disseminated disease. In localized disease, the predominant pattern of failure is local [12,34,35,43,47,52,53,62,63]. In patients treated with local radiation therapy, isolated recurrence outside of the radiation field is comparatively uncommon and has been reported to occur in 0% to 13% of patients [15,39,41,54,55]. Some early studies reported a benefit with the use of CSI, but these were largely before the MRI era and therefore occult spinal disease may have been present at diagnosis [47,53,64,65]. Most recent studies have not found a benefit with the use of CSI [12,13,15,33,37,40,43,50,54,56,66,67]. Schroeder et al [68] treated 22 patients with local radiation therapy, including gross tumor plus 1.3 to 2 cm margin, and noted that all of the six local recurrences were within the high-dose region. An autopsy series also demonstrated that recurrence is often within the high-dose radiation field [35]. Merchant et al treated patients with local radiation therapy (gross tumor or postoperative tumor bed or both) plus 1.3 to 1.5 cm margin and noted a recurrence rate outside the radiation field of 11.5% [36]. Schild et al [13] observed similar rates of spinal seeding in patients who received craniospinal radiation (7.3%) and those who received smaller radiation fields (6.4%). These same authors reported an actuarial 5-year rate of leptomeningeal failure of 41% with high-grade tumors versus 10% with low-grade tumors (p = 0.01). Of the 10 patients with high-grade disease, seven did not undergo CSI. The authors therefore recommended CSI for high-grade disease. Merchant et al [36] also reported a higher incidence of distant failure in patients with high-grade versus those with low-grade disease (17% versus 5% 7-year distant failure; p = 0.017). In contrast, Timmerman et al [66] found no advantage with the use of CSI compared with local radiation in 55 patients with anaplastic ependymoma, even if the tumor contacted or infiltrated the ventricular wall. An ongoing COG study (ACNS 0121) does not use craniospinal in patients with localized ependymoma. At this time, CSI is recommended only with documented cerebrospinal fluid/spinal dissemination.

Toxicity of Radiation Therapy

Toxicity of radiation therapy remains a significant concern, particularly in pediatric patients. Perhaps, most concerning is the potential for neurocognitive decline. Cognitive deficits have been reported even with the use of posterior fossa-only radiation therapy [69,70]. Merchant et al evaluated 82 children with intracranial ependymoma treated with localized radiation fields and noted a mean intelligence quotient (IQ) of 96 at 3 years after radiation. Younger age at the time of radiation and increasing volume of supratentorial brain treated with radiation correlated with lower IQ scores [71]. Although these results demonstrate an effect of radiation on IQ, the mean scores were within normal limits for the general population. In a prospective evaluation, Merchant et al did not observe a decline in IQ scores, Wechsler individual achievement scores, or Vineland adaptive behavior scale scores before versus 48 months after conformal radiation [72].

Doses about >20 Gy can result in hypoplasia of the treated bone in pediatric patients. Permanent alopecia can occur in children or adults. The hypothalamus and pituitary glands are particularly sensitive to radiation, and endocrine dysfunction can occur at doses as low as 20 Gy [12,73]. Growth hormone deficiency is most common and can be replaced through subcutaneous injection if necessary. Hearing deficits related to radiation therapy can occur, particularly in posterior fossa tumors [74]. Secondary malignancy is a rare but serious complication. Other late complications of radiation have been rarely reported, including cavernous malformation [40].

Modern radiation therapy techniques, including three-dimensional conformal radiation therapy and intensity-modulated radiation therapy, have improved the conformity of radiation therapy fields and decreased dose to normal structures compared with two-dimensional techniques used in the past [68]. An example of an intensity modulated radiation therapy plan is depicted in Figure 90.2.

Resection of infratentorial tumors can result in posterior fossa syndrome in about 8% of pediatric patients, with resultant speech disturbance/mutism, poor oral intake, personality changes, urinary retention, long tract signs, and/or decreased initiation of voluntary movements [39]. These symptoms are generally transient, lasting a median of 5 weeks, but there is no evidence that radiotherapy potentiates these toxicities [75]. Although there are no clear data for an enhanced incidence of cerebrospinal fluid leak with radiotherapy, the potential for this exists because radiotherapy can impair wound healing.

Chemoradiotherapy and Adjuvant Chemotherapy to Delay Radiotherapy

A randomized prospective study (COG 942) showed no benefit with the addition of chemotherapy (CCNU, vincristine, and prednisone) to radiation therapy [76]. Chemotherapy has been used in an attempt to avoid or delay radiation therapy in children. The French Society of Pediatric Oncology completed a prospective study using chemotherapy after gross or subtotal resection in pediatric ependymoma [77]. Chemotherapy consisted of alternating

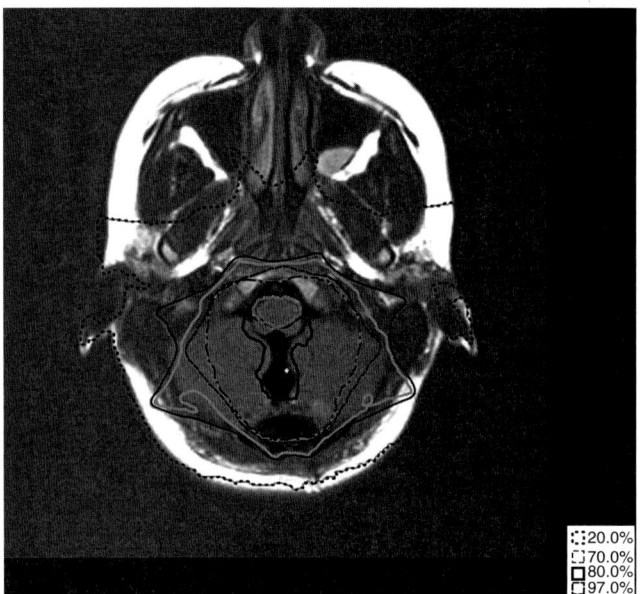

Figure 90.2 Intensity modulated radiation therapy planning for treatment of posterior fossa ependymoma. The resection cavity is outlined in solid, and the target volume (which includes the postoperative cavity plus 1.5 cm margin) is outlined in dashed lines. The 97% isodose surface in shown in dotted lines, and the target volume is completely encompassed by 97% of the prescribed dose. The radiation field conforms well to the shape of the target volume, thus minimizing dose to normal structures including the brain and cochlea.

courses of carboplatin/procarbazine, etoposide/cisplatin, and vincristine/cyclophosphamide. None of the 20 (of 73) patients with residual disease had a complete or partial response during chemotherapy, and all of the children with residual disease after surgery progressed. After relapse, 2-year overall survival was 49%. Only patients who underwent complete surgical resection plus radiation remained in complete remission after relapse; high-dose chemotherapy was not effective. Forty percent of patients were alive at 2 years after initiation of chemotherapy and did not need radiation, but by 4 years, only 23% were alive and did not need radiation. Among the 36 patients who eventually required radiation for salvage, radiation was deferred for a median of only 15 months. On multivariate analysis, a very high-risk subgroup was identified: posterior fossa tumor with incomplete resection. This population had a progression-free survival rate of 5% and an overall survival rate of 54% at 2 years. Given the poor response rates to chemotherapy and the nonrandomized nature of this study, it is difficult to determine whether the postoperative chemotherapy in fact delayed or prevented recurrence.

PROGNOSTIC VARIABLES

Overview

Survival rates and prognostic factors reported in various studies are summarized in Table 90.3. The factors of greatest current interest will be discussed in the following subsections.

Histologic Grade

The influence of histologic grade on outcome remains controversial, although high grade is generally believed to have worse prognosis. Some studies have shown no correlation between outcome and grade [12,15,24,38,39,42,54,78,79], whereas others have shown worse outcome with high grade compared with grade II (Table 90.4) [13,15,22,43,48,64]. These conflicting observations may be in part due to the small number of patients available for evaluation, many studies being insufficiently powered to show a difference. In addition, there is ambiguity in the assignment of grade. In a multi-institutional study, Horn et al [15] reported that histologic grade was altered in 24% of cases on central review. Finally, it is possible that grade influences outcome in the short term but not in the long term, as suggested by Mansur et al [14]. In their study, survival curves initially diverged for grade II versus grade III, but they converged again over time.

Some studies have shown higher rates of spinal failure with high-grade tumors. Schild et al reported that after treatment of localized ependymoma, actuarial 5-year rate of leptomeningeal failure was 41% with high-grade tumors versus 10% with low-grade tumors (p = 0.01) [13]. This study included spinal and intracranial ependymomas, making it difficult to extrapolate the results. However, 90% of their high-grade patients had intracranial disease. This study included patients treated in the pre-MRI era, and it is possible that some of these patients had subclinical metastases at diagnosis. Hukin et al [44] treated three patients with high-grade tumors with gross total resection alone, and none of these three patients have had disease recurrence. In the ongoing COG study of localized intracranial ependymoma (ACNS 0121), grade influences treatment for supratentorial tumors: patients with supratentorial nonanaplastic tumors treated with gross total resection are observed, and those with anaplastic histology undergo local field radiation. Infratentorial tumors are treated with local field radiation regardless of grade.

Extent of Resection

Gross total resection is associated with improvements in local control and overall survival in all but a few series [19,24,37–39,41,42,43,54,64,67,80] In a study by the Children's Hospital of Philadelphia, 5-year progression-free survival was 60% in those treated with complete resection versus 21% in those treated with partial resection or biopsy [80]. In another publication from this same group, 5-year overall survival was 80% with total resection versus 22% with a lesser resection [39]. Maximal safe resection is therefore recommended in all patients.

Disseminated Disease

Disseminated disease has a worse prognosis compared with localized disease, as expected [66,81,82]. Craniospinal radiation is recommended in these patients. Zacharoulis et al reported on 40 patients with metastatic disease at diagnosis from eight institutions. The 5-year event-free survival was 29%, and the 5-year overall survival was 43%. The majority (90%) had posterior fossa primary tumors,

Table 90.3 Ependymoma studies

Institute (N): Years of Study	5/10 year OS (%)	5/10 year EFS (%)	LR alone (%)	LR + DM (%)	DM alone (%)	Positive Prognostic Factors		
						OS	EFS	LC
Pittsburgh [39] (37): 1975–1993	57/45	45/36	41	5	5	GTR, Age >3, sx's > 1 mo	GTR, Age >3, sx's > 1 mo	
POG [15] (83): 1987–1991	57/46	46/33	39	16	11	LG	Age >3, GTR, LG	
Wash U [14] (60): 1964–2000	71/55	58/50	NR	NR	NR	ST, GTR[a,b]	IT[b]	
University of Iowa [37] (49): 1965–1997	69/63	69/63	40	9	0	LG[b]		LG, GTR, dose >45 Gy for GTR pts[b]
Multi-Institutional [22] (50): 1982–1999	NR	NR	24	8	0	LG	LG, no pre RT chemo	
Norway [20] (48): 1953–1974	24/13	NR	NR	NR	NR	Use of RT, LG, IT[b]		
Institute Gustave Roussy [41] (80): 1975–1989	56/NR	38/NR	25	4	13	GTR, LG[a], RT used[b]	GTR, RT used[b]	
University of Pennsylvania [42] (51): 1970–1998	30/NR	30/20	43	10	2	Age >4, IT[a], dose >45 Gy[b]		Dose >45 Gy[b]
Mayo Clinic [43] (33): 1963–1983	62/NR	61/NR	27	6	3	LG[b]	LG[b], female[a,b] no hydrocephalus[a,b], dose >45 Gy[a,b]	
Italy [38] (92): 1977–1993	55/55	38/35	NR	NR	NR	GTR[b]	GTR Use of RT[b]	
Gainesville [12] (31): 1966–1989	29(ST),[c] 58 (IT)[c] /20(ST), 45 (IT)	NR[d]	65	3	0	Grade[c]	None	
Barrow Neurological Institute [40] (45): 1983–2002	GTR 77/67 GTR + RT 83/83, STR 83/67	NR	GTR 50, GTR + RT 0, STR 64[e]	9	0	Younger age		Use of RT, GTR, Female[a], LG
St Judes [36] (153): 1997–2007	81 (7 year)	67 (7 years)	9	7	10	LG, GTR, white	LG, GTR, female	GTR, female, age > 3. LG had lower risk of DM.

Abbreviations: DM, distant metastasis; EFS, event-free survival; GTR, gross total resection; HG, high grade; IT, infratentorial; LC, local control; LG, low grade; LR, local recurrence; mo, months; N, number; NR, not reported; RT, radiation therapy; ST, supratentorial; Sx's > 1 mo, duration of symptoms before operation > 1 month; TTP, time to progression.

[a] Trend towards significant (p = 0.06–0.10)

[b] Multivariate analysis not performed. Results refer to univariate analysis.

[c] Significant on univariate analysis but not multivariate analysis.

[d] EFS at 10 years was 14% and 33% for pediatric and adult ST tumors, respectively. EFS at 10 years was 36% and 62% for pediatric and adult IT tumors, respectively. Differences did not reach statistical significance by age or location.

[e] Estimated from figure.

and most were younger than 36 months at diagnosis (72%). Timmerman et al reported that 3-year event-free survival was 0% in patients with metastatic disease compared with 66% in patients with localized disease (p = 0.0001) [66].

Age

Age at diagnosis <3 years has been associated with a more aggressive clinical course [15,19,22,38,39]. The poorer prognosis is possibly related to a predilection for posterior fossa location in young children [46], which in turn is associated with lower rates of gross total resection [15]. Furthermore, radiation therapy is more commonly omitted or delayed in young patients because of toxicity concerns, which may result in increased failures. The COG completed a prospective trial in children younger than 3 years in whom chemotherapy was used in an attempt to delay radiation. Results from this trial showed a 5-year overall survival rate of 63% if radiation was delayed for 1 year and 26% if radiation was delayed for 2 years, suggesting that the delay in radiation resulted in inferior survival. Pollack et al [39] showed a 5-year overall survival rate of 22% in 13 patients younger than 3 years, compared with 75% in older patients in whom radiation was generally not delayed. Similarly, a study by the St Judes Hospital showed a 3-year progression-free survival of 49% when radiation therapy was delayed compared with 84% when it was not delayed [22]. Although it is possible that younger patients have an inherently more aggressive disease, it seems more likely that differences in the aggressiveness of treatment account for differences in outcome.

Location

Infratentorial location has inferior outcome compared with supratentorial location in some studies and superior

Table 90.4 Effect of Grade on Outcome

Institute	Years	N	5-year OS HG (%)	5-year OS LG (%)	P value <0.05	5-year EFS HG (%)	5-year EFS LG (%)	P value <0.05
Pittsburgh [39]	1975–1993	37	57		no	45		No[a]
Pediatric Oncology Group [15]	1987–1991	83	36[a]	57[b]	yes	13	52	yes
Washington University [14]	1964–2000	60	66	74	no	52	62	no
University of Iowa [37]	1965–1997	49	46	76	yes	55 (LC)	70 (LC)	yes
Multi-Institutional [22]	1982–1999	50	NR	NR	–	28 (3 years)	84 (3 years)	yes
Norway [20]	1953–1974	48	17	25	NR	NR	NR	NR
Institute Gustave Roussy [41]	1975–1989	80	40	65	Trend	22	45	no
University of Pennsylvania [42]	1970–1998	51	42	47	no	31	27	no
Mayo Clinic [43]	1963–1983	33	29	71	yes	29	70	yes
Italian [38]	1977–1993	92	45	60	0.18[c]	0	45	yes[c]
Gainsville [12]	1966–1989	32	24 (10 year)	76 (10 year)	yes[d]	NR	NR	NR
St Judes [36,][c]	1997–2007	153	79	92	yes	61	86	yes

EFS, event-free survival; HG, high grade; LG, low grade; N, number; NR, not reported.

[a] The presence of necrosis was associated with inferior OS and EFS on univariate analysis (p=0.06 and 0.03, respectively), but not multivariate analysis
[b] Cumulative probability of survival.
[c] Significant on univariate but not multivariate analysis.
[d] High grade associated with higher 7 year distant failure rate (17% vs 5%, $p = 0.017$) but not local failure.

outcome in others [12,52,77]. A SEER database evaluation by McGuire et al demonstrated similar 5-year overall survival rates in the 193 patients with infratentorial disease versus the 106 patients with supratentorial disease (54% and 58%, respectively). Prospective data by Grill et al in 73 children younger than 5 years demonstrated superior survival in patients with supratentorial disease on univariate analysis, despite similar rates of complete resection. However, this finding lost statistical significance on multivariate analysis. Prospective data by Merchant et al did not identify site of ependymoma as a significant prognostic factor, although supratentorial disease had numerically superior 5-year overall survival compared with infratentorial disease (83% and 71%, respectively). Some studies have reported that infratentorial tumors are less likely to be high grade (10%–40%) compared with supratentorial tumors (50%–60%) [11,25,28]. The current literature does not clearly identify site of intracranial ependymoma as a reliable prognostic factor.

SURVEILLANCE AFTER TREATMENT

Close follow-up with serial MRI scans is essential after completion of planned therapy to diagnose disease, although it is relatively small and amenable to therapy. Surveillance is particularly important when radiation is not delivered as part of initial therapy. A majority of recurrences occur within the first 2 years after initial resection [43,54], but late recurrences can occur, and surveillance is recommended for a minimum of 10 years [14,42]. Because ependymomas are relatively slow-growing tumors, a scanning interval of 3 to 4 months may be reasonable in the first 2 years, extending to 6 months thereafter [44].

CONCLUSIONS

Ependymoma is a rare neoplasm that affects both children and adults. Gross total resection, the use of adjuvant radiation therapy, nonanaplastic histology, and the absence of spinal metastases have been correlated with improved outcome. Maximal safe resection is an essential component of therapy. Although prospective randomized data are lacking, radiation seems to improve local control after gross total resection, particularly for posterior fossa primaries, and survival after subtotal resection. Localized radiation therapy fields using conformal techniques are now standard and result in lower toxicity compared with earlier studies using large radiation fields and two-dimensional techniques. Further study is necessary to define the role of radiation dose escalation using hyperfractionation and/or stereotactic radiosurgery, as well as to better define the role of chemotherapy.

REFERENCES

1. Bailey P, Cushing H. *A Classification of the tumors of the glioma group on a histogenetic basis with a correlated study of prognosis*. Philadelphia: JB lippincott; 1926.
2. Healey EA, Barnes PD, Kupsky WJ, et al. The prognostic significance of postoperative residual tumor in ependymoma. *Neurosurgery*. 1991;28(5):666-671; discussion 671–662.
3. Merchant TE. Current management of childhood ependymoma. *Oncology (Williston Park)*. 2002;16(5):629–642, 644; discussion 645–626, 648.
4. Russell D, Rubenstein LJ. *Pathology of tumors of the nervous system*. 5th ed. Baltimore: Williams and Wilkins; 1989.
5. Louis DN, Ohgaki H, Wiestler OD, et al. The 2007 WHO classification of tumours of the central nervous system. *Acta Neuropathol*. 2007;114(2):97–109.
6. Furie DM, Provenzale JM. Supratentorial ependymomas and subependymomas: CT and MR appearance. *J Comput Assist Tomogr*. 1995;19(4):518–526.
7. Kulkarni AV, Drake, JM. Intracranial ependymomas. In: Kaye AH, Laws, ER Jr, eds. *Brain Tumors*. 2nd ed. London: Churchill Livingstone; 2001:541–550.
8. Schwartz TH, Kim S, Glick RS, et al. Supratentorial ependymomas in adult patients. *Neurosurgery*. 1999;44(4):721–731.
9. Schroder R, Firsching R, Kochanek S. Hemangiopericytoma of meninges. II. General and clinical data. *Zentralbl Neurochir*. 1986;47(3):191–199.
10. Warnick RE, Raisanen J, Adornato BT, et al. Intracranial myxopapillary ependymoma: case report. *J Neurooncol*. 1993;15(3):251–256.
11. Svien H, Mabou R, Kernohan JW, et al. Ependymoma of the brain: Pathologic aspects. *Neurology*. 1953;3:1–15.

12. McLaughlin MP, Marcus RB Jr, Buatti JM, et al. Ependymoma: results, prognostic factors and treatment recommendations. *Int J Radiat Oncol Biol Phys.* 1998;40(4):845–850.
13. Schild SE, Nisi K, Scheithauer BW, et al. The results of radiotherapy for ependymomas: the Mayo Clinic experience. *Int J Radiat Oncol Biol Phys.* 1998;42(5):953–958.
14. Mansur DB, Perry A, Rajaram V, et al. Postoperative radiation therapy for grade II and III intracranial ependymoma. *Int J Radiat Oncol Biol Phys.* 2005;61(2):387–391.
15. Horn B, Heideman R, Geyer R, et al. A multi-institutional retrospective study of intracranial ependymoma in children: identification of risk factors. *J Pediatr Hematol Oncol.* 1999;21(3):203–211.
16. Miller RW, Young JL Jr, Novakovic B. Childhood cancer. *Cancer.* 1995;75(1 suppl):395–405.
17. Kuratsu J, Ushio Y. Epidemiological study of primary intracranial tumors: a regional survey in Kumamoto Prefecture in the southern part of Japan. *J Neurosurg.* 1996;84(6):946–950.
18. Gurney JG, Severson RK, Davis S, Robison LL. Incidence of cancer in children in the United States. Sex-, race-, and 1-year age-specific rates by histologic type. *Cancer.* 1995;75(8):2186–2195.
19. Duffner PK, Krischer JP, Sanford RA, et al. Prognostic factors in infants and very young children with intracranial ependymomas. *Pediatr Neurosurg.* 1998;28(4):215–222.
20. Mork SJ, Loken AC. Ependymoma: a follow-up study of 101 cases. *Cancer.* 1977;40(2):907–915.
21. Barone BM, Elvidge AR. Ependymomas. A clinical survey. *J Neurosurg.* 1970;33(4):428–438.
22. Merchant TE, Zhu Y, Thompson SJ, Sontag MR, Heideman RL, Kun LE. Preliminary results from a Phase II trail of conformal radiation therapy for pediatric patients with localised low-grade astrocytoma and ependymoma. *Int J Radiat Oncol Biol Phys.* 2002;52(2):325–332.
23. McGuire CS, Sainani KL, Fisher PG. Incidence patterns for ependymoma: a surveillance, epidemiology, and end results study. *J Neurosurg.* 2009;110(4):725–729.
24. Robertson PL, Zeltzer PM, Boyett JM, et al. Survival and prognostic factors following radiation therapy and chemotherapy for ependymomas in children: a report of the Children's Cancer Group. *J Neurosurg.* 1998;88(4):695–703.
25. Coulon RA, Till K. Intracranial ependymomas in children: a review of 43 cases. *Childs Brain.* 1977;3(3):154–168.
26. Kricheff, II, Becker M, Schneck SA, Taveras JM. Intracranial Ependymomas: Factors Influencing Prognosis. *J Neurosurg.* 1964;21:7–14.
27. Van Tassel P, Lee YY, Bruner JM. Supratentorial ependymomas: computed tomographic and pathologic correlations. *J Comput Tomogr.* 1986;10(2):157–165.
28. Palma L, Celli P, Cantore G. Supratentorial ependymomas of the first two decades of life. Long-term follow-up of 20 cases (including two subependymomas). *Neurosurgery.* 1993;32(2):169–175.
29. Swartz JD, Zimmerman RA, Bilaniuk LT. Computed tomography of intracranial ependymomas. *Radiology.* 1982;143(1):97–101.
30. Armington WG, Osborn AG, Cubberley DA, et al. Supratentorial ependymoma: CT appearance. *Radiology.* 1985;157(2):367–372.
31. Centeno RS, Lee AA, Winter J, Barba D. Supratentorial ependymomas. Neuroimaging and clinicopathological correlation. *J Neurosurg.* 1986;64(2):209–215.
32. Phillips TL, Sheline GE, Boldrey E. Therapeutic Considerations in Tumors Affecting the Central Nervous System: Ependymomas. *Radiology.* 1964;83:98–105.
33. Vanuytsel L, Brada M. The role of prophylactic spinal irradiation in localized intracranial ependymoma. *Int J Radiat Oncol Biol Phys.* 1991;21(3):825–830.
34. Goldwein JW, Corn BW, Finlay JL, Packer RJ, Rorke LB, Schut L. Is craniospinal irradiation required to cure children with malignant (anaplastic) intracranial ependymomas? *Cancer.* 1991;67(11):2766–2771.
35. Wallner KE, Wara WM, Sheline GE, Davis RL. Intracranial ependymomas: results of treatment with partial or whole brain irradiation without spinal irradiation. *Int J Radiat Oncol Biol Phys.* 1986;12(11):1937–1941.
36. Merchant TE, Li C, Xiong X, Kun LE, Boop FA, Sanford RA. Conformal radiotherapy after surgery for paediatric ependymoma: a prospective study. *Lancet Oncol.* 2009;10(3):258–266.
37. Paulino AC, Wen BC, Buatti JM, et al. Intracranial ependymomas: an analysis of prognostic factors and patterns of failure. *Am J Clin Oncol.* 2002;25(2):117–122.
38. Perilongo G, Massimino M, Sotti G, et al. Analyses of prognostic factors in a retrospective review of 92 children with ependymoma: Italian Pediatric Neuro-oncology Group. *Med Pediatr Oncol.* 1997;29(2):79–85.
39. Pollack IF, Gerszten PC, Martinez AJ, et al. Intracranial ependymomas of childhood: long-term outcome and prognostic factors. *Neurosurgery.* 1995;37(4):655–666; discussion 666–657.
40. Rogers L, Pueschel J, Spetzler R, et al. Is gross-total resection sufficient treatment for posterior fossa ependymomas? *J Neurosurg.* 2005;102(4):629–636.
41. Rousseau P, Habrand JL, Sarrazin D, et al. Treatment of intracranial ependymomas of children: review of a 15-year experience. *Int J Radiat Oncol Biol Phys.* 1994;28(2):381–386.
42. Goldwein JW, Leahy JM, Packer RJ, et al. Intracranial ependymomas in children. *Int J Radiat Oncol Biol Phys.* 1990;19(6):1497–1502.
43. Shaw EG, Evans RG, Scheithauer BW, Ilstrup DM, Earle JD. Postoperative radiotherapy of intracranial ependymoma in pediatric and adult patients. *Int J Radiat Oncol Biol Phys.* 1987;13(10):1457–1462.
44. Hukin J, Epstein F, Lefton D, Allen J. Treatment of intracranial ependymoma by surgery alone. *Pediatr Neurosurg.* 1998;29(1):40–45.
45. Guyotat J, Signorelli F, Desme S, et al. Intracranial ependymomas in adult patients: analyses of prognostic factors. *J Neurooncol.* 2002;60(3):255–268.
46. McGuire CS, Sainani KL, Fisher PG. Both location and age predict survival in ependymoma: a SEER study. *Pediatr Blood Cancer.* 2009;52(1):65–69.
47. Garrett PG, Simpson WJ. Ependymomas: results of radiation treatment. *Int J Radiat Oncol Biol Phys.* 1983;9(8):1121–1124.
48. Stuben G, Stuschke M, Kroll M, Havers W, Sack H. Postoperative radiotherapy of spinal and intracranial ependymomas: analysis of prognostic factors. *Radiother Oncol.* 1997;45(1):3–10.
49. Chiu JK, Woo SY, Ater J, et al. Intracranial ependymoma in children: analysis of prognostic factors. *J Neurooncol.* 1992;13(3):283–290.
50. Shaw EG, Evans RG, Scheithauer BW, Ilstrup DM, Earle JD. Radiotherapeutic management of adult intraspinal ependymomas. *Int J Radiat Oncol Biol Phys.* 1986;12(3):323–327.
51. Kim YH, Fayos JV. Intracranial ependymomas. *Radiology.* 1977;124(3):805–808.
52. Salazar OM, Rubin P, Bassano D, Marcial VA. Improved survival of patients with intracranial ependymomas by irradiation: doseselection and field extension. *Cancer.* 1975;35(6):1563–1573.
53. Marks JE, Adler SJ. A comparative study of ependymomas by site of origin. *Int J Radiat Oncol Biol Phys.* 1982;8(1):37–43.
54. Merchant TE, Haida T, Wang MH, Finlay JL, Leibel SA. Anaplastic ependymoma: treatment of pediatric patients with or without craniospinal radiation therapy. *J Neurosurg.* 1997;86(6):943–949.
55. Carrie C, Mottolese C, Bouffet E, et al. Non-metastatic childhood ependymomas. *Radiother Oncol.* 1995;36(2):101–106.
56. Paulino AC, Wen BC. The significance of radiotherapy treatment duration in intracranial ependymoma. *Int J Radiat Oncol Biol Phys.* 2000;47(3):585–589.
57. Lo SS, Abdulrahman R, Desrosiers PM, et al. The role of Gamma Knife Radiosurgery in the management of unresectable gross disease or gross residual disease after surgery in ependymoma. *J Neurooncol.* 2006;79(1):51–56.
58. Stafford SL, Pollock BE, Foote RL, Gorman DA, Nelson DF, Schomberg PJ. Stereotactic radiosurgery for recurrent ependymoma. *Cancer.* 2000;88(4):870–875.
59. Mansur DB, Drzymala RE, Rich KM, Klein EE, Simpson JR. The efficacy of stereotactic radiosurgery in the management of intracranial ependymoma. *J Neurooncol.* 2004;66(1–2):187–190.
60. Kano H, Niranjan A, Kondziolka D, Flickinger JC, Lunsford LD. Outcome predictors for intracranial ependymoma radiosurgery. *Neurosurgery.* 2009;64(2):279–287; discussion 287–278.
61. Jawahar A, Kondziolka D, Flickinger JC, Lunsford LD. Adjuvant stereotactic radiosurgery for anaplastic ependymoma. *Stereotact Funct Neurosurg.* 1999;73(1–4):23–30.
62. Kovnar E, Curran W, Tomita. Hyper-fractionated irradiation for childhood ependymoma: improved local control in sub-totally resected tumors. *Childs Nerv Syst.* 1998;14(abstr):489.
63. Massimino M, Gandola L, Giangaspero F, et al. Hyperfractionated radiotherapy and chemotherapy for childhood ependymoma: final results of the first prospective AIEOP (Associazione Italiana di Ematologia-Oncologia Pediatrica) study. *Int J Radiat Oncol Biol Phys.* 2004;58(5):1336–1345.

64. Salazar OM, Castro-Vita H, VanHoutte P, Rubin P, Aygun C. Improved survival in cases of intracranial ependymoma after radiation therapy. Late report and recommendations. *J Neurosurg.* 1983;59(4):652–659.
65. Read G. The treatment of ependymoma of the brain or spinal canal by radiotherapy: a report of 79 cases. *Clin Radiol.* 1984;35(2):163–166.
66. Timmermann B, Kortmann RD, Kuhl J, et al. Combined postoperative irradiation and chemotherapy for anaplastic ependymomas in childhood: results of the German prospective trials HIT 88/89 and HIT 91. *Int J Radiat Oncol Biol Phys.* 2000;46(2):287–295.
67. Vanuytsel LJ, Bessell EM, Ashley SE, Bloom HJ, Brada M. Intracranial ependymoma: long-term results of a policy of surgery and radiotherapy. *Int J Radiat Oncol Biol Phys.* 1992;23(2):313–319.
68. Schroeder TM, Chintagumpala M, Okcu MF, et al. Intensity-modulated radiation therapy in childhood ependymoma. *Int J Radiat Oncol Biol Phys.* 2008;71(4):987–993.
69. Suc E, Kalifa C, Brauner R, et al. Brain tumours under the age of three. The price of survival. A retrospective study of 20 long-term survivors. *Acta Neurochir (Wien).* 1990;106(3–4):93–98.
70. Armstrong C, Ruffer J, Corn B, DeVries K, Mollman J. Biphasic patterns of memory deficits following moderate-dose partial-brain irradiation: neuropsychologic outcome and proposed mechanisms. *J Clin Oncol.* 1995;13(9):2263–2271.
71. Merchant TE, Kiehna EN, Li C, Xiong X, Mulhern RK. Radiation dosimetry predicts IQ after conformal radiation therapy in pediatric patients with localized ependymoma. *Int J Radiat Oncol Biol Phys.* 2005;63(5):1546–1554.
72. Merchant TE, Mulhern RK, Krasin MJ, et al. Preliminary results from a phase II trial of conformal radiation therapy and evaluation of radiation-related CNS effects for pediatric patients with localized ependymoma. *J Clin Oncol.* 2004;22(15):3156–3162.
73. Constine LS, Woolf PD, Cann D, et al. Hypothalamic-pituitary dysfunction after radiation for brain tumors. *N Engl J Med.* 1993;328(2):87–94.
74. Merchant TE, Gould CJ, Xiong X, et al. Early neuro-otologic effects of three-dimensional irradiation in children with primary brain tumors. *Int J Radiat Oncol Biol Phys.* 2004;58(4):1194–1207.
75. Ildan F, Tuna M, Erman T, Gocer AI, Zeren M, Cetinalp E. The evaluation and comparison of cerebellar mutism in children and adults after posterior fossa surgery: report of two adult cases and review of the literature. *Acta Neurochir (Wien).* 2002;144(5):463–473.
76. Evans AE, Anderson JR, Lefkowitz-Boudreaux IB, Finlay JL. Adjuvant chemotherapy of childhood posterior fossa ependymoma: craniospinal irradiation with or without adjuvant CCNU, vincristine, and prednisone: a Childrens Cancer Group study. *Med Pediatr Oncol.* 1996;27(1):8–14.
77. Grill J, Le Deley MC, Gambarelli D, et al. Postoperative chemotherapy without irradiation for ependymoma in children under 5 years of age: a multicenter trial of the French Society of Pediatric Oncology. *J Clin Oncol.* 2001;19(5):1288–1296.
78. Fokes EC Jr, Earle KM. Ependymomas: clinical and pathological aspects. *J Neurosurg.* 1969;30(5):585–594.
79. Ross GW, Rubinstein LJ. Lack of histopathological correlation of malignant ependymomas with postoperative survival. *J Neurosurg.* 1989;70(1):31–36.
80. Sutton LN, Goldwein J, Perilongo G, et al. Prognostic factors in childhood ependymomas. *Pediatr Neurosurg.* 1990;16(2):57–65.
81. Rezai AR, Woo HH, Lee M, Cohen H, Zagzag D, Epstein FJ. Disseminated ependymomas of the central nervous system. *J Neurosurg.* 1996;85(4):618–624.
82. Zacharoulis S, Ji L, Pollack IF, et al. Metastatic ependymoma: a multi-institutional retrospective analysis of prognostic factors. *Pediatr Blood Cancer.* 2008;50(2):231–235.

91 Vestibular Schwannoma

Bethany M. Anderson and Minesh P. Mehta

> If somebody had stated some twenty years ago that a technique involving irradiation would be used for the routine treatment of acoustic neurinomas that person would probably have been regarded as insane.
>
> G. Norén et al [1]

INTRODUCTION

Vestibular schwannoma, previously erroneously referred to as acoustic neuroma, is typically a benign neoplasm originating from the vestibular portion of the eighth cranial nerve. With time, progressive tumor growth may fill the internal auditory canal and extend into the cerebellopontine angle, causing compression of the brainstem and other nearby cranial nerves, and most commonly, the trigeminal and facial nerves. Magnetic resonance imaging (MRI) is the imaging method of choice for visualizing vestibular schwannomas, which typically appear as contrast-enhancing lesions on Time 1–weighted sequences (Figure 91.1). The majority of cases are unilateral and sporadic, although bilateral vestibular schwannoma is a pathognomonic feature of type 2 neurofibromatosis.

Although these tumors are rarely fatal, symptoms such as sensorineural hearing loss (Figure 91.2), tinnitus, imbalance, and cranial-nerve deficits can significantly impair quality of life. Management options include observation, surgical resection, stereotactic radiosurgery (SRS), or fractionated stereotactic radiation therapy (FSRT). There have been no true randomized, controlled trials published in patients with vestibular schwannoma, and interpretation of single institution series is limited by differences in factors such as patient selection, treatment techniques, and methods of assessing and reporting tumor control and treatment or tumor-related neurologic deficits. Currently, the choice of treatment modality is based on physician familiarity, bias and choice; patient characteristics, such as age, symptoms, location, and size of the lesion(s); and the availability of different technologies. Multidisciplinary evaluation, therefore, is a critical component of the management of vestibular schwannoma today.

MANAGEMENT OF VESTIBULAR SCHWANNOMA: A BRIEF HISTORICAL PERSPECTIVE

Sir Charles Ballance is credited with performing the first successful surgical resection of a vestibular schwannoma in 1894 [2]. Surgical resection became the mainstream approach to management of vestibular schwannomas over the following century, as techniques continued to evolve and the mortality risks decreased from 70% to 80% to the current rate of <1%.

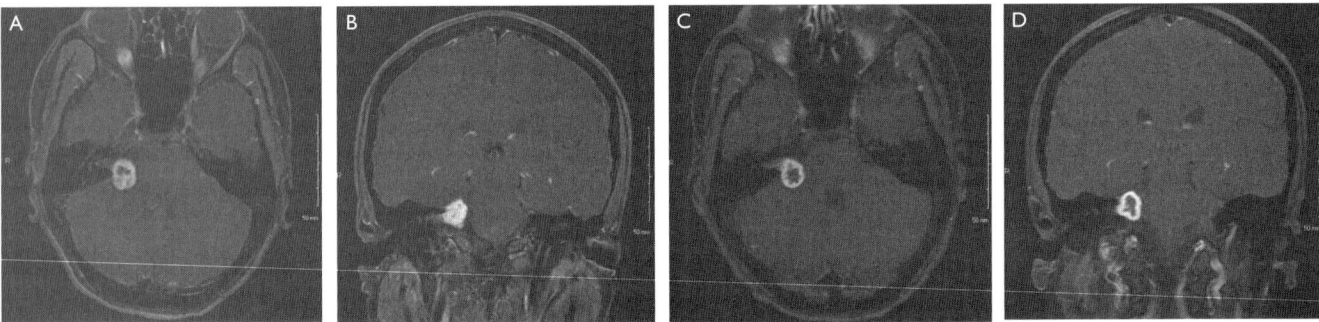

Figure 91.1 T1-weighted, contrast-enhanced MRI images from a 39-year-old woman with a right-sided vestibular schwannoma. She was treated with FSRT to 50.4 Gy at 1.8 Gy/F. Shown are representative pre-treatment axial (**A**) and coronal (**B**) images, and posttreatment axial (**C**) and coronal (**D**) images obtained 19 months after completing FSRT. Increased central necrosis is demonstrated in the posttreatment images.

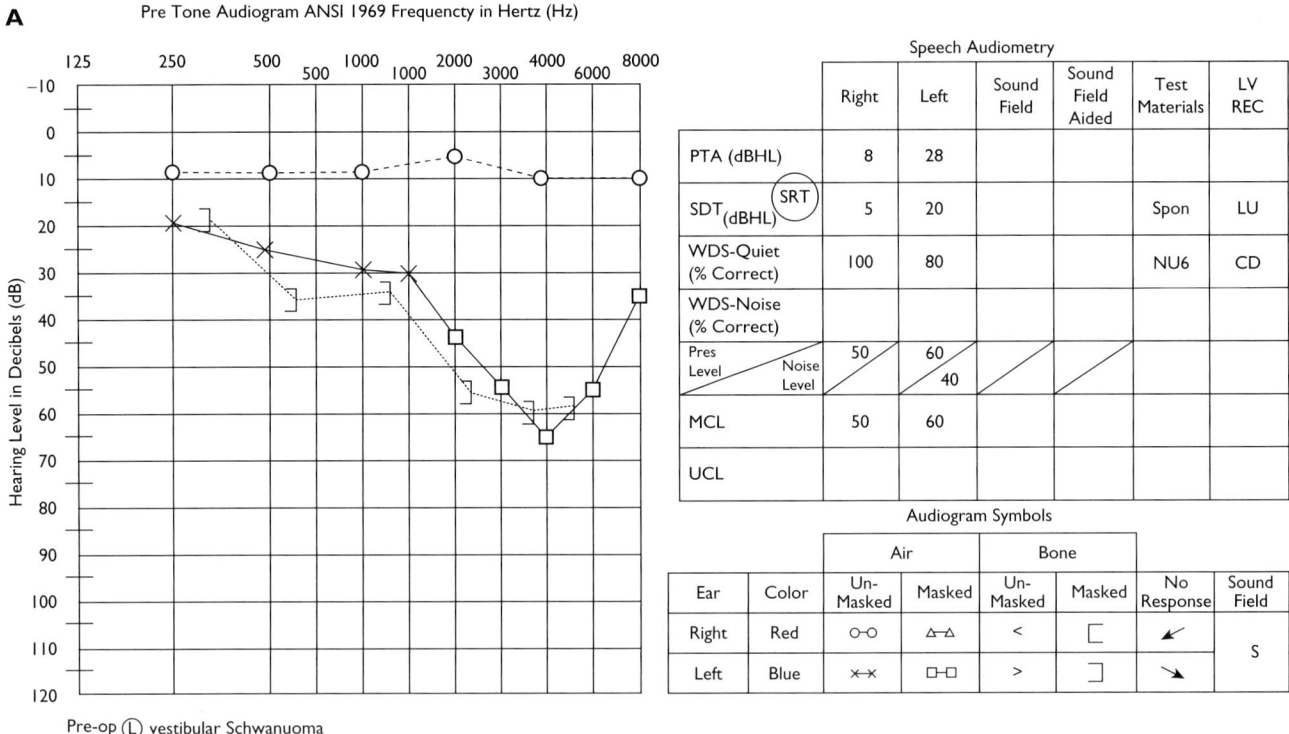

Figure 91.2 Pretreatment audiogram of vestibular schwannoma patient showing typical high-frequency sensorineural hearing loss **(A)**. Findings are used to classify hearing into varying grades of serviceable or nonserviceable hearing. The Gardner-Robertson [1] system assigned a grade of I to V, with grades I to II representing serviceable hearing **(B)**. The American Academy of Otolaryngology-Head and Neck Surgery (AAO-HNS [2]) system assigns a class of A–D, with A–B representing serviceable hearing **(C)**. As a rule of thumb, patients whose speech discrimination score is 50% or less at 50 decibels or more may not benefit from an approach focused on the preservation of hearing [11]. Each case must be considered individually, however, particularly in patients with bilateral vestibular schwanommas or other causes of contralateral hearing compromise.

The treatment landscape began to change, however, when the Swedish neurosurgeon Lars Leksell developed the first SRS system in the early 1950s [3] and treated the first vestibular schwannoma patient with SRS in 1969 [4]. As described in the following section, the relatively high SRS doses used in early experiences lead to higher-than-expected rates of hearing loss and other cranial-nerve toxicities. Major recent SRS advances have included reducing the prescription dose to 12 to 13 Gy and incorporating MRI for more accurate definition of the treatment target and adjacent critical structures. The excellent local control and low toxicity rates currently achieved with SRS, along with its potential benefit over microsurgery in terms of cost-effectiveness, have led some institutions to adopt SRS as the preferred primary treatment modality for vestibular schwannoma. It is not surprising that this paradigm shift was initiated by the Karolinska Institute in Stockholm, the birthplace of SRS [1].

Over the past 2 decades, FSRT techniques have also been developed that allow for precise target localization and highly conformal radiation delivery, with a significant corresponding reduction in the volume of adjacent normal tissues treated in a fractionated fashion. This approach offers a potential radiobiologic advantage with regards to normal tissue toxicity and has been utilized successfully at several major radiation oncology centers. Although the body of literature supporting the use of FSRT is currently less robust than that for SRS or surgical resection, reported rates of local control are excellent, and toxicity rates are consistently low with both hypofractionated and conventionally fractionated approaches. As highly accurate and conformal external beam radiation therapy technologies become more widespread, the role of FSRT for initial management of vestibular schwannoma may broaden within the neurootological community.

STEREOTACTIC RADIOSURGERY

Methods and Treatment Planning

In the modern era, either LINAC-based Gamma Knife or proton SRS may be employed to treat intracranial lesions with submillimeter precision. Due to the minimally invasive nature and excellent clinical outcomes achieved with SRS, practice patterns at some institutions are shifting to favor SRS over surgical resection. The ideal candidates have tumors less than 3 to 4 cm in size.

High-resolution MRI images should be used during treatment planning, either as the primary data set or through fusion with a treatment-planning computed tomography scan. Care should be taken when relying solely upon MRI, however, as spatial distortion may result in targeting errors with resulting compromise in local control [5]. The tumor is best visualized with contrast-enhanced T1 images, whereas the cochlea and semicircular canals are best seen with fast spin–echo T2 sequences.

Dose Selection and Toxicities

The ideal SRS prescription (marginal) dose is 12 to 13 Gy, as local control appears to be compromised with doses below this range [6,7], and cranial nerve toxicity increases with higher doses [8–11]. A recent retrospective analysis by Foote et al [6] found the 2-year incidence of any cranial neuropathy to be 2% with prescription doses of ≤12.5 Gy versus 24% with doses of >12.5 Gy. Facial, trigeminal, and auditory toxicities have also been shown to correlate with the length of nerve irradiated [9]. For example, in the early experience with higher-dose SRS, trigeminal and facial neuropathy rates were respectively higher in patients with extracanalicular tumor dimension >1 cm and sum of extracanalicular and intracanalicular diameter >2 cm [12]. Other factors that correlate with increased facial nerve preservation rates include age ≤60, tumor volume ≤1.5 cm^3, and marginal dose ≤13 Gy [13]. Most cranial neuropathies develop within 2 years of SRS, but hearing loss can occur much later.

Proposed mechanisms of post-SRS hearing loss (in the absence of progressive tumor growth) include transient conductive hearing loss due to serous otitis media and delayed sensorineural hearing loss due to direct radiation injury to the vestibulocochlear nerve or cochlea, compression of the vestibulocochlear nerve or internal auditory artery due to tumor edema, or thrombosis of the internal auditory artery. Patient-related factors that correlate with increased likelihood of hearing preservation after SRS include age <60, tumor volume <0.75 cm^3, intracanalicular tumor location, and better pretreatment hearing (class I Gardner-Robertson, speech discrimination score ≥80%, pure tone average <20 dB) [14,15]. Treatment-related factors that correlate with increased hearing preservation rates include MRI treatment planning techniques [9,16], marginal dose ≤12.5 to 13 Gy [15,17,18], cochlear dose <4.2 to 4.75 Gy [14,19], and cochlear nucleus dose <10 Gy [20]. Kondziolka et al [21] recommend prescribing 12 Gy for tumors >2 cm in extracanalicular diameter, 12.5 Gy for smaller tumors, 13 Gy for patients without serviceable hearing, and potentially up to 14 Gy for patients with hearing loss and facial weakness.

Radiation dose to the brainstem must also be carefully monitored. In 1994, Kihlstrom et al recommended limiting brainstem dose to ≤14 Gy with SRS, on basis of the development of adverse radiation imaging effects in 6/7 patients who received 14 to 35 Gy for low-grade gliomas of the tectal midbrain. In 2008, Sharma et al [22] demonstrated that adverse radiation imaging effects and new neurological deficits could develop after exposing ≥0.1 cm of brainstem to doses of >12 Gy. An example of an SRS treatment plan is shown in Figure 91.3.

Results

The results of single-institution experiences with SRS for vestibular schwannoma are shown in Table 91.1. Using modern techniques and doses, as described above, local

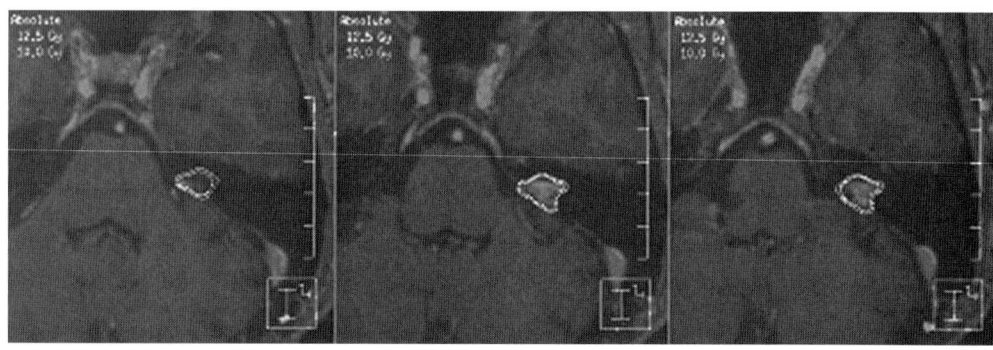

Figure 91.3 LINAC SRS treatment plan delivering 12.5 Gy to a small left-sided vestibular schwannoma using four isocenters.

Table 91.1 Single-Institution Outcomes of SRS for Vestibular Schwannoma

Series	No. pts	Dose	Local Control	Serviceable Hearing Preservation	CN VII Toxicity	CN V Toxicity
Fukuoka et al, 2009 [23]	152	12 Gy median (9–15 Gy)	92.4% at 8 years	71%	0%	2.6%
Pollock et al, 2009 [5]	293	13 Gy median (IQR 12–14 Gy)	94% at 7 years	NR	NR	NR
Lobato-Polo et al, 2009 [15][e]	55	13 Gy median (11–20 Gy)	96% at 5 years	93% at 10 years	1.8%	3.6%
Kalogeridi et al, 2009 [24]	20	11–12 Gy	100%	NA[a]	0%	0%
Chopra et al, 2007 [25]	216	13 Gy median (12–13 Gy)	98.3% at 10 years	44.5%	0%	5.1%
Rutten et al, 2007	26	12 Gy median (10–14 Gy)	94.7% at 5 years	90%	0%	8% (transient)
Friedman et al, 2006 [26]	390	12.5 Gy median (10–22.5 Gy)	90% at 10 years	NR	4.4%	3.6%
Lunsford et al, 2005 [27]	829	13 Gy (10–20 Gy)	98%	78.6%[d]	0%[d]	4%[d]
Chung et al, 2005 [7]	195	13 Gy median (11–18.2 Gy)	96.8% at 10 years[b]	60%	1.4% (transient)	1.1%
Muacevic et al, 2004 [28]	219	13 Gy median (10–15 Gy)	97% at 5 years	NR	0.5% (transient)	5.5%
Flickinger et al, 2001 [8]	190	13 Gy median (11–18 Gy)	97.1% at 5 years[c]	73.5% at 5 years	1.1%	2.6%
Foote et al, 2001 [6]	149	14 Gy mean (10–22.5 Gy)	87% at 5 years	NR	11.8% at 2 years	9.5% at 2 years
Spiegelmann et al, 2001 [29]	44	14.55 Gy mean (11–20 Gy)	98%	71%	8%	18%
Prasad et al, 2000 [30]	153	13 Gy median (9–20 Gy)	94%	40%	3.3%	2%
Ito et al, 2000 [31]	125	15.4 Gy mean (12–25 Gy)	NR	58%a	16%	25%
Miller et al, 1999 [32]	42 / 40	12–16 Gy / 16–20 Gy	97%	39% at 2 years	38% at 2 years / 8% at 2 years	29% at 2 years / 15% at 2 years
Kondziolka et al, 1998 [16]	162	16.6 Gy mean (12–20 Gy)	98%	47%	21%	27%
Ito et al, 1997 [33]	46	16.8 Gy mean (12–25 Gy)	95.6%	39%[f]	22%	30%
Flickinger et al, 1996 [9]	273	17 Gy mean (12–20 Gy) in CT planning era 14 Gy mean (12–19 Gy) in MRI planning era	96.4% at 7 years	51.8% at 7 years	17.2% at 3 & 7 years	22.6% at 3 & 7 years
Foote et al, 1995 [34]	36	16–20 Gy	100%	41.7% at 2 years	66.5% at 2 years (17.3% severe)	58.9% at 2 years (10.7% severe)
Kobayashi et al, 1994 [35]	44	14.8 Gy mean	NR	48% at 12 months[g]	16%	8% (transient)
Norén et al, 1993 [1]	254	10–20 Gy	84% NF2 94% unilateral	77%	17%	19%
Martens et al, 1994 [36]	22	16–20 Gy	100%	NR	4.5%	9%
Flickinger et al, 1993[37]	134	17 Gy median (12–20 Gy)	89.2% at 4 years	35.1% at 4 years	29.0% at 4 years	32.9% at 4 years
Flickinger et al, 1991[38]	85	18 Gy median (14–20 Gy)	98%	46% at 2 years	33% at 2 years	37% at 2 years

[a]No patients with serviceable hearing prior to treatment. [b]Intervention-free survival; radiologic control 93.6%. [c]Resection-free survival; radiologic control 91% at 5 years. [d]In subset of patients treated to 12–13 Gy. [e]Subset of patients age ≤40 from University of Pittsburgh experience. [f]Hearing loss defined as pure-tone average elevation ≥20 dB. [g]Method of discerning hearing preservation unknown.

Abbreviations: IQR, intra-quartile range; NR, not reported, or results incompatible with table format.

control rates with SRS are generally greater than 90%, and significant cranial nerve V and VII toxicity rates are less than 10%. Published hearing preservation rates are variable; 57% overall in a recent systemic review of patients treated with an average dose of 16 Gy [17]. Generally speaking, interpretation of the vestibular schwannoma literature is complicated by its overwhelmingly retrospective nature and wide variability in institutions' patient selection, treatment techniques, and methods of assessing and reporting tumor control and treatment-related neurologic deficits. For example, local control may be determined radiographically as a lack of tumor growth, progressive tumor growth, or need for further intervention. The natural history of vestibular schwannoma after SRS may be characterized by a transient increase in size [39], often with a necrotic-appearing center, followed by stability or regression. This type of MRI finding may confound the results of some published SRS series. Hearing deficits are also analyzed in multiple different fashions, including subjectively questioning (typically by querying patients on their ability to use the telephone with the affected ear), or using objective audiometric data. Facial function is typically scored using the House-Brackmann system (Table 91.2), but investigators differ in their method of defining "significant" facial and other cranial-nerve toxicity. Outcomes may also be reported as crude or actuarial rates, adding to the heterogeneity of published case series.

SRS Compared to Surgery

Six reports have been published comparing outcomes of patients treated with surgery versus SRS (Table 91.3) [40–46], demonstrating that both approaches achieve statistically equivalent local control rates in the order of 91% to 100% [42,44], but SRS produces equivalent or superior functional outcomes. A prospective analysis of 82 patients with small tumors (≤3 cm) eligible for either surgery or SRS at the Mayo Clinic found that patients who chose SRS subsequently had better preservation of normal facial movement and serviceable hearing [42]. A prospective analysis of 91 patients with small vestibular schwannomas (≤2.5 cm) treated with surgery ($n = 28$) or SRS ($n = 28$) at Haukeland University Hospital also showed better facial-nerve function and hearing preservation in patients who underwent radiosurgery [41]. A comparison of patients treated with surgery ($n = 110$) or SRS ($n = 100$) published by Régis et al [43] found better preservation of serviceable hearing and facial and trigeminal function with SRS. A retrospective analysis of 96 patients performed by Karpinos et al [44] showed better preservation of measurable (but not serviceable) hearing and lower rates of facial and trigeminal neuropathy in patients treated with SRS. Tumor size was larger in the surgical group, however. An early comparative study by van Roijen et al [45] identified meningitis, hydrocephalus, liquor cyst, urinary infection, and respiratory infection as acute treatment-related toxicities occurring in a minority of microsurgical patients (2–7%), which did not occur in SRS patients. Others have found hydrocephalus to occur infrequently after SRS, although the cause-effect relationship in this context is less clear [50].

Cost-Effectiveness Comparisons

The cost-effectiveness of surgical resection versus SRS has also been compared in at least 3 analyses [45,46,51,52]. The first two studies, published in the late 1990s, found SRS to have lower overall associated costs [46,45]. More recently, Banerjee et al determined that the mean cost of microsurgery was higher than that of SRS ($23 788 vs $16 143), but the follow-up costs after SRS tended to be higher due to factors such as increased use of MRI and audiograms. The authors concluded that SRS is likely to be less expensive than microsurgery from a societal perspective, provided that recurrence rates remain low over prolonged follow-up [51].

FRACTIONATED STEREOTACTIC RADIATION THERAPY

Methods and Treatment Planning

FSRT has been introduced into the treatment armamentarium for vestibular schwannoma at selected institutions over the past 10 to 20 years. Multiple localization systems have been developed, most of which achieve patient localization through infrared light-emitting diodes and are accurate to within 1 to 3 mm. Vestibular schwannomas are slowly proliferating tumors with a low estimated α/β ratio of 2.5 to 4. The hypothesized radiobiologic advantage of FSRT, therefore, is based on reducing late toxicity to surrounding normal structures, such as the cranial nerves and brainstem. Stereotactic localization techniques also contribute to reduction of normal toxicity by allowing reduction of treatment volumes. Typical candidates are those with tumors too large for radiosurgery, rare patients with malignant schwannomas, and patients for whom hearing preservation is a very high priority, although this last indication is highly controversial and subject to institutional preference. For example, at the University of British

Table 91.2 House-Brackmann Facial-Nerve Grading Scale [40]

Grade	Description	Characteristics
I	Normal	Normal facial function in all areas
II	Mild dysfunction	Gross: slight weakness noticeable on close inspection; may have very slight synkinesis At rest: normal symmetry and tone Motion: Forehead: moderate to good function Eye: complete closure with minimum effort Mouth: slight asymmetry
III	Moderate dysfunction	Gross: obvious but not disfiguring difference between two sides; noticeable but not severe synkinesis, contracture, and/or hemifacial spasm At rest: normal symmetry and tone Motion: Forehead: slight to moderate movement Eye: complete closure with effort Mouth: slightly weak with maximum effort
IV	Moderately severe dysfunction	Gross: obvious weakness and/or disfiguring asymmetry At rest: normal symmetry and tone Motion: Forehead: none Eye: incomplete closure Mouth: asymmetric with maximum effort
V	Severe dysfunction	Gross: only barely perceptible motion At rest: asymmetry Motion: Forehead: none Eye: incomplete closure Mouth: slight movement
VI	Total paralysis	No movement

Table 91.3 Single-institution analyses comparing outcomes of surgery, SRS, and FSRT

Series	Treatment (No. pts)	Serviceable-Hearing Preservation	CN VII Toxicity	CN V Toxicity
Surgery versus SRS				
Myrseth et al, 2009 [41]	SRS (63)	68%	1.6%	NR
	Surgery (28)	0%, $p < 0.001$	46%, $p < 0.001$	
Pollock et al, 2006 [42]	SRS (46)	63%	2%	NR
	Surgery (36)	5%, $p < 0.001$	17%, $p = 0.04$	
Régis et al, 2002 [43]	SRS (100)	40%	0%	4%
	Surgery (110)	5%, $p = 0.000001$	47%, $p = 0.00005$	29%, $p = 0.0009$
Karpinos et al, 2002 [44]	SRS (75)	44%	6.1%	12.2%
	Surgery (25)	40%	35.3%, $p = 0.008$	22%, $p = 0.009$
van Roijen et al, 1997 [45]	SRS (92)	NR	2%	0%
	Surgery (53)		10%	0%
Pollock et al, 1995 [46]	SRS (47)	75%	17%	14%
	Surgery (40)	14%, $p < 0.03$	37%, $p < 0.05$	11%
SRS versus FSRT				
Combs et al, 2009 [11]	SRS (30)	NR[a]	17%	7%
	FSRT (172)		2%	3%
Anderson et al, 2007 [47]	SRS (49)	33.3%	2%	10.2%
	FSRT or HypoFSRT (52)	65.4%, $p = .087$	2%,	0%, $p = .028$
Meijer et al, 2003 [48]	SRS (49)	75%	7%	8%
	HypoFSRT (80)	61%	3%	2%, $p = 0.048$
Andrews et al, 2001 [49]	SRS (69)	33%	2%	5%
	FSRT (56)	81%, $p = 0.0228$	2%	7%

Abbreviations: FSRT, fractionated stereotactic radiation therapy; HypoFSRT, hypofractionated FSRT; NR, not reported; SRS, stereotactic radiosurgery.

[a] Serviceable-hearing preservation rates not compatible with table format.

Columbia, patients with serviceable hearing (Gardner-Robertson grade 1–2) are treated with FSRT, whereas patients with unserviceable hearing receive SRS [53].

Dose Selection and Toxicities

Common regimens prescribed are on the order of 45 to 50 Gy at 1.8 to 2 Gy/F, or 20 to 25 Gy at 4 to 5 Gy/F. A recent retrospective analysis of 89 patients treated with FSRT to 46.8 Gy versus 50.4 Gy at 1.8 Gy/F found that patients treated to 46.8 Gy were more likely to have preservation of serviceable hearing; however, there was no statistically significant relationship between cochlear dose and serviceable hearing preservation [54]. In contrast, a prospective analysis of 34 patients treated with FSRT to 45 Gy at 1.8 Gy/F found that dose to the cochlea was the only significant prognostic factor for hearing deterioration [53]. In their experience, the median hearing loss was 10 dB for patients with <73.3% of the cochlea exposed to ≤90% of the prescription dose (45 Gy), as opposed to 25 dB for patients with a V_{90}% of ≤73.3%.

Results

Published single-institution outcomes of FSRT are summarized in Table 91.4. Results are essentially equivalent to those achieved with current, moderate-dose SRS, with local control rates greater than 90% and cranial-nerve toxicity rates at less than 10%. Serviceable hearing preservation rates may be higher than those achieved with SRS. It will be important to monitor local control rates with increasing follow-up to ensure that they remain high, considering the potential radiobiologic disadvantage of fractionated treatment for a slowly proliferating tumor.

FSRT Compared to SRS

Four single-institution analyses have been performed, comparing outcomes of SRS with those of FSRT (Table 91.3), all of which show equal rates of local control with both methods [11,48,49]. Meijer et al [48] conducted a prospective study of 129 patients with vestibular schwannomas who were allocated to SRS versus hypofractionated FSRT on the basis of dentition, with dentate patients ($n = 80$) receiving FSRT and edentulous patients ($n = 49$) receiving SRS. Toxicity rates were low for both groups, but trigeminal nerve preservation was slightly higher in the FSRT group (98% vs 92% at 5 years, $p = .048$). A review of 125 patients treated with SRS ($n = 69$) or conventional FSRT ($n = 56$) at Thomas Jefferson University also showed comparable outcomes, with the exception of functional-hearing preservation, which was better for patients treated with FSRT [49]. A recent analysis of 202 vestibular schwannomas treated with SRS ($n = 30$) versus conventional FSRT ($n = 172$) at the University of Heidelberg found equivalent outcomes between the two groups, with the exception of patients treated with SRS doses >13 Gy, who had lower rates of hearing preservation [11]. Finally, at the University of Wisconsin, patients treated with SRS ($n = 49$), conventional FSRT ($n = 32$), or hypofractionated FSRT ($n = 32$) were found to have equivalent 5-year progression-free rates of 92.3% overall, whereas FSRT produced lower rates of late trigeminal-nerve toxicity (0% vs 10.2%, $p = 0.028$) and

Table 91.4 Published Single-Institution Outcomes of FSRT for Vestibular Schwannoma

Series	No. pts	Dose	Local Control	Serviceable-Hearing Preservation	CN VII Toxicity	CN V Toxicity
McClelland et al, 2008 [55]	20	54 Gy at 1.8 Gy/F	100%	NR	0%	10%
Koh et al, 2007 [56]	60	50 Gy at 2 Gy/F	96.2% at 5 years	77.3%	0%	0%
Thomas et al, 2007 [53]	34	45 Gy at 1.8 Gy/F	95.7% at 4 years	63% at 3 years	0%	0%
Chan et al, 2005 [57]	70	54 Gy at 1.8 Gy/F	98% at 5 years	84% at 5 years	1%	4%
Combs et al, 2005 [18]	106	57.8 Gy at 1.8 Gy/F	93% at 5 years	94% at 5 years	2.3%	3.4%
Chang et al, 2005 [58]	61	18–21 Gy at 6–7 Gy/F daily	98%	74%	0%	0%
Sawamura et al, 2003 [59]	101	Median 48 Gy (40–50 Gy) at 2 Gy/F	91.4% at 5 years	71.7% at 5 years	0.9%	4%
Williams et al, 2002 [60]	125	25 Gy at 5 Gy/F for tumors <3 cm; 30 Gy at 3 Gy/F for tumors ≥3 cm	100%	83%	0%	1.6% (transient)
Szumacher et al, 2002 [61]	39	50 Gy at 2 Gy/F	95%	67.9%	NR	NR
Fuss et al, 2000 [62]	42	Mean 57.6 Gy at 1.8–2 Gy/F	95% at 5 years	85.2% at 5 years	0% at 5 years	4.8%
Kalapurakal et al, 1999 [63]	19[a]	30–36 Gy at 5–6 Gy/F weekly	100%	100%[b]	0%	0%
Poen et al, 1999 [64]	32	21 Gy at 7 Gy/F over 24 hours	93% at 2 years	77% at 2 years	3%	16%
Lederman et al, 1997 [65]	38	20 Gy at 5 Gy/F for tumors <3 cm; 20 Gy at 4 Gy/F for tumors ≥3 cm	100%	NR	2.6% (transient)	0%

Abbreviations: NR, not reported, or results incompatible with table format.

[a] All patients with large tumors.

[b] Detailed audiogram data not provided.

a trend toward better serviceable hearing preservation (65.4% vs 33.3%, $p = 0.087$) [47].

PROTON-BEAM THERAPY

Protons may be used to deliver either SRS or fractionated treatment. There is a paucity of published data on the use of protons for vestibular schwannoma, which parallels the limited availability of this technology at present. Weber et al [66] have published their experience treating 88 patients with proton-beam SRS at Harvard. The median dose was 12 cobalt Gy equivalents (CGE; range 10–18 CGE). Furthermore, 5-year actuarial outcomes showed 95.3% local control, 91.1% normal facial function, and 89.4% normal trigeminal-nerve function; however, the serviceable hearing rate was only 21.9%.

A hypofractionated FSRT approach was used to treat 51 patients with proton beam in South Africa [67]. The mean minimum tumor dose was 21.4 CGE in 3 fractions. The actuarial local control rate was 98% at 2 to 5 years, and 87% at 10 years. The actuarial facial-nerve and trigeminal-nerve preservation rates at 5 to 10 years were 90.5% and 93%, respectively. The actuarial serviceable-hearing rate was 74% at 2 years, and 42% at 5 to 10 years.

Investigators at Loma Linda reported their experience treating 29 patients with fractionated, conformal proton-beam therapy to total doses of 54 CGE in 30 fractions for patients with serviceable hearing, or 60 CGE in 30 to 33 fractions for patients without useful hearing [68]. Local control was 100% at a mean follow-up interval of 34 months, and no patient developed trigeminal- or facial-nerve toxicity; however, serviceable-hearing preservation was only 31%.

MANAGEMENT OF VESTIBULAR SCHWANNOMA IN THE PATIENT WITH NF2

Bilateral vestibular schwannomas, as mentioned above, occur commonly in patients with type 2 neurofibromatosis, a disorder with an estimated prevalence of 1/100 000 [69]. NF2 patients also have a predisposition to develop other tumors of the central nervous system (meningiomas, ependymomas, astrocytomas, neurofibromas), peripheral neuropathy, ocular findings (retinal hamartomas, epiretinal membranes, cataracts), and skin lesions (plaques and subcutaneous tumors), as recently reviewed by Asthagiri et al [70]

In comparison with sporadic tumors, vestibular schwannomas in patients with NF2 tend to grow more quickly and more aggressively surround or infiltrate the adjacent cochlear and facial nerves. Functional outcomes after treatment tend to be poorer in this population of patients. For example, in the experience of Combs et al [18], a diagnosis of NF2 was associated with significantly reduced likelihood of serviceable-hearing preservation in patients treated with FSRT (64% for NF2 versus 98% for sporadic tumors).

Mathieu et al [71] recently published the University of Pittsburgh's experience treating 74 vestibular schwannomas

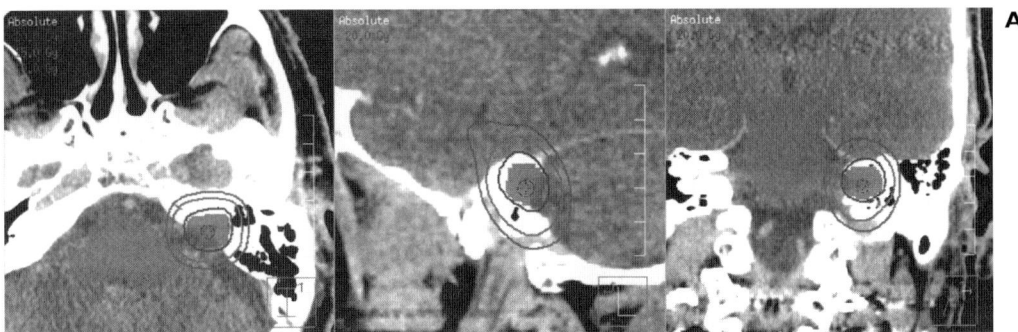
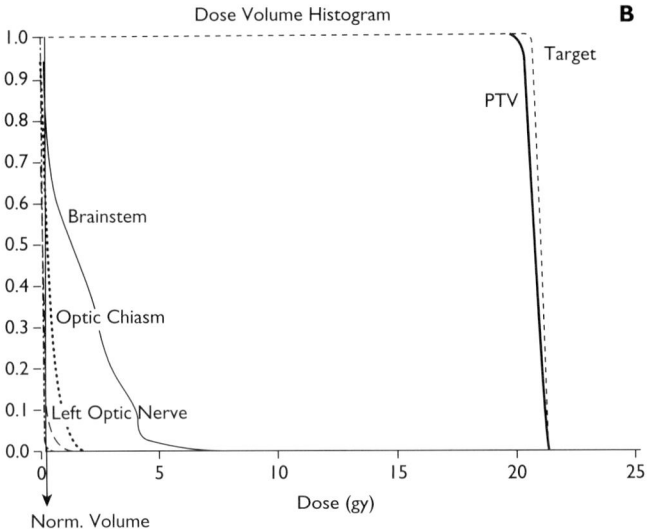

Figure 91.4 FSRT treatment plan delivering 20 Gy at 4 Gy/F weekly to a left-sided vestibular schwannoma. Representative axial (A), sagittal (B), and coronal (C) isodose lines are shown, along with the DVH (D) demonstrating good coverage of the GTV and PTV with minimal dose to adjacent normal structures.

in 62 NF2 patients with SRS, with a mean marginal dose of 14 Gy (range 11–20 Gy). The actuarial local control rate was 81% at 10 to 15 years. Margin dose was significantly related to serviceable-hearing preservation on multivariate analysis and the actuarial serviceable-hearing preservation rate of 48% at 5 years in patients treated with a marginal dose of ≤14 Gy. Tumor volume >5 cm^3 and maximum dose >28 Gy predicted for the development of other complications, such as facial weakness, trigeminal neuropathy, or neuralgia, and vestibular dysfunction. The authors recommend offering treatment only for large symptomatic tumors or tumors manifesting with progressive growth or hearing loss in order to maximize preservation of function and quality of life [71]. One advantage to earlier intervention may be the potential to spare function of the cochlear nerve, thereby allowing for future cochlear implantation (Figure 91.4).

CONCLUSIONS AND FUTURE DIRECTIONS

Patients with newly diagnosed vestibular schwannomas should ideally be evaluated by a multidisciplinary team with expertise in neurosurgery, SRS, and FSRT for discussion of the risks and benefits of treatment, as well as observation. Surgical resection may be performed for virtually any tumor, including large tumors causing brainstem compression or hydrocephalus. Hearing preservation rates may be lower with surgery than with radiation therapy, however. The ideal candidate for SRS is a patient with a small, intracanalicular tumor not approaching the brainstem; however, tumors ≤3 to 4 cm in size may be treated with marginal doses of 12 to 13 Gy. Conventional or hypofractionated FSRT may be a safer choice for tumors measuring 3 to 4 cm or larger and may result in higher hearing preservation rates. Randomized controlled trials comparing various treatment options would be very valuable.

REFERENCES

1. Norén G, Greitz D, Hirsch A, Lax I. Gamma knife surgery in acoustic tumours. *Acta Neurochir Suppl (Wien)*. 1993;58:104–107.
2. Ballance SC. Some Points in the Surgery of the Brain and its Membranes. 2nd ed. London: Macmillan; 1908.
3. Leksell L. The stereotaxic method and radiosurgery of the brain. *Acta Chir Scand*. 1951;102(4):316–319.
4. Leksell L. A note on the treatment of acoustic tumours. *Acta Chir Scand*. 1971;137(8):763–765.
5. Pollock BE, Link MJ, Foote RL. Failure rate of contemporary low-dose radiosurgical technique for vestibular schwannoma. *J Neurosurg*. 2009;111(4):840–844.
6. Foote KD, Friedman WA, Buatti JM, Meeks SL, Bova FJ, Kubilis PS. Analysis of risk factors associated with radiosurgery for vestibular schwannoma. *J Neurosurg*. 2001;95(3):440–449.
7. Chung WY, Liu KD, Shiau CY, et al. Gamma knife surgery for vestibular schwannoma: 10-year experience of 195 cases. *J Neurosurg*. 2005;102 suppl:87–96.
8. Flickinger JC, Kondziolka D, Niranjan A, Lunsford LD. Results of acoustic neuroma radiosurgery: an analysis of 5 years' experience using current methods. *J Neurosurg*. 2001;94(1):1–6.

9. Flickinger JC, Kondziolka D, Pollock BE, Lunsford LD. Evolution in technique for vestibular schwannoma radiosurgery and effect on outcome. *Int J Radiat Oncol Biol Phys*. 1996;36(2):275–280.
10. Chihara Y, Ito K, Sugasawa K, Shin M. Neurological complications after acoustic neurinoma radiosurgery: revised risk factors based on long-term follow-up. *Acta Otolaryngol Suppl*. 2007;559:65–70.
11. Combs SE, Welzel T, Schulz-Ertner D, Huber PE, Debus J. Differences in clinical results after LINAC-based single-dose radiosurgery versus fractionated stereotactic radiotherapy for patients with vestibular schwannomas. *Int J Radiat Oncol Biol Phys*. 2010;76(1): 193–200.
12. Linskey ME, Flickinger JC, Lunsford LD. Cranial nerve length predicts the risk of delayed facial and trigeminal neuropathies after acoustic tumor stereotactic radiosurgery. *Int J Radiat Oncol Biol Phys*. 1993;25(2):227–233.
13. Yang I, Sughrue ME, Han SJ, et al. Facial nerve preservation after vestibular schwannoma Gamma Knife radiosurgery. *J Neurooncol*. 2009;93(1):41–48.
14. Kano H, et al, Predictors of hearing preservation after stereotactic radiosurgery for acoustic neuroma. *J Neurosurg*. 2009;111(4): 863–873.
15. Lobato-Polo J, Kondziolka D, Zorro O, Kano H, Flickinger JC, Lunsford LD. Gamma knife radiosurgery in younger patients with vestibular schwannomas. *Neurosurgery*. 2009;65(2):294–300; discussion 300.
16. Kondziolka D, Lunsford LD, McLaughlin MR, Flickinger JC. Long-term outcomes after radiosurgery for acoustic neuromas. *N Engl J Med*. 1998;339(20):1426–1433.
17. Yang I, Aranda D, Han SJ, et al. Hearing preservation after stereotactic radiosurgery for vestibular schwannoma: a systematic review. *J Clin Neurosci*. 2009;16(6):742–747.
18. Combs SE, Volk S, Schulz-Ertner D, Huber PE, Thilmann C, Debus J. Management of acoustic neuromas with fractionated stereotactic radiotherapy (FSRT): long-term results in 106 patients treated in a single institution. *Int J Radiat Oncol Biol Phys*. 2005;63(1):75–81.
19. Timmer FC, Hanssens PE, van Haren AE, et al. Gamma knife radiosurgery for vestibular schwannomas: results of hearing preservation in relation to the cochlear radiation dose. *Laryngoscope*. 2009;119(6):1076–1081.
20. Paek SH, Chung HT, Jeong SS, et al. Hearing preservation after gamma knife stereotactic radiosurgery of vestibular schwannoma. *Cancer*. 2005;104(3):580–590.
21. Kondziolka D, Flickinger JC, Lunsford LD. The principles of skull base radiosurgery. *Neurosurg Focus*. 2008;24(5):E11.
22. Sharma MS, Kondziolka D, Khan A, et al. Radiation tolerance limits of the brainstem. *Neurosurgery*. 2008;63(4):728–732; discussion 732.
23. Fukuoka S, Takanashi M, Hojyo A, Konishi M, Tanaka C, Nakamura H. Gamma knife radiosurgery for vestibular schwannomas. *Prog Neurol Surg*. 2009;22:45–62.
24. Kalogeridi MA, Georgolopoulou P, Kouloulias V, Kouvaris J, Pissakas G. Long-term results of LINAC-based stereotactic radiosurgery for acoustic neuroma: the Greek experience. *J Cancer Res Ther*. 2009;5(1):8–13.
25. Chopra R, Dhingra N, Handa U, Mohan H. Ectomesenchymal chondromyxoid tumor of the tongue masquerading as pleomorphic adenoma on fine needle aspiration cytology smears: a case report. *Acta Cytol*. 2010;54(1):82–84.
26. Friedman WA, Bradshaw P, Myers A, Bova FJ. Linear accelerator radiosurgery for vestibular schwannomas. *J Neurosurg*. 2006;105(5):657–661.
27. Lunsford LD, Niranjan A, Flickinger JC, Maitz A, Kondziolka D. Radiosurgery of vestibular schwannomas: summary of experience in 829 cases. *J Neurosurg*. 2005;102 suppl:195–199.
28. Muacevic A, Jess-Hempen A, Tonn JC, Wowra B. Results of outpatient gamma knife radiosurgery for primary therapy of acoustic neuromas. *Acta Neurochir Suppl*. 2004;91:75–78.
29. Spiegelmann R, Lidar Z, Gofman J, Alezra D, Hadani M, Pfeffer R. Linear accelerator radiosurgery for vestibular schwannoma. *J Neurosurg*. 2001;94(1):7–13.
30. Prasad D, Steiner M, Steiner L. Gamma surgery for vestibular schwannoma. *J Neurosurg*. 2000;92(5):745–759.
31. Ito K, Shin M, Matsuzaki M, Sugasawa K, Sasaki T. Risk factors for neurological complications after acoustic neurinoma radiosurgery: refinement from further experiences. *Int J Radiat Oncol Biol Phys*. 2000;48(1):75–80.
32. Miller RC, Foote RL, Coffey RJ, et al. Decrease in cranial nerve complications after radiosurgery for acoustic neuromas: a prospective study of dose and volume. *Int J Radiat Oncol Biol Phys*. 1999;43(2):305–311.
33. Ito K, Kurita H, Sugasawa K, Mizuno M, Sasaki T. Analyses of neuro-otological complications after radiosurgery for acoustic neurinomas. *Int J Radiat Oncol Biol Phys*. 1997;39(5):983–988.
34. Foote RL, Coffey RJ, Swanson JW, et al. Stereotactic radiosurgery using the gamma knife for acoustic neuromas. *Int J Radiat Oncol Biol Phys*. 1995;32(4):1153–1160.
35. Kobayashi T, Tanaka T, Kida Y. The early effects of gamma knife on 40 cases of acoustic neurinoma. *Acta Neurochir Suppl*. 1994;62:93–97.
36. Martens F, Verbeke L, Piessens M, Van Vyve M. Stereotactic radiosurgery of vestibular schwannomas with a linear accelerator. *Acta Neurochir Suppl*. 1994;62:88–92.
37. Flickinger JC, Lunsford LD, Linskey ME, Duma CM, Kondziolka D. Gamma knife radiosurgery for acoustic tumors: multivariate analysis of four year results. *Radiother Oncol*. 1993;27(2):91–98.
38. Flickinger JC, Lunsford LD, Coffey RJ, et al. Radiosurgery of acoustic neurinomas. *Cancer*. 1991;67(2):345–353.
39. Meijer OW, Weijmans EJ, Knol DL, et al. Tumor-volume changes after radiosurgery for vestibular schwannoma: implications for follow-up MR imaging protocol. *AJNR Am J Neuroradiol*. 2008;29(5): 906–910.
40. House JW, Brackmann DE. Facial nerve grading system. *Otolaryngol Head Neck Surg*. 1985;93(2):146–147.
41. Myrseth E, Møller P, Pedersen PH, Lund-Johansen M. Vestibular schwannoma: surgery or gamma knife radiosurgery? A prospective, nonrandomized study. *Neurosurgery*. 2009;64(4):654–661; discussion 661.
42. Pollock BE, Driscoll CL, Foote RL, et al. Patient outcomes after vestibular schwannoma management: a prospective comparison of microsurgical resection and stereotactic radiosurgery. *Neurosurgery*. 2006;59(1):77–85; discussion 77.
43. Régis J, Pellet W, Delsanti C, et al. Functional outcome after gamma knife surgery or microsurgery for vestibular schwannomas. *J Neurosurg*. 2002;97(5):1091–1100.
44. Karpinos M, Teh BS, Zeck O, et al. Treatment of acoustic neuroma: stereotactic radiosurgery vs. microsurgery. *Int J Radiat Oncol Biol Phys*. 2002;54(5):1410–1421.
45. van Roijen L, Nijs HG, Avezaat CJ, et al. Costs and effects of microsurgery versus radiosurgery in treating acoustic neuroma. *Acta Neurochir (Wien)*. 1997;139(10):942–948.
46. Pollock BE, Lunsford LD, Kondziolka D, et al. Outcome analysis of acoustic neuroma management: a comparison of microsurgery and stereotactic radiosurgery. *Neurosurgery*. 1995;36(1):215–224; discussion 224.
47. Anderson BM, Khuntia D, Tomé WA, Bentzen S, Hayes L, Mehta MP. Single Institution Experience Treating 100 Vestibular Schwannomas with Fractionated Stereotactic Radiation Therapy of Stereotactic Radiosurgery. In: Proceedings of the 49th Annual ASTRO Meeting. 2007; Los Angeles, CA.
48. Meijer OW, Vandertop WP, Baayen JC, Slotman BJ. Single-fraction vs. fractionated linac-based stereotactic radiosurgery for vestibular schwannoma: a single-institution study. *Int J Radiat Oncol Biol Phys*. 2003;56(5):1390–1396.
49. Andrews DW, Suarez O, Goldman HW, et al. Stereotactic radiosurgery and fractionated stereotactic radiotherapy for the treatment of acoustic schwannomas: comparative observations of 125 patients treated at one institution. *Int J Radiat Oncol Biol Phys*. 2001;50(5):1265–1278.
50. Cauley KA, Ratkovits B, Braff SP, Linnell G. Communicating hydrocephalus after gamma knife radiosurgery for vestibular schwannoma: an MR imaging study. *AJNR Am J Neuroradiol*. 2009;30(5):992–994.
51. Banerjee R, Moriarty JP, Foote RL, Pollock BE. Comparison of the surgical and follow-up costs associated with microsurgical resection and stereotactic radiosurgery for vestibular schwannoma. *J Neurosurg*. 2008;108(6):1220–1224.
52. Verma S, Anthony R, Tsai V, Taplin M, Rutka J. Evaluation of cost effectiveness for conservative and active management strategies for acoustic neuroma. *Clin Otolaryngol*. 2009;34(5):438–446.
53. Thomas C, Di Maio S, Ma R, et al. Hearing preservation following fractionated stereotactic radiotherapy for vestibular schwannomas: prognostic implications of cochlear dose. *J Neurosurg*. 2007;107(5): 917–926.
54. Andrews DW, Werner-Wasik M, Den RB, et al. Toward dose optimization for fractionated stereotactic radiotherapy for acoustic

55. neuromas: comparison of two dose cohorts. *Int J Radiat Oncol Biol Phys.* 2009;74(2):419–426.
55. McClelland S 3rd, Dusenbery KE, Higgins PD, Hall WA. Treatment of a facial nerve neuroma with fractionated stereotactic radiotherapy. *Stereotact Funct Neurosurg.* 2007;85(6):299–302.
56. Koh ES, Millar BA, Ménard C, et al. Fractionated stereotactic radiotherapy for acoustic neuroma: single-institution experience at The Princess Margaret Hospital. *Cancer.* 2007;109(6):1203–1210.
57. Chan AW, Black P, Ojemann RG, et al. Stereotactic radiotherapy for vestibular schwannomas: favorable outcome with minimal toxicity. *Neurosurgery.* 2005;57(1):60–70; discussion 60.
58. Chang SD, Gibbs IC, Sakamoto GT, Lee E, Oyelese A, Adler JR Jr. Staged stereotactic irradiation for acoustic neuroma. *Neurosurgery.* 2005;56(6):1254–61; discussion 1261.
59. Sawamura Y, Shirato H, Sakamoto T, et al. Management of vestibular schwannoma by fractionated stereotactic radiotherapy and associated cerebrospinal fluid malabsorption. *J Neurosurg.* 2003;99(4):685–692.
60. Williams JA. Fractionated stereotactic radiotherapy for acoustic neuromas. *Int J Radiat Oncol Biol Phys.* 2002;54(2):500–504.
61. Szumacher E, Schwartz ML, Tsao M, et al. Fractionated stereotactic radiotherapy for the treatment of vestibular schwannomas: combined experience of the Toronto-Sunnybrook Regional Cancer Centre and the Princess Margaret Hospital. *Int J Radiat Oncol Biol Phys.* 2002;53(4):987–991.
62. Fuss M, Debus J, Lohr F, et al. Conventionally fractionated stereotactic radiotherapy (FSRT) for acoustic neuromas. *Int J Radiat Oncol Biol Phys.* 2000;48(5):1381–1387.
63. Kalapurakal JA, Silverman CL, Akhtar N, Andrews DW, Downes B, Thomas PR. Improved trigeminal and facial nerve tolerance following fractionated stereotactic radiotherapy for large acoustic neuromas. *Br J Radiol.* 1999;72(864):1202–1207.
64. Poen JC, Golby AJ, Forster KM, et al. Fractionated stereotactic radiosurgery and preservation of hearing in patients with vestibular schwannoma: a preliminary report. *Neurosurgery.* 1999;45(6):1299–1305; discussion 1305.
65. Lederman G, Lowry J, Wertheim S, et al. Acoustic neuroma: potential benefits of fractionated stereotactic radiosurgery. *Stereotact Funct Neurosurg.* 1997;69(1–4 Pt 2):175–182.
66. Weber DC, Chan AW, Bussiere MR, et al. Proton beam radiosurgery for vestibular schwannoma: tumor control and cranial nerve toxicity. *Neurosurgery.* 2003;53(3):577–86; discussion 586.
67. Vernimmen FJ, Mohamed Z, Slabbert JP, Wilson J. Long-term results of stereotactic proton beam radiotherapy for acoustic neuromas. *Radiother Oncol.* 2009;90(2):208–212.
68. Bush DA, McAllister CJ, Loredo LN, Johnson WD, Slater JM, Slater JD. Fractionated proton beam radiotherapy for acoustic neuroma. *Neurosurgery.* 2002;50(2):270–3; discussion 273.
69. Evans DG, Moran A, King A, Saeed S, Gurusinghe N, Ramsden R. Incidence of vestibular schwannoma and neurofibromatosis 2 in the North West of England over a 10-year period: higher incidence than previously thought. *Otol Neurotol.* 2005;26(1):93–97.
70. Asthagiri AR, Parry DM, Butman JA, et al. Neurofibromatosis type 2. *Lancet.* 2009;373(9679):1974–1986.
71. Mathieu D, Kondziolka D, Cooper PB, et al. Gamma knife radiosurgery in the management of malignant melanoma brain metastases. *Neurosurgery.* 2007;60(3):471–81; discussion 481.

92 Hemangioblastoma and Hemangiopericytoma

Malika L. Siker and Minesh P. Mehta

HEMANGIOBLASTOMA

Hemangioblastomas are uncommon benign vascular tumors that most often arise in the cerebellum and spinal cord. They are the most common primary cerebellar tumor in adults but account for only 1% to 2% of primary central nervous system (CNS) tumors in adults. They present during the third and fourth decades of life. Von Hippel-Lindau disease is an autosomal dominant disorder that may manifest with hemangioblastomas in the CNS and retina, pancreatic and renal cysts, and renal cell carcinoma. Although the majority of these tumors occur sporadically, an association with von Hippel-Lindau disease is noted in approximately 25% of patients [1]. The presence of multiple hemangioblastomas is suspicious for von Hippel-Lindau disease, although single tumors may occur in patients with von Hippel-Lindau disease. Histologically, the tumor consists of closely packed, thin-walled blood vessels in a stroma of large, oval foamy cells. The lesions are intensely enhancing on computed tomography and magnetic resonance imaging, and angiography confirms the vascular nature of the lesion. Imaging of the neuraxis should be considered in patients suspected to have von Hippel-Lindau disease. Clinically, patients may develop symptoms related to acute hemorrhage, local compression of neural structures, pain, or paraneoplastic syndromes such as erythrocytosis [2].

Treatment should be approached in a multidisciplinary setting including neurosurgery, radiation oncology, and interventional radiology. If feasible, complete resection should be attempted as it can be curative. Risks of surgery should be carefully considered, especially in patients with stable, asymptomatic lesions. Preoperative embolization of feeding arteries for larger tumors might decrease intraoperative hemorrhage and enhance the ease of resectability [3,4].

Fractionated adjuvant radiotherapy may be useful in patients with incomplete resections as recurrence rates can be as high as 25% [5]. Doses of at least 50 Gy should be considered from the results of a small study that showed that patients treated with 50 Gy or higher had improved local control (57% vs. 33%) [6]. At 5- and 15-years, recurrence-free survival was 76% and 42%, and overall survival was 85% and 58% [6]. Fractionated radiotherapy has also been used successfully in the setting of recurrent or extensive unresected disease [7].

Stereotactic radiosurgery has been evaluated for primary and recurrent disease but is associated with higher rates of recurrence [8–11]. Smaller lesions and treatment to higher doses are associated with improved local control [11]. Subsequent surgery may be required for expanding cystic components which are not always included in the treated field [9].

HEMANGIOPERICYTOMA

Hemangiopericytoma is a sarcomatous lesion developing from Zimmerman perictyes that surround capillaries typically found in the musculoskeletal system and skin. They occur rarely in the CNS, typically appearing along the base of the skull, although intraparenchymal lesions may also be seen. They occur more frequently in men during the fourth decade of life. In contrast to other primary CNS tumors, hemangiopericytomas commonly develop systemic metastases, most frequently to bone, liver, and lungs, and the natural history in terms of time to metastases can sometimes be very lengthy, spanning several years. They are locally aggressive tumors with a 90% 9-year actuarial risk for local failure following resection only. The majority of recurrences develop within 5 years [12].

Complete surgical resection is essential for disease control with retrospective studies showing improved local control and survival with gross total resection [12–14]. Because of the difficulty in controlling these tumors with surgery alone, postoperative radiotherapy has an important role in both completely and incompletely resected tumors. There are no prospective studies evaluating the impact of postoperative radiotherapy. Only retrospective studies are available and results have been mixed due to the small number of patients [12–15]. Most of these studies suggest that postoperative radiotherapy diminishes the probability of recurrence [12,14, 15]. Guthrie et al [12] demonstrated that radiotherapy after resection extended time before recurrence. Patients who receive complete resection followed by postoperative radiotherapy in these series have the best outcomes [12–15]. Tumor control is dose dependent, with doses greater than 50 Gy associated with superior outcomes [12]. Advanced technologies such as intensity-modulated radiotherapy and fractionated stereotactic radiotherapy have been shown to be safe and effective with good control rates [16]. Radiosurgery has been used for recurrent hemangiopericytomas with reported local control rates of approximately 80% following treatment [17,18].

REFERENCES

1. Neumann HP, Eggert HR, Weigel K, Friedburg H, Wiestler OD, Schollmeyer P. Hemangioblastomas of the central nervous system. A 10-year study with special reference to von Hippel-Lindau syndrome. *J Neurosurg.* 1989;70:24–30.
2. Waldmann TA, Levin EH, Baldwin M. The association of polycythemia with a cerebellar hemangioblastoma. The production of an erythropoiesis stimulating factor by the tumor. *Am J Med.* 1961;31:318–324.
3. Tampieri D, Leblanc R, TerBrugge K. Preoperative embolization of brain and spinal hemangioblastomas. *Neurosurgery.* 1993;33:502–505; discussion 5.
4. Georg AE, Lunsford LD, Kondziolka D, Flickinger JC, Maitz A. Hemangioblastoma of the posterior fossa. The role of multimodality treatment. *Arq Neuropsiquiatr.* 1997;55:278–286.
5. de la Monte SM, Horowitz SA. Hemangioblastomas: clinical and histopathological factors correlated with recurrence. *Neurosurgery.* 1989;25:695–698.
6. Smalley SR, Schomberg PJ, Earle JD, Laws ER Jr, Scheithauer BW, O'Fallon JR. Radiotherapeutic considerations in the treatment of hemangioblastomas of the central nervous system. *Int J Radiat Oncol Biol Phys.* 1990;18:1165–1171.
7. Koh ES, Nichol A, Millar BA, Menard C, Pond G, Laperriere NJ. Role of fractionated external beam radiotherapy in hemangioblastoma of the central nervous system. *Int J Radiat Oncol Biol Phys.* 2007;69:1521–1526.
8. Moss JM, Choi CY, Adler JR Jr, Soltys SG, Gibbs IC, Chang SD. Stereotactic radiosurgical treatment of cranial and spinal hemangioblastomas. *Neurosurgery.* 2009;65:79–85; discussion 85.
9. Wang EM, Pan L, Wang BJ, et al. The long-term results of gamma knife radiosurgery for hemangioblastomas of the brain. *J Neurosurg.* 2005;102 suppl:225–229.
10. Rajaraman C, Rowe JG, Walton L, Malik I, Radatz M, Kemeny AA. Treatment options for von Hippel-Lindau's haemangioblastomatosis: the role of gamma knife stereotactic radiosurgery. *Br J Neurosurg.* 2004;18:338–342.
11. Patrice SJ, Sneed PK, Flickinger JC, et al. Radiosurgery for hemangioblastoma: results of a multiinstitutional experience. *Int J Radiat Oncol Biol Phys.* 1996;35:493–499.
12. Guthrie BL, Ebersold MJ, Scheithauer BW, Shaw EG. Meningeal hemangiopericytoma: histopathological features, treatment, and long-term follow-up of 44 cases. *Neurosurgery.* 1989;25:514–522.
13. Soyuer S, Chang EL, Selek U, McCutcheon IE, Maor MH. Intracranial meningeal hemangiopericytoma: the role of radiotherapy: report of 29 cases and review of the literature. *Cancer.* 2004;100:1491–1497.
14. Kim JH, Jung HW, Kim YS, et al. Meningeal hemangiopericytomas: long-term outcome and biological behavior. *Surg Neurol.* 2003;59:47–53; discussion 53–54.
15. Dufour H, Metellus P, Fuentes S, et al. Meningeal hemangiopericytoma: a retrospective study of 21 patients with special review of postoperative external radiotherapy. *Neurosurgery.* 2001;48:756–762; discussion 62–63.
16. Combs SE, Thilmann C, Debus J, Schulz-Ertner D. Precision radiotherapy for hemangiopericytomas of the central nervous system. *Cancer.* 2005;104:2457–2465.
17. Sheehan J, Kondziolka D, Flickinger J, Lunsford LD. Radiosurgery for treatment of recurrent intracranial hemangiopericytomas. *Neurosurgery.* 2002;51:905–910; discussion 910–911.
18. Chang SD, Sakamoto GT. The role of radiosurgery for hemangiopericytomas. *Neurosurg Focus.* 2003;14:e14.

93 Radiation Therapy for Intracranial Meningiomas

C. Leland Rogers

INTRODUCTION

The earliest description of a meningioma has been attributed to Felix Plater, from an autopsy report in the early 17th century [1,2]. The early nomenclature was imprecise and varied, including such names as fungus of the dura mater, epithelioma, endothelioma, and meningoexotheliomas [3]. Harvey Cushing coined the simple name "meningioma," in a 1922 publication [4].

This chapter will examine the management of meningiomas and will appraise and contrast the varying therapeutic approaches. Emphasis will be given to benign (World Health Organization [WHO] grade I) meningiomas owing simply to a greater volume of information. Atypical (grade II) and anaplastic (grade III) meningiomas will also be reviewed. An overview of etiologic factors, epidemiology, molecular genetic and histopathology, clinical presentation, and imaging will supplement the discussion.

ETIOLOGY

Little is known about the etiology of most meningiomas. Associations have been made with endogenous factors, such as hormones, growth factors, and molecular genetics [5,6], and with exogenous influences, such as ionizing radiation and trauma [7,8,9,10]. However, the causative factors for the majority of these neoplasms remain elusive. Cushing and others considered trauma as a possible etiologic factor [11], but this has not found support in large epidemiologic studies [7,8].

An unambiguous relationship has been identified with ionizing radiation, including exposure to low, intermediate, and high doses of radiation [12]. Meningiomas are the most commonly reported radiation-associated neoplasm [13]. Our awareness of this association derives largely from populations with atomic bomb fallout, from cranial irradiation, and from scalp irradiation for tinea capitis [13,14–17]. The lag time is typically lengthy, ranging from about 10 to 35 years, proportional in part to the degree of radiation exposure [12,16]. Radiation-induced meningiomas occur at younger age, carry an increased risk of multifocality, and tend to have more aggressive histology and behavior [12,13,16]. Strojan and colleagues estimated that radiation-induced meningiomas occur at a rate of 0.53% at 5 years, escalating to 8.18% at 25 years following high-dose cranial irradition [16]. However, Flint-Richter and associates pointed out that less than 1% of individuals who are exposed to ionizing radiation develop meningiomas [18].

A role for sex hormones in meningioma induction is suggested by several findings. Meningiomas occur with greater abundance in females than in males (Figure 93.1). It has been reported that the relative risk is increased with postmenopausal hormone replacement therapy, with the use of long-acting hormonal contraceptives [19], and even with high-dose female hormone therapy in transsexual patients [20]. Furthermore, tumor size or symptoms may worsen during the luteal phase of menses or pregnancy [21,22]. The hazard ratio for meningiomas is increased in breast cancer patients, as is the risk of breast cancer in meningioma patients [21,22]. Obesity has also been correlated with a higher prevalence of meningiomas in males and females [21–23]. In spite of these observations, the precise role of hormones is unclear. Greater than 70% of meningiomas express progesterone receptors, up to 40% estrogen receptors [12,21], and nearly 40% androgen receptors as well [12]. These hormone receptor findings are true of both sexes.

Meningiomas occur with greater frequency in patients with certain rare genetic conditions such as type 2 neurofibromatosis (NF2) [24,25]. As will be discussed in greater detail in the subsequent section of this chapter, nearly all NF2-associated meningiomas, and many sporadic meningiomas, have mutations of the NF2 gene [6]. Nevertheless, phenotypic NF2 accounts for only a small minority of meningiomas. The majority develop with no known or discernible factor.

EPIDEMIOLOGY

Incidence and Prevalence

It has been long been acknowledged that meningiomas are the most common nonglial intracranial tumor [9,22,26–28]. Recent data from the Central Brain Tumor Registry of the United States now reveal that meningiomas are the most frequently reported primary intracranial neoplasm [5], with an estimated prevalence of 97.5 per 100,000 and with over 138,000 individuals currently diagnosed [29]. Meningiomas account for approximately 30% of all primary intracranial tumors [5,27,30]. There is no definitive evidence

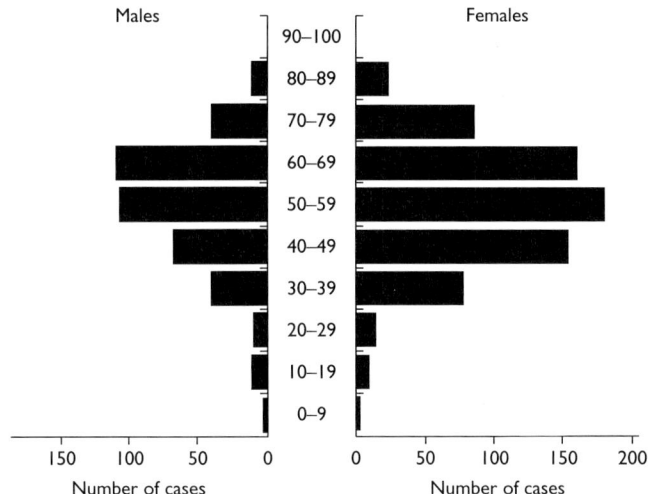

Figure 93.1 Age and gender distribution of meningiomas. Dual bar graph displaying age- and gender-related meningioma distributions. Based upon 1,078 cases treated at the University Hospital of Zurich. Reprinted with permission from Perry et al [12].

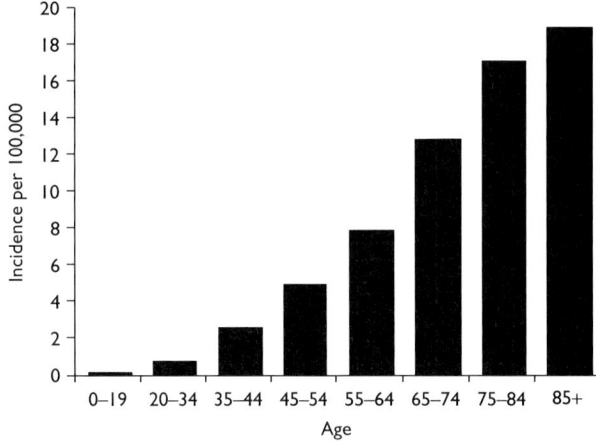

Figure 93.2 Age specific incidence of meningiomas. Age specific incidence of meningiomas, based upon data from the Central Brain Tumor Registry of the United States. Derived using data from Table 1 of Claus EB et al. [5].

that the actual incidence is rising. The apparent increase may reflect improved detection and reporting mandated by the Benign Brain Tumor Cancer Registries Amendment Act (HS5204) [5] as well as improved imaging.

Many meningiomas are identified solely on the basis of imaging. More intensive use of modern imaging may further increase detection. In this regard, investigators from the University of Pittsburgh reported that 35% of their meningioma patients treated with radiosurgery had been diagnosed on the basis of neuro-imaging alone. They maintained that an image-based diagnosis was reliable given a 2.3% 10-year rate of ultimately identifying a diagnosis other than meningioma [31]. In a University of Maryland report, the proportion of patients diagnosed radiographically was higher, at 62% [32]. When incidental meningiomas are considered, the numbers are greater. Vernooij et al [33] performed brain magnetic resonance imaging (MRI) among 2000 persons of at least 45 years of age (mean age 63.3 years) in the Netherlands and identified meningiomas in 0.9% of the sample. Moreover, meningiomas have been identified in as many as 2.3% of autopsies [34].

Gender, Age, and Race Distributions

As is evident in Figure 93.1, meningiomas occur more frequently in females [12]. The female to male ratio varies among large studies but is approximately 2 to 1 [5,9,35–38]. Interestingly, one autopsy study failed to find a difference in the gender distribution of meningiomas at autopsy [39]. There does not appear to be a female preponderance with malignant meningiomas [40].

Figure 93.1 demonstrates that the risk of developing a meningioma is proportional to age [12]. In absolute numbers, meningiomas are most often diagnosed during the fifth through seventh decades [38,41], but this should not be mistaken to imply that risk lowers thereafter. Age-specific incidence is still on the rise beyond 85 years of age [5]. The proportion of patients in older age groups is simply smaller. Figure 93.2, fashioned using data from the Central Brain Tumor Registry of the United States, illustrates a continued rise in age-specific incidence even beyond 85 year of age [5]. This purports that meningiomas will likely become more prevalent with increasing longevity.

Age-related incidence notwithstanding, meningiomas can occur at any age. Except in the setting of NF2 [24], they are infrequent in the pediatric population, accounting for only 1% to 4% of all pediatric brain tumors [9,24]. Although decidedly rare, meningiomas have been reported during fetal development and infancy [3,24,42–44]. Children and young adults have been noted to exhibit more aggressive clinical and histological features [25], and there is no gender predilection in pediatric patients [3,25]. Excepting these introductory comments, no specific focus on pediatric meningiomas in undertaken with this chapter. They have been recently and thoroughly reviewed elsewhere [25].

Even among adult patients, age may have prognostic relevance. Stafford and colleagues found inferior progression-free survival (PFS) in patients less than 40 years of age [36]. Jung and associates noted more rapid growth with subtotally resected meningiomas in patients less than 50 (7.51 cc per year) than in those 50 years or older (0.83 cc per year) [45].

A greater relative incidence among Africans and Americans of African descent [46] has previously been reported; however, recent data from the Central Brain Tumor Registry of the United States [47] indicates similar incidence rates for Caucasians, African Americans, and Hispanics.

MOLECULAR GENETICS AND HISTOPATHOLOGY

Molecular Genetics

As briefly aforementioned, meningiomas occur with greater frequency in patients with certain rare genetic conditions, such as NF2 [24,25]. Nearly all NF2-associated meningiomas have mutations of the NF2 gene on chromosome 22q12 [6], but phenotypic NF2 accounts for a small minority of meningiomas. It is notable, nevertheless, that most families identified as susceptible to meningiomas have alterations of the NF2 locus [6,48]. Monosomy of chromosome 22 is the most common cytogenetic alteration, along with mutations of NF2 and other members of its structural protein family. With atypical and anaplastic meningiomas, additional and more complex genetic alterations have been encountered, the most common being losses on chromosome 1p. Losses (6q, 10, 14q, 9p, 18q) and gains (1q, 9q, 12q, 15q, 17q, 20q) on several other chromosomes are found with atypical and anaplastic meningiomas. Adapted from Arie Perry and colleague's 2007 WHO classification of meningiomas [12], Figure 93.3 charts a genetic model for meningioma tumorigenesis and malignant progression.

Histogenesis

It was suggested over a century ago [49] that meningiomas derive from epithelioid cells on the outer surface of arachnoid villi, now known as arachnoid cap cells. These are generally accepted as the cell of origin, although this has never been categorically proven. The assertion is supported by several findings. Arachnoid cap cells are cytologically similar to most meningiomas; they are found in greater number at sites where meningiomas commonly occur, and they appear to increase with age, paralleling the age-related incidence of meningiomas [3].

Tumor Grade

Most meningiomas are benign and are projected to exhibit a protracted clinical course. Some meningiomas, particularly high-grade or multiply recurrent tumors, are aggressive and carry high rates of morbidity and mortality. Tumor grading is used to help make important clinicopathologic correlations and therapeutic decisions. WHO published updated grading criteria in 2007 [12]. These are updated from the preceding WHO 2000 criteria [50] and incorporate mitotic activity, sheet-like growth, hypercellularity, nucleolar prominence, nuclear to cytoplasmic ratio, spontaneous necrosis, brain invasion, and certain meningioma variants to assign a grade, I through III (Table 93.1). As shown in Figure 93.4, strong associations between grade, recurrence-free survival, and overall survival have been shown and confirmed in large series [51–54].

Most large studies agree that less than 5% are grade 3 [53–55], but there is much greater disparity in the proportion of patients allocated to grade II. A recent large epidemiologic analysis by Claus et al [5] reported that only 5% of meningiomas were categorized as atypical, whereas Perry and colleagues, whose work formed the basis for current WHO grading, found in a large combined series of patients from the Mayo Clinic and Washington University that over 20% were WHO grade II (Figure 93.4). In support of the latter contention, Willis et al [56] from Scotland regraded 314 patients using modern WHO guidelines and found that 20.4% had atypical (grade II) histology (Figure 93.5). Furthermore, 38% of patients assigned to grade I by older criteria were reclassified as grade II. Grading discrepancies remain an obstacle to progress.

Benign (WHO Grade I)

Approximately, 70% to 85% of intracranial meningiomas are WHO grade I. As will be reviewed in greater detail in subsequent sections, with definitive treatment, 80% or more of WHO grade I meningiomas remain in local control at 10 years [53,54,57].

Atypical (WHO Grade II)

Per current WHO standards, it appears that 15% to 25% of patients should be grade II [53,54,56]. Single-institution series have had smaller percentages of grade II patients, ranging from 4.7% [58] to 9.6% [59]. It is important to recognize grade II meningiomas since they carry a seven- to eightfold increased recurrence risk at 3 to 5 years [60].

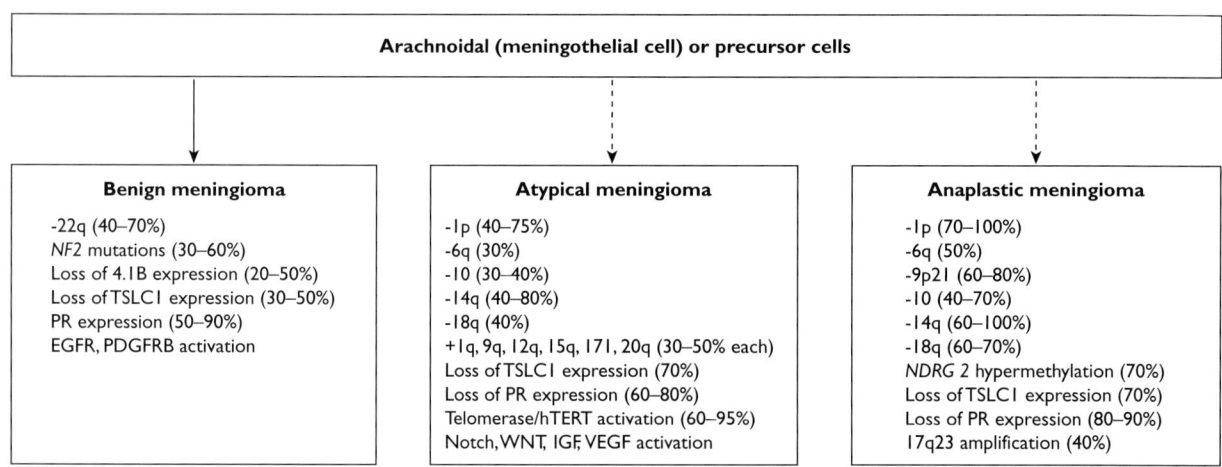

Figure 93.3 Model of meningioma tumorigenesis and malignant progression. Reprinted with permission from Perry et al [12].

Table 93.1 WHO 2007 Tumor Grade

Grade I (benign)	Grade II (atypical)	Grade III (anaplastic/malignant)

Any major variant other than clear cell, chordoid, papillary, or rhabdoid
Does not fulfill criteria for grades II or III
	Frequent mitoses (>4 per 10 hpf)
	or
	3 or more of the following:
	  Sheeting architecture
	  Hypercellularity (focal or diffuse)
	  Prominent nucleoli
	  Small cells with high nuclear cytoplasmic ratio
	  Foci of spontaneous necrosis
	or
	Additional subtypes / features
	  Chordoid meningioma
	  Clear cell meningioma
	  Brain invasion
		Excessive mitotic index (>20 per 10 hpf)
		or
		Frank anaplasia defined as focal or diffuse loss of meningothelial differentiation resembling:
		  Sarcoma
		  Carcinoma or
		  Melanoma
		or
		Additional subtypes / features
		  Papillary meningioma
		  Rhabdoid meningioma

The 2007 World Health Organization (WHO) criteria for meningioma grading. From ref. 12.
Abbreviation: hpf, high powered field.

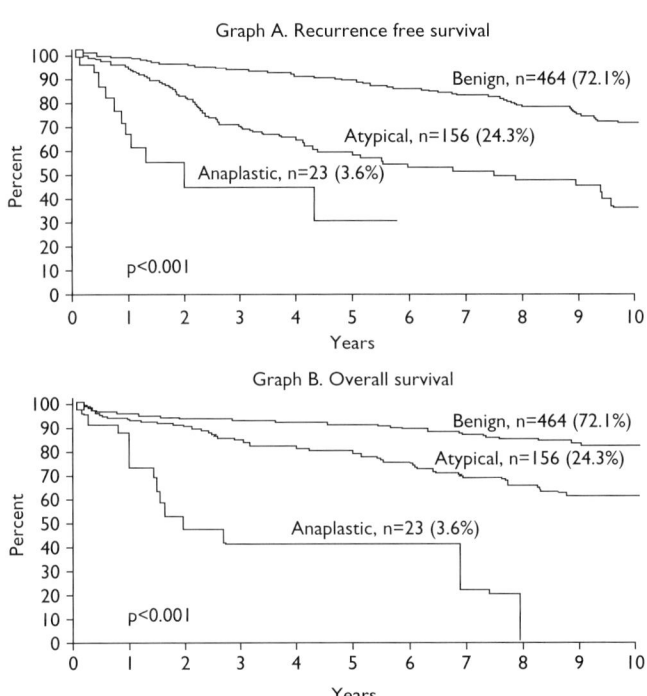

Figure 93.4 Recurrence-free survival by grade (643 patients). Kaplan-Meier recurrence free survival (graph A) and overall survival (graph B) for 643 meningioma patients stratified by tumor grade. The number of patients within each grade and the relative percentages are given. The grading criteria used from this analysis have been incorporated into the current (2007) WHO grading scheme. The percentages indicate the proportion of patients allocated to each grade. Reprinted with permission from Perry [3].

Even with definitive therapy, only about 40% to 60% of grade II patients are disease free at 10 years [53–55,61] (Figure 93.4). Brain invasion, previously considered evidence of malignancy, now consigns a meningioma to WHO grade II unless, of course, histologic anaplasia is found [60].

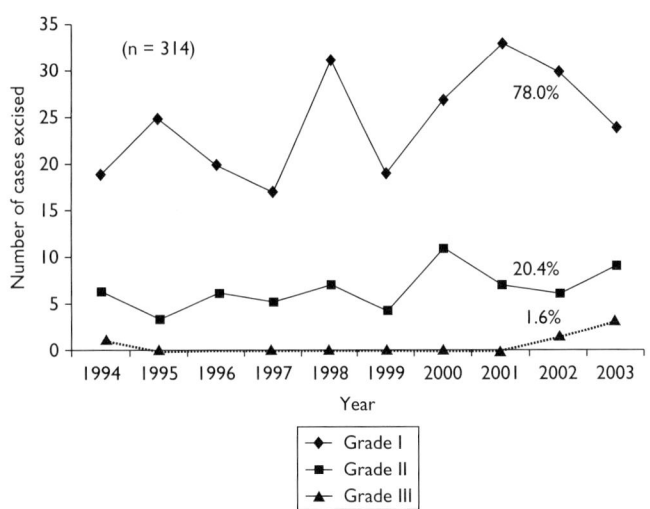

Figure 93.5 Proportion of meningiomas by grade Scottish Re-Grading Study. Frequency of grade I, II, and III meningiomas over a 10-year period (1994–2003), as re-graded per modern WHO grading criteria. Reprinted with permission from Willis et al [56].

Anaplastic/Malignant (WHO Grade III)

A minority of meningiomas, 1% to 5%, are malignant [53,54–56,62]. These are aggressive tumors, with a median recurrence-free survival less than 2 years and ultimately poor overall survival [53,54] (Figure 93.4). Therapeutic recommendations differ less among anaplastic meningiomas than their lower grade counterparts, and treatment typically entails surgery and radiation therapy (RT). Larger field external beam irradiation has been common, although stereotactic radiosurgery (SRS) has also been reported [63,64].

Histopathology—Histologic Subtypes and Variants

The current WHO classification sanctions the three aforementioned tumor grades as well as the 13 histologic variants [12]. The majority of histologic subtypes exhibit similar clinical behavior. Among these, meningothelial, fibrous, and transitional meningiomas are the most common. As listed in Table 93.1, four subtypes are more aggressive and by definition are placed in a higher grade category. Chordoid and clear cell variants are WHO grade II. Papillary and rhabdoid are grade III [12,65].

Clinical Presentation

As is the case with many intracranial mass lesions, patients with meningioma can present with a variety of signs and symptoms, depending largely upon tumor location. Table 93.2, compiled by Rockhill and colleagues, highlights patient history and physical exam findings obtained from a variety of publications and includes both low- and high-grade primaries [1,11,38,58,66–68]. In conformity with a common pattern of slow growth, the most common symptom is headache. Many patients have normal physical examinations. High-grade tumors are more likely to produce abrupt or critical physical findings, such as paresis, visual impairment, or altered consciousness.

Table 93.2 Intracranial Meningioma Signs and Symptoms

Signs and Symptoms	Number of Patients (%)	
	Low-Grade Meningioma	High-Grade Meningioma
Patient history		
Headache	70 (36)	5 (36)
Personality change/confusion	43 (22)	3 (21)
Paresis	37 (19)	6 (43)
Generalized seizures	36 (19)	1 (7)
Visual impairment	30 (16)	4 (29)
Focal seizures	29 (15)	2 (14)
Ataxia	28 (15)	3 (21)
Aphasia	19 (10)	2 (14)
Decreased level of consciousness	13 (7)	2 (14)
Paresthesia	11 (6)	0
Diplopia	6 (3)	0
Vertigo	2 (1)	0
Decreased hearing	2 (1)	0
Physical findings		
Paresis	57 (30)	7 (50)
Normal examination	51 (26)	2 (14)
Memory impairment	29 (15)	3 (21)
Visual field deficit	19 (10)	3 (21)
Other cranial nerve deficit	21 (12)	0
Paresthesia	17 (9)	3 (21)
Aphasia	17 (9)	1 (7)
Papilledema	15 (8)	2 (14)
Decreased visual acuity	12 (6)	7 (7)
Altered level of consciousness	9 (5)	2 (14)
Nystagmus	6 (3)	0
Decreased hearing	4 (2)	0

Reprinted with permission from Rockhill et al [2]. Compiled from ports by Bondy, Demonty, Jaaskelainen, Longstreth, Rutten, Sanson, Wilson, and their associates [Bondy 1996, DeMonte Oncology 95, Jaaskelainen 86, Longstreth 93, Rutten 07, Sanson 00, Wilson 94].

Neuro-Imaging

Before the advent of multiplanar imaging, meningiomas were often diagnosed via plain radiographs or angiography. At present, the most common modalities are computed tomography (CT) and MRI. MRI is generally considered superior, although CT is complementary in demonstrating orientation to bony landmarks, bone erosion, hyperostosis, and intratumoral calcifications [2,69–71]. Slower growth or improved outcome has been correlated with certain MRI and CT findings. Homogeneous enhancement [62], smooth tumor contour [40,69,72], iso to hypointense intratumoral T2 signal, and intratumoral calcifications have all been linked with slower growth [73–75]. Angiography may still be used to assess blood supply or to ascertain invasion or displacement of vasculature. Molecular imaging is yet the frontier, but may take on important roles in evaluating growth potential and treatment response [39,76], as may diffusion-weighted MRI [77], although further study is needed in both instances.

TREATMENT AND OUTCOME

Many retrospective studies have documented that resection, radiosurgery, and fractionated external beam irradiation result in excellent local control (LC) at 5 years for benign meningiomas. Indeed, meningiomas are often amenable to longer term control, and their treatment can thus be satisfying. However, occasionally owing to complex anatomical relationships with neurovascular structures, to recurrence or inexorable growth, they can also pose difficult challenges. The discussion of treatment and outcome emphasizes WHO grade I meningiomas, although a subsequent section will further address nonbenign meningiomas.

Surgery

Surgery remains the standard approach for meningiomas. Tumor control has consistently corresponded to the extent to which tumor and its attachments are removed. In 1957, Donald Simpson published an evaluation of 265 meningioma patients treated surgically in Oxford and London. His work formed the common characterization of resection extent [78]. As summarized in Table 93.3, this takes into account the degree of removal of tumor as well as any dural attachments or extradural extentions (e.g., hyperostotic bone). Dr. Simpson found that this classification correlated with the likelihood of clinically apparent tumor recurrence: 9% after a Simpson grade I resection, 19% after grade II, 29% following grade III, and 44% with grade IV. Dr. Simpson considered grades I and II to represent radical, gross total resections (GTRs) and grade III through V subtotal and "supposed that cases with grades III to V resection would inevitably develop symptomatic recurrence, soon or late [78]."

Nearly every subsequent surgical study has validated Simpson's grading system, and most have followed his lead by denoting Simpson grades I and II as gross total and grades III through V as subtotal. A University of Florida series by Condra et al, with 262 patients and a median follow-up of 8.2 years, casts further light on this. They did not

Table 93.3 Extent of Resection (Simpson's Grade)

Grade	Definition
I	Gross total resection of tumor, dural attachments, and abnormal bone
II	Gross total resection of tumor, coagulation of dural attachments
III	Gross total resection of tumor without resection or coagulation of dural attachments or extradural extensions (e.g., invaded or hyperostotic bone)
IV	Partial resection of tumor
V	Simple decompression (biopsy)

Graded resection extent based upon clinically apparent recurrence of intracranial meningioma in 265 patients from Radcliffe Infirmary in Oxford as well as patients. From Dr. Hugh Cairns in London; Simpson [78].

Table 93.4 Intracranial Meningioma Sites of Origin

Primary Site	Patients	Percent*
Parasagittal/Falx	448	22
Convexity	391	20
Sphenoid Wing/Petroclival	369	18
Posterior Fossa/CP Angle	290	14
Parasellar	215	11
Olfactory Groove/Planum	131	7
Multiple Sites	95	5
Other	48	2
Intraventricular	17	1
Total	2004	100

Sites of origin of intracranial meningiomas, as complied from four large series. From Mirimanoff, J Neurosurgery. 1985;62:18–24. Kallio, Neurosurgery. 1992;31:2–12. Condra, Int J Radiat Oncol Biol Phys. 1997;427–436. Stafford, Mayo Clin Proc. 1998;73:936–942.

* Percent=percent distribution by site of origin.

identify any significant difference in LC among Simpson grades I through III. Fifteen-year actuarial LC was 75% for grade I, 87% with grade II, and 71% in grade III patients. Patients with Simpson grades IV and V resections fared significantly worse, with 15-year LC of 30% ($P = 0.0001$). In conjunction with the surgeon's appraisal, it is now common to use postoperative MRI or CT. A definition of GTR, incorporating grade I through III, each of which entails gross total tumor removal, relates well to current practice. The likelihood of achieving a thorough resection, and thus the probability of recurrence after surgery alone, vary considerably by site of origin. Table 93.4 reviews sites of origin from 4 large series. Table 93.5 displays the likelihood of obtaining total excision by site or origin, and Table 93.6 the 5- and 10-year local recurrence risk by site.

Gross Total Resection

GTR is generally considered definitive; however, local recurrence is by no means obviated by it. Table 93.7 shows 5- to 15-year outcome after GTR alone in 923 patients from five retrospective series. Although LC is commonly maintained at 5-years, a greater risk of recurrence is manifest at later intervals. It is now acknowledged that meningiomas, even with excellent surgery, can and with ample follow-up often do recur [36,37,41,58,79–84]. With advances in neuroimaging, recurrences are now easier to recognize. It is notable in this regard that the highest rates of local recurrence were appreciated in the most recent study by Soyuer et al [83] (Table 93.7).

Even with excellent resection, approximately 20% to 60% of benign meningiomas will recur at 10 to 15 years (Table 93.7). This represents a relatively broad range, and further risk stratification would be constructive. Jaaskelainen and associates studied 657 benign intracranial meningioma patients, with median follow-up of 8 years. They identified three "strong risk factors" for recurrence after GTR: coagulation (rather then resection) of dura, bone invasion, and soft tumor. Stratifying outcome by these factors, the 20-year actuarial local recurrence risk was 11% for patients with none of the "strong risk factors," 15% to 24% with one factor, and 34% to 56% with two. They did not specify outcome in patients with all three factors but did note that even among the favorable subset of patients with benign convexity meningiomas, nearly all (96%) of whom had Simpson grade I resections, the 20-year recurrence risk was 18% [58].

Subtotal Resection

Table 93.8 comprises seven series describing local progression after subtotal resection (STR) alone. As has been confirmed by nearly every applicable study, STR results in higher rates of progression [85] than does GTR. As reviewed in Table 93.8, at 5 years, 37% to 62% of subtotally resected meningiomas progress; At 10 years, the rates increase to 52% to 82%, and at 15 years, to 70% to 91%. Condra and colleagues at the University of Florida found that cause-specific survival (CSS) was significantly superior with GTR than with STR, respectively 88% and 51% at 15 years ($P = 0.0003$). This data is displayed in Figure 93.6. As will be further discussed in a later section, this study also recognized that postoperative irradiation after STR improved both LC and CSS survival over STR alone.

Despite the high local progression risk following STR alone, observation remains common practice. In a large Mayo Clinic report, among 116 patients with STR, only 10 received postoperative irradiation [36]. In the above-referenced University of Florida study (Figure 93.6), only 17 of 72 patients with STR were irradiated postoperatively. This may be a function of the slow growth of most subtotally resected benign meningiomas. Soyuer and colleagues reported a 4.1-year median time to progression after STR alone [83]. It may also be related to questions regarding immediate versus delayed therapy following STR. Some have found either approach acceptable [57], while others have noted improved outcome with earlier postoperative irradiation. A prolonged natural history notwithstanding, many patients with meningioma have life expectancies beyond the anticipated time frames for recurrence, and recurrences themselves can result in morbidity and complex therapeutic challenges.

Radiation Therapy

Throughout much of the early and mid-20th century, meningiomas were considered insensitive to RT. More

Table 93.5 Likelihood of Total Excision by Site of Origin

Primary Site	Patients*	Percent
Parasagittal/falx	292/339	86
Convexity	280/292	96
Sphenoid wing/petroclival	153/266	58
Posterior fossa/CP angle	126/197	64
Parasellar	107/154	69
Olfactory groove/planum	98/116	84
Other	36/48	75
Intraventricular	8/11	73
Total	1100/1423	77

Likelihood of total excision of intracranial meningioma by site of origin, complied from three large series. From Mirimanoff, *J Neurosurgery.* 1985;62:18–24. Kallio, *Neurosurgery.* 1992;31:2–12. Condra, *Int J Radiat Oncol Biol Phys.* 1997;427–436).

* The numerator is the number of patients with total excision and the denominator, the number undergoing surgery.

Table 93.6 Likelihood of Local Recurrence by Site

			Recurrence Risk	
Tumor Location	n	GTR (%)	5-Year (%)	10-Year (%)
Spine	18	78	0	13
Convexity	47	96	3	25
Parasagittal area	38	76	18	24
Parasellar	28	57	19	35
Posterior fossa	31	32	23	38
Olfactory groove	22	77	30	41
Sphenoid ridge	36	28	34	54
Total	220	28–96	0–34	13–54

Likelihood of gross total resection (GTR) and local recurrence of intracranial meningiomas by site of origin. Adapted from text and graphs in Mirimanoff, *J Neurosurgery.* 1985;62:18–24.

Abbreiation: n, number of patients.

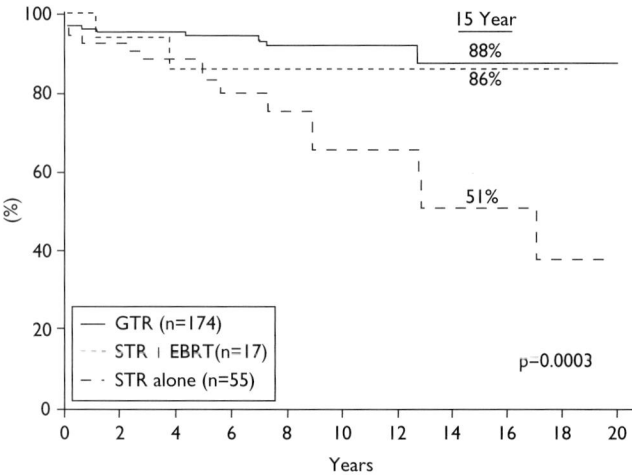

Figure 93.6 Cause-specific survival. Cause-specific survival from a University of Florida series comparing gross total resection alone (GTR alone), subtotal resection plus external beam radiation therapy (STR + EBRT), and subtotal resection alone (STR alone). Reprinted with permission from Condra et al., Benign meningiomas: Primary treatment selection affects survival, *Int J Radiation Oncology Biol Phys*, 1997;39(2):427–436.

Table 93.7 Local Recurrence After Gross Total Resection Alone

			Local Recurrence		
Author	Year	Patients	5-Year (%)	10-Year (%)	15-Year (%)
Mirimanoff	1985	145	7	20	32
Taylor [80]	1988	90	13[a]	25[a]	33[a]
Condra	1997	175	7	20	24
Stafford [36]	1998	465	12	25	–
Soyuer [83]	2004	48	23	39	60[a]
Total		923	7–23	20–39	24–60

Local recurrence risk at 5, 10, and 15 years following gross total resection alone.

[a] Actuarial data taken from graph.

Stereotactic Radiosurgery

SRS is a more recent development than EBRT and has been used with increasing frequency over the past two decades. SRS utilizes precise three-dimensional localization to accurately focus ionizing radiation upon a target. Radiation delivered in this manner blends the benefits of radiation physics and biology by permitting tight conformality, a steep dose gradient, and a higher, more ablative radiation dose. Indeed, as viewed in Table 93.9, 5-year PFS following SRS has exceeded 85% in all listed studies excepting a subset in one study treated with relatively lower single fractions doses of 10–12 Gy [85].

Radiosurgery is now an accepted form of treatment for meningiomas. LC have been impressive at 5 to 10 years, both with linear accelerator-based [90,91–95] and GammaKnife [32,96–106] systems. Pollock and coauthors reported on 188 benign meningioma patients treated with either surgery or SRS alone. After a median follow-up of 64 months, 7-year PFS rates between SRS and Simpson grade I surgery were equivalent at 95% and 96%. Additionally, they found that SRS was superior to less extensive surgery and concluded that it should be considered a primary management option when a Simpson grade I resection is unlikely or infeasible [105]. For many patients, SRS has been the primary treatment modality. Note the "no histology" column

recently, multiple retrospective studies have verified excellent LC from various forms of RT, including SRS (Table 93.9), fractionated external beam irradiation (Table 93.10), and brachytherapy [86–89]. RT was initially employed postoperatively for patients with STR or high-grade histology or for patients who were deemed inoperable. In publications of the last decade, many patients have received RT as primary treatment.

The various forms of RT each have merits in appropriately selected patients. Tables 93.9 and 93.10 display 50 studies with 5869 patients, showing the usefulness of RT in delaying or preventing recurrence, in both post-operative and primary settings. To date, RT remains the sole validated nonsurgical modality for the treatment of meningiomas. Both fractionated external beam irradiation and SRS will be reviewed.

of Table 93.9 identifying that 30% to 100% of patients in these studies were diagnosed and treated on the basis of radiographic and clinical criteria.

Target Volume and Dose

SRS is generally considered suitable for meningiomas less than 3 to 4 cm in maximum diameter, with distinct margins, with little or no surrounding edema, and with sufficient distance from critical normal tissues to allow for appropriate normal tissue dose restrictions [105,107]. Regarding tumor volume, DiBiase and coauthors reported 5-year disease-free survivals of 91.9% for patients with meningiomas <10 cc (equivalent diameter 2.7 cm) versus 68% for larger tumors [32]. Analyzing 203 patients, Kondziolka and colleagues described excellent outcomes (no tumor progression, no management morbidity, and no need for further treatment) in all patients with small tumors (<7.5 cc or 3 cm diameter), no prior surgery, and no neurologic deficit [107].

Figure 93.7 is a treatment planning MRI for a meningioma treated to 14 Gy at the 50% isodose. As depicted, most radiosurgery series have defined the planning target volume as the enhancing gross tumor volume (GTV). Nicolato and colleagues found no advantage to larger margins. With median follow-up of 4 years, they had 100% tumor growth control with a conformity index (ratio of prescription isodose volume to target volume) of <1.5 [103]. However, studies have encountered poorer outcome when a portion of the GTV is not encompassed within the prescription isodose.

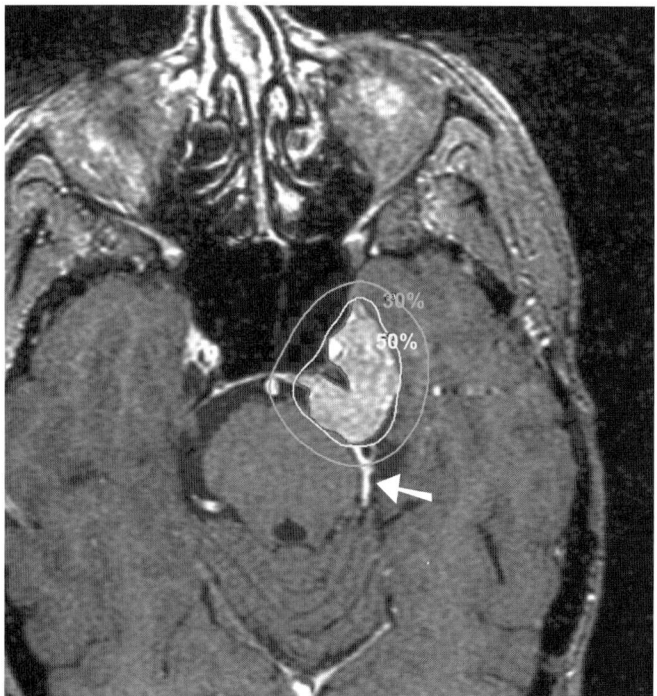

Figure 93.7 Stereotactic radiosurgery. Planning MRI for radiosurgery of a meningioma treated to 14 Gy at the 50% isodose. The prescription 50% and 30% isodose lines are included. The white arrow identifies a dural tail. *See color insert.*

Shin and associates reported increased progression risk when a portion of tumor was not targeted or received less than 10 to 12 Gy [85]. Malik et al found a comparatively low 87% 5-year rate of LC in 309 patients. In nearly half of their patients, the prescription isodose did not cover the entire target, principally with the intent of limiting dose to neural structures at risk, such as the optic apparatus [108].

As viewed in Table 93.9, tumor margin doses have ranged from 10 to 18 Gy and have trended somewhat downward without apparent decrement in LC, excepting those studies using the lowest doses—in the range of 10 Gy [85,109]. Ganz and associates noted that a minimum peripheral tumor dose of 10 Gy or less was associated with a higher risk of failure [109]. Morita et al [97] suggested tumor margin doses of 15 to 16 Gy. With extended follow-up, Stafford and coauthors reported no improvement in the 5-year LC of benign meningiomas using margin doses ≥16 Gy compared with doses <16 Gy [43]. Kondziolka et al [107] similarly reported no improvement with margin doses ≥15 Gy versus <15 Gy. More recently, large studies by Kollova [110], using a median margin dose of 12.6 Gy, reported a 5-year PFS of 97.9%. Another by Kriel [111], using a median 12 Gy, found a PFS of 98.5% at 5 years and of 97.2% at 10 years. Doses from 12 to 14 Gy to the tumor margin are now widely accepted [31,94,99,103,104,110–113] and have provided excellent tumor control with acceptable degrees of toxicity.

Toxicity

Early reports, often with higher doses to larger meningiomas, met with greater complications. Recent analyses, with more careful patient selection, have found less morbidity. Infrequent occurrences of radiation necrosis [103,114,115], peritumoral cyst formation [101], carotid stenosis [116], and hypothalamic dysfunction [93] have been described, but adverse events most frequently attributed to SRS have been cranial nerve deficits and edema.

Owing to anatomic proximity, cranial nerve deficits are a common feature with meningiomas involving the cranial base. With modern techniques and margin doses ranging from 14 to 16 Gy, four studies have identified new or worsened neurologic deficits in approximately 8% of patients [32,101,117]. These deficits, occasionally transient, can become apparent within 1 month [101] up to 2 or 5 years after treatment [112,118].

Sensory nerves are more susceptible to injury from SRS than motor nerves. Cranial neuropathies have been more common with the optic, cochlear, and trigeminal nerves. Sensory nerves of the anterior visual pathway are of particular concern, relating to the readily perceptible impact of even limited damage. Single doses of 10 Gy or less [97,118] carry a roughly 1% or 2% rate of optic neuropathy, and with higher doses complications rise steeply [118,119]. Motor nerves, including oculomotor nerves in the cavernous sinus, have demonstrated higher tolerance. In 80 patients with cavernous sinus meningioma, Roche and colleagues observed no new oculomotor deficits with a mean maximum prescription dose of 28 Gy (range 12–50 Gy), mean prescription isodose of 50%, and median follow-up of 30.5 months [98].

Cranial neuropathies are typically associated with skull base meningiomas, whereas edema is encountered more commonly with nonbasal primaries. Meningiomas produce vasoactive mediators [9,120–122], but this alone does not explain the higher rate of edema at nonbasal sites. A typically broader pial interface with nonbasal meningiomas may provide additional explanation, permitting vasogenic substrates greater access to adjacent brain [75,123]. A broader pial interface also permits a greater pial-cortical arterial supply and perhaps a greater degree of vascular steal. Basal primaries have more limited pial involvement [75,123,124]. Particularly with parasagittal meningiomas, for which edema has been frequently reported [107], sinus and/or venous occlusion may also contribute.

SRS-associated edema has been widely reported. Table 93.11 appraises postradiosurgery edema in 686 cases from nine series [106,107,109,125–131]. Edema developed in 25% to 100% of the nonbasal meningioma patients, compared to 0% to 22% of patients with basal primaries. Aside from tumor location (see "comments" column of Table 93.11), factors potentially associated with edema in these studies were as follows: higher margin dose (>15–18 Gy), integral dose, tumor size (e.g., volume >4 cc), and the presence of pretreatment edema or venous sinus occlusion. These data reflect the relative safety and the limits of safety for SRS and allow for a comparative analysis of fractionated external beam irradiation.

Fractionated External Beam Radiation Therapy

Until the mid-to-late 20th century, it remained open to question what role, if any, RT played in the treatment of patients with meningioma [41]. In the 1950s, Simpson accepted that EBRT was an appropriate consideration after incomplete resection but also felt that there was "little evidence of permanent benefit" [78]. Throughout the 1960s and 1970s, several studies found infrequent tumor regression and were unable to establish that EBRT improved outcome beyond short-term palliation [41,132–134]. Meningiomas were considered resistant to irradiation, and additional concerns were voiced on other fronts.

There was apprehension about the malignant degeneration of irradiated tumors, about the development of new, radiation-induced meningiomas, and about other potential adverse effects [16,132–137]. The probability of developing a meningioma after high-dose irradiation was assessed by Strojan et al [16], who found the actuarial risk after high-dose RT to be 0.53% at 5 years and 8.18% at 25 years. This risk appears to be less with lower doses irradiation. Flint-Richter and Sadetzki [18] reported that less than 1% of individuals irradiated for tinea capitis and followed for almost 40 years develop meningiomas. The current, more conformal methods of EBRT deliver lower doses to uninvolved tissues and may thus also convey a lower risk. RT-induced meningiomas have yet been rare in studies of fractionated stereotactic EBRT, as in reports of single-fraction radiosurgery, although prolonged follow-up will be needed to reach definitive conclusions. Malignant degeneration is widely felt to be interrelated with the natural history of recurrent or progressive meningiomas and has never been explicitly linked to RT. However, these issues have continued to guide patient care, and many inoperable or subtotally resected meningioma patients are observed rather than treated with RT [36,45,138].

Meningiomas typically remain stable or regress slowly following EBRT. Thus, studies with short-term follow-up are often uninformative. Series with long-term follow-up began to emerge in the 1970s and early 1980s and reached the conclusion that EBRT improved LC after incomplete resection or recurrence [79,84,139,140]. As included in Table 93.10, several reports have now compared STR alone with STR and EBRT, and have found consistent improvement in PFS with EBRT.

Postoperative EBRT

GTR is not always feasible. Many studies have documented excellent 5- to 10-year LC with STR and EBRT (Table 93.10). As viewed in Table 93.8, the likelihood of progression after incomplete resection exceeds 35% at 5 years and well exceeds 50% at 10 to 15 years. Retrospective studies have confirmed improvements in LC, CSS and possibly even survival [141]. It is notable from Table 93.10 that, since the turn of the recent century and with improvements in EBRT techniques, each publication analyzing outcome following STR + EBRT has found that 5- to 10-year PFS exceeds 90%. Figure 93.8 is a scatter plot comparing 5-year PFS following GTR alone, STR plus EBRT, and STR alone from each of the studies in Table 93.10. This intimates an upward trend in outcome following STR plus EBRT, possibly reflecting improvements in targeting and treatment delivery.

Primary EBRT

In publications through the 1980s and much of the 1990s, primary EBRT was the exception. Over the past decade, more patients have been diagnosed and treated on the basis of neuroimaging, without histologic confirmation, and results have been favorable. In an earlier era, Glaholm and colleagues found a 15-year, disease-free survival of 47% with primary EBRT, lower than the 61% rate with partial resection and EBRT, but surprisingly superior to the

Table 93.8 Local Progression After Subtotal Resection Alone

		Local Progression		
Author	Year	5-Year (%)	10-Year (%)	>15-Year (%)
Wara [84]	1975	47	63	75
Mirimanoff	1985	37	55	91
Barbaro§ [79]	1987	40	–	–
Mirabell§	1992	40	52[a]	–
Condra	1997	47	60	70
Stafford [36]	1998	39	61	–
Soyuer [83]	2004	62	82[b]	88[b]
Total		37–62	52–82	70–91

Local progression risk at 5, 10, and 15 years following subtotal resection alone.

[a] 8-year progression.

[b] Actuarial data taken from graph.

Abbreviation: Year: year published.

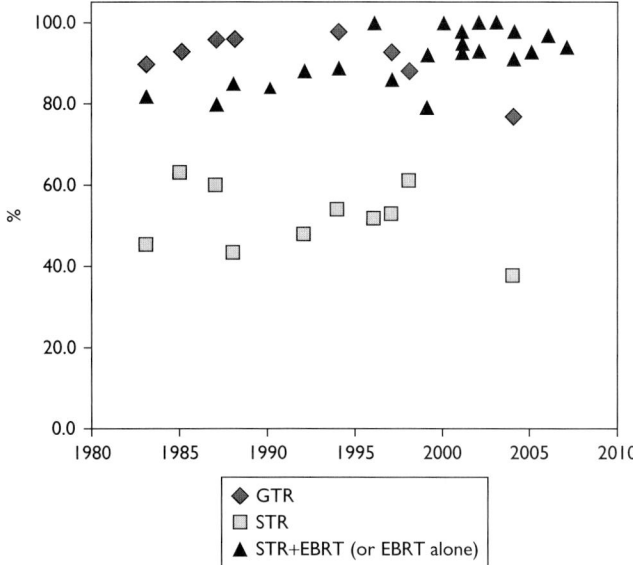

Figure 93.8 5-year progression-free survival fractionated external beam irradiation 26 retrospective studies (n = 3588). Scatter plot comparing 5-year progression-free survival following gross-total resection alone (GTR), subtotal resection alone (STR), and STR plus external beam radiation therapy (STR+EBRT). The x-axis is the year of publication. Some of the patients plotted as STR+EBRT were treated with primary EBRT without surgery or histologic confirmation.

40% 10-year rate following GTR and EBRT [135]. Rather than suggesting the inferiority of primary EBRT, or of GTR and EBRT, this likely reflects selection biases and outcomes before image-based planning. However, Carella and coauthors, reporting from a similar era, found uniform LC at 3 to 6 years with primary EBRT [139].

Recent reports by Henzel [142] and Milker-Zabel [59,140] included approximately 31% to 42% of patients treated with primary EBRT with excellent tumor control (Table 93.10). The latter study found similar LC with known WHO grade I tumors as with unknown histology and primary EBRT [143]. The former series, by Henzel and colleagues, reviewed 224 patients, 42% of whom received primary stereotactic fractionated EBRT. Five-year PFS was 97% [142]. In another recent analysis, Debus and coworkers had no recurrences in patients treated by radiotherapy alone and found no significant difference between primary stereotactic fractionated EBRT and similar EBRT postoperatively. In both subgroups, 10-year recurrence-free probabilities were 100% [144]. Several other publications over the past decade have corroborated excellent results with primary EBRT [145–148]. The "no histology" column of Table 93.10 indicates the percentage of patients in each study receiving EBRT.

Optic Nerve Sheath Meningioma

Optic nerve sheath meningiomas (ONSMs), although relatively uncommon, provide a superlative case in point for primary EBRT. ONSMs arise from the dura surrounding the optic nerve and have generally comprised only about 1% or 2% of meningiomas [149,150–153], although the incidence may be increasing with modern imaging [149]. Surgery plays a limited role in the management of ONSMs. Historically, as a consequence of supposed radioresistance, observation or resection of the tumor and optic nerve were common practices [149,151]. The former resulted in inexorable, although often gradual, loss of vision and the latter immediate blindness of the affected eye.

Attempts have been made to resect ONSMs while keeping the nerve in situ, but this has also carried a high risk of visual complications [154–157]. ONSMs are usually located between the optic nerve and its blood supply [149]. Resection commonly impairs this blood supply and results in blindness of the affected eye, even when the nerve is left grossly intact. The majority of ONSMs are thus not amenable to radical surgery, and less than radical resection has carried a high risk of local recurrence [155,158]. Resection has largely been abandoned as a primary treatment option, and even biopsies are unusual. Most patients are managed on the basis of clinical and imaging findings [149,150–153].

EBRT is now integral in the management of ONSMs [146,158]. In the same era that the efficacy of radiotherapy for meningiomas at other sites was coming to light, Smith and associates published a 1981 report documenting the successful treatment of five ONSM patients with EBRT [159]. Kennerdall et al subsequently reported on six patients. With 3 to 7 years of follow-up, five of the six patients had documented improvements in acuity or visual fields, and the remaining patient had stable vision. There were no observed complications [157].

In larger and more recent studies, the usefulness of EBRT for ONSMs has been confirmed. Turbin et al [158] reported 64 ONSM patients, with median follow-up of 8.3 years, and found that EBRT alone (40–55 Gy with standard fractionation) provided more favorable outcome than observation, surgery alone, or surgery plus EBRT. Narayan and colleagues, with median follow-up of 51.3 months, identified no radiographic progression in any of the 14 ONSM patients treated with conformal EBRT, 86% of whom had improved or stable vision [146]. Several other series using conformal or fractionated stereotactic EBRT have reached similar conclusions [146,150,160–164].

Table 93.12 compiles data from 12 ONSM studies [146,150,153,154,157,160,162,164–169]. In composite, these include 228 patients (244 affected eyes) with mean follow-up of 48 months. Tabulating all patients, whether treated with surgery and EBRT or EBRT alone, crude LC is 87% to 100%, and visual improvement or stability is often attained. If only patients managed with primary EBRT are analyzed [150,160,162,164,166,168–171], the results are more favorable: mean LC in 98%, improved vision in 75%, and stable vision in an additional 21% of patients (Table 93.12). Vision loss occurred in 4%, often with recurrence, but at times as a sequella of EBRT.

The natural history of ONSMs entails visual loss with progression to blindness of the affected eye in most cases [172]. With excellent results from EBRT, it has been suggested that earlier treatment may provide better visual outcome [149]. However, there is no uniform agreement as to whether ONSM patients with stable lesions should be approached with careful observation or early EBRT, particularly if vision is preserved.

Table 93.9 Stereotactic Radiosurgery (WHO Grade I; Often Presumptive)

Author	Year	n	f/u (months)	No Histo	Tumor Volume	Margin Dose	% Regression	5y-PFS
Chang (92)	1997	55	48	31%	7.3 cc	18 Gy	29%	98% (med f/u 48mo)
Hakim (94)	1998	127	31	54%	4.1 cc	15 Gy	NR	89%
Chang (93)	1998	24	46	33%	6.8 cc	17.7 Gy	37%	100% (median f/u 46 mo)
Liscak (97)	1999	53	19	64%	7.8 cc	12 Gy	52%	100% (median f/u 19 mo)
Kondziolka (114)	1999	99	all > 60	43%	4.7 cc	16 Gy	63%	93%
Morita (98)	1999	88	35	44%	10 cc	16 Gy	68%	95%
Shafron (91)	1999	70	23	NR	10 cc	12.7 Gy	28%	100% (mean f/u 23 mo)
Roche (99)	2000	80	31	63%	5.8 cc	14 Gy	31%	93%
Aichholzer (101)	2000	46	48	33%	23.5 mm (dia)	15.9 Gy	52%	96% (mean f/u 48 mo)
Stafford (102)	2001	168	40	41%	8.2 cc	16 Gy	56%	93%
Shin (90)	2001	15	42	30%	4.3 cc	10–12 Gy	38%	75% (5 & 10y)
"	"	22	"	"	"	14–18 Gy	"	100% (5 & 10y)
Nicolato (104)	2002	111	48	50%	8.4 cc	15 Gy	63%	96%
Lee (105)	2002	159	35	52%	6.5 cc	13 Gy	34%	93% (97% if SRS sole tx)
Spiegelmann (95)	2002	42	36	74%	8.2 cc	14 Gy	60%	97.5%
Pollock (106)	2003	62	64	46%	7.4 cc (All < 35 mm)	17.7 Gy	NR	95% (7y)
Roche (100)	2003	32	56	75%	2.3 cc	13 Gy	13%	100% (med f/u 56 mo)
Iwai (103)	2003	42	49	48%	14.7 cc	11 Gy	60%	92%
Flickinger (31)	2003	219	29	100%	5.0 cc	14 Gy	NR	93% (at 5 and 10 y)
Chuang (96)	2004	43	75	48%	5.7 cc	16 Gy	55%	90% 7y (100% SRS sole tx)
DiBiase (37)	2004	137	54	62%	4.5 cc	14 Gy	28%	86.2% (91.9% if <10 cc)
Kim (107)	2005	26	33	91%	4.7 cc	16 Gy	31%	95%
Kreil (111)	2005	200	95	51%	6.5 cc	12 Gy	57%	98.5% (97.2% at 10y)
Zachenhofer (115)	2006	36	103	31%	20 mm (dia)	16.8 Gy	83% (at 8y)	94% (at 5 and 8 y)
Kollova (112)	2007	325	60	70%	4.4 cc	12.6 Gy	70%	97.9%
Combined		2281	19–103	30–100%	4.1–14.7	10–18 Gy	13–83%	75–100%

5-year progression-free survival (5y-PFS) and other germane treatment factors.

Abbreviations: ": ditto; cc: cubic centimeters; dia, diameter; f/u, follow-up, mean or median follow-up unless otherwise specified; n, number of patients; No Histo, percentage of patients diagnosed without histopathologic confirmation (i.e., by imaging findings); NR, not reported; p, after; % Regression, percentage of patients with tumor regression following radiosurgery; Tumor Volume, mean or median tumor volume prior to radiosurgery; tx, treatment; y, year.

ONSMs underscore important issues pertaining to intracranial meningiomas generally. A diagnosis can be reached, and treatment given, on the basis of imaging findings. Carefully planned and delivered fractionated external beam irradiation is an effective primary therapy. Neurologic symptoms (in this case vision) commonly improve during or soon after EBRT. Limited side effects and long-term LC are frequently achieved.

Technical Factors

Technical improvements have favorably impacted the outcome and side-effect profile of postoperative EBRT. Treatment may now be delivered with more precision and conformality (Figure 93.9), and improved results expected [82,148,173]. Indeed, improvements in LC have been documented with CT- or MRI-based planning. Goldsmith [82] and Milosevic [174] each substantiated improved LC with modern imaging-based treatment planning. Goldsmith et al [35,82] found that with CT- and/or MRI-based target definition and appropriate immobilization, 10-year PFS improved from 77% to 98% ($P = 0.002$). These advances now represent a common standard.

Dose

Largely with benign (WHO grade I) meningiomas, the results outlined in Table 93.10 were generally attained with total doses of 50 to 55 Gy and fractions of 1.8 to 2.0 Gy. However, no definitive dose response has been established. Taylor [80], Miralbell [81], Condra, Maguire [145], Pourel [175], and Henzel [142] each were unable to clearly document a dose response, with the majority of patients treated in the relatively narrow range of 50 to 60 Gy. Winkler et al found no overt dose response in a broader range of 36 to 79.5 Gy (1.5–2.0 Gy per day) [176]. Goldsmith et al [82] did find that doses >52 Gy improved 10-year LC (93% vs 65% with lower doses, $P = 0.04$). This was a significant ($P = 0.04$) univariate factor, but significance was not retained on multivariate analysis.

Larger cohorts will likely be required to establish a dose response for varying patient subgroups; however, a dose schedule of 54 Gy in fractions of 1.8 to 2.0 Gy is common for benign meningiomas, excepting those anterior optic apparatus and optic nerve sheath where modestly lower biologic doses of 45 to 55 Gy with fractions of 1.6 to 1.8 Gy have been customary. Dose considerations for non-benign meningiomas are discussed in a separate section, including both atypical (WHO grade II) and anaplastic (WHO grade III) tumors.

Target Volume

The literature does not define the optimal margin breadth with certainty. Planning target volumes have varied from the GTV with a 4-cm margin [125], to GTV plus a 2-cm

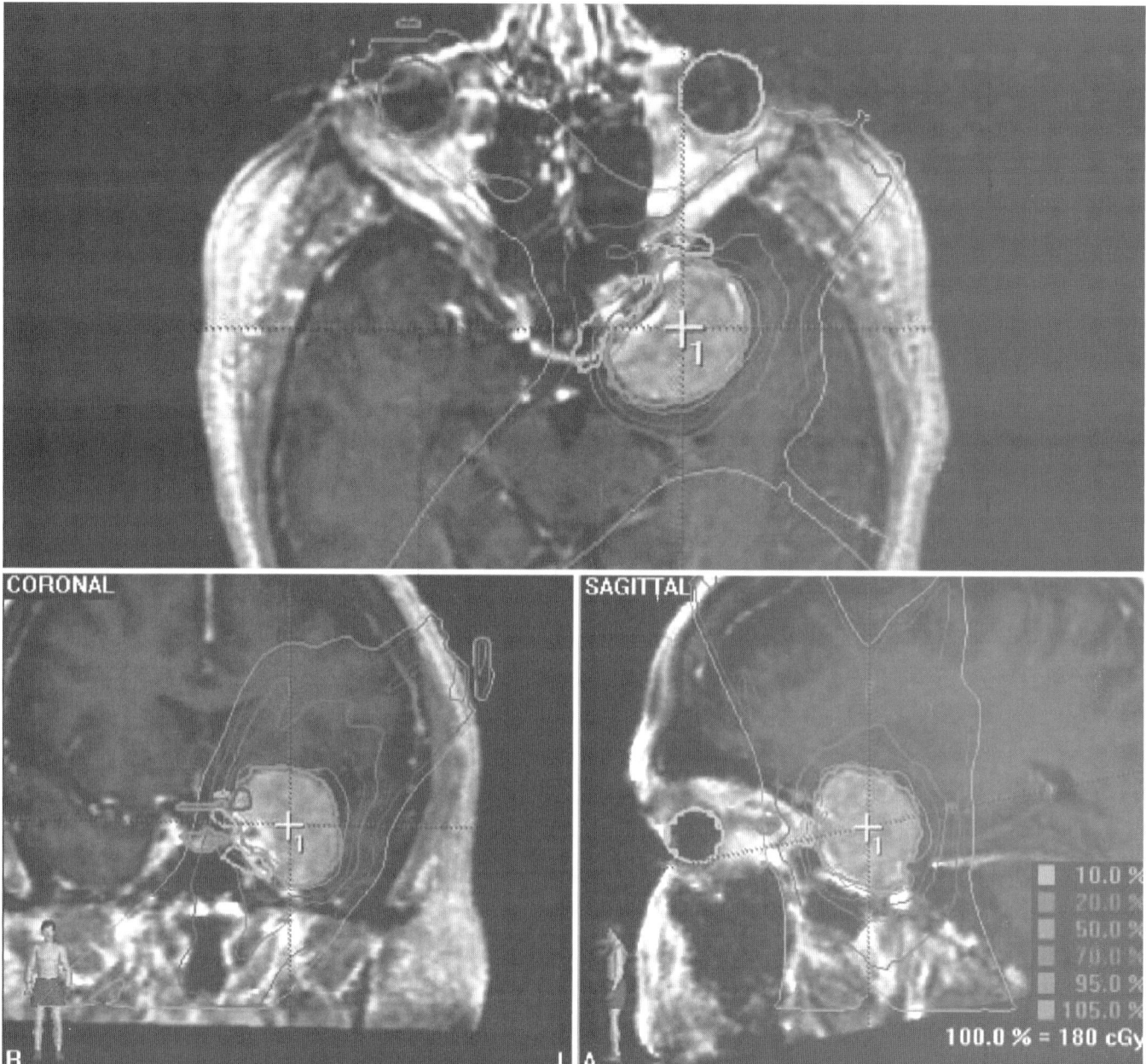

Figure 93.9 Fractionated stereotactic EBRT. Radiation therapy plan with isodoses. This paracavernous meningioma was treated to 54Gy in 30 fractions. The legend at the lower right hand corner illustrates percentage values for each of the pictured isodoses. Courtesy of Dennis Shrieve, MD, Chair of Radiation Oncology, Huntsman Cancer Institute, University of Utah. *See color insert.*

margin [177], GTV plus 1 cm [35], and as small as to GTV with a 1 to 2 mm margin in recent stereotactic fractionated EBRT series [142,141]. Others, such as Milker-Zabel and colleagues, describe varying margins of 1 to 2mm against normal brain, 3 mm against osseous structures, and 5 mm along dura [59]. Figure 93.9 displays a plan of fractionated stereotactic EBRT, 54 Gy in 30 fractions, for a paracavernous meningioma patient and who remains progression free at 4 years. Even with the tight conformity, marginal failures have been uncommon [103,141]. Using fractionated stereotactic radiotherapy with 2-mm margins, Debus et al [144] noted no marginal failures in 189 patients with 3-years median follow-up.

Dural Tail. A dural tail is a common feature with meningiomas; however, its inclusion within the treatment volume is controversial. The majority of meningiomas are attached to the dura and to varying degrees may invade it. Dura adjacent to the tumor may enhance in linear fashion, usually trailing off within a few millimeters to centimeters. The linear trailing enhancement is referred to as a "dural tail." In Figure 93.10, a petroclival and cavernous sinus meningioma with a large dural tail is shown. This feature

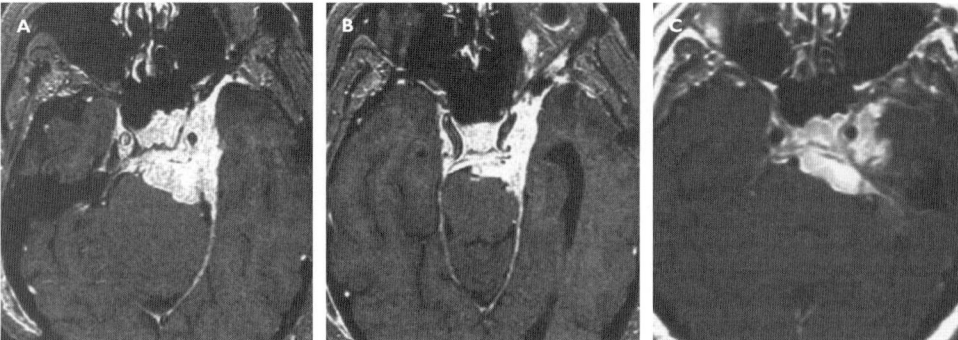

Figure 93.10 Dural tail. MRI before (images A & B) and after (image C) radiosurgery for a large petroclival and cavernous sinus meningioma, 14Gy to the 50% isodose to the enhancing tumor without a margin. The dural tail was not targeted. Images A and B show enhancing dura extending bilaterally around the tentorium. Image C is 1 year after treatment, showing modest shrinkage of the meningioma and near resolution of the untargeted dural tail. Courtesy of Kris Smith, Department of Neurosurgery, Barrow Neurological Institute, Phoenix, Arizona.

is not specific to meningiomas. It can be seen with other dural-based tumors but in the case of meningiomas is typically composed entirely or almost entirely of hypervascular dura [65,170,178,179]. Microscopic clusters of meningioma are occasionally observed but are also encountered in randomly selected dural strips [178]. Borovich and Doron [178] felt that the location of these aggregates, and their independence from blood vessels, precluded seeding and dural metastasis.

Ahmadi and colleagues assessed tissue changes responsible for dural enhancement in 73 patients with various neoplasms (29 with meningioma) undergoing surgery. Surgery included either en-bloc resection of tumor and surrounding dura or multiple dural biopsies. Two patterns of dural enhancement were identified: continuous and discontinuous. No patient with continuous enhancement had dural tumor invasion, whereas every instance of discontinuous enhancement was found to be invaded. In each case of discontinuous enhancement, tumor invasion was in direct continuity with the primary tumor rather than at a distance. Histologic examination of the dural tails revealed "proliferation, inflammation, and hypervascularity" predominantly involving the arachnoid membrane, but no invasion by meningioma [180].

A recent study suggested improved results by treating the dural tail [32], although in most studies the dural tail has not been targeted. It is noteworthy that the dural tail is an imaging finding, typically not visualized at surgery. Simpson's definitions predate CT and MRI, and it is not considered in the definition of resection extent according to Simpson's criteria (Table 93.3). Results with GTR alone (Table 93.4) have been obtained irrespective of removing the dural tail. Target volumes with single-fraction radiosurgery have tended to be contrast-enhanced tumor without a margin, often omitting the dural tail (Figure 93.7, white arrow) [36,90,112,125]. Figure 93.10 demonstrates near resolution of a large, nontargeted dural tail 1 year after radiosurgery. There is no evidence to suggest that recurrences are more likely within the dural tail than in any other portion of dura next to the tumor mass. This issue remains important. As aforementioned, irradiation of partial tumor volumes results in higher rates of progression [95,108]. Thus, accurately identifying tumor is critical. It may well be suitable not to target a dural tail as defined by thin linear enhancement (as in Figure 93.10) but to intentionally encompass more suspicious, thick, or nodular adjoining dura.

Hyperostosis. Hyperostosis can occur in association with meningiomas [181,182]. Pieper and coauthors performed a study correlating imaging to histopathology in 51 cranial base meningioma patients. Surgery included biopsies of adjacent hyperostotic and radiographically normal bone. Twenty-six patients had hyperostosis on preoperative imaging. Tumor invasion was present in all but one. However, 9 of 25 patients without hyperostosis were also found to have tumor invasion of bone. The authors suggested the removal of hyperostotic bone in order to achieve a complete resection; however, it remains unresolved whether resection of bone—or its inclusion within a RT target—is necessary for every patient. Simpson noted that bone invasion may be "of overrated importance.... When one recalls how frequently meningiomas are associated with hyperostosis, it is surprising how rare is a recurrence clearly arising from bone" [78]. In spite of this astute observation, Simpson required removal of abnormal bone for a grade I resection (Table 93.3).

Recurrence rates for patients with "gross total resections" not inclusive of hyperostotic bone have traditionally been low, as have recurrences after radiosurgery and EBRT whether or not neighboring bone was targeted. Expanding radiation portals to encompass all linear dural enhancement would likely escalate adverse events while providing minimal reward. However, hyperostotic bone more frequently contains tumor. Its location would generally have less impact on normal tissues, excepting hyperostosis near the anterior visual pathway or the petrous ridge near the acoustic nerve. Until further research illuminates the matter, it may be sensible to include hyperostotic bone when it can be accomplished safely.

Toxicity

The side effects of EBRT with current methods of planning and delivery are evidently few but are not negligible. Early publications identified no deleterious late effects [79,80] but, more recently, a small incidence of clinically important late effects is evident. A large recent series of fractionated irradiation by Debus et al reported 189 patients treated with a highly conformal stereotactic approach, using median daily fractions of 1.8 Gy to a mean cumulative dose (at isocenter) of 56.8 Gy. They identified clinically significant (grade 3) toxicity in four patients (2.2%), three (1.7%) in the absence of a preexisting deficit. These three were reduced vision, a visual-field deficit, and trigeminal neuropathy [144]. This is a substantial improvement over the 38% reported by Al-Mefty et al [183] with older methods of radiation delivery.

Goldsmith et al recognized complications attributable to EBRT in 5 of 140 patients (3.6%). These included cerebral necrosis, retinopathy, and optic neuropathy [82]. In a separate publication, Goldsmith and colleagues constructed a model to predict optic nerve tolerance and recommended a maximum dose of 890 optic ret (e.g., 54 Gy in 30 fractions) [184]. From this and other analyses, optic complications have been quite rare below this threshold, particularly with fractional doses of <2.0 Gy [81,135,147,185,186]. In the studies compiled in Table 93.12, retinopathy has been rare with total doses to the retina of 45 Gy or less. Nonocular cranial nerve deficits [144] have also been uncommon. Selch and colleagues found no treatment-related cranial neuropathies in 45 cavernous sinus meningioma patients treated to a median total dose of 50.4 Gy (fractions 1.7–1.8 Gy) [145].

Brain or brainstem necrosis is uncommon but has been observed by Goldsmith et al [184] and others [81,183]. Al-Mefty and coauthors reviewed post-EBRT toxicity in 58 adult patients with a variety of skull base, parasellar, or pineal region tumors. Seventeen (29%) developed late brain parenchymal changes, with latencies of 4 months to 23 years. These changes were encephalomalacia, cerebral atrophy, gliosis and/or necrosis, generalized, or involving the temporal lobes in 82% of cases [183]. Such occurrences are almost certainly related to outdated treatment techniques. Integral doses to untargeted brain are much lower with current methodologies.

Pituitary dysfunction [81,121,179,183], cerebrovascular events [121,135,147,148], second malignancy [57,183], orbital fibrosis [145], and other sporadic toxicities have been noted. In an older series, Glaholm et al found that all complications in their series occurred with former conventions of treating only a portion of the fields daily and with fractional doses >1.8 Gy (total doses of 50–55 Gy) [135].

Edema. Table 93.10 compiles and summarizes data from 26 EBRT series with 3588 patients. Only nine (0.2%) reportedly developed edema, and three of these nine were largely asymptomatic. This very low rate of edema from EBRT should be approached with some caution. Although there were likely few cases of clinically significant edema, 20 of the 26 studies did not specifically assess edema the possibility. Patients with asymptomatic edema, or with mild and transient symptoms such as headache or nausea, may have escaped detection. Even with this concession, Selch and colleagues did evaluate edema, and they noted none in 45 patients with 3-years median follow-up [148]. It appears evident that edema is a less likely consequence of fractionated EBRT than of single-fraction SRS.

Cognitive. Some studies have identified personality changes [185] and/or memory loss [57,81,145] as complications of EBRT. These studies included many patients treated with the less conformal techniques. Cognitive outcome has been prospectively evaluated by Steinvorth and associates who used highly conformal fractionated stereotactic radiotherapy. Neurocognitive outcome was studied using a comprehensive battery of tests before, after the first fraction, at completion, and 12 months subsequent to fractionated stereotactic radiotherapy. They observed a transient decline in memory after the first fraction, counterbalanced by an increase in attention. No cognitive deterioration was identified with further follow-up [187].

Comparative Outcomes: EBRT Versus SRS

Sibtain and Plowman published a comparison of EBRT with SRS for cavernous sinus meningiomas. They retrospectively evaluated 13 patients with tumors <3 cm in diameter, most of whom received radiosurgery, versus 15 patients with tumors >3 cm, most of whom had EBRT. They noted uniform LC for all patients at 12 to 83 months [177]. Nakamura et al, addressing dosimetric and technical concerns among 10 irregularly shaped skull base lesions, found that intensity-modulated radiation therapy provided target coverage and normal tissue sparing analogous to SRS. Intensity-modulated radiation therapy had an improved conformity index at the prescription isodose, although at times with less conformity at lower isodoses [74].

Multiple series now attest to the relative equivalence of EBRT and SRS with regard to PFS (see Tables 93.9 and 93.10). Table 93.13 encapsulates this data. Across all series, the 5-year PFS rates are remarkably similar between SRS or EBRT, and they remain similar with "recent" series (2002–2007). This "recent" time frame was chosen because it allows comparison of tumor volume and tumor regression data, not widely available in EBRT series prior to 2002. As shown in Table 93.13, EBRT has been used for larger meningiomas; mean tumor volumes in "recent" EBRT series have been 12 to 108 cc, compared to 2.3 to 8.2 cc with SRS. Tumor regression has been somewhat superior with SRS; however, there is no evidence for a better outcome with meningiomas based upon extent or rapidity of regression.

SPECIAL CIRCUMSTANCES

Nonbenign Meningiomas

Atypical (WHO grade II) and anaplasic (WHO grade III) tumors comprise the minority of meningiomas. Grade III primaries have consistently been identified in less than 5% of cases [5,53,54,56,58]. Although, as more thoroughly discussed in the "Molecular Genetics and Histopathology" section of this chapter, there has been considerable disparity with respect to grade II meningiomas. Classically,

Table 93.10 Fractionated External Beam Irradiation (WHO Grade I; Often Presumptive)

					5-year PFS					
Author	Year	n	f/u (mo)	No Histo (%)	GTR (%)	STR (%)	STR+EBRT (some 1° RT) (%)	Tumor Volume	% Regression	Any Late Complication (%)
Adegbite [41]	1983	114	10–276	0	90	45	82	NR	NR	NR
Mirimanoff	1985	225	65% >60	N/A	93	63		NR	NR	N/A
Barbaro [79]	1987	135	78	0	96	60	80	NR	NR	0
Taylor [80]	1988	132	60% >60	0	96	43	85	NR	NR	0
Glaholm [135]	1990	117	80	8			84	NR	NR	2
Miralbell [81]	1992	115	57	0		48	88 (8y PFS)	NR	NR	17
Mahmood [196]	1994	254	61	0	98	54		NR	NR	NR
Goldsmith [82]	1994	117	40	0			89 (98% p1980)	NR	NR	3.6
Peele [197]	1996	86	46	0		57	100	NR	NR	1
Condra	1997	262	98	3	93	53	86	4 cm (dia)	NR	14
Stafford [36]	1998	581	55	N/A	88	61		NR	NR	N/A
Nutting [57]	1999	82	108	0			92	NR	NR	21
Vendrely [198]	1999	156	40	49			79	NR	NR	12
Maguire [145]	1999	28	41	7			92	NR	NR	7
Wenkle	2000	46	53	20			100	34 cc	NR	17
Pourel [175]	2001	45	30	20			95	NR	NR	4
Dufour [199]	2001	31	73	45			93 (10y PFS)	NR	29	0
Debus [144]	2001	189	35	31			98	52.5 cc	14	2.1
Jalali [200]	2002	41	21	20			100 (3y PFS)	17.9 cc	27	9.8
Uy [185]	2002	40	30	38			93	20.2 cc	24	0.5
Pirzkall [147]	2003	20	36	20			100	108 cc	25	0
Soyuer [83]	2004	92	92	0	77	38	91	NR	NR	1
Selch [148]	2004	45	36	36			98 (3y PFS)	14.5 cc	18	2
Milker-Zabel [143]	2005	317	68	31			93	33.6 cc	23	2.5
Henzel [142]	2006	224	36	42			97	12 cc	46	2.5
Milker-Zabel [59]	2007	94	53	32			94	81.4 cc	20	1
Total:		3588	10–276 mo	0–49	77–98	38–63	79–100	12–108 cc	14–46	0–17

5-year progression-free survival (PFS) and other germane treatment factors.

Abbreviations: 1°, primary; 1° FRRT, primary fractionated external beam radiation therapy; cc, cubic centimeters; dia, diameter; f/u, follow-up, mean or median follow-up unless otherwise specified; GTR, gross total resection; mo, months; n, number of patients; No Histo, percentage of patients diagnosed without histopathologic confirmation (i.e., by imaging findings); NR, not reported; N/A, not applicable; p, after; % Regression, percentage of patients with tumor regression following EBRT; STR, sub-total resection; STR + EBRT, subtotal resection plus fractionated external beam radiation therapy; Tumor Volume, mean or median tumor volume prior to EBRT; y, year.

about 5% of meningiomas have been grade II [5]. Recent histopathologic studies have found that approximately 20% of cases should be atypical [53,54,56]. The inconsistency in identification of atypical tumors renders declarations about natural history, treatment, and outcome rather tenuous.

Compared to their benign counterparts, nonbenign meningiomas have an earlier peak incidence and a differing gender distribution [188]. A slight male predominance has even been suggested [12,188]. Some studies have found little if any variation in outcome among grade II and grade III patients [61,171], while others (see Figure 93.4) have identified significant differences in LC, median time to recurrence, and overall survival [53,54,159,189]. Even with these disparate results, some generalizations can be made.

Grade III meningiomas are aggressive. They tend to recur promptly even with radical resection. In two large surgery series, the 5-year recurrence rates were 72% to 78% [53–55] in spite of the common use of postoperative radiotherapy. Given such behavior, treatment is less controversial. Most patients are treated with surgery and adjuvant therapy. Radical surgery may improve LC and possibly overall survival [189], but this has not been a uniform finding [61,174]. This may be a matter of degree. Although Palma and colleagues found that a Simpson grade I resection did not significantly prolong survival for their entire cohort, among a small subset of four patients with anaplastic convexity meningiomas, each of whom had radical surgery, there were no recurrences after a mean of 11 years. Perhaps with extensive surgery including a large dural margin, as is feasible with convexity primaries, improved outcome can be appreciated with anaplastic tumors.

Regarding adjuvant radiotherapy, higher doses may improve outcome. Goldsmith [82] reported superior PFS, and Milosevic [174] reported better CSS with higher EBRT total doses. Coke et al reported a 5-year overall survival of 60% in eight patients with malignant meningioma treated to a mean total dose of 61 Gy [158]. Hug and associates noted an 8-year overall survival of 87% for patients receiving >60 CGE (cobalt gray equivalent) versus 15% with <60 Gy. About half of their patients were treated with photons and half with combined photons and protons [61]. Regarding SRS, using modern WHO grading criteria, Stafford and coworkers found that tumor margin dose (range of 12–36 Gy), although not allied with outcome for benign meningiomas, may have impact on LC for atypical and anaplastic tumors at doses >16 Gy. However, 5-year overall and CSS in this study were 0% for grade III patients. This may reflect their high proportion of patients with recurrent disease [160].

With such a high risk for recurrence and death, effective systemic therapy for malignant meningiomas would be desirable. When other treatments have failed, systemic therapy may be considered. Of the agents thus far studied, hydroxyurea appears to have the greatest effect. Tumor stability is reported in 50% to 88% of patients at 20 to 30 months [161,165], although tumor regression has been scarce. Multidrug regimens, including cyclophosphamide, adriamycin, and vincristine, as well as ifosfamide/mesna have been studied but not yet proven beneficial [2]. Hormonal agents, such as tamoxifen, medroxyprogesterone acetate, megestrol acetate (Megace), mifepristone (RU-486), have also been evaluated but have been generally been disappointing [2,190].

Atypical (WHO grade II) meningiomas appear to be underrecognized [56], and treatment guidelines are less uniform than for WHO grade I or III tumors. Many investigators, acknowledging that grade II tumors have a greater recurrence risk, recommend irradiation irrespective of resection extent [61,176], while others have advocated observation of gross totally resected atypical meningiomas [191]. Goyal and colleagues found grade II histology in 6.7% of patients. Among this group of 22 patients, 8 received postoperative EBRT (median 54 Gy). They reported that GTR achieved durable LC, 87% at 5 and 10 years, and that EBRT had no significant impact [191]. This highlights some of the difficulties in interpreting the literature respective to atypical tumors. The sample size is small; the percentage of grade II patients (6.7%) is too low to be representative of current WHO grading, and the doses used may be too low for grade II tumors.

Hug et al [61] found LC of atypical meningiomas to be superior with cumulative doses of >60 CGE (cobalt gray equivalent), 90% at 5 years as compared to 0% with doses <60 CGE. Similarly, Coke et al [171] reported excellent results with a group of grade II and III patients using a median total dose of 61 Gy. With respect to radiosurgery, Stafford and colleagues identified 93% 5-year actuarial LC for grade I meningiomas, compared with 68% for grade II [101]. This is very similar to the 64% reported by Condra et al with lower EBRT doses but inferior to the 90% rate with >60 CGE observed by Hug and coauthors [61].

Atypical meningiomas represent a prognostically heterogeneous group, which may relate in part to grading disparities. Many patients will fail with GTR alone, but precisely which patients remain unclear. There is relative consensus for irradiation following STR, and some studies suggest a benefit to higher doses of irradiation.

Recurrent Meningiomas

Local recurrence negatively impacts outcome. Recurrent meningiomas display a several fold increased rate of progression over newly diagnosed tumors [80,81]. This is understandable with tumors that have dedifferentiated to nonbenign histology but is also the case with tumors that remain low grade by WHO criteria. The available data are supportive of RT for recurrent meningiomas. Miralbell and coauthors found 78% 8-year PFS in patients treated with surgery and EBRT after first recurrence, versus 11% with surgery alone [81]. Taylor et al, also reporting of outcome after first recurrence, noted significantly better LC and determinant survival in patients who received salvage surgery and postoperative radiotherapy, as opposed to salvage surgery alone. Five-year LC was, respectively, 88% versus 30% and 5-year survival, 90% versus 45% [80]. These findings indicate that refractory meningiomas exhibit more aggressive biologic behavior and benefit from more aggressive treatment.

Incidental Meningiomas

Data concerning the diagnosis and treatment of meningiomas have traditionally derived from surgical series. This instills a bias toward symptomatic tumors. Asymptomatic tumors may have a differing natural history and, according to a recent screening study, are more common than symptomatic tumors. The Rotterdam Scan Study identified meningioma in 0.9% of 2,000 asymptomatic patients (median age 63 years). Studying the natural history of incidental meningiomas, Nakamura and coworkers analyzed 41 incidental patients approached conservatively. Mean annual growth was 0.8 cc, mean relative growth 14.6%, and mean doubling time 21.6 years. Shorter doubling times were found in young patients, in tumors without calcification, and in tumor with isointense or hypointense T2 signal. Intriguingly, growth rates were greater in six asymptomatic patients who underwent surgical excision, although factors other than surgery complicate interpretation.

Yoneoka and colleagues studied 37 incidental meningioma patients and also noted an annual growth rate of less than 1 cc. They confirmed that young age predicted for tumor progression. Among patients with tumor progression, the mean age was 53 [192]. They also suggested that larger tumor volume predicted progression, although other studies have not found an associated between tumor volume and growth [27,70]. Kuratsu et al reviewed 196 patients. Incidental meningiomas were more common in females and in individuals greater than 70 years of age. They agree with Nakamura's findings that incidental meningiomas with calcifications or hypointense intratumoral T2 signal had slower growth rates [27]. Niiro and associates further corroborated the impact of these imaging features on tumor growth [193].

Many patients with incidental meningiomas can be observed with serial clinical evaluations and imaging studies, particularly older patients with small, calcified tumors in a noneloquent locale. However, there are substantial variations in growth rate. Moreover, growth rate is not the sole factor for consideration. Incidental meningiomas are often smaller and thus lend themselves more readily to safe treatment with any modality. They may have a propensity to develop along the convexity or falx [194], precisely where they are more readily accessible to surgery. Tumor size, location, proximity to critical structures, edema, imaging parameters, patient age, and other factors may take precedence and add considerable complexity to the decision-making process.

Table 93.11 Stereotactic Radiosurgery and Edema

Author (year)	n (Basal/Nonbasal)	Edema (Basal vs. Nonbasal)	Method of Assessment	Comments
Ganz (1996) [109]	34 (27/7)	21% (7% vs. 71%)	Imaging	In 6 of 7 patients with edema, margin dose was >18 Gy Edema resolved in every case (timing not given)
Nakamura (1996) [126]	48 (32/16)	8% (0% vs. 25%)	Clinical and imaging	Edema occurred with margin dose 15–24 Gy
Kalapurakal (1997) [127]	43 (32/11)	35% (13% vs. 100%)	Imaging	SRS (n = 3), hypofx SRT (n = 33), standard EBRT (n = 7) Life threatening in 4 (steroids 1–3 yr) + fatal in 1 No edema with EBRT Predictive Factors: parasagittal, pre-treatment edema, and venous sinus occlusion ($P < 0.001$), dose >6 Gy/fx ($P = 0.043$)
Kondziolka (1998) [107]	203 all parasagittal	3 & 5y actuarial 16% "symptomatic edema"	Clinical	No association with margin dose No improvement in LC with margin dose >15Gy Edema occurred 1–23 mo after SRS, med duration 15mo More common if >3cm
Vermeulen (1999) [128]	95 (49/46)	32% (22% vs. 41%)	Imaging	1% (basal) versus 4% (nonbasal) had "deteriorating symptomatic edema" without tumor growth
Singh (2000) [201]	77 (50/27)	12% (6% vs. 22%)	Imaging	2/3rds of patients with edema are symptomatic Not association with dose, including dose to adjacent brain Only significant factor: tumor location Edema in 38% (6/16) parasagittal primaries Margin dose 10 to 15 Gy
Ramsey (2002) [130]	23 14/9	39% (22% vs. 78%)	Clinical and imaging	7 required steroids, 5 improved, 1 required surgery, 1 fatality Edema was symptomatic in 78% Predictive Factors: Parasagittal, Volume >4cc, Pre-tx edema Actuarial risk: 22% at 6 mo, 39% at 12 mo, 59% at 18 mo
Chang (2003) [131]	140 (79/61)	24% (5.1% vs. 50%)	Imaging	Edema symptomatic in 39% Imaging changes 3–49 mo (mean 8 mo) after SRS duration 3–28 mo (mean 14 mo) Multivariate analysis: only tumor location was significant
Kim (2005) [106]	23 all non-basal	43%	Imaging	Edema in 10 patients: 7 new edema, 3 aggravated edema Mean time to develop symptoms 3 mo, mean duration 9 mo All 10 resolved with steroids and/or analgesics Predictive factors: tumor volume >4.2 cc, integral dose
Total:	686	0 22% vs. 25–100%		

Nine series reporting on new or worsening edema following stereotactic radiosurgery.

Abbreviations: fx, radiotherapy fraction; Gy, Gray; mo, month(s); n, number of patients; Year, year of publication; Yr, year.

Table 93.12 Fractionated External Beam Irradiation (Optic Nerve Sheath Meningioma)

	Local Control (%)	Vision		
		Improved (%)	Stable (%)	Worse (%)
All studies	87–100	20–100	0–66	4
Mean 1° EBRT	98	75	21	4

Comments:

Visual improvement occurred during EBRT up to 10 months after

Some blind eyes regained vision

Visual improvement was durable, 3 to 7 years in these studies

RT recommended if VA or VFs worsen, or tumor grows

A dose limit to the retina of 45 Gy is commonly recommended

Local control and visual outcomes compiled from 12 studies with 228 patients (244 eyes). Mean follow-up 48 months. Range of external beam radiation therapy (EBRT) total doses 45 to 60 Gy, most commonly 50 to 54 Gy. Dose per fraction range 1.7 to 2.0 Gy. The "All Studies" row lists reported local control and visual outcome ranges from all studies, including patients treated with surgery and post-operative EBRT. The "Mean 1° EBRT" row refers to patients treated with primary external beam radiation therapy, without surgery.

Abbreviations: Gy, Gray; mo, months; VA, visual acuity; VFs, visual fields.

CONCLUSIONS

Meningiomas are now the most commonly reported primary intracranial tumor [5]. Owing to their characteristic protracted natural history, compounded by a lack of large cooperative group or randomized trials, standardized treatment recommendations are difficult to formulate. These limitations conceded, the data do permit some general recommendations. Small, incidental meningiomas can often be carefully observed. For most other patients, GTR is the benchmark. However, complete removal within the constraints of acceptable morbidity is not always achievable. Meningiomas frequently arise in proximity to critical neural or vascular structures or in sites with limited surgical access and remain among the most challenging of cases for surgeons [173,195].

When a GTR is not accomplished, postoperative RT is an important consideration. After STR, numerous retrospective studies document improvements in LC (Table 93.10, Figure 93.8). As shown in Figure 93.6, some have even found significant improvements in CSS. In spite of this, it remains controversial whether patients with subtotally resected meningiomas should be carefully observed

Table 93.13 Meningioma: SRS Versus EBRT (WHO Grade I; Often Presumptive)

	N	Mean or Median Follow-Up (months)	Mean Tumor Volumes (cc)	Mean Tumor Regression (%)	5-Year PFS (%)
SRS combined	2,281	19–103	2.3–10^a	13–83	75–100
EBRT combined	3,588	21–108	n/a	n/a	79–100
SRS recent	1,434	29–103	2.3–8.2^a	13–83	86–100
EBRT recent	8,37	21–92	12–108	18–46	91–100

Comparative analysis of the multiple series from Tables 93.9 and 93.10. Five-year progression-free survivals (PFS) are compared for all series combined, and for recent series. "Recent" applies to those series published from 2002–2007 for which volume and tumor regression data are available across the stereotactic radiosurgery (SRS) and external beam radiation therapy (EBRT) studies.

Abbreviations: n, number of patients; n/a, not applicable since limited data is available before the "recent" (2002–2007) grouping; WHO, World Health Organization.

^{a} 4.7 cc from Iwai [Iwai 03] excluded because 2 fraction radiosurgery was given if the tumor exceeded 4 cc.

and treated at progression or treated preemptively. Indeed, some patients do well for many years after STR alone, while others progress and develop larger, symptomatic tumors more promptly.

Experience with irradiation (EBRT or SRS) as an adjuvant or as a primary treatment modality is mounting. In the latter setting, the diagnosis is often based on imaging and clinical findings. This has been shown to be reliable, and results have been gratifying (Tables 93.9 and 93.10). Some series have even shown improved outcome for patients treated primarily with radiotherapy [105,107]. Results with fractionated external beam radiotherapy (EBRT) and SRS are remarkably similar (Table 93.13), and either can be recommended for many patients but not for all. EBRT is suitable for a broader range of patients, whereas excellent outcome with SRS has been realized among more distinct cohorts. Location—for instance, meningiomas involving the anterior visual pathway—can be a decisive factor. Tumor diameter or volume is also to be considered. Several studies have noted that radiosurgery offers improved LC and reduced toxicity when diameter or volume restrictions are applied. SRS entails a greater risk of treatment-related edema than EBRT, particularly for nonbasal meningiomas. As highlighted in Table 93.11, SRS entails a greater risk of treatment-related edema than EBRT, particularly for nonbasal tumor sites.

For benign meningiomas, these data indicate that radiosurgery is most judiciously applied to smaller meningiomas at an adequate distance from the optic apparatus and with less edema risk. Fractionated external beam irradiation does not bear these limitations. With currently accepted dose and fractionation guidelines, EBRT carries only small risks of optic neuropathy or edema, and with modern techniques, EBRT can be delivered in a highly conformal and reproducible fashion. Current outcomes with grade I meingiomas are commendable and promise to improve further with continuing developments in dose delivery and image guidance.

Anaplastic meningiomas engender less controversy. Postoperative RT is nearly always recommended. Atypical meningiomas, although less aggressive than their grade III counterparts, still carry high rate of recurrence after surgery alone, and postoperative radiotherapy is generally employed. There is still room for debate regarding a radically resected grade II meningioma, particularly if it is excised from the convexity where a larger rind of dura can often be removed as well. For nonbeningn meningiomas, the data support radiotherapy either as EBRT or SRS, but there is a strong suggestion that higher doses than those commonly used for benign lesions are warranted.

Further progress will derive from cooperative group trials and from more uniform histopathologic grading. Although the WHO 2007 grading standards are more straightforward, there are sizeable disparities in the rates with which grade is allocated, particularly with atypical meningiomas. Grade has consistently been a crucial prognostic factor, but it will remain difficult to interpret outcomes from single institution studies with the current 5% to 25% range of identifying grade II histology. Despite many important questions, no large cooperative group phase III trial has ever been completed with this common tumor. Such a study could address important clinical questions, help refine risk groups and grading, and perhaps identify imaging or molecular-genetic markers to help deduce outcome and direct a more individualized approach to patient care.

REFERENCES

1. Wilson CB. Meningiomas: genetics, malignancy, and the role of radiation in induction and treatment. The Richard C. Schneider Lecture. *J Neurosurg*. 1994;81(5):666–675.
2. Rockhill J, Mrugala M, Chamberlain MC. Intracranial meningiomas: an overview of diagnosis and treatment. *Neurosurg Focus*. 2007;23(4):E1.
3. Perry A. Meningiomas. In: McLendon R, Rosenblum M, Bigner DD, ed. *Russell & Rubinstein's Pathology of Tumors of the Nervous System*. 7th ed. London, England: Hodder Arnold; 2006:427–474.
4. Cushing H. The meningiomas (dural endotheliomas). Their source and favoured seats of origin. *Brain* 1922; 45:282–316.
5. Claus EB, Bondy ML, Schildkraut JM, Wiemels JL, Wrensch M, Black PM. Epidemiology of intracranial meningioma. *Neurosurgery*. 2005;57(6):1088–1095; discussion 1088.
6. Riemenschneider MJ, Perry A, Reifenberger G. Histological classification and molecular genetics of meningiomas. *Lancet Neurol*. 2006;5(12):1045–1054.
7. Annegers JF, Laws ER Jr, Kurland LT, Grabow JD. Head trauma and subsequent brain tumors. *Neurosurgery*. 1979;4(3):203–206.
8. Inskip PD, Mellemkjaer L, Gridley G, Olsen JH. Incidence of intracranial tumors following hospitalization for head injuries (Denmark). *Cancer Causes Control*. 1998;9(1):109–116.

9. McDermott MW, Quinones-Hinojosa A, Fuller GN, et al. Meningiomas. In: Levin, Victor A, ed. *Cancer in the Central Nervous System*. 2nd ed. New York, NY: Oxford University Press, Inc.; 2002:269–299.
10. Borggreven PA, de Graaf FH, van der Valk P, Leemans CR. Post-traumatic cutaneous meningioma. *J Laryngol Otol*. 2004;118(3):228–230.
11. DeMonte F. Current management of meningiomas. *Oncology* (Williston Park) 1995; 9:83–101.
12. Perry A, Louis DN, Scheithauer BW, Budka H, von Deimling A. Meningeal tumours. In: Louis DN, Ohgaki H, Wiestler OD, Cavenee WK, eds. *WHO Classification of Tumours of the Central Nervous System*. Lyon, France: IARC; 2007.
13. Al-Mefty O, Topsakal C, Pravdenkova S, Sawyer JR, Harrison MJ. Radiation-induced meningiomas: clinical, pathological, cytokinetic, and cytogenetic characteristics. *J Neurosurg*. 2004;100(6):1002–1013.
14. Regel JP, Schoch B, Sandalcioglu IE, et al. Malignant meningioma as a second malignancy after therapy for acute lymphatic leukemia without cranial radiation. *Childs Nerv Syst*. 2006;22(2):172–175.
15. Yousaf I, Byrnes DP, Choudhari KA. Meningiomas induced by high dose cranial irradiation. *Br J Neurosurg*. 2003;17(3):219–225.
16. Strojan P, Popovic M, Jereb B. Secondary intracranial meningiomas after high-dose cranial irradiation: report of five cases and review of the literature. *Int J Radiat Oncol Biol Phys*. 2000;48(1):65–73.
17. Salvati M, Cervoni L, Artico M. High-dose radiation-induced meningiomas following acute lymphoblastic leukemia in children. *Childs Nerv Syst*. 1996;12(5):266–269.
18. Flint-Richter P, Sadetzki S. Genetic predisposition for the development of radiation-associated meningioma: an epidemiological study. *Lancet Oncol*. 2007;8(5):403–410.
19. Wigertz A, Lönn S, Mathiesen T, Ahlbom A, Hall P, Feychting M. Risk of brain tumors associated with exposure to exogenous female sex hormones. *Am J Epidemiol*. 2006;164(7):629–636.
20. Gazzeri R, Galarza M, Gazzeri G. Growth of a meningioma in a transsexual patient after estrogen-progestin therapy. *N Engl J Med*. 2007;357(23):2411–2412.
21. Wahab M, Al-Azzawi F. Meningioma and hormonal influences. *Climacteric*. 2003;6(4):285–292.
22. DeMonte F, Marmor E, Al-Mefty O. Meningiomas. In Andrew K, Edward L, eds. *Brain Tumors*. 2nd ed. London: Churchill Livingstone; 2001:719–750.
23. Aghi MK, Eskandar EN, Carter BS, Curry WT Jr, Barker FG 2nd. Increased prevalence of obesity and obesity-related postoperative complications in male patients with meningiomas. *Neurosurgery*. 2007;61(4):754–760; discussion 760.
24. Perry A, Giannini C, Raghavan R, et al. Aggressive phenotypic and genotypic features in pediatric and NF2-associated meningiomas: a clinicopathologic study of 53 cases. *J Neuropathol Exp Neurol*. 2001;60(10):994–1003.
25. Perry A, Dehner LP. Meningeal tumors of childhood and infancy. An update and literature review. *Brain Pathol*. 2003;13(3):386–408.
26. Central Brain Tumor Registry in the United States (CBTRUS). Statistical report: Primary brain tumors in the Unites States, 1992–1997. In Central Brain Tumor Registry of the United States. Chicago: CBTRUS; 2000:11–26.
27. Kuratsu J, Kochi M, Ushio Y. Incidence and clinical features of asymptomatic meningiomas. *J Neurosurg*. 2000;92(5):766–770.
28. Kuratsu J, Ushio Y. Epidemiological study of primary intracranial tumors: a regional survey in Kumamoto Prefecture in the southern part of Japan. *J Neurosurg*. 1996;84(6):946–950.
29. Davis FG, Kupelian V, Freels S, McCarthy B, Surawicz T. Prevalence estimates for primary brain tumors in the United States by behavior and major histology groups. *Neuro-oncology*. 2001;3(3):152–158.
30. Central Brain Tumor Registry of the United States, CBTRUS Web site. http://www.cbtrus.org/cbtrus-bin/interactive/public/2005/search_incidence. Accessed November 28, 2007.
31. Flickinger JC, Kondziolka D, Maitz AH, Lunsford LD. Gamma knife radiosurgery of imaging-diagnosed intracranial meningioma. *Int J Radiat Oncol Biol Phys*. 2003;56(3):801–806.
32. DiBiase SJ, Kwok Y, Yovino S, et al. Factors predicting local tumor control after gamma knife stereotactic radiosurgery for benign intracranial meningiomas. *Int J Radiat Oncol Biol Phys*. 2004;60(5):1515–1519.
33. Vernooij MW, Ikram MA, Tanghe HL, et al. Incidental findings on brain MRI in the general population. *N Engl J Med*. 2007;357(18):1821–1828.
34. Nakasu S, Hirano A, Shimura T, Llena JF. Incidental meningiomas in autopsy study. *Surg Neurol*. 1987;27(4):319–322.
35. Goldsmith B. Meningioma. In: Steven L, Theodore P, eds. *Textbook of Radiation Oncology*. Philadelphia: WB Saunders;1998:324–340.
36. Stafford SL, Perry A, Suman VJ, et al. Primarily resected meningiomas: outcome and prognostic factors in 581 Mayo Clinic patients, 1978 through 1988. *Mayo Clin Proc*. 1998;73(10):936–942.
37. Wara WM, Bauman GS, Sneed PK, et al. Brain, brainstem, and cerebellum. In: Perez CA, Brady LW, Halperin EC, eds. *Principles and Practice of Radiation Oncology*. 3rd ed. Philadelphia: Lippincott-Raven, 1997:818–820.
38. Longstreth WT Jr, Dennis LK, McGuire VM, Drangsholt MT, Koepsell TD. Epidemiology of intracranial meningioma. *Cancer*. 1993;72(3):639–648.
39. Kurland LT, Schoenberg BS, Annegers JF, Okazaki H, Molgaard CA. The incidence of primary intracranial neoplasms in Rochester, Minnesota, 1935–1977. *Ann N Y Acad Sci*. 1982;381:6–16.
40. Rohringer M, Sutherland GR, Louw DF, Sima AA. Incidence and clinicopathological features of meningioma. *J Neurosurg*. 1989;71(5 pt 1):665–672.
41. Adegbite AB, Khan MI, Paine KW, Tan LK. The recurrence of intracranial meningiomas after surgical treatment. *J Neurosurg*. 1983;58(1):51–56.
42. Amirjamshidi A, Mehrazin M, Abbassioun K. Meningiomas of the central nervous system occurring below the age of 17: report of 24 cases not associated with neurofibromatosis and review of literature. *Childs Nerv Syst*. 2000;16(7):406–416.
43. Erdinçler P, Lena G, Sarioglu AC, Kuday C, Choux M. Intracranial meningiomas in children: review of 29 cases. *Surg Neurol*. 1998;49(2):136–140; discussion 140.
44. Zwerdling T, Dothage J. Meningiomas in children and adolescents. *J Pediatr Hematol Oncol*. 2002;24(3):199–204.
45. Jung HW, Yoo H, Paek SH, Choi KS. Long-term outcome and growth rate of subtotally resected petroclival meningiomas: experience with 38 cases. *Neurosurgery*. 2000;46(3):567–574; discussion 574.
46. DeMonte F, Al-Mefty O. Meningiomas. In: Andrew K, Edward Laws, eds *Brain Tumors*. London: Churchill Livingstone; 1995: 675–704.
47. Central Brain Tumor Registry of the United States, CBTRUS (2005). Statistical report: primary brain tumors in the United States, 1998–2002.
48. Louis DN, Ramesh V, Gusella JF. Neuropathology and molecular genetics of neurofibromatosis 2 and related tumors. *Brain Pathol*. 1995;5(2):163–172.
49. Cleland, J. Description of two tumours adherent to the deep surface of the dura mater. *Glasgow Medical Journal* 1864;11;148–159.
50. Louis DN, Scheithauer BW, Budka H. Meningiomas. In Kleihues P, Cavenee WK, eds *World Health Organization Classification of Tumours. Pathology and Genetics of Tumours of the Nervous System*. Lyon, France : IARC Press; 2000:176–184
51. Ho DM, Hsu CY, Ting LT, Chiang H. Histopathology and MIB-1 labeling index predicted recurrence of meningiomas: a proposal of diagnostic criteria for patients with atypical meningioma. *Cancer*. 2002;94(5):1538–1547.
52. Korshunov A, Shishkina L, Golanov A. Immunohistochemical analysis of p16INK4a, p14ARF, p18INK4c, p21CIP1, p27KIP1 and p73 expression in 271 meningiomas correlation with tumor grade and clinical outcome. *Int J Cancer*. 2003;104(6):728–734.
53. Perry A, Scheithauer BW, Stafford SL, Lohse CM, Wollan PC. "Malignancy" in meningiomas: a clinicopathologic study of 116 patients, with grading implications. *Cancer*. 1999;85(9):2046–2056.
54. Perry A, Stafford SL, Scheithauer BW, Suman VJ, Lohse CM. Meningioma grading: an analysis of histologic parameters. *Am J Surg Pathol*. 1997;21(12):1455–1465.
55. Jääskeläinen J, Haltia M, Servo A. Atypical and anaplastic meningiomas: radiology, surgery, radiotherapy, and outcome. *Surg Neurol*. 1986;25(3):233–242.
56. Willis J, Smith C, Ironside JW, Erridge S, Whittle IR, Everington D. The accuracy of meningioma grading: a 10-year retrospective audit. *Neuropathol Appl Neurobiol*. 2005;31(2):141–149.
57. Nutting C, Brada M, Brazil L, et al. Radiotherapy in the treatment of benign meningioma of the skull base. *J Neurosurg*. 1999;90(5):823–827.
58. Jääskeläinen J. Seemingly complete removal of histologically benign intracranial meningioma: late recurrence rate and factors predicting recurrence in 657 patients. A multivariate analysis. *Surg Neurol*. 1986;26(5):461–469.

59. Milker-Zabel S, Zabel-du Bois A, Huber P, Schlegel W, Debus J. Intensity-modulated radiotherapy for complex-shaped meningioma of the skull base: long-term experience of a single institution. *Int J Radiat Oncol Biol Phys*. 2007;68(3):858–863.
60. Perry A. Unmasking the secrets of meningioma: a slow but rewarding journey. *Surg Neurol*. 2004;61(2):171–173.
61. Hug EB, Devries A, Thornton AF, et al. Management of atypical and malignant meningiomas: role of high-dose, 3D-conformal radiation therapy. *J Neurooncol*. 2000;48(2):151–160.
62. Ayerbe J, Lobato RD, de la Cruz J, et al. Risk factors predicting recurrence in patients operated on for intracranial meningioma. A multivariate analysis. *Acta Neurochir (Wien)*. 1999;141(9):921–932.
63. Kano H, Takahashi JA, Katsuki T, et al. Stereotactic radiosurgery for atypical and anaplastic meningiomas. *J Neurooncol*. 2007;84(1):41–47.
64. Ojemann SG, Sneed PK, Larson DA, et al. Radiosurgery for malignant meningioma: results in 22 patients. *J Neurosurg*. 2000;93(suppl 3):62–67.
65. Perry A, Gutmann DH, Reifenberger G. Molecular pathogenesis of meningiomas. *J Neurooncol*. 2004;70(2):183–202.
66. Bondy M, Ligon BL. Epidemiology and etiology of intracranial meningiomas: a review. *J Neurooncol*. 1996;29(3):197–205.
67. Rutten I, Cabay JE, Withofs N, et al. PET/CT of skull base meningiomas using 2–18F-fluoro-L-tyrosine: initial report. *J Nucl Med*. 2007;48(5):720–725.
68. Sanson M, Cornu P. Biology of meningiomas. *Acta Neurochir (Wien)*. 2000;142(5):493–505.
69. Schubeus P, Schörner W, Rottacker C, Sander B. Intracranial meningiomas: how frequent are indicative findings in CT and MRI? *Neuroradiology*. 1990;32(6):467–473.
70. Nakamura JL, Pirzkall A, Carol MP, et al. Comparison of intensity-modulated radiotherapy with gamma knife radiosurgery for challenging skull base lesions. *Int J Radiat Oncol Biol Phys*. 2003;55(1):99–109.
71. Goldstein RA, Jorden MA, Harsh GR. Meningiomas: natural history, diagnosis, and imaging. In: Black PM, Loeffler JS, ed. *Cancer of the Nervous System*. 2nd ed. Philadelphia: Peter Lippincott, Williams & Wilkins; 2005:279–313.
72. Drape JL, Krause D, Tongio J. MRI of aggressive meningiomas. *J Neuroradiol*. 1992;19(1):49–62.
73. Kasuya H, Kubo O, Tanaka M, Amano K, Kato K, Hori T. Clinical and radiological features related to the growth potential of meningioma. *Neurosurg Rev*. 2006;29(4):293–6; discussion 296.
74. Nakamura M, Roser F, Michel J, Jacobs C, Samii M. The natural history of incidental meningiomas. *Neurosurgery*. 2003;53(1):62–70; discussion 70.
75. Ildan F, Tuna M, Göçer AP, et al. Correlation of the relationships of brain-tumor interfaces, magnetic resonance imaging, and angiographic findings to predict cleavage of meningiomas. *J Neurosurg*. 1999;91(3):384–390.
76. Lippitz B, Cremerius U, Mayfrank L, et al. PET-study of intracranial meningiomas: correlation with histopathology, cellularity and proliferation rate. *Acta Neurochir Suppl*. 1996;65:108–111.
77. Hakyemez B, Yildirim N, Gokalp G, Erdogan C, Parlak M. The contribution of diffusion-weighted MR imaging to distinguishing typical from atypical meningiomas. *Neuroradiology*. 2006;48(8):513–520.
78. Simpson D. The recurrence of intracranial meningiomas after surgical treatment. *J Neurol Neurosurg Psychiatr*. 1957;20(1):22–39.
79. Barbaro NM, Gutin PH, Wilson CB, Sheline GE, Boldrey EB, Wara WM. Radiation therapy in the treatment of partially resected meningiomas. *Neurosurgery*. 1987;20(4):525–528.
80. Taylor BW Jr, Marcus RB Jr, Friedman WA, Ballinger WE Jr, Million RR. The meningioma controversy: postoperative radiation therapy. *Int J Radiat Oncol Biol Phys*. 1988;15(2):299–304.
81. Miralbell R, Linggood RM, de la Monte S, Convery K, Munzenrider JE, Mirimanoff RO. The role of radiotherapy in the treatment of subtotally resected benign meningiomas. *J Neurooncol*. 1992;13(2):157–164.
82. Goldsmith BJ, Wara WM, Wilson CB, Larson DA. Postoperative irradiation for subtotally resected meningiomas. A retrospective analysis of 140 patients treated from 1967 to 1990. *J Neurosurg*. 1994;80(2):195–201.
83. Soyuer S, Chang EL, Selek U, Shi W, Maor MH, DeMonte F. Radiotherapy after surgery for benign cerebral meningioma. *Radiother Oncol*. 2004;71(1):85–90.
84. Wara WM, Sheline GE, Newman H, Townsend JJ, Boldrey EB. Radiation therapy of meningiomas. *Am J Roentgenol Radium Ther Nucl Med*. 1975;123(3):453–458.
85. Shin M, Kurita H, Sasaki T, et al. Analysis of treatment outcome after stereotactic radiosurgery for cavernous sinus meningiomas. *J Neurosurg*. 2001;95(3):435–439.
86. Ware ML, Larson DA, Sneed PK, Wara WW, McDermott MW. Surgical resection and permanent brachytherapy for recurrent atypical and malignant meningioma. *Neurosurgery*. 2004;54(1):55–63; discussion 63.
87. Obasi PC, Barnett GH, Suh JH. Brachytherapy for intracranial meningioma using a permanently implanted iodine-125 seed. *Stereotact Funct Neurosurg*. 2002;79(1):33–43.
88. Kumar PP, Patil AA, Syh HW, Chu WK, Reeves MA. Role of brachytherapy in the management of the skull base meningioma. Treatment of skull base meningiomas. *Cancer*. 1993;71(11):3726–3731.
89. Kumar PP, Patil AA, Leibrock LG, et al. Continuous low dose rate brachytherapy with high activity iodine-125 seeds in the management of meningiomas. *Int J Radiat Oncol Biol Phys*. 1993;25(2):325–328.
90. Shafron DH, Friedman WA, Buatti JM, Bova FJ, Mendenhall WM. Linac radiosurgery for benign meningiomas. *Int J Radiat Oncol Biol Phys*. 1999;43(2):321–327.
91. Chang SD, Adler JR Jr. Treatment of cranial base meningiomas with linear accelerator radiosurgery. *Neurosurgery*. 1997;41(5):1019–1025; discussion 1025.
92. Chang SD, Adler JR Jr, Martin DP. LINAC radiosurgery for cavernous sinus meningiomas. *Stereotact Funct Neurosurg*. 1998;71(1):43–50.
93. Hakim R, Alexander E 3rd, Loeffler JS, et al. Results of linear accelerator-based radiosurgery for intracranial meningiomas. *Neurosurgery*. 1998;42(3):446–453; discussion 453.
94. Spiegelmann R, Nissim O, Menhel J, Alezra D, Pfeffer MR. Linear accelerator radiosurgery for meningiomas in and around the cavernous sinus. *Neurosurgery*. 2002;51(6):1373–1379; discussion 1379.
95. Chuang CC, Chang CN, Tsang NM, et al. Linear accelerator-based radiosurgery in the management of skull base meningiomas. *J Neurooncol*. 2004;66(1–2):241–249.
96. Liscák R, Simonová G, Vymazal J, Janousková L, Vladyka V. Gamma knife radiosurgery of meningiomas in the cavernous sinus region. *Acta Neurochir (Wien)*. 1999;141(5):473–480.
97. Morita A, Coffey RJ, Foote RL, Schiff D, Gorman D. Risk of injury to cranial nerves after gamma knife radiosurgery for skull base meningiomas: experience in 88 patients. *J Neurosurg*. 1999;90(1):42–49.
98. Roche PH, Régis J, Dufour H, et al. Gamma knife radiosurgery in the management of cavernous sinus meningiomas. *J Neurosurg*. 2000;93(suppl 3):68–73.
99. Roche PH, Pellet W, Fuentes S, Thomassin JM, Régis J. Gamma knife radiosurgical management of petroclival meningiomas results and indications. *Acta Neurochir (Wien)*. 2003;145(10):883–888; discussion 888.
100. Aichholzer M, Bertalanffy A, Dietrich W, et al. Gamma knife radiosurgery of skull base meningiomas. *Acta Neurochir (Wien)*. 2000;142(6):647–652; discussion 652.
101. Stafford SL, Pollock BE, Foote RL, et al. Meningioma radiosurgery: tumor control, outcomes, and complications among 190 consecutive patients. *Neurosurgery*. 2001;49(5):1029–1037; discussion 1037.
102. Iwai Y, Yamanaka K, Ishiguro T. Gamma knife radiosurgery for the treatment of cavernous sinus meningiomas. *Neurosurgery*. 2003;52(3):517–524; discussion 523.
103. Nicolato A, Foroni R, Alessandrini F, Maluta S, Bricolo A, Gerosa M. The role of Gamma Knife radiosurgery in the management of cavernous sinus meningiomas. *Int J Radiat Oncol Biol Phys*. 2002;53(4):992–1000.
104. Lee JY, Niranjan A, McInerney J, Kondziolka D, Flickinger JC, Lunsford LD. Stereotactic radiosurgery providing long-term tumor control of cavernous sinus meningiomas. *J Neurosurg*. 2002;97(1):65–72.
105. Pollock BE, Stafford SL, Utter A, Giannini C, Schreiner SA. Stereotactic radiosurgery provides equivalent tumor control to Simpson Grade 1 resection for patients with small- to medium-size meningiomas. *Int J Radiat Oncol Biol Phys*. 2003;55(4):1000–1005.
106. Kim DG, Kim ChH, Chung HT, et al. Gamma knife surgery of superficially located meningioma. *J Neurosurg*. 2005;102(suppl):255–258.
107. Kondziolka D, Flickinger JC, Perez B. Judicious resection and/or radiosurgery for parasagittal meningiomas: outcomes from a multicenter review. Gamma Knife Meningioma Study Group. *Neurosurgery*. 1998;43(3):405–413; discussion 413.
108. Malik I, Rowe JG, Walton L, Radatz MW, Kemeny AA. The use of stereotactic radiosurgery in the management of meningiomas. *Br J Neurosurg*. 2005;19(1):13–20.

109. Ganz JC, Schröttner O, Pendl G. Radiation-induced edema after Gamma Knife treatment for meningiomas. *Stereotact Funct Neurosurg.* 1996;66(suppl 1):129–133.
110. Kollova A, Liscák R, Novotný J Jr, Vladyka V, Simonová G, Janousková L. Gamma Knife surgery for benign meningioma. *J Neurosurg.* 2007;107(2):325–336.
111. Kreil W, Luggin J, Fuchs I, Weigl V, Eustacchio S, Papaefthymiou G. Long term experience of gamma knife radiosurgery for benign skull base meningiomas. *J Neurol Neurosurg Psychiatr.* 2005;76(10):1425–1430.
112. Kondziolka D, Niranjan A, Lunsford LD, Flickinger JC. Stereotactic radiosurgery for meningiomas. *Neurosurg Clin N Am.* 1999;10(2):317–325.
113. Zachenhofer I, Wolfsberger S, Aichholzer M, et al. Gamma-knife radiosurgery for cranial base meningiomas: experience of tumor control, clinical course, and morbidity in a follow-up of more than 8 years. *Neurosurgery.* 2006;58(1):28–36; discussion 28.
114. Engenhart R, Kimmig BN, Höver KH, et al. Stereotactic single high dose radiation therapy of benign intracranial meningiomas. *Int J Radiat Oncol Biol Phys.* 1990;19(4):1021–1026.
115. Hudgins WR, Barker JL, Schwartz DE, Nichols TD. Gamma Knife treatment of 100 consecutive meningiomas. *Stereotact Funct Neurosurg.* 1996;66(suppl 1):121–128.
116. Stafford SL, Pollock BE, Foote, RL, et al. Stereotactic radiosurgery for meningioma. In: Pollock BE, ed. *Contemporary Stereotactic Radiosurgery: Technique and Evaluation.* Armonk, NY: Futura Publishing Company, Inc; 2002:157–171.
117. Subach BR, Lunsford LD, Kondziolka D, Maitz AH, Flickinger JC. Management of petroclival meningiomas by stereotactic radiosurgery. *Neurosurgery.* 1998;42(3):437–43; discussion 443.
118. Stafford SL, Pollock BE, Leavitt JA, et al. A study on the radiation tolerance of the optic nerves and chiasm after stereotactic radiosurgery. *Int J Radiat Oncol Biol Phys.* 2003;55(5):1177–1181.
119. Leber KA, Berglöff J, Pendl G. Dose-response tolerance of the visual pathways and cranial nerves of the cavernous sinus to stereotactic radiosurgery. *J Neurosurg.* 1998;88(1):43–50.
120. Kalkanis SN, Carroll RS, Zhang J, Zamani AA, Black PM. Correlation of vascular endothelial growth factor messenger RNA expression with peritumoral vasogenic cerebral edema in meningiomas. *J Neurosurg.* 1996;85(6):1095–1101.
121. Paek SH, Kim CY, Kim YY, et al. Correlation of clinical and biological parameters with peritumoral edema in meningioma. *J Neurooncol.* 2002;60(3):235–245.
122. Provias J, Claffey K, delAguila L, Lau N, Feldkamp M, Guha A. Meningiomas: role of vascular endothelial growth factor/vascular permeability factor in angiogenesis and peritumoral edema. *Neurosurgery.* 1997;40(5):1016–1026.
123. Alvernia JE, Sindou MP. Preoperative neuroimaging findings as a predictor of the surgical plane of cleavage: prospective study of 100 consecutive cases of intracranial meningioma. *J Neurosurg.* 2004;100(3):422–430.
124. Inamura T, Nishio S, Takeshita I, Fujiwara S, Fukui M. Peritumoral brain edema in meningiomas-influence of vascular supply on its development. *Neurosurgery.* 1992;31(2):179–185.
125. Kondziolka D, Lundsford LD, Flickinger JC. Stereotactic radiosurgery of meningiomas. In Lundsford LD, Kondziolka D, Flickinger JC, eds. *Gamma Knife Brain Surgery. Prog Neurol Surg,* vol. 14. Basel, Switzerland: Karger; 1998:104–113.
126. Nakamura S, Hiyama H, Arai K, et al. Gamma Knife radiosurgery for meningiomas: four cases of radiation-induced edema. *Stereotact Funct Neurosurg.* 1996;66(suppl 1):142–145.
127. Kalapurakal JA, Silverman CL, Akhtar N, et al. Intracranial meningiomas: factors that influence the development of cerebral edema after stereotactic radiosurgery and radiation therapy. *Radiology.* 1997;204(2):461–465.
128. Vermeulen S, Young R, Li F, et al. A comparison of single fraction radiosurgery tumor control and toxicity in the treatment of basal and nonbasal meningiomas. *Stereotact Funct Neurosurg.* 1999;72(suppl 1):60–66.
129. Singh VP, Kansai S, Vaishya S, Julka PK, Mehta VS. Early complications following gamma knife radiosurgery for intracranial meningiomas. *J Neurosurg.* 2000;93(suppl 3):57–61.
130. Ramsey AF, Blurton M, Ekstrand K, et al. Edema following gamma knife radiosurgery for intracranial meningiomas. *Int J Radiation Oncology Biol Phys.* 2002; 54(2) suppl: 146–147 (abst 250).
131. Chang JH, Chang JW, Choi JY, Park YG, Chung SS. Complications after gamma knife radiosurgery for benign meningiomas. *J Neurol Neurosurg Psychiatr.* 2003;74(2):226–230.
132. King DL, Chang CH, Pool JL. Radiotherapy in the management of meningiomas. *Acta Radiol Ther Phys Biol.* 1966;3:26–33.
133. Waga S, Yamashita J, Handa H. Recurrence of meningiomas. *Neurol Med Chir.* 1977;17:203–208 (Japan)
134. Yamashita J, Handa H, Iwaki K, Abe M. Recurrence of intracranial meningiomas, with special reference to radiotherapy. *Surg Neurol.* 1980;14(1):33–40.
135. Glaholm J, Bloom HJ, Crow JH. The role of radiotherapy in the management of intracranial meningiomas: the Royal Marsden Hospital experience with 186 patients. *Int J Radiat Oncol Biol Phys.* 1990;18(4):755–761.
136. Ron E, Modan B, Boice JD Jr. Mortality after radiotherapy for ringworm of the scalp. *Am J Epidemiol.* 1988;127(4):713–725.
137. Ron E, Modan B, Boice JD Jr, et al. Tumors of the brain and nervous system after radiotherapy in childhood. *N Engl J Med.* 1988;319(16):1033–1039.
138. Akeyson EW, McCutcheon IE. Management of benign and aggressive intracranial meningiomas. *Oncology (Williston Park, NY).* 1996;10(5):747–56; discussion 756.
139. Carella RJ, Ransohoff J, Newall J. Role of radiation therapy in the management of meningioma. *Neurosurgery.* 1982;10(3):332–339.
140. Chan RC, Thompson GB. Morbidity, mortality, and quality of life following surgery for intracranial meningiomas. A retrospective study in 257 cases. *J Neurosurg.* 1984;60(1):52–60.
141. McCarthy BJ, Davis FG, Freels S, et al. Factors associated with survival in patients with meningioma. *J Neurosurg.* 1998;88(5):831–839.
142. Henzel M, Gross MW, Hamm K, et al. Stereotactic radiotherapy of meningiomas: symptomatology, acute and late toxicity. *Strahlenther Onkol.* 2006;182(7):382–388.
143. Milker-Zabel S, Zabel A, Schulz-Ertner D, Schlegel W, Wannenmacher M, Debus J. Fractionated stereotactic radiotherapy in patients with benign or atypical intracranial meningioma: long-term experience and prognostic factors. *Int J Radiat Oncol Biol Phys.* 2005;61(3):809–816.
144. Debus J, Wuendrich M, Pirzkall A, et al. High efficacy of fractionated stereotactic radiotherapy of large base-of-skull meningiomas: long-term results. *J Clin Oncol.* 2001;19(15):3547–3553.
145. Maguire PD, Clough R, Friedman AH, Halperin EC. Fractionated external-beam radiation therapy for meningiomas of the cavernous sinus. *Int J Radiat Oncol Biol Phys.* 1999;44(1):75–79.
146. Narayan S, Cornblath WT, Sandler HM, Elner V, Hayman JA. Preliminary visual outcomes after three-dimensional conformal radiation therapy for optic nerve sheath meningioma. *Int J Radiat Oncol Biol Phys.* 2003;56(2):537–543.
147. Pirzkall A, Debus J, Haering P, et al. Intensity modulated radiotherapy (IMRT) for recurrent, residual, or untreated skull-base meningiomas: preliminary clinical experience. *Int J Radiat Oncol Biol Phys.* 2003;55(2):362–372.
148. Selch MT, Ahn E, Laskari A, et al. Stereotactic radiotherapy for treatment of cavernous sinus meningiomas. *Int J Radiat Oncol Biol Phys.* 2004;59(1):101–111.
149. Berman D, Miller NR. New concepts in the management of optic nerve sheath meningiomas. *Ann Acad Med Singap.* 2006;35(3):168–174.
150. Liu JK, Forman S, Hershewe GL, Moorthy CR, Benzil DL. Optic nerve sheath meningiomas: visual improvement after stereotactic radiotherapy. *Neurosurgery.* 2002;50(5):950–5; discussion 955.
151. Liu JK, Kan P, Karwande SV, Couldwell WT. Conduits for cerebrovascular bypass and lessons learned from the cardiovascular experience. *Neurosurg Focus.* 2003;14(3):e3.
152. Mendenhall WM, Amdur RJ, Morris CG, Friedman WA. Radiotherapy for optic nerve sheath meningiomas. *J Hong Kong College Radiologists.* 2003;6:183–186.
153. Smee R, Schneider M, Williams J. Optic nerve sheath meningiomas: the role of stereotactic radiotherapy. In: Kondziolka D, ed. *Radiosurgery.* Vol 6. Basel, Switzerland: Karger; 2006: 140–151.
154. Andrews BT, Wilson CB. Suprasellar meningiomas: the effect of tumor location on postoperative visual outcome. *J Neurosurg.* 1988;69(4):523–528.
155. Cristante L. Surgical treatment of meningiomas of the orbit and optic canal: a retrospective study with particular attention to the visual outcome. *Acta Neurochir (Wien).* 1994;126(1):27–32.

156. Ito M, Ishizawa A, Miyaoka M, Sato K, Ishii S. Intraorbital meningiomas. Surgical management and role of radiation therapy. *Surg Neurol.* 1988;29(6):448–453.
157. Kennerdell JS, Maroon JC, Malton M, Warren FA. The management of optic nerve sheath meningiomas. *Am J Ophthalmol.* 1988;106(4):450–457.
158. Turbin RE, Thompson CR, Kennerdell JS, Cockerham KP, Kupersmith MJ. A long-term visual outcome comparison in patients with optic nerve sheath meningioma managed with observation, surgery, radiotherapy, or surgery and radiotherapy. *Ophthalmology.* 2002;109(5):890–899; discussion 899.
159. Smith JL, Vuksanovic MM, Yates BM, Bienfang DC. Radiation therapy for primary optic nerve meningiomas. *J Clin Neuroophthalmol.* 1981;1(2):85–99.
160. Baumert BG, Villà S, Studer G, et al. Early improvements in vision after fractionated stereotactic radiotherapy for primary optic nerve sheath meningioma. *Radiother Oncol.* 2004;72(2):169–174.
161. Newton HB, Slivka MA, Stevens C. Hydroxyurea chemotherapy for unresectable or residual meningioma. *J Neurooncol.* 2000;49(2):165–170.
162. Pitz S, Becker G, Schiefer U, et al. Stereotactic fractionated irradiation of optic nerve sheath meningioma: a new treatment alternative. *Br J Ophthalmol.* 2002;86(11):1265–1268.
163. Richards JC, Roden D, Harper CS. Management of sight-threatening optic nerve sheath meningioma with fractionated stereotactic radiotherapy. *Clin Experiment Ophthalmol.* 2005;33(2):137–141.
164. Saeed P, Rootman J, Nugent RA, White VA, Mackenzie IR, Koornneef L. Optic nerve sheath meningiomas. *Ophthalmology.* 2003;110(10):2019–2030.
165. Mason WP, Gentili F, Macdonald DR, Hariharan S, Cruz CR, Abrey LE. Stabilization of disease progression by hydroxyurea in patients with recurrent or unresectable meningioma. *J Neurosurg.* 2002;97(2):341–346.
166. Becker G, Jeremic B, Pitz S, et al. Stereotactic fractionated radiotherapy in patients with optic nerve sheath meningioma. *Int J Radiat Oncol Biol Phys.* 2002;54(5):1422–1429.
167. Augspurger ME, The BS, Uhl BM, et al. Conformal intensity modulated radiation therapy for the treatment of optic nerve sheath meningioma. *Int J Radiat Oncol Biol Phys.* 1999;45(suppl):324 (abstract).
168. Tsao MN, Hoyt WF, Horton J, et al. Improved visual outcome with definitive radiation therapy for optic nerve sheath meningioma. *Int J Radiat Oncol Biol Phys.* 1999;45(3 suppl):324 (abstract).
169. Kupersmith MJ, Warren FA, Newall J, Ransohoff J. Irradiation of meningiomas of the intracranial anterior visual pathway. *Ann Neurol.* 1987;21(2):131–137.
170. Nägele T, Petersen D, Klose U, Grodd W, Opitz H, Voigt K. The "dural tail" adjacent to meningiomas studied by dynamic contrast-enhanced MRI: a comparison with histopathology. *Neuroradiology.* 1994;36(4):303–307.
171. Coke CC, Corn BW, Werner-Wasik M, Xie Y, Curran WJ Jr. Atypical and malignant meningiomas: an outcome report of seventeen cases. *J Neurooncol.* 1998;39(1):65–70.
172. Turbin RE, Pokorny K. Diagnosis and treatment of orbital optic nerve sheath meningioma. *Cancer Control.* 2004;11(5):334–341.
173. Schrieve DC, Loeffler JS. Radiotherapy in the treatment of meningiomas. In: Black PM, Loeffler JS, eds. *Cancer of the Nervous System.* 2nd ed. Philadelphia: Lippincott Williams & Wilkins; 2005:357–366.
174. Milosevic MF, Frost PJ, Laperriere NJ, Wong CS, Simpson WJ. Radiotherapy for atypical or malignant intracranial meningioma. *Int J Radiat Oncol Biol Phys.* 1996;34(4):817–822.
175. Pourel N, Auque J, Bracard S, et al. Efficacy of external fractionated radiation therapy in the treatment of meningiomas: a 20-year experience. *Radiother Oncol.* 2001;61(1):65–70.
176. Winkler C, Dornfeld S, Schwarz R, Friedrich S, Baumann M. [The results of radiotherapy in meningiomas with a high risk of recurrence. A retrospective analysis]. *Strahlenther Onkol.* 1998;174(12):624–628.
177. Sibtain A, Plowman PN. Stereotactic radiosurgery. VII. Radiosurgery versus conventionally-fractionated radiotherapy in the treatment of cavernous sinus meningiomas. *Br J Neurosurg.* 1999;13(2):158–166.
178. Borovich B, Doron Y. Recurrence of intracranial meningiomas: the role played by regional multicentricity. *J Neurosurg.* 1986;64(1):58–63.
179. Kawahara Y, Niiro M, Yokoyama S, Kuratsu J. Dural congestion accompanying meningioma invasion into vessels: the dural tail sign. *Neuroradiology.* 2001;43(6):462–465.
180. Ahmadi J, Hinton DR, Segall HD, Couldwell WT. Surgical implications of magnetic resonance-enhanced dura. *Neurosurgery.* 1994;35(3):370–7;discussion 377.
181. Cushing H, Eisenhardt L. Serial enumeration of meningiomas. In: *Meningiomas. Their Classification, Regional Behaviour, Life History, and Surgical End Results.* Springfield, IL: Charles C. Thomas; 1938:56–73.
182. Pieper DR, Al-Mefty O, Hanada Y, Buechner D. Hyperostosis associated with meningioma of the cranial base: secondary changes or tumor invasion. *Neurosurgery.* 1999;44(4):742–6; discussion 746.
183. Al-Mefty O, Kersh JE, Routh A, Smith RR. The long-term side effects of radiation therapy for benign brain tumors in adults. *J Neurosurg.* 1990;73(4):502–512.
184. Goldsmith BJ, Rosenthal SA, Wara WM, Larson DA. Optic neuropathy after irradiation of meningioma. *Radiology.* 1992;185(1):71–76.
185. Uy NW, Woo SY, Teh BS, et al. Intensity-modulated radiation therapy (IMRT) for meningioma. *Int J Radiat Oncol Biol Phys.* 2002;53(5):1265–1270.
186. Shrieve DC, Hazard L, Boucher K, Jensen RL. Dose fractionation in stereotactic radiotherapy for parasellar meningiomas: radiobiological considerations of efficacy and optic nerve tolerance. *J Neurosurg.* 2004;101(suppl 3):390–395.
187. Steinvorth S, Welzel G, Fuss M, et al. Neuropsychological outcome after fractionated stereotactic radiotherapy (FSRT) for base of skull meningiomas: a prospective 1-year follow-up. *Radiother Oncol.* 2003;69(2):177–182.
188. Mahmood A, Caccamo DV, Tomecek FJ, Malik GM. Atypical and malignant meningiomas: a clinicopathological review. *Neurosurgery.* 1993;33(6):955–963.
189. Palma L, Celli P, Franco C, Cervoni L, Cantore G. Long-term prognosis for atypical and malignant meningiomas: a study of 71 surgical cases. *Neurosurg Focus.* 1997;2(4):e3.
190. Ragel B, Jensen RL. New approaches for the treatment of refractory meningiomas. *Cancer Control.* 2003;10(2):148–158.
191. Goyal LK, Suh JH, Mohan DS, Prayson RA, Lee J, Barnett GH. Local control and overall survival in atypical meningioma: a retrospective study. *Int J Radiat Oncol Biol Phys.* 2000;46(1):57–61.
192. Yoneoka Y, Fujii Y, Tanaka R. Growth of incidental meningiomas. *Acta Neurochir (Wien).* 2000;142(5):507–511.
193. Niiro M, Yatsushiro K, Nakamura K, Kawahara Y, Kuratsu J. Natural history of elderly patients with asymptomatic meningiomas. *J Neurol Neurosurg Psychiatr.* 2000;68(1):25–28.
194. Kamiguchi H, Shiobara R, Toya S. Accidentally detected brain tumors: clinical analysis of a series of 110 patients. *Clin Neurol Neurosurg.* 1996;98(2):171–175.
195. Strang RD, Al-Mefty O. Comment on stereotactic radiosurgery for meningioma. In Pollock BE, ed. *Contemporary Stereotactic Radiosurgery: Technique and Evaluation.* Armonk, NY: Futura Publishing Company, Inc; 2002:172–180.
196. Mahmood A, Qureshi NH, Malik GM. Intracranial meningiomas: analysis of recurrence after surgical treatment. *Acta Neurochir (Wien).* 1994;126(2–4):53–58.
197. Peele KA, Kennerdell JS, Maroon JC, et al. The role of postoperative irradiation in the management of sphenoid wing meningiomas. A preliminary report. *Ophthalmology.* 1996;103(11):1761–6; discussion 1766.
198. Vendrely V, Maire JP, Darrouzet V, et al. [Fractionated radiotherapy of intracranial meningiomas: 15 years' experience at the Bordeaux University Hospital Center]. *Cancer Radiother.* 1999;3(4):311–317.
199. Dufour H, Muracciole X, Métellus P, Régis J, Chinot O, Grisoli F. Long-term tumor control and functional outcome in patients with cavernous sinus meningiomas treated by radiotherapy with or without previous surgery: is there an alternative to aggressive tumor removal? *Neurosurgery.* 2001;48(2):285–94; discussion 294.
200. Jalali R, Loughrey C, Baumert B, et al. High precision focused irradiation in the form of fractionated stereotactic conformal radiotherapy (SCRT) for benign meningiomas predominantly in the skull base location. *Clin Oncol (R Coll Radiol).* 2002;14(2):103–109.
201. Singh VP, Kansai S, Vaishya S, Julka PK, Mehta VS. Early complications following gamma knife radiosurgery for intracranial meningiomas. *J Neurosurg.* 2000;93(suppl 3):57–61.

94 Adult and Pediatric Brainstem Glioma

Carolyn R. Freeman

In children, tumors arising in the brainstem can be broadly grouped as the more favorable low-grade focal (solid and/or cystic), dorsal exophytic, and cervicomedullary tumors and the much more aggressive diffuse intrinsic (most commonly pontine) tumors. An algorithm for management that incorporates clinical and imaging findings is presented in Figure 94.1. In general, patients with favorable tumor types are managed similarly to those with low-grade astrocytomas at other sites. Thus, surgery is the mainstay of treatment for these lesions if they are accessible, and radiotherapy is reserved for patients with tumors that are not operable and for those that have progressive disease following surgery. In contrast, for patients who have typical diffuse intrinsic pontine tumors, radiotherapy is the treatment of choice.

It is important to appreciate, however, that within these broad groups there are clinical situations that require special consideration with respect to management in general and, when indicated, to radiotherapy. Thus, for example, third ventriculostomy alone may be an appropriate initial management for a patient with a nonenhancing focal lesion in the tectum presenting with hydrocephalus, with active intervention reserved for the small percentage of patients with lesions that on follow-up MRI are found to be enlarging and/or demonstrating changes in contrast enhancement. Patients with neurofibromatosis type I (NF-1) may be found, often incidentally, to have a variety of different types of lesions in the brainstem and for them, too, surveillance is also usually an appropriate initial management, with active intervention again reserved for patients with lesions showing evidence of clinical and/or radiological progression [1–3].

Tumors arising in the brainstem account for a smaller proportion of all CNS tumors seen in adult patients. They appear to be less frequently of the favorable clinicopathologic types seen in children. Surgery will less often be the treatment of choice, and most patients should probably be managed similarly to patients with supratentorial gliomas [4,5].

RADIOTHERAPY FOR FAVORABLE BRAINSTEM TUMORS

Indications for Treatment with Radiotherapy

Given the advances in neurosurgical techniques and peri-operative care, it is unusual now to see patients with favorable tumors considered at diagnosis to be inoperable. Consequently, most often now, the indication for treatment with radiotherapy is progressive disease following initial surgical resection, typically within the first 18 months to 2 years after surgery [6–8]. Although systemic chemotherapy could be considered an option, treatment of what is at this point usually a relatively small lesion using modern radiotherapy techniques is generally to be favored except in infants and very young children less than 6 or 7 years of age and those with NF-1, who are at greater risk for developing neurocognitive and other long-term sequelae of treatment.

Radiotherapy Target Volume

The majority of favorable tumors are pilocytic astrocytomas, which are generally well circumscribed with little invasion into surrounding normal brain. They are typically very well seen on contrast-enhanced CT scan or gadolinium-enhanced MRI. CT to MRI coregistration greatly aids radiotherapy treatment planning and permits the use of tighter margins than would have been considered standard practice in the past. Thus, the typical recommendation for the clinical target volume (CTV) using modern imaging and treatment planning and delivery techniques will be the tumor as seen on MRI at the time of treatment planning (the gross tumor volume, GTV) plus a margin of 0.5 to 0.8 cm, as per the current North American and European studies for low-grade gliomas in children. Until the results of these studies are available, larger margins for the CTV of 0.8 to 1.5 cm may be more appropriate for the less well-circumscribed WHO grade 2 tumors. The margin for the planning target volume (PTV) will depend on the immobilization system used and/or the availability of image guidance. Thus, with thermoplastic masks, it is necessary to add an additional 3 to 4 mm around the CTV to arrive at the PTV, but the use of rigid masks or stereotactic localization systems or image guidance may permit the use of an additional margin for the PTV of only 1 to 2 mm.

Radiotherapy Dose

In the absence of clear evidence for or against a dose response for low-grade gliomas, current studies in children with low-grade gliomas use 54 Gy given in 30 daily

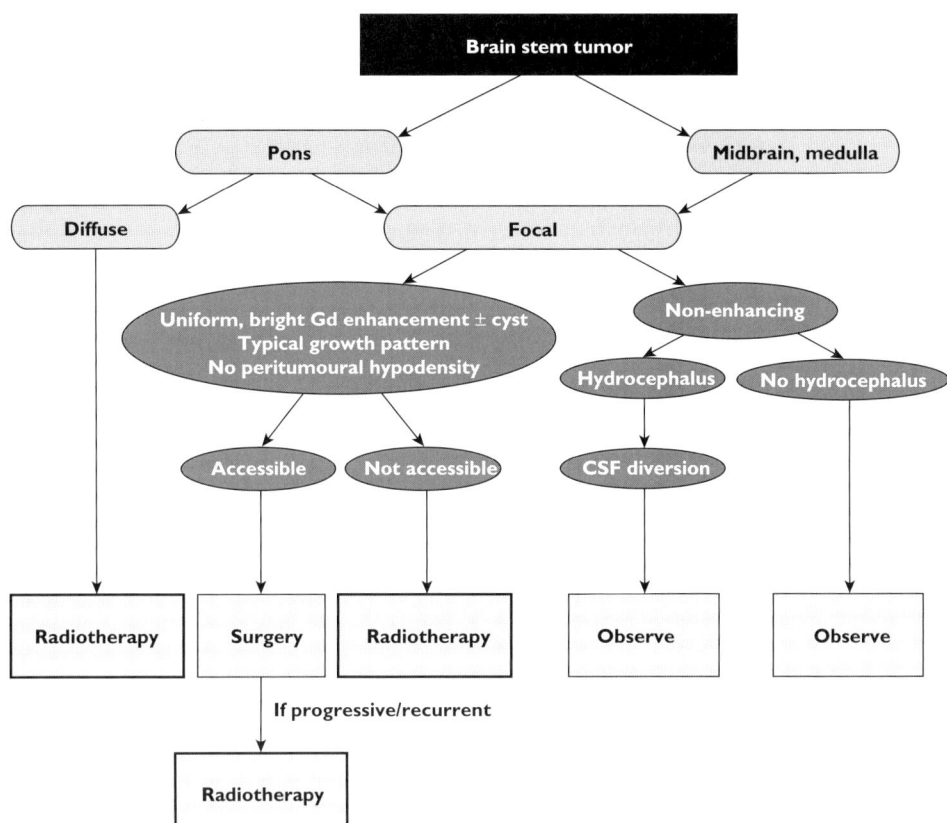

Figure 94.1 An algorithm for management of patients with brain stem tumors.

fractions over 6 weeks, and this should probably be considered for now the standard of care for all children over the age of 3 years and for adult patients.

Radiotherapy Delivery Techniques

For external beam radiotherapy, the technique used is that which provides homogeneous irradiation of the CTV and spares the greatest volume of normal tissue, in particular the supratentorial brain. Since the target volume for these tumors is relatively small, this can usually be accomplished with relatively simple 3D conformal techniques with careful attention to normal tissue sparing [9,10]. However, fractionated stereotactic irradiation may be a better option because of the reduced PTV margin and the reduced volume of normal tissue included in the treated volume as a result [11–13].

Radiosurgery using either the gamma knife or linac-based techniques is another option for focal brainstem gliomas because of the fact that they are usually relatively small at the time of radiotherapy and noninfiltrative. Doses used have ranged from 9 to 35 Gy, but because of the substantial morbidity seen with the higher doses used in older series, single doses between 10 to 18 Gy to the periphery of the tumor are now considered more appropriate [14,15].

Finally, brachytherapy with iodine-125 seeds has also been used with some success, particularly in European centers. Because of high efficacy and low treatment-related morbidity in experienced hands, brachytherapy is even considered by some to be the treatment of choice for tumors less than 4 cm in size in eloquent areas such as the brainstem [16–18].

Treatment Outcomes and Choice of Treatment Approach

As with low-grade gliomas at other sites, complete resection offers the best probability of long-term tumor control. Although this was rarely possible in the past, this is no longer the case. In one series, 25 of 30 patients with pilocytic astrocytoma underwent complete resection and the remaining 5 subtotal resection [19]. The available evidence would suggest that 80% to 95% of patients who undergo complete or subtotal resection will remain progression free without adjuvant treatment [7,8]. Results are less satisfactory for patients who undergo lesser degrees of resection, but since some 20% to 50% of patients will not progress [6–8], a management strategy consisting of close follow-up with radiotherapy at time of progression appears reasonable. Results using such an approach appear to be very good. The probability of tumor control is likely greater than 80% for patients with relatively small volume disease, regardless of the treatment technique used, that is, whether with 3D conformal radiotherapy [6,9], stereotactic radiotherapy [11,20], radiosurgery [14,15], or brachytherapy [17]. Of all of these, however, radiosurgery using single large doses or brachytherapy carry the greatest risk of treatment-related complications such as deterioration in neurological condition or necrosis requiring intervention and therefore are justifiable only in very specific situations. Results are less satisfactory for patients with bulkier disease (>4 cm) at the time of radiotherapy. For such patients, tumor control with external beam radiotherapy is likely not better than the 50% reported in older series in which radiotherapy was the primary treatment [6].

RADIOTHERAPY FOR DIFFUSE INTRINSIC BRAINSTEM GLIOMAS

Indications for Radiation Therapy

Radiation therapy is the mainstay of treatment for patients with diffuse intrinsic brainstem tumors. In the context of a typical clinical presentation with rapidly deteriorating neurological status and characteristic imaging findings, biopsy is not necessary and radiotherapy is usually started on a semiurgent basis.

Target Volume

Diffuse intrinsic tumors are best seen on T2-weighted or FLAIR MRI. The GTV is the extent of the disease as demonstrated on these studies. A margin of 1 to 1.5 cm is added for the CTV and an additional 0.3 to 0.5 cm for the PTV, depending on the immobilization system used and/or the availability of image guidance.

Radiotherapy Dose

The typical dose prescription for diffuse intrinsic brainstem tumors is 54 to 55.8 Gy given in 30 or 31 daily fractions over 6 weeks. Much higher doses have been explored with no significant improvement in survival.

Treatment Technique

Because of the typically rapid progression of neurological deficits and the need to achieve prompt symptomatic response, lateral opposed fields may be used, at least initially. A more complex conformal technique that reduces the dose to the auditory apparatus and temporal lobes may be considered as long as treatment will not be delayed.

Treatment Outcomes

A worthwhile improvement in neurological status is usually evident as early as 2 to 3 weeks into treatment with radiotherapy. Steroids, if used, can usually be discontinued at that point. This improvement is often impressive but of short duration. The outcome of treatment for patients with diffuse intrinsic brainstem tumors is dismal, with a median time to progression of 5 to 6 months, median survival of 11 to 12 months, and survival at 2 years of less than 20%.

Thus far, all attempts to improve the outcome for children with diffuse intrinsic brainstem tumors have proved futile. Hyperfractionated radiotherapy (HFRT) has been tested in a series of phase I-II studies using doses ranging from 64.8 to 78 Gy [21]. Time to progression and overall survival were not improved in comparison with conventional radiotherapy. Moreover, at the higher doses of HFRT of 75.6 and 78 Gy, morbidity was considerable. This included steroid dependency, vascular events, and white matter changes outside the radiation field as well as hearing loss, hormone deficiencies, and late-developing seizure disorders in the small number of long-term survivors [22–25]. Accelerated radiotherapy has also been tested in pediatric brainstem gliomas. In a study in the United Kingdom in which patients were treated to a total dose of 50.4 Gy given in 28 twice-daily fractions of 1.8 Gy over 3 weeks, progression-free and overall survival rates were not different from those seen in the HFRT studies [26].

Alternative approaches that use chemotherapy in combination with radiotherapy have also been disappointing. None of the many single agent and multiagent regimens or biological agents that have been tested in this patient population has been convincingly shown to result in any survival advantage compared with radiotherapy alone [27,28], although data compiled from the German HIT-GBM studies using a variety of different regimens show a small short-term advantage to the use of chemotherapy overall [29]. Current studies by the pediatric cooperative groups in North America and Europe are testing new agents and novel chemotherapy-radiotherapy combinations.

SPECIAL SITUATIONS

Brainstem Tumors in Patients with NF-1

As many as 20% of patients with NF-1 have lesions in the brainstem, some, but not all of which, are low-grade astrocytomas. Some even have lesions that have imaging characteristics of diffuse intrinsic tumors. However, the course of the disease is very different in patients with NF-1, and the majority of patients will not require any treatment. For those that do progress, surgery will be the treatment of choice for tumors that are resectable and chemotherapy for those that are not resectable or at the time of progression following surgery. Radiotherapy is considered a treatment to be avoided if possible but is useful, perhaps even at reduced doses of 45 to 50 Gy.

Unusual Pathologic Types

Other less common tumors seen in the brainstem include primitive neuroectodermal tumors, atypical teratoid/rhabdoid tumors, and medulloepithelioma. Management, including radiotherapy, is as for such tumors arising at other sites in the CNS.

REFERENCES

1. Farmer JP, Khan S, Khan A, et al. Neurofibromatosis type 1 and the pediatric neurosurgeon: a 20-year institutional review. *Pediatr Neurosurg*. 2002;37(3):122–136.
2. Pollack IF, Shultz B, Mulvihill JJ. The management of brainstem gliomas in patients with neurofibromatosis 1. *Neurology*. 1996;46(6):1652–1660.
3. Ullrich NJ, Raja AI, Irons MB, Kieran MW, Goumnerova L. Brainstem lesions in neurofibromatosis type 1. *Neurosurgery*. 2007;61(4):762–766.
4. Guillamo JS, Monjour A, Taillandier L, et al. Brainstem gliomas in adults: prognostic factors and classification. *Brain*. 2001;124 (Pt 12):2528–2539.

5. Mursch K, Halatsch ME, Markakis E, Behnke-Mursch J. Intrinsic brainstem tumours in adults: results of microneurosurgical treatment of 16 consecutive patients. *Br J Neurosurg.* 2005;19(2):128–136.
6. Farmer JP, Montes JL, Freeman CR, Meagher-Villemure K, Bond MC, O'Gorman AM. Brainstem Gliomas. A 10-year institutional review. *Pediatr Neurosurg.* 2001;34(4):206–214.
7. Pierre-Kahn A, Hirsch JF, Vinchon M, et al. Surgical management of brain-stem tumors in children: results and statistical analysis of 75 cases. *J Neurosurg.* 1993;79(6):845–852.
8. Sandri A, Sardi N, Genitori L, et al. Diffuse and focal brain stem tumors in childhood: prognostic factors and surgical outcome. Experience in a single institution. *Childs Nerv Syst.* 2006;22(9):1127–1135.
9. Merchant TE, Zhu Y, Thompson SJ, Sontag MR, Heideman RL, Kun LE. Preliminary results from a Phase II trial of conformal radiation therapy for pediatric patients with localised low-grade astrocytoma and ependymoma. *Int J Radiat Oncol Biol Phys.* 2002;52(2):325–332.
10. Perks JR, Jalali R, Cosgrove VP, et al. Optimization of stereotactically-guided conformal treatment planning of sellar and parasellar tumors, based on normal brain dose volume histograms. *Int J Radiat Oncol Biol Phys.* 1999;45(2):507–513.
11. Marcus KJ, Goumnerova L, Billett AL, et al. Stereotactic radiotherapy for localized low-grade gliomas in children: final results of a prospective trial. *Int J Radiat Oncol Biol Phys.* 2005;61(2):374–379.
12. Plathow C, Schulz-Ertner D, Thilman C, et al. Fractionated stereotactic radiotherapy in low-grade astrocytomas: long-term outcome and prognostic factors. *Int J Radiat Oncol Biol Phys.* 2003;57(4):996–1003.
13. Saran FH, Baumert BG, Khoo VS, et al. Stereotactically guided conformal radiotherapy for progressive low-grade gliomas of childhood. *Int J Radiat Oncol Biol Phys.* 2002;53(1):43–51.
14. Hadjipanayis CG, Kondziolka D, Gardner P, et al. Stereotactic radiosurgery for pilocytic astrocytomas when multimodal therapy is necessary. *J Neurosurg.* 2002;97(1):56–64.
15. Yen CP, Sheehan J, Steiner M, Patterson G, Steiner L. Gamma knife surgery for focal brainstem gliomas. *J Neurosurg.* 2007;106(1):8–17.
16. Mundinger F, Braus DF, Krauss JK, Birg W. Long-term outcome of 89 low-grade brain-stem gliomas after interstitial radiation therapy. *J Neurosurg.* 1991;75(5):740–746.
17. Peraud A, Goetz C, Siefert A, Tonn JC, Kreth FW. Interstitial iodine-125 radiosurgery alone or in combination with microsurgery for pediatric patients with eloquently located low-grade glioma: a pilot study. *Childs Nerv Syst.* 2007;23(1):39–46.
18. Voges J, Sturm VV. Interstitial irradiation with stereotactically implanted I-125 seeds for the treatment of cerebral glioma. *Crit Rev Neurosurg.* 1999;9(4):223–233.
19. Lesniak MS, Klem JM, Weingart J, Carson BS Sr. Surgical outcome following resection of contrast-enhanced pediatric brainstem gliomas. *Pediatr Neurosurg.* 2003;39(6):314–322.
20. Schulz-Ertner D, Debus J, Lohr F, Frank C, Hoss A, Wannenmacher M. Fractionated stereotactic conformal radiation therapy of brain stem gliomas: outcome and prognostic factors. *Radiother Oncol.* 2000;57(2):215–223.
21. Freeman CR. Hyperfractionated radiotherapy for diffuse intrinsic brain stem tumors in children. *Pediatr Neurosurg.* 1996;24(2):103–110.
22. Freeman CR, Bourgouin PM, Sanford RA, Cohen ME, Friedman HS, Kun LE. Long term survivors of childhood brain stem gliomas treated with hyperfractionated radiotherapy. Clinical characteristics and treatment related toxicities. The Pediatric Oncology Group. *Cancer.* 1996;77(3):555–562.
23. Freeman CR, Krischer JP, Sanford RA, et al. Final results of a study of escalating doses of hyperfractionated radiotherapy in brain stem tumors in children: a Pediatric Oncology Group study. *Int J Radiat Oncol Biol Phys.* 1993;27(2):197–206.
24. Packer RJ, Boyett JM, Zimmerman RA, et al. Outcome of children with brain stem gliomas after treatment with 7800 cGy of hyperfractionated radiotherapy. A Childrens Cancer Group Phase I/II Trial. *Cancer.* 1994;74(6):1827–1834.
25. Prados MD, Wara WM, Edwards MS, Larson DA, Lamborn K, Levin VA. The treatment of brain stem and thalamic gliomas with 78 Gy of hyperfractionated radiation therapy. *Int J Radiat Oncol Biol Phys.* 1995;32(1):85–91.
26. Lewis J, Lucraft H, Gholkar A. UKCCSG study of accelerated radiotherapy for pediatric brain stem gliomas. United Kingdom Childhood Cancer Study Group. *Int J Radiat Oncol Biol Phys.* 1997;38(5):925–929.
27. Freeman CR, Perilongo G. Chemotherapy for brain stem gliomas. *Childs Nerv Syst.* 1999;15(10):545–553.
28. Massimino M, Spreafico F, Biassoni V, et al. Diffuse pontine gliomas in children: changing strategies, changing results? A mono-institutional 20-year experience. *J Neurooncol.* 2008;87(3):355–361.
29. Wagner S, Warmuth-Metz M, Emser A, et al. Treatment options in childhood pontine gliomas. *J Neurooncol.* 2006;79(3):281–287.

95 Tumors of the Base of Skull

Kiran Devisetty, Robert S. Malyapa, and William M. Mendenhall

BACKGROUND

Etiology and Anatomy

Chordomas and chondrosarcomas are a group of locally invasive, slow-growing extra-axial neoplasms. Chordomas are presumed to arise from remnants of the primitive notochord, an embryonic precursor that is gradually replaced by mesodermal elements to form the vertebrae and skull base [1]. As the cartilage ossifies into vertebral bodies, the notochord is extruded into the intervertebral disk spaces to form the nucleus pulposus [2]. Thus, remnants can be found at any position along the neural axis. Chondrosarcomas, on the other hand, arise from embryonic rests of cartilaginous matrix that escape reabsorption during endochondral ossification [3].

At the base of the skull, chordomas are typically midline and originate within the clivus [1,3–6]. Off-midline chordomas are believed to originate from residual notochordal tissue within the nasopharynx, petrous apex, or Meckel's cave [7–9]. The location of chordomas could be histology-dependent, as Meyers et al [1] noted that three of four truly off-midline chordomas in their study were the chondroid variant. Chondrosarcomas, on the other hand, are commonly off-midline and originate within the temporal bone and petroclival fissure [2,10]. In a study of 200 cases of chondrosarcoma of the base of skull, the distribution was predominantly within the tempero-occipital junction (66%) followed by clivus (28%) and sphenoethmoid complex (6%) [11].

Epidemiology

Chordomas are an extremely rare tumor as a Survival, Epidemiology and End Results (SEER) database study identified only 400 cases from 1973 to 1995 [12]. The incidence of chordoma was 0.08 patients per 100,000 people and was more common in men (0.10) than in women (0.06). Of the cases with known race, 91.2% were found in whites, 2.2% in blacks, and 6.5% in others. The median age at diagnosis was 58.5 years (range 3–95) and was rarely diagnosed if less than 40 years (0.02 per 100,000). The distribution of chordomas was similar between cranial (32%), spinal (32.8%), and sacral (29.2%) sites; however, a small percent can occur in extra-axial and ill-defined locations (6%) [12] such as the nasopharynx, paranasal sinuses, and dura [8,9,13–15].

Historically, single institution series report predominance within the sacrum followed by the spheno-occipital region and rarely the spine; however, such studies are likely biased by referral patterns [12,16]. Cranial presentations tend to be more common in younger patients and women [12].

Chondrosarcomas are slightly more common than chordomas as a SEER analysis identified 2,890 cases from 1973 to 2003 with an incidence of 1 patient per 200,000 people [17]. The mean age at diagnosis was 51 years (range 1–102) and there was a slight male predominance (55%). Unlike chordomas, the majority of chondrosarcomas were classified as appendicular (44.5%) followed by axial (31.1%) and soft tissue (9.6%). Chondrosarcomas are considered to be a more indolent neoplasm than chordomas and associated with an improved median survival [12].

Pathology

Chordoma was first described by Virchow in 1846 when he discovered soft, jelly-like tissues arising from the spheno-occipital bone and believed it to be a cartilaginous tumor [18]. The lesion contained cells with large, vesicular, polygonal plant-like vacuoles containing mucin which he called *physaliferous cells*. They are characterized by an invasive lobular growth pattern with tumor cells arranged in cords, strands, and cohesive clusters surrounded by a mucinous matrix. Grossly, this tumor appears nodular with dense fibrous trabeculae surrounding a gelatinous center. The soft tissue masses are often surrounded by a pseudocapsule, but demarcation from adjacent normal bone is difficult [19].

Chordomas are histologically stratified into conventional, chondroid, and de-differentiated variants. The conventional variant is the same as described by Virchow, consisting of solid nests and cords of large epithelioid cells within a bubbly myxoid stroma. The chondroid variant was first described in 1973 as containing cartilaginous areas indistinguishable from chondrosarcoma. In that initial report, Heffelfinger et al [16] found that this chondroid variant had a favorable prognosis when compared to the conventional variant. Subsequently, many questioned whether chondroid chordoma was a distinct clinicopathologic entity or a misdiagnosed chondrosarcoma due to similar morphology. For example, in one study of 200 patients diagnosed with chondrosarcoma,

37% were originally classified as having chordoma [11]. The de-differentiated variant is a biphasic tumor showing areas of high-grade sarcoma with conventional or chondroid sarcoma components [20].

Researchers at the Massachusetts General Hospital (MGH) subsequently performed an immunohistochemical comparison of conventional chordoma, chondroid chordoma, and chondrosarcomas. They discovered that both variants of chordoma were universally positive for cytokeratin and the majority were positive for epithelial membrane antigen (EMA) and carcinoembryonic antigen (CEA). Chondrosarcomas, on the other hand, did not stain for any of these antigens. The authors concluded that chondroid chordoma was a distinct entity separate from chondrosarcoma [21].

The natural history of chondroid chordoma has also been an area of debate. Initially, the chondroid variant was described as having a favorable prognosis [16,19,22]. However, a histopathological study from the Mayo Clinic found no difference in survival between the classic and chondroid chordomas [23], and this has been confirmed in other series [24–26]. Instead, the more favorable prognosis with chondroid chordomas was attributed to the occurrence in younger patients [23].

Chondrosarcoma is histologically stratified into conventional (hyaline/myxoid), de-differentiated, clear cell, and mesenchymal variants. Chondrosarcomas are often hypercellular and infiltrate cancellous bone. The most common histology involving the base of skull is the conventional (hyaline/myxoid) variant. In a study of 200 patients with conventional chondrosarcoma of the base of skull, 63% were mixed hyaline/myxoid, 29.5% were myxoid, and 7.5% were hyaline subtypes [11]. In the hyaline subtype, neoplastic chondrocytes reside in lacunar spaces surrounded by hyaline matrix. It is not uncommon for these cells to have a bubbly or vacuolated appearance. In the myxoid subtype, lobular chondrocytes float in a mucinous matrix and form a honeycomb network of strands and cords of cells. It is this subtype that is most often confused with chordoma [11,21]. The mixed hyaline/myxoid subtype has appearances that range between the two. All chondrosarcomas are assigned a grade of 1 to 3 based on differentiation. On immunohistochemistry, 99% were positive for S-100, but none stained for keratin and only 8% stained for EMA [11].

Distinguishing chordomas from chondrosarcomas (especially the myxoid subtype of the conventional variant) on histology can be difficult. In the study of 200 patients with chondrosarcoma, of whom 37% were originally classified as chordoma, all were of the myxoid subtype. Because chordomas have a more unfavorable prognosis, it is important to distinguish them from low-grade chondrosarcomas.

Immunohistochemistry has helped elucidate differences between the two distinct entities. As mentioned above, Rosenberg et al and others reported that chordomas almost universally stained for cytokeratin, EMA, and CEA, whereas chondrosarcoma had essentially no reactivity to these antigens [11,21,27]. Juliao et al [28] analyzed 16 chordomas and 12 low-grade myxoid chondrosarcomas for galectin-3, a beta-galactoside binding protein, and found that 12 of 16 (75%) chordomas were positive compared with 1 of 12 (8%) chondrosarcomas. Naka et al [29] analyzed 15 chordomas and 8 chondrosarcomas for cell adhesion molecules (E-cadherin, α-catenin, β-catenin, γ-catenin, and neural cell adhesion molecules) and found that all, except α-catenin, were present significantly more often in chordomas than in chondrosarcomas.

Clinical Presentation

Both chordomas and chondrosarcomas are usually slow-growing, locally infiltrative, destructive lesions at the base of skull. However, occasionally these can demonstrate both rapid regrowth as well as metastatic potential. In a study of 97 patients, the average interval between first symptom and diagnosis was 14.6 months for chordoma and 23.5 months for chondrosarcoma [3]. Symptoms are dependent on location and can be insidious with progressive changes in neurologic functions. The majority of chordomas arise in the mid and upper portion of the clivus [2]. Superiorly, the chiasm and third ventricle can be displaced; inferiorly, the atlas can be invaded and adjacent foramen penetrated (e.g., jugular foramen, foramen lacerum); posteriorly, the brainstem can be compressed and the pontine cistern can be shifted anteriorly, the sella turcica and pituitary can be compressed or the nasopharynx invaded; laterally, the cavernous sinus can be encased [4].

Clinical findings from base of skull tumors are classified into generalized, ophthalmologic, and otolaryngologic symptoms [2]. Headache is the most common generalized symptoms and is present in at least 57% of patients [3], usually in the occipital and occipitocervical areas. These headaches can be aggravated by changes in neck position; this can reflect extent of local invasion, stretching of the dura, and possible hydrocephalus. Other general symptoms include facial pain, neck pain, torticollis, shoulder weakness, dysmenorrhea, decreased libido, galactorrhea, and pan-hypopituitarism [2].

Visual disturbances (61%) [3] are equally common to headaches due to involvement of the optic chiasm or cavernous sinus. The sixth cranial nerve (46%) is most commonly involved, although cavernous sinus invasion could also lead to cranial nerve III (14%), IV (4%), and V (9%) deficits [3]. Specific ophthalmologic symptoms include loss of vision, blurring of vision, ptosis, diplopia, visual field defects, papilledema, and optic atrophy [2]. Otolaryngologic symptoms are not as common, but include nasal obstruction, hearing loss, tinnitus, Eustachian tube obstruction, dizziness, ataxia, hoarseness, dysphagia, paresis of tongue and palate, and craniofacial pain [2].

Natural History

Chordomas exhibit locally destructive growth and most patients die from locally progressive or recurrent disease [19]. Recurrences may be observed many years after treatment and can occur along the surgical pathway [2,30,31]. Despite this, patients may survive for several years after recurrence. Distant metastases are extremely rare (6–22%) [19,30,32,33], but when present they usually occur in the craniospinal axis, bones, and lungs. Metastases have also been reported to lymph nodes, brain, and viscera [19,30]. The rate of metastases appears to be higher in the presence of locally recurrent disease [2].

Fagundes et al reported on the patterns of failure of 204 patients with base of skull and cervical spine chordomas treated at the MGH between 1975 and 1993. In total, 63 patients (31%) developed recurrent disease and the median time to local failure was 32 months. Of these 63 patients, 78% had local failure as initial site of relapse, but 95% eventually had a component of local failure. Regional lymph node relapses were present in 3% and surgical pathway recurrence in 5% (left neck, palate, nasal cavity). Distant metastases as the only site of failure was seen in 3%; however, 20% (or 6% of the entire population) eventually had a component of distant failure and this was observed most commonly in the lungs and bones. After any recurrence, the 3- and 5-year overall survival rates were 43% and 7%, respectively.

Chondrosarcomas of the base of skull are considered to be more indolent and associated with a much more favorable prognosis. In a separate study from MGH, of 200 patients with chondrosarcoma receiving a variety of surgical treatments followed by high-dose radiation therapy, only 3 patients developed a local recurrence and none developed distant metastases. The 10-year local control and disease-specific survival were both 99%. There was no relationship between outcome, histologic subtype, and grade [11]. This stands in stark comparison to the reported 5- and 10-year disease-free survival of 70% and 45%, respectively, in approximately 300 chordoma patients treated at the same institution [11].

DIAGNOSIS AND WORK-UP

Differential Diagnosis

Similar to other intracranial tumors, symptoms from base of skull tumors are dependent on the location and extent of disease. No one symptom is associated with chordoma or chondrosarcoma and they often present with the same constellation of findings. The differential diagnosis for tumors at this site includes chordoma, chondrosarcoma, chondroma, invasive pituitary adenoma, clivus meningioma, lymphoma, metastases, plasmacytoma, histiocytosis X, and fibrous dysplasia.

Work-Up and Staging

Initial work-up for base of skull tumors depends on the extent of invasion as determined by clinical symptoms and imaging (see below). Since many patients present with multiple neuroendocrine symptoms, they should have a full endocrine work-up and be referred for both visual and auditory testing. If dysphagia is present, patients should also be considered for a video swallowing evaluation with referral to speech therapy.

For management, patients should be referred to a neurosurgeon with a specialization in base of skull due to the delicate nature of surgery in this region. Several factors such as tumor location, the extent and pattern of tumor invasion, preoperative clinical status, and history of prior surgery have to be taken into account for surgical planning. As tumors rarely have a gross total resection in this region of the body, patients should also be referred to a radiation oncologist with access to particle therapy for treatment with high-dose radiation therapy. As will be discussed, particle radiation therapy offers a dosimetric advantage associated with both improved local control and less toxicity.

There is no formal staging system for base of skull chordoma or chondrosarcoma provided by either the American Joint Committee on Cancer or the Union Internationale Contre le Cancer. Al-Mefty et al proposed a surgical staging system based on tumor extent and the surgical procedures necessary to achieve a radical resection. Type I is a tumor restricted to one compartment of the base of skull, defined as a solitary anatomical area (e.g., sphenoid sinus, cavernous sinus, lower clivus, or occipital condyle). Type II is a tumor that extends to two or more contiguous areas of the base of skull and whose radical removal can be achieved using a single skull-based approach. Type III is a tumor that extends to several contiguous compartments of the base of skull and requires two or more skull-based procedures to achieve a radical surgical removal. In this series of 25 patients, 0% were Type I, 64% were Type II, and 12% were Type III; the remaining 24% had recurrent tumors [34]. The drawbacks of this staging system, though, are that stage may vary with the surgeon and a significant number of patients have lesions that are not amenable to radical resection.

Imaging

Radiographic findings of base of skull destruction, mainly within the clivus or temporal bone, should immediately raise the suspicion of chordoma or chondrosarcoma, respectively. Chordomas are generally considered midline lesions due to the position of notochordal remnants, but rarely can be found off midline. In the latter case, the histology is more likely the chondroid variant of chordoma [1] or chondrosarcoma [35]; however, differentiation of chordomas and chondrosarcomas based on radiologic findings is not reliable. It has been reported that chondrosarcomas can display linear, globular, or arclike calcifications that are uncommon in chordoma. Furthermore, chondrosarcomas can undergo progressive calcification after radiation therapy, which is not seen in chordomas [2].

In the past, skull x-rays and angiography provided an indirect assessment of the presence and extent of these lesions. Currently, computed tomography (CT) and magnetic resonance imaging (MRI) allow a more precise assessment of tumor extent and invasion critical to management.

Computed Tomography

High-resolution, thin-section CT scans with three-dimensional reconstructions are excellent for assessing both bone and, in most cases, soft tissue involvement. In the posterior fossa, CT may be limited in defining soft tissue structures due to beam-hardening artifacts [5,36]. Bone windows on CT axial and coronal projects allow for an accurate assessment of the degree of clival bony destruction. Chordomas typically cause lytic bone destruction without significant sclerosis.

On soft tissue windows, chordomas generally display a central, well-defined homogeneous mass with a density comparable to muscles but slightly more hyperdense than adjacent brain tissue. These tumors are heterogeneous with contrast and frequently demonstrate osteolytic changes. Intratumoral calcification is present in more than 50% of cases [5,6] and are thought to represent sequestra from destroyed bone rather than dystrophic calcification [2,37]. When used in concert, both bone and soft tissue windows are ideal for assessing paranasal sinus extension, that is, sphenoid sinus, posterior ethmoid sinuses, and orbit [2].

Magnetic Resonance Imaging

MRI is superior in delineating the exact boundaries of the soft tissue tumor intracranially and invasion into adjacent structures, such as the nasopharynx, brainstem, sella, and cavernous sinus [5]. MRI is also advantageous in examining the adjacent vasculature (e.g., petrous internal carotid artery, vertebrobasilar arteries) that can be displaced by base of skull tumors. Interestingly, MRI frequently demonstrates encasement of adjacent cerebral vessels; however, there is no associated narrowing of the vessel lumens [2,6]. Meningioma, on the other hand, typically causes luminal compromise [2].

T1-weighted MR images typically demonstrate low to moderate signal intensity within a background of the normal high-intensity signal of the fatty clivus. The tumors can also demonstrate high signal foci if intratumoral hemorrhage is present [1,38]. T2-weighted images, on the other hand, almost uniformly appear hyperintense and commonly with internal septations [38]. Some argue that this is due to the high fluid content of the vacuolated cellular components [1]; however, others believe this may be due to proteinaceous and mucinous material within the matrix [2,38]. Gadolinium-enhanced MRI scans clearly demonstrate the soft-tissue component of the tumor and appear heterogeneous with a "honeycomb" pattern [1,4]; fat-suppressed images accentuate the enhancing mass within the fatty clivus.

The chondroid variant of chordomas has been reported as having different signal characteristics, specifically shorter T1 and T2 signals. It is hypothesized that this is due to its composition of cartilaginous hyaline tissue and low water content [4,39]. However, others have argued that this difference in signal is not consistent and that MRI alone is not sufficient to discriminate histology [1,5].

Positron Emission Tomography

Fluorine-18-fluorodeoxyglucose positron emission tomography (FDG-PET) is not routinely used, but in recurrent and metastatic cases, may provide useful information. In musculoskeletal tumors, studies have suggested that FDG-PET may be able to discriminate between benign and malignant histologies [40,41], but the correlation is unclear for bone tumors [42]. At Washington University, using an SUV greater than 2.0, researchers were able to correctly classify 14 of 15 malignant bone tumors. These data could be extrapolated to chordoma; however, the use of FDG-PET has been limited to case reports [43–45] and should be used in conjunction with additional imaging and clinical history.

Tissue Diagnosis

Diagnosis can be made with fine needle aspiration [20,46] and may be associated with a lower rate of local recurrence when compared to open incisional biopsy [47]. The cytologic appearance typically demonstrates classic physaliferous cells arranged in small clusters and single cells. This is within the presence of a fibrillary, myxoid background and often with moderate to high cellularity. Biopsy may be performed by either interventional radiology or neurosurgery; however, in 20% to 36% of patients, chordomas may extend to the nasopharynx and a biopsy can easily be performed by otorhinolaryngology [1,34].

MANAGEMENT

Surgery

The general management of a patient with base of skull chordoma or chondrosarcoma is determined by the location and extent of spread. The principal treatment is surgery; however, complete surgical extirpation is unusual. Al-Mefty et al [34] reported on a series of 23 patients with cranial chordomas undergoing surgical resection of which 43% had a radical resection (absence of residual tumor), 48% had a subtotal resection (>90% resection of tumor), and 9% had a partial resection (<90% resection of tumor). Watkins et al [48] reported on 28 patients with cranial chordoma undergoing craniotomy of whom 89% had subtotal resection and 11% had a biopsy. Gay et al [22] reported on 60 patients with cranial chordomas or chondrosarcomas undergoing craniotomy of whom 47% had total, 20% near-total (questionable remnants), 23% subtotal (>90%), and 10% partial (<90%) resections. The surgery is often limited by the proximity of normal structures; thus, less than half are able to achieve a gross total resection.

The therapeutic role of surgical resection has not been defined in prospective trials; instead multiple retrospective series have suggested improved local control and survival in those patients with optimal surgical debulking. However, it is unclear whether this benefit is due to selection bias as treatment is guided by surgical expertise, patient comorbidities, and extent of tumor invasion.

Tai et al performed a comprehensive review of the literature and identified 159 patients with cranial chordomas treated by various therapeutic regimens. The patients were classified as having subtotal resection followed by adjuvant radiation therapy (53%), radiation therapy alone (27%), or varying degrees of surgery alone (20%). The median survival of these groups was not reached (i.e., >7.5 years), 7.5 years, and 0.25 years, respectively. Pairwise comparison demonstrated that subtotal resection followed by adjuvant radiation therapy had a significantly improved survival over surgery alone ($P = 0.011$); however, there was no difference when compared to radiation therapy alone ($P = 0.271$) [49]. Despite the lack of statistical difference between combined modality treatment and radiation therapy alone, the survival curves separate with follow-up and suggest a benefit to include surgery in management.

Photon Radiation Therapy: Conventional Fractionation (See Table 95.1)

Dose Response

The primary role for photon radiation therapy following maximal surgical resection is to improve local control as gross residual disease often remains. The initial data regarding the dose of radiation required originated from a series of papers in the 1960s and 1970s that suggested an improvement in symptomatic response and local control with increased dose [57–59]. There have been no randomized studies investigating optimal dose with photon therapy, and so these recommendations are drawn from retrospective series that are subject to many inherent biases. Specifically, these early papers used antiquated radiation techniques (e.g., orthovoltage, supervoltage, or low megavoltage) with suboptimal planning (i.e., non-CT-based planning). They also included tumors from multiple sites (base of skull, cervical vertebra, lumbar vertebra, and sacrum), small numbers of patients, selection/referral bias, poor radiographic localization, and variable treatment doses [60].

In 1970, Pearlman and Friedman were among the first to report a dose response with photon therapy in the treatment of chordoma. In this report, 15 patients treated at University Hospital in New York were combined with 81 patients acquired from a review of the literature. Chordomas were in the basi-sphenoid region, cervical vertebra, lumbar vertebra, and the sacrum. For those patients with known dosimetry, the authors noted a decrease in local failure with increasing dose (no p value was reported). For doses <40 Gy ($n = 47$), 40 to 60 Gy ($n = 18$), 60 to 80 Gy ($n = 8$), and >80 Gy ($n = 2$), the rates of failure were 85%, 60%, 43%, and 0%, respectively [57]. It must be noted that due to the time period of treatment, the majority of patients were treated with orthovoltage radiation (as opposed to megavoltage), thus causing uncertainty in the true dose distribution [50].

Romero et al reported a more contemporary photon dose response series of 18 patients with chordoma of the cranial, vertebral, and sacrococcygeal regions in which all were treated with megavoltage radiation following biopsy or subtotal resection. Fourteen patients were treated with conventional fractionation to a median 57.5 Gy (range 50–64.8) and eight patients were treated with hyperfractionation twice daily to a median 40.8 Gy (range 29.9–59.2). The authors noted a lower dose threshold than the aforementioned studies, as progression-free survival was statistically improved when >48 Gy versus <40 Gy (31% vs. 0%, $P = 0.04$). However, they also found a trend to worst progression-free survival with hyperfractionation versus conventional fractionation (0% vs. 38%, $P = 0.09$) [53]. At the Royal Marsden Hospital, Fuller et al [32] reported a similar dose response level at 55 Gy on a cohort of 25 patients.

No Dose Response

In a comprehensive review of the literature, Tai et al identified 47 patients with cranial chordoma treated with either adjuvant or definitive radiation therapy and known dosimetry. Since these patients were treated with various radiation therapy fractionation schemes, the regimens were normalized by calculating the biologically equivalent dose by assuming an α/β ratio of 2.1 for the brain and 7 for the tumor. The median dose delivered was 55 Gy (range 25–78)

Table 95.1 Summary of Results With Conventionally Fractionated Photon Therapy for Chordoma and Chondrosarcoma

Author	Period	N (Patients)	Site(s)	Tumor Dose (Gy)	% Local Control (Year)		% Overall Survival (Year)	
					5	10	5	10
Cummings et al, 1983 [50]	1958–1979	24	Multiple	25–67	–	–	62 (Ch)	28 (Ch)
Amendola et al, 1986 [51]	1962–1982	21	Multiple	50–66	–	–	50 (Ch)	20 (Ch)
Fuller et al, 1988 [32]	1952–1981	25	Multiple	30–70	33 (Ch)	20 (Ch)	44 (Ch)	17 (Ch)
Magrini et al, 1992 [52]	1955–1990	12	Multiple	35–60	17 (Ch)	17 (Ch)	58 (Ch)	35 (Ch)
Forsyth et al, 1993 [23]	1960–1984	39	BOS	23–67	39 (Ch)	31 (Ch)	51 (Ch)	35 (Ch)
Romero et al, 1993 [53]	1975–1990	18	Multiple	30–65	17 (Ch)	–	38 (Ch)	–
Catton et al, 1996 [54]	1958–1992	48	Multiple	25–60	23 (Ch)	15 (Ch)	54 (Ch)	20 (Ch)
Zorlu et al, 2000 [55]	1979–1997	18	BOS	50–64	23 (Ch)	–	35 (Ch)	–
Debus et al, 2000 [56]	1990–1997	45	BOS	Med. 66.6 (Ch) Med. 64.6 Gy (CS)	50 (Ch) 100 (CS)		82 (Ch) 100 (CS)	

Abbreviations: BOS, base of skull; Ch, Chordoma; CS, Chondrosarcoma.

of which 8 patients received >65 Gy. Using duration of symptom control as an end point, no dose response could be identified [49].

At the Princess Margaret Hospital, Cummings et al reported on a more heterogeneous population of 24 patients that included base of skull, cervical vertebra, lumbar vertebra, and sacrococcygeal chordomas. The median radiation dose was 50 Gy (range 25–66.6), and when comparing patients who received doses above and below the median, there was no difference in symptomatic response (the primary end point of the study). The authors also performed a review of the literature and identified an additional 32 patients with dosimetric data, but even then no dose response in symptomatic relief could be identified [50]. In an update from the same institution that now included 48 patients, there continued to be no evidence of dose response at 50 Gy. The authors also noted no difference in survival between clival and nonclival chordomas and no improvement in symptom control between hyperfractionated and conventionally fractionated radiation therapy [54].

In a series of 19 patients with chordoma of the base of skull, lumbar vertebra, and sacrococcygeal spine treated at M.D. Anderson Hospital, Saxton et al similarly questioned the presence of a radiation dose response. For patients with unresected tumors, no local control was achieved in patients treated up to 65 Gy, and one patient with a surgical resection had a local failure despite receiving 70 Gy. On the other hand, all the patients who received 50 to 58 Gy had no local failure. Despite any apparent correlation between radiation dose and local control, the authors did not rule out the need for escalating dose in the adjuvant setting, but in unresectable disease radiation is at best palliative [61].

Efficacy

The literature for conventionally fractionated photon therapy in the definitive or adjuvant treatment of chordoma extends over a prolonged period of time and includes a variety of techniques and management approaches. Interpretation of outcomes such as dose response and local control is difficult due to antiquated radiotherapy techniques and suboptimal imaging to provide an appropriate context with current technology. Many of these older series also relied on subjective assessments such as symptomatic response. A common theme, though, is that photon therapy rarely cured chordomas despite long median survivals. In the most recent update of the Princess Margaret Hospital experience, Catton et al noted that of the 48 patients reported, 96% were either dead from the disease (78%) or alive with disease persistence (17%) at last follow-up [54].

Even though these older, retrospective series did not provide conclusive evidence of a dose response with photon therapy, the lack of durable local control argues the need for dose escalation or use of radiation therapy with increased radiobiological effectiveness (RBE). This insight has led to the rapid evolution and application of new technologies, specifically stereotactic radiosurgery (SRS) and particle therapy, which allow for both dose escalation and improved sparing of adjacent normal tissue.

Photon Radiation Therapy: Stereotactic Radiosurgery (See Table 95.2)

SRS offers the benefit of more conformal radiation therapy through the use of multiple non-coplanar fields, sources, or arcs when compared to conventional external beam radiation therapy. SRS has been traditionally delivered with either a linear accelerator or Gamma Knife during which a single large fraction of radiation is delivered. The use of a large fraction increases the RBE when compared to conventional fractionation. SRS is often limited by the size of the lesion as dose heterogeneity can become prohibitive if the lesion is too large.

In the treatment of base of skull chordomas or chondrosarcomas, SRS has often been used to treat local recurrences or boost the tumor after patients have already received surgical resection and conventional radiation therapy. At the Mayo Clinic, Krishnan et al reported a series of 29 patients with chordoma ($n = 25$) or chondrosarcoma ($n = 4$) of which 11 patients were recurrent and 19 patients received prior conventional radiation therapy to a median 50.4 Gy (range 45–54 Gy). For SRS, the median margin dose was 15 Gy (range 10–20), the median maximum dose was 30 Gy (range 20–40), and the median volume treated was 14.4 cm^3 (range 0.6–65.1). There were seven local failures, of which four were out of field, for a 2- and 5-year local control rate of 89% and 32%, respectively. Notably, no patient with chondrosarcoma experienced a local failure. On subset analysis, there was a suggestion that dose >15 Gy was associated with improved local control in chordoma patients (100% vs. 50%, $P = 0.03$); however, the numbers were small. SRS was not without morbidity as 21% had cranial nerve dysfunction, 17% brain necrosis, and 10% anterior pituitary dysfunction. Interestingly, late toxicity only developed in those patients with prior radiation therapy [62].

Hasegawa et al reported their experience in Japan of 37 patients with chordoma ($n = 30$) or chondrosarcoma

Table 95.2 Summary of Results With Stereotactic Radiosurgery for Base of Skull Chordoma and Chondrosarcoma

Author	Period	N (Patients)	Tumor Dose (Gy)	% Local Control (Year)		% Overall Survival (Year)	
				5	10	5	10
Krishnan et al, 2005 [62]	1990–2002	29	10–20	32 (Ch/CS)	–	–	–
Hasegawa et al, 2007 [63]	1991–2006	37	9–20	76 (Ch/CS)	67 (Ch/CS)	80 (Ch/CS)	53 (Ch/CS)
Martin et al, 2007 [64]	1987–2004	28	10–25	53 (Ch) 80 (CS)	–	63 (Ch)	–

Abbreviations: Ch, Chordoma; CS, Chondrosarcoma; SRS, Stereotactic radiosurgery.

($n = 7$), of which 3 patients (8%) did not have a surgical intervention and 7 patients (19%) were recurrent after receiving prior conventional radiation therapy. The mean margin dose was 14 Gy (range 9–20), the mean maximum dose was 28 Gy (range 18–40), and the mean volume treated was 19.7 cm^3 (range 0.4–94.3). The 5- and 10-year local control rate was 76% and 67%, respectively, and only correlated to a tumor volume of 20 cm^3 on both univariate and multivariate analysis (but not dose). Due to the volume dependence, the authors argued that maximal surgical debulking should be pursued to minimize treatment volume and create space from adjacent normal critical structures. The 5- and 10-year overall survival was 80% and 53%, respectively, and none of the patients with prior radiation therapy experienced any late toxicity [63].

At University of Pittsburgh, Martin et al reported on 28 patients with chordoma ($n = 18$) and chondrosarcoma ($n = 10$), of which 15 and 7 patients had prior conventional photon (mean 65 Gy) or proton (mean 75 Gy) radiation therapy, respectively. The mean margin dose was 16.5 Gy (range 10.5–25), the mean maximum dose was 33 Gy (range 21–50), and the mean volume treated was 9.8 cm^3 (range 0.08–22). For chondrosarcomas, the 5-year local control was 80%, whereas for chordomas it was 53%, but it improved to 63% after repeat SRS. Toxicity was limited as three patients had changes on MRI, but only one presented with symptoms related to these changes [64].

At present, the role of SRS appears to be limited to adjuvant treatment or small local recurrences. SRS can be considered for the primary treatment of small, biopsy-proven disease; however, surgical resection must still be considered the standard of care.

Particle Radiation Therapy: Protons (See Table 95.3)

Physics and Radiobiology

Both photons and protons are considered low-energy transfer radiations, that is, the rate of energy transfer along the track of an ionizing particle is relatively low. However, due to the proton Bragg Peak, the confined area of rapid dose deposition and fall-off is believed to have increased RBE when compared to photons. This increased RBE has been speculated to be between 1.1 and 1.3 times the equivalent dose of photons [70–73], but most institutions like MGH have used an RBE of 1.1. Proton doses are expressed in cobalt gray equivalents (CGE), such that 1 CGE = proton Gray × 1.1 [66].

Outcomes

The clinical experience for proton therapy for base of skull chordomas and chondrosarcomas has been pioneered by institutions in the United States (Loma Linda University Medical Center [65], MGH [66]), Europe (Institut Curie Centre de Protonthérapie d'Orsay [67], Paul Sherrer Institute [74]), and Japan (Proton Medical Research Center [69]). None of the published series are prospective phase III randomized trials; however, collectively they represent the largest set of patient outcomes for base of skull tumors.

At Loma Linda University Medical Center, Hug et al reported on a series of 58 patients with base of skull chordoma (57%) or chondrosarcoma (43%). All patients underwent various limited surgical procedures (i.e., 91% had gross residual disease) followed by a mean 70.7 CGE (range 64.8–79.2) proton therapy. Only six patients had a combination of protons and megavoltage photons (36–50.4 Gy). As expected, chordoma had a worst 5-year local control of 59%, whereas for chondrosarcoma it was 75% ($P = 0.11$). The difference in local control translated to survival, as chondrosarcoma had a 5-year overall survival of 100% while for chordoma it was 79%. The majority of failures were in-field, but none was regional or distant. Subset analysis revealed that the size of the tumor was prognostic for local control, as lesions <25 mL had a 5-year local control of 100% versus 56% in those with >25 mL ($P = 0.02$). Brainstem involvement was present in all patients with local failure and associated with worst 5-year local control (53% versus 94%, $P = 0.04$). This decrease in local control showed a trend to worse overall survival ($P = 0.08$) [65].

Munzenrider et al reported the MGH experience with 621 patients with chordomas (60%) and chondrosarcomas (40%) of the base of skull (84%) and cervical spine (16%). Almost all patients received some portion of treatment with megavoltage photon therapy and the total prescribed dose ranged from 66 to 83 CGE. For base of skull tumors, chondrosarcomas had significant improvement in 5- and 10-year local recurrence-free survival (98% vs. 73% and 94% vs. 54%, respectively) and 5- and 10-year

Table 95.3 Summary of Results With Protons or Mixed Photons/Protons for Base of Skull Chordoma and Chondrosarcoma

Author	Period	N (Patients)	Tumor Dose (CGE)	% Local Control (Year)		% Overall Survival (Year)	
				5	10	5	10
Hug et al, 1999 [65]	1992–1998	58	64.8–79.2	59 (Ch) 75 (CS)	–	79 (Ch) 100 (CS)	–
Munzenrider et al, 1999 [66]	1975–1998	621	66–83	73 (Ch) 98 (CS)	54 (Ch) 94 (CS)	80 (Ch) 91 (CS)	54 (Ch) 88 (CS)
Noel et al, 2005 [67]	1993–2002	100	60–71	54 (Ch) (4-yr)	–	81 (Ch)	–
Ares et al, 2009 [68]	1998–2005	64	67–74 (Ch) 63–74 (CS)	81 (Ch) 94 (CS)	–	62 (Ch) 91 (CS)	–
Igaki et al, 2004 [69]	1989–2000	13	63–95	46 (Ch)	–	67 (Ch)	–

Abbreviaions: CGE, Cobalt gray equivalent; Ch, Chordoma; CS, Chondrosarcoma.

overall survival (91% vs. 80% and 88% vs. 54%, respectively) over chordomas. However, there was no statistical difference between cervical spine chondrosarcomas and chordomas. On subset analysis for base of skull tumors, male patients had improved 5- and 10-year local recurrence-free survival (81% vs. 65% and 65% vs. 42%, respectively) over female patients. This difference did not exist for cervical spine tumors as well [66].

At the Institut Curie Centre de Protonthérapie d'Orsay, Noel et al reported on a series of 100 patients with chordoma of the base of skull (90%) and cervical spine (10%) treated with mixed photon/proton radiation therapy. All patients had at least one surgical procedure followed by a median radiation dose of 67 CGE (range 60–71). The median photon dose was 45 Gy (range 29–55) and the median proton dose was 22 CGE (range 12–38). The 4-year local control rate was 54% and the median time to local failure was 26 months. Multivariate analysis revealed that unfavorable prognostic factors for local control were minimum tumor dose <56 CGE and when 95% of the GTV receives less than 95% of the total prescribed dose. The 5-year overall survival was 81% and multivariate analysis found local control was the only independent prognostic factor [67].

Ares et al reported the experience of the Paul Scherrer Institut on 64 patients with base of skull chordomas (66%) and chondrosarcomas (34%) [68]. This series was unique with its use of a novel technology in proton delivery. The other institutions presented here [65–67,69] used passive scattering, that is, use of an aperture, compensator, and range shifter wheel that conforms the dose distribution to the target volume laterally and at depth. The Paul Scherrer Institut used spot scanning, or rather the use of narrow pencil proton beams with a near monoenergetic Bragg peak that dynamically positions the dose along three dimensions throughout the target volume (i.e., active scanning or intensity-modulated proton therapy). This permits increased conformity when compared to passive scattering, which is limited by the fixed depth modulation of Bragg peaks across the treatment field [74]. Only five patients received mixed photon/proton therapy. Following at least one surgical procedure, patients with chordoma received a mean 73.5 CGE (range 67–74) and chondrosarcoma received a mean 68.4 Gy (range 63–74). The 5-year local control was 81% for chordoma and 94% for chondrosarcoma, and there were no regional or distant failures. On univariate analysis, brainstem compression and tumor volume >25 mL were negative prognostic factors for local control. The 5-year overall survival was 62% for chordomas and 91% for chondrosarcomas, and in an earlier subset analysis, there was a trend to worst progression-free survival for age >40 years [74].

Technique

There are some important considerations unique to proton therapy treatment planning. The devices used to immobilize patients for proton therapy must be "proton-friendly." The construction of these devices should be carefully evaluated for their physical properties to obtain homogeneous radiological lengths (accounting for attenuation and absorption) through potential paths of proton beams. Most often, patients are immobilized in the supine position on a carbon fiber skull-base frame with a mask and incorporated bite-block.

The prescribed dose for chordomas ranges from 73.8 to 79.2 CGE, whereas for chondrosarcomas the doses are lower between 68.4 and 72 CGE. Typically, the dose is delivered at 1.8 CGE per day. In all cases, the tolerance of adjacent critical structures, the brainstem, and the optic chiasm should be respected to avoid complications related to treatment. Three-dimensional treatment planning is generally carried out using a complex set of field arrangements (i.e., coplanar or non-coplanar) to cover the target. Due to the Bragg peak, the target can be partitioned and each component treated with individualized patch- and through- fields. In essence, this technique matches the 50% isodose line of the lateral penumbra of the through-field with the distal fall off of the patch-field (Figure 95.1). Such a field arrangement for a chordoma of the clivus, for example, allows sparing of the brainstem (Figure 95.2).

Proton Radiation Oncology Group 85–26

The MGH and Lawrence Berkeley Laboratory (LBL), with support from the National Cancer Institute and Radiation Therapy Oncology Group, initiated a randomized controlled trial in 1985 for patients with base of skull and cervical spine chordomas and chondrosarcomas. MGH used mixed photons/protons and LBL used helium ions, and the primary end points for the study were local control and normal tissue effects. Patients were initially randomized to 69.6 or 75.6 CGE; however, during the study researchers identified risk categories associated with local control. Low-risk patients were male base of skull chordomas or all base of skull chondrosarcomas, whereas high-risk patients were female base of skull chordomas or all cervical spine tumors. Researchers then changed the study design as low-risk patients continued to be randomized to 69.6 or 75.6 CGE, but high-risk patients were instead randomized to

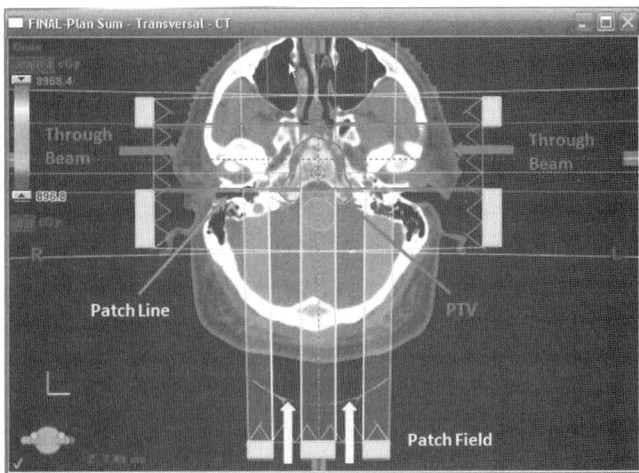

Figure 95.1 Example of proton therapy utilizing a combination of patch- and through-field techniques for treatment of clivus chordoma while sparing the brainstem. *See color insert.*

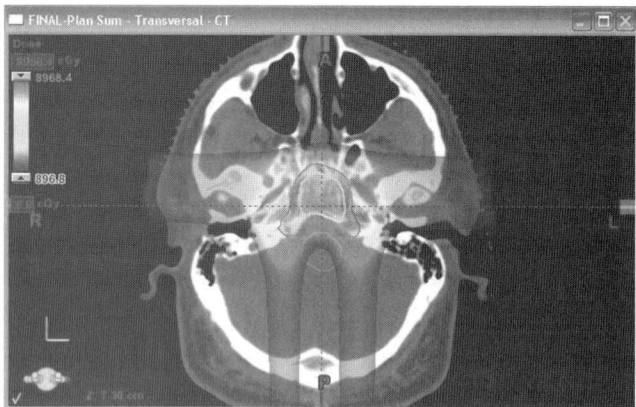

Figure 95.2 Color wash of the total dose delivered with proton therapy to treat a clivus chordoma. *See color insert.*

75.6 or 82.9 CGE [66,75]. Results from this study have not been published; however, patients enrolled in this trial have been reported in toxicity series [76] (see Toxicity section).

Particle Radiation Therapy: Carbon Ions (See Table 95.4)

An evolving technology in the treatment of chordomas is the use of heavy ion particles that have dosimetric properties similar to protons, but with the added advantage of increased RBE [81]. The initial experience with heavy particles in base of skull tumors focused on helium and neon ions [77,78]. Recently, carbon-12 ions have emerged as a viable treatment modality and have been actively explored in both Germany [79,82–85] and Japan [80,86,87]. Like protons, these ions demonstrate the "Bragg peak", that is an increase in dose with depth of penetration, such that the dose is constant until close to the end of the range when there is a sharp increase in deposited dose within the target. However, unlike protons, a tail of lighter fragments extend beyond the Bragg peak; thus, carbon ions do not share the advantage of the dose stopping sharply at the end of the particle range [88].

Carbon-12 ions also offer the unique advantage of *in vivo*, immediate post-treatment imaging as a by-product. When carbon ions penetrate a thick absorber, a fraction of the ions will undergo nuclear fragmentation to create positron-emitting isotopes carbon-11 and carbon-10. These isotopes travel approximately the same distance as the original ion, but as they have a short half-life, they annihilate to create gamma rays that can be detected in a PET scanner. Consequently, the location of the Bragg peak can be visualized immediately post therapy to verify accurate delivery of the heavy ion beam [88].

The Gesellschaft fur Schwerionenforschung in Darmstadt, Germany, has been using raster scanning carbon ion radiation therapy since 1997 and has published a series of experiences on the treatment of base of skull chordomas [79,82–85]. Using biologic plan optimization (i.e., creating an RBE of 3 within the target volume), researchers reported on 96 patients with base of skull chordomas that underwent at least one surgical procedure followed by a median 60 CGE (range 60–70) carbon ion radiotherapy. The 5-year local control and overall survival rates were 70% and 89%, respectively. Subset analysis revealed a dose response in 5-year local control as it improved from 63% for 60 CGE to 100% for >60 CGE. Late toxicity was primarily severe optic neuropathy (i.e., unilateral or bilateral blindness) in four patients (4.1%) in whom all of the affected optic nerves received a minimum dose of 60 CGE. Temporal lobe MRI changes were present in seven patients (7.2%) and increased in patients receiving >60 CGE; however, only two patients had clinically detectable toxicity [79].

Patterns of Failure

The primary pattern of failure in all base of skull chordoma and chondrosarcoma series is local despite aggressive surgical resection and adjuvant radiation therapy. As mentioned previously, gross total resection is rarely achieved due to adjacent critical structures. Similar constraints are applicable to radiotherapy planning as the risk of local recurrence is increased in regions of tumor inhomogeneity due to sparing of proximal normal structures. Solitary failures rarely occur in regional lymph nodes, surgical pathways, and distantly. More often, when these sites develop metastatic disease, they are associated with a concurrent local failure (see Natural History section) [30].

At MGH, Austin et al examined the patterns of failure of 141 patients with chordoma or chondrosarcoma of the base of skull and cervical spine treated with mixed

Table 95.4 Summary of Results With Heavy Ions for Base of Skull Chordoma and Chondrosarcoma

Author	Period	N (Patients)	Type of Particle	Tumor Dose (CGE)	% Local Control (Year)		% Overall Survival (Year)	
					5	10	5	10
Berson et al, 1988 [77]	1977–1986	45	Helium/Neon	36–80	59 (Ch/S)	–	62 (Ch/S)	–
Castro et al, 1994 [78]	1977–1992	80	Helium/Neon	60–80	63 (Ch) 78 (CS)	–	75 (Ch) 83 (CS)	–
Schulz-Ertner et al, 2007 [79]	1998–2005	96	Carbon	60–70	70 (Ch)	–	89 (Ch)	–
Mizoe et al, 2009 [80]	1995–2007	33	Carbon	48–61	85 (Ch)	64 (Ch)	88 (Ch)	67 (Ch)

Abbreviations: CGE, Cobalt gray equivalent; Ch, Chordoma; CS, Chondrosarcoma.

photon/proton radiation therapy. Local recurrence was identified in 26 patients (18%), of which 6 were completely in-field. The remainder of the failures occurred in regions of reduced dose at the margin of the target ($n = 3$), in surgical pathways not included in the target ($n = 2$), or in adjacent to critical normal structures ($n = 11$, brainstem or optic structures). Thus, the majority of failures were in regions restricted by dose constraints to the brainstem (53 CGE to center, 64 CGE to surface) and optic structures (60 CGE), suggesting that relative underdosing is the primary cause for local failure [89].

Terahara et al [90] reported on a series of 115 patients with base of skull chordomas undergoing surgical resection followed by mixed photon/proton radiation therapy. The median dose was 68.9 CGE (range 66.6–79.2) and the treatment volume included gross disease and areas with probable microscopic extension. The doses to the optic structures, brainstem surface, and brainstem center were limited to 60, 64, and 53 CGE, respectively. The 5- and 10-year local control was 59% and 44%, respectively. Gender was the strongest predictor of local control, as males had a 5-year local control of 70% compared to 53% for females. Using gender for stratification, multivariate analysis found the equivalent uniform dose, target volume, minimum tumor dose, and dose for the coolest 5 cm^3 of the tumor volume were all prognostic for local control. These dosimetric parameters suggest that tumor dose inhomogeneity and associated regional underdosage were most predictive for local control, and not for prescribed dose, median dose, maximum dose, and mean dose. In other words, lower probability of control in low-dose regions cannot be compensated by higher doses delivered to the rest of the target volume. This could also explain the lack of consistent dose response data in which the prescribed dose is often reported (not significant in this analysis) as opposed to the actual dose delivered and tumor inhomogeneity (i.e., low-dose regions) [90].

The risk for tumor inhomogeneity is directly related to the intimate contact of the tumor with normal critical structures. Some analyses have suggested tumor size is prognostic for local control [26,68,77,91], but it more likely serves as a surrogate for an inability to deliver uniform dose due to normal tissue constraints. As such, for tumors in contact with critical structures, initial or repeat surgical intervention should focus on creating space between the two to facilitate optimal radiation therapy delivery [67].

Salvage

Local recurrence portends a very poor prognosis as salvage treatment options are often limited to repeat surgical intervention or reirradiation. Chemotherapy use is rarely reported for these tumors and not routinely considered a viable option.

The Princess Margaret Hospital examined the outcomes of 15 patients with a local recurrence following adjuvant photon radiation. Six patients were treated with surgery alone (4 clival, 2 lumbar), 8 patients with reirradiation (2 clival, 5 sacral, 1 lumbar), and 1 patient with a sacral chordoma was treated with both surgery and reirradiation. The median reirradiation dose was 32 Gy (range 18–55) and the total cumulative dose was 78 Gy (range 44–105; 72 Gy and 75 Gy for the 2 clival tumors). The median survival after retreatment was 18 months (range 3–120) and none of the reirradiated patients suffered treatment-related complications; however, one patient died from surgical complications. Two patients with reirradiation had symptom control for 5 and 9 years [54].

Fagundes et al reported on 60 patients with local failure after mixed photon/proton radiotherapy, of which 49 received salvage therapy and 11 received supportive care. Among those who had salvage therapy, 46 patients had surgical resection (2 with additional radiation, another 2 with chemotherapy +/− radiation), 1 patient had radiation alone, 1 patient had chemotherapy alone, and 1 patient had chemotherapy and radiation. Following salvage, 14% had stable or improved symptoms without disease progression, 53% had initial stable or improved symptoms but eventual disease progression, and 33% did not respond to treatment. The 2- and 5- year survival for these patients was 63% and 6%, respectively, which compared favorably with the 2-year survival of 21% for those with supportive care only ($P = 0.0001$) [30].

TOXICITY

The primary challenge in the treatment of base of skull tumors is the preservation of multiple critical central nervous system structures. The clivus is situated in close proximity to the brainstem, cavernous sinus, optic chiasm, and pituitary gland, thus providing significant stereotactic and dosimetric challenges for both surgery and radiation, respectively. The morbidity and mortality from multidisciplinary treatments are defined by both the tumor bulk and location in addition to the techniques utilized. Due to these constraints, opinion strongly favors proton therapy as the optimal treatment of choice following organ-preserving surgical resection. However, even though particle therapy offers a superior dosimetric advantage over photon therapy, it is not without significant side effects as dose escalation is necessary to provide maximum local control.

Surgery

The incidence of postoperative complications following craniotomy is dependent on extent of the tumor, involvement of adjacent organs, surgical approach, and most importantly, surgeon experience. Al-Mefty et al reported in their series of 23 patients undergoing craniotomy that there was one postoperative death and two permanent neurologic deficits (visual field, cranial nerve III). Temporary complications included cerebrospinal fluid leak, meningitis, cranial nerve VII palsy, oronasal fistula, cranial nerve V palsy, and cranial nerve VI palsy [34].

At the University of Pittsburgh, in a series of 60 patients undergoing modern microsurgical techniques, Gay et al reported that 3 patients died within 3 months from the operation due to pulmonary embolism and myocardial infarction, of which one was recovering from quadriparesis. Two patients (3%) had postoperative myocardial infarcts and 3 patients (5%) had wound infections. Remarkably, 18 patients (30%) experienced cerebrospinal fluid leakage, of which 6 patients (10%) had associated meningitis. Also notable was that 48 patients (80%) suffered a new cranial nerve deficit. Cranial nerve VI palsy occurred in 28%, hearing loss in 15%, permanent facial paresis in 8%, and visual decline or loss in 8%. In total, there were 92 new cranial nerve deficits in this population of 60 patients [22].

Brain

Using patients enrolled into the prospective dose-searching study, the Proton Radiation Oncology Group protocol 85–26, Santoni et al investigated the incidence of temporal lobe toxicity in 96 patients with initial surgical intervention (biopsy or subtotal resection) followed by randomization to either 66.6 or 72 CGE combined photon/proton radiation therapy. The actual median total dose delivered was 68.4 CGE (range 64.8–72 CGE). The photon portion was delivered once per week with total dose ranging from 5.4 to 36 Gy (median 12.6), whereas the proton portion was delivered four times per week with total dose ranging from 30.6 to 66.2 CGE (median 30.6).

Based on clinical symptoms and MRI, 10 patients experienced temporal lobe damage for a 2- and 5-year incidence of 7.6% and 13.2%, respectively. Symptoms included deficits in mental status, memory, and motor function or new onset seizure disorders. Of 8 patients with severe toxicity, 3 required surgical resection of abnormal areas with pathology confirming radionecrosis. On univariate and stepwise Cox analysis, only male gender was predictive of late toxicity. Total dose and volume of temporal lobe receiving up to 50 Gy (in 10 Gy intervals) were not significant [76].

The functional impact of temporal lobe radiation was evaluated in a prospective study performed on 17 patients with base of skull tumors treated to a median 68.4 CGE (range 66.6–72) with mixed photon/proton radiation therapy [92]. The temporal lobes on average received a total of 50 to 60 CGE. A comprehensive battery of neurocognitive tests was utilized to assess intelligence/conceptual reasoning, language and visuospatial processing, memory, attention, motor function, and psychiatric function at four different time points. The findings were remarkable for a mild slowing of performance time and motor functions associated with increased radiation doses to the temporal lobes. Interestingly, there was actually an improvement in depression, mood, and anxiety. No interval change could be identified in intelligence, memory, rate of learning, fatigue, or cognitive efficiency [92].

Brainstem

In an experience from the MGH, researchers analyzed the incidence of brainstem toxicity in a series of 367 patients with chordomas and chondrosarcomas of the base of skull treated with combined megavoltage photon and proton radiotherapy. All patients initially had at least one surgical procedure followed by a mean target dose of 67.8 CGE (range 63–79.2). Multiple fields were used to minimize dose to adjacent critical structures, especially the brainstem. Dose to the brainstem was limited to ≤64 CGE to the surface and ≤54 CGE to the center, and the average maximum dose received was 62.2 CGE.

Brainstem symptoms were reported in 19 of 348 (5.5%) evaluable patients, of which 3 patients (0.9%) died from treatment-related toxicity. The mean time to symptoms was 17 months (range 4.5–92) and the 5- and 10-year freedom from high-grade brainstem toxicity was 94% and 88%, respectively. Presentation included complex neurologic findings with a combination of paresis, ataxia, motor, and sensory symptoms. On multivariate analysis, more than one surgical procedure, diabetes mellitus, and the brainstem volume receiving ≥60 CGE were associated with increased toxicity. Dosimetric analysis revealed that if the volume of brainstem receiving ≥60 CGE was ≤0.9 cc, the 10-year toxicity-free survival was 96%, whereas it was 79% if >0.9 cc ($P = 0.001$) [93].

Spinal Cord

The cervical spine is in the radiation field for patients with tumors of the lower clivus that extend inferiorly or primary tumors of the cervical vertebrae. Liu et al reported on a series of 78 patients treated with mixed photon/proton radiotherapy for chordomas and chondrosarcomas of the cervical spine. These patients were treated to a total dose of 64.5 to 79.2 CGE, and for treatment planning, dose constraints were ≤64 CGE to the surface and ≤55 CGE to the center of the spinal cord. During a mean follow-up of almost 4 years, four patients (5.1%) experienced high-grade late toxicity, with three patients developing sensory deficits without motor symptoms and one patient losing motor function of an upper extremity. This latter patient actually had prior radiation, and thus received greater cumulative dose than what was used as a constraint for treatment planning. Other reported toxicities included 6 patients (7.7%) with Lhermitte's syndrome and 1 patient (1.2%) with MRI changes but no symptoms. Analysis of risk factors suggested that the proton portion of tumor dose >55 CGE and spinal cord surface dose >60 CGE had increased the risk of cervical myelopathy [94].

Marucci et al reported a series of 85 patients treated for chordoma and chondrosarcoma of cervical vertebra tumors treated with mixed photon/proton radiotherapy. Patients were treated to a mean of 76.3 CGE (range 68.6–83.5) and limited the surface and center of the spinal cord to 67 to 70 and 55 to 58 CGE, respectively. With a median of 6 months (range 3–49) to developing toxicity, 13 patients (15.2%) experienced mild toxicity and 4 patients (4.7%) severe toxicity. The only significant factor predictive of toxicity was the number of preradiotherapy surgeries, and not any dosimetric factors such as total dose, cord length or volume, maximum dose, proton dose, or equivalent uniform dose. The authors recommended that 60 Gy in 1.5 Gy fractions or 52.5 Gy in 2 Gy fractions were considered safe doses for the cervical spinal cord [95].

Vision

Base of skull tumors are immediately adjacent to the optic chiasm and are often displaced or involved with tumors originating in the upper clivus. This proximity predisposes both the optic chiasm and optic nerves to be in regions of high-dose radiation. Habrand et al reported on a series of 15 patients with base of skull tumors who had known pretreatment neurovisual function. All were treated with surgery (biopsy or subtotal resection) followed by adjuvant radiation to a median 69.7 CGE (range 66.6–74.4). At a median follow-up of 52 months (range 30–68), the authors reported that two patients developed loss of vision with injury to both optic nerve and chiasm. Dosimetric analysis suggested that the risk of toxicity increased from 12.5% to 22% when the >20% of the optic nerve received 55 CGE and 60 CGE, respectively. The risk for optic chiasm injury was estimated to be 7.5% at 55 CGE [96].

In an updated series from the same institution, Kim et al identified 12 of 274 patients (4.4%) treated for base of skull tumors that eventually developed radiation-induced optic neuropathy. Patients were treated to a total dose of 61 to 76 CGE and the median time to presentation of visual loss was 12 months (range 7–40). The authors compared clinical and dosimetric factors to 24 matched patients who did not develop toxicity, and discovered the only factor significant on analysis was the "patch distance." The patch technique shapes dose around critical structures by using one portal to treat one segment and another portal to treat the remainder of the target. Areas of dose overlap subsequently lead to hot spots, and in this series, patients with optic neuropathy had significantly smaller patch distances (i.e., space between portals) [97].

A potential strategy to decrease the risk of radiation-induced optic neuropathy is with hyperfractionation. Bhandare et al analyzed a series of 273 patients with nasopharyngeal, paranasal, and nasal cavity cancers treated with radiation therapy and found 24 patients (9%) developed optic neuropathy at a median 2.5 years (range 0.9–6.5). Univariate analysis revealed total dose was predictive of optic neuropathy, as the 5-year freedom from neuropathy was 96% for ≤63 Gy vs. 83% for >63 Gy (P = 0.0021). For patients receiving >63 Gy, twice daily treatment (i.e., hyperfractionation) significantly improved the 5-year freedom from neuropathy over once daily treatment (91% vs. 78%, P = 0.0019) [98]. At the University of Florida Proton Therapy Institute, the proton therapy protocol for skull-base chordomas and chondrosarcomas uses a hyperfractionation scheme to reduce toxicity to both the optic nerves and the chiasm.

Hearing

Schoenthaler et al reported on a series of 25 patients with base of skull tumors with normal pretreatment audiograms and subsequent post-treatment evaluation. Moderate to severe hearing loss was identified in six patients (24%) and all had received >60 CGE to the cochlea and auditory nerve. The interval to hearing loss ranged from 8 to 60 months and the deficit was progressive, not acute. No dose response was observed in the range of 60 to 72 CGE; however, the authors suggested that the risk of hearing loss increased if 50% of the auditory nerve or cochlea received >60 CGE [99]. Similarly, Bhandare et al analyzed a series of 325 patients with nasopharyngeal, paranasal, and nasal cavity cancers treated with radiation therapy and found 49 patients (15%) developed sensorineural hearing loss at a median 1.8 years (range 0.5–5.9). Univariate analysis revealed total dose was predictive of auditory toxicity, as the 5-year incidence of sensorineural hearing loss was 3% for ≤60.5 Gy vs. 37% for >60.5 Gy ($P > 0.0001$) [100].

The dose constraint for the auditory nerve is similar to a prior analysis that examined the incidence of injury to all cranial nerves in patients treated for base of skull tumors. Urie et al reported on a series of 27 patients of which 5 patients developed various cranial neuropathies. Dosimetric analysis suggested that all the cranial nerves had equal sensitivity to radiation and the maximum dose was the best predictor for toxicity. For cranial nerves receiving >60 CGE, there was a 1% risk of complications, and it increased to 5% when dose >70 CGE [101].

Endocrine

For base of skull tumors of the upper clivus, both the pituitary gland and hypothalamus are often encompassed by the high doses of radiation therapy delivered to the target. Pai et al reported on the incidence of endocrine toxicity in a series of 107 patients with mostly chordomas and chondrosarcomas of the base of skull. Following biopsy or subtotal resection, patients received a median total dose 68.4 CGE (range 55.8–79) of adjuvant mixed photon/proton radiotherapy. The 5- and 10- year rates of endocrinopathy were 72% and 84% for hyperprolactinemia, 30% and 63% for hypothyroidism, 29% and 36% for hypogonadism, and 19% and 28% for hypoadrenalism. Growth hormone was not routinely checked, but it was notable that no patient developed diabetes insipidus secondary to vasopressin deficiency. Only 13% of patients had no evidence of endocrine sequelae at 10 years. Of those with an endocrine deficiency, 52% had one axis affected, 26% had 2, 15% had 3, and 6% had 4 axes affected.

Dosimetric analysis demonstrated that no patients developed an endocrine deficiency if the minimum dose (Dmin) to the pituitary gland was <50 CGE. However, for a Dmin >50 CGE, there was a statistically significant increase in hyperprolactinemia and number of endocrinopathies observed. If the maximum dose (Dmax) to the pituitary gland was >70 CGE, there was an increased incidence of hypogonadism and hypoadrenalism. The pituitary gland appeared to have a higher tolerance than the hypothalamus, as a Dmax >50 CGE for the latter was significantly associated with hypothyroidism with trends for hyperprolactinemia and hypoadrenalism. As pituitary dysfunction can present as late as 10 years post treatment, these patients must have lifelong endocrine follow-up [102,103].

CONCLUSIONS

Chordomas and chondrosarcomas have a generally slow rate of growth, are locally invasive, and often occur at the base of skull juxtaposed to the spheno-occiptial region. The complex shape of these tumors coupled with the proximity of critical structures provides a difficult management scenario. Optimal surgical debulking from surrounding critical structures followed by fractionated three-dimensional conformal high-dose proton therapy offers the best chance of local control and survival in these patients.

REFERENCES

1. Meyers SP, Hirsch WL Jr, Curtin HD, Barnes L, Sekhar LN, Sen C. Chordomas of the skull base: MR features. *AJNR Am J Neuroradiol.* 1992;13(6):1627–1636.
2. Weber AL, Liebsch NJ, Sanchez R, Sweriduk ST Jr. Chordomas of the skull base. Radiologic and clinical evaluation. *Neuroimaging Clin N Am.* 1994;4(3):515–527.
3. Volpe NJ, Liebsch NJ, Munzenrider JE, Lessell S. Neuro-ophthalmologic findings in chordoma and chondrosarcoma of the skull base. *Am J Ophthalmol.* 1993;115(1):97–104.
4. Doucet V, Peretti-Viton P, Figarella-Branger D, Manera L, Salamon G. MRI of intracranial chordomas. Extent of tumour and contrast enhancement: criteria for differential diagnosis. *Neuroradiology.* 1997;39(8):571–576.
5. Oot RF, Melville GE, New PF, et al. The role of MR and CT in evaluating clival chordomas and chondrosarcomas. *AJR Am J Roentgenol.* 1988;151(3):567–575.
6. Soo MY. Chordoma: review of clinicoradiological features and factors affecting survival. *Australas Radiol.* 2001;45(4):427–434.
7. Brown RV, Sage MR, Brophy BP. CT and MR findings in patients with chordomas of the petrous apex. *AJNR Am J Neuroradiol.* 1990;11(1):121–124.
8. Singh W, Kaur A. Nasopharyngeal chordoma presenting with metastases. Case report and review of literature. *J Laryngol Otol.* 1987;101(11):1198–1202.
9. Yuh WT, Flickinger FW, Barloon TJ, Montgomery WJ. MR imaging of unusual chordomas. *J Comput Assist Tomogr.* 1988;12(1):30–35.
10. Knott PD, Gannon FH, Thompson LD. Mesenchymal chondrosarcoma of the sinonasal tract: a clinicopathological study of 13 cases with a review of the literature. *Laryngoscope.* 2003;113(5):783–790.
11. Rosenberg AE, Nielsen GP, Keel SB, et al. Chondrosarcoma of the base of the skull: a clinicopathologic study of 200 cases with emphasis on its distinction from chordoma. *Am J Surg Pathol.* 1999;23(11):1370–1378.
12. McMaster ML, Goldstein AM, Bromley CM, Ishibe N, Parry DM. Chordoma: incidence and survival patterns in the United States, 1973–1995. *Cancer Causes Control.* 2001;12(1):1–11.
13. Mapstone TB, Kaufman B, Ratcheson RA. Intradural chordoma without bone involvement: nuclear magnetic resonance (NMR) appearance. Case report. *J Neurosurg.* 1983;59(3):535–537.
14. Richter HJ Jr, Batsakis JG, Boles R. Chordomas: nasopharyngeal presentation and atypical long survival. *Ann Otol Rhinol Laryngol.* 1975;84(3 Pt 1):327–332.
15. Shugar JM, Som PM, Krespi YP, Arnold LM, Som ML. Primary chordoma of the maxillary sinus. *Laryngoscope.* 1980;90(11 Pt 1):1825–1830.
16. Heffelfinger MJ, Dahlin DC, MacCarty CS, Beabout JW. Chordomas and cartilaginous tumors at the skull base. *Cancer.* 1973;32(2):410–420.
17. Giuffrida AY, Burgueno JE, Koniaris LG, Gutierrez JC, Duncan R, Scully SP. Chondrosarcoma in the United States (1973 to 2003): an analysis of 2890 cases from the SEER database. *J Bone Joint Surg Am.* 2009;91(5):1063–1072.
18. Halperin EC. Why is female sex an independent predictor of shortened overall survival after proton/photon radiation therapy for skull base chordomas? *Int J Radiat Oncol Biol Phys.* 1997;38(2):225–230.
19. Rich TA, Schiller A, Suit HD, Mankin HJ. Clinical and pathologic review of 48 cases of chordoma. *Cancer.* 1985;56(1):182–187.
20. Crapanzano JP, Ali SZ, Ginsberg MS, Zakowski MF. Chordoma: a cytologic study with histologic and radiologic correlation. *Cancer.* 2001;93(1):40–51.
21. Rosenberg AE, Brown GA, Bhan AK, Lee JM. Chondroid chordoma—a variant of chordoma. A morphologic and immunohistochemical study. *Am J Clin Pathol.* 1994;101(1):36–41.
22. Gay E, Sekhar LN, Rubinstein E, et al. Chordomas and chondrosarcomas of the cranial base: results and follow-up of 60 patients. *Neurosurgery.* 1995;36(5):887–896; discussion 896.
23. Forsyth PA, Cascino TL, Shaw EG, et al. Intracranial chordomas: a clinicopathological and prognostic study of 51 cases. *J Neurosurg.* 1993;78(5):741–747.
24. Colli B, Al-Mefty O. Chordomas of the craniocervical junction: follow-up review and prognostic factors. *J Neurosurg.* 2001;95(6):933–943.
25. Mitchell A, Scheithauer BW, Unni KK, Forsyth PJ, Wold LE, McGivney DJ. Chordoma and chondroid neoplasms of the spheno-occiput. An immunohistochemical study of 41 cases with prognostic and nosologic implications. *Cancer.* 1993;72(10):2943–2949.
26. O'Connell JX, Renard LG, Liebsch NJ, Efird JT, Munzenrider JE, Rosenberg AE. Base of skull chordoma. A correlative study of histologic and clinical features of 62 cases. *Cancer.* 1994;74:2261–2267.
27. Ishida T, Dorfman HD. Chondroid chordoma versus low-grade chondrosarcoma of the base of the skull: can immunohistochemistry resolve the controversy? *J Neurooncol.* 1994;18(3):199–206.
28. Juliao SF, Rand N, Schwartz HS. Galectin-3: a biologic marker and diagnostic aid for chordoma. *Clin Orthop Relat Res.* 2002;397:70–75.
29. Naka T, Oda Y, Iwamoto Y, et al. Immunohistochemical analysis of E-cadherin, alpha-catenin, beta-catenin, gamma-catenin, and neural cell adhesion molecule (NCAM) in chordoma. *J Clin Pathol.* 2001;54(12):945–950.
30. Fagundes MA, Hug EB, Liebsch NJ, Daly W, Efird J, Munzenrider JE. Radiation therapy for chordomas of the base of skull and cervical spine: patterns of failure and outcome after relapse. *Int J Radiat Oncol Biol Phys.* 1995;33(3):579–584.
31. Fischbein NJ, Kaplan MJ, Holliday RA, Dillon WP. Recurrence of clival chordoma along the surgical pathway. *AJNR Am J Neuroradiol.* 2000;21(3):578–583.
32. Fuller DB, Bloom JG. Radiotherapy for chordoma. *Int J Radiat Oncol Biol Phys.* 1988;15(2):331–339.
33. Lybeert ML, Meerwaldt JH. Chordoma. Report on treatment results in eighteen cases. *Acta Radiol Oncol.* 1986;25(1):41–43.
34. al-Mefty O, Borba LA. Skull base chordomas: a management challenge. *J Neurosurg.* 1997;86(2):182–189.
35. Grossman RI, Davis KR. Cranial computed tomographic appearance of chondrosarcoma of the base of the skull. *Radiology.* 1981;141(2):403–408.
36. Al-Mefty O, Colli B, Angtuaco EJ, Hug E. Chordomas and Chondrosarcomas of the Cranial Base. In: Berger MS, Prados MD, eds. *Textbook of Neuro-oncology.* 1st ed. Philadelphia: Elsevier Saunders; 2005:357–365.
37. Meyer JE, Oot RF, Lindfors KK. CT appearance of clival chordomas. *J Comput Assist Tomogr.* 1986;10(1):34–38.
38. Maclean FM, Soo MY, Ng T. Chordoma: radiological-pathological correlation. *Australas Radiol.* 2005;49(4):261–268.
39. Sze G, Uichanco LS 3rd, Brant-Zawadzki MN, et al. Chordomas: MR imaging. *Radiology.* 1988;166(1 Pt 1):187–191.
40. Adler LP, Blair HF, Makley JT, et al. Noninvasive grading of musculoskeletal tumors using PET. *J Nucl Med.* 1991;32(8):1508–1512.
41. Kern KA, Brunetti A, Norton JA, et al. Metabolic imaging of human extremity musculoskeletal tumors by PET. *J Nucl Med.* 1988;29(2):181–186.
42. Aoki J, Watanabe H, Shinozaki T, et al. FDG PET of primary benign and malignant bone tumors: standardized uptake value in 52 lesions. *Radiology.* 2001;219(3):774–777.
43. Lin CY, Kao CH, Liang JA, Hsieh TC, Yen KY, Sun SS. Chordoma detected on F-18 FDG PET. *Clin Nucl Med.* 2006;31(8):506–507.
44. Miyazawa N, Ishigame K, Kato S, Satoh Y, Shinohara T. Thoracic chordoma: review and role of FDG-PET. *J Neurosurg Sci.* 2008;52(4):117–121; discussion 121.
45. Park SA, Kim HS. F-18 FDG PET/CT evaluation of sacrococcygeal chordoma. *Clin Nucl Med.* 2008;33(12):906–908.
46. Kay PA, Nascimento AG, Unni KK, Salomão DR. Chordoma. Cytomorphologic findings in 14 cases diagnosed by fine needle aspiration. *Acta Cytol.* 2003;47(2):202–208.
47. Bergh P, Kindblom LG, Gunterberg B, Remotti F, Ryd W, Meis-Kindblom JM. Prognostic factors in chordoma of the sacrum and mobile spine: a study of 39 patients. *Cancer.* 2000;88(9):2122–2134.
48. Watkins L, Khudados ES, Kaleoglu M, Revesz T, Sacares P, Crockard HA. Skull base chordomas: a review of 38 patients, 1958–88. *Br J Neurosurg.* 1993;7(3):241–248.

49. Tai PT, Craighead P, Bagdon F. Optimization of radiotherapy for patients with cranial chordoma. A review of dose-response ratios for photon techniques. *Cancer*. 1995;75(3):749–756.
50. Cummings BJ, Hodson DI, Bush RS. Chordoma: the results of megavoltage radiation therapy. *Int J Radiat Oncol Biol Phys*. 1983;9(5): 633–642.
51. Amendola BE, Amendola MA, Oliver E, McClatchey KD. Chordoma: role of radiation therapy. *Radiology*. 1986;158(3):839–843.
52. Magrini SM, Papi MG, Marletta F, et al. Chordoma-natural history, treatment and prognosis. The Florence Radiotherapy Department experience (1956–1990) and a critical review of the literature. *Acta Oncol*. 1992;31(8):847–851.
53. Romero J, Cardenes H, la Torre A, et al. Chordoma: results of radiation therapy in eighteen patients. *Radiother Oncol*. 1993;29(1):27–32.
54. Catton C, O'Sullivan B, Bell R, et al. Chordoma: long-term follow-up after radical photon irradiation. *Radiother Oncol*. 1996;41(1):67–72.
55. Zorlu F, Gürkaynak M, Yildiz F, Oge K, Atahan IL. Conventional external radiotherapy in the management of clivus chordomas with overt residual disease. *Neurol Sci*. 2000;21(4):203–207.
56. Debus J, Schulz-Ertner D, Schad L, et al. Stereotactic fractionated radiotherapy for chordomas and chondrosarcomas of the skull base. *Int J Radiat Oncol Biol Phys*. 2000;47:591–596.
57. Pearlman AW, Friedman M. Radical radiation therapy of chordoma. *Am J Roentgenol Radium Ther Nucl Med*. 1970;108(2):332–341.
58. Higinbotham NL, Phillips RF, Farr HW, Hustu HO. Chordoma. Thirty-five-year study at Memorial Hospital. *Cancer*. 1967;20(11):1841–1850.
59. Tewfik HH, McGinnis WL, Nordstrom DG, Latourette HB. Chordoma: evaluation of clinical behavior and treatment modalities. *Int J Radiat Oncol Biol Phys*. 1977;2(9–10):959–962.
60. Tai PT, Bauman G. Photon Irradiation. In: Harsh G, Janecka IP, Mankin H, Ojemann R, eds. *Chordomas and Chondrosarcomas of the Skull Base and Spine*. 1st ed. New York: Thieme; 2003.
61. Saxton JP. Chordoma. *Int J Radiat Oncol Biol Phys*. 1981;7(7):913–915.
62. Krishnan S, Foote RL, Brown PD, Pollock BE, Link MJ, Garces YI. Radiosurgery for cranial base chordomas and chondrosarcomas. *Neurosurgery*. 2005;56(4):777–784; discussion 777.
63. Hasegawa T, Ishii D, Kida Y, Yoshimoto M, Koike J, Iizuka H. Gamma Knife surgery for skull base chordomas and chondrosarcomas. *J Neurosurg*. 2007;107(4):752–757.
64. Martin JJ, Niranjan A, Kondziolka D, Flickinger JC, Lozanne KA, Lunsford LD. Radiosurgery for chordomas and chondrosarcomas of the skull base. *J Neurosurg*. 2007;107(4):758–764.
65. Hug EB, Loredo LN, Slater JD, et al. Proton radiation therapy for chordomas and chondrosarcomas of the skull base. *J Neurosurg*. 1999;91(3):432–439.
66. Munzenrider JE, Liebsch NJ. Proton therapy for tumors of the skull base. *Strahlenther Onkol*. 1999;175(Suppl 2):57–63.
67. Noël G, Feuvret L, Calugaru V, et al. Chordomas of the base of the skull and upper cervical spine. One hundred patients irradiated by a 3D conformal technique combining photon and proton beams. *Acta Oncol*. 2005;44(7):700–708.
68. Ares C, Hug EB, Lomax AJ, et al. Effectiveness and safety of spot scanning proton radiation therapy for chordomas and chondrosarcomas of the skull base: first long-term report. *Int J Radiat Oncol Biol Phys*. 2009;75(4):1111–1118.
69. Igaki H, Tokuuye K, Okumura T, et al. Clinical results of proton beam therapy for skull base chordoma. *Int J Radiat Oncol Biol Phys*. 2004;60(4):1120–1126.
70. Proton therapy for base of skull chordoma: a report for the Royal College of Radiologists. The Proton Therapy Working Party. *Clin Oncol (R Coll Radiol)*. 2000;12:75–79.
71. Austin-Seymour M, Urie M, Munzenrider J, et al. Considerations in fractionated proton radiation therapy: clinical potential and results. *Radiother Oncol*. 1990;17(1):29–35.
72. Urano M, Verhey LJ, Goitein M, et al. Relative biological effectiveness of modulated proton beams in various murine tissues. *Int J Radiat Oncol Biol Phys*. 1984;10(4):509–514.
73. Powell SN, Harsh G. Radiobiology and the proton beam. In: Harsh G, Janecka IP, Mankin H, Ojemann R, eds. *Chordomas and Chondrosarcomas of the Skull Base and Spine*. 1st ed. New York: Thieme; 2003:287–298.
74. Weber DC, Rutz HP, Pedroni ES, et al. Results of spot-scanning proton radiation therapy for chordoma and chondrosarcoma of the skull base: the Paul Scherrer Institut experience. *Int J Radiat Oncol Biol Phys*. 2005;63(2):401–409.
75. Liebsch N, Munzenrider J. Proton radiotherapy for cranial base chordomas. In: Harsh G, Janecka IP, Mankin H, Ojemann R, eds. *Chordomas and Chondrosarcomas of the Skull Base and Spine*. 1st ed. New York: Thieme; 2003:307–314.
76. Santoni R, Liebsch N, Finkelstein DM, et al. Temporal lobe (TL) damage following surgery and high-dose photon and proton irradiation in 96 patients affected by chordomas and chondrosarcomas of the base of the skull. *Int J Radiat Oncol Biol Phys*. 1998;41(1):59–68.
77. Berson AM, Castro JR, Petti P, et al. Charged particle irradiation of chordoma and chondrosarcoma of the base of skull and cervical spine: the Lawrence Berkeley Laboratory experience. *Int J Radiat Oncol Biol Phys*. 1988;15(3):559–565.
78. Castro JR, Linstadt DE, Bahary JP, et al. Experience in charged particle irradiation of tumors of the skull base: 1977–1992. *Int J Radiat Oncol Biol Phys*. 1994;29(4):647–655.
79. Schulz-Ertner D, Karger CP, Feuerhake A, et al. Effectiveness of carbon ion radiotherapy in the treatment of skull-base chordomas. *Int J Radiat Oncol Biol Phys*. 2007;68(2):449–457.
80. Mizoe JE, Hasegawa A, Takagi R, Bessho H, Onda T, Tsujii H. Carbon ion radiotherapy for skull base chordoma. *Skull Base*. 2009;19(3):219–224.
81. Kraft G. RBE and its interpretation. *Strahlenther Onkol*. 1999;175(Suppl 2):44–47.
82. Schulz-Ertner D, Nikoghosyan A, Thilmann C, et al. Results of carbon ion radiotherapy in 152 patients. *Int J Radiat Oncol Biol Phys*. 2004;58(2):631–640.
83. Schulz-Ertner D, Nikoghosyan A, Thilmann C, et al. Carbon ion radiotherapy for chordomas and low-grade chondrosarcomas of the skull base. Results in 67 patients. *Strahlenther Onkol*. 2003;179(9): 598–605.
84. Schulz-Ertner D, Haberer T, Jäkel O, et al. Radiotherapy for chordomas and low-grade chondrosarcomas of the skull base with carbon ions. *Int J Radiat Oncol Biol Phys*. 2002;53(1):36–42.
85. Schulz-Ertner D, Haberer T, Scholz M, et al. Acute radiation-induced toxicity of heavy ion radiotherapy delivered with intensity modulated pencil beam scanning in patients with base of skull tumors. *Radiother Oncol*. 2002;64(2):189–195.
86. Takahashi S, Kawase T, Yoshida K, Hasegawa A, Mizoe JE. Skull base chordomas: efficacy of surgery followed by carbon ion radiotherapy. *Acta Neurochir (Wien)*. 2009;151(7):759–769.
87. Tsujii H, Mizoe JE, Kamada T, et al. Overview of clinical experiences on carbon ion radiotherapy at NIRS. *Radiother Oncol*. 2004;73(Suppl 2):S41-S49.
88. Hall EJ, Giaccia AJ. *Radiobiology for the Radiologist*. 6th ed. Philadelphia: Lippincott Williams & Wilkins; 2006.
89. Austin JP, Urie MM, Cardenosa G, Munzenrider JE. Probable causes of recurrence in patients with chordoma and chondrosarcoma of the base of skull and cervical spine. *Int J Radiat Oncol Biol Phys*. 1993;25(3):439–444.
90. Terahara A, Niemierko A, Goitein M, et al. Analysis of the relationship between tumor dose inhomogeneity and local control in patients with skull base chordoma. *Int J Radiat Oncol Biol Phys*. 1999;45(2): 351–358.
91. Noël G, Habrand JL, Jauffret E, et al. Radiation therapy for chordoma and chondrosarcoma of the skull base and the cervical spine. Prognostic factors and patterns of failure. *Strahlenther Onkol*. 2003;179(4):241–248.
92. Glosser G, McManus P, Munzenrider J, et al. Neuropsychological function in adults after high dose fractionated radiation therapy of skull base tumors. *Int J Radiat Oncol Biol Phys*. 1997;38(2): 231–239.
93. Debus J, Hug EB, Liebsch NJ, et al. Brainstem tolerance to conformal radiotherapy of skull base tumors. *Int J Radiat Oncol Biol Phys*. 1997;39(5):967–975.
94. Liu MCC, Munzenrider J, Finkelstein D, Liebsch N, Adams J, Hug E. Radiation tolerance of the cervical spinal cord: Incidence and dose-volume relationship of symptomatic and asymptomatic late effects following high dose irradiation of paraspinal tumors. *Int J Radiat Oncol Biol Phys*. 1997;39:1.
95. Marucci L, Niemierko A, Liebsch NJ, Aboubaker F, Liu MC, Munzenrider JE. Spinal cord tolerance to high-dose fractionated 3D conformal proton-photon irradiation as evaluated by equivalent uniform dose and dose volume histogram analysis. *Int J Radiat Oncol Biol Phys*. 2004;59(2):551–555.

96. Habrand IL, Austin-Seymour M, Birnbaum S, et al. Neurovisual outcome following proton radiation therapy. *Int J Radiat Oncol Biol Phys.* 1989;16(6):1601–1606.
97. Kim J, Munzenrider J, Maas A, et al. Optic neuropathy following combined proton and photon radiotherapy for base of skull tumors. *Int J Radiat Oncol Biol Phys.* 1997;39:1.
98. Bhandare N, Monroe AT, Morris CG, Bhatti MT, Mendenhall WM. Does altered fractionation influence the risk of radiation-induced optic neuropathy? *Int J Radiat Oncol Biol Phys.* 2005;62:1070–1077.
99. Schoenthaler R, Fullerton BC, Maas AV, et al. Relationship between dose to auditory pathways and audiological outcomes in skull-base tumor patients receiving high-dose proton-photon radiotherapy. *Int J Radiat Oncol Biol Phys.* 1996;36:1.
100. Bhandare N, Antonelli PJ, Morris CG, Malayapa RS, Mendenhall WM. Ototoxicity after radiotherapy for head and neck tumors. *Int J Radiat Oncol Biol Phys.* 2007;67(2):469–479.
101. Urie MM, Fullerton B, Tatsuzaki H, et al. A dose response analysis of injury to cranial nerves and/or nuclei following proton beam radiation therapy. *Int J Radiat Oncol Biol Phys.* 1992;23(1):27–39.
102. Pai HH, Thornton A, Katznelson L, et al. Hypothalamic/pituitary function following high-dose conformal radiotherapy to the base of skull: demonstration of a dose-effect relationship using dose-volume histogram analysis. *Int J Radiat Oncol Biol Phys.* 2001;49(4):1079–1092.
103. Slater JD, Austin-Seymour M, Munzenrider J, et al. Endocrine function following high dose proton therapy for tumors of the upper clivus. *Int J Radiat Oncol Biol Phys.* 1988;15(3):607–611.

96 Pituitary Tumors and Craniopharyngioma

Tim J. Kruser, Vinai Gondi, and Minesh P. Mehta

The differential diagnosis of lesions in the sella turcica includes pituitary adenomas (both functional and nonfunctional), craniopharyngioma, meningioma, chordoma, lymphoma, germ cell tumor, metastases, and nonmalignant lesions such as inflammatory processes and cysts. Pituitary adenomas can be further classified into tumors of the anterior or posterior pituitary. This chapter will focus on radiotherapy for anterior pituitary adenomas and craniopharyngiomas, the two most common pathologic entities of the sella turcica.

BACKGROUND

Pituitary Adenoma

Pituitary adenomas comprise 10% to 15% of all intracranial tumors. Roughly 70% of these tumors are hormone secreting, frequently presenting as microadenomas (size less than 1 cm). Goals of treatment in these instances are to normalize endocrine abnormalities and prevent further tumor growth. Nonsecretory (nonfunctioning) adenomas account for the remaining 30% of pituitary adenomas. These tumors are typically macroadenomas (greater than 1 cm) at presentation and become clinically apparent secondary to mass effect. This often manifests as bitemporal hemianopsia due to impingement of the optic chiasm and/or panhypopituitarism due to disruption of the hypothalamic-pituitary axis. In this case, goals of therapy focus on preservation of vision, control of further tumor growth, and maintenance of adequate endocrine function via the hypothalamic-pituitary axis. While medical therapy with dopamine agonists is the first-line approach in prolactin-secreting tumors, surgical resection, usually via transsphenoidal approach, is a mainstay in the management of most pituitary adenomas.

Craniopharyngioma

Despite their benign histology, craniopharyngiomas pose multiple challenges toward optimizing treatment. Arising from epithelial remnants of Rathke's pouch, they typically present in pediatric patients as partly cystic lesions with intra- and suprasellar components. Gross total resection, the standard treatment of choice, is associated with durable local control in 85% to 100% of patients [1]. However, the eloquent location of craniopharyngiomas, adjacent to the pituitary, hypothalamus, and optic apparatus, renders safe gross total resection achievable in only a subset of patients. By itself, however, subtotal resection leads to a 50% recurrence rate with further morbidity and mortality from tumor regrowth and repeat surgery [2–4]. After subtotal resection, radiotherapy plays an important role in mitigating recurrence risk and associated sequelae [4–12]. An alternative approach, especially in pediatric populations, is reserving radiotherapy as salvage therapy for recurrent disease, which allows for the omission of radiotherapy until recurrence is demonstrated [9]. Aggressive surgery, especially in the pediatric population, may permit avoidance of radiation toxicities altogether, but this benefit must be considered in the context of excessive mortality and morbidity associated with more aggressive resection.

RADIATION INDICATIONS

Pituitary Adenoma

Transsphenoidal resection is the preferred first-line therapy for definitive management of pituitary adenomas. Long-term control of microadenomas after resection is accomplished in 70% to 90% of cases, while macroadenomas are often incompletely resected, especially with extension into the cavernous sinus and/or suprasellar region. Tumor recurrence or new tumor growth from residual tissue occurs in 10% to 40% of cases. Medical management may prove sufficient for residual prolactinomas after debulking, while repeat surgery should also be considered for residual tumor or tumor recurrence. However, if no further medical or surgical options are available and if endocrine abnormalities persist or recur after surgery, postoperative radiation is warranted.

In nonfunctioning adenomas, adjuvant postoperative radiation should be strongly considered for residual disease, as regrowth of these tumors may threaten the eloquent adjacent structures such as the optic apparatus, cavernous sinus, or hypothalamus. Alternatively, if gross tumor resection is accomplished, adjuvant radiation can be deferred to avoid unnecessary toxicities, provided patients comply with close surveillance to enable for successful salvage surgery or radiation of recurrences [13].

Craniopharyngioma

Management of craniopharyngiomas should be tailored to the anatomic and symptomatic characteristics of each tumor. Generally, gross total resection should be attempted in tumors that are smaller, subdiaphragmatic in location, and/or without hypothalamic symptoms. Other patients at higher risk for surgical complications should be managed with biopsy, cyst decompression (if necessary), and adjuvant radiotherapy. Multiple large retrospective series, with long-term follow-up of patients treated with subtotal resection followed by adjuvant radiotherapy, have demonstrated local control and survival comparable to gross total resection and superior to subtotal resection alone. Ten- and 20-year local control rates following subtotal resection and adjuvant radiotherapy are 77% to 89% and 54% to 79%, respectively [5,14–21].

Whether radiotherapy should be offered immediately after subtotal resection or at the time of recurrence, remains controversial. Multiple pediatric series have suggested improved morbidity and local control with radiotherapy immediately after surgery, rather than at recurrence [8,15,17,20]. Similar reports in adult patients have shown equivalence in outcomes between these two options [18,19,21–23]. Based on these data, early postoperative radiotherapy is recommended for children with subtotal resections, whereas adults can be offered early postoperative radiotherapy or salvage radiotherapy at recurrence. The exception to this involves children younger than 3 years, in whom delaying radiotherapy may be warranted.

RADIOTHERAPY TECHNIQUES

Techniques for radiotherapy of pituitary adenomas and craniopharyngiomas are similar. One important distinction involves the use of cytostatic medical therapy with hormone secreting pituitary adenomas. In this case, multiple studies have demonstrated inferior outcomes with the concurrent use of radiotherapy with octreotide [24] or dopamine agonists [25,26]. If feasible from a symptomatic standpoint, these therapies should be discontinued in the weeks preceding and during radiotherapy.

Conventional Radiotherapy

Safe and efficacious delivery of conventional external beam radiotherapy using a linear accelerator (LINAC) is dependent on accurate image guidance and precise patient immobilization. Conventional radiotherapy has historically involved a three-field technique via 1) two wedged lateral fields through the temporal lobes, typically 5 × 5 cm fields, and 2) a coronal vertex field to mitigate dose to the orbits and lenses. Customized immobilization masks allow for setup accuracy in the range of 5 to 7 mm. Gross tumor volume (GTV) should be delineated using magnetic resonance images fused to computed tomography images of the brain. In the setting of cystic tumors, such as craniopharyngiomas, GTV should encompass both solid and cystic components. Planning target volume should encompass the GTV plus a 5 to 10 mm set-up margin, dependent on the technical uncertainty at an individual center. For pituitary adenomas, radiation doses of 45.0 to 50.4 Gy are delivered, with fraction sizes of 1.8 to 2.0 Gy daily. For craniopharyngiomas, 54.0 Gy in 1.8 Gy daily fractions is recommended.

Outcomes using these techniques have resulted in 5-year local control in approximately 90% of pituitary adenomas, using doses between 45 and 50.4 Gy [27–34] (Table 96.1), and in excess of 90% of craniopharyngiomas, using doses between 50 and 54 Gy [5,9,19,22,23,35] (Table 96.2). However, only 30% to 50% of pituitary adenomas achieve effective normalization of hormonal irregularities, defined as normal serum hormone levels in the absence of medical therapies. An additional proportion of patients with pituitary adenomas can expect a reduction in hormone irregularities that allow for a reduction in dosing of medications or enhanced response to administered medical therapies.

Table 96.1 Summary of Results on Published Series Using Conventional Radiotherapy for Pituitary Adenomas

Authors	Patients (N)	% Hormone Remission	% Tumor Control	Total Dose	Follow-Up (Years)	Visual Defects (%)
FSRT						
Snead [36]	100	NR	89	45	6.7	1
Minniti [37]	92	36	98	45	2.7	1
Colin [38]	110	42	99	50.4	4	1.8
Paek [39][a]	68	N/A*	98	50.4	2.5	3
Milker-Zabel	68	26	93	52.2	3.2	7.5
CRT						
Sasaki [31]	91	74	93	51	8.2	0
Mccord [29]	141	NR	94	47.2	10	3
Tsang [32]	145	40	96	50	7.3	0.7
Zierhut [34]	138	38	95	45.5	6.5	1.4
Zaugg [33]	89	NR	88	40–45	8.1	4.5
Hughes [27]	268	NR	81	widely variable	12.8	2.2
Salinger [30]	68	NR	90	50	5	0
McCullough [28]	105	NR	95	48.2	>5	1.8

Abbreviations: CRT, conventional radiotherapy; FSRT, fractionated stereotactic radiotherapy.

[a] Nonfunctioning adenomas only

For craniopharyngiomas, Regine et al [20] demonstrated a 44% relapse risk with doses less than 54 Gy, compared to a 16% relapse risk with doses greater than 54 Gy. Similar findings were reported by Habrand et al [15] although both studies involved a limited numbers of patients and seem to conflict with other series showing 5-year local control greater than 90% with doses of 50 to 54 Gy at 1.7 to 1.8 Gy per fraction [5,9,19,22,23,35]. Radiation doses in excess of 55 Gy have been shown to increase the risk of optic neuropathy [20,21].

More recently, conformal radiotherapy techniques have utilized multileaf collimators to shape the beams conformal to the tumor and shield normal structures. The use of 4 to 6 noncoplanar beam arrangements has reduced the volume of normal brain receiving high radiation doses. In addition, intensity-modulated therapy (IMRT) integrates multileaf collimators with inverse planning algorithms to allow for improved dose conformality and further sparing of critical structures, without compromise of target coverage. Despite promising results in pituitary adenomas [40], the use of IMRT has the potential to increase the volume of normal brain receiving low-dose radiation, a theoretical risk for radiation-induced secondary malignancies [41]. Given the absence of compelling clinical data for pituitary adenomas or craniopharyngiomas, the use of IMRT in these settings has, to date, not been widely adopted, except for situations where reducing the optic apparatus dose might not be feasible.

Stereotactic Techniques

The use of stereotactic techniques, including stereotactic radiosurgery (SRS) and fractionated stereotactic radiosurgery (FSRT), has become increasingly widespread for the radiotherapeutic management of pituitary adenomas and craniopharyngiomas.

SRS can conventionally be delivered using either a multisource cobalt-60 gamma knife unit or a LINAC although proton-based radiosurgery has also been developed [42]. Regardless of the radiation source, SRS patients are immobilized in a fixed frame with positioning accuracy of typically less than 1 mm. This allows for minimal GTV expansion and the delivery of radiation in a single, high-dose fraction. Compared to conventional fractionated radiotherapy, SRS is capable of delivering a higher biologically equivalent dose to a small target volume, while sparing adjacent normal tissue due to steeper dose gradients. In the setting of pituitary adenomas, retrospective data has demonstrated a shorter median time to complete hormonal response after single-fraction SRS (12–18 months) as compared to conventional fractionated radiotherapy [43–45]. In the setting of craniopharyngiomas, SRS has demonstrated an average local control rate of 90% for solid tumors, 88% for cystic tumors and 60% for mixed tumors, with no difference in outcomes between pediatric and adult patients [46–53] (Table 96.3). However, Ufarsson et al [52] observed a 95% recurrence rate for craniopharyngiomas that received a marginal dose of less than 6 Gy. While prescribing marginal dose to the GTV, dose to the optic chiasm and nerves must be kept below radiobiologic tolerance for optic neuropathy, estimated to be 8 to 10 Gy for single doses associated with SRS [54–56]. As a result, SRS is typically utilized for pituitary adenomas or craniopharyngiomas that are less than 3 cm in size and located greater than 3 to 5 mm from the optic apparatus.

In contrast, no size or location restrictions are necessary for image-guided FSRT, another relatively new technique that delivers high-dose, conformal radiation in multiple doses. Immobilization is achieved with a relocatable, noninvasive frame and mask, typically utilizing a bite tray. This allows for target accuracy of 1 to 2 mm. Radiation is delivered via 4 to 6 noncoplanar LINAC beams to a total dose of 45 to 50.4 Gy in 1.8 to 2 Gy fractions for pituitary adenomas and 54.0 Gy in 1.8 Gy fractions for craniopharyngiomas. These doses and dose-per-fraction remain below radiobiologic tolerance limits for neural tissue, including the optic apparatus. As a result, FSRT can be used for those tumors that are not amenable to SRS. Recent studies have demonstrated acceptable tumor control with minimal toxicities using this approach for pituitary adenomas (Table 96.1) [36–39,58] and craniopharyngiomas (Table 96.3) [22,23,57]. In addition, Snead et al [36] demonstrated that pituitary adenomas treated with FSRT technique had superior cause-specific survival compared to patients undergoing conventional radiotherapy.

Table 96.2 Summary of Results on Published Series Using Conventional Radiotherapy for Craniopharyngiomas

Authors	Patients	Median Dose (Gy)	Follow-up (Years)	Local Control (%)
Regine [20]	58	56–62	17	82 at 10 years
Rajan [19]	173	50	12	83 and 79 at 10 and 20 years
Hetelekidis [16]	37	54	4.1	86 at 10 years
Habrand [15]	37	50	N/A	78 and 56.5 at 5 and 10 years
Merchant [5]	15	54	6	94 at 5 years
Varlotto [21]	24	60	12	89 and 54 at 10 and 20 years
Stripp [9]	76	55	7.6	84 at 10 years
Moon [17]	50	54	12.8	96 and 91 at 5 and 10 years
Pemberton [18]	87	43	8	77 and 66 at 10 and 20 years
Merchant [35]	28	55	3	90 at 3 years

Data from Minniti G et al. Neurosurg Rev. 2009;32:125–132.

Table 96.3 Summary of Results on Published Series Using SRS or FSRT for Craniopharyngiomas

Authors	Patients	Marginal Dose (Gy)	Follow-Up (Years)	Tumor Size (cc)	Local Control (%)
SRS					
Prasad [46]	9	13	N/A	10	62.5
Mokry [47]	23	8–9.7	2	7	74
Chung [48]	31	12	3	8.9	87
Yu [49]	46	8–18	1.3	13.5	88
Chiou [50]	10	16	5.5	1.7	58
Amendola [51]	14	14	3.3	3.7	86
Ulfarsson [52]	21	3–25	17	8	34
Kobayashi [53]	98	11	5.4	3.5	61
FSRT					
Selch [57]	16	55	1.8	7.7	75 at 3 years
Combs [22]	40	52	8.2	13.7	100 at 10 yrs
Minniti [23]	39	50	3.3	10.2	92 at 5 years

Abbreviations: FSRT, fractionated stereotactic radiotherapy; SRS, stereotactic radiosurgery.
Data from Minniti G et al. Neurosurg Rev. 2009;32:125–132.

Intracavitary Radiotherapy

The vast majority of craniopharyngiomas have a cystic component to which symptoms are largely attributed. Multiple approaches to decreasing the cyst size, either at presentation or at the time of recurrence, can be pursued. These include intermittent aspiration by stereotactic puncture or placement of an Ommaya reservoir, sclerosis of the cyst wall by chemotherapeutic agents, and internal irradiation using radiocolloids. Beta-emitting isotopes, such as yttrium-90 (90Y), rhenium-186 (186Re), and phosphorus-32 (32P), delivering a tumoricidal dose (i.e., 200–300 Gy) to the cyst wall, are commonly employed due to the limited extent of their dose deposition and relative ease of handling [59–61]. However, the process of intracavitary injection of radioactive material can be technically challenging. Before injecting radioactive material into the catheter, contrast material should be injected to ensure that the catheter is well positioned in the cyst cavity and that the material does not leak outside the cyst. Retrospective series have demonstrated response rates in excess of 80% and improvement in or stability of visual symptoms in approximately 50% [59,60,62,63]. In patients whose total tumor bulk is more than 50% cystic but has three or fewer cysts, intralesional radiotherapy represents a reasonable option.

Proton Therapy

The superior dose distribution with protons compared to conformal or IMRT has rejuvenated interest in using proton therapy for pediatric central nervous system malignancies, including craniopharyngiomas. Single-institution series have demonstrated local control in excess of 90% using a combined photon-proton approach [64] or with proton therapy alone [65] for craniopharyngiomas, similar to the efficacy of photon-based treatments. However, the advantage of proton therapy arises from the lower integral radiation dose deposited in normal brain parenchyma. This has the potential to limit late toxicities in terms of neurocognitive function, endocrine effects, and secondary malignancies. Prospective outcome data are needed to corroborate this theoretical advantage.

Summary and Recommendations

Compared to conventional radiotherapy, stereotactic techniques offer the advantage of limiting the normal tissue radiation dose and thus minimizing the risk of late radiation side effects, including optic neuropathy, cognitive defects, cerebrovascular accidents (CVAs), and second malignancy risk. While prospective randomized comparisons have not been made, current radiotherapy recommendations include SRS for pituitary adenomas or craniopharyngiomas >3 to 5 mm from the optic apparatus utilizing marginal dose prescription of ≥25 Gy for hormone-secreting pituitary adenomas, 15 Gy for nonfunctioning pituitary adenomas, and 9.5 to 16.5 Gy for craniopharyngiomas. Optic nerve and chiasm dose ≤8 Gy must be maintained. For tumors in close proximity to the optic apparatus, FSRT delivered to 45 to 50.4 Gy for pituitary adenomas and 54.0 Gy for craniopharyngiomas, allows for equivalent tumor control while minimizing the risk for optic neuropathy.

RADIOTHERAPY-RELATED COMPLICATIONS

Optic Neuropathy

The most important factor when considering radiotherapy for pituitary lesions is their proximity to adjacent cranial nerves, especially the anterior visual pathway (optic chiasm and nerves). The risk of optic neuropathy is generally thought to be quite low with fractionated radiotherapy in the dose range used for pituitary adenomas (<1.5%) and craniopharyngiomas (<3%) [66,67]. However, this risk rises significantly with doses between 55 and 60 Gy [20,21] and with SRS, where high dose-per-fraction is utilized. Tishler et al [56] examined the tolerance of the cranial nerves in 62 patients treated for lesions within or near the cavernous sinus and observed visual complications in 24% of patients receiving greater than 8 Gy to the optic apparatus and in none of the patients receiving less than 8 Gy to the optic apparatus. Some series of SRS for pituitary lesions have shown rates of 4% to 7% for visual complications, though some of these patients had previous radiotherapy to the region [26,68,69]. The radiobiologic tolerance limit for a single-fraction dose to the optic chiasm has been established as 8 Gy [54,70]. To meet this dose constraint, SRS should be limited to tumors at least 3 to 5 mm from the chiasm or less than 3 cm in size, to allow for sufficient dose fall-off around the chiasm.

Other Cranial Neuropathies

Other cranial nerves, including the oculomotor, trochlear, trigeminal, and abducens nerves traverse the parasellar region. Retrospective series have identified a 1% risk of radiation-induced neuropathy of these nerves although the dose relationship for these events is poorly understood. In general, these nerves are felt to be more radioresistant than the optic chiasm and nerves, and SRS doses in the range of 19 to 23 Gy have been safely administered in this region [71,72]. The risk for radiation-induced cranial nerve neuropathy is predictably higher for salvage SRS after previous radiotherapy [69].

Cystic Enlargement

In the acute setting, radiotherapy for cystic craniopharyngiomas can lead to enlargement of their cystic portions due to accumulation of fluid. This acute complication occurs in 10% to 15% of patients [73] and, through mass effect, can manifest as visual deterioration or hydrocephalus during or within the first 2 to 3 months after radiotherapy. Early recognition of this complication is necessary to implement appropriate surgical intervention and prevent further neurologic compromise or even death.

Hypopituitarism

Given the proximity of the hypothalamic-pituitary axis to the pituitary, radiation-induced hypopituitarism (RIH) is the most common late complication of pituitary radiation, occurring in 50% to 100% of patients with pituitary adenomas [74] and 20% to 60% of patients with craniopharyngiomas [5,9,10,15,16,19,20]. For conventional radiotherapy, total doses >45 Gy and/or fraction size >2 Gy are associated with RIH [75]; RIH is also more common in patients with previous surgery to the region. In the craniopharyngioma literature, pediatric series have reported higher rates [5,15,16]. The growth hormone axis appears to be the most sensitive to radiation effects, with the gonadotropin and corticotropin axes also commonly affected and diabetes insipidus rarely caused. Some studies have suggested that SRS may result in lower rates of RIH, roughly 20% to 30% [76], although longer term follow-up have identified rates in excess of 70% [77]. RIH nearly doubles the rate of mortality [78], placing a greater emphasis on maintaining prolonged endocrine evaluation and instituting prompt management of hormone imbalances. Follow-up of such patients should be carefully coordinated with an endocrinologist.

Secondary Malignancies

Cranial irradiation, whether fractionated [79] or delivered via SRS [80], puts patients at a small but tangible risk for an intracranial radiation-induced secondary malignancy. Patients receiving radiotherapy for pituitary adenomas have consistently been demonstrated to have a risk for subsequent brain tumor of approximately 1.5% at 10 years and 2% to 3% at 15 to 20 years [66,81–83], placing them at 10 to 15 times the relative risk of the general population. Risk is not only highest for development of meningioma but also high for malignant gliomas. Meningeal and osteogenic sarcomas [84] have also been observed [85–90]. This risk should be discussed with patients, as it affects the necessity for long-term follow-up imaging.

Mortality

Patients with pituitary adenoma have also been demonstrated to be at an increased risk for all-cause mortality as compared to the general population. The factors involved in this risk are multiple, including local complications related to the pituitary tumors and their surgical removal, complex endocrine disturbances, and resultant excess cardiovascular, respiratory, and cerebrovascular sequelae [78]. Radiotherapy has also been implicated as a risk factor for long-term mortality [85], presumably because of an increased risk for CVAs in these patients. Brada et al [86] showed a 4-fold relative risk for CVA deaths in patients treated with surgery and radiotherapy for pituitary adenoma. An actuarial CVA incidence of 21% at 20 years has been demonstrated in this patient cohort, though the contribution of radiation to this risk cannot be fully defined given the potentially confounding effects of prior surgery and endocrine abnormalities in these patients [87].

Neurocognitive Effects

Patients with pituitary tumors have been demonstrated to have impairments of memory, executive function, and mental well-being [88,89]. With conventional radiation, areas vital to memory and emotion, such as the mammillary bodies, limbic system, and hippocampus receive substantial radiation doses. To date, however, radiotherapy for pituitary adenomas or craniopharyngiomas has not been clearly associated with neurocognitive deficits or reduced quality of life, partly due to the limited use of formal neuropsychological testing. In a phase II trial of conformal radiotherapy for craniopharygnioma, Merchant et al [35] tested 27 pediatric patients with serial neuropsychometic testing and observed a negative impact of surgical morbidity and brain volume receiving greater than 45 Gy on longitudinal IQ. In contrast, two retrospective series [90,91] have compared patients who underwent surgery alone versus surgery followed by radiation. Both studies were cross-sectional in nature and failed to convincingly demonstrate a detrimental impact of radiation on neurocognitive functioning utilizing a battery of functional and self-assessment measures. Van Beek et al [92] assessed quality of life measures in patients treated for nonfunctioning pituitary adenomas and found that radiotherapy was not associated with reduced quality of life or neurocognitive functioning. Further prospective analysis of neurocognitive effects, particularly in setting of small-volume irradiation, is needed.

RADIOTHERAPY FOR HISTOLOGIC SUBTYPES OF PITUITARY ADENOMA

Prolactinoma

The goals of treatment in prolactinoma include restoring sexual and reproductive function, stabilizing serum prolactin levels, and controlling galactorrhea. For macroadenomas, relief of mass effect and neurologic symptoms are also of importance. Currently, management of prolactinomas should begin with medical therapy in the form of a dopamine agonist, such as bromocriptine, cabergoline, or pergolide. Medical therapy can normalize prolactin levels and shrink tumors in 80% to 90% of cases. However, iatrogenic side effects can lead to the discontinuation of medical therapy, in which case disease recurrence occurs in roughly 90% of cases [93]. As a second-line intervention, transsphenoidal surgical resection provides durable cure of 75% to 90% microadenomas and 20% to 50% of macroadenomas.

Fractionated conventional radiotherapy has been investigated in the treatment of prolactinoma. Older studies examining conventional radiotherapy as a primary modality demonstrated inferior results compared to surgical series [27,94–97] and compared to other histologic subtypes of pituitary adenoma [27]. Though some series have demonstrated normalization in prolactin levels in approximately 50% of patients receiving 45 Gy in 1.8 Gy fractions, this process can take years to achieve, with the need for dopamine agonist use in the interim [98,99]. The efficacy of conventional radiotherapy can be limited by the significant radiation dose received by the hypothalamus. This leads to the inhibition of dopamine release and a resultant paradoxical increase in prolactin secretion [75]. In addition, conventional radiotherapy can induce high levels of postradiotherapy pituitary failure [100,101]. In contrast, FSRT and IMRT may minimize these adverse effects while still maintaining adequate radiation dose to the prolactinoma.

Series utilizing SRS demonstrate tumor control rates generally in excess of 90% (Table 96.4) [25,26,71,102–111]. However, hormone normalization is achieved in only 20% to 50% of patients. The majority of the remaining patients demonstrate improved prolactin levels but require continued dopamine agonist therapy, albeit at a lower dose. In contrast to other pituitary hormones, hypersecretion of prolactin is generally more difficult to control via SRS [111–113]. Retrospecive series have identified a possible radioprotective effect of concomitant use of dopamine agonists during SRS for prolactinomas [25,26]. Dopamine agonists are thought to inhibit the metabolic activity and cell cycle progression of prolactinoma cells, which may mitigate their radiosensitivity. A 2-month break from dopamine agonist therapy is recommended prior to SRS. At this point, SRS is recommended for use in patients who have already failed (or not tolerated) medical therapy and have had previous surgical resection.

Cushing Disease

Cushing syndrome is characterized by excess cortisol causing characteristic changes in body habitus (moon facies, a buffalo hump, central obesity) glucose intolerance, hypertension, hirsutism, and abdominal striae. Cushing disease refers to an adrenocorticotropic hormone (ACTH)-secreting adenoma and accounts for 70% of patients presenting with Cushing syndrome. If left untreated, the endocrine abnormalities associated with Cushing disease carry significant morbidity and mortality, more so than other pituitary adenomas. Historically, bilateral adrenalectomy was often pursued, resulting in high surgical morbidity and a substantial risk of Nelson syndrome (see section below). As a result, this approach has been replaced by transsphenoidal resection as first-line management, resulting in local control in 65% to 90% of patients [114]. Radiotherapy is typically reserved for postoperative adjuvant therapy for incompletely resected disease to mitigate recurrence risk or as salvage therapy for recurrent disease.

Table 96.4 Summary of Results on Published Series Using SRS for Prolactin-Secreting Pituitary Adenomas

Author	Patients (N)	% Hormone Remission	% Tumor Control	Marginal Dose (Gy)	Follow-Up (Months)
Castinetti [102]	15	46	100	26	>60
Kobayashi [107]	24	17	100	18.4	50
Wan [111]	176	23	90	22.4	67
Jezkova [106]	35	37	97	34	75
Ma [108]	51	39	100	26.1	37
Pouratian [26]	23	26	89[a]	18.6	55
Kuo [71]	15	87	NR	15	42
Choi [103]	21	24	100	28.5	42
Feigl [104]	18	NR	94	15	55
Landolt [25]	20	25	NR	25	29
Pan [110]	128	52	98	31.5	33
Izawa [105]	15	20	87	22	28

Abbreviation: SRS, stereotactic radiosurgery.

[a] 28 patients included for tumor control analysis, with median marginal dose of 18.9 Gy and median follow up of 48 months

Fractionated radiotherapy is an effective and well-tolerated option for residual or recurrent disease after transsphenoidal resection. Estrada et al [115] reported on 30 patients treated at a mean of 23 months after surgical resection with 48 to 54 Gy in 1.8 to 2 Gy fractions. Actuarial probability of remission of Cushing disease was 44% at 1 year and 83% at 3 years. New growth hormone deficiency developed in 57% of patients, but no visual impairment or radiation necrosis was noted. Minniti et al [116] demonstrated similar results in 40 postoperative patients treated with 45 to 50 Gy, with cortisol normalization observed in 28% of patients at 1 year, 73% at 3 years, and 84% at 10 years. Hypopituitarism was noted in 76% of patients 10 years after radiotherapy, but no other significant radiation sequelae were observed. For definitive treatment of Cushing's disease, however, retrospective series have demonstrated inferior control with conventional radiotherapy compared to transsphenoidal surgical resection for definitive treatment for Cushing disease [27,117–124]. Long-term control of hypercortisolism is achieved in 45% to 60% of patients treated with 45 to 50 Gy [27,117,122,124]. Therefore, primary fractionated radiotherapy should not replace transsphenoidal surgical resection as the initial intervention in Cushing disease.

Similarly, SRS has demonstrated efficacy in the postoperative and recurrent settings, offering a significant probability of hormone normalization and possibly a faster hormone response compared to fractionated radiotherapy (Table 96.5) [42,43,69,77,103,107,111,113,125,126]. Jagannathan et al [69] reported on 90 patients, of whom all but one had previous resection, and demonstrated cortisol normalization in 54%, at an average of 13 months after SRS; in addition, 92% of patients had tumor shrinkage. Sheehan et al [43] also reported on postoperative patients and demonstrated normalization of urinary-free cortisol in 63%, at an average of 12 months. Both of these studies noted disease recurrence in 10% to 20% of patients who achieved initial remission, and new hypopituitarism in approximately 20% of patients, highlighting the need for long-term follow-up. Similar to fractionated radiotherapy, primary management of Cushing's disease with SRS results in inferior rates (27%–28%) of hormone normalization [111,125].

Nelson Syndrome

Nelson syndrome may occur in 20% to 50% of patients following bilateral adrenalectomy, used historically as primary treatment for Cushing's disease. Currently, however, bilateral adrenalectomy is reserved as third-line salvage therapy for Cushing's disease, resulting in a considerably lower incidence of Nelson syndrome. Nelson syndrome is characterized by elevated serum ACTH levels, hyperpigmentation, and enlarging pituitary adenomas that are frequently invasive [127]. Given the invasive nature of tumors in Nelson syndrome, resection is often neither successful nor feasible.

Few series have reported on radiotherapy as primary management. Howlett et al [122] examined 15 patients treated with conventional fractionated radiotherapy (45 Gy in 25 fractions) for Nelson syndrome. Fourteen of the patients (93%) experienced a median decline of 84% of the plasma ACTH with accompanied progressive depigmentation. In addition, Jenkins et al [128] examined 20 patients who underwent prophylactic conventional radiotherapy following bilateral adrenalectomy, and only 5 patients developed subsequent Nelson syndrome. Conversely, 18 of 36 (50%) patients who did not receive prophylactic radiotherapy following bilateral adrenalectomy for Cushing disease developed Nelson syndrome at their center.

Reports on SRS for Nelson syndrome are scarce [42,113,129–131] (Table 96.6). The largest reported series examined 23 patients treated with SRS and demonstrated tumor shrinkage in more than 50% of patients, tumor control in 91% of patients, and improvement in ACTH in 67% of patients [129]. Forty percent of patients followed closely developed radiation-induced hypopituitarism. Petit et al [42] reported on 5 patients treated with proton-based SRS, and all patients had complete radiographic and hormonal remission.

Acromegaly

Similar to other secreting pituitary adenomas, transsphenoidal resection can often be curative, especially for microadenomas; medical therapy in the form of

Table 96.5 Summary of Results on Published Series Using SRS for Cushing Disease

Author	Patients (N)	% Hormone Remission	% Tumor Control	Marginal Dose (Gy)	Follow-Up (Months)
Wan [111]	68[a]	28	90	18.9 and 24.9[b]	67
Kobayashi [107]	25	35	100	28.7	64
Petit [42]	33	52	94	20 CGE	62
Jagannathan [69]	90	54	95	23	41
Castinetti [125]	40	43	NR	29.5	55
Voges [113]	17	53	88	16.4	59
Devin [126]	35	49	91	14.7	42
Choi [103]	9	56	86	28.5	42
Hoybye [77]	18	83		60–240[c]	204
Sheehan [43]	43	63	100	20	44

Abbreviation: SRS, stereotactic radiosurgery.

[a] ACTH secreting, does not distinguish between Cushings and Nelsons.

[b] Mean marginal dose of 18.9 for 21 microadenomas, and 24.9 for 47 macroadenomas.

[c] Maximal dose range reported.

Table 96.6 Summary of Results on Published Series Using SRS for Nelson Syndrome

Author	Patients (N)	% Hormone Remission	% Tumor Control	Marginal Dose (Gy)	Follow-Up (Months)
Vik-Mo (131)	10	10	100	26.2	84
Petit [42]	5	100	100	20 CGE	106
Mauermann [129]	23	20	91	25	50
Voges [113]	9	22	89	16.4	63
Pollock [130]	11	36	82	20	37

Abbreviation: SRS, stereotactic radiosurgery

somatostatin analogs are also useful as a second-line therapy. Several studies investigating conventional radiotherapy as treatment for acromegaly have recently been reported. In the largest experience, Jenkins et al [132] retrospectively analyzed 884 patients treated at 14 centers in the United Kingdom and demonstrated growth hormone normalization in 22%, 60%, and 77% at follow-up periods of 2, 10, and 20 years, respectively. Initial growth hormone levels significantly affected the time to normalization and ultimate efficacy. Other large series have shown similar results, with a substantial proportion of patients achieving hormone normalization more than 10 years after radiotherapy [133,134].

Reports on SRS for acromegaly have demonstrated excellent tumor control (97%–100%) over a wide range of doses and with 5-year remission rates comparing favorably to conventional radiotherapy series (Table 96.7) [102,107,111,113,135–141]. Similar comparisons are difficult to make for hormone remission rates, reported to be less than 60% after SRS, due to the absence of long-term follow-up in these SRS series. One study from Landolt et al reported on patients undergoing either SRS or conventional RT after unsuccessful resection with similar long-term follow-up of more than 7 years in each group. They reported a mean time to hormone normalization of 1.4 years in the SRS group versus 7.1 years in the conventional RT group [44]. Concurrent octreotide therapy at the time of SRS significantly lengthens time to hormone normalization after SRS. Thus medical therapy should be discontinued for 1 to 2 months prior to SRS [24].

Nonfunctioning Adenomas

Nonfunctioning adenomas (NFAs) account for 30% of all pituitary adenomas and are the most common among macroadenomas. These tumors typically present with decreases in visual acuity or visual field abnormalities secondary to mass effect on the optic nerves or chiasm. Therefore surgery is the most frequent initial treatment, even when complete resection is not anticipated, as immediate relief from compressive symptoms is achieved. However, while complete transsphenoidal resection may provide durable control in 80% to 90% of cases, gross total resection is often not attained due to the invasive nature of advanced NFAs. Recurrence rates up to 50% in patients with incomplete resection have been frequently reported. Unlike prolactinomas and growth hormone-secreting adenomas, medical therapy has little efficacy in NFAs. Therefore radiation is frequently utilized in the postoperative setting. In general, NFAs require lower doses than secreting adenomas for control, as hormone hypersecretion does not need to be controlled. Therefore SRS in the range of 15 Gy, or fractionated radiotherapy to 45 to 50 Gy, especially utilizing conformal arc or stereotactic techniques, represent reasonable treatment options for NFAs.

Gittoes et al [142] demonstrated the utility of fractionated conventional radiotherapy in the immediate postoperative setting. They compared results from one center where postoperative adjuvant radiotherapy was standard to another center where adjuvant radiotherapy was largely withheld. Actuarial progression-free survival was 68%, 47%, and 33% at 5, 10, and 15 years, respectively, in 63 patients who did not receive radiotherapy. Amongst the 63 patients who did receive immediate postoperative radiotherapy, progression-free survival was 93% at all three time points. Similar findings were reported elsewhere, with 95% local control at 10 years achieved with the use immediate postoperative radiotherapy for residual NFA. This compared favorably to the local control rate of 49% at 5 years and 22% at 10 years for patients who did not receive adjuvant radiotherapy for residual disease [143]. Other series are summarized in Table 96.8 [31,66,67,144–146]. However, most of those series analyzed patients in which imaging modalities were suboptimal for determining tumor size response to fractionated radiotherapy.

SRS is another reasonable treatment for NFAs following surgical resection (Table 96.8) [70,105,107,113,147–154]. The largest experience reported to date evaluated 90 patients who underwent Gamma Knife SRS [150]. Tumor control was 92%, and only 25% of patients with fully or partially functional pituitaries experienced new endocrine deficits. Doses as low as 12 Gy demonstrated efficacy for tumor control, with no benefit observed with doses greater than 20 Gy.

Follow-Up

Patients undergoing either fractionated radiotherapy or SRS for pituitary adenomas or craniopharyngiomas require long-term follow-up with serial imaging examinations. Initial posttherapy magnetic resonance imaging at 6 months with follow-up magnetic resonance imaging every year thereafter is a reasonable approach. Ophthalmologic and endocrine baseline evaluations should be documented before therapy and followed closely after radiotherapy. Clinical evaluation should include monitoring of height, weight, and pubertal status where appropriate. Prospective assessments of neurocognition are needed, and all patients

Table 96.7 Summary of Results on Published Series Using SRS for GH-Secreting Pituitary Adenomas

Author	Patients (N)	% Hormone Remission	% Tumor Control	Marginal Dose (Gy)	Follow-Up (Months)
Ronchi [139]	35	46	100	20	114
Castinetti [102]	43	42	100	24	>60
Kobayashi [107]	71	17	100	18.9	63
Wan [111]	103	37	95	21.4	67
Jagannathan [135]	95	53	98	22	57
Losa [137]	83	60	97	21.5	69
Pollock [138]	46	50	NR	20	63
Vik-Mo [140]	53	17	100	25	66
Jezkova [136]	96	50	100	35	54
Voges [113]	64	47	97	16.5	54
Gutt [141]	44	48	100	18	23

Abbreviations: GH, growth hormone; SRS, stereotactic radiosurgery.

Table 96.8 Summary of Results on Published Series Using SRS and CRT for Nonfunctioning Pituitary Adenomas

Author	Patients (N)	% Tumor Shrinkage	% Stable Tumor	% Tumor Growth	Marginal Dose (Gy)	Follow-up (Months)
Stereotactic Radiosurgery (SRS)						
Hoybye [147]	23	78	17	4	20	78
Kobayashi [107]	60	72	25	3	14.1	60
Pollock [148]	62	60	37	3[a]	16	64
Liscak [149]	79	89	11	0	20	60
Mingione [150]	90	66	27	8	18.5	45
Voges [113]	37	41	59	0	13.4	56
Iwai [151]	34	58	29	13	14	60
Losa [70]	54	42	54	4*	16.6	41
Petrovich [152]	56	100		0	15	36
Sheehan [153]	46	35	59	7	16	27
Wowra [154]	45	NR	NR	7	16	55
Izawa [105]	23	26	70	4	19.5	30
Conventional Radiotherapy (CRT)						
Langsenlehner [144]	61	93		7	50.4	127
van den Bergh [143]	76	95		4	45	93
Sasaki [31]	65	86	12	3	51	99
Gittoes [142]	63	93		6	45	109
Breen [146]	120	88		12	46.7	108
Grabenbauer [145]	50	94		6	48	54
Tsang [67]	160	87		13	45–50	100
Brada [66]	252	97		3	45–50	120

Abbreviations: CRT, conventional radiotherapy; GH, growth hormone; SRS, stereotactic radiosurgery.

[a]Represent recurrence outside of treatment area, not growth of treated tumor burden.

should be monitored for cognitive decline. In addition, clinicians should be aware of the increased risk for subsequent central nervous system malignancies and CVAs in these patients and should maintain lower thresholds for appropriate diagnostic evaluations when symptoms warrant.

REFERENCES

1. Yasargil MG, Curcic M, Kis M, Siegenthaler G, Teddy PJ, Roth P. Total removal of craniopharyngiomas. Approaches and long-term results in 144 patients. *J Neurosurg*. 1990;73(1):3–11.
2. Fahlbusch R, Honegger J, Paulus W, Huk W, Buchfelder M. Surgical treatment of craniopharyngiomas: experience with 168 patients. *J Neurosurg*. 1999;90(2):237–250.
3. Shi XE, Wu B, Fan T, Zhou ZQ, Zhang YL. Craniopharyngioma: surgical experience of 309 cases in China. *Clin Neurol Neurosurg*. 2008;110(2):151–159.
4. Wen BC, Hussey DH, Staples J, et al. A comparison of the roles of surgery and radiation therapy in the management of craniopharyngiomas. *Int J Radiat Oncol Biol Phys*. 1989;16(1):17–24.
5. Merchant TE, Kiehna EN, Sanford RA, et al. Craniopharyngioma: the St. Jude Children's Research Hospital experience 1984–2001. *Int J Radiat Oncol Biol Phys*. 2002;53(3):533–542.
6. Richmond IL, Wara WM, Wilson CB. Role of radiation therapy in the management of craniopharyngiomas in children. *Neurosurgery*. 1980;6(5):513–517.
7. Manaka S, Teramoto A, Takakura K. The efficacy of radiotherapy for craniopharyngioma. *J Neurosurg*. 1985;62(5):648–656.
8. Weiss M, Sutton L, Marcial V, et al. The role of radiation therapy in the management of childhood craniopharyngioma. *Int J Radiat Oncol Biol Phys*. 1989;17(6):1313–1321.
9. Stripp DC, Maity A, Janss AJ, et al. Surgery with or without radiation therapy in the management of craniopharyngiomas in children and young adults. *Int J Radiat Oncol Biol Phys*. 2004;58(3):714–720.
10. Karavitaki N, Brufani C, Warner JT, et al. Craniopharyngiomas in children and adults: systematic analysis of 121 cases with long-term follow-up. *Clin Endocrinol (Oxf)*. 2005;62(4):397–409.

11. Mark RJ, Lutge WR, Shimizu KT, Tran LM, Selch MT, Parker RG. Craniopharyngioma: treatment in the CT and MR imaging era. *Radiology*. 1995;197(1):195–198.
12. Lin LL, El Naqa I, Leonard JR, et al. Long-term outcome in children treated for craniopharyngioma with and without radiotherapy. *J Neurosurg Pediatr*. 2008;1(2):126–130.
13. Lillehei KO, Kirschman DL, Kleinschmidt-DeMasters BK, Ridgway EC. Reassessment of the role of radiation therapy in the treatment of endocrine-inactive pituitary macroadenomas. *Neurosurgery*. 1998;43(3):432–438; discussion 438.
14. Scott RM, Hetelekidis S, Barnes PD, Goumnerova L, Tarbell NJ. Surgery, radiation, and combination therapy in the treatment of childhood craniopharyngioma–a 20-year experience. *Pediatr Neurosurg*. 1994;21(suppl 1):75–81.
15. Habrand JL, Ganry O, Couanet D, et al. The role of radiation therapy in the management of craniopharyngioma: a 25-year experience and review of the literature. *Int J Radiat Oncol Biol Phys*. 1999;44(2):255–263.
16. Hetelekidis S, Barnes PD, Tao ML, et al. 20-year experience in childhood craniopharyngioma. *Int J Radiat Oncol Biol Phys*. 1993;27(2):189–195.
17. Moon SH, Kim IH, Park SW, et al. Early adjuvant radiotherapy toward long-term survival and better quality of life for craniopharyngiomas—a study in single institute. *Childs Nerv Syst*. 2005;21(8–9):799–807.
18. Pemberton LS, Dougal M, Magee B, Gattamaneni HR. Experience of external beam radiotherapy given adjuvantly or at relapse following surgery for craniopharyngioma. *Radiother Oncol*. 2005;77(1):99–104.
19. Rajan B, Ashley S, Gorman C, et al. Craniopharyngioma—a long-term results following limited surgery and radiotherapy. *Radiother Oncol*. 1993;26(1):1–10.
20. Regine WF, Mohiuddin M, Kramer S. Long-term results of pediatric and adult craniopharyngiomas treated with combined surgery and radiation. *Radiother Oncol*. 1993;27(1):13–21.
21. Varlotto JM, Flickinger JC, Kondziolka D, Lunsford LD, Deutsch M. External beam irradiation of craniopharyngiomas: long-term analysis of tumor control and morbidity. *Int J Radiat Oncol Biol Phys*. 2002;54(2):492–499.
22. Combs SE, Thilmann C, Huber PE, Hoess A, Debus J, Schulz-Ertner D. Achievement of long-term local control in patients with craniopharyngiomas using high precision stereotactic radiotherapy. *Cancer*. 2007;109(11):2308–2314.
23. Minniti G, Saran F, Traish D, et al. Fractionated stereotactic conformal radiotherapy following conservative surgery in the control of craniopharyngiomas. *Radiother Oncol*. 2007;82(1):90–95.
24. Landolt AM, Haller D, Lomax N, et al. Octreotide may act as a radioprotective agent in acromegaly. *J Clin Endocrinol Metab*. 2000;85(3):1287–1289.
25. Landolt AM, Lomax N. Gamma knife radiosurgery for prolactinomas. *J Neurosurg*. 2000;93(suppl 3):14–18.
26. Pouratian N, Sheehan J, Jagannathan J, Laws ER Jr, Steiner L, Vance ML. Gamma knife radiosurgery for medically and surgically refractory prolactinomas. *Neurosurgery*. 2006;59(2):255–266; discussion 255.
27. Hughes MN, Llamas KJ, Yelland ME, Tripcony LB. Pituitary adenomas: long-term results for radiotherapy alone and postoperative radiotherapy. *Int J Radiat Oncol Biol Phys*. 1993;27(5):1035–1043.
28. McCollough WM, Marcus RB Jr, Rhoton AL Jr, Ballinger WE, Million RR. Long-term follow-up of radiotherapy for pituitary adenoma: the absence of late recurrence after greater than or equal to 4500 cGy. *Int J Radiat Oncol Biol Phys*. 1991;21(3):607–614.
29. McCord MW, Buatti JM, Fennell EM, et al. Radiotherapy for pituitary adenoma: long-term outcome and sequelae. *Int J Radiat Oncol Biol Phys*. 1997;39(2):437–444.
30. Salinger DJ, Brady LW, Miyamoto CT. Radiation therapy in the treatment of pituitary adenomas. *Am J Clin Oncol*. 1992;15(6):467–473.
31. Sasaki R, Murakami M, Okamoto Y, et al. The efficacy of conventional radiation therapy in the management of pituitary adenoma. *Int J Radiat Oncol Biol Phys*. 2000;47(5):1337–1345.
32. Tsang RW, Brierley JD, Panzarella T, Gospodarowicz MK, Sutcliffe SB, Simpson WJ. Role of radiation therapy in clinical hormonally-active pituitary adenomas. *Radiother Oncol*. 1996;41(1):45–53.
33. Zaugg M, Adaman O, Pescia R, Landolt AM. External irradiation of macroinvasive pituitary adenomas with telecobalt: a retrospective study with long-term follow-up in patients irradiated with doses mostly of between 40–45 Gy. *Int J Radiat Oncol Biol Phys*. 1995;32(3):671–680.
34. Zierhut D, Flentje M, Adolph J, Erdmann J, Raue F, Wannenmacher M. External radiotherapy of pituitary adenomas. *Int J Radiat Oncol Biol Phys*. 1995;33(2):307–314.
35. Merchant TE, Kiehna EN, Kun LE, et al. Phase II trial of conformal radiation therapy for pediatric patients with craniopharyngioma and correlation of surgical factors and radiation dosimetry with change in cognitive function. *J Neurosurg*. 2006;104(2 suppl):94–102.
36. Snead FE, Amdur RJ, Morris CG, Mendenhall WM. Long-term outcomes of radiotherapy for pituitary adenomas. *Int J Radiat Oncol Biol Phys*. 2008;71(4):994–998.
37. Minniti G, Traish D, Ashley S, Gonsalves A, Brada M. Fractionated stereotactic conformal radiotherapy for secreting and nonsecreting pituitary adenomas. *Clin Endocrinol (Oxf)*. 2006;64(5):542–548.
38. Colin P, Jovenin N, Delemer B, et al. Treatment of pituitary adenomas by fractionated stereotactic radiotherapy: a prospective study of 110 patients. *Int J Radiat Oncol Biol Phys*. 2005;62(2):333–341.
39. Paek SH, Downes MB, Bednarz G, et al. Integration of surgery with fractionated stereotactic radiotherapy for treatment of nonfunctioning pituitary macroadenomas. *Int J Radiat Oncol Biol Phys*. 2005;61(3):795–808.
40. Mackley HB, Reddy CA, Lee SY, et al. Intensity-modulated radiotherapy for pituitary adenomas: the preliminary report of the Cleveland Clinic experience. *Int J Radiat Oncol Biol Phys*. 2007;67(1):232–239.
41. Hall EJ. The inaugural Frank Ellis Lecture–Iatrogenic cancer: the impact of intensity-modulated radiotherapy. *Clin Oncol (R Coll Radiol)*. 2006;18(4):277–282.
42. Petit JH, Biller BM, Yock TI, et al. Proton stereotactic radiotherapy for persistent adrenocorticotropin-producing adenomas. *J Clin Endocrinol Metab*. 2008;93(2):393–399.
43. Sheehan JM, Vance ML, Sheehan JP, Ellegala DB, Laws ER Jr. Radiosurgery for Cushing's disease after failed transsphenoidal surgery. *J Neurosurg*. 2000;93(5):738–742.
44. Landolt AM, Haller D, Lomax N, et al. Stereotactic radiosurgery for recurrent surgically treated acromegaly: comparison with fractionated radiotherapy. *J Neurosurg*. 1998;88(6):1002–1008.
45. Tinnel BA, Henderson MA, Witt TC, et al. Endocrine response after gamma knife-based stereotactic radiosurgery for secretory pituitary adenoma. *Stereotact Funct Neurosurg*. 2008;86(5):292–296.
46. Prasad D, Steiner M, Steiner L. Gamma knife surgery for craniopharyngioma. *Acta Neurochir (Wien)*. 1995;134(3–4):167–176.
47. Mokry M. Craniopharyngiomas: A six year experience with Gamma Knife radiosurgery. *Stereotact Funct Neurosurg*. 1999;72(suppl 1):140–149.
48. Chung WY, Pan DH, Shiau CY, Guo WY, Wang LW. Gamma knife radiosurgery for craniopharyngiomas. *J Neurosurg*. 2000;93(suppl 3):47–56.
49. Yu X, Liu Z, Li S. Combined treatment with stereotactic intracavitary irradiation and gamma knife surgery for craniopharyngiomas. *Stereotact Funct Neurosurg*. 2000;75(2–3):117–122.
50. Chiou SM, Lunsford LD, Niranjan A, Kondziolka D, Flickinger JC. Stereotactic radiosurgery of residual or recurrent craniopharyngioma, after surgery, with or without radiation therapy. *Neuro-oncology*. 2001;3(3):159–166.
51. Amendola BE, Wolf A, Coy SR, Amendola MA. Role of radiosurgery in craniopharyngiomas: a preliminary report. *Med Pediatr Oncol*. 2003;41(2):123–127.
52. Ulfarsson E, Lindquist C, Roberts M, et al. Gamma knife radiosurgery for craniopharyngiomas: long-term results in the first Swedish patients. *J Neurosurg*. 2002;97(5 suppl):613–622.
53. Kobayashi T, Kida Y, Mori Y, Hasegawa T. Long-term results of gamma knife surgery for the treatment of craniopharyngioma in 98 consecutive cases. *J Neurosurg*. 2005;103(6 suppl):482–488.
54. Leber KA, Berglöff J, Pendl G. Dose-response tolerance of the visual pathways and cranial nerves of the cavernous sinus to stereotactic radiosurgery. *J Neurosurg*. 1998;88(1):43–50.
55. Stafford SL, Pollock BE, Leavitt JA, et al. A study on the radiation tolerance of the optic nerves and chiasm after stereotactic radiosurgery. *Int J Radiat Oncol Biol Phys*. 2003;55(5):1177–1181.
56. Tishler RB, Loeffler JS, Lunsford LD, et al. Tolerance of cranial nerves of the cavernous sinus to radiosurgery. *Int J Radiat Oncol Biol Phys*. 1993;27(2):215–221.

57. Selch MT, DeSalles AA, Wade M, et al. Initial clinical results of stereotactic radiotherapy for the treatment of craniopharyngiomas. *Technol Cancer Res Treat.* 2002;1(1):51–59.
58. Milker-Zabel S, Debus J, Thilmann C, Schlegel W, Wannenmacher M. Fractionated stereotactically guided radiotherapy and radiosurgery in the treatment of functional and nonfunctional adenomas of the pituitary gland. *Int J Radiat Oncol Biol Phys.* 2001;50(5):1279–1286.
59. Derrey S, Blond S, Reyns N, et al. Management of cystic craniopharyngiomas with stereotactic endocavitary irradiation using colloidal 186Re: a retrospective study of 48 consecutive patients. *Neurosurgery.* 2008;63(6):1045–1052; discussion 1052.
60. Pollack IF, Lunsford LD, Slamovits TL, Gumerman LW, Levine G, Robinson AG. Stereotaxic intracavitary irradiation for cystic craniopharyngiomas. *J Neurosurg.* 1988;68(2):227–233.
61. Sadeghi M, Karimi E, Sardari D. Monte Carlo and analytical calculations of dose distributions in craniopharyngioma cysts treated with radiocolloids containing 32P or 186Re. *Appl Radiat Isot.* 2009;67(9):1697–1701.
62. Julow J, Backlund EO, Lányi F, et al. Long-term results and late complications after intracavitary yttrium-90 colloid irradiation of recurrent cystic craniopharyngiomas. *Neurosurgery.* 2007;61(2):288–295; discussion 295.
63. Voges J, Sturm V, Lehrke R, Treuer H, Gauss C, Berthold F. Cystic craniopharyngioma: long-term results after intracavitary irradiation with stereotactically applied colloidal beta-emitting radioactive sources. *Neurosurgery.* 1997;40(2):263–269; discussion 269.
64. Fitzek MM, Linggood RM, Adams J, Munzenrider JE. Combined proton and photon irradiation for craniopharyngioma: long-term results of the early cohort of patients treated at Harvard Cyclotron Laboratory and Massachusetts General Hospital. *Int J Radiat Oncol Biol Phys.* 2006;64(5):1348–1354.
65. Luu QT, Loredo LN, Archambeau JO, Yonemoto LT, Slater JM, Slater JD. Fractionated proton radiation treatment for pediatric craniopharyngioma: preliminary report. *Cancer J.* 2006;12(2):155–159.
66. Brada M, Rajan B, Traish D, et al. The long-term efficacy of conservative surgery and radiotherapy in the control of pituitary adenomas. *Clin Endocrinol (Oxf).* 1993;38(6):571–578.
67. Tsang RW, Brierley JD, Panzarella T, Gospodarowicz MK, Sutcliffe SB, Simpson WJ. Radiation therapy for pituitary adenoma: treatment outcome and prognostic factors. *Int J Radiat Oncol Biol Phys.* 1994;30(3):557–565.
68. Jagannathan J, Kanter AS, Sheehan JP, Jane JA Jr, Laws ER Jr. Benign brain tumors: sellar/parasellar tumors. *Neurol Clin.* 2007;25(4):1231–1249, xi.
69. Jagannathan J, Sheehan JP, Pouratian N, Laws ER, Steiner L, Vance ML. Gamma Knife surgery for Cushing's disease. *J Neurosurg.* 2007;106(6):980–987.
70. Losa M, Valle M, Mortini P, et al. Gamma knife surgery for treatment of residual nonfunctioning pituitary adenomas after surgical debulking. *J Neurosurg.* 2004;100(3):438–444.
71. Kuo JS, Chen JC, Yu C, et al. Gamma knife radiosurgery for benign cavernous sinus tumors: quantitative analysis of treatment outcomes. *Neurosurgery.* 2004;54(6):1385–1393; discussion 1393.
72. Liu AL, Wang C, Sun S, Wang M, Liu P. Gamma knife radiosurgery for tumors involving the cavernous sinus. *Stereotact Funct Neurosurg.* 2005;83(1):45–51.
73. Rajan B, Ashley S, Thomas DG, Marsh H, Britton J, Brada M. Craniopharyngioma: improving outcome by early recognition and treatment of acute complications. *Int J Radiat Oncol Biol Phys.* 1997;37(3):517–521.
74. Fernandez A, Brada M, Zabuliene L, Karavitaki N, Wass JA. Radiation-induced hypopituitarism. *Endocr Relat Cancer.* 2009;16(3):733–772.
75. Littley MD, Shalet SM, Beardwell CG, Ahmed SR, Applegate G, Sutton ML. Hypopituitarism following external radiotherapy for pituitary tumours in adults. *Q J Med.* 1989;70(262):145–160.
76. Jagannathan J, Yen CP, Pouratian N, Laws ER, Sheehan JP. Stereotactic radiosurgery for pituitary adenomas: a comprehensive review of indications, techniques and long-term results using the Gamma Knife. *J Neurooncol.* 2009;92(3):345–356.
77. Höybye C, Grenbäck E, Rähn T, Degerblad M, Thorén M, Hulting AL. Adrenocorticotropic hormone-producing pituitary tumors: 12- to 22-year follow-up after treatment with stereotactic radiosurgery. *Neurosurgery.* 2001;49(2):284–291; discussion 291.
78. Tomlinson JW, Holden N, Hills RK, et al. Association between premature mortality and hypopituitarism. West Midlands Prospective Hypopituitary Study Group. *Lancet.* 2001;357(9254):425–431.
79. Ron E, Modan B, Boice JD Jr, et al. Tumors of the brain and nervous system after radiotherapy in childhood. *N Engl J Med.* 1988;319(16):1033–1039.
80. Loeffler JS, Niemierko A, Chapman PH. Second tumors after radiosurgery: tip of the iceberg or a bump in the road? *Neurosurgery.* 2003;52(6):1436–1440; discussion 1440.
81. Brada M, Ford D, Ashley S, et al. Risk of second brain tumour after conservative surgery and radiotherapy for pituitary adenoma. *BMJ.* 1992;304(6838):1343–1346.
82. Minniti G, Traish D, Ashley S, Gonsalves A, Brada M. Risk of second brain tumor after conservative surgery and radiotherapy for pituitary adenoma: update after an additional 10 years. *J Clin Endocrinol Metab.* 2005;90(2):800–804.
83. Tsang RW, Laperriere NJ, Simpson WJ, Brierley J, Panzarella T, Smyth HS. Glioma arising after radiation therapy for pituitary adenoma. A report of four patients and estimation of risk. *Cancer.* 1993;72(7):2227–2233.
84. Bembo SA, Pasmantier R, Davis RP, Xiong Z, Weiss TE. Osteogenic sarcoma of the sella after radiation treatment of a pituitary adenoma. *Endocr Pract.* 2004;10(4):335–338.
85. Chang EF, Zada G, Kim S, et al. Long-term recurrence and mortality after surgery and adjuvant radiotherapy for nonfunctional pituitary adenomas. *J Neurosurg.* 2008;108(4):736–745.
86. Brada M, Ashley S, Ford D, Traish D, Burchell L, Rajan B. Cerebrovascular mortality in patients with pituitary adenoma. *Clin Endocrinol (Oxf).* 2002;57(6):713–717.
87. Brada M, Burchell L, Ashley S, Traish D. The incidence of cerebrovascular accidents in patients with pituitary adenoma. *Int J Radiat Oncol Biol Phys.* 1999;45(3):693–698.
88. Bülow B, Hagmar L, Ørbaek P, Osterberg K, Erfurth EM. High incidence of mental disorders, reduced mental well-being and cognitive function in hypopituitary women with GH deficiency treated for pituitary disease. *Clin Endocrinol (Oxf).* 2002;56(2):183–193.
89. Grattan-Smith PJ, Morris JG, Shores EA, Batchelor J, Sparks RS. Neuropsychological abnormalities in patients with pituitary tumours. *Acta Neurol Scand.* 1992;86(6):626–631.
90. Noad R, Narayanan KR, Howlett T, Lincoln NB, Page RC. Evaluation of the effect of radiotherapy for pituitary tumours on cognitive function and quality of life. *Clin Oncol (R Coll Radiol).* 2004;16(4):233–237.
91. Peace KA, Orme SM, Sebastian JP, et al. The effect of treatment variables on mood and social adjustment in adult patients with pituitary disease. *Clin Endocrinol (Oxf).* 1997;46(4):445–450.
92. van Beek AP, van den Bergh AC, van den Berg LM, et al. Radiotherapy is not associated with reduced quality of life and cognitive function in patients treated for nonfunctioning pituitary adenoma. *Int J Radiat Oncol Biol Phys.* 2007;68(4):986–991.
93. Platta CS, Mackay C, Welsh JS. Pituitary adenoma: a radiotherapeutic perspective. *Am J Clin Oncol.* 2009..
94. Grigsby PW, Stokes S, Marks JE, Simpson JR. Prognostic factors and results of radiotherapy alone in the management of pituitary adenomas. *Int J Radiat Oncol Biol Phys.* 1988;15(5):1103–1110.
95. Rush SC, Newall J. Pituitary adenoma: the efficacy of radiotherapy as the sole treatment. *Int J Radiat Oncol Biol Phys.* 1989;17(1):165–169.
96. Gómez F, Reyes FI, Faiman C. Nonpuerperal galactorrhea and hyperprolactinemia. Clinical findings, endocrine features and therapeutic responses in 56 cases. *Am J Med.* 1977;62(5):648–660.
97. Kleinberg DL, Noel GL, Frantz AG. Galactorrhea: a study of 235 cases, including 48 with pituitary tumors. *N Engl J Med.* 1977;296(11):589–600.
98. Grossman A, Cohen BL, Charlesworth M, et al. Treatment of prolactinomas with megavoltage radiotherapy. *Br Med J (Clin Res Ed).* 1984;288(6424):1105–1109.
99. Tsagarakis S, Grossman A, Plowman PN, et al. Megavoltage pituitary irradiation in the management of prolactinomas: long-term follow-up. *Clin Endocrinol (Oxf).* 1991;34(5):399–406.
100. Samaan NA, Vieto R, Schultz PN, et al. Hypothalamic, pituitary and thyroid dysfunction after radiotherapy to the head and neck. *Int J Radiat Oncol Biol Phys.* 1982;8(11):1857–1867.

101. Snyder PJ, Fowble BF, Schatz NJ, Savino PJ, Gennarelli TA. Hypopituitarism following radiation therapy of pituitary adenomas. *Am J Med.* 1986;81(3):457–462.
102. Castinetti F, Nagai M, Morange I, et al. Long-term results of stereotactic radiosurgery in secretory pituitary adenomas. *J Clin Endocrinol Metab.* 2009;94(9):3400–3407.
103. Choi JY, Chang JH, Chang JW, Ha Y, Park YG, Chung SS. Radiological and hormonal responses of functioning pituitary adenomas after gamma knife radiosurgery. *Yonsei Med J.* 2003;44(4):602–607.
104. Feigl GC, Bonelli CM, Berghold A, Mokry M. Effects of gamma knife radiosurgery of pituitary adenomas on pituitary function. *J Neurosurg.* 2002;97(5 suppl):415–421.
105. Izawa M, Hayashi M, Nakaya K, et al. Gamma knife radiosurgery for pituitary adenomas. *J Neurosurg.* 2000;93(suppl 3):19--22.
106. Jezková J, Hána V, Krsek M, et al. Use of the Leksell gamma knife in the treatment of prolactinoma patients. *Clin Endocrinol (Oxf).* 2009;70(5):732–741.
107. Kobayashi T. Long-term results of stereotactic gamma knife radiosurgery for pituitary adenomas. Specific strategies for different types of adenoma. *Prog Neurol Surg.* 2009;22:77--95.
108. Ma ZM, Qiu B, Hou YH, Liu YS. [Gamma knife treatment for pituitary prolactinomas]. *Zhong Nan Da Xue Xue Bao Yi Xue Ban.* 2006;31(5):714–716.
109 Pamir MN, Kilic T, Belirgen M, et al. Pituitary adenomas treated with gamma knife radiosurgery: volumetric analysis of 100 cases with minimum 3 year follow-up. *Neurosurgery.* 2007;61:270–280; discussion 280.
110. Pan L, Zhang N, Wang EM, Wang BJ, Dai JZ, Cai PW. Gamma knife radiosurgery as a primary treatment for prolactinomas. *J Neurosurg.* 2000;93(suppl 3):10–13.
111. Wan H, Chihiro O, Yuan S. MASEP gamma knife radiosurgery for secretory pituitary adenomas: experience in 347 consecutive cases. *J Exp Clin Cancer Res.* 2009;28(</Is>):36.
112. Pollock BE, Brown PD, Nippoldt TB, Young WF Jr. Pituitary tumor type affects the chance of biochemical remission after radiosurgery of hormone-secreting pituitary adenomas. *Neurosurgery.* 2008;62(6):1271–1276; discussion 1276.
113. Voges J, Kocher M, Runge M, et al. Linear accelerator radiosurgery for pituitary macroadenomas: a 7-year follow-up study. *Cancer.* 2006;107(6):1355–1364.
114. Biller BM, Grossman AB, Stewart PM, et al. Treatment of adrenocorticotropin-dependent Cushing's syndrome: a consensus statement. *J Clin Endocrinol Metab.* 2008;93(7):2454–2462.
115. Estrada J, Boronat M, Mielgo M, et al. The long-term outcome of pituitary irradiation after unsuccessful transsphenoidal surgery in Cushing's disease. *N Engl J Med.* 1997;336(3):172–177.
116. Minniti G, Osti M, Jaffrain-Rea ML, Esposito V, Cantore G, Maurizi Enrici R. Long-term follow-up results of postoperative radiation therapy for Cushing's disease. *J Neurooncol.* 2007;84(1):79–84.
117. Orth DN, Liddle GW. Results of treatment in 108 patients with Cushing's syndrome. *N Engl J Med.* 1971;285(5):243–247.
118. BOUCOT N, DOHAN FC, RAVENTOS A, ROSE E. Roentgen therapy in Cushing's syndrome without adrenocortical tumor. *J Clin Endocrinol Metab.* 1957;17(1):8–32.
119. Heuschele R, Lampe I. Pituitary irradiation for Cushing's syndrome. *Radiol Clin Biol.* 1967;36(1):27–31.
120. Edmonds MW, Simpson WJ, Meakin JW. External irradiation of the hypophysis for Cushing's disease. *Can Med Assoc J.* 1972;107(9):860–862.
121. Grigsby PW, Simpson JR, Stokes S, Marks JE, Fineberg B. Results of surgery and irradiation or irradiation alone for pituitary adenomas. *J Neurooncol.* 1988;6(2):129–134.
122. Howlett TA, Plowman PN, Wass JA, Rees LH, Jones AE, Besser GM. Megavoltage pituitary irradiation in the management of Cushing's disease and Nelson's syndrome: long-term follow-up. *Clin Endocrinol (Oxf).* 1989;31(3):309–323.
123. Littley MD, Shalet SM, Beardwell CG, Ahmed SR, Sutton ML. Long-term follow-up of low-dose external pituitary irradiation for Cushing's disease. *Clin Endocrinol (Oxf).* 1990;33(4):445–455.
124. Murayama M, Yasuda K, Minamori Y, Mercado-Asis LB, Yamakita N, Miura K. Long term follow-up of Cushing's disease treated with reserpine and pituitary irradiation. *J Clin Endocrinol Metab.* 1992;75(3):935–942.
125. Castinetti F, Nagai M, Dufour H, et al. Gamma knife radiosurgery is a successful adjunctive treatment in Cushing's disease. *Eur J Endocrinol.* 2007;156(1):91–98.
126. Devin JK, Allen GS, Cmelak AJ, Duggan DM, Blevins LS. The efficacy of linear accelerator radiosurgery in the management of patients with Cushing's disease. *Stereotact Funct Neurosurg.* 2004;82(5–6):254–262.
127. NELSON DH, MEAKIN JW, THORN GW. ACTH-producing pituitary tumors following adrenalectomy for Cushing's syndrome. *Ann Intern Med.* 1960;52:560–569.
128. Jenkins PJ, Trainer PJ, Plowman PN, et al. The long-term outcome after adrenalectomy and prophylactic pituitary radiotherapy in adrenocorticotropin-dependent Cushing's syndrome. *J Clin Endocrinol Metab.* 1995;80(1):165–171.
129. Mauermann WJ, Sheehan JP, Chernavvsky DR, Laws ER, Steiner L, Vance ML. Gamma Knife surgery for adrenocorticotropic hormone-producing pituitary adenomas after bilateral adrenalectomy. *J Neurosurg.* 2007;106(6):988–993.
130. Pollock BE, Young WF Jr. Stereotactic radiosurgery for patients with ACTH-producing pituitary adenomas after prior adrenalectomy. *Int J Radiat Oncol Biol Phys.* 2002;54(3):839–841.
131. Vik-Mo EO, Øksnes M, Pedersen PH, et al. Gamma knife stereotactic radiosurgery of Nelson syndrome. *Eur J Endocrinol.* 2009;160(2):143–148.
132. Jenkins PJ, Bates P, Carson MN, Stewart PM, Wass JA. Conventional pituitary irradiation is effective in lowering serum growth hormone and insulin-like growth factor-I in patients with acromegaly. *J Clin Endocrinol Metab.* 2006;91(4):1239–1245.
133. Barrande G, Pittino-Lungo M, Coste J, et al. Hormonal and metabolic effects of radiotherapy in acromegaly: long-term results in 128 patients followed in a single center. *J Clin Endocrinol Metab.* 2000;85(10):3779–3785.
134. Minniti G, Jaffrain-Rea ML, Osti M, et al. The long-term efficacy of conventional radiotherapy in patients with GH-secreting pituitary adenomas. *Clin Endocrinol (Oxf).* 2005;62(2):210–216.
135. Jagannathan J, Sheehan JP, Pouratian N, Laws ER Jr, Steiner L, Vance ML. Gamma knife radiosurgery for acromegaly: outcomes after failed transsphenoidal surgery. *Neurosurgery.* 2008;62(6):1262–1269; discussion 1269.
136. Jezková J, Marek J, Hána V, et al. Gamma knife radiosurgery for acromegaly–long-term experience. *Clin Endocrinol (Oxf).* 2006;64(5):588–595.
137. Losa M, Gioia L, Picozzi P, et al. The role of stereotactic radiotherapy in patients with growth hormone-secreting pituitary adenoma. *J Clin Endocrinol Metab.* 2008;93(7):2546–2552.
138. Pollock BE, Jacob JT, Brown PD, Nippoldt TB. Radiosurgery of growth hormone-producing pituitary adenomas: factors associated with biochemical remission. *J Neurosurg.* 2007;106(5):833–838.
139. Ronchi CL, Attanasio R, Verrua E, et al. Efficacy and tolerability of gamma knife radiosurgery in acromegaly: a 10-year follow-up study. *Clin Endocrinol (Oxf).* 2009.
140. Vik-Mo EO, Oksnes M, Pedersen PH, et al. Gamma knife stereotactic radiosurgery for acromegaly. *Eur J Endocrinol.* 2007;157(3):255–263.
141. Gutt B, Wowra B, Alexandrov R, et al. Gamma-knife surgery is effective in normalising plasma insulin-like growth factor I in patients with acromegaly. *Exp Clin Endocrinol Diabetes.* 2005;113(4):219–224.
142. Gittoes NJ, Bates AS, Tse W, et al. Radiotherapy for non-function pituitary tumours. *Clin Endocrinol (Oxf).* 1998;48(3):331–337.
143. van den Bergh AC, van den Berg G, Schoorl MA, et al. Immediate postoperative radiotherapy in residual nonfunctioning pituitary adenoma: beneficial effect on local control without additional negative impact on pituitary function and life expectancy. *Int J Radiat Oncol Biol Phys.* 2007;67(3):863–869.
144. Langsenlehner T, Stiegler C, Quehenberger F, et al. Long-term follow-up of patients with pituitary macroadenomas after postoperative radiation therapy: analysis of tumor control and functional outcome. *Strahlenther Onkol.* 2007;183(5):241–247.
145. Grabenbauer GG, Fietkau R, Buchfelder M, et al. [Hormonally inactive hypophyseal adenomas: the results and late sequelae after surgery and radiotherapy]. *Strahlenther Onkol.* 1996;172(4):193–197.

146. Breen P, Flickinger JC, Kondziolka D, Martinez AJ. Radiotherapy for nonfunctional pituitary adenoma: analysis of long-term tumor control. *J Neurosurg.* 1998;89(6):933–938.
147. Höybye C, Rähn T. Adjuvant Gamma Knife radiosurgery in nonfunctioning pituitary adenomas; low risk of long-term complications in selected patients. *Pituitary.* 2009;12(3):211–216.
148. Pollock BE, Cochran J, Natt N, et al. Gamma knife radiosurgery for patients with nonfunctioning pituitary adenomas: results from a 15-year experience. *Int J Radiat Oncol Biol Phys.* 2008;70(5): 1325–1329.
149. Liscák R, Vladyka V, Marek J, Simonová G, Vymazal J. Gamma knife radiosurgery for endocrine-inactive pituitary adenomas. *Acta Neurochir (Wien).* 2007;149(10):999–1006; discussion 1006.
150. Mingione V, Yen CP, Vance ML, et al. Gamma surgery in the treatment of nonsecretory pituitary macroadenoma. *J Neurosurg.* 2006;104(6):876–883.
151. Iwai Y, Yamanaka K, Yoshioka K. Radiosurgery for nonfunctioning pituitary adenomas. *Neurosurgery.* 2005;56(4):699–705; discussion 699.
152. Petrovich Z, Yu C, Giannotta SL, Zee CS, Apuzzo ML. Gamma knife radiosurgery for pituitary adenoma: early results. *Neurosurgery.* 2003;53(1):51–59; discussion 59.
153. Sheehan JP, Kondziolka D, Flickinger J, Lunsford LD. Radiosurgery for residual or recurrent nonfunctioning pituitary adenoma. *J Neurosurg.* 2002;97(5 suppl):408–414.
154. Wowra B, Stummer W. Efficacy of gamma knife radiosurgery for nonfunctioning pituitary adenomas: a quantitative follow up with magnetic resonance imaging-based volumetric analysis. *J Neurosurg.* 2002;97(5 suppl):429–432.

97 Primary Central Nervous System Germ Cell Tumors, Pineal Tumors, and Other Tumors of the Pineal and Sellar Regions

Kristin A. Bradley

PRIMARY CENTRAL NERVOUS SYSTEM GERM CELL TUMORS

Intracranial germ cell tumors (GCTs) arise from primordial germ cells in structures adjacent to the third ventricle. They are rare, accounting for less than 1% of adult brain tumors and for approximately 3% to 6% of primary pediatric brain tumors, with a higher incidence reported in Asia than in the United States and Europe [1–3] The World Health Organization (WHO) classification of central nervous system (CNS) GCTs includes: germinomas (60%–70%); teratomas (20%); and nongerminomatous GCTs (NGGCTs; 15%–20%), composed of embryonal carcinoma, yolk sac tumor (endodermal sinus tumor), choriocarcinoma, and mixed GCTs [4,5].

Management of germinomas and NGGCTs varies, and therefore, proper diagnosis is necessary to guide treatment decisions. Although the diagnosis of some NGGCTs can empirically be made on the basis of increased tumor markers, biopsy is imperative to establishing a diagnosis in the absence of increased tumor markers or if β-human chorionic gonadotropin (hCG) is only modestly increased. Once the diagnosis of an intracranial GCT is made, gadolinium-enhanced magnetic resonance imaging (MRI) of the head and spine and lumbar cerebrospinal fluid (CSF) for cytology are required to evaluate for CNS dissemination because 10% to 15% of patients have leptomeningeal spread at diagnosis.

Although there are multiple subtypes of intracranial GCTs with diverse clinical presentations and disease extents, the approach to treatment is based on whether the tumor is a CNS germinoma or an NGGCT. Germinomas are radio- and chemosensitive with high cure rates, whereas NGGCTs are less responsive to therapy. Surgery is needed in patients presenting with hydrocephalus and clinical symptoms of increased intracranial pressure. An aggressive surgery with attempted gross total resection is not warranted for germinomas, given their sensitivity to radiation and chemotherapy. Attempts at gross total resection of NGGCTs, which have lower control rates than germinomas, with chemotherapy and radiation, are sometimes made at diagnosis or after neoadjuvant chemotherapy. Different institutions and study groups advocate either approach, and this remains an area of debate [6–9].

Radiation Therapy for Germinomas

Using radiation therapy alone, germinomas are highly curable, and long-term survival rates exceed 80% [10–14]. Radiotherapy approaches have varied in terms of volumes and doses and have included craniospinal irradiation, whole brain irradiation, whole ventricle irradiation, and localized fields. Historical doses have ranged from 30 to 36 Gy followed by a boost to the primary site to a total dose of 45 to 50 Gy.

A debate continues over the appropriate volume to irradiate. Some series report increased neuraxis failures after more localized radiation volumes compared with CSI. From 1981 to 2002, 21 patients with germinomas treated at The University of Texas MD Anderson Cancer Center achieved a 10-year local control rate of 59% in the brain when receiving focal irradiation compared with 100% when receiving CSI ($P = .08$). The rate of distant control in the spine at 5 years was 62% for patients who received focal irradiation and 100% for patients who received CSI ($P = .04$) [15]. However, other series report that in patients with histologically confirmed germinomas and negative MRI and CSF staging of the neuraxis, isolated spinal failures after whole ventricle or whole brain radiation occur in less than 10% of patients [12,14,16,17].

Because of the concern over significant late toxicities seen in children receiving craniospinal irradiation, alternative treatment strategies have been investigated with the goal of maintaining the excellent cure rates seen with larger field and higher dose radiation for intracranial germinomas while trying to reduce the potential neurocognitive, endocrine, and quality-of-life late effects. One such strategy has been to try chemotherapy alone for CNS germinomas, and two International Central Nervous System Germ Cell Tumor Study Group protocols have investigated this approach [18,19]. In the first, 71 patients (45 germinoma and 26 NGGCT) received six cycles of combination chemotherapy. A complete response (CR) without irradiation was achieved in 84% of germinomas and 78% of NGGCTs. Despite the high initial response rates, 49% of patients recurred at a median time of 13 months, nearly two-thirds of surviving patients required radiation therapy for salvage, and the 2-year survival rate was only 84% for patients with germinoma and 62% for patients with NGGCT [18].

Another strategy has been a combined modality approach with chemotherapy followed by radiotherapy using lower doses and treatment volumes. This approach has been tested in several small studies using a variety of cisplatin- or carboplatin-based regimens 20–24]. In the largest trial, a French study of 57 patients with CNS germinoma, four cycles of carboplatin/etoposide alternating with ifosfamide/etoposide were followed by 40 Gy of localized radiotherapy (CSI for the six patients with leptomeningeal dissemination). With a median follow-up of 42 months, the estimated 3-year overall survival and event-free survival were excellent at 98% and 96.4%, respectively [21].

On the basis of the promising results of these pilot studies, a phase III randomized trial of radiation alone versus combined modality therapy is being conducted by the Children's Oncology Group (COG) for patients with histologically confirmed primary CNS germinoma with serum and CSF β-hCG ≤ 50 IU/dL, serum AFP ≤ 10 IU/L, and CSF AFP ≤ 2.0 IU/L. This study will evaluate overall and event-free survival, recurrence patterns, quality of life, and neuropsychological function between patients receiving radiotherapy alone and patients receiving pre-radiotherapy chemotherapy. The schema and treatment plan are complicated, with radiation therapy volumes and doses based on disease extent at diagnosis, randomization arm, and response to chemotherapy (Table 97.1). Although there is no universally accepted standard radiotherapy volume and dose, the contemporary approach has moved to more limited fields, and patients randomized to radiotherapy alone in this study will receive whole ventricular irradiation to 24 Gy for localized disease and CSI to 24 Gy for disseminated disease, with an involved field boost of 21 Gy after the whole ventricle or craniospinal irradiation. Patients randomized to combined modality therapy will receive two cycles of carboplatin and etoposide followed by radiotherapy in complete responders, and additional chemotherapy with radiotherapy in patients without a CR. The radiation volumes and doses are based on disease extent at diagnosis, staging evaluation, response to chemotherapy, and number of chemotherapy cycles administered. Radiation treatment planning should use image-guided, 3D conformal techniques, and intensity-modulated radiation therapy is permitted for whole ventricle and involved field radiation to achieve lower doses to uninvolved brain than possible with lateral opposed fields [25]. As shown in the axial computed tomography slices in Figure 97.1, the normal brain adjacent to the ventricles receives 100% of the prescribed dose using opposed lateral fields. When an intensity-modulated radiation therapy plan is used, there is a steep dose gradient from the 100% to 50% isodose curves, thus reducing the dose to the uninvolved brain.

In addition to evaluating whether chemotherapy followed by response-based reductions in radiation dose and volume is able to maintain the excellent cure rates achieved by radiation alone, the COG study will compare

Table 97.1 Radiation Volumes and Doses for Children's Oncology Group ACNS0232 Study of Radiotherapy Alone versus Chemotherapy Followed by Response-based Radiotherapy for Newly Diagnosed Primary CNS Germinoma

Response	Chemotherapy Cycles	Stage	Initial Field Volume	Initial Field Dose (Gy)	Boost Field Volume	Boost Field Dose (Gy)	Total Dose (Gy)
Radiation	**Only arm**						
—	—	Local	WV[a]	24	IF[b]	21	45
—	—	Occult multifocal	WV[a]	24	IF[b]	21	45
—	—	Disseminated	CSI[c]	24	IF[b]	21	45
Combined	**Modality arm**						
CR[d]	2	Local	IF[a]	30	None	0	30
		Occult multifocal	WV[a]	21	IF[b]	9	30
		Disseminated	CSI[c]	21	IF[b]	9	30
CR[d] or MRD[e]	4	Local	IF[b]	30	None	0	30
		Occult multifocal	WV[a]	21	IF[b]	9	30
		Disseminated	CSI[c]	21	IF[b]	9	30
PR[f], SD[g], or PD[h]	4	Local	WV[a]	24	IF[b]	21	45
		Occult multifocal	WV[a]	24	IF[b]	21	45
		Disseminated	CSI[c]	24	IF[b]	21	45

Adapted from Tables 17.1 and 17.2 of Protocol ACNS0232, Children's Oncology Group Website.

[a] Whole ventricular.

[b] Involved field.

[c] Craniospinal.

[d] Complete response.

[e] Minimal residual disease.

[f] Partial response.

[g] Stable disease.

[h] Progressive disease.

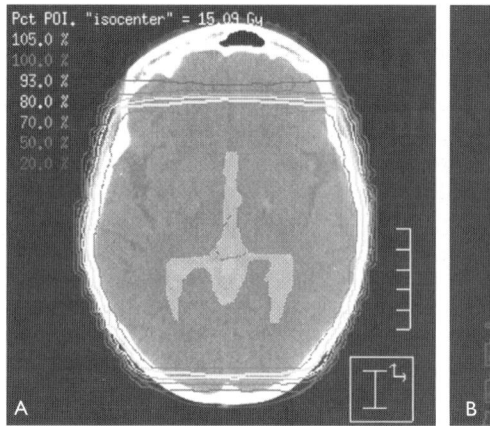 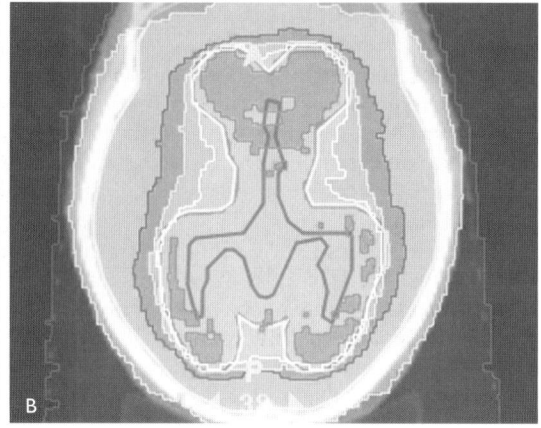

Figure 97.1 Comparison of whole ventricular treatment using opposed lateral fields **(A)** or with a tomotherapy IMRT plan **(B)**. See color insert.

the treatment-related morbidity as measured by verbal learning and memory, executive functioning, and quality of life between the randomization arms. Previous reports that have assessed neuropsychological outcome of children treated for CNS germinomas document the late toxicities in small numbers of survivors. In general, these studies do not report a significant decline in neurocognitive functioning, although the studies are limited by few numbers of survivors and often only evaluated intelligence, a single measure of neuropsychological functioning [26–29]. In one study, Sands et al. reported that psychosocial and physical health scores and intelligence positively correlated with age at diagnosis. Survivors who received CNS radiotherapy reported significantly worse physical health, but similar psychosocial health, compared with those treated without radiation [30]. The COG hopes to expand on these previous efforts with the current study.

Radiation Therapy for NGGCTs

Although NGGCTs include several different histological subtypes, as a group, they are less radiosensitive than germinomas, and the prognosis after radiation therapy alone is poor, with reported long-term survival rates of 10% to 35% [4,31–34]. On the basis of the success of chemotherapy in the treatment of gonadal nonseminomatous GCTs, chemotherapy was incorporated into the treatment of primary intracranial NGGCTs. The previously mentioned International Central Nervous System Germ Cell Tumor Study Group protocols included 26 patients with NGGCT in the first study and 20 in the second study. Patients received chemotherapy alone with radiation therapy reserved for salvaging recurrences. The 2-year survival rate was 62% for patients with NGGCT in the first trial, and the 5-year overall and event-free survival rates were 75% and 36%, respectively, in the second trial [18,19].

Reports from the United States, Europe, and Japan demonstrate that combination therapy with surgery, chemotherapy, and radiotherapy for NGGCTs yield long-term survival rates of more than 50% [35–38]. A French retrospective analysis reported on a trial that included 27 patients with NGGCTs who received six to eight cycles of chemotherapy followed by focal radiation to 55 Gy (CSI if disseminated disease). Resection of residual tumor was recommended before starting radiotherapy, and 52% of patients underwent a second-look surgery. At a median follow-up of 53 months, 8 of 27 patients had relapsed, and 74% of patients were alive [35]. Similar to the treatment of CNS germinomas, a debate exists regarding the recommended radiation treatment volume for disease that is localized at presentation. The results of a prospective German study supports the use of craniospinal irradiation—patients who received protocol therapy of cisplatin-based chemotherapy and resection of residual tumor followed by CSI had a 5-year relapse-free survival rate of 74% compared with 38% in patients who were not treated according to protocol recommendations [8].

The current COG study for NGGCTs is a phase II trial that will evaluate the response rate to induction chemotherapy with the goal of improving progression-free and overall survival in these patients. Eligible patients have a histologically confirmed NGGCT, a histologically unconfirmed pineal or suprasellar tumor with serum/CSF β-hCG > 50 IU/dL or AFP > 10 IU/L, or a histologically confirmed germinoma with serum/CSF β-hCG > 50 IU/dL or AFP > 10 IU/L. On study, patients receive six cycles of neoadjuvant chemotherapy, alternating between carboplatin/etoposide and ifosfamide/etoposide. Patients who demonstrate a CR to chemotherapy then receive CSI with involved field boost radiation. For patients not obtaining CR after neoadjuvant chemotherapy, second-look surgery is strongly encouraged, and for patients with persistent positive tumor markers, residual malignant elements (histologically), or residual unresectable disease, an attempt to increase survival will be made by using high-dose chemotherapy with peripheral blood stem cell rescue before CSI. All patients will receive 36 Gy to the entire neuraxis followed by a localized boost to the prechemotherapy gross tumor volume, tumor bed, and any residual tumor with a specified margin to a total dose of 54 Gy.

PINEAL REGION TUMORS

Pineal region tumors comprise up to 1% of adult brain tumors and 2% to 8% of pediatric brain tumors in the United States. However, in Asia, up to 15% of pediatric CNS tumors are pineal region tumors. In adults, GCTs are the most common histology at 30% to 40% followed by nongerminomatous GCTs at 10% to 20%. In children, roughly one-half of pineal region tumors are GCTs (30%–80% reported), 10% to 20% are pineal parenchymal tumors, and approximately 15% are astrocytomas. Gliomas account for most of the remainder, but ependymomas, meningiomas, and metastases are also seen [1,2,32,39–41]. Treatment and prognosis is determined by histological diagnosis. The previous section discussed GCTs, and this section will discuss the role of radiation therapy in other pineal region tumors.

Pineal Parenchymal Tumors

Pineal parenchymal tumors (PPTs) are derived from pinealocytes, which are specialized neurons of the pineal gland that produce and secrete melatonin, or their embryonal precursors. According to the WHO classification of pineal tumors, there are three main categories: 1) pineocytoma; 2) pineoblastoma; and 3) pineal parenchymal tumor of intermediate differentiation. Mixed tumors can be seen, and prognosis depends on histological classification [42]. In addition, in the most recent 2007 WHO classification, a new entity, papillary tumor of the pineal region, has been added [43].

Pineocytomas

Slightly less than half of PPTs are pineocytomas, a slow-growing tumor composed of mature cells resembling normal pinealocytes. Mitoses are rarely present, and pineocytomas are classified as WHO grade II. They can be diagnosed across many ages, but present most commonly in older adolescents and adults, with the peak incidence in the 30- to 35-year-old age group. Neuraxis dissemination has been reported, but is rare [44].

The recommended treatment for pineocytomas is surgical resection for tumors without evidence of leptomeningeal spread. Tumors that are amenable to gross total resection have low recurrence rates after surgery alone without adjuvant therapy [7,42]. Although the literature regarding adjuvant therapy is retrospective and is limited by few number of patients, postoperative radiation therapy to reduce local recurrences is generally recommended for pineocytomas that are subtotally resected or undergo biopsy alone. Not all studies, however, have found a clear relationship between the extent of radiotherapy and survival [42]. If radiation therapy is delivered, localized fields should be used, targeting the gross tumor volume with a 1- to 2-cm margin for microscopic extension and daily positioning variability. CSI is reserved for patients with overt leptomeningeal spread. Doses of 50 to 55 Gy are generally delivered, with excellent outcomes reported. In a multiinstitutional cohort of 135 patients with histologically confirmed pineal tumors and other GCTs, 9 pineocytomas were included, and the 5-year survival rate was 86% for pineocytomas [45].

Stereotactic radiosurgery is being investigated as primary, adjuvant, or salvage therapy in the treatment of newly diagnosed and focally recurrent PPTs and other pineal region tumors [46–48]. The group from Pittsburgh retrospectively evaluated 16 patients who had undergone radiosurgery for pineal parenchymal tumors. Ten patients had pineocytomas, four had pineoblastomas, and two had mixed tumors. The mean marginal dose was 15 Gy, and the mean tumor volume was 5.0 cm^3. With a mean follow-up of 52 months from treatment, the local tumor control rate (complete remission, partial remission, or no change) was 100%. One patient with a pineocytoma and three patients with pineoblastomas died secondary to leptomeningeal or extracranial tumor spread. Two patients developed adverse radiation effects after radiosurgery [46]. In another series, pineocytomas had a 100% control rate, but pineoblastomas did poorly with 50% response and progression rates [47]. From these initial experiences, stereotactic radiosurgery shows promise for pineocytomas; however, further investigation is needed.

Pineoblastomas

Pineoblastomas, which are classified as a WHO grade IV tumor, are embryonal primitive neuroectodermal tumors with highly aggressive clinical behavior. They are composed of sheets of densely packed, poorly differentiated cells with a high mitotic rate and frequent necrosis. Infants and young children are most frequently diagnosed with pineoblastomas, and these tumors account for approximately 45% of PPTs. Clinical symptoms are generally short in duration, with patients presenting with manifestations of increased intracranial pressure. Five to ten percent of patients with bilateral ocular retinoblastoma will be diagnosed with a pineoblastoma, a disease referred to as "trilateral retinoblastoma." Most commonly, these patients have familial retinoblastoma, although it is seen in sporadic bilateral disease as well, and do poorly with most patients dying within 1 year of diagnosis [49,50]. Compared with pineocytomas, pineoblastomas typically are larger and multilobulated. On MRI, they demonstrate heterogenous contrast enhancement. Leptomeningeal spread is common—it is reported in 20% to 50% of patients at diagnosis and is the dominant mode of failure [51–53].

Unlike pineocytomas, pineoblastomas frequently infiltrate adjacent structures, and attempts at surgical resection are often incomplete 44,45]. Given the propensity for CSF dissemination, a treatment approach with craniospinal irradiation and chemotherapy has been based on that used for other supratentorial primitive neuroectodermal tumors and is used in all patients except very young infants. A dose of 30 to 36 Gy to the neuraxis followed by a boost to the primary site to 50 to 55 Gy is recommended. Gross spinal metastases receive 45 to 50.4 Gy. By using a combination of CSI and chemotherapy, the reported 3- to 5-year survival rates are in the range of 40% to 70% for older kids and adults [39,44,45,52–57]. In the previously mentioned report of

135 patients with biopsy-proven pineal region tumors, the 5-year survival rate was 49% for PPTs other than pineocytomas. In this study cohort, patients not receiving craniospinal irradiation and patients receiving total doses less than 50 Gy had increased leptomeningeal and local failures, respectively. In a multicenter, retrospective study of 56 adult patients who received postoperative radiotherapy (chemotherapy was administered to 34 patients), the median overall survival was 100 months, and factors that significantly influenced survival were the extent of disease (localized vs disseminated), differentiation (pineal parenchymal tumor of intermediate differentiation vs pineoblastoma), and residual disease (≥50% vs <50% reduction in size) [55]. However, not all investigators have found residual posttreatment disease to be predictive of outcome [53].

Because of concerns about developmental delay, neuroendocrine and neurocognitive deficits, and growth retardation in children younger than 3 years treated with large-volume radiation, two trials were conducted by the Children's Cancer Group and Pediatric Oncology Group to prospectively evaluate postoperative multiagent chemotherapy without radiation for infants [53,58]. Both studies reported dismal results for patients with pineoblastomas, with all patients experiencing disease progression. Median time to progression was 4 months from the start of treatment in the Children's Cancer Group study. In the Baby Pediatric Oncology Group study, all patients died within 13 months of diagnosis.

Pineal Parenchymal Tumors of Intermediate Differentiation

These tumors are rare, making up 10% or less of PPTs. Because they are so rare, the optimal therapy is not known, and treatment recommendations vary from surgical resection alone to postoperative CSI and chemotherapy.

OTHER PINEAL AND SELLAR REGION TUMORS

GCTs and pineal parenchymal tumors originate from the pineal gland. Other pineal region tumors, including gliomas, ependymomas, choroid plexus papillomas, and meningiomas are extrapineal and arise from tissues adjacent to the pineal gland. Dorsally exophytic brainstem and tectal gliomas are distinct from the more common intrinsic pontine gliomas and demonstrate more indolent progression and have a better prognosis. Locally progressive and symptomatic dorsally exophytic gliomas are typically amenable to resection [59–61]. Radiation therapy provides good local control in the setting of multiply recurrent and symptomatic disease [60,62,63]. Radiation therapy for other tumors that can occur in the pineal and sellar regions, such as low-grade gliomas, high-grade gliomas, ependymomas, and meningiomas, follows the same principles as those used to treat these tumors in their more typical intracranial locations. The role of radiation therapy for these tumors is discussed in preceding chapters.

REFERENCES

1. Freeman C, Farmer J, Taylor R. Central nervous system tumors in children. In: Halperin E, Perez C, Brady L, eds. *Principles and Practice of Radiation Oncology*. 5th ed. Philadelphia: Lippincott Williams & Wilkins; 2008:1822–1849.
2. Kun LE. Supratentorial brain tumors except ependymomas; brain tumors in babies and very young children. In: Halperin EC, Constine LS, Tarbell NJ, eds. *Pediatric Radiation Oncology*. 4th ed. Philadelphia: Lippincott Williams & Wilkins; 2005:41–88.
3. Wong TT, Ho DM, Chang KP, et al. Primary pediatric brain tumors: statistics of Taipei VGH, Taiwan (1975–2004). *Cancer*. 2005;104(10):2156–2167.
4. Jennings MT, Gelman R, Hochberg F. Intracranial germ-cell tumors: natural history and pathogenesis. *J Neurosurg*. 1985;63(2):155–167.
5. Louis DN, Ohgaki H, Wiestler OD, et al. The 2007 WHO classification of tumours of the central nervous system. *Acta Neuropathol*. 2007;114(2):97–109.
6. Borg M. Germ cell tumours of the central nervous system in children-controversies in radiotherapy. *Med Pediatr Oncol*. 2003;40(6):367–374.
7. Bruce JN, Ogden AT. Surgical strategies for treating patients with pineal region tumors. *J Neurooncol*. 2004;69(1–3):221–236.
8. Calaminus G, Bamberg M, Jürgens H, et al. Impact of surgery, chemotherapy and irradiation on long term outcome of intracranial malignant non-germinomatous germ cell tumors: results of the German Cooperative Trial MAKEI 89. *Klin Padiatr*. 2004;216(3):141–149.
9. Sawamura Y, de Tribolet N, Ishii N, Abe H. Management of primary intracranial germinomas: diagnostic surgery or radical resection? *J Neurosurg*. 1997;87(2):262–266.
10. Bamberg M, Kortmann RD, Calaminus G, et al. Radiation therapy for intracranial germinoma: results of the German cooperative prospective trials MAKEI 83/86/89. *J Clin Oncol*. 1999;17(8):2585–2592.
11. Chitapanarux I, Lorvidhaya V, Kamnerdsupaphon P, Goss B, Ford J. CNS germ cell tumors: pattern of failure and effects of radiation volume. *J Med Assoc Thai*. 2006;89(4):415–421.
12. Haas-Kogan DA, Missett BT, Wara WM, et al. Radiation therapy for intracranial germ cell tumors. *Int J Radiat Oncol Biol Phys*. 2003;56(2):511–518.
13. Maity A, Shu HK, Janss A, et al. Craniospinal radiation in the treatment of biopsy-proven intracranial germinomas: twenty-five years' experience in a single center. *Int J Radiat Oncol Biol Phys*. 2004;58(4):1165–1170.
14. Ogawa K, Shikama N, Toita T, et al. Long-term results of radiotherapy for intracranial germinoma: a multi-institutional retrospective review of 126 patients. *Int J Radiat Oncol Biol Phys*. 2004;58(3):705–713.
15. Nguyen QN, Chang EL, Allen PK, et al. Focal and craniospinal irradiation for patients with intracranial germinoma and patterns of failure. *Cancer*. 2006;107(9):2228–2236.
16. Shirato H, Nishio M, Sawamura Y, et al. Analysis of long-term treatment of intracranial germinoma. *Int J Radiat Oncol Biol Phys*. 1997;37(3):511–515.
17. Shibamoto Y, Sasai K, Oya N, Hiraoka M. Intracranial germinoma: radiation therapy with tumor volume-based dose selection. *Radiology*. 2001;218(2):452–456.
18. Balmaceda C, Heller G, Rosenblum M, et al. Chemotherapy without irradiation–a novel approach for newly diagnosed CNS germ cell tumors: results of an international cooperative trial. The First International Central Nervous System Germ Cell Tumor Study. *J Clin Oncol*. 1996;14(11):2908–2915.
19. Kellie SJ, Boyce H, Dunkel IJ, et al. Primary chemotherapy for intracranial nongerminomatous germ cell tumors: results of the second international CNS germ cell study group protocol. *J Clin Oncol*. 2004;22(5):846–853.
20. Allen JC, DaRosso RC, Donahue B, Nirenberg A. A phase II trial of preirradiation carboplatin in newly diagnosed germinoma of the central nervous system. *Cancer*. 1994;74(3):940–944.
21. Bouffet E, Baranzelli MC, Patte C, et al. Combined treatment modality for intracranial germinomas: results of a multicentre SFOP experience. Société Française d'Oncologie Pédiatrique. *Br J Cancer*. 1999;79(7–8):1199–1204.
22. Buckner JC, Peethambaram PP, Smithson WA, et al. Phase II trial of primary chemotherapy followed by reduced-dose radiation for CNS germ cell tumors. *J Clin Oncol*. 1999;17(3):933–940.

23. Kretschmar C, Kleinberg L, Greenberg M, Burger P, Holmes E, Wharam M. Pre-radiation chemotherapy with response-based radiation therapy in children with central nervous system germ cell tumors: a report from the Children's Oncology Group. *Pediatr Blood Cancer.* 2007;48(3):285–291.
24. Sawamura Y, Shirato H, Ikeda J, et al. Induction chemotherapy followed by reduced-volume radiation therapy for newly diagnosed central nervous system germinoma. *J Neurosurg.* 1998;88(1):66–72.
25. Roberge D, Kun LE, Freeman CR. Intracranial germinoma: on whole-ventricular irradiation. *Pediatr Blood Cancer.* 2005;44(4):358–362.
26. Aoyama H, Shirato H, Ikeda J, Fujieda K, Miyasaka K, Sawamura Y. Induction chemotherapy followed by low-dose involved-field radiotherapy for intracranial germ cell tumors. *J Clin Oncol.* 2002;20(3):857–865.
27. Kiltie AE, Gattamaneni HR. Survival and quality of life of paediatric intracranial germ cell tumour patients treated at the Christie Hospital, 1972–1993. *Med Pediatr Oncol.* 1995;25(6):450–456.
28. Merchant TE, Sherwood SH, Mulhern RK, et al. CNS germinoma: disease control and long-term functional outcome for 12 children treated with craniospinal irradiation. *Int J Radiat Oncol Biol Phys.* 2000;46(5):1171–1176.
29. Sutton LN, Radcliffe J, Goldwein JW, et al. Quality of life of adult survivors of germinomas treated with craniospinal irradiation. *Neurosurgery.* 1999;45(6):1292–1297; discussion 1297.
30. Sands SA, Kellie SJ, Davidow AL, et al. Long-term quality of life and neuropsychologic functioning for patients with CNS germ-cell tumors: from the First International CNS Germ-Cell Tumor Study. *Neuro-oncology.* 2001;3(3):174–183.
31. Dearnaley DP, A'Hern RP, Whittaker S, Bloom HJ. Pineal and CNS germ cell tumors: Royal Marsden Hospital experience 1962–1987. *Int J Radiat Oncol Biol Phys.* 1990;18(4):773–781.
32. Fuller BG, Kapp DS, Cox R. Radiation therapy of pineal region tumors: 25 new cases and a review of 208 previously reported cases. *Int J Radiat Oncol Biol Phys.* 1994;28(1):229–245.
33. Hoffman HJ, Otsubo H, Hendrick EB, et al. Intracranial germ-cell tumors in children. *J Neurosurg.* 1991;74(4):545–551.
34. Matsutani M, Sano K, Takakura K, et al. Primary intracranial germ cell tumors: a clinical analysis of 153 histologically verified cases. *J Neurosurg.* 1997;86(3):446–455.
35. Baranzelli MC. Carboplatin-based chemotherapy (CT) and focal irradiation (RT) in primary cerebral germ cell tumors (GCT): A French Society of Pediatric Oncology (SFOP) experience. *Proc Am Soc Clin Oncol.* 1999;538.
36. Calaminus G, Bamberg M, Harms D, et al. AFP/beta-HCG secreting CNS germ cell tumors: long-term outcome with respect to initial symptoms and primary tumor resection. Results of the cooperative trial MAKEI 89. *Neuropediatrics.* 2005;36(2):71–77.
37. Ogawa K, Toita T, Nakamura K, et al. Treatment and prognosis of patients with intracranial nongerminomatous malignant germ cell tumors: a multiinstitutional retrospective analysis of 41 patients. *Cancer.* 2003;98(2):369–376.
38. Robertson PL, DaRosso RC, Allen JC. Improved prognosis of intracranial non-germinoma germ cell tumors with multimodality therapy. *J Neurooncol.* 1997;32(1):71–80.
39. Blakeley JO, Grossman SA. Management of pineal region tumors. *Curr Treat Options Oncol.* 2006;7(6):505–516.
40. Freeman CR, Farmer JP, Taylor RE. Central nervous system tumors in children. In: Halparin EC, Perez CA, Brady LW, eds. *Principles and Practice of Radiation Oncology.* 5th ed. Philadelphia: Lippincott Williams & Wilkins; 2008:1822–1849.
41. Lassman AB, Bruce JN, Fetell MR. Metastases to the pineal gland. *Neurology.* 2006;67(7):1303–1304.
42. Fauchon F, Jouvet A, Paquis P, et al. Parenchymal pineal tumors: a clinicopathological study of 76 cases. *Int J Radiat Oncol Biol Phys.* 2000;46(4):959–968.
43. Roncaroli F, Scheithauer BW. Papillary tumor of the pineal region and spindle cell oncocytoma of the pituitary: new tumor entities in the 2007 WHO Classification. *Brain Pathol.* 2007;17(3):314–318.
44. Schild SE, Scheithauer BW, Schomberg PJ, et al. Pineal parenchymal tumors. Clinical, pathologic, and therapeutic aspects. *Cancer.* 1993;72(3):870–880.
45. Schild SE, Scheithauer BW, Haddock MG, et al. Histologically confirmed pineal tumors and other germ cell tumors of the brain. *Cancer.* 1996;78(12):2564–2571.
46. Hasegawa T, Kondziolka D, Hadjipanayis CG, Flickinger JC, Lunsford LD. The role of radiosurgery for the treatment of pineal parenchymal tumors. *Neurosurgery.* 2002;51(4):880–889.
47. Kobayashi T, Kida Y, Mori Y. Stereotactic gamma radiosurgery for pineal and related tumors. *J Neurooncol.* 2001;54(3):301–309.
48. Reyns N, Hayashi M, Chinot O, et al. The role of Gamma Knife radiosurgery in the treatment of pineal parenchymal tumours. *Acta Neurochir (Wien).* 2006;148(1):5–11; discussion 11.
49. Kivelä T. Trilateral retinoblastoma: a meta-analysis of hereditary retinoblastoma associated with primary ectopic intracranial retinoblastoma. *J Clin Oncol.* 1999;17(6):1829–1837.
50. Antoneli CB, Ribeiro Kde C, Sakamoto LH, Chojniak MM, Novaes PE, Arias VE. Trilateral retinoblastoma. *Pediatr Blood Cancer.* 2007;48(3):306–310.
51. Duffner PK, Cohen ME, Sanford RA, et al. Lack of efficacy of postoperative chemotherapy and delayed radiation in very young children with pineoblastoma. Pediatric Oncology Group. *Med Pediatr Oncol.* 1995;25(1):38–44.
52. Jakacki RI. Pineal and nonpineal supratentorial primitive neuroectodermal tumors. *Childs Nerv Syst.* 1999;15(10):586–591.
53. Jakacki RI, Zeltzer PM, Boyett JM, et al. Survival and prognostic factors following radiation and/or chemotherapy for primitive neuroectodermal tumors of the pineal region in infants and children: a report of the Childrens Cancer Group. *J Clin Oncol.* 1995;13(6):1377–1383.
54. Cohen BH, Zeltzer PM, Boyett JM, et al. Prognostic factors and treatment results for supratentorial primitive neuroectodermal tumors in children using radiation and chemotherapy: a Childrens Cancer Group randomized trial. *J Clin Oncol.* 1995;13(7):1687–1696.
55. Lutterbach J, Fauchon F, Schild SE, et al. Malignant pineal parenchymal tumors in adult patients: patterns of care and prognostic factors. *Neurosurgery.* 2002;51(1):44–55; discussion 55.
56. Lee JY, Wakabayashi T, Yoshida J. Management and survival of pineoblastoma: an analysis of 34 adults from the brain tumor registry of Japan. *Neurol Med Chir (Tokyo).* 2005;45(3):132–141; discussion 141.
57. Konovalov AN, Pitskhelauri DI. Principles of treatment of the pineal region tumors. *Surg Neurol.* 2003;59(4):250–268.
58. Duffner PK, Horowitz ME, Krischer JP, et al. The treatment of malignant brain tumors in infants and very young children: an update of the Pediatric Oncology Group experience. *Neuro-oncology.* 1999;1(2):152–161.
59. Hoffman HJ. Dorsally exophytic brain stem tumors and midbrain tumors. *Pediatr Neurosurg.* 1996;24(5):256–262.
60. Pollack IF, Hoffman HJ, Humphreys RP, Becker L. The long-term outcome after surgical treatment of dorsally exophytic brain-stem gliomas. *J Neurosurg.* 1993;78(6):859–863.
61. Stark AM, Fritsch MJ, Claviez A, Dörner L, Mehdorn HM. Management of tectal glioma in childhood. *Pediatr Neurol.* 2005;33(1):33–38.
62. Kihlström L, Lindquist C, Lindquist M, Karlsson B. Stereotactic radiosurgery for tectal low-grade gliomas. *Acta Neurochir Suppl.* 1994;62:55–57.
63. Wang C, Zhang J, Liu A, Sun B, Zhao Y. Surgical treatment of primary midbrain gliomas. *Surg Neurol.* 2000;53(1):41–51.

98 Primary Central Nervous System Lymphoma

Christopher J. Schultz and Joseph Bovi

INTRODUCTION

Primary central nervous cell lymphoma (PCNSL) is an uncommon neoplasm of the brain, leptomeninges, and rarely the spinal cord. Initially thought to be characteristically associated with congenital, iatrogenic, or acquired immunosuppression, PCNSL is now recognized with increasing frequency in immunocompetent individuals. PCNSL most often occurs in middle-aged and elderly individuals. It is rarely encountered in immunocompetent children or young adults. The role of surgery is limited to establishing diagnosis, as PCNSL is often multifocal with a propensity to involve the subarachnoid space. Steroids can provide temporary tumor regression and palliation of presenting symptoms, though if instituted prior to tumor biopsy, the use of steroids can interfere with the establishment of a definitive pathologic diagnosis. Historically, whole brain radiation therapy (WBRT) has been the treatment of choice. This approach was largely based on the successful use of involved field radiation therapy in the treatment of other organ-confined extranodal malignant lymphomas. A whole brain volume has empirically been used to adequately address multifocal tumor frequently encountered at the time of PCNSL diagnosis. Despite high rates of response following WBRT, rapid recurrence is common and long-term survival is the exception. Chemotherapy alone or in combination with whole brain has more recently become the treatment of choice. Most effective regimens contain high-dose methotrexate and/or other agents that are capable of penetrating the blood–brain barrier. High response rates and improved survival with the use of chemotherapy have lead to treatment strategies that defer or eliminate WBRT in hopes of lessening the risk of neurotoxicity attributed to WBRT. Unfortunately, elimination of WBRT is also associated with a higher rate of relapse. Combined chemotherapy and WBRT regimens are now being explored, which use lower total doses of radiation and altered fractionation schedules in hopes of maintaining high rates of tumor control while minimizing neurotoxicity. Novel pre- and post-WBRT chemotherapeutic agents and treatment schedules that include a maintenance component are being explored as well. Pretreatment, multifactor prognostic indices have recently been described, which may allow selection of treatment regimens that strike an appropriate balance of risk and benefit for the individual PCNSL patient.

EPIDEMIOLOGY

It is estimated that PCNSL accounts for less than 1% to 2% of all non-Hodgkin's lymphomas and 3% to 6% of all primary brain tumors [1]. The annual incidence rate of PCNSL in the United States is approximately 0.04 to 0.06 per 100,000 person-years [1,2]. The incidence of PCNSL has been increasing over the past several decades in the United States [3], the United Kingdom [4], the Netherlands [5], Norway [6], and Japan [7] but has remained stable in Canada [8], Denmark [9], Scotland [10], Hong Kong [11], and India [12]. No single factor has been identified to explain this increase. The increase has been more pronounced than that noted for either primary brain tumors or non-Hodgkin's lymphomas. The trend cannot be attributed entirely to the increase in acquired or iatrogenic immunosuppression related to human immunodeficiency syndrome (HIV) and solid organ transplant, respectively, as increases are apparent in immunocompetent individuals as well. In some reports, the increase antedates the development of, and widespread implementation of, improved diagnostic imaging technologies and changes in pathologic classification schemes, which suggests that the increase is real and not an artifact related to improved detection or changes in PCNSL nosology.

According to the Central Brain Tumor Registry of the United States 1998 to 2002 statistical report, the median age of immunocompetent patients diagnosed with PCNSL is 60 years of age with the peak incidence rate occurring in the eighth decade [2]. The male-to-female ratio for immunocompetent PCNSL patients is approximately 2:1. Over 90% of HIV-related PCNSL patients are males, the majority of whom have used intravenous drugs. The median age of diagnosis in HIV-related PCNSL patients is 35 years. The risk of developing PCNSL is 2% to 6% in AIDS patients. This risk may increase as the length of survival is extended in AIDS patients with the use of highly active antiretroviral therapy (HAART). Solid organ transplant patients have an overall risk of 1% to 5% of developing a PCNSL. The risk is 1% to 2% for renal and 2% to 7% for cardiac, lung, or liver transplant recipients. Patients with congenital immune deficiency have a risk of 4% [13].

NATURAL HISTORY

The typical presentation of PCNSL in an immunocompetent patient involves progressive focal symptoms associated with a mass lesion. Nonspecific mental status changes frequently can herald the diagnosis of PCNSL. In a large series of 248 immunocompetent PCNSL patients, 70% presented on admission with a focal neurologic deficit, 43% with mental status changes, 33% with signs of increased intracranial pressure, 14% with seizures, and 4% with visual symptoms related to vitreous involvement [14]. The diagnosis of PCNSL can be difficult in both immunocompetent and immunocompromised patients who present with isolated brain, ocular, or meningeal tumors. Such patients often give a vague history of blurred vision, headache, and cranial nerve dysfunction or spinal nerve root symptoms. Remitting symptoms lasting several months to a year or more may delay the diagnosis of PCNSL. Empiric administration of corticosteroids may cause prolonged remission of clinical signs and symptoms, as well as radiographic findings; however, clinical and radiographic remission can also occur spontaneously [15]. Progressive dementia or stupor without focal signs is more common in patients with AIDS who have PCNSL. Unusual and uncommon PCNSL variants such as intravascular malignant lymphomatosis can mimic stroke or neurolymphomatosis; the latter, which characteristically includes lymphomatous involvement of both the central and peripheral nervous systems at presentation, can also confuse and/or delay diagnosis of PCNSL [16].

DIAGNOSTIC WORKUP

The diagnosis of PCNSL is predicated on the exclusion of the presence of systemic lymphoma. A subcommittee of the International PCNSL Collaborative Group recently reported a consensus opinion regarding the recommended baseline evaluation for all immunocompetent patients with PCNSL [17]. The recommended workup for PCNSL patients is summarized in Table 98.1.

History and Physical

A comprehensive baseline physical and neurologic examination should be performed on all patients. Age and performance status must be documented, as these two variables are established prognostic variables for PCNSL. Particular attention should be paid to the examination of peripheral lymph node regions, liver, spleen, and the testes, as primary testicular lymphoma can present with isolated brain involvement. An assessment of baseline neuropsychological function is recommended. No consensus has been established as to what test battery is most appropriate, though at a minimum a mini-mental status examination should be preformed as part of the baseline neurologic assessment. A more comprehensive test battery for the assessment of neuropsychological function and quality of life has recently been proposed for PCNSL patients. This comprehensive assessment incorporates multiple domains including attention and executive functions, verbal memory function, motor function, premorbid IQ estimation, and quality of life [18]. A complete ophthalmologic examination including dilatation and comprehensive (slit-lamp) fundoscopic examination is required in all patients to exclude vitreous, retinal, and optic nerve involvement. Cerebrospinal fluid (CSF) evaluation by lumbar puncture should be obtained for cytologic evaluation either preoperatively or at least 1 week following surgery. If an Ommaya reservoir is present, a separate ventricular CSF sample should also be obtained. Other CSF studies are optional and include flow cytometry, glucose, protein, and β2-microglobulin. Immunoglobulin gene rearrangement studies using the polymerase chain reaction can be useful in distinguishing reactive vs clonal populations of lymphocytes [19,20]. In HIV-positive patients for whom a biopsy is not advisable, detection of Epstein-Barr virus DNA in CSF lymphocytes can be helpful in establishing the diagnosis of PCNSL [21–23].

Laboratory Studies

HIV testing is suggested for all patients given the high risk of developing PCNSL in the HIV-positive patient population. Serum lactate dehydrogenase has been identified as a prognostic factor in extranodal lymphomas and should be obtained at baseline. Adequate liver, renal, and hematologic function should be established for patients who will be receiving chemotherapy. For patients receiving high-dose methotrexate, a creatinine clearance of 50 to 60 mL/min is also required to ensure adequate methotrexate excretion.

Radiographic Studies

Computed Tomography

Whole body computed tomography (CT) should be obtained to exclude the presence of systemic lymphoma. CT imaging of the primary brain lesion(s) is less informative than magnetic resonance imaging (MRI) and is typically used only in the setting of medical contraindication to the use of MRI. If CT imaging is obtained, PCNSL lesions are typically hyperdense or isodense. Nearly all lesions enhance following administration of contrast. Calcification and hemorrhage are rarely seen in immunocompetent patients [24]. In HIV patients a wider spectrum CT imaging characteristics can be seen, including a greater likelihood of detecting nonenhancing or ring-enhancing lesions. Hemorrhage and necrosis is also more common in HIV-associated PCNSL [25].

Magnetic Resonance Imaging

In a series of 100 immunocompetent patients with PCNSL, characteristic pretreatment MRI findings included contrast enhancement, tumor diameter of at least 15 mm, and contact with the subarachnoid space. The most frequent tumor locations were the cerebral hemisphere, the basal ganglia, and the corpus callosum. The mean number of lesions at presentation was 1.7 with a range of 1 to 8 [26]. Coulon et al. reported that most PCNSL lesions are hypointense or isointense on T1-weighted MRI images and approximately 50% are hyperintense on T2-weighted images. Uniform enhancement is common in immunocompetent patients. Modest edema and mass effect are present. Calcification,

Table 98.1 Baseline Evaluation for Newly Diagnosed Immunocompetent PCNSL Patients

Clinical Evaluation	Laboratory Evaluation	Evaluation of Extent of Disease	CNS Evaluation
Comprehensive physical examination emphasizing: peripheral lymph nodes, liver, spleen, and testes in male patients	Liver function tests	CT scans Chest Abdomen Pelvis	MRI with gadolinium contrast Brain Spine only if spinal symptoms present
Comprehensive neurologic examination including assessment of cognitive function	Renal function Creatinine BUN Creatinine clearance for patient who are to receive high-dose MTX	Positron emission tomography if CT imaging negative	CT scan in contrast may be substituted for patients in whom MRI is medically contraindicated (eg, cardiac pacemaker) Brain Spine only if spinal symptoms present
Recording of: Age Performance status Corticosteroid dose MMSE	Hematologic function CBC with differential platelets	Ophthalmologic evaluation Dilated fundoscopic exam (slit-lamp exam) assessing vitreous, retina, and optic nerve Fluorescein angiography helpful if retinal involvement suspected	CSF obtained preoperative or 1 week postoperative via lumbar puncture (and ventricular system if Ommaya reservoir present) Cytology Cell count (optional) Flow cytometry (optional) Protein (optional) Glucose (optional) β2-microglobulin (optional) Immunoglobulin gene rearrangement (optional)
	LDH HIV infection testing	Bone marrow biopsy Testicular ultrasound	

Abbreviations: BUN, blood urea nitrogen; LDH, lactate dehydrogenase; MMSE, mini-mental status examination; MTX, methotrexate.
Adapted from Abrey et al. [17].

hemorrhage, or necroses are scarcely seen [24]. The typical appearance of a PCNSL lesion in an immunocompetent patient is illustrated in Figure 98.1. Proton magnetic spectroscopy in PCNSL characteristically includes loss of N-acetylaspartate, a decrease in creatine, dramatic increase in choline, lactate, and lipids/macromolecules [27]. As noted with CT, MRI imaging in HIV patients has greater variability. Nonenhancing lesions and irregular enhancement patterns in addition to hemorrhage and necrosis are more commonly seen in HIV-related PCNSL patients [25].

Positron Emission Tomography

F^{18}-Fluorodeoxyglucose (FDG) positron emission tomography (PET) can be helpful in distinguishing MRI lesions that are suspicious for PCNSL from inflammatory and infectious processes. In HIV-positive patients, the standard uptake value (SUV) ratio for subjects found to have cerebral infections was significantly lower than the SUV for PCNSL patients. No overlap was seen between the range of SUV ratios for infection (0.3–0.7) and the range of SUV ratios for patients with lymphoma (1.7–3.1) [28]. In a recent retrospective analysis of immunocompetent PCNSL patients, FDG-PET was reported to be useful as part of initial staging and restaging. FDG avid foci were identified in 12 of 53 patients during the course of their disease. Nineteen percent had positive FDG-PET findings at initial diagnosis and 36% at relapse. Of note, in 8% of the patients FDG-PET was the only abnormal test suggestive of lymphoma [29]. FDG-PET is also useful in monitoring therapeutic response, especially in patients with persistent equivocal posttreatment MRI findings. It has been reported

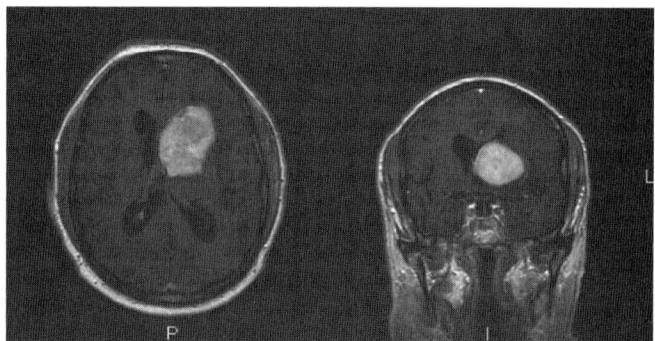

Figure 98.1 Coronal and axial gadolinium enhanced T1-weighted MRI images demonstrating homogeneously enhancing deep hemispheric periventricular mass characteristic of PCNSL in an immunocompetent patient.

that early FDG-PET response during or shortly after completion of chemotherapy can accurately predict long-term outcome in a small series of PCNSL patients [30].

PATHOLOGY

First described by Baily in 1929 as a "perithelial small cell sarcoma" and thereafter as a reticulum cell sarcoma and microglioma, respectively, PCNSL is now recognized as histologically identical to a systemic (typically) B-cell lymphoma [31]. Accordingly, the tumor cells express B-cell antigens, such as CD-20, with T-cell antigens restriction to small reactive lymphocytes. Further histological classification of PCNSL is possible using the Kiel classification (mainly used in Europe), the Working Formulation of non-Hodgkin's Lymphoma for Clinical Usage (mainly used in the United States), or the more recently proposed Revised European American Lymphoma classification that was developed to represent a compromise between the former two systems. All of these classification systems were developed for the purpose of grouping nodal lymphomas into useful clinical pathologic entities with distinct prognostic characteristics. Unfortunately, despite sharing similar histologic features with nodal lymphomas, further classification of PCNSL using any of these classification schemes is not useful, as correlative clinical prognostic significance for PCNSL is missing for these classification schemes. Practically, the majority of PCNSL can be REAL classified either as a small cell variant (high-grade B-cell lymphoma, Burkitt-like) or as a large cell variant (diffuse large B-cell lymphoma) [32].

The pathogenesis of PCNSL is not known and is potentially different in immunocompetent and immunocompromised patients. The consistent detection of EBV in HIV-related PCNSL implicates a possible viral cause for this immunosuppressed cohort. Detection of EBV is substantially less common in immunocompetent PCNSL patients suggesting that EBV infection is not necessarily central to the development of PCNSL in immunocompetent patients [33,34]. A variety of oncogenes and tumor suppressor genes known to be involved in the pathogenesis of nodal lymphomas have been assessed in small cohorts of immunocompetent PCNSL cases. Single mutations have been found in genes encoding p15, p16, and p53, whereas no alterations have been detected in common proto-oncogenes coding for cdk4, mdm2, rel, bcl-1, bcl-2, and c-myc. The most common abnormality reported thus far appears to involve down-regulation of p16 by homozygous deletion and more rarely methylation of the CDKN2A gene [32].

PROGNOSTIC FACTORS

Patient-Related Prognostic Factors

The prognosis of AIDS-associated PCNSL is inferior to PCNSL arising in immunocompetent individuals prompting similar though distinct treatment strategies [35]. With improved therapy for HIV since the introduction of HAART over the last decade, the merit of using similar treatment strategies for HIV-positive PCNSL patients and immunocompetent PCNSL patients is being reconsidered [36]. For both immunocompetent and immunocompromised PCNSL patients, age and performance status are the dominant prognostic factors. In the first prospective clinical trial, RTOG 83-15, age and Karnofsky performance status (KPS) were identified as independent prognostic factors [37]. Since that time, several prospective phase II cooperative group clinical trials have consistently confirmed the prognostic importance of age and performance status [38–40]. The importance of these patient-related variables is magnified by the inability to complete randomized clinical trial for PCNSL. For example, it has been suggested that the superior results reported for combined chemotherapy and radiotherapy reflect patient selection bias rather than treatment approach [41]. More recently, three prognostics scoring schemes have been proposed. The Nottingham/Barcelona prognostic score is based on age, performance status, multifocal, or meningeal disease [42]. The power of this scheme to detect important prognostic factors is questioned as it is based on a rather small cohort of 77 patients. Using this prognostic score, two significantly different prognostic groups can be identified. The International Extranodal Lymphoma Study Group has devised a 5-point scoring system that includes Eastern Cooperative Oncology Group performance status, lactate dehydrogenase, CSF total protein concentration, and involvement of deep structures [43]. This score was derived from retrospective analysis of 105 patients with complete data form a total of cohort of 378 patients treated at 48 different centers. The International Extranodal Lymphoma Study Group identifies three separate risk groups based on the presence of 0–1, 2–3, or 4–5 of the factors. Most recently, the Memorial Sloan-Kettering Cancer Center prognostic model for PCNSL has been described [44]. Two hundred eighty two patients from Memorial Sloan-Kettering Cancer Center were analyzed using the recursive partitioning analysis (RPA) method. Three distinct prognostic classes were identified: class 1: age ≤50, class 2: age >50 and KPS ≥70, and class 3: age >50 and KPS <70. The median failure-free survival for classes 1, 2, and 3 were 2.0, 1.8, and 0.6 years, respectively. The Memorial Sloan-Kettering Cancer Center PCNSL prognostic score was validated using an external data set of 152 patients treated on RTOG PCNSL trials, thereby confirming the validity of this prognostic scheme. Use of these prognostic scores may allow for more meaningful comparison of available phase II data and aid in the design of future prospective trials.

Tumor-Related Factors

Up until recently the only known prognostic factors of importance for PCNSL were clinical features, specifically: age, performance status, and immune status as described earlier. It is only recently that phenotypic and genetic markers have become the subject of investigation. Morphologic, immunophenotypic, and molecular genetic studies of PCNSL suggest that the cell of origin is related to the germinal center [45]. Bcl-6 protein is expressed almost exclusively in normal lymphoid germinal center B cells as well as in nodal lymphoma cells that arise from germinal center cells. Braaten and colleagues have identified Bcl-6 as a potentially promising prognostic marker for PCNSL [46]. Patients treated with high-dose intravenous methotrexate, who expressed Bcl-6, had a median survival of 101 months as compared with 14.7 months for those not expressing Bcl-6. Importantly, this finding held up in statistical analysis controlling for age, a powerful clinical prognostic factor as previously noted. In a much smaller series of patients, Chang and colleagues were not able to confirm the usefulness of Bcl-6 as a prognostic marker [47]. However, in this later analysis, an interesting observation of extremely poor survival was identified for immunocompetent PCNSL patients coexpressing p53 and c-Myc. Further work will be needed to validate these findings and to identify other useful tumor-related prognostic markers.

TREATMENT

Surgery

The role of surgical management on PCNSL is to establish a tissue diagnosis. Given the multifocality and propensity for subarachnoid space involvement, aggressive resections are rarely indicated. Typically, if PNCSL is suspected on clinical and radiographic grounds, a stereotactic biopsy is sufficient. As noted previously, CSF analysis including immunoglobulin gene rearrangement studies using the polymerase chain reaction can identify clonal lymphocytic populations, which may be sufficient to establish a diagnosis of PCNSL. In HIV-positive patients for whom a biopsy is not advisable, detection of Epstein-Barr virus DNA in CSF lymphocytes can be helpful in establishing the diagnosis of PCNSL [21–23].

Radiotherapy

Involved field radiation therapy alone is highly successful in the treatment of low volume early stage (organ-confined) extranodal lymphomas. Extrapolating this experience with the more common extranodal lymphomas, radiation therapy alone for PCNSL was the empiric treatment of choice for several decades. Paradoxically, the ability to achieve a complete response of PCNSL to WBRT alone in the majority of cases has not assured long-term control, as is often the case with other extranodal lymphomas.

Treatment Volume

The current RT treatment volume for PCNSL patients is a whole brain field empirically chosen to address the multifocal nature of PCNSL. A left and right lateral equally weighted, opposed field arrangement using 6 to 10 Mv photon is most often used. Custom cerrobend blocks or a multileaf collimation is used to shape the fields. The field shaping at the skull base must be carefully considered to avoid inadvertent shielding of the meninges/subarachnoid space in the region of the anterior temporal lobes and the cribriform plate. Most often, the posterior one third of the orbits are included in the treatment volume. The anterior edge of the field is typically made coplanar via a gantry rotation so as to avoid exposure of the contralateral eye due to anterior divergence of the lateral beam. The anterior, posterior, and superior field borders include 1 to 2 cm of "fall off" to insure adequate dosimetric coverage of the meninges/subarachnoid space. The inferior border is usually the C1–2 or C2–3 vertebral body interspace. When ocular involvement is evident and WBRT alone is to be given or if there is a desire to boost the eyes after initial response to "up-front" chemotherapy, the entirety of both eyes are included for a portion of the treatment up to a dose of 20 to 30 Gy. For some patients, a scalp block may be added after 18 to 20 Gy to minimize the likelihood of developing permanent convexity alopecia. Representative dosimetric profiles and collimation patterns for WBRT and WBRT/whole orbit field arrangements used to treat PCNSL patients are provided in Figures 98.2 and 98.3, respectively.

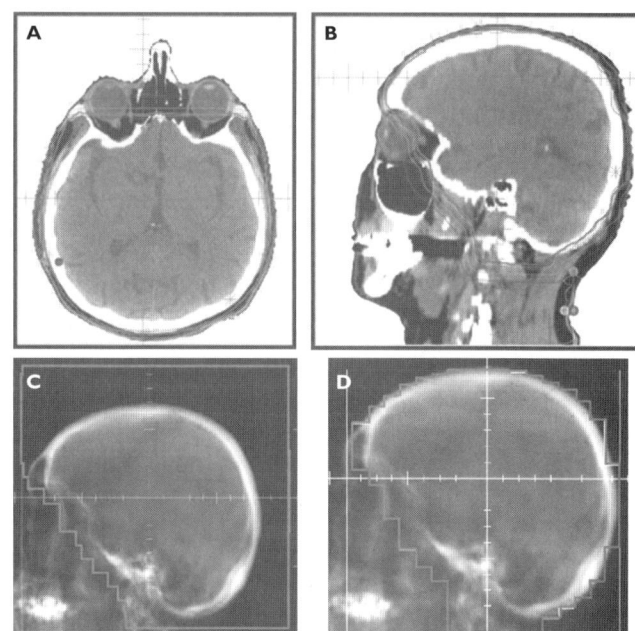

Figure 98.2 Isodose plots superimposed on the treatment planning CT images for a parallel opposed shaped WBRT PCNSL field arrangement (100% isodose line shown in red). The axial plot **(A)** demonstrates the desired coplanar anterior field edge in region of the posterior orbit, thereby avoiding divergence into contralateral orbit. Adequate coverage of the subarachnoid space is demonstrated on the sagital plot **(B)**. Typical WBRT multileaf collimation is demonstrated in image **(C)**. A "scalp block" multileaf collimation pattern is shown in image **(D)** that may be considered after 18 to 20 Gy has been delivered to the initial WBRT fields. Use of such a "scalp block" allows for adequate dose to subarachnoid space while lowering the probability of permanent convexity alopecia. *See color insert.*

Dose

Based on a comprehensive review of the literature, Murray reported a dose response for PCNSL patients treated with WBRT alone [48]. A significant improvement in survival time for PCNSL patients who received a total dose of ≥50 Gy was identified in 188 cases selected from published series. This finding framed the hypothesis for the first prospective cooperative group trial, RTOG 83–15. In this trial, immunocompetent PCNSL patients received fractionated WBRT to 40 Gy followed by a boost to the initial tumor site(s) of 20 Gy. The treatment was delivered using 2 Gy fractions. This trial failed to show a significant improvement in survival with the use of "high-dose" WBRT as a median survival of 11.6 months was achieved, not substantially different from survival reported for historical controls that received lower WBRT doses. Importantly, this trial was the first completed prospective cooperative group trial of any kind for patients with PCNSL. Although no survival advantage was identified with the escalation of WBRT in RTOG trial 83–15, age and performance status were identified for the first time as significant prognostic factors [37].

In the second RTOG trial 88–06, the role of nonpenetrating CHOD (cyclophosphamide, adriamycin, vincristine,

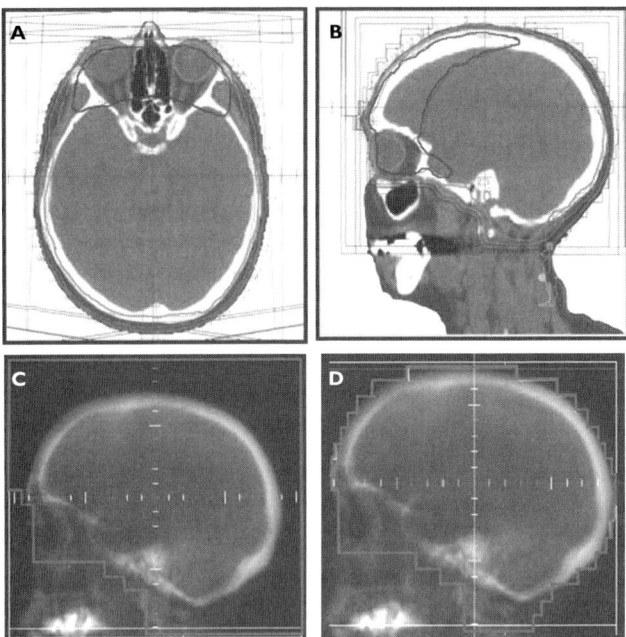

Figure 98.3 Isodose plots superimposed on treatment planning CT images for a parallel opposed shaped WBRT and whole orbit PCNSL field arrangement used when there is ocular involvement. The axial **(A)** and sagital **(B)** plots illustrate the dose inhomogeneity (volume encompassed by 110% isodose line shown in blue, 100% isodose line shown in green) that can occur when using typical WBRT arrangements. Compensating filters or "wedges" can be used to improve the homogeneity of dose in such cases. In addition, the total dose and fractionation scheme can be modified to lessen the risk of acute and late toxicity associated with such dosimetric inhomogeneity. Typical WBRT/orbit multileaf collimation pattern and WBRT/orbit "scalp block" multileaf collimation pattern are shown in images **(C)** and **(D)**, respectively. See color insert.

and decadron) chemotherapy was tested [39]. The WBRT treatment regimen was intentionally identical to that used in RTOG trial 83–15 so as to allow for historical comparison of the phase II trials isolating the effect of the "experimental" chemotherapy. No difference was identified between the two studies. A secondary analysis of these two studies was performed by Corn et al. and revealed that complete tumor response was achieved in approximately 80% of treated patients. Complete response was associated with statistically improved median survival, 2 years vs 0.5 years; however, the majority of patients including those achieving complete response failed to survive 4 years. The authors concluded that additional dose escalation strategies to improve the rate of complete response were not warranted [49]. The third RTOG trial 93–10 tested the role of penetrating chemotherapy using a combined chemotherapy regimen initially piloted by DeAngelis et al. [50]. In this trial, the dose of WBRT was 45 Gy delivered 25 fractions of 1.8 Gy. No field reduction or "boost" was given. This regimen was the first prospective multi-institutional cooperative group trial to demonstrate improved survival using combined chemotherapy and radiation therapy. A median progression-free survival of 24 months and median overall survival of 36.9 months were achieved far superior to the median survival of 11 to 12 months achieved in the two previous RTOG trials [40]. In RTOG trial 93–15, a subset of the patients achieving a complete response to pre-WBRT chemotherapy were treated with a hyperfractionated regimen of 36 Gy delivered at 1.2 Gy bid. This approach was chosen to begin to test whether the use of smaller doses per fraction and a lower total dose could be used in a sequential chemotherapy and WBRT regimen with the goal of reducing treatment-related neurotoxicity. In a secondary analysis of this subset reported by Fisher et al., there was no statistical difference in progression-free survival or overall survival for the patients receiving hyperfractionated WBRT despite a 25% reduction in the estimated biological effective tumor dose of the hyperfractionated regimen. The hyperfractionated regimen delayed but did not eliminate the development of severe neurotoxicity associated with combined chemoradiation [51]. The fourth RTOG trial 02–27 is ongoing and is a phase I/II trial testing the efficacy of pre-WBRT chemotherapy that includes high-dose intravenous methotrexate, rituximab, and temozolomide and post-WBRT maintenance temozolomide. The WBRT hyperfractionated regimen piloted in RTOG trial 93ñ10 is being used in this trial in hopes of further defining the role of dose-reduced WBRT.

Two other studies have been published, which used reduced-dose WBRT. Bessell and colleagues reported their experience using WBRT to total doses of 30.6 Gy vs 45 Gy (plus a 10 Gy boost in five fractions, to site of a single lesion) delivered in once daily 1.8 Gy fractions in patient's achieving a complete response to pre-WBRT chemotherapy. The overall 3-year survival for those patients receiving 45 Gy vs 30.6 Gy was 92% vs 60%, respectively, a difference that reached statistical significance. Their results suggest that when using the chemotherapy regimen as delivered in this trial, it may be necessary to deliver WBRT doses above 30.60 Gy [52]. In distinction to this finding, the use of reduced-dose WBRT of 23.4 Gy in a cohort of 17 patients following complete response to pre-WBRT chemotherapy (using a similar chemotherapy regimen tested in RTOG trial 93–10 plus rituximab) was not associated with a decrease in progression-free survival when compared with historical results for patients receiving WBRT to 45 Gy. Importantly, no neurocognitive decline has developed in the reduced WBRT cohort [53]. Future studies will be necessary to further define the optimal WBRT dose in the setting of combined modality treatment of PCNSL.

Chemotherapy

Lack of long-term efficacy of WBRT alone has prompted the investigation of combined chemotherapy and radiation therapy approaches, again in fashion analogous to the evolution of treatment of locally advanced systemic nodal and extranodal lymphomas. Many of the initial combined modality therapy approaches, including the first completed phase II prospective combined modality intergroup group trial, tested agents commonly used for systemic lymphoma such as cyclophosphamide, adriamycin, vincristine, and prednisone. Other trials using similar regimens that tested the so-called nonpenetrating chemotherapy were subsequently completed. These trials collectively have failed to identify any improvement in survival over the use of WBRT alone. Use of agents that are not capable of penetrating the intact blood–brain barrier is thought to be the major reason for the failure of these nonpenetrating chemotherapy approaches [54]. In contrast, combined regimens that incorporate agents capable of penetrating the intact blood–brain barrier (such as high-dose methotrexate and cytosine arabinoside) or hybrid regimens contain both penetrating and nonpenetrating chemotherapy have resulted in substantial improvement in survival, particularly for patients younger than 50 to 60 years of age. In many trials, WBRT is delivered following initial chemotherapy so as to allow for assessment of chemotherapy response. High rates of initial response in these trials have also prompted, treatment strategies, which defer WBRT, with the hope that delayed neurotoxicity, largely attributed to WBRT can be avoided. In most trials when WBRT is used, radiation doses are similar to the doses employed when radiation therapy alone is used. Mixed long-term results using deferred WBRT have been reported. A significant number of patients treated with "up-front" chemotherapy will require deferred or salvage WBRT. In addition to these patients who fail to achieve an initial complete response or who later progress, patients with initial poor renal function or deteriorating renal function following initiation of chemotherapy (particularly those receiving potentially renal toxic high-dose methotrexate) are often not able to receive or cannot complete the desired "up-front" chemotherapy. These patients will often require "salvage" WBRT. A representative summary of recent phase II clinical trials that have tested WBRT alone, penetrating and nonpenetrating chemotherapy administered alone or in combination with WBRT for immunocompetent PCNSL patients is provided in Table 98.2 [37–40,42,51,55–67].

Intrathecal Chemotherapy

High-dose methotrexate is the most effective single agent in the treatment of PCNSL. Recognizing the propensity for PCNSL to involve the subarachnoid space, intrathecal chemotherapy, most often, methotrexate is prophylactically administered together with high-dose intravenous methotrexate or multiagent chemotherapy to insure adequate CSF drug levels. A recent case matched retrospective comparison of high-dose intravenous methotrexate with or without intrathecal methotrexate failed to demonstrate a difference in survival, disease control, or neurotoxicity [68]. The authors contend that adequate CSF methotrexate levels can be achieved when adequate doses and infusion rates are utilized when administering intravenous methotrexate alone. Other intrathecal agents used in PCNSL regimens include Ara-C and hydrocortisone. Similar outcomes have been reported from single institutional and cooperative group studies using penetrating systemic chemotherapy with or without intrathecal therapy (see Table 98.2). In distinction to the use of prophylactic intrathecal chemotherapy, there is little doubt that intrathecal chemotherapy is necessary when treating PCNSL patients with positive CSF cytology at diagnosis or at relapse.

Intra-Arterial Chemotherapy

Intra-arterial chemotherapy delivered with mannitol blood–brain barrier disruption has been used in the treatment of PCNSL. This technique allows enhanced delivery of chemotherapeutic agents that do not readily cross the blood–brain barrier when administered intravenously. Neuwelt et al. reported prolonged survival with preservation of cognitive function in a pilot single institutional study [69]. A select subset of patients who received osmotic blood–brain barrier enhanced intra-arterial chemotherapy alone had complete tumor clearance and had stable or improved neurocognitive function 1 to 7 years posttreatment. The authors point out that this approach is more aggressive, costly, and requires considerable experience to administer safely than standard intravenous chemotherapy. This approach is currently being explored further in the Blood–Brain Barrier Consortium.

High-Dose Chemotherapy with Stem Cell Support

High-dose chemotherapy supported with autologous peripheral blood stem cell transfusion is another strategy that has recently been investigated for patients with PCNSL. This approach may allow drug dose escalation, which overcomes the blood–brain barrier constraints for drugs that do not penetrate the blood–brain barrier in sufficient concentrations when given at conventional lower doses. In addition, the strategy may allow dose intensification of "penetrating" chemotherapeutic agents, thereby eliminating the need for WBRT and the associated neurocognitive toxicity attributed to WBRT. Two recent phase II multi-institutional trials have tested this approach and have established feasibility [70,71]. Although feasible, the event-free survival for both trials was not superior to that achieved with conventional chemotherapy and WBRT. Interestingly, the more intensive chemotherapy regimens did not produce better complete response rates. A complete response rate of 44% (OSHO) and 70% (GOELOMS) for the two trials was in fact similar to that achieved with conventional chemotherapy. Despite the intent to defer or eliminate the need for WBRT with this approach, all patients in the GOELOMS trial and 9 or 23 patients who failed to achieve a complete response in the OSHO trial received WBRT. Induction regimen toxicity remains a potential pitfall of this approach as one death occurred during induction in the GOELOMS trial and three deaths occurred in the OSHO trial. The authors conclude this approach is best considered for patients with refractory disease, in relapse, or partially responding to conventional chemotherapy.

Salvage Chemotherapy

Sixty percent of patients who achieve an initial complete response following treatment for PCNSL will relapse [72]. Survival after relapse of PCNSL without treatment is approximately 2 months; however, salvage regimens have been shown to significantly improve this outcome [72–77]. Isolated systemic location and good KPS are

Table 98.2 Representative Summary of the Recent Clinical Trials for Immunocompetent PCNSL Patients

	References	Median Age	Chemotherapy	Penetrating vs Nonpenetrating		IT/IO Therapy	Radiation WBRT (Boost)	XRT at Relapse	PFS	OS	Neuro-Tox
				Pen	Non						
XRT alone	Nelson et al. [37]	66	None			None	40 Gy (20 Gy)		NS	1 year 48% 2 years 28%	None
Chemo + XRT	DeAngelis et al. [40]	56.5	MTX, Vin, Pro, Leu, Dex, ARA-C after XRT			IO MTX	45 Gy		24 months	2 years 64% 3 years 52% 5 years 32%	53% Gr 3, 4/w chemo, 15% leu[a], no change in MMSE[b]
	Poortmans et al. [55]	51	MBVP	X		IT MTX ARA-C Hydrocortisone	40 Gy		NS	2 years 69% 3 years 58%	None
	Gavrilovic et al. [56]	65	MTX, Vin, Pro	X		IO MTX	45 Gy		Not reached	Pts ≥ 60 years 29 months	26% <60 years 75% ≥60 years
	Fisher et al. [51]	NS	MTX, Vin, Pro, Leu, Dex, ARA-C after XRT	X		IO MTX	45 Gy 25 fx (STD) or 36 Gy 30 fx 3 weeks (HFX)		24.5 months STD FX 23.3 months HFX	Median 36.9 months	10% grade 5
	O'Brien et al. [57]	58	MTX	X		None	45 Gy (5.4)		2 years 65%	2 years 65% 2 years 70%	22% at 30 months
	Blay et al. [58]	51	C5R	X		IT MTX Hydrocortisone	20 Gy (30 Gy)		NS	3 years 56%	None
	Abrey et al. [59]	65	MTX Leu Pro Vin, ARA-C	X		IO MTX	45 Gy		NS	Median 60 months	25% overall 83% in pts >60 years
	Abrey et al. [60]	59	MTX Leu ARA-C	X		IO MTX	40 Gy (14.4 Gy)		NS	5 years 22.3%	2 pts <50 years 80% >60 years
	Bessell et al. [42]	59	CHOD/BVAM	X		None	45 Gy (10 Gy)		NS	5 years 31%	8% in pt <60 62% in pt >60
	O'Neill et al. [38]	63.5	CHOP/HDAC		X	None	50.4 Gy		1 year 35% 3 years 11%	1 year 44% 3 years 14%	Higher in pt >60
	Schultz et al. [39]	NS	CHOD		X	None	41.4 Gy		Median 9.2 months	2 years 42%	1 encephalomalacia
	Brada et al. [61]	51	MACOP-B		X	None	40 Gy (15 Gy)		5 years 32%	5 years 36%	1 pt unclear if treatment related
Chemotherapy alone	Pels et al. [62]	62	MTX, Vin, Ifos, Dex Pred, ARA-C	X		IT MTX		28%	NS	2 years 69% 5 years 43%	35% MRI white matter changes, asymptomatic
	Gerstner et al. [63]	60	MTX	X		None		52%	Median 12.8 months	Median 55.4 months	No leu[a] reported
	Batchelor et al. [64]	60	MTX	X		None		52%	Median 12.8 months	Not reached	NS
	Hoang-Xuan et al. [65]	72	MTX Lom Pro methylpred	X		IT MTX cytarabine		NS	1 year 40% Median 6.8 months	Median 14.3 months	8% MMSE[b] decrease
	Sandor et al. [66]	57	MTX Leu Thio Vin Dex	X		IT MTX ARA-C		57%	Median 16.5 months 57 months 34.3%	4.5 years 68.8%	2 pt w/ grade 3 leu[a]
	Dahlborg et al. [67]	52.3	CMPD	X		None		31%	NS	Median 40 months	No neuropsych deficit reported
	Gavrilovic et al. [56]	65	MTX Vin Pro	X		IO MTX		NS	7 months	3 years 55% 5 years 31%	1 pt

Abbreviations: ARA-C, cytarabine; C5R, cyclophosphamide, vincristine, methotrexate, hydrocortisone, methylprednisolone, adriamycin, cytarabine; CHOD/BVAM, cyclophosphamide, doxorubicin, vincristine, dexamethasone, carmustine, vincristine, cytarabine, methotrexate; CHOP/HDAC, cyclophosphamide, adriamycin, vincristine, prednisone, high-dose cytarabine; CMPD, cyclophosphamide, methotrexate, procarbazine, dexamethasone; Dex, dexamethasone; HFX, hyperfractionation; Ifos, ifosfamide; IO MTX, intra-ommaya methotrexate; IT MTX, intrathecal methctrexate; Leu, leucovorin; Lom, lomustine; MACOP-B, methotrexate, doxorubicin, cyclophosphamide, vincristine, prednisolone; MBVP, methotrexate, teniposide, carmustine, methylprednisolone; Methylpred, methylprednisolone; MTX, Methotrexate; Pred, prednisone; Pro, procarbazine; STD, standard fractionation; Thio, thiotepa; Vin, vincristine.

[a] Leukoencephalopathy.
[b] Mini-mental status examination.
NS—Not stated.

associated with favorable response to salvage chemotherapy [78]. Tumor responses are achieved with a variety of salvage regimens although no regimen has been established as a standard of care. High-dose methotrexate has been examined as salvage therapy in patients who had a complete response to initial therapy [74]. Overall response rates were 91% for first salvage and median survival was 61.9 months after first relapse. Both single agent temozolomide and topotecan have been examined [77,79]. Topotecan was given for five consecutive days for each 21-day cycle in patients with relapsed PCNSL. The overall response rate to this regimen was 40%. This benefit was at the cost of significant myelotoxicity with over two third of the patients having grade 3 or 4 neutropenia [77]. Temozolomide was much better tolerated without any major toxicity. There was a 26% objective response noted in those patients who were treated with temozolomide at relapse and those who achieved a complete response and maintained the response for a median duration of 6+ months [79].

Multidrug regimens have been used for relapsed PCNSL including procarbazine, lomustine, and vincristine (PCV). Results of this regimen showed an 86% overall response rate and 57% of patients with a complete response or stable disease for more than 1 year out from treatment. More recently, temozolomide and rituximab have been used as salvage treatment for relapsed PCNSL. Response rates of greater than 50% and a median survival ranging from 8 to 14 months have been reported in small single institutional trial [80,81]. A far more intensive regimen of high-dose chemotherapy followed by stem cell rescue has also been employed with promising results [82].

Salvage therapies have clearly shown improvement over supportive care alone in median survival and duration of response in patients with relapsed PCNSL. Further study is warranted to determine the most effective regimen for this patient population.

TREATMENT OF AIDS-RELATED PCNSL

Patients with HIV who develop PCNSL in general have had inferior survival as compared with non-HIV-related PCNSL patients. The use of conventional treatment strategies used for non-HIV patients in the era before HAART was in routine use, resulted in only modest prolongation of survival over supportive care alone [35]. As an example, the median survival for patients treated on an intergroup trial that combined sequential chemotherapy and an accelerated WBRT was 2.4 months [83]. Forty percent of patients failed to complete the protocol therapy. Four of 34 patients survived more than 12 months. In contrast, HIV patients receiving HAART therapy and treatment for PCNSL appear to have improved survival [84]. It is assumed that this is a consequence of recovery of the immune system; however, it has been suggested that the improved survival may at least be in part related to the radiosensitizing effects of HAART therapy [85]. In a review of 111 patients with HIV-related PCNSL, the use of HAART and WBRT to doses ≥30 Gy had an additive positive effect on survival [86]. The authors suggest that use of HAART and WBRT RT to ≥30 Gy might serve as a standard of care for future trials of novel therapy and quality of life.

The association between EBV infection and HIV-related PCNSL has led investigators to consider antiviral therapy for immunocompromised PCNSL patients. Raez et al. proposed that the use of interleukin, ganciclovir, and HAART therapy might be a novel treatment strategy for HIV-related PCNSL [87]. Anecdotal responses have been reported using this approach lending support to the notion that antiviral therapy and reconstitution of the immune system can be effective in EBV-related PCNSL [88]. The use of ganciclovir has been shown to decrease the EBV DNA load in the CSF of patients with HIV-related PCNSL. This finding lends support to the hypothesis that EBV is in fact replicating in HIV patients with PCNSL and therefore may be a therapeutic target [89].

RT TREATMENT EFFECTS

Acute Treatment Effects

Acute effects are defined as effects that develop ≤90 days from the start of WBRT. All patients are likely to develop total scalp alopecia, erythema, and dry desquamation of the scalp within the treatment portal. Some PCNSL patients may experience fatigue, anorexia, mild nausea, or headache. Inflammation of the external auditory canal (rarely progressing to external otitis media) complicating dry desquamation of the external auditory canal skin or accumulation of middle ear fluid associated with eustation tube dysfunction is not uncommon. Patients requiring treatment to the entire eye are likely to experience conjunctival irritation and may note dry eyes. All of the above-described acute effects are typically reversible with resolution 4 to 6 weeks from completion of WBRT. If middle ear congestion persists, it may be associated with conductive hearing loss. Patients with such persistence, who fail to respond to oral decongestants, may require myringotomy tube placement.

Late Treatment Effects

Late effects occur >90 days from completion of WBRT. Patients receiving WBRT to doses greater than 30 Gy delivered in conventional fractions of 1.8 to 2 Gy will likely experience permanent, total or partial, scalp alopecia. Chronic middle ear effusions are rare. Sensory neural hearing loss is uncommon in patients who receive 45 Gy or less to the inner ear. All patients are at a high risk of developing cataracts that may or may not require treatment. Patients receiving steroids, chemotherapy, and/or WBRT, which includes the entire eye, are at the highest risk of developing cataracts. All patients receiving WBRT are at risk of developing neurocognitive dysfunction. The risk of developing neurocognitive decline following WBRT increases with age (particularly age >60), total WBRT dose, co-administration of chemotherapy, and sequence of chemotherapy delivery (highest risk with concurrent or post-WBRT chemotherapy administration). Post-WBRT cognitive decline may be associated with urinary incontinence and gait

Table 98.3 Several Fundamental Challenges yet to be Addressed in Future PCNSL Trials

1. What is the best MTX-based chemotherapy for PCNSL?
2. What is the best administration schedule for high-dose MTX?
3. Is combined chemotherapy superior to high-dose MTX regimens?
4. Is intrathecal chemotherapy necessary for all patients with PCNSL?
5. What is the role for blood–brain barrier disruption, what agents?
6. What is the role for high-dose chemotherapy with autologous stem cell transplant?
7. Is WBRT necessary for all patients with PCNSL?
8. Has the optimal total dose and fractionation scheme for WBRT?
9. What is the best treatment for ocular involvement in patients with PCNSL?
10. What is the best treatment for meningeal lymphoma?
11. What is the optimal salvage therapy for progressive or relapsed PCNSL patients?

Abbreviations: MTX, methotrexate; PCNSL, primary central nervous system lymphoma.

Adapted from Ferreri et al. [91].

abnormalities similar to that seen with normal pressure hydrocephalus [90].

FUTURE DIRECTIONS

Optimal therapy for PCNSL remains to be defined. The uncommon nature of PCNSL hampers the ability to perform large randomized single institutional or cooperative group trials. International intergroup trials will be required to convincingly address fundamental unanswered questions. Several of the challenges yet to be addressed in future PCNSL trials are summarized in Table 98.3. Additional research strategies, which may compliment formal prospective clinical trials, have been suggested and include the creation of a shared historical database, which would pool information from multiple studies that incorporates identical patient entry criteria and similar end point reporting that necessarily includes cognitive function and quality of life information. Creation of an international PCNSL tissue bank may also provide an additional resource to identify pivotal biological information that may hasten the development of novel and effective PCNSL therapy [91].

REFERENCES

1. U.S. Cancer Statistics Working Group. United States Cancer Statistics: 1999–2004 Incidence and Mortality Web-based Report. Atlanta: U.S. Department of Health and Human Services, Centers for Disease Control and Prevention and National Cancer Institute; 2007–2008.
2. CBTRUS. Statistical Report: Primary Brain Tumors in the United States, 1998–2002. Published by the Central Brain Tumor Registry of the United States; 2005.
3. Olson JE, Janney CA, Rao RD, et al. The continuing increase in the incidence of primary central nervous system non-Hodgkin lymphoma: a surveillance, epidemiology, and end results analysis. *Cancer.* 2002;95:1504–1510.
4. Lutz JM, Coleman MP. Trends in primary cerebral lymphoma. *Br J Cancer.* 1994;70:716–718.
5. van der Sanden GA, Schouten LJ, van Dijck JA, et al. Primary central nervous system lymphomas: incidence and survival in the Southern and Eastern Netherlands. *Cancer.* 2002;94:1548–1556.
6. Salvesen Haldorsen I, Aarseth JH, Hollender A, Larsen JL, Espeland A, Mella O. Incidence, clinical features, treatment and outcome of primary central nervous system lymphoma in Norway. *Acta Oncol.* 2004;43:520–529.
7. Makino K, Nakamura H, Kino T, Takeshima H, Kuratsu J. Rising incidence of primary central nervous system lymphoma in Kumamoto, Japan. *Surg Neurol.* 2006;66:503–506.
8. Hao D, DiFancesco LM, Brasher PM, et al. Is primary CNS lymphoma really becoming more common? A population based study of incidence, clinicopathologic features and outcome in Alberta from 1975 to 1996. *Ann Oncol.* 1999;10:65–70.
9. Clinicopathological features, survival and prognostic factors of primary central nervous system lymphomas: trends in incidence of primary central nervous system lymphomas and primary malignant brain tumors in a well-defined geographical area. Population-based data from the Danish Lymphoma Registry, Lyfo, and the Danish Cancer Registry. *Leuk Lymphoma.* 1995;19:223–233.
10. Yau YH, O'Sullivan MG, Signorini D, Ironside JW, Whittle IR. Primary lymphoma of the central nervous system in immunocompetent patients in south-east Scotland. *Lancet.* 1996;348:890.
11. Au WY, Chan AC, Srivastava G, Leung SY, Liang R. Incidence and pathology of primary brain lymphoma in Hong Kong Chinese patients. *Leuk Lymphoma.* 2000;37:175–179.
12. Sarkar C, Sharma MC, Deb P, Singh R, Santosh V, Shankar SK. Primary central nervous system lymphoma—a hospital based study of incidence and clinicopathological features from India (1980–2003). *J Neurooncol.* 2005;71:199–204.
13. Schabet M. Epidemiology of primary CNS lymphoma. *J Neurooncol.* 1999;43:199–201.
14. Bataille B, Delwail V, Menet E, et al. Primary intracerebral malignant lymphoma: report of 248 cases. *J Neurosurg.* 2000;92:261–266.
15. Partap S, Spence AM. Spontaneously relapsing and remitting primary CNS lymphoma in an immunocompetent 45-year-old man. *J Neurooncol.* 2006;80:305–307.
16. Shenkier TN. Unusual variants of primary central nervous system lymphoma. *Hematol Oncol Clin North Am.* 2005;19:651–664.
17. Abrey LE, Batchelor TT, Ferreri AJ, et al. Report of an international workshop to standardize baseline evaluation and response criteria for primary CNS lymphoma. *J Clini Oncol.* 2005;23:5034–5043.
18. Correa D, Maron L, Harder H, et al. Cognitive functions in primary central nervous system lymphoma: literature review and assessment guidelines. *Ann Oncol.* 2007;18:1145–1151.
19. Ekstein D, Ben-Yehuda D, Slyusarevsky E, Lossos A, Linetsky E, Siegal T. CSF analysis of IgH gene rearrangement in CNS lymphoma: relationship to the disease course. *J Neurol Sci.* 2006;247:39–46.
20. Wildemann B, Jansen O, Haas J, Vogt-Schaden ME, Storch-Hagenlocher B. Rapid distinction of acute demyelinating disorders and central nervous system lymphoma by molecular analysis of cerebrospinal fluid cells. *J Neurol.* 2001;248:127–130.
21. Cinque P, Brytting M, Vago L, et al. Epstein-Barr virus DNA in cerebrospinal fluid from patients with AIDS-related primary lymphoma of the central nervous system. *Lancet.* 1993;342:398–401.
22. Yu H, Xie Y, Wang G. [The clinical features and prognostic factors of 22 patients with primary central nervous system lymphoma]. *Chung-Hua Nei Ko Tsa Chih Chin J Int Med.* 2001;40:325–328.
23. De Luca A, Antinori A, Cingolani A, et al. Evaluation of cerebrospinal fluid EBV-DNA and IL-10 as markers for *in vivo* diagnosis of AIDS-related primary central nervous system lymphoma. *Br J Haematol.* 1995;90:844–849.
24. Coulon A, Lafitte F, Hoang-Xuan K, et al. Radiographic findings in 37 cases of primary CNS lymphoma in immunocompetent patients. *Eur Radiol.* 2002;12:329–340.
25. Thurnher MM, Rieger A, Kleibl-Popov C, et al. Primary central nervous system lymphoma in AIDS: a wider spectrum of CT and MRI findings. *Neuroradiology.* 2001;43:29–35.
26. Kuker W, Nagele T, Korfel A, et al. Primary central nervous system lymphomas (PCNSL): MRI features at presentation in 100 patients. *J Neurooncol.* 2005;72:169–177.
27. Raizer JJ, Koutcher JA, Abrey LE, et al. Proton magnetic resonance spectroscopy in immunocompetent patients with primary central nervous system lymphoma. *J Neurooncol.* 2005;71:173–180.
28. Villringer K, Jager H, Dichgans M, et al. Differential diagnosis of CNS lesions in AIDS patients by FDG-PET. *J Comput Assist Tomogr.* 1995;19:532–536.

29. Mohile NA, DeAngelis LM, Abrey LE. The utility of body FDG PET in staging primary central nervous system lymphoma. *Neuro-oncology.* 2008;10:223–228.
30. Palmedo H, Urbach H, Bender H, et al. FDG-PET in immunocompetent patients with primary central nervous system lymphoma: correlation with MRI and clinical follow-up. *Eur J Nucl Med Mol Imaging.* 2006;33:164–168.
31. Baily P. Intracranial sarcomatous tumors of leptomeningeal origin. *Arch Surg.* 1929;18:1359–1399.
32. Paulus W. Classification, pathogenesis, and molecular pathology of primary CNS lymphomas. *J Neurooncol.* 1999;43:203.
33. DeAngelis LM, Wong E, Rosenblum M, Furneaux H. Epstein-Barr virus in acquired immune deficiency syndrome (AIDS) and non-AIDS primary central nervous system lymphoma. *Cancer.* 1992;70:1607–1611.
34. Rao CR, Jain K, Bhatia K, Laksmaiah KC, Shankar SK. Association of primary central nervous system lymphomas with the Epstein-Barr virus. *Neurol India.* 2003;51:237–240.
35. Kasamon YL, Ambinder RF. AIDS-related primary central nervous system lymphoma. *Hematol Oncol Clin North Am.* 2005;19:665–687.
36. Persad GC, Little RF, Grady C. Including persons with HIV infection in cancer clinical trials. *J Clin Oncol.* 2008;26:1027–1032.
37. Nelson DF, Martz KL, Bonner H, et al. Non-Hodgkin's lymphoma of the brain: Can high dose, large volume radiation therapy improve survival? Report on a prospective trial by the Radiation Therapy Oncology Group (RTOG): RTOG 8315. *Int J Radiat Oncol Biol Phys.* 1992;23:9–17.
38. O'Neill BP, O'Fallon JR, Earle JD, Colgan JP, Brown LD, Krigel RL. Primary central nervous system non-Hodgkin's lymphoma: survival advantages with combined initial therapy? *Int J Radiat Oncol Biol Phys.* 1995;33:663–673.
39. Schultz CJ, Scott C, Sherman W, et al. Preirradiation chemotherapy with cyclophosphamide, doxorubicin, vincristine, and dexamethasone for primary CNS lymphomas: initial report of radiation therapy oncology group protocol 88-06. *J Clin Oncol.* 1996;14:556–564.
40. DeAngelis LM, Seiferheld W, Schold SC, Fisher B, Schultz CJ, Radiation Therapy Oncology Group Study, 93-10. Combination chemotherapy and radiotherapy for primary central nervous system lymphoma: Radiation Therapy Oncology Group Study 93 10. *J Clin Oncol.* 2002;20:4643–4648.
41. Corry J, Smith JG, Wirth A, Quong G, Liew KH. Primary central nervous system lymphoma: age and performance status are more important than treatment modality. *Int J Radiat Oncol Biol Phys.* 1998;41:615–620.
42. Bessell EM, Graus F, Lopez-Guillermo A, et al. Primary non-Hodgkin's lymphoma of the CNS treated with CHOD/BVAM or BVAM chemotherapy before radiotherapy: long-term survival and prognostic factors. *Int J Radiat Oncol Biol Phys.* 2004;59:501–508.
43. Ferreri AJM, Blay J, Reni M, et al. Prognostic scoring system for primary CNS lymphomas: The International Extranodal Lymphoma Study Group Experience. *J Clin Oncol.* 2003;21:266–272.
44. Abrey LE, Ben-Porat L, Panageas KS, et al. Primary central nervous system lymphoma: the Memorial Sloan-Kettering Cancer Center prognostic model. *J Clin Oncol.* 2006;24:5711–5715.
45. Larocca LM, Capello D, Rinelli A, et al. The molecular and phenotypic profile of primary central nervous system lymphoma identifies distinct categories of the disease and is consistent with histogenetic derivation from germinal center-related B cells. *Blood.* 1998;92:1011–1019.
46. Braaten KM, Betensky RA, de Leval L, et al. BCL-6 expression predicts improved survival in patients with primary central nervous system lymphoma. *Clin Cancer Res.* 2003;9:1063–1069.
47. Chang CC, Kampalath B, Schultz C, et al. Expression of p53, c-Myc, or Bcl-6 suggests a poor prognosis in primary central nervous system diffuse large B-cell lymphoma among immunocompetent individuals. *Arch Pathol Lab Med.* 2003;127:208–212.
48. Murray K, Kun L, Cox J. Primary malignant lymphoma of the central nervous system: results of the treatment of 11 cases and review of the literature. *J Neurosurg.* 1986;65:600–607.
49. Corn BW, Dolinskas C, Scott C, et al. Strong correlation between imaging response and survival among patients with primary central nervous system lymphoma: a secondary analysis of RTOG studies 83-15 and 88-06. *Int J Radiat Oncol Biol Phys.* 2000;47:299–303.
50. DeAngelis LM, Yahalom J, Thaler HT, Kher U. Combined modality therapy for primary CNS lymphoma. *J Clin Oncol.* 1992;10:635–643.
51. Fisher B, Seiferheld W, Schultz C, et al. Secondary analysis of Radiation Therapy Oncology Group study (RTOG) 9310: an intergroup phase II combined modality treatment of primary central nervous system lymphoma. *J Neurooncol.* 2005;74:201–205.
52. Bessell EM, Lopez-Guillermo A, Villa S, et al. Importance of radiotherapy in the outcome of patients with primary CNS lymphoma: an analysis of the CHOD/BVAM regimen followed by two different radiotherapy treatments. *J Clin Oncol.* 2002;20:231–236.
53. Shah GD, Yahalom J, Correa DD, et al. Combined immunochemotherapy with reduced whole-brain radiotherapy for newly diagnosed primary CNS lymphoma. *J Clin Oncol.* 2007;25:4730–4735.
54. Ott RJ, Brada M, Flowers MA. Measurements of blood–brain barrier permeability in patients undergoing radiotherapy and chemotherapy for primary cerebral lymphoma. *Eur J Cancer.* 1991;27:1356–1361.
55. Poortmans PMP, Kluin-Nelemans HC, Haaxma-Reiche H, et al. High-dose methotrexate-based chemotherapy followed by consolidating radiotherapy in non-AIDS-related primary central nervous system lymphoma: European Organization for Research and Treatment of Cancer Lymphoma Group Phase II Trial 20962. *J Clin Oncol.* 2003;21:4483–4488.
56. Gavrilovic IT, Hormigo A, Yahalom J, DeAngelis LM, Abrey LE. Long-term follow-up of high-dose methotrexate-based therapy with and without whole brain irradiation for newly diagnosed primary CNS lymphoma. *J Clin Oncol.* 2006;24:4570–4574.
57. O'Brien PC, Roos DE, Pratt G, et al. Combined-modality therapy for primary central nervous system lymphoma: long-term data from a phase II multicenter study (Trans-Tasman Radiation Oncology Group). *Int J Radiat Oncol Biol Phys.* 2006;64:408–413.
58. Blay J, Bouhour D, Carrie C, et al. The C5R protocol: a regimen of high-dose chemotherapy and radiotherapy in primary cerebral non-Hodgkin's lymphoma of patients with no known cause of immunosuppression [see comments]. *Blood.* 1995;86:2922–2929.
59. Abrey LE, Yahalom J, DeAngelis LM. Treatment for primary CNS lymphoma: the next step. *J Clin Oncol.* 2000;18:3144–3150.
60. Abrey LE, DeAngelis LM, Yahalom J. Long-term survival in primary CNS lymphoma. *J Clin Oncol.* 1998;16:859–863.
61. Brada M, Hjiyiannakis D, Hines F, Traish D, Ashley S. Short intensive primary chemotherapy and radiotherapy in sporadic primary CNS lymphoma (PCL). *Int J Radiat Oncol Biol Phys.* 1998;40:1157–1162.
62. Pels H, Schmidt-Wolf IG, Glasmacher A, et al. Primary central nervous system lymphoma: results of a pilot and phase II study of systemic and intraventricular chemotherapy with deferred radiotherapy. *J Clin Oncol.* 2003;21:4489–4495.
63. Gerstner ER, Carson KA, Grossman SA, Batchelor TT. Long-term outcome in PCNSL patients treated with high-dose methotrexate and deferred radiation. *Neurology.* 2008;70:401–402.
64. Batchelor T, Carson K, O'Neill A, et al. Treatment of primary CNS lymphoma with methotrexate and deferred radiotherapy: a report of NABTT 96-07. *J Clin Oncol.* 2003;21:1044–1049.
65. Hoang-Xuan K, Taillandier L, Chinot O, et al. Chemotherapy alone as initial treatment for primary CNS lymphoma in patients older than 60 years: a multicenter phase II study (26952) of the European Organization for Research and Treatment of Cancer Brain Tumor Group. *J Clin Oncol.* 2003;21:2726–2731.
66. Sandor V, Stark-Vancs V, Pearson D, et al. Phase II trial of chemotherapy alone for primary CNS and intraocular lymphoma. *J Clin Oncol.* 1998;16:3000–3006.
67. Dahlborg SA, Henner WD, Crossen JR, et al. Non-AIDS primary CNS lymphoma: first example of a durable response in a primary brain tumor using enhanced chemotherapy delivery without cognitive loss and without radiotherapy. *Cancer J Sci Am.* 1996;2:166–174.
68. Khan RB, Shi W, Thaler HT, DeAngelis LM, Abrey LE. Is intrathecal methotrexate necessary in the treatment of primary CNS lymphoma? *J Neurooncol.* 2002;58:175–178.
69. Neuwelt E, Goldman D, Dahlborg S, et al. Primary CNS lymphoma treated with osmotic blood–brain barrier disruption: prolonged survival and preservation of cognitive function. *J Clin Oncol.* 1991;9:1580–1590.
70. Montemurro M, Kiefer T, Schuler F, et al. Primary central nervous system lymphoma treated with high-dose methotrexate, high-dose busulfan/thiotepa, autologous stem-cell transplantation and response-adapted whole-brain radiotherapy: results of the multicenter Ostdeutsche Studiengruppe Hamato-Onkologie OSHO-53 phase II study. *Ann Oncol.* 2007;18:665–671.

71. Colombat P, Lemevel A, Bertrand P, et al. High-dose chemotherapy with autologous stem cell transplantation as first-line therapy for primary CNS lymphoma in patients younger than 60 years: a multicenter phase II study of the GOELAMS group. *Bone Marrow Transplant.* 2006;38:417–420.
72. Soussain C, Suzan F, Hoang-Xuan K, et al. Results of intensive chemotherapy followed by hematopoietic stem-cell rescue in 22 patients with refractory or recurrent primary CNS lymphoma or intraocular lymphoma. *J Clin Oncol.* 2001;19:742–749.
73. Enting RH, Demopoulos A, DeAngelis LM, Abrey LE. Salvage therapy for primary CNS lymphoma with a combination temozolomide and rituximab. *Neurology.* 2004;40:1682–1688.
74. Plotkin SR, Betensky RA, Hochberg F. Treatment of relapsed central nervous system lymphoma with high dose methotrexate. *Clin Cancer Res.* 2004;10:5643–5646.
75. Herrlinger U, Brugger W, Bamberg M, Kuker W, Dichgans J, Weller M. PCV salvage chemotherapy for recurrent primary CNS lymphoma. *Neurology.* 2000;54:1707–1708.
76. Nguyen P, Chakravarti A, Finkelstein D, Hochberg F, Batchelor TT, Loeffler J. Results of whole brain radiation as salvage of methotrexate failure for immunocompetent patients with primary CNS lymphoma. *J Clin Oncol.* 2005;23:1507–1513.
77. Voloschin AD, Betensky RA, Wen PY, Hochberg F, Batchelor T. Topotecan as salvage therapy for relapsed or refractory primary central nervous system lymphoma. *J Neurooncol.* 2008;86:211–215.
78. Jahnke K, Thiel E, Martus P. Relapse of primary central nervous system lymphoma: clinical features, outcome, and prognostic factors. *J Neurooncol.* 2006;80:159–165.
79. Reni M, Mason WP, Zaja F, Perry J. Salvage chemotherapy with temozolomide in primary CNS lymphoma: preliminary results of a phase II trial. *Eur J Cancer.* 2004;40:1682–1688.
80. Wong ET, Tishler R, Barron L, Wu JK. Immunochemotherapy with rituximab and temozolomide for central nervous system lymphomas. *Cancer.* 2004;101:139–145.
81. Enting RH, Demopoulos A, DeAngelis LM, Abrey LE. Salvage therapy for primary CNS lymphoma with a combination of rituximab and temozolomide [see comment]. *Neurology.* 2004;63:901–903.
82. Soussain C, Hoang-Xuan K, Levy V. [Results of intensive chemotherapy followed by hematopoietic stem-cell rescue in 22 patients with refractory or recurrent primary CNS lymphoma or intraocular lymphoma]. *Bull Cancer.* 2004;91:189–192.
83. Ambinder RF, Lee S, Curran WJ, et al. Phase II intergroup trial of sequential chemotherapy and radiation therapy for AIDS-related primary central nervous system lymphoma. *Cancer Therapy.* 2003;1:215–221.
84. Hoffmann C, Tabrizian S, Wolf E, et al. Survival of AIDS patients with primary central nervous system lymphoma is dramatically improved by HAART-induced immune recovery. *AIDS.* 2001;15:2119–2127.
85. Pajonk F, McBride WH. Survival of AIDS patients with primary central nervous system lymphoma may be improved by the radiosensitizing effects of highly active antiretroviral therapy. *AIDS.* 2002;16:1195–1196.
86. Newell ME, Hoy JF, Cooper SG, et al. Human immunodeficiency virus-related primary central nervous system lymphoma: factors influencing survival in 111 patients. *Cancer.* 2004;100:2627–2636.
87. Raez L, Cabral L, Cai J, et al. Treatment of AIDS-related primary central nervous system lymphoma with zidovudine, ganciclovir, and interleukin 2. *AIDS Res Hum Retroviruses.* 1999;15:713–719.
88. Aboulafia DM. Interleukin-2, ganciclovir, and high-dose zidovudine for the treatment of AIDS-associated primary central nervous system lymphoma. *Clin Infect Dis.* 2002;34:1660–1662.
89. Bossolasco S, Falk KI, Ponzoni M, et al. Ganciclovir is associated with low or undetectable Epstein-Barr virus DNA load in cerebrospinal fluid of patients with HIV-related primary central nervous system lymphoma. *Clin Infect Dis.* 2006;42:e21–e25.
90. Abrey LE, Correa DD. Treatment-related neurotoxicity. *Hematol Oncol Clin North Am.* 2005;19:729–738.
91. Ferreri AJ, Abrey LE, Blay JY, et al. Summary statement on primary central nervous system lymphomas from the Eighth International Conference on Malignant Lymphoma, Lugano, Switzerland, June 12 to 15, 2002. *J Clin Oncol.* 2003;21:2407–2414.

99 Neurocytoma

Sayana Rachel Thomas and Deepak Khuntia

INTRODUCTION

Central neurocytomas were first indentified as a distinct clinicopathologic entity in 1982 by Hassoun et al [1]. These tumors are typically benign and associated with a favorable prognosis. Not infrequently, however, neurocytomas are mistaken for other central nervous system (CNS) tumors associated with less favorable outcomes, including oligodendrogliomas, ependymomas, and meningiomas [2]. Neurocytomas have been increasingly recognized over the past two decades, now with more than 500 cases reported, as their microscopic appearance and immunohistochemical staining properties are becoming better understood [3]. Despite this, these tumors continue to be a relatively uncommon entity, representing only 0.25% to 0.5% of all primary brain tumors [4]. They are most frequently recognized in young adults during the second and third decade of life and seem to be equally distributed between both genders [2].

Neurocytomas are confined to the CNS and are usually seen arising from the septum pellucidum, fornix, or walls of the lateral ventricles, straddling the lateral and third ventricles [2]. These tumors often manifest with signs and symptoms of raised intracranial pressure from obstructive hydrocephalus, such as seizures, headaches, nausea, vomiting, vision changes, and memory disturbances. Less commonly, extraventricular neurocytomas have been observed, which have been documented in nearly every lobe of the cerebrum, cerebellum, thalamus, hypothalamus, pons, spinal cord, and retina [5]. Although somewhat controversial, most believe that neurocytomas arise from bipotential cells in the periventricular matrix [2]. A subgroup of neurocytomas have been defined, which demonstrate increased mitotic activity, focal necrosis, vascular endothelial proliferation, and MIB-1 labeling index >2%. These tumors, termed "atypical neurocytomas," are associated with an increased likelihood of recurrence and worse prognosis [3].

DIAGNOSIS

Close examination of the radiologic, pathologic, and immunohistochemical staining features of neurocytomas must be performed to avoid misdiagnosis as other CNS tumors. The differential diagnosis includes oligodendrogliomas, astrocytomas, meningiomas, ependymomas, subependymomas, choroid plexus papillomas, colloid cysts, craniopharyngiomas, and germ cell tumors [6]. Differentiating neurocytomas from other tumors is particularly important as the former often have a more favorable prognosis. On computed tomography scan, these lesions are either isodense or mildly hyperdense, with generally uniform contrast enhancement, calcifications, and often cystic changes [2]. On magnetic resonance imaging, high signal is seen on both T1- and T2-weighted images, with moderate to strong enhancement following gadolinium administration. Light microscopy of neurocytomas reveals clusters of uniform, round cells, a central round nucleus, finely stippled chromatin, eosinophilic and fibrillary cytoplasm, perivascular pseudorossettes, occasional perinuclear halos, and fixation artifacts resulting in cytoplasmic vacuoles, which resemble a "fried-egg" appearance [6] (see Figure 99.1). Many of the morphologic features resemble those of oligodendrogliomas, but these tumors are clearly genetically distinct, as neurocytomas are devoid of any association with 1p19q [3]. These tumors uniformly demonstrated synaptophysin immunoreactivity [6]. They have also been reported to express a variety of other markers including glial fibrillary acidic protein, neuron-specific enolase, neuron-associated class III β-tubulin, tau, microtubule-associated protein-2, calcineurin, α-synuclein, neuron-specific antigen L1, and embryonal form of neural cell adhesion molecule [2].

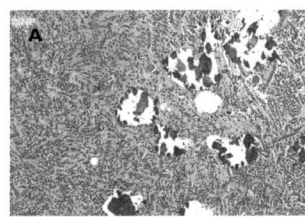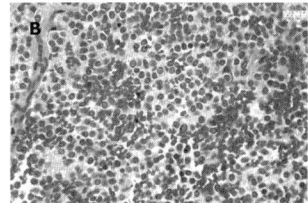

Figure 99.1 **(A)** Central neurocytoma. H&E stained slide demonstrating a cellular lesion composed of monomorphous small, round cells in a fibrillar background containing arborizing capillaries. Coarse calcifications are present. **(B)** Central neurocytoma. Higher power view demonstrating monomorphous, round nuclei with finely stippled chromatin, and inconspicuous nucleoli. Courtesy of Stephanie Koplin, MD, and Shahriar Salamat, MD, PhD, University of Wisconsin Department of Pathology. *See color insert.*

TREATMENT

Gross total resection (GTR) is the mainstay of therapy for neurocytomas, as most are intraventricular in location, without any invasion into the surrounding brain parenchyma [2]. However, sometimes only a subtotal resection (STR) can be achieved due to adhesions to eloquent structures, profuse intraoperative bleeding, and excessive calcifications. These patients often receive postoperative radiotherapy (RT) and, rarely, treatment with chemotherapeutic agents has also been reported. It is difficult to define the best therapy for neurocytomas and the magnitude of benefit from postoperative irradiation because most articles regarding these tumors have been case reports. However, Rades and Schild [7] recently reviewed and published the data of 438 neurocytoma patients documented since this tumor was first reported in 1982. They compared local control (LC) and overall survival (OS) for all patients who received GTR ± RT and STR ± RT. Also, the authors performed subgroup analysis of those with typical versus atypical neurocytomas as well as children versus adults. The addition of RT to GTR did not significantly improve LC or OS, but the administration of postoperative RT to patients who received STR significantly improved both 5- and 10-year LC (41% and 35% vs. 83% and 76%, respectively) and 5- and 10-year OS (82% and 82% vs. 89% and 89%, respectively). These findings held true in subgroup analysis of typical versus atypical neurocytomas. Further analysis performed comparing STR followed by RT with ≤54Gy versus >54 Gy, revealed that >54 Gy significantly improves LC. In children, RT provided no added benefit to GTR, but significantly improved 5- and 10-year LC when added to STR (52% and 39% vs. 94% and 94%, respectively). Of note, dose escalating above 54 Gy did not improve LC or OS in children. Patients with atypical histologies or MIB-1 labeling index greater than 2% should also be considered for adjuvant radiation therapy.

Other less frequently used treatment modalities for neurocytomas include radiosurgery and chemotherapy, either as primary treatment or secondarily in patients with residual or recurrent tumor. Radiosurgery (SRS), which involves treatment with a single, high dose fraction of radiation with a steep drop-off, is in some ways uniquely suited to treat neurocytomas, as these lesions are typically well-circumscribed and located within the ventricular system. A recent report by Kim et al [8] described the use of gamma knife radiosurgery, both as a primary and secondary treatment modality in 13 patients. All patients demonstrated a partial response (tumor volume reduction >25%), but two patients treated with secondary SRS suffered a recurrence, stemming from residual tumor that was nonenhancing due to cutoff of blood supply by surgery.

The role of chemotherapy in treatment of neurocytomas is unclear, as it has most often been given in the salvage setting or closely with radiation, making it difficult to determine the effect of chemotherapy on tumor control [9]. Regardless, reduction in tumor size has been seen with a combination of a variety of agents including etoposide, cisplatin, cyclophosphamide, carboplatin, vincristine, lomustine, and carmustine.

CONCLUSION

Given the limited data above, the standard treatment recommendation for neurocytomas should be GTR, if possible. If GTR is not achievable, STR should be performed in conjunction with postoperative RT, with the total dose >54 Gy in cases of atypical neurocytomas and <54 Gy in children. Both SRS and chemotherapy have shown some efficacy but should be used primarily in cases where surgical resection cannot be performed or used to treat recurrent or residual tumor, as insufficient experience with these modalities to recommend them as primary treatments. Neurocytomas continue to be increasingly recognized as primary CNS tumors and fortunately are associated with a more favorable prognosis. However, with increasing recognition, both the need and opportunity to conduct more studies to further define the best treatment modalities is necessary.

REFERENCES

1. Hassoun J, Soylemezoglu F, Gambarelli D, Figarella-Branger D, von Ammon K, Kleihues P. Central neurocytoma: a synopsis of clinical and histological features. *Brain Pathol.* 1993;3:297–306.
2. Sharma MC, Deb P, Sharma S, Sarkar C. Neurocytoma: a comprehensive review. *Neurosurg Rev.* 2006;29:270–285; discussion 85.
3. Leenstra JL, Rodriguez FJ, Frechette CM, et al. Central neurocytoma: management recommendations based on a 35-year experience. *Int J Radiat Oncol Biol Phys.* 2007;67:1145–1154.
4. Yeh IB, Xu M, Ng WH, Ye J, Yang D, Lim CC. Central neurocytoma: typical magnetic resonance spectroscopy findings and atypical ventricular dissemination. *Magn Reson Imaging* 2008;26(1):59 64.
5. Kowalski RJ, Prayson RA, Lee JH. Skull base neurocytoma: case report and review of the literature of extraventricular neurocytomas. *Skull Base.* 2002;12:59–65.
6. Goergen SK, Gonzales MF, McLean CA. Interventricular neurocytoma: radiologic features and review of the literature. *Radiology.* 1992;182:787–792.
7. Rades D, Schild SE. Treatment recommendations for the various subgroups of neurocytomas. *J Neurooncol.* 2006;77:305–309.
8. Kim CY, Paek SH, Jeong SS, et al. Gamma knife radiosurgery for central neurocytoma: primary and secondary treatment. *Cancer.* 2007;110:2276–2284.
9. von Koch CS, Schmidt MH, Uyehara-Lock JH, Berger MS, Chang SM. The role of PCV chemotherapy in the treatment of central neurocytoma: illustration of a case and review of the literature. *Surg Neurol.* 2003;60:560–565.

100 Radiation Therapy of Primary Spinal Cord Tumors

Volker Wilhelm Walter Stieber

TECHNIQUES OF RADIATION THERAPY

Definitions of Treatment Volumes

Treatment planning should be three dimensional, based on ICRU volumes [1,2]. Gross tumor volume (GTV) represents the grossly visible disease burden. Typically, this is the T1-enhancing abnormality on magnetic resonance imaging (MRI) or nonenhancing tumor seen on T2 or fluid attenuated inversion recovery images. If there is no residual abnormality after a surgical resection, the tumor resection cavity is defined to be the GTV. Surrounding edema is not considered part of the GTV. Clinical target volume is the T2 or fluid attenuated inversion recovery abnormality (which does include edema) on MRI as well as any areas potentially containing microscopic disease. Suggested definitions of and doses to be delivered to GTV and clinical target volume are listed in Table 100.1 by histologic diagnosis. The planning target volume adds a dosimetric margin that takes into account uncertainties in daily treatment setup and physiologic variations that are difficult or impossible to control, such as (potential) fluctuations in the mass effect from cord edema that may occur over the course of treatment. Organs at risk typically include the thyroid and salivary glands, esophagus, lungs, heart, stomach, small bowel, liver, kidneys, bladders, ovaries, testicles, and the uninvolved portions of the spinal cord itself.

Treatment Techniques

The most common treatment approaches include a single posterior field (PA), opposed lateral fields, a PA field with opposed laterals, and oblique wedge-pair fields [3,4]. They are typically designed to treat the clinical target volume and GTV. For tumors in the cervicothoracic region, a split-beam approach is often used. The central axis is placed just above the shoulders. Opposed lateral fields are used to treat the upper spine, whereas a PA field is used for the area of the spine below. Tumors in the thoracic region are often treated with a three-field approach using a PA field and opposed lateral beams. In the lumbar region, care must be taken to minimize dose to the kidneys; a four-field approach using AP/PA and opposed lateral beams with the AP/PA beams preferentially weighted may be useful. Comparison of differing treatment setups by means of dose-volume histograms (as described above) is strongly recommended.

Certain neoplasms require treatment to the entire craniospinal axis. Several modifications of this approach are used in clinical practice [5]. Patients may be treated either in the supine or prone position, often in an immobilization cast to ensure daily positional reproducibility. The intracranial contents, including the upper one or two segments of the cervical cord, are treated through opposed lateral fields. Customized blocks protect the normal head and neck tissues from the primary radiation beam. The spine is treated through one or two PAs, depending on the size of the patient. In one method, the collimator for the lateral cranial fields is angled to match the divergence of the upper border of the adjacent spinal field and the treatment couch is angled so that the inferior border of the cranial field is perpendicular to the superior edge of the spinal field. Alternatively, one may dispense with collimator and couch angles by calculating appropriate gaps. The gap is calculated so that the 50% isodose lines meet at the level of the anterior spinal cord. All junction lines are moved 0.5 to 1.0 cm every 8 to 10 Gy to avoid overdosing or underdosing segments of the cord. This is accomplished by shortening the inferior margin of the lateral cranial fields, symmetrically lengthening the superior and inferior margins of the posterior spine field, and shortening the cranial margin of the caudal spinal field; a fixed block is placed at the inferior margin of the caudal spinal field to keep the lower margin of the irradiated volume at the same location.

Stereotactic radiosurgery of primary spinal cord tumors remains experimental at this time [6,7].

Tolerance of the Spinal Cord and Lumbosacral Nerve Roots

A dose of 45 to 50.4 Gy in 25 to 28 fractions over 5 to 5½ weeks usually is considered to be safe, the risk of myelopathy being less than 1%, well below the steep portion of the dose-response curve [6,8–10]. It is estimated that with conventionally fractionated irradiation (1.8–2.0 Gy per fraction, five fractions per week), at five years the incidence of myelopathy is 5% for doses in the range of 57 to 61 Gy (tolerance dose $TD_{5/5}$) and 50% for doses of 68 to 73 Gy ($TD_{50/5}$) [10]. There is no convincing evidence that the cervical and thoracic cord differ in their radiosensitivity, and

Table 100.1 Suggested Definitions of ICRU Volumes Based on MRI and Dose Ranges (in Gray) Delivered to Volumes

Diagnosis	Definition of Initial Treatment Field (CTV)	Dose to CTV	Definition of Final Field (to GTV)	Dose to GTV	Dose to Craniospinal axis (if indicated)
WHO grade I glioma	(n/a)	(n/a)	Enhancing tumor (T1 + C) 1 cm margin	45–50.4 Gy	(n/a)
WHO grade II glioma	Enhancing tumor (T1 + C) Edema (T2/FLAIR) 2 cm margin	45 Gy	Enhancing tumor (T1 + C) 2 cm margin	50.4 – 54 Gy	(n/a)
WHO grade III–IV glioma	Enhancing tumor (T1 + C) Edema (T2/FLAIR) 2 cm margin	45–50.4 Gy	Enhancing tumor (T1 + C) 2 cm margin	55.8–59.4 (60) Gy	Leptomeningeal spread on MRI: 30–39.6 Gy Bulky disease: 55.8–59.4 Gy
Ependymoma	Enhancing tumor (T1 + C) Edema (T2/FLAIR) 2 cm margin	45 Gy	Enhancing tumor (T1 + C) 2 cm margin	50.4–55.8 Gy	Negative CSF: 30 Gy Positive CSF: 36 Gy Leptomeningeal spread on MRI: 39.6 Gy Bulky disease: 54 Gy
Meningioma, benign/atypical	(n/a)	(n/a)	Enhancing tumor (T1 + C) 1 cm margin	52.2 – 55.8 Gy	(n/a)
Meningioma, malignant	Enhancing tumor (T1 + C) Edema (T2/FLAIR) 2 cm margin	45–50.4 Gy	Enhancing tumor (T1 + C) 2 cm margin	55.8–59.4 Gy	(n/a)
Chordoma	Enhancing tumor (T1 + C) Tumor Bed 2 cm margin	50 Gy	Enhancing tumor (T1 + C) 2 cm margin	60–76 Gy	(n/a)
Chondrosarcoma	Enhancing tumor (T1 + C) Tumor Bed 2 cm margin	50 Gy	Enhancing tumor (T1 + C) 2 cm margin	60–76 Gy	(n/a)
Sarcoma	Enhancing tumor (T1 + C) Tumor bed Surgical track, including scar 2 cm margin	50 Gy	Enhancing tumor (T1 + C) 2 cm margin	60–70 Gy	(n/a)
Vertebral hemangioma	Enhancing vascular lesion Entire involved vertebral body ≥ 1 cm margin	(n/a)	(n/a)	36–45 Gy	(n/a)

Abbreviations: CSF, cerebrospinal fluid; CTV, clinical target volume; +C, with contrast; FLAIR, fluid attenuated inversion recovery; GTV, gross tumor volume.

there appears to be little change in tolerance with variations in the length of cord irradiated [10]. Table 100.2 shows a range of isomorbid fractionation schemes, all of which carry a 5% risk of radiation myelopathy.

The tolerance of the lumbosacral nerve roots appears to be somewhat higher than that of the spinal cord. Most series report a 0% complication rate if patients are treated to doses of 70 Gy (or equivalent) as long as fraction sizes are kept at or below 2 Gy [22–24].

INDICATIONS AND OUTCOMES BY TUMOR TYPE

Astrocytoma

The treatment of choice for intramedullary astrocytomas is complete excision of the tumor, when it can be accomplished without neurologic compromise. Otherwise, an incomplete excision is typically performed for grade I lesions and biopsy alone is the surgical strategy for the nonexophytic component of an infiltrative glioma. In patients with favorable prognostic factors (low-grade histology, good performance status, and young age), observation with serial imaging studies, reserving radiation therapy for local recurrence, is an appropriate management option, particularly for young children [25,26]. In the remainder of patients, adjuvant radiation therapy is usually recommended as progression of tumor in the spinal cord may lead to significant neurological impairment [27–32]. Doses have traditionally been based on the experience with cerebral tumors, with lower grade tumors typically receiving 45 to 54 Gy and high-grade tumors receiving higher doses [33–35].

The overall outcomes are similar for patients with low-grade gliomas of the spinal cord treated either by gross total resection or subtotal resection/biopsy followed by radiation therapy, with most series reporting overall survival

Table 100.2 Fractionation Schemes with a 5% Risk of Radiation-Induced Spinal Cord Myelopathy

Dose Per Fraction	Number of Fractions	Total Dose
2.00	29	58.00
3.00	13	39.00
3.30	11	33.00
4.00	7	28.00
5.00	5	25.00
10.00	1	10.00

From refs. [8, 11–21].

rates at 5 and 10 years in the ranges of 55% to 88% and 39% to 83%, respectively, and disease-free survival rates of 38% to 75% and 26% to 55% at 5 and 10 years, respectively. Postoperative radiation therapy has shown a survival benefit for patients with infiltrative gliomas (24 vs 3 months) but not with pilocytic tumors [34,36]. Overall, long-term local control rates for gliomas range from 31% to 100%, with grade being the strongest predictor [4,28,34,36–45]. A comparison of survival and local control rates is shown in Table 100.3.

With high-grade tumors in adults and children, median survival time is quite poor (4–10 months) despite surgery and radiation therapy; approximately two-thirds of patients die of both local and disseminated disease [4,39,46–51]. One small series suggested a survival benefit for patients with high-grade tumors treated with craniospinal axis irradiation [52].

Ependymoma

Postoperative radiation therapy appears to improve local control in patients with subtotally resected ependymomas, for all high-grade lesions, and for patients with craniospinal axis dissemination (positive cerebrospinal fluid or MRI scan), though not all authors agree on this, with many series showing increasing age to be the most significant predictor [36,53–61]. In most series, the outcome for subtotal resection followed by radiation therapy appears to be similar to that of complete excision. Typically, the dose given to the tumor bed is 49 to 56 Gy whereas the craniospinal axis (if indicated) receives 30 to 36 Gy [62–65]. Low-grade lesions with low risk of seeding are typically treated with limited fields to 50.4 to 55.8 Gy in 1.8 Gy daily fractions. In patients with tumors at high risk of seeding, when pretreatment cerebrospinal fluid cytology studies reveal malignant cells, or if the spinal MRI scan shows evidence of leptomeningeal disease, the craniospinal axis should be treated to 36 Gy in 1.5 to 1.8 Gy daily fractions. Subsequently, the primary tumor site is boosted to a total dose of 50.4 to 55.8 Gy. If gross leptomeningeal spread is evident, the craniospinal axis dose should be 39.6 Gy (1.8 Gy/fraction) or 40.5 Gy (1.5 Gy/fraction), with the same boost dose to primary as previously discussed.

In those patients undergoing incomplete resection followed by radiation therapy, overall survival rates at 5, 10, and 15 years are 67% to 100%, 67% to 100%, and 75%, respectively [34,61,64–67]. Cause-specific survival rates at 5, 10, and 15 years for all tumors are 74% to 93%, 50% to 93%, and 35% to 46%, respectively [28,36,61,68]. By tumor grade, cause-specific survival rates at 5 years are 87% to 97% for myxopapillary and low-grade lesions and 27% to 71% for high-grade tumors [65,67]. Disease-free survival rates at 5 and 10 years are 59% and 59%, respectively [61]. Local control rates are 88% to 100% [62–64,67,69].

Meningioma

The role of radiation therapy is not well understood due to the small number of cases reported in the literature, and most clinicians extrapolate from the data on irradiation of intracranial meningiomas [70–72]. The expected outcome of radiation therapy is long-term stabilization of disease [73]. Patients who undergo complete resection should be observed. Even those with subtotally resected disease who either have improvement of their neurological status or are asymptomatic postoperatively can be closely followed. When patients are irradiated, the dose delivered is typically 52.2 to 54 Gy, based on the data from the treatment of intracranial meningioma [73]. Single-fraction spinal stereotactic radiosurgery must be considered investigational at this time [6].

Chordoma

Although en bloc gross total resection has traditionally been advocated for these lesions, it is rarely possible. As such, most patients undergo subtotal resection or biopsy, followed by radiation therapy. In most series, patients have been treated with conventional photon radiation therapy, typically to doses of 55 to 70 Gy in 2 Gy fractions, with 5-year actuarial survival rates of 38% to 58% [20,74–80]. Although radiation therapy prolongs the disease-free interval [75], the majority of tumors still recur unless they have also undergone complete resection [75,80], and local progression is the most common cause of death. In an older series, the local control rate of sacrococcygeal tumors was 0% with either surgery or radiation therapy as monotherapy but 40% when the two were combined [79].

Some treatment series using conventional photon radiation therapy suggest that local control rates improve with increasing radiation doses. With doses of <40, >48, <50, and >55 Gy, 5-years disease-free survival rates are approximately 0%, 13%, 31%, and 41%, respectively [20,78]. However, not all authors have found that increased dose improves outcome [81].

To improve the therapeutic ratio when treating residual or recurrent disease, most authors now advocate a combination of photon and charged particle therapy (typically protons) [82–90]. When patients are treated either immediately after maximum resection or at the time of recurrence, with median doses of 65 to 76 Gy equivalent using charged particle radiation therapy (with or without photons), local control rates at 3, 5, and 10 years are 67% to 71%, 40% to 75%, and 54%, respectively, with overall survival rates at 3, 5, and 10 years at 88% to 97%, 75% to 80%, and 54%, respectively [22,85–87,91].

Radiosurgery has also been used in the treatment of residual and recurrent cervical spine chordoma. A mean dose of 19 Gy in a single fraction prescribed at the tumor margin resulted in a 4-year local control rate of 80% without neurologic sequelae in one series [92]. The experience with interstitial irradiation is minimal and this modality has fallen out of favor with the advent of charged particle therapy and radiosurgery [93–95].

Chondrosarcoma

Surgical resection is the mainstay of treatment of these lesions. After complete resection, the local control rate is 97%, with a 90% 10-year overall survival rate and an 84%

Table 100.3 Outcomes of the Most Common Spinal Cord Tumors by Treatment Modality

Histology	Treatment	S_{med} (months)	OS_5 (%)	OS_{10} (%)	OS_{15} (%)	CSS_5 (%)	DFS_5 (%)	DFS_{10} (%)	DFS_{15} (%)	LC_3 (%)	LC_5 (%)	LC_{10} (%)	Overall LC (%)
Low-grade glioma (WHO Gr. I–II)	GTR or STR + XRT	98–479 (Gr I); 33–68 (Gr II)	47–100	47–83	32–60	50–79	38–93	29–80	15		100		31–100
High-grade glioma (WHO Gr. III–IV)	Sx + XRT	10–15	20	15–35		30	20						
Ependymoma	GTR	104	80	64									55–100
	STR + XRT	77–135	60–95	51–84	64	96	53–80	39–80	35–80			72	66–100
	GTR or STR + XRT						93	80	68				96
	STR alone						63	45	09				94
Chordoma	Surgery + XRT		87–38 (at 3 years)			68	63			67–71	40–78	54	69
Chondrosarcomas	Surgery + XRT	72					63			85	78		36

The numbers in subscript denote the number of years. References are found in the text.

Abbreviations: CSS, cause-specific survival; DFS, disease-free survival; GTR, gross total resection; LC, local control; OS, overall survival; STR, subtotal resection; XRT, radiation therapy.

disease-free survival rate [96]. Radiation therapy after incomplete resection has been shown to lengthen the disease-free interval from 16 to 44 months in one series.

Miscellaneous Primary Spinal Tumors

The most effective treatment of chloroma (*aka* granulocytic sarcoma) appears to be multimodality therapy coupled with early diagnosis. Options include surgical decompression, intravenous and/or intrathecal chemotherapy, radiation therapy at doses of 2000 to 3000 cGy, or any combination of these treatments. Patient survival ranges from 18 days to 9.5 years after diagnosis [97].

After decompressive laminectomy, subtotal tumor resection, and spinal irradiation, the local control rate of lymphoma is 60% with a median duration of survival of 42 months [98].

Central neurocytoma has been reported to arise in the spine [99–101]. Because this tumor arises centrally in the spinal cord, observation or radiation may be primary management strategies with resection reserved for those with progressive neurologic deficits.

Surgical debulking of sarcoma, followed by postoperative radiation therapy to approximately 60 Gy in 1.8 to 2.0 Gy fractions represents the typical treatment approach described in the literature [102,103]. The 5-year survival rate of patients with high-grade lesions is significantly worse at 28% than the 83% reported with low-grade lesions.

Surgical resection is the treatment of choice for schwannoma [104–106]. Only 3% of these tumors are malignant [107] in which case adjuvant radiation therapy has been used. Outcomes are mixed [106,107].

Early surgical resection of teratoma is recommended to preserve neurological status. Although there is no well-defined role for radiation therapy, it is generally reserved for multiply recurrent, subtotally resected disease.

Treatment of vertebral hemangioma is initiated only when progressive symptoms, including focal pain or progressive neurologic deficit, develop. Radiation therapy is an effective treatment option. A meta-analysis demonstrated that a total dose of 30 Gy given in 2 Gy fractions resulted in a 57% complete and 32% partial improvement of pain [108]. A second, smaller analysis showed an apparent dose response. Patients treated with the biologic equivalent 36 to 44 Gy in 2 Gy fractions had significantly better complete pain relief than those treated with 20 to 34 Gy (82% vs 39%, respectively) [109].

There is no well-defined role for radiation therapy in the treatment of primary spinal epidermoid tumor, hemangioblastoma, lipoma, and melanoma.

COMPLICATIONS OF TREATMENT

Radiation myelopathy may present as a transient early delayed or as a late delayed reaction. Transient radiation myelopathy is clinically manifested by momentary, electrical shock-like paresthesias or numbness radiating from the neck to the extremities, precipitated by neck flexion (Lhermitte sign) [110]. The syndrome typically develops 3 to 4 months after treatment and spontaneously resolves over the following 3 to 6 months without therapy. It is attributed to transient demyelination caused by radiation-induced inhibition of myelin-producing oligodendroglial cells in the irradiated spinal cord segment [110–112].

Irreversible radiation myelopathy usually is not seen earlier than 6 to 12 months after completion of treatment. Typically, half of the patients who develop radiation-induced myelopathy in the cervical or thoracic cord region will do so within 20 months of treatment, and 75% of the cases will occur within 30 months [113]. The signs and symptoms are typically progressive over several months, but acute onset of plegia over several hours or a few days is possible. It is thought to be multifactorial in origin, involving demyelination and white matter necrosis ultimately due to oligodendroglial cell depletion and microvascular injury. The diagnosis of radiation myelopathy is one of exclusion, which first requires a history of radiation therapy in doses sufficient to result in injury. The region of the irradiated cord must lie slightly above the dermatome level of expression of the lesion, the latent period from the completion of treatment to the onset of injury must be consistent with that observed in radiation myelopathy, and local tumor progression must be ruled out. There are no pathognomonic laboratory tests or imaging studies that conclusively diagnose radiation myelopathy. MRI findings include swelling of the spinal cord with hyperintensity on the T2-weighted images with or without areas of contrast enhancement [87,114]. There is no known consistently effective treatment for radiation myelitis [115,116]. The probability of dying from radiation myelopathy is approximately 70% in cervical lesions and 30% with thoracic spinal cord injury [117].

Radiation side effects in children include growth abnormalities, such as decreased vertebral height, kyphosis, and scoliosis [118]. Secondary malignancies, including bone or soft tissue sarcomas and glioblastomas multiforme, have been reported after irradiation of spinal cord tumors [54,119,120].

REFERENCES

1. International Commission on Radiation Units and Measurements I. *ICRU Report 50, Prescribing, Recording, and Reporting Photon Beam Therapy*. Bethesda, MD: Nuclear Technology Publishing; 1993.
2. International Commission on Radiation Units and Measurements I. *ICRU Report 62: Prescribing, Recording and Reporting Photon Beam Therapy (Supplement to ICRU Report 50)*. Wambersie A, Landberg T, eds. Journal of the ICRU 62. Bethesda, MD: Nuclear Technology Publishing; 1999.
3. Michalski JM. Spinal canal. In: Leibel SA, Phillips TL, eds. *Textbook of Radiation Oncology*. 1st ed. Philadelphia: WB Saunders; 1998:860–875.
4. Minehan KJ, Shaw EG, Scheithauer BW, Davis DL, Onofrio BM. Spinal cord astrocytoma: pathological and treatment considerations. *J Neurosurg*. 1995;83(4):590–595.
5. Shiu AS, Chang EL, Ye JS, et al. Near simultaneous computed tomography image-guided stereotactic spinal radiotherapy: an emerging paradigm for achieving true stereotaxy. *Int J Radiat Oncol Biol Phys*. 2003;57(3):605–613.
6. Ryu SI, Chang SD, Kim DH, et al. Image-guided hypo-fractionated stereotactic radiosurgery to spinal lesions. *Neurosurgery*. 2001;49(4):838–846.
7. Yin FF, Ryu S, Ajlouni M, et al. A technique of intensity-modulated radiosurgery (IMRS) for spinal tumors. *Med Phys*. 2002;29(12):2815–2822.

8. Marcus RB Jr, Million RR. The incidence of myelitis after irradiation of the cervical spinal cord. *Int J Radiat Oncol Biol Phys.* 1990;19(1):3–8.
9. Ryu S, Fang Yin F, Rock J, et al. Image-guided and intensity-modulated radiosurgery for patients with spinal metastasis. *Cancer.* 2003;97(8):2013–2018.
10. Leber KA, Berglöff J, Pendl G. Dose-response tolerance of the visual pathways and cranial nerves of the cavernous sinus to stereotactic radiosurgery. *J Neurosurg.* 1998;88(1):43–50.
11. Schultheiss TE, Kun LE, Ang KK, Stephens LC. Radiation response of the central nervous system. *Int J Radiat Oncol Biol Phys.* 1995;31(5):1093–1112.
12. Ang KK, Jiang GL, Feng Y, Stephens LC, Tucker SL, Price RE. Extent and kinetics of recovery of occult spinal cord injury. *Int J Radiat Oncol Biol Phys.* 2001;50(4):1013–1020.
13. Benzil DL, Saboori M, Mogilner AY, Rocchio R, Moorthy CR. Safety and efficacy of stereotactic radiosurgery for tumors of the spine. *J Neurosurg.* 2004;101(suppl 3):413–418.
14. McCunniff AJ, Liang MJ. Radiation tolerance of the cervical spinal cord. *Int J Radiat Oncol Biol Phys.* 1989;16(3):675–678.
15. Cohen L, Creditor M. An iso-effect table for radiation tolerance of the human spinal cord. *Int J Radiat Oncol Biol Phys.* 1981;7(7):961–966.
16. Jeremic B, Djuric L, Mijatovic L. Incidence of radiation myelitis of the cervical spinal cord at doses of 5500 cGy or greater. *Cancer.* 1991;68(10):2138–2141.
17. Macbeth FR, Wheldon TE, Girling DJ, et al. Radiation myelopathy: estimates of risk in 1048 patients in three randomized trials of palliative radiotherapy for non-small cell lung cancer. The Medical Research Council Lung Cancer Working Party. *Clin Oncol (R Coll Radiol).* 1996;8(3):176–181.
18. Nieder C, Milas L, Ang KK. Tissue tolerance to reirradiation. *Semin Radiat Oncol.* 2000;10(3):200–209.
19. Niewald M, Feldmann U, Feiden W, et al. Multivariate logistic analysis of dose-effect relationship and latency of radiomyelopathy after hyperfractionated and conventionally fractionated radiotherapy in animal experiments. *Int J Radiat Oncol Biol Phys.* 1998;41(3):681–688.
20. Schultheiss TE. The radiation dose response of the human cervical spinal cord. *Int J Radiat Oncol Biol Phys.* 1999;45:174.
21. Wara WM, Phillips TL, Sheline GE, Schwade JG. Radiation tolerance of the spinal cord. *Cancer.* 1975;35(6):1558–1562.
22. Fuller DB, Bloom JG. Radiotherapy for chordoma. *Int J Radiat Oncol Biol Phys.* 1988;15(2):331–339.
23. Pieters RS, O'Farrell D, Fullerton B. Cauda equina tolerance to radiation therapy. *Int J Radiat Oncol Biol Phys.* 1996;36:359.
24. Schoenthaler R, Castro JR, Petti PL, Baken-Brown K, Phillips TL. Charged particle irradiation of sacral chordomas. *Int J Radiat Oncol Biol Phys.* 1993;26(2):291–298.
25. Jallo GI, Freed D, Epstein F. Intramedullary spinal cord tumors in children. *Childs Nerv Syst.* 2003;19(9):641–649.
26. Mottl H, Koutecky J. Treatment of spinal cord tumors in children. *Med Pediatr Oncol.* 1997;29(4):293–295.
27. Constantini S, Miller DC, Allen JC, Rorke LB, Freed D, Epstein FJ. Radical excision of intramedullary spinal cord tumors: surgical morbidity and long-term follow-up evaluation in 164 children and young adults. *J Neurosurg.* 2000;93(2 suppl):183–193.
28. Linstadt DE, Wara WM, Leibel SA, Gutin PH, Wilson CB, Sheline GE. Postoperative radiotherapy of primary spinal cord tumors. *Int J Radiat Oncol Biol Phys.* 1989;16(6):1397–1403.
29. McLaughlin MP, Buatti JM, Marcus RB Jr, Maria BL, Mickle PJ, Kedar A. Outcome after radiotherapy of primary spinal cord glial tumors. *Radiat Oncol Investig.* 1998;6(6):276–280.
30. Nishio S, Morioka T, Fujii K, Inamura T, Fukui M. Spinal cord gliomas: management and outcome with reference to adjuvant therapy. *J Clin Neurosci.* 2000;7(1):20–23.
31. Rodrigues GB, Waldron JN, Wong CS, Laperriere NJ. A retrospective analysis of 52 cases of spinal cord glioma managed with radiation therapy. *Int J Radiat Oncol Biol Phys.* 2000;48(3):837–842.
32. Shirato H, Kamada T, Hida K, et al. The role of radiotherapy in the management of spinal cord glioma. *Int J Radiat Oncol Biol Phys.* 1995;33(2):323–328.
33. Katoh N, Shirato H, Aoyama H, et al. Hypofractionated radiotherapy boost for dose escalation as a treatment option for high-grade spinal cord astrocytic tumor. *J Neurooncol.* 2006;78(1):63–69.
34. Minehan KJ, Brown PD, Scheithauer BW, Krauss WE, Wright MP. Prognosis and treatment of spinal cord astrocytoma. *Int J Radiat Oncol Biol Phys.* 2009;73(3):727–733.
35. Robinson CG, Prayson RA, Hahn JF, et al. Long-term survival and functional status of patients with low-grade astrocytoma of spinal cord. *Int J Radiat Oncol Biol Phys.* 2005;63(1):91–100.
36. Abdel-Wahab M, Etuk B, Palermo J, et al. Spinal cord gliomas: a multi-institutional retrospective analysis. *Int J Radiat Oncol Biol Phys.* 2006;64(4):1060–1071.
37. Bouffet E, Pierre-Kahn A, Marchal JC, et al. Prognostic factors in pediatric spinal cord astrocytoma. *Cancer.* 1998;83(11):2391–2399.
38. Cervoni L, Salvati M, Celli P, Caruso R, Gagliardi FM. Gliomas of the conus medullaris. *Tumori.* 1996;82(3):249–251.
39. Huddart R, Traish D, Ashley S, Moore A, Brada M. Management of spinal astrocytoma with conservative surgery and radiotherapy. *Br J Neurosurg.* 1993;7(5):473–481.
40. Jyothirmayi R, Madhavan J, Nair MK, Rajan B. Conservative surgery and radiotherapy in the treatment of spinal cord astrocytoma. *J Neurooncol.* 1997;33(3):205–211.
41. Lee HK, Chang EL, Fuller GN, et al. The prognostic value of neurologic function in astrocytic spinal cord glioma. *Neuro-oncology.* 2003;5(3):208–213.
42. Przybylski GJ, Albright AL, Martinez AJ. Spinal cord astrocytomas: long-term results comparing treatments in children. *Childs Nerv Syst.* 1997;13(7):375–382.
43. Rossitch E Jr, Zeidman SM, Burger PC, et al. Clinical and pathological analysis of spinal cord astrocytomas in children. *Neurosurgery.* 1990;27(2):193–196.
44. Sandler HM, Papadopoulos SM, Thornton AF Jr, Ross DA. Spinal cord astrocytomas: results of therapy. *Neurosurgery.* 1992;30(4):490–493.
45. Zorlu F, Ozyigit G, Gurkaynak M, Soylemezoglu F, Akyol F, Lale Atahan I. Postoperative radiotherapy results in primary spinal cord astrocytomas. *Radiother Oncol.* 2005;74(1):45–48.
46. Allen JC, Aviner S, Yates AJ, et al. Treatment of high-grade spinal cord astrocytoma of childhood with "8-in-1" chemotherapy and radiotherapy: a pilot study of CCG-945. Children's Cancer Group. *J Neurosurg.* 1998;88(2):215–220.
47. Cohen AR, Wisoff JH, Allen JC, Epstein F. Malignant astrocytomas of the spinal cord. *J Neurosurg.* 1989;70(1):50–54.
48. Epstein FJ, Farmer JP, Freed D. Adult intramedullary astrocytomas of the spinal cord. *J Neurosurg.* 1992;77(3):355–359.
49. Kim MS, Chung CK, Choe G, Kim IH, Kim HJ. Intramedullary spinal cord astrocytoma in adults: postoperative outcome. *J Neurooncol.* 2001;52(1):85–94.
50. Merchant TE, Nguyen D, Thompson SJ, Reardon DA, Kun LE, Sanford RA. High-grade pediatric spinal cord tumors. *Pediatr Neurosurg.* 1999;30(1):1–5.
51. Santi M, Mena H, Wong K, Koeller K, Olsen C, Rushing EJ. Spinal cord malignant astrocytomas. Clinicopathologic features in 36 cases. *Cancer.* 2003;98(3):554–561.
52. Ciappetta P, Salvati M, Capoccia G, Artico M, Raco A, Fortuna A. Spinal glioblastomas: report of seven cases and review of the literature. *Neurosurgery.* 1991;28(2):302–306.
53. Akyurek S, Chang EL, Yu TK, et al. Spinal myxopapillary ependymoma outcomes in patients treated with surgery and radiotherapy at M.D. Anderson Cancer Center. *J Neurooncol.* 2006;80(2):177–183.
54. Garcia DM. Primary spinal cord tumors treated with surgery and postoperative irradiation. *Int J Radiat Oncol Biol Phys.* 1985;11(11):1933–1939.
55. Hulshof MC, Menten J, Dito JJ, Dreissen JJ, van den Bergh R, González González D. Treatment results in primary intraspinal gliomas. *Radiother Oncol.* 1993;29(3):294–300.
56. Lin YH, Huang CI, Wong TT, et al. Treatment of spinal cord ependymomas by surgery with or without postoperative radiotherapy. *J Neurooncol.* 2005;71(2):205–210.
57. McGuire CS, Sainani KL, Fisher PG. Both location and age predict survival in ependymoma: a SEER study. *Pediatr Blood Cancer.* 2009;52(1):65–69.
58. Sgouros S, Malluci CL, Jackowski A. Spinal ependymomas—the value of postoperative radiotherapy for residual disease control. *Br J Neurosurg.* 1996;10(6):559–566.
59. Shaw EG, Evans RG, Scheithauer BW, Ilstrup DM, Earle JD. Radiotherapeutic management of adult intraspinal ependymomas. *Int J Radiat Oncol Biol Phys.* 1986;12(3):323–327.

60. Wahab SH, Simpson JR, Michalski JM, Mansur DB. Long term outcome with post-operative radiation therapy for spinal canal ependymoma. *J Neurooncol.* 2007;83(1):85–89.
61. Whitaker SJ, Bessell EM, Ashley SE, Bloom HJ, Bell BA, Brada M. Postoperative radiotherapy in the management of spinal cord ependymoma. *J Neurosurg.* 1991;74(5):720–728.
62. Kochbati L, Nasr C, Frikha H, et al. [Primary intramedullary ependymomas: retrospective study of 16 cases]. *Cancer Radiother.* 2003;7(1):17–21.
63. Lee TT, Gromelski EB, Green BA. Surgical treatment of spinal ependymoma and post-operative radiotherapy. *Acta Neurochir (Wien).* 1998;140(4):309–313.
64. McLaughlin MP, Marcus RB Jr, Buatti JM, et al. Ependymoma: results, prognostic factors and treatment recommendations. *Int J Radiat Oncol Biol Phys.* 1998;40(4):845–850.
65. Waldron JN, Laperriere NJ, Jaakkimainen L, et al. Spinal cord ependymomas: a retrospective analysis of 59 cases. *Int J Radiat Oncol Biol Phys.* 1993;27(2):223–229.
66. Hanbali F, Fourney DR, Marmor E, et al. Spinal cord ependymoma: radical surgical resection and outcome. *Neurosurgery.* 2002;51(5):1162–1172; discussion 1172.
67. Schild SE, Nisi K, Scheithauer BW, et al. The results of radiotherapy for ependymomas: the Mayo Clinic experience. *Int J Radiat Oncol Biol Phys.* 1998;42(5):953–958.
68. Gomez DR, Missett BT, Wara WM, et al. High failure rate in spinal ependymomas with long-term follow-up. *Neuro-oncology.* 2005;7(3):254–259.
69. Wen BC, Hussey DH, Hitchon PW, et al. The role of radiation therapy in the management of ependymomas of the spinal cord. *Int J Radiat Oncol Biol Phys.* 1991;20(4):781–786.
70. Gezen F, Kahraman S, Canakci Z, Bedük A. Review of 36 cases of spinal cord meningioma. *Spine.* 2000;25(6):727–731.
71. Roux FX, Nataf F, Pinaudeau M, Borne G, Devaux B, Meder JF. Intraspinal meningiomas: review of 54 cases with discussion of poor prognosis factors and modern therapeutic management. *Surg Neurol.* 1996;46(5):458–463; discussion 463.
72. Schiebe ME, Hoffmann W, Kortmann RD, Bamberg M. Radiotherapy in recurrent malignant meningiomas with multiple spinal manifestations. *Acta Oncol.* 1997;36(1):88–90.
73. Goldsmith BJ, Wara WM, Wilson CB, Larson DA. Postoperative irradiation for subtotally resected meningiomas. A retrospective analysis of 140 patients treated from 1967 to 1990. *J Neurosurg.* 1994;80(2):195–201.
74. Kaiser TE, Pritchard DJ, Unni KK. Clinicopathologic study of sacrococcygeal chordoma. *Cancer.* 1984;53(11):2574–2578.
75. Klekamp J, Samii M. Spinal chordomas–results of treatment over a 17-year period. *Acta Neurochir (Wien).* 1996;138(5):514–519.
76. Magrini SM, Papi MG, Marletta F, et al. Chordoma-natural history, treatment and prognosis. The Florence Radiotherapy Department experience (1956–1990) and a critical review of the literature. *Acta Oncol.* 1992;31(8):847–851.
77. Rich TA, Schiller A, Suit HD, Mankin HJ. Clinical and pathologic review of 48 cases of chordoma. *Cancer.* 1985;56(1):182–187.
78. Romero J, Cardenes H, la Torre A, et al. Chordoma: results of radiation therapy in eighteen patients. *Radiother Oncol.* 1993;29(1):27–32.
79. Saxton JP. Chordoma. *Int J Radiat Oncol Biol Phys.* 1981;7(7):913–915.
80. Sundaresan N, Galicich JH, Chu FC, Huvos AG. Spinal chordomas. *J Neurosurg.* 1979;50(3):312–319.
81. Cummings BJ, Hodson DI, Bush RS. Chordoma: the results of megavoltage radiation therapy. *Int J Radiat Oncol Biol Phys.* 1983;9(5):633–642.
82. Austin-Seymour M, Munzenrider JE, Goitein M, et al. Progress in low-LET heavy particle therapy: intracranial and paracranial tumors and uveal melanomas. *Radiat Res Suppl.* 1985;8:S219-S226.
83. Benk V, Liebsch NJ, Munzenrider JE, Efird J, McManus P, Suit H. Base of skull and cervical spine chordomas in children treated by high-dose irradiation. *Int J Radiat Oncol Biol Phys.* 1995;31(3):577–581.
84. Berson AM, Castro JR, Petti P, et al. Charged particle irradiation of chordoma and chondrosarcoma of the base of skull and cervical spine: the Lawrence Berkeley Laboratory experience. *Int J Radiat Oncol Biol Phys.* 1988;15(3):559–565.
85. Hug EB, Loredo LN, Slater JD, et al. Proton radiation therapy for chordomas and chondrosarcomas of the skull base. *J Neurosurg.* 1999;91(3):432–439.
86. Munzenrider JE, Liebsch NJ. Proton therapy for tumors of the skull base. *Strahlenther Onkol.* 1999;175(suppl 2):57–63.
87. Noël G, Habrand JL, Jauffret E, et al. Radiation therapy for chordoma and chondrosarcoma of the skull base and the cervical spine. Prognostic factors and patterns of failure. *Strahlenther Onkol.* 2003;179(4):241–248.
88. Noël G, Habrand JL, Mammar H, et al. Combination of photon and proton radiation therapy for chordomas and chondrosarcomas of the skull base: the Centre de Protonthérapie D'Orsay experience. *Int J Radiat Oncol Biol Phys.* 2001;51(2):392–398.
89. Rutz HP, Weber DC, Sugahara S, et al. Extracranial chordoma: Outcome in patients treated with function-preserving surgery followed by spot-scanning proton beam irradiation. *Int J Radiat Oncol Biol Phys.* 2007;67(2):512–520.
90. Slater JM, Slater JD, Archambeau JO. Proton therapy for cranial base tumors. *J Craniofac Surg.* 1995;6(1):24–26.
91. Castro JR, Linstadt DE, Bahary JP, et al. Experience in charged particle irradiation of tumors of the skull base: 1977–1992. *Int J Radiat Oncol Biol Phys.* 1994;29(4):647–655.
92. Chang SD, Martin DP, Lee E, Adler JR Jr. Stereotactic radiosurgery and hypofractionated stereotactic radiotherapy for residual or recurrent cranial base and cervical chordomas. *Neurosurg Focus.* 2001;10(3):E5.
93. Bernstein M, Gutin PH. Interstitial irradiation of skull base tumours. *Can J Neurol Sci.* 1985;12(4):366–370.
94. Gutin PH, Leibel SA, Hosobuchi Y, et al. Brachytherapy of recurrent tumors of the skull base and spine with iodine-125 sources. *Neurosurgery.* 1987;20(6):938–945.
95. Kumar PP, Good RR, Skultety FM, Leibrock LG. Local control of recurrent clival and sacral chordoma after interstitial irradiation with iodine-125: new techniques for treatment of recurrent or unresectable chordomas. *Neurosurgery.* 1988;22(3):479–483.
96. Bergh P, Gunterberg B, Meis-Kindblom JM, Kindblom LG. Prognostic factors and outcome of pelvic, sacral, and spinal chondrosarcomas: a center-based study of 69 cases. *Cancer.* 2001;91(7):1201–1212.
97. Mostafavi H, Lennarson PJ, Traynelis VC. Granulocytic sarcoma of the spine. *Neurosurgery.* 2000;46(1):78–83; discussion 83.
98. Lyons MK, O'Neill BP, Kurtin PJ, Marsh WR. Diagnosis and management of primary spinal epidural non-Hodgkin's lymphoma. *Mayo Clin Proc.* 1996;71(5):453–457.
99. Martin AJ, Sharr MM, Teddy PJ, Gardner BP, Robinson SF. Neurocytoma of the thoracic spinal cord. *Acta Neurochir (Wien).* 2002;144(8):823–828.
100. Tatter SB, Borges LF, Louis DN. Central neurocytomas of the cervical spinal cord. Report of two cases. *J Neurosurg.* 1994;81(2):288–293.
101. Tatter SB, Borges LF, Louis DN. Correction: central neurocytomas of the cervical spinal cord. *J Neurosurg.* 1995;82(4):706.
102. Merimsky O, Lepechoux C, Terrier P, Vanel D, Delord JP, LeCesne A. Primary sarcomas of the central nervous system. *Oncology.* 2000;58(3):210–214.
103. Oliveira AM, Scheithauer BW, Salomao DR, Parisi JE, Burger PC, Nascimento AG. Primary sarcomas of the brain and spinal cord: a study of 18 cases. *Am J Surg Pathol.* 2002;26(8):1056–1063.
104. Konno S, Yabuki S, Kinoshita T, Kikuchi S. Combined laminectomy and thoracoscopic resection of dumbbell-type thoracic cord tumor. *Spine.* 2001;26(6):E130-E134.
105. Seppälä MT, Haltia MJ, Sankila RJ, Jääskeläinen JE, Heiskanen O. Long-term outcome after removal of spinal schwannoma: a clinicopathological study of 187 cases. *J Neurosurg.* 1995;83(4):621–626.
106. Shadmehr MB, Gaissert HA, Wain JC, et al. The surgical approach to "dumbbell tumors" of the mediastinum. *Ann Thorac Surg.* 2003;76(5):1650–1654.
107. Seppälä MT, Haltia MJ. Spinal malignant nerve-sheath tumor or cellular schwannoma? A striking difference in prognosis. *J Neurosurg.* 1993;79(4):528–532.
108. Heyd R, Strassmann G, Filipowicz I, Borowsky K, Martin T, Zamboglou N. [Radiotherapy in vertebral hemangioma]. *Rontgenpraxis.* 2001;53(5):208–220.
109. Rades D, Bajrovic A, Alberti W, Rudat V. Is there a dose-effect relationship for the treatment of symptomatic vertebral hemangioma? *Int J Radiat Oncol Biol Phys.* 2003;55(1):178–181.
110. Esik O, Csere T, Stefanits K, et al. A review on radiogenic Lhermitte's sign. *Pathol Oncol Res.* 2003;9(2):115–120.
111. Nieder C, Ataman F, Price RE, Ang KK. Radiation myelopathy: new perspective on an old problem. *Radiat Oncol Investig.* 1999;7(4):193–203.

112. Okada S, Okeda R. Pathology of radiation myelopathy. *Neuropathology*. 2001;21(4):247–265.
113. Schultheiss TE, Higgins EM, El-Mahdi AM. The latent period in clinical radiation myelopathy. *Int J Radiat Oncol Biol Phys*. 1984;10(7):1109–1115.
114. Wang PY, Shen WC, Jan JS. MR imaging in radiation myelopathy. *AJNR Am J Neuroradiol*. 1992;13(4):1049–1055; discussion 1056.
115. Feldmeier JJ, Lange JD, Cox SD, Chou LJ, Ciaravino V. Hyperbaric oxygen as prophylaxis or treatment for radiation myelitis. *Undersea Hyperb Med*. 1993;20(3):249–255.
116. Liu CY, Yim BT, Wozniak AJ. Anticoagulation therapy for radiation-induced myelopathy. *Ann Pharmacother*. 2001;35(2):188–191.
117. Schultheiss TE, Stephens LC, Peters LJ. Survival in radiation myelopathy. *Int J Radiat Oncol Biol Phys*. 1986;12(10):1765–1769.
118. Mayfield JK. Postradiation spinal deformity. *Orthop Clin North Am*. 1979;10(4):829–844.
119. Nadeem SQ, Feun LG, Bruce-Gregorios JH, Green B. Post radiation sarcoma (malignant fibrous histiocytoma) of the cervical spine following ependymoma (a case report). *J Neurooncol*. 1991;11(3):263–268.
120. Rappaport ZH, Loven D, Ben-Aharon U. Radiation-induced cerebellar glioblastoma multiforme subsequent to treatment of an astrocytoma of the cervical spinal cord. *Neurosurgery*. 1991;29(4):606–608.

101 Metastatic Disease

Carsten Nieder and Dirk Rades

BRAIN METASTASES

The clinical problems associated with development of brain metastases in advanced-stage solid tumors and the number of patients with this serious condition has not decreased over the past years. Some data, for example, in breast cancer even point to increasing rates over time [1]. Breast cancer patients with secondary brain metastases incurred significantly more health care resources following diagnosis compared to those with breast cancer but no brain metastases. Patients with brain metastases had more than double the costs than patients without brain metastases at 6 and 12 months. In general, brain metastases patients might present with variable numbers, sizes, and locations of brain metastases, with different pattern and activity of extracranial disease and with differing comorbidity and performance status. Therefore, they represent an inhomogeneous group with large variations in survival. The number of available treatment options has increased since the era of corticosteroids with or without whole-brain radiotherapy (WBRT), allowing now for individually tailored regimens. The aim might range from palliation of symptoms to effective long-term control of brain metastases over several years.

PALLIATIVE WHOLE-BRAIN RADIOTHERAPY

Effects on Symptom Relief and Quality of Life

Uncontrolled data on the efficacy of palliative radiotherapy via two opposing lateral fields (Figure 101.1) have already been published more than 50 years ago, for example, describing palliation in 64% of patients [2]. More systematic, prospective data were generated by the Radiation Therapy Oncology Group (RTOG) in the trials 69–01 and 73–61. Their reports suggest that the median survival of patients treated with WBRT is longer (3–6 months) than that of patients managed with steroids without radiotherapy (1–2 months). The Medical Research Council has recently embarked on a large-scale randomized trial of steroids/best supportive care alone versus the same treatment plus WBRT in patients with primary non–small cell lung cancer. The aforementioned RTOG reports describe that 43% to 64% of patients experienced neurologic response by week 2 [3,4]. More recently, various groups reported responses in the same range, for example, after 30 Gy in 38% of the patients [5] and a symptomatic relief after ≥25 Gy in 66%, allowing a steroid dose reduction [6], and radiographic responses were observed in comparable proportions of patients [7]. Radiographic responses after WBRT with 30 Gy in 10 fractions are more likely in brain metastases from lung and breast cancer [8]. Responders were found to have significantly longer overall survival in many series. WBRT-induced tumor shrinkage correlated with better survival and neurocognitive function preservation also in a cohort of 135 patients from a phase III trial of WBRT plus the sensitizing agent motexafin-gadolinium [9]. Previous RTOG data also suggest that patients with controlled brain metastases after WBRT tend to experience stable mini-mental status examination (MMSE) scores, while those with uncontrolled lesions had an average drop of 6 at 3 months [10]. The 6-months survivors from the WBRT arm of the randomized RTOG radiosurgery (RS) trial had improved mental status in 40% and decreased steroids in 45% of those with available data [11]. The WBRT dose was 37.5 Gy in 2.5 Gy fractions in that study. Overall, no correlation between radiation dose and palliation could be established in the trials that compared different fractionation schedules. The same holds true for subgroup analyses of patients with better prognosis or separate trials for this population [12,13].

Despite the difficulties in separating the palliative effect of dexamethasone from that of WBRT itself, many durable clinical responses for the remaining lifetime were seen in different studies. This type of effect would be unlikely in the case of unirradiated metastases, which could continue to grow and produce increasing deficits. Acute side effects of WBRT typically are self-limiting, mild to moderate changes and might include skin erythema, dry desquamation, hair loss, fatigue, and increased vascular permeability, which might give raise to edema. Late effects such as cataract, endocrine disturbances and brain atrophy, leucencephalopathy, and neurocognitive decline have been observed in long-term survivors and are discussed in the sections dealing with combined WBRT and surgery or RS.

Fractionation and Total Dose

The large RTOG trials and a smaller randomized trial from the United Kingdom with 544 patients suggest that

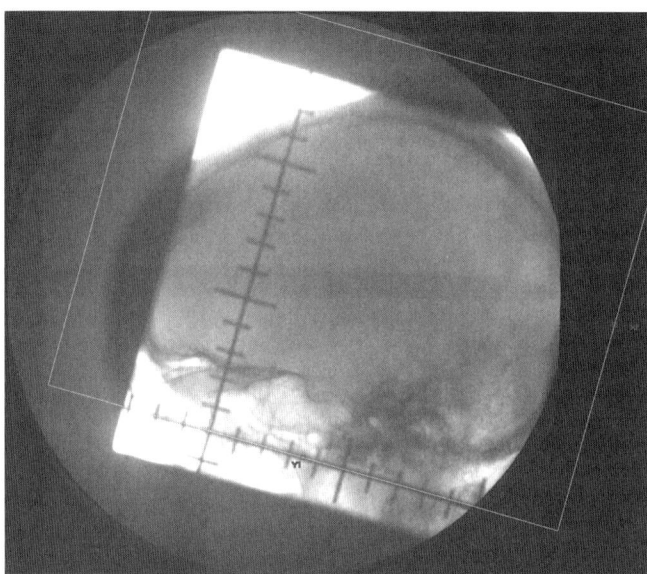

Figure 101.1 Whole-brain radiotherapy is typically administered via 2 lateral opposing photon beams as shown on the simulation film and fixation of the head in a thermoplastic mask.

fractionation is not important with regard to palliation and survival. The doses, which were investigated, range from 12 Gy in 2 fractions to 50 Gy in 20 fractions. The U.K. trial (2 fractions of 6 Gy vs. 10 fractions of 3 Gy) points to better survival with 30 Gy in the good prognostic group [14]. Overall responses were seen in 39% of those given 2 fractions and 44% of patients receiving 10 fractions. Recent multi-institutional analyses are in accordance with previous recommendations of short-course treatment (maximum 5 fractions of 4 Gy) for patients with limited life expectancy [15]. Ten fractions of 3 Gy or 15 fractions of 2.5 Gy might be considered for patients with longer life expectancy, also with regard to avoidance of neurotoxicity, which might occur after high doses per fraction. Estimation of prognosis is possible by using the RTOG recursive partitioning analysis (RPA) classes, first described by Gaspar et al (1997) and afterwards validated by several groups (Table 101.1). In breast cancer patients, lymphopenia and negative hormone receptor status might also be considered [23]. With WBRT to 30 Gy, very few lesions that measure more than 1 cm^3 are locally controlled after 1 year [7]. This provides arguments in favor of dose escalation in patients where brain control impacts on survival. Doses of 40 to 45 Gy were found not to improve local control or survival [15]. Attempts to improve the results by dose escalation to more than 50 Gy, for example, with bid radiotherapy by the RTOG, were not successful either [24].

Treatment Intensification by Surgical Resection or Radiosurgery

Of three relatively small randomized trials that compared WBRT with WBRT and surgical resection of single brain metastases (25–27), two found improved results. The third trial failed to demonstrate significantly better survival after surgery [27]. However, this trial included patients with lower performance status and a higher proportion of patients with progressive extracranial tumors. To date, intensified local treatment is mainly justified in patients with controlled extracranial disease. The combination of WBRT and RS as a better method to escalate the dose also led to significant progress in the field (Figure 101.2). In a small randomized study, patients with two to four brain metastases (all ≤25 mm diameter) either received WBRT alone (30 Gy in 12 fractions) or WBRT plus RS [28]. The study was stopped at an interim evaluation. Twenty-seven patients were randomized at that time. The rate of local failure at 1 year was 100% after WBRT alone but only 8% in patients who had boost RS. Patients who received WBRT alone lived a median of 7.5 months, while those who received WBRT plus RS lived 11 months ($P = 0.22$). A different randomized study by the RTOG enrolled 333 patients with one to three brain metastases [11]. Maximum diameter of the largest lesion was 4 cm and additional lesions could not exceed 3 cm. Minimum Karnofsky performance status was 70. WBRT dose was 37.5 Gy in 15 fractions in both groups. RS boost dose was adjusted to lesion size (15 Gy in lesions larger than 3 cm, 24 Gy in those up to 2 cm, and 18 Gy in others). Median survival was significantly better after RS boost in patients with single brain metastasis. By multivariate analysis, survival was also improved in RPA class I patients. RS patients were more likely to have a stable or improved performance status at 6 months (43% vs. 27%, $P = 0.03$). Central imaging review showed higher response rates at 3 months and better control of the treated lesions at 1 year, $P = 0.01$. The risk of developing a local recurrence was 43% greater with WBRT alone. In the United States, a new randomized trial is currently comparing WBRT plus RS with or without additional Temozolomide.

Combining Drugs and Whole-Brain Radiotherapy

Relatively few patients with multiple brain metastases, which are not suitable for RS, might be candidates for studies of combined WBRT and drug treatment (radiation sensitizers, chemotherapy) to increase the efficacy of standard WBRT. The aim of maximizing local control within the brain is reasonable only in case of controlled extracranial disease and good performance status. A small randomized study with only 52 patients evaluated WBRT with 20 fractions of 2 Gy versus combined WBRT and temozolomide 75 mg/m^2 day^{-1} [29]. In the combined modality arm, temozolomide continued for six more cycles (200 mg/m^2 day^{-1} for 5 days every 4 weeks). There was a significantly higher response rate in the temozolomide arm resulting from increased numbers of PR (96% vs. 67%). The influence on overall survival was not significant (7 vs. 8.6 months). A second randomized trial of temozolomide (75 mg/m^2 day^{-1} and two additional cycles with 200 mg/m^2 day^{-1} for 5 days every 4 weeks) plus WBRT (30 Gy) was designed as phase II study with 82 patients and therefore also does not allow to draw definitive conclusions [30]. Overall survival and response rates were similar, whereas progression-free survival (PFS) at 90 days was better for combined treatment (72% vs. 54%; $P = 0.03$). Death from brain metastases was more common after WBRT alone (69% vs. 41%; $P = 0.03$).

Table 101.1 Prognostic Value of Recursive Partitioning Analysis (RPA) Classes. Median Survival in Months From Different Publications

Reference	Number of Patients	RPA Class I	RPA Class II	RPA Class III
16	1,200	7.1	4.2	2.3
17	916	8.2	4.9	1.8
				(IIIA 3.2)
18	528	10.5	3.5	2.0
19	125 (resected brain met.)	14.8	9.9	6.0
20	271 (resected single brain met.)	21.4	9.0	8.9
21	110 (RS)	27.6	10.7	2.8
22	268 (RS only)	14.0	8.2	5.3
	301 (RS+WBRT)	15.2	7.0	5.5

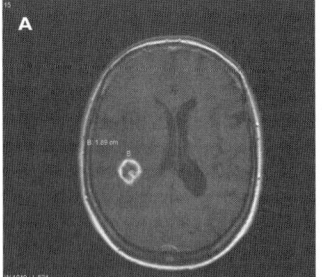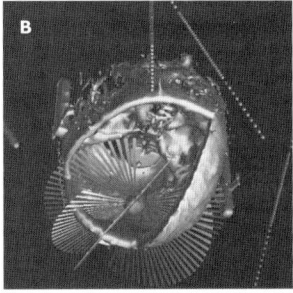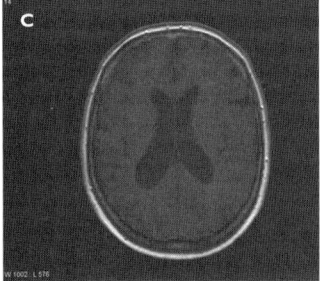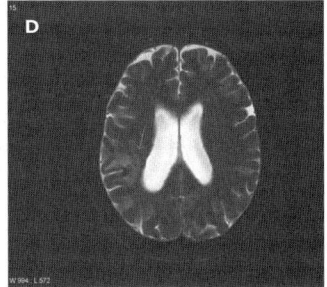

Figure 101.2 **(A)** Single-fraction stereotactic radiosurgery for a single brain metastasis from kidney cancer. **(B)** Immobilization is achieved with a stereotactic head ring fixed to the patient's skull. Treatment planning is based on CT/MRI image fusion. Small, well circumscribed lesions with very limited brain infiltration, such as brain metastasis, represent ideal targets for radiosurgery. In this case, a dose of 20 Gy was prescribed to the 45% isodose, which encloses the target volume. The lesion volume was 5 cc. Radiosurgery is characterized by a highly conformal dose distribution with very steep dose gradients toward the normal tissues. In this case, treatment was administered with a gamma knife. **(C)** The follow-up MRI scans were taken 3 years after successful radiosurgery. **(D)** Slight white matter changes are present in the irradiated region. *See color insert.*

A nonrandomized phase II trial with 33 patients reported objective responses in just below 60%, while median survival was 12 months (temozolomide 60 mg/m^2 day^{-1} [days 1–16] concomitantly with WBRT [36 Gy/12 fractions given in 16 days]). One month after the end of radiotherapy, six cycles of temozolomide were administered (200 mg/m^2 day^{-1} for 5 consecutive days every 28 days). The large differences in outcome between these studies point to the influence of patient selection and emphasize the need for prospective randomized trials with sufficient numbers of patients. Topotecan daily IV in addition to WBRT has been evaluated in two phase I/II trials [31,32]. Median survival was 5 and 3 months, respectively, and CR + PR rate in assessable patients was 58% or lower. To date, outside of prospective clinical trials, no firm role for chemotherapy or radiochemotherapy of brain metastases has been established.

Other recent approaches for radiosensitization of tumor cells in conjunction with WBRT investigated the drugs efaproxiral, which modifies tumor oxygenation [33], and motexafin gadolinium (MGd), a paramagnetic redox active drug [34]. In a large randomized phase III study, efaproxiral significantly improved the survival of the patient subgroup with breast cancer [33]. Therefore, a confirmatory trial in this population was started. However, development of the drug has been discontinued in 2007. MGd concentrates in tumor cells and is visible by magnetic resonance imaging (MRI). Its interactions lead to oxidative damage by generation of reactive oxygen species. MGd displays catalytic activity by accepting electrons from various cellular-reducing metabolites and regenerating the MGd molecule through futile redox cycling [35]. In a randomized trial of MGd with 401 patients, which used the coprimary endpoint of time to neurologic progression, the subgroup with non–small cell lung cancer (NSCLC, $n = 251$) had significantly longer time to neurologic progression [34]. A new phase III trial in NSCLC patients has recently been completed. It included 554 patients with brain metastases from NSCLC and a Karnofsky performance status of ≥70 [36]. Patients were excluded if they had liver metastases, ≥2 sites of extracranial metastases, and leptomeningeal or subarachnoid metastases. All patients received WBRT (30 Gy/10 fractions), or WBRT with MGd, 5 mg/kg day^{-1}, 2 to 5 hours prior to each WBRT fraction. The primary endpoint was time to neurologic progression or death with evidence of neurologic progression. The intent-to-treat analysis of all 554 patients showed a strong trend favoring the MGd group in the primary endpoint. The median time to neurologic progression was 10.0 months for WBRT and 15.4 months for MGd, $P = 0.122$. Stepwise Cox model analysis demonstrated that performance status, histology, and region were also independent predictors of time to neurologic progression. Among these variables, a statistically significant treatment interaction was only found for geographic region. In North America, the median time to neurologic progression was 8.8 months for WBRT and 24.2 months for MGd, $P = 0.004$, HR = 0.53. Analyses to identify baseline factors that differed by region showed that treatment delay and the use of chemotherapy for the initial treatment of brain metastases varied by region. Patients in North America received treatment more promptly than patients in Europe and Australia. Certain sites used chemotherapy alone as initial therapy for brain metastases. This was responsible for delayed use of WBRT in many patients. Cox proportional hazard models were used to estimate the benefit of MGd in patients treated promptly. A significant MGd treatment benefit was seen in patients treated within 28 days of brain metastasis diagnosis ($n = 435$, $P = 0.032$, HR = 0.68). There was no significant difference in survival or PFS. The median survival was 5.8 months in the WBRT group and 5.1 months in the MGd group. This might result, among other factors, from statistically significantly greater use of salvage surgery or RS in the WBRT group. The Federal Drug Administration has not approved MGd for patients with brain metastases from NSCLC.

WHOLE-BRAIN RADIOTHERAPY AFTER SURGICAL RESECTION

While WBRT might reduce the risk of in-brain-recurrence, it might also cause certain adverse events. In this context, neurocognitive decline is of particular concern. Both local tumor cell kill (and thus ultimate local control) and normal tissue effects are dose dependent. An optimal balance between high local control and minimal toxicity requires detailed analysis of the dose-response relationships. Nieder et al [37] have recently published a review of related articles. The analysis included patients treated with WBRT and different types of local "partial brain" radiotherapy. Patients from 10 studies were included. After surgery alone ($n = 94$ from three studies, all had complete resection) 38 patients developed a local relapse at the original site (40%). After additional radiotherapy ($n = 224$ from three studies, all had complete resection) 28 patients developed this type of failure (12.5%, $P < 0.01$). No significant difference was found between local relapse rates after WBRT and local "partial brain" RT, respectively. The local relapse rate also was significantly reduced in patients with unknown resection status. Within the dose range of 30 to 60 Gy, no significant dose-response relationship was observed. Development of new brain metastases away from the originally resected lesion ("new distant lesions") occurred in 32% after surgery alone (74 cases) and 45% after surgery plus local radiotherapy (66 cases). It was significantly reduced to 19% by WBRT (291 cases), $P < 0.01$. With the given WBRT dose range (30–50.4 Gy) no significant dose-response relationship was observed. Very few data related to late side effects were available. Neurotoxicity > grade I was observed in 1/66 patients after WBRT [38]. Patchell et al [39] noted that the length of functional independence was similar between patients treated by surgery alone and those that received surgery plus WBRT. Aoyama et al [40] found leucencephalopathy in 3/65 patients after WBRT in their study of radiosurgery (RS) alone versus RS plus WBRT. There were no significant differences between the two groups regarding longitudinal development of MMSE results and Karnofsky performance status. Murray et al [41] have previously suggested that 16% of patients had a MMSE score of less than 23, indicating possible dementia, prior to treatment.

Compared to a large prospective randomized trial, pooled data might have the disadvantage of variations in inclusion criteria, staging examinations, treatment, and follow-up protocols in the individual trials. However, they suggest that both local and whole-brain radiotherapy significantly reduce local recurrence at the original site and that WBRT also reduces the development of new lesions. The latter finding has also been confirmed in a randomized trial of RS with or without WBRT [40]. As mentioned above, a dose-response relationship was not observed in the pooled analysis. Possible conclusions are that a dose-response relationship does indeed not exist or that confounding factors prevent its detection. It is, for example, known that many patients die from extracranial disease progression before a cerebral relapse can be detected. There is also no reliable method to account for the effect of continuous reseeding from extracranial sites, which will create a nonpreventable type of brain failure.

The risk of serious toxicity after WBRT appears rather low. Furthermore, one must acknowledge that any type of cancer treatment might cause measurable neurocognitive decline [42,43] and that some postradiation symptoms might be caused by certain drugs rather than radiation itself [44,45]. Given these facts, can a general recommendation for routine moderate-dose WBRT after surgery be given? Importantly, the randomized trials were not able to demonstrate a prolongation of survival by WBRT after either surgery or RS [39,40]. Survival is largely dependent on other factors, such as performance status and extent of extracranial disease. Survival was not the endpoint of the pooled analysis, given the inhomogeneity of prognostic factors in the studies available. However, if one looks at 1-year survival rates from the nonrandomized studies in order to explore survival trends and their consistency with the findings from the randomized trials, the survival rate of patients from the surgical series is 46%, compared to 47% after resection plus WBRT. The ongoing, but slowly recruiting, randomized trials by the European Organisation for Research and Treatment of Cancer (EORTC 22952) and the neuro-oncological working group of the German Cancer Society (NOA-06) will hopefully provide further high-quality data on the subject of postoperative WBRT. In addition, a Japanese group is randomizing patients between postoperative WBRT and salvage RS at relapse. The pooled data discussed here do not support high-dose WBRT or local boost treatment, unless incomplete resection was performed. This finding is unfortunately in disagreement with another recently published analysis. Rades et al [46] performed a retrospective analysis of pooled data from

201 patients with different inclusion criteria, that is, patients with one to two brain metastases in RPA class 1 to class 2. Patients underwent either resection of the metastases plus WBRT with 10 fractions of 3 Gy each or 20 fractions of 2 Gy each (99 patients) or the same treatment plus boost to the metastatic site (10 fractions of 3 Gy each plus 5 fractions of 3 Gy each or 20 fractions of 2 Gy each plus 5 fractions of 2 Gy each) (102 patients). Boost patients had better 1-year survival (66% vs. 41%; $P < 0.001$). On multivariate analysis, treatment regimen (relative risk of 1.94; $P < 0.001$), extent of surgical resection, and interval from tumor diagnosis to WBRT were found to be statistically significant. On multivariate analysis of brain control, the same three factors emerged. For local control at the resected site(s), treatment regimen and extent of surgical resection were found to be statistically significant. On RPA class subgroup analyses, outcome was found to be significantly better with a boost in both RPA class 1 and class 2 patients. A boost resulted in better outcome after both complete and incomplete surgical resection. Therefore, the issue of radiation dose is currently unsettled.

Very high brain control rates were found in a small study where 25 patients underwent craniotomy for a single brain metastasis, and carmustine polymer wafers were placed in the tumor resection cavity [47]. Patients then received WBRT. The local recurrence rate was 0%. Four patients (16%) relapsed elsewhere in the brain, and two patients (8%) relapsed in the spinal cord. Median survival was 33 weeks, and 33% of patients survived 1 year. Two patients had severe adverse events thought to be related to wafer placement, one with seizures alone and one with seizures and subsequent respiratory compromise.

RADIOSURGERY

Local control of a limited number (mostly one to three) of brain metastases can effectively be achieved by surgical resection or RS with or without adjuvant WBRT (Table 101.2). The number of patients dying from uncontrolled brain metastases despite intensive local treatment ranges from 20% to 30%. There is no indication toward significant differences in outcome with the use of different technologies for RS. If the radiation dose would have to be reduced because a lesion is located in close vicinity to sensitive structures, for example, optic nerve and chiasm or brain stem, and even a low probability for radionecrosis cannot be accepted, it should be considered whether fractionated stereotactic radiotherapy offers a better therapeutic ratio (Figure 101.3). The radiobiologic effects of fractionation allow for additional sparing of normal tissue beyond the physical advantages of precise targeting and steep dose gradients that characterize RS. In general, RS doses have varied with lesion size although it is counterintuitive to treat larger tumors with lower doses of radiation. While small lesions typically receive minimum doses of 20 to 24 Gy to the margin of the lesion, those that measure between 2 and 3 cm are treated with 18 to 20 Gy and those that measure between 3 and 4 cm with 15 to 16 Gy. A retrospective analysis of 375 lesions suggests that 1-year local control after 18 Gy or less is in the range of 45% to 49% as opposed to 85% after 24 Gy [54]. In the Japanese RS study with 132 patients, which is discussed in greater detail in the next paragraph, only four patients (3%) developed radionecrosis [40]. Prognosis of RS patients might be assessed either by RPA classes or the score index for radiosurgery (SIR) [21,55]. The most favorable SIR group contains patients with age ≤50 years, Karnofsky performance status >70%, no evidence of systemic disease at the time of RS, limited number of brain lesions, and largest RS-treated lesion <13 ml.

RS might also be performed for small lesions in the brainstem, as indicated by the results in 42 consecutive patients with brainstem metastases that had Gamma Knife RS to 44 lesions (7 midbrain, 31 pontine, and 6 medullary) in 42 sessions [56]. The median survival time was 9 months. Longer survival was associated with single metastasis, nonmelanoma histology, and extracranial disease control. The median target volume was 0.26 ml (max. 2.8 ml) and the median prescribed dose was 16.0

Table 101.2 Results of Surgery and Stereotactic Radiosurgery for Brain Metastases

Reference	n (Patients and Lesions)	Prescribed dose (Median; Range [Gy])[a]	Median OS	1-year PFS (%)
25	25/25	Surgery	9.5	80
39	49/49	Surgery	11.0	82
48	236/311	20; 10–30	5.5	89
49	73/136	17.5; 6–50	7.8	80
50	106/157	20; 12–25	8.0	85
51	62/118[b]	18; 15–22	11.3	80
	43/117[c]	17.5; 15–22	11.1	86
52	137/208	16; 12–25	Not given	90
11	164/269[d]	Not given; 15–24	6.5	82
53	205/4–18 lesions each[e]	16; 12–20	8.0	71

OS: overall survival in months; PFS: progression-free survival; ?: data not reported

[a] Prescription isodose or point varied, some series included RS plus WBRT

[b] RS only

[c] RS plus WBRT (no significant difference in OS and PFS between both groups)

[d] RS plus WBRT

[e] RS plus/minus WBRT

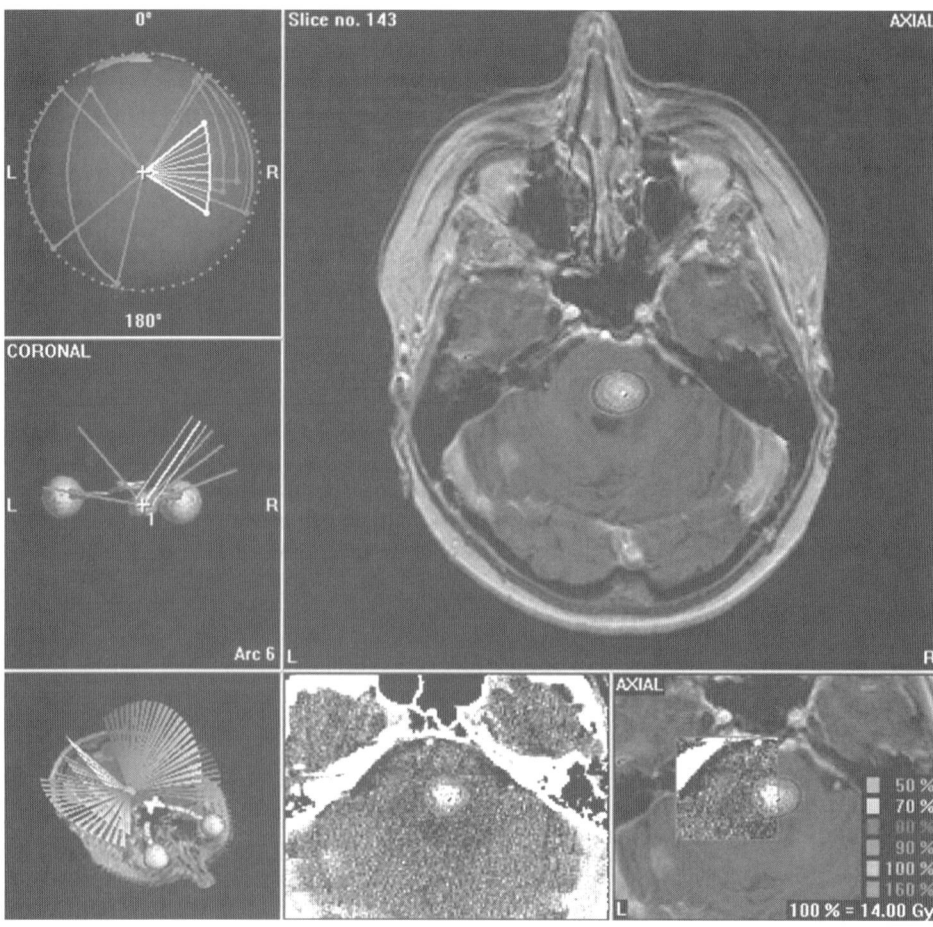

Figure 101.3 A situation with a rather large metastasis in the brain stem, where the therapeutic ratio of radiosurgery is small. The long-term tumor control probability with a margin dose of 14 Gy, as displayed here, is not satisfactory. Under such circumstances, fractionated stereotactic radiotherapy might be considered. The total dose will thus be administered in 5–7 fractions. Fractionated treatment requires the use of a removable non-invasive immobilization system attached to a stereotactic localization device rather than a classic stereotactic ring. See color insert.

Gy (10.0–19.8 Gy). Brainstem lesion freedom from progression was 90% at 6 months and 77% at 1 year. Four patients had brainstem complications following treatment. Poor brainstem outcome was associated with melanoma and renal cell histology as well as brainstem lesion volume ≥1 ml.

Patients with four or more lesions were treated with RS during one session by a number of groups [57]. Among 205 such patients, only 17% received RS as sole management, while the others also were treated with WBRT or had failed after previous WBRT. Better survival was observed in the subgroup with <7 brain metastases and total treatment volume of <7 ml (median 13 months). Patients without these two variables survived for a median of 6 months.

In the absence of published randomized trial data, four retrospective analyses have compared RS and surgical resection. Rades et al [58] (186 patients) suggest that patients in RPA class I or II with 1 to 2 brain metastases can be treated with either approach, without significant differences in overall survival and local control. The studies by the other groups point into the same direction (59–61). RS, however, is a minimally invasive procedure, which in many health care systems reduces the cost of treatment. Surgical resection might be required if rapid decompression must be achieved, a tissue diagnosis is mandatory, or RS is not feasible (Table 101.3).

Table 101.3 Key Questions When Selecting Between the Different Treatment Options for Brain Metastases

Is the patient's performance status after initiation of steroid treatment at a level that justifies initiation of radiation therapy?
Are extracranial disease sites absent or controlled and if so, do we expect rapid extracranial progression?
Do laboratory tests point to advanced disease status and poor compliance to further therapy?
Will brain control impact on the survival of the patient or is treatment focused on palliation of symptoms?
Will surgical intervention lead to rapid symptom improvement or effective local control, if co-morbidity and other factors allow for consideration of invasive measures? Could the same goals be achieved without surgery?
Can the patient participate in a prospective clinical trial?
Does the risk of microscopic brain metastases justify whole-brain radiotherapy in addition to focal treatment?

RADIOSURGERY PLUS WHOLE-BRAIN RADIOTHERAPY

After many years of controversy about the role of combining WBRT with RS and considerable variation in practice, comparable to the discussion around WBRT after surgical resection of brain metastases, a Japanese group has recently published the results of a prospective randomized multicenter phase III study of RS alone versus combined

RS and WBRT [40]. The primary endpoint was survival with an expected difference of 30%. The trial included adult patients with Karnofsky performance score of >60% and maximum four brain metastases up to 3 cm in diameter. The patients were stratified for number of lesions (1 vs. 2–4), extracranial tumor activity (active vs. stable, i.e., controlled for at least 6 months), and primary tumor (lung cancer vs. others). WBRT was given in 10 fractions of 3 Gy. RS dose varied with size of the lesion (up to 2 cm: 22–25 Gy, >2 cm: 18–20 Gy margin dose). This dose was reduced by 30% if additional WBRT was given. Overall, the mean dose was 21.9 Gy in the RS-alone arm and 16.6 Gy in the combined arm. The combined arm contained 65 patients, the RS arm 67 patients. However, only 57 patients received WBRT plus RS (6 had WBRT only, and 2 RS only). In the RS arm, 2 patients did not receive RS for medical reasons. Almost 50% of patients had a single lesion. The RS group contained slightly more patients with performance status of 90% to 100% (66% vs. 52%) and patients without neurological symptoms (70% vs. 59%). However, the differences were not significant. Median survival was 7.5 months after RS plus WBRT and 8 months after RS alone. One-year survival in the combined-treatment arm was increased by 36% (38.5% vs. 28.4%, $P > 0.05$). There was no significant difference in the percentage of patients who died from predominantly neurologic causes (23% vs. 19%). In multivariate analysis, age, performance status, extracranial disease activity, and status of the primary tumor were significant prognostic factors. After RC alone, two patients developed serious late complications (radionecrosis and grade 4 seizures, respectively). After RC plus WBRT, three patients developed a radionecrosis and three signs of leukencephalopathy. The trial revealed statistically significant differences in local control (Table 101.4). For all brain metastases relapses together, actuarial rate of failure at 1 year was 47% after combined treatment but 76% after RS alone ($P < 0.001$). New lesions developed in 42% versus 64% ($P = 0.003$). The risk was significantly higher in patients presenting with two to four lesions before treatment, those with active extracranial metastases, and those with KPS of 70% to 80%. WBRT reduced the risk of failure at the site of RS from 27% to 11% after 1 year ($P = 0.002$).

Quality of life was not examined in greater detail. Relatively few patients ($n = 92$) had a MMSE during follow-up. Their values were largely comparable (median 28 vs. 27 pretreatment, 27 vs. 28 at last follow-up). In the baseline MMSE analyses, statistically significant differences were observed for total tumor volume, extent of tumor edema, age, and performance status. Of the 92 patients who underwent the follow-up MMSE, 39 had a baseline MMSE score of ≤27 (17 in the WBRT + RS group and 22 in the RS-alone group). Improvements of ≥3 points in the MMSE of 9 WBRT + RS patients and 11 RS-alone patients ($P = 0.85$) were observed. Of the 82 patients with a baseline MMSE score of ≥27 or whose baseline MMSE score was ≤26 but had improved to ≥27 after the initial brain treatment, the 12-, 24-, and 36-month actuarial free rate of the three-point drop in the MMSE was 76%, 69%, and 15% in the WBRT + RS group and 59%, 52%, and 52% in the RS-alone group, respectively. The average duration until deterioration was 16.5 months in the WBRT + RS group and 7.6 months in the RS-alone group ($P = 0.05$). These findings suggest that, for most patients, brain control is the most important factor for stabilizing neurocognitive function. However, occasional patients will develop long-term adverse effects of WBRT.

While important improvements in local control were achieved by adding WBRT, this study confirms that survival is a problematic endpoint in patients with brain metastases. Improved local control from WBRT at the site of RS might result from compensation of difficulties in target volume delineation or biologic effects of fractionation and their influence on reoxygenation and redistribution of tumor cells. Both institutions that practice RS without planned WBRT and those that combine the two modalities will find arguments that support their approach from this randomized study. However, patients with two or more lesions have a probability of developing new lesions after RC alone that exceeds 40% already at 6 months, suggesting that WBRT should be considered in such cases. Retrospective data from patients treated with RS alone also demonstrate 1-year actuarial risk of distant brain failure of 61% [62]. Significant multivariate predictors of distant failure included more than three metastases (hazard ratio, 3.30; $P = 0.004$), stable or poorly controlled extracranial disease (hazard ratio, 2.16; $P = 0.04$), and melanoma histologic characteristics (hazard ratio, 2.14; $P = 0.02$). In the United States, the ACOSOG has embarked on a new randomized trial comparing RS with RS plus WBRT in patients with one to three brain metastases.

Current treatment planning studies are trying to reduce the dose to the hippocampus, aiming at selective sparing of this neural stem cell-containing area in order to reduce the risk of toxicity of WBRT [63]. By using helical tomotherapy, the hippocampus dose was limited to <6 Gy. The whole brain dose was prescribed at 32.25 Gy to 95% in 15 fractions, and the simultaneous boost doses to individual brain metastases were 63 Gy to lesions ≥2.0 cm in the maximal diameter and 70.8 Gy to lesions <2.0 cm. Clinical data on such approaches are not available yet.

FRACTIONATED STEREOTACTIC RADIOTHERAPY

A normal brain tissue dose recommendation in RC planning is to limit the volume receiving 10 Gy or more to 10 to 12 cm^3. If the complication probability is to be minimized, sufficiently high tumor doses are difficult to obtain both

Table 101.4 Results of Focal Treatment With or Without Whole-Brain Radiotherapy

Therapy	All Brain Metastases Relapses	Relapse At The Original Site Only	Distant Brain Relapse Only
RS (40)	76%	27%	64%
RS plus WBRT [40]	47%	11%	42%
OP [39]	70%	68%	50%
OP plus WBRT [39]	24%	21%	18%
RS plus WBRT [11]	Not available	18%	Not available
WBRT [11]	Not available	29%	Not available

in larger lesions and in those located very close to sensitive structures. In such cases, fractionated high-precision treatment with stereotactic localization and mask fixation of the head might offer a solution. Currently, relatively small patient series on this topic are available. Total doses ranged from 28 to 42 Gy administered in four to seven fractions. Fahrig et al [64] studied three different regimens in 150 patients with 228 lesions. Local control was inferior with 10 fractions of 4 Gy as compared to 7 fractions of 5 Gy or 5 fractions of 6 to 7 Gy. Overall 1-year survival rate was 66%. With a median follow-up of 28 months in surviving patients, local control was obtained in 93% of the lesions. Higher doses, for example, 5 fractions of 8 Gy, do not improve the outcome, as demonstrated in a series of 47 patients where local control was 84% [65]. However, 2 patients developed radionecrosis. More than 80% of the patients died from extracranial metastases.

BRACHYTHERAPY

After the advent of stereotactic external beam radiotherapy, the number of publications on brachytherapy, for example, with ^{125}I seeds, has decreased. Other techniques of brachytherapy include a miniature X-ray generator that can stereotactically irradiate brain metastases (Photon Radiosurgery System) and the GliaSite brachytherapy system. In the most recent report on seed brachytherapy, newly diagnosed single brain metastases were treated [66]. Twenty-six patients underwent gross-total resection and placement of seeds. With a median follow-up of 12 months, the local tumor control rate was 96%. Distant metastases occurred in three patients within 3 months and in six patients more than 3 months after treatment (overall 35%). Two patients who suffered radiation necrosis required operative intervention. The GliaSite study reported on 62 patients with solitary lesions, which received postoperative brachytherapy by injecting a ^{125}I containing liquid into a balloon placed within the resection cavity [67]. Actuarial local control at 1 year was 79%. Twenty-four patients (44%) developed new brain metastases. Nine patients developed radionecrosis, prompting the authors to reduce the radiation dose in their next study protocol.

RETREATMENT

Patients with recurrent lesions should preferentially be treated with stereotactic high-precision techniques. RTOG study 90–05 has defined the maximum tolerable RC dose after previous WBRT [68]. While small lesions <2 cm can be treated with up to 24 Gy to the margin of the lesion, those that measure between 2 and 3 cm might receive 18 Gy and those that measure between 3 and 4 cm, 15 Gy. Fractionated treatment might be an alternative in cases with unfavorable therapeutic ratio. In a Canadian study, RS was used in smaller lesions (n = 35), while a split dose was used in larger ones (29.7 Gy at the 90% isodose surface in two fractions, n = 69) [69]. The median time from WBRT was 30 weeks. Median survival after retreatment was 16 weeks after RS and 30 weeks after two fractions. A repeat course of WBRT is rarely used to date. Limited experience with two courses of WBRT in 72 patients suggests that 31% of patients experienced a partial clinical response after reirradiation [70]. In responders, the mean duration of response was 5.1 months. The median survival after reirradiation was 4.1 months. One patient was reported as having memory impairment and pituitary insufficiency after 5 months of PFS. The most frequent dose used for the initial radiotherapy was 20 Gy in five fractions. The most common doses of reirradiation were 25 Gy in 10 fractions, 20 Gy in 10 fractions, and 15 Gy in 5 fractions. Largely comparable results were published in 86 reirradiated patients in 1996 by Wong et al (median dose of initial WBRT 30 Gy and of repeat WBRT 20 Gy) [71].

SPINE METASTASES

With regard to treatment of spine metastases without manifest or impending cord compression, several recent reviews and meta-analyses have summarized the results of multiple prospective randomized trials that included such patients but were not limited to spine metastases. A systematic review of radiotherapy trials in bone metastases was performed by the Swedish Council of Technology Assessment in Health Care (SBU) [72]. Their report is based on data from 16 randomized trials and 20 prospective studies. The results were compared with those of a similar overview from 1996 including 13,054 patients and provide strong evidence that radiotherapy of skeletal metastases gives an overall complete and partial pain relief in up to 80% of patients. The duration of pain relief in at least 50% of patients lasts for ≥6 months. There is convincing evidence that pain relief, in terms of degree and duration, does not depend on the fractionation schedules applied. Irrespective of the fractionation schedule used at irradiation, the number of later complications, such as spinal cord compression or pathological fractures, at the index fields is low. There is strong evidence that the radionuclides ^{89}Sr and ^{153}Sm are efficient when they are used as a systemic treatment of generalized bone pain due to metastasis from carcinomas of the prostate and breast. Overall bone pain relief occurs in about 60% to 80% of patients with median response duration of 2 to 4 months.

In 2004, a Cochrane review and meta-analysis of single-fraction radiotherapy versus multifraction radiotherapy for metastatic bone pain relief and prevention of bone complications was published [73]. Eleven trials that involved over 3,000 patients were analyzed. The results support those already described by the Swedish group. Patients treated by single-fraction radiotherapy had a higher retreatment rate with 21.5% requiring retreatment compared to 7.4% of patients in the multifraction radiotherapy arm (odds ratio 3.44 [95% CI: 2.67–4.43]). The pathological fracture rate was also higher in single-fraction radiotherapy arm patients. Three percent of patients treated by single-fraction radiotherapy developed pathological fracture compared to 1.6% for those treated by multifraction radiotherapy (odds ratio 1.82 [95% CI: 1.06–3.11]). The spinal cord compression rates were similar for both arms. In 2007, the previous meta-analyses were updated with a systematic review of randomized palliative radiotherapy trials comparing single fractions versus multiple fractions by Chow et al No significant differences were found in response rates. Trends showing an increased risk for single-fraction treatment in terms of pathological fractures and spinal cord compressions were observed, but neither was statistically significant. The likelihood of retreatment was 2.5 fold higher (95% CI: 1.76 to 3.56).

The Dutch group reviewed 342 patients with painful spinal metastases without neurologic impairment who were treated conservatively within a large, prospectively randomized radiotherapy trial [74]. Response to radiotherapy and prognostic factors for survival were studied. Responses were noted in 73% of patients. In 3% of patients, spinal cord compression was reported a mean of 3.5 months after randomization. The median survival was 7 months, and significant predictors for survival were Karnofsky performance score, primary tumor, and the absence of visceral metastases. The best prognostic group (median survival 19 months, 18% of all patients) was comprised of patients with breast carcinoma, a good performance status, and no visceral metastases. The Dutch model was validated by Chow et al [75] in a total of 231 patients with spinal bone metastases. Overall, the majority of patients with spinal metastases can safely be treated with single-fraction radiotherapy without compromising pain improvement, quality of life, survival, or other outcome parameters.

METASTATIC SPINAL CORD COMPRESSION (MSCC)

MSCC occurs in 5% to 10% of all cancer patients during the course of their disease [76,77]. The most common tumors are breast cancer, prostate cancer, and lung cancer, which each account for 15% to 20% of the cases, followed by myeloma and renal cell carcinoma, which each account for about 10% of the cases [78]. MSCC was first described in 1925 [79] and defined as "comprehensive indentation, displacement, or encasement of the thecal sac that surrounds spinal cord or cauda equina by spinal epidural metastases." If a mass is touching the spinal cord but is not yet associated with neurological deficits, the situation should be called "impending" MSCC. Spinal cord compression is mostly caused by posterior extension of a vertebral body mass or by anterior extension of a mass arising from the dorsal elements of the spine [80] (Figure 101.4). A mass of the vertebral body can impinge on the thecal sac, the spinal cord, and the epidural venous plexus. Pathological vertebral body fractures may also occur with dislocation of bony fragments into the epidural space. Rarely, MSCC may be caused by growth of a mass that invades through the vertebral foramen from the paraspinal region or by metastases of the epidural space. According to animal studies reported 20 to 30 years ago, MSCC is associated with white-matter edema and axonal swelling, which may result in necrosis and gliosis of the white matter (81–83). Disrupted blood flow was observed for both venous and arterial circulation. The white-matter changes vary with the speed at which MSCC develops. A slower development leads to venous congestion and vasogenic edema of the white matter resulting in mostly reversible neurological

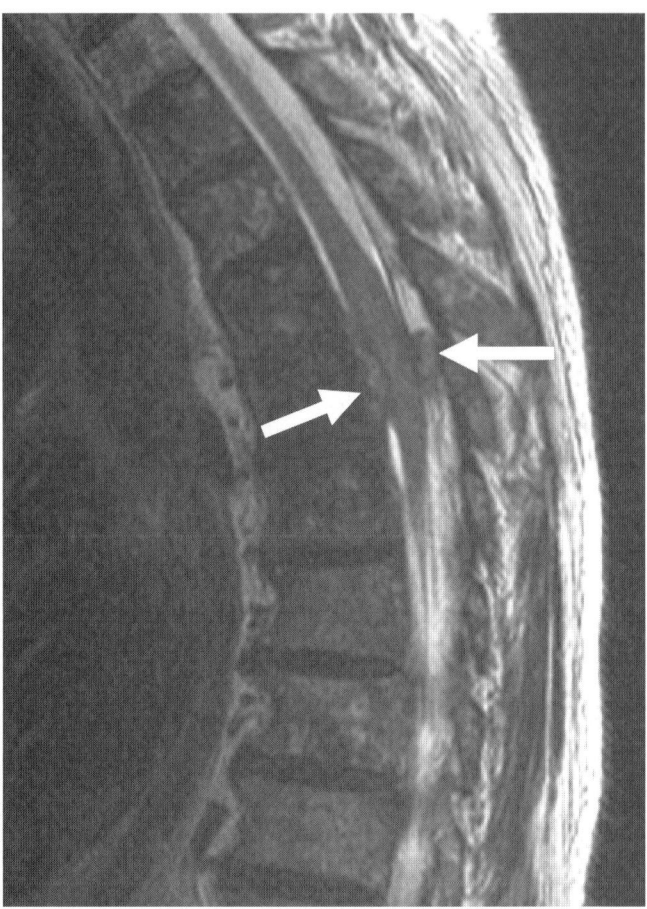

Figure 101.4 Spinal MRI (T2-weighed image): Metastatic spinal cord compression at levels Th 4 to Th 5 in a 75-year old patient with prostate cancer. MSCC is caused by both posterior extension of a vertebral body mass (left arrow) and anterior extension of a mass arising from the dorsal elements (right arrow).

deficits. A faster development may result in a disruption of the arterial blood flow followed by ischemia or spinal cord infarction. In the latter case, the damage to the spinal cord and the subsequent neurological deficits are mostly not reversible. The impact of the time of developing MSCC was demonstrated in animal studies already more than 50 years ago [84,85]. It was suggested that the rapid development of MSCC required decompression within 8 to 10 hours to achieve a significant improvement in neurological function. After slower development of MSCC, decompression could reverse the neurological dysfunction when performed much later, that is, within 7 days. A prospective study demonstrated that significantly more patients irradiated for MSCC improved motor function after a slower development of motor deficits before radiotherapy compared to those with a faster development of motor deficits (86% vs. 20%, $P < 0.001$) [86].

Back pain usually is the first and the most common symptom of MSCC (70%-96%), followed by motor deficits (61%-91%), sensory deficits (46%-90%), and autonomic dysfunction (40%-57%) [76,87,88]. If pain is the only symptom, the situation is better described as "impending" MSCC. If neurological deficits develop, pain has usually been present for several weeks or even months. The major goal of treatment is to regain and maintain the ambulatory function. In the 1990s, more than 50% of the patients were not ambulatory at presentation [89,90]. Because of greater awareness of physicians of MSCC, the proportion of patients who are ambulatory at presentation increased during the past decade [78]. Sensory deficits are little less frequent than motor deficits but may not infrequently be missed because they are much less noticeable to patients than motor dysfunction [76,91]. Dysfunction of bladder and bowel control (autonomic dysfunction) occurs relatively late and less frequently when compared to the other symptoms [80]. Because its presence is associated with a poor functional outcome following radiotherapy alone, patients with autonomic dysfunction should be considered for immediate surgical intervention whenever medically reasonable. Immediate decompressive surgery mostly is the appropriate treatment option to improve or restore neurological function in these patients.

Spinal MRI is the diagnostic procedure of choice, the diagnostic "gold standard" (92–94). The rates of sensitivity, specificity, and diagnostic accuracy regarding the detection of MSCC are 93%, 97%, and 95%, respectively [92]. Spinal MRI also is an excellent method to detect multiple sites of MSCC and the degree of spinal cord compression. Motor dysfunction can be appropriately graded with several systems. The available grading systems include a 5-point scale reported in 1983 [95] : 0 = normal strength, 1 = ambulatory without aid, 2 = ambulatory with aid, 3 = not ambulatory, and 4 = complete paraplegia. The Tomita score is similar to the 5-point Frankel scale: A = complete paraplegia, B = sensory function only, C = nonambulatory, D = ambulatory, and E = no neurological symptoms or signs. About 30 years ago, Gilbert et al [87] presented a 4-point scale: 1 = ambulatory (with or without weakness), 2 = not ambulatory but able to lift the legs against gravity, 3 = unable to lift the legs against gravity, and 4 = complete paraplegia. If a more differentiated grading system is required, the 8-point scale according to the American Spinal Injury Association and the International Medical Society of Paraplegia [96] can be used: 0 = complete paraplegia, 1 = palpable or visible muscle contractions, 2 = active movement of the leg without gravity, 3 = active movement of the leg against gravity, 4 = active movement of the leg against mild resistance, 5 = active movement of the leg against moderate resistance, 6 = active movement of the leg against severe resistance, and 7 = normal strength.

MSCC patients are most commonly treated with radiotherapy. The patients should initially be evaluated also by a neurosurgeon in order to decide whether the patient is a better candidate for decompressive surgery followed by radiotherapy than radiotherapy alone. However, the indications for surgery are usually limited to selected patients with a good performance status, involvement of only one segment of the spinal cord, no very radiosensitive tumors such as myeloma or lymphoma, and a comparably good survival prognosis. Thus, the majority of MSCC patients are not surgical candidates, and radiotherapy alone remains the most common treatment. However, it has to be supplemented by administration of glucocorticosteroids. The most common corticosteroid in MSCC treatment is dexamethasone, which has been reported to inhibit the production and the activity of prostaglandin PEG2 and vascular endothelial growth factor (VEGF) resulting in a decrease in ischemic spinal cord edema. The efficacy of glucocorticosteroids in MSCC treatment is well recognized, in particular regarding improvement or maintaining of the functional status. However, the appropriate dose schedule is still controversial [97]. In the literature, loading doses ranged from 10 to 100 mg and were followed by single doses of 4 to 24 mg up to 4 times per day. A randomized trial compared high-dose dexamethasone (96 mg daily) to no glucocorticosteroid administration during radiotherapy. Ambulatory status was maintained following radiotherapy in 81% of the patients who had received high-dose dexamethasone and in 63% of those patients not receiving glucocorticosteroids [98]. Another prospective study compared initial high-dose (100 mg) followed by low-dose (16 mg daily) dexamethasone versus initial low-dose (10 mg) followed by low-dose (16 mg daily) dexamethasone [99]. Improvement of motor function was observed in 25% and 8% of the patients, respectively ($P = 0.22$). In a historical case-control series that compared high-dose dexamethasone (96 mg IV loading dose, decreasing doses to zero in 14 days) to moderate-dose dexamethasone (16 mg daily, reduced to zero in 14 days), a significantly higher rate of serious glucocorticosteroid-induced side effects, such as gastric ulcers, gastrointestinal bleeding, and perforation, occurred after the high-dose regimen (14 % vs. 0 %) [100]. If one considers both the effect on motor function and the acute toxicity associated with glucocorticosteroid administration, it appears reasonable to start with dexamethasone at an intermediate dose level (24–40 mg daily) followed by tapering down over several weeks after the completion of radiotherapy.

Radiotherapy Alone

Radiotherapy alone is the most frequently administered therapy for MSCC. However, the most appropriate regimen for the individual MSCC patient is still controversial. Due to their markedly reduced life expectancy of only a few months [80], for most MSCC patients a radiotherapy program with a short overall treatment time (short-course radiotherapy, treatment time: 1–5 days) is preferable to standard radiotherapy with 10 × 3 Gy (treatment time: 2 weeks). However, short-course radiotherapy can only be recommended if it provides similar functional outcome as more protracted regimens such as 10 × 3 Gy. Studies comparing different radiation schedules with respect to post-treatment functional outcome are presented and discussed below. Regardless of the radiotherapy schedule, the first radiation fraction should be delivered as soon as possible but no later than 24 hours from the first patient presentation to a radiation oncologist. Irradiation is performed most often with 6 to 10 MV linear accelerators. If a linear accelerator is not available, a cobalt-60 unit may be used despite the less adequate dose distribution. The radiation dose is delivered either through a single posterior field or through parallel opposed fields depending on the depth of the spinal cord. If the distance between the patient's skin and the spinal cord exceeds 5.5 cm, the maximum dose may exceed 115% of the dose prescribed at depth. This is not optimal because it may result in fibrosis of the subcutaneous tissue. The dose distribution is generally more favorable for parallel-opposed fields than for a single posterior field. The radiation dose is usually prescribed to the midplane when using parallel opposed fields or the posterior edge of the vertebral body when using a single posterior field. Treatment volumes usually encompass one normal vertebra above and below the metastatic lesions. If the radiation field includes the cervical spine, usually two cervical vertebrae are included. Because of the palliative situation, conventional simulation can be considered sufficient for most patients with MSCC (Figure 101.5).

Prognostic factors may guide the radiation oncologist to select the appropriate radiation schedule for the individual MSCC patient. In a multivariate analysis of 1,304 retrospectively evaluated MSCC patients, improved motor function following radiotherapy was significantly associated with younger age (≤63 vs. ≥64 years, $P = 0.026$), better performance status (Eastern Cooperative Oncology Group performance status 1–2 vs. 3–4, $P < 0.001$), involvement of only one to two vertebrae (vs. ≥three vertebrae, $P = 0.001$), ambulatory status before radiotherapy (vs. nonambulatory, $P < 0.001$), an interval from tumor diagnosis to MSCC >24 months (vs. ≤24 months, $P < 0.001$), and a slower development of motor deficits before radiotherapy (>14 vs. 8–14 and 1–7 days, $P < 0.001$) [101]. In contrast, gender and the radiation schedule (1 × 8 Gy vs. 5 × 4 Gy vs. 10 × 3 Gy vs. 15 × 2.5 Gy vs. 20 × 2 Gy) had no significant impact on functional outcome. The prognostic value of primary tumor type, ambulatory status, and time of developing motor deficits has been previously described [86,88,89,102].

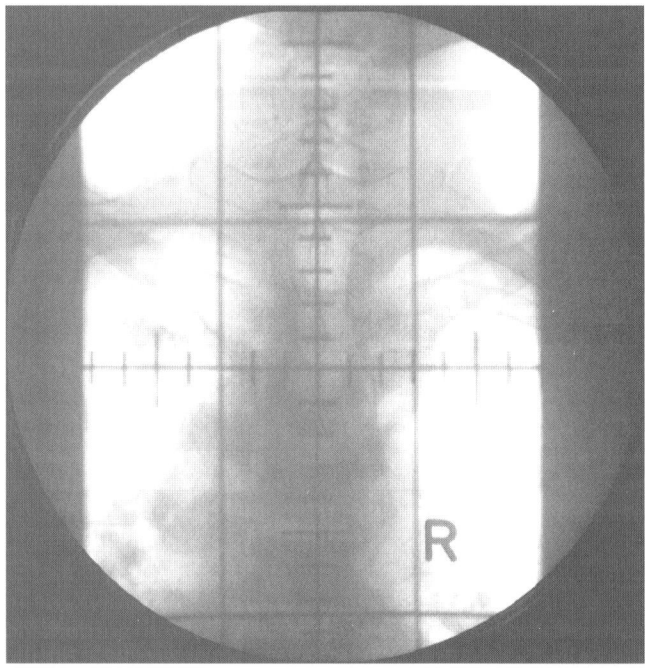

Figure 101.5 Conventional simulation of a single posterior field including the spinal area from Th 2 to Th 7 (MSCC affected Th 3 to Th 6).

Functional Outcome After Radiotherapy Alone

The appropriate radiation schedule for MSCC is still controversial. Many different radiation schedules are used, including single-fraction programs, such as 1 × 8 Gy or 1 × 10 Gy; multifraction short-course programs given in about 1 week, such as 4 × 4 Gy, 5 × 4 Gy, 5 × 5 Gy, and 6 × 4 Gy; long-course programs given in 2 to 4 weeks, such as 10 × 3 Gy, 15 × 2.5 Gy, and 20 × 2 Gy; and split-course regimens, such as 3 × 5 Gy followed by 4 days rest and another 5 × 3 Gy. Considering the limited life span of MSCC patients and the fact that the patient's transport to the radiotherapy department and positioning on the treatment couch may cause discomfort to the often debilitated patients, a program with a short overall treatment time (short-course radiotherapy) appears preferable if it provides similar results as long-course programs.

Following pain, motor dysfunction is the second most common symptom from MSCC and usually marks the threshold between impending and manifest MSCC. The success rates of radiotherapy alone in the treatment of MSCC depend on its definition as well as on the endpoint investigated. For example, Klimo et al [103] presented a review of different therapeutic approaches and defined success of therapy as the ability to walk after treatment (i.e., gait function was maintained, improved, or regained). In that review, the success rates after radiotherapy alone ranged between 34% and 73% (mean 47%, median 47%) and were comparable to those after posterior decompressive laminectomy followed by radiotherapy (43%-57%, mean 47%, median 46%) and higher than those after decompressive laminectomy alone (14%-58%, mean 30%, median 30%). However, in more recent series, the ambulatory rates after radiotherapy alone were better and ranged between 63% and 74% [101,104,105].

Only a few studies compared different radiation schedules for posttreatment motor function of MSCC patients (101,104–108). A retrospective study did not reveal a difference in functional outcome between 10 × 3 Gy, 15 × 2.5 Gy, and 40 Gy [106]. Improvement of motor function was observed in 32%, 33%, and 34% of the patients, respectively ($P = 0.99$). In another retrospective study, 1 × 8 Gy and 10 × 3 Gy resulted in similar postradiotherapy functional outcome [108]. Of the initially nonambulatory patients, 37% and 32% regained the ability to walk after radiotherapy, respectively ($P = 0.82$). In a more recently published retrospective study of 1,304 patients comparing five different fractionation schedules (1 × 8 Gy, 5 × 4 Gy, 10 × 3 Gy, 15 × 2.5 Gy, and 20 × 2 Gy), improvement of motor function occurred in 28% of patients and no further progression of motor dysfunction in another 57% [101]. The type of the fractionation schedule had no significant impact on posttreatment functional outcome. Despite the heterogeneity of the fractionation schedules used for MSCC worldwide and despite a lack of standards, only two prospective studies comparing different fractionation schedules have been performed so far to better define the appropriate radiotherapy regimen. Both prospective studies compared different fractionation schedules with regard to posttreatment functional outcome. The first prospective study was not randomized and compared two long-course programs (10 × 3 Gy in 2 weeks vs. 20 × 2 Gy in 4 weeks) [107]. In this study, both investigated fractionation schedules resulted in similar posttreatment motor function and ambulatory status. Motor function improved in 43% of the patients after 10 × 3 Gy and in 41% of the patients after 20 × 2 Gy ($P = 0.80$). Postradiotherapy ambulatory rates were 60% and 64%, respectively ($P = 0.71$). The other prospective study was a randomized phase III trial that compared 2 × 8 Gy (1 × 8 Gy followed by 1-week rest and another 1 × 8 Gy) and a split-course regimen (3 × 5 Gy followed by 4 days rest and 5 × 3 Gy) [105]. After radiotherapy, 56% and 59% patients had back pain relief (P = NS), and 68% and 71% were able to walk (P = NS). The various tumor entities differ with respect to biological behavior and radiosensitivity [80]. Thus, it appears reasonable to consider each tumor entity separately. The comparison between long-course and short-course radiotherapy for several tumor entities regarding functional outcome are given in Table 101.5. The improved functional outcome with long-course compared to short-course radiotherapy in myeloma patients became significant at 6 months (P = 0.043) and 12 months (P = 0.003) following radiotherapy [109].

Recalcification Following Radiotherapy Alone and Bisphosphonates

A randomized trial from Germany including 107 patients with bone metastases demonstrated long-course radiotherapy with 10 × 3 Gy to result in better recalcification of the osteolytic bone/vertebra compared to 1 × 8 Gy [117].

The recalcification rates according to computed tomography-based bone density assessment were 173% and 120%, respectively ($P < 0.001$). However, the authors did not provide any data regarding the clinical relevance of their findings. In another randomized trial that included patients with painful bone metastases, a significantly higher rate of pathological fractures was observed after 1 × 8 Gy than after 6 × 4 Gy [118]. However, clinically relevant recalcification can only be expected several months following radiotherapy and is therefore not important for most MSCC patients because of their markedly reduced life expectancy ranging between 2.3 and 6 months in most reported series (89,102,104,105,119–121). Recalcification after radiotherapy can be further improved with the administration of bisphosphonates. In patients with bone metastases, prospective studies have demonstrated a significant effect of bisphosphonates regarding the prevention from skeletal-related events such as retreatment, pathologic fractures, and MSCC (122–124). A phase III trial including 422 prostate cancer patients with bone metastases found a risk reduction by 22% (49% vs. 38%, P = 0.028) with administration of 4-mg zoledronate every 3 weeks [124]. Thus, MSCC patients with an expected survival of 6 months or longer should be considered for bisphosphonate therapy. A prospective comparative study demonstrated zoledronate to be more effective than pamidronate in decreasing the risk of skeletal-related events in 528 breast cancer patients with at least one osteolytic lesion [123]. The rates of skeletal-related events were 48% and 58%, respectively (P = 0.058).

Table 101.5 Comparison of Short-Course to Long-Course Radiotherapy with Respect to Functional Outcome, Related to Different Primary Tumors

Primary Tumor Type	Improvement N(%)	No Change N(%)	Deterioration N(%)	P
Breast Cancer (N = 335)				0.81
Short-course radiotherapy	44(34)	74(57)	12(9)	
Long-course radiotherapy	61(30)	118(58)	26(12)	
Prostate Cancer (N = 281)				0.83
Short-course radiotherapy	52(34)	70(50)	25(16)	
Long-course radiotherapy	40 (32)	72(57)	14(11)	
NSCLC (N = 252)				0.87
Short-course radiotherapy	16 (15)	58(55)	31(30)	
Long-course radiotherapy	19 (13)	78(53)	50(34)	
Myeloma (N = 172)				0.10
Short-course radiotherapy	34 (39)	35(58)	2(3)	
Long-course radiotherapy	66 (59)	43(39)	2(2)	
Unknown Primary (N = 143)				0.74
Short-course radiotherapy	5 (7)	49(72)	14(21)	
Long-course radiotherapy	10 (13)	32(43)	33(44)	
Renal cell carcinoma (N = 87)				0.91
Short-course radiotherapy	10 (27)	24(65)	3(8)	
Long-course radiotherapy	15 (30)	28(56)	7(14)	
Colorectal cancer (N = 81)				0.50
Short-course radiotherapy	5 (16)	21(68)	5(16)	
Long-course radiotherapy	6 (12)	34(68)	10(20)	
Bladder cancer (N = 32)				0.12
Short-course radiotherapy	1 (6)	13 (76)	3 (18)	
Long-course radiotherapy	1 (7)	12 (80)	2 (13)	
Ovarian cancer (N = 7)				0.61
Short-course radiotherapy	0 (0)	1 (50)	1 (50)	
Long-course radiotherapy	3 (60)	2 (40)	0 (0)	

Data from refs. 109–116.

In-Field Recurrences of MSCC and Spinal Reirradiation

In the largest series of MSCC patients including 1,852 patients, an in-field recurrence (recurrence of MSCC in the previously irradiated spinal region) following radiotherapy was observed in 144 patients (8%) after median 7 months (range: 2–62 months) [78]. The in-field recurrence rate at 1 year was 11%. In the multivariate analysis of that study, long-course radiotherapy with either 10 × 3 Gy, 15 × 2.5 Gy, or 20 × 2 Gy resulted in significantly fewer recurrences than short-course radiotherapy with 1 × 8 Gy or 5 × 4 Gy. The 1-year recurrence rates were 7% and 18%, respectively ($P < 0.001$). Long-course radiotherapy has been reported to result in better local control of MSCC than short-course radiotherapy, in particular in breast cancer, prostate cancer, and myeloma patients (109–111). Long-course radiotherapy appears to be better option for any MSCC patients with a comparably favorable survival prognosis, regardless of the primary tumor type, because these patients may live long enough to develop a recurrence of MSCC. Patients with a poor survival prognosis may be considered for short-course radiotherapy, as these patients would spend less time of their limited life span receiving treatment.

However, occasionally reirradiation is the only available treatment option. The risk of radiation-induced myelopathy depends on the cumulative (primary radiotherapy plus reirradiation) biologically effective dose (BED), the interval between the two radiation courses, and the BED of each radiation course [125,126]. The risk of radiation myelopathy appears small for a cumulative BED of 135.5 Gy_2 or less, an interval between both radiation courses of at least 6 months, and a BED of each course of 98 Gy_2 or less. Reirradiation can be considered safe if the cumulative BED does not exceed 100 Gy_2 [127]. The BED can be calculated with the equation BED = D × [1 + (d/α/β)], as derived from the linear-quadratic model; D = total dose, d = dose per fraction, α = linear (first-order dose-dependent) component of cell killing, β = quadratic (second-order dose-dependent) component of cell killing, α/β ratio = dose at which both components of cell killing are equal. The α/β ratio suggested for radiation myelopathy is 2 Gy.

A second course with 1 × 8 Gy, 5 × 3 Gy, or 5 × 4 Gy following primary radiotherapy with 1 × 8 Gy or 5 × 4 Gy proved to be effective and resulted in an improvement of motor function in 40% and in prevention from further progression in another 45% of patients [127]. If reirradiation is required after primary long-course radiotherapy, high-precision techniques can be used to reduce the cumulative BED delivered to the spinal cord, in particular if the cumulative BED exceeds 135.5 Gy_2 [128,129] (Figure 101.6).

Survival After Radiotherapy Alone

In the multivariate analysis of survival of 1,852 MSCC patients treated with radiotherapy alone, improved overall survival was associated with favorable primary tumor type (myeloma/lymphoma, breast cancer, and prostate cancer) ($P < 0.001$), absence of other bone metastases ($P = 0.018$) and absence of visceral metastases ($P < 0.001$) before radiotherapy, a longer interval between tumor diagnosis

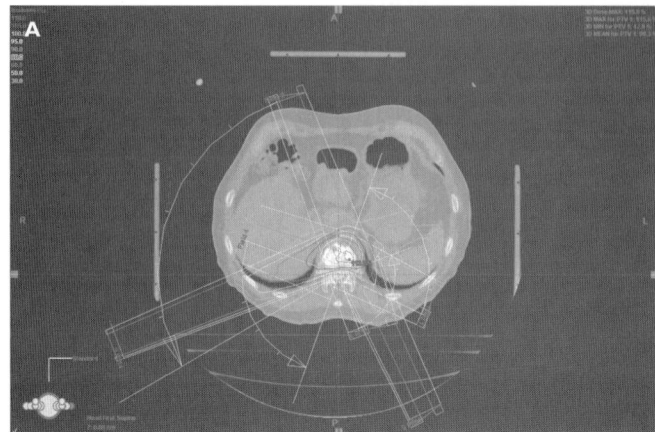
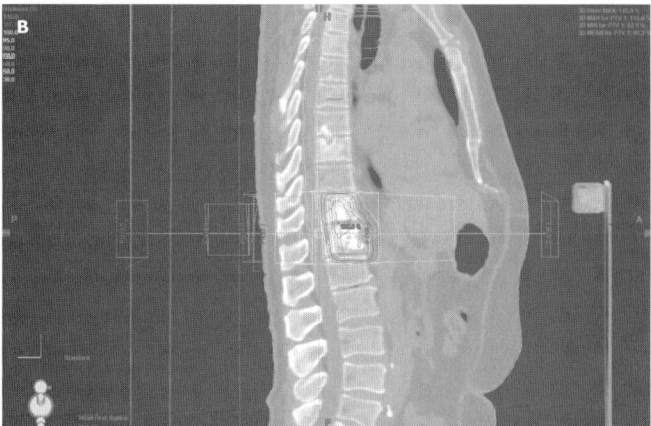
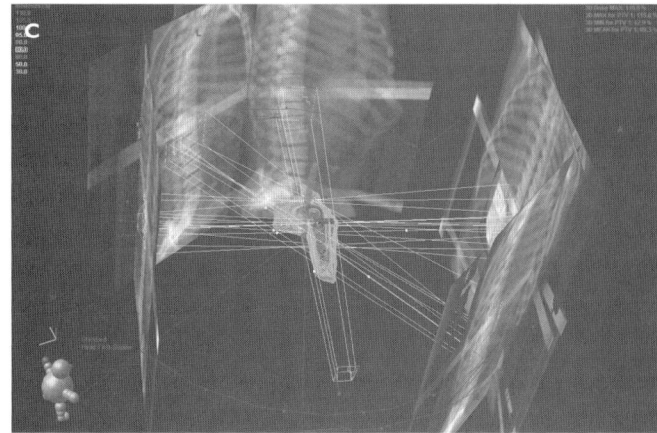

Figure 101.6 High-precision irradiation with fractionated stereotactic radiotherapy. The maximum dose delivered to the spinal cord was 27% of the prescribed dose. *See color insert.*

and MSCC (>15 months vs. ≤15 months, $P < 0.001$), ability to walk before radiotherapy ($P < 0.001$), and slower development of motor deficits before RT (>14 days vs. ≤14 days, $P < 0.001$) [78]. The 1-year survival rate was 43%. The impact of visceral metastases, other bone metastases, and the preradiotherapy ambulatory status on survival has been previously described [80,88,89,104,130]. Based on the above-mentioned multivariate analysis of 1,852 patients, a new scoring system was developed to predict the survival of MSCC patients [131]. This scoring system included the six prognostic factors that were significantly associated with survival in the multivariate analysis. The score for each prognostic factor was determined by dividing the 6-month survival rate (given in %) by 10. The total score represented the sum of the six scores obtained for each prognostic factor. The total scores ranged between 20 and 45 points. Five groups were defined according to the total scores: 20 to 25 points, 26 to 30 points, 31 to 35 points, 36 to 40 points, and 41 to 45 points. The 6-month survival rates for each group were 4%, 11%, 48%, 87%, and 99% ($P < 0.001$). Subgroup analyses were performed for each of the five groups comparing short-course to long-course radiotherapy with respect to survival. In the patients who achieved scores of 36 or more points, long-course radiotherapy resulted in significantly better overall survival compared to short-course radiotherapy. In contrast, the patients with scores of less than 36 points had similar survival with either short- or long-course radiotherapy. Thus, patients with scores of <36 points appear well treated with short-course programs, whereas the patients with scores of ≥36 points should receive long-course radiotherapy.

Radiotherapy Alone for Patients with Oligometastatic Disease

Oligometastatic disease can be defined as involvement of one to three vertebrae and no other bone or visceral metastases. Patients with oligometastatic disease have an extraordinarily favorable prognosis with radiotherapy alone. In a series of 521 MSCC patients with oligometastatic disease, motor function improved in 40% and remained stable in another 54% of patients after radiotherapy alone[132]. Of the nonambulatory patients, 54% regained the ability to walk, and 94% of the initially ambulatory patients remained ambulatory. Local control rates at 1st and 2nd years were 92% and 88%, respectively, and survival rates at 1st and 2nd years were 71% and 58%, respectively.

RADIOTHERAPY SUPPLEMENTED BY CHEMOTHERAPY OR PRECEEDING DECOMPRESSIVE SURGERY

Chemotherapy

Chemotherapy has a very limited role in the treatment of MSCC. It may be applied in addition to radiotherapy in case of chemo-sensitive tumors, such as myeloma, lymphoma, or germ cell tumors (133–135). In a small series of 48 lymphoma patients who received either radiotherapy alone, chemotherapy alone, or radiochemotherapy, neurological recovery was similar in the three groups [135]. The 10-year local control was nonsignificantly better after radiochemotherapy when compared to radiotherapy alone or chemotherapy alone (76% vs. 50% and 46%). In another series of 48 lymphoma and myeloma patients who received radiotherapy or radiochemotherapy, no further progression of neurological symptoms was observed in 58% and 75% of patients ($P = NS$) [134]. Further studies are required to define the potential role of chemotherapy in the treatment of MSCC.

Decompressive Surgery

The indications for spinal surgery are intraspinal bony fragment with bony compression, spinal instability, impending or present sphincter dysfunction, no response to radiotherapy, and a recurrence of MSCC after long-course radiotherapy with a high BED [80,136]. The advantages of spinal surgery are immediate decompression of the spinal cord and direct mechanic stabilization of the spine. Laminectomy may be indicated in case of MSCC due to anterior extension of a mass arising from the dorsal elements. However, it should not be performed in case of compression due to posterior extension of a vertebral body mass [137,138]. Because in that situation laminae and spinosus processes represent the last "pillar" responsible for the stability of the vertebral segment, laminectomy most likely results in further decrease of stability. The appropriate surgical option is anterior decompression, which includes a resection of the vertebral body and the tumor mass followed by replacement by cement and fixation of the involved vertebral segment [139,140].

The benefit of surgery in addition to radiotherapy is still controversial. Klimo et al [103] defined success of treatment as being ambulatory after treatment. In their review article, mean success rates were 47% after radiotherapy alone (11 reports, $N = 841$), 47% after surgery followed by radiotherapy (9 reports, $N = 866$), and 30% after surgery alone (13 reports, $N = 1,003$) in patients treated between 1957 and 1990. Surgery must be considered inadequate because it was performed as posterior decompressive laminectomy and not as anterior decompression plus stabilization. A more recent meta-analysis by the same group included also patients treated with "modern" surgical techniques for MSCC. In this meta-analysis, 999 patients (24 reports) who received surgery (mainly in conjunction with radiotherapy) were compared to 543 patients from four reports who received radiotherapy alone [141]. The posttreatment ambulatory rates were 85% for patients receiving surgery and 64% for those having radiotherapy alone. In the surgery group, 228 of 384 (59%) nonambulatory patients regained ambulatory status versus 79 of 265 (30%) patients in the radiotherapy-alone group. However, the results most likely have been confounded due to selection bias. Patients in the surgery group had more favorable prognostic factors known to affect functional outcome, such as higher proportion of ambulatory patients before treatment, better performance status, younger age, and involvement of fewer vertebrae. The distribution of other relevant prognostic factors, such as the time of developing motor deficits and the interval from tumor diagnosis to MSCC, was not even stated. Thus, the results of the meta-analysis by Klimo et al suggesting an advantage for surgery must be regarded with great caution.

A randomized trial using appropriate surgical techniques found a benefit for surgery followed by long-course radiotherapy (10 × 3 Gy) compared to long-course radiotherapy (10 × 3 Gy) alone [142]. The study was stopped after an interim analysis of 101 patients. Significantly, more patients in the surgery group were ambulatory after treatment (84% vs. 57%, $P = 0.001$), maintained the ability to walk longer (122 days vs. 13 days, $P = 0.003$), and had better overall survival (126 days vs. 100 days, $P = 0.033$). Of the initially nonambulatory patients, 10/16 and 3/16 patients regained ambulatory status ($P = 0.01$). However, major concerns were addressed suggesting that the results may have been confounded due to methodological problems [143,144]. Because it took 10 years to accrue the relatively small number of 101 patients, it was questioned if really all eligible patients have been included. One institution included about 70% of the patients. The average inclusion rate of each other institution was only about one patient every 2 years. It was also criticized that the functional results after radiotherapy alone appeared extraordinarily poor when compared to the results of other series. Regarding the small number of patients, in particular of those not ambulatory before treatment ($n = 32$), the study appeared statistically underpowered. Only patients with an expected survival of ≥3 months, a Karnofsky performance Score of ≥70, and involvement of only a single spinal area were considered eligible. Patients with very radiosensitive tumors were excluded. Furthermore, the patients could not have had brain metastases, complete paraplegia for >48 hours, cauda equina compression, or previous radiotherapy to the area of MSCC. Thus, the criteria regarding suitability for surgery are only applicable to a minority of MSCC patients. A retrospective study of 345 patients compared radiotherapy alone ($n = 149$), surgery alone ($n = 105$), and surgery plus radiotherapy ($n = 91$) [145]. The posttreatment ambulatory rates were 38%, 34%, and 53%, respectively ($P = 0.001$). Patients treated with surgery plus radiotherapy seemed to respond better than those treated with radiotherapy or surgery alone. However, when pretreatment motor function was considered, no significant difference was found between the three treatments. In that study, surgery was usually performed as laminectomy, which is not the appropriate surgical technique for most MSCC patients. This has to be taken into account when interpreting the results. If one summarizes the few available studies that compared radiotherapy alone to surgery plus radiotherapy, decompressive surgery followed by long-course radiotherapy appears beneficial for selected patients. However, there is an urgent need for randomized studies with appropriate methodology and a number of patients large enough to provide an adequate statistical power to properly define the role of surgery in the treatment of MSCC.

RADIOSURGERY

RS, that is, delivery of a single, large radiation dose to a localized tumor using a stereotactic approach, has recently also been studied in patients with spinal metastases. The spine is considered a suitable site for RS because there is minimal or no breathing-related organ movement. Treatment is typically delivered with image-guided and intensity-modulated approaches and with a noninvasive positioning device. The accuracy for the isocenter was within 1.36 mm ± 0.11 mm [128]. The radiation dose to the spinal cord is relatively low. The maximum dose to the anterior edge of the spinal cord within a transverse section, on average, was 50% of the prescribed dose [128]. These authors reported on 49 patients with 61 solitary spinal metastases treated with 10 to 16 Gy of RS [146]. Complete and partial pain relief was achieved in 85% of the lesions treated. Relapse of pain at the treated site was noted in 7%. Radiologically, lesions progressively metastasized to the immediately adjacent vertebrae in 5%. In 2007, the same group reported on 230 spine lesions in 177 patients treated with RS of 8 to 18 Gy, prescribed to the 90% isodose line that encompassed the target volume [147]. Spinal cord volume was defined as 6 mm above and below the RS target volume. Spinal cord dose was calculated from the dose-volume histogram and correlated with complications (median follow-up 6.4 months). The average spinal cord volume defined at the treated spinal segment was 5.9 ± 2.2 mL. The average dose to the 10% spinal cord volume was 9.8 ± 1.5 Gy, calculated from the dose-volume histogram in the group of 18 Gy prescribed dose. The spinal cord volume that received higher than 80% of the prescribed dose was 0.07 ± 0.10 mL, which represented $1.3 \pm 1.8\%$ of the cord volume. Among the 86 patients who survived longer than 1 year, there was one case of radiation-induced cord injury after 13 months of RS. According to their experience, partial volume tolerance is at least 10 Gy to 10% of the spinal cord volume defined as 6 mm above and below the RS target.

The largest cohort of 500 cases of spinal metastases treated with RS was reported by Gerszten et al. 2007. Lesion location included 73 cervical, 212 thoracic, 112 lumbar, and 103 sacral. The maximum intratumoral dose ranged from 12.5 to 25 Gy (mean 20). Tumor volume ranged from 0.20 to 264 mL (mean 46). Long-term pain improvement occurred in 290 of 336 cases (86%). Long-term tumor control was demonstrated in 90% of lesions treated with RS as a primary treatment modality and in 88% of lesions treated for radiographic tumor progression. Twenty-seven of 32 cases (84%) with a progressive neurologic deficit before treatment experienced at least some clinical improvement. Gibbs et al [148] described the experience at Stanford University from 1996 to 2005, where 74 patients with 102 spinal metastases were treated. Sixty-two (84%) patients were symptomatic. Using the CyberKnife, 16 to 25 Gy in one to five fractions was delivered. With mean follow-up of 9 months, 84% of symptomatic patients experienced improvement or resolution of symptoms after treatment. Three patients developed treatment-related spinal injury. Analysis of dose-volume parameters and clinical parameters failed to identify predictors of spinal cord injury. Chang et al [149] treated 15 patients within a phase I trial, where each patient received five fractions. A dose of 30 Gy was attempted; however, the total dose was constrained by limiting the spinal cord to a maximum dose of 10 Gy. No neurologic toxicity was observed in any patient. The median follow-up time was 9 months. The positional setup error was determined to be within 1 mm of planning isocenter. In the absence of published randomized trials, the role of RS for spinal metastases remains undefined. The same holds true for long-term tolerance doses of the cord to such high doses per fraction. However, RS or SFRT appear to offer an important treatment option for patients previously treated to high doses of external beam radiotherapy.

RADIOPHARMACEUTICALS

While external beam radiotherapy remains the mainstay of pain palliation of spine lesions, bone-seeking radiopharmaceuticals have entered the therapeutic armamentarium for the treatment of multiple painful osseous lesions. ^{32}P has been used for >three decades in the treatment of multiple osseous metastases. The myelosuppression caused by this agent has led to the development of other bone-seeking radiopharmaceuticals, including ^{89}SrCl, ^{153}Sm-ethylenediaminetetramethylene phosphonic acid (^{153}Sm-EDTMP), (179m)SnCl, and ^{166}Ho-Labeled 1,4,7,10-tetraazacyclododecane-1,4,7,10-tetramethylenephosphonate (^{166}Ho-DOTMP). Randomized and controlled clinical trials of radionuclide therapy that compared treatment with radioisotopes and placebo, and where the major outcome was either pain or complications of bone metastases (e.g., hypercalcaemia, bone fracture, spinal cord compression), were recently analyzed [150]. Four trials (325 patients) provided data that suggest a small effect of radioisotopes on pain control both at short and medium term (1 to 6 months). No evidence was available to assess long-term effects (12 months). Only one study provided data on analgesia use and concluded that patients when given either radioisotopes or placebo showed similar levels of analgesic use when compared to baseline use. Currently, a multinational placebo-controlled, double-blind randomized trial with a new α-emitting agent based on ^{223}Ra in patients with bone metastases from hormone-refractory prostate cancer is underway.

LEPTOMENINGEAL METASTASES

Leptomeningeal metastases might arise from solid tumors (breast cancer, lung cancer, malignant melanoma, etc.), primary brain tumors (glioblastoma, medulloblastoma, etc.), or leukemias and lymphomas. The best prognosis has been reported for patients with acute leukaemia. The extent of treatment is often individualized on the basis of prognostic factors, for example, unfavorable performance status, higher age, cranial nerve palsies, bulky CNS disease, abnormal CSF flow, low CSF glucose, and high CSF protein levels [151]. While initial clinical, radiological, and cytological responses might be obtained in most patients with haematological malignancies and a large proportion of patients with breast cancer or medulloblastoma, the ultimate outcome in adult patients is often dismal, and median survival of 6 months or less commonly has been reported (152–156). Patients with hydrocephalus might require shunt placement before administration of oncologic treatment.

The palliative role of radiotherapy is limited by the facts that focal treatment is unable to control disease spread outside of the radiation portals, while craniospinal-axis irradiation to higher total doses has a small therapeutic index, which might seriously interfere with the ability to tolerate chemotherapy administration. In a German series of 16 patients with different types of solid tumors, six received craniospinal-axis irradiation with 36 Gy, while the others received intrathecal methotrexate in addition [157]. Median survival was 8 weeks with radiotherapy alone and 16 weeks with combined treatment. Regression of symptoms was achieved in 68% of patients including seven who regained their ability to walk. Comparable palliation and survival was reported with local radiotherapy. In a series of 67 breast cancer patients treated in Poland between 2000 and 2005, 85% received intrathecal chemotherapy, 61% intravenous chemotherapy, and 64% whole-brain or local spinal radiotherapy [158]. Forty percent of patients were treated with all three modalities. Clinical response was achieved in 49 patients (76%). Median survival was 4 months. In multivariate analysis of prognostic factors, radiotherapy was not associated with prolongation of survival. No prospective randomized trials on the role of radiotherapy have yet been published. In patients with spread from solid tumors and favorable prognostic factors, intrathecal methotrexate treatment might be followed by radiotherapy to sites of symptomatic and macroscopic disease, for example, whole-brain radiotherapy to 30 Gy, typically with lateral opposing fields that include the first two segments of the cervical spine [159]. Care should be taken to include all of the anterior and medial parts of the base of skull, for example, the lamina cribrosa. Palliative local radiotherapy might also be administered to spinal cord segments that harbor macroscopic disease. In long-term survivors, leukencephalopathy, brain atrophy, and neurocognitive deficits might develop. The prognosis of patients that failed to respond to intrathecal chemotherapy is too unfavorable to justify administration of radiotherapy. Whether a patient qualifies for systemic chemotherapy depends on extracranial disease status, performance status, age, pretreatment, bone marrow reserve, kidney and liver function. Special aspects of treatment for primary leukemias and lymphomas include, for example, the role of administration of antibodies such as rituximab and CNS prophylaxis [160]. Radiotherapy for CNS recurrence of leukemia might provide excellent CNS control, as reported by Sanders et al [161], who treated 16 patients with a median dose of 24 Gy to the cranium and 18 Gy to the spine. Fifteen patients also received intrathecal chemotherapy. Thirteen patients achieved a complete remission and two were long-term survivors. However, median survival was 4 months from the start of craniospinal-axis irradiation and 9 months from the diagnosis of CNS recurrence. The role of craniospinal-axis irradiation in medulloblastoma and the possible advantages of intensity-modulated treatment and proton beam treatment [162,163] are discussed elsewhere in this volume.

REFERENCES

1. Pelletier EM, Shim B, Goodman S, Amonkar MM. Epidemiology and economic burden of brain metastases among patients with primary breast cancer: results from a US claims data analysis. *Breast Cancer Res Treat.* 2008;108(2):297–305.
2. Chao JH, Phillips R, Nickson JJ. Roentgen-ray therapy of cerebral metastases. *Cancer.* 1954;7(4):682–689.
3. Borgelt B, Gelber R, Kramer S, et al. The palliation of brain metastases: final results of the first two studies by the Radiation Therapy Oncology Group. *Int J Radiat Oncol Biol Phys.* 1980;6(1):1–9.
4. Borgelt B, Gelber R, Larson M, Hendrickson F, Griffin T, Roth R. Ultra-rapid high dose irradiation schedules for the palliation of brain metastases: final results of the first two studies by the Radiation Therapy Oncology Group. *Int J Radiat Oncol Biol Phys.* 1981;7(12):1633–1638.

5. Antoniou D, Kyprianou K, Stathopoulos GP, et al. Response to radiotherapy in brain metastases and survival of patients with non-small cell lung cancer. *Oncol Rep.* 2005;14(3):733–736.
6. Sundström JT, Minn H, Lertola KK, Nordman E. Prognosis of patients treated for intracranial metastases with whole-brain irradiation. *Ann Med.* 1998;30(3):296–299.
7. Nieder C, Berberich W, Schnabel K. Tumor-related prognostic factors for remission of brain metastases after radiotherapy. *Int J Radiat Oncol Biol Phys.* 1997;39(1):25–30.
8. Stea B, Suh JH, Boyd AP, Cagnoni PJ, Shaw E; REACH Study Group. Whole-brain radiotherapy with or without efaproxiral for the treatment of brain metastases: Determinants of response and its prognostic value for subsequent survival. *Int J Radiat Oncol Biol Phys.* 2006;64(4):1023–1030.
9. Li J, Bentzen SM, Renschler M, Mehta MP. Regression after whole-brain radiation therapy for brain metastases correlates with survival and improved neurocognitive function. *J Clin Oncol.* 2007;25(10):1260–1266.
10. Regine WF, Scott C, Murray K, Curran W. Neurocognitive outcome in brain metastases patients treated with accelerated-fractionation vs. accelerated-hyperfractionated radiotherapy: an analysis from Radiation Therapy Oncology Group Study 91–04. *Int J Radiat Oncol Biol Phys.* 2001;51(3):711–717.
11. Andrews DW, Scott CB, Sperduto PW, et al. Whole brain radiation therapy with or without stereotactic radiosurgery boost for patients with one to three brain metastases: phase III results of the RTOG 9508 randomised trial. *Lancet.* 2004;363(9422):1665–1672.
12. Gelber RD, Larson M, Borgelt BB, Kramer S. Equivalence of radiation schedules for the palliative treatment of brain metastases in patients with favorable prognosis. *Cancer.* 1981;48(8):1749–1753.
13. Chatani M, Matayoshi Y, Masaki N, Inoue T. Radiation therapy for brain metastases from lung carcinoma. Prospective randomized trial according to the level of lactate dehydrogenase. *Strahlenther Onkol.* 1994;170(3):155–161.
14. Priestman TJ, Dunn J, Brada M, Rampling R, Baker PG. Final results of the Royal College of Radiologists' trial comparing two different radiotherapy schedules in the treatment of cerebral metastases. *Clin Oncol (R Coll Radiol).* 1996;8(5):308–315.
15. Rades D, Haatanen T, Schild SE, Dunst J. Dose escalation beyond 30 grays in 10 fractions for patients with multiple brain metastases. *Cancer.* 2007;110(6):1345–1350.
16. Gaspar L, Scott C, Rotman M, et al. Recursive partitioning analysis (RPA) of prognostic factors in three Radiation Therapy Oncology Group (RTOG) brain metastases trials. *Int J Radiat Oncol Biol Phys.* 1997;37(4):745–751.
17. Lutterbach J, Bartelt S, Stancu E, Guttenberger R. Patients with brain metastases: hope for recursive partitioning analysis (RPA) class 3. *Radiother Oncol.* 2002;63(3):339–345.
18. Nieder C, Nestle U, Motaref B, Walter K, Niewald M, Schnabel K. Prognostic factors in brain metastases: should patients be selected for aggressive treatment according to recursive partitioning analysis (RPA) classes? *Int J Radiat Oncol Biol Phys.* 2000;46(2):297–302.
19. Agboola O, Benoit B, Cross P, et al. Prognostic factors derived from recursive partition analysis (RPA) of Radiation Therapy Oncology Group (RTOG) brain metastases trials applied to surgically resected and irradiated brain metastatic cases. *Int J Radiat Oncol Biol Phys.* 1998;42(1):155–159.
20. Tendulkar RD, Liu SW, Barnett GH, et al. RPA classification has prognostic significance for surgically resected single brain metastasis. *Int J Radiat Oncol Biol Phys.* 2006;66(3):810–817.
21. Lorenzoni J, Devriendt D, Massager N, et al. Radiosurgery for treatment of brain metastases: estimation of patient eligibility using three stratification systems. *Int J Radiat Oncol Biol Phys.* 2004;60(1):218–224.
22. Sneed PK, Suh JH, Goetsch SJ, et al. A multi-institutional review of radiosurgery alone vs. radiosurgery with whole brain radiotherapy as the initial management of brain metastases. *Int J Radiat Oncol Biol Phys.* 2002;53(3):519–526.
23. Le Scodan R, Massard C, Mouret-Fourme E, et al. Brain metastases from breast carcinoma: validation of the radiation therapy oncology group recursive partitioning analysis classification and proposition of a new prognostic score. *Int J Radiat Oncol Biol Phys.* 2007;69(3):839–845.
24. Murray KJ, Scott C, Greenberg HM, et al. A randomized phase III study of accelerated hyperfractionation versus standard in patients with unresected brain metastases: a report of the Radiation Therapy Oncology Group (RTOG) 9104. *Int J Radiat Oncol Biol Phys.* 1997;39(3):571–574.
25. Patchell RA, Tibbs PA, Walsh JW, et al. A randomized trial of surgery in the treatment of single metastases to the brain. *N Engl J Med.* 1990;322(8):494–500.
26. Noordijk EM, Vecht CJ, Haaxma-Reiche H, et al. The choice of treatment of single brain metastasis should be based on extracranial tumor activity and age. *Int J Radiat Oncol Biol Phys.* 1994;29(4):711–717.
27. Mintz AH, Kestle J, Rathbone MP, et al. A randomized trial to assess the efficacy of surgery in addition to radiotherapy in patients with a single cerebral metastasis. *Cancer.* 1996;78(7):1470–1476.
28. Kondziolka D, Patel A, Lunsford LD, Kassam A, Flickinger JC. Stereotactic radiosurgery plus whole brain radiotherapy versus radiotherapy alone for patients with multiple brain metastases. *Int J Radiat Oncol Biol Phys.* 1999;45(2):427–434.
29. Antonadou D, Paraskevaidis M, Sarris G, et al. Phase II randomized trial of temozolomide and concurrent radiotherapy in patients with brain metastases. *J Clin Oncol.* 2002;20(17):3644–3650.
30. Verger E, Gil M, Yaya R, et al. Temozolomide and concomitant whole brain radiotherapy in patients with brain metastases: a phase II randomized trial. *Int J Radiat Oncol Biol Phys.* 2005;61(1):185–191.
31. Kocher M, Eich HT, Semrau R, Güner SA, Müller RP. Phase I/II trial of simultaneous whole-brain irradiation and dose-escalating topotecan for brain metastases. *Strahlenther Onkol.* 2005;181(1):20–25.
32. Mirmiran A, McClay E, Spear MA. Phase I/II study of IV topotecan in combination with whole brain radiation for the treatment of brain metastases. *Med Oncol.* 2007;24(2):147–153.
33. Suh JH, Stea B, Nabid A, et al. Phase III study of efaproxiral as an adjunct to whole-brain radiation therapy for brain metastases. *J Clin Oncol.* 2006;24(1):106–114.
34. Mehta MP, Rodrigus P, Terhaard CH, et al. Survival and neurologic outcomes in a randomized trial of motexafin gadolinium and whole-brain radiation therapy in brain metastases. *J Clin Oncol.* 2003;21(13):2529–2536.
35. Sessler JL, Tvermoes NA, Guldi DM, et al. Pulse radiolytic studies of metallotexaphyrins in the presence of oxygen: relevance of the equilibrium with superoxide anion to the mechanism of action of the radiation sensitizer motexafin gadolinium (Gd-Tex^{2+}, Xcytrin). *J Phys Chem.* 2001;B1452-B1457.
36. Mehta MP, Shapiro WR, Phan SC, et al. Motexafin gadolinium combined with prompt whole brain radiotherapy prolongs time to neurological progression in non-small-cell lung cancer patients with brain metastases: results of a Phase III trial. *Int J Radiat Oncol Biol Phys.* 2009;73:1069–1076.
37. Nieder C, Astner ST, Grosu AL, Andratschke NH, Molls M. The role of postoperative radiotherapy after resection of a single brain metastasis. Combined analysis of 643 patients. *Strahlenther Onkol.* 2007;183(10):576–580.
38. Nieder C, Schwerdtfeger K, Steudel WI, Schnabel K. Patterns of relapse and late toxicity after resection and whole-brain radiotherapy for solitary brain metastases. *Strahlenther Onkol.* 1998;174(5):275–278.
39. Patchell RA, Tibbs PA, Regine WF, et al. Postoperative radiotherapy in the treatment of single metastases to the brain: a randomized trial. *JAMA.* 1998;280(17):1485–1489.
40. Aoyama H, Shirato H, Tago M, et al. Stereotactic radiosurgery plus whole-brain radiation therapy vs stereotactic radiosurgery alone for treatment of brain metastases: a randomized controlled trial. *JAMA.* 2006;295(21):2483–2491.
41. Murray KJ, Scott C, Zachariah B, et al. Importance of the mini-mental status examination in the treatment of patients with brain metastases: a report from the Radiation Therapy Oncology Group protocol 91–04. *Int J Radiat Oncol Biol Phys.* 2000;48(1):59–64.
42. Rugo HS, Ahles T. The impact of adjuvant therapy for breast cancer on cognitive function: current evidence and directions for research. *Semin Oncol.* 2003;30(6):749–762.
43. Heflin LH, Meyerowitz BE, Hall P, et al. Cancer as a risk factor for long-term cognitive deficits and dementia. *J Natl Cancer Inst.* 2005;97(11):854–856.
44. Nieder C, Leicht A, Motaref B, Nestle U, Niewald M, Schnabel K. Late radiation toxicity after whole brain radiotherapy: the influence of antiepileptic drugs. *Am J Clin Oncol.* 1999;22(6):573–579.

45. Klein M, Heimans JJ, Aaronson NK, et al. Effect of radiotherapy and other treatment-related factors on mid-term to long-term cognitive sequelae in low-grade gliomas: a comparative study. *Lancet.* 2002;360(9343):1361–1368.
46. Rades D, Pluemer A, Veninga T, Dunst J, Schild SE. A boost in addition to whole-brain radiotherapy improves patient outcome after resection of 1 or 2 brain metastases in recursive partitioning analysis class 1 and 2 patients. *Cancer.* 2007;110(7):1551–1559.
47. Ewend MG, Brem S, Gilbert M, et al. Treatment of single brain metastasis with resection, intracavity carmustine polymer wafers, and radiation therapy is safe and provides excellent local control. *Clin Cancer Res.* 2007;13(12):3637–3641.
48. Pirzkall A, Debus J, Lohr F, et al. Radiosurgery alone or in combination with whole-brain radiotherapy for brain metastases. *J Clin Oncol.* 1998;16(11):3563–3569.
49. Cho KH, Hall WA, Gerbi BJ, Higgins PD, Bohen M, Clark HB. Patient selection criteria for the treatment of brain metastases with stereotactic radiosurgery. *J Neurooncol.* 1998;40(1):73–86.
50. Kocher M, Voges J, Müller RP, et al. Linac radiosurgery for patients with a limited number of brain metastases. *J Radiosurg.* 1998;1:9–15.
51. Sneed PK, Lamborn KR, Forstner JM, et al. Radiosurgery for brain metastases: is whole brain radiotherapy necessary? *Int J Radiat Oncol Biol Phys.* 1999;43(3):549–558.
52. Varlotto JM, Flickinger JC, Niranjan A, et al. Analysis of tumor control and toxicity in patients who have survived at least one year after radiosurgery for brain metastases. *Int J Radiat Oncol Biol Phys.* 2003;57:452–464.
53. Bhatnagar AK, Flickinger JC, Kondziolka D, Lunsford LD. Stereotactic radiosurgery for four or more intracranial metastases. *Int J Radiat Oncol Biol Phys.* 2006;64(3):898–903.
54. Vogelbaum MA, Angelov L, Lee SY, Li L, Barnett GH, Suh JH. Local control of brain metastases by stereotactic radiosurgery in relation to dose to the tumor margin. *J Neurosurg.* 2006;104(6):907–912.
55. Weltman E, Salvajoli JV, Brandt RA, et al. Radiosurgery for brain metastases: who may not benefit? *Int J Radiat Oncol Biol Phys.* 2001;51(5):1320–1327.
56. Kased N, Huang K, Nakamura JL, et al. Gamma knife radiosurgery for brainstem metastases: the UCSF experience. *J Neurooncol.* 2008;86(2):195–205.
57. Bhatnagar AK, Kondziolka D, Lunsford LD, Flickinger JC. Recursive partitioning analysis of prognostic factors for patients with four or more intracranial metastases treated with radiosurgery. *Technol Cancer Res Treat.* 2007;6(3):153–160.
58. Rades D, Bohlen G, Pluemer A, et al. Stereotactic radiosurgery alone versus resection plus whole-brain radiotherapy for 1 or 2 brain metastases in recursive partitioning class 1 and 2 patients. *Cancer.* 2007;109(12):2515–2521.
59. O'Neill BP, Iturria NJ, Link MJ, Pollock BE, Ballman KV, O'Fallon JR. A comparison of surgical resection and stereotactic radiosurgery in the treatment of solitary brain metastases. *Int J Radiat Oncol Biol Phys.* 2003;55(5):1169–1176.
60. Schöggl A, Kitz K, Reddy M, et al. Defining the role of stereotactic radiosurgery versus microsurgery in the treatment of single brain metastases. *Acta Neurochir (Wien).* 2000;142(6):621–626.
61. Muacevic A, Kreth FW, Horstmann GA, et al. Surgery and radiotherapy compared with gamma knife radiosurgery in the treatment of solitary cerebral metastases of small diameter. *J Neurosurg.* 1999;91(1):35–43.
62. Sawrie SM, Guthrie BL, Spencer SA, et al. Predictors of distant brain recurrence for patients with newly diagnosed brain metastases treated with stereotactic radiosurgery alone. *Int J Radiat Oncol Biol Phys.* 2008;70(1):181–186.
63. Gutiérrez AN, Westerly DC, Tomé WA, et al. Whole brain radiotherapy with hippocampal avoidance and simultaneously integrated brain metastases boost: a planning study. *Int J Radiat Oncol Biol Phys.* 2007;69(2):589–597.
64. Fahrig A, Ganslandt O, Lambrecht U, et al. Hypofractionated stereotactic radiotherapy for brain metastases–results from three different dose concepts. *Strahlenther Onkol.* 2007;183(11):625–630.
65. Lindvall P, Bergström P, Löfroth PO, Henriksson R, Bergenheim AT. Hypofractionated conformal stereotactic radiotherapy alone or in combination with whole-brain radiotherapy in patients with cerebral metastases. *Int J Radiat Oncol Biol Phys.* 2005;61(5):1460–1466.
66. Dagnew E, Kanski J, McDermott MW, et al. Management of newly diagnosed single brain metastasis using resection and permanent iodine-125 seeds without initial whole-brain radiotherapy: a two institution experience. *Neurosurg Focus.* 2007;22(3):E3.
67. Rogers LR, Rock JP, Sills AK, et al.; Brain Metastasis Study Group. Results of a phase II trial of the GliaSite radiation therapy system for the treatment of newly diagnosed, resected single brain metastases. *J Neurosurg.* 2006;105(3):375–384.
68. Shaw E, Scott C, Souhami L, et al. Single dose radiosurgical treatment of recurrent previously irradiated primary brain tumors and brain metastases: final report of RTOG protocol 90–05. *Int J Radiat Oncol Biol Phys.* 2000;47(2):291–298.
69. Davey P, Schwartz ML, Scora D, Gardner S, O'Brien PF. Fractionated (split dose) radiosurgery in patients with recurrent brain metastases: implications for survival. *Br J Neurosurg.* 2007;21(5):491–495.
70. Sadikov E, Bezjak A, Yi QL, et al. Value of whole brain re-irradiation for brain metastases–single centre experience. *Clin Oncol (R Coll Radiol).* 2007;19(7):532–538.
71. Wong WW, Schild SE, Sawyer TE, Shaw EG. Analysis of outcome in patients reirradiated for brain metastases. *Int J Radiat Oncol Biol Phys.* 1996;34(3):585–590.
72. Falkmer U, Järhult J, Wersäll P, Cavallin-Ståhl E. A systematic overview of radiation therapy effects in skeletal metastases. *Acta Oncol.* 2003;42(5–6):620–633.
73. Wai MS, Mike S, Ines H, Malcolm M. Palliation of metastatic bone pain: single fraction versus multifraction radiotherapy - a systematic review of the randomised trials. *Cochrane Database Syst Rev.* 2004;(2):CD004721.
74. van der Linden YM, Dijkstra SP, Vonk EJ, Marijnen CA, Leer JW; Dutch Bone Metastasis Study Group. Prediction of survival in patients with metastases in the spinal column: results based on a randomized trial of radiotherapy. *Cancer.* 2005;103(2):320–328.
75. Chow E, Harris K, Fung K. Successful validation of a survival prediction model in patients with metastases in the spinal column. *Int J Radiat Oncol Biol Phys.* 2006;65(5):1522–1527.
76. Bach F, Larsen BH, Rohde K, et al. Metastatic spinal cord compression. Occurrence, symptoms, clinical presentations and prognosis in 398 patients with spinal cord compression. *Acta Neurochir (Wien).* 1990;107(1–2):37–43.
77. Loblaw DA, Laperriere NJ, Mackillop WJ. A population-based study of malignant spinal cord compression in Ontario. *Clin Oncol (R Coll Radiol).* 2003;15(4):211–217.
78. Rades D, Fehlauer F, Schulte R, et al. Prognostic factors for local control and survival after radiotherapy of metastatic spinal cord compression. *J Clin Oncol.* 2006;24(21):3388–3393.
79. Spiller WG. Rapidly progressive paralysis associated with carcinoma. *AMA Arch Neurol Psychiatry.* 1925;13:471–477.
80. Prasad D, Schiff D. Malignant spinal-cord compression. *Lancet Oncol.* 2005;6(1):15–24.
81. Ushio Y, Posner R, Posner JB, Shapiro WR. Experimental spinal cord compression by epidural neoplasm. *Neurology.* 1977;27(5):422–429.
82. Kato A, Ushio Y, Hayakawa T, Yamada K, Ikeda H, Mogami H. Circulatory disturbance of the spinal cord with epidural neoplasm in rats. *J Neurosurg.* 1985;63(2):260–265.
83. Manabe S, Tanaka H, Higo Y, Park P, Ohno T, Tateishi A. Experimental analysis of the spinal cord compressed by spinal metastasis. *Spine.* 1989;14(12):1308–1315.
84. Tarlov IM, Klinger H, Vitale S. Spinal cord compression studies. I. Experimental techniques to produce acute and gradual compression. *AMA Arch Neurol Psychiatry.* 1953;70(6):813–819.
85. TARLOV IM, KLINGER H. Spinal cord compression studies. II. Time limits for recovery after acute compression in dogs. *AMA Arch Neurol Psychiatry.* 1954;71(3):271–290.
86. Rades D, Heidenreich F, Karstens JH. Final results of a prospective study of the prognostic value of the time to develop motor deficits before irradiation in metastatic spinal cord compression. *Int J Radiat Oncol Biol Phys.* 2002;53(4):975–979.
87. Gilbert RW, Kim JH, Posner JB. Epidural spinal cord compression from metastatic tumor: diagnosis and treatment. *Ann Neurol.* 1978;3(1):40–51.
88. Helweg-Larsen S, Sørensen PS, Kreiner S. Prognostic factors in metastatic spinal cord compression: a prospective study using multivariate analysis of variables influencing survival and gait function in 153 patients. *Int J Radiat Oncol Biol Phys.* 2000;46(5):1163–1169.

89. Maranzano E, Latini P. Effectiveness of radiation therapy without surgery in metastatic spinal cord compression: final results from a prospective trial. *Int J Radiat Oncol Biol Phys.* 1995;32(4):959–967.
90. Husband DJ. Malignant spinal cord compression: prospective study of delays in referral and treatment. *BMJ.* 1998;317(7150):18–21.
91. Gilbert H, Apuzzo M, Marshall L, et al. Neoplastic epidural spinal cord compression. A current perspective. *JAMA.* 1978;240(25):2771–2773.
92. Li KC, Poon PY. Sensitivity and specificity of MRI in detecting malignant spinal cord compression and in distinguishing malignant from benign compression fractures of vertebrae. *Magn Reson Imaging.* 1988;6(5):547–556.
93. Colletti PM, Siegel HJ, Woo MY, Young HY, Terk MR. The impact on treatment planning of MRI of the spine in patients suspected of vertebral metastasis: an efficacy study. *Comput Med Imaging Graph.* 1996;20(3):159–162.
94. Rades D, Bremer M, Goehde S, Joergensen M, Karstens JH. Spondylodiscitis in patients with spinal cord compression: a possible pitfall in radiation oncology. *Radiother Oncol.* 2001;59(3):307–309.
95. Tomita T, Galicich JH, Sundaresan N. Radiation therapy for spinal epidural metastases with complete block. *Acta Radiol Oncol.* 1983;22(2):135–143.
96. Baskin DS. Spinal cord injury. In: Ewans RW, ed. *Neurology and Trauma.* Philadelphia, Saunders; 1996:276–299.
97. Loblaw DA, Laperriere NJ. Emergency treatment of malignant extradural spinal cord compression: an evidence-based guideline. *J Clin Oncol.* 1998;16(4):1613–1624.
98. Sørensen S, Helweg-Larsen S, Mouridsen H, Hansen HH. Effect of high-dose dexamethasone in carcinomatous metastatic spinal cord compression treated with radiotherapy: a randomised trial. *Eur J Cancer.* 1994;30A(1):22–27.
99. Vecht CJ, Haaxma-Reiche H, van Putten WL, de Visser M, Vries EP, Twijnstra A. Initial bolus of conventional versus high-dose dexamethasone in metastatic spinal cord compression. *Neurology.* 1989;39(9).1255–1257.
100. Heimdal K, Hirschberg H, Slettebø H, Watne K, Nome O. High incidence of serious side effects of high-dose dexamethasone treatment in patients with epidural spinal cord compression. *J Neurooncol.* 1992;12(2):141–144.
101. Rades D, Stalpers LJ, Veninga T, et al. Evaluation of five radiation schedules and prognostic factors for metastatic spinal cord compression. *J Clin Oncol.* 2005;23(15):3366–3375.
102. Kim RY, Smith JW, Spencer SA, Meredith RF, Salter MM. Malignant epidural spinal cord compression associated with a paravertebral mass: its radiotherapeutic outcome on radiosensitivity. *Int J Radiat Oncol Biol Phys.* 1993;27(5):1079–1083.
103. Klimo P Jr, Kestle JRW, Schmidt MH. Treatment of metastatic spinal epidural disease: a review of the literature. *Neurosurg Focus* 2003;15:1–9.
104. Hoskin PJ, Grover A, Bhana R. Metastatic spinal cord compression: radiotherapy outcome and dose fractionation. *Radiother Oncol.* 2003;68(2):175–180.
105. Maranzano E, Bellavita R, Rossi R, et al. Short-course versus split-course radiotherapy in metastatic spinal cord compression: results of a phase III, randomized, multicenter trial. *J Clin Oncol.* 2005;23(15):3358–3365.
106. Rades D, Karstens JH, Alberti W. Role of radiotherapy in the treatment of motor dysfunction due to metastatic spinal cord compression: comparison of three different fractionation schedules. *Int J Radiat Oncol Biol Phys.* 2002;54(4):1160–1164.
107. Rades D, Fehlauer F, Stalpers LJ, et al. A prospective evaluation of two radiotherapy schedules with 10 versus 20 fractions for the treatment of metastatic spinal cord compression: final results of a multicenter study. *Cancer.* 2004;101(11):2687–2692.
108. Rades D, Stalpers LJ, Hulshof MC, et al. Comparison of 1 x 8 Gy and 10 x 3 Gy for functional outcome in patients with metastatic spinal cord compression. *Int J Radiat Oncol Biol Phys.* 2005;62(2):514–518.
109. Rades D, Hoskin PJ, Stalpers LJ, et al. Short-course radiotherapy is not optimal for spinal cord compression due to myeloma. *Int J Radiat Oncol Biol Phys.* 2006;64(5):1452–1457.
110. Rades D, Veninga T, Stalpers LJ, et al. Prognostic factors predicting functional outcomes, recurrence-free survival, and overall survival after radiotherapy for metastatic spinal cord compression in breast cancer patients. *Int J Radiat Oncol Biol Phys.* 2006;64(1):182–188.
111. Rades D, Stalpers LJ, Veninga T, Rudat V, Schulte R, Hoskin PJ. Evaluation of functional outcome and local control after radiotherapy for metastatic spinal cord compression in patients with prostate cancer. *J Urol.* 2006;175(2):552–556.
112. Rades D, Stalpers LJ, Schulte R, et al. Defining the appropriate radiotherapy regimen for metastatic spinal cord compression in non-small cell lung cancer patients. *Eur J Cancer.* 2006;42(8):1052–1056.
113. Rades D, Walz J, Stalpers LJ, et al. Short-course radiotherapy (RT) for metastatic spinal cord compression (MSCC) due to renal cell carcinoma: results of a retrospective multi-center study. *Eur Urol.* 2006;49(5):846–852; discussion 852.
114. Rades D, Fehlauer F, Veninga T, et al. Functional outcome and survival after radiotherapy of metastatic spinal cord compression in patients with cancer of unknown primary. *Int J Radiat Oncol Biol Phys.* 2007;67(2):532–537.
115. Rades D, Walz J, Schild SE, Veninga T, Dunst J. Do bladder cancer patients with metastatic spinal cord compression benefit from radiotherapy alone? *Urology.* 2007;69(6):1081–1085.
116. Rades D, Schild SE, Dunst J. Radiotherapy is effective for metastatic spinal cord compression in patients with epithelial ovarian cancer. *Int J Gynecol Cancer.* 2007;17(1):263–265.
117. Koswig S, Budach V. [Remineralization and pain relief in bone metastases after after different radiotherapy fractions (10 times 3 Gy vs. 1 time 8 Gy). A prospective study]. *Strahlenther Onkol.* 1999;175(10):500–508.
118. Steenland E, Leer JW, van Houwelingen H, et al. The effect of a single fraction compared to multiple fractions on painful bone metastases: a global analysis of the Dutch Bone Metastasis Study. *Radiother Oncol.* 1999;52(2):101–109.
119. Sørensen S, Børgesen SE, Rohde K, et al. Metastatic epidural spinal cord compression. Results of treatment and survival. *Cancer.* 1990;65(7):1502–1508.
120. Helweg-Larsen, Hansen SW, Sørensen PS. Second occurrence of symptomatic metastatic spinal cord compression and findings of multiple spinal epidural metastases. *Int J Radiat Oncol Biol Phys.* 1995;33:595–598.
121. Rades D, Heidenreich F, Bremer M, Karstens JH. Time of developing motor deficits before radiotherapy as a new and relevant prognostic factor in metastatic spinal cord compression: final results of a retrospective analysis. *Eur Neurol.* 2001;45(4):266–269.
122. Rosen LS, Gordon D, Tchekmedyian S, et al. Zoledronic acid versus placebo in the treatment of skeletal metastases in patients with lung cancer and other solid tumors: a phase III, double-blind, randomized trial–the Zoledronic Acid Lung Cancer and Other Solid Tumors Study Group. *J Clin Oncol.* 2003;21(16):3150–3157.
123. Rosen LS, Gordon DH, Dugan W Jr, et al. Zoledronic acid is superior to pamidronate for the treatment of bone metastases in breast carcinoma patients with at least one osteolytic lesion. *Cancer.* 2004;100(1):36–43.
124. Saad F, Gleason DM, Murray R, et al.; Zoledronic Acid Prostate Cancer Study Group. Long-term efficacy of zoledronic acid for the prevention of skeletal complications in patients with metastatic hormone-refractory prostate cancer. *J Natl Cancer Inst.* 2004;96(11):879–882.
125. Nieder C, Grosu AL, Andratschke NH, Molls M. Proposal of human spinal cord reirradiation dose based on collection of data from 40 patients. *Int J Radiat Oncol Biol Phys.* 2005;61(3):851–855.
126. Nieder C, Grosu AL, Andratschke NH, Molls M. Update of human spinal cord reirradiation tolerance based on additional data from 38 patients. *Int J Radiat Oncol Biol Phys.* 2006;66(5):1446–1449.
127. Rades D, Stalpers LJ, Veninga T, Hoskin PJ. Spinal reirradiation after short-course RT for metastatic spinal cord compression. *Int J Radiat Oncol Biol Phys.* 2005;63(3):872–875.
128. Ryu S, Fang Yin F, Rock J, et al. Image-guided and intensity-modulated radiosurgery for patients with spinal metastasis. *Cancer.* 2003;97(8):2013–2018.
129. Gerszten PC, Burton SA, Ozhasoglu C, Welch WC. Radiosurgery for spinal metastases: clinical experience in 500 cases from a single institution. *Spine.* 2007;32(2):193–199.
130. Brown PD, Stafford SL, Schild SE, Martenson JA, Schiff D. Metastatic spinal cord compression in patients with colorectal cancer. *J Neurooncol.* 1999;44(2):175–180.

131. Rades D, Dunst J, Schild SE. The first score predicting overall survival in patients with metastatic spinal cord compression. *Cancer.* 2008;112(1):157–161.
132. Rades D, Veninga T, Stalpers LJ, et al. Outcome after radiotherapy alone for metastatic spinal cord compression in patients with oligometastases. *J Clin Oncol.* 2007;25(1):50–56.
133. Higgins SA, Peschel RE. Hodgkin's disease with spinal cord compression. A case report and a review of the literature. *Cancer.* 1995;75(1):94–98.
134. Wallington M, Mendis S, Premawardhana U, Sanders P, Shahsavar-Haghighi K. Local control and survival in spinal cord compression from lymphoma and myeloma. *Radiother Oncol.* 1997;42(1):43–47.
135. Avilés A, Fernández R, González JL, et al. Spinal cord compression as a primary manifestation of aggressive malignant lymphomas: long-term analysis of treatments with radiotherapy, chemotherapy or combined therapy. *Leuk Lymphoma.* 2002;43(2):355–359.
136. Rades D, Schild SE. Spinal cord compression. *Eur J Cancer Suppl.* 2007;5:359–370.
137. Findley GF. The role of vertebral body collapse in the management of malignant spinal cord compression. *J Neurol Neurosurg Psychiatry.* 1987;50:151–154.
138. Klimo P Jr, Dailey AT, Fessler RG. Posterior surgical approaches and outcomes in metastatic spine-disease. *Neurosurg Clin N Am.* 2004;15(4):425–435.
139. Pigott KH, Baddeley H, Maher EJ. Pattern of disease in spinal cord compression on MRI scan and implications for treatment. *Clin Oncol (R Coll Radiol).* 1994;6(1):7–10.
140. Yen D, Kuriachan V, Yach J, Howard A. Long-term outcome of anterior decompression and spinal fixation after placement of the Wellesley Wedge for thoracic and lumbar spinal metastasis. *J Neurosurg.* 2002;96(1 Suppl):6–9.
141. Klimo P Jr, Thompson CJ, Kestle JR, Schmidt MH. A meta-analysis of surgery versus conventional radiotherapy for the treatment of metastatic spinal epidural disease. *Neuro-oncology.* 2005;7(1):64–76.
142. Patchell RA, Tibbs PA, Regine WF, et al. Direct decompressive surgical resection in the treatment of spinal cord compression caused by metastatic cancer: a randomised trial. *Lancet.* 2005;366(9486):643–648.
143. Kunkler I. Surgical resection in metastatic spinal cord compression. *Lancet.* 2006;367(9505):109; author reply 109–109; author reply 110.
144. Knisely J, Strugar J. Can decompressive surgery improve outcome in patients with metastatic epidural spinal-cord compression? *Nat Clin Pract Oncol.* 2006;3(1):14–15.
145. Sørensen PS, Borgesen SE, Rohde K, et al. Metastatic epidural spinal cord compression: results of treatment and survival. *Cancer.* 1990b;65:1502–1508.
146. Ryu S, Rock J, Rosenblum M, Kim JH. Patterns of failure after single-dose radiosurgery for spinal metastasis. *J Neurosurg.* 2004;101(Suppl 3):402–405.
147. Ryu S, Jin JY, Jin R, et al. Partial volume tolerance of the spinal cord and complications of single-dose radiosurgery. *Cancer.* 2007;109(3):628–636.
148. Gibbs IC, Kamnerdsupaphon P, Ryu MR, et al. Image-guided robotic radiosurgery for spinal metastases. *Radiother Oncol.* 2007;82(2):185–190.
149. Chang EL, Shiu AS, Lii MF, et al. Phase I clinical evaluation of near-simultaneous computed tomographic image-guided stereotactic body radiotherapy for spinal metastases. *Int J Radiat Oncol Biol Phys.* 2004;59(5):1288–1294.
150. Roqué M, Martinez MJ, Alonso P, Català E, Garcia JL, Ferrandiz M. Radioisotopes for metastatic bone pain. *Cochrane Database Syst Rev.* 2003;(4):CD003347.
151. Grossman SA, Finkelstein DM, Ruckdeschel JC, Trump DL, Moynihan T, Ettinger DS. Randomized prospective comparison of intraventricular methotrexate and thiotepa in patients with previously untreated neoplastic meningitis. Eastern Cooperative Oncology Group. *J Clin Oncol.* 1993;11(3):561–569.
152. Chamberlain MC, Kormanik PA. Non-AIDS-related lymphomatous meningitis: combined modality therapy. *Neurology.* 1997;49(6):1728–1731.
153. Glantz MJ, Jaeckle KA, Chamberlain MC, et al. A randomized controlled trial comparing intrathecal sustained-release cytarabine (DepoCyt) to intrathecal methotrexate in patients with neoplastic meningitis from solid tumors. *Clin Cancer Res.* 1999;5(11):3394–3402.
154. Glantz MJ, LaFollette S, Jaeckle KA, et al. Randomized trial of a slow-release versus a standard formulation of cytarabine for the intrathecal treatment of lymphomatous meningitis. *J Clin Oncol.* 1999;17(10):3110–3116.
155. Saito R, Kumabe T, Jokura H, Shirane R, Yoshimoto T. Symptomatic spinal dissemination of malignant astrocytoma. *J Neurooncol.* 2003;61(3):227–235.
156. Lassman AB, Abrey LE, Shah GD, et al. Systemic high-dose intravenous methotrexate for central nervous system metastases. *J Neurooncol.* 2006;78(3):255–260.
157. Hermann B, Hültenschmidt B, Sautter-Bihl ML. Radiotherapy of the neuroaxis for palliative treatment of leptomeningeal carcinomatosis. *Strahlenther Onkol.* 2001;177(4):195–199.
158. Rudnicka H, Niwinska A, Murawska M. Breast cancer leptomeningeal metastasis-the role of multimodality treatment. *J Neurooncol.* 2007;84(1):57–62.
159. Bruno MK, Raizer J. Leptomeningeal metastases from solid tumors (meningeal carcinomatosis). *Cancer Treat Res.* 2005;125:31–52.
160. Nolan CP, Abrey LE. Leptomeningeal metastases from leukemias and lymphomas. *Cancer Treat Res.* 2005;125:53–69.
161. Sanders KE, Ha CS, Cortes-Franco JE, Koller CA, Kantarjian HM, Cox JD. The role of craniospinal irradiation in adults with a central nervous system recurrence of leukemia. *Cancer.* 2004;100(10):2176–2180.
162. Parker W, Filion E, Roberge D, Freeman CR. Intensity-modulated radiotherapy for craniospinal irradiation: target volume considerations, dose constraints, and competing risks. *Int J Radiat Oncol Biol Phys.* 2007;69(1):251–257.
163. Yuh GE, Loredo LN, Yonemoto LT, et al. Reducing toxicity from craniospinal irradiation: using proton beams to treat medulloblastoma in young children. *Cancer J.* 2004;10(6):386–390.

Index

Note: Page references followed by "*f*" and "*t*" denote figures and tables, respectively.

Accelerated hyperfractionated (AH)
 radiotherapy, 639
Acquired evasive resistance, 135
Acromegaly, 291, 629–630
 clinical manifestations of, 293*t*
 management of, 447
 radiotherapy for, 867–868
Acrylamide, 19
Acrylonitrile, 20
Actinomycin-D, for infant tumors, 772
Active immunotherapy, 693–694
Acupuncture, 714
Acute lymphoblastic leukemia (ALL), 27
Acute radiation encephalopathy, 326
ADAMTS-5 protease, 115
Adaptive equipment, 345
Adaptor molecules, 116–117
Adeno-associated virus vectors
 (AAV), 698
Adenohypophysis, 294
Adenoid cystic carcinomas, 287
Adenomas. *See also* Astrocytomas; Cancer;
 Carcinomas; Ependymomas;
 Gliomas; Meningiomas; Metastases;
 Neurofibromas; Papillomas;
 Sarcomas; Tumors
 atypical pituitary adenoma, 450–451
 clinically functioning adenomas, 178
 clinically nonfunctioning
  adenomas, 179
 Crooke cell adenoma, 179
 endocrinologically inactive pituitary
  adenomas, 630
 functional adenomas, 445
 gonadotropin-producing
  adenomas, 179, 449–450
 hormonally active pituitary
  adenomas, 292
 hormone-inactive adenomas, 628*t*
 hormone-secreting adenomas, 628*t*
 invasive pituitary adenoma, 848
 lactotroph adenomas, 178
 macroadenomas, 447
 mammosomatotroph adenomas, 178
 mixed gangliocytoma-adenoma, 625
 nonfunctioning adenomas, 445
 null-cell adenoma, 179, 450
 pituitary adenoma, 522–523, 628*t*, 861
 plurihormonal adenomas, 179–180
 prolactin-secreting adenomas, 178, 291,
  293, 445–446
 somatotroph adenomas, 178
Adenomatous pituitary-derived sellar
 masses, 627
 acromegaly, 629–630
 Cushing disease, 628–629
 endocrinologically inactive pituitary
  adenomas, 630
 pituitary carcinoma, 630–631
 prolactinoma, 629
 TSH-secreting pituitary tumors, 630
Adenomatous polyposis coli (APC)
 gene, 16, 242
Adenoviral vectors, 698
Adherent stem cell cultures, 82*t*
Adjuvant postoperative radiation, 861
Adjuvant radiation therapy, primary
 spinal tumors, 454
Adjuvant therapy
 in astrocytoma, 473
 in ependymoma, 473
 in hemangioblastomas, 473–474
 in intramedullary spinal cord
  metastasis, 474
 in low-grade gliomas (LGGs), 482–483
 in pineal gland tumors, 491–492
Adoptive cellular immunotherapy, 693
Adrenocorticotropin (ACTH)-secreting
 adenomas, 179, 291, 447–449
Adriamycin, 634
Adult brainstem glioma, 842
 management algorithm, 843*f*
 radiotherapy
  delivery techniques, 843
  dose, 842–843
  indications for treatment, 842
  target volume for, 842
  treatment outcomes and approach,
   843–844
Adult medulloblastoma, 789
Adult pilocytic astrocytoma (PA), 797
AEE788, 680
Affymetrix U95A GeneChips, 94
Aflibercept (VEGF-Trap)
Age-adjusted incidence rate
 (AAIR), 59*f*
AIDS-related PCNSL, 650, 657
AKT activation, 91
AKT pathway, 84
Aldolase A, 108
Alendronate, 306
Alfacalcidiol, 712
ALK oncogene, amplification and
 mutation of, 231
Allergies and glioma, 1, 39
 allergy-related cytokines, 40–41
 antibodies' role against tumor
  antigens, 43
 IL-10
  in allergic conditions, 41
  in glioma, 41
  and glioma survival time, 42
  paradoxical role, 43
 immunosuppression, 41
 immunosuppressive regulatory
  T-cells, 42
 regulatory T-cells and glioma
  survival time, 42–43
 reverse causality, 43–44
 TGF-β
  in allergic conditions, 42
  in glioma, 42
  and glioma survival time, 42
  paradoxical role, 43
All-trans retinoic acid (ATRA),
 704, 705, 706
Alpha fetoprotein (AFP), 661
10alpha-hydroxycholecalciferol, 712
α/β ratio, 723
α particles, 731
α-synuclein, 892
α-tocopherol, 322, 330
ALPL gene, 72
Alproic acid, 707
Alternative therapies, 710, 713
 biologically based therapies,
  710–713
 body-based therapies, 713
 CAM in patients with brain
  tumor, 710
 mind-body therapies, 713
Amino acid positron emission
 tomography (AA-PET), 365
Aminoglutethimide, 628

5-aminolevulinic acid (5-ALA), 422
　fluorescence-guided resections
　　dosage and time of ALA
　　　application, 423
　　efficacy, 422–423
　　equipment, 424
　　implementation during surgery,
　　　424–425
　　light protection, 423–424
　　photobleaching, 425
　　pitfalls, 425–426
　　safety profile, 423
　-induced fluorescent porphyrins, 426
Aminolevulinic acid dehydratase
　(ALAD), 76
Anaplastic (WHO grade III)
　meningomas, 823
Anaplastic astrocytomas (AAs), 7, 101f,
　205, 569–570, 579, 754–755
　adjuvant chemotherapy in patients
　　with, 754
　RTOG recursive partitioning
　　analysis for patients with, 752t
　temozolomide, use of, 755
Anaplastic ependymoma, 210f
Anaplastic gliomas
　chemoradiotherapy trails for
　　patient with, 754–755
　conclusion of, 757–758
　and median survival, 752
　molecular genetics, importance of,
　　752–753
　　chemotherapy, 753
　　enzyme O6-methylguanine-DNA
　　　methyltransferase (MGMT),
　　　importance, 753
　　1p and 19q, alterations involving, 752
　　temozolomide and
　　　bischloroethylnitrosourea
　　　(BCNU), treatment with, 753
　occurrence of, 752
　prognostic factors of, 752
　treatment approach, 753–754
　　adjuvant radiotherapy, maximal
　　　surgical resection followed by,
　　　753–754
　　chemotherapy, 754
　　GBM, patients with, 753
　　radiotherapy and chemotherapy
　　　modifiers, 757
　　re-irradiation of, 757
Anaplastic meningiomass, 600
Anaplastic oligoastrocytoma, 7, 755–757
Anaplastic oligodendroglioma (AO), 9,
　570–572, 755–757
　chemotherapy with PCV, second trial
　　RTOG 9402, 753
　1p and 19q, combined codeletions
　　at, 752, 753
　PCV chemotherapy, 571, 756
　phase III trials examining median
　　progression-free survival, 753t
　prognostic factors of, 752
　progression-free survival rate, 756
　radiotherapy alone and salvage
　　therapy, 756
　temozolomide chemotherapy, 571–572

Anatomical imaging, 407
Ang-2 expression, 125
Angiocentric glioma, 58, 205, 206f
Angiogenesis, 93, 122, 669
　antiangiogenic agents
　　AZD2171, 673
　　bevacizumab, 670–671
　　enzastaurin, 671–672
　　sorafenib, 672
　　sunitinib, 672–673
　　thalidomide, 672
　escape mechanisms and treatment
　　strategies, 670
　in gliomas, 122
　　angiopoietins and VEGFs, 125–128
　　c-Met, 128
　　in CNS ontogeny and oncogeny, 130t
　　endogenous antiangiogenic
　　　factors, 128
　　epigenetic alterations, 129
　　genetic alterations, 128–129
　　"glioma stem cells" and tumor
　　　neovascularization, 129
　　molecular pathology, 122–123
　　scatter factor (SF), 128
　　SDF-1α, 128
　　by tumor hypoxia and
　　　metabolism, 123–125
　　and vasculogenesis, 129–130
　therapies, 670
　toxicities associated with
　　antiangiogenic therapy, 670
Angiopoietin-2 (Ang-2), 123
Angiopoietins and VEGFs, 125–128
Animal models
　neurofibromatosis 1, 151
　neurofibromatosis 2, 151
　peripheral nerve tumors, specific
　　mouse models of, 151
　specific mouse glioma models, 148
　transgenic and knockout mice,
　　strategies using, 148–150
　transgenic mouse models, potential
　　use of, 151
　viral and transgenic mice,
　　strategies using, 150
Animal neurocarcinogens, 18
Anterior fossa syndrome, 288
Anterior interhemispheric transcallosal
　approach, 497–498
Anterior longitudinal ligament (ALL), 457
Antiangiogenic agents
　AZD2171, 673
　bevacizumab, 670–671
　enzastaurin, 671–672
　in gliomas patients
　　case illustration, 134f
　　clinical trials, 133
　　clinical vignette, 133–135
　　complications, 135–137
　　molecular signaling pathways, 136f
　　rationale, patient selection, and
　　　outcome measure, 132–133
　　resistance to, 135
　sorafenib, 672
　sunitinib, 672–673
　thalidomide, 672

Antiapoptotic protein, 92
Antibodies, 43
Antiepileptic drugs (AEDs), 304, 306t, 326
Antigrowth signals, insensitivity to, 91–92
Antihistamines, 22–23
Antiinflammatory agents, 711
Antioxidant genes, 64–65
Antioxidants, 21–22, 711
Antitumor immune responses, 692–693
Anti-VEGF antibody, 137
Antoni A area, 168
Antoni B area, 168, 169
ANXA2 gene, 601
APC gene, 242, 243
Apoptosis, evasion of, 92
Apparent diffusion coefficient (ADC), 355
Arachnoid cap cells, 159f
　age-related meningiomas incidence, 822
Arachnoid cyst, 627
Arm weakness, 258
Arterial input function, 363
Aryl hydrocarbon nuclear translocator
　(ARNT), 124
Aryl hydrocarbon receptor interacting
　protein (AIP) gene, 175
Ashworth Scale, 347, 347t
Asians, glioma in, 7
Aspirin, 22, 404
Assistance Scale, 347, 347t
Astroblastomas, 58
Astrocytic tumors, 6, 88
　anaplastic astrocytoma, 205
　angiocentric glioma, 205, 206f
　in children, 9
　diffuse astrocytoma, 205, 207f
　glioblastoma, 205–206
　growth patterns of, 100–101
　pilocytic astrocytoma, 204, 205f
　pilomyxoid astrocytoma, 204–205, 206f
　pleomorphic xanthoastrocytoma
　　(PXA), 206
Astrocytic tumors, classification of, 760
　infiltrative low-grade, 760
　pilocytic, 760, 762f
　survival rates, 764f
Astrocytomas, 6, 7, 88–89, 148t,
　465, 635, 895–896. See also
　Adenomas; Cancer; Carcinomas;
　Ependymomas; Gliomas;
　Meningiomas; Metastases;
　Neurofibromas; Papillomas;
　Sarcomas; Tumors
　adjuvant therapy in, 473
　adult pilocytic astrocytoma, 797
　anaplastic astrocytomas, 7, 101f, 205,
　　569–570, 579, 754–755
　cerebellar astrocytomas, 268, 275, 528
　in children, 9
　desmoplastic infantile astrocytoma,
　　211, 212f
　diffuse astrocytomas, 7, 205, 207f, 278
　vs. ependymoma, 468
　fibrillary astrocytoma, 582
　gemistocytic astrocytomas, 105
　grades I and II, 775
　grades III and I, 775
　granular cell astrocytomas, 105

high-grade astrocytomas, 216, 217f
juvenile pilocytic astrocytoma, 216
IMSCT genetics, 466
low-grade astrocytoma, 771, 772, 773
NOS, 7
oligoastrocytoma, 90
origins of, 200–201
pediatric pilocytic astrocytoma, 795
pediatric grade II, radiation therapy
 for, 775–778
pediatric spinal cord astrocytoma, 467
pilomyxoid astrocytoma, 204–205, 206f
presentation, 466–467
and radiation therapy, 895–898
subependymal giant cell
 astrocytomas, 58, 253, 274
survival rate for, 10
Asymptomatic tumors, 275
Ataxia-telangiectasia mutant gene
 (ATM), 73
ATF5 (activating transcription
 factor 5), 108
Atypical (WHO Grade II), intracranial
 meningiomass, 822–823
Atypical choroid plexus papilloma, 58
Atypical neurofibroma, 188
Atypical pituitary adenoma, 450–451
Atypical teratoid/rhabdoid tumor
 (ATRT), 58, 209, 209f, 267, 844
Autologous stem cell rescue (ASCR), 595
Autologous stem-cell transplantation
 (ASCT), 655
 AIDS-related PCNSL, 657
 immunotherapy, 656–657
 investigational therapy, 657
Autonomy, respect for, 311
Autophagy, decrease of, 93
Avastin, 670
Average risk patients, of PNETs
 current standard of care, 784
 hyperfractionated radiotherapy
  trials, 784
 neoadjuvant chemotherapy trials,
  782–783
 postradiotherapy chemotherapy
  trials, 784
 reduced dose radiotherapy trials, 782
 reduced radiotherapy volume trials, 784
Awake technique, 395–396
AZD2171, 609, 673
Aziridinylbenzoquinone, 635

^{10}B, 729, 730
Babinski signs, 300
Baby-POG I, 592
Baclofen, 347
BAD gene, 601
Basal temporal language area
 (BTLA), 378
BB SFOP protocol, 594
B-cells, 2, 43
BCL-2, 233
BCNU, 85
BDNF, 64
Beclin 1, 93
Beneficence, 311

Benign (WHO Grade I), intracranial
 meningiomass, 822
Benign nonperipheral nerve sheath
 tumors, 536
Benign peripheral nerve sheath
 tumors, 535–536
Benzamides, 707
Benzidine-based dyes, 19
Benzodiazepines, 347
Benzotriazole, 18
Beta-emitting isotopes, 864
Beta-human chorionic gonadotropin
 (B-HCG), 661
Beta plus decay, 720
Bevacizumab (Avastin), 40, 133, 135, 549,
 568, 570, 581, 609, 670–671, 680, 684
Biochanin A, 711
Biologically based therapies, 710
 copper depletion, 712–713
 dietary restriction, 712
 marijuana, 711
 miscellaneous supplements, 712
 nutritional supplements, 711
  antiinflammatory agents, 712
  antioxidants, 712
  fatty acids, 711–712
  flavonoids, 712
  phytoestrogens, 711
  polysaccharide peptides, 711
  selenium, 712
  vitamin D, 712
Biologics, 692
 general principles, 692
 gene therapy, 695
 immunotherapy, 692–693
  active immunotherapy (vaccination),
   693–694
  adoptive cellular immunotherapy, 693
  cell-mediated immunotherapy, 693
  humoral-mediated immunotherapy,
   694–695
 multimodal biologic therapy, 700
  immunogene therapy, 700–701
  immunotherapy with chemotherapy
   and radiation, 700
 strategies to enhance efficacy of gene
  therapy and virotherapy for brain
  tumors, 699–700
 viruses, 695
  measles virus, 697
  newcastle disease virus (NDV), 697
  oncolytic adenovirus, 696–697
  oncolytic HSV-1, 696
  poliovirus, 697
  replication-competent (oncolytic)
   viruses, 696
  replication-defective viruses, 698
  transgene strategies, 698–699
Bioluminescence imaging (BLI), effect of,
 155–156
Biopsy, definition of, 400
Bischloroethyl-nitrosourea, 711
Bithalamic glioma, 58
BK virus, 62
Blacks, glioma in, 7
 survival rate for, 11
Bladder management, 346–347

Bleeding problems, 345
Blood-brain barrier (BBB), 547
 anatomy and physiology, 547–548
 osmotic disruption, 550
 pathology, 547
Blood oxygenation level dependent
 (BOLD) contrast fMRI, 364, 372
BMI-1, 84
Body-based therapies, 713
Bone marrow-derived proangiogenic
 cells, mobilization and
 recruitment of, 131f
Bone mineral density (BMD), 292
Bone morphogenic proteins (BMPs), 85
Bone pain relief, metastatic, 910
Bone scan, primary spinal tumors, 454
Boron neutron capture therapy (BNCT),
 730–731, 732t
Bortezomib (Velcade), 92, 681
Boswellic acid, 548–549
Bowel management, 347
Brachial plexus tumor, 534
 management of selected lesions
  affecting the brachial plexus
  benign peripheral nerve sheath
   tumors, 541
  desmoid tumors, 542
  extraneural lesions, 542
  hyperplastic lesions, 542
  lipomatous lesions of nerve, 542
  malignant peripheral nerve sheath
   tumors, 542–543
  malignant tumors of nonneural
   sheath origin, 543–544
  nonneural sheath origin intraneural
   lesions, benign lesions of, 542
  syndromes (NF-1, NF-2, segmental
   forms of NF, schwannomatosis),
   541–542
 MRI of specific lesions
  benign nonperipheral nerve sheath
   tumors, 536
  benign peripheral nerve sheath
   tumors, 535–536
  decision on whom to operate,
   539–540
  malignant peripheral nerve and
   nonperipheral nerve sheath
   tumors, 537–539
  other benign lesions affecting
   nerve, 536–537
  percutaneous biopsy, 539
 operative evaluation, 540
 postoperative evaluation, 540–541
 preoperative evaluation
  electromyography/nerve
   conduction study, 534
  history, 534
  imaging, 534–535
  physical examination, 534
Brachytherapy, 724–726
 for GBM, 745
Bragg Peak, 731
Brain-derived neurotrophic factor
 (BDNF), 232
Brain herniation, 283
Brain invasion, 823

Brain metastases, 638
  brachytherapy, 909
    other techniques of, 909
    recurrent lesion, retreatment for, 909
  clinical presentation, diagnosis, and imaging, 262–263
  epidemiology, 262
  fractionated stereotactic radiotherapy, 908–909
  incidence, 638
    diagnosis and prognosis, 638–639
    from kidney cancer, single-fraction stereotactic radiosurgery for, 904f
  and leptomeningeal disease (LMD), 645
    intrathecal chemotherapy for, 646
    palliative treatments, 645–646
    presentation and diagnosis, 645
    systemic therapy options, 646
  palliative whole-brain radiotherapy, 902–905
    combining drugs and, 903–905
    fractionation and total dose, 902–903
    surgical resection or radiosurgery, treatment intensification by, 903
    symptom relief and quality of life, effects on, 902
  pathological diagnosis-special stains, 263–264
  prognostic factors, 263–264
  radiosurgery (RS), one to three brain metastases, 906–907
    plus whole-brain radiotherapy, 907–908
  RTOG RPA classification, 264t
  supportive treatment, 265
  surgical resection, whole-brain radiotherapy after, 905–906
  systemic disease, correlation to, 263–264
  theories of spread, migration, propensities, 264–265
  treatment
    efaproxiral, 640
    gefitinib and erlotinib, 644–645
    lapatinib, 645
    motexafin gadolinium, 640
    options, key questions for selecting, 907t
    other regimens, 644
    platinum agents alone/in combination, 643
    radiation therapy, 639
    stereotactic radiosurgery (SRS), 640–641
    surgery vs. stereotactic radiosurgery, 641
    surgical resection alone/with radiotherapy, 639–640
    systemic chemotherapy alone/in combination with WBRT, 641–642
    temozolomide (TMZ), 642–643
    topotecan, 643–644
    whole-brain radiation therapy with/without radiosensitizers, 640
    whole-brain radiotherapy alone/with SRS, 641
Brain shift, 408
  and deformation, 394

Brainstem, 343, 380
  cranial nerve circuitry, 380–381
  long white matter tracts, 381
  reticular circuitry, 381
Brainstem gliomas, 216f, 268, 275
Brainstem metastases, radiosurgery for, 906–907
Brainstem tumors, 278
  as cause of cognitive deficits, 326–327
  clinical presentation, 278
  diagnostic evaluation, 280
  imaging of. See Imaging of brain tumors
  pathology, 278
  radiographic appearance, 278–280
  serial assessment of
    initial assessment, 366
    post-treatment response assessment, 367
    two-dimensional methods, 366
    volumetric methods, 367
  unique impact of, 316
  targeted therapy for, 667
Brainstem tumors, medical management for, 608
  in adults, 612
  in children
    cervicomedullary gliomas, 610–611
    diffuse brainstem gliomas, 608–610
    dorsally exophytic gliomas, 610
    focal brainstem tumors, 610
    midbrain tumors, 611
  and NF 1, 611–612
Brain tumor initiating cells
  aberrant signaling pathways in, 84–85
  definition, 82–83
  isolation methods, 82t
  markers of, 83–84
  multipotency, 81t, 82
  origin of, 82
  proliferation, 81t, 84, 85
  self-renewal, 81t, 82, 84, 85
  stem cell hypothesis, 81
  treatment, 85
    limitations, 85
Brain tumor polyposis syndrome
  type 1, 242
  type 2, 242
Brain Tumor Study Group (BTSG), 744
Braking radiation, 721
Branchial motor nuclei, 380
"Breaking energy," 720f
Breast cancer, 264
  and meningiomas, association between, 71–72
  metastasis, 539f
  patients and meningiomass, 820
  screening for, 15–16
Bremsstrahlung, 719, 721
Brinstem tumors, in patients with NF1, 844
Broca, Paul, 377
Bromocriptine, 629, 630
Bromodeoxyuridine (BrdU), 640
Bromoethane, 18
Busulfan, 655
Bystander effect, 698
1,3-Butadiene, 18–19

C5 quadriplegia, 345
C8-T1 quadriplegia, 345
Cabergoline, 629
Cadherin family, 115
Café-au-lait macules, 249
Calcarine sulcus, 499
Calcineurin, 892
Camptothecan, 657
Camptothecin, 707
Cancer. See also Adenomas; Astrocytomas; Carcinomas; Ependymomas; Gliomas; Meningiomas; Metastases; Neurofibromas; Papillomas; Sarcomas; Tumors
  breast cancer, 15–16, 71–72, 264, 539f, 820
  hereditary nonpolyposis colorectal cancer, 242
  non-small cell lung cancer, 642, 643, 645, 685
  small cell lung cancer, 638
Cancer Genome Atlas (TCGA), 54, 79, 95
Cancer patients, exercise guidelines and precautions for, 346t
Cancer rehabilitation, 342
Cancer stem cells (CSC), 129, 200, 233
  vs. BTSC, 200f
  hypothesis, 79, 81, 85, 596
  neuroblastoma development, genetic model of, 233
  spontaneous regression, 234
  tumor initiation and progression, 233–234
Cannabinoid, 711
Carbamazepine, 305, 330
Carboplatin, 473, 583, 584, 586, 586, 595, 609, 635, 662
  for average-risk PNET, 783
  and etoposide
    for NGGCTs, 876
  and procarbazine
    for ependymomas, 802–803
Carcinogen metabolism genes, 48, 64
Carcinomas, 58. See also Adenomas; Astrocytomas; Cancer;; Ependymomas; Gliomas; Meningiomas; Metastases; Neurofibromas; Papillomas; Sarcomas; Tumors
  adenoid cystic carcinomas, 287
  pituitary carcinoma, 174, 180, 450–451, 630–631
  choroid plexus carcinoma, 210, 664
  squamous cell carcinomas, 287
Caregivers, 316, 317
  communication, 318
  issues, 351
  roles and responsibilities, 318
  support, 318
Carmustine (BCNU), 330, 566, 618, 635
Carmustine wafer (Gliadel®), 695
Carney syndrome, 168
Carotenoids, 22, 712
  consumption, 22
Caucasian children, 267
Cavernous angiomas, 386
Cavernous sinus, 294
  meningiomass, 285

CCND1 gene, 601
CCNU, 473, 773
CD44, 115
   expression, 190
CD46, 697
CD133, 81, 83, 84, 84*t*
   tumor cells, 106
CDK4 gene, 92
CDK6 gene, 92
CDKN2A gene, 232
CDNK1A, 92
Cediranib (AZD2171, Recentin), 680, 684
Celecoxib, 640
Cell/tissue-specific transgenesis, 146–147
Cell culture–based methods, 154
Cell cycle dysregulation, 92
Cell-mediated immunity, 692, 693
Cell of origin
   for pediatric brain tumors, 196
      anatomical sites, 201*f*
      astrocytoma, origins of, 200–201
      ependymoma, origins of, 199–200
      medulloblastoma, origins of, 196–199
   of solid tumors, 79
Cell surface receptors, changes in expression of, 114–115
Cellular heterogeneity, 105
   differentiation patterns, 105–106
   proliferative/apoptotic heterogeneity, 106–107
   stem cells/glioma progenitor cells, 106
Cellular neurofibroma with atypia, 188
Cellular schwannoma, 169–170, 170*f*
Cellular Src, 116
Central Brain Tumor Registry of the United States (CBTRUS), 4, 6, 7, 59
"Central necrosis," 104
Central nervous system (CNS), 43, 79–80
   brachytherapy, 724–726
   neurotoxicity to, 330
   tumors, 27, 125
Central nervous system (CNS) tumors, rehabilitation of, 342
   approach to, 342
      dietician, 343
      nurse, 343
      occupational therapist, 343
      physiatrist, 342–343
      physical therapist, 343
      physicians, 342
      psychologist, 343
      social worker/case manager, 343
      speech therapist, 343
      vocational counselors, 343
   deficits related to treatment, 344@3
      steroids, 344
      chemotherapy, 344
      endocrine deficiencies, 344
      myelopathy, 344
      postsurgical sequelae, 344
      radiation therapy, 344
   functional deficits, 343
      brainstem, 343
      frontal lobe tumors, 343
      parietal lobe, 343
      temporal lobe, 343
   general effects of cancer on function, 344
      bleeding problems, 345
      joint contractures, 345
   overview, 342
   rehabilitation interventions, 345
      adaptive equipment, 345
      bladder management, 346–347
      bowel management, 347
      cognitive-perceptual interventions, 345
      functional outcomes, 348
      hemiparesis and hemiplegia, 345
      malignant epidural cord compression, patients with, 348
      spasticity, 347
      spinal cord involvement, 345–346
      therapeutic exercises, 345
      treatment, 347–348
Central nervous system (CNS) tumors, transgenic mouse models of, 145
   animal models
      neurofibromatosis 1, 151
      neurofibromatosis 2, 151
      peripheral nerve tumors, specific mouse models of, 151
      specific mouse glioma models, 148
      transgenic and knockout mice, strategies using, 148–150
      transgenic mouse models, potential use of, 151
      viral and transgenic mice, strategies using, 150
   mouse transgenesis, techniques for, 145
      cell/tissue-specific transgenesis, 146–147
      ES cell-mediated transgenesis, 146
      homologous recombination, 145, 146*f*
      pronuclear injection, 145–146
      somatic gene transfer, using RCAS-tva system, 147–148
Central nervous system (CNS) tumors, transplantation mouse models of, 153
   bioluminescence imaging, effect of, 155–156
   human tumor xenograft models, 154
      cell culture–based methods, 154
      orthotopic vs. heterotopic tumor cell growth, 155
      xenograft-based tumor propagation, 154–155
   human tumor panels and high-throughput preclinical testing, 156
   immunocompetent hosts
      chemically induced tumor cells, 153
      transgenic models, 153–154
Central neurocytoma, 524–525
   and radiation therapy, 898
Central sulcus, 373
Cephalosporins, 551
Cerebellar astrocytomas, 268, 275, 528
   medical management for, 584–585
Cerebellar gliomas, 268
Cerebellar medulloblastoma, 208*f*
Cerebellar neural stem cells (c-Myc), 242
"Cerebellar neuroblastomas," 197
Cerebral abscess, 261
Cerebral blood volume (CBV), stereotactic brain biopsy, 403
Cerebral hemispheres
   gliomas of, 274
   neoplasms of, 258–259
Cerebral low-grade glioma, 583
Cerebrospinal fluid (CSF) flow, 349
   fistula, 472
Cerebrum, 6
Cereport® RMP-7, 550
Cervicomedullary gliomas, 610–611
Cetuximab, 91
Chang system, 781
CHAPs, 707
CHEK2, 48, 243
Chemically induced tumor cells, 153
Chemodectomas, 635
   general considerations, 287
   glomus jugulare tumors, 287
Chemotherapy, 275–276, 344
   alone or in combination WBRT, primary central nervous system lymphoma (PCNSL), 880
   with BCNU, anaplastic gliomas, 754
   for cerebral low-grade glioma, 583
   for choroid plexus tumors, 665
   for ependymomas, 586
   in gangliomas, use of, 770
   for GBM, 564–566
   for high-grade gliomas, 579–580
   for low-grade gliomas (LCGs), 558–561
   metastatic spinal tumors, 459–460
   oligodendrogliomas and, 762
   for optic pathway glioma, 584
   for PCNSL, 654
   PCV chemotherapy, 754
   for pediatric pilocytic astrocytoma (PA), 797
   primary spinal tumors, 454
   spinal cord tumors, 473
   for tumors of skull base and cranial nerves, 615, 615*t*
      chondrosarcoma, 617
      chordoma, 616–617
      esthesioneuroblastoma, 618–619
      malignant peripheral nerve sheath tumors, 619–620
      paraganglioma, 617–618
Childhood brain tumors, 57
   classification, 57
      embryonal tumors, 58
      glioneuronal tumors, 58–59
      neuroepithelial tumors, 58
   definition, 57–58
   descriptive epidemiology, 59
      distribution by gender, race/ethnicity, and age, 59
      trends, 59–60
   suggested causes of
      antioxidant genes, 64–65
      carcinogen metabolism genes, 64
      chromosomal gain, 63
      chromosomal loss, 63
      constitutive genetic variation, 64
      developmental genes, 65

Childhood brain tumors (cont.)
  diet and vitamin supplementation, 61–62
  DNA repair genes, 65
  electromagnetic fields (EMFs), 60
  environmental risk factors, 60
  epigenetic alterations, 63–64
  head injury, 62
  immune function genes, 65
  infectious agents, 62
  ionizing radiation, 60
  molecular genetic and epigenetic characteristics, 63
  nitroso compounds, 61
  nonionizing radiation, 60
  occupational exposure, 60–61
  pesticides, 61
  population exposure to NOC, 61
  predisposing genetic syndromes and familial occurrence, 62–63
  tobacco, 62
Childhood Cancer Survivor Study, 27
Children's Oncology Group (COG), 234
  risk stratification schema, 228t
Chitinase-3-like-1 gene (*CHI3L1*), 94
Chloroethane, 18
Choline, 279–280, 363, 402
Choline-to-*N*-acetylaspartate index (CNI), 364
Chondroid variant, chordomas, 846, 847
  magnetic resonance imaging (MRI) of, 849
  prognosis of, 847
Chondrosarcomas, 287, 615t, 617
  clinical presentation of, 847
  cytotoxic chemotherapy, 617
  diagnosis and work-up, 848–849
    differential diagnosis, 848
    imaging, 848–849
    tissue diagnosis, 849
    work-up and staging, 848
  epidemiology of, 846
    age and gender distribution, 846
  etiology and anatomy of, 846
  gender, age and race distributions, 846
  natural history of, 848
  pathology of, 846–847
    conventional variants, 847
    physaliferous cells, 846
  radiation sensitizers, 617
  and radiation therapy, 896–898
  management of patient with, 849–855
    particle radiation therapy, carbon ions, 854–855
    particle radiation therapy, protons, 852–854
    photon radiation therapy, conventional fractionation, 850–851
    photon radiation therapy, stereotactic radiosurgery, 851–852
    surgery, 849–850
  toxicity and particle therapy, 855–857
    brain, 856
    brain stem, 856
    endocrine deficiency, 857
    hearing loss, 857
    postoperative complications, 855–856
    spinal cord, 856
    vision, 856–857
Chordoid gliomas, 58
Chordoid meningiomas, 160, 160f, 600, 823t
Chordomas, 287, 616, 615t, 634
  clinical presentation of, 847
  cytotoxic chemotherapy, 616
  diagnosis and work-up, 848–849
    differential diagnosis, 848
    imaging, 848–849
    tissue diagnosis, 849
    work-up and staging, 848
  epidemiology of, 846
    age and gender distribution, 846
  etiology and anatomy of, 846
    off–midline chordomas, 846
  management of patient with, 849–855
    particle radiation therapy, carbon ions, 854–855
    particle radiation therapy, protons, 852–854
    photon radiation therapy, conventional fractionation, 850–851
    photon radiation therapy, stereotactic radiosurgery, 851–852
    surgery, 849–850
  molecularly targeted agents, 616
  natural history of, 847–848
    progressive or recurrent disease, death by, 847
  pathology of, 846–847
    conventional variants, 846
    physaliferous cells, 846
  radiation sensitizers, 617
  toxicity and particle therapy, 855–857
    brain, 856
    brain stem, 856
    endocrine deficiency, 857
    hearing loss, 857
    postoperative complications, 855–856
    spinal cord, 856
    vision, 856–857
Choroid plexus, anatomy of, 500
Choroid plexus carcinoma (CPC), 210, 664
Choroid plexus neoplasms, 58
Choroid plexus papilloma (CPP), 210, 211f, 664, 878
Choroid plexus tumors, 361, 523–524
  medical management for, 664
    chemotherapy, 665
    radiation therapy, 664–665
    surgery, 664
Chromatin helicase-binding domain 5 (*CHD5*) gene, 231–232
Chromosomal gain, 63
Chromosomal loss, 63
Chromosome 1p, 162
Chromosome 6 polymorphism, 229
Chromosome 9p, 163
Chromosome 10, 163
Chromosome 10q, loss of heterozygosity on, 48
Chromosome 14q, 163
Chromosome 17, 163
Chromosome 17p, 63
Chromosome 17q gain, 229
Chromosome 19q, 54
Chromosome 22q, 162
Chronic inflammatory demyelinating polyneuropathy (CIDP), 536
Chronic myelogenous leukemia (CML), 676
Cilengitide, 94
Circulating endothelial cells in glioma neovascularization, 130–131
Cisplatin, 85, 344, 473, 580, 586, 591, 593, 595, 609, 610, 616, 619, 634, 635, 643, 661, 707
  for average-risk PNET, 782
Classic medulloblastoma, 206
Classification systems, of glioma, 4–6
Clear-cell ependymoma, 58
Clear cell meningiomas, 160, 160f, 600, 823t
Clinical and demographic characteristics, of glioma
  distribution of glioma, by site and histological type, 6
  frequency by gender and race, 7
  primary gliomas, frequency of, 6
Clinically functioning adenomas, 178
Clinically nonfunctioning adenomas, 179
Clinically silent ACTH-producing adenomas, 179
Clinical target volume (CTV), 786
Clinoidal meningiomas, 284
Clival chordoma, 626–627
Clival meningiomas, 284
Clivus meningiomas
  diagnosis of, 848
  proton therapy and, 853f
Clonal evolution model, 81
Clonality, 180
Cluster headaches, 260
c-Met, 128
Co-60, 719
Cognitive deficits, 326
  brain tumor as cause of, 326–327
  late encephalopathy
    in extracranial malignancies, 329–330
    in high-grade glioma patients, 329
    in low-grade glioma patients, 328–329
  medical therapy as cause of
    antiepileptic drugs, 330
    chemotherapy, 330–331
    steroids, 331
  mood disorder as cause of, 331
  radiotherapy as cause of, 327–328
  surgery as cause of, 327
Cognitive-perceptual interventions, 345
Combined-modality therapy for PCNSL, 654
Communication, of caregivers, 318
Comparative genomic hybridization (CGH), 228
Complementary and alternative medicine (CAM), 710
  in patients with brain tumor, 710
Completely endoscopic intra-axial tumor resection, 441–443
Computed tomography (CT), 279, 326, 353
  -based simulation, 746

Brachial plexus tumor, 535
and chordomas, 849
-guided biopsy of spine, 459
for meningomas, 602
metastatic spinal tumors, 459
primary spinal tumors, 453
scanner, 440
stereotactic brain biopsy, 401
Conformal radiation therapy, 454
Connecticut children, with
  CNS tumors, 62
Consequentialism, 311
Constitutive genetic polymorphisms and
  glioma survival, 48, 49–53t
Constitutive genetic variation, 64
Convection-enhanced delivery
  (CED), 397, 695
Conventional variants, chordomas, 846
  immunohistochemical comparison
    of, 847
Copper depletion, 712–713
Copy-number variation (CNV), 228
Coriolus versicolor, 711
Coronal/paramedian plane, 438
Corticosteroids, 305–306, 331, 459,
  548, 549t
Corticotrophin-releasing hormone
  (CRH), 448
  -producing tumors, 293
Coumestans (coumestrol), 711
Cowden disease, 244
  animal models, 245
  clinical features and diagnostic
    criteria, 244
  molecular pathogenesis, 244
  therapy and prognosis, 245
Cranial chordomas, 287
Cranial irradiation, 820
Cranial irradiation therapy (CRT), 336
Cranial nerve circuitry, 380–381
Cranial neuropathies,
  radiation-induced, 865
Cranial radiation, 276
Craniofacial immobilization device, 728
Craniopharyngioma, 59, 213, 213f, 286,
  291, 336, 391, 520–521, 623
  conventional radiotherapy, 862
  intracavitary radiotherapy, 864
  proton therapy, 864
  radiotherapy
    cranial neuropathies, 865
    cystic enlargement, 865
    follow-up, 868–869
    hypopituitarism, 865
    mortality, 865
    neurocognitive effects, 865–866
    optic neuropathy, 864–865
    secondary malignancies, 865
    techniques, 862–864
  radiation indications, 861
  stereotactic techniques
    fractionated stereotactic
      radiosurgery (FSRT), 863
    stereotactic radiosurgery (SRS), 863
Craniospinal irradiation (CSI), 646
Craniospinal irradiation (CSI), for
  PNETs, 786

boost fields, 787
radiotherapy-chemotherapy
  interactions, 788–789
techniques of, 787
  boost fields, 788
  dose of, 788
  electron therapy, 788
  intensity-modulated
    radiotherapy, 788
  photon irradiation, 787–788
  in prone position, 788f
  proton therapy, 788
Craniospinal meningiomass, 285
Creatine, 279, 363
Cre-loxP recombinase system, 147, 147f
Cre recombinase, 198
crk gene, 116
Crooke cell adenoma, 179
CT-on-Rails, 730t
Cushing disease (CD), 291, 292–293,
  447–448, 628–629
  clinical manifestations of, 293t
  radiotherapy for, 866–867
Cutaneous schwannomas, 167, 168f
CXCL12. See SDF-1α
CXCL13, 43, 653
CXCR4, 43, 128
CyADIC (cyclophosphamide, doxorubicin,
  and dacarbazine), 618
CyberKnife, 459, 730t
Cyclic tetrapeptides (trapoxin, apicidin,
  and depsipeptide), 707
Cyclin a1, 64
Cyclin-dependent kinase (CDK), 89
Cyclin-dependent kinase inhibitor 1B
  (CDKN1B) gene, 174
Cyclooxygenase (COX) inhibitors, 680–681
Cyclooxygenase 2 (COX-2) inhibitors, 22
Cyclophosphamide, 344, 580, 586, 591,
  592, 593, 595, 609, 616, 619, 620,
  634, 635, 655, 662, 707
  for average-risk PNET, 783, 784
  for high-risk PNET, 786
  for infant medulloblastoma, 790
Cyclophosphamide, 642-flourouracil, and
  prednisone (CFP), 644
Cyclophosphamide, adriamycin,
  vincristine, and etoposide
  (CAVE), 644
Cyclophosphamide, doxorubicin,
  vincristine, and prednisone
  (CHOP), 654
Cyclophos-phamide/doxorubicin/
  5-fluorouracil (CAF), 644
Cyclophosphamide/methotrexate/
  5-fluorouracil (CMF), 644
Cyclosporine, 551
CYP1B1, 64
Cystic degeneration, radiation
  therapy, 773
Cystic enlargement, radiation-
  induced, 865
Cytarabine (Ara-C), 85, 344, 580,
  595, 635, 657, 646
  for average-risk PNET, 782
Cytochrome p450 enzymes
  (CYP450s), 64

Cytochrome P450 polypeptide 2E1
  (CYP2E1), 64, 73
Cytokeratin 7, 263
Cytokine, 323
Cytomegalovirus (CMV), 694
Cytoplasmic kinases, role of, 115–116
Cytostatic medical therapy with
  hormone secreting pituitary
  adenomas, 862

Dacarbazine, 616, 617, 620, 634, 635
Daclizumab, 700
Dactinomycin, 634
Daidzein, 711
Dantrolene, 347
Dasatinib, 617, 677
De-differentiated variant,
  chordomas, 846, 847
Deep venous thrombosis
  (DVT), 306–307
Delirium, 350
Dendritic cells (DCs), 692, 693
Densely ionizing, 721
39-deoxy-39-18F-fluorothy-midine
  (FLT), 403
DepoCyt, 646, 657
Dermal neurofibroma (DNF), 185
Dermoid and epidermoid tumors, 625
Descriptive epidemiology of glioma.
  See Epidemiology of glioma
Desmoid tumors, 536, 538f
Desmoplastic infantile astrocytoma
  (DIA), 211, 212f
Desmoplastic infantile ganglioglioma
  (DIG), 211, 212f, 274
Desmopressin, 448
Developmental genes, 65
Development and progression, of
  glioma, 89f
Dexamethasone, 265, 305, 306, 349,
  423, 459, 657, 672
Dibromodulcitol, 773
Diencephalic gliomas, 274–275
Diencephalic syndrome, 772
Diet, 21
  N-nitroso compound exposure, 21
  supplementation, for childhood
    brain tumors, 61–62
  vitamins and antioxidants, 21–22
Dietary restriction, 712
Dietician, 343
Differential diagnosis of MPNST, 192
Differentiated neurons, 197f
Diffuse adult gliomas, 88
Diffuse astrocytomas, 7, 205, 207f, 278
Diffuse brainstem gliomas, 608–610
Diffuse fibrillary astrocytoma, survival
  rates of, 764f
Diffuse intrinsic brainstem tumors
  radiotherapy
    dose, 844
    indications for treatment, 844
    target volume for, 844
    treatment outcome, 844
    treatment technique, 844
Diffusely infiltrative pontine glioma, 279

Diffuse pontine brainstem glioma (DIPG), 215
　molecular genetics, 215–216
　translational therapies, 216
Diffusion tensor image (DTI), 280, 372, 428–429, 481
　tractography, 375
Diffusion weighted imaging (DWI), 353–355
Diplopia, 258
Distribution of glioma, by site and histological type, 6
DNA ligase IV (Lig4), 244
DNA methylation, 63
DNA mutation, 22
DNA repair genes, 65
Docosahexanoic acid, 711, 712
Doctrine of substituted judgment, 311
Donepezil, 322
Dopamine, 629
Dopamine agonists (bromocriptine, cabergoline), 447
Dorsally exophytic gliomas, 610
Dose rate, 724
Dose-response relationship, 27–28
Doxorubicin, 616, 619, 634, 635, 707
Drinking water, 61
Dumbbell tumor, 299, 302f
DuraGen, 439, 442
Dying patient, care of, 350–351
Dynamic contrast enhancement (DCE), 362–363
Dynamic susceptibility contrast imaging (DSCI), 356–362
Dysembryoplastic neuroepithelial tumors (DNET), 211–212, 212f, 518
Dysphagia and swallowing disorders, 307–308
Dyspnea, 350

Early-responding tissues, 723
E-cadherin, 115
Edema, assessing, 344
EF5, 103
　intratumoral heterogeneity, 105f
Efaproxiral, 640
"Effective dose," 26
EGFR gene, 47, 48, 108
EGFRvIII, 47–48, 91, 108, 149, 150
Eicosapentaenoic acid, 711
"Eight drugs in 1 day," 782, 785
8q24, 11q23 (PHLDB1), 1
Electrocortical stimulation mapping (ESM), 372
Electrocorticography (ECoG), 432
Electroencephalography (EEG), 371
Electromagnetic fields (EMFs), 60
Electron capture, 720
Electron microscopy, 170
　of neurofibroma, 189
Embryonal form of neural cell adhesion molecule, 892
Embryonal tumors, 58
　atypical teratoid/rhabdoid tumor (ATRT), 209, 209f
　choroid plexus carcinoma (CPC), 210

choroid plexus papilloma (CPP), 210
classic medulloblastoma, 206
ependymoblastoma, 208–209
ependymomas, 209, 210f
medulloblastoma, 206
　variants, 206–207
medulloepithelioma, 208–209
supratentorial primitive neuroectodermal tumors (sPNETs), 208, 208f
Embryonic stem (ES) cell-mediated transgenesis, 146, 147f
"En bloc" resection, of primary spinal tumors, 456
Encephalopathy, 331
　acute radiation encephalopathy, 326
　late encephalopathy, 328–330
　leukoencephalopathy, 329, 331
Endocrine deficiencies, 344
Endocrinologically inactive pituitary adenomas, 630
Endocrinopathies, 276
End-of-life planning
　caregiver issues, 351
　hospice, 351
Endogenous and exogenous influences, meningiomass, 820
Endogenous antiangiogenic factors, 128
Endoscopic endonasal approaches (EEAs), 435, 436f
　transplanum/transcribriform, 437
　transsellar, 436–437
Endoscopic third ventriculostomy (ETV), 525, 526, 529
Endoscopy, 435
　skull-base surgery, 435–436
　　coronal/paramedian-plane approach, 438–439
　　exposure, general considerations of, 436
　　sagittal midline approaches, 436–438
　transcranial endosopic approaches
　　completely endoscopic intra-axial tumor resection, 441–443
　　endoscopic intraventricular Surgery, 439–441
Endothelial progenitor cells (EPCs), 130, 131
Enoxaparin, 307
En plaque meningiomass, 282
Environmental chemical exposure, 18
Enzastaurin (ENZ), 671–672, 680
Enzastaurin (LY317615), 684
Enzyme-inducing antiepileptic drugs (EIAEDs), 670, 671
Eosinophilic granular bodies (EGBs), 204
Eosinophilic granuloma, 634
Ependymal tumors, 6, 7
Ependymoblastoma, 208–209
Ependymomas, 6, 7, 58, 209, 210f, 269, 297, 528, 465, 635, 878. *See also* Adenomas; Astrocytomas; Cancer; Carcinomas; Gliomas; Meningiomas; Metastases; Neurofibromas; Papillomas; Sarcomas; Tumors
adjuvant therapy in, 473

after treatment surveillance, 805
anaplastic ependymoma, 210f
vs. astrocytoma, 468
clear-cell ependymoma, 58
in children, 9
epidemiology, 799
histology and grading, 799
imaging of, 799–800
IMSCT genetics, 466
location of, 799
medical management for, 585–586
myxopapillary, 58, 635, 799
origins of, 199–200
presentation, 466
prognostic variables, 803
　age, 804
　disseminated disease, 803–804
　histologic grade, 803
　location of, 804–805
　resection extent, 803
and radiation therapy, 896
signs and symptoms of, 800
subependymoma, 58, 799
survival rate for, 10
treatment of
　altered fractionation, 801–802
　radiation therapy, 800–801
　stereotactic radiosurgery, 801
　surgery, 800
Eph family of cell adhesion receptors, 115
Epidemiological studies, on relationship between chemical exposure and glioma risk, 18
Epidemiology of glioma
clinical and demographic characteristics
　distribution, by site and histological type, 6
　frequency by gender and race, 7
　primary gliomas, frequency of, 6
definitions and classification systems, 4–6
incidence rates
　in childhood, 9
　by gender, 7–9
　by histological type, 7
　overall incidence rates, ethnicity, and age, 7
　trends in, 9
survival rates, 10–12
Epidermal growth factor (EGF), 48
Epidermal growth factor receptor (EGFR), 63, 82, 84, 88, 91, 149, 187, 215, 605, 616, 676, 733
　amplification, 154
　inhibitors, 676–677
Epidermoid/dermoid, 286–287
Epigenetic alterations, in childhood brain tumors, 63–64
Epigenetics, 129
　and medulloblastoma, 222
Epilepsy, 326
Epileptic seizures, 330
Epithelial membrane antigen (EMA), 189, 205
"Equivalent dose," 26
Erlotinib (Tarceva), 91, 583, 644–645, 672, 683, 684

Esthesioneuroblastoma, 287, 615t, 618, 627
  cytotoxic chemotherapy, 618–619
Ethylene oxide, 20
Ethylnitrosourea (ENU), 20, 61
Etoposide, 580, 586, 592, 593, 595, 609, 616, 619, 634, 635, 657, 662, 707
  for average-risk PNET, 782, 783
  and cisplatin
    for ependymomas, 802–803
European Organisation for Research and Treatment of Cancer (EORTC) trial 26951, anaplastic gliomas, 752
Everolimus, 91
Ewing's sarcoma, 634
Exercise guidelines and precautions for cancer patients, 346t
Exophytic brainstem, 878
Exophytic chiasmatic-hypothalamic gliomas, 275
External beam radiotherapy (EBRT), 454, 599, 603, 719, 724, 726–728, 734
External granule layer (EGL), 198
Extracellular matrix (ECM), 93, 94, 112–114
Extracranial malignancies, late encephalopathy in, 329–330
Extradural neoplasms, 633
  biphosphonate therapy, 633
  metastasis, 633
  pain management, 633
  systemic chemotherapy/hormonal therapy, 633
Extramedullary tumors, of spinal canal, 302–303
Extraventricular neurocytoma, 59
Extreme capsule, 378

Facial nerve schwannomas, 286, 387
Facial sensation, 379
Familial adenomatous polyposis (FAP), 16, 242
Familial aggregation of glioma, 14
  case-control and cohort studies, 14
  case reports, 14
Famotidine, 306
Farnesyltransferase inhibitors (FTIs), 677, 679
Fas expression, 107
FasL expression, 107
Fast neutrons, 731
Favorable brainstem tumor
  management algorithm, 843f
  radiotherapy
    delivery techniques, 843
    dose, 842–843
    indications for treatment, 842
    target volume for, 842
    treatment outcomes and approach, 843–844
F-deoxyglucose (FDG), 403
Fenretinide (4-hydroxyphenyl-retinamide), 704–705, 706
FET-PET, 366
FGFR4 gene, 182
Fibrillary astrocytoma, 582
Fibroblast growth factor (FGF), 669
Fibroblastic meningiomass, 160f

Fibrous dysplasia, diagnosis of, 848
Fixation device (FD), 395
5p15.33 (TERT), 1
FLAIR MRI, 479f
Flavonoids, 22, 92, 711, 712
Flow cytometry, 82t
Flp recombinase, 147
Fluid attenuation inversion recovery (FLAIR) images, 353
Fluorescein, 421
Fluorescence-guided resections, 421
  using 5-aminolevulinic acid, 422
    dosage and time of ALA application, 423
    efficacy, 422–423
    equipment, 424
    implementation during surgery, 424–425
    light protection, 423–424
    photobleaching, 425
    pitfalls, 425–426
    safety profile, 423
Fluorescent in situ hybridization (FISH), 163f
Fluorodeoxyglucose positron emission tomography (FDG PET), 280
18-Fluorodeoxyglucose (18F-FDG), 365, 454
Fluorouracil, 617
Focal adhesion kinase (FAK), 113, 115
Focal brainstem tumors, 610
Focal gliomas, 278
Focal radiotherapy, 331
Focal tectal glioma, 612
Foramen magnum meningiomas, 390f
Foramen of Monro, 501
Forehead melanoma, 264f
Formononetin, 711
Fossa meningiomas, 158f
Foster-Kennedy syndrome, 283
Fotemustine, 712
FOXM1 gene, 94
FOXO, 680
Fractional anisotropy (FA) maps, 355
Fractionated adjuvant radiotherapy, for hemangioblastoma, 818
Fractionated stereotactic radiosurgery (FSRT), 728–729, 863
  for vestibular schwannoma
    compared to SRS, 813–814
    dose selection and toxicities, 813
    methods and treatment planning, 812–813
    results of, 813
Frame/frameless stereotaxy, 392
Frameless stereotaxy, 407
Frameless vs. frame-based SBB, 404
Free thyroxine (FT4), 449
Frequency of glioma, by gender and race, 7
Frontal eye fields, 377
Frontal lobe, 6
  functional neuroanatomy of, 372
    Broca's area, 377–378
    frontal eye fields, 377
    insula, 378
    presupplementary motor, 375–377

  primary motor cortex, 372–375, 373f
  supplementary motor area (SMA), 375–377
  tumors, 343
Fruits, intake of, 61
FSH/LH deficiency, 292
5-FU, 707
Functional adenomas, 445
  adrenocorticotropin-secreting adenomas, 447–449
  GH-producing adenomas, 446–447
  PRL-secreting adenomas, 445–446
  thyrotropin (TSH)-secreting adenomas, 449
Functional magnetic resonance imaging (fMRI), 364, 372, 380
Functional neuroanatomy. See Neuroanatomy, functional
Functional outcomes, 348
Fundoscopy, 274

G47delta, 696
Gabapentin, 305, 305, 330
GADD45γ, 182
Gadolinium texaphyrin (Gd-Tex), 749
Galectin-1, 112
  expression, 113
Galectin-3, 112
Galectins, 112
Gamma Knife (GK), 730t
  radiosurgery, 628
  treatment, 728, 729f
Gamma-linolenic acid (GLA), 711
γ ray, 721
Gangliocytomas, 625
  "WHO grade I," 210
Ganglioglioma, 58, 210–211, 212f, 518, 771
  imaging features of, 469
Gangliomas
  overview and natural history of, 769
  pathology of, 769
  radiographic appearance of, 769
    T1-weighted MRI, 769
    T2-weighted MRI, 769
  treatment and outcomes, 769–770
    epileptic symptoms, 770
    surgical resection, 769
Ganglioneuroblastoma, 208
Gastrointestinal stromal tumors (GIST), 676
157Gd 112, 729, 730
Gefitinib, 91, 644–645, 646, 684
Gemcitabine, 635
Gemistocytic astrocytomas, 105
Gender, frequency of glioma by, 7
General principles, of medical therapy
  blood-brain barrier (BBB), 547
    anatomy and physiology, 547–548
    pathology, 548
  chemotherapy, delivery of, 549
    BBB, osmotic disruption of, 550
    Cereport RMP-7, 550
    convection-enhanced delivery, 551
    drug manipulation, 550
    implantable polymers, 551
    intra-arterial delivery, 550

General principles, of medical
    therapy (cont.)
  intranasal delivery, 550–551
  intrathecal delivery, 550
  chemotherapy, toxicity of, 552–553
  drug resistance and susceptibility,
    551–552
  measurement of effects, 552
  tumoral vasogenic edema,
    treatment of, 548
    bevacizumab, 549
    boswellic acid, 548–549
    corticosteroids, 548
    diuretics, 549
    osmotherapy, 549
    Xerecept, 548
Gene therapy, 666–667, 695, 696t
Genetic heterogeneity, 107–108
Genistein, 711
Germ cell tumors (GCTs), 486,
    491, 526, 625–626, 771
Germinomas, 661–662, 874
  radiotherapy for, 874–876
Germline, 79
Gli, 84
Gli1, 84
Gliadel, 570
Glial fibrillary acidic protein
    (GFAP), 195, 205, 892
Glial tumors, 526
Glioblastoma (GBM), 1, 6, 7, 9,
    22, 61, 101f, 205–206, 563
  cells, 116f
  chemotherapy, 564–566
  in elderly, 566–567
  heterogeneity, 108
  molecularly targeted therapies,
    567–568
  radiotherapy (RT), 564
  radiation for, 744
    brachytherapy for, 745
    dose-limiting structures, 747–748
    doses, 744–745
    in elderly/poor performance patients,
      748–749
    follow-up, 749
    future directions, 749–750
    re-irradiation, 749
    sensitizers, 749
    simulation, 746
    toxicity, 748
    treatment volume/margins,
      745–746, 747f
  recurrent, 557
  proliferation within, 106
  surgery, 563
  survival, 47
    rate for, 10
  tumor cells, 129
  tumors, 112–113, 113t
  in Turcot syndrome, 16
Glioblastoma multiforme (GBM),
    80, 81, 83, 85, 122, 145, 154,
    200, 215, 305, 579, 719
  hypoxic and metabolic
    heterogeneity in, 103–104
  vascular heterogeneity in, 101–102

Gliomas, 518, 626, 878. See also Adenomas;
    Astrocytomas; Cancer; Carcinomas;
    Ependymomas; Meningiomas;
    Metastases; Neurofibromas;
    Papillomas; Sarcomas; Tumors
  adult brainstem glioma, 842
  anaplastic gliomas. See Anaplastic
    gliomas
  angiocentric glioma, 58, 205, 206f
  bithalamic glioma, 58
  brainstem gliomas, 216f, 268, 275, 842
  cerebellar gliomas, 268
  chordoid gliomas, 58
  definitions, 4–6
  diencephalic gliomas, 274–275
  diffuse adult gliomas, 88
  diffuse brainstem gliomas, 608–610
  diffusely infiltrative pontine
    glioma, 279
  diffuse pontine brainstem glioma, 215
  dorsally exophytic gliomas, 610
  exophytic chiasmatic-hypothalamic
    gliomas, 275
  focal gliomas, 278
  focal tectal glioma, 612
  hemispheric gliomas, 274
  high-grade gliomas, 7, 326, 562
  hypothalamic glioma, 626
  low-grade gliomas, 273, 275,
    477, 556, 557f
  malignant glioma, 6, 273, 363
  mouse models, 148
  oligodendroglioma, 2, 7, 9, 58, 88,
    89–90, 479f, 480f, 570
  optic nerve glioma, 16, 626
  optic pathway glioma, 250, 771
  orthotopic gliomas, 123
  paraganglioma, 615t, 617, 635
  pediatric grades II–IV (non-JPA)
    and radiation therapy in, 775–778
  pontine glioma, 58
  relapsed malignant glioma, 705–706
  risk, increase in, 1
  stem cells and tumor
    neovascularization, 129
  supratentorial gliomas, 16, 257,
    258, 518, 519f, 583
  survival time, 42–43
    and IL-10, 42
    and TGF-β, 42
  tectal gliomas, 278, 878
  thalamic gliomas, 525
Glioma NOS, 7
Glioma progenitor. See Tumor stem cells
Gliomatosis cerebri, 561–562
Glioneuronal tumors, 58–59
Gliosarcoma, 106
"Glomeruloid bodies," 102
Glomus jugulare tumors, 287
Glomus tumors. See Chemodectomas
Glucocorticoids, 653
GLUT1, 108
Glutamate, 363
Glutamine, 305, 363
Glutathione S-transferase (GST), 64, 338
Glutathione S-transferase Mu 1 (GSTM1)
    polymorphisms, 338

Glyceraldehyde-3-phosphate
    dehydrogenase, 108
Glycidol, 18
Gonadotroph adenoma cells, 179
Gonadotropin-producing adenomas, 179,
    449–450
Gorlin syndrome, 65, 219, 220, 267.
    See also Nevoid basal cell
    carcinoma syndrome (NBCCS)
Graded Prognostic Assessment (GPA), 639
Grading tumors, 355
Granular cell astrocytomas, 105
Granular cell tumors, 624–625
Granule neuron precursors (GNPs),
    198–199
Granulocytic sarcoma, and radiation
    therapy, 898
Gross total resection (GTR), 469–470, 473
  for choroid plexus tumors, 664
  for high-grade gliomas, 579
Gross tumor volume (GTV), 786, 862
Growth hormone (GH)
  hypersecretion, 293
  producing adenomas, 178,
    291, 293, 446–447
  receptor antagonism, 178
Growth signals, self-sufficiency in, 90
GSI018, 596
GSI in Germany, 732
Gsα point mutations, 180
Gyrus, 84

Hallmarks of malignant gliomas. See
    Malignant gliomas, hallmarks of
Haloperidol, 306
Hamartomas, 771
Handicap, 342
Hands-free equipment, use of, 31
Haploinsufficiency, 186
hCHK2 gene, 15
Headache, 257, 260, 283, 349
Head injury, 62
Head tumor, 34
Heavy ions, 732
Hedgehog (Hh) pathway, 241
HEF1, 116
Hemangioblastoma, 465, 467, 635–636
  adjuvant therapy in, 473–474
  imaging features, 468–469
  IMSCT genetics, 466
  occurrence of, 818
  treatment approach for, 818
    fractionated adjuvant
      radiotherapy, 818
    stereotactic radiosurgery, 818
  tumor structure of, 818
  von Hippel-Lindau disease,
    association with, 818
Hemangiomas studies, 27
Hemangiopericytoma (HPC), 192, 600, 602
  age and gender distribution of, 818
  treatment approach for, 818
    complete surgical resection, 818
    postoperative radiotherapy,
      use of, 818
Hemiparesis, 345

Hemiparetic weakness, 258
Hemiplegia, 345
Hemispheric gliomas, 274
Hepatocyte growth factor (HGF).
  See Scatter factor (SF)
Hereditary nonpolyposis colorectal
  cancer (HNPCC), 242
Hereditary syndromes, for primary
  brain tumors (PBTs), 15
Heschl's transverse gyri, 378–379
HIC1 (hypermethylated in cancer), 64
HIC-1 tumor suppressor gene, 63
Hierarchical model. See Cancer stem
  cell (CSC) hypothesis
HIF-1α, 124
HIF-1β, 124
HIF-1 transcriptional complex, 123
HIG2 (hypoxia-inducible protein-2), 108
High-grade astrocytomas, 216, 217f
  clinical overview, 216
  molecular genetics, 216
    chromosomal alterations, 216–219
    translational therapies, 219
High-grade glial neoplasms, 771
High-grade gliomas, 7, 326, 562
  anaplastic astrocytomas (AAs), 569–570
  anaplastic oligodendroglioma (AO),
    570–572
  in children, 9
  definitive treatment, 570–572
  glioblastoma (GBM), 563
    chemotherapy, 564–566
    in elderly, 566–567
    molecularly targeted therapies,
      567–568
    radiotherapy (RT), 564
    recurrent, 557
    surgery, 563
  malignant, 273
  medical management for
    future direction for, 581
    radiation and chemotherapy, 579–580
    recurrent, 581
    surgery, 579
    in very young children, 581
  molecular and genetic alterations
    in, 582t
  patients, late encephalopathy in, 329
  survival rate for, 10
Highly active antiretroviral therapy
  (HAART), 657
  and HIV-positive PCNSL patients, 883
High risk patients, of PNETs
  concurrent radiotherapy and
    chemical trials, 785–786
  current standard of care, 786
  hyperfractionated radiotherapy
    trials, 786
  neoadjuvant chemotherapy
    trials, 784–785
  postradiotherapy chemotherapy
    trials, 785
  radiotherapy dose escalation trials, 786
HIMAC and HARIMAC, in Japan, 732
Hippocampal formation, 379
Hirschsprung disease, 228
Hispanics, glioma in, 7

Histamine, 22
Histiocytosis X, diagnosis of, 848
Histogenesis, meningiomass and, 822
*Histological Groups for Comparative
  Studies*, 4
Histological type, distribution of
  glioma by, 6
Histologic grade, 47
Histologic subtypes and variants,
  meningiomas, 823–824
Histone acetyltransferases (HATs), 681
Histone deacetylase inhibitors
  (HDACs), 222, 681
  inhibitors, 706–707
HIV-positive PCNSL patients,
  HAART and, 883
HK2 (hexokinase 2), 108
HLA-A*32, 54
HLA-B*55, 54
hMLH1 gene, 16
hMSH2 gene, 16
hMSH6 gene, 16
Hoffman signs, 300
Homologous recombination, 145, 146f
Hook effect, 446
Hormonally active pituitary adenomas
  Cushing disease, 292–293
  GH-secreting adenomas, 293
  PRL-secreting adenomas, 293
Hormone-inactive adenomas, 628t
Hormone-secreting adenomas, 628t
Hospice, 351
  care, implementation of, 314
Hounsfield units (HUs), 401
House-Brackmann Facial-Nerve
  Grading Scale, for vestibular
  schwannoma, 812t
hPMS gene, 16
H-ras mutation, 180
hSNF5/INI-1 gene, 58
Hsp90, 683
HSV-1, 696
HSV-TK/ganciclovir system, 701
hTERT gene, 54
Human fibroblast interferon (HFIF), 561
Human glioblastoma, intratumoral
  heterogeneity in, 104f
Human gliomas, expression
  profiling of, 94
Human leukocyte antigen (HLA), 54
Human tumor panels and high-
  throughput preclinical testing, 156
Human tumor xenograft models, 154
  cell culture–based methods, 154
  orthotopic vs. heterotopic
    tumor cell growth, 155
  xenograft-based tumor
    propagation, 154–155
Humoral immunity, 692
Humoral-mediated immunotherapy
  ligand-toxin conjugates, 694–695
  passive antibody transfer, 694
Hydrocephalus, 286, 287, 521, 528–529
Hydrocortisone, 306
Hydroxamic acids, 707
Hydroxyurea, 605, 635, 677
Hypercalcemia, 344

Hyperfractionated craniospinal
  radiotherapy (HFRT), 591, 594
  trials, for high-risk PNET, 786
Hyperplastic lesions, 542
Hyperprolactinemia, 178
  causes of, 446t
Hypoglossal schwannomas, 286
Hypopituitarism, radiation-induced, 865
Hypoplasia
  radiation therapy toxicity, in
    ependymoma, 802
Hypothalamic glioma, 626
Hypothalamic hamartoma, 627
Hypothalamus, 286
Hypoxia, 103
Hypoxia-inducible factor-1 (HIF-1), 101
Hypoxia-response elements (HREs), 124
Hypoxic GBM cells, 101

^{125}I, 725, 726
^{131}I-81C6 (anti-tenascin monoclonal
  antibody), 734
^{131}I-m81C6, 694
Idarubicin, 586
Ifosfamide, 473, 580, 586, 595, 634, 635
  for average-risk PNET, 782
Ifosfamide/etoposide
  for NGGCTs, 876
Ik6 isoform, 182
Ikaros (Ik), 182
IL4R gene, 54
Image-guided radiation therapy
  (IGRT), 728
Imaging of brain tumors, 353
  computed tomography, 353
  magnetic resonance imaging, 353
    assessing edema, 355
    diffusion weighted imaging
      (DWI), 353–355
    dynamic contrast enhancement
      (DCE), 362–363
    dynamic susceptibility contrast
      imaging (DSCI), 356–362
    functional magnetic resonance
      imaging (fMRI), 364
    grading tumors, 355
    magnetic resonance spectroscopy
      (MRS), 363
    mobile lipids, 363–364
    novel contrast agents, 364, 365t
    perfusion MRI, 356
    postoperative injury, 355
    white matter tracts, assessing
      integrity of, 355–356
  PET imaging, 365
    FET-PET, 366
    indications, 365
    MET-PET, 365–366
    single-photon emission
      tomography (SPECT), 366
  multichannel magnetoencephalography
    (MEG), 366
  serial assessment
    initial assessment, 366
    post-treatment response
      assessment, 367

Imaging of brain tumors (cont.)
  two-dimensional methods, 366
  volumetric methods, 367
Imaging techniques and
  meningiomass, 821
Imatinib mesylate (Gleevec), 90,
  605, 616, 617, 676, 677, 682
Imidazole carboxamide, 620
Immune function genes, 65
Immunocompetent hosts
  chemically induced tumor cells, 153
  transgenic models, 153–154
Immunoglobulin E (IgE)
  elevated, 54
  levels and glioma growth, 39
Immunohistochemistry, 189
  chordomas and chondrosarcomas
    comparison, 847
  of MPNST, 192
Immunosuppression, 41
Immunosuppressive regulatory
  T-cells, 42
Immunotherapeutic strategies,
  for brain tumors, 692
Incidence and mortality rates, of glioma, 1
Incidence and prevalence,
  meningiomas, 820–821
  age and gender distribution, 821f
Incidence rates, of glioma
  in childhood, 9
  by gender, 7–9
  by histological type, 7
  overall incidence rates, ethnicity,
    and age, 7
  trends in, 9
Incisural meningiomass, 284
Infant medulloblastoma, 790
Infectious agents causing brain tumors, 62
Inferior parietal lobule, functional
  neuroanatomy of, 379–380
Infiltrating astrocytomas,
  microenvironment of, 101f
Infiltrating gliomas, molecular
  subtypes of, 94
  non-mRNA based markers, 95
Infratentorial neoplasms, 530
Inherited brain tumor predisposition
  syndromes, 249t, 252f
Inherited susceptibility to glioma, 14–17
INK4A gene, 190
Insula
  functions, 505
  normal anatomy, 505–506
Insular tumors, 505
  classifications, 507–508
  clinical presentation, 508
  complication avoidance, surgical
    considerations for, 509
    internal capsule injury, 511
    MCA manipulation, 510–511
    opercular retraction, 509–510
    perforating vessels, 511
  intraoperative adjuncts, 514
  pathological anatomy, 506
  surgical anatomy, 511f
  surgical method, 511
    MCA exposure, 512

peri-insular sulcus dissection,
  512–513
position and craniotomy, 511
sylvian fissure dissection, 511–512
tumor devascularization, 513–514
tumor mass removal, 514
surgical decision making, 508–509
surgical outcomes, 514
  neurologic function, 514–515
  resection, extent of, 515–516
types, 506
Insulin-like growth factor I (IGF-1), 447
Integrin inhibitors, 681
Integrin-linked kinase, 113
Integrin receptor coordination with
  growth factor receptors, 114
Intelligence quotient (IQ) test, 335
Intensity-modulated radiation
  therapy (IMRT), 454, 728,
  744–745, 746, 788, 863
Intercessory prayer, 714
Interferon-a2b, 635
Interferon alpha, 634
Interferon α-2a, 474
Interferon-β, 604
Interferons (IFNs), 700
Interleukin (IL)-101
  in allergic conditions, 41
  in glioma, 41
  and glioma survival time, 42
  paradoxical role, 43
Interleukin (IL)-4
  receptor alpha (IL-4Rα), 40, 41
Interleukin (IL)-6, 54
Interleukin (IL)-8, 101
  expression, 102
Interleukin (IL)-13, 40, 41
International Classification of
  Childhood Cancer (ICCC), 4
*International Classification of Diseases for
  Oncology, Third Edition* (ICD-O-3), 4
International Neuroblastoma Pathology
  Classification System (INPC), 234
International Neuroblastoma Staging
  System (INSS), 225
Intracavitary radiotherapy, 864
Intracranial germ cell tumors (GCTs), 874
Intracranial meningiomass, 599
  clinical presentation of, 824
  EBRT vs. SRS, 833
    (WHO Grade I), 837t
  epidemiology of, 820–821
    gender, age, and race
      distributions, 821
    incidence and prevalence, 820–821
    etiologic factors of, 820
  molecular genetics and
    histopathology of, 821–824
    histogenesis, 822
    histologic subtypes and
      variants, 823–824
    molecular genetics, 821–822
    recurrence-free survival, 822, 823
    tumor grade, 822–823
  molecular neuropathology, 600–602
  neuroimaging and, 602–603, 824
  neuropathology, 599–600

sites of origin of, 826t
special circumstances, 833–836
  incidental meningiomass, 835–836
  nonbenign meningiomass, 833–835
  recurrent meningiomass, 835
treatment, 603
  drug therapies, 604–605
  radiotherapy, 603–604
  surgery, 603
treatment and outcome, 824–833
  fractionated external beam
    radiation therapy, 828–833
  gross total resection, 825
  radiation therapy, 825–826
  stereotactic radiosurgery, 826–828
  subtotal resection, 825
  surgery, 824–825
Intracranial pressure (ICP), 349
Intracranial tumors, 6
Intracranial xenograft bioluminescence
  signal variation, 155f, 156f
Intradural-extramedullary neoplasms
  ependymoma myxopapillary, 635
  meningiomas, 634
  nerve sheath tumors of the spine,
    634–635
  paraganglioma, 635
Intramedullary spinal cord metastasis,
  adjuvant therapy in, 474
Intramedullary spinal cord tumors
  (IMSCT), 465, 635
  astrocytoma, 635
  ependymoma, 466, 635
  functional evaluation, 472t
  hemangioblastoma, 466, 635–636
  metastasis, 636
Intramedullary tumors, of spinal
  canal, 301–302
Intraocular lymphoma (IOL),
  650, 651, 652
  primary IOL, 657–658
Intraoperative anatomical imaging, 407
  brain shift, 408
  technologies
    contrast agents, 416–417
    future developments, 417
    high-field iMRI approaches, 412
    image quality, 408–409
    iMRI-based neuronavigation, 417
    intraoperative CT, 410–411
    intraoperative MRI, 411
    intraoperative ultrasound, 408
    iUS and neuronavigation systems, 409
    iUS, applications of, 409
    length of surgery, effect on, 414
    low-field iMRI approaches, 411–412
    mid-field iMRI approaches, 412
    resection, effect on, 412–413
    surgical instruments, effect on,
      414–416
    3-dimensional iUS, applications, and
      future developments, 409–410
  tumor invasion, 407–408
Intraoperative computed tomography
  (iCT), 407, 410–411
Intraoperative consultation, 189
  of MPNST, 192

Intraoperative functional mapping, 428
  language function mapping during
      awake craniotomy
    indications, 430–431
    neuroanesthetic regimen, 431
    preoperative functional imaging, 431
    preoperative neurological
        evaluation, 431
    surgical technique, 431–433
  motor-function mapping during
      asleep craniotomy, 428
    indications, 428
    preoperative functional
        imaging, 428–429
    preoperative neurological
        evaluation, 428
    surgical technique, 429–430
Intraoperative molecular imaging
    (ioMRI), 404–405, 411–412, 421, 481
  fluorescence-guided surgery using
      5-aminolevulinic acid, 422
    dosage and time of ALA
        application, 423
    efficacy, 422–423
    equipment, 424
    implementation during surgery,
        424–425
    light protection, 423–424
    photobleaching, 425
    pitfalls, 425–426
    resection, 425
    safety profile, 423
  previously used fluorescent
      agents, 421–422
  rationale for, 421
Intraoperative ultrasound (iUS), 407
  applications of, 409
  and neuronavigation systems, 409
  3-dimensional iUS, 409–410
Intraparenchymal schwannomas, 167
Intraparietal sulcus/superior parietal
    lobule approach, 499–500
Intrathecal (IT) chemotherapy, 646
Intratumoral heterogeneity, in human
    glioblastoma, 104f
Intraventricular cytosine arabinoside
    (IVT Ara-C), 646
Intraventricular tumors, 496
  anterior interhemispheric
      transcallosal approach, 497–498
  in children, 523
    choroid plexus tumors, 523–524
    central neurocytoma, 524–525
    endoscopy in, 525
    thalamic gliomas, 525
  fourth ventricle, surgical approaches
      to, 502–503
  interforniceal approach, 501–502
  intraparietal sulcus/superior parietal
      lobule approach, 499–500
  lateral ventricles, surgical approaches
      to, 496
  middle fronal gyrus/superior frontal
      sulcus approach, 500
  middle temporal gyrus/superior
      temporal sulcus, 498
  occipitotemporal sulcus approach, 499

  pertinent anatomy, 500–501
  posterior interhemispheric
      transcingular approach, 498–499
  subfrontal approach, 502
  third ventricle, surgical approaches
      to, 500
  transchoroidal approach, 501
  transforaminal approach, 501
Intrinsic resistance, 135
Invasion, 93–94
Invasive behavior of glioma, 112
  mechanisms
    adaptor molecules, 116–117
    cell surface receptors, changes in
        expression of, 114–115
    changes in ECM, 112–114
    cytoplasmic kinases, role of, 115–116
    phosphatidylinositol-3-hydroxyl
        kinase (PI3K), 117
    protease/protease receptor
        expression, changes in, 115
    protein kinase C, 117
    PTEN, 117
  process of invasion, 112
Invasive pituitary adenoma,
    diagnosis of, 848
3-123I-Iodo-alpha-methyl-l-tyrosine
    SPECT (IMT-SPECT), 366
Ionizing radiation, 2, 26, 60, 721
  case-control studies, 28
  case reports, 26
  and meningiomass, 820
  prospective studies, 26
    ALL studies, 27
    Childhood Cancer Survivor Study, 27
    dose-response relationship, 27–28
    hemangiomas studies, 27
    occupational exposure, 28
    relative risk variance, 28
    tinea capitis cohorts, 26–27
Irinotecan (Camptosar), 305, 564,
    580, 586, 680, 685
Isocitrate dehydrogenase-1 (IDH1), 150
Isoflavones, 711
Isoprene, 18–19
Isotopes for brachytherapy, 725

JC virus, 62, 222
Job-exposure matrix (JEM), 36
Johrei, 714
Joint contractures, 345
Jugular foramen meningiomass, 285
Jugular foramen syndrome, 288
"Jumping ahead" by glioma cells, 112
Juvenile pilocytic astrocytoma (JPA), 216

Kadish stage A/B/C disease, 618–619
Kaplan-Meier analyses, 422
Karnofsky Performance Status
    (KPS), 313, 552
  anaplastic gliomas, 752
Ketoconazole, 628
Ki-67/MIB-1 antibody, 106
Ki-67 antigen, 178
Ki-67 labeling index, 600

KIF1 beta, 232
Krestin (PSK), 711

Lactate, 363
Lactotroph adenomas, 178
Laminin-8, 113, 114
Lamotrigine, 330
Lamustine, 591
Language function mapping
    during awake craniotomy
  indications, 430–431
  neuroanesthetic regimen, 431
  preoperative functional imaging, 431
  preoperative neurological
      evaluation, 431
  surgical technique, 431–433
Language surface functional
    anatomy, 374f
Lanreotide (Somatuline), 630
Lapatinib, 645
Late encephalopathy
  in extracranial malignancies, 329–330
  in high-grade glioma patients, 329
  in low-grade glioma patients, 328–329
Laterality of mobile phone use, 34
Lateral ventricles, surgical
    approaches to, 496
Late-responding tissues, 723
Latinos, incidence rates for
    glioblastomas in, 7
l-dopa, 392
Lenalidomide, 672
Lentiviral vectors, 698
Leptomeningeal carcinomatosis, 645
Leptomeningeal disease (LMD), 645
  intrathecal chemotherapy for, 646
  palliative treatments, 645–646
  presentation and diagnosis, 645
  systemic therapy options, 646
Leptomeningeal metastases
    (LMM), 645, 917
Lesion momentum, 320
Letrozole, 646
Leukemia
  acute lymphoblastic leukemia, 27
  chronic myelogenous leukemia, 676
  risk for, 28
Leukoencephalopathy, 329, 331
Level of alertness (LOA), 307–308
Levetiracetam, 305, 330
Lhermitte-Duclos disease (LDD), 244, 244f
Lifestyle, chemical exposure mediated
    through, 18
Li–Fraumeni-like syndrome
    (LFL), 15, 243
Li-Fraumeni syndrome (LFS),
    15t, 15–16, 219–220
  animal models, 244
  clinical features and diagnostic
      criteria, 243
  molecular pathogenesis, 243
  therapy and prognosis, 244
LIG1 gene, 601
Ligand-toxin conjugates, 694–695
Lignins, 711
Linear-quadratic (LQ) model, 722–723

Lomustine (CCNU), 330, 549, 586, 618
Lonafarnib (Sarasar), 91, 679
Long-term mobile phone use, 34
    according to laterality of phone use, 35t
    epidemiological studies, 33t
Long white matter tracts, 381
Lonidamine, 640
Loss of heterozygosity (LOH), 63, 185
    LOH 1p/19q, 760, 761
    LOH 10q, 63
    in CDKN2A gene, 190
Low-grade astrocytoma, 771, 772, 773
Low-grade gliomas (LGG), 273, 275, 477, 556, 557f
    adjuvant treatment, 482–483
    biopsy, 479–481
    chemotherapy for, 558–561
    in children, 9
    classification, 478t
    clinical presentation of, 762–763
    clinical signs and symptoms, 478
    common symptoms of, 762–763
        headache, 763
        motor deficit, occurrence of, 763
        seizure, 762
    FLAIR MRI, 479f
    grade and prognostic factors, 760
    imaging, 478–479
    introduction to, 760
        age and gender distribution, 760
        common molecular genetic alterations, 760
        pilocytic astrocytoma, 760
    medical management for, 582
        cerebellar astrocytomas, 584–585
        cerebral low-grade glioma, 583
        ependymomas, 585–586
        optic pathway glioma, 583–584
    p53 function, loss of, 761
    pathology, 477–478
        classifications, 760
    patients, late encephalopathy in, 328–329
    PFS rates and, 763
    prognostic factors and, 760–762
        clinical, 760–761
        molecular, 761–762
        poor prognosis, indicators of, 761
    prospective neurocognitive trials of, 763t
    radiological features of, 762
    recurrent disease, 765–766
    resection and outcome, extent of, 482
    surgery, 481–482, 557–558
        management, strategies for, 479
    survival rate for, 10, 11
    treatment options
        chemotherapy in combination with radiotherapy, 765
        observation, 763
        radiotherapy, 764–765
        surgery, 763–764
Low-molecular-weight heparin (LMWH), 307
loxP recombination, 147
Lycopene, 712

Lymphoma, 626
    diagnosis of, 848
    intraocular lymphoma, 650, 651, 652
    neurolymphoma, 539f
    Non-Hodgkin's lymphoma, 43–44, 650
    primary central nervous system lymphoma, 306, 650
    primary cerebral lymphoma, 361

Macdonald Criteria, 366
Macroadenomas, surgical management of, 447
Magnetic resonance imaging (MRI), 16, 297, 326, 353, 421, 616
    assessing edema, 355
    benign nonperipheral nerve sheath tumors, 536
    benign peripheral nerve sheath tumors, 535–536
    brachial plexus tumor, 535
    and chordomas, 849
    decision on whom to operate, 539–540
    diffusion weighted imaging (DWI), 353–355
    dynamic contrast enhancement (DCE), 362–363
    dynamic susceptibility contrast imaging (DSCI), 356–362
    functional magnetic resonance imaging (fMRI), 364
    fusion, 746, 748f
    grading tumors, 355
    guided therapy machines, 730t
    magnetic resonance spectroscopy (MRS), 363
    malignant peripheral nerve and nonperipheral nerve sheath tumors, 537–539
    medulloblastoma, 527
    for meningomas, 602–603
    metastatic spinal tumors, 458–459
    mobile lipids, 363–364
    novel contrast agents, 364, 365t
    other benign lesions affecting nerve, 536–537
    percutaneous biopsy, 539
    perfusion MRI, 356
        stereotactic brain biopsy, 403
    postoperative injury, 355
    primary spinal tumors, 453
    spinal cord tumors, 467
    stereotactic brain biopsy, 401–402
    white matter tracts, assessing integrity of, 355–356
Magnetic resonance perfusion, 280
Magnetic resonance simulators, 746
Magnetic resonance spectroscopy (MRS), 363
    in glioma grading, 363
    stereotactic brain biopsy, 402–403
Magnetic source imaging (MSI), 371, 428, 429f
Magnetoencephalography (MEG), 428
    and transcranial magnetic stimulation, 371–372

Major histocompatibility complexes (MHC), 692
Male-to-female ratios, of incidence rates for glioma, 7
Malignant central nervous system (CNS) tumors, 57
Malignant epidural cord compression, patients with, 348
Malignant glioma (MG), 6, 273, 363
    in children, 9
    growth factor receptor expression in, 114t
    hallmarks of, 90, 90f
        angiogenesis, 93
        antigrowth signals, insensitivity to, 91–92
        apoptosis, evasion of, 92
        autophagy, decrease of, 93
        cell cycle dysregulation, 92
        EGFR, 91
        growth signals, self-sufficiency in, 90
        invasion, 93–94
        MAPK pathway, 91
        mitogenic signaling pathways, 91
        p53 pathway, 92
        PDGF/PDGFR, 90
        PI3K pathway, 91
        Rb pathway, 92
        TGF-β, 91
        unlimited replicative potential, 93
    incidence, 9f
    integrin expression in, 114t
    survival rate for, 10
Malignant glioma (MG) therapy, signal transduction pathways inhibitors in, 676
    growth factor receptor signaling pathways in, 679f
    investigational targeted molecular agents for, 678t
    NOS, 7
    targeted molecular agents, 676
        cyclooxygenase inhibitors, 680–681
        epidermal growth factor receptor inhibitors, 676–677
        farnesyltransferase inhibitors, 677, 679
        histone deacetylase inhibitors, 681
        mammalian target of rapamycin inhibitors, 679–680
        matrix metalloproteinase and integrin inhibitors, 681
        phosphatidylinositol-3 kinase inhibitors, 680
        platelet-derived growth factor receptor inhibitors, 677
        proteasome inhibitors, 681
        protein kinase C inhibitors, 680
        VEGFR and VEGFR inhibitors, 680
    targeted molecular agents, improving efficacy of, 681, 685–686
        addressing multiple targets simultaneously, 682
        agents that inhibit multiple targets, 682–683
        combinations of targeted molecular agents, 683–684

combining targeted molecular agents with chemotherapy, 684–685
combining targeted molecular agents with RT, 684
reliable animal models, creating, 682
target selection, optimizing, 682
Malignant nerve sheath tumors (MNSTs), 634, 635
Malignant peripheral nerve sheath tumors (MPNST), 185, 191f, 250, 542–543, 615t, 619–620, 635
background, 185, 189
cytotoxic chemotherapy, 620
histopathology, 190–192
with mesenchymal differentiation, 191
molecular pathogenesis, 189–190
molecularly targeted agents, 620
Malignant triton tumor (MTT), 191
Mammalian target of rapamycin (mTOR)
inhibitors, 679–680
signaling, 250
Mammography, 16
Mammosomatotroph adenomas, 178
MAPK pathway, 91
Marijuana, 711
Matairesinol, 711
Matrix metalloproteinases (MMP), 91, 94, 115, 187, 681
McCune-Albright syndrome, 174
MCT3 (monocarboxylate tansporter3), 64
MDM2 gene, 92
MDM4 gene, 92
Measles virus, 697
Meat consumption, 21
Mechlorethamine, oncovin-vincristin, procarbacine, and prednisone (MOPP), 592
Median-nerve schwannoma, 541f
Medical therapy as cause of cognitive deficits
antiepileptic drugs, 330
chemotherapy, 330–331
steroids, 331
Medical treatment primary cns germ cell tumors, 661
germinomas, 661–662
nongerminomatous germ cell tumors, 662
Medicare, 314
Medications, 22
antihistamines, 22–23
COX-2 inhibitors, 22
Medullablastoma, 16, 58, 62, 206, 219, 220f, 239, 242, 267, 527–528, 781. *See also* Primitive neuroectodermal tumors (PNETs)
association with T-antigen of JC virus, 222
cerebellar, 208f
chromosomal alterations, 220
classic, 206
clinical overview, 219
clinical presentation, 268–269
dissemination, 271
and epigenetics, 222
etiology, 267–268
evaluation of, 781

familiar cancer syndromes, 219
Gorlin syndrome, 219
Li-Fraumeni syndrome, 219–220
Turcot syndrome, 219
incidence, 267
medical management of, 589
chemotherapy, 591
late effects, 592
radiation therapy, 590–591
staging and risk stratification, 589–590
surgical resection, 590
in very young child, 592–593
molecular genetics, 219
neuroradiographic findings, 269–271
origins of, 196–199
radiotherapy complications
acute side effects, 790
late complications, 790–791
radiotherapy technique, 786–789
radiotherapy treatment evolution, clinical trials, 781–782
re-treatment of, 791
risk groups, 781
selected clinical trials, 782t
signaling pathways, 220, 221f
Notch pathway, 221
sonic hedgehog (SHH) pathway, 220–221
Wnt/B-catenin pathway, 221
staging, 271
translational therapies, 222
variants, 206–207
treatment volumes, 786
Medulloblastoma variants, 206–207
Medulloepithelioma, 208–209, 844
Megestrol acetate, 646
Melanoma-associated antigen A3 gene (*MAGE-A3*) gene, 182
Melanotic neurofibroma, 187
Melanotic schwannomas, 170
Meningiomass, 59, 71, 158, 252, 282, 283, 297, 298, 361, 385, 387, 388, 389, 389f, 390f, 625, 634, 878. *See also* Adenomas; Astrocytomas; Cancer; Carcinomas; Ependymomas; Gliomas; Metastases; Neurofibromas; Papillomas; Sarcomas; Tumors
arachnoid cap cells, 159f
anaplastic meningiomas, 600
breast cancer, association with, 71–72
cavernous sinus meningiomas, 285
chordoid meningiomas, 160, 160f, 600, 823t
clear cell meningiomas, 160, 160f, 600, 823t
clinoidal meningiomas, 284
clival meningiomas, 284
clivus meningiomas, 848, 853f
craniospinal meningiomas, 285
environment, interaction with, 73–76
epidemiology, 71
en plaque meningiomas, 282
family history, 71
fibroblastic meningiomas, 160f
foramen magnum meningiomas, 390f

fossa meningiomas, 158f
general considerations, 283
genetic polymorphisms, 73
genetics, 161
background, 161
chromosome 1p, 162
chromosome 9p, 163
chromosome 10, 163
chromosome 14q, 163
chromosome 17, 163
chromosome 22q, 162
radiation, 164
telomere stability, 163–164
grading, 158
incidence, 158
incisural meningiomas, 284
intracranial meningiomas, 599
jugular foramen meningiomas, 285
location, 158
meningothelial meningiomas, 159f
metaplastic meningiomas, 160f
microarray analyses, 76
microcystic meningiomas, 159, 160f
middle fossa meningiomas, 158f
molecular genetics, 72–73
olfactory groove meningiomas, 159f, 282, 283
optic nerve meningiomas, 283
papillary meningiomas, 160, 823t
parasagittal meningiomas, 828
pathology
immunohistochemistry and electron microscopy, 161
macroscopic, 158
microscopic, 158–161
petroclival meningiomas, 284–285
posterior pyramid meningiomas, 285
psammomatous meningiomas, 159, 160f, 167
and radiation therapy, 896
rhabdoid meningiomas, 160, 823t
secretory meningiomas, 159, 160f, 161
sphenoid wing meningiomas, 284, 388f
suprasellar meningiomas, 283–284
transitional meningiomas, 160f
trigeminal meningiomas, 284
tuberculum sellae meningiomas, 390f
Meningothelial meningiomas, 159f, 160f
Meningothelial tumors, 159
Merlin, 170, 252
Mesenchymal tumors, 59
Mesna, 634
Metaiodobenzylguanidine (MIBG), 227f, 618
Metalloproteinases-1 inhibitors, 711
Metaplastic meningiomas, 160f
Metastases. *See also* Adenomas; Astrocytomas; Cancer; Carcinomas; Ependymomas; Gliomas; Meningiomas; Neurofibromas; Papillomas; Sarcomas; Tumors
brain metastases, 638
diagnosis of, 848
leptomeningeal metastases, 645, 917
skull base hematogenous metastases, 287
spine metastases, 909

Metastatic brain tumor (MBT), 304
Metastatic disease
  brain metastases, clinical problems
      associated with, 902
    brachytherapy, 909
    fractionated stereotactic
        radiotherapy, 908–909
    palliative whole-brain
        radiotherapy, 902–905
    plus whole-brain radiotherapy,
        907–908
    radiosurgery, 906–907
    recurrent lesion, retreatment for, 909
    surgical resection, whole-brain
        radiotherapy (WBRT) after, 905–906
  leptomeningeal metastases, 917
  spine metastases
    metastatic spinal cord compression
        (MSCC), radiotherapy alone and,
        910–915
    radiopharmaceuticals for, 917
    radiosurgery, 916
Metastatic epidural spinal cord
    compression (MESCC), 458
Metastatic spinal cord compression
    (MSCC), 910–911
  backpain caused by, 910–911
  chemotherapy, radiotherapy
      supplemented by, 915
  decompressive surgery, 915–916
  functional outcome after radiotherapy
      alone, 912–913
  glucocorticosteroids in treating, 911
  "impending" MSCC, 910
  patients with oligometastatic disease,
      radiotherapy alone for, 915
  radiotherapy alone, 911–912
  radiotherapy alone and
      bisphosphonates, recalcification
      following, 913
  and spinal reirradiation, in-field
      recurrences of, 914
  spinal MRI for, 911
  survival after radiotherapy alone,
      914–915
  white-matter edema and axonal
      swelling, associations with, 910
Metastatic spinal tumors, 458
  chemotherapy and radiation
      therapy, 459–460
  clinical presentation and
      workup, 458–459
  surgical management, 460–461
Metastatic tumors, 288
Methotrexate (MTX), 305, 306, 331, 344,
    580, 595, 646, 654–655, 657
  for average-risk PNET, 782
  for high-risk PNET, 784
Methylnitrosourea (MNU), 20, 21
Methylphenidate (Ritalin), 322, 339
MET-PET, 365–366
Metronidazole, 640
Metyrapone, 628
Meyer's loop, 379
MGMT gene, 54
MIB1/Ki67 immunohistochemistry, 161
Microcystic meningiomass, 159, 160*f*

Microinjection, 145
Micro-RNAs (miRNAs), 95
Microsatellite instability (MSI), 16, 217
Microtubule-associated protein-2, 892
Microvascular hyperplasia, 100
Midbrain tumors, 611
Middle cerebral artery (MCA),
    510–511, 512
Middle fossa syndrome, 288
Middle fronal gyrus/superior frontal
    sulcus approach, 500
Middle temporal gyrus/superior
    temporal sulcus, 498
Migraine headaches, 260
Mind-body therapies, 713
Minimal access craniotom, 394–395
miR-21, 95
miRNAs, 129
Misonidazole, 640
Missense mutations, families with, 15
Mitogenic growth signals, 90
Mitogenic signaling pathways, 91
Mitogens, 84
Mitotane, 628–629
Mixed gangliocytoma-adenoma
    (MGA), 625
Mixed oligo-astrocytoma,
    survival rates of, 764*f*
MLN518, 677
MNS16A, 54
Mobile lipids, 363–364
Mobile phone use
  and glioma risk, 32
    laterality of mobile phone use, 34
    long-term mobile phone use, 34
    short-term mobile phone use, 32–34
  health effects of, 2
  laterality of, 34
  long-term, 34
  short-term, 32–34
Modafinil, 322
Molecular genetic and epigenetic
    characteristics, 63
Molecular genetics and
    meningiomass, 821–822
Molecular heterogeneity and
    tumor microenvironment, 100
  astrocytic neoplasms, growth
      patterns of, 100–101
  cellular heterogeneity, 105
    differentiation patterns, 105–106
    proliferative/apoptotic
        heterogeneity, 106–107
    stem cells/glioma progenitor
        cells, 106
  glioblastoma multiforme
    hypoxic and metabolic
        heterogeneity in, 103–104
    vascular heterogeneity in, 101–102
  proton magnetic resonance
      spectroscopy imaging of tumor
      metabolites, 104–105
  genetic heterogeneity, 107–108
Molecular neuro-oncology, essentiality, 79
Molecular pathogenesis of glioma, 88
  cells of origin, 88
  glioma classification, 88

  human gliomas, expression
      profiling of, 94
  infiltrating gliomas, molecular
      subtypes of, 94
  non-mRNA based markers, 95
  malignant gliomas, hallmarks of, 90
    angiogenesis, 93
    antigrowth signals, insensitivity
        to, 91–92
    apoptosis, evasion of, 92
    autophagy, decrease of, 93
    cell cycle dysregulation, 92
    EGFR, 91
    growth signals, self-sufficiency in, 90
    invasion, 93–94
    MAPK pathway, 91
    mitogenic signaling pathways, 91
    p53 pathway, 92
    PDGF/PDGFR, 90
    PI3K pathway, 91
    Rb pathway, 92
    TGF-β, 91
    unlimited replicative potential, 93
  malignant progression, pathways of
    astrocytoma, 88–89
    oligoastrocytoma, 90
    oligodendrogliomas, 89–90
Molecular pathology of gliomas, 122–123
Monoclonal antibodies (mAbs), 666
Mood disorder as cause of cognitive
    deficits, 331
MOPP (mechlorethamine, oncovin-
    vincristin, procarbacine, and
    prednisone), 592
Mortality
  and radiotherapy, 865
  rates, of glioma, 1
Motexafin gadolinium (MGd), 640, 749
Motor evoked potential (MEP)
    monitoring, 514, 515
Motor-function mapping during
    asleep craniotomy, 428
  indications, 428
  preoperative functional imaging,
      428–429
  preoperative neurological
      evaluation, 428
  surgical technique, 429–430
Mouse transgenesis, techniques for, 145
  cell/tissue-specific transgenesis, 146–147
  ES cell-mediated transgenesis, 146
  homologous recombination, 145, 146*f*
  pronuclear injection, 145–146
  somatic gene transfer, using RCAS-tva
      system, 147–148
MRI/x-ray/OR suite (MRXO), 412, 415*f*
mRNA editing, 186
M-tetrahydroxyphenylchlorin, 421
Müller glia cells, 196
Multichannel magnetoencephalography
    (MEG), 366
Multidrug resistance genes, 232
Multiple cranial nerve abnormalities, 343
Multiple endocrince neoplasia (MEN)
  animal models, 245
  clinical features and diagnostic
      criteria, 245

molecular pathogenesis, 245
therapy and prognosis, 245
Multiple schwannoma syndromes, 167–168
Multipotent neural progenitors, 82
Multireceptor tyrosine kinase
inhibitors, 93
Multitarget model, 722
Musashi-1, 84, 84*t*
Mustard/vincristine/procar-bazine
(MOP) therapy, 561
Mutism, 529–530
MYCN amplification, 230–231, 233, 234
MYCN-amplified neuroblastomas, 229
MYC oncogene, 220
Myelopathy, 297, 344
Myxopapillary ependymoma, 58, 635, 799

N-acetyl aspartate (NAA), 279, 363, 402
Naproxen, 22
National Cancer Act, 342
National Cancer Institute, 54, 342
National Center for Complementary
and Alternative Medicine
(NCCAM), 710
National Human Genome Research
Institute, 54
Navigation-directed brain biopsy, 396
NDRG2, 72
Neck tumor, 34
Necrosis, microscopic foci of, 100
Needle electrode technique, 103
Nelson syndrome, radiotherapy
for, 867, 868*t*
Neoadjuvant chemotherapy, 454
Neovascularization of glioma
tumors, 122, 124*f*
angiogenesis in gliomas, 122
angiopoietins and VEGFs, 125–128
c-Met, 128
endogenous antiangiogenic
factors, 128
epigenetic alterations, 129
genetic alterations, 128–129
"glioma stem cells" and tumor
neovascularization, 129
molecular pathology, 122–123
scatter factor (SF), 128
SDF-1α, 128
by tumor hypoxia and metabolism,
123–125
antiangiogenic therapies in gliomas
patients
clinical trials, 133
clinical vignette, 133–135
complications, 135–137
rationale, patient selection, and
outcome measure, 132–133
resistance to, 135
vasculogenesis in gliomas
and angiogenesis, 129–130
circulating endothelial cells in glioma
neovascularization, 130–131
proangiogenic cells in glioma
neovascularization, 131
potential molecular and cellular
biomarkers, 132

Nerve sheath tumors of spine, 634–635
Nervous system tumors, 79, 80
Nestin, 81, 82, 83, 84*t*
Neural cell adhesion molecule
(NCAM), 733
Neural stem cells (NSCs), 106
Neurilemmomas. *See* Schwannomas
Neurinomas. *See* Schwannomas
Neuroanatomy, functional, 371
brainstem, 380
cranial nerve circuitry, 380–381
long white matter tracts, 381
reticular circuitry, 381
frontal lobe, 372
Broca's area, 377–378
frontal eye fields, 377
insula, 378
presupplementary motor, 375–377
primary motor cortex, 372–375, 373*f*
supplementary motor area (SMA),
375–377
inferior parietal lobule, 379–380
occipital lobe, 380
primary visual cortex, 380
parietal lobe, 379
primary somatosensory, 379
preoperative functional mapping
diffusion tensor imaging, 372
functional magnetic resonance
imaging, 372
magnetoencephalography and
transcranial magnetic stimulation,
371–372
spinal cord, 381
ascending tracts, 381–382
descending tracts, 381
temporal lobe, 378
basal temporal language area, 378
hippocampal formation, 379
optic radiations, 379
primary auditory, 378–379
Wernicke's area, 378
Neuroblastomas, molecular
pathogenesis of, 225, 226*f*
cancer stem cells, 233
neuroblastoma development,
genetic model of, 233
spontaneous regression, 234
tumor initiation and progression,
233–234
chromosomal abnormalities, 228
chromosome 6 polymorphism, 229
chromosome 17q gain, 229
clinical presentation, 225
deletion or allelic loss at 1p and 11q,
228–229
disease staging, 225–226
neuroblastoma predisposition, 226–228
oncogene amplification and
activation, 230
abnormal gene expression, 232
ALK oncogene, amplification and
mutation of, 231
BCL-2, 233
CDKN2A gene, 232
chromatin helicase-binding domain
5 (*CHD5*) gene, 231–232

DNA content, 233
KIF1 beta, 232
multidrug resistance genes, 232
MYCN amplification, 230–231
neurotrophin receptors, 232
p53, 231
p73, 231
RAS activation, 231
telomerase activity, 232–233
tumor-suppressor inactivation,
231–232
risk stratification, 234–235
tumors, histopathology of, 227*f*
Neurocarcinogens, 1, 18
Neurocognitive correlates, 337–338
Neurocognitive dysfunction, 320
contributions to, 320
effect of, on function, 320–321
interventions, 321
cognitive rehabilitation, 321–322
education, 324
emotional distress and fatigue,
323–324
pharmacologic strategies, 322–323
prophylactic treatment
approaches, 323
Neurocytoma, 892
diagnosis of, 892
treatment of, 893
NEUROD1, 64
NEUROD2, 64
Neuroendocrine tumors, 617
Neuroepithelial tumors, 5*t*, 58
astrocytic tumors
anaplastic astrocytoma, 205
angiocentric glioma, 205, 206*f*
diffuse astrocytoma, 205, 207*f*
glioblastoma, 205–206
pilocytic astrocytoma, 204, 205*f*
pilomyxoid astrocytoma,
204–205, 206*f*
pleomorphic xanthoastrocytoma, 206
embryonal tumors
atypical teratoid/rhabdoid
tumor, 209, 209*f*
choroid plexus carcinoma, 210
choroid plexus papilloma, 210
classic medulloblastoma, 206
ependymoblastoma, 208–209
ependymomas, 209, 210*f*
medulloblastoma, 206
medulloblastoma variants, 206–207
medulloepithelioma, 208–209
supratentorial primitive
neuroectodermal tumors
(sPNETs), 208, 208*f*
incidence of, 7, 8*t*, 9*f*
neuronal and mixed neuroglial
tumors, 210
desmoplastic infantile astrocytoma/
ganglioglioma (DIA/G),
211, 212*f*
dysembryoplastic neuroepithelial
tumor (DNET), 211–212, 212*f*
ganglioglioma, 210–211, 212*f*
nonneuroepithelial tumors, 213
craniopharyngioma, 213, 213*f*

Neurofibromas, 59, 145, 185, 188f, 302
　atypical neurofibroma, 188
　background, 185
　cellular neurofibroma, 188
　dermal neurofibroma, 185
　histopathology, 187–189
　melanotic neurofibroma, 187
　molecular pathogenesis, 185–187
　pigmented neurofibroma, 187
　plexiform neurofibroma, 185, 250
Neurofibromatosis
　patients, 228
　segmental forms of, 541–542
Neurofibromatosis 1 (NF-1) syndrome, 15t, 16, 151, 185, 249–251, 273, 541–542, 620, 771
　and brainstem tumors, 611–612
　diagnostic criteria for, 250t
　nervous system tumors in, 251f, 252f
　-related plexiform neurofibroma, 536f
Neurofibromatosis 2 (NF-2) syndrome, 15t, 16, 72, 151, 252–253, 536, 541
　diagnostic criteria for, 252t
　and meningiomass, 820, 822
Neurohypophysis, 294
Neurolymphoma, 539f
Neuromelanin granules, 187
Neuronal and mixed neuroglial tumors, 210
　desmoplastic infantile astrocytoma/ganglioglioma (DIA/G), 211, 212f
　dysembryoplastic neuroepithelial tumor (DNET), 211–212, 212f
　ganglioglioma, 210–211, 212f
Neuron-associated class III β-tubulin, 892
Neurons in supplementary motor area, 375
Neuron-specific antigen L1, 892
Neuron-specific enolase, 892
Neuro-oncology
　ethical issues in, 311
　　decision to stop therapy, 313–314
　　discussing diagnosis and prognosis, 311–312
　　hospice care, implementation of, 314
　　QOL during and after therapy, 313
　　treatments, 312–313
　palliative care in. See Palliative care, in neuro-oncology
　supportive care in, 304
　　corticosteroids, 305–306
　　dysphagia and swallowing disorders, 307–308
　　gastric acid inhibitors, 306
　　seizures and anticonvulsant therapy, 304–305
　　thromboembolic complications and anticoagulation, 306–307
　unsolved problem in, 47
Neuropil, 112
Neuropsychological decline, biologic foundations of, 338
Neuropsychological deficits, risk factors for, 335
　diagnosis, age at, 335
　pre-RT factors, impact of, 337

RT treatment
　age at, 335–336
　impact of, 336
　tumor location, 336–337
Neurosphere assays, 82t
Neurosphere culture, 195, 196f
Neurotoxicity to CNS, 330
Neurotrophin receptors, 232
Neutron capture therapy (NCT), 729–731
Nevoid basal cell carcinoma syndrome (NBCCS)
　animal models, 241–242
　clinical features and diagnostic criteria, 240
　molecular pathogenesis, 240–241
　therapy and prognosis, 241
New Approaches to Brain Tumor Therapy (NABTT), 746
Newcastle disease virus (NDV), 697
NF1 gene, 16, 151
NF2 gene, 16, 72, 76, 151, 162, 170, 601
　inactivation, 170
　in neurofibromatosis 2, 171
　in schwannomatosis, 171
　in sporadic schwannomas, 170
9p21.3 (CDKN2B), 1
19q deletions, anaplastic gliomas, 752
2-Nitroimidazoles, 103
Nitrosamides, 20, 61
Nitroso compounds, 61
Nitrosoureas, 305, 564, 579
N-methyl d-aspartate (NMDA), 305
N-Myc, 242
　amplification, 230f
N-nitroso compounds (NOCs), 20, 21, 61
　exposure to, 21, 61
N-nitrosomethylurea (MNU), 153
NOD-SCID mice, 85
Nonadenomatous pituitary-derived sellar masses, 623–625
　craniopharyngiomas, 623
　dermoid and epidermoid tumors, 625
　gangliocytomas, 625
　granular cell tumors, 624–625
　pituicytomas, 624
　Rathke cleft cysts, 624
Nonenhancing brain tumors, managing, 510f
Nonfunctioning adenomas (NFAs), 445
　gonadotropin-secreting adenomas, 449–450
　null-cell adenoma, 450
　radiotherapy for, 868
　treatment, 450
Nongerminomatous germ cell tumors (NGGCTs), 662, 874
　radiation therapy for, 876
Nonglial tumors, 361
　imaging features of, 469
Non-Hispanic whites, glioma in, 7
Non-Hodgkin's lymphoma (NHL), 43–44, 650
Nonionizing radiation, 60
Non-Latinos, incidence rates for glioblastomas in, 7
Nonmaleficence, 311
Nonmalignant brain tumors, 4

Nonmalignant glioma, incidence rate for, 7
Non-mRNA based markers, 95
Non-neoplastic disorders, clinical presentation of, 261
Nonneural sheath origin, malignant tumors of, 543–544
Nonneuroepithelial tumors, 213
　craniopharyngioma, 213, 213f
Nonpituitary derived sellar masses, 625–627
　clival chordoma, 626–627
　esthesioneuroblastoma, 627
　germ cell tumors, 625–626
　gliomas, 626
　hypothalamic hamartoma, 627
　lymphoma, 626
　meningiomass, 625
　metastases, 627
　schwannoma, 627
Non-small cell lung cancer (NSCLC), 642, 643, 645, 685
Nonsteroidal anti-inflamatory drugs (NSAIDs), 22
Non-Tmz Chemotherapies, 564
Nonviral vectors, 695
Normal neuroglial stem cells (NSCs), 82
Notch pathway, 84, 221, 265, 595–596
Not otherwise specified (NOS), 7
Novalis, 730t
Novel contrast agents, 364, 365t
NRP receptors, 125
Null-cell adenoma, 179, 450
Nutritional supplements, 711
　antiinflammatory agents, 712
　antioxidants, 712
　fatty acids, 711–712
　flavonoids, 712
　phytoestrogens, 711
　polysaccharide peptides, 711
　selenium, 712
　vitamin D, 712
Nystagmus, 274

O2A progenitor cells, oligodendrogliomas, 760
O6-(4-bromothenyl)-guanine (PaTrin-2), 685
O6-benzylguanine (O6BG), 580, 685
O6-methylguanine-DNA methyltransferase (MGMT), 551, 565, 566, 580, 618, 681, 685
　low-grade gliomas (LGGs) and, 761
Obesity and meningiomass, 820
Occipital condyle syndrome, 288
Occipital lobe, functional neuroanatomy of, 380
　primary visual cortex, 380
Occipital-transtentorial (OTT) approach, 490
Occipitotemporal sulcus, 499
Occupation, chemical exposure mediated through, 18, 19t
　acrylamide, 19
　acrylonitrile, 20
　animal studies, evidence from, 18

benzidine-based dyes, 19
epidemiological and animal studies, evidence from, 18
ethylene oxide, 20
isoprene, 18–19
N-nitroso compounds, 20
1,3-butadiene, 18–19
polycyclic aromatic hydrocarbons (PAHs), 20
Occupational exposure, 28
as risk factor for childhood brain tumors, 60–61
Occupational therapist, 343
OCT6, 64
Octreotide, 618, 630
Odds ratio (OR), 34
Off Therapy Registry, 27
Olfactory groove meningiomas, 159f, 282, 283
Olfactory neuroblastoma. *See* Esthesioneuroblastoma
OLIG2 (oligodendrocyte transcription factor 2), 108
Oligoastrocytoma, 90
anaplastic oligoastrocytoma, 7, 755–757
Oligodendrocytes, 327
Oligodendroglial tumor, 6, 10
Oligodendroglioma, 2, 7, 9, 58, 88, 89–90, 479f, 480f, 570
anaplastic oligodendroglioma, 9, 570–572, 755–757
and chemosensitivity and, 762
MR images of temporal lobe grade II, 762f
survival rate for, 10, 764f
Omeprazole, 306
Oncogene activation in pituitary tumors, 180–181
Oncogene amplification and activation, 5
abnormal gene expression, 232
ALK oncogene, amplification and mutation of, 231
BCL-2, 233
CDKN2A gene, 232
chromatin helicase-binding domain 5 (*CHD5*) gene, 231–232
DNA content, 233
KIF1 beta, 232
multidrug resistance genes, 232
MYCN amplification, 230–231
neurotrophin receptors, 232
p53, 231
p73, 231
RAS activation, 231
telomerase activity, 232–233
tumor-suppressor inactivation, 231–232
Oncolytic adenovirus, 696–697
Oncolytic HSV-1, 696
"Oncomirs," 95
1p deletions
anaplastic gliomas, 752
in neuroblastoma, 229
ONYX-015, 696–697
Opsoclonus-myoclonus syndrome, 225
Optic nerve glioma, 16, 626
Optic nerve meningiomass, 283

Optic nerve sheath meningiomass (ONSMs), 829–830
Optic neuropathy, radiation-induced, 864–865
Optic pathway glioma (OPG), 250, 771
clinical presentation of, 771–772
medical management for, 583–584
pathology, 771
radiographic findings of, 771
treatment and outcome, 772
chemotherapy, 772–773
radiation therapy, 773
surgery, 772
Optic radiations, 379
Orbital syndrome, 288
Orbital tumors, 386
Orthotopic gliomas, 123
Orthotopic vs. heterotopic tumor cell growth, 155
Osseous tumors, 386
Osteoid osteoma, 634
Osteosarcoma, 634
Oxamflatin, 707
Oxidants, 21
Oxidative DNA lesions, 22
Oxygen enhancement ration (OER), 724

$p14^{ARF}$ gene, 92, 190
$p16^{INK4A}$, 190
p21-Ras activity, 149
$p27^{Kip1}$, 190
p53 gene, 72, 231, 242, 243
germline mutations, 15
p53 mutation, 63, 150
p53 pathway, 92
p53 protein, 92
p53-regulated cell cycle pathways, 148
p73, 72, 231
p130CAS, 116
P311 polypeptide, 118
Paclitaxol, 305
Paired-like homeobox 2B (PHOX2B), 228
Palliative care, in neuro-oncology, 349
end-of-life planning
caregiver issues, 351
hospice, 351
delirium, 350
dying patient, care of, 350–351
dyspnea, 350
treatment-related side effects, 350
tumor-related side effects, 349–350
Palliative rehabilitation, 342
Palliative whole-brain radiotherapy (WBRT), single brain metastasis, 902–905
administration of, 903f
after surgical resection, 905–906
carmustine polymer wafers placement, 906
neurocognitive decline, 905
survival rate, 905
toxicity, 905
combining drugs and, 903–905
nonrandomized phase II trial, 904
NSCLC patients, phase III trial in, 904

tumor cells, motexafin gadolinium (MGd) concentration in, 904
fractionation and total dose, 902–903
Radiation Therapy Oncology Group (RTOG) trails, 902–903
results of focal treatment with or without, 908t
surgical resection or radiosurgery, treatment intensification by, 903
symptom relief and quality of life, effects on, 902
overall survival rate, 902
Radiation Therapy Oncology Group (RTOG) trails, 902
Papillary glioneuronal tumor, 59
Papillary meningiomass, 160, 823t
Papillomas, 58. *See also* Adenomas; Astrocytomas; Cancer; Carcinomas; Ependymomas; Gliomas; Meningiomas; Metastases; Neurofibromas; Sarcomas; Tumors
choroid plexus papilloma, 210, 211f, 664, 878
Paraganglioma, 615t, 617, 635. *See also* Chemodectomas
cytotoxic chemotherapy, 617–618
molecularly targeted agents, 618
radioisotope treatment, 618
Paraoxonase 1 (*PON1*), 64
Parasagittal meningiomass, 828
Parasympathetic nuclei, 380
Parasympathomimetic agent, 345
Parietal lobe, 343
functional neuroanatomy of, 379
primary somatosensory, 379
Parinaud syndrome, 260
Parsonage-Turner syndrome, 536–537
Particle radiation therapy, skull base tumors
carbon ions, 854–855
failure, patterns of, 854–855
protons, 852–854
outcomes of, 852–853
physics and radiobiology, 852
techniques unique to, 853
Passive antibody transfer, 694
Paternalism, 311
Pazopanib (GW786034), 677, 680
PCNU, 586
PCTH gene, 219
PD098059, 605
PDGF/PDGFR, 90
PDGFRA, 616
PDGFRB, 616
Pediatric astrocytoma, 200
Pediatric brainstem glioma, 842
management algorithm, 843f
radiotherapy
delivery techniques, 843
dose, 842–843
indications for treatment, 842
target volume for, 842
treatment outcomes and approach, 843–844
Pediatric brain tumors
'cell of origin' for. *See* 'cell of origin' for pediatric brain tumors, 196
histopathological features of, 204–213

Pediatric brain tumor syndromes and murine models, 239
　Cowden disease, 244
　　animal models, 245
　　clinical features and diagnostic criteria, 244
　　molecular pathogenesis, 244
　　therapy and prognosis, 245
　Li-Fraumeni syndrome
　　animal models, 244
　　clinical features and diagnostic criteria, 243
　　molecular pathogenesis, 243
　　therapy and prognosis, 244
　multiple endocrince neoplasia
　　animal models, 245
　　clinical features and diagnostic criteria, 245
　　molecular pathogenesis, 245
　　therapy and prognosis, 245
　nevoid basal cell carcinoma syndrome
　　animal models, 241–242
　　clinical features and diagnostic criteria, 240
　　molecular pathogenesis, 240–241
　　therapy and prognosis, 241
　Turcot syndrome
　　animal models, 243
　　clinical features and diagnostic criteria, 242
　　molecular pathogenesis, 242–243
　　therapy and prognosis, 243
　von-Hippel Lindau (VHL)
　　animal models, 240
　　clinical features and diagnostic criteria, 239–240
　　molecular pathogenesis, 240
　　therapy and prognosis, 240
Pediatric gliomas, 273
　classification, 273
　late sequelae, 276
　presentation and clinical features, 273
　　brainstem gliomas, 275
　　cerebellar astrocytomas, 275
　　cerebral hemispheres, gliomas of, 274
　　diencephalic (visual pathway) gliomas, 274–275
　treatment, 275–276
Pediatric gliomas, medical management for, 579
　high-grade gliomas
　　future direction for, 581
　　molecular and genetic alterations in, 582t
　　radiation and chemotherapy, 579–580
　　recurrent, 581
　　surgery, 579
　　in very young children, 581
　low-grade glioma, 582
　　cerebellar astrocytomas, 584–585
　　cerebral low-grade glioma, 583
　　ependymomas, 585–586
　　optic pathway glioma, 583–584
Pediatric grade II–IV (Non-JPA) gliomas, radiation therapy in
　future directions of, 4
　proton therapy, 778
　introduction to, 775
　review of data in, 775–776
　　high-grade gliomas, 776
　simulation, 776
　toxicity, 777–778
　treatment planning, 776–777
　　clinical target volume, 776, 777
　　gross tumor volume, 776, 777
　　planning target volume, 776
Pediatric medulloblastoma, 269
Pediatric neuropsychology, during the last four decades, 334–335
　incidence and survival rate for, 334t
Pediatric pilocytic astrocytoma (PA)
　clinical presentation of, 795
　introduction and epidemiology, 795
　pathology and radiographic findings of, 795
　　computed tomography, 795
　　magnetic resonance imaging, 795
　treatment and outcome
　　chemotherapy, 797
　　complete resection, 796
　　incomplete resection, 796
　　radiation therapy, postoperative period, 796–797
Pediatric spinal cord astrocytoma, 467
Pediatric tumor surgery, 518
　clinical pearls, 530
　　infratentorial neoplasms, 530
　　neonates and infants, 530
　　supratentorial neoplasms, 530
　intraventricular tumors, 523
　　central neurocytoma, 524–525
　　choroid plexus tumors, 523–524
　　endoscopy in, 525
　　surgical considerations, 524
　　thalamic gliomas, 525
　pineal region tumors, 525
　　classification, 525–526
　　germ cell tumors, 526
　　glial tumors, 526
　　hydrocephalus treatment and tissue diagnosis, 526
　　management, 526
　　microsurgical approaches, 526–527
　　miscellaneous tumors, 526
　　outcomes, 527
　　pineal parenchymal tumors, 526
　posterior fossa tumors, 527
　　cerebellar astrocytoma, 528
　　ependymoma, 528
　　medulloblastoma, 527–528
　　posterior fossa syndrome and mutism, 529–530
　　surgical considerations, 528–529
　　surgical positioning, 529
　　surgical technique, 529
　supratentorial tumors, 518
　　dysembryoplastic neuroepithelial tumors, 518
　　functional imaging, 519–520
　　gangliogliomas, 518
　　gliomas, 518
　　neuronavigation, 519
　　surgical considerations, 519
　suprasellar tumors, 520
　　craniopharyngioma, 520–522
　　pituitary adenoma, 522–523
Peer-facilitated groups, 317
Pegvisoman, 630
Pentero™ system, 424
Perfusion MRI, 356
Pericyte progenitor cells (PPCs), 132
Perifosine, 91, 92
Peri-insular sulcus dissection, 512–513
Perineurioma, 536, 537f
Periodic acid-Schiff (PAS), 179
Peripheral nerve sheath tumors, 59
　specific mouse models of, 151
Peripheral nervous system (PNS), 79, 80
Peripheral neurofibromatosis. See Neurofibromatosis-1 (NF-1)
Peritumoral edema, 305, 355
Permanent alopecia
　radiation therapy toxicity, in ependymoma, 802
Personalized gene therapy/immunotherapy, 700
Pesticides, 61
Petroclival meningiomass, 284–285
P-glycoprotein (Pgp), 551, 686
4-Phenylbutyrate, 707
Phenytoin, 305, 330
Phosphatase and tensin homolog (PTEN) protein, 88
Phosphatidyl inositide, 733
Phosphatidylinositol-3-hydroxyl kinase (PI3K), 117
　inhibitors, 680
　pathway, 91
Phosphocreatine, 279, 363
Phosphoglycerate kinase, 108
Phosphorus-32 (32P), 864
Photobleaching, 425
Photon, 721
Photon irradiation therapy
　for PNETs
　　in prone position, 787
　　in supine position, 787–788
　skull base tumors
　　conventional fractionation, 850–851
　　efficacy of, 851–852
　　failure, patterns of, 854–855
　　stereotactic radiosurgery, 851–852
Photons, 731
Physiatrist, 342–343
Physical Medicine and Rehabilitation (PMR), 342
Physical therapist, 343
Physicians, 342
Phytoestrogens, 711
PI3K/AKT pathway, 605
PI3K-AKT/PKB pathway, 92
Pigmented neurofibroma, 187
Pilocytic astrocytoma (PA), pediatric
　clinical presentation of, 795
　introduction and epidemiology, 795
　pathology and radiographic findings of, 795
　treatment and outcome
　　chemotherapy, 797
　　complete resection, 796
　　incomplete resection, 796

radiation therapy, postoperative period, 796–797
Pilocytic astrocytoma, 4, 9, 58, 204, 205f, 582, 760, 762, 771
  in children, 9, 795
  survival rate for, 10
Pilomyxoid astrocytoma, 204–205, 206f
  WHO grade II, 760
Pimonidazole, 103
Pineal gland tumors, 485
  classification, 486f
  clinical considerations
    hydrocephalus management, 487
    preoperative workup, 486–487
  historical review of pineal region surgery, 485–486
  pathology, 486
  pineal region, anatomy of, 485
  surgical decision making
    objectives, 487–488
  surgical procedures, 488
    adjuvant therapy, 491–492
    craniospinal evaluation, 492–493
    endoscopy, 489
    microsurgery, 490–491
    specific pathologies, role of surgery for, 491
    stereotactic biopsy, 488–489
    stereotactic radiosurgery, 489–490
Pineal parenchymal tumors (PPTs), 174, 175f, 445t, 486, 491, 526
Pineal region tumor, 59, 259–260, 525, 877
  classification, 525–526
  germ cell tumors, 526
  glial tumors, 526
  hydrocephalus treatment and tissue diagnosis, 526
  management, 526
  microsurgical approaches, 526–527
  miscellaneous, 526
  outcomes, 527
  pineal parenchymal tumors, 526, 877
    intermediate differentiation, 878
    pineoblastomas, 877–878
    pineocytomas, 877
Pirfenidone, 635
Pit-1 gene, 176
Pituicytomas, 624
Pituitary adenoma, 522–523, 628t, 861
  atypical pituitary adenoma, 450–451
  classification, 175–178
  clinicopathological classification of, 176t
  conventional radiotherapy, 862
  definition, 174
  endocrinologically inactive pituitary adenoma, 630
  epidemiology, 174–175
  familial syndromes involving, 176t
  histopathology, 178
    ACTH-producing adenomas, 179
    clinically functioning adenomas, 178
    clinically nonfunctioning adenomas, 179
    clinically silent ACTH-producing adenomas, 179
    GH-producing adenomas, 178

gonadotropin-producing adenomas, 179
    null cell adenoma, 179
    pituitary carcinomas, 180
    plurihormonality, 179–180
    PRL-producing adenomas, 178
    prognosis, 180
    TSH-producing adenomas, 179
  hormonally active pituitary adenomas, 292
  immunohistochemical classification, 177t
  invasive pituitary adenoma, 848
  intracavitary radiotherapy, 864
  molecular pathogenesis, 180
    clonality, 180
    epigenetic changes, 181–182
    growth and angiogenic factors, 181
    hereditary syndromes, 181
    hormones and their receptors, 181
    pituitary tumors, oncogene activation in, 180–181
    TSG inactivation in pituitary tumors, 181
  and pituitary carcinoma, 450–451
  proton therapy, 864
  radiation indications, 861
  radiotherapy
    for acromegaly, 867–868
    cranial neuropathies, 865
    for Cushing syndrome, 866–867
    cystic enlargement, 865
    follow-up, 868–869
    hypopituitarism, 865
    for Nelson syndrome, 867, 868t
    mortality, 865
    neurocognitive effects, 865–866
    for nonfunctioning adenomas (NFAs), 868
    optic neuropathy, 864–865
    for prolactinoma, 866
    secondary malignancies, 865
    techniques, 862–864
  stereotactic techniques
    fractionated stereotactic radiosurgery (FSRT), 863
    stereotactic radiosurgery (SRS), 863
Pituitary and sellar region, tumors of, 291
  clinical presentation and diagnostic evaluation, 291–292
  epidemiology, 291
  hormonally active pituitary adenomas
    Cushing disease, 292–293
    GH-secreting adenomas, 293
    PRL-secreting adenomas, 293
  sellar region and diagnostic imaging, surgical anatomy of, 294–295
  sellar lesions, diagnostic evaluation of, 293–294
  sellar masses, 623
    adenomatous pituitary-derived sellar masses, 627–631
    arachnoid cyst, 627
    clival chordoma, 626–627
    craniopharyngiomas, 623
    dermoid and epidermoid tumors, 625
    differential diagnosis, 624t

esthesioneuroblastoma, 627
    gangliocytomas, 625
    germ cell tumors, 625–626
    gliomas, 626
    granular cell tumors, 624–625
    hypothalamic hamartoma, 627
    lymphoma, 626
    meningiomass, 625
    metastases, 627
    nonpituitary derived sellar masses, 625
    pituicytomas, 624
    Rathke cleft cysts, 624
    schwannoma, 627
Pituitary carcinoma/tumors, 174, 180, 282, 450–451, 630–631
  oncogene activation in, 180–181
  TSG inactivation in, 181
Pituitary tumortransforming gene (PTTG), 180
Placental alkaline phosphatase, 733
Plasmacytoma, diagnosis of, 848
Platelet-derived growth factor (PDGF), 669, 676
  signaling, 88
Platelet-derived growth factor-B (PDGF-B) gene, 42
Platelet-derived growth factor receptor (PDGFR), 82, 84, 88, 616, 676
  inhibitors, 677
Cis-platinum, 592
Platinum compounds, 580
Pleomorphic xanthoastrocytoma (PXA), 58, 206, 760
Plexiform neurofibroma (PNF), 185, 250
Plexiform schwannoma, 169, 169f
PLOD2 (procollagen hydroxylase 2), 108
Plurihormonal adenomas, 179–180
Pneumocystis carinii pneumonia (PCP), 306
Pneumocystis jiroveci pneumonia, 350
POFUT2 (protein-o-fucosyltransferase 2), 108
PoleStar iMRI, 414
Poliovirus, 697
Poly(ADP-ribose) polymerase (PARP) system, 565, 685
Polycyclic aromatic hydrocarbons (PAHs), 18, 20
Polymers, implantable, 551
Polymethylmethacrate (PMMA) cement, 461
Polysaccharide peptides, 711
Pontine glioma, 58
Population exposure to NOC, 61
Positron emission tomography (PET), 103, 365, 403, 616, 720
  amino acid positron emission tomography, 365
  Brachial plexus tumor, 535
  FET-PET, 366
  fluorodeoxyglucose positron emission tomography, 280
  indications, 365
  MET-PET, 365–366
  primary spinal tumors, 454
  single-photon emission tomography, 366

Posterior fossa syndrome, 288
Posterior fossa tumors, 527
　cerebellar astrocytoma, 528
　ependymoma, 528
　medulloblastoma, 527–528
　mutism, 529–530
　surgical considerations, 528–529
　surgical positioning, 529
　surgical technique, 529
Posterior inferior cerebellar arteries (PICAs), 502
Posterior interhemispheric transcingular approach, 498–499
Posterior longitudinal ligament (PLL), 457
Posterior pyramid meningiomass, 285
Postmenopausal hormone replacement therapy and meningiomass, 820
Postoperative injury, 355
Postsurgical sequelae, 344
Precentral cerebellar vein, 502
Predisposing genetic syndromes and familial occurrence, of brain tumors, 62–63
Predisposition syndromes, 249–253
Prednisone, 306, 579, 586, 635
Prehabilitation model, 323
Preoperative functional mapping, functional neuroanatomy of
　diffusion tensor imaging, 372
　functional magnetic resonance imaging (fMRI), 372
　magnetoencephalography and transcranial magnetic stimulation, 371–372
Pre-SMA, 376
Presupplementary motor, 375–377
Preventative rehabilitation, 342
Primary bone lesions
　benign, 634
　malignant, 634
　pediatry, 634
Primary brain tumors (PBTs), 304
　hereditary syndromes predisposing for, 15
　　inherited syndrome, 15t
　　Li-Fraumeni Syndrome, 15–16
　　neurofibromatosis type 1, 16
　　neurofibromatosis type 2, 16
　　Turcot syndrome, 16–17
Primary central nervous system germ cell tumors, 874
　radiation volume and dose, 875t
Primary central nervous system lymphoma (PCNSL), 306, 650
　AIDS-related PCNSL, treatment of, 888
　autologous stem-cell transplantation (ASCT), 655
　　AIDS-related PCNSL, 657
　　immunotherapy, 656–657
　　investigational therapy, 657
　clinical features and presentation, 650
　clinical prognostic factors, 652
　diagnosis and clinical evaluation, 650–652
　diagnostic workup of
　　history and physical examination, 881
　newly diagnosed immunocompetent patients, baseline evaluation for, 882t
　epidemiology of, 880
　　congenital immune deficiency, patients with, 880
　　immunocompetent patients, median age of, 880
　and future directions
　　Future PCNSL Trials and fundamental challenges, 889t
　　immunocompetent PCNSL patients, clinical trails for, 887t
　intrarterial chemotherapy, 886
　intrathecal chemotherapy, 886
　　high-dose methotrexate, use of, 886
　introduction to, 880
　　age and gender distribution of, 880
　　occurrence, 880
　　treatment choice, 880
　laboratory studies of, 881
　natural history of, 880–881
　nonpenetrating CHOD chemotherapy, role of, 885
　pathology and prognosis in, 652–653, 883
　prognostic factors and
　　patient related, 883
　　tumor-related, 883
　primary IOL, 657–658
　radiographic studies of
　　computed tomography (CT), 881
　　F^{18}-fluorodeoxyglucose (FDG) positron emission tomography (PET), 882–883
　　magnetic resonance imaging, 881–882
　risk factors for, 652
　salvage chemotherapy, 886–888
　stem cell support, high-dose chemotherapy with, 886
　therapy
　　chemotherapy, 654
　　combined-modality therapy, 654
　　glucocorticoids, 653
　　high-dose methotrexate, 655
　　immunocompetent PCNSL, 653
　　intrathecal methotrexate, 654–655
　　radiation therapy, 653–654
　treatment
　　of AIDS-related PCNSL, 888
　　chemotherapy, 885–887
　　late treatment effects, 888–889
　　radiotherapy, 884
　　radiotherapy, effects of, 888
　　surgery, 884
　　treatment volume and dosage, 884–885
　whole brain radiation therapy (WBRT) for, 880
Primary cerebral lymphoma (PCL), 361
Primary gliomas, frequency of, 6
Primary intraspinal tumors, symptoms and signs of, 299t
Primary malignant glioma, 10t
　incidence rate for, 7
Primary Meckel cave meningiomass, 284
Primary motor cortex, 372–375, 373f
Primary site for glioma, 6
Primary somatosensory, 379
Primary spinal cord tumors, radiation therapy of
　miscellaneous tumors
　　central neurocytoma, 898
　　granulocytic sarcoma, 898
　　sarcoma, surgical debulking of, 898
　　schwannoma, 898
　　teratoma, 898
　　vertebral hemangioma, 898
　spinal cord and lumbosacral nerve roots, tolerance of, 894–895
　techniques, 894
　treatment complications, 898
　　radiation myelopathy, 898
　treatment volumes, definition of, 894
　tumor type, indications and outcomes by, 895–898
　　astrocytoma, 895–896
　　chondrosarcoma, 896–898
　　ependymoma, 896
　　meningiomas, 896
Primary spinal tumors
　chemotherapy and radiation therapy, 454
　clinical presentation and workup, 453–454
　surgical management, 454–456
　surgical technique, 456–458
Primary visual cortex, 380
Primitive neuroectodermal tumors (PNETs), 219, 526, 781, 844.
　See also Medullablastoma
　evaluation of, 781
　M staging in, 782t
　risk groups, 781
　treatment volumes, 786
Primitive neuroectodermal tumors (PNETs), medical management of
　future directions, 595–596
　medulloblastoma, 589
　　chemotherapy, 591
　　late effects, 592
　　radiation therapy, 590–591
　　staging and risk stratification, 589–590
　　surgical resection, 590
　　in very young child, 592–593
　radiotherapy complications
　　acute side effects, 790
　　late complications, 790–791
　radiotherapy technique, 786–789
　radiotherapy treatment evolution, clinical trials, 781–782
　　average risk patients, 782–784
　　high-risk patients, 784–786
　supratentorial PNETs (sPNETs), 593
　　chemotherapy, 594–595
　　radiation therapy, 594
　　staging and prognostic factors, 593–594
　　surgical resection, 594
Proangiogenic cells in glioma neovascularization, 131
Proapoptotic Bax protein, 92
Proapoptotic protein, 92

Procarbazine, 549, 580, 635, 654, 773
  for average-risk PNET, 782
  for high-risk PNET, 784, 785, 786
  for infant medulloblastoma, 790
  vincristine
Prodrug-suicidal gene therapy, 698–699
Progenitor cells, 82
Prognosis and survival, of glioma. *See*
    Survival and prognosis, of glioma
Prolactin (PRL)-secreting adenomas, 178,
    291, 293, 445–446
Prolactinoma, 174, 522, 629
  clinical manifestations of, 294t
  radiotherapy for, 866
Pronuclear injection technique,
    145–146, 146f
Proopiomelanocortin, 176
Protease/protease receptor expression,
    changes in, 115
Proteasome inhibitors, 681
Protein kinase C (PKC) inhibitors, 117, 680
Proteomic-based studies, 79
Proton beam therapy, 454, 731
  for vestibular schwannoma, 814
Proton magnetic resonance
    spectroscopy, 279
  of tumor metabolites, 104–105
Protons and heavy particles, 731–732
Proton therapy, 864
Psammomatous meningiomass,
    159, 160f, 167
Pseudo-Cushing syndrome, 293
Pseudopalisades, 101, 102f, 108
Pseudopalisading cells, 102
Pseudoprogression, 566
Pseudopsammoma, 159
Psychologist, 343
PTCH, 241
PTDSR (phosphatidylserine receptor), 108
PTEN, 63, 117
PTEN gene, 244
Pulmonary embolism (PE), 306–307
Putative tumor suppressor genes, 89
PV-RIPO, 697
Pyk2 expression, 115, 116
Pyroxamide, 707
Pyruvate kinase, 108

Qigong, 714
Quality of life (QOL), 313, 314, 320, 326
  impact of neuropsychological
    functioning on, 338–339

Race
  frequency of glioma by, 7
  -specific survival rates for glioma, 11
Radiation, 164
  -associated neoplasm, 820
Radiation therapy (RT), 27, 276, 312,
    313, 323, 329, 331, 344, 653–654,
    671, 677, 719
  accelerated hyperfractionated
    radiotherapy, 639
  anaplastic oligodendroglioma
    plus BCNU, 754
    plus PCV, 752
  basic physics, 719
    interaction of photons with
      matter, 720
    radioactivity, 719–720
    structure of matter, 719
    X-rays, 719
  as cause of cognitive deficits, 327–328
  cerebellar astrocytomas, 585
  for cerebral low-grade glioma, 583
  for choroid plexus tumors, 664–665
  in combination with chemotherapy,
    low-grade gliomas, 765
    oral alkylating agent
      temozolomide, 765
  craniopharyngiomas. *See*
    Craniopharyngiomas
  for ependymomas, 585–586
    chemoradiotherapy and adjuvant
      chemotherapy, for delaying of, 802
    dose of, 801
    duration of, 802
    field size of, 802
    gross total resection, 800–801
    subtotal resection, 801
    toxicity of, 802
  external beam radiotherapy, 454, 599,
    603, 719, 724, 726–728, 734
  focal radiotherapy, 331
  fractionated adjuvant radiotherapy, 818
  gangliomas and, 770
  general radiobiological principles,
    720–724
  for glioblastoma multiforme, 564
  for high-grade gliomas, 579–580
  hyperfractionated craniospinal
    radiotherapy, 591, 594
  -induced glioma, 16
  intracavitary radiotherapy, 864
  for low-grade gliomas (LCGs), 557–558,
    764–765
  metastatic spinal tumors, 459–460
  for optic pathway glioma, 584
  palliative whole-brain radiotherapy,
    902–905
  for patients with anaplastic
    oligodendroglioma, 752
  for PCNSL, 653–654
  for pediatric pilocytic astrocytoma (PA),
    postoperative period, 796–797
  pituitary adenomas. *See* Pituitary
    adenomas
  and primary central nervous system
    lymphoma (PCNSL), 888
  for primary spinal cord tumors, 454,
    894–898
    spinal cord and lumbosacral nerve
      roots, tolerance of, 894–895
    techniques, 894
    treatment volumes, definition of, 894
    tumor type, indications and outcomes
      by, 895–898
  radiation delivery mechanism, 724
    brachytherapy, 724–726
    external beam radiation, 726–728
    neutron capture therapy (NCT),
      729–731
    protons and heavy particles, 731–732
    stereotactic radiosurgery and
      fractionated stereotactic
      radiotherapy, 728–729
    targeted radionuclide
      radiotherapy, 732–739
    whole-brain radiation therapy,
      638, 639, 640
Radiation therapy, intracranial
    meningiomass and
  clinical presentation, 824
  EBRT vs. SRS, 833
    WHO Grade I, 837t
  epidemiology, 820–821
    gender, age, and race
      distributions, 821
    incidence and prevalence, 820–821
  etiologic factors, 820
  molecular genetics and
    histopathology, 821–824
    histogenesis, 822
    histologic subtypes and variants,
      823–824
    molecular genetics, 821–822
    tumor grade, 822–823
  neuroimaging and, 824
  special circumstances, 833–836
    incidental meningiomass, 835–836
    nonbenign meningiomass, 833–835
    recurrent meningiomass, 835
  treatment and outcome, 824–833
    fractionated external beam radiation
      therapy, 828–833
    gross total resection, 825
    radiation therapy, 825–826
    stereotactic radiosurgery, 826–828
    subtotal resection, 825
    surgery, 824–825
Radiation Therapy Oncology Group
    (RTOG) recursive partitioning
    analysis (RPA), anaplastic
    gliomas, 752
Radiofrequency fields and glioma risk, 31
  exposure assessment, 31–32
  mobile phone use and glioma risk, 32
    laterality of mobile phone use, 34
    long-term mobile phone use, 34
    short-term mobile phone use, 32–34
  occupational studies, 34–36
  selection bias, 32
Radiologic diagnosis, 260
Radionuclides for TRT, 733t
Radiosurgery, 728–729
  for recurrent hemangiopericytomas, 819
Radio transmitter, 31
Radium (^{226}Ra) treatment, 27
RAF kinase inhibitor, 605
Ranitidine hydrochloride, 306
Rapamycin, 91
RAS, 186
  activation, 231, 679
  activity in gliomas, 91
Ras-association domain 1A gene
    (*RASSF1A*), 182
RASSF1 methylation, 64
Rathke's pouch, 291, 294
Rathke cleft cysts, 624

Rb pathway, 92
RCAS-*tva* system, 150
  somatic gene transfer using, 147–148, 148f
Receptor tyrosine kinase (RTK) activation, 91
Recombinant interferon-α, 604
Recurrence
  gangliomas, 770
  of hemangiopericytoma, 819
  lipoma, 537f
  low-grade gliomas (LGGs) and, 765–766
    treatment options, 766
Recursive partitioning analysis (RPA), 264
Reference signal, 363
Regulatory T-cells and glioma survival time, 42–43
Rehabilitation of CNS tumors. *See* CNS tumors, rehabilitation of
Reiki, 714
Re-irradiation, for GBMs, 749
Relapsed malignant glioma, 705–706
Relative biological effective-ness (RBE), 721, 731
Relative cerebral blood volume (rCBV), 357
Relative risk variance, 28
Replication-competent (oncolytic) viruses, 696
Replication-defective viruses, 698
Repopulation, 723–724
Resident normal neuroglial stem cells, 197f
Respect for autonomy, 311
Respect for persons, 311
Response Evaluation Criteria in Solid Tumors (RECIST), 366
Restorative rehabilitation, 342
Restricted glial progenitors, 82
Restricted neural progenitors, 82
Reticular circuitry, 381
Retinoblastoma (*Rb*), 15t, 244
Retinoblastoma protein (pRb), 92
Retinoic acids (RAs), 704
13-cis-Retinoic acid, 570
Retroperitoneal schwannoma, 168f
Retroviral vectors, 698
Reversible posterior leukoencephalopathy syndrome (RPLS), 137
Rhabdoid meningiomas, 160, 823t
Rhabdomyosarcoma, 59, 287
Rheb (Ras homolog expressed in brain), 253
Rhenium-186 (186Re), 864
Risedronate, 306
Rituximab, 657
RMP-7, 610
Romberg sign, 300
Rosette-forming glioneuronal tumor of the 4th ventricle, 59
Rous sarcoma virus family, 150
RTOG 9802, 558

S6kinase gene, 73
SAHA (vorinostat), 707
S allele of MNS16, 54

Sarcomas. *See also* Adenomas; Astrocytomas; Cancer; Carcinomas; Ependymomas; Gliomas; Meningiomas; Metastases; Neurofibromas; Papillomas; Tumors
  chondrosarcomas, 287, 615t, 617
  Ewing's sarcoma, 634
  gliosarcoma, 106
  granulocytic sarcoma, 898
  osteosarcoma, 634
  rhabdomyosarcoma, 59, 287
  surgical debulking of and radiation therapy, 898
Scalp irradiation, 820
Scatter factor (SF), 128
Schwann cell, 186, 187
Schwannoma, 145, 167, 252, 285, 389, 390f, 535f, 627
  bilateral vestibular, 16
  chondrosarcomas, 287
  chordomas, 287
  clinical features, 167
  craniopharyngiomas, 286
  cutaneous schwannoma, 168f
  epidermoid/dermoid, 286–287
  facial schwannoma, 286
  general considerations, 285
  gross appearance, 168f
  histology, 168f, 169f
  hypoglossal schwannomas, 286
  molecular biology, 170
    NF2 gene, 170
    NF2 gene in neurofibromatosis 2, 171
    NF2 gene in schwannomatosis, 171
    NF2 gene in sporadic schwannomas, 170
    NF2 inactivation, 170
    SMARCB1/INI1 gene in schwannomas, 171
    SMARCB1/INI1 gene, 171
  multiple schwannoma syndromes, 167–168
  neuroimaging, 167
  pathology, 168
    cellular schwannoma, 169–170, 170f
    electron microscopy, 170
    histology, 168–169
    macroscopy, 168
    melanotic schwannomas, 170
    plexiform schwannoma, 169, 169f
  and radiation therapy, 898
  retroperitoneal schwannoma, 168f
  sites, 167
  trigeminal schwannomas, 286
  tumors, 302
  vestibular schwannomas, 285–286
Schwannomatosis, 541t
SDF-1/CXCL12, 43
SDF-1α, 128
Secoisolariciresinol, 711
Secondary malignancies, radiation-induced, 865
Secretory meningiomass, 159, 160f, 161
Segregation analysis, 14
Selection bias, 32
Selenium, 712

Sellar lesions, diagnostic evaluation of, 293–294
Sellar masses, 623
  adenomatous pituitary-derived sellar masses, 627–631
  arachnoid cyst, 627
  differential diagnosis, 624t
  nonadenomatous pituitary-derived sellar masses, 623
    craniopharyngiomas, 623
    dermoid and epidermoid tumors, 625
    gangliocytomas, 625
    granular cell tumors, 624–625
    pituicytomas, 624
    Rathke cleft cysts, 624
  nonpituitary derived sellar masses, 625
    clival chordoma, 626–627
    esthesioneuroblastoma, 627
    germ cell tumors, 625–626
    gliomas, 626
    hypothalamic hamartoma, 627
    lymphoma, 626
    meningiomass, 625
    metastases, 627
    schwannoma, 627
Sellar-parasellar syndrome, 288
Sellar region and diagnostic imaging, surgical anatomy of, 294–295
Semustine (MeCCNU), 744
Sensorimotor functional anatomy, 374f
7560 cGy, 608–609
Sex hormones and meningiomass, 820
Shh antagonists, 242
Shh signaling pathway, 241f
Short-term mobile phone use, 32–34
  epidemiological studies, 33t
Shunting, 645–646
Signs and symptoms, intracranial meningiomas, 824
Simian sarcoma virus, 150
Simpson's grading system, meningiomass, 824–825
Sin/Efs, 116
Single-nucleotide polymorphisms (SNPs), 64, 73, 74–75t, 215, 228
"Single-phase" treatment volume, 746
Single photon emission computed tomography (SPECT), 366, 652
Sinonasal tumors, 385–386
Site, distribution of glioma by, 6
Skinfold freckling, 250
Skull base, tumors of
  clinical presentation of, 847
    generalized symptoms of, 847
    headache, 847
    ophthalmologic symptoms of, 847
    otolaryngologic symptoms of, 847
    visual disturbances, 847
  diagnosis and work-up, 848–849
    differential diagnosis, 848
    imaging, 848–849
    tissue diagnosis, 849
    work-up and staging, 848
  epidemiology of, 846
  etiology and anatomy of, 846
  generalized symptoms of, 847
  management of patient with, 849–855

particle radiation therapy, carbon ions, 854–855
particle radiation therapy, protons, 852–854
photon radiation therapy, conventional fractionation, 850–851
photon radiation therapy, stereotactic radiosurgery, 851–852
surgery, 849–850
natural history of, 847–848
ophthalmologic symptoms of, 847
otolaryngologic symptoms of, 847
pathology of, 846–847
positron emission tomography, use of, 849
toxicity and particle therapy, 855–857
brain, 856
brain stem, 856
endocrine deficiency, 857
hearing loss, 857
postoperative complications, 855–856
spinal cord, 856
vision, 856–857
Skull base anatomy, 385
anterior fossa, 385f
meningiomass, 385
orbital tumors, 386
osseous tumors, 386
sinonasal tumors, 385–386
surgical approaches, 386–387
central skull base, 385f
chordoma/chondrosarcoma/fibrous dysplasia, 389–390
meningiomass, 389
schwannoma, 389, 390f
surgical approaches, 391
middle fossa
facial nerve schwannomas, 387
glomus tympanicum, 387
meningiomass, 387
surgical approaches, 387–388
posterior fossa, 385f
meningiomass, 388
posterior cranial base, surgical approaches to, 389
vestibular schwannomas, 388
Skull base and cranial nerves tumors, 282, 615, 615t
clinical presentation
general considerations, 282–283
special considerations, 283–288
chondrosarcoma, 617
cytotoxic chemotherapy, 617
radiation sensitizers, 617
chordoma, 616
cytotoxic chemotherapy, 616–616
molecularly targeted agents, 616
radiation sensitizers, 617
epidemiology, 282
esthesioneuroblastoma, 618
cytotoxic chemotherapy, 618–619
malignant peripheral nerve sheath tumors (MPNSTs), 619–620
cytotoxic chemotherapy, 620
molecularly targeted agents, 620
paraganglioma, 617
cytotoxic chemotherapy, 617–618

molecularly targeted agents, 618
radioisotope treatment, 618
Skull base hematogenous metastases, 287
anterior fossa syndrome, 288
general considerations, 287–288
jugular foramen syndrome, 288
middle fossa syndrome, 288
occipital condyle syndrome, 288
orbital syndrome, 288
posterior fossa syndrome, 288
sellar-parasellar syndrome, 288
Skull-base surgery, endoscopic
coronal/paramedian-plane approach, 438–439
exposure, general considerations of, 436
sagittal midline approaches, 436–438
Skull base technique, 385
Small cell lung cancer (SCLC), 638
Smallest-region of overlap (SRO), 229
Small-molecule inhibitors (SMI), 666
Small molecule tyrosine kinase inhibitors, 644–645
SMARCB1/INI1 gene, 171
in schwannomas, 171
SMOH gene, 221
Smoking, 20–21
Social worker/case manager, 343
Somatic gene transfer, using RCAS-tva system, 147–148
Somatic sensation, 380–381
Somatosensory evoked potentials (SEPs), 373
Somatostatin analogues, 447
Somatotroph adenomas, 178
Somatotrophinomas, 174
Sonic hedgehog (Shh), 595
Sonic hedgehog pathway (SHH), 220–221
Sorafenib (Nexavar), 581, 672, 605, 680, 683, 684
SOX2, 81, 82
Sparc, 113
Sparsely ionizing, 721
Spasticity, 347
Spectral editing, 363
Speech therapist, 343
Sphenoid sinus, 294
Sphenoid wing meningiomas, 284, 388f
Spiegel-Wycis apparatus, 400
Spinal cord, 381
ascending tracts, 381–382
descending tracts, 381
Spinal cord involvement, 345–346
Spinal cord levels, 346t
Spinal cord tumors, 297, 465
astrocytoma, 465
clinical presentation 299–301
compartments and anatomy, 298–299
ependymoma, 465
epidemiology, 465
etiology, 299
functional outcome, 472
hemangioblastoma, 465
history, 465
imaging characteristics, 467
ependymoma vs. astrocytoma, 468
gangliogliomas, imaging features of, 469

hemangioblastoma, imaging features of, 468–469
magnetic resonance imaging, 467
nonglial tumor, imaging features of, 469
operative vs. nonoperative lesions, evaluating, 467–468
surgical planning, 468
IMSCT genetics, 466
astrocytoma, 466
ependymoma, 466
hemangioblastoma, 466
incidence and tumor histology, 297–298
metastasis, 466
miscellaneous tumors, 466
neuroradiographic findings, 301
extramedullary tumors, 302–303
intramedullary tumors, 301–302
outcomes and adjuvant therapy, 472
astrocytoma, adjuvant therapy in, 473
chemotherapy, 473
conventional radiation, 472–473
ependymoma, adjuvant therapy in, 473
hemangioblastomas, adjuvant therapy in, 473–474
intramedullary spinal cord metastasis, adjuvant therapy in, 474
long-term survival, 472
postoperative care and complications, 471
CSF fistula, 472
postoperative disability, 471
prevention and correction of spinal deformity, 471–472
presentation, 466
astrocytoma, 466–467
ependymoma, 466
miscellaneous tumors, 467
pediatric spinal cord astrocytoma, 467
preoperative evaluation, 469
surgical strategy
intraoperative monitoring, 470
operative technique, 470–471
surgical objective, 469–470
Spinal cord tumors, medical treatment of, 633
extradural, 633
biphosphonate therapy, 633
metastasis, 633
pain management, 633
systemic chemotherapy/hormonal therapy, 633
intradural-extramedullary
ependymoma myxopapillary, 635
meningiomas, 634
nerve sheath tumors of the spine, 634–635
paraganglioma, 635
intramedullary, 635
astrocytoma, 635
ependymoma, 635
hemangioblastoma, 635–636
metastasis, 636
primary bone lesions
benign, 634
malignant, 634
pediatry, 634

Spinal gliomas, survival rate for, 10
Spinal lesions, 349
Spinal neoplasms, 453
   metastatic spinal tumors, 458
      chemotherapy and radiation therapy, 459–460
      clinical presentation and workup, 458–459
      surgical management, 460–461
   primary spinal tumors
      chemotherapy and radiation therapy, 454
      clinical presentation and workup, 453–454
      surgical management, 454–456
      surgical technique, 456–458
Spine metastases, 909
   without impending cord compression, 909–910
      radiotherapy trails, 910
   metastatic spinal cord compression, 910–911
      backpain caused by, 910–911
      chemotherapy, radiotherapy supplemented by, 915
      decompressive surgery, 915–916
      functional outcome after radiotherapy alone, 912–913
      glucocorticosteroids in treating, 911
      "impending" MSCC, 910
      patients with oligometastatic disease, radiotherapy alone for, 915
      radiotherapy alone, 911–912
      radiotherapy and bisphosphonates, recalcification following, 913
      spinal MRI for, 911
      and spinal reirradiation, in-field recurrences of, 914
      survival after radiotherapy alone, 914–915
      white-matter edema and axonal swelling, associations with, 910
   radiopharmaceuticals for, 917
   radiosurgery, 916
SPlit Anterior Tibial Transfer (SPLATT) procedure, 347
Sporadic merlin (schwannomin) inactivation, 162
Squamous cell carcinomas, 287
Squamous metaplasia, 286
SQUIDs (superconducting quantum interference devices), 371
Src family of cytoplasmic tyrosine kinases, 116
SSEA-1, 84, 84t
Standard fractionation, 723
Stem cell hypothesis, 81
Stereotactic, definition of, 400
Stereotactic biopsy, 488–489
Stereotactic brain biopsy (SBB), 400
   complications, 405
   computerized tomography, 401
   frameless vs. Frame-Based SBB, 404
   lexicon, 400
   magnetic resonance imaging, 401–402
   magnetic resonance spectroscopy, 402–403

   MR perfusion, 403
   positron emission tomography, 403
   procedure, 405
   surgical navigation technology, 404–405
   surgical stereotaxis, 400–401
   targets
      accessing, 404
      location, 401
Stereotactic radiosurgery (SRS), 489–490, 603, 604, 640–641, 728–729, 863
   in gangliomas, use of, 770
   for hemangioblastoma, 818
   meningiomas, 826–828
      vs. EBRT, 833
      and edema, 828, 836t
   for vestibular schwannoma vs. surgery, comparison, 812
Stereotactic techniques
   fractionated stereotactic radiosurgery (FSRT), 863
   stereotactic radiosurgery (SRS). See Stereotactic radiosurgery (SRS)
Steroid dementia, 331
Steroids, 265, 645–646
Stochastic model, 81, 81f
Strabismus, 274
SU 5416, 474
Subcutaneous schwannomas, 167
Subependymal giant cell astrocytomas (SEGAs), 58, 253, 274
   WHO grade I, 760
Subependymoma, 58, 799
Suberoylanilide hydroxamic acid (SAHA), 704
Substituted judgment, doctrine of, 311
Subtotal resection (STR), 473
   for choroid plexus tumors, 664
Subventricular zone (SVZ), 82
SUFU gene, 221
Sunitinib (Sutent), 93, 605, 636, 672–673, 680
Superconducting quantum interference devices (SQUIDs), 371
Supplementary motor area (SMA), 375–377
   syndrome, 375
Support groups' role, in neuro-oncology, 316
   facilitation, 317
   format, 317
   location, 316–317
Supportive rehabilitation, 342
Suprasellar meningiomass, 283–284
Suprasellar tumors, 287, 520
   craniopharyngioma, 520–521
      surgical considerations, 521
   hydrocephalus, 521
   intracavitary therapy, 522
   postoperative care, 522
   radiation therapy, 522
   surgical resection, 521–522
   pituitary adenoma, 522–523
      surgical considerations, 523
Supratentorial gliomas, 16, 257, 258, 518, 519f
   dysembryoplastic neuroepithelial tumors, 518

   functional imaging, 519–520
   gangliogliomas, 518
   gliomas, 518
   neuronavigation, 519
   surgical considerations, 519
Supratentorial gliomas, medical management of, 556
   high-grade gliomas, 562
      anaplastic astrocytomas (AAs), 569
      anaplastic oligodendroglioma, 570–572
      definitive treatment, 569–572
      glioblastoma, 563–568
   low-grade gliomas (LGG), 556
      chemotherapy for, 558–562
      surgery, 557–558
Supratentorial gliomas in adults, 257, 258t
   cerebral hemispheres, neoplasms of, 258–259
   common diagnostic dilemmas, 260–261
   pineal region, neoplasms of, 259–260
   presenting signs and symptoms, 257
      neurological signs, 257–258
      neurological symptoms, 257
   radiologic diagnosis, 260
   thalamus and basal ganglia, neoplasms of, 259
Supratentorial low-grade gliomas, 583
   cerebellar astrocytomas, 584–585
   cerebral low-grade glioma, 583
   ependymomas, 585–586
   optic pathway glioma, 583–584
Supratentorial neoplasms, 530
Supratentorial primitive neuroectodermal tumors (sPNETs), 208, 208f, 781, 789–790
   medical management of, 593
      chemotherapy, 594–595
      radiation therapy, 594
      staging and prognostic factors, 593–594
      surgical resection, 594
Surgery as cause of cognitive deficits, 327
Surgically created resection cavity (SCRC), 734
Surgical navigation (SN), 392
   biopsy, 396
   brain shift and tissue deformation, 394
   coregistration, 393, 394f
   craniotomy for tumor, 394
      awake technique, 395–396
      general SNS-assisted craniotomy technique, 395
      minimal access craniotomy, 394–395
      resection control, 395
   frame stereotaxy, 392
   future uses, 397
   related procedures, 397
   technology, 404–405
   types, 392–393
Surgical navigation system (SNS), 394
   awake technique, 395–396
   types, 392–393
Surgical stereotaxis, history of, 400–401
Surveillance, Epidemiology, and End Results (SEER) data, 7
Survival and prognosis, of glioma, 47

constitutive genetic polymorphisms and glioma survival, 48, 49–53t
serologic and immunologic factors, 54
tumor markers, studies of, 47
  insights from expression array studies, 48
Survival rates, 10–12
SV40, 62
Sylvian fissure, 379
  dissection, 511–512
"Synaptic transmission," 8

Tamoxifen, 549, 609, 635, 646
Targeted molecular agents, 676
  cyclooxygenase inhibitors, 680–681
  efficacy, improving, 681, 685–686
    addressing multiple targets simultaneously, 682
    agents that inhibit multiple targets, 682–683
    combinations of targeted molecular agents, 683–684
    combining targeted molecular agents with chemotherapy, 684–685
    combining targeted molecular agents with RT, 684
    reliable animal models, creating, 682
    target selection, optimizing, 682
  epidermal growth factor receptor inhibitors, 676–677
  farnesyltransferase inhibitors, 677, 679
  histone deacetylase inhibitors, 681
  mammalian target of rapamycin inhibitors, 679–680
  matrix metalloproteinase and integrin inhibitors, 681
  phosphatidylinositol-3 kinase inhibitors, 680
  platelet-derived growth factor receptor inhibitors, 677
  proteasome inhibitors, 681
  protein kinase C inhibitors, 680
  VEGFR and VEGFR inhibitors, 680
Targeted radionuclide therapy (TRT), 719, 732–739
Targeted therapies, general principles of, 666
  clinical trials, 667–668
  for brain tumors, 667
  mechanism of action, 666
  molecular pathways in, 666
  types, 666–667
Targeting Construct, 734t
T-cell, 2, 41
Tectal gliomas, 278, 878
Television transmitter, 31
Telomerase activity, 54, 232–233
Telomerase expression, 93
Telomere stability, 163–164
Temozolamide (TMZ), 93, 135, 305, 330, 344, 350, 549, 560–561, 564–566, 567, 568, 569–570, 580, 583, 586, 606, 617, 618, 642–643, 646, 657, 671, 677, 685, 694, 700, 705, 707, 750

Temporal lobe, 6, 343
  and auditory surface functional anatomy, 375f
  functional neuroanatomy of, 378
    basal temporal language area (BTLA), 378
    hippocampal formation, 379
    optic radiations, 379
    primary auditory, 378–379
    Wernicke's area, 378
  gliomas, 259
  tumor location, 336
Temsirolimus (Torisel), 672, 680
Tenascin, 733
Tension headaches, 260
Teratoma, 59, 874
  and radiation therapy, 898
TGF-β, 91
  in allergic conditions, 42
  in glioma, 42
  and glioma survival time, 42
  paradoxical role, 43
Thalamic gliomas, 525
Thalamic tumors, 259
Thalamus and basal ganglia, neoplasms of, 259
Thalidomide, 635, 672
Thallium, 366
T-helper type 2 (Th2) cells, 40
Therapeutic exercises, 345
Therapeutic touch, 714
6-Thioguanine, 773
Thiotepa (TT), 646, 655
Third ventricle, surgical approaches to, 500
Three-dimensional conformal radiation, 727
Three-dimensional magnetic resonance spectroscopy (3DMRS), 363–364
Thromboembolic complications and anticoagulation, 306–307
Thyroid transcription factor-1 positivity, 263
Thyrotropin (TSH)
  -secreting adenomas, 179, 449
  -secreting pituitary tumors, 630
TI571 (Gleveec), 635
Tie2-expressing monocytes (TEMs), 132
Tinea capitis cohorts, 26–27
Tipifarnib (Zarnestra), 672, 679, 683
Tipifarnib, 91, 187
Tobacco, 62
Todd's postictal paralysis, 258
Tomotherapy HI-ART, 730t
Tomotherapy proton therapy system, 732
Topiramate, 305
Topotecan, 580, 643–644, 657
Total en bloc spondylectomy (TES), 456, 461
Toxoplasma gondii, 62
TP53 gene, 48, 73
TP53 mutations, 63, 88, 107–108
  low-grade gliomas (LGGs) and, 1
Tpit function, 176
Transcranial endoscopic approaches
  completely endoscopic intra-axial tumor resection, 441–443

endoscopic intraventricular surgery, 439–441
Transcranial magnetic stimulation, 372
Transgenic and knockout mice, strategies using, 148–150, 159t
Transgenic models, 153–154
Transgenic mouse models, potential use of, 151
Transitional meningiomass, 160f
Transplanum/transcribriform, 437
Transsphenoidal, 445
  atypical pituitary adenoma and pituitary carcinoma, 450–451
  clinical presentation, 445
  functional adenomas, 445
    adrenocorticotropin-secreting adenomas, 447–449
    GH-producing adenomas, 446–447
    PRL-secreting adenomas, 445–446
    thyrotropin (TSH)-secreting adenomas, 449
  nonfunctioning adenomas, 449
    gonadotropin-secreting adenomas, 449–450
    null-cell adenoma, 450
  treatment, 450
Transsphenoidal adenomectomy, 448
Transsphenoidal resection
  pituitary adenomas, 861
Treatment, 347–348
  related side effects, 350
Treatment and outcome, meningiomass, 824–833
  gross total resection, 825
  radiation therapy, 825–826
  subtotal resection, 825
    local progression after, 828t
  stereotactic radiosurgery, 826–828
    target volume and dose, 827
    toxicity, 827–828
  fractionated external beam radiation therapy, 828–833
    postoperative EBRT, 828
    primary EBRT, 828–830
    target volume and dose, 830–832
    toxicity, 833
Triazolam, 306
Trigeminal meningiomass, 284
Trigeminal neuralgia, 284
Trigeminal schwannomas, 286
Tri-iodothyronine (T3), 449
Trimethoprim–sulphamethoxazole (TMP-SMX), 306
Trizanadines, 347
TrkB (NTRK2), 232
Trustbuilding, of caregivers, 318
Truth-telling, 311
TSA, 707
TSG Rb, 182
TSLC1 (tumor suppressor in lung cancer 1), 72
TSP-1 expression, 113
Tuberculum sellae meningiomas, 390f
Tuberous sclerosis, 15t
Tuberous sclerosis complex (TSC), 253
  diagnostic criteria for, 253t

Tumor antigens, antibodies'
role against, 43
Tumor-associated seizures (TASs), 305
Tumor grading, meningiomas,
822, 823, 823t
anaplastic/malignant
(WHO grade III), 823
atypical (WHO Grade II), intracranial
meningiomass, 822–823
benign (WHO Grade I), intracranial
meningiomass, 822
Tumor histology, 234
Tumor hypoxia and metabolism,
angiogenesis and its regulation
by, 123–125, 126–127f
Tumor-initiating cells (TICs). See
Brain tumor initiating cells;
Tumor stem cells
Tumor markers, studies of, 47–48
Tumor neovascularization and "glioma
stem cells," 129
Tumor-related side effects, 349–350
Tumors. See also Adenomas;
Astrocytomas; Cancer; Carcinomas;
Ependymomas; Gliomas;
Meningiomas; Metastases;
Neurofibromas; Papillomas;
Sarcomas
astrocytic tumors, 6, 88
asymptomatic tumors, 275
atypical teratoid/rhabdoid tumor (atrt),
58, 209, 209f, 267, 844
benign nonperipheral nerve sheath
tumors, 536
benign peripheral nerve sheath
tumors, 535–536
brachial plexus tumor, 534
brainstem tumors, 278, 608
central nervous system tumors.
See Central nervous system
(cns) tumors
childhood brain tumors, 57
dermoid and epidermoid tumors, 625
desmoid tumors, 536, 538f
diffuse intrinsic brainstem tumors, 844
dumbbell tumor, 299, 302f
dysembryoplastic neuroepithelial
tumors, 211–212, 212f, 518
embryonal tumors. See Embryonal
tumors
ependymal tumors, 6, 7
extramedullary tumors, 302–303
favorable brainstem tumor, 842
focal brainstem tumors, 610
gastrointestinal stromal tumors, 676
germ cell tumors, 486, 491, 526,
625–626, 771
glial tumors, 526
glioneuronal tumors, 58–59
glomus jugulare tumors, 287
glomus tumors. See Chemodectomas
grading tumors, 355
granular cell tumors, 624–625
head tumor, 34
insular tumors, 505
intramedullary spinal cord
tumors, 465, 635

intramedullary tumors, 301–302
intraventricular tumors, 496, 523
malignant peripheral nerve sheath
tumors, 185, 191f, 250, 542–543,
615t, 619–620, 635
malignant triton tumor, 191
meningothelial tumors, 159
mesenchymal tumors, 59
midbrain tumors, 611
neck tumor, 34
nerve sheath tumors of spine, 634–635
nervous system tumors, 79, 80
neuroepithelial tumors, 58
neuronal and mixed neuroglial
tumors, 210
nonglial tumors, 361
nonneuroepithelial tumors, 213
oligodendroglial tumor, 6, 10
orbital tumors, 386
osseous tumors, 386
papillary glioneuronal tumor, 59
peripheral nerve sheath tumors, 59
pineal gland tumors, 485
pineal parenchymal tumors,
174, 175f, 445t, 486, 491, 526
pineal region tumor, 59, 259–260,
525, 877
pituitary and sellar region,
tumors of, 291
posterior fossa tumors, 527
primary brain tumors, 304
primitive neuroectodermal
tumors, 526, 781
schwannomas tumors, 302
sinonasal tumors, 385–386
spinal cord tumors, 297, 465, 633
suprasellar tumors, 287, 520
supratentorial primitive
neuroectodermal tumors,
208, 208f, 781, 789–790
thalamic tumors, 259
wilm's kidney tumor, 64
Tumor size and sex hormones,
meningiomass, 820
Tumor stem cells, 106
Tumor suppressor genes (TSG), 174
inactivation in pituitary tumors, 181
Tumor-suppressor inactivation, 231–232
Tumor-treating fields, 714
Tumor type, distinctive image findings
by, 354t
Turcot syndrome, 15t, 16–17, 219
animal models, 243
clinical features and diagnostic
criteria, 242
molecular pathogenesis, 242–243
therapy and prognosis, 243
20q13.3 (RTEL1), 1
Two-dimensional radiation, 726
Tyrosine kinase inhibitors (TKI), 666
^{235}U, 729, 730
decay of, 720

Ultrasound, 16
Ultrastructural examination of
MPNST, 192

Unique impact, of brain tumors, 316
University of California, Los Angeles
(UCLA) group, 95
Unlimited replicative potential, 93
Urokinase plasminogen activator
(uPA), 94, 115
uPAR, 115
Utah cancer registry data base, 14
Utilitarianism, 311

Vaccination. See Active immunotherapy
Valproate (valproic acid), 305, 330
Vandetanib (ZD6474, Zactima), 680, 684
Vascular endothelial growth factor
(VEGF), 93, 101, 102, 123, 135,
187, 568, 605, 669
and angiopoietins, 125–128
mRNA, 125
Vascular epidermal growth factor
(VEGF) Trap, 581
Vascular endothelial growth factor
receptor (VEGFR) inhibitors,
568, 605, 680
VEGFR-2 kinase inhibitors, 137
Vascular proliferation in brain
tumors, 122
Vasculogenesis, 122
in gliomas
and angiogenesis, 129–130
circulating endothelial cells in
glioma neovascularization, 130–131
in CNS ontogeny and
oncogeny, 130t
potential molecular and cellular
biomarkers, 132
proangiogenic cells in glioma
neovascularization, 131
Vasogenic edema, 265
Vatalanib (PTK787), 93, 684
Vegetables, intake of, 61
Vena cava filter (VCF), 307
Ventricular zone (VZ) stem cells, 197–198
Verapamil, 551
Verocay bodies, 168
Vertebral hemangioma, and radiation
therapy, 898
Vertigo, 285
Vestibular schwannoma, 808
fractionated stereotactic radiotherapy
compared to SRS, 813–814
dose selection and toxicities, 813
methods and treatment planning,
812–813
results of, 813
future directions of, 815
management of, 808–810
in patient with NF2, 814–815
proton-beam therapy, 814
stereotactic radiosurgery
dose selection and toxicities, 810
methods and treatment
planning, 810
results of, 810–811
vs. surgery, comparison, 812
Vestibular schwannomas, 167, 285–286,
388, 389f

Vincristine, 344, 473, 549, 579, 580, 583, 584, 586, 591, 592, 593, 595, 609, 616, 619, 620, 634, 635, 654, 662
  for infant tumors, 772, 773
  and cyclophosphamide
    for ependymomas, 802–803
Viral and transgenic mice, strategies using, 150
Viral vector-mediated gene therapy, 699t
Viruses, 695
  measles virus, 697
  newcastle disease virus (NDV), 697
  oncolytic adenovirus, 696–697
  oncolytic HSV-1, 696
  poliovirus, 697
  replication-competent (oncolytic) viruses, 696
  replication-defective viruses, 698
  transgene strategies, 698–699
Visceral sensory system, 380
Visual pathway gliomas. See Diencephalic gliomas
Visual surface functional anatomy, 375f
Vitamins, 21–22
  supplementation, for childhood brain tumors, 61–62
  vitamin C, 21, 22

vitamin D, 712
vitamin E, 322
Vocational counselors, 343
Volumetric arc therapy, 730t
von-Hippel Lindau (VHL) disease, 278
  animal models, 240
  clinical features and diagnostic criteria, 239–240
  molecular pathogenesis, 240
  therapy and prognosis, 240
von Hippel-Lindau (VHL) gene, 299
von Recklinghausen disease. See Neurofibromatosis 1 (NF1) syndrome
Vorinostat (suberoy-lanilide hydroxamic acid [SAHA]), 681, 707
VP-16, 580, 662

Walkers, 345
Weber's meningiomas model, 73f
Wernicke's area, 378
White-matter abnormalities, 327
White matter tracts, assessing integrity of, 355–356
Whites, glioma in, 7
  survival rate for, 11

Whole-brain radiation therapy (WBRT), 638, 639, 640
  for primary central nervous system lymphoma (PCNSL), 880
  late treatment effects, 888–889
  vs. WBRT with SRS, 641
Whole-brain radiotherapy alone/with SRS, 641
Wilm's kidney tumor, 64
Wnt/B-catenin pathway, 221
Wnt pathway genes, 65

Xenograft-based tumor propagation, 154–155, 154f
Xenograft-enabled research, 155
Xenotransplantation, 85
XERECEPT®, 548
X-ray, 721, 719

YKL-40 expression, 117
Yttrium-90 (90Y), 864

ZD-6474, 605
Zonisamide, 305